P9-DVR-901

Occupational Therapy FOR Children AND Adolescents

Occupational Therapy FOR Children AND Adolescents

SEVENTH EDITION

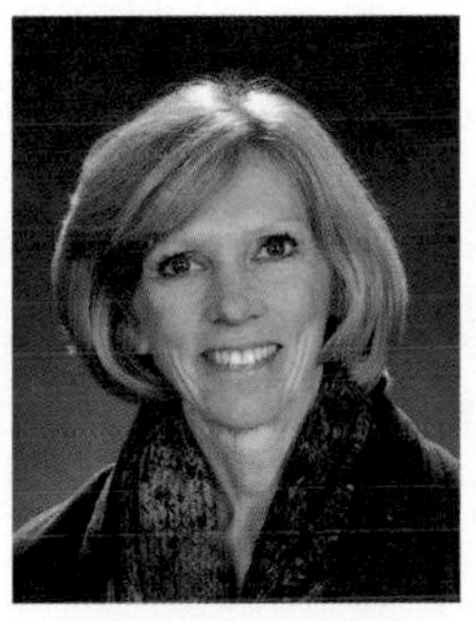

Jane Case-Smith
EdD, OTR/L, FAOTA (deceased)
Professor and Chair
Division of Occupational Therapy
School of Health and Rehabilitation Sciences
The Ohio State University
Columbus, Ohio

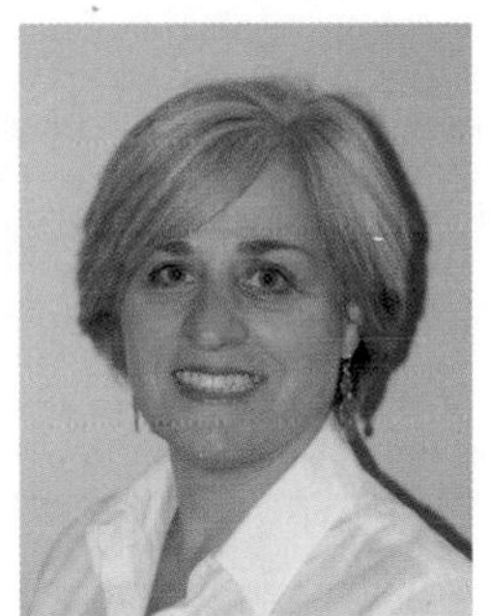

Jane Clifford O'Brien
PhD, MS, EdL, OTR/L, FAOTA
Associate Professor
Occupational Therapy Program Director
Occupational Therapy Department
Westbrook College of Health Professions
University of New England
Portland, Maine

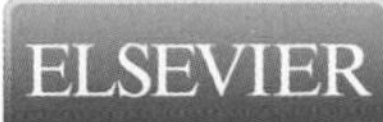

ELSEVIER
MOSBY

3251 Riverport Lane
St. Louis, Missouri 63043

OCCUPATIONAL THERAPY FOR CHILDREN AND ADOLESCENTS, SEVENTH EDITION ISBN: 978-0-323-16925-7

Library of Congress Cataloging-in-Publication Data
Occupational therapy for children
Occupational therapy for children and adolescents / [edited by] Jane Case-Smith, Jane Clifford O'Brien.—Seventh edition.
p. ; cm.
Preceded by: Occupational therapy for children / [edited by] Jane Case-Smith, Jane Clifford O'Brien. 6th ed. c2010.
Includes bibliographical references and index.
ISBN 978-0-323-16925-7 (hardcover : alk. paper)
I. Case-Smith, Jane, 1953- , author, editor. II. O'Brien, Jane Clifford, author, editor. III. Title.
[DNLM: 1. Occupational Therapy. 2. Adolescent. 3. Child, Exceptional. 4. Child. 5. Developmental Disabilities—rehabilitation. 6. Disabled Children—rehabilitation. WS 368]
RJ53.O25
615.8515083—dc23

2014033094

Professional Reference Director: Penny Rudolph
Content Development Manager: Jolynn Gower
Publishing Services Manager: Jeff Patterson
Project Manager: Tracey Schriefer
Design Direction: Karen Pauls/Renee Duenow

Printed in Canada.

Last digit is the print number: 9 8 7 6 5 4 3 2 1

Dr. Jane Case-Smith was soft spoken, thoughtful, and a brilliant scholar,
who consistently reinforced respect for children and their families.
She developed personal and professional relationships with each author, helping them
to produce chapters that would lead students, practitioners, and educators in their best practice.
Jane also believed strongly in using science as a foundation for intervention,
while never overlooking the art of therapy.
Her ability to integrate these two important aspects of occupational therapy will forever influence
the profession and help many children and their families participate in daily occupations.
Her spirit is infused throughout the pictures and words of this book.

I dedicate this book to my friend Dr. Jane Case-Smith.

Contributors

Leslie Altimier, DNP, RNC, NE-BC
Fellow, Nursing
Northeastern University
Boston, Massachutsetts

Beth Ball, MS (Allied Medicine), BS (Occupational Therapy)
Member, Occupational Therapy Section
Ohio Occupational Therapy, Physical Therapy and Athletic Trainers Board
Columbus, Ohio;
Member, Occupational Therapy Advisory Board
The Ohio State University
Columbus, Ohio

Susan Bazyk, PhD, OTR/L, FAOTA
Professor, Occupational Therapy
School of Health Sciences
Cleveland State University
Cleveland, Ohio

Matthew E. Brock, PhD
Department of Education Studies and Crane Center
The Ohio State University
Columbus, Ohio

Susan Cahill, PhD, OTR/L
Assistant Professor
Occupational Therapy Program
Midwestern University
Downers Grove, Illinois

Erik Carter, PhD
Associate Professor
Department of Special Education
Vanderbilt University
Nashville, Tennessee

Jane Case-Smith, EdD, OTR/L, FAOTA (deceased)
Professor and Chair
Division of Occupational Therapy
School of Health and Rehabilitation Sciences
The Ohio State University
Columbus, Ohio

Jana Cason, DHS, OTR/L, FAOTA
Associate Professor
Auerbach School of Occupational Therapy
Spalding University
Louisville, Kentucky

Elizabeth Chapelle
Occupational Therapy
Seattle Children's Hospital
Seattle, Washington

Dennis Cleary, BA, BS, MS, OTD, OTR/L
Assistant Professor
Division of Occupational Therapy
The Ohio State University
Columbus, Ohio

Patty C. Coker-Bolt, PhD, OTR/L, FAOTA
Assistant Professor
Department of Health Professions
Medical University of South Carolina
Charleston, South Carolina

Sharon Cosper, MHS, OTR/L
Assistant Professor
Department of Occupational Therapy
College of Allied Health Sciences
Georgia Regents University
Augusta, Georgia

Laura Crooks, OTR, MHA
Director, Rehabilitation Services
Seattle Children's Hospital
Seattle, Washington

Melissa Demir, MSW, LICSW
Department of Occupational Therapy
Boston University
Boston, Massachutsetts

Jenny Dorich, MBA, OTR/L, CHT
Occupational Therapist II
Program Lead, Hand Therapy
Division of Occupational Therapy, Physical Therapy and Therapeutic Recreation
Cincinnati Children's Hospital Medical Center
Cincinnati, Ohio

Brian J. Dudgeon, PhD, OTR, FAOTA
Professor and Chair, Department of Occupational Therapy School of Health Professions
University of Alabama at Birmingham
Birmingham, Alabama

M. Louise Dunn, ScD, OTR/L
Associate Professor
School of Occupational Therapy
Brenau University
Gainesville, Georgia

Charlotte E. Exner, PhD, OT/L, FAOTA
Executive Director
Hussman Center for Adults with Autism
Towson University
Towson, Maryland

Kaity Gain, PhD, MSc, OT
Health and Rehabilitation Science
Western University
London, Ontario
Canada

Rebecca E. Argabrite Grove, MS, OTR/L
Governance, Leadership Development & International Liaison
Professional Affairs Division
American Occupational Therapy Association
Bethesda, Maryland

Karen Harpster, PhD, OTR/L
Director of Occupational Therapy Research
Occupational Therapy, Physical Therapy and Therapeutic Recreation
Cincinnati Children's Hospital Medical Center
Cincinnati, Ohio

Claudia List Hilton, OTR, Phd, MBA, SROT, FAOTA
Assistant Professor
Occupational Therapy & Rehabilitation Sciences
School of Health Professions
University of Texas Medical Branch
Galveston, Texas

Brooke Howard, MS, OTR/L
Transition Coordinator
Ivy Street School
Brookline, Massachutsetts

Jan Hunter, MA, OTR
Assistant Professor
School of Health Professions
University of Texas Medical Branch
Galveston, Texas;
Neonatal Clinical Specialist
Clear Lake Regional Medical Center
Webster, Texas

Lynn Jaffe, ScD, OTR/L, FAOTA
Professor Emerita
Department of Occupational Therapy
College of Allied Health Sciences
Georgia Regents University
Augusta, Georgia

Susan H. Knox, PhD, OTR, FAOTA
Director Emeritus
Therapy in Action
Tarzana, California

Kimberly Korth, MEd, OTR/L
Occupational Therapist
Feeding and Swallowing Coordinator
Children's Hospital Colorado
Denver, Colorado

Jessica Kramer, PhD, OTR/L
Assistant Professor
Department of Occupational Therapy & PhD Program in Rehabilitation Sciences
Boston University
Boston, Massachutsetts

Anjanette Lee, MS, CCC/SLP
Speech-Language Pathologist
Infant Development Specialist
Neonatal Intensive Care Unit
Memorial Hermann Hospital Southwest
Houston, Texas

Kendra Liljenquist, MS
ScD Program in Rehabilitation Sciences
Boston University
Boston, Massachutsetts

Kathryn M. Loukas, OTD, MS, OTR/L, FAOTA
Clinical Professor
Occupational Therapy Department
Westbrook College of Health Professions
University of New England
Portland, Maine

Amber Lowe, MOT, OTR/L
Occupational Therapist
Division of Occupational Therapy, Physical Therapy and Therapeutic Recreation
Cincinnati Children's Hospital Medical Center
Cincinnati, Ohio

Zoe Mailloux, OTD, OTR/L, FAOTA
Adjunct Associate Professor
Department of Occupational Therapy
Jefferson School of Health Professions
Thomas Jefferson University
Philadelphia, Pennsylvania

Angela Mandich, PhD, MSc, OT
School of Occupational Therapy
Western University
London, Ontario
Canada

Heather Miller-Kuhaneck, PhD, OTR/L, FAOTA
Assistant Professor
Occupational Therapy
Sacred Heart University
Fairfield, Connecticut

Christine Teeters Myers, PhD, OTR/L
Associate Professor and Coordinator, OTD Program
Department of Occupational Science and Occupational Therapy
Eastern Kentucky University
Richmond, Kentucky

Erin Naber, PT, DPT
Senior Physical Therapist
Fairmount Rehabilitation Programs
Kennedy Krieger Institute
Baltimore, Maryland

Patricia S. Nagaishi, PhD, OTR/L
Occupational Therapy Specialist
Preschool Assessment Team
Pasadena Unified School District
Special Education-Birth to 5 and Clinic Services
President, Occupational Therapy Association of California
Pasadena, California

Jane Clifford O'Brien, PhD, MS EdL, OTR/L, FAOTA
Associate Professor
Occupational Therapy Program Director
Occupational Therapy Department
Westbrook College of Health Professions
University of New England
Portland, Maine

L. Diane Parham, PhD, OTR/L, FAOTA
Professor
Occupational Therapy Graduate Program
School of Medicine
University of New Mexico
Albuquerque, New Mexico

Andrew Persch, PhD, OTR/L
Assistant Professor
Division of Occupational Therapy
The Ohio State University
Columbus, Ohio

Teressa Garcia Reidy, MS, OTR/L
Senior Occupational Therapist
Fairmount Rehabilitation Programs
Kennedy Krieger Institute
Baltimore, Maryland

Lauren Rendell, OTR/L
Occupational Therapist
Spalding Rehabilitation Hospital
Aurora, Colorado

Pamela K. Richardson, PhD, OTR/L, FAOTA
Acting Associate Dean
College of Applied Sciences and Arts
San Jose State University
San Jose, California

Zachary Rosetti, PhD
Assistant Professor of Special Education
Boston University
Boston, Massachutsetts

Colleen M. Schneck, ScD, OTR/L, FAOTA
Professor and Chair
Department of Occupational Therapy
Eastern Kentucky University
Richmond, Kentucky

Judith W. Schoonover, MEd, OTR/L, ATP, FAOTA
Occupational Therapist/Assistive Technology Professional
Loudoun County Public Schools
Ashburn, Virginia

Patti Sharp, OTD, MS, OTR/L
Occupational Therapist II
Department of Occupational, Physical Therapy and Therapeutic Recreation
Cincinnati Children's Hospital Medical Center
Cincinnati, Ohio

Jayne Shepherd, MS, OTR/L, FAOTA
Assistant Chair, Associate Professor
Director of Fieldwork
Department of Occupational Therapy
Virginia Commonwealth University
Richmond, Virginia

Karen Spencer, PhD, OTR (retired)
Associate Professor
Department of Occupational Therapy
Colorado State University
Fort Collins, Colorado

Kari J. Tanta, PhD, OTR/L, FAOTA
Program Coordinator
Children's Therapy Department
UW Medicine—Valley Medical Center
Renton, Washington;
Clinical Assistant Professor
Division of Occupational Therapy
University of Washington
Seattle, Washington;
Adjunct Faculty
Department of Occupational Therapy
University of Puget Sound
Tacoma, Washington

Carrie Thelen, MSOT, OTR/L
Occupational Therapist II
Division of Occupational Therapy, Physical Therapy and Therapeutic Recreation
Cincinnati Children's Hospital Medical Center
Cincinnati, Ohio

Kerryellen Vroman, PhD, OTR/L
Associate Professor and Department Chair
Occupational Therapy
College of Health and Human Services
University of New Hampshire
Durham, New Hampshire

Beth Warnken, MOT, OTR/L, ATP
Occupational Therapist II
Division of Occupational Therapy, Physical Therapy and Therapeutic Recreation
Cincinnati Children's Hospital Medical Center
Cincinnati, Ohio

Renee Watling, PhD, OTR/L, FAOTA
Clinical Assistant Professor
Division of Occupational Therapy
Department of Rehabilitation Medicine
University of Washington
Seattle, Washington;
Autism Services Lead
Children's Therapy Center
Dynamic Partners
Kent, Washington

Jessie Wilson, PhD, OT Reg. (Ont.)
Discipline of Occupational Therapy
School of Public Health, Tropical Medicine & Rehabilitation Services
James Cook University, Douglas Campus
Townsville, Queensland
Australia

Christine Wright-Ott, OTR/L, MPA
Occupational Therapy Consultant
The Bridge School
Hillsborough, California

Preface

Organization

The current edition is organized into four sections to reflect the knowledge and skills needed to practice occupational therapy with children and to help readers apply concepts to practice. The first section describes foundational knowledge and includes chapters on theories and practice models, child and adolescent development, and family-centered care. In Chapters 1 and 2 Dr. Case-Smith describes theories of child development and learning and specific models of practice used in occupational therapy. These theories and models of practice range from those that originated in psychology, education, and basic sciences to ones that were proposed and developed by occupational therapy scholars and practitioners. With this theoretic grounding, children's development of occupations is presented in two chapters: Chapter 3 explains occupational development in infants, toddlers, and children, and Chapter 4 describes how occupations continue to emerge and mature in youth and young adults. Chapter 5 describes families, illustrates family occupations across the life span, discusses experiences of families who have children with special needs, and explains the importance of family-centered care.

The second section of the book begins with an explanation of the use of standardized tests, including how to administer a standardized test, score items, interpret test scores, and synthesize the findings. Chapters 7 through 20 cover a variety of intervention approaches (e.g., motor control/motor learning, sensory integration, assistive technology). The authors describe interventions to target performance areas (e.g., hand skills) and occupations (e.g., feeding, activities of daily living, play, social participation). The chapters explain both the theory and science of occupational therapy practice and discuss practical issues that frequently occur in practice. Together these chapters reflect the breadth and depth of occupational therapy with children and adolescents.

The fourth section (Chapters 21 through 30) of the book describes practice arenas for occupational therapy practice with children. These chapters illustrate the rich variety of practice opportunities and define how practice differs in medical versus education systems and institutions. Only by understanding the intervention context and the child's environments can occupational therapists select appropriate intervention practices.

Chapters 25 through 30 provide readers with intervention strategies for specific populations. For example, Chapter 25 examines factors influencing a child's transition to adulthood. Other chapters illustrate how practitioners help children with visual impairments or blindness, autism, cerebral palsy, hand conditions, or trauma-induced conditions engage in occupations.

Distinctive Features

Although the chapters contain related information, each chapter stands on its own, such that the chapters do not need to be read in a particular sequence. Each chapter begins with key questions to guide reading. Case reports exemplify concepts related to the chapter and are designed to help the reader integrate the material. Research literature is cited and used throughout. The goal of the authors is to provide comprehensive, research-based, current information that can guide practitioners in making optimal decisions in their practice with children.

Distinctive features of the book include the following:

- Research Notes boxes
- Evidence-based summary tables
- Case Study boxes

Ancillary Materials

The *Occupational Therapy for Children and Adolescents* text is linked to an Evolve website that provides a number of learning aids and tools. The Evolve website provides resources for each chapter, including the following:

- Video clips with case study questions
- Additional case studies with guiding questions to reinforce chapter content
- Learning activities
- Multiple choice questions for students and faculty
- Resources (such as forms and handouts)
- Glossary

The Evolve learning activities and video clip case studies relate directly to the text; it is hoped that readers use the two resources together. In addition, readers are encouraged to access the Evolve website for supplemental information.

Acknowledgments

We would like to thank all the children who are featured in the video clips and case studies:

Adam	Emily	Luke	Peggy
Ana	Emily	Matt	Samuel
Annabelle	Faith	Micah	Sydney
Camerias	Isabel	Nathan	Teagan
Christian	Jessica	Nathaniel	Tiandra
Christina	Jillian	Nicholas	William
Eily	Katelyn	Paige	Zane
Ema			

A special thank you to the parents who so openly shared their stories with us:

Charlie and Emily Adams	Lori Chirakus	Sandra Jordan	Ann Ramsey
Robert and Carrie Beyer	Joy Cline	Joanna L. McCoy	Teresa Reynolds-Armstrong
Freda Michelle Bowen	Sondra Diop	Maureen P. McGlove	Tuesday A. Ryanhart
Nancy Bowen	Lisa M. Grant	Jill McQuaid	Julana Schutt
Kelly Brandewe	Ivonne Hernandez	Stephanie L. Mills	P. Allen Shroyer
Ernesty Burton	Shawn Holden	David J. Petras	Douglas Warburton
Ruby Burton	Luann Hoover	Theresa A. Philbrick	

We are very appreciative of the siblings and buddies who agreed to help us out:

Aidan	Robert
Lori	Todd and Keith
Megan	Tommy, Owen, and Colin

We thank all the therapists and physicians who allowed us to videotape their sessions and provided us with such wonderful examples:

Chrissy Alex	Katie Finnegan	Lisa A. King	Julie Potts
Sandy Antoszewski	Karen Harpster	Dara Krynicki	Ann Ramsey
Mary Elizabeth F. Bracy	Terri Heaphy	Marianne Mayhan	Suellen Sharp
Amanda Cousiko	Katherine Inamura	Taylor Moody	Carrie Taylor
Emily de los Reyes			

A special thanks to Matt Meindl, Melissa Hussey, David Stwarka Jennifer Cohn, Stephanie Cohn, and all the authors who submitted videotapes. Thank you to Emily Krams, Alicen Johnson, Britanny Peters, Katherine Paulaski, Kate Loukas, Scott McNeil, Jan Froehlich, MaryBeth Patnaude, Molly O'Brien, Keely Heidtman, Greg Lapointe, Caitlin Cassis, Judith Cohn, Jazmin Photography, and Michelle Lapelle. A special thanks to Mariana D'Amico, Peter Goldberg, and Carrie Beyer for all their expertise with videotaping. Jolynn Gower, Penny Rudolph, Tracey Schriefer, and Katie Gutierrez were instrumental in developing and completing this text and were a pleasure with whom to work. Jane O'Brien would like to thank her family—Mike, Scott, Alison, and Molly—for their continual support. She would also like to thank her colleagues and students at the University of New England, all the authors, and Jane Case-Smith.

Jane Case-Smith thanks her family—Greg, David, and Stephen—for their support and patience. She also thanks her colleagues in the Division of Occupational Therapy, The Ohio State University, for their support. We both thank all the authors for their willingness to share their expertise and their labor and time in producing excellent chapters.

Contents

CHAPTER 1

An Overview of Occupational Therapy for Children

Jane Case-Smith

KEY TERMS

- Child-centered and family-centered practice
- Strength-based approaches
- Inclusion, integrated services, and natural environments
- Cultural competence
- Evidence-based practice
- Therapeutic relationships
- Occupation-based models
- Ecologic models
- Assistive technology
- Environmental modification/universal access
- Consultation, coaching, and education

GUIDING QUESTIONS

1. Which concepts describe occupational therapy services for children and families?
2. How do occupational therapists use individualized, child-centered, and family-centered interventions and strength-based models?
3. How do occupational therapists use inclusive and integrated practices?
4. How do occupational therapists embrace diversity and value cultural differences?
5. How do occupational therapists use research evidence and science-based reasoning to make intervention decisions?
6. How does comprehensive evaluation guide clinical reasoning and lead to efficacious interventions?
7. What are the elements of the intervention process, and how do occupational therapy practitioners combine these elements to improve performance and participation of children and youth?
8. How are ecologic models that include task adaptation, environmental modification, and consultation/coaching used to promote the child's full participation in natural environments?

Occupational therapy practitioners develop interventions based on assessment of the occupations in which the child or youth engages, understanding of his or her natural contexts, and analysis of performance. When evaluating a child's performance, the occupational therapist determines how performance is influenced by impairment and how the environment supports or constrains performance. The occupational therapist also identifies discrepancies between the child's performance and activity demands and interprets how to overcome or minimize those discrepancies. Analysis of the interrelationships among environments, occupations, and persons and the goodness-of-fit of these elements is the basis for sound clinical decisions. At the same time that occupational therapists systematically analyze the child's occupational performance and social participation, they acknowledge that the child's spirit and family's support highly influence the outcome.

This text describes theories, practice models, principles, and strategies that are used in occupational therapy with children. It presents evidence-based interventions designed to help children and families cope with disability and master occupations that have meaning to them. Although this theoretical and technical information is important to occupational therapy practice with children, it is childhood itself that creates meaning for the practitioner. Childhood is hopeful, joyful, and ever new. The spirit, the playfulness, and the joy of childhood create the context for occupational therapy with children. This chapter describes the primary themes in occupational therapy practice with children and adolescents that are illustrated throughout the text.

Essential Concepts in Occupational Therapy for Children and Adolescents

Using the research literature and their own expertise, the book's authors illustrate the role of occupational therapy with children and adolescents in specific practice areas and settings. Certain themes flow through many, if not most, of the chapters, suggesting their importance to occupational therapy. Four overarching themes (Box 1-1), briefly described in this chapter, are ubiquitous throughout practice and are well illustrated throughout the chapters of this book.

Individualized Therapy Services

A child or adolescent is referred to occupational therapy services because he or she has a specific diagnosis (e.g., autism or cerebral palsy) or because he or she exhibits a particular functional problem (e.g., poor fine motor skills or poor attention). Although the diagnosis or problem is the reason for therapy services, the occupational therapist always views the child or youth as a person first. Client-centered intervention has many implications for how the occupational therapist designs intervention. Primary implications of client-centered practice are listed in Table 1-1.

TABLE 1-1 Principles of Client-Centered Intervention

Area of Intervention	Principles
Assessment	Child or adolescent and family concerns and interests are assessed in a welcoming and open interview.
	Child or adolescent and family priorities and concerns guide assessment of the child.
Team interaction	Child or adolescent and family are valued members of the intervention team.
	Communication among team members is child- and family-friendly.
	Relationships among team members are valued and nourished.
Intervention	Child or adolescent with caregivers guide intervention.
	Families choose level of participation they wish to have.
	Family and child or adolescent interests are considered in developing intervention strategies.
	When appropriate, intervention directly involves other family members (e.g., siblings, grandparents).
Life span approach	As child transitions to preadolescence and adolescence, he or she becomes the primary decision maker for intervention goals and activities.

BOX 1-1 Themes That Characterize Occupational Therapy Practice with Children and Adolescents

Individualized therapy services
- Client-centered services
- Strength-based approaches
- Family-centered services

Inclusive and integrated services
- Natural environments
- Integrated services

Cultural competence

Evidence-based practice and scientific reasoning

As illustrated throughout the book, client-centered evaluation involves first identifying concerns and priorities of the child and family. Initially and throughout therapy services, occupational therapists prioritize and make specific efforts to learn about the child and family's interests, goals, daily routines, and preferred activities. What is important to the child and caregivers frames the goals and activities of the intervention. Fit of occupational therapy recommendations to family goals and interests is revisited throughout the intervention period to ensure that services are meeting the priorities of the child or adolescent and family.

Child-Centered Practices

As described by Law, Baptiste, and Mills,[73] client-centered occupational therapy is an approach to service that embraces a philosophy of respect for and partnership with people receiving services. Tickle-Degnen[128] further explains that practitioners form a therapeutic alliance with their clients in which they build rapport and collaborate to develop common goals and shared responsibility for achieving those goals. According to Parham et al.,[96] a primary feature of sensory integration intervention is "fostering therapeutic alliance." They describe this alliance as one in which the occupational therapist "respects the child's emotions, conveys positive regard toward the child, seems to connect with the child and creates a climate of trust and emotional safety"[96] (see Chapter 9). This relationship with the child is a priority for the occupational therapist and is believed to be instrumental to achieving positive intervention outcomes.

Philosophically, theoretically, and practically, client-centeredness is ubiquitous to occupational therapy interventions This concept means that occupational therapists provide choices, allow the child or youth to make activity choices, and broadly consider the child's culture and context when designing interventions. In child-centered practice, practitioners use activities that are meaningful to and preferred by the child, knowing that they engage the child's efforts. Children are motivated to take on skill challenges that the occupational therapist embeds in preferred activities. It is also implied that the occupational therapist selects activities that are developmentally appropriate, suitable to the child's environment, and aligned with the child's expressed or understood goals.

Occupational therapists invite children and youth to participate actively in the evaluation process and goal setting using developmentally appropriate methods.[87] Measures have been developed to assess the child's perspective on his or her ability to participate in desired occupations. For example, when using the Canadian Occupational Performance Measure (COPM), the family and child rate the importance of self-identified performance problems. By administering the COPM as part of the initial evaluation, the occupational therapist can prioritize the child's goals and begin a collaborative relationship with the family. The Perceived Efficacy and Goal Setting System (PEGS) is another example of a measure that uses the child as the primary informant.[88] These assessments are explained further in Chapters 11, 15, and 23. The information gathered from measuring children's thoughts and feelings about their participation in childhood roles can complement results obtained from functional assessments. In addition, occupational therapists may consider gathering information about the child's life satisfaction. Often the best strategy for gathering information about the child's or adolescent's interests and perspectives is to ask open-ended questions about his or her play preferences, favorite activities, best friends, special talents, and greatest concerns.

The occupational therapist monitors the fit of intervention activities to the child's daily routines by asking parents and teachers. The occupational therapist seeks ways to adapt recommendations to match the child's evolving interests and routines and to ensure that therapy is directed to current priorities of the child and family. Continually assessing which therapeutic activities are most appropriate given the child's developmental levels, current performance, and interests, the practitioner

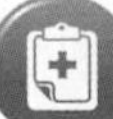

CASE STUDY 1-1 A Strength-Based Approach with a Child Who Has High Functioning Autism

Victor is a 10-year-old boy with high functioning autism. He has extraordinary visual perceptual skills and visual memory; he also has significant delays in social skills. In particular, he has difficulty knowing how to interact with his peers on the playground or in unstructured social activities. The therapist, Amy, suggests that he video record his peers when they are playing together or talking on the playground. Using these videos, Victor has examples of appropriate social interactions. He and Amy analyze the videos together, discussing how the children initiate and respond to social interaction; he practices some of the interactions with Amy. Amy encourages him to watch the examples of positive social interactions a number of times.

Using the videos, Victor makes and labels photographs of different examples of social interactions. With Amy's help, Victor organizes the photographs into stories that he uses to learn how to engage with others socially. Amy also helps him organize the photographs into a social story; she creates a visual step-by-step procedure for initiating a social interaction.

The other children were interested in his videos and stories; they read the stories and praised Victor's skills in video recording and photography. His interest in and talents for photography resulted in a sequence of naturally occurring social interactions that allowed Victor to practice the social skills. By using a strength-based approach, he not only had used his talents to learn new skills, but also his peers recognized and appreciated his talent, establishing enhanced contexts for social participation.

Adapted from Bianco, Carothers, & Smiley.[10]

selects activities that are most useful for obtaining the child and family's goals.[128]

Strength-Based Approaches

Using holistic approaches, occupational therapists begin intervention by considering the strengths of a child or youth. With a full understanding of the child's strengths and interests, practitioners develop a plan to increase participation by building on those strengths. By identifying the positive aspects of a child's behavior and areas of greatest competence as well as performance limitations, the occupational therapist can access these strengths to overcome the challenges to participation. The strength-based model contrasts with the traditional medical model, in which the focus of intervention is on identifying the health or performance problem and resolving that problem. As explained in many chapters of this book, focusing on a child's performance problem does not always lead to optimal participation and improved quality of life. Because occupational therapists are concerned with a child's full participation in life activities, focusing solely on impairment narrows the vision of what the child can become and do.

Children and youth with disabilities often have unique strengths that are overlooked by professionals, but if these strengths are identified and encouraged, they can lead to increased participation. For example, a youth with high functioning autism may have excellent visual memory or analytic abilities. For this youth, cognitive approaches that engage the youth in problem solving and in determining how to structure social activities can help him overcome social skill limitations. For a child with spastic quadriparesis cerebral palsy who has a joyous sense of humor, encouraging his sense of humor in a social group can help to build peer supports and friendships that increase his participation in school activities.

As explained in numerous chapters, strength-based approaches can lead to increased self-efficacy and self-determination. When an occupational therapist acknowledges a child's strengths and competence, the child becomes more self-efficacious and motivated, and he or she may be more willing to take on performance challenges. A child with positive self-efficacy is more likely to make repeated and sustained efforts to achieve his or her goals, despite lack of immediate success.[7] Case Study 1-1 illustrates use of a strength-based approach with a child who has high functioning autism spectrum disorder. Chapter 12 explains how an occupational therapist's emphasis on strength-based approaches can facilitate increased self-determination and skills in self-advocacy in youth with disabilities. Identifying an adolescent's strengths can be particularly potent in interventions to promote social participation and friendship networks because it helps peers and family members recognize and acknowledge the adolescent's talents and interest and establish these as the basis for social interaction. Kramer and colleagues (Chapter 12) describe a community service program, EPIC Service Warriors, in which youth with disabilities serve others by cleaning up parks and making food at homeless shelters. This program expands the social networks of youth with disabilities, demonstrates a model of community inclusion, and changes the way these adolescents think about themselves. Envisioning roles for youth and adults with disabilities to serve others can enhance self-efficacy and change society's view of potential roles for people with disabilities.

A strength-based approach when offering parent supports and education is equally important. By identifying positive characteristics in the child, occupational therapists can help relieve parents' stress and can improve parents' engagement.[49,121] Steiner[121] found that when occupational therapists acknowledged the strengths of parents of children with autism (versus noting their deficits), parents demonstrated more positive affect and physical affection toward their child. When occupational therapists made positive statements about a child, parents repeated their statements and, less expected, demonstrated more playful behaviors and physical affection.[121]

Family-Centered Practices

In a family-centered approach, the occupational therapist is invested in establishing a relationship with the family characterized by open communication, shared decision making, and parental empowerment.[12] An equal partnership with the family is desired, where each partner values the knowledge and opinions of the other.[53,130] Trust building between professionals and family members is a first step in building a relationship. Demonstrating mutual respect, being positive, and maintaining a nonjudgmental position with a family appear to be important to establishing trust (see Chapter 5). Trust building can be particularly challenging with certain families—for example, families whose race, ethnicity, culture, or socioeconomic status may differ from that of the occupational therapist. These families may hold strong beliefs about child rearing, health care, and disabilities that are substantially different from those of the occupational therapist. However, establishing a relationship of mutual respect is essential to the therapeutic process.

Jaffe and Cosper (Chapter 5) explain that occupational therapists cultivate positive relationships with families when they establish open and honest communication and encourage participation of parents in their child's program to the extent that they desire. When asked to give advice to occupational therapists, parents stated that they appreciated (1) specific, objective information; (2) flexibility in service delivery; (3) sensitivity and responsiveness to their concerns[83]; (4) positive, optimistic attitudes[24]; and (5) technical expertise and skills.[12]

In a qualitative study in which 29 families were interviewed about their experiences in parenting a child with disabilities and working with the intervention systems, four themes emerged.[42] (1) Parents need professionals to recognize that parenting a child with a disability is a "24/7" job with continual and often intensive responsibilities. (2) Both internal (coping and resilience) and external (e.g., extended family) resources are needed to raise a child with a disability; these should be bolstered and encouraged. (3) Parents ask that professionals respect them as the experts on their child. (4) Parents also ask that professionals accept their family's values. Although this study's qualitative findings do not constitute rigorous evidence of intervention effects, the findings concur with other descriptive studies of family-centered intervention. When combined, these studies suggest that respecting parents' knowledge of their child, acknowledging their resilience, accepting their values, and facilitating the building of a network of social resources are important components of family-centered intervention.[40]

In Chapter 22, on early intervention services, Myers, Case-Smith, and Cason explain methods for partnering with families. Recommended activities most likely to be implemented by and most helpful to the family are activities that are directly relevant to the family's lifestyle and routines. When interventions make a family's daily routine easier or more comfortable, the intervention can have an immediate positive effect and is more likely to be sustained and generalized to other routines and environments.

In a meta-analysis of family-centered practice in early intervention service, two types of family-centered services were identified: (1) services that fostered positive professional-family relationships and (2) services that enabled the family's participation in intervention activities.[40] In relationship building practices, occupational therapists actively listen, show compassion and respect, and believe in the family's capabilities. Occupational therapists enable and promote the family's participation by individualizing their services, demonstrating flexibility in meeting family needs, and being responsive to family concerns. Dunst, Trivette, and Hamby[41] found that the provision of family-centered services was highly related to the family's self-efficacy beliefs, parents' satisfaction with the program, parenting behaviors, and child behavior and functioning.

Inclusive and Integrated Services

Practitioners of occupational therapy are strong advocates for inclusion of all persons with disabilities. They embrace the vision that children and youth with disabilities fully participate in the community and take on roles to facilitate full participation. Inclusion of people with disabilities into communities involves transforming attitudes and assumptions, through education but primarily through demonstration that children and youth with disabilities can fully participate. To support inclusion of children and youth with disabilities in environments with children without disabilities, practitioners may recommend modifications to increase physical access, accommodations to increase social participation, or strategies to improve the child's ability to meet the performance and behavioral expectations. For example, occupational therapists often have roles in evaluating physical access in schools or jobs and recommending assistive technology or task modification. Occupational therapists have been leaders in promoting inclusion throughout their history,[54,65] providing services that enable full inclusion of persons with mental, physical, and cognitive disabilities.

In current practice, legal mandates necessitate that services to children with disabilities be provided in environments with children who do not have disabilities. The Individuals with Disabilities Education Act requires that services to infants and toddlers be provided in "natural environments" and that services to preschool and school-aged children be provided in the "least restrictive environment." The infant's natural environment is most often his or her home, but it may include any place that the family defines as the child's natural environment. This requirement shifts when the child reaches school age, not in its intent but with recognition that community schools and regular education classrooms are the most natural and least restrictive environments for services to children with disabilities. Inclusion in natural environments or regular education classrooms succeeds only when specific supports and accommodations are provided to children with disabilities. Occupational therapists are often important team members in making inclusion successful for children with disabilities. (This concept is discussed further in Chapters 22 and 23.)

Early Intervention Services in the Child's Natural Environment

The Division of Early Childhood of the Council for Exceptional Children supports the philosophy of inclusion in natural environments with the following statement: "Inclusion, as a value, supports the right of all children, regardless of their diverse abilities, to participate actively in natural settings within their communities. A natural setting is one in which the child would spend time if he or she had not had a disability."[36]

As explained by Myers, Case-Smith, and Cason (Chapter 22), the philosophy of inclusion extends beyond physical inclusion to mean social and emotional inclusion of the child and family.[26,131] The implications for occupational therapists are that they provide opportunities for expanded and enriched natural learning with typically developing peers. A natural environment can be any setting that is part of the everyday routine of the

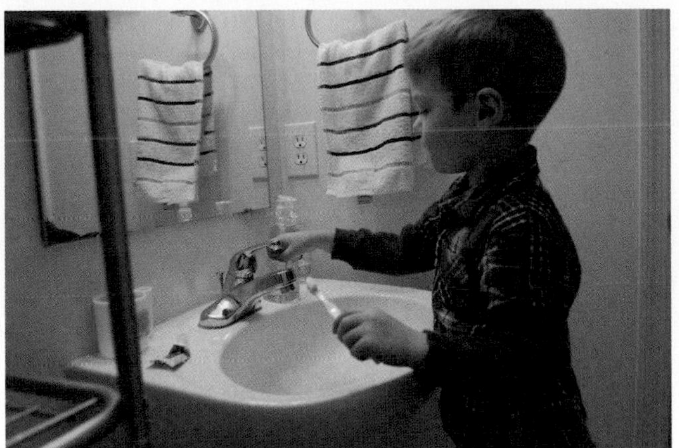

FIGURE 1-1 When occupational therapy is provided in the child's home, the practitioners and child have easy access to practice of self-care activities.

child and family where incidental learning experiences occur.[42] Intervention and consultation services can occur in a childcare center, at a grandmother's house, or in another place that is part of a family's routine. Social, play, and self-care learning opportunities in these environments are plentiful. Figure 1-1 shows an example of a child's natural environment in which the occupational therapist could intervene.

When occupational therapy occurs in a natural environment such as the home, the intervention activities are embedded in naturally occurring interactions and situations. In incidental learning opportunities, the occupational therapist challenges the child to try a different approach or to practice an emerging skill during typical activities. The occupational therapist follows the young child's lead and uses natural consequences (e.g., a smile or frown, a pat or tickle) to motivate learning (Figure 1-2).

Research has shown that intervention strategies that occur in real-life settings produce greater developmental change than those that take place in more contrived, clinic-based settings.[18,42] In addition, generalization of skills and behaviors occurs more readily when the intervention setting is the same as the child's natural environments.[58,59]

Early intervention therapy services in natural environments require the occupational therapist to be creative, flexible, and spontaneous.[41] The occupational therapist must accept and use the toys, objects, and environmental spaces in the family's home as those are most important and culturally relevant to the child's development (Figure 1-3). The occupational therapist must think through many alternative ways to reach the established goals and adapt those strategies to whichever situation is presented.[52] Recognizing and accepting the family's uniqueness in cultural and child-rearing practices enables the occupational therapist to facilitate the child's participation in his or her natural environments.

Integrated Service Delivery Models

In school-based services, inclusion refers to integration of the child with disabilities into the regular classroom with support to accomplish the regular curriculum. Box 1-2 lists the desired outcomes of inclusive school environments. In schools with well-designed inclusion, every student's competence in diversity and tolerance for differences increases. To promote the child's participation across school environments, occupational therapy practitioners integrate their services into multiple environments (e.g., within the classroom, on the playground, in the cafeteria, on and off the school bus). The occupational therapist's presence in the classroom benefits the instructional staff members, who observe the occupational therapy intervention. As explained by Bazyk and Cahill (Chapter 23), integrated therapy ensures that the occupational therapist's focus has high relevance to the performance expected within the classroom. It also increases the likelihood that adaptations and therapeutic techniques will be carried over into classroom activities,[8,117,137]

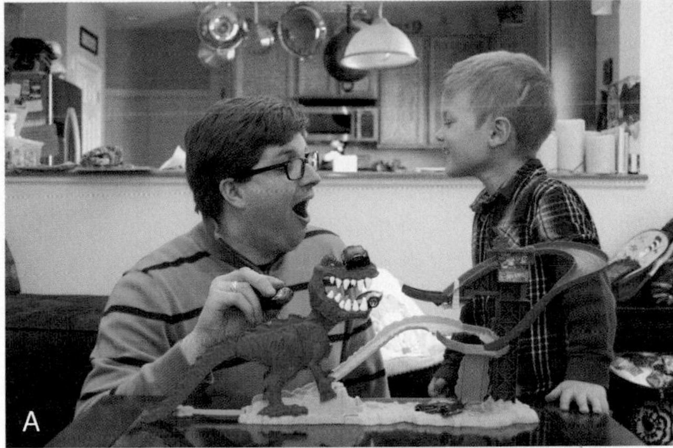

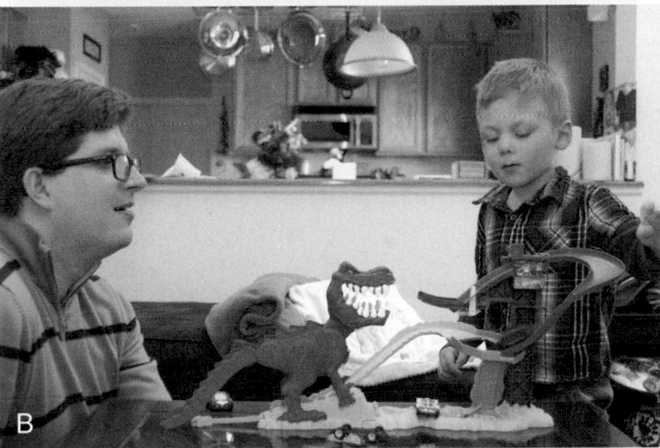

FIGURE 1-2 A and B, Therapist and child rapport is demonstrated by sharing pleasure and clowning around.

BOX 1-2 Desired Inclusion Outcomes

- Children with disabilities are full participants in school, preschool, and childcare center activities.
- Children with disabilities have friends and relationships with their peers.
- Children with disabilities learn and achieve within the general educational curriculum to the best of their abilities.
- All children learn to appreciate individual differences in people.
- All children learn tolerance and respect for others.
- Children with disabilities participate to the fullest extent possible in their communities.

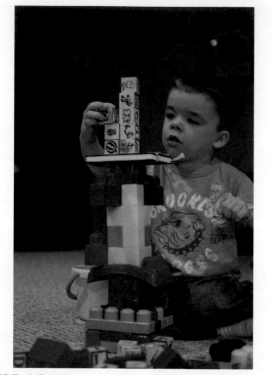

FIGURE 1-3 The occupational therapist uses the child's own toys in the home to challenge and practice his or her emerging skills with the high probability that the child will continue to practice these skills.

and it allows the occupational therapist to link his or her goals and activities to the curriculum and the classroom priorities.

Children with disabilities benefit when therapy is provided as both direct and consultative services. Occupational therapists provide these services in the context of an interprofessional team, where communication about the child's strengths and limitations, expected performance, and contextual barriers and resources enables a cohesive plan and the likelihood of positive outcomes. Because children constantly change and the environment is dynamic, frequent team communication and planning are needed. With opportunities to interact directly with the child and experience the classroom environment, the occupational therapist can best support the child's participation and guide the support of other adults.

In a fluid service delivery model, therapy services increase when naturally occurring events create a need—for example, when the child obtains a new adapted device, when the child has surgery or casting, or when a new baby brother creates added stress for a family. Similarly, therapy services should be reduced when the child has learned new skills that primarily need to be repeated and practiced in his or her daily routine or the child has reached a plateau on therapy-related goals.

Models for school-based service delivery that offer the possibility for greater flexibility[21] include block scheduling[99] and co-teaching.[22] These models of flexible scheduling allow occupational therapists to move fluidly between direct and consultative services. In block scheduling, occupational therapists spend 2 to 3 hours in the early childhood classroom working with the children with special needs one on one and in small groups, while supporting the teaching staff (see Chapter 22). Block scheduling allows occupational therapists to learn about the classroom, develop relationships with the teachers, and understand the curriculum so that they can design interventions that are easily integrated into the classroom. By being present in the classroom for an entire morning or afternoon, the occupational therapist can find natural learning opportunities to work on a specific child's goals. Using the child's self-selected play activity, the occupational therapist employs strategies that are meaningful to the child, fit into the child's preferred activities, and are likely to be practiced.[119] During the blocked time, the occupational therapist can run small groups, coach the teacher and assistants,[21,109] evaluate the child's performance, and monitor the child's participation in classroom activities.

Another integrated model of service delivery is co-teaching.[31,37] This model emphasizes preventive approaches in that children at risk for disabilities as well as children in individualized education programs receive occupational therapy services. In this model, the occupational therapist and teacher plan and implement the sessions together. Collaborative planning allows interdisciplinary perspectives on student issues and behaviors; enables the occupational therapist to align interventions closely with the curriculum; and ensures that interventions can be feasibly implemented in the classroom, with consideration given to the teacher's goals and curricular expectations. Co-teaching models have been successfully implemented for handwriting programs, in which occupational therapists take on teaching roles while providing individualized supports and interventions for students who have handwriting difficulties.[23] Benefits of co-teaching are that occupational therapy services are embedded into the classroom instruction; students at risk receive more intensive instruction with individualized supports; and students with individualized education programs receive integrated services that support performance throughout their school day.

Cultural Competence That Embraces Diversity

To achieve full inclusion, all team members and systems must demonstrate cultural competence.[29] With increasing diversity within all communities, respecting and honoring the culture of the child and family are important to enable full inclusion and facilitate full participation. Cross-cultural competence can be defined as "the ability to think, feel, and act in ways that acknowledge, respect, and build upon ethnic, [socio]cultural, and linguistic diversity."[79] Cultural competence in health care refers to behaviors and attitudes that enable an individual to function effectively with culturally diverse families.[29] Cross-cultural competence is salient to occupational therapists who work with children and youth given that:

1. Cultural diversity of the United States continues to increase.
2. A child's occupations, including social participation, are embedded in the cultural practices of his or her family and community.

Cultural Diversity in the United States

The diversity and heterogeneity of American families continue to increase each year. The latest census numbers[132] show that the fastest growing populations in the United States are multiracial Americans, Asians, and Hispanics and that non-Hispanic white Americans will become a minority group within the next 3 decades. The United States has become a multicultural

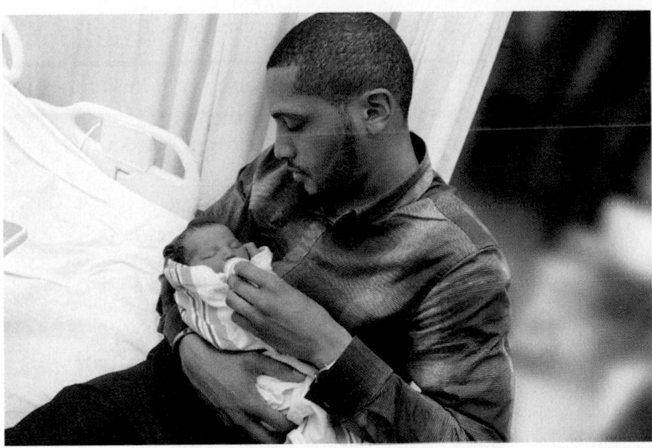

FIGURE 1-4 A father bonds with his just-born son. (Photo © istock.com.)

nation, and today's children will become adults in this environment that is rich with cultural and racial diversity. In 2011, the United States was home to 74 million children. Of these, 53% were white, 14% were African American, 4.5% were Asian, and 23.5% were Hispanic.[3]

Diversity of ethnicity and race can be viewed as a risk or as a resource to child development.[45] Low birthrate, preterm delivery, and infant mortality are higher in African American families, suggesting that these families frequently need early childhood intervention programs. Race can also be a resource; for example, African American families are well supported by their communities and focused on their children (Figure 1-4). Studies also show that African Americans are child-centered and highly invested in child development.[55] Parents often perceive discipline and politeness as positive attributes and instill these in their children.[134] Children are taught to be obedient and respectful of adults. In addition, many African American families emphasize the importance of spirituality and religion.[126] Occupational therapists who work with African American families find many positive attributes in their family interactions and parenting styles. Families from other cultures, such as Hispanic families, have similar beliefs and child-rearing practices.[102]

Poverty has a pervasive effect on children's developmental and health outcomes.[28] Despite overall prosperity in the United States, a significant number of children and families live in poverty. Although children younger than 18 years old represent only 23% of the U.S. population, they account for 34% of all people in poverty. Among all children, 45% live in low-income families, and approximately 20% live in poor families.[62] In 2014, the Children's Defense Fund reported that 1 in every 5 children, or 16.1 million, was poor and that 40% of these lived in extreme poverty. These children are disproportionately black, American Indian, and Hispanic. Often these children live in families with a single parent. Families in poverty often have great need for, yet limited access to, health care and educational services.

Many families who are served by early intervention and special education systems are of low socioeconomic status. When families lack resources (e.g., transportation, food, shelter), their priorities and concerns orient to these basic needs. Responsive occupational therapists provide resources to assist with these basic needs, making appropriate referrals to community agencies. They also demonstrate understanding of the family's priorities as these relate to the child's occupational performance goals and the family's participation in the community. Chapter 5 describes helpful practices for families with limited resources.

Influence of Cultural Practices on a Child's Development of Occupations

To support and improve a child's participation in the home, school, and community, occupational therapists need to understand the multitude of ways that cultural practices influence a child's occupations. Table 1-2 lists questions to elicit information about the cultural practices and values that may influence a child's development of occupations. For certain cultures, performance goals of interdependence may be more appropriate than goals for independence, particularly at certain ages. Cultural groups vary in their perception of giving and receiving help, communication styles, and child-rearing beliefs. The literature is replete with examples of the influence of culture on children's occupations.[27,34,45,61,108]

Cultural values in families often influence their routines, daily activities, and expectations for child participation in family routines. For example, Middle Eastern families often do not emphasize early independence in self-care; skills such as self-feeding may not be a family priority until ages well beyond the normative expectations.[115] Interventions to promote self-feeding during early childhood may not be a priority for Middle Eastern families. In Hispanic cultures, holding and cuddling are highly valued, even in older children.[138] Mothers hold and carry their preschool children. Recommending a wheelchair for a young child may be unacceptable to families who value close physical contact and holding.

In some cultures (e.g., Polynesian), parents delegate child-care responsibilities to older siblings. In established families, siblings care for the infants. Young children in Polynesian cultures tend to rely on their older siblings rather than their parents for structure, assistance, and support. Being responsible for a younger sibling helps the older sibling mature quickly by learning responsibility and problem solving.[108] Primary care by an older sibling is challenging when the younger child has a disability and needs additional or prolonged assistance.

Because the focus of occupational therapy is to enhance a child's ability to participate in his or her natural environment and everyday routines, the occupational therapist must appreciate, value, and understand those environments and routines. Recommendations that run counter to a family's cultural values are not likely to be implemented by family members and may be detrimental to the professional-family relationship. By asking open-ended questions, occupational therapists can elicit information about the family's routines, rituals, and traditions to provide an understanding of the cultural context.

A culturally competent occupational therapist demonstrates an interest in understanding the family's culture, an acceptance of diversity, and a willingness to participate in traditions or cultural patterns of the family. In home-based services, cultural competence may mean removing shoes at the home's entryway, accepting foods when offered, scheduling therapy sessions around holidays, and accommodating language differences. In center-based services, cultural sensitivity remains important, although a family's cultural values may be more difficult to ascertain outside the home.

TABLE 1-2 Cultural Values and Styles That Influence Children's Development of Occupations

Value or Style	Guiding Questions
Family composition	Who are the members of the family? How many family members live in the same house? Is there a hierarchy in the family based on gender or age?
Decision making	Who makes the decisions for the family?
Primary caregiver	Who is the primary caregiver? Is this role shared?
Independence/interdependence	Do family members value independence?
Feeding practices	Who feeds the infant or child? What are the cultural rules or norms about breastfeeding, mealtime, self-feeding, and eating certain foods? When is independence in feeding expected?
Sleeping patterns	Do children sleep with parents? How do parents respond to the infant during the night? What are appropriate responses to crying?
Discipline	Is disobedience tolerated? How strict are the rules governing behavior? Who disciplines the child? How do the parents discipline the child?
Perception of disability	Do the parents believe that the disability can improve? Do they feel responsible for the disability? Do family members feel that they can make a difference in improving the disability? Are spiritual forms of healing valued?
Help seeking	From whom does the family seek help? Does the family actively seek help, or do family members expect help to come to them?
Communication and interaction	Does the family use a direct or an indirect style of communication? Do family members share emotional feelings? Is most communication direct or indirect? Does the family value socializing?

Adapted from Wayman, K. I., Lynch, E. W., & Hanson, M. J. (1990). Home-based early childhood services: cultural sensitivity in a family systems approach. *Topics in Early Childhood Special Education, 10,* 65–66.

A culturally competent occupational therapist inquires about family routines, cultural practices, traditions, and priorities; demonstrates a willingness to accommodate to these cultural values; and integrates intervention recommendations into the family's cultural practices. The occupational therapist's appreciation of the influence of culture on children's occupations facilitates the development of appropriate priorities and the use of strategies that are congruent with the family's values and lifestyle.

In summary, occupational therapy services can be characterized as child-centered and family-centered, integrated into the natural environment of the child or youth, and culturally competent. These concepts guide the practitioner's decision making about which interventions and service delivery models are most appropriate. Clinical reasoning is also guided by the research evidence. As explained in the following section, occupational therapy interventions are grounded in occupation-based models that are supported by research evidence.

Evidence-Based Practice and Scientific Reasoning

Occupational therapists have fully moved into the era of evidence-based practice (EBP). Historically, practice techniques were handed down from practitioner to practitioner.[56] Beginning in the 1940s and 1950s, intervention strategies and activities were described in journals and textbooks; however, measures and data were rarely included in these descriptions. Occupational therapy was considered to be a "craft" in which the therapist viewed each client as unique and designed an intervention plan based on his or her experience and expertise. Although research was recognized to be important to the profession, the art of therapy and the uniqueness of each client were emphasized. In the second half of the twentieth century, scholars in occupational therapy realized that professional reasoning needed to be guided by practice models. An understanding of critical reasoning and theory-based practice developed in the 1960s and 1970s.[106] At that time, theories of occupation,[67] play,[100] and sensory integration[5] were organized into practice models and became widely accepted by the profession. These theory-based practice models, described by Parham[94] as "tools for thinking," were guided by hypotheses about how individuals perform occupations, develop occupational roles, and function in their environments.[66] These models included postulates on how interventions can improve occupational performance and function.[106] Although theory-based models resulted in more systematic clinical reasoning and improved coherence in intervention methods, the field had little evidence of its efficacy, and practitioners made decisions with mostly personal knowledge of intervention outcomes.

Beginning in the 1990s and continuing into the twenty-first century, the profession has been highly invested in evaluating intervention outcomes and in researching its practice models to establish evidence for their effectiveness.[74] In the past 25 years, researchers in occupational therapy and related professions have focused their efforts on creating trials and studies that examine the effectiveness of interventions. As a result, hundreds of efficacy studies on occupational therapy interventions for children have been published.[70,98] Many of these studies are cited in the chapters of this book and are incorporated in the explanations of interventions.

With extensive availability of research on pediatric practice, competent practitioners read, appraise, and use this evidence when making clinical decisions about intervention. The Institute of Medicine defines health care quality as the extent to which health services are consistent with current professional knowledge.[60] However, despite wide agreement among professionals regarding the importance of EBP, studies have shown

BOX 1-3 Steps in Evidence-Based Practice

Step 1
- Convert the need for information (about intervention effects, prognosis, therapy methods) into an answerable question.

Step 2
- Search the research databases using the terms in the research question.
- Track down the best evidence to answer that question.

Step 3
- Critically appraise the evidence for its:
  - validity (truthfulness)
  - impact (level of effect)
  - clinical meaningfulness

Step 4
- Critically appraise the evidence for its applicability and usefulness to your practice.

Step 5
- Implement the practice or apply the information.
- Evaluate the process.

that research findings are not routinely integrated into everyday practice.[111,127] Barriers to implementing research findings fully into daily practice include practitioners' limited time to read and consume all the available evidence and lack of administrative support to develop systems for routinely using evidence in practice.

With the proliferation of published research related to pediatric occupational therapy,[9,70] organizations, including the American Occupational Therapy Association, have supported the development of EBP guidelines.[20] EBP guidelines are developed by a group of experts who synthesize the research on a particular intervention or diagnosis to formulate recommendations for practice. These guidelines translate the research evidence to practice by making specific recommendations for evaluations and interventions that prioritize the recommendations using a grading system.[48,92]

Hospitals and medical systems are aggressively promoting use of EBP guidelines to improve the consistency and effectiveness of medical intervention.[1] Schools and educational systems also are calling for research evidence to be used to guide educational practices and policies.[118] Clinical guidelines enable efficient consumption of efficacy research; however, implementing the guidelines consistently also requires commitment, system and environmental supports, and consensus among the agency's or program's team. EBP clinical guidelines have been adopted by children's hospitals and medical systems as tools to promote quality improvement and patient outcomes.[30] When EBP guidelines are implemented within quality improvement processes, they also are embedded in existing processes that include monitoring and examining outcomes. Numerous steps are needed to ensure that use of EBP guidelines results in improved outcomes (Box 1-3).

Using evidence is part of the occupational therapist's scientific reasoning (Figure 1-5). With scientific reasoning,[112] the occupational therapist uses clinical guidelines that have

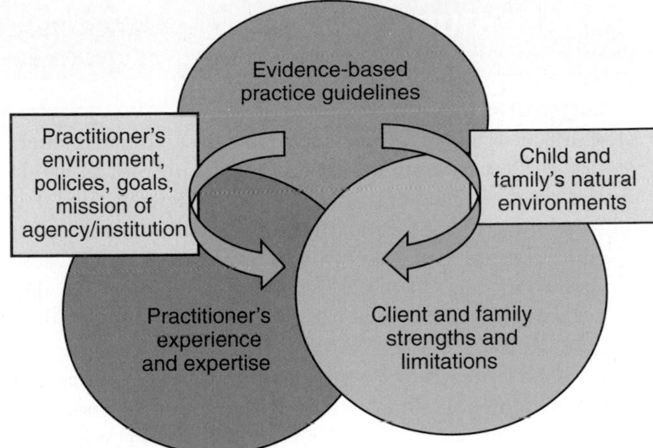

FIGURE 1-5 Scientific reasoning using evidence-based practice guidelines.

synthesized the research evidence, science-based knowledge about the diagnosis, and past experience in all steps of the assessment and intervention process. These resources are accessed, interpreted for the practice context and the child's and family's needs, and used to guide intervention. Case Study 1-2 describes using an EBP guideline in clinical decision making for a young child with autism spectrum disorder.

There are benefits to using the recommendations from EBP guidelines; they:

1. Are relevant because experts in the diagnosis or type of intervention determine the scope and methods for developing the recommendations.
2. Represent synthesis of current research that is appraised and evaluated.
3. Incorporate appraisal of available evidence by grading the recommendations based on the rigor of the research; these grades determine the importance and priority of the recommendations.
4. Represent the consensus of the experts.

Following clinical guidelines has the potential of increasing the consistency of practice and its efficacy. The likelihood of positive outcomes is high when occupational therapists (1) select EBP guidelines with optimal fit to their clientele and environment, (2) adapt the guidelines to fit their work environment, (3) modify them into user-friendly protocols, (4) examine and resolve barriers to implementation, and (5) establish systems to monitor their outcomes.[19] All of the chapters in this book use research evidence in describing evaluation and intervention.

In summary, the occupational therapy process is grounded in research evidence. Occupational therapists select assessments with evidence of validity and reliability and interventions that demonstrate positive effects for performance and participation goals of relevance to their clients. The following sections briefly describe the occupational therapy process of evaluation and intervention as it is presented throughout the book.

Comprehensive Evaluation

The chapter authors recommend using a *top-down* approach to assessment—that is, the occupational therapist begins the

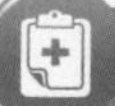

CASE STUDY 1-2 Using Evidence-Based Practice Guidelines for Restricted Eating in Autism Spectrum Disorder

Background

Meg, a school-based occupational therapist, initiated intervention for Rebecca, a 5-year-old girl with autism with highly restricted eating. Meg evaluated Rebecca and determined that she eats eight to nine foods throughout the day as snacks. She does not participate in mealtime with the family because she has a tantrum when foods that are not part of her diet are presented. Rebecca eats crackers, cereals, chips, noodles, and French fries, and she occasionally eats yogurt, milk, and cheese. She interacts with her caregiver using gestures and two-word sentences. She also uses jargon that does not have communicative intent. She is very skilled in computer tablet games, puzzles, and Lego blocks. She is independent in eating and dressing but continues to require some assistance with bathing, and she dislikes water and soap. Rebecca's parents have prioritized her eating as a first occupational therapy goal.

Meg accessed the BESt evidence statement from *Behavioral and oral motor interventions for feeding problems in children* (Cincinnati Children's Hospital and Medical Center, 2013) to guide her intervention planning. Listed in order of evidence strength, the following BESt recommendations seemed relevant, appropriate given Rebecca's age and behaviors, and feasible to implement at home and school. These recommendations were particularly applicable because Rebecca exhibited significant behavioral rigidity and stereotypic behaviors, and she did not appear to have sensory processing problems.

- It is recommended that the following behavioral interventions within a treatment package may be used to increase intake for children with feeding problems:
  - Differential attention
  - Positive reinforcement
  - Escape extinction/escape prevention
  - Stimulus fading
  - Simultaneous presentation
- It is recommended that a child (4 months to 7 years old) with feeding difficulties be exposed 10 to 15 times to a previously unfamiliar or nonpreferred food to increase intake (Cincinnati Children's Hospital Medical Center, 2013).

An intervention was designed in which a nonpreferred food was placed on Rebecca's plate with her preferred foods twice a day. The teacher or occupational therapist implemented the intervention at school, and the mother implemented it once each day at home. The occupational therapist, teacher, or parent gave Rebecca praise and attention when she touched, played with, or tasted the nonpreferred foods. The occupational therapist and parent ate some of the nonpreferred food with her, modeling for her and having fun with that food. The same nonpreferred food was presented at least 10 times. The occupational therapist and parent used highly positive affect during the meal, and although Rebecca was allowed to eat her preferred foods, she was praised and reinforced only when she ate a nonpreferred food. The table was arranged to make escape very difficult, and she was encouraged to stay at the table.

In the first week, Rebecca did not eat any nonpreferred foods, but she touched and played with these foods (fruits, cream cheese, peanut butter, and pita bread). In the second week, she took several bites of nonpreferred foods each week, and by the third week, her regular diet had increased to 11 foods, including fruit, cream cheese, and peanut butter. Meg, the teacher, and Rebecca's mother recorded and tracked her eating and mealtime behavior each day to decide which foods to try and which reinforcement seemed most effective.

Summary

This guideline on feeding problems effectively improved Rebecca's eating and diet because:

- Rebecca's mother and teacher were invested in implementing mealtime interventions.
- The occupational therapist created a protocol from the feeding guideline that worked both at home and at school.
- The occupational therapist, teacher, and mother were committed to implementing the protocol consistently.
- A system for routinely assessing Rebecca's intake and behavior was developed and implemented.

Adapted from Cincinnati Children's Hospital Medical Center (2013). *Best evidence statement (BESt). Behavioral and oral motor intervention for feeding problems in children.* <http://www.guideline.gov/content.aspx?id=47062&search=autism%2c+eating> Accessed March 10, 2014.

evaluation process by gaining an understanding of the child's level of participation in daily occupations and routines with family, other caregiving adults, and peers. Initially, the occupational therapist surveys multiple sources to acquire a sense of the child's ability to participate and to develop an occupational profile for the child that includes his or her interests and priorities.[3] Table 1-3 lists attributes of occupational therapy evaluation of children.

Ecologic Assessment

Ecologic assessment allows the occupational therapist to consider how the environment influences performance and to design interventions that are easily implemented in the child's natural environment. By considering the child's performance in the context of physical and social demands, ecologic assessment helps to determine the discrepancy between the child's performance and expected performance (Figure 1-6). Ecologic assessment uses a top-down model that considers cultural influences, resources, and value systems of the child's environment. Bazyk and Cahill (Chapter 23) advocate for ecologic assessment of what the child "needs and wants to do across a variety of occupational performance areas and settings." In ecologic assessment, the occupational therapist considers the fit or match between the performance of the child or youth and the demands and expectations of the environment (e.g., in school-based practice, the relationship between the child's performance and the educational context and curriculum).

TABLE 1-3 Description of Comprehensive Evaluation of Children

Evaluation Component	Description of Occupational Therapist's Role—Tools, Informants
Occupational profile	Obtains information about child's developmental and functional strengths and limitations. Emphasis on child's participation across environments. Interview with parents, teachers, and other caregivers. Informal interview and observation.
Assessment of performance	Carefully assesses multiple areas of developmental performance and functional behaviors and underlying reasons for limitations. Standardized evaluations, structured observation, focused questions to parents and caregivers.
Analysis of performance	Analyzes underlying reasons for limitations in performance and behavior. In-depth structured observations, focused standardized evaluations.
Environment	Assessment and observation of environment, focused on supports and constraints of child's performance. Focused observations, interview of teachers and parents.

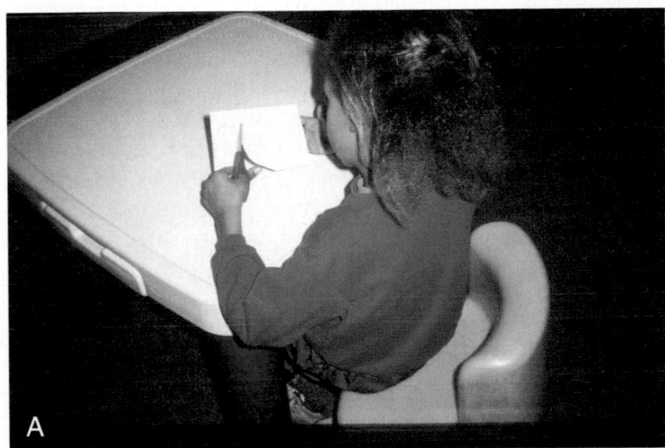

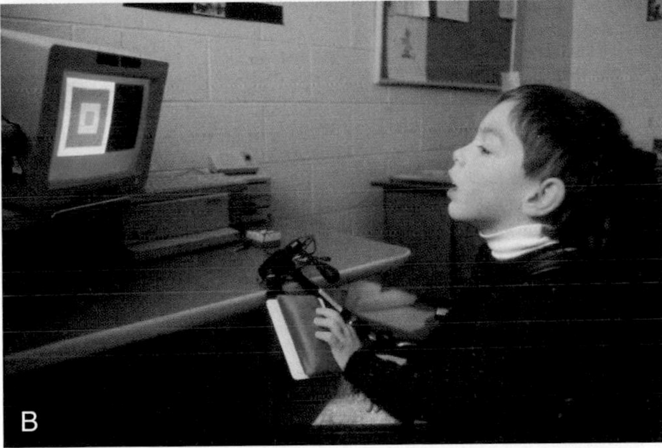

FIGURE 1-6 **A,** Cutting skills are assessed using the classroom art activity. **B,** The child's ability to access an instructional activity is assessed in the computer lab.

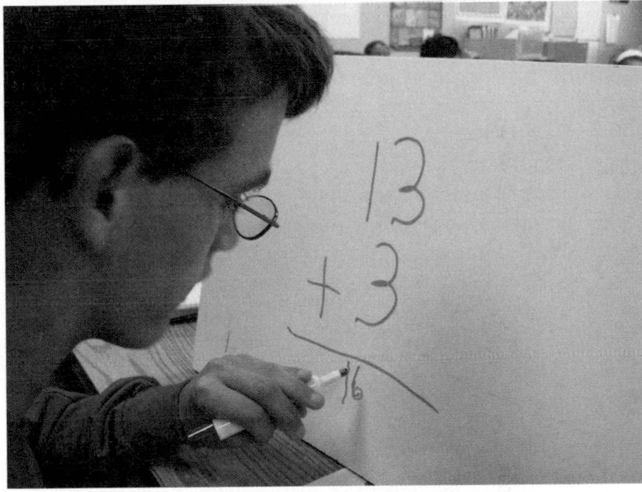

FIGURE 1-7 Through observation of writing activity at school, the occupational therapist gains an understanding of the child's performance and the accommodations and supports needed.

Two examples of standardized ecologic assessments are the School Function Assessment (SFA)[33] and the Participation and Environment Measure—Children and Youth (PEM-CY).[32] Both of these assessments are comprehensive measures of children's functioning in the context of school, home, and community. As described in Chapter 23, the SFA measures the child's performance in functional tasks that support participation in academic and social aspects of school. To rate the SFA, the teacher or occupational therapist judges the child's performance compared with the performance of other students in his or her class or grade. Performance is rated in the natural context of the classroom. Figure 1-7 shows an example of an activity observed to complete the SFA. As described in Chapters 11 and 16, the PEM-CY assesses participation and environment across home, school, and community environments. The parent rates the frequency and intensity of participation of the child or youth in activities, defines whether or not he or she desires the level of participation to change, and identifies which features of the environment promote or constrain the child's participation. Both the SFA and the PEM-CY allow the occupational therapist to assess performance and context as they influence the child's participation.

To support adolescents preparing for employment, occupational therapists use ecologic assessment of the adolescent's performance as it relates to job tasks and work environments. Through in-depth task analysis and performance analysis, the occupational therapist identifies the skills required for the job tasks and the discrepancy between the task requirements and the youth's performance. If the team seeks to identify the student's interests and abilities as they relate to future community living, an ecologic assessment would take place in the community and the home. Cleary, Persch, and Spencer

(Chapter 25) explain ecologic assessment in which the demands of the environment and job tasks are compared with the person's skills and limitations to determine the fit between person and context. By identifying job and task demands that are too challenging for the client, the occupational therapist can focus intervention on specific performance skills and task or environment accommodations. Ecologic approaches allow occupational therapists to optimize job matching and to focus interventions where performance problems are most likely to occur.

Evaluating Context

Occupational therapists also evaluate the contexts in which the child learns, plays, and interacts. Evaluating performance in multiple contexts (e.g., homes, schools, childcare centers, other relevant community settings) allows the occupational therapist to appreciate how different contexts affect the child's performance and participation.

Contexts particularly important to consider when evaluating children include *cultural, physical,* and *social.* Assessment of cultural context was described in an earlier section. The physical space available to the child can facilitate or constrain exploration and play. Family is the primary social context for the young child, then peers and other adult caregivers become important in the social context at preschool and school ages. Few standardized assessments of context are available, and most often the occupational therapist evaluates physical and social contextual factors informally, guided by the following questions:

- Does the environment allow safe physical access?
- Are materials to promote the child's development and participation available?
- Does the environment provide an optimal level of supervision and adult assistance?
- Are a variety of spaces and sensory experiences available?
- Is the environment conducive to social interaction, and does it provide opportunities for social interaction?
- Are opportunities for exploration, play, and learning available?
- Is positive adult support available, readily accessed, and developmentally appropriate?

Practitioners evaluate how environmental and activity demands facilitate or constrain the child's performance. The family culture, lifestyle, parenting style, and values have a profound influence on the child's development, and an understanding and appreciation of this influence form a foundation for intervention planning. Chapters 3 and 4 explain how these variables influence the child's development of occupations. Using ecologic assessments to frame the evaluation and establish the priorities, the occupational therapist further assesses specific performance areas.

Analyzing Performance

With priorities identified, the occupational therapist completes a performance analysis to gain insight into the reasons for the child's performance limitations (e.g., neuromuscular, sensory processing, visual perceptual). This analysis allows the occupational therapist to refine the goals and to design intervention strategies likely to improve functional performance. Richardson (Chapter 6) describes the use of standardized assessments in analyzing performance. Assessment of multiple performance areas is essential to understanding a child's strengths and limitations for developing a focused intervention plan to improve performance. Many of the chapters in this book describe the evaluation process and identify valid tools that help to analyze a child's performance and behavior. For example in Chapter 8, Case-Smith and Exner explain that comprehensive evaluation of fine motor (hand) skills includes assessment of developmental and functional skills (e.g., Bruininks-Oseretsky Test of Motor Proficiency [BOT-2], Bayley Scales of Infant and Toddler Development, Assisting Hand Assessment, work task performance) and analysis of performance components (e.g., range of motion, strength, sensitivity, stereognosis, visual motor integration). Evaluation also includes assessment of related performance components that may influence fine motor skills, such as postural stability, visual perception, or motor planning.

When a child exhibits evidence of sensory problems, the occupational therapist uses standardized parent report and observational measures to identify patterns of behavior and performance that infer sensory integration or sensory modulation difficulties. The practitioner interprets these patterns in the context of the original concerns and resources available to make recommendations for therapy services. Parham and Mailloux (Chapter 9) describe assessment of sensory integration and praxis skills as these influence a child's performance. Sensory integration and praxis are assessed using multiple standardized tests that are scored and analyzed to reveal performance patterns that infer specific sensory difficulties.[4] Sensory processing difficulties (i.e., hyperreactivity and hyporeactivity) are often identified through parent report of the child's behaviors and sensory preferences (see Chapter 9).[84]

In Chapters 11 and 12, measures of social participation are described. Assessment of social interaction skills often includes a parent's or teacher's report of the child's communication skills, behaviors (including disruptive behaviors), and social initiation and responsiveness as key features of social participation. The occupational therapist also analyzes individual performance factors that may influence social participation, such as nonverbal communication, social awkwardness, turn-taking, voice volume, interest in others, and understanding of nonspoken rules of social interaction.

Through comprehensive evaluation, the occupational therapist analyzes the discrepancies between performance, expectations for performance, and activity demands. He or she identifies potential outcomes that fit the child's and family's story. By moving from assessment of participation to analysis of performance and contexts, the occupational therapist gains a solid understanding of the strengths, concerns, and resources of the individuals involved (e.g., child, parent, or caregiver; family members; teachers). The occupational therapist also understands how to interact with the child to build a trusting and positive relationship.

Occupational Therapy Intervention Process

Much of this book describes interventions for children. Occupational therapists improve children's performance and participation (1) by providing interventions to enhance performance; (2) by recommending activity adaptations and environmental modifications; and (3) through consultation, coaching, and

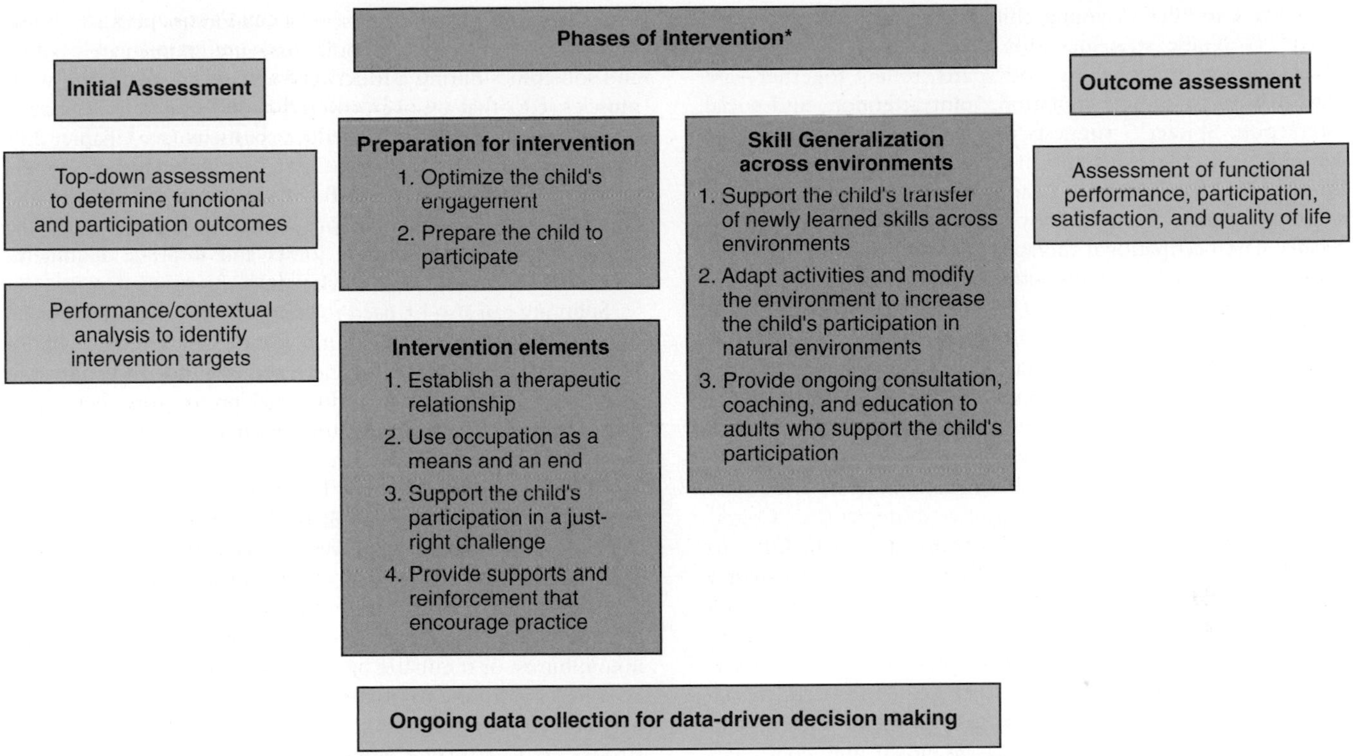

Phases of Intervention*

Initial Assessment

Top-down assessment to determine functional and participation outcomes

Performance/contextual analysis to identify intervention targets

Preparation for intervention

1. Optimize the child's engagement
2. Prepare the child to participate

Intervention elements

1. Establish a therapeutic relationship
2. Use occupation as a means and an end
3. Support the child's participation in a just-right challenge
4. Provide supports and reinforcement that encourage practice

Skill Generalization across environments

1. Support the child's transfer of newly learned skills across environments
2. Adapt activities and modify the environment to increase the child's participation in natural environments
3. Provide ongoing consultation, coaching, and education to adults who support the child's participation

Outcome assessment

Assessment of functional performance, participation, satisfaction, and quality of life

Ongoing data collection for data-driven decision making

FIGURE 1-8 Phases of the occupational therapy process. *The intervention phases are generally overlapping—that is, provided both concurrently and sequentially.

education roles. These intervention strategies complement each other and in best practice are applied together to support optimal growth and function in the child.

Interventions to Enhance Performance

This section illustrates the chapter themes that explain how the occupational therapist interacts with, challenges, and supports the child and develops interventions that promote and reinforce the child's participation. Occupational therapists understand that specific interventions or supports may be needed to enable a child to participate fully in learning activities or intervention sessions.

Children with motor limitations may need postural supports that promote alignment or provide additional stability to perform an activity optimally. Children with autism spectrum disorder may benefit from a visual schedule to orient them to the sequence of activities in which they are expected to participate. Figure 1-8 presents the phases of interventions and elements that characterize the goals and activities for each phase. Although illustrated as phases, occupational therapists typically provide the intervention goals and activities concurrently as well as sequentially.

Optimize Child's Engagement

The child's engagement in an activity or a social interaction is an essential component of a therapy session. This engagement funnels the child's energy into the activity, helps him or her sustain full attention, and implies that the child has adopted a goal and purpose that fuels his performance in the activity. When children are given supports that enable them to focus on and engage fully in a learning activity, they are more likely to persevere and attempt challenging aspects of the activity. Children engage in an activity and sustain engagement when they are motivated to participate, share positive affect with others (peers and adults) involved in the activity, and respond to and initiate interaction.[64,82] These elements promote learning.[44,85,95,107] The child's readiness to engage and self-regulation are foundational to his or her readiness to learn or participate in a therapy session (see Chapter 9).[81] Occupational therapists often facilitate a child's self-regulation of behavior—that is, promote attentive, focused, calm behavior—using sensory strategies, social-emotional supports, or cognitive cues. Teachers more frequently use cognitive strategies or cues to promote a student's focus, whereas occupational therapists often use physiologic or sensory approaches that consider the child's arousal level, sensory modulation, attention, and comfort within the learning or intervention environment. They also provide social-emotional supports (e.g., relate to the child on a personal level) to promote motivation, self-efficacy, and interest in participation (see Chapters 11 and 23).

Parham and Mailloux (Chapter 9) propose that soliciting the child's active engagement and tapping the child's inner drive are key features of the sensory integration intervention. Engagement is essential because the child's brain responds differently and learns more effectively when he or she is actively involved in a task rather than merely receiving passive stimulation. Children integrate their sensory experiences and make adaptive responses when they are actively and fully engaged in participating.[5]

Engagement can be difficult to obtain when the child has an autism spectrum disorder. Sensory strategies (e.g., strategies that apply deep touch or rhythmic movement) that elicit a physiologic response of pleasure can be particularly useful for engaging a toddler or young child with autism spectrum disorder.[81,107] These strategies—for example, hugging and giggling, singing and touching body parts, rolling together—are playful ways to initiate imitation, joint attention, and social interaction. Spitzer[119] suggests that an occupational therapist can engage a child with autism by beginning with his or her immediate interest, even if it appears as nonpurposeful (e.g., spinning a wheel, lining up toy letters, lying upside down on a ball). The occupational therapist may begin with the child's obsessive interest (i.e., trains, letters, or balls) and create a more playful, social interaction using these objects. By engaging in the child's preferred activity, the occupational therapist can foster and sustain social interaction, at the same time making the activity more playful and purposeful. Hilton (Chapter 11) further describes these intervention strategies to support positive social participation outcomes.

In Chapter 10, Mandich, Wilson, and Gain describe how the occupational therapist uses cognitive strategies (i.e., Cognitive Orientation to Occupational Performance [CO-OP]) to engage the child and build his or her motivation to master everyday occupations. The occupational therapist and child identify a performance goal of interest to the child. By guiding the child to identify the performance problem and then a feasible goal and plan for reaching that goal, the occupational therapist encourages the child's own problem solving and investment in achieving that goal. Mandich and colleagues explain how engaging the child as a collaborator in the intervention process enhances the child's motivation, best efforts to improve performance, and sustained engagement. There is emerging positive evidence for use of cognitive strategies to engage the child and improve occupational performance in children with developmental coordination disorder, high functioning autism, and attention-deficit disorder.[85,103,124]

Prepare the Child to Participate

Occupational therapists prepare the child to participate in multiple ways, according to the type of disorder the child exhibits and the context in which he or she is performing. When children have motor challenges, various strategies are needed to enable the child to participate fully and perform optimally. For children with neuromotor disorders, occupational therapists select and arrange activities and environment supports to optimize postural alignment, postural stability, and motor control. The occupational therapist selects a positioning device or seating that supports midline and upright spinal alignment, offers a firm base of support, and facilitates postural stability for optimal eye-hand and bimanual manipulation skills. For example, using a prone stander can enable functional positioning for using eyes and hands together to manipulate objects in a well-aligned, weight-bearing posture. Caregivers report that when adaptive seating that supports posture well and gives the child a biomechanical advantage is used, the child's participation in eating, self-care, play, and recreational activities increases.[101] Chapters 7 and 19 explain the importance of biomechanical principles to position and support a child with neuromotor disorders for optimal participation in daily tasks and play activities.

Other therapeutic techniques are used to prepare a child with a neuromotor disorder to participate in intervention activities designed to increase strength and motor control. Coker-Bolt, Reidy, and Nabor (Chapter 28) describe use of electrical stimulation to improve muscle activation to perform a fine motor activity. Electrical stimulation is used immediately before and sometimes during a functional activity to strengthen weak muscles (e.g., that are overpowered by the antagonist muscles), increase range of motion, or reduce spasticity (see Chapter 28). Another technique that can facilitate or inhibit specific muscle groups is kinesiology taping. Emerging evidence suggests that kinesiology tape, applied before and during performing fine motor activities, can support joints and improve alignment, improve circulation, and reduce pain.[135]

Splinting can also be used to support weak joints and, when used to support wrist or thumb joints, can give the child a biomechanical advantage for increased strength and control in manipulation or tool use. Additional preparatory techniques using biomechanical and neuromuscular principles are discussed in Chapters 28, 29, and 30.

In the acute care setting for children following trauma, preparatory activities may focus on pain reduction, improving the child's physiologic stability, or preventing secondary problems from extended periods of immobility. In Chapter 30, Lowe, Sharp, Thelen, and Warnken describe preparatory methods for children who are in acute care units for spinal cord injury, burns, or traumatic brain injury. The occupational therapist may contribute to nonpharmaceutical strategies to reduce pain and to provide more comfort. In Chapter 24, Dudgeon, Crooks, and Chappelle describe interventions to prevent loss of skills and potential injuries in children hospitalized following acute trauma who are not yet sufficiently stable to participate in purposeful activities. Occupational therapists along with nursing staff use preventive measures, including splinting and positioning, to ensure that range of motion and skin integrity are maintained during acute care or until the child is sufficiently stable to participate in activities.[136]

Establish a Therapeutic Relationship

The occupational therapist establishes a relationship with the child that encourages, supports, and motivates. The occupational therapist first establishes a relationship of trust (Figure 1-9).[15,129] The occupational therapist becomes invested in the child's success and reinforces the importance of the child's efforts. Although the occupational therapist presents challenges and asks the child to take risks, the occupational therapist also supports and facilitates the performance so that the child succeeds or feels okay when he or she fails. This trust enables the child to feel safe and willing to take risks. The occupational therapist shows interest in the child, makes efforts to enjoy his or her personality, and values his or her preferences and goals. The child's unique traits and behaviors become the basis for designing activities that will engage the child and provide the just-right challenge.

To establish a therapeutic relationship, occupational therapists demonstrate a positive affect, show personal interest in the child, and seek opportunities for personal connection. The occupational therapist collaborates with the child to select an activity of interest, makes the activity fun and playful, and gives the child choices.[11,14,119] Fostering a therapeutic relationship involves respecting the child's emotions, conveying positive regard toward the child, attempting to connect with the child, and creating a climate of trust and emotional safety (see Chapters 9 and 11). The occupational therapist encourages positive affect by attending to and imitating the child's actions

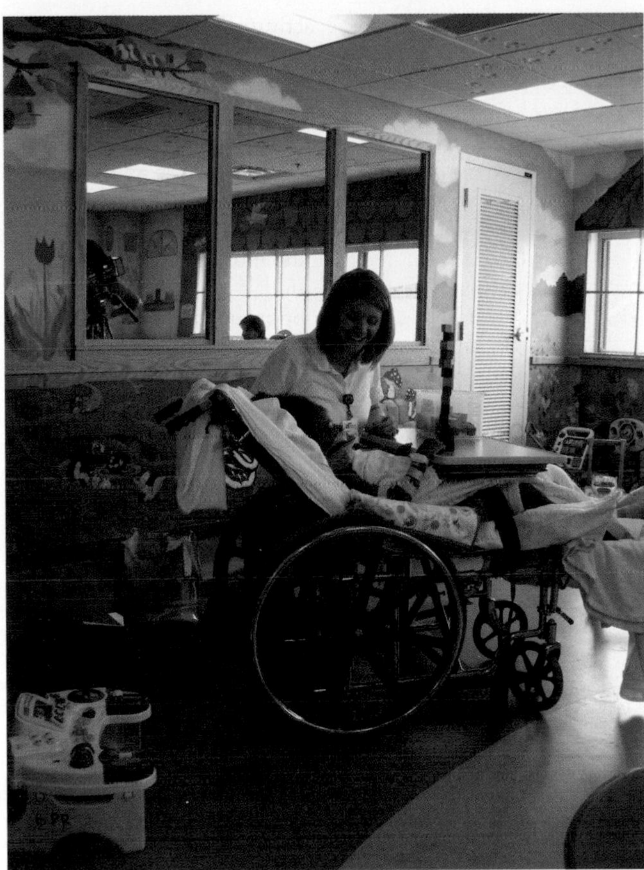

FIGURE 1-9 Conversation helps to establish the occupational therapist's relationship with the child. (Courtesy of Suellen Sharp.)

and communication attempts, waiting for the child's response, establishing eye contact, using gentle touch, and making non-evaluative comments. By choosing activities that allow the child to feel important and by grading the activity to match the child's abilities, the occupational therapist gives the child the opportunity to achieve mastery and a sense of accomplishment. Generally, the intrinsic sense of mastery is a stronger reinforcement to the child and youth with greater probability of sustained effects than external rewards, such as verbal praise or other contingent reward systems.[6] The occupational therapist vigilantly attends to the child's performance during an activity to provide precise levels of support that enable the child to succeed. A child's self-esteem and self-image are influenced by skill achievement and by success in mastering a task (see Chapters 2 and 3).[7] This concept is illustrated in many chapters.

Research evidence suggests that interventions in which the occupational therapist establishes a relationship with the child and emphasizes playful social interaction within the therapy session have positive effects on children's development.[50,120,133] Studies of the effectiveness of relationship-based interventions have found that they promote communication and play,[50] social-emotional function,[51,80,120] and learning.

The occupational therapist remains highly sensitive to the child's emerging self-actualization and helps the team and family provide activities and environments that support the child's sense of self as an efficacious person. Self-actualization, as defined by Fidler and Fidler,[43] occurs through successful coping with problems in the everyday environment. It implies more than the ability to respond to others: self-actualization means that the child initiates play activities, investigates problems, and initiates social interactions. A child with a positive sense of self seeks experiences that are challenging, responds to play opportunities, masters developmentally appropriate tasks, and forms and sustains relationships with peers and adults. In therapeutic relationships, the occupational therapist focuses on fostering the self-actualization of the child or youth. Vroman (Chapter 4) defines self-esteem, self-image, and self-worth and explains how teenagers' self-concepts influence health and activity. In Chapter 12, Kramer and colleagues describe how occupational therapists can support adolescents' participation in self-advocacy activities, leading to increased social participation and enhanced quality of life. In Chapter 16, Loukas and Dunn discuss the importance of therapeutic relationships for fostering self-determination in adolescents with significant disabilities. The practitioner's therapeutic relationship with the child appears to be a consistent feature of efficacious interventions.[69]

Use Occupation as a Means and an End

As illustrated throughout this text, occupation-based models are core to occupational therapy practice with children and youth. The profession is uniquely skilled in understanding the interaction of person, his or her occupations, and contextual influences on those occupations.[105] As stated by Law,[72] "Occupational therapy focuses on enabling individuals and groups to participate in everyday occupations that are meaningful to them, provide fulfillment, and engage them in everyday life with others." For young children, play occupations serve as the means and the end for interventions, and playfulness is part of interventions across age groups.[11,95] Occupation-based models emphasize the interaction of person, environment, and occupation; use purposeful activities with goals that are meaningful to the child (and family); and incorporate holistic methods that consider the child's sensory, motor, social-emotional, and cognitive abilities. Occupation-based approaches are well researched, and the evidence consistently supports positive effects on performance. In a systematic review of occupation-based therapy, Lee[77] found 29 outcomes studies that demonstrate positive effects across a wide variety of ages and populations. In a systematic review of occupation-based interventions for children, Kreider, Bendixen, Huang, and Lim[70] found that in almost a third (12 of 38) of the studies, the researchers focused on the child's participation in occupations within natural contexts using interventions that adapted the environment or used occupational task practice, demonstrating the importance of linking context, occupation, and person in pediatric occupational therapy research.

One occupation-based intervention with emerging evidence of effectiveness is CO-OP (see Chapter 10). CO-OP is a task-oriented, problem-solving approach that engages the child or youth in setting goals and planning strategies to improve performance. This approach was originally designed for children with strong cognitive skills and motor limitations to improve in motor tasks[85]; however, it has been used more recently with children who have high functioning autism.[103,104] This occupation-based approach has shown positive effects in multiple single-subject design studies.[85,86,97,104]

Motor learning approaches are also task-oriented interventions, acknowledging the importance of engaging children in meaningful, purposeful activities to harness their motivation and full efforts (see Chapter 7). Whole activities with multiple steps and a meaningful goal (versus repetition of activity components) elicit the child's full engagement and participation. Repeating a single component (e.g., squeeze the Play-Doh or place pennies in a can) has minimal therapeutic value. By engaging in an activity with a meaningful goal (e.g., cooking or an art project), children use multiple systems and organize their performance around that goal. For example, if a game requires that a preschool child attend to a peer, wait for his turn, and correctly place a game piece, the child is developing the joint attention that he needs to participate in circle time or a family meal. Functional magnetic resonance imaging studies indicate that more areas of the brain are activated when individuals engage in meaningful whole tasks versus parts of tasks (see Chapter 7).[68] Children and youth participate for more extended time and stay engaged in skills practice when the activity is meaningful.[47] In addition, the quality of movement improves when the activity has meaning to the child.[122] Research supporting functional, task-oriented approaches has consistently resulted in positive effects.[89]

Occupation-based models are illustrated throughout the text, including interventions for feeding (Chapter 14), activities of daily living (Chapters 15 and 16), play (Chapters 9, 17, and 22), school tasks (Chapters 18 and 23), and work occupations (Chapter 25). Chapters on social participation (Chapters 11, 12, 13, and 23) also emphasize occupation-based approaches, often involving groups of children and youth engaging in meaningful activities that facilitate social interaction.

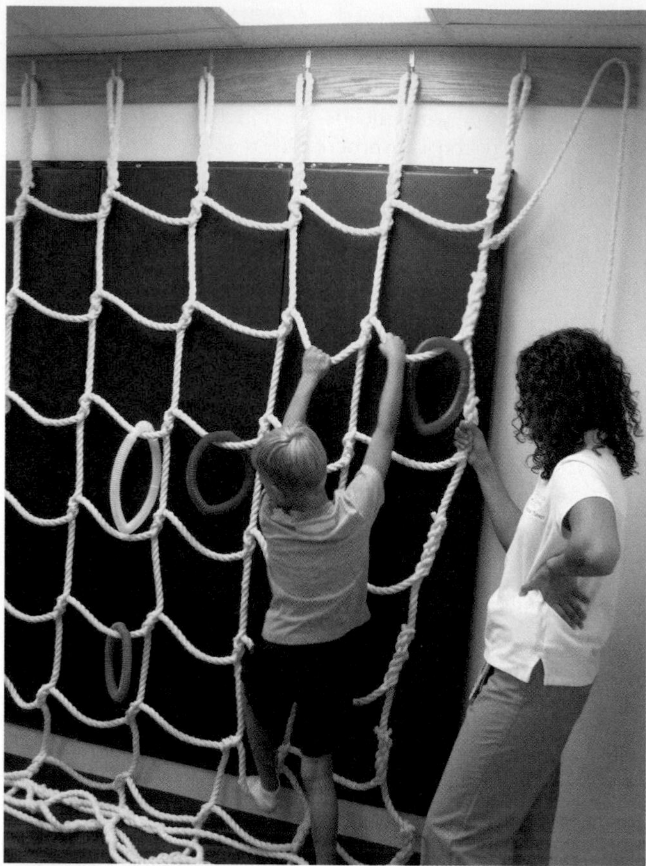

FIGURE 1-10 A climbing wall activity challenged this child's motor planning, bilateral coordination, strength, and postural stability.

Provide a Just-Right Challenge

A child's active participation and efforts to achieve a task are elicited when therapeutic activities are at just the right level of complexity—that is, where the child not only feels comfortable and nonthreatened but also experiences some challenge that requires effort. An activity that is a child's "just-right" challenge has the following elements: the activity (1) matches the child's developmental skills and interests, (2) provides a reasonable challenge to current performance level, (3) engages and motivates the child, and (4) can be mastered with the child's focused effort.

Based on careful analysis of performance and behavior, the occupational therapist selects an activity that matches the child's strengths and limitations across performance domains. The analysis allows the occupational therapist to individualize the difficulty, the pace, and the supports needed for a child to accomplish a task. Generally, the occupational therapist selects highly adaptable activities that can be modified to increase or decrease the difficulty level based on the child's performance. To promote change in the child, the activity must be challenging and create a degree of stress. The stress is meant to elicit a higher level of response. Figure 1-10 provides an example of an activity challenging to a child with sensory integration problems. The interactions of the occupational therapist and the child are like a dance: The occupational therapist poses a problem or challenge to the child, who is then motivated by that challenge and responds. The occupational therapist facilitates or supports the action to prompt the child to respond at a higher level. The occupational therapist gives feedback regarding the action and presents another problem of greater or lesser difficulty, based on the success of the child's response. Cognitive, sensory, motor, perceptual, or social aspects of the activity may be made easier or more difficult (Case Study 1-3). By precisely assessing the adequacy of the child's response, the occupational therapist finds the just-right challenge.

Parham and Mailloux (Chapter 9) explain that occupational therapy sessions typically begin with activities that the child can engage in comfortably and competently and then move toward increasing challenges. For example, the occupational therapist may initially provide a child who has gravitational insecurity (i.e., fear of and aversion to being on unstable surfaces or heights with immature postural balance) with therapy activities that begin close to the ground and provide close physical support to help the child feel secure during a game played while sitting on a ball. Gradually, in subsequent sessions, the occupational therapist designs activities that require the child to walk on unstable surfaces and to swing with his or her whole body suspended (Figure 1-11). These graded activities pose a just-right level of challenge, while respecting the child's need to feel secure and in control. This gradual approach is key to maximizing the child's active involvement and to eliciting and practicing higher level skills.

Myers, Case-Smith, and Cason (Chapter 22) suggest that occupational therapists design and employ play activities that engage and challenge the child across domains (e.g., activities

CASE STUDY 1-3 Grading an Activity: Challenging and Eliciting Full Participation

Aaron, a 10-year-old boy with autism, participated in a cooking activity with the occupational therapist and three peers. The children were proceeding in an organized manner—sharing cooking supplies and verbalizing each step of the activity. As they proceeded, Aaron had great difficulty participating in the task; the materials were messy, and the social interaction was frequent and unpredictable. He performed best when the activity was highly structured, the instructions were very clear, and the social interaction was kept at a minimum. To help him participate at a comfortable level, the occupational therapist suggested that his contribution to the activity be to put away supplies and retrieve new ones. The other children were asked to give him specific visual and verbal instructions as to what they needed and what should be replaced in the refrigerator or cupboard. With this new rule in place, the children gave simple and concrete instructions that Aaron could follow. An important element of this strategy was that it included the support of his peers to elicit an optimal level of participation and could be generalized to other small-group activities involving Aaron and his peers.

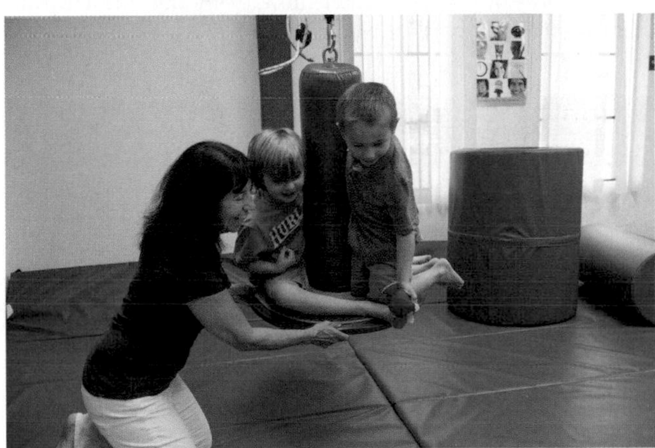

FIGURE 1-11 Applying a sensory integration approach, the occupational therapist gradually introduced a child with gravitational insecurity to unstable surfaces and higher levels of vestibular input.

that are slightly higher than the child's developmental level in motor, cognitive, and social domains). When a task challenges both cognitive and motor skills, the young child becomes fully engaged, and the activity has high therapeutic potential for improving the child's developmental level of performance.

Provide Supports and Reinforcement That Encourage Practice

Research evidence cited throughout this book indicates that more intense intervention has greater positive effects on performance.[35,46,125] One intervention, constraint-induced movement therapy (CIMT), has been shown to have strong positive effects (see Chapter 8). This intervention uses a specific protocol with a specific population of children. In CIMT, the non-affected hand and arm of a child with hemiparesis cerebral palsy is casted, and the child practices specific skills with the affected hand and arm. CIMT also provides an intensive dosage of therapy (Figure 1-12). The "shaping" intervention is provided 3 to 6 hours a day for 21 days. Across time, trials of CIMT have demonstrated improvement in the child's upper extremity movement and function.[25,57,110]

Although this level of therapy is not typical and may be impractical in most situations, these research findings suggest that intensive services have clear benefit. Schertz and Gordon[113] conclude that intensive interventions that involve repeated practice and progressive challenge can produce positive changes in functional performance. O'Brien (Chapter 7) explains the importance of repeated practice in skill attainment. She notes that children learn new skills with frequent practice and various types of practice. Motor learning studies have shown that intense (blocked) practice is helpful when first learning a new skill but that the child also needs variable and random practice to generalize and transfer the newly learned skill to a variety of situations. When distributed practice (i.e., practicing a task

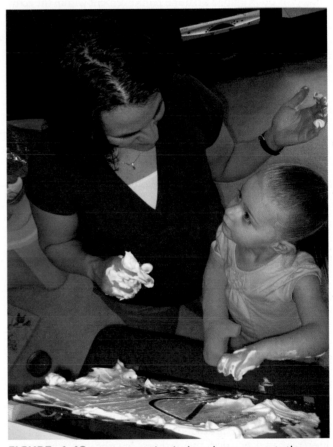

FIGURE 1-12 In constraint-induced movement therapy, the child's less involved arm was casted, and she received intensive therapy to build skills in the involved arm and hand.

alternating with periods of rest) is compared with blocked practice, distributed practice results in superior long-term learning.[139]

Research has also demonstrated that interventions in which the child is rewarded for performing well have positive effects.[16,123] Burtner et al.[16] demonstrated that children with cerebral palsy and typical children who practiced with 100% feedback consistently demonstrated better performance on a complex motor task compared with children who had intermittent feedback. Feedback may be more important when learning a complex skill versus a simple task.

Based on a behavioral model, most occupational therapy interventions include reinforcement of the child's efforts. This reinforcement can range from hugs and praises to more tangible objects, such as a prize or piece of candy. Occupational therapists often embed a natural reinforcement within the activity. For example, the occupational therapist designs a session in which a group of four 12-year-olds with Asperger's syndrome bake cookies. The natural reinforcement includes eating cookies and enjoying socialization with others during the activity. Positive reinforcement includes both intrinsic (e.g., feeling competent or sense of success) and extrinsic (e.g., adult praise or a treat) feedback. O'Brien (Chapter 7) explains that feedback can be most effective when it is given on a variable schedule, with initially high-frequency feedback that is lessened as the skill is mastered. External feedback appears to be effective when it provides specific information to the child about performance and when it immediately follows performance.[116] In summary, research evidence supports that children's performance improves with intense practice of emerging skills and with a system of rewards for higher level performance.

Support the Child's Transfer of Newly Learned Skills across Environments

Occupational therapists carefully plan strategies for children to generalize newly learned skills. Recognizing that transfer of new skills to natural environments does not always automatically follow performance of that skill in an intervention session, occupational therapists plan multiple ways for children to practice new skills in various tasks. They also recommend supports for performance that will ensure success. To support the generalization of new skills, occupational therapists educate caregivers and teachers to support and reinforce that practice. They suggest strategies to support the child's practice of skills in a variety of tasks. For example, in Chapters 24 and 30 on hospital-based practice, the authors describe how children in rehabilitation units after trauma spend a weekend at home before discharge so that they can try newly learned skills in their natural environments with the support of family members. Based on feedback from the visit home, the occupational therapist solves the problem of how to improve function in the home and school environments. Education and coaching methods are illustrated throughout the text; see Chapters 22, 23, and 25 for examples of consultation to promote skill transfer. These methods are also briefly described in the sections that follow.

Many research-based interventions include specific components to help the child generalize newly learned skills. Often these are home programs carefully developed in collaboration with parents to ensure that they are a good fit. Novak[91] describes the components of an effective home program. She defines a "partnership home program" as one that includes (1) establishing a collaborative partnership between the parent, child, and occupational therapist; (2) establishing parent and child goals; (3) selecting therapeutic activities that focus on achieving family goals; (4) supporting parents to implement the program through education, home visiting, and progress updates; and (5) evaluating outcomes. These elements are important to promoting the child's ability to generalize emerging skills to home activities. Approaching home programs first as a partnership, checking progress and supporting parents throughout, has demonstrated efficacy for improving parent efficacy and the child's function.[93] In summary, occupational therapists thoughtfully promote skill transfer by strategizing how and when children can practice new skills in different environments, by planning with teachers and parents how to phase out supports that were available during the intervention sessions, and by recommending how to modify the environment to enable successful performance.

Activity Adaptation and Environmental Modifications

The emphasis of intervention is often on implementing adapted methods or applying assistive technology to increase the child's participation despite performance problems. The following sections and many of the subsequent chapters explain how occupational therapists use task adaptation, assistive technology, and environmental modification to improve a child's participation in home, school, and community activities.

Interventions Using Assistive Technology

Occupational therapists often help children with disabilities participate by adapting activities and applying assistive technology (Figure 1-13). Chapter 19 provides an in-depth explanation of assistive technology. In Chapter 15, Shepherd offers many examples of adapted techniques to increase a child's independence in self-care and activities of daily living.

Technology is pervasive throughout society, and its increasing versatility makes it easily adaptable to an individual child's

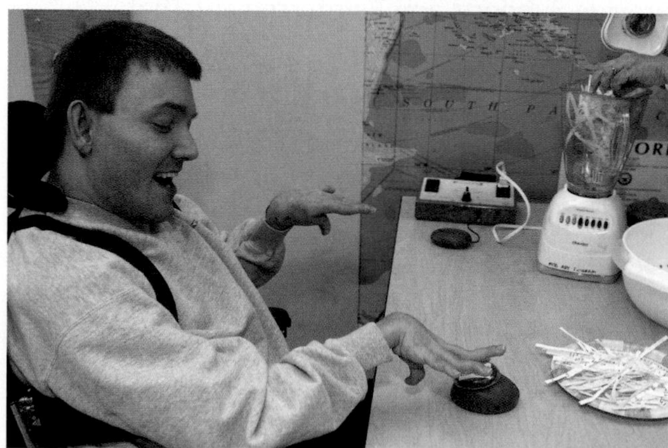

FIGURE 1-13 The occupational therapist designed an adaptive switch so that the adolescent can activate a blender. (Photo © istock.com.)

needs. Low-technology solutions are often applied to increase the child's participation in activities of daily living. Adapted techniques can be used to increase independence and reduce caregiver assistance in eating, dressing, or bathing. Examples include built-up handles on utensils, weighted cups, elastic shoelaces, and electric toothbrushes (see Chapter 16). Low technology solutions can also be used to support participation in play activities.[71] Adapted techniques for play activities may include switch toys, battery-powered toys, enlarged handles on puzzle pieces, or magnetic pieces that can easily fit together.

High-technology solutions are often used to increase mobility or functional communication. Examples are power wheelchairs, augmentative communication devices, and computers. High technology is becoming increasingly available and typically involves computer processing and switch or keyboard access (e.g., augmentative communication devices) (see Chapter 19). As stated by Schoonover and Argabrite Grove, "Assistive technologies may unlock human potential and optimize human performance throughout the life span and across contexts and allow individuals to assume or regain valued life roles." Occupational therapists frequently support the use of assistive technology by identifying the most appropriate device or system and features of the system. They often help families obtain funding to purchase the device, set up or program the system, train others to use it, and monitor its use. Occupational therapists also make themselves available to problem-solve the inevitable technology issues that arise.

The role of assistive technology with children is not simply to compensate for a missing or delayed function; it is also used to promote development in targeted performance areas. Research has demonstrated that increased mobility with the use of a power wheelchair increases social and perceptual skills (see Chapter 20).[63,90] Based on synthesis of the research and expert consensus, Livingstone and Paleg[78] concluded that for children with minimal mobility, a power mobility device can promote overall development. When introduced to power mobility, children particularly improve in psychosocial function.[78]

The occupational therapist selects assistive technology not only to enable the child to participate more fully in functional or social activities but also to enhance the development of skills related to a specific occupational area. The use of an augmentative communication device can enhance language and social skills and may prevent behavioral problems common in children who have limited means of communicating.[17] For example, to develop preliteracy skills, a child who has a physical disability with severe motor impairments can access a computer program that simulates reading a book; to promote computer skills, the child can use an expanded keyboard (Figure 1-14). The computer programs used in schools to promote literacy, writing, and math skills with all children are particularly beneficial to children who have learning and physical disabilities. Because schools have invested in universal design and appropriate accommodations for all learners, many students with disabilities can access computer programs that promote their literacy and writing skills. In Chapter 19, Schoonover and Argabrite Grove describe currently available technologies designed to promote children's functional performance.

Assistive technology solutions continually change as devices become more advanced and more versatile. Although an occupational therapist can extensively train a student to use power mobility, an augmentative communication device, or an adapted computer, the child's skills with the technology will not generalize into everyday routines unless parents, teachers, and aides are sufficiently comfortable with and knowledgeable about the technology. Because it is important that the adults closest to the child be able to implement the technology and troubleshoot when necessary, the occupational therapist educates them extensively about how to apply the technology and remains available to solve problems that inevitably arise. Often, it is necessary to talk through and model each step in the use of the technology. Strategies for integrating the technology into a classroom or home environment (e.g., discussing the ways the device can be used throughout the day) help to achieve the greatest benefit.[17] All team members need to update their skills routinely so that they have a working knowledge of emerging technology.

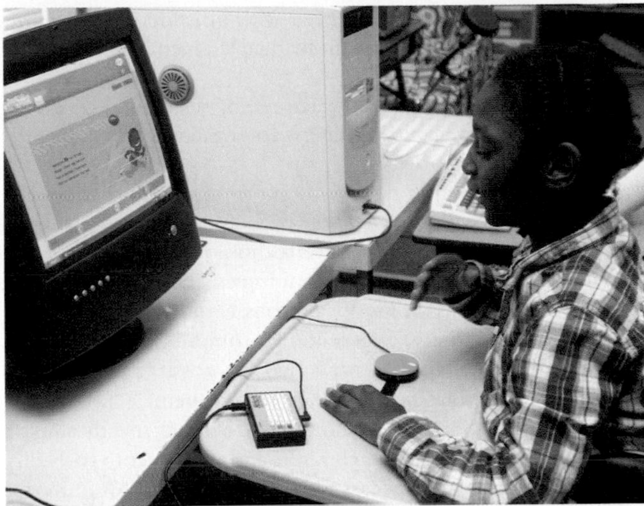

FIGURE 1-14 A switch activates a computer program that simulates a storybook. (Photo © istock.com.)

In many school systems, the occupational therapist serves as an assistive technology consultant or becomes a member of a district-wide assistive technology team. Assistive technology teams have been formed to provide support and expertise to school staff members in applying assistive technology with students. These teams make recommendations to administrators on equipment to order, train students to use computers and devices, troubleshoot technology failures, determine technology needs, and provide ongoing education to staff and families. Use of assistive technology is particularly helpful to adolescents preparing for supported employment (see Chapter 25).

Technologic solutions are described throughout this text and are the focus of Chapters 15, 19, 20, and 25. These chapters offer the following themes on the use of assistive technology:

- Assistive technology is carefully selected according to the individual abilities of the child or youth (intrinsic variables), task demands or desired activities, and environmental supports and constraints (extrinsic variables).
- Techniques and technology should be adaptable and flexible so that devices can be used across environments and over time as the child develops.

- Technology should be selected with a future goal in mind and a vision of how the individual and environment will change.
- The strategy and technology should be selected in consultation with all caregivers, teachers, and other professionals and adults who support its use.
- Extensive training, ongoing monitoring to adjust the technology for optimal use, and outcome evaluation should accompany the use of assistive technology.

In summary, assistive technologies have significantly improved the quality of life for persons with disabilities. Computers, power mobility, augmentative communication devices, and environmental control units make it possible for children to participate in roles previously closed to them.

In addition to assistive technology designed specifically for children with impairments, children and adolescents with disabilities also have more access to technology through universal access. The concept of universal access, now widespread, refers to the movement to develop devices and design environments that are accessible to everyone. When schools invest in universal access for their learning technology, all students can access any or most of the school's computers, and adaptations for visual, hearing, motor, or cognitive impairment can be made on all or most of the school's computers. Universal access means that the system platforms can support software with accessibility options and that a range of keyboards, "mice" (tracking devices), and switches are available for alternative access. The concepts of universal design and access are well illustrated in Chapter 19.

Environmental Modification

To succeed in a specific setting, a child with disabilities often benefits from modifications to the environment. Goals include not only enhancing a child's participation but also increasing safety (e.g., reducing barriers on the playground) and improving comfort (e.g., improving ease of wheelchair use by reducing the incline of the ramp). Children with physical disabilities may require specific environmental adaptations to increase accessibility or safety. For example, although a school's bathroom may be accessible to a child in a wheelchair, the occupational therapist may recommend the installation of a handlebar beside the toilet so that the child can safely perform a standing pivot transfer. Desks and table heights may need to be adjusted for a child in a wheelchair. See Chapter 15 for additional examples.

Environmental adaptations, such as modifying a classroom or a home space to accommodate a specific child with a disability, can be accomplished only through partnership with the adults who manage the environment. High levels of collaboration are needed to create optimal environments for the child to attend and learn at school and at home. Environmental modifications often affect everyone in that space, so the modifications must be appropriate for all children in that environment. The occupational therapist articulates the rationale for the modification and negotiates the changes to be made by considering what is most appropriate for all, including the teacher and other students. Through discussion, the occupational therapist and teacher reach agreement as to what the problems are.

With consensus regarding the problems and desired outcomes, often the needed environmental modification logically follows. It is essential that the occupational therapist follow through by evaluating the impact of the modification on the targeted child and others. The Americans with Disabilities Act provides guidelines for improving accessibility to schools and community facilities.

Often the role of the occupational therapist is to recommend adaptations to the sensory environment that accommodate children with sensory processing problems.[38] Preschool and elementary school classrooms usually have high levels of auditory and visual input. Classrooms with high noise levels may be overwhelmingly disorganizing to a child who is hypersensitive to auditory stimulation. Young children who need calming techniques or quiet times during the day may need their own physical space in the corner of the room where they are allowed to "take a break" intermittently throughout the school day. The occupational therapist may suggest that a preschool teacher implement a quiet time with lights off to provide a period to calm children. Contextual modifications to accommodate a child who has sensory processing problems are described in Chapters 9, 11, 13, and 22.

Other environmental modifications can improve arousal and attention in children. Sitting on movable surfaces (e.g., liquid-filled cushions) can improve a child's posture and attention to classroom instruction.[114] The intent of recommendations regarding the classroom environment is often to maintain a child's arousal and level of alertness without overstimulating or distracting the child. Modifications should enhance the child's performance; make life easier for the parent or teachers; and have a neutral or positive effect on siblings, peers, and others in the environment. Owing to the dynamic nature of the child and the environment, adaptations to the environment may require ongoing assessment to evaluate the goodness-of-fit between the child and the modified environment and determine when adjustments need to be made.

In a study of children with sensory processing challenges, Dunn et al.[39] used an intervention in which occupational therapists made recommendations for changing the family's contexts based on analysis of the child's sensory processing and sensory characteristics of the environment. This contextually focused intervention resulted in improvements in children's participation and parent's sense of competence. Law et al.[76] also examined the effects of intervention that focused on adapting the environment to promote function for children with cerebral palsy. A 6-month period of context-focused therapy was as effective as traditional occupational therapy in improving function in self-care, mobility, and participation.[76] Ecologic approaches that focus on use of adaptive equipment, assistive technology, and environmental modification are often achieved through consultation, coaching, and education.

Consultation, Coaching, and Education Roles

Pediatric occupational therapy involves working intimately with caregivers and teachers to create opportunities for the child to participate optimally across environments. This aspect of service delivery is challenging and fulfilling because it requires a complementary skill set to assess, plan, implement, and evaluate the effects of parent and teacher consultation, coaching, and education.

Consultation and Coaching

Services "on behalf of" children complement and extend direct service delivery. Occupational therapists provide these indirect services by consulting with, coaching, and educating parents, assistants, childcare providers, and any adults who spend a significant amount of time with the child. Through these models of service delivery, the occupational therapist helps to develop solutions that fit into the child's natural environment and promotes the child's transfer of new skills into various environments.

In Chapter 9, Parham and Mailloux explain that a first step in consultation is "demystifying" the child's disorder.[14] By explaining the child's behaviors as a sensory processing problem to teachers and parents, occupational therapists foster a better understanding of the reasons for the child's behavior (e.g., constant bouncing in a chair or chewing on a pencil), which gives adults new tools for helping the child change behavior. Reframing the problem for caregivers and teachers enables them to identify new and different solutions to the problem and often makes them more open to the occupational therapist's intervention recommendations.[13] For a situation in which a highly specific, technical activity is needed to elicit a targeted response in the child, teaching others may not be appropriate, and a less complex and less risky strategy should be transferred to the caregivers to implement. To implement routinely a strategy recommended by the occupational therapist, teachers and caregivers need to feel confident that they can apply it successfully.

A major role for school-based occupational therapists is to support teachers in providing optimal instruction to students and helping children succeed in school (see Chapter 23). Occupational therapists accomplish this role by promoting the teacher's understanding of the physiologic and health-related issues that affect the child's behavior and helping teachers apply strategies to promote the child's school related performance. Occupational therapists also support teachers in adapting instructional activities that enable the child's participation and collaborate with teachers to collect data on the child's performance. This focus suggests that, in the role of consultant, the occupational therapist sees the teacher's needs as a priority and focuses on supporting his or her effectiveness in the classroom.[53] Consultation is most likely to be effective when occupational therapists understand the curriculum, academic expectations, and classroom environment.

Effective consultation or coaching also requires that the teacher or caregiver be able to assimilate and adapt the strategies offered by the occupational therapist and make them work in the classroom or the home. The occupational therapist asks the teacher how he or she learns best and accommodates that learning style.[53] Teachers need to be comfortable with suggested interventions, and occupational therapists should offer strategies that fit easily in the classroom routine. The occupational therapist and teacher can work together to determine which interventions would benefit the child and be least intrusive to other students.

Education Roles

Occupational therapists also educate administrators and policymakers about the need to improve accessibility of recreational, school, or community activities. They work directly with school curriculum committees to modify curriculum materials and develop educational materials that align with the core curriculum and use universal design. They educate the public to improve attitudes toward disabilities (see Chapters 12 and 25). By participating in curriculum revision or course material selection, occupational therapists can help establish a curriculum that meets required standards but has sufficient flexibility to meet the needs of children and youth with disabilities. Often a system problem that negatively affects one child is problematic to others as well. The occupational therapist needs to recognize which system problems can be changed and how these changes can be encouraged. For example, if a child has difficulty reading and writing in the morning, he or she may benefit from physical activity before attempting to focus on deskwork. The occupational therapist cannot change the daily schedule and move recess or physical education to the beginning of the day, but he or she may convince the teacher to begin the first period of the day with warm-up activities. The occupational therapist can educate teachers on the benefits of using a simplified, continuous stroke handwriting curriculum, which can benefit children with motor-planning problems but also benefit all children beginning to write. Education on accessible playgrounds can promote greater participation and safety on the playground for all children, regardless of skill levels.

Ecologic models recognize the powerful influence of home, school, and community environments on child and youth outcomes (see Chapter 25).[75] Occupational therapists educate others about and advocate for environments that are both physically accessible and welcoming to children with disabilities. With an extensive background on which elements create a supportive environment, occupational therapists can help design physical and social environments that facilitate participation of every child. To change the system on behalf of all children, including children with disabilities, requires communication with stakeholders or persons who are invested in the change. The occupational therapist needs to share confidently the rationale for change, appreciate the views of others invested in the system, and change and negotiate when needed.

A system change through education is most accepted when the benefits appear high and the costs are low. Can all children benefit? Which children are affected? If administrators and teachers in a childcare center are reluctant to enroll an infant with a disability, the occupational therapist can advocate for accepting the child by explaining specifically the care that the child would need, the resources available, the behaviors and issues to expect, and the benefits to other families.

Convincing a school to build an accessible playground or establish a completely accessible computer lab are examples of how a focused education effort can create system change. Occupational therapists are frequently involved in designing playgrounds that are accessible to all and promote the development of sensory motor skills. Another example is helping school administrators select computer programs that are accessible to children with disabilities (see Chapter 19). The occupational therapist can serve on the school committee that selects computer software for the curriculum and advocate for software that is easily adaptable for children with physical or sensory disabilities. A third example is helping administrators and teachers select a handwriting curriculum to be used by regular and special education students. The occupational therapist may advocate for classroom instruction that emphasizes prewriting skills or one that takes a multisensory approach to teaching handwriting (see Chapter 18). The occupational therapist may also advocate for adding sensory-motor-perceptual activities to an early childhood curriculum. In Chapter 23, Bazyk and Cahill describe the role of occupational therapists in promoting positive behavioral supports to improve school mental health outcomes. These examples of proactive roles to create system change illustrate how occupational therapy practitioners take leadership roles in promoting participation of all children and youth, preventing disability among children at risk, and promoting healthy environments where all children and adolescents can learn and grow.

Summary

This chapter introduces the book by describing concepts that characterize occupational therapy practices with children. All chapters of this book emphasize evidence-based interventions for children and youth across practice settings. The occupational therapy process was briefly explained and is illustrated in depth in the subsequent chapters of the book. Occupational therapy practice with children has matured in recent decades from a profession that relied on basic theories and practice models to drive decision making to one that uses scientific evidence in clinical reasoning. A primary goal of this book is to define and illustrate the application of research evidence in clinical reasoning. The subsequent chapters expand on the basic concepts presented in this chapter by exploring the breadth of occupational therapy for children, explaining theories that guide practice, illustrating practice models in educational and medical systems, and describing interventions with evidence of effectiveness.

Summary Points

- Occupational therapists provide child-centered services to ensure that intervention is developmentally appropriate, meaningful and motivating to the child, and well aligned with the child's goals.
- In family-centered services, occupational therapists develop positive relationships with families, demonstrate compassion, exhibit responsiveness and sensitivity, and foster parental self-efficacy.
- Occupational therapists advocate for inclusion and recognize the value of services within the child's natural environments.
- Collaborative models of services delivery, such as classroom-embedded services or co-teaching, allow occupational therapy services to be integrated into the child's goals for participating in the curriculum and functioning in the school environment.
- Culturally competent occupational therapists respect the child and family's culture and design services that demonstrate respect for the family's culture.
- Occupational therapists access, interpret, and use evidence to make clinical decisions; high-quality, efficacious intervention uses evidence-based practice guidelines.
- Occupational therapists use top-down, ecologic assessment with performance analysis to determine how context, task demands, and performance strengths and limitations influence the participation of the child or adolescent.
- The intervention process includes specific methods to prepare the child or adolescent for participating in intervention.
- Evidence-based occupation-based models include establishing a therapeutic relationship, using occupation as a means and an end, providing a just-right challenge, providing appropriate supports for and reinforcement of performance, and supporting generalization of newly learned skills to natural environments.
- Ecologic models that include application of assistive technology and environmental modifications increase the participation of the child or adolescent in activities for daily living, play, school functions, and work.
- Occupational therapists have important roles in consulting with, coaching, and educating caregivers, teachers, and other professionals who support the participation of children and adolescents with disabilities.

REFERENCES

1. American Hospital Association. (2010). Long-range policy committee. In John W. Bluford III, Chair (Ed.), *A call to action: Creating a culture of health.* Chicago: American Hospital Association. January 2011.
2. American Occupational Therapy Association. (2014). Occupational therapy practice framework: Domain and process. *American Journal of Occupational Therapy, 68*(Suppl. 1), S1–S48.
3. America's Children. (2013). Key national indicators of well-being, 2013. Forum on child and family statistics, retrieved June 3, 2014, from <childstats.gov>.
4. Ayres, A. J. (1989). *Sensory Integration and Praxis Test Manual.* Los Angeles: Western Psychological Services.
5. Ayres, A. J. (1972). Improving academic scores through sensory integration. *Journal of Learning Disabilities, 5*, 339–343.
6. Ayres, A. J. (1979). *Sensory integration and the child.* Los Angeles: Western Psychological Services.
7. Bandura, A. (1997). *Self-efficacy: The exercise of control.* New York: Freeman.
8. Bazyk, S., Goodman, G., Michaud, P., et al. (2009). Integration of occupational therapy services in a kindergarten curriculum: A look at the outcomes. *American Journal of Occupational Therapy, 63*, 160–171.
9. Bendixen, R., & Kreider, C. M. (2011). Centennial Vision—review of occupational therapy research in the practice area of children and youth. *American Journal of Occupational Therapy, 65*, 351–359.
10. Bianco, M., Carothers, D. E., & Smiley, L. R. (2009). Gifted students with Asperger syndrome: Strategies for strength-based programming. *Intervention in School and Clinic, 44*, 206–215.
11. Blanche, E. (2008). Play in children with cerebral palsy: Doing with and not

doing to. In L. D. Parham & L. Fazio (Eds.), *Play in occupational therapy for children* (2nd ed., pp. 395–412). St. Louis: Mosby.
12. Blue-Banning, M., Summers, J. A., Frankland, H. C., et al. (2004). Dimensions of family and professional partnerships: Constructive guidelines for collaboration. *Exceptional Children, 70*(2), 167–184.
13. Bundy, A. (2002). Using sensory integration theory in schools: Sensory integration and consultation. In A. C. Bundy, S. J. Lane, & E. A. Murray (Eds.), *Sensory integration: Theory and practice* (2nd ed., pp. 141–165). Philadelphia: F. A. Davis.
14. Bundy, A. C. (2002). Play theory and sensory integration. In A. C. Bundy, S. Lane, & E. Murray (Eds.), *Sensory integration: Theory and practice* (2nd ed., pp. 228–240). Philadelphia: F. A. Davis.
15. Bundy, A., & Koomar, J. A. (2002). Orchestrating intervention: The art of practice. In A. Bundy, S. J. Lane, & E. A. Murray (Eds.), *Sensory integration: Theory and practice* (2nd ed., pp. 242–260). Philadelphia: F. A. Davis.
16. Burtner, P. A., Leinwand, R. O., Sullivan, K. J., et al. (2014). Motor learning in children with hemiplegic cerebral palsy: Feedback effects on skill acquisition. *Developmental Medicine and Child Neurology, 56*, 259–266.
17. Cafiero, J. M. (2001). The effect of an augmentative communication intervention on the communication, behavior, and academic program of an adolescent with autism. *Focus on Autism and Other Developmental Disabilities, 16*, 179–189.
18. Campbell, P. H. (2004). Participation-based services: Promoting children's participation in natural settings. *Young Exceptional Children, 8*, 20–29.
19. Carey, M., Buchan, H., & Sanson-Fisher, R. (2009). The cycle of change: Implementing best-evidence clinical practice. *International Journal for Quality in Health Care, 21*, 37–43.
20. Case-Smith, J., & Arbesman, M. (2008). Evidence-based review of interventions for autism used in or of relevance to occupational therapy. *American Journal of Occupational Therapy, 62*, 416–429.
21. Case-Smith, J., & Holland, T. (2009). Making decisions about service delivery in early childhood program. *Language, Speech, and Hearing Services in School, 40*, 416–423.
22. Case-Smith, J., Holland, T., & Bishop, B. (2011). Effectiveness of an integrated handwriting program for first-grade students: A pilot study. *American Journal of Occupational Therapy, 65*, 670–678.
23. Case-Smith, J., Holland, T., & White, S. (2014). Effectiveness of a co-taught handwriting program for first grade students. *Physical and Occupational Therapy in Pediatrics, 34*, 30–43.
24. Case-Smith, J., Sainato, D., McQuaid, J., et al. (2007). IMPACTS project: Preparing therapists to provide best practice early intervention services. *Physical and Occupational Therapy in Pediatrics, 27*(3), 73–90.
25. Case-Smith, J., Holland, T., & Bishop, B. (2011). Effectiveness of an integrated handwriting program for first-grade students: A pilot study. *American Journal of Occupational Therapy, 65*, 670–678.
26. Chai, A. Y., Zhang, C., & Bisberg, M. (2006). Rethinking natural environment practice: Implications from examining various implications and approaches. *Early Childhood Education Journal, 34*(3), 203–208.
27. Chen, X., & Eisenberg, N. (2012). Understanding cultural issues in child development: Introduction. *Child Development Perspectives, 6*, 1–14.
28. Children's Defense Fund. (2014). *The State of American's Children, 2014.* At: <http://www.childrensdefense.org/child-research-data-publications/state-of-americas-children/> Accessed on March 18, 2014.
29. Chin, J. L. (2000). Viewpoint on cultural competence. *Public Health Reports, 115*, 25–34.
30. Cincinnati Children's Evidence-Based Care Recommendations. (n.d.). At: <http://www.cincinnatichildrens.org/service/j/anderson-center/evidence-based-care/recommendations/default/> Accessed on March 29, 2014.
31. Cook, L., & Friend, M. (1991). Principles for the practice of collaboration in schools. *Preventing School Failure, 35*(4), 6–9.
32. Coster, W., Bedell, G., Law, M., et al. (2011). Psychometric evaluation of the participation and environment measure for children and youth (PEM-CY). *Developmental Medicine and Child Neurology, 53*, 1030–1037.
33. Coster, W., Deeney, T., Haltiwanger, J., et al. (1998). *School Function Assessment.* San Antonio: Psychological Corporation.
34. Deater-Deckard, K., Dodge, K. A., Bates, J. E., et al. (1996). Physical discipline among African American and European American mothers: Links to children's externalizing behaviors. *Developmental Psychology, 6*, 1065–1072.
35. DeLuca, S. C., Echols, K., Law, C. R., et al. (2006). Intensive pediatric constraint-induced therapy for children with cerebral palsy. *Journal of Child Neurology, 21*, 931–938.
36. Division of Early Childhood/National Association for the Education of Young Children. (2009). *Early childhood inclusion: A joint position statement of the Division of Early Childhood (DEC) and the National Association for the Education of Young Children (NAEYC).* Chapel Hill: The University of North Carolina, FPG Child Development Institute.
37. Duchardt, B., Marlow, L., Inman, D., et al. (2010). Collaboration and co-teaching: General and special education faculty. *The Clearing House: A Journal of Educational Strategies, Issues, and Ideas, 72*, 186–190.
38. Dunn, W. (2007). Supporting children to participate successfully in everyday life by using sensory process knowledge. *Infants and Young Children, 20*(2), 84–101.
39. Dunn, W., Cox, J., Foster, L., et al. (2012). Impact of a contextual intervention on child participation and parent competence among children with autism spectrum disorders: A pretest-posttest repeated measures design. *American Journal of Occupational Therapy, 66*, 520–528.
40. Dunst, C. J., & Dempsey, I. (2007). Family-professional partnerships and parenting competence, confidence, and enjoyment. *International Journal of Disability, Development and Education, 54*, 305–318.
41. Dunst, C. J., Trivette, C. M., & Hamby, D. W. (2007). Meta-analysis of family-centered helpgiving practices research. *Mental Retardation and Developmental Disabilities Research Reviews, 13*, 370–378.
42. Dunst, C. J., Trivette, C. M., Humphries, T., et al. (2001). Contrasting approaches to natural learning environment interventions. *Infants and Young Children, 14*, 48–63.
43. Fidler, G. S., & Fidler, J. W. (1978). Doing and becoming: Purposeful action and self-actualization. *American Journal of Occupational Therapy, 32*, 305–310.
44. Freeman, S., & Kasari, C. (2013). Parent-child interactions in autism: Characteristics of play. *Autism: The International Journal of Research and Practice, 17*, 147–161.
45. Garcia Coll, C., & Magnuson, K. (2000). Cultural differences as sources of developmental vulnerabilities and resources. In S. J. Meisels & J. P. Shonkoff (Eds.), *Handbook of early childhood intervention* (2nd ed., pp. 94–114). Cambridge: Cambridge University Press.

46. Gordon, A. M., Hung, Y.-C., Brandao, M., et al. (2011). Bimanual training and constraint-induced movement therapy in children with hemiplegic cerebral palsy: A randomized trial. *Neurorehabilitation and Neural Repair, 25,* 292.
47. Gordon, A., Schneider, J., Chinnan, A., et al. (2007). Efficacy of a hand-arm bimanual intensive therapy (HABIT) in children with hemiplegic cerebral palsy: A randomized control trial. *Developmental Medicine and Child Neurology, 49,* 830–839.
48. GRADE (Grade of Recommendation, Assessment, Development, and Evaluation) Working Group. (2004). Grading quality of evidence and strength of recommendation. *BMJ (Clinical Research Ed.), 328,* 1490–1494.
49. Gray, D. E. (2006). Coping over time: The parents of children with autism. *Journal of Intellectual Disability Research, 50,* 647–654.
50. Greenspan, S. L., & Wieder, S. (1997). Developmental patterns and outcomes in infants and children with disorders in relating and communicating. A chart review of 200 cases of children with autistic spectrum diagnoses. *Journal of Developmental and Learning Disorders, I,* 87–141.
51. Gutstein, S. E., Burgess, A., & Monfort, K. (2007). Evaluation of the Relationship Development Intervention program. *Autism, 11,* 397–411.
52. Hanft, B. E., & Piklington, K. O. (2000). Therapy in natural environment: The means or end goal for early intervention? *Infants and Young Children, 12,* 1–13.
53. Hanft, B., Rush, D. D., & Sheldon, M. L. (2004). *Coaching families and colleagues in early childhood.* Baltimore: Paul H. Brookes.
54. Hansen, R., Hinojosa, J., & Commission on Practice. (2009). Occupational therapy's commitment to nondiscrimination and inclusion. *American Journal of Occupational Therapy, 63,* 819–820.
55. Hill, S. A. (2000). Class, race, and gender dimensions of child rearing in African American families. *Journal of Black Studies, 31,* 494–508.
56. Holmes, M. (2000). Our mandate for the new millennium: Evidence-based practice. *American Journal of Occupational Therapy, 54,* 575–585.
57. Huang, H. H., Fetters, L., Hale, J., et al. (2009). Bound for success: A systematic review of constraint-induced movement therapy in children with cerebral palsy supports improved arm and hand use. *Physical Therapy, 89,* 1126–1141.
58. Humphry, R. (2002). Young children's occupations. *American Journal of Occupational Therapy, 56,* 171–179.
59. Humphry, R., & Wakeford, L. (2006). An occupation-centered discussion of development and implications for practice. *American Journal of Occupational Therapy, 60,* 258–267.
60. Institute of Medicine. (2011). Finding what works in health care: Standards for systematic reviews. At: <http://www.iom.edu/Reports/2011/Finding-What-Works-in-Health-Care-Standards-for-Systematic-Reviews.aspx> Accessed on March 24, 2014.
61. Jarrett, R. (1996). African American family and parenting strategies in impoverished neighborhoods. *Qualitative Sociology, 20,* 275–288.
62. Jiang, Y., Ekono, M., & Skinner, C. (2014). *Basic facts about low-income children: Children under 3 years, 2012.* Columbia University, New York City: National Center for Children in Poverty.
63. Jones, M. A., McEwen, I. R., & Hansen, L. (2003). Use of power mobility for a young child with spinal muscular atrophy. *Physical Therapy, 83,* 253–262.
64. Kasari, C., Freeman, S., & Paparella, T. (2006). Joint attention and symbolic play in young children with autism: A randomized controlled intervention study. *Journal of Child Psychology and Psychiatry, 47,* 611–620.
65. Kellegrew, D. H., & Allen, D. (1996). Occupational therapy in full-inclusion classrooms: A case study from the Moorpark model. *American Journal of Occupational Therapy, 50,* 718–724.
66. Kielhofner, G., & Burke, J. P. (1980). A model of human occupation, Part 1. Conceptual framework and content. *American Journal of Occupational Therapy, 34,* 572–581.
67. Kielhofner, G., Burke, J. P., & Igi, C. H. (1980). A model of human occupation, Part 4. Assessment and intervention. *American Journal of Occupational Therapy, 34,* 777–788.
68. Klingberg, T., Forssberg, H., & Westerberg, H. (2002). Increased brain activity in frontal and parietal cortex underlies the development of visuospatial working memory capacity during childhood. *Journal of Cognitive Neuroscience, 14*(1), 1–10.
69. Kramer, P., Luebben, A. J., & Hinojosa, J. (2010). Contemporary legitimate tools of pediatric occupational therapy. In P. Kramer & J. Hinosoja (Eds.), *Frames of reference for pediatric occupational therapy* (3rd ed., pp. 50–66). Philadelphia: Lippincott Williams & Wilkins.
70. Kreider, C. M., Bendixen, R. M., Huang, Y. Y., et al. (2014). Review of occupational therapy intervention research in the practice area of children and youth 2009–2013. *American Journal of Occupational Therapy, 68,* e61–e73.
71. Lane, S. J., & Mistrett, S. (2002). Let's play!: Assistive technology interventions for play. *Young Exceptional Children, 5,* 19–27.
72. Law, M. (2002). Participation in the occupations of everyday life, 2002 Distinguished Scholar Lecture. *American Journal of Occupational Therapy, 56,* 640–649.
73. Law, M., Baptiste, S., & Mills, J. (1995). Client-centred practice: What does it mean and does it make a difference? *Canadian Journal of Occupational Therapy, 62,* 250–257.
74. Law, M., & MacDermid, J. (2008). *Evidence-based rehabilitation: A guide to practice.* Thorofare, NJ: SLACK Inc.
75. Law, M., Petrenchik, T., Zivinani, J., et al. (2006). Participation of children in school and community. In S. Rodger & J. Ziviani (Eds.), *Occupational therapy with children: Understanding children's occupations and enabling participation* (pp. 67–90). Oxford: Blackwell Publishing.
76. Law, M. C., Darrah, J., Pollock, N., et al. (2011). Focus on function: A cluster, randomized controlled trial comparing child- versus context-focused intervention for young children with cerebral palsy. *Developmental Medicine & Child Neurology, 53,* 621–629.
77. Lee, J. (2010). Achieving best practice: A review of evidence linked to occupation-focused practice models. *Occupational Therapy in Health Care, 24,* 206–224.
78. Livingstone, R., & Paleg, G. (2014). Practice considerations for the introduction and use of power mobility for children. *Developmental Medicine & Child Neurology, 56,* 210–221.
79. Lynch, E., & Hanson, M. (1993). Changing demographics: Implications for training in early intervention. *Infants and Young Children, 6*(1), 50–55.
80. Mahoney, G., & Perales, F. (2005). The impact of relationship focused intervention on young children and children with disabilities. *Topics in Early Childhood Special Education, 18,* 5–17.
81. Mailloux, Z., & Roley, S. S. (2010). Sensory integration. In H. Miller Kuhaneck & R. Watling (Eds.), *Autism: A comprehensive occupational therapy approach* (3rd ed.). Bethesda, MD: American Occupational Therapy Association, Inc.
82. Malone, D. M., & Langone, J. (1998). Variability in the play of preschoolers with cognitive delays across different toy

sets. *International Journal of Disability, Development and Education, 45*, 127–142.
83. McWilliam, R. A., Tocci, L., & Harbin, G. L. (1998). Family-centered services: Service providers' discourse and behavior. *Topics in Early Childhood and Special Education, 18*(4), 206–221.
84. Miller Kuhaneck, H., Ecker, C., Parham, L. D., et al. (2010). *Sensory Processing Measure—Preschool (SPM-P): Manual.* Los Angeles: Western Psychological Services.
85. Miller, L. T., Politajko, H. J., Missiuna, C., et al. (2001). A pilot trial of a cognitive treatment for children with developmental coordination disorder. *Human Movement Science, 20*, 183–210.
86. Missiuna, C., DeMatteo, C., Hanna, S., et al. (2010). Exploring the use of cognitive intervention for children with acquired brain injury. *Physical and Occupational Therapy in Pediatrics, 30*(3), 205–219.
87. Missiuna, C., & Pollock, N. (2000). Perceived efficacy and goal setting in young children. *Canadian Journal of Occupational Therapy, 67*, 101–109.
88. Missiuna, C., Pollock, N., & Law, M. (2004). *The perceived efficacy and goal setting system.* San Antonio, TX: Psychological Corporation.
89. Niemeijer, A. S., Smits-Engelman, B. C., & Schoemaker, M. M. (2007). Neuromotor task training for children with developmental coordination disorder: A controlled trial. *Developmental Medicine and Child Neurology, 49*, 406–522.
90. Nilsson, L., & Nyberg, P. (2003). Driving to learn: A new concept for training children with profound cognitive disabilities in a powered wheelchair. *American Journal of Occupational Therapy, 57*(2), 229–233.
91. Novak, I. (2011). Parent experience of implementing effective home programs. *Physical and Occupational Therapy in Pediatrics, 31*, 198–213.
92. Novak, I., McIntyre, S., Morgan, C., et al. (2013). A systematic review of interventions for children with cerebral palsy: State of the evidence. *Developmental Medicine and Child Neurology, 55*, 885–910.
93. Novak, I., Cusick, A., & Lannin, N. (2009). Occupational therapy home programs for cerebral palsy: Double-blind, randomized, controlled trial. *Pediatrics, 124*, e606–e614.
94. Parham, L. D. (1987). Toward professionalism: The reflective therapist. *American Journal of Occupational Therapy, 41*, 555–561.
95. Parham, D. (2008). Play and occupational therapy. In L. D. Parham & L. Fazio (Eds.), *Play in occupational therapy for children* (2nd ed., pp. 3–40). St. Louis: Mosby.
96. Parham, L. D., Cohn, E. S., Spitzer, S., et al. (2007). Fidelity in sensory integration intervention research. *American Journal of Occupational Therapy, 61*, 216–227.
97. Phelan, S., Steinke, L., & Mandich, A. (2009). Exploring a cognitive intervention for children with pervasive developmental disorder. *Canadian Journal of Occupational Therapy, 76*(1), 23–28.
98. Ramey, S. L., DeLuca, S. C., Reidy, T. G., et al. (2013). Key findings from original research articles with functional and occupational outcomes of pediatric CIMT and related componential interventions. In S. L. Ramey, P. Coker-Bolt, & S. D. DeLuca (Eds.), *Handbook of pediatric constraint-induced movement therapy (CIMT)*. Bethesda, MD: AOTA Press.
99. Rainforth, B., & York-Barr, J. (1997). *Collaborative teams for students with severe disabilities: Integrating therapy and education* (2nd ed.). Baltimore: Paul H. Brookes.
100. Reilly, M. (Ed.), (1974). *Play as exploratory learning.* Beverly Hills, CA: Sage Publications.
101. Rigby, P. J., Ryan, S. E., & Campbell, K. A. (2009). Effect of adaptive seating devices on the activity performance of children with cerebral palsy. *Archives of Physical Medicine and Rehabilitation, 90*, 1389–1396.
102. Rodriguez, B. L., & Olswang, L. B. (2003). Mexican-American and Anglo-American mothers' beliefs and values about child rearing, education, and language impairment. *American Journal of Speech-language Pathology, 12*, 454–462.
103. Rodger, S., Ireland, S., & Vun, M. (2008). Can Cognitive Orientation to daily Occupational Performance (CO-OP) help children with Asperger's syndrome to master social and organisational goals? *British Journal of Occupational Therapy, 71*(1), 23–32.
104. Rodger, S., & Brandenburg, J. (2009). Cognitive Orientation to (daily) Occupational Performance (CO-OP) with children with Asperger's syndrome who have motor-based occupational performance goals. *Australian Occupational Therapy Journal, 56*, 41–50.
105. Rodger, S., Ashburner, J., Cartmill, L., et al. (2010). Helping children with autism spectrum disorders and their families: are we losing our occupation-centered focus? *Australian Occupational Therapy Journal*, 57, 276–280.
106. Rogers, J. (1983). Clinical reasoning: The ethics, science and art. *American Journal of Occupational Therapy, 37*, 601–616.
107. Rogers, S., & Dawson, G. (2010). *Early Start Denver Model for young children with autism: Promoting language, learning, and engagement.* New York: Guilford Press.
108. Rogoff, B. (2003). *The cultural nature of human development.* New York: Oxford University Press.
109. Rush, D. D., Shelden, M. L., & Hanft, B. E. (2003). Coaching families and colleagues: A process for collaboration in natural settings. *Infants and Young Children, 16*(1), 33–47.
110. Sakzewski, L., Ziviani, J., & Boyd, R. (2009). Systematic review and meta-analysis of therapeutic management of upper limb dysfunction in children with congenital hemiplegia. *Pediatrics, 123*, e111–e1122.
111. Salls, J., Kolhi, C., Silverman, L., et al. (2009). The use of evidence-based practice by occupational therapist. *Occupational Therapy in Health Care, 23*, 134–145.
112. Schell, B. A. (2014). Professional reasoning in practice. In B. B. Schell, G. Gillen, & M. E. Scaffa (Eds.), *Willard and Spackman's occupational therapy* (12th ed.). Philadelphia: Lippincott Williams & Wilkins.
113. Schertz, W., & Gordon, A. (2008). Changing the model: A call for a re-examination of intervention approaches and translational research in children with developmental disabilities. *Developmental Medicine and Child Neurology, 51*(1), 6–7.
114. Schilling, D. L., Washington, K., Billingsley, F. F., et al. (2003). Classroom seating for children with attention deficit hyperactivity disorder. *American Journal of Occupational Therapy, 57*, 534–541.
115. Sharifzadeh, V. S. (1997). Families with Middle Eastern roots. In E. W. Lynch & M. Hanson (Eds.), *Developing cross-cultural competence* (2nd ed., pp. 441–482). Baltimore: Brookes.
116. Shepherd, J. J. (2008). Using motor learning approaches for treating swallowing and feeding disorders: A review. *Language, Speech, and Hearing Services in Schools, 39*, 227–236.
117. Silverman, F. (2011). Promoting inclusion with occupational therapy: A coteaching model. *Journal of Occupational Therapy, Schools, and Early Intervention, 4*, 100–107.
118. Slavin, R. E. (2002). Evidence-based education policies: Transforming educational practice and research. *Educational Researcher, 31*, 15–21.

119. Spitzer, S. L. (2008). Play in children with autism: Structure and experience. In L. D. Parham & L. S. Fazio (Eds.), *Play in occupational therapy for children* (pp. 351–374). St. Louis: Mosby.
120. Stagnitti, K., O'Connor, C., & Sheppard, L. (2012). Impact of the Learn to Play program on play, social competence and language for children aged 5-8 years who attend a specialist school. *Australian Occupational Therapy Journal, 59*, 302–311.
121. Steiner, A. M. (2011). A strength-based approach to parent education for children with autism. *Journal of Positive Behavior Interventions, 13*, 178–190.
122. Steultjens, E. M. J., Dekker, J., Bouter, L. M., et al. (2005). Evidence of the efficacy of occupation therapy in different conditions: An overview of systematic reviews. *Clinical Rehabilitation, 19*, 247–254.
123. Sullivan, K. J., Kantak, S. S., & Burtner, P. A. (2008). Motor learning in children: Feedback effects on skill acquisition. *Physical Therapy, 88*, 720–732.
124. Taylor, S., Fayed, N., & Mandich, A. (2007). CO-OP Intervention for young children with developmental coordination disorder. *OTJR: Occupation, Participation and Health, 27*, 124–130.
125. Taub, E., Ramey, S. L., DeLuca, S., et al. (2004). Efficacy of constraint-induced movement therapy for children with cerebral palsy with asymmetric motor impairment. *Pediatrics, 113*, 305–312.
126. Thomas, A. J. (2000). Impact of racial identity on African American child rearing beliefs. *Journal of Black Psychology, 26*, 317–329.
127. Thomas, A., & Law, M. (2013). Research utilization and evidence-based practice in occupational therapy: A scoping study. *American Journal of Occupational Therapy, 67*, e55–e65.
128. Tickle-Degnen, L. (2002). Client-centered practice, therapeutic relationship, and the use of research evidence. *American Journal of Occupational Therapy, 56*, 470–474.
129. Tickle-Degnen, L., & Coster, W. (1995). Therapeutic interaction and the management of challenge during the beginning minutes of sensory integration treatment. *Occupational Therapy Journal of Research, 15*, 122–141.
130. Trivette, C. M., & Dunst, C. J. (2005). DEC recommended practices: Family-based practices. In S. Sandall, M. L. Hemmeter, B. J. Smith, & M. E. McLean (Eds.), *DEC recommended practices: A comprehensive guide for practical application in early intervention/early childhood special education* (pp. 107–126). Missoula, MT: Division for Early Childhood.
131. Turnbull, A. P., Turnbull, H. R., & Blue-Banning, M. J. (1994). Enhancing inclusion of infants and toddlers with disabilities and their families: A theoretical and programmatic analysis. *Infants and Young Children, 7*(2), 1–14.
132. United States Census 2010. (n.d.). At: <http://www.census.gov/2010census/data/> Accessed on April 3, 2014.
133. Vismara, L. A., & Rogers, S. J. (2010). Behavioral treatments in autism spectrum disorder: What do we know? *Annual Review of Clinical Psychology, 6*, 447–468.
134. Willis, W. (1997). Families with African American roots. In E. W. Lynch & M. Hanson (Eds.), *Developing cross-cultural competence* (2nd ed., pp. 165–208). Baltimore: Brookes.
135. Yasukawa, A., Patel, P., & Sisung, C. (2006). Pilot study: Investigating the effects of kinesiotaping in an acute pediatric rehabilitation setting. *American Journal of Occupational Therapy, 60*, 723–727.
136. Ylvisaker, M., Adelson, D., Braga, L. W., et al. (2005). Rehabilitation and ongoing support after pediatric TBI: Twenty years of progress. *Journal of Head Trauma Rehabilitation, 20*, 95–109.
137. York, J., Giangreco, M. F., Vandercook, T., et al. (1992). Integrating support personnel in inclusive classrooms. In S. Stainback & W. Stainback (Eds.), *Curriculum considerations in inclusive classrooms: Facilitating learning for all students* (pp. 101–116). Baltimore: Brookes.
138. Zuniga, M. E. (1997). Families with Latino roots. In E. W. Lynch & M. Hanson (Eds.), *Developing cross-cultural competence* (2nd ed., pp. 209–250). Baltimore: Brookes.
139. Zwicker, J. G., & Harris, S. R. (2009). A reflection on motor learning theory in pediatric occupational therapy practice. *Canadian Journal of Occupational Therapy, 76*, 29–37.

CHAPTER

2

Foundations and Practice Models for Occupational Therapy with Children

Jane Case-Smith

KEY TERMS

World Health Organization International Classification System
Ecologic theories
Person-environment-occupation model
Client-centered and family-centered practice
Strength-based approaches
Practice models
Learning/acquisition
Behavioral theories
Cognitive orientation
Social participation
Motor learning/motor acquisition
Neurodevelopmental
Sensory integration
Coaching/consultation
Prevention and primary care

GUIDING QUESTIONS

1. What overarching theoretical concepts guide occupational therapy practice with children?
2. What are primary theoretical models that define children's *occupation and participation* in the context of the cultural, social, and physical environments?
3. How are ecologic theories used in occupational therapy?
4. What is meant by person-environment-occupation congruence?
5. What are the implications of client-centered and family-centered practice?
6. Which major practice models and principles guide occupational therapy practice with children?
7. How do occupational therapists make intervention decisions using specific theories, conceptual models of practice, and principles?
8. What is the research evidence for major theories and practice models used by occupational therapists?
9. Using practice examples, how do intervention activities derived from different theoretical approaches and practice models compare?

Occupational therapists have developed and used theory as the basis for professional practice for many years. Early developers of occupational therapy focused on the theories of occupation and the use of time.[113,161] As stated by Meyer,

> Our conception of man is that of an organism that maintains and balances itself in the world of reality and actuality by being in active life and active use, i.e., using and living and acting its time in harmony with its own nature and the nature about it. It is the use that we make of ourselves that gives the ultimate stamp to our [being] (p. 64).[113]

Meyer posited that humans maintain rhythms of work, play, rest, and sleep that need to be balanced and that "the only way to attain balance in all this is actual doing, actual practice" (p. 64).[113] Current practices with children build on many of the original concepts of the profession's founders that children learn and develop through their participation in activities and occupations. Social engagement (with family and friends) enables children to develop a sense of belonging and self-esteem that contributes to health and well-being. Since the time of Meyer, occupational therapists have continued to develop models of practice based on an understanding of humans as occupational beings. They have also integrated the theories and science of psychology, neuroscience, and other disciplines into their practices. This chapter describes overarching theoretical concepts, practice models, and principles commonly used in occupational therapy for children and youth. The chapter also provides examples of evidence for the practice models.

In the first section, we explain five overarching theoretically based concepts or models common to occupational therapy practice: (1) occupation and participation as these relate to health; (2) ecologic theories and person-environment-occupation (PEO) models; (3) International Classification of Functioning, Disability, and Health (ICF); (4) client-centered and family-centered models; and (5) strength-based approaches. In the following sections, specific practice models that align with the conceptual theories are explained. These sections are organized by cognitive, social, motor, and sensory outcomes, recognizing that the models are used to attain various client goals across performance areas.

Occupational therapists make decisions and select strategies using their synthesized knowledge of practice theories, including evidence for those theories, their own experiences, and their perceptions of the client's priorities. Through the use of theory, assessment, and professional reasoning, occupational therapists hypothesize and develop interventions to improve the performance and participation of children. Practice models and the theories from which they are developed provide a guide and rationale for occupational therapy intervention.

As noted earlier, *theoretically based conceptual models* for occupational therapy practice with children have defined practice since the profession's inception[113] and have evolved with continual refinement over the ensuing decades.[8,71,89,121] *Practice models* more specifically define interventions for different types of children and settings and guide the day-to-day delivery of occupational therapy services. A practice model provides occupational therapists with specific principles, methods, and guidelines for decision making when evaluating, planning, and implementing intervention.

This chapter also explains the research evidence for occupational therapy models of practice. Evidence-based practice models and interventions are ones that have been tested through research that examined the theory's inherent relationships or assumptions. Intervention practices are often tested in controlled studies with inference to original theory. Testing of theoretical propositions about practice (i.e., which interventions promote children's performance, participation, and well-being) allows the profession to refine, revise, or expand practice models.

Overarching Conceptual Models

This section describes the overarching theoretically based concepts and models that influence the profession's core focus on occupation and participation of children and youth with disabilities. Ecologic theories are described as the foundation for PEO models. The ICF and the occupational therapy practice framework[2] are essential models for understanding how the environment and occupation are determinants of an individual's health, societal participation, and well-being. Family-centered and strength-based approaches, as cornerstones for occupational therapy practice with children, are defined.

Occupation and Participation

Throughout the 1920s and into the 1930s, the focus of occupational therapy was the development of the idea of occupation as a cure for disease and disability. The occupations best suited to cure specific medical problems were identified. The original focus of the profession was on the fundamental activities of human life: "work and play and rest and sleep" (p. 8).[113] Occupational therapists continue to use the principles of graded, purposeful activity and a balance of work, rest, and play as the basis for intervention methods.[111,161] As originally conceived, occupation has a dual role in the profession: the focus of intervention and the medium through which occupational therapists intervene.

Because occupations are everyday activities, they may appear to be simple; occupations are the basic activities that people perform each day for self-care, to care for others, to be productive, and to enjoy life. Engagement in occupation is driven by an intrinsic need for mastery, competence, and self-identity. Dunton,[53] a founder of occupational therapy, expressed his belief that occupation is as necessary to life as food and drink. The definition of occupation becomes more complex with the inclusion of its meaning or purpose. The meaning and value of an occupation are determined by the individual's culture and values. Occupations have many layers, relate to and are defined by one's roles, and are central to the human experience.

Although the original focus was on the therapeutic effect of occupation on mental health, this focus shifted during and after the world wars as a result of the escalating demand for physical rehabilitation of soldiers and veterans. In the 1960s through 1980s, new knowledge from neuroscience and increased understanding of critical reasoning promoted the development of a science-based profession. Emphasizing work and play as the contexts for developing competency, Reilly[141,142] developed a theory of occupational behavior in which the individual inherently strives to develop and achieve skill mastery. Her view of occupational therapy, "that man through the use of his hands as they are energized by mind and will, can influence the state of his own health" (p. 2),[140] has inspired generations of practitioners. In the 1970s, Fidler and Fidler[58] focused on the importance of purposeful activity, or *doing*, in the development of self and the prevention of disability. Yerxa et al.[194] followed Reilly's work, stating that in "authentic occupational therapy," the occupational therapist commits to the client's goals, offers activity choices that are meaningful, and engages the client in meaningful and purposeful activity. Also building on Reilly's theories, Kielhofner and Burke[82] developed a model of human occupation that incorporated a systems view of the nature of occupation. In the model of human occupation, the motivation for occupation, the routine patterning of occupations, skilled performance, and the influence of the environment systematically and continually interact. This model expanded the understanding of life roles and the powerful influence they have on daily life and health.

Wilcock described occupation as a "synthesis of doing, being, and becoming."[185] Humans need to use time in a purposeful way to develop and flourish.[183] Occupational science, using primarily qualitative methods of analysis, integrates social, cultural, and historical views of how people live and act in everyday life. Studies have explored the relationships among activity, participation, and health; social views of disability; and quality of life and human experience of persons with disabling conditions.[72,185] Both physical and mental health can be strongly influenced by a person's engagement in meaningful occupations, and, conversely, the absence of meaningful occupation can have dire health consequences.[184]

For children, occupation and doing enable skill development, personality formation, and self-identity development. Occupations are linked to roles and evolve over the life span. Children's occupations are largely determined for them in the beginning of life, and they gradually become more independent and more responsible for how they use their time and in which activities they participate. The shift in responsibility for and independence in daily occupations is often delayed, uneven, and less predictable for children with disabilities. Occupational science studies have promoted understanding of how occupations develop,[76] the complexity of engagement in occupation, and the relationship between occupation and human health.

Development of Occupations

During the 1960s and 1970s, occupational therapists working with children had a strong developmental perspective. These theories attempted to explain the functioning and growth of children and adolescents from an occupational therapy perspective. Llorens[99] identified a developmental practice model that focused on the physical, social, and psychological aspects of life tasks and relationships. She viewed the role of the occupational therapist to be one of facilitating development, assisting in the mastery of life tasks, and enabling children to cope with life expectations. Gilfoyle, Grady, and Moore[65] created a spatiotemporal adaptation model that views development as a spiraling process, moving from simple to complex. Adaptation is a continuous process of interaction involving the individual, time, and space. This model became central to occupational therapists' views of child development and fostered the development of intervention models.

In recent years, occupational therapy researchers have suggested a dynamic system perspective of developmental processes.[74,75] A child's occupational development is based on complex, reciprocal, and nonlinear relationships involving the child's innate characteristics and environmental factors. Children develop in the context of interpersonal and social opportunities (e.g., interaction with other children). They learn by observing others perform activities, through play with other children and adults, and through adults teaching and modeling for them. These social mechanisms are the catalyst for much of a child's learning. Building on the work of Vygotsky[178] and Bandura et al.,[6] Humphry[75] posited that occupations develop through vicarious learning when observing others. For example, children learn through shared occupations, such as circle time or group activities in preschool.

In addition to vicarious learning in social situations, children learn directly by engaging in novel activities. Through new play activities, the child reorganizes learned skills, adapts skills on the basis of trial and error, and tries new actions to accomplish the activity. Fully engaging in an activity is an important catalyst to learning. To engage completely, the child must find the activity to be meaningful, fun, and challenging. These concepts about development of occupational performance imply that children learn in social contexts and that engagement in activity results in learning. Various adult roles are implicated by these concepts, including designing group activities, creating learning environments, modeling, encouraging, supporting, and guiding.

At the broadest level, communities invest in children's learning by developing programs, places, and opportunities for social engagement that enable children to participate in community life. Examples of community investment in children with diverse developmental needs include childcare centers that welcome the attendance of children with disabilities, play spaces that use universal design allowing all children to use them, and educational programs that encourage the participation of families with young children. Communities that invest in child development support human resources, childcare centers, educational programs, and spaces that encourage healthy development and learning in children of all abilities. These influences are explained further in the later section on ecologic theories and PEO models. Chapter 3 further explains developmental theories used in occupational therapy.

Participation of Children and Youth with Disabilities

The goal of an occupation-based model of practice is the child's achievement of optimal occupational performance and participation. Participation (i.e., being involved and sharing in activities)[91] meets a basic human need and contributes positively to health.[23] What do professionals know about the participation of children with special needs? Children with special needs have lower rates of participation in ordinary daily activities.[11] Young adolescents with physical disabilities need supports to participate in household chores, cooking, and managing their laundry (see Chapter 16).[57] Researchers have also documented that children with disabilities are more restricted in active recreation and community socialization activities.[10] Numerous researchers have found that children with disabilities participate less frequently in community activities than children without disabilities.[11,108] Specifically, Bedell and Dumas[11] found that children with acquired brain injury were most restricted in participating in structured community events, managing daily routines, and socializing with peers, and they were least restricted in physical mobility. Youth with cerebral palsy have fewer opportunities to participate in community activities compared with children without disabilities.[96,156] In their systematic review of studies of leisure activities in children and youth with physical disabilities, Shikako-Thomas et al.[157] found that children with disabilities participate more in informal activities (e.g., activities that require little or no planning and are often self-initiated, such as reading or playing with toys) than in formal activities (e.g., activities with a formally designated coach or instructor, such as music or art lessons or organized sports). These researchers later found that adolescents with cerebral palsy spend most of their leisure time in sedentary, informal recreation, such as watching TV or listening to music (Research Note 2-1).

Australian[105] and Canadian[95] studies found an inverse relationship in children with disabilities between the amount

RESEARCH NOTE 2-1

Shikako-Thomas, K., Shevell, M., Lach, L., Law, M., Schmitz, N., Poulin, C., Majnemer, A., & the QUALA group (2013). Picture me playing—a portrait of participation and enjoyment of leisure activities in adolescents with cerebral palsy. Research in Developmental Disabilities, 34, *1001–1010.*

Picture Me Playing—A Portrait of Participation and Enjoyment of Leisure Activities in Adolescents with Cerebral Palsy

Shikako-Thomas, Shevell, Lach, Law, Schmitz, Poulin, Majnemer, the QUALA group (2013). This descriptive study by a Canadian group of researchers examined the level of participation and enjoyment in leisure activities among adolescents with cerebral palsy. Participants were 175 adolescents 12 to 20 years old with a range of cerebral palsy severity. The participants completed the Children's Assessment of Participation and Enjoyment (CAPE). Occupational therapists complete the Manual Ability Classification System (MACS) and the Gross Motor Function Classification System (GMFCS) from parent report.

Results: The adolescents reported that their most frequent activity was watching TV or a rented movie or listening to music. When with peers, the participants "hung out" or visited. Older adolescents (>15 years old) engaged in few recreational activities and completed them less often. Adolescents who were ambulatory and had high manual ability participated in more activities and at higher frequency than adolescents who were nonambulatory and had low manual ability.

Implications for Occupational Therapy

- Adolescents with cerebral palsy most frequently participate in informal, passive recreational activities such as watching TV or listening to music.

of physical activity and age, with a significant decline in active leisure participation from childhood to adolescence. Although healthy children are less physically active as adolescents, they continue to participate in a wide range of leisure activities. In contrast, adolescents with disabilities engage in fewer leisure and social activities, and their activities tend to be more often home-based than community-based.[157] These studies conclude that greater efforts among community organizations are needed to support the participation of children and youth with disabilities.

Community participation appears to vary by type of disability and is higher for children with functional communication and social behavior. The most important determinant of participation is adaptive behavior (i.e., can the child express needs, follow instructions, and interact appropriately?).[130] Children who have sustained traumatic brain injury and have behavioral problems or executive functioning impairments may have more difficulty in structured activities than children with cerebral palsy, who can more often fully participate in structured activities.[13] Adolescents with autism spectrum disorder (ASD) have limited social participation as they transition into young adulthood; almost 50% do not receive phone calls from friends or are not invited to activities with friends.[128] Limited social participation often continues into adulthood; more than 50% of adults with ASD do not have close friendships.[98] See Chapters 4 and 12 for discussions of adolescent participation.

Both intrinsic (personal) and environmental (family and community) factors influence the diversity of activities and the intensity of participation. As noted earlier, intrinsic factors include communication skills, adaptive behavior, motor function,[129] personality, and social skills. Social participation appears to be most influenced by the child's conversational ability and functional cognitive skills.[128] Girls tend to participate more in arts and social activities, and boys participate more in group activities involving physical activity and sports.[54,157] Family support can have a positive or negative effect. Children's activities may be restricted by family time constraints, financial burden, and lack of supportive mechanisms (e.g., babysitting).[95,176] Participation for children with disabilities is positively influenced by high levels of family cohesion, high incomes, strong family coping skills, and low levels of stress.[95,157] Parents of children with disabilities report that barriers to participation are access to the physical environment; the physical, cognitive, and social demands of the activity; attitudes; peer relations; and safety.[11,13] Encouraging participation in the typical activities of childhood needs to be the major focus of pediatric occupational therapy. Bedell et al.[13] recommended that occupational therapists advocate for modification of the physical and social environments for community activities in ways that support full participation by children and youth with disabilities. In her seminal article, Law[91] defined occupational therapy intervention principles that promote participation in everyday life (Box 2-1).

Ecologic Theories

Human ecology is the study of human beings and their relationships with their environments. *Environments* are the contexts and situations that occur outside individuals and elicit responses from them, including personal, social, institutional, and physical factors. Environmental factors can facilitate or limit engagement in occupation. A concept prevalent in the human development literature and more recently in health care is person-environment congruence, or *environmental fit* (i.e., the congruence between individuals and their environments).[162] Over the past 3 decades, occupational therapy scholars have stressed the importance of the interaction between individual and environment, and most occupational therapy models of practice embrace the importance of cultural, social, institutional, and physical environments in the transactional relationship between people and the environments in which they live, work, and play.[46,82,93,192]

Psychologists who created theories and models about the relationship between humans and their environments that have influenced occupational therapy include Bronfenbrenner,[18,19] E. Gibson,[63] and J. Gibson.[64] Bronfenbrenner[18] developed an ecologic model to explain how social and cultural environments influence a child's development. In his model, interdependent relationships between a child and his or her social and cultural environments have an important influence on the child's outcomes. Different levels of social support and social interactions surround the individual, including informal (e.g., family and friends) and formal (e.g., occupational therapists and teachers). Levels of the environment are defined by their proximity to the individual—family is most important, then friends and extended family, and then the community and society. Children and their families interact with and are influenced by all levels of the social environment. Changes at any level of the environment influence a person's behavior. Throughout the course of life, a person constantly adapts to and influences changes in his or her social environment.

According to Bronfenbrenner's theories of social development,[18] occupational therapists are part of a person's social environment, and the occupational therapist's influence on the systems that closely surround the child may be as important as direct interventions to the child. Although social contexts change over the life span, family, community, and societal interrelationships continue, influencing outcomes for the individual. The interdependence between a person and the social environment implies that occupational therapists expand intervention strategies to include families and communities.

Ecologic psychologists E. Gibson[63] and J. Gibson[64] considered the interdependence of a person with his or her

BOX 2-1 Best Practice Principles of Occupational Therapy to Promote Participation in Everyday Life

Occupational therapy:

- Is evidence-based and client-centered.
- Focuses on occupations important to each person within his or her environment.
- Acknowledges the power of engagement in occupation.
- Recognizes the force of the environment as a means of intervention.
- Has a broad intervention focus.
- Measures outcomes of participation.
- Focuses on occupations important to each person within his or her environment.

From Law, M. (2002). Participation in the occupation of everyday life. *American Journal of Occupational Therapy, 56*, 640–649.

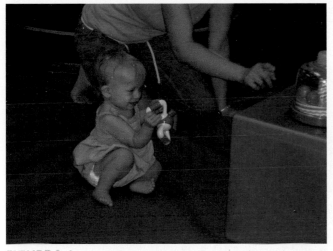

FIGURE 2-1 The infant uses sensorimotor play with mouth and hands to explore an object.

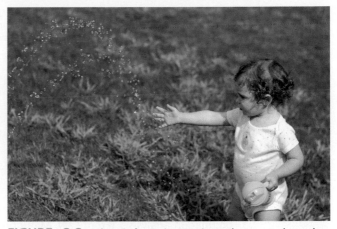

FIGURE 2-2 The infant is motivated to explore her environment.

environment to be an explanation of *perceptual* development. E. Gibson[63] understood that manipulative play had a key role in the infant's cognitive development and that a child's intrinsically motivated exploratory actions lead to perceptual, motor, and cognitive development. She defined an *affordance* as the quality of an object or an environment that allows an individual to perform an action. Action and perception are tightly linked: the child's first actions are to gather new information about the environment, and those actions form the basis for perceptual development (the child's understanding of the environment) (Figure 2-1). "As new action systems mature, new affordances open up and new experiments on the world can be undertaken" (p. 7).[63] As explained by E. Gibson:

> The young organism grows up in the environment (both physical and social) ..., one that imposes demands on his actions for his individual survival. To accommodate to his world, he must detect the information for these actions—that is, perceive the affordances it holds ... evolution has provided [the child] with action systems and sensory systems that equip him to discover what the world is all about. He is "programmed" or motivated to use these systems, first by exploring the accessible surround, then acting on it ... extending his explorations further. The exploratory systems emerge in an orderly way that permits an ever-spiraling path of discovery. The observations made possible via both exploratory ... actions provide the material for his knowledge of the world—a knowledge that does not cease expanding, whose end (if there is an end) is understanding (p. 37).[63]

Successful adaptation to the environment occurs when a person matches his or her activities to the affordances of the environment or when the person modifies the environment to achieve successful completion of an activity. The Gibsons' theories emphasize the importance of understanding a child's development in the context of daily surroundings and activities. Occupational therapists are encouraged to provide activities (based on their understanding of the activity's inherent affordances) that allow a child to explore and learn about the environment, enabling achievement of the child's goals. In Figure 2-2, an infant shows motivation to explore objects within her environment.

Person-Environment-Occupation Models

PEO ecologic theories gave rise to occupational therapy models that situate a child's participation in the context of his or her social, cultural, and physical environment. Occupational therapy practitioners are concerned not only with the child's performance in everyday activities but also the environmental influences that enable a child's engagement and participation in activities.[186] Occupational therapy practitioners recognize that health is supported and maintained when clients engage in occupations and activities that allow desired or needed participation in home, school, workplace, and community life.[2]

Most occupational therapy practice models explain the interaction of person, occupation, and environment, recognizing the premise that human performance cannot be understood outside of context.[46] In earlier models (e.g., person-environment-performance, person-task-environment[145]), the focus of primary intervention is on the person, with relatively less emphasis on changing environments. Law et al.[93] developed the PEO model, which focuses equally on facilitating change in the person, occupation, or environment.

The PEO model was developed using theoretical foundations from the *Canadian Guidelines for Occupational Therapy,* environmental-behavioral theory, and theories about optimal experience as proposed by Csikszentmihalyi and Csikszentmihalyi.[37] Csikszentmihalyi[38] explained that optimal experience, or "flow," occurs when a person's activity is an optimal challenge for his or her skill level; the person is focused on his or her actions and goals; time passes without awareness; and the activity becomes an end in itself. The PEO model suggests that optimal fit of the activity (occupation) and environment to a person's goals, interests, and skills can lead to optimal participation and health. The PEO model outlines the concepts of person, environment, and occupation as follows[93]:

- *Person:* A unique being who, across time and space, participates in various roles important to him or her.
- *Environment:* Cultural, socioeconomic, institutional, physical, and social factors outside a person that affect his or her experiences.
- *Occupation:* Any self-directed, functional task or activity in which a person engages over the life span.

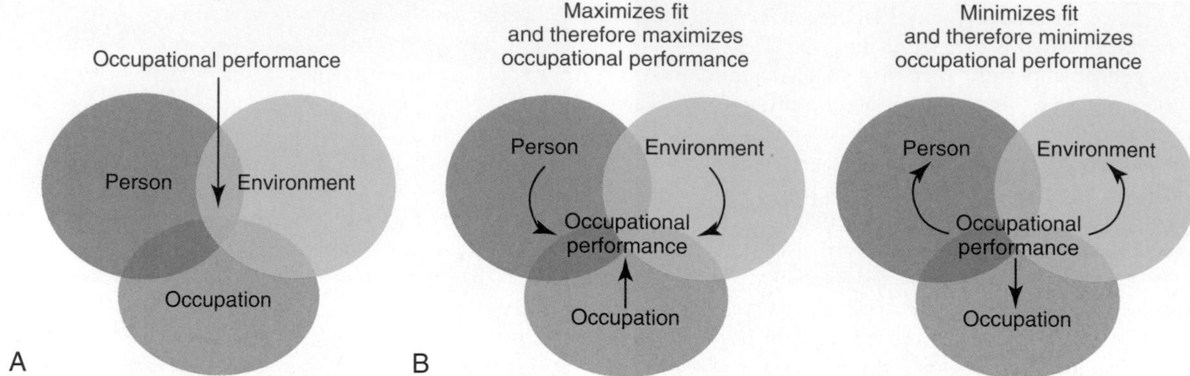

FIGURE 2-3 **A,** Person-environment-occupation model. **B,** Person-environment-occupation analysis. (From Law, M., Cooper, B., Strong, S., Stewart, D., Rigby, P., & Letts, L. [1996]. The person-environment-occupation model: A transactive approach to occupational performance. *Canadian Journal of Occupational Therapy, 63*[1], 9–23.)

The PEO model suggests that occupational performance is the result of the dynamic, transactive relationship involving person, environment, and occupation (Figure 2-3, *A*). Across the life span and in different environments, the three major components—person, environment, and occupation—interact continually to determine occupational performance. Increased congruence, or fit, among these components represents more optimal occupational performance (Figure 2-3, *B*).

The PEO model can be used as an analytic tool to identify factors in the person, environment, or occupation that facilitate or hinder the performance of occupations chosen by the person. Using this model, occupational therapy intervention focuses on facilitating change in any of these three dimensions to improve occupational performance. Specific models of practice, as defined in later sections, can be used in conjunction with the PEO model to address specific performance limitations or environmental conditions that impede occupational performance.

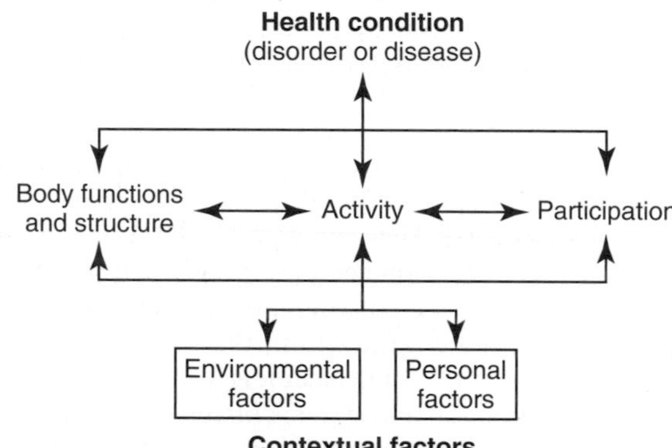

FIGURE 2-4 The International Classification of Functioning, Disability, and Health (ICF). According to ICF terminology, problems with body functions and structure are called impairments; activity limitations are difficulties in executing tasks or actions; and participation restrictions describe problems with involvement in life situations. (From World Health Organization [2002]. *Towards a Common Language for Functioning, Disability and Health: ICF*. Geneva: WHO.)

Occupational Therapy Practice Framework and World Health Organization International Classification of Functioning, Disability, and Health

The American Occupational Therapy Association[2] occupational therapy practice framework and World Health Organization[193] ICF are essential frames of reference for occupational therapists. The practice framework defines the domain and process of occupational therapy and has been internationally adopted by occupational therapists to guide the scope and process of practice.[2] The ICF is a classification system for health and health-related domains. Recognizing that the experience of disability is a universal human experience, the ICF views human functioning at three levels: the body (structure and function), the person (activities), and society (participation) (Figure 2-4). It also includes the domain of environmental factors, which can have a significant influence on a person's functioning and health. The ICF model of functioning, disability, and health depicts the dynamic interaction between a person and his or her environment at all levels of functioning. An extension of the ICF, the International Classification of Functioning, Disability, and Health for Children and Youth has been developed to address the unique concerns of developing children.[100] The American Occupational Therapy Association has acknowledged the strong connection between its practice framework and the ICF by establishing the domain of the profession as "supporting health and participation in life through engagement in occupation" (pp. 626-627).[2]

The classification of levels and definition of occupational therapy domains offer a framework for explaining top-down and bottom-up approaches. Although occupational therapists traditionally focused on underlying performance or performance impairments—that is, a "bottom-up" approach—more recently developed interventions follow a "top-down" approach that focuses on changing the environment and adapting activities to increase the child's participation.

The occupational therapist may design bottom-up interventions to reduce impairment (e.g., by increasing strength, improving balance, or reducing social anxiety). The advantage of a bottom-up approach is that by gaining specific new skills, the child's higher level performance may generalize to a broad range of activities (e.g., increased motor coordination may improve the child's handwriting, typing, cutting, and buttoning). A top-down approach allows the occupational therapist to think about multiple aspects of the child's performance, including the environment, the routine, activity patterns, contextual supports, and opportunities for participation, bringing a broader lens to the child's restricted participation. When using a top-down approach, the occupational therapist recommends modifications to the environment (e.g., social supports or assistive technology) to enhance the child's participation. Practitioners often use both approaches or use them sequentially. Systems (e.g., medical versus educational), occupational therapy roles (e.g., consultant versus direct therapy), resources (e.g., to purchase technology or modify the environment), expected outcomes (i.e., improved performance or increased participation), and the individual child (e.g., age, level of disability) influence the type of approach used. Using the practice models defined later in this chapter, Table 2-1 gives examples of top-down and bottom-up assessments and interventions.

Occupational therapy measures align with the ICF and enable practitioners to assess children at multiple levels. The School Function Assessment (SFA) is a scale that reflects a top-down approach rating the child's function at two levels, activities and participation.[34] Similarly, the Participation and Environment Measure for Children and Youth (PEM-CY)[12,31] assesses the effect of home, school, and community environments on children's participation. The PEM-CY identifies the factors that support or limit a child's participation across contexts, identifying factors that the family can modify to increase the child's participation.[32] Both the SFA and the PEM-CY take a top-down approach that identifies the environments and tasks that can be modified to accommodate increased performance and participation in specific contexts. Chapters 8, 11, 13, 16, and 17 provide additional examples of interventions using a top-down approach that emphasize task and environment modification.

Child-Centered and Family-Centered Service

Client-centeredness has always been an essential tenet of occupational therapy. In pediatric occupational therapy the client is

TABLE 2-1 Examples of Occupational Therapy Assessments and Interventions Categorized by the World Health Organization International Classification of Functioning, Disability, and Health (ICF) and the American Occupational Therapy Association Occupational Therapy Practice Framework*

Type of Approach	ICF Level	Occupational Therapy Practice Framework Domain	Assessment Examples	Intervention Example
Bottom-up	Body function and body structures	Client factors: Values, beliefs, and spirituality Body functions Body structures	Range of motion Muscle strength Motor coordination (Bruininks Oseretsky–2; M-Fun) Sensory processing (Sensory Processing Measure) Visual perception (Motor Free Visual Perception Test)	Biomechanical interventions, active range of motion Shaping and practice of motor skills Sensory integration intervention Action imitation Motor planning activities
	Activity and participation	Performance skills Performance patterns	School function (School Function Assessment; School AMPS) Self Care (PEDI-CAT; Wee-FIM) Social skills (Social Skills Rating Scale) Leisure and recreation (Children's Assessment of Participation and Enjoyment; Pediatric Activity Card Sort)	Handwriting interventions Self-regulation strategies Visual schedules for increasing activities of daily living Social skills groups Eating interventions Peer modeling
Top-down	[illegible]nvironmental and personal factors	Context and environment Activity demands	Environmental assessment (Home Observation for Measurement of the Environment [HOME]) Family preferences	Consult with school in developing a playground Recommend a Social Story for going to a restaurant with family Fit child in ultra-lightweight wheelchair for sports activities Modify work space for job internship

*Data from American Occupational Therapy Association. (2014). Occupational therapy practice framework: Domain and process (3rd ed.). *American Journal of Occupational Therapy, 68*(Suppl.1), S1–S48. http://dx.doi.org/10.5014/ajot.2014.682006; World Health Organization. (2001).

expanded to encompass the family in recognition that child and family are inextricably linked. In services for children and youth, this focus shifts from the parents of the young infant to the individual youth as he or she matures in decision making and self-determination. Client-centered occupational therapy practice emphasizes the importance of activities that are meaningful to the child, match the child or family's goals and priorities, provide choice, and elicit intrinsic motivation. During the past 30 years, families of children with disabilities have increased their roles in determining and implementing services for their children. Families have been leaders in promoting family-centered service, a philosophy of service provision that emphasizes the central role of families in making decisions about the interventions their children receive. Challenged by the changes in the health services field and an increased demand by consumers for involvement in the services they receive, health care providers have made great strides in implementing family-centered service.

The term *family-centered service* arose from early intervention programs. Three important concepts define the rationale for family-centered service: (1) parents know their children best and want the best for their children; (2) families are different and unique; and (3) optimal child functioning occurs in a supportive family and community context. Chapters 5 and 22 further explain the rationale for and application of family-centered practice.

In family-centered service, the family's right to make autonomous decisions is honored. The relationship between the family and professionals is a partnership in which the family defines the priorities for intervention and, with the service providers, helps direct the intervention process.[52] In working with families, service providers emphasize education to enable parents to make informed choices about the therapeutic needs of their child. Comprehensive education about services and community resources can help families understand the disability, acquire tools to manage behavior, and develop strategies for obtaining community resources. In family-centered practice, intervention is based on the family's visions and values; service providers recognize their own values and do not impose them on the family. The family's roles and interests, the environments in which the family members live, and the family's culture make up the context for service provision. Individualization of both the assessment and the intervention processes is essential to family-centeredness. Intervention is viewed as a dynamic process in which clients and parents work together as partners to define the therapeutic needs of the child with a disability. Services are designed to fit the needs of the family, rather than forcing the family to fit the needs of the service providers or the intervention policies already in place. DeGrace explains that occupational therapy intervention needs to fit into a family daily routine because how a family participates in daily routines "defines who that family is and plays a key role in determining its health" (p. 348).[41] Because each family is unique, practitioners need to ask about and learn how each family defines its routines, habits, and values and to adapt their services to this family-constructed definition. The overriding goal of intervention is to empower families by enhancing their capacity to manage the care of their child, to participate fully in desired roles and activities, and to pursue desired family goals.[48,50]

The later section on coaching and consulting conceptual models defines approaches that occupational therapists use to support families in problem solving and transfer therapy activities into family routines. Other examples of family-centered practice include helping families find social supports and network with other families[14] and supporting families in gathering needed resources.[69]

Parenting roles are strengthened and outcomes are improved when service providers solicit and value parental participation.[48] Increasing evidence in the literature indicates that interdisciplinary, family-centered services for children with disabilities lead to increased family satisfaction and may lead to greater functional improvement in children with disabilities.[106,149] Parents are less likely to act on behalf of their child when practitioners are unresponsive to the family's needs, are paternalistic, or fail to recognize and accept family decisions.[51] In a qualitative study of families participating in early intervention, parents asked for flexibility in how services are delivered. Parents vary in the extent to which they are willing and able to participate in interventions; it is inappropriate to give parents responsibilities for delivering intervention unless this model fits their preferences and abilities to manage.[70]

Intervention programs and occupational therapy practice need mechanisms for families to provide feedback about their experience and satisfaction with services. The findings of a large survey distributed at Canadian children's rehabilitation centers indicate that parental satisfaction with service is primarily determined by the family-centered culture of the organization and by parental perceptions of family-centered service.[94] Family satisfaction with services also decreases feelings of distress and depression and improves feelings of well-being.[83] Using qualitative methods, Hiebert-Murphy et al.[70] confirmed previous findings that families desire professionals who work collaboratively to identify and meet the family's goals. Occupational therapists enhance the effectiveness of their services when they practice from a family-centered perspective.

Strength-Based Approaches

A child's motivation, attitude, and self-perception are core to his or her initiative to attempt new skills and responsiveness to environmental demands. The relationship between learning and other affective components is complex. It is widely accepted that children's motivation to perform occupations is influenced by their perceptions of self-efficacy, regardless of whether these perceptions are correct.[10] Learning and competence are also enhanced through positive and supportive relationships.[88,150] When children experience success in learning situations, they gain perceived competence and internal control, gain support from significant others, and show pleasure at mastering the task. The assumption is made that with success, a child is more likely to seek new optimal challenges.[6] The corollary of this theory is that a child who experiences repeated failure begins to avoid challenges and is less likely to seek new learning situations.

In a strength-based approach to intervention, the strengths of the child and family are identified and become the building blocks for skill development and optimal participation. At the foundation of a strength-based approach is the belief that children and families have unique talents and skills that often are not recognized by professionals.[55] Implied in this approach is a positive, respectful relationship between the child and family and the occupational therapist. A focus on child and family resources and strengths and building on a positive therapist-client relationship imply different approaches to performance deficits. For example, a child with ASD who is cognitively proficient but is nonverbal may benefit from alternative methods of communication, rather than a focus on developing speech. A child with cerebral palsy who has communication and social competence but few functional fine motor skills may best participate in school by using a "buddy" whom he or she directs to perform required motor tasks.

A strength-based approach means that the occupational therapist:

1. Recognizes the strengths of the child or youth and accesses strengths to attain new levels of participation.
2. Gives the child or youth meaningful choices.
3. Collaborates with the child or youth in defining intervention goals.

Therapy goals that focus only on the child's deficits and missing skills miss the opportunity to use the child's strengths to promote function and participation. Strength-based approaches lead to increased self-determination. When children feel self-efficacious, they are motivated to try harder and to improve performance; they take initiative in attempting new activities and have greater facility to problem solve when they meet barriers. Self-efficacy beliefs contribute to motivation in several ways. A child with self-efficacy tries harder to attain a goal, expends more effort, perseveres in the face of difficulties, and is willing to try again when failing.[10]

Occupational therapists need to be aware of the importance of emphasizing a child's strengths, providing successful learning opportunities, and supporting the child or youth in challenging situations. Child strengths known to promote growth and participation include strong self-esteem, positive mental health, and positive communication skills.[9,181,182] Other child attributes that are associated with positive outcomes include intelligence, emotion regulation, temperament, coping strategies, and attention.[172] Children and youth who can effectively process information and problem solve can use these abilities in adverse situations.[84] Children who can regulate their emotions can monitor and modify the intensity and duration of their emotional reactions, enabling them to function better at school and in social relationships. An easygoing temperament is also a protective factor because it may evoke more positive attention from adults. Coping skills are also important because children with strong coping skills can moderate the impact of a difficult situation.[190]

The family, extended family, and environment can provide supports and resources that enhance the child's ability to cope with challenges and optimize the child's participation. Table 2-2 lists protective factors in the social environment that foster optimal child development. Family resources such as love, nurturance, and a sense of safety and security increase the child's resilience. Attributes of the family that influence positive outcomes include family cohesion and harmony. Researchers have shown that a high-quality relationship with at least one parent, characterized by high levels of warmth and openness and low levels of conflict, is associated with positive outcomes across level of risk and stages of development.[102]

Protective factors in the community also contribute to the child's development. These are specified in Chapter 4. Neighborhood quality, youth community organizations, quality of school programs, and after-school activities all can influence a child's ability to cope with risk factors and overcome adversity.[172] Attributes of the social environment that promote resilience include extended social support and availability of external

TABLE 2-2 Protective Factors in Families and Communities That Promote Health and Well-Being in Children

Protective Factor	Strategies That Promote Parenting Roles to Enhance the Child's Well-Being
Nurturing and attachment	Emphasize bonding and attachment throughout childhood. Support fathers in nurturing roles. Encourage play, particularly pretend and creative play. Support families in using positive discipline methods.
Knowledge of parenting and child development	Encourage parents to guide and reinforce appropriate child behaviors. Model desirable behaviors. Recommend nonpunitive disciplinary techniques.
Parental resilience	Teach or recommend stress management techniques. Suggest community resources and supports, such as faith communities. Participate in programs that offer family-to-family help. Suggest community supports for mental health if these are indicated. Guide, model, and encourage problem solving.
Societal connections	Help family overcome transportation, childcare, or other barriers to participate in a social network. Encourage the parent to join a parent's group or play group.
Concrete supports for parents	When appropriate, link parents with community leaders or disability groups to organize support and advocacy. Give parents suggestions on how to advocate for their interests and needs.
Social and emotional competence of children	Teach or model responsive interactions with the child. Praise the parents' nurturing behaviors; acknowledge the child's assets and positive traits. Encourage the parents to share their child with extended family and friends.

Adapted from U.S. Department of Health and Human Services, Administration for Children and Family, Child Welfare Information Gateway. *Protecting Children/Strengthening Families* (n.d.). <https://www.childwelfare.gov/preventing/preventionmonth/factors.cfm> Accessed January 3, 2014.

resources. Environmental factors, such as family-centered service delivery, acceptance of community attitudes, supportive home environments, and mentoring relationships with adults, have been shown to have a positive influence on child development.[178,182] The concepts discussed in this section share the common goal of promoting participation in social and physical roles, enhancing quality of life, and increasing self-efficacy. Figure 2-5 shows the theoretical constructs and intervention principles described in this section that promote an individual's self-efficacy and self-determination.

Conceptual Practice Models Specific to Performance Areas

Most conceptual practice models used by occupational therapists who work in pediatrics are concerned with change, specifically enhancement of children's behaviors, skills, and life participation. This section describes practice models that form intervention principles and guide practice in the following areas: (1) cognitive performance, (2) social participation, (3) sensory and motor performance, (4) task and environment adaptation, and (5) coaching and consultation. Practice models can be used across and within different *phases of intervention*: (1) preparation—interventions to promote self-regulation, sensory modulation; (2) behavioral change and skill development; and (3) generalization or transfer of learning. See Figure 2-6 for examples of practice models appropriate for different phases of intervention.

Cognitive Performance

Occupational therapists apply learning theories and principles when teaching children basic life skills, often embedding

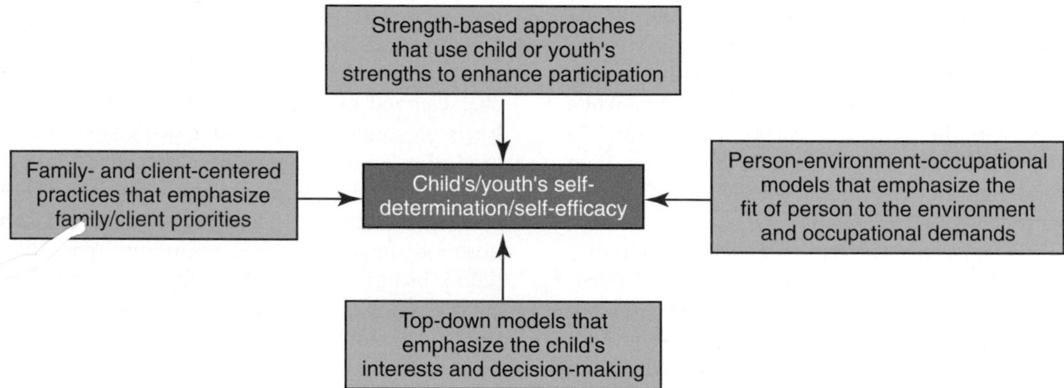

FIGURE 2-5 Relationship of theoretical constructs to a common goal of self-determination and self-efficacy.

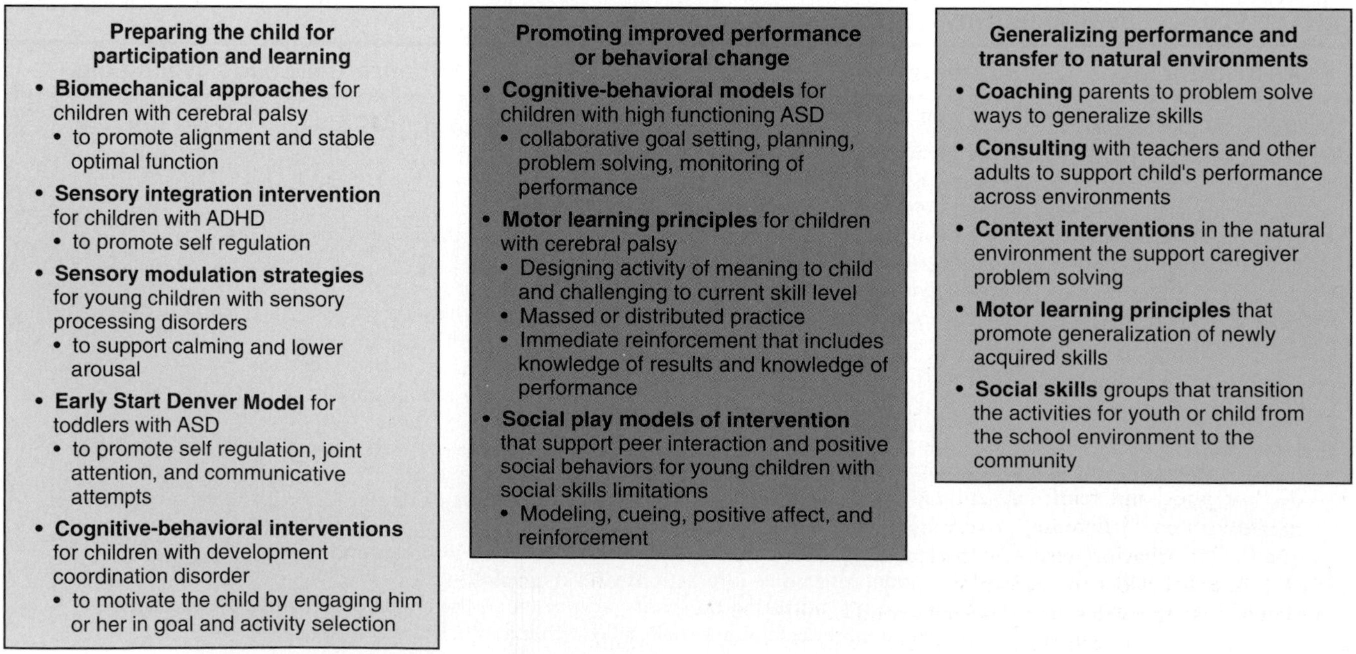

Preparing the child for participation and learning

- **Biomechanical approaches** for children with cerebral palsy
  - to promote alignment and stable optimal function
- **Sensory integration intervention** for children with ADHD
  - to promote self regulation
- **Sensory modulation strategies** for young children with sensory processing disorders
  - to support calming and lower arousal
- **Early Start Denver Model** for toddlers with ASD
  - to promote self regulation, joint attention, and communicative attempts
- **Cognitive-behavioral interventions** for children with development coordination disorder
  - to motivate the child by engaging him or her in goal and activity selection

Promoting improved performance or behavioral change

- **Cognitive-behavioral models** for children with high functioning ASD
  - collaborative goal setting, planning, problem solving, monitoring of performance
- **Motor learning principles** for children with cerebral palsy
  - Designing activity of meaning to child and challenging to current skill level
  - Massed or distributed practice
  - Immediate reinforcement that includes knowledge of results and knowledge of performance
- **Social play models of intervention** that support peer interaction and positive social behaviors for young children with social skills limitations
  - Modeling, cueing, positive affect, and reinforcement

Generalizing performance and transfer to natural environments

- **Coaching** parents to problem solve ways to generalize skills
- **Consulting** with teachers and other adults to support child's performance across environments
- **Context interventions** in the natural environment the support caregiver problem solving
- **Motor learning principles** that promote generalization of newly acquired skills
- **Social skills** groups that transition the activities for youth or child from the school environment to the community

FIGURE 2-6 Examples of practice models and principles that can be used in phases of intervention.

learning concepts into the child's daily routine and natural contexts. Learning is the acquisition of knowledge, skills, and occupations through experience that leads to a permanent change in behavior and performance. Learning to perform at higher levels and adapting to performance difficulties reflect neuroplasticity (i.e., the ability of the central nervous system [CNS] to adapt to and assimilate novel information or tasks). Learning theories foundational to occupational therapy practice models include behavioral theories and social cognitive learning. This section includes a description of the cognitive orientation to daily occupational performance approach, in which a child or youth uses cognitive (and metacognitive) skills to establish goals and apply learning techniques to overcome functional deficits.

Behavioral Theories

The past 60 years have witnessed tremendous progress in the field of learning theories. Early learning theorists, such as Thorndike, emphasized the association between a behavior and the resulting reward or punishment as a simple explanation of behavioral change. More than 60 years ago, Skinner[159] developed learning theories based on his belief that the environment shapes all human behaviors and that behaviors may be randomly emitted in response to an environmental stimulus. Learning occurs when a person tries a behavior that worked in a previous situation and the behavior is reinforced by environmental consequences that follow. Learning can also occur when a person exhibits an involuntary, reflexive response to an environmental stimulus and is subsequently reinforced by a consequence. This sequence—stimulus situation, behavioral response, and environmental consequence—constitutes a *contingency of behavior*, the mechanism by which the environment shapes behavior.

Through natural occurrences in the environment, a child's adaptive behaviors are reinforced, and behaviors that are not adaptive are ignored or punished.[160] The Skinnerian concept that became fundamental to interventions for children is *instrumental* or *operant learning*, or the use of reinforcement to modify behavior. Behavior is strengthened and maintained when it results in positive reinforcement (rather than punishment). If reinforcement is absent (i.e., not given and therefore negative), positive behaviors may be extinguished. Behavioral interventions are explained further in Chapters 13 and 15.

Applied behavior analysis has been well developed in the fields of education and psychology. Applied behavioral interventions primarily use operant conditioning in highly controlled environments in which an occupational therapist or teacher gives the child an instruction and rewards the child for an appropriate response (reinforcement). Components of the approach are in-depth analysis of behavior to understand when and why a behavior occurs and development of strategies to modify the targeted behavior. The child is presented with a stimulus that prompts a new behavior that is rewarded or reinforced. Prompting and reinforcement are repeated until the behavior is learned.[122] Extensive research has confirmed that when particular behaviors result in specific, consistent consequences, these behaviors are learned.[33]

Occupational therapists using operant conditioning techniques can help a child achieve a higher level of performance or to refine an existing skill through a process called *shaping*.[136] Shaping involves breaking down a complex behavior into components and reinforcing each component of the behavior individually and systematically until it approximates the desired behavior (Box 2-2). Although this technique is structured, the occupational therapist implements shaping techniques into the child's play, and play activities are used to motivate the child's actions (Figure 2-7).

BOX 2-2 Example of Shaping Techniques

Shaping is a systematic process of progressive acquisition of a new behavior through performance of successive acts that collectively represent a more advanced skill. In this process, the occupational therapist (1) defines behavior as a series of incremental steps or parts, (2) prompts and cues the child to demonstrate the steps, and (3) rewards each successive approximation of the skill. Shaping is appropriate for multicomponent skills that have a developmental progression in which the skills can be divided into steps and a progression in performance can be elicited. It is implemented within the child's play activities and within natural interaction. The small steps can be modeled, cued, or prompted. The child's responses and actions are immediately reinforced. During this repetition, a higher level skill is prompted and when performed it is reinforced.

For example, 5-year-old Anne has left hemiparesis with limited reach and grasp in her left arm. The occupational therapist initiated building a castle with large Lego pieces. She initially positioned the castle so that Anne used her left hand to place blocks on the left side and at midline. The occupational therapist praised her successful placement of blocks, encouraging her to build a taller and bigger castle. Seeing repeated successes in block placement, the occupational therapist moved the castle to a position that required Anne to reach with her left hand across midline. As the castle grew bigger, Anne had to reach overhead with her left hand, at which time the occupational therapist provided physical support at her left shoulder with continued positive verbal reinforcement. Because overhead movement was an emerging skill, Anne and the occupational therapist practiced this movement repeatedly before moving on to another activity.

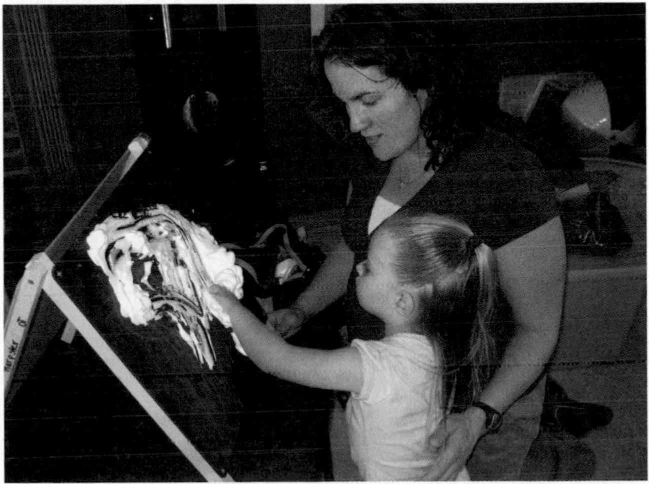

FIGURE 2-7 In this example, the child selected the activity (finger painting) and the medium (shaving cream). The occupational therapist reinforces the child's efforts to reach overhead with praise and touch.

TABLE 2-3 Comparison of Discrete Trial Training and Incidental Teaching in Early Childhood Programs

Discrete Trial Training	Incidental Teaching
Occupational therapist plans highly structured sessions with planned stimulus and reward.	Occupational therapist plans a loosely structured session with environment designed to elicit specific responses, but directives are not used.
Occupational therapist gives instructions to direct the child's actions.	Child initiates and paces the activity.
The training session is generally one-on-one in a clinic or the home.	The session generally takes place in the classroom, childcare center, or home, in the child's natural environment.
The same stimuli are used repeatedly.	A variety of stimuli selected from the natural environment is used.
Occupational therapist uses artificial reinforcers and often the same reinforcers.	A variety of reinforcers selected from the natural environment is used. The goal is that these reinforcers be available to the child without the presence of the occupational therapist.

Adapted from Cowan, R. J., & Allen, K. D. (2007). Using naturalistic procedures to enhance learning in individuals with autism: A focus on generalized teaching within the school setting. *Psychology in the Schools, 44*, 701–715.

In recent years, learning and behavioral theories used with young children have evolved into approaches that can be applied broadly across settings. Applied behavioral interventions are successful in developing skills; however, skills learned in an isolated setting, as in discrete trial training, do not always generalize into new or higher level behaviors across all settings. Educators have developed behavioral approaches that also use Skinner's framework of instrumental (operant) learning and can be implemented in the child's natural environment to teach children adaptive behaviors that generalize across environments.[87] Educators in early childhood programs have advocated for naturalistic teaching procedures that can be implemented in minimally structured sessions in various locations and contexts with a variety of stimuli. Although educators and occupational therapists who used naturalistic teaching procedures hold the same developmental goals for children as professionals who use classical behavioral theory, their procedures tend to be more flexibly structured, incorporate peers, and use naturalistic conditions and reinforcers.[35] Two types of these naturalistic learning procedures, incidental teaching and pivotal response training, are frequently used by occupational therapists with young children in early childhood programs and are described subsequently. A third evolution of behavioral theories, positive behavioral supports, uses functional behavioral assessment to identify antecedents to behavior that can be removed from or modified with the environment. Positive behavior supports are implemented school-wide by teams of teachers, aides, and occupational therapists to promote positive student behavior and prevent harmful, inappropriate behavior. This preventive model is described in Chapter 23.

In *incidental teaching*, a play environment is created to stimulate the young child's interest and curiosity. It is important that toys used be developmentally appropriate and include both novel and familiar toys. The goal is for the child to select an activity and spontaneously begin to play. The occupational therapist builds on the child's play selection by expanding the play scenario so that it becomes more challenging or creates a problem for the child to solve. The occupational therapist may cue the child to perform a different action and reward the child for attempting more challenging actions. These teaching sessions take a different approach than behavioral interventions, which use discrete trial training in which the child is given specific directives and rewarded for a specific response. Table 2-3 compares incidental teaching and discrete trial training.

Pivotal response training is also a naturalistic teaching and learning approach used with young children.[86] The goal of pivotal response training is to teach children a set of pivotal behaviors believed to be central to learning. The desired outcomes of pivotal response training include increasing (1) the child's motivation to learn, (2) attention to learning tasks, (3) persistence in tasks, (4) initiation of interactions, and (5) positive affect.[107] Procedures that are used in pivotal behavioral training are similar to procedures used in incidental teaching with emphasis on methods to promote generalization of learning. When applying pivotal response training, the occupational therapist gives the child a choice in play materials, uses natural reinforcers, intersperses mastered tasks with learned tasks, and reinforces attempts at new learning (Figure 2-8).[35]

Social Cognitive Theories

In general, social cognitive theory explains learning that occurs in a social context. The initial acquisition of highly complex and abstract behaviors was difficult for learning theorists to explain until the advent of the social cognitive theory proposed by Bandura et al.[6] Children learn by observing the behavior of others.[75] This learning may not be immediately observed in behavior but becomes part of the child's general understanding of the world. In contrast with the behavioralists, who believe that all learning produces behavioral change, social cognitive theorists believe that learning can occur without observable behavioral changes. A child can learn by observing the behavior of others, such as subtle nonverbal gestures that are used in conversation. These are observed and stored in memory and may not be demonstrated by the child until a much later time, when the child may exhibit similar gestures but with his or her own unique style.

In social cognitive theory, people determine their own learning by seeking certain experiences and focusing on their own goals. Children do not simply learn random elements from the environment; they direct their own learning and are goal-oriented in what they learn. Social cognitive theorists also believe that children learn indirectly by observing how their peers' behaviors are rewarded or punished. Direct reinforcement is not always needed when learning new behaviors.[127]

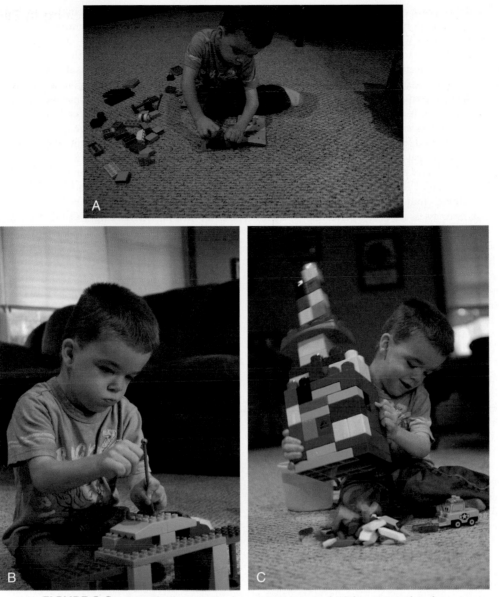

FIGURE 2-8 **A-C,** Challenging tasks are interspersed with mastered tasks.

These principles do not always apply in the case of children with ASD, for whom learning often needs to be more explicit, structured, and directed.

With some exceptions, children frequently learn by observing the consequences of behaviors of individuals around them. Learning that occurs when observing the behaviors of others also depends on the child's goals, interests, and relationship to the observed individual. Children's learning increases when they are given an incentive to learn a new behavior (e.g., an anticipated valued outcome or reward). Learning is also promoted when the child establishes his or her own goals, is given opportunities to work on those goals, and evaluates whether the goal was accomplished. When children set their own goals, they direct their behavior in a specific way; they are more likely to persist in the behavior to achieve the goal; and they are often more satisfied with the outcome. Practice models that use social cognitive and cognitive theories are described in the next section.

Cognitive Approaches

Cognitive approaches are "top-down" or occupation-based approaches because the emphasis in occupational therapy is on assisting the child to identify, develop, and use cognitive strategies to perform daily occupations effectively. These models build on Bandura's research[6] supporting the importance of self-efficacy and establishing goals to motivate individual achievement.

In cognitive approaches, the occupational therapist designs interventions to increase a child's repertoire of cognitive strategies and improve the child's ability to select, monitor, and evaluate his or her use of these strategies during the performance of a task. The inherent assumption is that improved performance results from the dynamic interaction of the child's skills with the parameters of the task in the context in which it needs to be performed. The child discovers, applies, and evaluates cognitive strategies during task performance in his or her typical environments.[119]

In a cognitive model of practice, the occupational therapist identifies and uses a global problem-solving strategy, which provides a consistent framework within which the child discovers specific strategies applicable to tasks that he or she either needs or wants to perform. This global strategy is based on the five-stage problem-solving structure first outlined by Luria.[101] Using occupational therapy terminology, these steps include (1) task analysis, (2) anticipation of the child's difficulties, (3) exploration and selection of task-specific strategies, (4) application of a strategy to the task, and (5) evaluation of the strategy's effectiveness.[118] The occupational therapist guides the child to develop his or her own cognitive strategies based on the problems encountered during tasks. The task-specific strategies a child discovers are unique to him or her.

Using cognitive skills to assess his or her performance, identifying successful and unsuccessful actions, the child learns to become more efficient in functional activities. The occupational therapist supports the child's goals and self-evaluation. The occupational therapist can also cue, prompt, or model the task, aligning these supports to the child's goals. The atmosphere in the therapy session is one of acceptance and support for taking risks. Although the child guides the selection of activities, the occupational therapist is always aware of the generalization and task-specific strategies that the child needs to learn and creates opportunities for the child to discover these.[119,138]

Because the selection of tasks is critical to the approach, a client-centered tool must be used that allows the child to identify goals for intervention. An appropriate goal-setting instrument for use with children older than 9 years of age is the Canadian Occupational Performance Measure[95]; for children 5 to 9 years old, the Perceived Efficacy and Goal Setting system can be used.[120] The cognitive approach is probably not a suitable model of practice for children younger than 5 years old because of its emphasis on the development of metacognitive skill and knowledge.

One of the key features of a cognitive model of practice is the way in which the occupational therapist helps the child explore strategies, make decisions, apply strategies, and evaluate their use. The occupational therapist does not give instructions. Rather, occupational therapists use questions to help children (1) discover the relevant aspects of the task, (2) examine how they are currently performing the task, (3) identify where they are getting "stuck," (4) creatively think about alternative solutions, and (5) try out these solutions and evaluate them in a supportive environment. When a strategy is found to be helpful, the occupational therapist uses questions to help the child "bridge" or generalize the strategy, eliciting from the child other times and situations in which that strategy may apply.[138]

In recent years, a particular cognitive approach, the Cognitive Orientation to daily Occupational Performance (CO-OP),[137] has been developed and researched systematically (see Chapter 10). The CO-OP approach is most appropriate for children who demonstrate cognitive strengths and a range of performance problems. The components include (1) working with the child to establish the goals, (2) analyzing performance, (3) identifying cognitive strategies to use, (4) guiding the child to discover solutions to the performance problem, (5) enabling the child to improve performance relative to the goal, and (6) promoting generalization and transfer. The child is asked to apply a global executive strategy, "Goal, Plan, Do, Check,"[112] to guide his or her problem solving. CO-OP has been successfully applied to children with developmental coordination disorders,[15,180] attention-deficit/hyperactivity disorder, traumatic brain injury,[117] and high functioning autism.[128]

Evidence is accumulating that CO-OP is effective at enabling skill acquisition and that it results in generalization and transfer of learned skills.[138] A randomized clinical trial comparing CO-OP with an equivalent number of sessions of direct skill training found that although children in both groups improved and achieved motor goals, the gains in the CO-OP group were greater; long-term maintenance both of the motor goals and of the cognitive strategies was significantly stronger in the CO-OP group, which led parents to report greater satisfaction with this treatment approach.[115]

Various cognitive strategies have been identified that seem to be helpful when using CO-OP to remediate occupational performance difficulties. Videotape analysis has been used to identify systematically and describe some of these strategies.[109] Verbalization and repetition of the strategy, "Goal, Plan, Do, Check"[112] to guide problem solving appears to be important to maintaining goal-directed action. In addition, specific strategies seem to be useful for improving performance, including verbal self-guidance (child talks himself or herself through the motor sequence), feeling the movement (drawing attention to an aspect of the sensation of movement as it is performed), motor mnemonic (labeling a body position or motor sequence), body position (verbalizing or directing attention to the body position or body parts relative to the task), and task specification (discussing specific parts of the task or actions to change the task).[109] Chapter 10 summarizes the research on the CO-OP approach with various diagnoses.

In summary, occupational therapists who use a cognitive model of practice (1) focus on the occupations a child wishes to perform rather than on foundational skill building; (2) use a general problem-solving framework that guides the child to discover, select, apply, and evaluate the use of specific cognitive strategies; (3) use process questions to increase the child's awareness of the use of strategies during the performance of daily tasks; and (4) plan for transfer and generalization of the strategies that the child has learned.[118,138]

Social Participation

Occupational therapists use various psychosocial approaches when working with children and adolescents experiencing problems in occupational performance because of social, emotional, or behavioral issues or difficulties with relationships. Several of these approaches, such as a cognitive approach or the compensatory and environmental approach, were described in the previous section. These approaches are grounded in theories that focus on the development of self, on family and peer relationships, and on the aspects of the social and cultural environment that influence each of these. Although the number of occupational therapists who work with children with chronic mental health issues is relatively small, all occupational therapists who work in pediatrics use the concepts of psychological and social development implicitly and explicitly because developing the ability to maintain relationships with peers and significant others is an essential part of the occupational performance of childhood and adolescence.

Several chapters (e.g., Chapters 11, 12, and 23) describe the models of practice that focus on social behavior and the development of self. Personal attributes, such as temperament, self-esteem and self-efficacy, problem-solving ability, and social skills, are considered important determinants of healthy functioning. Environmental influences on behavior and social development suggest the need to consider the expectations and social elements of the home, school, and community environments and to recognize the importance of friends in a young person's life.

Given the complex nature of behavior and social relationships, occupational therapists often draw on numerous intervention approaches to promote a child's social skills and peer relationships. The occupational therapist's knowledge of normal behavior, vulnerabilities associated with particular disabilities, attachment, coping skills, and compatibility of temperaments may guide intervention with a parent-child dyad (see Chapter 3). Cognitive-behavioral strategies may be used by occupational therapists to help young people who are depressed or socially withdrawn develop strategies that encourage participation in social situations (see Chapters 11 and 12).

Coping Model

The coping model addresses psychosocial function, uses cognitive-behavioral strategies, and is congruent with the PEO model.[189,194] Occupational therapists who use this model emphasize the use of coping resources that enable the child to meet challenges posed by the environment. The goal is to improve the child's ability to cope with stress in personal, social, and other occupational performance areas. When children are successful in coping with their own personal needs and the demands of the environment, they feel good about themselves and their place in the world. Coping strategies are learned, and children build on previous successful experiences in coping with environmental expectations.[194]

All children experience stress when faced with physical, cognitive, and emotional challenges. When these challenges are successfully met by the child's inner resources and caregiving supports, the result is a sense of motivation, learning, and mastery. Stress can evoke negative feelings when the child's resources are poorly matched to the environment's demands.

Developmental skills and competence are the internal resources a child brings to a task. Often a child with disabilities is placed in situations that match the child's chronologic age (e.g., a preschooler play group) but not necessarily the developmental age. When environmental demands do not match developmental skills (e.g., to sit quietly and attend), children experience stress and generally seek external coping supports.

Parents and other primary caregivers are the most significant external resources for coping in the child's early years.[189] Parents buffer the child's exposure to stress, make demands, model coping behaviors, encourage and assist the child in coping efforts, and give contingent feedback. Environmental supports are the spaces and materials available to the child and may include adapted equipment and technology associated with comfort and functional support.

The child successfully copes with new challenges when (1) he or she has underlying resources that enable a successful response to an environmental demand or new situation; (2) human supports are provided to facilitate his or her performance (e.g., the occupational therapist gives the child a visual or verbal cue); and (3) environmental supports are provided that enable the child to feel safe and comfortable, be attentive and engaged, and feel calm and organized (e.g., a classroom that is quiet and well organized and that has a comfortable lighting level and temperature). The occupational therapist continually evaluates whether the child's skills (internal resources) and environmental supports (external resources) are adequate to meet the demands of the activity. When the child exhibits ineffective coping strategies, the occupational therapist adjusts the task demands and provides more human or environmental support to enable the child to succeed in his or her coping efforts. Table 2-4 provides examples of interventions using the coping model (Figure 2-9).[189]

Social Play Interactions

When working with young children, occupational therapists often foster social skill development in play interactions. Occupational therapists establish developmentally appropriate play activities that promote sharing, fun, and creativity. To support the play of children with disabilities, peer models with higher level skills and similar interests are selected to participate. The occupational therapist offers support to the play activity without being directive. Social play interventions reflect theories about play occupations, child development, and behavioral interventions. One practice model, the Early Start Denver Model (ESDM),[40] which targets toddlers and preschoolers with ASD, is based on principles from Pivotal Response Training[85] and developmental, relationship-based intervention.[67] ESDM practices and principles are defined in Table 2-5. ESDM is implemented in the toddler's natural environment (preschool setting or home), and occupational therapists can use the principles in play activities, group eating activities (snack time), or throughout the child's daily routines. ESDM is child-centered, meaning that the occupational therapist selects a play activity known to be of interest to the child, shares control of the play by selecting objects that are appropriate choices for the child, models and reinforces specific child actions, and sequences activities to increase the challenge. Every social interaction is considered to be a teaching opportunity in which the occupational therapist is modeling, cueing, reinforcing, and supporting generalization. Whether ESDM is implemented in an early childhood program or at home, the parents are important participants. Parents are taught the same interaction techniques (see Table 2-5) to promote the child's social development and to manage difficult or undesired behaviors.

Early studies of ESDM provided in the classroom resulted in improved symbolic play and social communication.[146] With success in improving social competence using therapist-child interactions, Vismara and Rogers[177] developed a parent-coaching model for ESDM, demonstrating that parents can be trained to implement ESDM with fidelity. After this pilot study, a randomized controlled trial of home-based ESDM resulted in positive effects for children with ASD 18 to 30 months old.[146] The intervention comprised sessions in the home led by the occupational therapist twice a day (average 15 hours/week), and parents were asked to use ESDM strategies throughout the day. These strategies included consistent use of positive affect during interpersonal exchanges with the child, responsivity and sensitivity to child cues, and developmentally appropriate communication. Imitating the child's actions is a strategy that encourages interaction. After 2 years of home-based intervention, children who received ESDM improved more than

TABLE 2-4 Principles of the Coping Model and Examples of Interventions

Coping Model Principles	Intervention Examples
Occupational therapist grades or modifies the environmental demands to ensure that they are congruent with the child's adaptive capabilities.	The environment of a child with attention-deficit/hyperactivity disorder is adapted by reorganizing materials to reduce visual demands and enhance visual attention. For a child with ASD, a picture board is organized that indicates the sequence of activities in the preschool day to promote easy transitions between activities.
Occupational therapist designs intervention activities to enhance the child's internal and external coping resources. Intervention focuses on the child's resources, including coping style, physical and affective states, developmental skills, human supports, and material and environmental supports. The occupational therapist fosters a positive sense of self and can involve the child in activities that promote self-efficacy.	For older children, the occupational therapist can facilitate group discussions of personal goals and plans for reaching these goals. Personal social skills may be emphasized by practice of social skills in the context of games with peers. Activities that emphasize group skills, such as problem solving, sharing, and communication, can help older children develop improved personal social skills that can be generalized to school and extracurricular activities.
Occupational therapist provides appropriate, contingent responses to the child's coping efforts. Timely, positive, and explicit feedback to coping efforts helps the child experience a sense of mastery. Feedback that effectively enhances coping efforts emphasizes self-directed, purposeful behaviors. The occupational therapist supports child-initiated activity and provides feedback that encourages the extension and elaboration of emerging skills.	When the child with ASD initiates a social interaction with peers, the occupational therapist cues and encourages the peers' responsiveness and promotes the interactions by showing interest and promoting the "fun" of the play activity. When a child with dyspraxia initiates a puzzle but cannot fit the pieces, the occupational therapist gestures to indicate the correct placement or suggests a game of turn-taking so that the therapist can model correct puzzle piece placement for the child.

ASD, Autism spectrum disorder.
Adapted from Williamson, G., & Szczepanski, M. (1999). Coping frame of reference. In P. Kramer & J. Hinojosa (Eds.). *Frames of reference in pediatric occupational therapy* (pp. 431–465). Baltimore, MD: Williams & Wilkins.

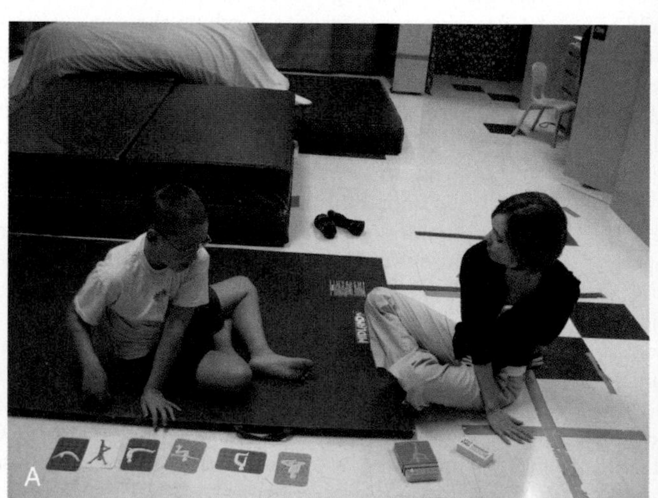

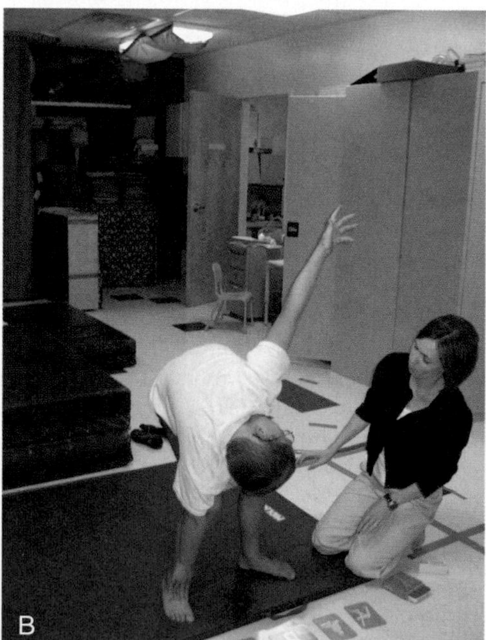

FIGURE 2-9 **A** and **B,** Therapist guides child through a yoga routine. She encourages the child to perform the yoga routine learned in therapy daily to reduce stress and improve his physical agility and coordination.

TABLE 2-5 Principles of the Denver Model

Principle	Description
1. Occupational therapist helps the child modulate arousal, affect, and attention.	Often using sensory input, occupational therapist may provide input to calm or regulate the child, increase arousal, engage the child's attention, or eliminate distraction. Occupational therapist attempts to modulate arousal through deep pressure, vestibular, or tactile input so that the child is in an alert, attentive state.
2. Occupational therapist uses positive affect.	Occupational therapist models fun, laughs, smiles, and makes full eye contact when possible.
3. Occupational therapist models and encourages turn-taking and dyadic engagement.	Occupational therapist selects activities that allow turn-taking and sharing. Occupational therapist models turn-taking, demonstrates reciprocity. The child's turn-taking and reciprocity are reinforced.
4. Occupational therapist responds sensitively and immediately to the child's communication and gestures.	Occupational therapist reads and acknowledges the child's cues, including gestures or utterances. Occupational therapist may respond empathetically, may imitate child's behavior; occupational therapist clearly acknowledges any attempt that the child makes to communicate.
5. Occupational therapist creates multiple and varied communication opportunities.	Occupational therapist models communication with gestures, expressions, and speech. Occupational therapist uses developmentally appropriate language.
6. Occupational therapist scaffolds the child's skill practice and elaboration of new skills.	Occupational therapist encourages child to perform new skills in various activities. Occupational therapist encourages practice of new skills using different materials and in a variety of settings.
7. Occupational therapist uses developmentally appropriate language and communication.	Occupational therapist gestures, uses 1- to 2-word sequences. Occupational therapist carefully selects simple language and combines language with gesture. Occupational therapist emphasizes pragmatics, i.e., facial and body expressions that accompany language.
8. Occupational therapist supports the child's transitions.	Occupational therapist helps the child shift attention from one activity to another. Occupational therapist uses visual schedules, visual cards, or social stories to help child with the transition.

Adapted from Rogers, R. J., & Dawson, G. (2010). *Early Start Denver Model for Young Children with Autism.* New York: Guilford Press.

children who received community intervention in cognitive ability, language, and adaptive behaviors.[148]

In a later study, using a sample of young children, aged 12 to 24 months, Rogers et al.[149] examined the efficacy of a brief period of ESDM (12 weeks) provided at a lower dosage (1 hour/week) of parent training. Occupational therapists coached parents in using ESDM techniques, and parents were responsible for providing the ESDM intervention. A comparison group received community-based interventions. Child outcomes for the group receiving ESDM provided by the parents were not significantly different from outcomes for children who received community-based interventions; however, the parents developed strong alliances with the primary occupational therapist. Developmental gains during the 12 weeks related to the number of intervention hours received and the child's age (younger children improved more). Coaching models that ask parents to implement the intervention may have varied effects that are influenced by family culture, time, work schedules, values, priorities, and resources.

Another child-centered, play-based intervention model that occupational therapists use, reciprocal imitation training (RIT),[77] appears to benefit social skill development in young children with ASD. This intervention, led by the occupational therapist and implemented by the parent, emphasizes parent-child joint attention and imitation in naturalistic play. The occupational therapist contingently imitates the child's actions and describes them for the child to reinforce their meaning or models variations of the child's actions.[78] To teach social imitation, the occupational therapist prompts the child to imitate his or her actions. In a randomized controlled trial, young children (27 to 47 months old) with ASD who received RIT improved more in spontaneous, social use of imitation and in elicited imitation skills than a control group.[78] In RIT, the occupational therapist selects play activities that are developmentally appropriate, fun, and interesting and that embed natural social opportunities. Within these well-designed play activities, the occupational therapist can use opportunities to enhance the child's social skills by imitating his or her actions; responding to, reinforcing, and expanding the child's communicative cues and gestures; and scaffolding interactions between peers. These interventions have evidence of efficacy for promoting social competence, joint attention, and communication skills in young children with ASD.[77,78]

Peer-Mediated Approaches

Learning to interact positively with peers is an important social skill that is typically acquired during early childhood. Peer relationships are also inherently of value in promoting healthy social-emotional development. Interventions to promote peer interaction are commonly implemented in early childhood programs and are often used with children who have ASD. Peer-mediated interventions involve a typically developing peer interacting with a targeted child and combine behavioral and social-behavioral theories. The peer is trained to serve as a model and to encourage interaction and reinforce the targeted child's actions. The occupational therapist encourages these peer-to-peer interactions in routine activities and play interactions that occur naturally during the preschool day. A practitioner trains the peer by introducing the peer to the targeted child, explaining what is expected of him or her, practicing with the peer, and prompting the peer to interact with the child.[66] For example, an occupational therapist may prompt the peer to invite the targeted child to play, offer to share, or offer help. The occupational therapist carefully selects a peer to interact with the targeted child and trains the peer to engage with that particular child, giving the peer information about the targeted child's interests and how best to initiate and sustain an interaction.

Karasi et al.[79] taught peers to how to engage children with ASD, 6 to 11 years old, on the playground by asking them to play. The peers were taught strategies to support social interaction with children who appeared to be having difficulty making friends (the targeted children were not specifically identified to the peers). The children who received the peer supports decreased their solitary play and demonstrated increased engagement in games and conversation. Although teachers reported the children in the peer-mediated intervention showed increased social participation, the children did not report more friendships, suggesting that additional supports are needed to create and sustain friend relationships. Peer-mediated interventions have also resulted in children with ASD interacting in closer proximity and sustaining play for longer periods.[30] Based on a synthesis of research on peer-mediated interventions, Goldstein et al.[66] recommended that a consistent peer be used, that the strategies taught to the peer be simple to learn, and that the occupational therapist encourage peer interactions throughout the day. A combination of strategies may be needed to produce optimal results, including combining peer-mediated strategies with social stories, visual cueing, or specific verbal scripts.

Social Skills Training

As described in the previous section, young children can learn social skills through well-designed play interactions with adults and peers. When older children continue to have delayed social skills, they may benefit from structured social groups designed to promote positive peer interactions and appropriate social behaviors. Social skills groups are based on learning and acquisition theories, self-efficacy theories, and occupation models. Social skills groups allow young people to master social communication in a safe and supportive environment. Goals for social skills groups vary according to the types of children involved and the context for the group. Occupational therapists may include strategies to promote emotional regulation; modeling and reinforcing specific social behaviors (e.g., greetings, introducing oneself, asking for a favor); or discussing dating, friendships, and online relationships. Occupational therapists create occupation-based groups, in which members share a goal and activities that focus on a theme. Activities that provide an appropriate context for the development of social-emotional skills encourage positive peer interaction; allow for modeling, sharing, and reciprocal interaction; are creative rather than competitive; and enable give and take that can lead to relationship building. The occupational therapist models for group members, encourages interactions, maintains a safe atmosphere, monitors behaviors to prevent inappropriate or escalating behaviors, and collects data on members' social behaviors. See Table 2-6 for examples of venues for social groups.

Social skills training groups have shown positive effects with school-age children and adolescents with autism. Gutman, Raphael-Greenfield, and Rao[68] implemented a weekly small-group intervention with children with high functioning autism. This intervention emphasized motor imitation as a key element of social behaviors and focused on the children role playing specific social skills, practicing the skills with peers, and learning both the verbal and the nonverbal aspects of social interaction. The children were paired with a social partner with similar but higher level social skills to practice targeted social behaviors in the school setting and later in the community. Using a multiple baseline design, all of the participants improved in their targeted social behaviors, making the greatest gains in the first 7 weeks. The Program for the Education and Enrichment of Relational Skills (PEERS) social group intervention was developed to promote social skills in adolescents with ASD.[90] In the highly structured PEERS intervention, occupational therapists teach specific social skills; group members practice and receive feedback about their performance; and repetition is reinforced through homework. Social cognitive techniques are used through discussion of the role playing and by members identifying their own social etiquette rules. The PEERS intervention includes the parents, who meet separately to discuss the content that their adolescent is learning. Using standardized scales of social responsiveness and social behaviors, the PEERS intervention resulted in improvement in social awareness, social cognition, communication, and social motivation. Friendship skills improved after the 14-week session and at follow-up.[91] Social skills groups with adolescents can also promote improvement in initiating, maintaining, and closing conversations.[17] Groups that meet regularly and allow relationships to develop can improve self-esteem and confidence.[17] Social networks have been shown to help a person establish positive attitudes, improve self-esteem, and develop moral and social values.

Other occupational therapy studies have identified the interactive, protective factors in child, family, and social environment that support social participation of children with brain injuries. Bedell, Cohn, and Dumas[10] described a "Building Friendship Approach" in which collaborative student-centered school teams (student, school personnel, family, and friends) identify strategies to improve the social opportunities of students with brain injury. The team helps the student generate his or her own solutions and set goals to improve his or her social opportunities. This approach appears to be effective, but the outcomes need to be monitored to ensure that they are maintained. When occupational therapists embed well-designed, interactive, and meaningful activities that facilitate reciprocity and creativity, social skills groups can enhance social participation and social emotional competence in children and youth.

Sensorimotor Performance

From infancy through childhood, sensorimotor systems develop rapidly, resulting in competent and coordinated sensorimotor performance. Children move constantly in direct response to the environment or on their own initiative, and by exploring, manipulating, and moving through the environment, a child quickly attains competent motor skills. When children, such as children with cerebral palsy or developmental coordination disorder, demonstrate motor delays or impairment, occupational therapists have key roles in supporting the development

TABLE 2-6 Occupational Therapy Social Skills Groups to Improve Social Participation and Peer Relationships

Therapeutic Activity	Description	Targeted Group
Yoga dyads	Occupational therapist provides yoga sessions for small groups. Children hold hands and cooperate with a partner to perform yoga poses and actions. They experience touch, movement, and mindfulness in a group setting. Emphasis on movement, balance, breathing, meditation.	School-age children with behavioral problems; children at risk who experience increased stress (e.g., disadvantaged homes).
Arts and crafts groups	Occupational therapist develops arts and crafts groups, often related to holidays, seasons, or school themes. These groups work together cooperatively, sharing materials and conversation. Usually they work together to create one product.	School-age children with low social skills; can include children with Asperger's syndrome, children with behavioral problems, children at risk.
After-school groups	Occupational therapist organizes after-school groups. These meet to plan projects and events. Social participation is modeled and encouraged. The groups are organized to promote turn-taking, sharing of ideas, and joint activities. These groups generally have themes that can be determined by the group (e.g., sharing information on favorite music bands).	Middle school or high school youth with delayed social skills; can include youth Asperger's syndrome, high functioning autism, intellectual impairment.
Cooking groups	Occupational therapist embeds cooking groups into weekly therapy sessions. These groups often plan a meal, budget the meal, shop for the food items, prepare the meal together, and then eat together.	Middle school or high school youth with delayed social skills; can include youth with high functioning autism or intellectual impairment.
Special interest clubs	Occupational therapist leads the development of a club in middle school or high school that supports the special interests of a targeted cohort of youth. Examples of special interests are video or music, extreme Legos, weird animals and reptiles, cartoons, and comedy.	Youth or young adults with autism or intellectual impairment who have low social participation and no or few friends.

of sensorimotor skills. Chapters 7, 8, and 9 describe motor development, diagnoses that involve the sensorimotor systems, and interventions that are helpful in remediating sensorimotor problems. This section describes five primary theories and practice models that guide evaluation and intervention to promote sensorimotor performance: (1) dynamic systems theory, (2) motor learning, (3) biomechanical models, (4) neurodevelopmental therapy (NDT), and (5) sensory integration therapy (SIT).

Dynamic Systems Theory

Dynamic systems theory[166] contrasts with a hierarchical model of neural organization, originally thought to explain how movement developed.[62] This theory proposes that the CNS functions with flexible and dynamic organization and that the control of movement is distributed among many elements of the CNS rather than vested in a single hierarchical level.[174] It follows that the CNS controls groups of muscles (not individual muscles) and that these groups can potentially change motor behavior without CNS control. Motor control can emerge spontaneously from relationships among kinematics (muscles) and biomechanics (joints and bones) that naturally limit the degrees of freedom of movement, implying that the motor system is self-organizing.

Dynamic systems theorists emphasize that learning not only occurs in the brain but also reflects body and environment variables that constantly change and simultaneously influence each other.[173] In this theoretical approach, instead of viewing behavior (e.g., sensorimotor skills) as predetermined in the CNS, systems theory views motor behavior as emerging from the dynamic cooperation of the many subsystems in a task-specific context. It implies that all factors contributing to motor behavior are important and exert an influence on the outcome by either facilitating performance or constraining it. It also implies that a child's actions organize and reorganize over time into a series of dynamically stable behavioral patterns (i.e., occupations). Although a child acquires a specific skill, performance of the skill varies based on the social and physical variables in the environment. The child performs the skill flexibly based on his or her goal and fluctuating internal variables (e.g., fatigue, arousal, motivation) and external variables (e.g., parental encouragement, perceived desired goal, comfort and safety of the environment).[60]

Dynamic systems theory is an ecologic approach that assumes that a child's functional performance depends on the interactions of the child's inherent and emerging skills, the characteristics of the desired task or activity, and the environment in which the activity is performed. System variables that facilitate learning and drive a child's transition from one level to another change over time.[20,166] Physical growth and biomechanics may be highly important for motor learning in infancy, whereas experience, practice, and motivation may be more influential in the learning of motor activities in an older child.[165] Self-organization is optimal in a functional task that has a meaningful goal and outcome. Most functional tasks (e.g., eating and drinking) elicit a predictable pattern of movement; the task itself can organize the movements attempted. These features suggest that dynamic systems theory aligns well with occupational therapy.

Research in dynamic systems theory has focused on explaining the ways new skills are learned.[56,167,168] The learning of new movements or ways of completing an activity requires that previously stable movements be broken down or become unstable. New movements and skills emerge when a critical change occurs in any of the components that contribute to motor behavior. These periods of change are called *transitions*. Motor change in young children is envisioned as a series of events during which destabilization and stabilization of movement take place before the transitional phase movement becomes stable and functional.[136]

The period of instability that occurs in a transitional phase is seen as the optimal time to effect changes in movement behavior. The sequential transitional stages are as follows[136]:

1. Variability in motor performance increases. The child experiments with different movement patterns.
2. Through these exploratory movements, the child determines which pattern is the most adaptive.
3. The child selects the movement that is most adaptive, the movement that meets his or her goals given environmental demands and constraints (e.g., which pattern makes it easiest to rise from sit to stand given the effects of gravity and available supports). During this phase, the child repeatedly practices the new movement pattern.

In children with impairments such as cerebral palsy, constraints hinder the emergence of motor functions. Such *constraints* are limitations imposed on motor behaviors by the child's physical, social, cognitive, and neurologic characteristics. The constraint that traditionally has received most attention is the integrity of the CNS; less frequently, other biomechanical constraints are considered, such as biomechanical forces, muscle strength, or a disproportionate trunk-to-limb ratio. *Environmental constraints* include physical, social, and cultural factors not related to a specific task. One example of a physical constraint is a suboptimal surface for the child's activity (e.g., a soft, unstable couch or inclined surface); a social constraint could be a parent's lack of reinforcement of the acquisition of motor behaviors. *Task constraints* are restrictions on motor behavior imposed by the nature of the task. Established motor behaviors may be altered by specific task requirements. For example, when faced with the task of crawling on rough terrain, infants may alter motor behavior by straightening the knees and "bear walking." When a child reaches for a ball, the ball's size influences the shape of the child's hand and the approach taken (e.g., one hand versus two). The unique features of these tasks have shaped the child's motor behavior. See Table 2-7 for a list of dynamic systems theory principles.

TABLE 2-7 Principles of Dynamic Systems Theory Applied to Motor Development

Dynamic System Theory Principle	Application to Motor Development
Sensory perception and motor systems are coupled. These systems continually interact in learning new motor skills. The infant's perceptions guide his or her movements, which create the infant's perception of the world.	Haptic sense, discrimination of the physical properties of objects through touch, is acquired through object manipulation. Sensory information is gained as the infant's fingers move over the object's surfaces.
Functional synergies are the basis of motor behavior. Movement synergies are based on kinematic (e.g., muscles) and biomechanical (e.g., joints) constraints and are the basic units that control movement. The basic units of motor behavior are functional synergies or coordinated structures rather than specific muscle actions. These functional synergies are "soft"—assembled (i.e., they are highly adaptable and highly reliable).	Similar synergies are used for eating and drinking that involve shoulder internal rotation and adduction, elbow extension followed by flexion, forearm pronation followed by slight supination, and neutral wrist position. This functional synergy is also used with slight modification in combing one's hair and cleansing face and teeth. This is a stable but flexible synergy.
Transition to new movement patterns involves exploration, selection, and practice phases. The infant or child first explores many different patterns and exhibits high variability in movement. The infant then selects an optimal pattern to achieve his or her goal. This pattern is practiced and becomes more adaptable to various environmental demands.	When first learning to eat with a spoon, the infant exhibits various patterns with the spoon, including banging, stabbing, and waving. The infant then selects a functional pattern that successfully meets the environmental demand (e.g., the toddler learns to supinate the forearm when bringing the spoon to mouth so that the food reaches the mouth rather than spilling down the chest). This adaptive pattern is repeatedly practiced as the toddler insists on always self-feeding.
The infant's unique motor patterns are the result of input from multiple systems that interact in dynamic ways both to facilitate and to constrain movement. Behavior is multiply determined, and children develop in context. Behavior is determined by an integrated system of perception, action, and cognition. These elements are integrated over time to form a child's unique developmental trajectory.	The pattern an infant uses to reach for an object is determined by many variables. Variables that may influence reaching include biomechanical and kinematic factors such as weight of his or her arm, stiffness of joints, strength, and eye-hand coordination. However, the reaching pattern is also influenced by how successful the child was in previous reach and grasp (did the object move before the child could obtain it?), how motivated the child is to attain the object, general energy level, and curiosity.

Adapted from Case-Smith, J. (1996). Analysis of current motor development theory and recently published infant motor assessments. *Infants and Young Children, 9*(1), 29–41; Spencer, J. P., Corbetta, D., Buchanan, P., Clearfield, M., Ulrich, B., & Schoner, G. (2006). Moving toward a grand theory of development: A memory of Esther Thelen. *Society for Research in Child Development, 77,* 1521–1538.

Dynamic systems theory has many similarities to the emerging occupational therapy theories that focus on person, environment, and occupation relationships. This theory is explained further in Chapter 7.

Occupational therapists approach intervention with a child by first gaining an understanding of the environmental, family, and child factors that influence the performance of specific activities. From the literature that discusses the application of systems theory or dynamic systems theory to occupational therapy intervention, the following principles emerge:

- Assessment and intervention strategies must recognize the inherent complexity of task performance. The most useful assessment strategy is to develop a "picture" or "profile" of the ways performance components and environmental and task factors affect performance of the tasks the child wants to accomplish. Assessment of only one or a few components (e.g., balance, mood, strength) is not likely to lead to the most effective identification of constraints.
- The focus of assessment and intervention is on the interaction of the person, the environment, and the occupation. Therapy begins and ends with a focus on the occupational performance tasks a child or youth wants to, needs to, or is expected to perform. When a child shows readiness and motivation to attempt a task or activity, the focus of intervention on that particular activity can effect changes in his or her performance.[95]
- The therapy process focuses on identification and change of child, task, or environmental constraints that prevent the achievement of the desired activity. Some of these factors may be manipulated to enhance the functional motor task or goal; others may be managed by providing the missing component during the execution of the task. Parts of activities can be changed (e.g., different toy sizes, different position for child or activity).
- Activities should be practiced in various environments that can facilitate completion of the task and promote the flexibility of movement patterns. Activities incorporated into the child's daily routine provide opportunities for finding solutions for functional motor challenges (Figure 2-10).
- When preparing therapeutic activities, the occupational therapist identifies playful activities that appear to motivate the child, are developmentally appropriate, match the child's and family's goals, provide a challenge to current skills levels, and match an expected or hoped for outcome.
- With intervention through the systems approach, the focus on changing environments and occupations is at least as great as the focus on changing the inherent skills of the child or adolescent. Intervention is best accomplished in natural, realistic environments.
- The accomplishment of complete occupations, not parts of them, is emphasized. The goal in therapy is to enable a child to accomplish an identified activity, rather than promote change in a developmental sequence or improve the quality of the movement.
- Therapeutic effect and positive outcomes are determined by the child's engagement in the activity, the match between the intervention activities and the child's skill levels, the meaningfulness of the activity, the amount of practice, and the opportunities to transfer and generalize the newly learned skill to a variety of contexts. Positive effects relate to how well the interventions enable the child to perform well across his or her natural environments given age and role expectations.

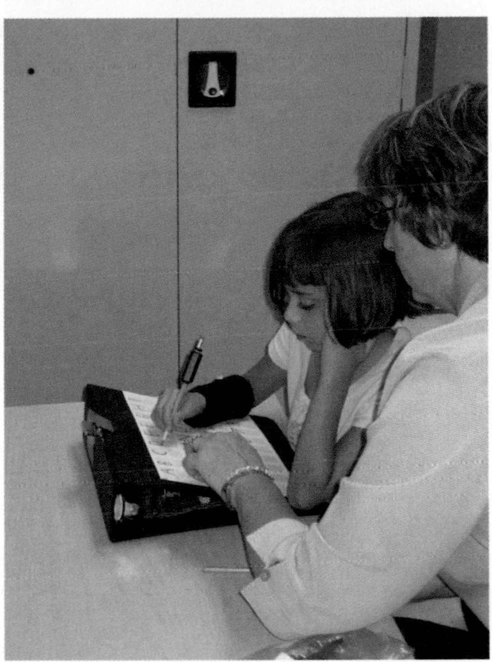

FIGURE 2-10 For written work at home and at school, the child uses a slant board to promote improved posture and grasp of the pencil. A weight on the pencil provides added proprioceptive input.

Research on interventions based on dynamic systems theory is beginning to emerge. In a study of 55 children receiving either functional therapy based on dynamic systems theory or therapy aimed at developing "typical" movement patterns, Ketelaar et al.[80] found that children in the functional therapy group demonstrated significantly more functional skills (mobility and self-care). Law et al.[97] and Darrah et al.[39] developed an intervention model, context therapy approach, for children with cerebral palsy using dynamic systems theory to guide the therapy principles. Context therapy is a functional, task-oriented, activity-focused, top-down approach to assessment and intervention. Occupational therapists explicitly manipulate characteristics of the task and the environment to achieve the goals (i.e., therapy activities are not directed toward changing the child's performance). Underlying this approach is the tenet of the dynamic system that motor behavior is organized around functional tasks and goals. The occupational therapist encourages the parents and child to develop their own solution to an environmental challenge. Primary roles of the occupational therapist and parents are to eliminate barriers to the child's function, enabling greater participation. Another tenet of dynamic systems theory is that new motor behaviors are learned by experimenting with different actions that can accomplish a new goal. The new skill or performance goal that a child is attempting or exploring becomes an appropriate intervention focus. Occupational therapists help the child accomplish the new goal by modifying environment barriers and adapting the task to make goal accomplishment possible.[39]

In a randomized controlled trial that compared context therapy with child-focused therapy, preschool children improved equally; effect sizes for self-care and gross motor function pre to post were large for both groups. This study demonstrated that children with cerebral palsy can improve in performance when intervention focuses on modifying tasks and the environment to promote function and goal achievement.[97] These findings validate the theoretical concept of dynamic systems theory as a basis for intervention principles and strategies.

Motor Learning and Skill Acquisition

Motor learning as a model of practice focuses on helping the child achieve goal-directed functional actions. It may initially appear to be a skill-building approach because the focus is on the acquisition of skills involved in movement and balance. However, motor learning is an occupation-based approach because it is directed toward the search for a motor solution that emerges from an interaction of the child with the task and the environment.

When a child is learning a new functional task, a general movement structure is brought into place that takes into consideration the relationship involving the child's movement capabilities, the environmental conditions, and the action goal. When the task is performed repeatedly, these correspondences become more refined, and the goal is achieved more successfully. Specific processes, such as muscle contraction patterns, stabilization and positioning of joints, and response to gravity and other forces, are only crudely organized at first. However, with continued practice, these become more organized and fine-tuned.[61] These patterns are called *movement synergies*, or *coordinative structures*, and they represent the child's preferred strategy for solving a task in the most energy-efficient way.[165]

Children with motor programming and motor control deficits often have difficulty establishing the timing and sequencing of functional synergies. Task and activity demands may vary, and each of these dimensions is relevant to the way in which tasks are learned. These characteristics of a task determine which motor learning strategies are used to improve performance.

1. *Simple-complex*. Simple tasks, such as reaching for an object, require a decision followed by a sequenced response. Complex tasks, such as handwriting, require the integration of information from a variety of sources and the application of underlying rules that guide performance.
2. *Open loop–closed loop*. In an open-loop task, a motor program is put into place before the action begins and is not modified during the performance of a task. An example of an open-loop task is throwing a ball. In a closed-loop task, the child continues to monitor and respond to feedback that he or she receives intrinsically from the body and extrinsically from the environment. An example of a closed-loop task is cutting out a shape using scissors.[1]
3. *Environment changing–environment stationary*. The difficulty of learning a task is tremendously influenced by the extent to which the task is predictable. When the environment is changeable or variable, the child has to learn the movement and learn to monitor the environment to adapt to change. Running on rough terrain and playing soccer are examples of tasks in which the environment is constantly changing. This concept is not to be confused with the open-loop and closed-loop features of the task previously described. Brushing the teeth and playing the piano are tasks during which the child must monitor sensory feedback (closed loop), but the environment remains stationary.[163]
4. *Task characteristics*. The ease or difficulty of learning a task depends on the match between the way the task is presented and the preferred learning style of the child. Some children learn best through auditory or visual methods; others prefer movement and touch.

Different types of feedback contribute to the motor learning process.[196] Feedback is ***intrinsic*** when it is produced by the child's sensory systems and is inherent in a task. An example of intrinsic feedback is information available to the child through vision, proprioception, sensation, or kinesthesia. The occupational therapist observing the child's performance provides two types of ***extrinsic*** feedback: ***knowledge of results*** and ***knowledge of performance***.[124] In ***knowledge of results***, the occupational therapist provides information to the child about the relationship between the actions and the goal. For example, a child who is throwing a basketball toward the hoop may be told that the ball is not going high enough and is missing the hoop. To provide extrinsic feedback that allows ***knowledge of performance***, the occupational therapist emphasizes the pattern of movement and its relationship to achievement of the task. In the same example, the child may be told that he is not extending his arms far enough before releasing the ball. In both cases, the occupational therapist's feedback focuses on the outcome of the action, not on the child's effort. These terms are explained further in Chapter 7.

Research on the scheduling, frequency, and amount of feedback that best promote learning can guide application of motor learning theories.[164,190] Studies have shown that immediate extrinsic feedback may prevent the learner from paying attention to the intrinsic sources of feedback that are always available, such as vision and proprioception. This lack of attention to intrinsic feedback may make the learner dependent on information from the person providing instruction.[155]

Few research studies have focused on the effect of different types of feedback on task performance in children experiencing occupational performance difficulties. However, research investigating motor learning principles in children with movement difficulties has suggested that they may not solve movement problems in the same way that adults do. Sullivan et al.[164,196] found that children perform best when they receive constant and immediate feedback compared with reduced and intermittent feedback, which is shown to improve performance in adults. Extrinsic sources of feedback that focus a child's attention on specific aspects of the task and on important sensory cues may be important.

Another important concept in motor learning is the influence of different types of practice on learning and performance.[158] Although we know that task practice results in learning, research findings differ in regard to whether practice of the ***whole task*** or practice of ***task components*** results in optimal learning. The benefits of practicing either the whole task or parts of the task may depend on the inherent goals of the task. If coordination or timing of the parts is important to the task, whole-task practice is more effective for learning.[104] Examples of these continuous types of tasks are walking, swinging at a ball, and bicycling. If a task contains distinct parts that can be performed in a serial manner, these can be practiced as parts of the task. A child learning to don his jacket can be taught how to zip it as a first step. Most occupations involving movement are a combination of continuous and discrete tasks (Figure 2-11). Consequently, doing the whole task must follow

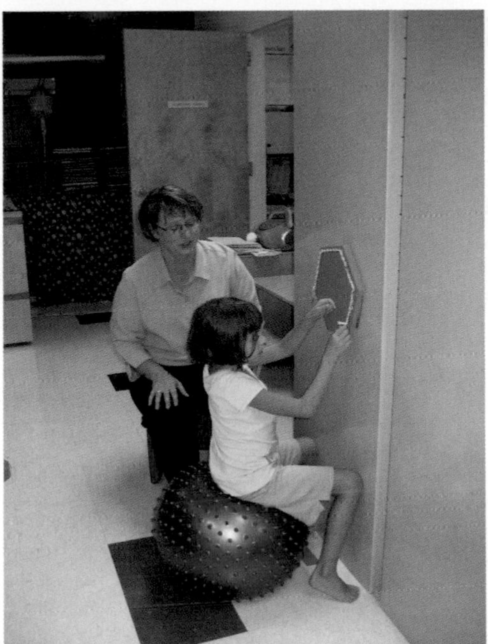

FIGURE 2-11 This activity of threading a string through hooks to create a design involves eye-hand coordination, dexterity, and control of arm in space (strength). It requires multiple steps to achieve a completed product.

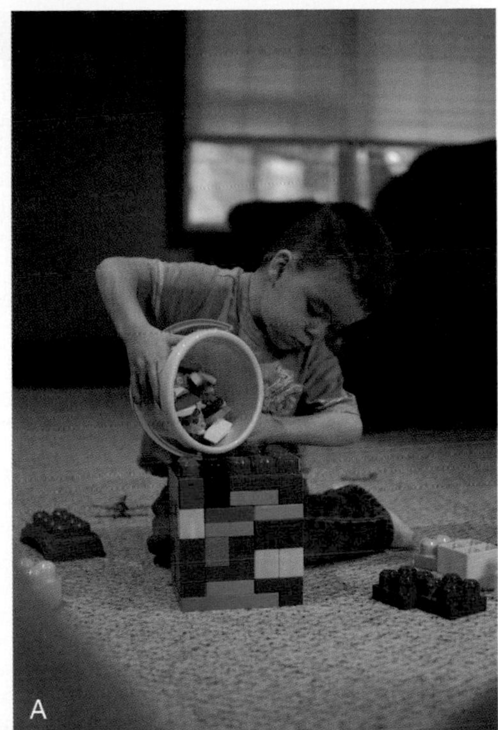

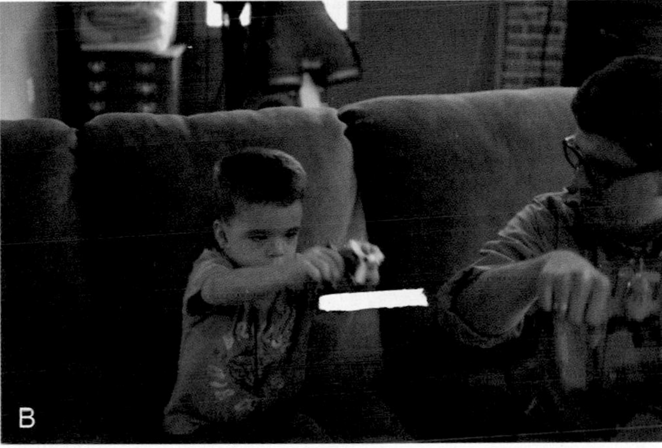

FIGURE 2-12 **A** and **B**, The occupational therapist emphasizes the child's understanding of relationships among objects in achieving functional goals.

learning its parts. For example, in learning to ride a tricycle, the child can focus on learning to pedal separately from steering, but he or she must then combine them.

Another important consideration in planning practice sessions is the use of random versus blocked practice. During random practice, the environmental conditions vary slightly each time; blocked practice involves drilling the task over and over in the same way. In most cases, random practice produces better learning because practice in variable contexts allows the child to solve a slightly different movement "problem" every time.

Some of the key techniques that occupational therapists use in this model of practice are giving verbal instructions and demonstrating movement strategies. Verbal instructions focus on the relationship between the child and the objects in the environment and emphasize key movement features directly related to achievement of the functional goal (Figure 2-12).[61] Physical or manual guidance can be helpful during the initial teaching of a movement because it may clarify the goal, guide selective attention, and help the child organize and plan the movement. Researchers stress that guidance or facilitation of movement should be removed as soon as possible, arguing that the occupational therapist rapidly becomes part of the environment, which alters the performance context and the intrinsic feedback available to the child.[61]

Motor learning researchers[126,161,191] recognize that learning has occurred when there is evidence of a relatively permanent change in the child's ability to respond to a movement problem or to achieve a movement goal. The learning of a new motor skill needs to be evaluated through tests of retention and transfer, not just immediate changes in performance.[103] Occupational therapists who use a motor learning model of practice must create opportunities for the child to demonstrate learning during a subsequent therapy session (retention), on a closely related task (transfer), or in a different setting (generalization). Case Study 2-1 and Table 2-8 apply motor learning concepts and compare motor learning with adaptation approaches.

Occupational therapists use theories about motor learning to promote development in areas of function that involve learning complex skills and behaviors. Self-care and handwriting are examples of areas of occupational performance to which occupational therapists have applied a motor learning approach. Researchers and practitioners have advocated for acquisitional and motor learning approaches to help children achieve handwriting competence (see Chapter 18). Many remedial or practice-based handwriting programs are commercially available. Several studies have demonstrated that the use of acquisitional principles by occupational therapists and educators in

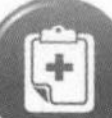

CASE STUDY 2-1 Reggie; Cerebral Palsy

Reggie is a 5-year-old girl who has cerebral palsy with moderate quadriplegia. She has difficulty controlling the movement of her arms and hands and functions at Manual Ability Classification System (MACS) level III (to manipulate objects, she needs help to prepare and modify activities). Isolated finger movements are limited. Reggie walks short distances using a walker. With limited arm strength, she can wheel her wheelchair only 4 to 5 feet. She has no other form of independent mobility. Her parents have set current goals for Reggie that include participation in dressing tasks and drawing and cutting skills in kindergarten activities. They also would like her to become more independent in mobility because she currently needs personal assistance to travel to the playground, cafeteria, and bus. Goals include increased participation and independence in dressing, drawing, cutting, and mobility.

TABLE 2-8 Occupational Therapy Evaluation and Intervention

Problem Definition and Intervention Goals	Description of Intervention	Expected Outcome
Motor Learning Theory		
Reggie lacks the motor skills needed to perform motor tasks through her day. Often the feedback she receives from movement is negative (e.g., she fails to reach her goal). Goals include that Reggie will: • Pull up her pants and fasten with minimal assistance. • Orient and don her shirt with moderate assistance in buttoning. • Cut a straight line using regular Fiskars scissors independently • Push her manual chair 20 feet without taking a break.	The intervention for Reggie focuses on improving coordination and strengthening her upper extremities. The occupational therapist identifies specific movement patterns that become the focus of intervention and whole task-related action to practice. To enhance dressing performance, she decides to practice in Reggie's bedroom in a large chair with arm rests and a firm seat. Easy clothing is selected first, and practice is repeated. Then Reggie practices with a variety of pants and shirts; she also attempts to don and doff clothes when sitting on the bed. Both the occupational therapist and the mother reinforce her efforts with praise. To improve her cutting and mobility skills, the occupational therapist selects the kindergarten classroom. The occupational therapist provides cueing and guidance during cutting with feedback on how to hold the scissors and paper. Reggie first cuts a strip of paper into small pieces and then cuts a large piece of paper. To practice mobility, Reggie practices wheeling her manual chair in the hallway. The occupational therapist encourages her, gives her cues to move in a straight line, and times her as if in a race.	Reggie's strength and coordination improve. Her endurance improves. She dresses with less caregiver assistance. She uses scissors to cut straight lines. Her wheelchair mobility improves. Reggie's intrinsic motivation improves because she is more independent and successful in these activities. Her parents are less anxious about her entering first grade and are satisfied with the gains that she has made in dressing and mobility.
Adaptation of Task and Environment		
The demands of Reggie's kindergarten classroom and home environment surpass her abilities. Task demands are often higher than her current abilities. She would benefit from adapted equipment or technology to enhance her function. Goals include that Reggie will: • Pull up her elastic band pants with Velcro fastener independently. • Orient and don her open neck sweatshirt independently. • Cut a straight line using adapted scissors independently. • Use a joystick to maneuver her power wheelchair independently from her classroom to the playground.	The occupational therapist and family focus on selecting and trialing adapted equipment and technology. The occupational therapist recommends types of clothing that are easier to don, and the family selects attractive clothing that they think Reggie will enjoy wearing. The occupational therapist practices with Reggie's new clothing and instructs the family in how to support her donning and doffing until she becomes independent. The kindergarten class has different adapted scissors available. The occupational therapist first selects loop scissors for Reggie to use in cutting activities. After practicing with straight-line cutting, the occupational therapist gives Reggie spring-release scissors to use in cutting activities. The occupational therapist encourages the family to consider power mobility as an optimal way for Reggie to explore her environment, become independent in mobility, and manage the longer traveling distances required in elementary grades. They select a power chair with joystick. The occupational therapist trains Reggie to use the joystick to drive her chair. Together they practice in a range of natural environments.	The adaptation approach improves Reggie's function and participation at home and school. With the adapted clothing and scissors and power wheelchair, her participation is markedly improved. She becomes almost completely independent in dressing, easing the parent's burden in preparing her for school. She participates in arts and crafts activities, cutting simple shapes with straight lines. With her power wheelchair, she moves independently in the school environment. The family engages in more community activities because Reggie is more independent in mobility.

a positive, interesting, and dynamic learning environment promotes the development of handwriting.[43] Further research is needed to determine the effectiveness of this approach with children who have challenges in sensorimotor and occupational performance.

To summarize, an occupational therapist using a motor learning model of practice:

1. Analyzes the movement synergies the child uses to achieve the functional action goal.
2. Considers the child's stage of learning and determines how best to facilitate the provision of both extrinsic and intrinsic feedback to improve the efficiency of the movement.
3. Provides opportunities for optimal practice of the goal and encourages practice in the natural environment.
4. Emphasizes practice of whole tasks, massed or distributed, according to the skill to be learned, child's developmental level, and context.
5. Establishes an activity that provides both intrinsic and extrinsic feedback. When appropriate, the occupational therapist provides knowledge of results and knowledge of performance by praising the child and giving specific information about the child's performance.
6. Promotes independent performance and decision making as soon as possible and evaluates whether the motor learning has been acquired, transferred, and generalized.[195]

Biomechanical Approaches

Biomechanical approaches require the understanding of anatomy and physiology related to posture and movement and the mechanics (i.e., kinetics and kinematics) that define movement. Through biomechanical approaches, occupational therapists use an understanding of the internal and external forces that act on and affect the body—that is, the musculoskeletal system. Specifically, occupational therapists analyze the relationships between musculoskeletal systems and body function to optimize body (trunk and neck) alignment as a basis for the child or youth to move and control extremities.

Joints and posture can be in poor alignment or misalignment when a child has low or high muscle tone, paralysis, or significant weakness. When muscles do not support joints, the forces of gravity or forces from the weight-bearing surface can create misalignment.[29] Poor alignment of joints affects movement, and when alignment is not corrected, contractures or deformity can result.

Methods for achieving joint alignment include passive range of motion, active range of motion, and strengthening. Achieving joint alignment may require that muscles or ligaments are relaxed or stretched; that joints are held in position by an external means, such as a splint or positioner; or that muscles around the joint are strengthened to maintain correct alignment. Gravity and its effects on weak muscles or low postural tone need to be considered when positioning or seating a child because gravity can negatively affect posture. Appropriate alignment of the trunk that includes a stable neck and trunk with the head directly over the pelvis allows the eyes to scan and visualize the environment, the mouth and throat structures to eat and breathe safely, the eyes to visualize hands and the hands to come to midline, and the pelvis to support an upright trunk that allows controlled arm movement through full range of motion.

Biomechanical principles are important when designing seating systems for a wheelchair or other positioner, making a splint or cast, or positioning a child for a functional task. Principles for attaining correct postural alignment when seated have been established; these are described further in Chapter 20. General guidelines for selecting appropriate seating that allows optimal function (i.e., coordinating eyes and hands, reaching, eating) include the following:

1. The head aligns over the shoulders that align with the pelvis.
2. The hip angle is approximately 90 to 95 degrees. The pelvis is secured with a strap.
3. The trunk is at midline with symmetric weight bearing on buttocks.
4. The arms are forward toward midline and can move freely.
5. Muscle tone is sufficiently relaxed to allow movement of the head and extremities.
6. The feet are supported, and the legs are well supported.

Often biomechanical approaches are combined with other practice models (e.g., motor learning). Biomechanical approaches are often preparatory for interventions that promote functional performance (see Figure 2-6). When alignment has been achieved, skill building, strengthening, and practice of functional tasks become easier for the child. Range of motion exercises and splinting are often helpful techniques for hand trauma or hand surgery. The use of biomechanical approaches in hand therapy is described in Chapter 29.

Neurodevelopmental Therapy

NDT may follow biomechanical approaches and targets children with cerebral palsy. Also similar to and expanding biomechanical approaches, NDT focuses on attainment of normal postural reactions that promote normal movement.[16] Although this intervention approach continues to focus on problems in postural control and motor coordination, as seen in cerebral palsy, the principles underlying the treatment approach have expanded to include motor learning and dynamic systems theories. In addition, NDT principles have shifted to recognize the importance of the environment and to place more emphasis on activities that are clearly functional and meaningful to the child.[73]

When using this approach to evaluate a child, the occupational therapist analyzes the child's movements to identify missing or atypical musculoskeletal elements that create functional limitations. These missing elements become one focus of intervention and are used to select the developmental level of therapeutic activities. Therapeutic handling is integral to the NDT approach and is used to facilitate postural control and movement synergies and to inhibit or constrain motor patterns that, if practiced, would lead to secondary deformities and dysfunction.[73] An occupational therapist applying NDT strategies focuses on changing movement patterns to achieve the most energy-efficient performance for the individual in the context of age-appropriate tasks.

As the occupational therapist manually guides and handles the child in the context of an activity, these elements are always combined with the child's active participation. With the occupational therapist's guidance, the child practices sequences of movements in slightly different ways to reinforce learning of the task. This practice is important for making a movement strategy functional and automatic. Occupational therapists emphasize quality of movement (e.g., accuracy, quickness, adaptability, fluency). Although therapeutic handling remains an integral part of NDT, practitioners use many treatment methods, "manipulating the individual task or the environment in order to positively influence function" (p. 63).[73]

Acknowledging that NDT principles have changed over the years to incorporate theories of motor learning and dynamic systems theory, clinical evaluation studies of the NDT approach (many of which were completed >10 years ago) have raised questions about its efficacy. Comparison studies of the NDT approach for children with cerebral palsy have been conducted over the past 30 years. In these studies, the NDT approach has been compared with functional therapy,[154] infant stimulation,[131] Vojta therapy, and differing intensities of therapy.[92,110] The results of these trials have been mixed, with two demonstrating no difference,[93] two supporting NDT,[110,154] and two supporting alternative treatments.[131] The more rigorous randomized clinical trials have generally produced results that do not support the efficacy of the NDT approach.[135]

A systematic review of NDT concluded that "the preponderance of results ... do not confer any advantage to NDT over alternatives to which it was compared" (p. 789).[21] The only consistent effect of NDT that was statistically significant was an immediate effect on range of motion. In contrast to NDT methods, the motor-based interventions that produce meaningful improvements in functional outcomes for children with disabilities incorporate three essential elements: (1) intensive task repetition, (2) progressive challenges to the learner with increasing difficulty, and (3) the presence of motivators and rewards.[153] Novak et al.[125] completed a systematic review on interventions for cerebral palsy and concluded that NDT was not a recommended intervention for children with cerebral palsy. However, despite lack of evidence on efficacy,[125,153] NDT remains a widely used approach with children who have cerebral palsy and CNS dysfunction affecting motor performance. Because the conceptual basis of NDT has evolved over the past decade, a first step in additional research on its efficacy would be to operationalize the new concepts into treatment protocols that can be measured and replicated for research purposes. Despite this recommendation, many of the principles of NDT are widely implemented and appear to be helpful; core concepts and specific principles of NDT may be integrated into other approaches. For example, key concepts on the importance of postural stability to functional movement suggest that good alignment and positioning are beneficial when a child with cerebral palsy performs fine motor play activity.

Sensory Integration Therapy

The theory of sensory integration, together with the intervention approach derived from that theory, grew from the work of Ayres.[3] Ayres developed her theory in an effort to explain behaviors observed in children with learning difficulties based on neural functioning. Specifically, she hypothesized that some children with learning difficulties experience problems in "organizing sensory information for use."[3] She named this neural process *sensory integration.*

Much of Ayres' work and that of her colleagues was devoted to the development of evaluation tools that could clearly identify individuals with sensory integrative problems. The Sensory Integration and Praxis Tests (SIPT) are the result of this work.[5] Included in this area of identification and evaluation are numerous studies aimed at describing different subtypes of sensory integrative problems (see Chapter 9 for a summary). Parham and Mailloux (Chapter 9) identify five sensory integrative patterns based on behavioral observation and assessment beyond the SIPT: (1) sensory modulation problems, (2) sensory seeking behavior, (3) sensory discrimination and perception problems, (4) vestibular-bilateral functional problems, and (5) praxis problems.

Although these disorders overlap, each suggests a specific type of intervention. The work of Dunn and Brown[45] identifying children with a sensory modulation disorder has shown that these children have patterns of poor registration of sensation, are hypersensitive to stimuli, avoid certain sensations, or seek particular inputs. These sensory processing patterns may be present in children with various developmental disorders, and they are often described in children with ASD.[7,170] Evaluation tools for identifying sensory processing problems in children and adults are widely used by occupational therapists.[52,54,116]

Ayres[3] also developed interventions that she believed would help to resolve sensory integration problems. She proposed an intervention approach based on assumptions drawn from neuromaturation theory and systems theory. Neuromaturation concepts, such as hierarchical organization of cortical and subcortical areas, developmental sequence of learning and skill acquisition, and neural plasticity, are essential to an understanding of the mechanisms of sensory integration. Systems theory also underlies sensory integration because the focus is on the child seeking sensory input and using adaptive behavior as an organizer of the input. Intervention sessions are playful and child-directed. The occupational therapist and child collaborate to select activities that are of interest to the child and provide a "just-right challenge" to the child's skill level (Figure 2-13). SIT seeks to provide the child with enhanced opportunities for controlled sensory input, with a particular emphasis on vestibular, proprioceptive, and tactile input, in the context of

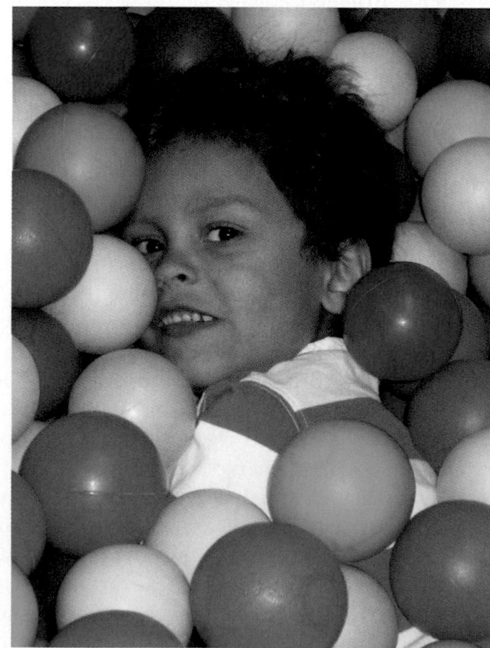

FIGURE 2-13 The child's selection of jumping into a ball pit helps to meet his need for proprioceptive input.

meaningful activity. In intervention, the occupational therapist facilitates an adaptive response, which requires the child to integrate the sensory information (Figure 2-14). Sensory integration is hypothesized to improve through this process. SIT is widely used by occupational therapists. In a survey of occupational therapists working with children with autism, 99% of the occupational therapists reported using sensory integration techniques with their clients.[179] See Case Study 2-2 for an example of a child with developmental coordination disorder and Table 2-9 to compare sensory integration intervention and the CO-OP approach.

Many authors have proposed intervention programs specifically to address sensory modulation disorders.[151,188] Sensory modulation difficulties can limit a child's participation in activities of daily living, and this is often the case for children with ASD. Sensory integration strategies are often integrated into interventions that promote play and activities of daily living, including eating[171] and sleeping.[143] In addition, primary autism interventions, such as Floortime[67] and ESDM,[40] have adopted sensory integration principles. Sensory strategies can promote a child's self-regulation and optimal arousal level, allowing engagement in interaction, attention to activity, and learning from social contexts (see Figure 2-6).

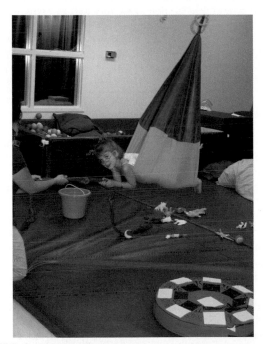

FIGURE 2-14 The child exhibits an adaptive response by pulling on the rope to control her movement through space.

Research of sensory integration intervention with various diagnoses has been published. The original research of Ayres and later Miller, Coll, and Schoen[114] demonstrated benefit with children with learning disabilities and sensory processing disorder (see Chapter 9). Early work by Ayres[4] and others[8] reported positive changes resulting from SIT for outcomes such as motor, academic, and language performance. Studies in the late 1980s and the 1990s evaluated the efficacy of sensory integration intervention using more rigorous methods, including randomized controlled trials. Using meta-analysis techniques, Vargas and Camilli[175] concluded that children who received SIT improved in performance, particularly educational and motor outcomes, compared with children who received no therapy. When sensory integration intervention was compared with alternative therapies, the outcomes were no different across groups.

In the past decade, a group of scholars examined the research literature on sensory integration to develop a fidelity measure for sensory integration intervention.[132,133] Based on a comprehensive review of the research literature, observation of master clinicians, and critique by master clinicians, the fidelity measure defines the active ingredients or core elements for sensory integration intervention. The fidelity measure has been used in more recent trials (Table 2-10).

Studies using rigorous methods have shown positive effects of sensory integration interventions. In a randomized trial comparing sensory integration intervention with an activity protocol or no treatment, Miller et al.[114] assigned children with sensory modulation disorders to one of three groups. The children in the sensory integration group and the activity group received intervention twice a week for 10 weeks, and the control group children were placed on a waitlist for intervention. Children in the sensory integration intervention group made significant gains on goal attainment scaling and in attention and cognitive and social performance as measured by the Leiter International Performance Scale. Other measures of child behavior, sensory processing, and electrodermal reactivity improved in the sensory integration group but did not differ when the sensory integration group was compared with the activity and control groups.[114]

Trials of SIT have focused on effects for children with ASD. In two randomized controlled trials with young children with ASD, one examined the effects of clinic-based SIT compared with usual care,[152] and one examined SIT effects compared with a fine motor activity intervention.[134] Both trials used the Ayres sensory integration fidelity measure (see Table 2-9)[133] to standardize the intervention procedures. Following 6 weeks of SIT or fine motor activities, Pfeiffer et al.[134] found that the children with ASD who received SIT improved more in their individualized goals (as measured by Goal Attainment Scaling) and

CASE STUDY 2-2 John; Developmental Coordination Disorder

John is an 8-year-old boy with developmental coordination disorder. As an infant, he was delayed in development of motor skills, and as a preschooler, he was described as clumsy and awkward. At 8 years old, he rarely participates in physical activities with his peers. He has great difficulty in learning new motor tasks and motor planning complex motor tasks. He has struggled to learn handwriting. He is in second grade, and key issues for the teacher are (1) his handwriting is illegible and his written work is highly disorganized, and (2) he does not participate in recess activities but stands on the side watching the other children play.

TABLE 2-9 Core Elements of Sensory Integration Therapy

Element	Description
1. Ensures physical safety	Occupational therapist anticipates physical hazards and attempts to ensure that the child is physically safe through manipulation of protective and therapeutic equipment and the therapist's physical proximity and actions.
2. Presents sensory opportunities	Occupational therapist presents the child with 2 of 3 types of sensory opportunities—tactile, vestibular, and proprioceptive—to support the development of self-regulation, sensory awareness, or movement in space.
3. Helps child to attain and maintain appropriate levels of alertness	Occupational therapist helps the child to attain and maintain appropriate levels of alertness and an affective state that supports engagement in activities.
4. Challenges postural, ocular, oral, or bilateral motor control	Occupational therapist supports and challenges postural control, ocular control, or bilateral development. At least 1 of these types of challenges is intentionally offered: postural challenges, resistive whole-body challenges, ocular-motor challenges, bilateral challenges, oral challenges, projected action sequences.
5. Challenges praxis and organization of behavior	Occupational therapist supports and presents challenges to the child's ability to conceptualize and plan novel motor tasks and to organize his or her own behavior in time and space.
6. Collaborates in activity choice	Occupational therapist negotiates activity choices with the child, allowing the child to choose equipment, materials, or specific aspects of an activity. Activity choices and sequences are not determined solely by the occupational therapist.
7. Tailors activity to present just-right challenge	Occupational therapist suggests or supports an increase in complexity of challenge when the child responds successfully. These challenges are primarily tailored to the child's postural, ocular, or oral control; sensory modulation and discrimination; or praxis developmental level.
8. Ensures that activities are successful	Occupational therapist presents or facilitates challenges that focus on sensory modulation or discrimination; postural, ocular, or oral control; or praxis in which the child can be successful in making an adaptive response to challenge.
9. Supports child's intrinsic motivation to play	Occupational therapist creates a setting that supports play as a way to engage the child fully in intervention.
10. Establishes a therapeutic alliance	Occupational therapist promotes and establishes a connection with the child that conveys a sense of working together toward one or more goals in a mutually enjoyable partnership. Relationship of occupational therapist and child goes beyond pleasantries and feedback on performance such as praise or instruction.

From Parham, L. D., Roley, S. S., May-Benson, T. A., Koomar, J., Brett-Green, B., Burke, J. P., et al. (2011). Development of a fidelity measure for research on the effectiveness of the Ayres sensory integration intervention. *American Journal of Occupational Therapy, 65,* 133–142.

demonstrated fewer autistic mannerisms; the groups did not differ in adaptive behaviors or sensory processing. In the trial by Schaaf et al.,[152] children with ASD received 10 weeks of SIT or usual care. Children in the SIT group improved more in individualized goals and required less caregiver assistance in self-care and social functions. In a systematic review of sensory interventions for children with ASD, Case-Smith, Weaver, and Fristad[25] concluded that SIT results in "meaningful positive effects" on individualized goals and overall moderate effects on parent-reported and teacher-reported assessments.

Qualitative research has explored parents' perceptions of change in their children and in themselves as a result of occupational therapy that used sensory integration intervention.[27,28] Parents reported positive changes in their children's social participation, perceived competence, and self-regulation. The parents valued the new understanding of the child's behavior and used this perspective to support and advocate for the child more effectively. Ayres' work has had a significant impact on occupational therapy practice with children and has led to an increased sophistication and rigor in the scholarly work accomplished in the field of occupational therapy.

Task and Environment Adaptation

Occupational performance is successful when the demands of the task, the skills of the child, and the features of the environment are congruent. When the skills of the child or youth do not meet the demands of the task in the environment, occupational performance becomes less successful. Most of the models of practice in occupational therapy, particularly with children who are developing, focus on increasing the child's performance and participation; however, often the task and environment are modified or adapted to optimize participation. The adaptation approach can be combined with remedial intervention or may be the focus of occupational therapy services.

To implement an adaptation approach, the occupational therapist first completes an in-depth task and environment analysis. This analysis identifies the following:

1. What is the goal of the task, and what are the task demands?
2. Which performance components required for the task are difficult for the child, and which is the child unable to perform?
3. How can the task or environment be modified to increase the child's function?
4. Which resources, technologies, and methods are needed to enable the child to accomplish this task (or the goal of the task)?

The goal of the adaptation model of practice is to modify the demands of the task and environment so that they are congruent with the child's ability level. Adaptations may involve modifying the occupation so that it is easier to perform, using assistive technology devices, or changing the physical or social

TABLE 2-10 Occupational Therapy Evaluation and Intervention

Problem Definition and Goals	Description of Intervention	Expected Outcome
Cognitive Orientation to Occupational Performance		
Services are provided by the school-based occupational therapist. Through a discussion with John about his handwriting and his participation in playground activities, the occupational therapist identifies his frustration with his performance and his feeling of isolation that he is limited in participating in physical activities with his peers. Together they establish two goals: John will: • Improve his handwriting so that his teacher and his parents can read his stories. • Improve the neatness of his paper to earn a gold star from the teacher. • Participate in playground activities 4 of 5 days.	Based on an analysis of John's handwriting, the occupational therapist targets letter formation and letter alignment. She and John agree to work on handwriting together by making picture books about his pets. Throughout the sessions, the occupational therapist guides him in letter formation. Together they select the handwriting aids that help him most. They select a pencil grip and an alphabet strip. They also practice on paper with highlighted lines. They agree to make two copies of the book, the first one just for practice. John is motivated to make his pet book neat and readable. The occupational therapist also analyzes his performance on the playground and determines that his difficulty with motor coordination creates anxiety in using the equipment, and he is embarrassed to use the equipment in front of his peers. The occupational therapist gets permission for John to practice using the playground equipment with her at times other than recess. They practice on simple and then more difficult equipment. The occupational therapist models for him and sometimes cues him, but she does not often offer praise as his achieving the motor tasks is sufficient (intrinsic) reinforcement.	Having followed the Goal, Plan, Do, Check strategy, the occupational therapist asks John if he is pleased with his pet book. He indicates to the occupational therapist which supports were most helpful and which he would like to continue to use. John realizes that he needs to practice his handwriting and to take his time when writing. The teacher is pleased with his improvement in handwriting legibility. The occupational therapist and John check his participation on the playground. He prefers to stay with the swings, which are easiest to use. The occupational therapist and he agree that the swings are a good activity for recess. Later in the school year, they will create a new goal to use other pieces of playground equipment.
Sensory Integration Intervention		
Services are provided by a clinic-based occupational therapist. John appears to have a sensory integration disorder, specifically somatosensory dyspraxia. This means that his somatosensory perception (touch and movement) is limited; he does not receive accurate or sufficient feedback from movement to learn new motor skills easily. His coordination will improve if his sensory integration improves and he gains increased perception of his body's movement. The goals for therapy: John will: • Increase the accuracy of his tactile and proprioceptive perception as measured on the Sensory Integration and Praxis Tests (SIPT). • Demonstrate improved motor planning skills as measured on the Bruininks Oseretsky Test of Motor Proficiency (BOT-2) and the Evaluation Tool of Children's Handwriting	Based on the results of the SIPT, John shows low tactile discrimination and very low praxis skills. Intervention focuses on enhancing sensory integration of the tactile and proprioceptive systems and improving motor planning. The occupational therapist provides a sensory-rich environment with a variety of swings, unstable surfaces, crawling surfaces, and equipment that provides deep pressure. She and John collaborate in selecting activities that are fun but challenging, and the occupational therapist offers supports and guidance as needed for John to master the activities. Although the occupational therapist allows John to repeat fun activities, she also changes the activities so that they are more challenging. She often asks John if he can think of ways to make the activity harder. Together they plan activities that simulate the playground equipment at school so that he becomes more proficient and confident in performing these activities. To improve motor planning, the therapist devises obstacle courses for him to complete in the clinic. They spend some of the session practicing visual motor integration activities, such as games and handwriting practice.	John's scores on the SIPT and the BOT-2 improve. At the end of 6 months, he scores within normal limits on many of the subtests. His improvement in sensory integration and motor planning translates to his participation and performance at school. His handwriting improves and becomes more legible. His family helps him generalize skills that he gained in occupational therapy by taking him to the playground twice a week. With this support in generalizing his new skills, John participates with his peers on the playground equipment at school.

environment.[36] Often when children have significant impairments, task modification is needed to maximize the child's participation. For example, a child with cerebral palsy may require an adapted spoon and cup to eat dinner with his family. A child with autism may require a picture exchange card system to communicate his need to use the bathroom.

When skills are insufficient to enable performance, task adaptation is used to modify the demands of a task to bring it to the competence level of the child. An example in school-based practice would be adapting the writing surface by using a slant board so that the child's written work is more easily visualized and the child's hand and arm posture are supported in a posture that promotes writing. A child with a learning disability may be able to complete a page of arithmetic problems when the font is enlarged and the paper has a color tint.

Often adaptive equipment or assistive technology is used to modify or adapt the task. Campbell, Milbourne, and Wilcox[22] view assistive technology as a bridge or mediator between the skills that a child can currently perform and the requirements of the task. Assistive technology may be as simple as adaptive brushes or crayons that allow a preschool child to participate in art activities. A wide variety of assistive technology devices can enable children with significant motor impairments to access their environment better. For example, assistive technology devices can help position the child to perform an activity (e.g., a prone stander) or provide postural support (e.g., wheelchair straps). "High-tech" technology is also available to provide a method for written communication (e.g., a laptop computer) or augmentative communication (e.g., a device for synthesized speech). Chapters 15, 19, and 20 describe assistive technology devices that use this approach to increase children's participation in their natural environments.

With children, the compensatory approach often complements other approaches that focus on skill building. Methods for adapting tasks are selected not only so that the child succeeds at a particular task but also to promote skills in similar tasks and in other environments. For example, a child with poor drawing skills can create a picture using peel-off stickers of animals. Although this adaptation allows him or her to create a picture more easily than drawing with markers, peeling off and placing the stickers provide practice of fine motor skills—specifically, bilateral coordination, isolated finger movements, spatial relations, and use of force. Practice in these skills may generalize to other art activities, and the easy success the child achieves when using colorful animal stickers may encourage him or her to attempt other art activities.

More recent research has used adaptation approaches as the primary occupational therapy intervention to optimize the child's function and participation. Research by Law et al.,[97] described in the section on dynamic systems theory, and Dunn et al.,[47] described in the next section, demonstrates the effectiveness of interventions that focus on adapting activities and the environment to enhance the child's participation.

Coaching and Consultation Models

Virtually all occupational therapy interventions for children involve coaching and consulting. Theory-based conceptual models guide how occupational therapists approach and implement these aspects of practice. Service delivery using coaching and consultation is particularly relevant for preventive interventions; they also support generalization or transfer of new skills (see Figure 2-6). Often, but not always, these approaches to service delivery are provided in combination with direct interventions. The role of occupational therapy in prevention is emerging and promises to be an important part of practice.

Coaching models have evolved in recent years into essential elements of health care service delivery and therapeutic intervention. Coaching models vary in educational and medical models of service delivery, reflecting philosophical differences, top-down versus bottom-up approaches, and the targeted goal (health, development, function, relationships). Fundamental to coaching models are theories of self-efficacy and family-centered approaches.[48,49] The positive outcomes of coaching are that parents can identify their own solutions; parents can fully participate in intervention; and parents' competence increases.[47]

Coaching and Consulting Models in Early Childhood and Educational Settings

Researchers and practitioners have advocated for the use of coaching models in early intervention and early childhood programs.[49] Coaching can be defined as a reciprocal process between a coach (occupational therapist) and learner (parent), comprising a series of conversations focused on child outcomes that allow the learner to discovery his or her own solutions for achieving the agreed outcomes. In coaching, the practitioner recognizes that when clients are informed and make their own decisions, they are more likely to participate fully, to maintain participation over time, and to be satisfied with services. It is an interactive process that supports the parents' observations and reflections about the child's behaviors. Because it is built on trust, respect, and open communication, this interaction facilitates the development of a therapist-caregiver relationship that sustains the intervention process and increases caregiver competence and satisfaction with services. An occupational therapist can apply the following steps in the coaching process: (1) use reflective statements and questions to invite parents to discuss the child's problem or desired goal; (2) guide the parents to become more aware of the problem and possible reasons for the problem; (3) help the parents analyze the problem; (4) suggest possible alternative solutions or guide the parent into identifying solutions; (5) identify with the parent an action, then encourage and support that action; and (6) ask questions to guide the parent in identifying potential outcomes that would determine goal achievement.[47] Coaching principles are listed in Table 2-11 and are described further in Chapter 22. Case Study 2-3 presents a brief example of coaching.

Coaching strategies have been used to promote parent-child interaction in home visits of early intervention professionals.[107] They have also been used to support parents in providing teaching opportunities to their children. Education and occupational therapy researchers have found positive effects when implementing coaching models.[47,169] Coaching of teachers has resulted in positive outcomes for classroom management and teachers' support of student social-emotional development.[24,144] Teaching children with ASD self-management of behavior allows them to be more self-directed, self-reliant, and independent and less dependent on external supervision.[187] Self-management is considered to be a pivotal skill that can generalize to adaptive behavior and promote autonomy for

TABLE 2-11 Coaching Principles and Examples

Coaching Principle	Explanation	Example
Coaching is a voluntary process based on collaborative relationship.	It is important that the professional does not approach the relationship with a sense of power over the family. The focus is on potential outcomes and not fixing a problem.	The occupational therapist asks: How would you like me to help you? What goals for your child are important to you?
The process involves small steps toward positive change.	Small steps are important. When problems arise, these can be reframed as opportunities for change.	The occupational therapist praises small accomplishments, helps the parent recognize the child's progress, even if it is short of the hoped-for outcome.
Occupational therapist creates opportunities for the learner to master new competencies.	Occupational therapist can suggest that the parent practice a new skill in different settings and context. This allows problem solving when context-specific problems arise.	The occupational therapist suggests that the parent try a strategy that was successful at home in the community. The occupational therapist suggests that the mother teach her spouse the strategy as way of reinforcing her learning.
Occupational therapist provides ongoing support and encouragement.	This support and trust enhances the positive relationship between the coach and parent.	Rather than giving the parent solutions, the occupational therapist guides the parent into identifying solutions and may give the parent additional resources.
Occupational therapist and parent together analyze situations and problem solve solutions.	Ideas and resources are shared. This process leads to self-discovery of solutions and establishes where more support is needed.	The occupational therapist asks: What happened when you tried ... ? What changes would you make the next time? What have you learned from this process?
Occupational therapist and parent reflect on the outcome of the strategy.	The parent and occupational therapist review experiences, discuss what worked, check perceptions, and analyze strategies.	The occupational therapist asks for the parent's perceptions of outcome. The occupational therapist asks about the parent's satisfaction with the child's outcome and the coaching process.

Adapted from Rush, D. D., Shelden, M. L., Hanft, B. E. (2003). Coaching families and colleagues: A process for collaboration in natural settings. *Infants and Young Children, 16*(1), 33–47.

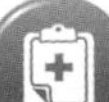

CASE STUDY 2-3 Examples of Coaching in School-Based Practice

Michael is struggling at school to fulfill his role as a student successfully because he has high functioning autism spectrum disorder (ASD). Michael struggles with his academic occupations because he becomes anxious in social situations, requires high structure to engage in academic activities, and has limited social skills. His social participation is characterized by interest in his peers but limited ability to read the social cues of his peers and anxiety about initiating a social interaction.

Thom, the occupational therapist, evaluates the school activities in which Michael is expected to participate and determines what personal and environmental factors are influencing his performance. School occupations with high social interaction become the focus of intervention; for example, Thom helps the teacher structure the classroom environment to allow for nonsocial activities to be interspersed with social activities. Thom coaches Michael to use strategies that help him interpret social cues and gestures and make appropriate social responses. Thom creates opportunities for him to interact with peers in safe and structured environments. Scaffolding the child's participation in social activities with peers at school is likely to develop skills that generalize to other opportunities for social participation. This brief example illustrates intervention principles that enable participation of children in everyday occupations (see Research Note 2-1).[90]

children with high functioning ASD.[87] To promote self-management of behavior, the occupational therapist meets with the child or youth to develop a plan and to identify goals. The occupational therapist and child determine how and when the targeted behaviors will be recorded and how positive behavior will be rewarded. The occupational therapist and child meet regularly to evaluate behavior and progress, and the occupational therapist provides rewards; this process is faded as the child becomes more independent, and behaviors become consistent.[187]

Most occupational therapy interventions for children include a coaching or consultation component with direct intervention, making it difficult to separate the effects of consultation versus direct intervention. However, a few studies have examined consultation or coaching as the primary intervention model. In a comparison study, Dreiling and Bundy[44] found that consultation services were equal in effectiveness to direct services. Dunn et al.[47] examined the effects of a contextual intervention in which occupational therapists coached parents to develop strategies that supported participation of their children with sensory processing problems. The occupational therapists provided home-based reflective coaching to support parent problem solving. Ten sessions of coaching resulted in improved child participation as measured on the Canadian Occupational Performance Measure and based on individualized goals. In addition, the parents who participated in the contextual intervention improved in self-efficacy, resulting in gains that were well above normative data for parent self-efficacy. In addition, occupational therapists using context intervention[39] apply coaching and consultation methods. Context intervention is a strength-based approach specifically designed to enhance parents' competence to problem solve and adapt task and environment barriers that limit the child's participation.[97] The occupational therapists encourage the parents to find solutions, using a trial-and-error approach to discovering what works best. In this intervention, the occupational therapists make specific recommendations for adapting tasks and environment, collaborate with families to implement the modifications, and are open to parent suggestions to ensure that the adaptations are congruent with the family's daily routine.

Coaching and Consultation in Medical Settings

Medical models of coaching focus on shifting the power from health professional to the client or family and recognizing the family's stage of readiness to change behavior. Core constructs for the coaching models that have been developed in medical systems follow the theories of Prochaska[139] on behavioral change and self-management—the therapist's coaching methods follow the family's readiness for behavioral change. The continuum of readiness is (1) precontemplation, (2) contemplation, (3) preparation, (4) action, and (5) maintenance. This continuum is relevant to the occupational therapist giving a family a home program, asking the parents to implement specific strategies or change their routine. Without considering this continuum, occupational therapists may overwhelm parents, may be unrealistic in their expectations, or may not provide sufficient resources to enable participation of parents in their child's intervention. The factors that influence behavioral change or a parent's readiness to participate in intervention include:

1. The pros and cons for the desired behavior change.
2. Self-efficacy or confidence in their ability to change.
3. Cognitive process including self-image.
4. Social norms for expected behavior.
5. Behavior process such as making a commitment.
6. Social resources available to support behavioral change.

Interventions focused on prevention and primary care frequently use consultation models of service delivery. For example, interventions to prevent skin ulcers in children in wheelchairs focus on coaching families to support the child's activity level, encourage the child to spend time out of the wheelchair, maintain the cushion and seating supports, and encourage weight shifts during sedentary activity.[81] Occupational therapy programs to prevent weight gain in children with diabetes and to maintain activity levels for children with asthma also involve primarily family consultation and coaching.[42] More recently developed coaching models that use telehealth technology have increased the range of occupational therapy services available to families with limited access to services.[26]

Occupational therapists, nurses, and physicians have successfully used coaching and consultation models to promote self-management of treatment for children with diabetes and asthma.[59] Occupational therapists can coach families on healthy lifestyles and healthy habits to help them manage these chronic conditions. In a study to promote parents' management of their child's asthma, Nelson et al.[123] used the transtheoretical model of behavioral change. The coaches assessed the parents' level of readiness and motivation to change and adjusted the coaching to match each stage. Parents made significant progress in moving forward in their stage of readiness. Parents were more engaged and made greater progress when contacts with the coaches were frequent and consistent.[123] The transtheoretical model of behavioral change is useful when parents face a sudden change in their child's health status (e.g., a head injury) and they are unprepared for the major changes in their daily routine and home environment that are necessary to accommodate a child with significant medical problems or disability. Using this frame of reference can guide how the occupational therapist coaches the parent, which information and resources to provide to the parent, the pace of coaching, and the level of support needed for transfer of care from the rehabilitation professionals to the family. Coaching is a strength-based and family-centered model of service delivery with the potential to build self-efficacy and self-determination in families and children.

Summary

Occupational therapists who provide services to children and youth use theory-based practice models. These models originated in the fields of psychology, education, and medicine and have been adapted using the lens of occupation and occupational therapy. They provide a framework for clinical decision making and reasoning. They also guide occupational therapists to consider the child, his or her occupations, the environment, and the interactions of these elements. Practitioners recognize that theories are overlapping and complementary. To meet the individual needs of the children they serve, they use theoretical concepts specific to certain problems as well as in combination. Occupational therapists apply different practice models as the child grows and experiences different contexts. Research studies have examined the effectiveness of practice models, assessing their benefits and for whom they are most beneficial and investigating how they should be staged across the life span. Research evidence has helped occupational therapists in refining practice models and using them appropriately in various contexts.

Summary Points

- Occupational therapy practice models have evolved from learning, development, occupation, and ecological theories.
- Outcomes of occupational therapy interventions include children's engagement in occupations—meaningful, goal-directed activities and participation across a balance of life activities.
- Ecological theories explain the influence of the environment on human behavior and function. Environment fit is the congruence between individuals and their environments, and optimal congruence allows for optimal participation.

- The person-environment-occupation model explains the dynamic, transactive relationship of person, environment, and occupation across the life span.
- The International Classification of Functioning, Disability, and Health and the occupational therapy practice framework define the relationships among body structures and functions, activities, and participation, suggesting that health directly relates to participation.
- Occupational therapy practice is child-centered, family-centered, and strength-based; these concepts are directly linked to enhancing self-efficacy and self-determination.
- Occupational therapy interventions based on behavioral theories, such as shaping, incidental teaching, pivotal response training, motor learning, and social skills training, use performance analysis, apply learning principles, access the natural environment and play activities, promote practice and repetition, challenge mastered skills and support emerging skills, and provide positive reinforcement.
- Cognitive-behavioral interventions, such as CO-OP, use a collaborative, strength-based approach to establish goals with the child, analyze performance, identify strategies to reach goals, guide the child in discovery of solutions for performance problems, enable the child to improve performance relative to goals, and promote generalization.
- Interventions to promote social behaviors and participation often use social play, occupation-based social groups, and peer-mediated models. There is positive evidence for use of these models with children and youth with ASD.
- Interventions to improve motor skills use dynamic systems theory and motor learning principles to identify the variables that influence the child's sensorimotor performance, focus on goals that allow reorganization of performance, identify contexts and activities optimal for sensorimotor practice, apply multiple dimensions of reinforcement, and specifically design strategies to promote generalization.
- Occupational therapists use collaborative models of coaching and consultation to promote parents' sense of competence, self-efficacy, and partnership in promoting child outcomes. These models are useful in preventive interventions for children with chronic health problems and are beneficial to families who are responsible for managing their child's health care and intervention long-term.

REFERENCES

1. Adams, J. A. (1971). A closed-loop theory of motor learning. *Journal of Motor Behavior, 3*, 111–149.
2. American Occupational Therapy Association. (2014). Occupational therapy practice framework: Domain and process (3rd ed.). *American Journal of Occupational Therapy, 68*(Suppl. 1), S1–S48.
3. Ayres, A. J. (1972). *Sensory integration and learning disorders.* Los Angeles: Western Psychological Services.
4. Ayres, A. J. (1978). Learning disabilities and the vestibular system. *Journal of Learning Disabilities, 11*, 18–29.
5. Ayres, A. J. (1989). *Sensory Integration and Praxis Tests.* Los Angeles: Western Psychological Services.
6. Bandura, A., Barbaranelli, C., Caprara, G. V., et al. (1996). Multifaceted impact of self-efficacy beliefs on academic functioning. *Child Development, 67*, 1206–1222.
7. Baranek, G. T., Foster, L. G., & Berkson, G. (1997). Sensory defensiveness in persons with developmental disabilities. *Journal of Autism and Developmental Disorders, 29*, 213–224.
8. Baum, C., & Christiansen, C. (2004). Occupation-based framework for practice. In C. Christiansen, C. M. Baum, & J. Bass-Haugen (Eds.), *Occupational therapy: Performance, participation and well-being* (3rd ed., pp. 242–259). Thorofare, NJ: SLACK Inc.
9. Bazyk, S. (2011). *Mental health promoting, prevention, and intervention with children and youth: A guiding framework for occupational therapy.* Bethesda, MD: AOTA Press.
10. Bedell, G. M., Cohn, E. S., & Dumas, H. M. (2005). Exploring parents' use of strategies to promote social participation of school-age children with acquired brain injuries. *American Journal of Occupational Therapy, 59*, 65–75.
11. Bedell, G. M., & Dumas, H. M. (2004). Social participation of children and youth with acquired brain injuries discharged from inpatient rehabilitation: A follow-up study. *Brain Injury, 18*, 65–82.
12. Bedell, G. M., Khetani, M. A., Cousins, M. A., et al. (2011). Parent perspectives to inform development of measures of children's participation and environment. *Archive of Physical Medical and Rehabilitation, 92*, 765–773.
13. Bedell, G., Coster, W., Law, M., et al. (2013). Community participation, supports, and barriers of school-age children with and without disabilities. *Archives of Physical Medicine and Rehabilitation, 94*(2), 315–323.
14. Bernheimer, L. P., & Weisner, T. S. (2007). "Let me just tell you what I do all day …": The family story at the center of intervention research and practice. *Infants and Young Children, 20*(3), 192–201.
15. Bernie, C., & Rodger, S. (2004). Cognitive strategy use in school-aged children with developmental coordination disorder. *Physical and Occupational Therapy in Pediatrics, 24*, 23–45.
16. Bobath, K. (1980). *A neurophysiological basis for the treatment of cerebral palsy.* London: Heinemann Books.
17. Broderick, C., Caswell, R., Gregory, S., et al. (2002). "Can I join the club?": A social integration scheme for adolescents with Asperger syndrome. *Autism: The International Journal of Research and Practice, 5*, 427–431.
18. Bronfenbrenner, U. (1977). Toward an experimental ecology of human development. *American Psychologist, 32*, 513–531.
19. Bronfenbrenner, U. (1979). *The ecology of human development.* Cambridge, MA: Harvard University.
20. Burton, A. W., & Miller, D. E. (1998). *Movement skill assessment.* Champaign, IL: Human Kinetics.
21. Butler, C., & Darrah, J. (2001). Effects of neurodevelopmental treatment (NDT) for cerebral palsy: An AACPDM evidence report. *Developmental Medicine and Child Neurology, 43*(11), 778–790.
22. Campbell, P. H., Milbourne, S., & Wilcox, M. J. (2008). Adaptation interventions to promote participation in natural settings. *Infants and Young Children, 21*, 94–106.
23. Canadian Association of Occupational Therapists (CAOT). (1997). *Enabling*

occupation: An occupational therapy perspective. Ottawa, ON: Canadian Association of Occupational Therapists (CAOT).

24. Cappella, E., Hamre, B. K., Kim, H. Y., et al. (2012). Teacher consultation and coaching within mental health practice: Classroom and child effects in urban elementary school. *Journal of Consulting and Clinical Psychology, 80*, 597–610.
25. Case-Smith, J., Weaver, L., & Fristad, M. A. (2014). A systematic review of sensory processing interventions for children with autism spectrum disorder. *Autism: The International Journal of Research and Practice*, doi:10.1177/1362361313517762.
26. Cason, J. (2011). Telerehabilitation: An adjunct service delivery model for early intervention services. *International Journal of Telerehabilitation, 3*(1), 19–28.
27. Cohn, E. S. (2001). Parent perspectives of occupational therapy using a sensory integration approach. *American Journal of Occupational Therapy, 55*, 285–294.
28. Cohn, E., Miller, L. J., & Tickle-Degnen, L. (2000). Parental hopes for therapy outcomes: Children with sensory modulation disorders. *American Journal of Occupational Therapy, 54*, 36–43.
29. Colangelo, C. A., & Shea, M. (2008). A biomechanical frame of reference for positioning children for functioning. In P. Kramer & J. Hinojosa (Eds.), *Frames of reference for pediatric occupational therapy* (3rd ed., pp. 489–569). Philadelphia: Lippincott Williams & Wilkins.
30. Conroy, M. A., Boyd, B. A., Asmus, J. M., et al. (2007). A functional approach for ameliorating social skills deficits in young children with autism spectrum disorders. *Infants and Young Children, 20*, 242–254.
31. Coster, W., Bedell, G., Law, M., et al. (2011). Psychometric evaluation of the participation and environment measure for children and youth. *Developmental Medicine & Child Neurology, 53*, 103–107.
32. Coster, W., Law, M., Bedell, G., et al. (2012). Development of the participation and environment measures for children and youth: Conceptual basis. *Disability and Rehabilitation, 34*, 238–246.
33. Cooper, J. O., Heron, T. E., & Heward, W. L. (2007). *Applied behavior analysis*. Upper Saddle River, NJ: Pearson Merrill Prentice Hall.
34. Coster, W., Deeny, T., Haltiwanger, J., et al. (1998). *School Function Assessment*. San Antonio, TX: Psychological Corporation.
35. Cowan, R. J., & Allen, K. D. (2007). Using naturalistic procedures to enhance learning in individuals with autism: A focus on generalized teaching within the school setting. *Psychology in the Schools, 44*, 701–715.
36. Crepeau, E. B., & Schell, B. A. B. (2008). Analyzing occupations and activity. In E. B. Crepeau, E. S. Cohn, & B. A. B. Schell (Eds.), *Willard and Spackman's occupational therapy* (11th ed., pp. 359–374). Philadelphia: Lippincott Williams & Wilkins.
37. Csikszentmihalyi, M., & Csikszentmihalyi, I. S. (1988). *Optimal experience: Psychological studies in flow in consciousness*. Cambridge, UK: Cambridge University Press.
38. Csikszentmihalyi, M. (1997). *Finding flow: The psychology of engagement with everyday life*. New York: Basic Books.
39. Darrah, J., Law, M. C., Pollock, N., et al. (2011). Context therapy: A new intervention approach for children with cerebral palsy. *Developmental Medicine and Child Neurology, 53*, 615–620.
40. Dawson, G., Rogers, S., Munson, J., et al. (2010). Randomized, controlled trial of an intervention for toddlers with autism: The Early Start Denver Model. *Pediatrics, 125*, e17–e23.
41. DeGrace, B. W. (2003). Occupation-based and family centered care: A challenge for current practice. *American Journal of Occupational Therapy, 57*, 347–350.
42. Dieterle, C., Fanchiang, S., Farmer, M., et al. (2012). OT and diabetes: Understanding our role in chronic care management. American Occupational Therapy Association Annual Conference, Long Beach, CA, April 26, 2012.
43. Denton, P., Cope, S., & Moser, C. (2006). Effects of sensorimotor-based intervention versus therapeutic practice on improving handwriting performance in 6-to-11-year-old children. *American Journal of Occupational Therapy, 60*, 16–27.
44. Dreiling, D. S., & Bundy, A. C. (2003). Brief report—a comparison of consultative model and direct-indirect intervention with preschoolers. *American Journal of Occupational Therapy, 57*, 566–569.
45. Dunn, W., & Brown, C. (1997). Factor analysis on the sensory profile from a national sample of children without disabilities. *American Journal of Occupational Therapy, 51*, 490–495.
46. Dunn, W., Brown, C., & McGuigan, A. (1994). The ecology of human performance: A framework for considering the effect of context. *American Journal of Occupational Therapy, 48*, 595–607.
47. Dunn, W., Cox, J., Foster, L., et al. (2012). Impact of a contextual intervention on child participation and parent competence among children with autism spectrum disorders: A pretest-posttest repeated measures design. *American Journal of Occupational Therapy, 66*, 520–528.
48. Dunst, C. J. (2002). Family-centered practices: Birth through high school. *Journal of Special Education, 36*, 139–147.
49. Dunst, C. J., Trivette, C. M., & Hamby, D. W. (2007). Meta-analysis of family-centered helpgiving practices research. *Mental Retardation and Developmental Disabilities Research Reviews, 13*, 370–378.
50. Dunst, C. J., & Trivette, C. M. (2009). Capacity-building family systems intervention practices. *Journal of Family Social Work, 12*, 119–143.
51. Dunst, C. J., Trivette, C. M., Davis, M., et al. (1988). Enabling and empowering families of children with health impairments. *Children's Health Care: Journal of the Association for the Care of Children's Health, 17*, 71–81.
52. Dunst, C., Trivette, C., & Deal, A. (1994). *Supporting and strengthening families: Methods, strategies and practices*. Cambridge, MA: Brookline Books.
53. Dunton, W. R. (1919). *Reconstruction therapy*. Philadelphia: Saunders.
54. Engel-Yeger, B., Jarus, T., Anaby, D., et al. (2009). Differences in patterns of participation between youths with cerebral palsy and typically developing peer. *American Journal of Occupational Therapy, 63*, 96–104.
55. Epstein, M. (1999). The development and validation of a scale to assess the emotional and behavior strengths of children and adolescents. *Remedial and Special Education, 5*, 258–262.
56. Evans, J. L. (2002). Variability in comprehension strategy use in children with SLI: A dynamical systems account. *International Journal of Language and Communication Disorders, 37*(2), 95–116.
57. Evans, J., McDougall, J., & Baldwin, P. (2006). An evaluation of the "Youth En Route" program. *Physical and Occupational Therapy in Pediatrics, 26*, 63–87.
58. Fidler, G. S., & Fidler, J. W. (1978). Doing and becoming: Purposeful action and self-actualization. *American Journal of Occupational Therapy, 32*, 305–310.
59. Fisher, E. B., Strunk, R. C., Highstein, G. R., et al. (2009). A randomized controlled evaluation of the effects of community health workers on hospitalization for asthma: The

asthma coach. *Archives of Pediatric and Adolescent Medicine, 163*, 225–232.
60. Fogel, A. (2011). Theoretical and applied dynamic systems research in developmental science. *Child Development Perspectives, 5*, 267–272.
61. Gentile, A. M. (1998). Implicit and explicit processes during acquisition of functional skills. *Scandinavian Journal of Occupational Therapy, 5*, 7–16.
62. Gesell, A. (1945). *The embryology of behavior: the beginnings of the human mind.* New York: Harper & Brothers.
63. Gibson, E. (1988). Exploratory behavior in the development of perceiving, acting and acquiring of knowledge. *Annual Review of Psychology, 39*, 1–41.
64. Gibson, J. (1979). *The ecological approach to visual perception.* Boston: Houghton-Mifflin.
65. Gilfoyle, E. M., Grady, A. P., & Moore, J. C. (1990). *Children adapt* (2nd ed.). Thorofare, NJ: SLACK Inc.
66. Goldstein, H., Schneider, N., & Thiemann, K. (2007). Peer-mediated social communication intervention: When clinical expertise informs treatment development and evaluation. *Topics in Language Disorders, 27*, 182–199.
67. Greenspan, S. I., & Wieder, S. (1997). Developmental patterns and outcomes on infants and children with disorders of relating and communicating: A chart review of 200 cases of children with autistic spectrum diagnoses. *Journal of Developmental and Learning Disorders, 1*, 87–141.
68. Gutman, S. A., Raphael-Greenfield, R., & Rao, A. K. (2012). Effect of a motor-based role-play intervention on the social behaviors of adolescents with high-functioning autism: Multiple-baseline single-subject design. *American Journal of Occupational Therapy, 66*, 529–537.
69. Hanft, B. E., Rush, D. D., & Shelden, M. L. (2004). *Coaching families and colleagues in early intervention.* Baltimore, MD: Brookes Publishing.
70. Hiebert-Murphy, D., Trute, B., & Wright, A. (2011). Parents' definition of effective child disability support services: Implications for implementing family-centered practice. *Journal of Family Social Work, 14*, 144–158.
71. Hinojosa, J., & Segal, R. (2012). Build intervention from theory: From Legos and Tinkertoys to skyscrapers. In S. J. Lane & A. C. Bundy (Eds.), *Kids can be kids: A childhood occupations approach* (pp. 161–179). Philadelphia: F. A. Davis.
72. Hocking, C. (2011). Occupational science: A stock take of accumulated insights. *Journal of Occupational Science, 7*, 58–67.
73. Howle, J. M. (2002). *Neurodevelopmental treatment approach: Theoretical foundations and principles of clinical practice.* Laguna Beach, CA: Neuro-Developmental Treatment Association.
74. Humphry, R. (2002). Young children's occupations: Explicating the dynamics of developmental processes. *American Journal of Occupational Therapy, 56*, 171–179.
75. Humphry, R. (2009). Occupation and development: A contextual perspective. In E. B. Crepeau, E. S. Cohn, & B. A. B. Schell (Eds.), *Willard and Spackman's occupational therapy* (pp. 22–32). Philadelphia: Lippincott Williams & Wilkins.
76. Humphry, L., & Wakeford, L. (2006). An occupation-centered discussion of development and implications for practice. *American Journal of Occupational Therapy, 60*, 258–267.
77. Ingersoll, B., & Gergans, S. (2007). The effect of a parent-implemented imitation intervention on spontaneous imitation skills in young children with autism. *Research in Developmental Disabilities, 28*, 163–175.
78. Ingersoll, B. (2010). Pilot randomized controlled trial of Reciprocal Imitation Training for teaching elicited and spontaneous imitation to children with autism. *Journal of Autism and Developmental Disorders, 40*, 1154–1160.
79. Kasari, C., Rotheram-Fuller, E., Locke, J., et al. (2012). Making the connection: Randomized controlled trial of social skills at school for children with autism spectrum disorders. *Journal of Child Psychology and Psychiatry, 53*, 431–439.
80. Ketelaar, M., Vermeer, A., Hart, H., et al. (2001). Effects of a functional therapy program on motor abilities of children with cerebral palsy. *Physical Therapy, 81*, 1534–1545.
81. Kids Health, The Children's Hospital at Westmead. (n.d.). Pressure ulcers. At: <http://kidshealth.schn.health.nsw.gov.au/fact-sheets/pressure-ulcers> Retrieved on January 4, 2014.
82. Kielhofner, G., & Burke, J. (1980). A model of human occupation. Part 1. Conceptual framework and content. *American Journal of Occupational Therapy, 34*, 572–581.
83. King, G., King, S., Rosenbaum, P., et al. (1999). Family-centred care-giving and wellbeing of parents of children with disabilities: Linking process with outcome. *Journal of Pediatric Psychology, 24*, 41–53.
84. Kinnealey, M., Koenig, K. P., & Shoener, R. F. (2008). You can know me now if you listen: Sensory, motor, and communication issues in a nonverbal person with autism. *American Journal of Occupational Therapy, 72*, 547–553.
85. Koegel, R., Koegel, L. K., & Brookman, L. I., 2003). Empirically supported pivotal response interventions for children with autism. In A. E. Kazdin (Ed.), *Evidence-based psychotherapies for children and adolescents* (pp. 241–257). New York: Guilford Press. Yale University School of Medicine and Child Study Center.
86. Koegel, R. L., & Koegel, L. K. (2006). *Pivotal response treatment for autism: Communication, social, and academic development.* Baltimore, MD: Brookes.
87. Koegel, R. L., Koegel, L. K., & Carter, C. M. (1999). Pivotal teaching interactions for children with autism. *School Psychology Review, 28*, 576–594.
88. Kopp, C. B. (2009). Emotion-focused coping in young children. Self and self-regulatory processes. In E. A. Skinner & M. J. Zimmer-Gembeck (Eds.), *Coping and the development of regulation* (Vol. 124, pp. 33–46). San Francisco: New Directions for Child and Adolescent Development.
89. Kramer, P., & Hinojosa, J. (2008). *Frames of reference for pediatric occupational therapy* (3rd ed.). Philadelphia: Lippincott Williams & Wilkins.
90. Laugeson, E. A., Frankel, R., Gantman, A., et al. (2012). Evidence-based social skills training for adolescents with autism spectrum disorders: The UCLA PEERS program. *Journal of Autism and Developmental Disorders, 42*, 1025–1036.
91. Law, M. (2002). Participation in the occupations of everyday life. *American Journal of Occupational Therapy, 56*, 640–649.
92. Law, M., Cadman, D., Rosenbaum, P., et al. (1991). Neurodevelopmental therapy and upper extremity casting: Results of a clinical trial. *Developmental Medicine and Child Neurology, 33*, 334–340.
93. Law, M., Cooper, B., Strong, S., et al. (1996). The person-environment-occupation model: A transactive approach to occupational performance. *Canadian Journal of Occupational Therapy, 63*(1), 9–23.
94. Law, M., Hanna, S., King, G., et al. (2003). Factors affecting family-centred service delivery for children with disabilities. *Child: Care, Health and Development, 29*, 41–53.
95. Law, M., King, G., Kind, S., et al. (2006). Patterns of participation in

recreation and leisure activities among children with complex physical disabilities. *Developmental Medicine and Child Neurology, 48,* 337–342.

96. Law, M., Petrenshik, T., King, G., et al. (2007). Perceived environmental barriers to recreational, community, and school participation for children and youth with physical disabilities. *Archives of Physical Medicine and Rehabilitation, 88,* 1636–1642.
97. Law, M. C., Darrah, J., Pollock, N., et al. (2011). Focus on function: A cluster, randomized controlled trial comparing child- versus context-focused intervention for young children with cerebral palsy. *Developmental Medicine and Child Neurology, 53,* 621–629.
98. Liptak, G. S., Kennedy, J. A., & Dosa, N. P. (2011). Social participation in a nationally representative sample of older youth and young adults with autism. *Journal of Developmental and Behavioral Pediatrics, 32,* 277–283.
99. Llorens, L. A. (1991). Performance tasks and roles throughout the life span. In C. Christiansen & C. Baum (Eds.), *Occupational therapy: Overcoming human performance deficits* (pp. 45–68). Thorofare, NJ: SLACK Inc.
100. Lollar, D. J., & Simeonsson, R. J. (2005). Diagnosis to function: Classification for children and youths. *Developmental and Behavioral Pediatrics, 26,* 323–330.
101. Luria, A. R. (1961). *The role of speech in the regulation of normal and abnormal behaviors.* New York: Liveright.
102. Luthar, S. S. (2006). Resilience in development: A synthesis of research across five decades. In D. Cicchetti & D. Cohen (Eds.), *Developmental psychopathology: Risk, disorder, and adaptation* (2nd ed., Vol. 3, pp. 739–795). Hoboken, NJ: John Wiley & Sons, Inc.
103. Ma, H., Trombly, C. A., & Robinson-Podolski, C. (1999). The effect of context on skill acquisition and transfer. *American Journal of Occupational Therapy, 53,* 138–144.
104. Ma, H. I., & Trombly, C. A. (2001). The comparison of motor performance between part and whole tasks in elderly persons. *American Journal of Occupational Therapy, 55,* 62–67.
105. Maher, C. A., Williams, M. T., Olds, T., et al. (2007). Physical and sedentary activity in adolescents with cerebral palsy. *Developmental Medicine and Child Neurology, 29,* 450–457.
106. Mahoney, G., & Bella, J. M. (1998). An examination of the effects of family-centered early intervention on child and family outcomes. *Topics in Early Childhood Special Education, 18,* 83–94.
107. Mahoney, G., & Perales, F. (2005). Relationship-focused early intervention with children with pervasive developmental disorders and other disabilities: A comparative study. *Developmental and Behavioral Pediatrics, 26,* 77–85.
108. Majnemer, A., Shevell, M., Law, M., et al. (2008). Participation and enjoyment of leisure activities in school-aged children with cerebral palsy. *Developmental Medicine and Child Neurology, 50,* 751–758.
109. Mandich, A. D., Polatajko, H., Missiuna, C., et al. (2001). Cognitive strategies and motor performance in children with developmental coordination disorder. *Physical and Occupational Therapy in Pediatrics, 20*(2–3), 125–143.
110. Mayo, N. E. (1991). The effect of physical therapy for children with motor delay and cerebral palsy. *American Journal of Physical Medicine and Rehabilitation, 70,* 258–267.
111. McColl, M., Law, M., Stewart, D., et al. (2003). *Theoretical basis of occupational therapy* (2nd ed.). Thorofare, NJ: SLACK Inc.
112. Meichenbaum, D. (1977). *Cognitive-behavior modification: An integrative approach.* New York: Plenum Press.
113. Meyer, A. (1922). The philosophy of occupational therapy. *Archives of Occupational Therapy, 1,* 1–10.
114. Miller, L. J., Coll, J. R., & Schoen, S. A. (2007). A randomized controlled pilot study of the effectiveness of occupational therapy for children with sensory modulation disorder. *American Journal of Occupational Therapy, 61,* 228–238.
115. Miller, L., Polatajko, H., Missiuna, C., et al. (2001). A pilot trial of a cognitive treatment for children with developmental coordination disorder. *Human Movement Science, 20,* 183–210.
116. Miller-Kuhaneck, H., Henry, D., & Glennon, T. (2007). *Sensory Processing Measure.* San Antonio, TX: Therapy Skill Builders.
117. Missiuna, C., DeMatteo, C., Hanna, S., et al. (2010). Exploring the use of cognitive intervention for children with acquired brain injury. *Physical and Occupational Therapy in Pediatrics, 30*(3), 205–219.
118. Missiuna, C., Malloy-Miller, T., & Mandich, A. (1998). Mediational techniques: Origins and application to occupational therapy in pediatrics. *Canadian Journal of Occupational Therapy, 65,* 202–209.
119. Missiuna, C., Mandich, A., Polatajko, P., et al. (2001). Cognitive orientation to daily occupational performance (CO-OP). Part 1. Theoretical foundations. *Physical and Occupational Therapy in Pediatrics, 20*(2–3), 69–81.
120. Missiuna, C., & Pollock, N. (2000). Perceived efficacy and goal setting in young children. *Canadian Journal of Occupational Therapy, 67,* 101–109.
121. Mosey, A. C. (1970). *Three frames of reference for mental health.* Thorofare, NJ: SLACK Inc.
122. Mullick, J. A. (2006). Positive behavior support and applied behavior analysis. *Behavior Analyst, 29,* 51–74.
123. Nelson, K. A., Highstein, G., Garbutt, J., et al. (2012). Factors associated with attaining coaching goals during an intervention to improve child asthma care. *Contemporary Clinical Trial, 33,* 912–919.
124. Nicholson, D. E. (1996). Motor learning. In C. M. Fredericks & L. K. Saladin (Eds.), *Pathophysiology of the motor systems: Principles and clinical presentations* (pp. 238–254). Philadelphia: F. A. Davis.
125. Novak, I., McIntyre, S., Morgan, C., et al. (2013). A systematic review of interventions for children with cerebral palsy: State of the evidence. *Developmental Medicine & Child Neurology, 55,* 885–910.
126. Nudo, R. J. (2006). Plasticity. *NeuroRx: The Journal of the American Society for Experimental NeuroTherapeutics, 3,* 420–427.
127. Ormrod, J. E. (2006). *Educational psychology: Developing learners* (5th ed.). Upper Saddle River, NJ: Prentice Hall.
128. Orsmond, G. I., Shattuck, P. T., Cooper, B. P., et al. (2013). Social participation among young adults with an autism spectrum disorder. *Journal of Autism and Development Disorders, 43,* 2710–2719.
129. Palisano, R. J., Copeland, W. P., & Galuppi, B. E. (2007). Performance of physical activities by adolescents with cerebral palsy. *Physical Therapy, 87,* 77–87.
130. Palisano, R. J., Orlin, M., Chiarello, L. A., et al. (2011). Determinants of intensity of participation in leisure and recreational activities by youth with cerebral palsy. *Archives of Physical Medicine and Rehabilitation, 92,* 1468–1476.
131. Palmer, F. B., Shapiro, B. K., Wachtal, R. C., et al. (1988). The effects of physical therapy on cerebral palsy: A controlled trial in infants with spastic diplegia. *New England Journal of Medicine, 318,* 903–908.
132. Parham, L. D., Cohn, E. S., Spitzer, S., et al. (2007). Fidelity in sensory integration intervention research. *American Journal of Occupational Therapy, 61,* 216–227.

133. Parham, L. D., Roley, S. S., May-Benson, T. A., et al. (2011). Development of a fidelity measure for research on the effectiveness of the Ayres sensory integration intervention. *American Journal of Occupational Therapy, 65*, 133–142.
134. Pfeiffer, E., Koenig, K., Kinnealey, M., et al. (2011). Effectiveness of sensory integration interventions in children with autism spectrum disorders: A pilot study. *American Journal of Occupational Therapy, 65*, 78–85.
135. Piper, M. C. (1990). Efficacy of physical therapy: Rate of motor development in children with cerebral palsy. *Pediatric Physical Therapy, 2*, 126–130.
136. Piper, M. C., & Darrah, J. (1994). *Motor assessment of the developing infant.* Philadelphia: Saunders.
137. Polatajko, H. J., Mandich, A. D., Miller, L. T., et al. (2001). Cognitive orientation to daily occupational performance (CO-OP). Part 2. The evidence. *Physical and Occupational Therapy in Pediatrics, 20*(2–3), 83–106.
138. Polatajko, H. J., Mandich, A. D., Missiuna, C., et al. (2001). Cognitive orientation to daily occupational performance (CO-OP). Part 3. The protocol in brief. *Physical and Occupational Therapy in Pediatrics, 20*(2–3), 107–123.
139. Prochaska, J. O. (1994). Strong and weak principles for progressing from precontemplation to action based on twelve problem behaviors. *Health Psychology, 13*, 47–51.
140. Reilly, M. (1969). The educational process. *American Journal of Occupational Therapy, 23*, 299–307.
141. Reilly, M. (1974). *Play as exploratory learning.* Beverly Hills, CA: Sage Publications.
142. Reilly, M. (1974). Occupational behavior: A perspective on work and play. *American Journal of Occupational Therapy, 25*, 291–296.
143. Reynolds, S., Lane, S., & Thacker, L. (2012). Sensory processing, physiological stress, and sleep behaviors in children with and without autism spectrum disorders. *OTJR: Occupation, Participation and Health, 32*, 246–257.
144. Rimm-Kaufman, S. E., & Sawyer, B. E. (2004). Primary-grade teachers' self-efficacy beliefs, attitudes toward teaching and discipline and teaching practice priorities in relation to the "Responsive Classroom" approach. *The Elementary School Journal, 104*, 321–241.
145. Rogers, J. C., & Holm, M. B. (2009). The occupational therapy process. In E. B. Crepeau, E. S. Cohn, & B. A. B. Schell (Eds.), *Willard and Spackman's occupational therapy* (pp. 22–32). Philadelphia: Lippincott Williams & Wilkins.
146. Rogers, S., & DiLalla, D. (1991). A comparative study of the effects of a developmentally based instructional model on young children with autism and young children with other disorders of behavior and development. *Topics in Early Childhood Special Education, 11*, 29–48.
147. Rodger, S., Ireland, S., & Vun, M. (2008). Can Cognitive Orientation to daily Occupational Performance (CO-OP) help children with Asperger's syndrome to master social and organizational goals? *British Journal of Occupational Therapy, 71*(1), 23–32.
148. Rogers, S. J., Estes, A., Lord, C., et al. (2012). Effects of a brief Early Start Denver Model (ESDM)–based parent intervention on toddlers at risk for autism spectrum disorders: A randomized controlled trial. *Journal of the American Academy of Child and Adolescent Psychiatry, 51*, 1052–1065.
149. Rosenbaum, P., King, S., Law, M., et al. (1998). Family-centred service: A conceptual framework and research review. *Physical and Occupational Therapy in Pediatrics, 18*, 1–20.
150. Ryan, R. M., & Deci, E. L. (2000). Self-determination theory and the facilitation of intrinsic motivation, social development and well-being. *American Psychologist, 55*, 68–78.
151. Schaaf, R. C., & Nightlinger, K. M. (2007). Occupational therapy using a sensory integrative approach: A case study of effectiveness. *American Journal of Occupational Therapy, 61*, 239–246.
152. Schaaf, R., Benevides, T., Mailloux, Z., et al. (2013). Occupational therapy using sensory integration for children with autism: A randomized trial. *Journal of Autism and Developmental Disorders*, doi:10.1007/s10803-013-1983-8.
153. Schertz, M., & Gordon, A. M. (2009). Changing the model: A call for a re-examination of intervention approaches and translational research in children with developmental disabilities. *Developmental Medicine and Child Neurology, 51*, 6–7.
154. Scherzer, A. L., Mike, V., & Ilson, J. (1976). Physical therapy as a determinant of change in the cerebral palsied infant. *Pediatrics, 53*, 47–52.
155. Schmidt, R. A. (1988). *Motor control and learning: A behavioral emphasis.* Champaign, IL: Human Kinetics.
156. Shikako-Thomas, K., Shevell, M., Lach, L., et al. (2013). Picture me playing—a portrait of participation and enjoyment of leisure activities in adolescents with cerebral palsy. *Research in Developmental Disabilities, 34*, 1001–1010.
157. Shikako-Thomas, K., Majnemer, A., Law, M., et al. (2008). Determinants of participation in leisure activities in children and youth with cerebral palsy: Systematic review. *Physical and Occupational Therapy in Pediatrics, 28*, 155–170.
158. Shumway-Cook, A., & Woollacott, M. H. (2011). *Motor control: Translating research into clinical practice* (4th ed.). Baltimore: Lippincott Williams & Wilkins.
159. Skinner, B. F. (1953). *Science and human behavior.* New York: Free Press.
160. Skinner, B. F. (1976). *Walden two.* New York: Macmillan.
161. Slagle, E. C. (1922). Training aides for mental patients. *Archives of Occupational Therapy, 1*, 11–17.
162. Stewart, D., & Law, M. (2003). The environment: Paradigms and practice in health, occupational therapy and inquiry. In L. Letts, P. Rigby, & D. Stewart (Eds.), *Using environments to enable occupational performance* (pp. 3–15). Thorofare, NJ: SLACK, Inc.
163. Sugden, D. A., & Sugden, L. (1990). *The assessment and management of movement skill problems.* Leeds, UK: School of Education.
164. Sullivan, K. J., Kantak, S. S., & Burtner, P. A. (2008). Motor learning in children: Feedback effects on skills acquisition. *Physical Therapy, 88*, 720–732.
165. Thelen, E. (1995). Motor development: A new synthesis. *American Psychologist, 50*(2), 79–95.
166. Thelen, E. (2005). Dynamic systems theory and the complexity of change. *Psychoanalytic Dialogues, 15*, 255–283.
167. Thelen, E., Schoner, G., Scheier, C., et al. (2001). The dynamics of embodiment: A field theory of infant preservative reaching. *Behavioral and Brain Sciences, 24*, 1–86.
168. Thelen, E., & Spencer, J. P. (1998). Postural control during reaching in young infants: A dynamic systems approach. *Neuroscience and Behavioral Reviews, 22*, 507–514.
169. Timmer, S. G., Zebell, N. M., Culver, M. A., et al. (2010). Efficacy of adjunct in home coaching to improve outcomes in parent-child interaction therapy. *Research on Social Work Practice, 20*, 36–45.
170. Tomchek, S. D., & Dunn, W. (2007). Sensory processing in children with and without autism: A comparative study using the Short Sensory Profile. *American Journal of Occupational Therapy, 61*, 190–200.

171. Twachtman-Reilly, J., Amaral, S. C., & Zebrowski, P. P. (2008). Addressing feeding disorders in children on the autism spectrum in school-based settings: Physiological and behavioral issues. *Language, Speech, and Hearing Services in Schools*, *39*, 261–272.
172. Vanderbilt-Adriance, E., & Shaw, D. S. (2008). Conceptualizing and re-evaluating resilience across levels of risk, time, and domains of competence. *Clinical Child and Family Psychology Review*, *11*, 30–58.
173. Van Gelder, T. (1995). What might cognition be, if not computation? *Journal of Philosophy*, *91*, 345–381.
174. VanSant, A. F. (1991). Neurodevelopmental treatment and pediatric physical therapy: A commentary. *Pediatric Physical Therapy*, *3*, 137–141.
175. Vargas, S., & Camilli, G. (1999). A meta-analysis of research on sensory integration treatment. *American Journal of Occupational Therapy*, *53*, 180–198.
176. Verschuren, O., Wiart, L., Hermans, D., et al. (2012). Identification of facilitators and barriers to physical activity in children and adolescents with cerebral palsy. *Journal of Pediatrics*, *161*, 488–494.
177. Vismara, L. A., & Rogers, S. J. (2008). Treating autism in the first year of life: A case study of the Early Start Denver Model. *Journal of Early Intervention*, *31*, 91–108.
178. Vygotsky, L. S. (1978). *Mind in society: The development of higher mental processes.* Cambridge, MA: Harvard University Press.
179. Wallander, J., & Varni, J. (1989). Social support and adjustment in chronically ill and handicapped children. *American Journal of Community Psychology*, *17*(2), 185–201.
180. Ward, A., & Rodger, S. (2004). The application of Cognitive Orientation to daily Occupational Performance (CO-OP) with children 5-7 years with developmental coordination disorder. *British Journal of Occupational Therapy*, *67*(6), 256–264.
181. Watling, R., Deitz, J., Kanny, E. M., et al. (1999). Current practice of occupational therapy for children with autism. *American Journal of Occupational Therapy*, *53*, 498–505.
182. Werner, E. E. (1989). High-risk children in young adulthood: A longitudinal study from birth to 32 years. *American Journal of Orthopsychiatry*, *59*, 72–81.
183. Werner, E. E. (1994). Overcoming the odds. *Developmental and Behavioral Pediatrics*, *15*, 131–136.
184. Wilcock, A. A. (1993). A theory of human need for occupation. *Occupational Science: Australia*, *1*, 17–24.
185. Wilcock, A. A. (1998). Reflections on doing, being, becoming. *Canadian Journal of Occupational Therapy*, *65*, 248–256.
186. Wilcock, A. A. (2001). Occupational science: The key to broadening horizons. *British Journal of Occupational Therapy*, *64*, 412–417.
187. Wilcock, A. A., & Townsend, E. (2008). Occupational justice. In E. B. Crepeau, W. S. Cohn, & B. B. Schell (Eds.), *Willard and Spackman's occupational therapy* (11th ed., pp. 192–199). Baltimore, MD: Lippincott Williams & Wilkins.
188. Wilkinson, L. (2008). Self-management for children with high-functioning autism spectrum disorder. *Intervention in School and Clinic*, *43*, 150–157.
189. Williams, M. S., & Shellenberger, S. (1994). *How does your engine run? A leader's guide to the alert program for self-regulation.* Albuquerque, NM: Therapy Works.
190. Williamson, G., & Szczepanski, M. (1999). Coping frame of reference. In P. Kramer & J. Hinojosa (Eds.), *Frames of reference in pediatric occupational therapy* (pp. 431–465). Baltimore, MD: Williams & Wilkins.
191. Winstein, C. J., & Schmidt, R. A. (1990). Reduced frequency of knowledge of results enhances motor skills learning. *Journal of Experimental Psychology. Learning, Memory, and Cognition*, *16*, 677–691.
192. Winstein, C. J., Merians, A. S., & Sullivan, K. J. (1999). Motor learning after unilateral brain damage. *Neuropsychologia*, *37*, 975–987.
193. World Health Organization (2001). *International Classification of Functioning, Disability and Health.* Geneva: Author.
194. Yerxa, E. J., Clark, F., Frank, G., et al. (1989). Occupational science: The foundation for new models of practice. *Occupational Therapy in Health Care*, *6*, 1–17.
195. Zeitlin, S., & Williamson, G. G. (1994). *Coping in young children: Early intervention practices to enhance adaptive behavior and resilience.* Baltimore, MD: Brookes.
196. Zwicker, J. G., & Harris, S. R. (2009). A reflection on motor learning theory in pediatric occupational therapy practice. *Canadian Journal of Occupational Therapy*, *76*, 29–37.

CHAPTER

3 Development of Childhood Occupations

Jane Case-Smith

KEY TERMS

Stages of cognitive development
Zone of proximal development
Scaffolding
Neuromaturational theory
Dynamical systems theory
Perceptual-action coupling
Functional synergies
Temperament
Attachment
Emotion regulation
Risk and resiliency
Self-determination and self-efficacy
Cultural practices
Occupations within cultural, social, and physical contexts
Development of play occupations

GUIDING QUESTIONS

1. What are historical and current theories of child development?
2. How do a child's unique characteristics influence skill development?
3. Using an occupational therapy perspective, how do occupations develop?
4. How do individual biologic systems and cultural, social, and physical contexts contribute to a child's occupational performance in the first 10 years of life?
5. How do child performance and contextual variables contribute to the development of play?

An understanding of child development is foundational knowledge for pediatric occupational therapists. Researchers from many disciplines, including medicine, psychology, anthropology, education, sociology, and occupational therapy, have contributed to the literature on human development, and the different perspectives they provide should be woven into a holistic and comprehensive understanding of how children become adults.

Occupational therapists ask *what* developmental changes occur in children and *how* children develop their unique personhood. The answers to these questions provide essential knowledge for evaluating children and for determining the appropriate materials, activities, and environments to support children's skill development and participation in their communities. They are also interested in how human occupations develop over the life span.

This chapter focuses on child development theories, with emphasis on concepts that have emerged in the past 3 decades. The first section discusses concepts that explain how children develop and which variables and interactions influence developmental outcomes. In the second part of the chapter, a model for the development of childhood occupations is applied to children's development of play in the first 10 years of life. Chapter 4 describes the development of preadolescent and adolescent occupations in the second decade of life.

Developmental Theories and Concepts

Developmental theories have guided education and therapy for children with developmental disorders for the past 60 years. Researchers of the 1930s and 1940s identified a sequence of skill maturation that defined the steps of normal development. Gesell and colleagues[52-54] and McGraw[96] assumed that normal development followed a specific skill sequence that reflected maturation of the central nervous system (CNS). These scholars believed that the sequence of motor, cognitive, social-emotional, and language skill development was relatively unaffected by the infant's experiences. The sequence of normal development is an important frame of reference for creating developmental assessment tools that identify children with disabilities. Gesell and Amatruda[53] believed that variations in the normal sequence of development indicate CNS dysfunction. Identifying children with developmental deficits or significant delays remains an important role of physicians, nurses, occupational therapists, and others who provide early intervention services. Since the 1940s, theories of child development have evolved from observational and longitudinal research that identify the stages of child development and define key developmental milestones to studies that reveal the complexity of child development as it relates to cultural, physical, and social environments. This section describes theories that relate primarily to (1) cognitive development, (2) motor development, (3) social-emotional development, (4) self-identity and self-determination development, and (5) ecologic models.

Cognitive Development

In contrast to the first theories of child development that proposed a predetermined step-by-step process,[9,53] scholars and researchers in the twentieth century understood that child development was influenced by the child's cultural, social, and physical contexts. They explained that development can be represented by a pyramid, meaning that new skills are built on foundational abilities.[62,109] The concept of a pyramid suggested that each new stage builds on specific foundational skills. Children move between more advanced or more primitive behaviors in different contexts, and new behaviors depend on not only neurologic maturation but also the demands, challenges, supports, and learning opportunities in the environment.[81]

Interplay of Intrinsic and Environmental Factors

One of the first scholars to describe this interactive nature of cognitive development was Jean Piaget. Piaget[109] expanded our understanding of a child's maturation by emphasizing that development occurs through the interaction between the environment and the child's innate abilities. Children adapt and grow developmentally through social and physical relationships. Piaget[109] introduced the idea that children are intrinsically motivated to learn from their surroundings and that they act on, rather than simply react to, their environment. Beginning in infancy, children develop *cognitive structures,* or *schemas,* to represent objects, events, and relationships in their minds.[98] Piaget emphasized the maturation of cognitive structures that enable the child to understand the environment, language, and social action. Every interaction is an opportunity either to assimilate new knowledge into existing structures or to adapt existing structures to accommodate new information. The influence of the environment on the child's development changes as the child becomes increasingly able to assimilate the complexities of physical and social events.

Piaget documented the child's maturation through stages of sensorimotor exploration to the acquisition of symbolic thought and formal cognitive operations. The developmental stages follow a predictable sequence but vary to the extent that they reflect genetic endowment and the child's experiences. Children's cognition matures from the simple to the complex, from the concrete to the abstract, and from personal to worldly concerns. Piaget specified four maturational levels or periods of cognitive function—sensorimotor, preoperational, concrete operational, and formal operational[46,86,97,98]—that lead to the cognitive maturity of adulthood. Through these stages, children develop mental representations of the world that they use to understand and respond to events. The culmination of these levels is a person who has values, goals, and purpose (i.e., has become an occupational being). At the present time, most child researchers agree that the child is an active learner but do not view development in discrete stages.

This interplay between the child's abilities and his or her experience can be appreciated in the early development of tool use. Children at 8 to 10 months of age can manipulate two objects and can move an obstacle to reach an interesting or novel object (sensorimotor stage). By 12 months, infants can relate an object to other objects, in addition to relating the objects to themselves. At this stage, infants use a stick to rake in an object out of reach and place objects into containers (sensorimotor). By 18 months of age, infants begin to use trial-and-error to solve problems (preoperational). At 24 months of age, children no longer exclusively need physical manipulation to solve problems and begin to demonstrate use of mental manipulation (preoperational).[96,110,111]

Research studies in the 1990s demonstrated that cognitive structures develop at earlier ages than Piaget assumed; they also demonstrated that child development has more continuity and integration across the stages of development.[21,46] At 1 month of age, infants demonstrate the ability to associate learning from one sensory system with another sensory system. For example, they recognize objects with their eyes that they previously felt in their mouths.[93] Researchers found that 9-month-old infants can remember an event 1 week after it happened.[99]

Problem solving also appears to develop earlier than believed; developmental studies show that toddlers can manipulate and use tools and can solve problems such as how to grasp and use a spoon. After grasping a spoon awkwardly, children 9 to 14 months old can adjust the spoon's orientation to get the food into the mouth.[96] Children 19 months old can plan how to grasp and orient the spoon to get the food before acting, avoiding the use of an awkward grasp that required adjusting. At 19 months of age, children can solve problems without physical manipulation and trial-and-error to handle a tool accurately. By this age, the child can scoop food, fill the spoon, and correctly angle it toward the mouth,[71] signifying the early emergence of tool use.

Scholars have critiqued and expanded Piaget's original theories to appreciate fully how the environment influences development. For example, Piaget's theories lack full appreciation of the influence of culture, society, and technology on development of children. Current occupational therapy theories consider these variables to have important roles in a child's development.[11,150] In addition, Piaget's theories did not address the development of emotions and did not have a coherent explanation for individual differences, individuality, or variability.[46,97] The importance of variability has been highlighted in the work of other psychologists[133,136] and by occupational therapy researchers.[74]

An understanding of Piaget's theory is important to occupational therapists who provide interventions for children. Regardless of the therapeutic approach used in treatment, the occupational therapist interacts with a thinking child who is continually learning from his or her environment. It is essential that the selection and structure of an activity be in accordance with the child's cognitive development.

Influence of Social Interaction on Learning

Following Piaget, another developmental theorist, Vygotsky,[143] proposed new concepts that explained how children learn through interacting with their environment. Similar to his predecessors (e.g., Gesell, Piaget), he understood that genetics has unequivocal influence on development; however, Vygotsky theorized that the child develops by internalizing the social interactions that he experiences. Social interaction has a fundamental influence on the child's development of cognition and language. A child's cognitive processing first requires the assistance of another being within a social interaction before the child can mentally process on his or her own. Cognitive processing is a social process before it is an internal process, and a child's development and learning are critically dependent on social interaction. Learning is essentially culturally determined, and culturally valued activities are the context of a child's development.[143]

Vygotsky defined a "*zone of proximal development*" to explain how learning occurs through social interaction. The zone of proximal development is "the distance between the actual developmental level as determined by independent problem solving and the level of potential development as determined through problem solving under adult guidance or collaboration with more capable peers" (p. 86).[143] What a child can achieve and learn with the assistance of another is the zone of proximal development and defines the area in which adults can work with the child to promote the child's development and independence in a particular skill.[143] What children can do with the assistance of others may be more indicative of their mental development than what they could do independently. When presented with a *just-right* challenge (e.g., a task that is slightly more difficult than the tasks the child has currently mastered), the child generally attempts and succeeds in this challenge, learning the next step in skill development.

The mechanism through which children learn in social interaction is termed *scaffolding*—the support provided by caregivers and teachers. Scaffolding performance within the child's zone of proximal development is the process by which an occupational therapist supports or guides a child's actions to improve competence. Appropriate guidance is the just right amount of support that enables the child to perform at a higher level. When using scaffolding to facilitate the child's learning, the adult gradually decreases the amount of support provided such that the child performs more independently. Through this process, actions that are externally supported become internalized. The child's help-seeking in an activity can be as important to his learning as receiving assistance By asking questions and help-seeking, the child becomes more self-directed in his learning; he also develops an understanding about his own learning and how to direct social interactions that can lead to his learning. When the occupational therapist understands a child's zone of proximal development and perceives methods for scaffolding his learning, the therapist can design an optimal activity to promote the child's learning.

When an adult creates a learning opportunity that is an optimal balance between the child's existing skills and the challenge of the task, the adult can model language and behavior to help the child progress. Vygotsky's emphasis on the interactions between a child's learning, his or her environment, and the type of instruction provided was a precursor to many of the system models that influence learning theory today.

Vygotsky and many subsequent developmental theorists have examined how human development transpires through a dynamic interplay involving the child and the child's cultural, social, and physical environments. For example, rates of development appear different according to the family's economic status,[16,89] cultural groups, and generations,[16] in part because of differences in nutrition and childcare practices. In human development research, the emphasis currently is on the variations expressed by individual infants and on how human systems and environmental constraints contribute to these variations.

Motor Development

Neuromaturation

In neuromaturational theory, the essential sequence in which children attain developmental milestones is linear and consistent across children. Skills emerge sequentially according to the maturation of CNS structures.[41,100] Brainstem structures develop first, as evidenced by the reflexive responses of the newborn (e.g., automatic grasp, asymmetric tonic neck reflex) that are controlled by neural pathways originating in the brainstem. Cortical structures appear to develop later, as evidenced by the coordinated and planned actions of the child. The infant's increasing control of action and skill indicates not only development and myelination of the midbrain and cortical structures but also simultaneous inhibition of brainstem control of movement. Using neuromaturational theory, motor development is explained by the following principles:

1. Movement progresses from primitive reflex patterns to voluntary, controlled movement. In newborn and young infants, motor reflexes provide the first methods of interaction with the environment (e.g., reflexive grasp) and are essential to life (e.g., the sucking and swallowing reflexes). Because early reflexive movements serve functional needs, the newborn appears surprisingly competent. These reflex patterns subside as balance, postural reactions, and voluntary motor control emerge (i.e., when the infant learns to roll, sit, creep, stand, and walk).
2. The sequence and rate of motor development are consistent among infants and children. The developmental scales of Gesell and Amatruda,[53,75,76] Bayley,[10] and others are based on a typical rate and sequence of development. By assuming that the sequence of milestones (i.e., major motor accomplishments) is constant and predictable, the normative developmental sequence can be used to diagnose neurologic impairment and disability.[10]
3. Low-level skills are prerequisites for certain high-level skills. Infants develop motor control in a cephalocaudal direction, with head control maturing first, followed by trunk control sufficient for independent sitting, and, finally, pelvic control sufficient for standing and walking (Figure 3-1).

In assuming a hierarchy of CNS function, the neuromaturational theory limits our understanding of how a child learns

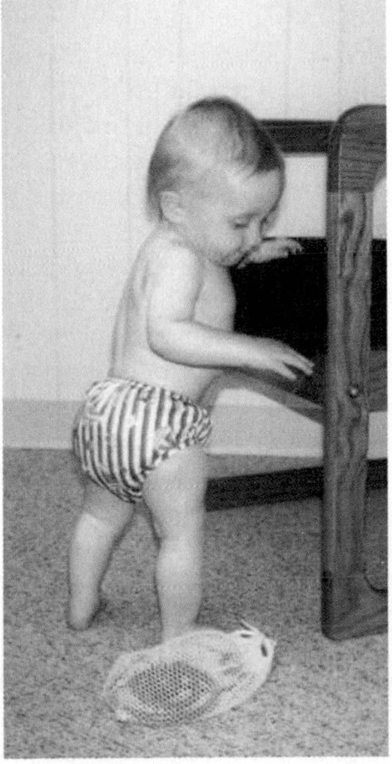

FIGURE 3-1 Infants play in supported standing for extended periods, gaining postural stability and balance when holding onto a stable surface.

to act in the environment. It particular, this theory does not explain how children learn new motor skills and ignores that the CNS has vast plasticity that allows humans to adapt to their environments. Gottlieb[63] defines plasticity as a fusion of the child and the environment. Through both experience and development, new structures (e.g., cellular) and functions (e.g., performance) emerge. The child's experiences produce new neurologic connections and structural changes, and development of the relationships among components is important. Acknowledgment of the system's plasticity places the focus on the child's potential for change and on the contextual features that promote or limit a child's performance. Using current research models,[58,60,133,134] occupational therapists and others recognize that multiple variables at different levels influence the child's skill development. The child learns occupations through interaction with his or her environment rather than through the emergence of a predetermined scenario reflecting neuromaturational principles.[72]

Dynamical Systems Theory

Dynamical systems theory refers to performance or action patterns that emerge from the interaction and cooperation of many systems, both internal and external to the child.[134] In the context of child development, performance patterns emerge from the interaction of an individual's systems and performance contexts as the child strives to achieve a functional goal.[94,95,103] The dynamical systems theory is useful in describing how specific motor and process skills develop.

Humans are complex biologic systems comprising many subsystems (e.g., motor sensory, perceptual, skeletal, and psychological subsystems). These subsystems are in constant flux, interacting according to the task at hand and conditions in the environment. The child's actions during the performance of a task are the result of the subsystems' interaction with each other and with the environment.[130] These individual systems come together and self-organize in a coordinated way to achieve the child's goal.[131] For example, initially a child is interested in exploring the sensory characteristics of a toy. As the child reaches for the toy, grasps it, and brings it to midline in hand-to-hand play and then finally to the mouth, the child's attention and cognitive focus are not on planning each of these actions. Instead, they are on assimilating the toy's actions and perceptual features (Figure 3-2).

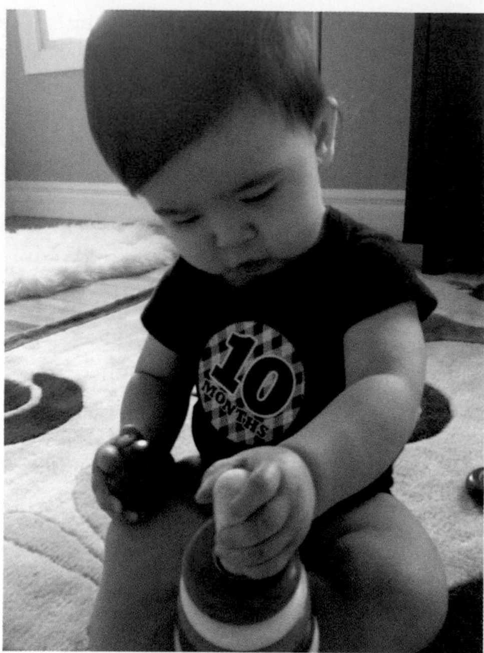

FIGURE 3-2 The infant explores a toy, assimilating its action and perceptual features.

Longitudinal studies reveal that children demonstrate unique trajectories of development and that variations in functional performance among children persist into adulthood. Thelen, Corbetta, and Spencer[135] demonstrated the uniqueness of motor development in a study of reaching in 4- and 5-month-old infants. Each 5-month-old infant was able to reach toward an object, but the patterns demonstrated were unique. Some infants demonstrated a slow, cautious first approach to the object, whereas others made ballistic arm movements in an attempt to reach it. Although all first reaches tended to be circuitous, the amount of correction made to obtain the object, the speed at which the attempt was made, and the angle at which arms were held differed across infants. These investigators concluded that the development of reaching represented more than development of eye-hand coordination; rather, in the simple act of reaching and grasping an object, the infant demonstrated (1) motivation to obtain the object, (2) ability to localize the object in space, (3) understanding that the object was reachable, (4) planning of the reach trajectory, (5) correction of the movement as the hand approached the toy, (6) lift and stabilization of the arm in space, and (7) successful grasp of the object. How a 5-month-old infant manages all of these components to reach and grasp a toy successfully varies among infants and for different reasons. Reach and grasp, as an example of developmental skill, is best understood as the outcome of the interaction of multiple systems, intrinsic and extrinsic to the child.

In a similar way, between 8 and 10 months of age, most infants acquire the motivation to be independently mobile. The need to self-initiate movement from place to place emerges as an important task, or goal, to accomplish. This goal reflects the infant's curiosity about the environment, a desire to explore space, and a determination to reach a specific play object. Although mobility becomes a common goal for the infant toward the end of the first year, the method used to achieve that mobility varies greatly. Some infants roll to another space in the room, whereas others scoot on their buttocks in a sitting position. Some infants push backward while lying in a prone position, and others creep forward to explore their environment. How the infant achieves mobility is influenced by many contributing body systems (e.g., strength, coordination, and sense of balance and movement).

Conditions in the environment also influence an infant's mobility (e.g., the surfaces on which the infant plays, the encouragement provided by caregivers, and the way in which the task is presented). The infant's energy level, motivation, and curiosity about the environment influence when independent mobility is achieved. In addition to the factors that influence the maturation of mobility skills, becoming mobile influences the development of skills in other performance domains. When an infant achieves mobility, he or she becomes more independent in initiating a social interaction or in seeking help. Independent mobility contributes to the acquisition of social skills, self-determination, problem solving, and motivation to explore. A child learns perceptual skills, spatial relations, form perception, and object relations by moving through the environment.

Perceptual Action Reciprocity

Perception and action are interdependent and inextricably linked. This relationship is particularly observed in infants and is useful in understanding motor development. An individual's perception of the environment informs action, and the individual's actions provide feedback about movement, performance, and consequences in the environment. Initially, many of the child's actions are exploratory in nature—the child moves fingers over the surfaces of objects to learn their shape, texture, and consistency. The child waves an object in the air to hear the sounds it makes and feel its weight. These actions help the child perceive sensory and perceptual features (affordances) of objects. *Affordance* is the fit between the child and his or her environment.[57,59,61] The environment and objects in it offer the child opportunities to explore and act. This action is based on what the environment affords as well as the child's perceptual capability to recognize affordances in that environment. For example, colorful noise-making toys afford manipulation because they have movable parts and rounded surfaces and fit easily into an infant's hand. Learning about affordances entails exploratory activities. Individual finger movements, thumb opposition, hand-to-hand transfer, and eye-hand coordination are facilitated by the physical characteristics of the toy.

Manipulation in the infant initially is guided by visual, tactile, and kinesthetic input.[114,123] Exploration of objects begins with visual exploration and mouthing.[115] By 6 months of age, infants prefer exploring with their eyes and hands.[114] Fingering and manipulation skills increase substantially between 6 and 12 months of age, enabling infants to gather more precise information about objects. By 12 months of age, infants detect object properties with increasing specificity and learn to adjust their exploratory action.[1] For example, to perceive the consistency of a soft, squishy object, a child squeezes it, and to perceive the texture of velvet or corduroy, the child runs the fingers back and forth over it.

Through object manipulation, the child develops haptic perception (i.e., an understanding of shape, texture, and mass of objects). Table 3-1 explains perceptual-action reciprocity in the development of object manipulation. Bushnell and Boudreau[19] propose that specific motor skills are required to develop haptic perception. They note that infants learn to identify an object's sensory qualities (e.g., texture, consistency, temperature, contour) only when they develop the motor skills to explore each different sensory quality. For example, an infant does not accurately discriminate texture until he or she can explore texture by moving the fingers back and forth (at about age 6 months). The infant also cannot discriminate hardness until 6 months, when he or she can tighten and lessen the grip while holding an object.[19] Because configural shape requires that two hands be involved in exploring an object's surfaces, children typically cannot accurately perceive shape until 12 months of age. By 2½ years, children can identify common objects through their haptic sense, and by 5 years, children recognize common objects using active touch (without vision).[25] By 5 years, the child has also fully developed in-hand manipulation skills,[107] suggesting that haptic perception develops in association with the child's development of manipulation skills. Maturation of haptic perception and manipulation underlies the child's ability to use tools for written communication (e.g., handwriting and keyboarding) and activities of daily living.

Functional Performance: Adaptive and Flexible

As mentioned, the infant begins life with few constraints on performance, which permits the greatest variability in the system for the generation of spontaneous movements. This variability permits flexibility for exploration of the environment and rapid perceptual and cognitive learning. The infant quickly selects functional synergistic movement patterns. For example, from birth, the infant demonstrates a pattern of hand-to-mouth movement (e.g., for self-calming by sucking on a fist) (Figure 3-3). Only minimal adaptive changes are made in this synergistic pattern (shoulder rotation and horizontal adduction, elbow flexion and forearm pronation, followed by supination and neutral wrist position) as the child learns to self-feed with various utensils.

Because synergies that enable tool use are softly assembled around the goal of the task at hand, they are stable but flexible units. Synergies have specific consistent characteristics, such as the sequence of movements and the ratio of joint movement, which can be adjusted to accommodate each new situation. This *adaptable stability* is a hallmark of normal movement.[29] Soft assembly is critical to allow the child to act in changing and variable environments. It also allows the child to explore and select a response to the environment because his or her

TABLE 3-1 Perceptual-Action Reciprocity in the Development of Perceptual and Object Manipulation Skills

Age	Perceptual Skill	Object Manipulation Skill
<6 months	Visually explores and mouths objects	Brings object to mouth
	Explores object textures by moving fingers back and forth	Begins to extend and move fingers together
6-12 months	Explores objects with eyes and hands	Fingers and manipulates objects
	Discriminates hardness of object	Can tighten and loosen grip while holding an object
12 months-3 years	Adjusts manipulation according to the object property	Moves an object from hand to hand
	Perceives object shape by moving between hands	Uses two hands to manipulate object
>3 years	Identifies common objects using haptic perception (active touch)	Begins to demonstrate in-hand manipulation skills
		Uses dynamic grasping patterns

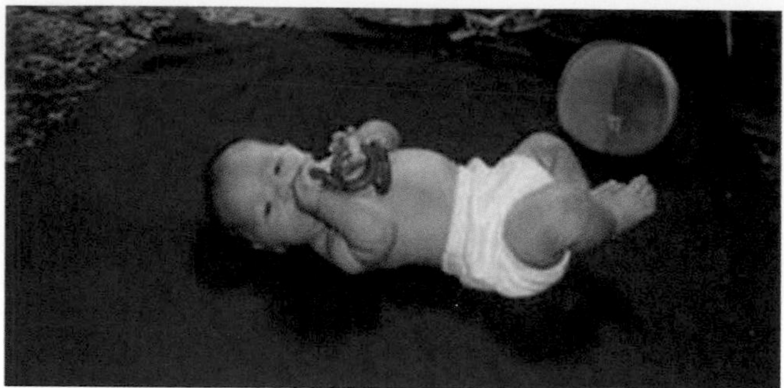

FIGURE 3-3 Hand-to-mouth movement is observed throughout the first year, first for sensory exploration of the mouth and hand and then as a feeding behavior. (From Henderson, A., & Pehoski, C. [2006]. *Hand function in the child: Foundations for remediation* [2nd ed.]. St. Louis: Mosby.)

response patterns are variable and flexible.[131] See Figure 3-4 for examples of fluid exploration of objects and a child exploring and manipulating shapes.

The functional synergies that characterize a child's development of occupations are highly adaptable and reliable. The child self-organizes these synergies around tasks and goals, and his or her first goals are embedded in and organized around play (as described later in this chapter).

How does a child learn new performance skills? Although learning new skills is not limitless and is constrained by biologic and contextual factors, human development is believed to have relative *plasticity*.[85] This concept has importance to occupational therapists, who provide intervention services designed to change and promote children's performance. Gottlieb[63] defines plasticity as a fusion of the organism (the child) and the environment (including its cultural, physical, and socioeconomic characteristics).[64] Individual development involves the emergence of new structural (e.g., cellular) and functional (e.g., body systems) components. The child's experiences produce new neurologic connections (i.e., new associations) and structural changes (e.g., physical growth), and the relationships among components, not the components themselves, are most important to development. Acknowledgment of the system's plasticity places the focus on the child's potential for change and on the contextual features that promote or limit the child's performance.

Stages of Motor Learning

How does motor competence develop during childhood? Children generally pass through three stages of learning to acquire a new skill.[59,111,136] The first stage involves *exploratory activity*. The first year of life is primarily a period of sensorimotor exploration. Exploration occurs naturally in all human beings, generally when an individual is presented with a new object or task. Through exploration, a child learns about self and the environment. In this stage, the child experiments with objects and activities using different systems, new combinations of perception and movement, and new sequences of action. In this exploratory stage or when challenged by a new and difficult task, a child tends to demonstrate primitive movement. New challenges tend to elicit lower levels of skills because these can be accessed more easily than the child's highest level skills, which demand more energy and effort.[66] By using lower level skills to address new problems, the child can focus on perceptual learning about the task before beginning to use higher level skills, which ultimately allow more success in performing the task. Gilfoyle, Grady, and Moore[62] noted that when children are first challenged with a new and difficult performance task (e.g., a first step), they use primitive movement patterns (e.g., balance by stiffening the legs and trunk) before progressing to integrated skill.

In the second stage of learning, *perceptual learning,* the child begins to use the feedback and reinforcement received from his or her exploration. In this transitional stage, the child exhibits more consistency in the movement patterns used to accomplish tasks. Because this second stage is a phase of perceptual learning, certain actions that were tried initially are discarded as ineffective. Interest in the activity remains high as perceptual learning continues and is inherently motivating and meaningful to the child. In this stage, the child appears focused on learning and attempts activities multiple times. The child may fluctuate between higher and lower levels of skill. Connolly and Dalgleish[33] found considerable variability when toddlers attempted to use a spoon. Greer and Lockman[68] found similar variability when 3-year-olds attempted to use a writing tool. See Figure 3-5 for an example of a transitional marker grip. At times, the children grasped the tool using an adult gripping pattern, and at other times, they used a primitive, full-hand grasp. Mature patterns are selected more often as children enter the third stage of skill learning.

In the third stage of learning, *skill achievement,* the child selects the action pattern that works best for achieving a goal. The pattern selected is comfortable and efficient for the child. Selection of a single pattern indicates both perceptual learning and increased self-organization. During this end stage of learning, the child demonstrates flexible consistency in performance. He or she uses the same pattern and approach to the task but easily adapts the pattern according to task requirements. High adaptability is always characteristic of a well-learned task. Another attribute of learned performance is the use of action patterns that are orderly and economical. Children continue to practice performance when given opportunities in the environment. The third stage of learning leads to exploration of new and different activities; a child's learning continues into new performance arenas, expanding his or her occupations (Figure 3-6).

For most children, new experiences and new learning are sought and are a source of pleasure. Learning occurs when children seek opportunities for skill development; it also occurs when children adapt to the natural environment and daily activities in which they participate. Ayres[3,4] explains that children make adaptive responses to the environment. An adaptive response is one in which the child responds to an environmental change in "a creative or useful way" (p. 14).[4] These adaptive responses allow skill mastery and help to organize the child's CNS. An adaptive response helps to integrate the child's sensory and perceptual systems to respond more skillfully to new challenges to the sensory system. For example, once an infant can pull herself up to her mother's lap to ask to be held, she no longer needs to cry to solicit her mother's attention.

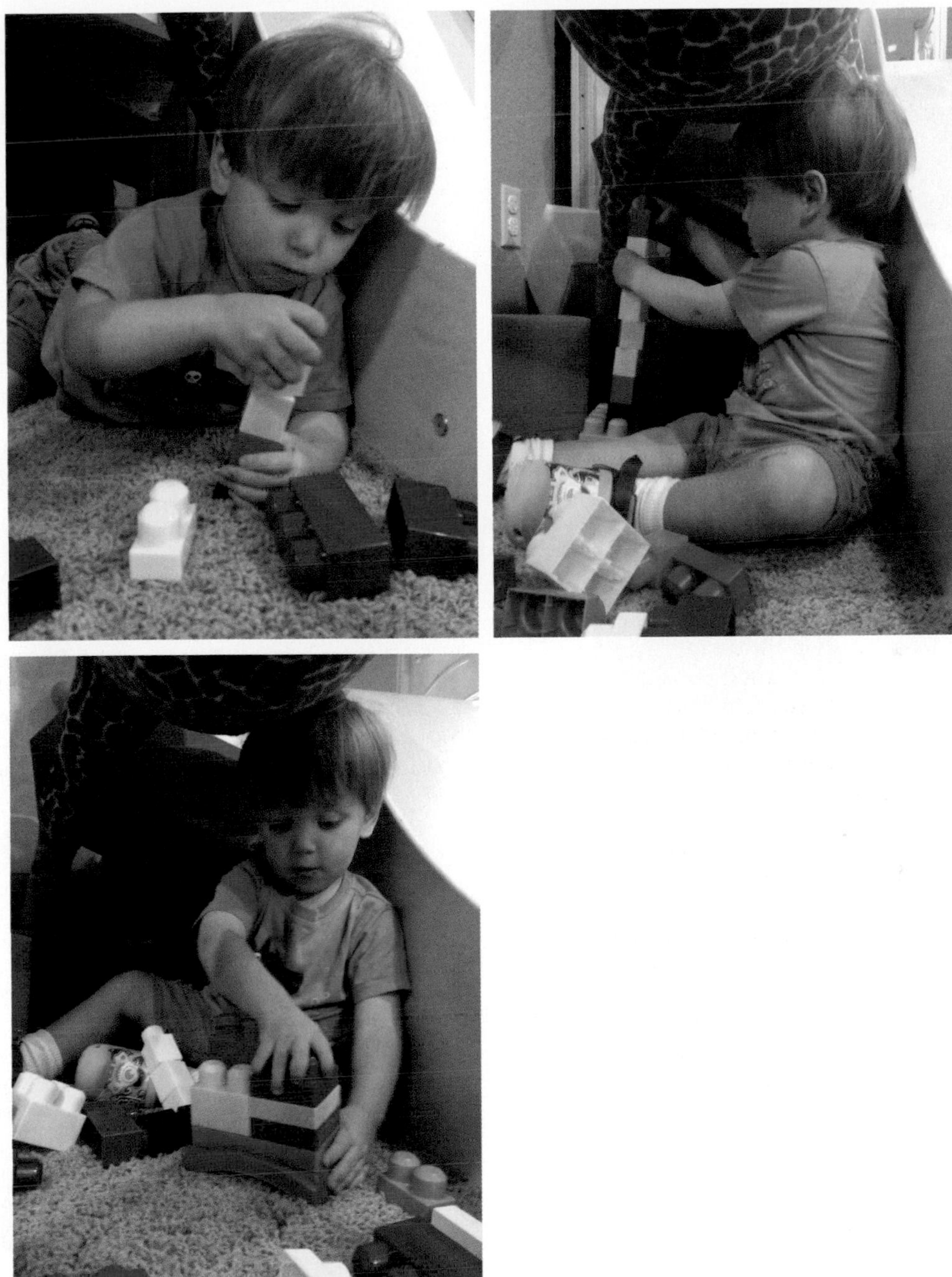

FIGURE 3-4 The child's movement patterns in exploring objects and the environment are variables and flexible.

Social-Emotional Development

Theories on temperament, attachment, and emotion regulation explain how a child's social-emotional behaviors develop and how social-emotional function affects performance across domains. These theories explain individual differences among children based on genetic endowment and social environmental influences.

Emotions play an important part in the child's appraisal of his or her experience and in the child's readiness for action in response to contextual change. Emotions relate to how a child evaluates the meaning of an experience in relation to his or her goals. If a child engages in an activity with the goal of succeeding but does not, the child may become disappointed or frustrated. If a child engages in an activity simply to participate and without expectation for success, he or she may experience pleasure regardless of success. Emotions and temperament influence the child's interest in attempting new activities, the amount of effort demonstrated, and attempts to engage others. These variables influence how a child approaches an activity (e.g., joyfully, reluctantly) and influence its social nature (e.g., whether the child solicits the involvement of others).

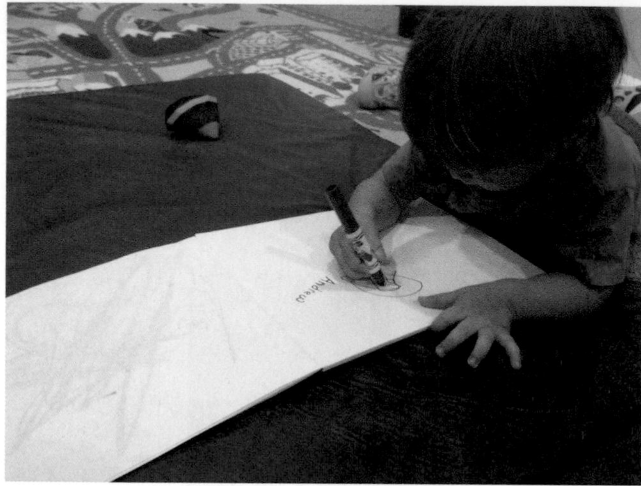

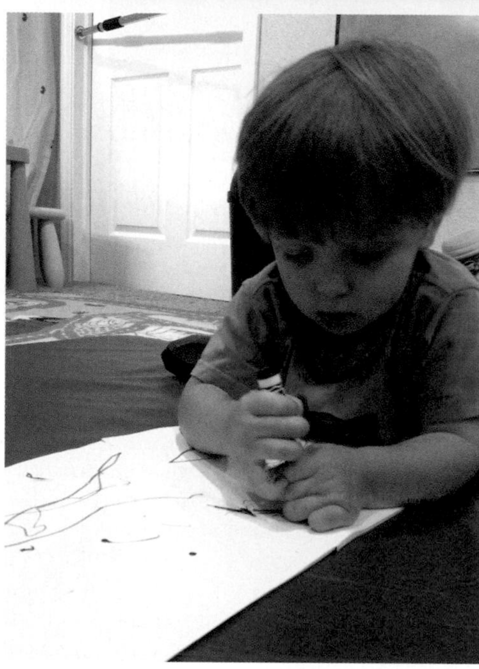

FIGURE 3-5 The child experiments with writing utensil grasping patterns.

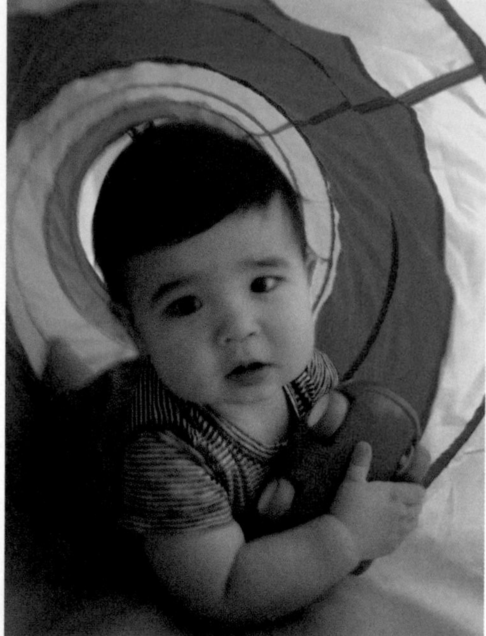

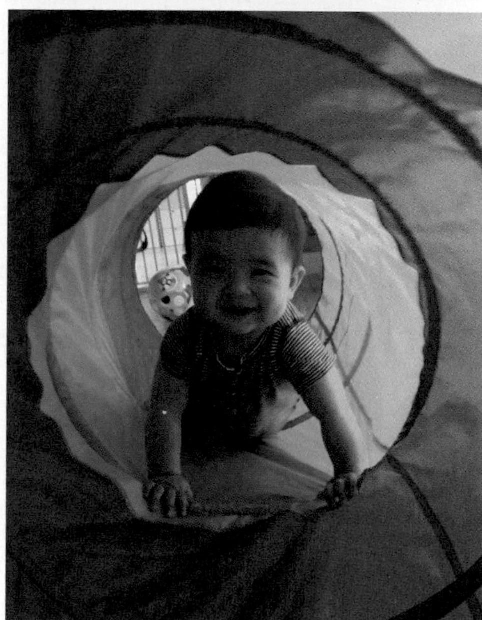

FIGURE 3-6 The infant's learning demonstrates high adaptability. The third stage of learning leads to exploration of new and different activities, expanding learning into new occupations.

Temperament

Temperament reflects relatively stable traits that influence how individuals process and respond to the environment. These characteristics contribute to personality and everyday functioning. The child's temperament is an important determinant in how well a child matches the caregiver and the caregiving environment.[86] Temperament also influences the child's style of social interaction. Nine areas of temperament have been identified: (1) activity level, (2) approach or withdrawal, (3) distractibility, (4) intensity of response, (5) attention span and persistence, (6) quality of mood, (7) rhythmicity, (8) threshold of response, and (9) adaptability. Each of these areas contributes uniquely to the child's preferences, interests, and style in forming social relationships and responding to the social environment.[137]

Taken together, these areas of temperament have their own continuum. Extreme temperament levels are associated with problematic behaviors, and moderate levels are related to easy and appropriate behaviors. Children who exhibit extreme temperament characteristics (e.g., children who are highly active, moody, or irritable) have been identified as *difficult*. The difficult child may not fit with the expectations and schedules of caregivers. Others with happy moods and moderate intensity of response are considered *easy*. A child with an easy temperament may easily establish routines (exhibiting regular sleep/wake cycles) and have positive moods and may have a better fit with caregivers. A match of parent and child temperament can facilitate strong attachment, just as a mismatch can create difficulties in attachment.

TABLE 3-2 Emotion Regulation Development

Phases	Approximate Ages	Characteristics	Examples
Neurophysiologic modulation	Birth to 2-3 months	Modulation of arousal, activation of organized patterns of behavior.	Infant is can self-soothe (e.g., with nonnutritive sucking) or respond quickly when soothed by parents. May be fussy, calm. Different routines of awake/sleeping cycles.
Sensorimotor modulation	3-9 months	Behavior depends on social or environmental stimuli or events.	Infant derives pleasure from sensorimotor play; infants seek sensory exploration. Some infants have difficulty modulating sensory behaviors (e.g., may be sensory seeking).
Control	12-18 months	Behavior demonstrates awareness of social demands. Toddler demonstrates compliance and self-initiated monitoring.	Toddler's behavior is goal-directed. May show different levels of inhibition and compliance according to understanding of consequences.
Self-control	24 48 months	Child's behaviors are in accordance with social expectations; developing a sense of identity. Behavior becomes more internally monitored.	Child demonstrates knowledge of social rules and conventions. Has limited flexibility in adapting to new demands. May visually check in with parent before acting.
Self-regulation	≥36 months	Child develops behavioral flexibility according to demands of the situation; develops strategies for managing different situations. Has self-awareness and can self-evaluate	Child may self-initiate clean-up. Adaptability increases, such that child can adapt to unexpected events (e.g., parent leaving for a long time), primarily because communication and language have increased.

Adapted from Kopp, C.B. (1982). Antecedents of self-regulation: A developmental perspective. *Developmental Psychology, 18,* 199–214.

Chess and Thomas[27,28] asserted that if a child's characteristics provide a good fit (or match) with the demands of a particular setting, adaptive outcomes result. The congruence, or *goodness of fit,* between the child and his or her social and physical context determines the quality of development, influencing which occupations are reinforced and which are hindered. *Positive goodness of fit,* meaning that the social and physical environment support the child's skill development, can increase the child's developmental trajectory. Lack of goodness of fit can create disruption of psychological development and may put the child at risk for behavioral or academic problems.

To illustrate how temperament affects goodness of fit, children with arrhythmic, poorly regulated sleep/wake cycles were reported to be difficult to manage by European American families in which the parents worked and needed a consistent routine of sleeping patterns. Puerto Rican parents did not have difficulty in accommodating children with poorly regulated sleep/wake cycles because they molded their schedules around them and allowed their children to sleep when they wanted. In the Puerto Rican families, the incidence of child behavior problems was very low, particularly before school age when a school schedule was imposed.[85] These studies and many others suggest that the child's temperament and behavior affect goodness of fit between the caregiver and the child, which influences developmental outcomes.[28]

Emotion Regulation

Emotion regulation is related to temperament and can be influenced by caregivers, the environment, and experience. It refers to the modulation of emotional reactions, including its inhibition, activation, and grading.[121] Emotion regulation includes the child's ability to control his or her emotions and use adaptive behaviors when frustrated or experiencing negative emotions, that is, "processes used to manage and change if, when and how intensely one experiences emotion and emotion-related motivational and physiological states and how emotions are expressed as behaviors."[40] Similar to other skill sets, emotion regulation increases with age and shifts from external sources of control to internal child factors. As presented in Table 3-2, a child's self-regulation of emotion emerges from socialization with primary caregivers and others and is linked to language and cognitive development. In early emotion regulation, physiologic and sensory modulation determines behavior; however, as toddlers learn self-control, between 2 and 3 years of age, the child's behaviors become more influenced by social demands. The self-control learned in the second and third years becomes more flexible and adaptable as rules are learned and remembered.[80] Children who have achieved self-regulation of emotions can use multiple strategies flexibly to cope with stressful events. For example, a child can shift attention away from a distressing event to decrease arousal or can focus attention on positive aspects of an event. A child's positive affect appears to increase emotion regulation, and children who have had frequent positive experiences appear better able to cope with negative experiences or stressful events.[140]

Attachment as a Basis for Social-Emotional Development

One aspect of early social-emotional development, attachment to a primary caregiver, can potentially influence social relationships and intimacy throughout life. Attachment can be defined as a bond that develops between the infant and his or her caregiver over the first year of life.[12,14] Infants are genetically programmed to seek and maintain proximity to an attachment figure. In an early study of attachment, infants 2 to 4 months old orient to adults, grasping and reaching for them, smiling and babbling. They appear to have indiscriminate attachments and respond similarly to any caregiver. Infants increasingly orient to familiar persons after 3 months. Infants 3 to 6 months old actively seek proximity exclusively to familiar caregivers and use them as a secure basis from which to explore. Social responses are greater and more positive for familiar people, particularly primary caregivers. After 6 months, the infant prefers the primary caregiver with whom he or she has formed an attachment, and the infant develops separation anxiety, signaling that the relationship with the attachment figure has become more intense and exclusive. The primary caregiver becomes a base from which the infant explores. When the infant is mobile (1 to 2 years of age), he or she demonstrates attachment behaviors designed to maintain proximity to the attached parent. By age 3, the child has developed a greater understanding of what the parent means by stating that she will return soon. At this age, the child becomes more flexible about his or her relationship with attached caregivers.[15,36]

Attachment to caregivers provides the child with an understanding of emotions and social relationships. Successful accomplishment of attachment results in a sense of security, and separation from the attachment figure leads to infant distress. Five patterns of attachment have been identified in infants: (1) a secure pattern that results from interactions with a caregiver who is sensitively responsive to the infant's signals, reading them accurately and responding appropriately; (2) an anxious pattern characterized by clinginess or need for constant reassurance, related to a parent who is excessively protective; (3) an insecure-avoidance pattern of minimal emotional expression related to a less responsive, slightly rejecting caregiver; (4) an insecure-ambivalent pattern related to a caregiver who appears to be overinvolved, inconsistent, or neglectful in his or her responses to the child; and (5) a disorganized pattern that results from parents who are intrusive, withdrawn, negative, or abusive.[15,17] A parent's (typically mother's) sensitive responses can heighten a child's positive emotions and inhibit negative emotions. Secure attachment facilitates a child's formation of a coherent and organized relationship with the parent, including an ability to predict the parent's responsiveness. These patterns suggest that the parent-child relationship has a primary role in a child's representation of his or her social world and that the attachment relationship shapes that child's understanding of self.[15]

Self-Identity and Self-Determination Development

Although attachment, temperament, and emotion regulation explain certain aspects of a child's social participation, other theories describe how self-identity and self-determination develop and contribute to participation. Erikson[42,43] described the stages of psychosocial development as conflicts and explained that resolution of these conflicts directly influences the child's self-identity, motivation, and personality. Of equal influence at this time, Maslow[91] developed a hierarchy of human needs to explain what motivates behavior and which needs must be met to reach self-actualization.

Self-Identity and Motivation

According to Erikson, the first stage that characterizes infants, birth to 1 year, is the development of trust.[43] Because the infant is dependent on caregivers in the first year, trust is based on dependability and responsiveness of caregivers. If the infant develops trust, he or she feels safe and secure; failure to develop trust results in fear and insecurity. Through the first four stages, children have opportunities to develop hope (trust), will (autonomy), purpose (initiative), and competence (industry). These qualities and virtues are important to the child becoming an occupational being. Erikson's psychosocial stages are defined in Table 3-3.

TABLE 3-3 Erikson's Psychosocial Stages, 0-12 Years

Stage/Age (Approximate)	Outcomes	Examples of Key Related Developmental Activities
Basic Trust vs. Mistrust Birth-2 years	Infant develops trust, believes the world is dependable. When parents are not sensitive or responsive, the infant becomes insecure, lacks trust, withdraws from others.	Infant is regularly fed; caregivers respond when he cries; caregivers give comfort when distressed.
Autonomy vs. Shame and Doubt 2-4 years	Child develops autonomy and will, attempts new challenges, becomes more self-sufficient. When parents are restrictive, the child can feel doubt and become reluctant to attempt new challenges.	Child feeds self, begins to dress self; becomes toilet trained; moves about the environment; caregivers support the child's performance, allow some choice.
Initiative vs. Guilt 4-5 years	Child begins to take initiative, plans activities, accomplishes tasks. When parents are dismissive, the child may feel ashamed or become overly dependent.	Child directs own play; attempts to assert control over others. Demonstrates imaginative and dramatic play.
Industry vs. Inferiority 5-12 years	Child develops a sense of pride in his accomplishments. Child strives to master new skills; when encouraged he develops a feeling of competence and self-confidence. When adults do not encourage, he does not believe in his skills and doubts that he will be successful. Child feels inferior.	Child participates in school and school-related activities. Social play and sports become important. Games, sports, and school work give the child opportunities to accomplish and demonstrate competence.

From Erikson, E.H. (1950). *Childhood and society.* New York: Norton.

Another psychologist who followed Erikson also developed a developmental hierarchy that explained how behaviors were based on a hierarchy of human needs. Maslow, sometimes considered the father of humanistic psychology in the United States,[70] outlined a hierarchy of basic human needs that is believed to follow a longitudinal sequence.[91,92] An individual's most basic needs, those at the base of this hierarchy, are *physiologic needs,* such as food, water, rest, air, and warmth, that are necessary to basic survival. The next level is characterized by the *need for safety,* broadly defined as the need for both physical and physiologic security. The *need for love and belonging* promotes the individual's search for affection, emotional support, and group affiliation. The *need for a sense of self-esteem,* which is defined as the ability to regard the self as competent and of value to society, is evidenced as an individual grows. The *need for self-actualization,* which represents the highest level, is attained through achievement of personal goals.

Maslow proposed that each of these needs serves as a motivator to achieve a higher level of human potential. Throughout development, individuals must satisfy their most basic needs before they are motivated by or interested in other life goals. Foundational biologic and egocentric needs must be satisfied before an individual has social interests and can fully participate in social relationships. With important social relationships established, an individual becomes interested in the broader community and has a broader sense of commitment and responsibility to others within the community. If the lower level needs are not met, the individual is unable to direct his or her energies toward higher levels. For example, a child who comes to school hungry finds it difficult to concentrate on the classroom learning activities. Recognition of a child's needs and the hierarchy of development of these basic needs helps the occupational therapist understand behaviors that indicate that basic needs are not met and identify needs that should become the focus of goals and interventions.

Self-Efficacy and Self-Determination

Understanding what motivates action and learning and how children develop personal well-being has expanded since the time of Maslow. Concepts explaining what intrinsic and extrinsic factors influence a child's development of self-identity, personal well-being, and self-determination are well integrated into client-centered occupational therapy approaches. Bandura[5] explained that children are inherently self-organizing and goal-directed; they typically have interest in new events and activities, initiate new tasks, and persevere in those tasks. When they succeed, positive self-efficacy is reinforced, and they attempt other challenges. When they do not succeed, they are at risk for developing poor self-efficacy and eventually do not attempt new or challenging activities. Self-efficacy is highly linked to learning and occupational development because it influences levels of motivation, initiative, and perseverance.[5-7]

Ryan and Deci[124] further developed the theory of self-efficacy by explaining that the key elements of self-determination are competence, autonomy, and relatedness. When children feel competent, they believe that if they persist in an activity, they will succeed. A child who has succeeded in performing is more likely to persist and to continue to succeed. A child who repeatedly fails when performing an activity may discontinue attempting it and may feel a sense of failure. Children who perceive themselves to be autonomous are intrinsically motivated to explore, learn, perform well, persist, show interest, and act energetically. Children with high autonomy and intrinsic motivation are likely to be self-directed and to have high self-esteem and general well-being. When children are externally pressured to act, they lose initiative and learn less effectively.[125] Parents and occupational therapists who promote a child's autonomy and competence are likely to instill intrinsic motivation. Competence and autonomy appear to be linked, in that feelings of competence do not enhance intrinsic motivation unless accompanied by a sense of autonomy.[125] Autonomous, intrinsically motivated pursuits are characterized by curiosity, meaningfulness, interest, and enjoyment.

A third factor, relatedness, also influences the development of intrinsic motivation. For example, intrinsic motivation is easily observed in the exploratory behavior of infants, and it is most evident in infants who are securely attached to a parent. When children are asked to perform a task or learn a new behavior, they become more competent and successful in the presence of a caring adult or interested caregiver.[126] Secure relationships form a foundation for emotional growth, increased autonomy, and intrinsic motivation and, by extension, increased participation.

Occupational therapists assess and facilitate a child's inner motivation to engage in occupations (tasks with meaning and purpose). Children fully participate when the fit among child, task, and environment is optimal; this fit becomes the occupational therapist's goal.[73,84] When a child has a disability, motivation to learn and attempt new activities may be lower, and the match among child, occupation, and environment may be suboptimal. In this case, a child may not learn independently, and adult support may be needed to motivate, provide a just-right challenge, support actions, and reinforce performance. Self-determination and self-efficacy are of high importance to occupational therapists, who understand that intrinsic motivation underlies a child's interest in learning from the environment and in participating in occupations. Intrinsic motivation is discussed further in other chapters, including Chapters 4, 12, and 25.

Resiliency

Children develop self-efficacy when they are raised in a supportive environment and learn that they are competent, autonomous, and supported by caregivers.[111] *Resiliency* refers to a child's internal characteristics that enable him or her to thrive and develop despite high-risk factors in the environment. The concept of resiliency emerged from studies of child development in which the context included risk factors known to have negative effects (e.g., child abuse, parental mental illness or substance abuse, socioeconomic hardship).[142,146] A resilient child has protective factors that enable him or her to develop positive interpersonal skills and general competence despite stressful or traumatic experiences or social environments known to limit developmental potential (e.g., that of an adolescent, single parent). Both child protective factors (e.g., intelligence, prosocial behavior, and social competence) and family protective factors (e.g., material resources; love, nurturance, and sense of safety and security; quality of parent-child relationship) are important to positive child outcomes. Researchers have demonstrated that a high-quality relationship with at least one parent, characterized by high levels of warmth and openness and low levels of conflict, is associated with positive outcomes across levels of risk and stages of development.[147]

A child's ***resiliency versus vulnerability*** also seems to relate to basic physiologic and regulatory characteristics. Children with low cardiovascular reactivity and high immune competence cope better with stressful situations and are less vulnerable to illness when stressed.[146] In middle childhood, well-developed problem solving and communication skills are important to a child's ability to deal with stress. Resilient boys and girls tend to be reflective rather than impulsive, demonstrate an internal locus of control, and use flexible coping strategies in overcoming adversity.[146] In addition to intelligence and competence, emotional regulation—that is, being able to monitor, evaluate, and modify the intensity and duration of emotional reactions—is important to positive outcomes.[142]

These concepts suggest that in the interpretation of the influence of environmental factors on a child's development, variables internal to the child can overcome negative contextual variables, including variables believed to have a profound influence (e.g., poor caregiving). Although the evidence suggests that children with strong resilience can overcome a high-risk environment (e.g., abusive situations, poverty), a research synthesis of risk and resilience studies found that both internal (e.g., child's intelligence, positive affect, emotional regulation) and contextual (e.g., supportive family relationships) protective factors are needed for positive outcomes (e.g., school success, positive relationships).[141] Taken together, the theories that explain how children grow and develop into competent adults and full participants in the community suggest that a child's development of occupations must always be understood as an interaction between the child's biologic being and his or her cultural, social, and physical contexts.

Development of Occupations

Occupations can be defined as the "patterns of action that emerge through transaction between the child and environment and are the things the child wants to do or is expected to do" (p. 22).[73] Although most children accomplish certain occupations and their corresponding tasks in a known sequence, the way these tasks are accomplished is unique for each child. A child learns new occupations based on the facility that the child brings to the activity. Motor and praxis, sensory-perceptual, emotion regulation, cognitive, and communication and social skills contribute to occupational performance.[2] These skill areas are interdependent; that is, they work together in such a way that the strengths of one system (e.g., visual) can support limitations in others (e.g., kinesthetic). Which systems are recruited for a task varies according to the novelty of the activity and the degree to which the task has become automatic.

Eating a meal illustrates the interdependence of the above-described developmental areas. Research has shown that self-feeding using a spoon involves visual-perceptual, kinesthetic, visual-motor, and cognitive systems.[32,55,71] Eating also relates to emotion regulation and social-emotional development.[127] As previously described, grasp of the spoon initially is guided by vision, and the child uses trial-and-error to hold the spoon so that he or she can scoop the food. With practice and maturation, grasp of the spoon is guided primarily by the kinesthetic system, and correct grasp becomes automatic; vision plays a lesser role. When food is in the mouth, chewing skills require primarily oral motor skills and somatosensory perception of food texture and food location within the mouth. The skills involved in occupational performance vary not only according to the learning phase but also according to the child's learning preferences and styles. Eating also relates to emotion regulation that may affect whether or not the child approaches the spoon. A child may resist eating because of past negative experiences with food or mealtime, anxiety about new foods, need for highly structured routines at mealtime, and difficulty coping with the social demands inherent in a mealtime. The complexity of the occupation of eating, often viewed as a simple occupation, reveals the level of understanding and analysis required when a child experiences eating challenges.

Humphry[73] suggests that children learn through both direct and indirect social participation. A young child often first learns about an occupation through observing parents, siblings, and other adults or peers. The first representational pretend play is typically imitation of the mother's actions when cleaning and cooking. Children imitate their parents' gestures and speech without being explicitly taught to do so. They also learn the consequences of actions by observing how their parents respond to each other or to their siblings. They can learn that an action is wrong by observing punishment of a peer for that action. Vicarious learning appears to be particularly important to a child's assuming cultural beliefs and values. Children learn the traditions and rituals of a culture by observing their family's participation in these. Inclusive models of education are believed to be effective learning environments for children with disabilities based on the known benefit of observing and interacting with typical peer models.[37,38] When in a child's presence, occupational therapists should always be conscious that their actions and words influence children's learning and whether these actions are directed toward the child.

Learning is generally more vigorous when the child actively participates in an occupation. Children's play with each other is an integrated learning experience in which the child acts, observes, and interacts. Play involves most or all performance areas, including affective, sensory, motor, communicative, social, and cognitive. When children play together, they learn from, model for, challenge, and reinforce each other. This flow of interactions occurs in meaningful activities that generally bring pleasure and intrinsic reinforcement and enable learning.

To learn a specific skill, the child must actively practice it. Specific scaffolding, guidance, cueing, prompting, and reinforcement by an occupational therapist can assist the child in learning to perform a skill. This direct support from a caregiver or other adult can facilitate performance at a higher level or at a more appropriate level so that the fit between the child and desired occupations and context becomes optimal. In the case of a child with disabilities, a more intensive level of direct support and scaffolding may be necessary for learning new skills. Adult guidance and support of the child during play can facilitate a successful strategy, help the child evaluate his or her performance, and encourage and reinforce continued practice. Occupational therapists can also optimize the environment to support and reinforce the child's performance. Participation in play occupations in a natural environment results in integrated learning across performance areas (e.g., including sensory, motor, cognitive, and affective learning) (Figure 3-7).

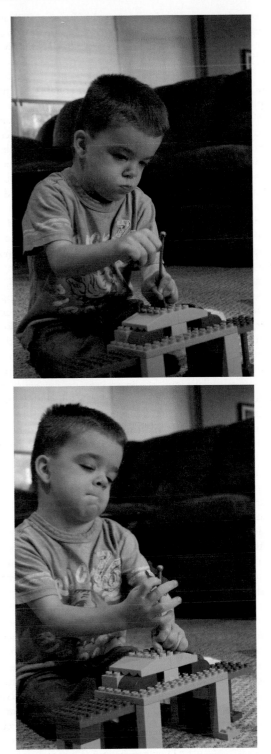

FIGURE 3-7 This child engages in meaningful play occupations based on his interest in airplanes in a natural environment (home).

The child's play and actions are always within a social, cultural, and physical context.[112] To understand the development of occupational performance, the occupational therapist must understand the child's play and actions as coherent occupations within specific contexts.

Ecologic Models and Contexts for Development

Children develop occupations through participation in family activities and cultural practices. As a child participates in the family's cultural practices, the child learns occupations and performance skills that enable him or her to become a full participant in the community. Rogoff et al. explain, "People develop as participants in cultural communities. Their development can be understood only in light of the cultural practices and circumstances of their communities."[116] Variations in the child's play activities (e.g., how he builds with wooden blocks, draws a picture of himself, or sings a song) reflect the child's biologic abilities and the influence of cultural, social, and physical contexts.

The ecologic model, developed by Bronfenbrenner,[18] situates child development in the center of the child's community. In this model, children are most influenced by their families and their home environment, termed the microsystem.[18] The child is also an integral part of a neighborhood and community, and this broader community has indirect but important influence by providing opportunities and cultural context for the child's development. Bronfenbrenner's ecologic model defines the importance of the physical and social context on child development and explains the interactions among family, cultural, and societal influences. The broadest influence on a child's occupations is the community in which the child is raised. Communities and society in general have invested in children's occupations by providing playgrounds, preschools, child-oriented music, child-oriented restaurants, and soccer fields. A community's orientation toward children determines available opportunities to play organized sports, learn about art and music, play safely in neighborhoods, and develop friendships with diverse peers. Communities that value organized sports and outdoor activities may have soccer or baseball teams, horseback riding, and swimming specifically designed for children with disabilities (e.g., Special Olympics, Miracle League Baseball, therapeutic horseback riding). Characteristics of the community become barriers or opportunities for the child and family and their desired occupations. As advocates for children with disabilities, occupational therapists can influence the development of programs that are accessible and appropriate for children with a wide range of abilities. They can emphasize the importance of supporting the participation of all children in community activities, recognizing the different levels of support and accommodation needed.

A child's cultural, social, and physical contexts change through the course of development and tend to expand as the child matures. The environment surrounds and supports the child's action; it also forces the child to adapt and assists or accommodates that adaptation. As a child perceives the affordances of the environment, he or she learns to act on those affordances, expanding a repertoire of actions. At the same time, the child's understanding of how the world responds to his or her actions increases. Rogoff[116,117] argued that culture affects every aspect of the child's development, which cannot be understood outside this context. The child is nested in his or her family, culture, and community, which have influenced the child's genetic makeup and continue to provide the learning environment.[117] By recognizing this influence, occupational therapists view each child in his or her cultural context and work as change agents within that context.

Cultural Contexts

Cultural practices are the routine activities common to a people of a culture and may reflect religion, traditions, economic survival, community organization, and regional ideology. A child's learning is highly influenced by participation in these cultural practices. Reciprocally, the child's participation in the occupations and cultural practices of his or her family and community contributes to that community.

Cultures vary in many aspects, such as the roles of women and children, values and beliefs about family and religion, family traditions, and the importance of health care and education. The continuum of interdependence versus autonomy of individuals varies in cultural groups and is a significant determinant of childhood occupations. The value an ethnic group or a community places on interdependence among its members versus individual autonomy creates differences in child-rearing practices and different experiences for developing children.[12] Most middle-class European Americans value independence as a primary goal for their children. Parents in the United States encourage individuality, self-expression, and independence in their children's actions and thoughts. Families from Asian and Hispanic backgrounds often value interdependence and reliance on family members throughout the life span. Cultures that value interdependence over independence also value cooperation over competition. For example, children of Asian and Hispanic backgrounds have been found to be more cooperative in play than children from European American backgrounds.[116]

To illustrate, parents in the United States, in part to foster early independence in children, do not co-sleep with their infants; instead infants sleep in their own room or crib. Co-sleeping may be more common among cultures in which parents value interdependence, promote high reciprocity with their children, and encourage the primacy of family relationships.[116] For example, it is prevalent across other societies in the world, such as Asia, Africa, and South America, where infants sleep in their parents' bed or room.[149] Mayan infants and toddlers sleep in the same room with their parents, often in the mother's bed.[75] Asian and Middle Eastern parents tend to sleep with their infants because they believe that these sleeping arrangements are important to nurturing and bonding. In the United States, co-sleeping is four times more common in Asian and African American families than in white families.[149] Close physical contact at night and into the day can foster interdependence within families.[56]

One consequence of infants sleeping in their own crib, separated from their parents, is that middle-class U.S. parents often engage in elaborate and time-consuming bedtime routines (e.g., reading books, lullabies). Black and Hispanic parents are less likely to establish an interactive bedtime routine with their young children.[69] Parents of these ethnic groups may not value an interactive bedtime routine. In addition, a routine to separate at bedtime may not be needed when infants sleep with the parents. These examples briefly illustrate how cultural beliefs and values influence the ways parents raise their children.

Social Contexts

Culture influences the social relationships that envelop the child, yet certain aspects of the child's social context appear to be independent of cultural influences and are consistent across cultures. The most important relationships formed during infancy are the relationships with parents or primary caregivers.[101] When caregivers are sensitive and responsive to the infant, healthy social-emotional development results.[39,87] Infants' interactions with parents serve to enhance the infants' basic physiologic and regulatory systems. When parents attune to the infant's sensory modulation and arousal needs and support these needs, the infant develops secure attachment. Mothers who modulate their behaviors to match their infants' needs for stimulation and comfort also promote the infants' abilities to self-regulate. A child's interaction with a caregiver gives the child essential information about how self and other are related, which becomes important to engaging in future relationships. Attachment patterns seem to influence the child's style of interaction and engagement in later years. Sensitive responding consolidates the infant's sense of efficacy and provides a foundation of security for confident exploration of the environment.[39,101]

Csikszentmihalyi and Rathunde[35] describe parenting as a dance between supporting and challenging the child. Supporting the child enables him or her to assimilate or explore the environment—to play. Parental challenge requires a child to accommodate and conform. Parenting provides a combination of these supports and challenges. All parents use some measure of support to bolster children's attempts to master skills and some degree of challenge to move children toward higher levels of mastery.[101,116] These elements are subtly provided by parents in the ways they present tasks and select when and how they instruct or intervene. Effective guidance relies on careful observation of the child's cues. Sensitivity and responsivity to the child's needs appear to be among the most important variables in the promotion of child development.[85]

In typical situations, infants receive care from multiple care providers, including childcare providers, grandparents, and other adults. The infant may or may not attach to caregivers other than the parents or primary caregivers; however, these social relationships are important to the infant's emotional development and provide opportunities for the development of social skills. About 55% of children 3 to 5 years of age participate in nonparent childcare, including center-based and family childcare.[141] A study for the National Institute of Child Health and Human Development revealed that positive caregiving occurred when children were in small groups; child-to-adult ratios were low; caregivers did not use an authoritarian style; and the physical environment was safe, clean, and stimulating.[104] Family factors predicted child outcomes even for children who spent many hours in childcare. The family environment appears to have a significantly greater effect on a child's development than the childcare environment.[47,88]

Physical Contexts

The physical environment surrounds and supports the child's actions; it forces the child to adapt his or her actions to meet the demands and constraints of the physical surroundings. As a child perceives the affordances of the environment, the child learns to act on those affordances, expanding a repertoire of actions. At the same time, the child's understanding of how the world responds to his or her actions increases. Gibson[58] explained how a child's exploration of physical surfaces and objects allows the child to develop and practice mobility and manipulation skills. Examples of the interactions of a child and his or her physical environments and the developmental consequences are presented next.

Children's Occupations, Performance Skills, and Contexts

This section describes a child's development of play occupations as enabled by the child's performance skills and cultural, physical, and social contexts. For three age groups—infancy, early childhood, and middle childhood—typical play occupations and activities are described. The contribution of motor, sensory, emotional, cognitive, and social abilities and contexts to the development of play occupations is described. Although children's occupations are similar within a particular age level, the contexts, individual abilities, and activities are varied and diverse, resulting in a unique occupational performance for each child. Recognition of the uniqueness of a child's development and of how these components contribute to performance within individuals is key to analysis of occupational performance.

Although the child learns occupations other than play (e.g., occupations related to activities of daily living or school functions), occupational therapists are invested in play outcomes and most often use play activities to engage the child in the therapeutic process. Play activities serve as the means to improve performance because they are self-motivating and offer goals around which the child can self-organize.[106] Play also serves as the end or goal of therapy services.[112] Children put effort and energy into play activities because they are inherently interesting and fun. (A more detailed description of play as a goal and modality of therapy is provided in Chapter 17.) Descriptions of a child's development of feeding, self-care, activities of daily living, instrumental activities of daily living, and school function are presented in other chapters (see Chapters 14, 15, 16, and 23). The child's ability to communicate, although essential to the development of play and other childhood occupations, is not specifically described in this chapter because language and communication are the domain of speech-language pathologists and are well described in many other texts.

Infants: Birth to 2 Years

Play Occupations

The play occupations of infants in the first 12 months are exploratory and social—they are related to bonding with caregivers (Boxes 3-1 and 3-2). As in every stage, these occupations overlap (e.g., bonding occurs during exploratory play with the parent's hair and face, and the parent's holding supports the infant's play with objects). Much of the infant's awake and alert time is spent in exploratory play, often play that occurs in the caregiver's arms or with the caregiver nearby.

Exploratory play is also called *sensorimotor play*. Rubin[121] defined *exploratory play* as an activity performed simply for the enjoyment of the physical sensation it creates. It includes repetitive movements to create actions in toys for the sensory experiences of hearing, seeing, and feeling. The infant places toys in the mouth, waves them in the air, and explores their surfaces with the hands. These actions allow for intense perceptual learning and bring delight to the infant (without any more complex purpose). Research Note 3-1 explains Gibson's ecologic theories on how the infant learns through exploration of object affordances.

In the second year of life, the infant engages in *functional*, or *relational, play*; an object's function is understood, and that function determines the action (Boxes 3-3 and 3-4). Initially, children use objects on themselves (e.g., pretending to drink from a cup or to comb the hair). These self-directed actions signal the beginning of *pretend play*.[110] The child knows cause and effect and repeatedly makes the toy telephone ring or the battery-powered doll squeal to enjoy the effect of the initial action.

By the end of the second year, play has expanded in two important ways. First, the child begins to combine actions into play sequences (e.g., he or she relates objects to each other by stacking one on the other or by lining up toys beside each other). These combined actions show a play purpose that

BOX 3-1 Development of Play Occupations: Infants—Birth to 6 Months

Play Occupations

Exploratory Play
Sensorimotor play predominates
Social play
Focused on attachment and bonding with parents

Performance Skills

Regulatory/Sensory Organization
Quiets when picked up
Shows pleasure when touched and handled
Relaxes, smiles, and vocalizes when held
Cuddles
Listens to a voice
Uses hands and mouth for sensory exploration of objects

Fine Motor/Manipulation
Follows moving person with eyes
Develops accurate reach to object
Uses variety of palmar grasping patterns
Secures object with hand and brings to mouth
Transfers objects hand to hand
Examines objects carefully with eyes
Plays with hands at midline

Gross Motor/Mobility
Lifts head (3-4 months), raises trunk when prone (4-6 months)
Kicks reciprocally when supine
Sits propping on hands
Plays (bounces) when standing with support from parents
Rolls from place to place

Cognitive
Repeats actions for pleasurable experiences
Uses hands and mouth to explore objects
Searches with eyes for sound
Bangs object on table
Integrates information from multiple sensory systems

Social
Coos, then squeals
Smiles, laughs out loud
Expresses discomfort by crying
Communicates simple emotions through facial expressions

Data from Parks, S. (2007) *HELP Strands*. Palo Alto, CA: VORT Corp; Gesell, A., & Amatruda, G. (1947). *Developmental diagnosis* (2nd ed.). New York: Harper & Row.

BOX 3-2 Development of Play Occupations: Infants—6 to 12 Months

Play Occupations

Exploratory Play
Sensorimotor play evolves into functional play
Functional Play
Begins to use toys according to their functional purpose
Social Play
Attachment to parents and caregivers
Social play with parents and others

Performance Skills

Regulatory/Sensory Organization
Enjoys being held up in the air and moving rapidly through the air
Listens to speech without being distracted
Finger-feeds self, including a variety of food textures
Cooperates with dressing
Fine Motor/Manipulation
Mouths toys
Uses accurate and direct reach for toys
Plays with toys at midline; transfers hand to hand
Bangs objects together to make sounds
Waves toys in the air
Releases toys into container
Rolls ball to adult
Grasps small objects in fingertips
Points to toys with index finger, uses index finger to explore toys
Crudely uses tool
Gross Motor/Mobility
Sits independently
Rolls from place to place
Independently gets into sitting position
Pivots in sitting position
Stands, holding on for support
Plays in standing when leaning on support
Crawls on belly initially, then crawls on all fours (10 months)
Walks with hand held (12 months)
Cognitive
Responds to own name
Recognizes words and family members' names
Responds with appropriate gestures
Listens selectively
Imitates simple gestures
Looks at picture book
Begins to generalize from past experiences
Acts with intention on toys
Takes objects out of container
Social
Shows special dependence on mother
May show stranger anxiety
Lifts arms to be picked up
Plays contentedly when parents are in room
Interacts briefly with other infants
Plays give and take
Responds playfully to mirror (laughs or makes faces)

Data from Parks, S. (2007). *HELP Strands.* Palo Alto, CA: Vort; Linder, T. (2008). *Transdisciplinary play-based assessment* (rev. ed.). Baltimore: Brookes; Gesell, A., & Amatruda, G. (1947). *Developmental diagnosis* (2nd ed.). New York: Harper & Row.

RESEARCH NOTE 3-1

Gibson, E.J. (2000). Perceptual learning in development: Some basic concepts. Ecological Psychology, 12, *295–302.*

Gibson eloquently presents her theory of perceptual learning in this research synthesis. These concepts can explain early perceptual-motor development:

- Infants learn by exploring their environment and selecting the movements that optimally fit environmental affordances.
- Through perception of objects and their surfaces, shapes, actions, and function, the infant learns which movements are most effective and efficient for exploring and activating the object.
- When the infant grasps an object in view and brings it to his mouth, he learns what is within reaching distance, how long his arm is, how large the object is, how much it weighs when transported, and how it feels in his mouth. From this action, the infant learns how far he needs to extend his arm, how much force is needed to hold the object, and how to turn the object to bring it to his mouth. The result is the infant selects the most efficient movements and action for reaching, grasping, and mouthing an object.
- The infant quickly learns that proprioceptive information from his arm in carrying an object to his mouth matches perfectly visual information from watching the object travel to his mouth. This match of visual and proprioceptive information is redundant and invariant, allowing the infant to select only one sensory system to guide his movements, and he generally selects the proximal sensory (proprioceptive) system as the most efficient.
- Economy of action and reduction of perceptual information are principles that the infant uses to develop coordinated and efficient movements.
- These principles of perceptual-motor reciprocity can be easily observed in the refining of grasping patterns and actions applied to objects in the first 2 years of life.

matches the function of the toy. Second, 2-year-old children now direct actions away from themselves. The objects used in play generally resemble real-life objects.[86] The child places the doll in a toy bed and then covers it. The child pretends to feed a stuffed animal or drives toy cars through a toy garage. At 2 years of age, play remains a very central occupation of the child, who now has an increased attention span and the ability to combine multiple actions in play. The emergence of ***symbolic,*** or ***imaginary, play*** with toys and objects offers the first opportunities for the child to practice the skills of living.[102]

The child also engages in gross motor play throughout the day. As the child becomes mobile, exploration of space, surfaces, and large action toys becomes a primary occupation. Movement is enjoyed simply as movement; the child delights in swinging and running or attempting to run and moving in water or sand. Deep pressure and touch are craved and requested. As in exploratory play, the child's exploration of space involves simple, repeated actions in which the goal appears to be sensation. Often, extremes in sensation seem to be enjoyed and are frequently requested. Repetition of these

BOX 3-3 Development of Play Occupations: Infants—12 to 18 Months

Play Occupations

Relational and Functional Play

Engages in simple pretend play directed toward self (pretend eating, sleeping)
Links two or three schemas in simple combinations
Demonstrates imitative play from an immediate model

Gross Motor Play

Explores all spaces in the room
Rolls and crawls in play close to the ground

Social Play

Begins peer interactions
Parallel play

Performance Skills

Regulatory/Sensory Organization

Enjoys messy activities
Reacts to extreme sensations, such as warm, cold, sweet

Fine Motor/Manipulation

Holds crayon and makes marks; scribbles
Holds two toys in hand and toys in both hands
Releases toys inside containers, even small containers
Stacks blocks and fits toys into form space (places pieces in board)
Attempts puzzles
Opens and shuts toy boxes or containers
Points to pictures with index finger
Uses two hands in play, one to hold or stabilize and one to manipulate

Gross Motor/Mobility

Sits in small chair
Plays in standing
Walks well, squats, picks up toys from the floor
Climbs into adult chair
Flings ball
Pulls toys when walking
Begins to run
Walks upstairs with one hand held
Pushes and pulls large toys or boxes on floor

Cognitive

Acts on object using variety of schemas
Imitates model
Symbolic play with real props (e.g., pretends to drink with cup)
Understands how objects work
Understands function of objects
Uses trial-and-error in problem solving
Recognizes names of various body parts

Social

Moves away from parent
Shares toys with parent
Responds to facial expressions of others

Data from Parks, S. (2007). *HELP Strands.* Palo Alto, CA: Vort; Linder, T. (2008). *Transdisciplinary play-based assessment* (rev. ed.). Baltimore: Brookes; Gesell, A., & Amatruda, G. (1947). *Developmental diagnosis* (2nd ed.). New York: Harper & Row.

BOX 3-4 Development of Play Occupations: Toddlers—18 to 24 Months

Play Occupations

Functional Play

Multischema combinations
Performs multiple related actions together

Gross Motor Play

Enjoys sensory input of gross motor play

Pretend or Symbolic Play

Makes inanimate objects perform actions (dolls dancing, eating, hugging)
Pretends that objects are real or that they symbolize another object

Social Play

Participates in parallel play
Imitates parents and peers in play
Participates in groups of children
Watches other children
Begins to take turns

Performance Skills

Regulatory/Sensory Organization

Enjoys solitary play for a few minutes
Uses Play-Doh
Enjoys rough and tumble play

Fine Motor/Manipulation

Completes 4- to 5-piece puzzle
Builds towers (e.g., 4 blocks)
Holds crayon in fingertips and draws simple figures (straight stroke or circular stroke)
Strings beads
Begins to use simple tools (e.g., play hammer)
Participates in multipart tasks
Turns pages of book

Gross Motor/Mobility

Runs, squats, climbs on furniture
Climbs on jungle gym and slides
Moves on ride-on toy without pedals (kiddy car)
Kicks ball forward
Throws ball at large target
Jumps with both feet (in place)
Walks up and down stairs

Cognitive

Links multiple steps together
Has inanimate object perform action
Begins to use nonrealistic objects in pretend play
Continues to use objects according to functional purpose
Object permanence is completely developed

Social

Expresses affection
Shows wide variety of emotions: fear, anger, sympathy, joy
Can feel frustrated
Enjoys solitary play, such as coloring, building
Engages in parallel play
Laughs when someone does something silly

Data from Parks, S. (2007). *HELP Strands.* Palo Alto, CA: Vort; Linder, T. (2008). *Transdisciplinary play-based assessment* (rev. ed.). Baltimore: Brookes.

full-body kinesthetic, vestibular, and tactile experiences appears to be organizing to the CNS (Figure 3-8). In addition, this repetition is important to the child's development of balance, coordination, and motor planning. The occupational goal of movement and exploration becomes the means for development of multiple performance areas.

In the first year, the goal of an infant's *social play* is attachment, or bonding, to the parents. As described by Greenspan,[67] this is a period in which the infant falls in love with the parents and learns to trust the environment because of the care and attention provided by the parents or caregivers. These

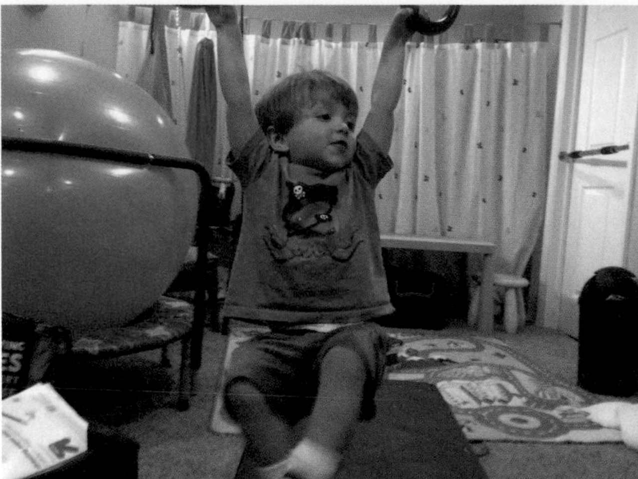

FIGURE 3-8 Gross motor fun of a 2-year-old.

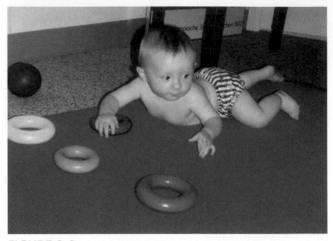

FIGURE 3-9 In prone position, the infant shifts his weight from side to side when playing with toys; later he learns to pivot while prone to expand where he can reach and what he can visualize.

BOX 3-5 Emergence of Self-Efficacy

Infants develop an initial sense of efficacy through cause-and-effect actions (e.g., crying brings adult attention). Infants who experience success in controlling environment events become more attentive to their own behavior and more competent in learning. In addition to seeing the effects of their actions, infants develop self-efficacy when they can differentiate themselves from others. Infants learn that their actions produce effects different from others' actions, and they begin to perceive themselves as distinct selves, differentiated from others.[6] When parents make remarks, such as "look what Audrey did, isn't she cute," or "You are such an ornery baby," the infant gains self-knowledge and begins to understand that she is a distinct individual. From this knowledge, self-efficacy emerges.

From Bandura, A. (1993). Perceived self-efficacy in cognitive development and functioning. *Educational Psychologist, 28,* 117–148.

occupations are critical foundations to later occupations that involve social relating and demonstration of emotions. At 1 year of age, infants play social games with parents and others to elicit responses. As the toddler gains competence and is supported by parental responsiveness, he or she gains a sense of personal agency and self-efficacy. See Box 3-5 for an example of how Bandura[6] explains the emergence of self-efficacy early in life. Although infants at this age engage readily with individuals other than family, they require their parents' presence as an emotional base and return to them for occasional emotional refueling before returning to play.[138]

By the second year, children exhibit social play in which they imitate adults and peers. Imitation of others is a first way to interact and socially relate.[8] Both immediate and deferred imitation of others are important to social play as children enter preschool environments and begin to relate to their peers.

Performance Skills

Sensory Functions

The newborn can interpret body sensations and respond reflexively. He enjoys and needs a consistent caregiver's physical contact and tactile stimulation. The neonate turns his head when touched on the cheek, relaxes in his mother's arms, and expresses discomfort from a wet diaper. Self-regulation of sleep/wake cycles, feeding, and display of emotions and arousal emerge in early infancy. The infant molds himself to the parent's embrace, clinging to the parent's arms and chest. The newborn's vestibular system is also quite mature as he calms from rocking and enjoys the motion of a parent walking him about the room. The neonate demonstrates orientation and attention to visual, auditory, and tactile stimuli. An important fact is that the newborn also exhibits *habituation,* or the ability to extinguish incoming sensory information (e.g., ability to sleep by blocking out sound in a noisy nursery). Chapter 9 further describes sensory development of infants and young children.

Gross Motor and Mobility

The first movements of newborns appear to be reflexive; however, on closer examination, they reveal the ability to process and integrate sensory information. The neonate's movements contribute to perceptual development and organization and initiate his learning about the world. In the first month of life, the infant moves the head side to side when in a prone position and rights the head when supported in sitting. By 4 months, the prone infant lifts the head to visualize activities in the room. This ability to lift and sustain an erect-head position appears to relate to the infant's interest in watching the activities of others as well as improved trunk strength and stability. As the infant reaches 6 months, he or she demonstrates increased ability to lift the head and trunk when in a prone position to visualize the environment. When prone, the infant can also move side to side on the forearms, then on the hands (Figure 3-9). When supine, the infant actively kicks and brings the feet to the mouth. Over the next 6 months, this dynamic, postural stability prepares the infant to become mobile.

Rolling is normally the infant's first method of becoming mobile and exploring the environment. Initially, rolling is an automatic reaction of body righting; usually the infant first rolls from the stomach to the side and then from the stomach to the back. By 6 months, the infant rolls sequentially to move across the room. Heavy or large infants may initiate rolling several months later, and infants with hypersensitivity of the vestibular system (i.e., overreactivity to rotary movement) may avoid rolling entirely.

Most infants enjoy supported sitting at a very early age. As their vision improves in the first 4 months, they become more eager to view their environment from a supported sitting position. The newborn sits with a rounded back; the head is erect only momentarily. Head control emerges quickly. By 4 months, the infant can hold the head upright with control for long periods, moving it side to side with ease. Most 6-month-old infants sit alone by propping forward on the arms, using a wide base of support with the legs flexed. However, this position is precarious, and the infant easily topples when tilted. Many 7-month-old infants sit independently. Often their hands are freed for play with toys, but they struggle to reach beyond arm's length.

By 8 to 9 months, the infant sits erect and unsupported for several minutes. At that time, or within the next couple of months, the infant may rise from a prone posture by rotating (from a side-lying position) into a sitting position. This important skill gives the infant the ability to progress by creeping to a toy and then, after arriving at the toy, to sit and play. By 12 months, the infant can rise to sitting from a supine position, rotate and pivot when sitting, and easily move in between positions of sitting and creeping (Figure 3-10).

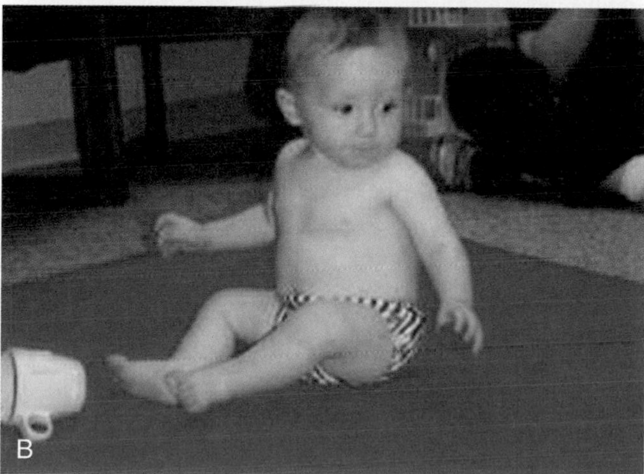

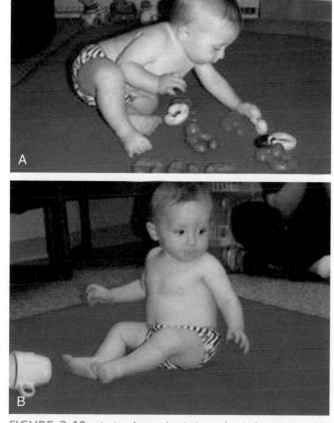

FIGURE 3-10 **A,** In dynamic sitting, the infant has sufficient postural stability to reach in all directions. **B,** By 10 months of age, the infant easily moves into and out of sitting positions.

After experimenting with pivoting and backward crawling in a prone position, the 7-month-old infant crawls forward. The infant may first attempt belly crawling using both sides of the body together. However, reciprocal arm and leg movements quickly emerge as the most successful method of forward progression. Crawling in a hands-and-knees posture (sometimes called *creeping*) requires more strength and coordination than belly crawling. The two sides of the body move reciprocally. In addition, shoulder and pelvic stability are needed for the infant to hold the body weight over the hands and knees. Mature, reciprocal hands-and-knees crawling also requires slight trunk rotation (Figure 3-11). Through the practice of crawling in the second 6 months of life, the child develops trunk flexibility and rotation. Most 10- to 12-month-old infants crawl rapidly across the room, over various surfaces, and up and down inclines.

Infants at 5 and 6 months of age delight in standing, and they gleefully bounce up and down while supported by their parents' arms. The strong vestibular input and practice of patterns of hip and knee flexion and extension are important to the development of full upright posture after 1 year. The infant also prepares for a full upright posture by standing against furniture or the parent's lap. A 10-month-old infant practices rising and lowering in upright postures while holding onto the furniture. By pulling up on furniture to standing, the infant can reach objects previously unavailable. This new level of exploration and increase in potential play objects motivates infants to practice standing and motivates parents to place breakable objects on higher shelves (Figure 3-12). At 12 months, the infant learns to shift the body weight onto one leg and to step

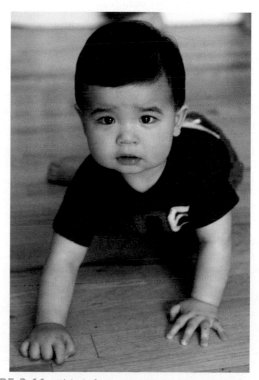

FIGURE 3-11 This infant transitions into crawling, allowing him to explore new spaces. Crawling on all fours promotes the rotational patterns needed for ambulation.

to the side with the other leg. The infant soon takes small steps forward while holding onto furniture or the parent's finger.

The infant's first efforts toward unsupported forward movement through walking are short, erratic steps with a wide-based gait and arms held in high guard. All these postural and mobility skills contribute to the infant's ability to explore space and obtain desired play objects. By 18 months, the infant prefers walking to other forms of mobility, but balance remains immature, and the infant falls frequently. The infant continues to use a wide-based gait and has difficulty with stopping and turning. However, infants remain highly motivated to practice this new skill because walking brings new avenues of exploration and a sense of autonomy, and the parent must now protect the infant from objects that previously could not be reached and from spaces that have not yet been explored.

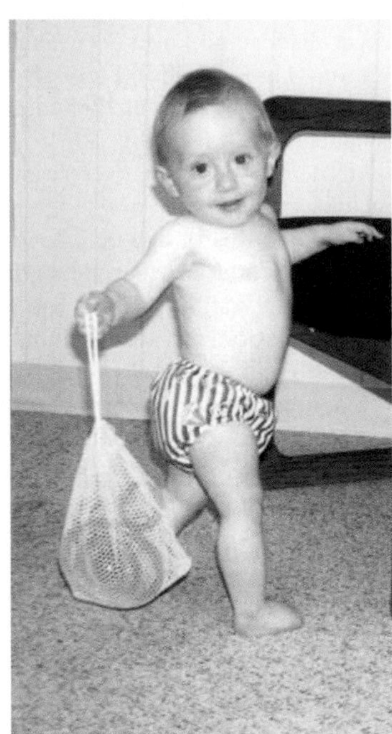

FIGURE 3-12 Supported stance is a favorite play position for infants 8 to 11 months old.

Fine Motor and Manipulation

The newborn moves the arms in wide ranges, mostly to the side of the body. In the first 3 months, the infant contacts objects with the eyes more than with the hands. By age 3 months, the infant follows his mother's face in a smooth arc, crossing midline. By 1 to 2 months of age, an infant learns to swipe at objects placed at his or her side. This first pattern of reaching is inaccurate, but by 5 months, the accuracy of reaching toward objects increases greatly.[119] The infant struggles to combine grasp with reach and may make several efforts to grasp an object held at a distance. As postural stability increases, the infant also learns to control arm and hand movements as a means of exploring objects and materials in the environment. By the time an infant is 6 months old, direct unilateral and bilateral reaches are observed, and the infant smoothly and accurately extends the arm toward a desired object.[143] Table 3-4 describes how the stages of motor learning are exemplified by the development of reach and grasp.

Grasp changes dramatically in the first 6 months (Figure 3-13). Initially, grasping occurs automatically (when anything is placed in the hand) and involves mass flexion of the fingers as a unit. The object is held in the palm rather than distally in the fingers or fingertips. Infants 3 to 4 months of age squeeze objects within their hands, and the thumb does not appear to be involved in this grasp. At 4 to 5 months of age, the infant exhibits a palmar grasp in which flexed fingers and an adducted

TABLE 3-4 Stages of Motor Learning for Reach and Grasp

Stage/Age	Motor Pattern
Reach	
I. Exploratory 1-3 months	Swipes at objects, reach is inaccurate; infant cannot combine reach and grasp.
II. Perceptual learning/ transitional stage 3-6 months	Reaching becomes more accurate, becomes more direct; infant reaches to midline. By 6 months, combines reach and grasp with two hands.
III. Skill achievement/adaptability and flexibility 6-9 months	Reaches with one or two hands; accurate and direct reach; can change direction of reach midstream. By 8-9 months, infant can reach in all directions. Reach is smooth and efficient. Infant easily combines reach and grasp. Infant carries object through space.
Grasp	
I. Exploratory 3-5 months	First voluntary grasp begins between 2 and 3 months. Infant squeezes object with all fingers, thumb does not participate. Release is random, without voluntary control. Grasp is inefficient and infant cannot move object in his hand.
II. Perceptual learning/ transitional stage 6-12 months	Radial palmar and radial digital grasping patterns emerge. Infant actively uses thumb to grasp objects. Infant is unable to move an object within his hands but can transfer hand to hand and explore in his mouth. Voluntary release begins at 6-7 months. Infant awkwardly prehends small objects.
III. Skill achievement/adaptability and flexibility 12 months-2 years	By 12 months, infant demonstrate a pincer grasp; this grasp is precise by 18 months. By 18 months, demonstrates precision release. By 2 years, grasp is dynamic, allowing tool use; the child can use an object while holding it (toothbrush, spoon). Blended grasping patterns develop—the child can move an object while maintaining his grasp of the object.

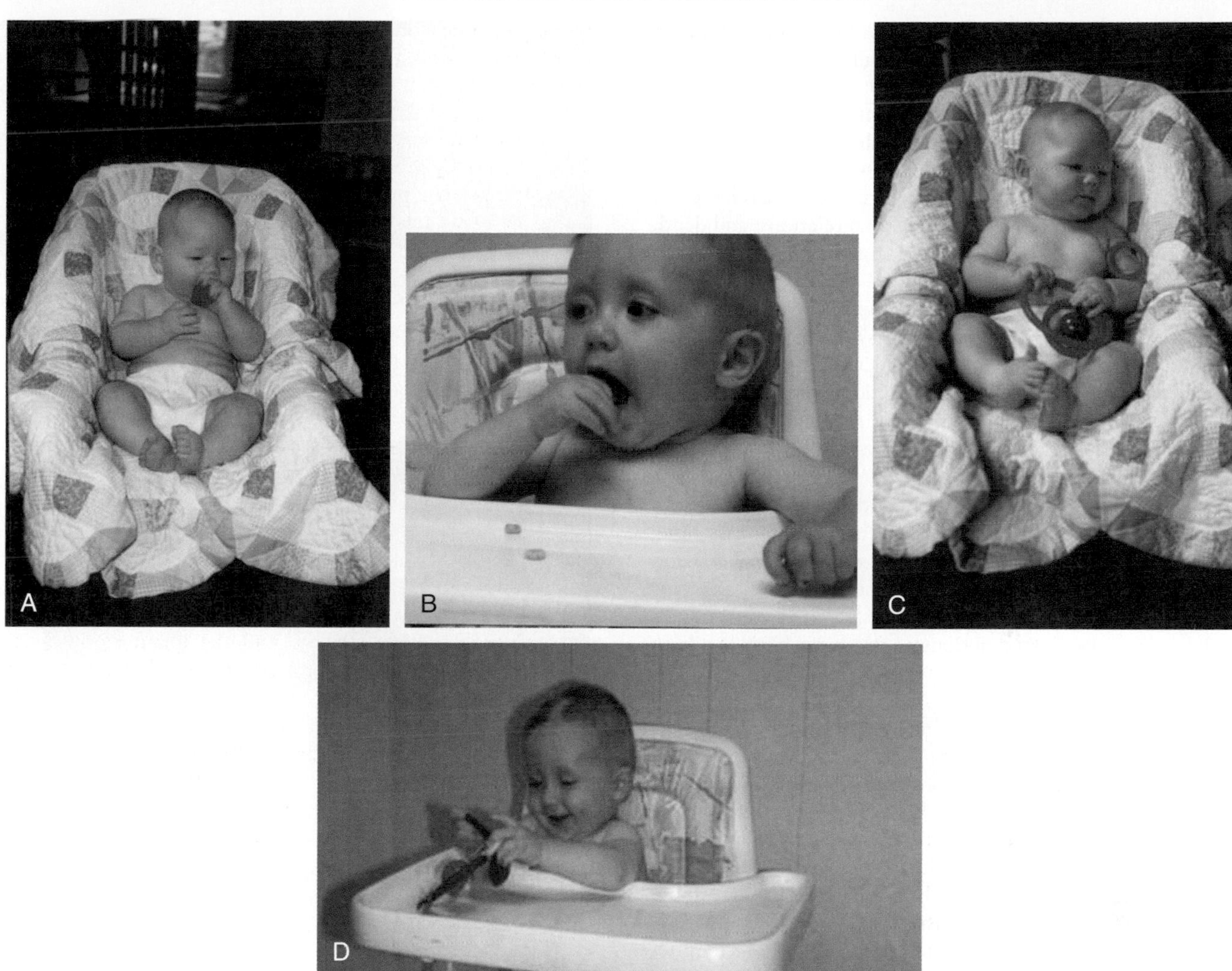

FIGURE 3-13 **A and B,** Grasping patterns evolve from palmar grasp without active thumb use **(A)** to radial digital grasp **(B)**. **C,** At 4 months, the infant holds the object tight against the palm, with all fingers flexing as a unit. **D,** At 8 months, the infant holds objects in the radial digits.

thumb press the object against the palm (Figure 3-13, *C*). At 6 months, the infant uses a radial palmar grasping pattern in which the first two fingers hold the object against the thumb. This grasp enables the infant to orient the object so that it can be easily seen or brought to the mouth (Figure 3-13, *D*). The infant secures small objects using a raking motion of the fingers, with the forearm stabilized on the surface.

Grasp continues to change rapidly from 7 to 12 months.[22,34] A radial digital grasp emerges in which the thumb opposes the index and middle finger pads. At approximately 9 months, wrist stability in extension increases, and the infant is better able to use the fingertips in grasping (e.g., the infant can use fingertips to grasp a small object, such as a cube or cracker). By holding objects distally in the fingers, the infant can move the object while it is in the hand; movement of objects within the hands allows the infant to explore them and use objects for functional purposes. A pincer grasp, with which the infant holds small objects between the thumb and finger pads, develops by 10 to 11 months. A 12-month-old infant uses various grasping patterns, often holding an object in the radial fingers and thumb. The infant may also grasp a raisin or piece of cereal with a mature pincer grasp (i.e., the thumb opposes the index finger).

In the second year of life, grasping patterns continue to be refined. The child holds objects distally in the fingers, where holding is more dynamic. By the end of the second year, a tripod grasp on utensils and other tools may be observed. Other grasping patterns may also be used, depending on the size, shape, and weight of the object held. For example, tools are held in the hand using first a palmar grasp and then a digital grasp. Blended grasping patterns develop toward the end of the second year, allowing the child to hold a tool securely in the ulnar digits while the radial digits guide its use.

Voluntary release of objects develops around 7 to 8 months of age. The first release is awkward and is characterized by full extension of all fingers. The infant becomes interested in dropping objects and practices release by flinging them from the highchair. By 10 months of age, objects are purposefully released into a container, one of the first ways the infant relates separate objects. As the infant combines objects in play, release becomes important for stacking and accurate placement. For example, the play of 1-year-old children includes placing objects in containers, dumping them out, and beginning the activity again.

By 15 to 18 months of age, the infant demonstrates release of a raisin into a small bottle and the ability to stack two cubes. Stacking blocks is part of relational play because the infant now has the needed control of the arm in space, precision grasp without support, controlled release, spatial relations, and depth perception. The infant can also place large, simple puzzle pieces and pegs in the proper areas. At the same time, the infant acquires the ability to discriminate simple forms and shapes. The infant's learning of perceptual skills is supported by improved manipulative abilities, and increased perceptual discrimination promotes the infant's practice of manipulation.[107] Perception of force increases, enabling the infant to hold an object with the just-right amount of pressure (e.g., so cookies are not crushed before eaten).

The complementary use of both hands to play with objects develops between 12 months and 2 years. During this time, one hand is used to hold the object, while the other hand manipulates or moves the object. It is not until the third year that children consistently demonstrate use of two hands in simultaneous, coordinated actions (e.g., using both hands to string beads or button a shirt).[44]

Cognitive

In the first 6 months, the infant learns about the body and the effects of its actions. Interests are focused on the actions with objects and the sensory input these actions provide. The infant's learning occurs through the primary senses: looking, tasting, touching, smelling, hearing, and moving. The infant enjoys repeating actions for their own sake, and play is focused on the action that can be performed with an object (e.g., mouthing, banging, shaking), rather than the object itself.[86] By 8 to 9 months of age, the infant has an attention span of 2 to 3 minutes and combines objects when playing (e.g., placing a favorite toy in a container). At this age, children begin to understand object permanence; that is, they know that an object continues to exist even though it is hidden and cannot be seen.[30] They can also find a hidden sound and actively try to locate new sounds.

By 12 months of age, the infant's understanding of the functional purpose of objects increases. Play behaviors are increasingly determined by the purpose of the toy, and toys are used according to their function. The infant also demonstrates more goal-directed behaviors, performing a particular action with the intent of obtaining a specific result or goal. Tools become important at this time because the infant uses play tools (e.g., hammers, spoons, shovels) to gain further understanding of how objects work. At the same time, the infant begins to understand how objects work (e.g., how to activate a switch or open a door).

In the second year, the child can put together a sequence of several actions, such as placing small "people" in a toy bus and pushing it across the floor. The sequencing of actions indicates increasing memory and attention span. Some of the first sequential behaviors illustrate the child's imitation of parent or sibling actions; increased ability to imitate and increased play sequences appear to develop concurrently (Figure 3-14).

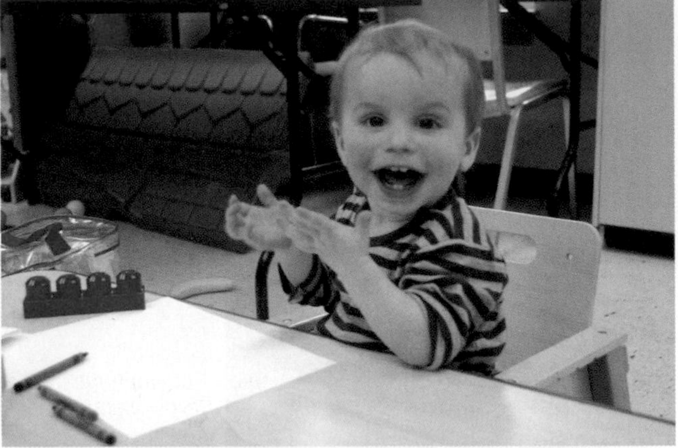

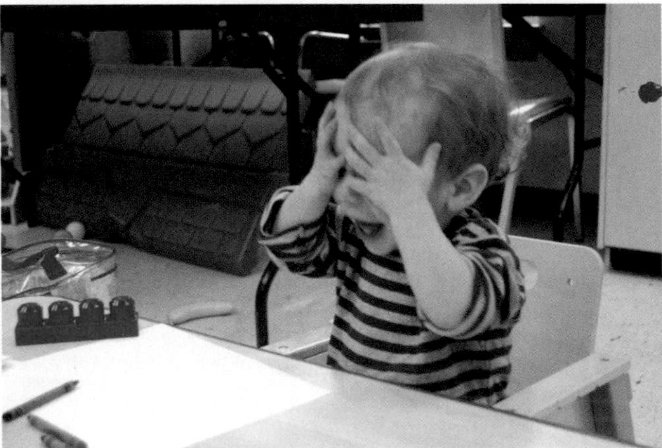

FIGURE 3-14 This 1½-year-old boy engages in social play, imitating an adult, sequencing action, taking turns, and demonstrating understanding of object permanence on self.

Social

The infant's emotional transition from the protective, warm womb to the moment of birth is a dramatic change. The primary purpose of the newborn's system is to maintain body functions (i.e., cardiovascular, respiratory, and gastrointestinal systems). However, as the infant matures, the focus shifts to increasing competence in interaction with the environment. The sense of basic trust or mistrust becomes a main theme in the infant's affective development and is highly dependent on the relationship with the primary caregivers. According to Erikson,[42] the first demonstration of an infant's social trust is observed in the ease with which he or she feeds and sleeps (see Table 3-3).

The basic trust relationship has varying degrees of involvement. Parent-infant bonding is not endowed but is developed from experiences shared between parent and child over time. These feelings are seen in the progression of physical contact between parent and infant. The infant shows a differentiated response to the parent's voice, usually quieting and calming. Although infants are capable of crying from birth, they begin to express other emotions by 2 months, such as smiling and laughing.

By 5 to 6 months, the infant becomes very interested in a mirror, indicating a beginning recognition of self. By 4 to 5 months, he or she vocalizes in tones that indicate pleasure and displeasure. In the second year of life, the parents (or caregivers) remain the most important people in the child's life. The 2-year-old infant likes to be in constant sight of the parents and expresses emotions by hugging and kissing them.

TABLE 3-5 Development of Emotion Regulation and Related Social Behaviors

Age	Emotion Regulation	Social Interaction Skills
0-12 months	Self-soothes Learns to modulate reactivity Regulates attention Relies on caregiver for support during stressful situations	Discriminates others' expressions Shows expressive responsiveness to stimuli Demonstrates different facial expressions
12-30 months	Shows increasing self-awareness Shows emerging consciousness of own emotional responses Can be irritable because of constraints and limits imposed when desiring to explore	Expresses self-consciousness, shows shame, pride, coyness Understands more language and more emotions Expresses affective state

Adapted from Saarni, C. (1999). *The development of emotional competence* (pp. 18–19). New York: Guilford Press; Kopp, C. (1982). Antecedents of self-regulation: A developmental perspective. *Developmental Psychology, 18*, 199–214.

Although toddlers practice their autonomy around parents, they have no intention of giving up reliance on them and may become upset or frightened when the parents leave. Children at age 2 are interested in other children, but they tend to watch them rather than verbally or physically interacting with them. In a room of open spaces, 2-year-olds are likely to play next to each other. Their side-by-side play often involves imitation, with few verbal acknowledgments of each other. As discussed in the section on emotion regulation, Table 3-5 describes how the development of emotion regulation influences social interaction during infancy.

Contexts of Infancy

Cultural Contexts

The family's cultural beliefs and values influence caregiving practices and determine many of the child's earliest experiences. Breastfeeding practices influence the infant's development. Breastfeeding and bottle-feeding practices vary across different cultures and ethnic groups. In the United States, breastfeeding rates in the first 6 months for all ethnic groups is 73%; however, among women of Hispanic background, it is 80%, and among black mothers, it is 54%. Hispanic mothers tend to seek breastfeeding advice from their families; in contrast, white mothers tend to rely on advice from their health care providers.[24] In the United Kingdom, black and Asian mothers have the highest breastfeeding rates compared with white mothers.[77] Culture (as well as education) interacts with race and ethnicity in determining breastfeeding rates. Factors that contribute to a woman's decision to breastfeed include social and cultural norms, social support, guidance and support from health care providers, work environment, and the media,[24,88] illustrating Bronfenbrenner's ecologic model of social influences. The mother's decision to breastfeed can affect the child's nutrition, health, eating habits, and growth.

Race and ethnicity also influence how attentive parents are, how often they hold the infant,[50] how quickly a crying infant is consoled,[139] and many other aspects of infant caregiving.[13] For example, Chinese parents are often very attentive, carrying and holding their infants throughout the day, even during naps. When infants are not held, they are kept nearby and picked up immediately if they cry.[26]

Physical Contexts

Although many infants have a supplemental play area in a childcare center, the home provides the infant's first play environment. The crib is often a play environment, providing a place for comforting toys (e.g., music boxes, colorful mobiles). Other early play spaces include a playpen, infant seat, and swing. The infant also spends time playing on the floor's carpeted surface or on a blanket. Because the infant is not yet mobile, safety is not as much of a concern as it will be in the next 2 years of life. Early play also occurs in the parent's or caregiver's arms. Exploratory play and attachment occupations are pursued on the parent's lap, and the infant is fascinated by the parent's face and clothing. At the same time, the infant feels safe and comforted by the parent's presence.

In the second 6 months, the infant requires less support to play, and a major role of the parent becomes one of protector from harm. As the infant becomes more mobile, spaces are closed, and objects now within reach are removed. Exploration of all accessible spaces becomes an infant's primary goal.

In the second year of life, the child's environment may expand to the yard, to neighbors' homes and yards, and to previously unexplored spaces in the home. Most children have opportunities for play in their home's yard or in the fenced-in areas of their childcare centers. Although the child's increasing interest in visiting outdoor spaces provides important opportunities for sensory exploration, it also creates certain safety concerns. Parents invest in gates and other methods of restricting the child's mobility to safe areas.

Early Childhood: Ages 2 to 5 Years

Play Occupations

The three types of play that predominate in early childhood are (1) *pretend,* or *symbolic, play*; (2) *constructive play*; and (3) *rough-and-tumble,* or *physical, play* (Boxes 3-6 and 3-7). Similar changes are observed in each type of play. First, the child's play becomes more elaborate—the child now combines multiple steps and multiple schemas. Short play sequences become long scripts involving several characters or actors in a story.[79,86] Second, play becomes more social. The preschool-age child orients play toward peers, involving one or two peers in the story and taking turns playing various roles. When preschool-age children play with peers, the interaction appears to be as important as the activity's goal. As the child approaches 5 years of age, all play becomes increasingly social, generally involving a small group of peers.[79,132]

Beginning at 2 years of age and continuing through the early childhood years, the child's play is symbolic and imaginative.

BOX 3-6 Development of Play Occupations: Preschoolers—24 to 36 Months

Play Occupations

Symbolic Play

Links multiple schema combinations into meaningful sequences of pretend play
Uses objects for multiple pretend ideas
Uses toys to represent animals or people
Plays out drama with stuffed animals or imaginary friends
Plays house, assigning roles to others, taking on specific roles

Constructive Play

Participates in drawing and puzzles
Imitates adults using toys

Gross Motor Play

Likes jumping, rough-and-tumble play
Makes messes

Social Play

Associative, parallel play predominates

Performance Skills

Regulatory/Sensory Organization

Handles fragile items carefully
Enjoys interesting tactile surfaces
Plays with water and sand
May experience difficulty with transitions

Fine Motor/Manipulation

Snips with scissors
Traces form, such as a cross
Colors in large forms
Draws circles accurately
Builds towers and lines up objects
Holds crayon with dexterity
Completes puzzles of 4-5 pieces
Plays with toys with moving parts

Gross Motor/Mobility

Rides tricycle
Catches large ball against chest
Jumps from step or small height
Begins to hop on one foot

Cognitive

Combines actions into entire play scenario (e.g., feeding doll, then dressing in nightwear, then putting to bed)
Shows interest in wearing costumes; creates entire scripts of imaginative play
Matches pictures
Sorts shapes and colors
Plays house

Social

Cooperative play, takes turns at times
Shows interest in peers, enjoys having companions
Begins cooperative play and play in small groups
Shy with strangers, especially adults
Engages in dialog of few words
Can be possessive of loved ones

Data from Parks, S. (2007). *HELP Strands*. Palo Alto, CA: Vort; Linder, T. (2008). *Transdisciplinary play-based assessment* (rev. ed.). Baltimore: Brookes.

BOX 3-7 Development of Play Occupations: Preschoolers—3 to 4 Years

Play Occupations

Complex Imaginary Play

Creates scripts for play in which pretend objects have actions that reflect roles in real or imaginary life
May use complex scripts for pretend sequences; portrays multiple characters with feelings

Constructive Play

Creates art product with adult assistance
Works puzzles and blocks

Rough-and-Tumble Play

Enjoys physical play, swinging, sliding board at playground, jumping, running

Social Play

Participates in circle time, games, drawing, and art time at preschool
Engages in singing and dancing in groups
Associative play: plays with other children, sharing and talking about play goal

Performance Skills

Fine Motor/Manipulation

Uses precision (tripod) grasp on pencil or crayon
Colors within lines
Copies simple shapes; begins to copy letters
Uses scissors to cut; cuts simple shapes
Constructs three-dimensional design (e.g., 3-block bridge)
Manipulates objects within the hand

Gross Motor/Mobility

Jumps, climbs, runs
Begins to skip and hop
Rides tricycle
Stands briefly on one foot
Alternates feet walking upstairs
Jumps from step with 2 feet

Cognitive

Uses imaginary objects in play
Makes dolls and action figures carry out roles and interact with other toys
Categorizes and sorts objects
Shows a sense of humor

Social

Attempts challenging activities
Prefers play with other children; group play replaces parallel play
Follows turn-taking in discourse and is aware of social aspects of conversation
Shows interest in being a friend
Prefers same-sex playmates

Data from Knox, S. (2008). Development and current use of the Knox Preschool Play Scale. In L. D. Parham & L. Fazio (Eds.), *Play in occupational therapy for children* (2nd ed., pp. 55–70). St. Louis: Mosby; Folio, M. R., & Fewell, R. R. (2000). *Peabody Developmental Motor Scales* (rev. ed.). Austin, TX: Pro-Ed.

The child pretends that dolls, figurines, and stuffed animals are real. The child may also imitate the actions of parents, teachers, and peers. At ages 3 and 4, pretend play becomes more abstract, and objects, such as a block, can be used to represent something else. Pretend play now involves many steps that relate to each other. Children develop scripts as a basis for their play (e.g., one child is the father and one is the mother). They base these scripts on real-life events and play their roles with enthusiasm and imagination, creating their own stories and enjoying the power of their imaginary roles (Figure 3-15). Their dramatic play is quite complex at this time. However, when they are in small groups, their interaction with their peers seems to be more important than the play goal, and they can easily turn to new activities suggested by one member of the group.

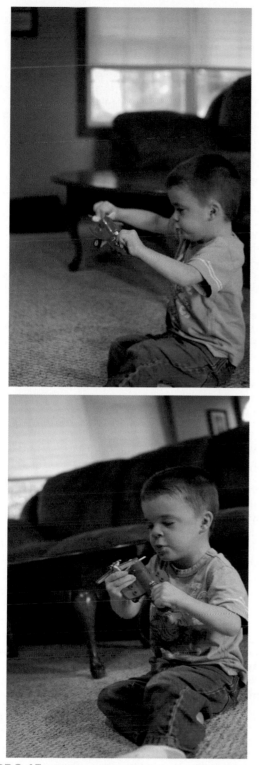

FIGURE 3-15 Pretend play of this 4-year-old focuses on his interests.

BOX 3-8 Development of Play Occupations: Preschoolers—4 to 5 Years

Play Occupations

Games with Rules

Begins group games with simple rules
Engages in organized play with prescribed roles
Participates in organized gross motor games such as kickball or "duck, duck, goose"

Constructive Play

Takes pride in products
Shows interest in the goal of the activity
Constructs complex structures

Social Play/Dramatic Play

Participates in role play with other children
Participates in "dress up"
Tells stories
Continues with pretend play that involves scripts with imaginary characters

Performance Skills

Fine Motor/Manipulative

Draws using a dynamic tripod grasp
Copies simple shapes
Completes puzzles of up to 10 pieces
Uses scissors to cut out squares and other simple shapes
Colors within the lines
Uses two hands together well, one stabilizing paper or object and the other manipulating object
Draws stick figure or may begin to draw trunk and arms
Copies own name
Strings small beads

Gross Motor/Mobility

Jumps down from high step; jumps forward
Throws ball
Hops for long sequences (4-6 steps)
Climbs on playground equipment, swinging from arms or legs
Throws ball and hits target
Skips for a long distance
Walks up and down stairs reciprocally

Cognitive

Understands rules to a game
Remembers rules with a few reminders
Makes up stories that involve role playing with other children
Participates in goal-oriented, cooperative play with two or three other children
Participates in planning a play activity
Begins abstract problem solving

Social

Enjoys clowning
Sings whole songs
Role plays based on parents' roles

Data from Linder, T. (2008). *Transdisciplinary play-based assessment* (rev. ed.). Baltimore: Brookes.

By 5 years of age, this imaginary play is predominantly social, as small groups of two and three join in cooperative play. A 5-year-old child engages in pretend play about one third of the time.[122] However, this pretend play is based on imitation of real life and dressing up to play certain roles (e.g., firefighter, police officer, ballerina). Although children of this age demonstrate some understanding of adult roles, they erroneously assume that roles are one-dimensional (e.g., a firefighter has one role, that of putting out fires). Through pretending, children develop creativity, problem solving, and an understanding of another person's point of view (Boxes 3-8 and 3-9).[129] Case Study 3-1 presents an example of applying Vygotsky's theories to a preschooler's learning the skills that support pretend play.

BOX 3-9 Development of Play Occupation: Kindergartners—5 to 6 Years

Play Occupations

Games with Rules
Board games
Computer games
Competitive and cooperative games

Dramatic Play
Elaborate imaginary play
Role plays stories and themes related to seasons or occupations
Emphasis is on reality
Reconstructs real world in play

Sports
Participates in ball play

Social Play
Participates in group activities
Organized play in groups
Goal of play (winning) may compete with social interaction at times

Performance Skills

Fine Motor/Manipulation
Cuts with scissors
Prints name from copy
Copies triangle; traces diamond
Completes puzzles of up to 20 pieces
Traces letters, begins to copy letters
Manipulates tiny objects in fingertips without dropping
Uses two hands together in complementary movements

Gross Motor/Mobility
Hops well for long distances
Skips with good balance
Catches ball with two hands
Kicks with accuracy
Stands on one foot for 8-10 seconds

Cognitive
Reasons through simple problems
Bases play more on real life than on imaginary world
Participates in organized games
Uses complex scripts in play
Demonstrates deferred imitation
Sorts objects in different ways
Copies elaborate block structures

Social
Participates in groups of two to four that play in organized, complex games
Has friends (same sex)
Enjoys singing and dancing; reflects meaning of words and music
Demonstrates understanding of others' feelings

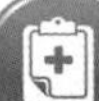

CASE STUDY 3-1 Example of Vygotsky: Scaffolding and the Zone of Proximal Development

Sarah is a 4-year-old girl with autism spectrum disorder. She demonstrates age-appropriate development in motor skills; however, she has difficulty with motor planning and sequencing a series of movements. Her communication, play, and activities of daily living skills appear to be at a 2-year-old level. She also has difficulty with perceptual skills and often confuses concepts such as up-down, right-left, and spatial awareness. Teresa, an occupational therapist, selected a dress-up activity to promote Sarah's self-care, self-identity, and pretend play development. Teresa, who has collaborated with the speech-language pathologist, also tries to elicit simple questions and use of action verbs in this play scenario.

Teresa sets up the activity by inviting Sarah to come explore the large bin of dress-up clothes in the preschool classroom. As Teresa holds up a fireman's jacket and a doctor's coat, she asks Sarah to identify the top and bottom and to state what part of the body it fits. When Teresa asks Sarah what she wants to be ("Would you like to be a princess, a nurse, a superhero?"), Sarah's pretend skills are not sufficiently developed to choose. Teresa suggests that she be a princess, wearing a gown, princess shoes, and a crown. Teresa asks, "How will you get on your gown?" Sarah is hesitant, so Teresa points to the top and bottom, shows the zipper, and indicates that she can step into the gown. Sarah hesitates, and Teresa holds her hand to encourage her to step into the gown. She verbally cues her to slide her arms through the sleeves and models the action with an imaginary dress. Physical assistance is unnecessary as Sarah dons the gown with this cueing.

Throughout the activity, Teresa helps Sarah learn and integrate body awareness, saying, "Where are your toes? Let me see your hands and fingers." When Sarah has her gown, shoes, and crown on, Teresa suggests that she dance in front of a mirror to see how the gown flows and to imagine being a princess. They parade through the preschool classroom so that the other children can see her gown. When it is time to go outside and Sarah must take off the gown, Teresa decides to allow Sarah to sequence the undressing activity without verbal or physical cueing. She kneels by Sarah, prepared to help or give guidance, but knowing that undressing is easier, she hopes that Sarah can accomplish it on her own. Although Teresa begins the zipper, Sarah removes her princess clothing independently. Teresa reminds her of top and bottom, right and left during the undressing to reinforce those concepts.

Although this is a simple play scenario, common in preschool classrooms, Teresa has applied principles of Vygotsky's theories. She selected an activity within Sarah's proximal zone of development that she could achieve with a minimal amount of support. Teresa was prepared at each step to provide assistance (e.g., physical assistance in donning), but she first observed what support was needed to give the just-right amount of support. She promoted Sarah's development of pretend play, self-care, and self-identity by selecting an appropriate activity, providing just-right cues and guidance, and reinforcing perceptual concepts.

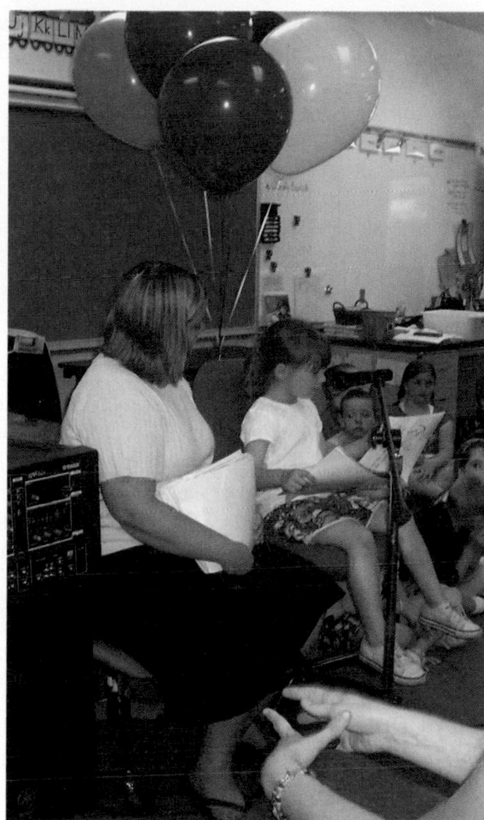

FIGURE 3-16 Children enjoy reading and writing activities at school. Molly is proud of her first book!

Play that involves building and construction also teaches the child a variety of skills during early childhood. At first, these skills are demonstrated in the completion of puzzles and toys with fit-together pieces (Figure 3-16). However, with mastery of simple pegs and puzzles, the child becomes more creative in construction. For example, a 4-year-old child can develop a plan to build a structure with blocks and then carry out the steps to complete the project. With instructions and a model, a 5-year-old child can make a simple art project or create a three-dimensional design. A 5-year-old child can also put together a 10-piece puzzle. The final product has become more important, and the child is motivated to complete it and show others the final result. The planning and designing involved in building and construction play help the child acquire an understanding of spatial perception and object relationships. This activity also appears to be foundational to academic performance in school.

Children 2 to 5 years of age are extremely active and almost always readily engage in rough-and-tumble play. They continue to delight in movement experiences that provide strong sensory input. Activities such as running, hopping, skipping, and tumbling are performed as play without any particular goal. Although rough-and-tumble play generally involves other children, it is generally noncompetitive and rarely organized. Children enjoy this activity for the simple, simultaneous pleasure of movement as they play together.[23]

In associative physical play, children are generally more interested in being with other children than in the goal of the activity. However, some children enjoy primarily social play, whereas others enjoy solitary play. These differences do not relate to ability as much as they relate to preferences and temperament.[138]

Performance Skills

Gross Motor and Mobility

Young children are amazingly competent individuals, and their repertoire of motor function leaps forward during the preschool years (see Performance Skills in Boxes 3-6, 3-7, 3-8, and 3-9). By age 2 years, the child walks with an increased length of stride and an efficient, well-coordinated, and well-balanced gait. Although children begin to run by 2 years, they do not exhibit true running (characterized by trunk rotation and arm swing) until 3 to 4 years of age. The 4-year-old child demonstrates a walking pattern similar to that of an adult. By 5 to 6 years of age, the mature running pattern has developed, and children test their speed by challenging each other to races.

As mobility develops, children gain access to spaces previously unavailable to them. By 2 years of age, a child walks up stairs without holding onto a parent's hand, and at 2½ years, the child can walk down stairs without support. A child 3½ years old walks up and down stairs by alternating the feet and without needing to hold onto a rail.

Running and stair climbing become possible, in part, because the child's balance and strength increase. Emerging balance can be observed as the 2-year-old child briefly stands on one foot to kick a ball. By 5 years of age, the child can balance on one foot for several seconds and walk on a curb without falling.[49] Between 3 and 5 years, the child may successfully attempt to use skates or roller blades.

Jumping is first observed in 2-year-old children. This skill requires strength, coordination, and balance. By 3 years of age, the child can jump easily from a step. Hopping requires greater strength and balance than jumping and is first observed at 3½ years. Skipping is the more difficult gross motor pattern because it requires sequencing of a rhythmic pattern that includes a step and a hop. A coordinated skipping pattern is not observed until 5 years of age.[78]

A 2-year-old child can begin to pedal a tricycle and move small riding toys. By 3 years of age, the child can pedal a tricycle but may run into objects. A 4-year-old child can steer and maneuver a tricycle around obstacles.

By 2½ years, most children can catch a 10-inch ball. This pattern of maturity enables the 4-year-old child to catch a much smaller ball, such as a tennis ball, successfully.[49] The first pattern of throwing involves a pushing motion, with the elbow providing the force for the throw. The 4-year-old child demonstrates more forward weight shift with throwing, increasing the force of the ball and the distance thrown. Kicking emerges in the 2- to 3-year-old child, with accurate kicking to a target exhibited by 6 years of age. Ball skills become increasingly important as the child begins participating in organized sports during the primary grades.

Fine Motor and Manipulation

Early childhood is a time of rapid improvement in fine motor and manipulation performance. By 4 years of age, children learn to move small objects efficiently within one hand (i.e., in-hand manipulation). A 4-year-old child can hold several small objects in the palm of the hand while moving individual pieces with the radial fingers.[107] In-hand manipulation indicates that isolated finger movement is well controlled and that the thumb easily moves into opposition for pad-to-pad prehension. These skills also indicate that the child can modulate force and that he or she has an accurate perception of the gentle force needed to handle small objects with the fingertips.[107]

With efficient in-hand manipulation, the preschool child also learns the functional use of drawing and cutting tools. Most 3-year-old children hold a pencil with a static tripod grasp (i.e., with the pencil resting between the thumb and first two fingers) and use forearm and wrist movement to draw; however, by 5 years, a child demonstrates a mature, dynamic tripod. In this grasp pattern, the pencil is held in the tips of the radial fingers and is moved using finger movement. By controlling the pencil using individual finger movements, the child can make letters and small forms.

Drawing skills progress from drawing circles to lines that intersect and cross in a diagonal (e.g., an X). The 5-year-old child can draw a person with multiple and recognizable parts. Drawing is often a strong interest at this age and contributes to the child's imaginative play.[148] He or she can also draw detailed figures created in the imagination (i.e., monsters, fairies, and other fanciful creatures) (Table 3-6).

The development of scissors skills follows the development of controlled pencil use. The first cutting skill, observed at 3 years, is snipping with alternating full-finger extension and flexion. Between 4 and 6 years, bilateral hand coordination, dexterity, and eye-hand coordination improve, enabling the child to cut out simple shapes. Mature use of scissors is not achieved until 5 to 6 years because it requires isolated finger movements, simultaneous hand control, and well-developed eye-hand coordination for cutting accuracy.[49,103]

Other fine motor skills acquired during the preschool years are important to the child's constructive and dramatic play. Activities such as putting puzzles together, building towers, stringing small beads, using keys, and cutting out complex designs usually require dexterity, bilateral coordination, and motor planning.

Cognitive

Preschool-age children create symbolic representations of real-life objects and events during play. In addition, they begin to plan pretend scenarios in advance, organizing who and what are needed to complete the activity. Play becomes an elaborate sequence of events that is remembered, acted out, and later described for others. For example, the child may act out the role of an adult, imitating action remembered from an earlier experience. This form of role play demonstrates the child's understanding of how roles relate to actions and how actions relate to each other (e.g., the child may role play a grocery store clerk, displaying items for sale, taking money from the customer, and placing the money in a toy cash register).

Abstract thinking begins in the preschool years as the child pretends that an object is something else. For example, the

TABLE 3-6 Dynamical Systems Theory Perspective on Development of Drawing Skills (4-6 Years)

Stages of Drawing Development

Age	Developmental Skills
2-3 years	Makes scribbling marks on paper that are without symbolic meaning (exploratory phase). Repetitious marks.
3-4 years	Interprets drawing after it has been produced. Shapes emerge from scribbling.
4-5 years	Draws an image, draws with intent a picture that represents an object, person, or event. Has shapes and distinct elements, may be disordered, incorrect sizing, but has some semblance to intent.

Dynamical Systems Influencing Drawing Skill, 3-5 Years

Performance	Intrinsic Factors (Individual)	Extrinsic Factors (Environment)
Dynamic grasp of pencil or marker	Haptic perception of pencil in hand. Moves object in hand while holding (efficient intrinsic muscle use). Demonstrates dynamic tripod grasp.	Experience holding different drawing utensils, e.g., crayons, markers. Experience drawing on different surfaces. Experience in manipulating small objects, e.g., puzzles, blocks, small figurines.
Eye-hand coordination	Visual acuity. Visual perception. Motor coordination. Coordination of arm, hand, and finger action.	Experience in eye-hand coordination, e.g., stringing beads, stacking, puzzles. Available colors, contrasts, lighting, sizing of drawing utensils.
Draws shapes	Motor planning skills. Visual motor coordination.	Experience moving through the environment, handling objects with different shapes. Available colors, contrast, shapes in 2 and 3 dimensions. Cues from adults or others. Feedback from adults.
Draw figures and forms	Motor planning skills. Spatial relation skills.	Cues that guide drawing, e.g., models, examples. Adult reinforcement. Available color, lighting, surfaces, utensils.
Drawing represents an action, person, object, or event	Cognitive skills of attributing symbolic meaning, demonstrating representational thinking.	Play opportunities. Adult guidance. Peer models. Experience with books, pictures, stories, art.

From Ziviani, J., & Wallen, M. (2006). The development of graphomotor skills. In A. Henderson & C. Pehoski (Eds.), *Hand function in the child* (2nd ed., pp. 217–238). St. Louis: Mosby.

child may pretend a block is a doll bed; later the same block may become a telephone receiver or a train car.

In construction play (e.g., constructing train sets or building castles with Lego blocks), the child discriminates object size and shape. Building in three dimensions also requires spatial understanding and problem-solving skills. When building from a set of blocks, the child usually must first categorize and organize the blocks. Next, the child must solve the problem of how to fit them together to replicate a model or create the imagined structure.

In a similar way, the emergence of drawing skills reflects cognitive abilities, motor planning, and perceptual skills. The 3-year-old child makes crude attempts to represent people and objects in drawings. By 4 years of age, a child can draw a recognizable person, demonstrating the ability to select salient features and represent them on a two-dimensional surface. The 4-year-old child not only identifies the parts of a person but also relates them correctly, although the size of the parts is rarely proportional to real life. At 5 years, the child's drawing is more refined, more realistic, and better proportioned. By this age, pictures begin to tell stories and reflect the child's emotions (see Table 3-6).[86,148]

Social

In early childhood, interaction and play with peers take on increasing importance. Children become social beings and identify themselves as individuals (i.e., separate from parents). Autonomy dominates psychosocial development from 2 to 4 years as the toddler shows his or her independence by moving away from the parent. The child is adamant about making personal decisions. The development of trust in the environment and improvements in language bring forth control over self, strengthening the child's autonomous nature.

The discovery of the body and how to control it promotes independence in self-care. Success in acting independently instills a sense of confidence and self-control. The child also begins to perceive that now all of his independent actions meet the approval of adults. See previous section on self-identity development.

Children need to achieve a balance between initiative to act independently and the responsibility they feel for their own actions. Children 4 to 5 years old explore beyond the environment, discovering new activities. They seek new experiences for the pleasure of learning about the environment and for the opportunities they offer for exploration. If the child's learning experiences are successful and effective and his or her actions meet parental approval, a sense of initiative is developed. Through these activities, the child learns to question, reason, and find solutions to problems.

Adult-child relationships and early home experiences also influence later peer relations. According to research, children whose attachments to their mothers are rated as secure tend to be more responsive to other children in childcare settings. They are also more curious and competent.[80] Peer play becomes an important avenue for the child's development of social and cognitive abilities. With their peers, they practice social roles, engage in dramatic play, and enjoy rough-and-tumble play.[109]

The development of autonomy provides a foundation for the child's imagination. The young child explores the world not only through the use of his or her senses but also by thinking and reasoning. Although play can be reality based, it usually includes fantasy, wishes, and role play. Words, rhymes, and songs also complement this type of play.[108]

Contexts

Cultural and Social Contexts

The social roles of young children are influenced by cultures, ethnicity, and community. In the United States, the importance of interaction with peers is stressed at young ages. Most American children begin to interact with their peers (same age group) at about 3 years of age. Same-age peers become increasingly important through elementary school and dominate the social life of a teenager. In the United States and much of the world, children are grouped exclusively by age. These age groupings may provide more opportunities for play, but they also diminish opportunities for older children to teach and nurture younger children. Younger children have fewer opportunities to imitate older children.

Children in other parts of the world play and socialize with people of different ages. Cultural influences on social play behaviors are time and space to play, access to objects and materials, adult behavior and attitudes, and the availability of play partners.[45] For example, in Hispanic communities, children spend almost all of their time with siblings and other young relatives of a wide range of ages and primarily play with family members, including extended family. They socially participate in mixed-age groups, playing "on the edge" and watching intently until they can join in the play. Toddlers play with children of various ages, and they often play with older siblings. This "enduring social network" remains in place over time to care for, teach, and discipline children to adulthood.[116] When children spend their days with people of various ages, they have many opportunities to imitate and learn from older children and adults. Interaction with children of varying ages provides older children the opportunity to practice teaching and nurturance with young children and provides young children the opportunity to imitate older children.[148]

At very young ages, Mayan children play within their parents' work activities.[11] For example, children engage in play activities while helping their mothers wash clothes. The children's play in the Mayan culture is tolerated during daily work activities but is not specifically encouraged.[11] Bazyk and colleagues[11] found that children's work was playful, blurring the European American distinction between work and play. When children play in work activities, they are learning skills that will serve them well in adulthood. In contrast, the age-based groupings used in U.S. childcare centers and preschools provide children with opportunities to play with same-age peers but reduce their opportunities to play within adult work activities.

Families in the United States specifically design and encourage their children's play and at times become playmates with children. Although play is emphasized as the primary occupation for young children, children demonstrate interest in helping parents accomplish their work. Parents may encourage young children (e.g., 5 to 6 years old) to participate in household tasks, such as picking up their own toys. When children begin school, parents usually expect them to participate more in household tasks such as cleaning and meal preparation (see Chapter 16).[83]

Physical Contexts

By the age of 5, a child's outdoor environment has expanded beyond the areas around the home and childcare center. A variety of outdoor environments offer space for rough-and-tumble play, and expanded social and physical environments give the child new opportunities for learning (and generalizing) the skills he or she has achieved. Although adult supervision remains essential, the entire neighborhood may become the child's playground.

The availability of new indoor environments is also to be expected. Preschool classrooms usually have centers for different types of activities (e.g., creating art, listening to stories, playing games). In addition, community groups often sponsor a variety of indoor activities (e.g., preschool gymnastics, organized play programs) in which the child can participate.

Expanded environments offer children the opportunity to adapt play skills learned at home to the constraints of new spaces. For example, the child who climbs and slides down the stairs at home learns to climb a 6-foot ladder and slide down the slide in the neighborhood park. Parks and playgrounds also provide the child with new surfaces that challenge balance and equipment that offers intense vestibular experiences.

Cultural and socioeconomic differences can influence a child's physical environment. Inner-city parents frequently confine their children to the immediate household and forbid them to go outside after school, particularly to play. These protective strategies limit children's exposure to dangerous neighborhood influences, but they also restrict the physical context available for play.[20,51,144,145]

Most preschool-age children also enjoy spending time in quiet spaces. Quiet spaces can be organizing and calming after a day in a childcare center (Figure 3-17). Based on sensory preferences, arousal levels, and activity levels, other children may seek stimulating environments that are full of activity, or they may create their own high activity in an otherwise quiet space.

When placed in new environments, children often respond by instinctively exploring the new spaces (e.g., hallways, cupboards, corners, furniture). Exploring the features of an environment can help orient children to the spaces that surround them, promote perceptual learning, and provide an understanding of the play possibilities in that environment.

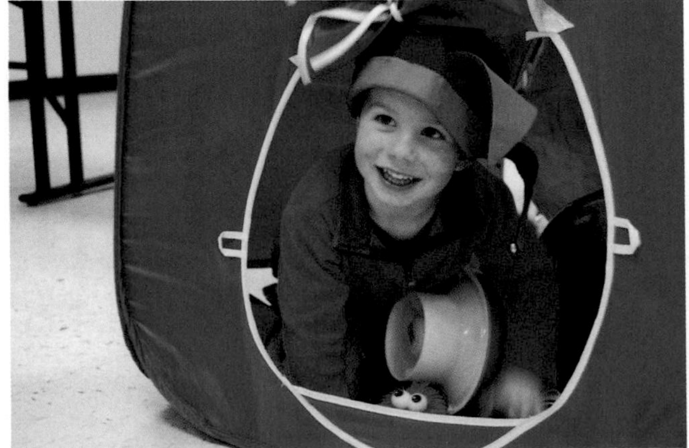

FIGURE 3-17 Children enjoy pretend play and creating fun games that may challenge balance, strength, postural stability, and coordination.

Middle Childhood: Ages 6 to 10 Years

Play Occupations

Although 6-year-old children continue to enjoy imaginative play, they begin increasingly to structure and organize their play. Box 3-10 describes Piaget's classification of games that correspond to stages of cognitive development. By the time a child is 7 or 8 years old, structured games and organized play predominate (Box 3-11). *Games with rules* are the primary mode for physical and social play. Groups of children organize themselves, assign roles, and explain (or create) rules to guide the game they plan to play. The goal of the game now competes with the reward of interacting with peers, and children become fascinated with the rules that govern the games they play.

At 7 or 8 years of age, children do not understand that rules apply equally to everyone involved in the game, and they are often unable to place the rules of the game above the personal need to win.[48] However, breaking the rules may incur the criticism of peers, who also acknowledge the importance of rules at this time. By 9 and 10 years of age, children are more conscientious about obeying rules. They also learn to negotiate the rules of a game and construct their own rules.

BOX 3-10 Piaget's Stages of Cognitive Development as Expressed in Children's Games

Dimitri's Favorite Games

Dimitri, who is 5 years old, loves games, and although he has spastic diplegia cerebral palsy, he fully engages in games that match different cognitive levels as defined by Piaget.

Practice (Sensorimotor Exploratory) Games

Dimitri loves to wrestle with his brother on the living room rug. In this game, Dimitri pulls his 7-year-old brother to the floor. Mostly they roll on top of each other vying for the top position. This game does not have rules or structure, and, most often, the wrestling ends without a victor, when Dimitri tires or his mother intervenes.

Symbolic Games

Dimitri also loves playing with his dinosaurs, doing battles, roaming for food, and running over hills and valleys in the sandbox. The dinosaurs can talk and often bargain with each other for dominion of the sand mountain. This game also lacks structure. Dimitri plays with his friend Samuel or alone, and the dinosaurs' play scenarios are often the same.

Games with Rules

Dimitri also plays "Go Fish" and "Candyland" with his brother. Dimitri knows most of the rules, plays cooperatively and takes turns, and knows how the game ends. At 5, he does not always figure out when his older brother breaks the rules to gain the lead in the game.

Although these classifications of play reflect different cognitive levels, children play at all three levels over an extended period of time.

These play categories also have different goals and outcomes for the child's performance across developmental domains.

All three play categories can be social play, object play, or both.

From Parham, L.D. (2008). Play and occupational therapy. In L.D. Parham & L.S. Fazio (Eds.), *Play in occupational therapy for children*. St. Louis: Mosby.

BOX 3-11 Development of Play Occupations: Middle Childhood—6 to 10 Years

Play Occupations

Games with Rules

Computer games, card games that require problem solving and abstract thinking

Crafts and Hobbies

Has collections

May have hobbies

Organized Sports

Cooperative and competitive play in groups or teams of children

Winning and skills are emphasized

Social Play

Play includes talking and joking

Peer play predominates at school and home

Plays with consistent friends

Performance Skills

Fine Motor/Manipulation

Good dexterity for crafts and construction with small objects

Bilateral coordination for building complex structure

Precision and motor planning evident in drawing

Motor planning evident in completion of complex puzzles

Gross Motor/Mobility

Runs with speed and endurance

Jumps, hops, skips

Throws ball well at long distances

Catches ball with accuracy

Cognitive

Abstract reasoning

Performs mental operations without need to try physically

Demonstrates flexible problem solving

Solves complex problems

Social

Cooperative, less egocentric

Tries to please others

Has best friend

Is part of cliques

Is less impulsive, is able to regulate behavior

Has competitive relationships

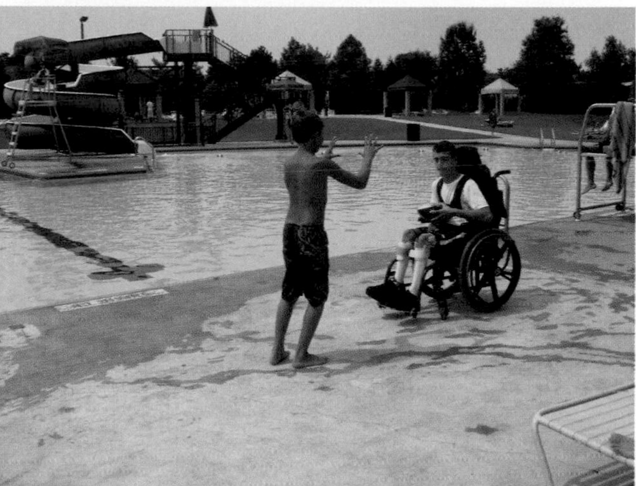

FIGURE 3-18 Favorite play activities for all children include swimming, ball play, and outdoor sports.

Children who are 8 or 9 years old become interested in sports, and parents are generally supportive of sports activities. Although a form of play, organized sports can assume a serious nature (i.e., intrinsic motivation and the internal sense of control are overridden by the external demands of practice and serious competition with peers). In addition to organized sports, physical play is a favorite interest, including climbing, rollerblading, skipping rope, and skateboarding (Figure 3-18).

Interest in creating craft and art projects continues into middle childhood. During this time, the child shows an increased ability to organize, solve problems, and create from abstract materials. However, the completion of craft and art projects continues to require the support of adults to organize materials and identify steps. The final product, which is relatively unimportant to younger children, is now valued. Computer play and video games are popular and may dominate play in middle childhood into adolescence (see Chapter 4).[128]

In middle childhood, children play in cooperative groups and value interaction with their peers. Increasingly, social contact is virtual, through e-mail, texting, and social media websites. When friends come together, almost all activity is play and fun. Simply talking and joking become playful and entertaining. Children spend more than 40% of their waking hours with peers.[31] In these peer groups, children learn to cooperate but also to compete.[48] They are now interested in *achievement* through play; they recognize and accept an outside standard for success or failure and criteria for winning or losing. With competition in play comes risk taking and strategic thinking. Children who compete in sports and other activities exhibit courage to perform against an outside standard.[113]

Performance Skills

Gross Motor and Mobility

During the elementary school years, gross motor development reflects the refinement of previously acquired skills with increases in speed, precision of movement, and strength. To achieve this refinement, children spend hours in repetition of favorite physical activities, including sports, to attain mastery. Children ride bicycles, scale fences, swim, skate, and jump rope (Figure 3-19). Although motor capabilities are highly varied for this age group, balance and coordination improve throughout the middle childhood years, providing children with the agility to dance and play sports with proficiency. Research indicates that children who struggle with physical skills have lower self-esteem and are very socially marginalized.[90] Not only does self-esteem improve as children master physical skills, but also peer acceptance improves.

Fine Motor and Manipulation

By middle childhood, children become increasingly efficient in tool use (e.g., scissors, tweezers) and demonstrate precise drawing skills. Children handle and manipulate materials (fold, sort, adhere, cut) with competency. The drawing skills of 8- and 9-year-old children demonstrate appropriate proportions and accuracy, and handwriting skills improve in speed and accuracy as children learn manuscript and then cursive writing.[65] These improvements provide evidence of increased dexterity and coordination. Construction skills, manipulation, and abilities to use tools continue to generalize across performance areas, with increases in speed, strength, and precision.

FIGURE 3-19 Children enjoy playing and swimming at the beach.

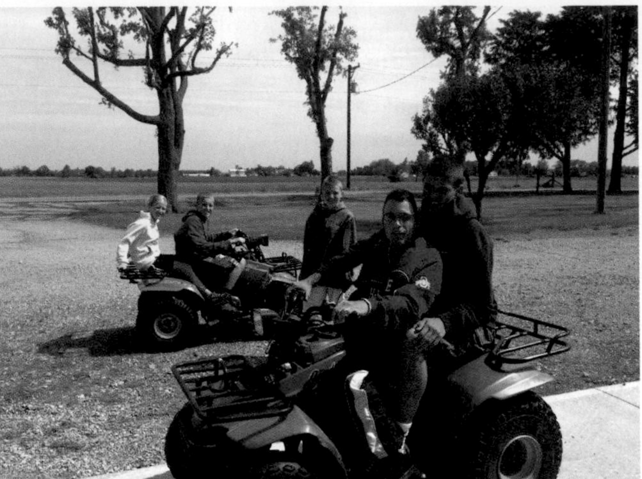

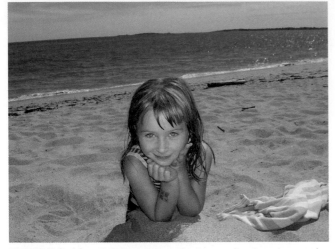

FIGURE 3-20 Brothers and cousins enjoy outdoor activities at their family farm, including tractor rides.

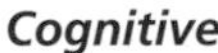

Cognitive

In middle childhood, concepts and relationships in the physical world are understood and applied. The child relates past events to future plans and comprehends how situations change over time. Thinking has become more flexible and abstract. The child has become a reasoning individual who can solve problems by understanding variables and weighing pertinent factors before making decisions. The child now has a clear understanding of the difference between fantasy and reality, and he or she chooses to move from one to the other.

At younger ages, children could apply only one solution, and they often were stuck when the solution of choice did not work. However, by 8 and 9 years of age, children recognize that different solutions can be tried, and they arrive at answers through abstract reasoning rather than through concrete trial-and-error. At this age, children can also pay attention to more than one physical characteristic at a time and can systematically put elements together.

In play, children order objects by size or shape, demonstrating the ability to discriminate perceptual aspects of objects and to order them accurately. They also understand the relationship of the whole to the parts, and they imagine pieces as parts of a whole. With this understanding, they become more competent in organizing tasks and organizing time. Children 9 to 10 years of age can give instructions to others and tell stories in detail.

By middle childhood, children learn to combine tasks and routines into complex games and competitive sports. Because numerous rules are needed to play sports, such as baseball or hockey, the child understands the need to combine the rules into a complete game. To participate in the activity successfully, the child also understands when rules apply and when rules can be negotiated. Most children also know rules can be implemented with flexibility and can be negotiated with adults.[109] The child's progression from games with some structure and flexible rules to highly competitive games demonstrates progression in moral development.

Social

Children 6 to 10 years old form close friendships and "belong" to one or more peer groups that greatly influence their decisions, how they spend their time, and what they value. Florey and Greene explain, "In the beginning of middle childhood, friendships are characterized by sharing of interests. Toward the end of this period, children tend to organize around common values, commitment, loyalty, and mutual support" (p. 282).[48]

Children in middle childhood focus on meeting challenges in themselves as well as challenges presented by others. Children appreciate the recognition that comes with successful completion of assignments or projects. Comparison with peers is increasingly important during this time. If a child's schoolwork is compared with the work of a more successful student, a negative evaluation can reduce his or her sense of mastery and may produce feelings of inferiority.

School-age children seek independence of identity. They are not as egocentric as young children and demonstrate a more objective view of themselves. Children at this age have a definite subculture, or clique, that includes only certain friends (Figure 3-20). At this age, children are quick to criticize others who do not conform to the group esthetic. Rejection by the child's peers may result from a lack of conformity in dress or physical appearance. Children who have difficulty communicating or who do not know how to initiate relationships are less likely to have close friendships. Children who are socially able and positive are more accepted and have more close friendships. At this age, children develop a peer culture and derive self-worth from their group of peers.[48]

During middle childhood, children become disinterested in adults, including their parents. The values of peers become significantly more important than those of adults. Data indicate that children 7 to 10 years old are highly compliant with and easily shift in the direction of their peers.[48]

Contexts

Cultural Contexts

Expectations for children to work vary across cultures. These expectations determine the timing and type of occupations children develop and the balance between work and play. Examples for countries other than the United States and countries of Europe illustrate these differences. In a study of 50 communities, children at 5 to 7 years of age were given responsibility for caring for younger children, for tending animals, and for carrying out household chores.[118] Larsen and Verma[82] reported that in nonindustrial populations, work during middle childhood exceeds 5 hours per day. In the United States, chores are rarely given to children younger than 8 or 9 years old. Many American families do not expect children to take responsibility for chores until the age of 10 or 11. In contrast, Polynesian children develop household skills by 3 or 4 years, at which time they gather wood, sweep, or run errands to the store. In West Africa, children have duties and run errands when they are 3 years old. In Kenya, 8-year-old girls perform most of the housework.[116]

Mayan children are continuously at their parents' side during work days. At early ages, they participate in work tasks, such as running errands and helping with cleanup. Bazyk et al.[11] found that although Mayan children began work activities at a very early age, they embedded play in these chores. Children in Central Africa acquire work experience from toddler age, and by age 12 they can trap animals, kill game, make medicines, and garden.[116] In Nigeria, young children are taught to be helpful, responsible, and respectful. Before age 5, Nigerian girls are taught to perform household chores such as washing, sweeping, cooking, and caring for their younger siblings, and by middle childhood, the girls take full responsibility for these work roles. The number of errands a child was required to run and cognitive performance were significantly related, indicating that having children participate in work tasks at an early age may enhance cognitive competence.[105]

In the United States, most children and youth have very few opportunities to work with adults. By one estimate, children contribute about 15% of all labor in households.[63] Rogoff et al.[116] believe that American children are missing valuable opportunities for learning and gaining self-satisfaction. Compared with practices in societies outside the United States, the lack of work opportunities for American children limits their practice of skills important to their future and may delay their entry into adult work roles. Through experiences in school and guided participation in household work, children may develop work skills and learn social rules and cultural values.[83] Children who participate in household chores have higher self-esteem, are more responsible, and can cope more easily with frustrations. One of the best predictors of success as an adult is participation in household tasks during childhood.[120]

Physical Contexts

In middle childhood, the child's play environment is now large and complex; more activities take place in the neighborhood and at school. The school's playground supports both social and physical play of small groups (or pairs) of children. Play occurs on ball fields and in community centers, amusement parks, and sports arenas. Organized activities are often sponsored by churches or by groups such as the Young Men's Christian Association (YMCA). By middle childhood, children have the mobility skills to maneuver through all environments (e.g., rough terrain, busy city streets). The society of school-age children dominates neighborhood streets and backyards, with bicycle races and spontaneous street hockey games. These children explore the woods and go on adventures in nearby parks to find areas unexplored by others. Although supervision by adults is still needed at times, intermittent supervision usually suffices.

Children spend many of their waking hours in school. Schools offer complex environments (e.g., playgrounds, computer rooms, libraries, classrooms, lunchrooms) with many social and learning opportunities.

Summary

The development of occupational performance is influenced by many systems and variables in the individual child and in the environment. The various patterns observed in children provide insight into how and why a child follows a certain developmental trajectory. Sensory, motor, cognitive, and social skills support the child's performance in play occupations. At the same time, a child's activities are highly influenced by his or her cultural, social, and physical contexts. As an essential occupation of childhood, play provides a means of understanding and appreciating children's performance and a means for enhancing functional performance when development is delayed. The ability to play is also an important outcome of occupational therapy, one that reflects the being of childhood.

Summary Points

- Cognitive development reflects the interaction of genetic endowment and experience. Piaget and Vygotsky theorized that children learn through interaction with the environment and are particularly influenced by their social environment.
- Occupational therapists understand that children acquire new skills within their zone of proximal development through adult scaffolding of the just-right challenge to the child's learning.
- In dynamical systems theory, children acquire new skills through the interaction of intrinsic and extrinsic factors that are flexibly assembled to meet goals that are meaningful to the child.
- Children actively explore their environment. Manipulation skills emerge from perceptual exploration of objects and surfaces. Tactile, proprioceptive, and haptic perception develops from active manipulation of objects.
- Attachment, temperament, and emotion regulation contribute to social-emotional development. Children who develop emotion regulation can cope with stressful events by flexibly using multiple strategies.
- Children develop self-determination by attaining a sense of autonomy, competence, and relatedness. When a child can act independently and competently with the support of others, the child develops intrinsic motivation and self-determination.
- Children develop occupations through participation in family activities and cultural practices. Cultural context influences the child's self-identity, motivations, values, and interests and determines the range of activities and occupations in which the child can participate.
- Occupational therapists working with children must be knowledgeable about the child's development of play and its related performance skills.

REFERENCES

1. Adolf, K. E., Eppler, M. A., & Gibson, E. J. (1993). Development of perception of affordances. In C. Rovee-Collier & L. P. Lipsitt (Eds.), *Advances in infancy research* (Vol. 8, pp. 51–98). Norwood, NJ: Ablex.
2. American Occupational Therapy Association. (2014). Occupational therapy practice framework: Domain and process (3rd ed.). *American Journal of Occupational Therapy, 68*(Suppl. 1), S1–S48. <http://dx.doi.org/10.5014/ajot.2014.682006>.
3. Ayres, A. J. (1979). *Sensory integration and the child.* Los Angeles: Western Psychological Services.
4. Ayres, A. J. (2005). *Sensory integration and the child: Understanding hidden sensory challenges. 25th anniversary edition.* Los Angeles: Western Psychological Services.
5. Bandura, A. (1978). The self system in reciprocal determinism. *American Psychologist, 33,* 344–358.
6. Bandura, A. (1993). Perceived self-efficacy in cognitive development and functioning. *Educational Psychologist, 28,* 117–148.
7. Bandura, A. (1999). A social cognitive theory of personality. In L. Pervin & O. John (Eds.), *Handbook of personality* (2nd ed., pp. 154–197). New York: Guilford Press.
8. Bandura, A., & Walters, R. H. (1963). *Social learning and personality development.* New York: Holt Rinehart & Winston.
9. Bayley, N. (1933). Mental growth during the first three years. *Genetic Psychology Monograph, 14,* 1–12.
10. Bayley, N. (2005). *Bayley Scales of Infant Development* (3rd ed.). San Antonio: Psychological Corporation.
11. Bazyk, S., Stalnaker, D., Llerena, M., et al. (2003). Play in Mayan children. *American Journal of Occupational Therapy, 57,* 273–283.
12. Bhavnagri, N. P., & Gonzalez-Mena, J. (1997). The cultural context of infant caregiving. *Childhood Education, 74,* 2–8.
13. Bornstein, M. H., & Putnick, D. L. (2012). Cognitive and socioemotional caregiving in developing countries. *Child Development, 83,* 46–61.
14. Bowlby, J. (1978). *Attachment and loss* (Vol. 1). New York: Penguin Books.
15. Bowlby, J. (1982). *Attachment* (2nd ed.). New York: Basic Books.
16. Bradley, R. H., & Corwyn, R. F. (2002). Socioeconomic status and child development. *Annual Reviews in Psychology, 53,* 371–399.
17. Bretherton, I., & Monholland, K. A. (2008). Internal working models in attachment relationships. Elaborating a central construct in attachment theory. In J. Cassidy & P. R. Shaver (Eds.), *Handbook of attachment* (2nd ed.). New York: Guilford.
18. Bronfenbrenner, U. (1979). *The ecology of human development: Experiments by nature and design.* Cambridge, MA: Harvard University Press.
19. Bushnell, E. W., & Boudreau, J. P. (1993). Motor development and the mind: the potential role of motor abilities as a determinant of aspects of perceptual development. *Child Development, 64,* 1005–1021.
20. Carver, A., Timperio, A., & Crawford, D. (2008). Playing it safe: The influence of neighbourhood safety on children's physical activity—a review. *Health and Place, 14,* 217–227.
21. Case, R. (1999). Conceptual development in the child and the field: A personal view of the Piagetian legacy. In E. Scholnick, K. Nelson, S. Gelman, & P. Miller (Eds.), *Conceptual development: Piaget's legacy* (pp. 23–51). Mahwah, NJ: Lawrence Erlbaum.
22. Case-Smith, J. (2006). Hand skill development in the context of infants' play: Birth to 2 years. In A. Hendersen & P. Pehoski (Eds.), *Hand function in the child: Foundations for remediation* (pp. 117–142). St. Louis: Mosby.
23. Case-Smith, J., & Kuhaneck, H. (2008). Play preferences of typically developing children and children with developmental delays between ages 3 and 7 years. *OTJR: Occupation, Participation and Health, 28,* 19–29.
24. Centers for Disease Control and Prevention. (2010). Racial and ethnic differences in breastfeeding initiation and duration, by state: National immunization survey, United States, 2004-2008. Retrieved on December 18, 2013 at: <http://www.cdc.gov/mmwr/preview/mmwrhtml/mm5911a2.htm>.
25. Cermak, S. (2006). Perceptual functions of the hand. In A. Hendersen & P. Pehoski (Eds.), *Hand function in the child: Foundations for remediation* (pp. 63–88). St. Louis: Mosby.
26. Chan, S. (1998). Families with Filipino roots. In E. W. Lynch & M. J. Hanson (Eds.), *Developing cross-cultural competence* (2nd ed., pp. 355–408). Baltimore: Brookes.
27. Chess, S., & Thomas, A. (1984). *The origins and evolution of behavior disorders: Infancy to early adult life.* New York: Brunner/Mazel.
28. Chess, S., & Thomas, A. (1999). *Goodness of fit: Clinical applications from infancy through adult life.* New York: Brunner/Mazel.
29. Cioni, G., Ferrari, F., Einspieler, C., et al. (1997). Comparison between the observation of spontaneous movements and neurologic examination in preterm infants. *Journal of Pediatrics, 130,* 704–711.
30. Cohen, L. B., & Cashon, C. H. (2003). Infant perception and cognition. In R. M. Lerner, M. A. Easterbrooks, & J. Mistry (Eds.), *Handbook of psychology: Vol. 6. Developmental psychology* (pp. 65–90). New York: John Wiley & Sons.
31. Cole, M., & Cole, S. (1989). *The development of children.* New York: Scientific American Books.
32. Connolly, K., & Dalgleish, M. (1989). The emergence of a tool-using skill in infancy. *Developmental Psychology, 25,* 894–912.
33. Connolly, K. J., & Dalgleish, M. (1993). Individual patterns of tool use by infants. In A. F. Kalverboer, B. Hopkins, & R. Geuze (Eds.), *Motor development in early and later childhood: Longitudinal approaches* (pp. 174–204). Cambridge: Cambridge University Press.
34. Corbetta, D., & Mounoud, P. (1990). Early development of grasping and manipulation. In C. Bard, M. Fleury, & L. Hay (Eds.), *Development of eye-hand coordination across the life span.* Columbia, SC: University of South Carolina Press.
35. Csikszentmihalyi, M., & Rathunde, K. (1998). The development of the person: An experiential perspective on the ontogenesis of psychological complexity. In W. Damon & R. M. Lerner (Eds.), *Handbook of child psychology: Vol 1. Theoretical models of human development* (5th ed., pp. 635–684). New York: John Wiley & Sons.
36. Driscoll, A., & Nagel, N. G. (2008). *Early childhood education: Birth-8: The world of children, families, and educators.* Upper Saddle River, NJ: Prentice-Hall, Inc.
37. Dunst, C. J. (2001). Participation of young children with disabilities in community learning activities. In M. J. Guralnick (Ed.), *Early childhood inclusion: Focus on change* (pp. 307–333). Baltimore: Paul H. Brookes.
38. Dunst, C. J., Bruder, M. B., Trivette, C. M., et al. (2001). Natural learning opportunities for infants, toddlers and preschoolers. *Young Exceptional Children, 4,* 18–25.

39. Easterbrooks, M. A., & Biringen, Z. (2000). Mapping the terrain of emotional availability and attachment. *Attachment and Human Development, 2*, 123–129.
40. Eisenberg, N., Hofer, C., & Vaughan, J. (2007). Effortful control and its socioemotional consequences. In J. J. Gross (Ed.), *Handbook of emotion regulation* (pp. 287–306). New York, NY: Guilford.
41. Ellison, P. H. (1994). *The INFANIB: A reliable method for the neuromotor assessment of infants.* Tucson, AZ: Therapy Skill Builders.
42. Erikson, E. H. (1950). *Childhood and society.* New York: W.W. Norton.
43. Erikson, E. H. (1963). *Childhood and society* (2nd ed.). New York: W.W. Norton.
44. Fagaard, J. (1990). The development of bimanual coordination. In C. Bard, M. Fleury, & L. Hay (Eds.), *Development of eye-hand coordination across the life span.* Columbia, SC: University of South Carolina Press.
45. Farver, J. M., Kim, Y. K., & Lee, Y. (1995). Cultural differences in Korean-and Anglo-American preschoolers' social interaction and play behavior. *Child Development, 66*, 1088–1099.
46. Feldman, D. H. (2003). Cognitive development in childhood. In R. M. Lerner, M. A. Easterbrooks, & J. Mistry (Eds.), *Handbook of psychology, Vol. 6. Developmental psychology* (pp. 195–210). Hoboken, NJ: John Wiley & Sons.
47. Fitzgerald, H., Munn, T., Cabrera, N., et al. (2003). Diversity in caregiving contexts. In R. M. Lerner, M. A. Easterbrooks, & J. Mistry (Eds.), *Handbook of psychology: Vol. 6. Developmental psychology* (pp. 135–169). New York: John Wiley & Sons.
48. Florey, L. L., & Greene, S. (2008). Play in middle childhood. In L. D. Parham & L. Fazio (Eds.), *Play in occupational therapy for children* (2nd ed., pp. 279–300). St. Louis: Mosby.
49. Folio, M. R., & Fewell, R. R. (2000). *Peabody Developmental Motor Scales* (rev. ed). Austin, TX: Pro-Ed.
50. Franco, F., Rogetl, A., Messinger, D. S., et al. (1996). Cultural differences in physical contact between Hispanic and Anglo mother-infant dyads living in the United States. *Early Development and Parenting, 5*, 119–127.
51. Garcia Coll, C., & Magnuson, K. (2000). Cultural differences as sources of developmental vulnerabilities and resources. In J. P. Shonkoff & S. J. Meisels (Eds.), *Handbook of early childhood intervention* (2nd ed., pp. 94–114). Cambridge: Cambridge University Press.
52. Gesell, A. (1945). *The embryology of behavior: The beginnings of the human mind.* New York: Harper & Brothers.
53. Gesell, A., & Amatruda, G. (1947). *Developmental diagnosis* (2nd ed.). New York: Harper & Row.
54. Gesell, A., Halverson, H. M., Thompson, H., et al. (1940). *The first five years of life.* New York: Harper & Row.
55. Gesell, A., & Ilg, F. (1937). *Feeding behavior of infants.* Philadelphia: Lippincott.
56. Bhavnagri, N. P., & Gonzalez-Mena, J. (1997). The cultural context of infant caregiving. *Childhood Education, 74*, 2–8.
57. Gibson, E. J. (1988). Exploratory behavior in the development of perceiving, acting, and the acquiring of knowledge. *Annual Reviews Psychology, 39*, 1–42.
58. Gibson, E. J. (1995). Exploratory behavior in the development of perceiving, acting, and the acquiring of knowledge. In L. P. Lipsitt & C. Rovee-Collier (Eds.), *Advances in infancy* (pp. xxi–lxi). Norwood, NJ: Ablex.
59. Gibson, E. J. (1997). An ecological psychologist's prolegomena for perceptual development: A functional approach. In C. Dent-Read & P. Zukow-Goldring (Eds.), *Evolving explanations of development: Ecological approaches to organisms-environment systems.* Washington, DC: American Psychological Association.
60. Gibson, E. J. (2000). Perceptual learning in development: Some basic concepts. *Ecological Psychology, 12*, 296–302.
61. Gibson, J. J. (1979). *The ecological approach to visual perception.* Boston: Houghton-Mifflin.
62. Gilfoyle, E., Grady, A., & Moore, J. (1990). *Children adapt* (2nd ed.). Thorofare, NJ: SLACK, Inc.
63. Gottlieb, G. (1997). *Synthesizing nature-nurture: Prenatal roots of instinctive behavior.* Hillsdale, NJ: Lawrence Erlbaum.
64. Goldscheider, F., & Waite, L. (1991). *New families, no families?* Los Angeles: University of California Press.
65. Graham, S., & Weintaub, N. (1996). A review of handwriting research: Progress and prospects from 1980 to 1994. *Educational Psychology Review, 8*, 7–87.
66. Granott, N. (2002). How microdevelopment creates macrodevelopment: Reiterated sequences, backward transitions, and the zone of current development. In N. Granott & J. Parziale (Eds.), *Microdevelopment: Transition processes in development and learning* (pp. 213–242). Cambridge: Cambridge University Press.
67. Greenspan, G. (1990). *Infancy and early childhood: The practice of clinical assessment and intervention with emotional and developmental challenges.* New York: International Universities Press.
68. Greer, T., & Lockman, J. J. (1998). Using writing instruments: Invariances in young children and adults. *Child Development, 69*, 888–902.
69. Hale, L., Berger, L. M., LeBourgeoi, M. K., (2009). Social and demographic predictors of preschoolers' bedtime routines. *Journal of Developmental and Behavioral Pediatrics, 30*, 394–402.
70. Hall, C. S., & Lindzey, G. (1978). *Theories of personality* (3rd ed.). New York: John Wiley & Sons.
71. Henderson, A. (2006). Self care and hand skill. In A. Henderson & C. Pehoski (Eds.), *Hand function in the child* (2nd ed.). St. Louis: Mosby.
72. Humphry, R. (2002). Young children's occupations: Explicating the dynamics of developmental processes. *American Journal of Occupational Therapy, 56*, 172–179.
73. Humphry, R. (2009). Occupation and development: A contextual perspective. In E. B. Crepeau, E. S. Cohn, & B. A. B. Schell (Eds.), *Willard & Spackman's occupational therapy* (pp. 22–32). Philadelphia: Lippincott Williams & Wilkins.
74. Humphry, R., & Wakeford, L. (2006). An occupation-centered discussion of development and implications for practice. *American Journal of Occupational Therapy, 60*, 258–268.
75. Illingworth, R. S. (1966). The diagnosis of cerebral palsy in the first year of life. *Developmental Medicine and Child Neurology, 8*, 178–194.
76. Illingworth, R. S. (1984). *The development of the infant and young child.* Edinburgh: Churchill Livingstone.
77. Kelly, Y. J., Watt, R. G., & Nazroo, J. Y. (2006). Racial/ethnic differences in breastfeeding initiation and continuation in the United Kingdom and comparison with findings in the United States. *Pediatrics, 118*, e1428–e1435.
78. Knobloch, H., & Pasamanick, B. (1974). *Gesell & Amatruda's developmental diagnosis* (3rd ed.). New York: Harper & Row.
79. Knox, S. (2008). Development and current use of the Knox Preschool Play Scale. In L. D. Parham & L. Fazio (Eds.), *Play in occupational therapy for*

children (2nd ed., pp. 55–70). St. Louis: Mosby.
80. Kopp, C. B. (2009). Emotion-focused coping in young children. Self and self-regulatory processes. In E. A. Skinner & M. J. Zimmer-Gembeck (Eds.), Coping and the development of regulation. *New Directions for Child and Adolescent Development, 124*, 33-46
81. Kramer, P., & Hinojosa, J. (2010). Developmental perspective: Fundamentals of developmental theory. In P. Kramer & J. Hinojosa (Eds.), *Frames of reference for pediatric occupational therapy* (3rd ed., pp. 23–30). Baltimore: Wolters Kluwer.
82. Larsen, R., & Verma, S. (1999). How children and adolescents spend time across cultural setting of the world: Work, play and developmental opportunities. *Psychological Bulletin, 125*, 701–736.
83. Larson, E. A. (2004). Children's work: The less-considered childhood occupation. *American Journal of Occupational Therapy, 58*, 369–379.
84. Law, M., Cooper, B., Strong, S., et al. (1996). The person-environment-occupation model: A transactive approach to occupational performance. *Canadian Journal of Occupational Therapy, 63*(1), 9–23.
85. Lerner, R. M., Anderson, P. M., Balsano, A. B., et al. (2003). R. M. Lerner, M. A. Easterbrooks, & J. Mistry (Eds.), *Handbook of psychology, Vol. 6. Developmental psychology* (pp. 535–558). New York: John Wiley & Sons.
86. Linder, T. (2008). *Transdisciplinary play-based assessment* (rev. ed). Baltimore: Brookes.
87. Luthar, S. S., & Latendresse, S. J. (2005). Comparable "risks" at the socioeconomic status extremes: Preadolescents' perceptions of parenting. *Development and Psychopathology, 17*, 207–230.
88. Maholmes, V., & King, R. B. (2012). *The Oxford Handbook of Poverty and Child Development*. New York: Oxford University.
89. Mandich, A., Polatajko, H., & Rodger, S. (2003). Rites of passage: Understanding participation of children with developmental coordination disorder. *Human Movement Science, 22*, 583–595.
90. Mandler, J. M. (1990). A new perspective on cognitive development in infancy. *American Scientist, 78*, 236–243.
91. Maslow, A. H. (1968). *Toward a psychology of being*. Princeton, NJ: Van Nostrand.
92. Maslow, A. H. (1970). *Motivation and personality*. New York: Harper & Row.
93. Mathiowetz, V., & Haugen, J. (1994). Motor behavior research: Implications for therapeutic approaches to central nervous system dysfunction. *American Journal of Occupational Therapy, 48*, 733–745.
94. Mathiowetz, V., & Haugen, J. (1995). Evaluation of motor behavior: Traditional and contemporary views. In C. A. Trombly (Ed.), *Occupational therapy for physical dysfunction* (4th ed., pp. 157–186). Baltimore: Williams & Wilkins.
95. McCarty, M. E., Clifton, R. K., & Collard, R. R. (2001). The beginnings of tool use by infants and toddlers. *Infancy, 2*, 233–256.
96. McGraw, M. (1945). *The neuromuscular maturation of the human infant*. New York: Macmillan.
97. McLeod, S. A. (2009). Jean Piaget. Retrieved from: <http://www.simlypsychology.org/piaget.html> Accessed April 4, 2014.
98. Metzoff, A. N., & Moore, M. K. (1992). Early imitation within a functional framework: The importance of person identity, movement, and development. *Infant Behavior and Development, 15*, 470–505.
99. Milani-Comparetti, A., & Gidoni, E. A. (1967). Pattern analysis of motor development and its disorders. *Developmental Medicine and Child Neurology, 9*, 625–630.
100. Morris, A. S., Silk, J. S., Steinberg, L., et al. (2007). The role of the family context in the development of emotion regulation. *Social Development, 16*, 361–390.
101. Munier, V., Myers, C. T., & Pierce, D. (2008). The power of object play for infants and toddlers. In L. D. Parham & L. Fazio (Eds.), *Play in occupational therapy for children* (2nd ed., pp. 219–250). St. Louis: Mosby.
102. Myers, C. A. (2006). A fine motor program for preschoolers. In A. Henderson & C. Pehoski (Eds.), *Hand function in the child* (2nd ed., pp. 267–292). St. Louis: Mosby.
103. National Institute of Child Health and Human Development (NICHD), Early Child Care Research Network. (2000). Characteristics and quality of child care for toddlers and preschoolers. *Applied Development Science, 4*, 116–135.
104. Ogunnaike, O. A., & Houser, R. F. (2002). Yoruba toddlers' engagement in errands and cognitive performance on the Yoruba Mental Subscale. *International Journal of Behavioral Development, 26*, 145–153.
105. Parham, L. D. (2008). Play and occupational therapy. In L. D. Parham & L. Fazio (Eds.), *Play in occupational therapy for children* (pp. 2–22). St. Louis: Mosby.
106. Pehoski, C. (2006). Object manipulation in infants and children. In A. Henderson & C. Pehoski (Eds.), *Hand function in the child* (pp. 143–160). St. Louis: Mosby.
107. Pelligrini, A. D. (2009). *The role of play in human development*. New York: Oxford University Press.
108. Petty, K. (2009). Using guided participation to support young children's social development. *Young Children, 64*, 80–86.
109. Piaget, J. (1952). *The origins of intelligence in children* M. Cook, Trans. New York: International Universities Press.
110. Piper, M. C., & Darrah, J. (1994). *Motor assessment of the developing infant*. Philadelphia: W.B. Saunders.
111. Poulson, A. A., Rodger, S., & Ziviani, J. M. (2006). Understanding children's motivation from a self-determination theoretical perspective: Implications for practice. *Australian Occupational Therapy Journal, 53*, 78–86.
112. Reilly, M. (Ed.), (1974). *Play as exploratory learning*. Beverly Hills, CA: Sage Publications.
113. Rochat, P. (1989). Object manipulation and exploration in 2- to 5-month-old infants. *Developmental Psychology, 25*, 871–884.
114. Rochat, P., & Gibson, E. J. (1985). Early mouthing and grasping: Development and cross-modal responsiveness to soft and rigid objects in young infants. *Canadian Psychology, 26*, 452.
115. Rogoff, B. (2003). *The cultural nature of human development*. New York: Oxford University Press.
116. Rogoff, B., Mosier, C., Mistry, J., et al. (1993). Guided participation in cultural activity by toddlers and caregivers. *Monographs of the Society for Research in Child Development, 58*, 1–179.
117. Rogoff, B., Selless, M. J., Pinotta, S., et al. (1975). Age of assignment of roles and responsibilities to children: A cross-cultural survey. *Human Development, 18*, 353–369.
118. Rosblad, B. (2006). Reaching and eye-hand coordination. In A. Henderson & C. Pehoski (Eds.), *Hand function in the child* (pp. 89–100). St. Louis: Mosby.
119. Rossman, M. (2002). Involving children with household tasks: Is it worth the effort? University of Minnesota. Driven to discover. Retrieved on December 23, 2013 at: <http://www.cehd.umn.edu/research/highlights/Rossmann/>.

120. Rothbart, M. K., & Sheese, B. E. (2007). Temperament and emotion regulation. In J. J. Gross (Ed.), *Handbook of emotion regulation* (pp. 3–26). New York: Guilford Press.
121. Rubin, K. (1984). *The Play Observation Scale.* Ontario, Canada: University of Waterloo Press.
122. Ruff, H. A. (1989). The infant's use of visual and haptic information in the perception and recognition of objects. *Canadian Journal of Psychology, 43,* 302–319.
123. Ryan, R. M., & Deci, E. L. (2000). Intrinsic and extrinsic motivation: Classic definitions and new directions. *Contemporary Educational Psychology, 25,* 54–67.
124. Ryan, R. M., & Deci, E. L. (2000). Self-determination theory and the facilitation of intrinsic motivation, social development and well-being. *American Psychologist, 55,* 68–78.
125. Ryan, R. M., Deci, E. L., Grolnick, W. S., et al. (2006). The significance of autonomy support in psychological development and psychopathology. In D. Cicchetti & D. J. Cohen (Eds.), *Developmental psychopathology, Vol. 1: Theory and method* (2nd ed., pp. 795–849). Hoboken, NJ: John Wiley & Sons.
126. Schreck, K. A., Williams, K. E., & Smith, A. F. (2004). A comparison of eating behaviors between children with and without autism. *Journal of Autism and Developmental Disorders, 34,* 433–438.
127. Singer, D. G., & Singer, J. L. (2005). *Imagination and play in the electronic age.* Cambridge, MA: Harvard University Press.
128. Singer, D. G., & Singer, J. L. (1990). *The house of make-believe: Play and the developing imagination.* Cambridge, MA: Harvard University Press.
129. Smith, L., & Thelen, E. (2003). Development as a dynamic system. *Trends in Cognitive Sciences, 7,* 343–348.
130. Spencer, J. P., Corbetta, D., Buchanan, P., et al. (2006). Moving toward a grand theory of development: In memory of Esther Thelen. *Child Development, 77,* 1521–1538.
131. Takata, N. (1974). Play as a prescription. In M. Reilly (Ed.), *Play as exploratory learning* (pp. 209–246). Beverly Hills, CA: Sage Publications.
132. Thelen, E. (1995). Motor development: A new synthesis. *American Psychologist, 50,* 79–95.
133. Thelen, E. (2002). Self-organization in developmental processes: Can systems approaches work? In M. Johnson & Y. Munakata (Eds.), *Brain development and cognition: A reader* (2nd ed., pp. 544–557). Malden, MA: Blackwell Publishers.
134. Thelen, E., Corbetta, D., Kamm, K., et al. (1993). The transition to reaching: Mapping intention and intrinsic dynamics. *Child Development, 64,* 1058–1098.
135. Thelen, E., Corbetta, D., & Spencer, J. P. (1996). The development of reaching during the first year. The role of movement speed. *Journal of Experimental Psychology. Human Perception and Performance, 22,* 1059–1076.
136. Thomas, A., & Chess, S. (1977). *Temperament and development.* New York: Brunner/Mazel.
137. Thompson, R. A., Easterbrooks, M. A., & Padilla-Walker, L. M. (2003). Social and emotional development in infancy. In R. M. Lerner, M. A. Easterbrooks, & J. Mistry (Eds.), *Handbook of psychology: Vol. 6. Developmental psychology* (pp. 91–112). New York: John Wiley & Sons.
138. Toselli, M., Agostini, A., & Bukaci, L. (2011). Maternal responses to infant crying: cultural differences, context newborns. *Interdisciplinary Journal of Family Studies*: Disability and the family, vol XVI 1/2011.
139. Tugade, M. M., & Fredrickson, B. L. (2007). Regulation of positive motions: Emotion regulation strategies that promote resilience. *Journal of Happiness Studies, 8,* 311–333.
140. U.S. Department of Education, Institute of Education Sciences, National Center for Education Statistics. National Household Education Surveys Program (NHES). (2007). Retrieved on December 16, 2013 at <http://nces.ed.gov/nhes/dataproduct.asp#2007dp>.
141. Vanderbilt-Adriance, E., & Shaw, D. S. (2008). Conceptualizing and re-evaluating resilience across levels of risk, time, and domains of competence. *Clinical Child and Family Psychology Review, 11,* 30–58.
142. von Hofsten, C. (1993). Studying the development of goal-directed behaviour. In A. F. Kalverboer, B. Hopkins, & R. Geuze (Eds.), *Motor development in early and later childhood: Longitudinal approaches.* New York: Cambridge Press.
143. Vygotsky, L. S. (1978). *Mind in society: The development of higher psychological processes.* Cambridge, MA: Harvard University Press.
144. Weir, L. A., Etelson, D., & Brand, D. A. (2006). Parents' perceptions of neighborhood safety and children's physical activity. *Preventive Medicine, 43,* 212–217.
145. Werner, E. E. (2000). Protective factors and individual resilience. In J. P. Shonkoff & S. J. Meisels (Eds.), *Handbook of early childhood intervention* (pp. 115–134). Cambridge: Cambridge University Press.
146. Werner, E. E., & Smith, R. S. (1992). *Overcoming the odds: High risk children from birth to adulthood.* Ithaca, NY: Cornell University Press.
147. Whiting, B., & Edwards, C. P. (1988). A cross-cultural analysis of sex differences in the behavior of children aged 3 through 11. In G. Handel (Ed.), *Childhood socialization* (pp. 281–297). Cambridge, MA: Harvard University Press.
148. Willinger, M., Ko, C.-W., Hoffman, H. J., et al. (2003). Trends in infant bed sharing in the United States, 1993–2000. The National Infant Sleep Position Study. *Archives of Pediatrics and Adolescent Medicine, 157,* 43–49.
149. Ziviani, J., & Rodger, S. (2006). Environmental influences on children's participation. In S. Rodger & J. Ziviani (Eds.), *Occupational therapy with children: Understanding children's occupations and enabling participation* (pp. 41–66). Oxford, UK: Blackwell Publishing.
150. Ziviani, J., & Wallen, M. (2006). The development of graphomotor skills. In A. Henderson & C. Pehoski (Eds.), *Hand function in the child* (2nd ed., pp. 217–238). St. Louis: Mosby.

CHAPTER 4

Adolescent Development: Transitioning from Child to Adult

Kerryellen Vroman

KEY TERMS

Adolescents
Physical development
Psychosocial development
Peer relationships
Body image
Identity

GUIDING QUESTIONS

1. What are the typical physical, psychological, and social developmental processes of adolescence?
2. What are the milestones of healthy adolescent development?
3. How do occupations promote and support development of adolescents?
4. What is the interrelationship between mental health, a sense of well-being, and adolescent psychosocial development?
5. How do adolescents' developmental issues influence and guide the occupational therapist's choice of therapeutic activities and interventions?
6. How can parents and occupational therapists promote self-determination and healthy autonomy for all adolescents?
7. What are the challenges of adolescents with disabilities, and how do these challenges influence their development?
8. What are community opportunities for adolescents, including adolescents with physical disabilities, chronic illness, and behavioral and emotional disorders, to engage in social participation to promote healthy development?
9. What are the roles and responsibilities of occupational therapists in facilitating social participation and community engagement in age-related activities by adolescents with disabilities?

This chapter focuses on cognitive, physical, and psychosocial development of adolescents and explains how the developmental process of adolescence influences participation in occupations and occupational performance. In particular, the chapter explores the effect of disabilities and chronic health conditions on adolescents' experiences and participation in age-related occupations that promote healthy development. The information in this chapter comes with the caveat that occupational therapists need to see each adolescent as an individual and apply knowledge of typical development judiciously, cognizant that variability in development is normal. An adolescent's strengths, goals, needs, priorities, context (e.g., sociopolitical, economic, cultural), and current developmental status are integral in a comprehensive client-centered evaluation and occupation-based intervention plan.

Adolescence

> Of all the stages of life adolescence is the most difficult to describe. Any generalization about teenagers immediately calls forth an opposite one. Teenagers are maddeningly self-centered, yet capable of impressive acts of altruism. Their attention wanders like a butterfly, yet they can spend hours concentrating on seemingly pointless involvements. They are lazy and rude, yet when you least expect it they can be loving and helpful.[23]

Adolescents live mostly in the moment. They have moments of joy and pleasure, overwhelming loneliness and isolation, laughter and fun, unbearable emotional pain, anger, frustration, and embarrassment, which are equal to moments of supreme confidence and perceived immortality. They want the security of family but push back on the boundaries set by parents, demanding to be seen as grown up at the same time expecting and wanting unquestioned support. They desire and experience the closeness of peer friendships; they experience the pleasure and anxiety of exploring intimacy; and they have intense and seemingly eternal passion for clothes, music, sports, or other interests, which for a week, a month, or a year are all-absorbing. More than anything, they wish to belong, to fit in, to be seen the same as others, while at the same time wishing to be seen as unique. These are the experiences of all American teenagers. In Case Study 4-1, Caroline, whose teenage sister is intellectually developmentally disabled, speaks to the universality of being a teenager. The universality of the experiences and desires of adolescents is also the foundational principle of the I Am Norm campaign (http://iamnorm.com).

Adolescent Development

Adolescence is generally viewed as the developmental stage occurring between the ages of 12 and 18 years. Early adolescence encompasses the middle school years between ages 10 and 13, middle adolescence is the high school years between ages 14 and 17, and late adolescence is 17 through 21 years, which are typically the first years of work or college.[4,99]

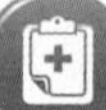

CASE STUDY 4-1 My Sister Is a Teenager

In the 6th edition of Occupational Therapy for Children, *Caroline Glass, a college student at Wake Forest University, wrote the following excerpt about her sister Corinne, an adolescent who is moderately developmentally disabled.*

My younger sister, Corinne, was born with Noonan's syndrome, a genetic disorder. Corinne is lucky to have few of the characteristic physical problems of her disorder; however, her speech and cognitive abilities are delayed. As a 17-year-old girl, Corinne is meeting many of the same decisions and difficulties that "typical" teenagers face (Figure 4-1).

Corinne goes to a public school and takes a mixture of classes. Some are integrated with regular students, and others are only with other teenagers with disabilities. High school is a trial for everyone, and my sister is no exception. Seeing people's reactions to Corinne's differences is always interesting, and many times disappointing. She is subject to teasing, bullying, and, perhaps worst of all, pity. Many people do not regularly interact with people who are mentally retarded and do not understand that Corinne wants no special treatment; she simply wants to be like everyone else.

Just like everyone else, Corinne has to tackle the teenage years. As she gets older, she desires more independence, just as I did at her age. When Corinne's disability presents her with situations in which she is forced to accept help, she becomes frustrated and angry. Her mood swings are like those of any other adolescent, easy to trigger and quick to pass. Her adolescence is complicated by the fact that logical explanations do not always satisfy her. Corinne has an incomplete understanding of time and events, which can make it difficult to relate to her way of thinking.

When faced with such daunting challenges, it is easy for Corinne to forget her strengths. Our family tries to remind Corinne of her abilities every day, and we find that in frustrating situations, it is often helpful to distract her with what she can do, instead of focusing on what she cannot do. Corinne has an incredibly detailed memory and has the ability to locate missing keys or beat anyone in a matching card game. However, her greatest strength is her unwavering ability to love. The kids at school wave to Corinne while passing in the hallway and she responds with unrivaled enthusiasm. In fact, everywhere we go, people recognize her. That's because Corinne is never afraid to say hello to new people, give them a hug, or call them her friend. Even when she is made fun of or excluded, she never judges. As Corinne's older sister, I thought it would be my job to teach her. However, I have come to realize that Corinne has much more to teach me.

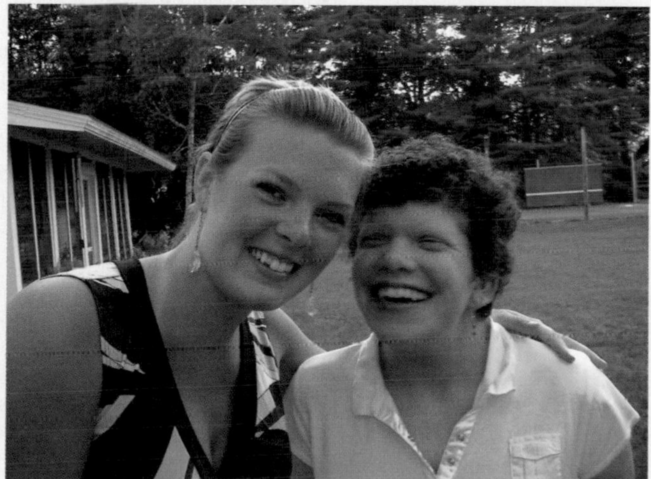

FIGURE 4-1 Sisters: Corinne and Caroline.

Today, Caroline and her sister as young adults have both left home. For this 7th edition, Caroline updates Corinne's story and shares with us her path into early adulthood.

2014 Update

In recent months, Corinne has experienced many changes, mostly positive, to her daily routine. At 21 years old, she exited the public school system in Virginia. She graduated from high school at age 18, but stayed in the public school system in an extended special education class, called Reaching Educational and Career Hopes (REACH). The REACH program worked on vocational and social participation skills and community involvement. It was not an academic class, but a program designed to help students from special education programs find and integrate into postschool opportunities.

The REACH program turned out to be an ideal way for Corinne to transition into adult life. After aging out of the program at 21, she received a Medicaid Intellectual Disability (ID) waiver from the Commonwealth of Virginia. Thousands of people are assessed as eligible to receive an ID waiver, yet only a few are granted each year. Corinne was fortunate to be awarded one of them, and with an ID waiver she was eligible to join a day support program and live in a residential placement. Attending the program 5 days a week, Corinne engages in a variety of educational services while having the opportunity to interact socially with the others and make friends. The length of the day and the structure of the schedule are similar to her experiences in high school and REACH, and Corinne has responded enthusiastically to participating in the program.

A more difficult transition has been our family's decision to move Corinne into a supported living arrangement. Corinne moved into a residential placement with a full-time care provider 6 months after being enrolled in the day support program. She lives with one other boy with special needs. Her care provider is someone our family has known for years and whom Corinne knew as a substitute teacher in middle school as well as a part-time care provider. Her familiarity with Corinne's personality and needs and her long-term participation in the special needs community were major factors in my parents' decision to move Corinne into her home. We liked the fact that Corinne would receive highly individualized care, which is more difficult to achieve in larger group homes. It was important for my parents that Corinne would have the flexibility to come to her family home and to participate in family holidays and activities as she and they wanted.

We chose to wait until Corinne had acclimated to the day support program before changing her living situation because

Continued

CASE STUDY 4-1 My Sister Is a Teenager—cont'd

too many new things at once can be overwhelming—both for her and for us. In the weeks leading up to the move, we spoke to her at length about what this change would mean. Ultimately, referring to her new home as her "apartment" is what helped Corinne to understand this step—she compared her "apartment" with my apartment in Baltimore, where I currently live, and our brother's apartment in Washington, D.C. Seeing her life following our typical transitions, such as moving away from home and getting an apartment, helped her to understand that some of her things would stay at our parents' house, for when she returns home to visit, and some things would be moved permanently to her apartment. However, there were still some difficult moments; a new home means new rules and routines. Like any new living arrangement, Corinne has had moments of frustration with her care provider and her roommate. In addition, she has faced many new challenges and the need to develop other life skills, such as packing to come home (my mother previously had always packed for her) and remembering which items are at which house. Mostly, these small trials are beneficial because they push Corinne to become more independent and expose her to new things. The challenges have not only been Corinne's; at times it has been difficult for my family members and me to have Corinne in the care of another person. Knowing decisions and plans can change and that we will continue to think critically and work with Corinne about which of her choices are the best for her well-being makes it easier to embrace change and move forward.

Courtesy Caroline Glass, 2008, updated 2014.

BOX 4-1 Facts About American Teenagers

- There are 64 million teenagers in the United States between the ages of 10 and 24 years (United States Census Bureau, 2010).
- Adolescents between 10 and 24 years old are more racially and ethnically diverse than the general population: 52.2% are white, 16.5% are Hispanic, 13.6% are black non-Hispanic, 3.9% are Asian/Pacific Islander, and 0.9% are American Indian/Alaskan Native.
- Two thirds of teenagers live in suburban areas, with the highest percentage in the South (35.6%) followed by the Midwest (23.5%), West (22.7%), and East (18.1%).
- Two thirds of teenagers between the ages of 12 and 17 years live with both parents. Black adolescents are the least likely to live in a two-parent home (2006 data).
- Of young people, 24% live in immigrant families (2008 data).
- Approximately 94.6% of teenagers 16 to 17 years old are enrolled in school (2006 data). More girls than boys are enrolled in school. The high school dropout rate is highest among Hispanics (22.5%), blacks (10.8%), and whites (6%) (2005 data). One third of high school students also work.
- Of children and adolescents younger than age 17, 17% live below the federal poverty line. Black and Hispanic adolescents are more likely to experience poverty.
- Although there has been a decline in mortality rates over the last 20 years, male teens continue to have a higher mortality rate than female teens. Significant racial and ethnic disparities exist, with American Indian/Alaskan Native and African Americans experiencing the highest death rate among teens.
- More than 5 million children and adolescents (8%) between the ages of 5 and 20 years have a disability.

Data from the National Adolescent Health Information Center. *2008 fact sheet on demographics: adolescents and young adults.* <http://nahic.ucsf.edu/downloads/Demographics08.pdf>; *Morbidity and mortality among adolescents and young adults in the United States: fact sheet 2011.* <www.jhsph.edu/research/centers-and-institutes/center-for-adolescent-health/az/_images/US Fact Sheet_FINAL.pdf>.

During this period of life, a child prepares for adulthood. This intense period of physical and physiologic (biologic) maturation and psychosocial development influences an adolescent's ability to think, relate, and act as a competent adult. A period of learning, experimentation, and experiences, adolescence influences an individual's choice of long-term occupation, social participation, and his or her physical and psychological well-being. Box 4-1 lists facts about teenagers in the United States.

In observing the developmental process of adolescence, occupational therapists observe adolescents' physical growth and his or her physiologic, emotional, and psychological changes. They are cognizant that it is important to evaluate how adolescents perform common age-related tasks. This evaluation includes developing an occupational profile of the teen, including his or her occupational choices, interests, personal causation (i.e., how competent he or she feels in performing in age-related skills), and how he or she participates in social contexts. Also relevant is how the adolescent seeks out new and novel experiences, self-regulates impulsive behavior, and expresses emerging values. These age-related tasks and experiences are crucial to the process of adolescents gaining physical and financial independence and redefining their psychological and emotional relationships with their parents. As they develop, adolescents establish norms and lifestyles congruent with the values and culture of their peers and their families. They accept and explore the physical and sexual development of their bodies. They work to establish their gender, personal, moral, and occupational identity. Successfully navigated, adolescence culminates in an overall state of well-being and a positive transition to adulthood and adult roles. Failure to integrate and engage in the roles and tasks of adolescence can result in ongoing physical and psychosocial difficulties that potentially affect an adolescent's future occupational performance and roles.[54]

A working knowledge of adolescent development and awareness of occupations that facilitate age-appropriate development are fundamental to effective occupational therapy with adolescents. Effective occupational therapy interventions begin with an evaluation of physical, cognitive, and psychosocial factors associated with adolescents' development and the quality of their occupational performance. This process includes standardized criterion-referenced (based on performance expected of an adolescent) or norm-referenced (based on actual performance of other adolescents) assessments that evaluate client factors and performance. Ideally, the evaluation process is occupation-based. Only interventions based on thorough evaluation are likely to be age-appropriate, promote healthy development, and foster performance skills. This chapter provides an overview of adolescent development intended to guide occupational therapy evaluations and interventions with adolescents.

Physical Development and Maturation

Adolescence is characterized by the biologic and physiologic changes of puberty, dramatic increases in height and weight, and changes in body proportion. The age for the onset of puberty is variable, and a child may begin to notice these changes from ages 8 to 14 years. The stimulus for this physical growth and physiologic maturation of reproductive systems is a complex interaction of hormones. It involves the hypothalamus and the pituitary gland that releases hormones that control growth and stimulate the release of sex-related hormones from the thyroid, adrenal glands, and the ovaries and testes (collectively referred to as the gonads).[110]

The growth- and sex-related hormones initiate a period of rapid physical growth, which varies in intensity, onset, and duration. In this growth phase, people gain approximately 50% of their adult weight and 20% of their adult height. This process, which generally lasts about 4 years, can start at 9 years of age and may continue in some adolescents to age 17. In the United States, the average peak of growth occurs around age 11 for girls and age 13 for boys.

Growth of the skeletal system is not even; head, hands, and feet reach their adult size earliest. Bones become longer and wider. Calcification, which replaces the cartilaginous bone composition of childhood, makes bones denser and stronger. Muscles also become stronger and larger. This process of skeletal growth and muscle development culminates in increased overall strength and endurance for physical activities. Increases in strength are greatest about 12 months after adolescents' height and weight have reached their peak and are associated with an overall improvement in motor performance, including better coordination and endurance. Increases in muscle mass and heart and lung function are typically greater in boys than in girls. This growth is the basis of the difference in strength and gross motor performance between males and females.[20] Motor performance peaks for males in late adolescence around 17 to 18 years of age.[17] Girls typically show an increase in motor performance, including enhancements in speed, accuracy, and endurance, around age 14. However, the changes in motor performance in girls are highly variable and are influenced by a complex interaction of physical and social factors, such as their musculoskeletal development, onset of menses, personal interests, motivation, and participation in physical activities.[17]

An adolescent finds security and social confidence in fitting within the "norm" for physical development, and perceived physical competency in activities such as sports builds self-esteem, particularly for adolescent boys. Self-confidence in early maturing teens benefits from enhanced physical performance and enhanced social status. However, expectations of coaches, parents, and peers to excel at sports can add unwelcome pressure and anxiety. These adolescents are more concerned with being liked and are likely to adhere to rules and routines. Adolescents who achieve the "desired standard" for physical appearance or level of physical performance (e.g., high school sports teams with high visibility such as football, cheerleading, or basketball) receive validation and approval from their peers and from adults. During adolescence, early-maturing boys are reportedly more popular, described as better adjusted, more successful in heterosexual relationships, and more likely to be leaders at school. Conversely, late maturing boys are reported to feel self-conscious about their lack of physical development.[45]

Physical Activities and Growth: Teenagers with Disabilities

Physical activity is important for the health of all teens, including individuals with physical, emotional, or cognitive disabilities. Participation in physical activities maintains functional mobility, enhances well-being and overall health, and provides opportunities for social interaction with peers. However, compared with teens without disabilities, adolescents with disabilities are less likely to engage in regular physical activity.[47] For example, adolescents with cerebral palsy report walking less than they did as children.[2]

Scholars have frequently reported that physical functioning (e.g., mobility) deteriorates in adolescents with congenital physical disabilities because of secondary musculoskeletal impairments associated with adolescent growth.[2,110] These secondary impairments include an inability of muscles to lengthen in proportion to bone growth, deterioration of joint mobility because of contractures, fatigue, overuse syndromes, obesity, and early joint degeneration. However, evidence does not support that such deterioration in performance is inevitable.[92] Studies have shown maintenance or improvement in teens with disabilities who engage in physical fitness or therapy programs.[3,92] Activity and exercise programs have resulted in adolescents' improving and maintaining gross motor function and walking speed. The achieved independence promotes self-efficacy.[64] For example, Darrah et al.[24] reported that teens with cerebral palsy who participated in a community-based fitness program showed significant gains in strength and reported improved psychosocial skills at school.

Occupational therapists take an active role in assisting teens to identify opportunities for physical activity within supportive environments (e.g., teams and physical fitness programs that accommodate and welcome adolescents with disabilities). Occupational therapists work with the teen's education team to facilitate inclusion in junior high and high school sports and fitness programs as specified as goals in a teen's individual education program. Physical activities can also include programs outside of school, such as summer camps and community activities. All such activities strengthen occupational performance skills and promote physical and emotional health.

Physical growth in adolescents with disabilities can lead to performance difficulties that require occupational therapy interventions. For example, changes in height and weight often require reassessment at the level of client factors (e.g., positioning, balance, strength, and coordination) that affect clients' occupational performance and activities of daily living (ADLs). Clients may need new or modified assistive devices or mobility aids (e.g., a wheelchair); they may also need new adaptive strategies, strengthening, and endurance training to ensure full participation in their occupations. With new environmental and activity demands,[1] such as transitioning between classrooms in high school, some teens elect to conserve their energy and use a wheelchair instead of crutches or replace a manual chair with a powered chair.

Teens with progressive disorders (e.g., spinal muscular atrophy, Friedreich's ataxia, and muscular dystrophy) may require ongoing therapy as their functional abilities deteriorate. For example, boys with Duchenne's muscular dystrophy, the most common type of muscular dystrophy, use wheelchairs by early adolescence for functional mobility because of their progressive muscle weakness. Their ability to use their hands and fingers for eating, writing, and keyboarding becomes weaker throughout adolescence. Respiratory and trunk muscles become progressively weaker, and scoliosis and other skeletal deformities, including joint contractures at the ankles, knees, elbows, and hips, are common. With these adolescents, occupational therapists have an active role in facilitating adaptation to the progressive loss of motor function. Often they implement compensatory strategies such as wheelchair seating to maintain skeletal alignment, splinting to prevent deformities, and assistive technology (e.g., voice recognition software for computers) to maintain occupational performance.

Primary caregivers must also adjust to the physical growth and physiologic maturation of the adolescent. Adolescence can be challenging, especially for parents and caregivers of adolescents with moderate to severe physical disabilities or intellectual disability because of the continued and, at times, increased levels of care required. For example, transferring small children into and out of vehicles, lifting them into the shower, and dressing them are relatively easy. As the adolescent grows and gains weight, these caregiving tasks become more difficult. Significant household modifications may be needed to accommodate to the changes, and additional adapted equipment, such as the use of a commode chair or hoists for transfers, may be required for basic ADLs.

In other situations, such as when an adolescent is developmentally disabled, the family's challenge is to encourage more autonomy and independence in self-care to prepare for a transition to semi-independent settings such as a group home. This situation can require that parents reduce supervision and the adolescent develop independence in new self-care routines, such as shaving or managing menses.

Although the occupational therapist effectively addresses practical needs with adolescents and parents, it is equally important that the therapist be aware of the emotional adjustment for parents. With each new developmental stage that has a universally recognized marker of progress (e.g., going to junior high school, first date, learning to drive), parents may revisit their grief as they adapt to the realization that their child may not have the opportunity to enjoy many of these activities. Adolescence can heighten parents' awareness of the barriers and limitations that exist for their children.[52] An effective, empathetic occupational therapist is sensitive to the meaning of adolescence for teens and their families and acknowledges the experience and concerns that this period brings.

Puberty

Puberty is the term used to define the maturation of the reproductive system. The onset of puberty has typically been viewed as the marker that indicates the adolescent developmental stage; however, studies show that puberty may and does occur in preadolescence.[43] During puberty, primary and secondary sex characteristics develop in conjunction with significant physical growth. This period involves both biologic and psychosocial development. A complex interaction/feedback loop involving the pituitary gland, hypothalamus, and gonads (ovaries in females and testes in males) controls biologic development. In healthy adolescents, full sexual development may vary 3 years from the average age. The average age at onset of puberty for American girls is 8 to 13 years, with occurrence of the first period (menarche) between 12 and 13 years of age.[8,83] For boys, puberty generally begins later than it does in girls, on average between 11 and 12 years of age.

Changes in the sex organs involved in reproduction (e.g., menarche in girls and the growth of penis and testicles in boys) are the hallmark of puberty. In girls, race, socioeconomic status, heredity, and nutrition influence the time of menarche. Ovulation usually occurs 12 to 18 months after the onset of menarche.[100] Breasts, areolar size, and adult pubic hair patterns develop over a 3- to 4-year period. This is also a period of peak growth in height, and a girl usually reaches her full height 2 years after she begins menstruating.

Puberty has additional challenges for adolescents with developmental and physical disabilities. Minimal information about puberty in this population is available to guide these adolescents, their caregivers, or health professionals.[98] Some research suggests that in girls with moderate to severe cerebral palsy, sexual maturation begins earlier or ends much later than it does on average in the general population.[128] A retrospective study involving women with autism spectrum conditions reported menarche either 8 months earlier than is typical (i.e., around the age of 13 years) or later.[66]

In boys, development of primary sex characteristics, such as an increase in the size of the testicles and the penis (length and circumference), coincides with overall physical growth. Changes include growth of the larynx, causing a deepening of the voice, and the ability to obtain an erection and ejaculate. First ejaculations (spermarche) occur on average between the ages of 12 and 13 years, but the seminal fluid does not contain mature sperm until later (around age 15). In this process, referred to as adrenarche, the adrenal glands are largely responsible for the secondary sex characteristics such as the growth of axillary and pubic hair, axillary perspiration, and body odor. Also, many adolescents, especially boys (70% to 90%), develop acne because of the effect of testosterone.[41,88]

For adolescents with disabilities, puberty can present additional practical and psychosocial issues. For example, misperceptions exist about the capacity of an adolescent with a disability to be in a sexual relationship, experience sexual desire, and reproduce successfully.[44] Many adolescents with disabilities report that others ignore or avoid their emerging sexuality. Consequently, they receive minimal education about contraception or sexually transmitted diseases or how their disability may affect their sexuality or reproductive capacity.[44,62] Sexual development and the individuation process can be difficult for parents, especially when the child requires extensive caregiving.[62] Adults with disabilities describe the ambivalence and difficulties that their parents had in acknowledging them as sexual beings.[48,114] Mary Stainton poignantly describes the demands associated with managing her menses, the emotional strain this task posed for her mother, and the decisions that denied her womanhood. In the following excerpt, she describes her mother's response to her menses: "Frustration ripped through her as she cleaned between my legs and pulled up the Kotex pad. She felt she constantly needed to be with me when I went to the bathroom. I felt guilty for making a mess: for bleeding at all."[114] Her menarche was not celebrated as a coming of age as a woman; instead, she writes, "Around the time I was 12 or 13, we started talking about options. She [her mother] took me to doctors. I was put on the pill, then, given shots to stop or at least curtail my menstrual flow. A normal body process was now a huge problem, we had to control."[114]

A meta-analysis of 36,284 adolescents in the seventh through twelfth grades with visible (e.g., physical) and nonvisible (e.g., deafness) disabilities found no differences between adolescents with or without disabilities with respect to the proportion who have had intercourse, age at first sexual experience, pregnancy, contraceptive use, or sexual orientation.[119] However, a significant number of girls with invisible conditions reported a history of sexual abuse. A similar finding was reported in a study of children and adolescents with mobility impairments in which more girls with visible conditions reported a history of a sexually transmitted disease.[57] The conclusion drawn in these studies is that adolescents with chronic conditions and disabilities are at least as sexually involved as other teens. However, these teens are significantly more likely to be sexually abused.

Occupational therapists working with adolescents with disabilities and chronic conditions need to be receptive to teen-initiated discussions and open to dialog with adolescents and their parents on topics ranging from physical development, sexual expression, and contraception. They also need to be aware of signs of sexual abuse.

TABLE 4-1 Normal Development of Body Image

Stage of Adolescence	Healthy Behaviors and Concerns
Early adolescents	Are preoccupied with self Are self-evaluative about their attractiveness Make comparisons between their own body and appearance and that of other teens Have an interest and anxiety about their sexual development
Middle adolescents	Have achieved pubertal changes Are developing an acceptance of their bodies Are less preoccupied with their physical changes and shift their interest to their appearance, grooming, and "trying to be attractive" Are more apt at this age to develop eating disorders and other body image–related disorders (e.g., anorexia nervosa or body dysmorphic disorder)

Modified from Radizik, M., Sherer, S., & Neinstein, L. (2002). Psychosocial development in normal adolescents. In L. S. Neinstein (Ed.), *Adolescent health: A practical guide* (4th ed.). Philadelphia: Lippincott Williams & Wilkins.

Psychosocial Development of Puberty and Physical Maturation

Adolescents regard the physical changes in their bodies and their emerging sexuality with a combination of anxiety and pride. These changes can cause confusion, excessive anxiety, or emotional turmoil. With changes in physical stature and the development of secondary sex characteristics, physical appearance becomes increasingly important. Sexuality and the development of healthy relationships are critical to positive personal adjustment.[49] How an adolescent views his or her own physical and sexual development influences self-esteem.[107] Adolescence involves integrating these significant physical and physiologic changes into a healthy self-concept that includes a positive body image (Table 4-1).

Body image, a dynamic perception of one's body, affects a person's emotions, thoughts, and behaviors and influences both public and intimate relationships.[97] Adolescents need support to learn about their bodies and to understand that their feelings and thoughts about their bodies are universal among their peers. Such support significantly reduces the anxiety associated with physical and sexual development. Support from family and friends and the availability of information positively influence adolescents' adjustment to their bodies' physical and physiologic changes.

Self-esteem, self-worth, and the perceived evaluations of others influence perceptions of and attitudes toward one's body.[22] Teenage girls pepper their conversations with remarks about their appearance (e.g., "Do you think my thighs are too big?" or "I'm too fat."). Negative body image is associated with both low self-esteem and mental health problems, including anxiety, depression, and eating disorders, all disorders with a peak onset in adolescence. It is estimated that 50% to 80% of girls, especially in early adolescence, are dissatisfied with two or more aspects of their appearance.[42] Studies show that body dissatisfaction is universal. Girls of all ethnicities express a desire to be thin.[74] Peer attitudes and perceptions in relation to body image concerns are a factor among girls' weight-related behavior. Peer weight-related attitudes and behaviors in early adolescence have been shown to be predictive of individual girls' level of body image concern, dieting, extensive weight loss behaviors, and binge eating.[56]

Boys also compare their internalized perceptions of masculinity with the image they see of themselves in the mirror. This ideal body image is defined by characteristics such as height, muscle mass, broadness of the upper body, and strength.[135] Boys dissatisfied with their bodies generally want to gain weight and develop muscle mass in their upper body (i.e., shoulders, arms, and chest),[37] and such desires can lead to excessive weight training and use of steroids. However, concerns about being overweight are also becoming prevalent among boys.[36] Research shows that by 18 years of age, boys and girls are more satisfied with their bodies than they were in early adolescence and mid adolescence.[34]

Socially constructed views of femininity and masculinity affect how a teenager develops a body image. One powerful social influence is the media (e.g., advertisements, magazines, music videos, video games, movies, and the fashion industry). The media markets a physical appearance that represents little of the diverse population of teens in the United States. They portray an "ideal" that bears little resemblance to the "average" teen. It is not surprising that many adolescents are critical of their bodies.[16] When girls compare themselves with the media's images of slim, large-breasted, small-waisted women with perfect skin or when boys try to measure up to the lean, strong, attractive, acne-free men, they inevitably feel inadequate compared with these illusions of perfection. The media's portrayal often includes proximity of equally "perfect" members of the opposite sex, and possessions such as cars and consumer goods equating attractiveness with success.[22]

Because the process of healthy body image development involves comparison with peers and the media's "ideal" image, one might expect that developing a healthy body image would be even more challenging for adolescents with visible disabilities or conditions (e.g., spina bifida, cerebral palsy, Tourette's syndrome, or congenital limb abnormalities). However, the research in this area is contradictory. Stevens et al.[115] reported no significant differences between adolescents with and without disabilities in self-esteem or satisfaction with physical appearance, and Meeropol[80] found that most adolescents with spina bifida and cerebral palsy surveyed felt they are attractive to other people. However, other studies report that adolescents with physical disabilities view themselves as different from their peers and unattractive to others.[50]

Body image can also be difficult for a teen who develops a disorder or illness (e.g., cancer, diabetes, epilepsy) in adolescence; their previously healthy bodies "fail" them. Research indicates that teens experiencing long-term effects (e.g., impaired organ function, scars, skeletal deformities) from serious illness have a negative body image and impaired emotional functioning.[14]

As with physical growth and development, sexual maturation has social implications. Adolescents who outwardly appear sexually mature and seem older than their actual age can encounter demands and expectations (including sexual) that they are not psychologically equipped to navigate. In contrast to boys, early-maturing girls often demonstrate lower self-esteem and poor self-concept associated with body image, and they engage in more risky behaviors (e.g., unprotected sex).[126] They also experience more psychological difficulties (e.g., eating disorders and depression) than more slowly developing girls do. They are more likely to have lower grades, engage in substance abuse (alcohol, drugs), and have behavioral issues. Late maturation in boys is associated with inappropriate dependence and insecurity, disruptive behaviors, and substance abuse.[41] Some late-maturing boys find validation in academic pursuits and nonphysical competitive activities, especially boys from middle and upper socioeconomic status families that value such achievements.[45]

Adolescents use appearance to express their individuality or make a statement of belonging (e.g., fashionable clothes similar to those of friends, gang colors and insignia). Since the 1990s, body piercing and tattoos have emerged as forms of self-expression among adolescents. Whatever the "body project" (e.g., clothes, jewelry, hairstyles, make-up, tattoos), these activities related to appearance are within the adolescent's control and are consistent with practices within Western countries.[12] Experimentation with appearance is healthy for most adolescents and is integral to developing self-identity. It promotes a level of satisfaction and connectedness with peers. However, adolescents with psychological difficulties may abuse their bodies by engaging in activities such as cutting, excessive piercings and tattoos, or extreme weight loss; others adopt clothing and make-up that marginalizes them. All such actions further alienate vulnerable teens from mainstream society. Piercing and tattooing of minors is regulated in many states, and the struggle for autonomy can be an act of rebellion or a public display of "I own my body; I can do to it what I choose."[12]

Adolescents who have a disability may depend on others for their self-care, may not have their own discretionary money from part-time work, and may lack independence in mobility. Their opportunities to participate in activities of self-expression, experimentation, and expressing personal control are limited. For example, adolescents with disabilities are not always encouraged or offered opportunities to experiment with appearance (clothes, hairstyles) or interests that differ from those sanctioned by family and caregivers. Sometimes, it is more comfortable for parents and others to prolong the childhood of teens with disabilities. Because making choices about appearance and experimentation are part of the adolescent experience that contributes to self-identity, self-esteem, and healthy body image, occupational therapists have a role in working with both teens and parents as they navigate these adolescent changes.

Cognitive Development

Cognition is the term used to define the mental processes of construction, acquisition, and use of knowledge as well as perception, memory, and use of symbolism and language.[91] Advances in magnetic resonance imaging have enhanced understanding of the neurobiologic processes that enable these higher level cognitive functions and the changes that occur in the brain during adolescence. For example, the prefrontal lobe matures later than other regions, and its development is reflected in increased abilities in abstract reasoning as well as processing speed and response inhibition.[133]

The quality of an adolescent's thinking changes during adolescence. Piaget[96] referred to this cognitive development as logical thinking (formal operations), which involves functions such as symbolic thought and hypothetical-deductive reasoning.[60,135] Adolescents' ability to think becomes more creative, complex, and efficient in both speed and adeptness. Thinking is more thorough, organized, and systematic than it was in late childhood, and problem solving and reasoning become increasingly sophisticated. In developing the capacity to think abstractly, adolescents rely less on concrete examples. For example, hypothetical-deductive reasoning does not require actual situations. Instead, a person identifies and explores many imagined possible outcomes to determine the most likely outcome to a particular situation or problem as well as the relationship between present actions and future consequences. Hypothetical-deductive reasoning is essential for problem solving and for the process of arguing. Preadolescents have difficulty considering possibilities as generalizations of actual real events, whereas adolescents appreciate that the actual world is one of many possibilities.[91]

The development of cognitive abilities enables adolescents to achieve independence in thought and action.[19] They develop a perspective of time and become interested in the future. Cognitive development is also central to the development of personal, social, moral, and political values that denote membership in adult society. The development of moral and social reasoning is seen in the adolescent's newly acquired ability to deal with concepts such as justice, truth, identity, and a sense of self.[91]

Because of this cognitive development, teens come to understand the consequences of their actions and the values influencing their decision making. They also become future oriented. They increasingly evaluate their behaviors and decisions in relation to the future they desire. The impulsive behaviors of a middle school or early high school student are replaced by decisions and actions that anticipate the consequences. This emerging self-regulation means that the adolescent gains the ability to control emotions and to moderate behavior appropriately relative to both situation and social cues.

Adolescents with cognitive impairments have difficulties comprehending the consequences of their actions and moderating their behavior accordingly. Because of the lack of hypothetical-deductive reasoning, problem solving in relation to future, or responsiveness to subtleness of social cues, self-evaluation that typically informs judgment is lacking. Instead, their impulsive decisions and actions are more consistent with a cognitive level arrested at the preformal stage, and their occupational performance skills are limited. Adolescents with autism spectrum disorders, teens with developmental disabilities whose abilities are classified in the moderate to higher functioning levels of intellectual disability, and teens who have had a traumatic brain injury at this stage may find that the academic demands of high school markedly exceed their abilities. Their peers' increasing psychosocial maturity and independence accentuate the long-term implications of their cognitive and social disabilities. At this phase of their education, they often transition into prevocational programs and programs that better align with their skills and facilitate an optimal level of independence in adulthood.

Psychosocial Development

It is useful to view adolescent psychosocial development in three phases (Table 4-2). The middle years of adolescence are the most intense period of psychosocial development. In this phase, peers displace parents as the significant influence in the adolescent's life. Conformity with peer groups is desirable, and the opinions of friends and peers matter.

Late adolescence is about consolidation; adolescents ideally are developing into responsible young adults who can make decisions, have a stable and consistent value system, and can successfully take on adult roles, such as an employee or a contributing member of the community. A stable, positive sense of self and self-knowledge of ability enable late adolescents and young adults to establish healthy relationships.

Difficulties navigating psychosocial development can have adverse health and social outcomes, such as psychological problems (e.g., eating disorders, depression, substance abuse) and psychopathology with behavioral problems (e.g., oppositional defiance disorder, criminal activity). Psychological problems do not result in difficulties in adult life, although disorders can increase the vulnerability for further psychological and life challenges. However, some adolescent disorders, such as conduct disorder, are associated with adverse outcomes (e.g., dropping out of school, lower employment rates, substance abuse).[21,79]

Search for Identity: Identity Formation

Research suggests identity is a key variable in adolescent development.[81] Self-identity has two components. One is an individualistic component: Who am I? A healthy individualistic sense of identity is an internalized, stable self-concept from which a person interacts effectively with the physical and social world around them.[76] The other component of identity is contextual: Where and how do I fit in my world?[69] The contextual component is the position from which a person understands his or her values, beliefs, interests, and commitments to a job or career and social roles, such as daughter or friend.[76] The contextual dimension of self-identity is more visible to others and is shaped by external influences (i.e., peers, family, and society) (Box 4-2).

Identity formation is regarded as the optimal outcome of the "psychosocial crisis" and a crucial psychosocial task during adolescence. The hallmark of identity formation is developing problem-solving strategies, a sense of responsibility for one's actions, a capacity to self-regulate emotions and behaviors, and commitment to a set of values and beliefs congruent with the social norms and values of one's community. Exploration and experimentation is believed to lead to a positive sense of identity (i.e., an investment in a set of values, beliefs, interests, and an occupation).[36] In this complex process, adolescents identify

BOX 4-2 Being Disabled Is Not an Identity

Social acceptance is highly valued and important to identity. Adolescents with disabilities or chronic health disorders have additional challenges. Teens are acutely self-aware and want to be "like everyone else," that is, like other teens in their social groups. Teens with disabilities or health conditions must also constructively integrate their disabilities or health problems into a healthy self-concept that does not make their disabilities or health problems their identities. Adults (e.g., teachers, occupational therapists) and friends in their lives who refer to them as "disabled teens" or by any other label (e.g., autistic, disruptive) reinforce and shape an adolescent identity based on the disability rather than on the adolescent's unique qualities (e.g., personality characteristics, interests, values, and abilities).

The occupational therapist has a role in:

- Modeling appropriate use of first-person language. For example, rather than saying, "Steve, who has arthrogryposis ...," it would be preferable to identify Steve by qualities or characteristics other than his disability (e.g., "Steve with red hair ...").
- Avoiding the use of emotive language that marginalizes and assumes that disability is always a negative experience (e.g., "Lisa, who suffers from cerebral palsy.").
- Assisting teens to identify abilities, interests, and positive qualities that will be the primary characteristics of their identity.

TABLE 4-2 Typical Characteristics of Psychosocial Development

Stage of Adolescence	Typical Psychosocial Development Characteristics
Early adolescents	Are engrossed with self (e.g., interested in personal appearance) Separate from parents emotionally (e.g., reduced participation in family activities) Display less overt affection to parents Comply less with parents' rules or limits as well as challenge other authority figures (e.g., teachers, coaches) Question adults' opinions (e.g., are critical of and challenge their parents' opinions, advice, and expectations); begin to see parents as having faults Have changeable moods and behavior Have mostly same-sex friendships with strong feelings toward these peers Demonstrate abstract thinking Fantasize idealistically about careers; think about possible future self and roles Need privacy (e.g., they have their own bedrooms with doors closed, write in diaries, and have private telephone conversations) Become interested in experiences related to personal sexual development and exploration of sexual feelings (e.g., masturbation) Self-consciously display modesty (blushing, awkwardness about self and body) Display an ability to self-regulate emotional expression and can limit behavior but do not think beyond immediate want or need and are susceptible to peer pressure May experiment with drugs (cigarettes, alcohol, and marijuana)
Middle adolescents	Continue to move toward psychological and social independence from parents Increase their involvement in peer group culture, displayed by adopting peer value system, codes of behavior, style of dress, and appearance, all of which demonstrate in an overt way individualism and separation from family Are involved in formal and informal peer group activities, such as sports teams, clubs, gangs Accept body development, engage in sexual expression, and experiment with sex (e.g., dating, sexual activity with partner) Explore and reflect their feelings and feelings of other people Become more realistic in career/vocational aspirations Show increased creative and intellectual abilities and interest in intellectual activities and capacity to do work (e.g., mentally and emotionally) Use risk-taking behaviors to minimize or alleviate feelings of omnipotence (sense of being powerful) and immortality (e.g., reckless driving, unprotected sex, high alcohol consumption, drug use) Experiment with drugs (cigarettes, alcohol, marijuana, and other illicit drugs)
Late adolescents	Become more stable as the sense of self becomes stable in opinions, values, and beliefs Strengthen relationships with parents (e.g., seek out and value parental advice and assistance) Increase their independence in decision making and the ability to express ideas and opinions Have increased interest in their future and consider the consequences of current actions and decisions on the future, leading to delayed gratification, setting personal limits, monitoring their own behavior, and reaching compromises Resolve their earlier angst regarding puberty, physical appearance, and attractiveness Feel diminished peer influence and increased confidence in personal values and sense of self Show a preference for one-to-one relationships and start to select an intimate partner Become realistic in vocational choice or employment, establishing worker role and financial independence Develop a value system (e.g., moral, belief system, religious affiliation, and sexual values) that becomes increasingly stable

Data from Radizik, M., Sherer, S., & Neinstein, L. (2002). Psychosocial development in normal adolescents. In L. S. Neinstein (Ed.), *Adolescent health care: A practical guide* (4th ed.). Philadelphia: Lippincott Williams & Wilkins; and American Academy of Child and Adolescent Psychiatry. <http://www.aacap.org/publications> Accessed September 7, 2004.

their spiritual and religious beliefs; intellectual, social, and political interests; and a vocational or career path. It also involves exploration of friendships and intimate relationships, gender orientation (i.e., awareness and acceptance of one's male or female identity and sexual orientation), culture, ethnicity, and perceptions of one's personality traits (e.g., introverted, extroverted, open, conscientious).

To achieve a sense of identity, adolescents daydream and fantasize about their real and imagined selves. These images energize and motivate. Adolescents actively attempt to make sense of their world and find meaning in what happens to them and their life experiences by exploring different roles, expressing a variety of opinions and preferences, making choices, and seeking to interpret their experiences. They engage in various activities and try different lifestyles before settling on a viewpoint, set of values, or life goals. Adolescents are reflective and introspective. They spend time thinking about themselves, making social comparisons between self and peers, and evaluating how others view them. They set goals, take action, learn to resolve conflicts and problems,[69] and, through this process, identify what makes them individual and how to interact effectively with the world with a stable sense of self.

Adolescents' behaviors, thoughts, and emotions can seem contradictory, especially between ages 13 and 15. For example, a teen might have body piercings, break parental rules, and attend school erratically but at the same time responsibly hold a job and dress appropriately for the work setting. Similarly, adolescents may choose healthy behaviors such as vegetarianism or sports participation but also experiment with alcohol, drugs, or tobacco. Adolescents can be fickle and contrary; they may be interested in different religions and political systems, arguing passionately with their parents on political views or outwardly dismissing parental values. One day they express disinterest in relationships with the opposite sex, but the next day is spent exclusively with a girlfriend or boyfriend.

Erikson[35,36] was the first to propose that acquiring a sense of identity is a critical task of adolescence characterized by one of two states, *identity resolution* or *identity confusion*. This theory of how identity develops through recognition of one's abilities, interests, strengths, and weaknesses by the self and others continues to be the basis of how identity formation is viewed in research and clinical practice. Significantly expanding on Erikson's developmental theory of adolescents, Marcia[76] in his *identity status model* argues that identity development is understood by examining the extent to which an adolescent explores and commits to an identity in a variety of life domains, such as occupation, religion, friendships, gender roles, and intimate relationships. *Exploration* and *commitment* are two key components of this process that lead to identity formation. Exploration is when adolescents actively consider and investigate a variety of alternatives in many domains of their lives. By exploring and evaluating options and making choices, they identify their preferred choices and commit to them. The commitment to their choices becomes a stable investment in values, beliefs, goals, politics, and interests that define their sense of self and their way of seeing the world. Marcia[76] describes four states of identity formation: *identity diffusion, moratorium, identity foreclosure,* and *identity achievement*. Other developmental theorists have criticized Marcia, claiming his description of identity as "states" implies the existence of a final ideal state of identity formation, rather than the reality one observes among adolescents, which is a complex ongoing process of negotiation, adaptation, and decision making that extends into and throughout adulthood.

The identity states model continues to be used and can be helpful when working with adolescents to understand behaviors. *Identity diffusion,* most frequently associated with early adolescence, is a state characterized by an ill-defined sense of identity. In this state, adolescents have little or no interest in exploring their options. They have not made any commitments to choices, interests, or values and have little interest in the question, "Who am I?"[9] However, adolescents who continue to experience identity diffusion into their middle and late teen years can have difficulty meeting the psychosocial demands of adolescence. They may demonstrate an "I don't care" attitude of impulsivity, disorganized thinking, and immature moral reasoning resulting in poor choices in many domains of their lives.[20] Identity diffusion is associated with lower self-esteem; a negative attitude; and dissatisfaction with life, parents' lifestyle, and school.[20,59] In this state, adolescents seldom anticipate and think about their future and have difficulties meeting day-to-day demands of life, such as completing schoolwork or participating in sports or extracurricular activities. Consequences of prolonged identity diffusion can be unhappiness and loneliness, and finding employment can be a problem later because of a lack of exploration of interests and awareness of personal strengths.[8]

Moratorium is a state in early and middle adolescence that involves actively exploring and developing a sense of identity. In a state of identity diffusion, adolescents avoid or ignore exploring and experimenting, whereas the opposite mindset characterizes moratorium. Developing one's identity is a project that is pursued vigorously. Teens in moratorium (searchers) openly investigate alternatives. They strive for autonomy and a sense of individuality. Prolonged moratorium that extends into late adolescence or early adulthood is problematic. Indecision about life goals, course of study, or future career can cause anxiety, self-consciousness, impulsiveness, and depression.[20]

Identity foreclosure is associated with achieving a sense of identity prematurely without having engaged adequately in self-exploration and experimentation. An adolescent making premature decisions about career, relationships, and interests characterizes foreclosure by committing to an identity early in adolsecence.[68] Adolescents demonstrating identity foreclosure commonly accept their parents' values and beliefs and follow family expectations regarding career choices without considering other possibilities, personal interests, or possible options. Such adolescents are conventional in their moral reasoning, less autonomous than their peers, less flexible in their thinking regarding opinions about what is "right," and more comfortable with a structured environment.[68] Research has found foreclosure is associated with approval-seeking behaviors, avoidance of new experiences, and a high respect for authority. These teens are less self-reflective, less intimate in personal relationships, and less open to experiences than peers, but foreclosure on identity makes these adolescents less anxious than many of their peers (see Box 4-2).[20]

Identity achievement, also referred to as identity formation and described earlier, occurs in the latter years of adolescence. Gains in identity achievement are often seen in college years because students have opportunities to explore career choices, ideas, and different lifestyles and cultures and commit to interests, values, gender orientation, political views, careers or jobs, and moral stances after exploring the possibilities. Identity achievement represents coherence between a person's identity and his or her self-expression and behaviors and is associated with autonomy and independence, especially in decision making.[68,107]

More recent thinking on identity development is moving away from viewing it as a progressive process from identity diffusion leading to identity achievement. Meta-analysis of longitudinal identity research strongly supports a pattern of continuity as well as identity progression as a lifelong process that extends into adulthood.[68,81] Developmental researchers propose that breadth and depth of exploration contribute differently to identity achievement. Breadth in exploration has been found to be negatively associated with making commitments to choices in an active manner, whereas depth of exploration is positively associated with actively maintaining a commitment to existing choices.[81] Although this concept is similar to Marcia's model, the dual-cycle model of identity formation assumes adolescents have more stability of identity than previously thought. It is proposed that we view adolescents as starting with a set of commitments, not yet strongly established, that are related to their existing ideological and personal identities. The process is one of gradually working toward making commitments to the values, interests, and occupations that will be the basis of one's identity.[81]

Self-Identity and Well-Being

Adolescents' quest for self-identity is the material of films, TV shows, and literature, and the "angst" of adolescence is found in lyrics of popular music targeted at this age group and is reflected in Facebook and YouTube postings and blogs. However, research suggests that the reality is less dramatic, and most adolescents navigate this psychosocial developmental stage with minimal distress.[60] Adolescents who have a stable sense of identity are able to adapt and respond to personal and social demands without undue anxiety. Studies show that adolescents who are committed to a sense of identity (identity achiever) report higher levels of well-being.[81] A relatively stable sense of self is associated with self-esteem and efficacy in one's abilities. Adolescents who have a commitment to their values, occupations, and interests are less self-absorbed, less self-conscious, and less susceptible to pressure from peers. They can be open and creative in their thinking and have a capacity for intimacy. They are able to self-regulate emotions, and they demonstrate mature (postconventional) moral reasoning.

Adolescents who are unable to develop a stable and distinct sense of self may have difficulties, such as a lack of confidence and lower self-esteem. They are more likely to experience depression or anxiety and report a poor sense of well-being than their peers who demonstrate strong commitments.[81] Adolescents who continue to search and fail to make a commitment are not adapting or developing lifelong skills required for the future. As adults, they may have problems with work, establishing and maintaining intimate relationships, and meeting the responsibilities of life, such as parenting or being a contributing member of their community. Identity formation enables adolescents and young adults to integrate contradictory aspects of the self into a global self-concept, which enables them to meet different situational (contextual) demands.

The study of identity development continues to expand interdisciplinary perspectives, including the effect of external barriers and culture on adolescents' exploration and commitment to identity.[131] Occupational therapists observe identity exploration in the activities adolescents choose, the roles they take on, and the desires they express about their futures. Occupational therapists promote psychosocial development, including identity formation, by emotionally supporting adolescents, working with them to develop abilities in their chosen activities and roles, and offering opportunities for self-directed exploration through participation in age-related activities. Occupational therapy sessions develop and explore work and leisure activities, promote the acquisition of social and life skills, promote participation and self-determinism, and address barriers to community access. Occupational therapy sessions can create an environment that supports identity achievement.

Sexual Orientation: Gender Identity

Sexual orientation refers to an individual's pattern of physical and emotional arousal toward other persons of either the opposite or the same sex.[39] Awareness of sexual orientation generally occurs during adolescence, a time of sexual exploration, dating, and romance. Most adolescents identify their sexual orientation as heterosexual, although about 15% of teens in mid-adolescence experience an emotional or sexual attraction to their own gender. Approximately 5% of teens identify their sexual orientation as gay or lesbian,[102] although they often delay openly identifying their sexual orientation until late adolescence or early adulthood. Reasons for this delay include a lack of support among their peers and experiences of verbal and physical harassment in high school.[39,59] Openness and a willingness to discuss emerging sexuality with all adolescents is important for all occupational therapists working with them. Occupational therapists need to use gender-neutral language (e.g., partner rather than boyfriend or girlfriend; protection rather than birth control), inquire if they suspect violence in intimate relationships, and provide nonjudgmental support to adolescents as they develop their sexuality and sexual orientation.[39]

Self-Concept and Self-Esteem

As adolescents define their identity, their self-concept (the feelings and perception of one's identity consisting of stable values, beliefs, and abilities) becomes differentiated.[100] Self-concept is multifaceted. It includes self-acceptance, which is associated with many areas of the adolescent's life (e.g., sports and athletic competence, parent and peer relationships, academic competence, social acceptance, and physical appearance). In adolescence, self-concept develops from a self-absorbed description based on social roles and personality characteristics in early adolescence to an integrated self-concept that reflects development in cognition, moral reasoning, and social awareness.

A significant aspect of self-concept is self-esteem, the global self-evaluation of values and positive and negative qualities (i.e., how a person feels about oneself). In early adolescence, self-esteem tends to decline, partly because of an increased self-awareness and a tendency to compare oneself with the ideal and realize a discrepancy between one's actual self and desired ideal self.[100] However, self-esteem usually improves throughout adolescence. Table 4-3 provides an outline of the behavioral characteristics of positive and negative self-esteem throughout adolescence. Persistent low self-esteem is associated with serious psychological difficulties (e.g., depression; anxiety disorders such as social phobia, bulimia, and self-abuse). Self-abuse may take the form of cutting or harming oneself, excessive use of alcohol and drugs, or engaging in risky behaviors such as unprotected sex. Behaviors such as frequent negative self-critical statements, fears of anticipated failure, and difficulty coping with perceived failure also indicate poor self-esteem. Teens with poor self-esteem are hypersensitive to negative comments from peers and adults alike and to a lack of responsiveness or overreaction from others, and they can be defensive to constructive criticism. In a desire to belong or "fit in" by seeking social approval, they are more susceptible to peer-group influence.

Factors contributing to self-esteem of adolescents with disabilities are similar to factors that affect teens without disabilities, especially the value-laden self-assessment of one's own attributes and limitations.[5] A stereotypic view of adolescents with disabilities infers that self-esteem is low. However, a

TABLE 4-3 Behavioral Indicators of Self-Esteem

Self-Esteem	Behavioral Indicators
Teen with positive self-esteem	Expresses opinions
	Mixes with other teens (e.g., interacts socially with groups of teens)
	Initiates friendly interactions with others
	Makes eye contact easily when speaking
	Faces others when speaking to them
	Observes comfortable, socially determined space between self and others
	Speaks fluently in first language without pauses or visible discomfort
	Participates in group activities
	Assumes leadership role among peers
	Works collaboratively with others
	Gives directions or instructions to others
	Volunteers for tasks and activities
Teen with negative self-esteem	Avoids eye contact
	Appears overly confident (e.g., brags about achievements or skills to mask a lack of self-efficacy in performance skills)
	Expresses self-criticism, makes self-deprecating comments, makes fun of self as a form of humor
	Speaks loudly or dogmatically to avoid others responding
	Is submissive and overly agreeable to others' requests or demands, even if he or she does not wish to do them
	Gives opinions or views reluctantly, especially if it will draw attention to himself or herself
	Monitors behaviors (e.g., hypervigilant of surroundings and other people)
	Makes excuses for performance, seldom evaluates personal performance as satisfactory or good
	Engages in putting others down, name calling, gossiping, and, at worst, bullying
	Reports a lack of emotional support from parents and friends

Modified from Santrock, J. W. (2003, 2012). *Adolescence*. New York: McGraw-Hill.

meta-analysis of studies examining self-esteem in teens with minor physical disabilities reported that they had lower self-esteem about physical competencies compared with their peers without disabilities, but the effect on their general, social, and physical appearance self-esteem was only moderate.[82] This analysis did find a relationship between the severity of physical disability and level of general self-esteem. Miyahara and Register[83] found that this low self-esteem was related to misunderstanding by peers and adults and poor performance that reflected lack of effort rather than disability. A study of self-esteem and self-consciousness among adolescents with spina bifida found that their perception of being treated by parents in an age-appropriate manner and parents' tolerance of social participation contributed positively to self-esteem, whereas school problems and the perceptions of disability by others contributed negatively.[127] Similarly, positive peer attitudes and inclusion contribute to an adolescent's self-esteem and sense of worth. Occupational therapists need to recognize potential obstacles to positive self-esteem and incorporate strategies and experiences that validate and facilitate self-recognition of one's strengths and abilities as part of the therapeutic process.

Adolescence and Mental Health

Mental health is defined as the "successful performance of mental functions, resulting in productive activities, fulfilling relationships with others, and the ability to change and cope with adversity."[117] Adolescents who have good mental health generally have better physical health than peers who have poor mental health; they demonstrate positive social behaviors and are less likely to participate in risky behaviors (Box 4-3).[67] However, there is an increased vulnerability to mental health disorders in adolescence and early adulthood. Most diagnosable mental health disorders, associated with altered thinking, mood, or changes in behavior causing distress or impaired cognitive functioning, begin in adolescence, many before the age of 14. Adolescents who have mental health disorders (e.g., depression, substance abuse) are likely to have difficulties learning and developing social and life skills and are more likely than peers to engage in risky health behaviors. Engaging in risky behaviors can further heighten the vulnerability to mental health problems or are a precursor.

"The Mental Health of Adolescents: A National Profile" report estimates that 1 in 5 adolescents experiences symptoms of emotional distress and that 1 in 10 is emotionally impaired.[67] The most common disorders are depression, anxiety disorders, substance use/abuse, and attention-deficit disorder (with and without hyperactivity). The Youth Risk Behavior Surveillance System study reported that 35.9% of female and 21.5% of male high school students answered "yes" to the question "Have you ever felt so sad or hopeless every day for two weeks in a row that you couldn't do some of your usual activities?"[31] This depression in young people (15 to 20 years of age) is often comorbid with other mental health disorders, such as addictions, anxiety disorders, and conduct disorder. Suicide, the third leading cause of death in adolescents, is significantly associated with depression. In 2011, 15.8% of high school students (ninth to twelfth grades) reported seriously considering suicide in the previous 12 months, 7.8% attempted suicide, and 2.4% required medical treatment.[31] Although suicide attempts were more frequent among female students, especially in the ninth grade, the number of deaths among boys 10 to 14 years old

BOX 4-3 Critical Health Behaviors of American Adolescents

Alcohol Use

Alcohol is the most widely used substance by adolescents (more than tobacco or illicit drugs).

- Typical initial drug use for boys is alcohol.
- The proportions of eighth, tenth, and twelfth graders who reported drinking an alcoholic beverage in the 30-day period before being surveyed were 10%, 26%, and 39%, respectively.
- Binge drinking has continued to decline from its peak level in the 1990s.
- Alcohol is a factor in approximately 41% of all deaths from motor vehicle accidents.

Drug Use

The annual prevalence of adolescents using any illicit drug including marijuana has continued to increase. In 2013, it increased by 1.3 percentage points (eighth, tenth, and twelfth grades combined). Marijuana use remains relatively stable. *Psychotherapeutic* (prescription) drugs are increasingly a more significant problem than in the previous decade. This trend is due in part to the fact that adolescents perceive them as safer than street drugs, and the availability of street drugs has declined.

- Among twelfth graders, 15% reported misusing prescription drugs in the previous year.
- Marijuana and alcohol use are positively correlated at the individual level.
- Rural teens have equal access to drugs as urban teens.

Tobacco Use

- Every day, approximately 4000 adolescents 12 to 17 years old try their first cigarette. Typically, initial drug use for girls is cigarettes. Lifetime prevalence for cigarette use is declining owing to fewer students initiating smoking. The 2013 prevalence was 15% of eighth graders, 26% of tenth graders, and 38% of twelfth graders.
- About one fourth of ninth through twelfth graders (18.5% of girls and 28.1% of boys) reported they smoked a cigarette or cigar or used other forms of tobacco on at least one day during the past 30 days.
- Boys are more likely than girls to have engaged in tobacco use (cigarettes, chewing tobacco, cigars, little cigars, and snuff).

Injury and Violence (Including Suicide)

- Injury and violence are the leading cause of death among youth aged 10 to 24 years: motor vehicle crashes (26% of all deaths), all other unintentional injuries (17%), homicide (16%), and suicide (13%).
- Nationwide 5.4% of students (ninth to twelfth grade inclusive) report carrying a gun; more boys than girls reported they brought their guns onto school property.
- Almost one third (32.8%) of students report being in a physical fight in the past 12 months.

Nutrition

- Healthy eating is associated with reduced risk for many diseases, including the three leading causes of death: heart disease, cancer, and stroke. In 2011, 62.3% of high school students reported eating vegetables and 64% reported eating fruit or drinking fruit juices one or more times per day during the past 7 days. Consumption was slightly higher for boys.
- Among adolescents, 19% drank a bottle, can, or glass of soda one or more times per day during the 7 days before the Youth Risk Behavior Surveillance System survey.

Physical Activity

- Nationwide, 13% of adolescents are obese, and 15% are overweight.
- The 2012 Youth Risk Behavior Surveillance System survey found 32.4% of ninth to twelfth graders had participated in a physical education class 1 or more days per week when in school.
- More than half (58.4%) participated in at least one sports team during the past 12 months.
- Approximately half of American adolescents (12 to 21 years old) are vigorously active on a regular basis. Inactivity is more common among girls (14%) than boys (7%) and among black girls (21%) than white girls (12%).

Sexual Behaviors

- Approximately 50% of high school students are sexually active; by graduation, two thirds will have had sexual intercourse.
  - Less than 2% of adolescents have had sex by age 12 years.
  - Almost 33% have had sex by age 15 years.
  - Nearly 50% have had sex by age 17 years. The average teen has his or her first sexual experience at age 17.
- The first experience was reported to be with a steady partner by 70% of girls and 56% of boys.
- Most teens used contraception the first time they had sex and continue to use conception.[78] However, European teens have higher use and use more effective methods than U.S. teens.[106]
- Approximately half of the 19 million new sexually transmitted infections in the United States affect adolescents 15 to 24 years old. In 2007, 39% of sexually active high school students did not use a condom during last sexual intercourse.
- The teenage pregnancy rate is decreasing, most markedly between 2010 and 2011, when teen pregnancies decreased by 8%. The live birth rate was 31.3 per 1000 girls 15 to 19 years old.[86]

Sources: *Monitoring the Future National Survey results on drug use: Overview 2013 key findings of adolescents drug use. Monitoring the Future National Survey Results on drug use 1975-2013.* <http://www.monitoringthefuture.org/pubs/monographs/mtf-overview2013.pdf>.

Youth Risk Behavior Surveillance System (YRBSS). *Selected 2011 national health risk behaviors and health outcomes by sex.* <http://www.cdc.gov/healthyyouth/yrbs/brief.htm>.

<http://www.cdc.gov/TeenPregnancy/AboutTeenPreg.htm>.

<http://www.cdc.gov/HealthyYouth/healthtopics/index.htm>.

Neinstein, L. S. (2002). *Adolescent healthcare: A practical guide* (4th ed.). Philadelphia: Lippincott Williams & Wilkins.

was 2.5% higher than deaths among girls and among boys 15 to 19 years old was 3.5% higher.[31] Programs designed to reduce suicide among adolescents offer essential resources for health care practitioners and educators working with adolescents.

Other mental health disorders include eating disorders (e.g., anorexia nervosa and bulimia), learning disorders, and behavioral disorders (e.g., conduct disorder and oppositional defiance disorder). Schizophrenia and bipolar disorder are serious but less common disorders. The onset of schizophrenia (excluding paranoid schizophrenia) in males is typically in late adolescence. Both schizophrenia and bipolar disorder have significant implications for teens because they disrupt participation in typical developmental activities, and these lost opportunities can contribute to lifelong disability.

Occupational therapists can assist with early identification of children and adolescents with mental health disorders because initially (e.g., in early adolescence) these individuals may receive therapy services for related difficulties such as learning and behavioral problems. Occupational therapists also are among the professionals involved in interdisciplinary teams providing early detection and intervention for teens with mental health disorders such as schizophrenia and bipolar disorder.

Areas of Occupation: Performance Skills and Patterns

In the American Occupational Therapy Association (AOTA) Practice Framework, activities that humans engage in are categorized into domains. These are ADLs, instrumental ADLs (IADLs), rest and sleep, education, work, play, leisure, and social participation.[1] Participation in all of these areas develops self-efficacy (confidence in one's abilities to achieve desired outcomes), peer acceptance, and promotion of social status and self-esteem. Adolescents are likely to adopt the values that are associated with the work, play, leisure, and social activities in which they participate.[32] In this section, adolescent development and participation in four domains (work, IADLs, leisure and play, and social participation) are described.

Work: Paid Employment and Volunteer Activities

Work is a general term associated with a job (work undertaken as a means of earning money) or a career (an organized life path that often involves a formal occupation or vocation). Studies of working patterns in teenagers in the United States report that approximately 70% of adolescents older than age 16 work while also attending school.[6] The age at which teens may work is 14 years; however, the hours they may work are regulated. Beyond the age of 16, teens attending school cannot work more than 4 hours on a day that they attend school and are restricted on the evening hours they may work. Although working can be beneficial for adolescents, excessive working (i.e., >20 hours a week) for high school students can be detrimental. It is associated with emotional distress, early onset of sexual activity, and substance abuse.[118] Work takes time away from schoolwork, recreational activities, social activities, and participation in sports, and it may expose teens to work-related injuries.[103] Despite these adverse consequences, approximately 18% of high school students work 20 hours or more per week.[90]

Work includes unpaid work such as volunteerism. The 2000 edition of "America's Children: Key National Indicators of Well-being" reported that 55% of high school students participated in volunteer activities. Educators and organizations such as sports teams and church groups encourage participation in community service. Similar to adults, the reasons teens cited for participating in volunteer activities included a desire to help others, social interaction, and recognition of contributions.[109] An adolescent's personal future goals also influence his or her participation in volunteer activities. Students with higher grade point averages and higher academic self-esteem who have plans for higher education volunteer in their communities.[58]

Work (both paid and unpaid) significantly contributes to healthy adolescent development. In work settings, adolescents interact with adults on a more equal level, have opportunities to assume responsibilities and learn social behaviors, shape values, and develop knowledge of their possible preferences for an adult career/work.[65] Participating in paid employment and volunteerism also develops life and social skills beyond the work environment, such as managing money, organizing time, developing routines, developing skills in collaboration, and negotiating relationships with other people. It also provides opportunities to learn from and communicate with more diverse social and racial groups than in their family and school contexts.[103] The disposable income earned from paid employment gives some adolescents discretionary spending money and a sense of economic independence, whereas others need to work to support themselves financially or contribute to their families. Whatever the circumstances, work helps adolescents assume adultlike responsibilities.

Occupational therapy programs for adolescents focus on strategies that develop work skills and behaviors that assist in their transition from school to work. These skills and behaviors constitute the performance dimension of work required for adult employment. In addition to these skills and behaviors, another significant aspect of engaging in work is the development of an occupational identity.

Occupational identity combines interests, values, and abilities into a realistic choice of a job or career path. It begins in early adolescence with the development of abstract thinking and a capacity for future-oriented thinking. Adolescents start to fantasize about their future work occupations. Initially, these daydreams are idealistic aspirations about a possible adult self. By mid-adolescence, such fantasies become more realistic, and by late adolescence, aspirations have a realism based on interests, values, and a match between performance abilities and actual job demands. Pursuing postsecondary education (college or university) delays the transition to full-time work, and settling on an occupational identity may be deferred. Professional academic programs of study that begin with undergraduate degrees (e.g., nursing, occupational therapy, and engineering) proactively facilitate and shape occupational identity generally earlier than postsecondary degrees in other sciences or liberal arts.

Full-time employment is a tangible marker of the transition from adolescent to adult. The worker role with accompanying financial independence replaces the student role. The successful transition to the worker role involves a choice of occupation that integrates personal identity and interests with individual occupational performance skills and job requirements. Occupational therapy programs start to explore occupational identity early in adolescence and combine this process with skill development, ensuring future work options.

Work Opportunities and Outcomes for Adolescents with Disabilities

Opportunities for paid employment have increased for teens with physical, cognitive, and learning disabilities, but they still significantly lag behind their peers without disabilities, and early work experiences remain elusive for adolescents with severe disabilities.[15,51] Occupational therapists work to foster skills and strategies that assist adolescents to transition from school to work (see Chapter 25). Successful work experiences for teens with disabilities are contingent on strong social networks, formal and informal support within the work setting, support of supervisors, and a workplace culture that positively supports inclusion and diversity in hiring practices.[13]

Positive work experience and exploration are critical for adolescents with high incidence disabilities (i.e., learning disabilities, emotional disorders, and speech and language impairments). They are among the students who have significant difficulties transitioning from high school. Although children with high incidence disabilities often receive occupational therapy services, they no longer receive such services at the high school level. Because adolescents with high incidence disabilities have higher dropout rates from high school and lower postsecondary education enrollment than their peers, additional supports and services are needed during these transition years.[105,123] Factors that contribute to their pattern of lower achievement include lower self-esteem, poor awareness of the expectations and requirements of the workplace, delays in career maturity, and reduced capacity and judgment for making and attaining realistic career goals.[101] Intervention can mitigate self-imposed lower occupational aspirations that limit their postsecondary work and education choices.

Instrumental Activities of Daily Living

IADLs support daily life within the home and the community, and although the tasks can appear mundane, competency in the performance skills associated with everyday living is essential. Developing independence and interdependence in IADLs establishes the foundation of physical and financial independence.

Adolescents take on more responsibility for IADLs; for example, the chores and simple routines of childhood increase from cleaning one's room to tasks that contribute to the household (e.g., mowing lawns, doing laundry, cleaning the car, cooking). As autonomy increases, teens gain experience with most IADLs. They learn to drive or use public transport so they can move about the community without adult supervision. Although continuing to receive parental oversight, they take on their own health management, such as taking medications, learning about health risks, and making decisions about health behaviors (e.g., smoking, having protected sex, nutrition, and personal hygiene routines). They learn money management associated with IADLs, such as shopping, planning how and when to spend money, saving for the future, and managing a credit card and bank account.

By middle adolescence, teens may also take on responsibilities of caring for children by babysitting and assisting with coaching or lifeguarding. With these tasks, they develop a knowledge and awareness of safety and emergency procedures. These roles and associated responsibilities further extend their repertoires of skills. Positive role models such as adult family members and other significant adults facilitate the gradual development of multiple and complex IADLs.

Adolescents initiate communication and use a wide variety of communication technologies to interact with peers. Of adolescents between the ages of 12 and 17, 87% interact through online social networks.[72] Consequently, they have almost 24-hour connection with peers through text messaging, cell phones, instant messaging, and increased contact with adults such as teachers and coaches via e-mail; this is particularly true of girls, and their contact increases with age. These social networks are equally available to teens with and without disabilities. Adolescents' use of the Internet has intensified and broadened: they log on more often and do more things when they are online. They shop online, play games, and research information for school assignments. Girls dominate most content created online by teens; 35% of girls blog, whereas only 20% of boys blog; 54% of girls post photos compared with 40% of boys; but more boys post video content.[73] In a Canadian study, adolescents' reported use of technologies could be seen as a continuum from highly interactive to fixed information sources that fell within one of four domains. These were personal communication (telephone, cell phone, and pager), social communication (e-mail, instant messaging, chat, and bulletin boards), interactive environments (websites, search engines, and computers), and unidirectional sources (television, radio, and print).[112] Consequently, teens have access to a vast amount of information and connect with people beyond their known social networks and geographic locations.

The enjoyment of social network sites and the use of social applications, such as Facebook or Twitter, are tempered with risks. Teens are making moral decisions about the information accessed and the people with whom they interact, often outside of parental or adult oversight. Discerning use of technology integrates cognitive skills, values and interests, and knowledge of the need to protect personal identity and privacy, all at an age when risk taking is more likely, the anticipation of consequences is underdeveloped, and problem-solving skills are inconsistent. The Internet and communication technologies, which provide a complex virtual, social, and physical world for children and adolescents, are increasingly becoming an area of research in child and adolescent development.[46] In the future, this research will expand the understanding of how these technologies influence and facilitate cognitive, psychological, and social development.

Achieving Competencies in Instrumental Activities of Daily Living with a Disability

Adolescents with disabilities and their families face an array of challenges in the area of IADLs. They deal with the paradox of achieving emotional and psychological independence and developing identity as a self-determining individual (which in society is represented overtly by work and autonomy in IADLs), while remaining physically dependent on their parents or caregivers. These teens may always require the assistance or oversight of other people for many IADLs. Although teens with developmental delays eventually learn skills to optimize their autonomy, most have semidependent relationships with their care providers, who make executive life decisions with them.

However, it is a different scenario for cognitively able teens with physical disabilities. To enter adult life, these teens must learn to apply their executive cognitive skills and emotional self-regulation to IADLs. They need opportunities to develop decision-making and problem-solving skills applicable to IADLs, such as health management, money management, and community access (maybe driving an adapted vehicle), all decisions previously undertaken by parents. They need these experiences because eventually as adults they will instruct and oversee attendant caregivers. It is the responsibility of the adults in their lives (occupational therapists, family members, and other caregivers) to augment this learning. As caregivers gradually transfer such responsibilities to the teen, they simultaneously change their roles in relation to their child.

Parents as primary caregivers have different demands and new emotional strains as their child enters adolescence. Similar to parents of teens without disabilities, they are seeking the balance of "letting go," while still being supportive. Yet they and their adolescent also manage additional life challenges that are psychologically and socially demanding. This transition is difficult for parents, and retrospective studies report that adults with disabilities say that, as adolescents, their parents tended to be overprotective.[85]

Although adolescents with physical and developmental disabilities may struggle to become autonomous self-determining individuals, at-risk, emotionally troubled teens often find themselves prematurely independent. Although they continue to need the support and nurturing of a stable family, these teens, because of personal and socioeconomic circumstances, have a pseudoindependence that they are not developmentally ready to manage. They may lack adequate cognitive development and performance skills to meet their IADL and ADL needs. Sometimes, they are even caregivers of their own children. Adolescents in such circumstances often deal with issues such as violence, poverty, homelessness, school failure, and discrimination, while struggling through normal developmental processes.[133]

Leisure and Play

"We must be careful not to discourage our twelve-year-olds by making them waste the best years of their lives preparing for examinations."

—Freeman John Dyson, Infinite in All Directions

Leisure and play activities are the discretionary, spontaneous, and organized activities that provide enjoyment, entertainment, or diversion in social environments that may be different from school and work settings.[93,129] These activities account for more than 50% of American adolescents' waking hours.[70] In an occupational therapy study, teens reported that leisure provided enjoyment, freedom of choice, and "time-out."[94] The use of this free time may seem like "time-out," but it can have a significant role in development. In this free time, teens explore and engage in new behaviors and roles, are exposed to different interests, establish likes and dislikes, and socialize with an array of social groups, developing skills, patterns of behavior, and self-identity.

Unstructured use of time, particularly passive activities (e.g., watching television and playing computer games), have few positive benefits. The main criticism of passive activities is that they contribute to boredom, which is associated with a greater risk of dropping out of school, drug use, and antisocial or delinquent activities.[125] Alternatively, constructive use of non-school hours in nonacademic extracurricular and leisure activities such as sports is linked with positive adolescent health and well-being and development of physical, intellectual, and social skills.[33] These extracurricular school programs (e.g., sports teams, school band or orchestra, drama club) and community-based activities such as scouts, music, or dance classes typically include goal-directed activities as well as a sense of belonging to a peer group (Figure 4-2).

An additional benefit of these activities is relationships with nonfamilial adults. Positive interactions with coaches, adult leaders, and teachers facilitate problem solving, provide social support (sometimes compensating for a lack of parental validation and support), increase self-esteem, and promote skill acquisition and competency.[33] Participation in these extracurricular activities is also associated with higher academic performance and occupational achievement such as the likelihood of attending college.[10] Male students with lower academic achievement or from lower socioeconomic backgrounds who play sports are more likely to finish high school, be involved in the community, and have better interpersonal skills. They also have lower rates of alcohol and drug use or antisocial behaviors.[33,48,77]

An area of concern is the decline of physical extracurricular and leisure activities, which is linked to an increased risk for poor health among adolescents, including obesity and chronic health conditions such as diabetes.[61] The national public health initiatives to promote adolescents' participation in physical extracurricular and leisure activities, which have not been successful, have significant implications. Adolescent physical leisure activity patterns predict adult physical activity levels.[122] Males are more likely to continue to participate in and have a positive attitude toward physical activities than females, perhaps because of the relationship between masculinity and vigorous sports, competition, and sports achievement.[122] The stereotypes of bodily contact, face-to-face opposition, and endurance associated with male sports and esthetics or gracefulness associated with female sports may explain why some girls drop out of sports and physical activities[50] and why girls are more likely to participate in dance and gymnastics, which do not compromise their femininity. Although stereotypes and other influences such as parents and teachers affect participation in physical activity, the strongest influence is peer participation.[122]

Participation in popular adolescent activities that are transferable beyond the context of occupational therapy develops performance skills and facilitates social behaviors that enhance self-efficacy and autonomy. The outcome of developing leisure skills in occupational therapy can be successful participation in peer activities and increased social inclusion. Having the skills to engage successfully in leisure activities contributes to healthy and perceived quality of life by providing a social network and enjoyment and promoting constructive use of time. Developing competence in leisure skills can have additional value, especially for adolescents who may not gain employment.

Social Participation

Social activities, friendships, and the behaviors associated with these activities and roles that characterize and define individuals within society are salient to adolescents' development of social

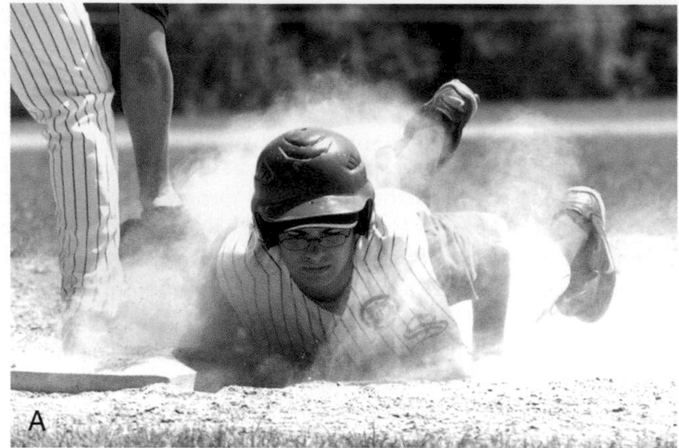

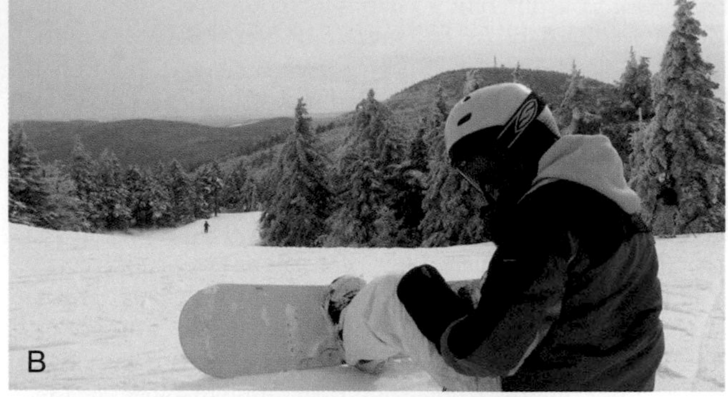

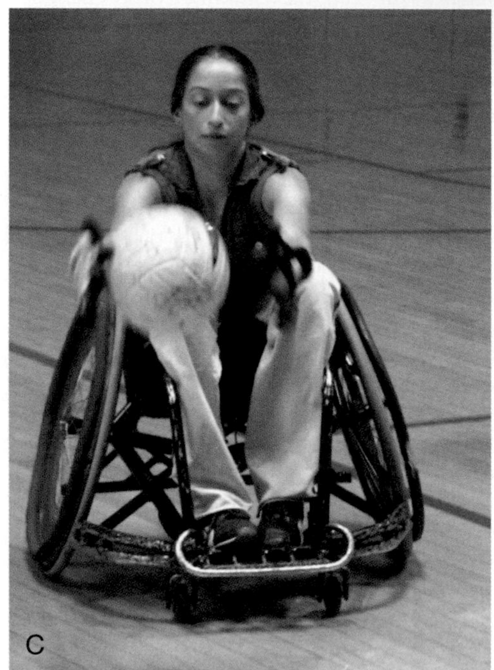

FIGURE 4-2 Examples of goal-directed activities. **A,** Baseball. **B,** Snowboarding. **C,** Basketball.

participation. Social roles and relationships are explored and developed by engaging in a variety of social activities, especially peer group activities.[94] In middle and high school, teens strive to "fit in" and make friends. Peer-focused social interactions and relationships formed in school through leisure activities provide social status and develop adolescents' social identity.[52] This emerging identity may differ from the teen's identity in his or her family. The changes represent moving from family members as the primary source of emotional and social support to a reliance on friends, peers, and nonfamily adults.[7,53]

Peer Relationships

Having friends significantly contributes to social and emotional adjustment in adolescents.[132,134] A Norwegian longitudinal study found the frequency of meeting friends and subjective well-being were the strongest predictors of psychosocial functioning in early adulthood.[28] Peer relationships offer social integration and a sense of belonging or acceptance. Initially, these relationships develop around cliques that are small, cohesive groups of teens that have a flexible membership, meet personal needs, and have common activities. Participation in peer cliques provides a normative reference for comparison with peers and influences adolescents' developing social attitudes and behaviors as well as their academic adjustment.[7] Making the shift from middle school to high school can be easier with membership in supportive and peer-recognized cliques. Initially, in early and middle adolescence, membership in cliques develops spontaneously around common interests, school activities, or even neighborhood affiliations. In junior high, cliques are usually same sex; by middle to late adolescence, these groups expand to include the opposite sex. In late adolescence, cliques weaken, and they are replaced by loose associations between groups that consist of couples.[53] Lack of participation in peer groups or exclusion from cliques comes with a cost (e.g., a sense of rejection, a lack of opportunity to participate in peer activities, social isolation, a lack of social status). Adolescents who do not find their niche in cliques are more likely to be depressed and lonely and have other psychological problems.[19] Exclusion from cliques and the resulting lack of choices are suggested as the reason some adolescents join less constructive peer groups such as gangs or groups who engage in illegal or antisocial activities.

Most adolescents also have lasting stable friendships that differ from the relationships within cliques. Initially, they are same-sex friendships that develop around sharing activities and a closeness of mutual understanding. They can be emotionally intense, involve openness and shared confidences, and depend less on social acceptance; however, these same-sex friendships also imply a heightened vulnerability.[19] Girls' friendships are interdependent and reflect a preference of intimacy, whereas boys' friendships are congenial relationships established around shared interests such as sports, music, or computer games. These friendships evolve with social and cognitive development. In middle adolescence, the basis of friendships is shared loyalty and an exchange of ideas; in late adolescence, friendships progress to incorporate autonomy and interdependence, and as intimate relationships develop in late adolescence, the salience of these friendships lessens.

Navigating Social Participation with a Disability

Because teens strive for conformity and identification with their peers, making and maintaining friendships can be particularly difficult for teens with disabilities (Case Study 4-2). The data

CASE STUDY 4-2 Friendship: Sam's Experience

"Intimacy, companionship, closeness and low levels of conflict" typify a friendship.[120] However, when you grow up with an intellectual or developmental disability, friendship, as just described, becomes harder to come by as you transition into adolescence. Studies show that adolescents with intellectual or developmental disabilities experience friendship differently compared with their typically developing counterparts. These differences include warmth and closeness and positive reciprocity.[120] They spend less time outside of school, or school-based activities, with their friends and are less likely to have a consistent group of close friends.

I have seen firsthand the change in friendships as a child with an intellectual or developmental disability grows into adolescence and then adulthood. My younger sister, Sam, has Down syndrome (Figure 4-3). She has always been very friendly and eager to meet new people. She is the definition of a people person. So why is it that, over time, her friendships with peers disintegrated as she aged? In elementary school, Sam was surrounded by friends and often was invited to play dates or had friends over our house. She was having typical friendships, for her age, with her peers. At this age, parents are still involved in peer-related activities (e.g., coordinating play dates and supervising extracurricular activities), which may have contributed to her ability to participate in activities with her friends.

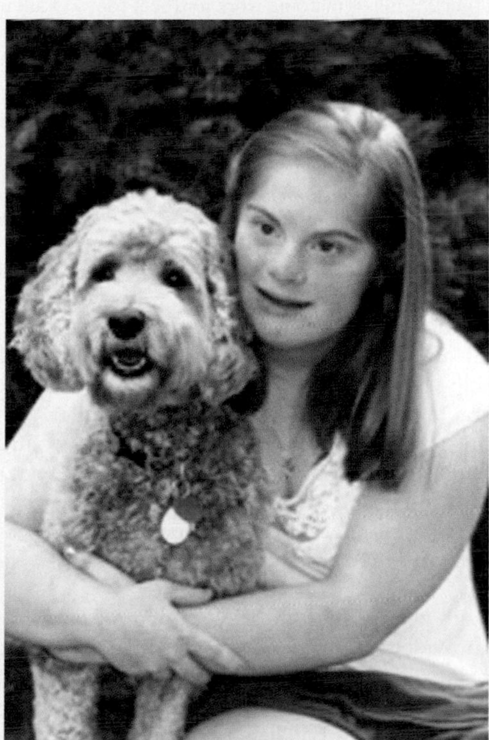

FIGURE 4-3 Sam and her dog.

As Sam grew into a preteen and entered middle school, a change in her friendships was evident. She began getting fewer calls from friends and spending less time with friends outside of school. Where she might have had 10 or more friends in elementary school, she now had, maybe, 4 or 5 friends who were regularly in touch with her. Although she may not have noticed the significance of the change, she did begin to spend more time on her own or with our immediate family. She frequently asked to call friends and ask them to come over, but more often than not that friend was busy.

In high school, the decrease in time with friends was more marked than in middle school. She frequently talked about friends from school but rarely had anyone over or went to any friend's houses. She began getting involved in extracurricular activities, such as being the freshman field hockey manager. Even though she was participating in after-school activities alongside her peers, she was still very isolated outside of these activities. As high school came to an end, she maintained maybe one or two friendships and still keeps in touch with these people today.

Now 21 years old, Sam has developed friendships with peers who also have developmental or intellectual disabilities. These friendships have developed through programs such as Friends in Action, Camp Pals, and Best Buddies UNH, and she has been able to form and maintain relationships in a supportive environment. I have come to believe, through observation and conversation with my sister, that her sense of self-identity, her social skills, and social behaviors have developed further since high school because of the opportunities, experiences, and relationships brought about by programs designed to provide social opportunities in an environment that supports positive social interactions and social behaviors while participating in functional activities.

Resources

For more information on Best Buddies, please visit: bestbuddies.org

For more information of Friends in Action, please visit: friendsinactionnh.org

For more information on Camp Pals, please visit: palsprograms.org

By Alexandra Cousins, Sam's sister and graduate occupational therapy student.

on the social life of adolescents with disabilities provide contradictory information. A national Canadian study found that adolescents with physical disabilities reported good self-esteem; strong family relationships; and positive attitudes toward school, teachers, and many close friends.[115] However, other studies found that because teens with disabilities lack the "qualities" that bestow social status among adolescents (e.g., excellence in sports or physical attractiveness), they often are not included socially in peer groups.[116] Teens with disabilities reported more loneliness, participation in fewer social activities, fewer intimate relationships, and more social isolation than their peers without disabilities reported.[29,116] Even teens with disabilities with good social relationships in school had less contact with friends outside the school setting than their peers without disabilities.[40,115] Factors that affect social acceptance of teens with physical disabilities include role marginalization (lacking a clear role and the inability to undertake the tasks of typical adolescent roles), lower social achievement, and limited contact with peers.[84] Adolescents without disabilities consider their peers with physical disabilities as less socially attractive and report that they are less likely to interact with them in social settings.[40] An asset for teens with disabilities is academic achievement because high academic achievement is shown to promote better social acceptance.[84] See Chapter 12 for a comprehensive examination of social participation.

Understanding the interaction between adolescents and their environments helps the occupational therapist facilitate social participation on multiple levels. The World Health Organization's International Classification of Functioning, Disability, and Health (ICF) model provides a way to interpret this interaction of individual and environment. The ICF has replaced the concepts of disability and handicap with the constructs capacity and performance. Performance is defined as what an adolescent does (performs) in the environmental context in which he or she actually lives, and capacity refers to an adolescent's ability to execute a task or action, usually in a standardized evaluation setting such as a clinic.[87] Capacity and motivation to engage in an activity produce performance (Fig. 4-4). Teens with disabilities may experience a gap between their capacity and performance because of social and physical environmental barriers that limit their access and opportunities to engage with peers. In other situations, they may lack performance skills for inclusion in age-related social activities. For example, in early and middle adolescence, play and leisure activities frequently involve physical skills, which can exclude adolescents with physical disabilities.[5] Later in adolescence, peers have a driver's license, independently move about the community, and have earned discretionary income to spend on activities. In comparison, teens with disabilities may have limited participation because of lack of transportation, accessibility challenges, limited opportunities to work, negative peer attitudes, and parental concerns.[62] Regardless of the personal challenges in mobility, communication, and cognitive skills, it is the assumptions and discrimination of others that most often widen the gap between capacity for friendship and actual ability to form friendships.[119]

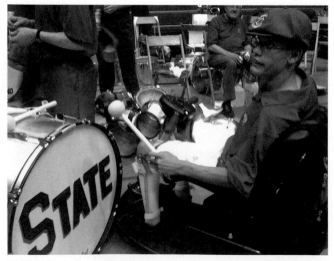

FIGURE 4-4 Matt plays the drums for the high school assembly.

When adolescents with disabilities are with teens without disabilities, they deal with their differences in a variety of ways. Some attempt to mask or make fun of their disabilities, attempting to make their peers without disabilities feel more comfortable. Self-image and self-esteem of teens with disabilities can create barriers to social acceptance and integration. If they internalize the negative societal attitudes, they will limit their social participation and lower their expectations. However, some teens find alternative ways for inclusion that capitalize on their strengths rather than weaknesses and on their ability rather than disability. Doubt and McColl[30] describe one student's approach to forging friendships with his peer group:

> I approached the [hockey team] about being a statistician because I really wanted to get involved in the team. This is probably the closest [to the team] without playing … that I could [get] … plus I'm doing work for them too, so I am useful and that's a good way to get involved … and it really gives me a chance to be one of the guys, finally; a secondary guy but one of the guys nonetheless.

Evolution of Adolescent-Parent Relationships

Adolescents are apt to claim, "Parents don't understand." As increased social participation with peers and close friendships provide intimacy and reflect adolescents' social and emotional adjustment and self-knowledge, the child-parent relationship shifts. Through an almost constant stream of communication among adolescents (being together, e-mailing, and texting), they share their concerns and fears with friends rather than with parents. This reframing of the parent-child relationship and peer friendships facilitates self-identity. It is an important transition because close friendships are associated with better self-esteem and social skills and less anxiety and depression.[20]

Although peer relationships are significant, the stability and security provided by relationships with parents or significant adults are equally important. Contrary to popular belief, major conflict between parents and adolescents is not a normal part of adolescence, and if conflicts exist, they are mostly during early adolescence.[71] When adolescents' relationships with parents are stable, periods of physical and emotional distancing from parents and of questioning parents' values and beliefs eventually evolve into positive adolescent-parent relationships.

Environments of Adolescence

The environment is a significant determinant of an adolescent's choice of activities and success.[48] The social (e.g., friends, team members, family, and social groups), cultural (e.g., race, religion), and socioeconomic and physical (e.g., home, school, and community) environments in which the adolescent lives influence his or her development. Environments can encourage positive behaviors and provide opportunities or conversely fail to provide the adolescent the support and resources needed for healthy development. One example is the influence of membership in social groups. Social groups have cultures, belief systems, and norms that shape values and participation[63] and can offer both social status and privileges. Psychosocial development involves the ability to recognize the expectations of social groups and an ability to develop behaviors and values that are congruent with the norm. In disadvantaged communities, excelling in school sports activities may be linked with the identity of "good student," resulting in opportunities and status among peers and within a community. In higher socioeconomic status communities, where academic achievement is highly valued, other types of extracurricular activities, such as music, science clubs, theater, and volunteerism, are also associated with the "good student" and are positively reinforced.[48]

Environments that are unsafe, lack resources, or are unhealthy can be a barrier to growth and development. Membership in less desirable social groups (e.g., recent immigrants, less popular high school groups, low socioeconomic status) can marginalize teens and make them more susceptible to adverse outcomes and negative influences (e.g., behaviors such as drug use, criminal activity, dropping out of school, or being a victim of bullying). These teens lack opportunities such as access to high-quality education, adequate health care, and the expectation of personal safety. Disenfranchised youth are more likely to seek a sense of belonging in groups such as gangs.

The occupational therapist's understanding of the nuances of an adolescent's social environment and cultural context is vital to the development of an intervention plan.[111] The culturally competent occupational therapist is cognizant of the norms and expectations of ethnic and sociocultural contexts and how these shape adolescents' perceptions of themselves and the development of constructive self-esteem.[113] These factors influence adolescents' choices of activities, interests, the expectations of their families, and the values they develop. Likewise, the adolescent's social peer context shapes "adaptive social and emotional development."[7]

Context can have adverse consequences on an adolescent's development. Lower socioeconomic status and family disorganization increase the likelihood that a child or adolescent will exhibit deviant and high-risk behaviors leading to adverse outcomes.[77] These environments can limit access of adolescents (often minority adolescents) to information and to resources and limit their opportunities to develop self-esteem, personal mastery, and complex cognitive development.[77] Experiences in school, occupational therapy, and extracurricular activities can have a compensatory role in meeting a teen's needs and ameliorating the effect of an inadequate social and home environment.

The multidimensional influence of context is considered in all intervention programs. Family contexts that value and facilitate the development of peer partnerships, participation in extracurricular activities, and mentoring by caring adults promote healthy adolescents. Conversely, school or community contexts that pose barriers to participation, limit positive opportunities, or encourage involvement in unhealthy groups need to be discouraged. For example, in a client-centered approach, the occupational therapist provides choices, opportunities for decision making, and autonomy, all of which provide a sense of personal control and efficacy. Similarly, a therapeutic milieu offers the adolescent opportunities for self-directed exploration and experimentation within a safe, supportive environment. Box 4-4 lists some of the characteristics of contexts that support and foster adolescent self-development and acquisition of skills.

BOX 4-4 Environmental and Contextual Factors of Healthy Adolescent Development

Support

- Family support that includes positive parent-adolescent communication
- Parental involvement in school activities (e.g., schoolwork, sports activities)
- Constructive relationships with adults (e.g., friends, coaches, teachers)
  - Adolescents who report they have good communication and relationships with an adult are less likely to engage in risky behaviors
- Caring, inclusive neighborhood and school environments

Empowerment

- Community that values youth
- Useful and valued roles in community
- Involvement in community service activities that value their contribution and opinions
- Safe home and community environment

Boundaries and Expectations of Adolescents

- Family boundaries that include realistic and fair rules and consequences
- School and neighborhood boundaries that include rules, consequences, and community monitoring of behavior
- Positive and varied adult role models
- Positive peer influences
- High and positive expectations: family, friends, and school personnel expect adolescent to do well

Modified from Search Institute (2014). *40 Developmental assets for adolescents: External assets.* <http://www.search-institute.org/content/40-developmental-assets-adolescents-ages-12-18> Accessed February 2014.

Occupational Therapy to Facilitate Adolescent Development

Improving the quality of life of adolescents with disabilities is a major goal of the national health promotion and prevention initiative Healthy People 2020. The 23% to 35% of adolescents in the United States who have chronic health conditions, disabilities, or special health care needs have the same developmental needs as other adolescents, but because of their special needs or dependence on parents and other caregivers, they have fewer opportunities to explore and develop a sense of their own abilities.[89] Their successful transition from adolescence to adulthood requires that they have the same experiences as teens without disabilities (Case Study 4-3). They need to have opportunities to resolve the psychosocial issues of adjusting to the physical changes of puberty and to develop psychological, if not physical, independence from parents or caregivers. They need opportunities to build social and intimate relationships with peers to establish a sense of identity and skills that will equip them to navigate adult life. These developmental tasks are prerequisites for choosing a job, completing school, finding meaningful work, and developing adult relationships.[26]

Adolescents with disabilities have fewer opportunities to engage in typical adolescent experiences; to make their own choices; to engage in social relationships; or to explore the world of ideas, values, and cultures different from those of their

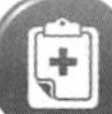

CASE STUDY 4-3 Bullying: Nick's Story

"I am a 14-year-old student in eighth grade. I don't like going to school because I have problems with the kids there. Sometimes my classmates yell at me, and sometimes they hit me. One time when I was in the locker room a kid punched me and tore my sweatshirt. Another time, I was punched in the face and thrown into a locker. In gym class, people throw balls at me and hit me with lacrosse sticks. In my class, a girl yells at me and calls me names. She gets other students to join her. Since I've been diagnosed with Tourette's and Asperger's, students call me Tourette's Man and Twitchy. I don't like to go to school because kids don't treat me very nice. I don't feel like I have very many friends. When I'm at school, I feel like I'm alone, and I feel sad. I wish school was better and I had more friends."

School can become an unhappy place, a daily experience of harassment, alienation, and victimization. Adolescents with Asperger's syndrome are among students who are vulnerable to discrimination. Both teachers and other students can be intolerant toward students with interpersonal and learning challenges, especially when learning and classroom work involve collaboration.[104] Adolescents with disabilities are vulnerable and at heightened risk of victimization compared with their peers without disabilities.[121,124] They report rejection by other students, bullying, or being ignored and treated negatively when working in groups.[124] Nick's story highlights bullying and the experiences of adolescents who are susceptible to bullying.[18] The passage he wrote for this case study resonates with the frustration, disappointment, hurt, and isolation that he and other teens experience at the hands of peers.

The level of verbal abuse is consistent across educational levels, whereas physical bullying increases in elementary school, peaks in middle school, and declines in high school.[55] Students subjected to bullying are at risk of mental health problems (e.g., depression). They report being lonely, show deterioration in performance (grades), and avoid school or drop out.[27] Bullying increases the likelihood that victims will commit acts of violence.[25]

Cyberbullying is increasing with serious consequences for adolescents. A 2010 study in which cyberbullying was defined as when a "person repeatedly harasses, mistreats, or makes fun of another person online or while using cell phones or other electronic devices" reported that approximately 20% of a sample of 4441 adolescents reported they had experienced cyberbullying in their lifetimes. Online was the most commonly cited form of cyberbullying experienced.[95] This frequently anonymous form of bullying is cruel and devastating and has long-term effects because the exposure is wider than the immediate social network. A University of New Hampshire study for the National Center for Missing and Exploited Children reported that online bullying increased by 50% between 2000 and 2005.[130]

Bullying is often underreported, minimized, or unacknowledged in schools. Student surveys have shown that teachers seldom discuss bullying in class or intervene effectively. When adults do intervene, students often see the interventions as ineffective or as worsening the situation.[55] In combating bullying, it is important to empower all students, especially students with disabilities, through a mastery-focused school climate. The U.S. Department of Education issued an official statement regarding disability harassment in school. In the same year, the National Center on Secondary Education and Transition provided advice and strategies on school interventions and educational programs to address and deter bullying (http://www.ncset.org). Specifically targeting the prevention of disability harassment, the U.S. Department of Education makes the following recommendations[125]:

- Create a campus environment that is aware of and sensitive to disability concerns and harassment.
- Weave discussion and awareness of bullying into the curriculum or extracurricular programs.
- Encourage parents, students, employees, and community members to discuss disability harassment and report it when they become aware of its occurrence.
- Publicize antiharassment statements and procedures for addressing discrimination complaints.
- Provide appropriate training for staff and students regarding harassment.
- Counsel both victims and perpetrators of harassment.
- Implement monitoring programs to follow up on resolved issues of disability harassment.
- Assess and modify existing disability harassment policies and procedures to ensure effectiveness.

Acknowledgment

Thanks to Nick for writing about his experiences. His frankness about being bullied offers us insight into the experience of being bullied. Thanks also to Nick's mother for her perspective as a parent. This fall, Nick started at a high school that has a zero tolerance policy for bullying that includes consequences for bullies. Nick's grades have improved, and he says school is okay.

family.[11] As outlined earlier in this chapter, exploration and experimentation provide teens with experiences of success and failure, both of which are required if they are to develop a sense of the boundaries of their competence.[134] Adolescents with disabilities face many additional challenges, including their own and others' negative perceptions and lower expectations of them.[75] They also face barriers such as lack of resources, problems related to mobility and environmental access, discrimination, and the stigma of disability.[30]

Flexibility, a sense of humor, a capacity to see strengths and potential before identifying problems, and the ability to set clear and consistent boundaries are ideal attributes in occupational therapists working with teens. It is essential that the occupational therapist integrate typical adolescent developmental needs into the occupational therapy evaluation process and interventions. However, the occupational therapist needs to keep in mind that most teens, including teens with mental health, developmental, or physical disabilities, successfully navigate adolescence.[108] This knowledge means that the occupational therapist can convey an encouraging attitude grounded in a realistic, yet positive, outcome for most adolescents.

Occupational therapists provide evaluation and interventions that help adolescents address their difficulties and disabilities, acquiring skills and fully participating in the social and academic opportunities provided in school and the community. Occupational therapy services within the public school system are available to many adolescents up to the age of 21 years under the Individuals with Disabilities Education Act. The transition from high school to work or secondary education is a significant time for students to receive occupational therapy reassessment and interdisciplinary programs that develop life and prevocational skills. Occupational therapists work collaboratively with students, families, and teachers to identify each student's strengths so that the student can develop the basic life skills and emotional resources needed to move forward into adulthood. Case Study 4-4 presents an example of occupational

CASE STUDY 4-4 Understanding That Development Is the Foundation of Effective Occupational Therapy Practice

Jeremiah, a 15-year-old boy with Down syndrome, is living at home with his parents. His two older siblings have left home to work and attend college. Psychological test scores classify Jeremiah as mildly mentally retarded under the guidelines of the DSM IV-TR. Before high school, Jeremiah had participated in mainstream school activities, with some accommodations within the classroom. He has good social skills and enjoys being with others. However, as the cognitive abilities required to achieve academically in high school have increased, the gap between his functioning and that of his peers has widened. He now spends most of his day in an alternative class that has a vocational emphasis. Jeremiah's recent individual educational program (IEP) prioritized goals to facilitate his transition from high school to the community. His goals are to live in a group home and have a job.

The Individuals with Disabilities Education Act (IDEA) of 1997 recognized the need to facilitate the transition from high school for students with disabilities with an amendment that required an individualized transition plan (ITP). The IDEA requires that the IEP team carefully consider post school goals when the student is about to enter high school at age 14 because the highest dropout rate occurs in the first 2 years of high school. Beginning at age 16 (or younger, if appropriate), a statement of transition services needed must be included in a student's IEP. Jeremiah's goals might be that he would achieve semi-independence and a personal sense of autonomy, understand and accept his physical changes, form and maintain friendships, and achieve independence in his community mobility to transition from an educational setting to a community and a work environment. Occupational therapy for adolescents such as Jeremiah requires that a occupational therapist understand the extent to which an adolescent's biologic development (e.g., cognition and motor skills) will support development of social competencies and daily living skills associated with adolescence. Based on the findings of his functional evaluation and specific assessments of client factors, realistic goal setting and intervention planning can be determined. An occupational therapist selects evidence-based interventions to help students such as Jeremiah acquire the life and social skills they need to live and work in the community with support or oversight.

For example, when working with adolescents with cognitive disabilities, the occupational therapist needs to understand the developmental functional level of their cognitive abilities. This information can identify the types of difficulties the adolescent may have in processing information and how these limitations in understanding and using information will influence the ability to do and acquire everyday skills. This is crucial information in optimizing learning and determining accommodations that need to be implemented to support functioning. In Jeremiah's case, recognizing that his cognitive assessment scores indicate that he processes information at a preformal (i.e., concrete) operational level, the occupational therapist might use a cognitive disability approach to formulate an intervention plan. Jeremiah has a stable condition that influences how he learns, how much information he can handle at one time, how well he remembers and recalls information, and the complexity of instructions he can follow. The occupational therapist may use a direct, skill-teaching approach to ensure that Jeremiah acquires activities of daily living, instrumental activities of daily living, work, and social participation performance skills. An example would be a visual list to provide the sequence of activities to ensure safety in the kitchen or to improve accessibility. The information about his cognitive abilities and developmental level also helps determine the level of interdependence he will require in his group home; it also helps others understand how to adapt his environment to support his optimal level of independent functioning and, most important, his well-being and life satisfaction. The skilled occupational therapist develops expectations specific to the adolescent that include the "just-right" challenge to meet his goals and to promote his successes.

therapy that supports adolescents with cognitive deficits; sensory impairments; and physical, communicational, or behavioral disabilities in their school-to-work transition.[29,116]

Summary

Adolescence is a distinct developmental stage characterized by growth and maturation, the refinement of skills, self-determinism, relative individuation, and development of a sense of identity that culminates in a positive self-concept as a healthy adult. Many of these qualities and skills are achieved through critical tasks in all areas of development. An adolescent's development of critical thinking and reasoning skills is integral to acquiring personal values and beliefs, a sense of accountability, and a burgeoning understanding of one's responsibilities and actions that extends beyond the egocentric concerns for self.

Summary Points

- Adolescent cognitive competencies support enhanced communication and interpersonal skills, including a capacity for meaningful relationships with peers and adults and, ultimately, intimate adult relationships.
- The social development of adolescents results in an understanding of their rights and responsibilities as members of society.
- In addition to significant cognitive and social development, adolescents experience and adjust to the physical changes and maturation of puberty.
- Adolescents need to develop a healthy body image that incorporates acceptance of these physical changes. The exploration of physical skills and participation in sports, leisure activities, and work enhances and builds knowledge of one's skills, interests, and performance competency that contribute to identity and occupational choice. An important goal is that healthy lifestyle patterns (e.g., physical fitness and nutrition) become life habits.
- The desired outcomes of adolescence are a sense of personal identity, autonomy, independent decision making, and adequate life skills for adulthood.
- Occupational therapists who work with adolescents use clinical reasoning to integrate discipline-specific expertise, knowledge of adolescent development and associated disorders, and occupation-based practice to facilitate healthy development. They forge therapeutic relationships with each teen, his or her family, and the interdisciplinary team members to facilitate a successful transition to adulthood.

To conclude this chapter, an occupational therapist who is a mother of a daughter with significant developmental and physical disabilities shares some advice:

> The best thing I can tell occupational therapy practitioners and students is that every parent and every child/adolescent, like our daughter Brie, has his or her own values and unique story. Occupational therapy practitioners can facilitate relationships and friendships, promote full participation in regular classes, and assist in developing a future. As a parent and occupational therapist, I hope each occupational therapist, through his or her actions, is recognized and remembered by the adolescents they work with as "someone who really made a difference in their lives."—Ann Donoghue Dillon, MEd, OTRL.

REFERENCES

1. American Occupational Therapy Association. (2008). Occupational therapy practice framework: Domain and process. *The American Journal of Occupational Therapy, 62*, 609–639.
2. Anderson, C., & Mattersson, E. (2001). Adults with cerebral palsy: A survey describing problems, needs and resources with special emphasis on locomotion. *Developmental Medicine and Child Neurology, 43*, 76–82.
3. Andrew, M., Penny, P., Simpson, D., et al. (2004). Functional changes in adolescents with physical disabilities receiving school based physiotherapy over one year. *Journal of Physiotherapy, 32*, 3–9.
4. Arnett, J. J. (2000). Emerging adulthood: A theory of development from the late teens through the twenties. *American Psychologist, 55*, 469–480.
5. Arnold, P., & Chapman, M. (1992). Self-esteem, aspirations and expectations of adolescents with physical disability. *Developmental Medicine and Child Neurology, 34*, 97–102.
6. Bachman, J. G., & Schulenberg, J. (1993). How part-time work intensity relates to drug use, behavior, time use and satisfaction among school seniors: Are these consequences or merely correlates. *Developmental Psychology, 29*, 220–235.
7. Bagwell, C. L., Coie, J. D., Terry, R. A., et al. (2000). Peer clique participation and social status in preadolescence. *Merrill-Palmer Quarterly, 46*, 280–305.
8. Berger, K. S., & Thompson, R. A. (1998). *The developing person through the life span* (4th ed.). New York: Worth Publishers.
9. Berzonsky, M. D., & Kuk, L. S. (2005). Identity style, psychosocial maturity, and academic performance. *Personality and Individual Differences, 38*, 235–247.
10. Broh, B. A. (2002). Linking extracurricular programming to academic achievement: Who benefits and why? *Sociology of Education, 75*, 69–91.
11. Brollier, C., Shepherd, J., & Markey, K. F. (1994). Transition from school to community living. *American Journal of Occupational Therapy, 48*, 346–354.
12. Brumberg, J. J. (1997). *The body project: An intimate history of American girls.* New York: Vantage Books, Random House.
13. Butterworth, J., Hagner, D., Helm, D. T., et al. (2000). Workplace culture, social interactions, and supports for transition-age young adults. *Mental Retardation, 38*, 342–353.
14. Calaminus, G., Weinspach, S., Teske, C., et al. (2007). Quality of survival in children and adolescents after treatment for childhood cancer: The influence of reported late effects on health related quality of life. *Klinische Pädiatrie, 219*, 152–157.
15. Carter, E. W., Austin, D., & Trainor, A. A. (2011). Factors

associated with the early work experiences of adolescents with severe disabilities. *Intellectual and Developmental Disabilities, 49*, 233–247.

16. Cash, T. F., & Putzinsky, T. (Eds.), (2002). *Body image*. New York: Guilford Press.
17. Cech, D. J., & Martin, S. (2002). *Functional movement development across the life span* (2nd ed.). Philadelphia: W.B. Saunders.
18. Chamberlain, B., Kasari, C., & Rotherman-Fuller, E. (2007). Involvement or isolation? The social networks of children with autism in the regular classroom. *Journal of Autism and Developmental Disorders, 37*, 230–242.
19. Coleman, J. C. (2011). *The nature of adolescence* (2nd ed.). Hove, UK: Routledge.
20. Conger, J. J., & Galambos, N. L. (1997). *Adolescence and youth: Psychological development in a changing world* (5th ed.). New York: Longman.
21. Copeland, W. E., Miller-Johnson, S., Keeler, G., et al. (2007). Childhood psychiatric disorders and young adult crime: A prospective, population-based study. *The American Journal of Psychiatry, 164*, 1668–1675.
22. Croll, J. (2005). Body image and adolescents. In J. Strang & M. Story (Eds.), *Guidelines for Adolescent Nutrition Services, Center for Leadership, Education, and Training in Maternal and Child Nutrition* (pp. 155–166), Division of Epidemiology and Community Health, School of Public Health, University of Minnesota. Retrieved from: <http://www.epi.umn.edu/let/pubs/adol_book.htm>.
23. Csikszentmihayli, M., & Larson, R. (1984). *Being adolescent: Conflict and growth in the teenage years.* New York: Basic Books.
24. Darrah, J., Wessel, J., Nearingburg, P., et al. (1999). Evaluation of a community fitness program for adolescents with cerebral palsy. *Pediatric Physical Therapy, 11*, 18–32.
25. Davis, J. L., Nelson, C. S., & Gauger, E. S. (2000). *The Boys Town Model: Safe and effective secondary schools.* Boys Town, NE: Boys Town Press.
26. Davis, S. E. (1985). Developmental tasks and transitions of adolescents with chronic illness and disabilities. *Rehabilitation Counseling Bulletin, 29*, 69–80.
27. Deshler, D., Schumaker, J., Bui, Y., et al. (2005). High schools and adolescents with disabilities: Challenges at every turn. Retrieved June 2008 from: <http://www.corwinpress.com/upm-data/10858_Chapter_1.pdf>.
28. Derdikman-Eiron, R., Hjemdal, O., Lydersen, S., et al. (2013). Adolescent predictors and associates of psychosocial functioning in young men and women: 11 year follow-up findings from the Nord-Trøndelag Health Study. *Scandinavian Journal of Psychology, 54*, 95–101.
29. Dirette, D., & Kolak, L. (2004). Occupational performance needs of adolescents in alternative education programs. *American Journal of Occupational Therapy, 58*, 337–341.
30. Doubt, L., & McColl, M. A. (2003). A secondary guy: Physically disabled teenagers in secondary schools. *Canadian Journal of Occupational Therapy, 70*, 139–150.
31. Eaton, D. K., Kann, L., Kinchen, S., et al. (Eds.), (2011). *Youth risk behavior surveillance—United States. Department of Health and Human Services, National Center for Disease Control and Prevention.* <http:// www.cdc.gov/mmwr/preview/mmwrhtml/ss6104al.htm>. Accessed June 23, 2014.
32. Eccles, J. S., & Barber, B. L. (1999). Student council, volunteering, basketball or marching band: What kind of extracurricular involvement matters? *Journal of Research on Adolescence, 14*, 10–43.
33. Eccles, J. S., Barber, B. L., Stone, M., et al. (2003). Extracurricular activities and adolescent development. *Journal of Social Issues, 59*, 865–889.
34. Eisenberg, M., Neumark-Sztainer, D., Haines, J., et al. (2006). Weight-teasing and emotional well-being in adolescents: Longitudinal findings from Project EAT. *Journal of Adolescent Health, 38*, 675–683.
35. Erikson, E. (1968). *Identity, youth, and crisis.* New York: Norton.
36. Erickson, E. H. (1980). *Identity and the life cycle.* New York: W. W. Norton.
37. Field, A. E., Austin, B., Camargo, C., et al. (2005). Exposure to the mass media, body shape concerns, and use of supplements to improve weight and shape among male and female adolescents and among girls. *Pediatrics, 16*, 214–220.
38. Finer, L. B., & Philbin, J. M. (2013). Sexual initiation, contraceptive use, and pregnancy among young adolescents. *Pediatrics, 131*, 886–891.
39. Frankowski, B. L. (2004). Sexual orientation and adolescents. *Pediatrics, 113*, 1827–1832.
40. Frederickson, N., & Turner, J. (2002). Utilizing the classroom peer group to address children's social needs: An evaluation of the circle of friends' intervention approach. *Journal of Special Education, 30*, 234–245.
41. Ge, X., Conger, R., & Elder, G. (2001). The relation between puberty and psychological distress in adolescent boys. *Journal of Research on Adolescence, 11*, 49–70.
42. Gilligan, C., Lyons, N. P., & Hanmer, T. J. (1990). *Making connections: The relational worlds of adolescent girls at Emma Willard School.* Cambridge, MA: Harvard University Press.
43. Gluckman, P. D., & Hanson, M. A. (2006). Evolution, development and timing of puberty. *Trends in Endocrinology and Metabolism, 17*, 7–12.
44. Gordon, P. A., Tschopp, M. K., & Feldman, D. (2004). Addressing issues of sexuality with adolescents with disabilities. *Child and Adolescent Social Work Journal, 21*, 1573–2797.
45. Graber, J., Seeley, J., Brooks-Gunn, J., et al. (2004). Is pubertal timing associated with psychopathology in young adulthood? *Journal of the American Academy of Child & Adolescent Psychiatry, 43*, 718–726.
46. Greenfield, P., & Yan, Z. (2006). Children, adolescents, and the Internet: A new field of inquiry in developmental psychology. *Developmental Psychology, 42*, 391–394.
47. Grunbaum, J. A., Kann, L., Kinchen, S. A., et al. (2002). Youth risk behavior surveillance—United States, 2001. *Journal of School Health, 72*, 313–328.
48. Guest, A., & Schneider, B. (2003). Adolescents' extracurricular participation in context: The mediating effects of schools, communities, and identity. *Sociology of Education, 76*, 89–109.
49. Guest, V. (2000). Sex education: A source for promoting character development in young people with physical disabilities. *Sexuality and Disability, 18*, 137–142.
50. Guillet, E., Sarrazin, P., Fontayne, P., et al. (2006). Understanding female sport attrition in a stereotypical male sport within the framework of Eccles expectancy-value. *Psychology of Women Quarterly, 30*, 358–368.
51. Hallum, A. (1995). Disability and the transition to adulthood: Issues for the disabled child, the family, and the pediatrician. *Current Problems in Pediatrics, 25*, 12–50.
52. Harris, S. L., Glasberg, B., & Delmino, L. (1998). Families and the developmentally disabled adolescent. In V. B. Van Hasselt & C. M. Hersen (Eds.), *Handbook of psychological treatment protocols for children and*

adolescents (pp. 519–548). Mahwah, NJ: Lawrence Erlbaum Assoc.
53. Heiman, T. (2000). Friendship quality among children in three educational settings. *Journal of Intellectual Disability, 25*, 1–12.
54. Hooker, K. (1991). Developmental tasks. In R. M. Lerner, A. C. Petersen, & T. Brooks-Gunn (Eds.), *Encyclopedia of adolescence* (Vol. 1). London: Garland Publishing.
55. Hoover, J., & Stenhjem, P. (2003). Bullying and teasing of youth with disabilities: Creating positive school environments for effective inclusion. Retrieved February 2014 from: <http://www.ncset.org/publications/issue/NCSETIssueBrief_2.3.pdf>.
56. Hutchinson, D. M., & Rapee, R. M. (2007). Do friends share similar body image and eating problems? The role of social networks and peer influences in early adolescence. *Behaviour Research and Therapy, 45*, 1557–1577.
57. Jemtå, L., Fugl-Meyer, K. S., & Oberg, K. (2008). On intimacy, sexual activities and exposure to sexual abuse among children and adolescents with mobility impairment. *Acta Paediatrica, 97*, 641–646.
58. Johnson, M. K., Beebe, T., Mortimer, J. T., et al. (1998). Volunteerism in adolescence: A process perspective. *Journal of Research on Adolescence, 8*, 309–332.
59. Kail, R., & Cavanaugh, J. C. (2006). *Human development: A life-span perspective* (4th ed.). Belmont, CA: Thomson Wadsworth.
60. Keating, D. P. (1991). Cognition, adolescents. In R. M. Lerner, A. C. Petersen, & T. Brooks-Gunn (Eds.), *Encyclopedia of adolescence* (pp. 981–991). London: Garland Publishing.
61. Kemper, H. C. G. (2002). The importance of physical activity in childhood and adolescence. In L. Haynan, M. M. Mahon, & J. R. Turner (Eds.), *Health behavior in childhood and adolescence* (pp. 105–142). New York: Springer Publishing.
62. Kewman, D., Warschausky, S., Engel, L., et al. (1997). Sexual development of children and adolescents. In M. L. Sipski & C. J. Alexander (Eds.), *Sexual function in people with disabilities and chronic illness: A health professional's guide* (pp. 355–378). Gaithersburg, MD: Aspen Publishers.
63. Kielhofner, G. (2008). *Model of human occupation* (4th ed.). Baltimore: Lippincott Williams & Wilkins.
64. King, G., Schultz, I., Steel, K., et al. (1993). Self-evaluation and self-concept of adolescents with physical disabilities. *American Journal of Occupational Therapy, 47*, 132–140.
65. Kirkpatrick, J. M. (2002). Social origins, adolescents' experiences and work value trajectories during the transition to adulthood. *Social Forces, 80*, 32–37.
66. Knickmeyer, R. C., Wheelwright, S., Hoekstra, R., et al. (2006). Age of menarche in females with autism spectrum conditions. *Developmental Medicine and Child Neurology, 48*, 1007–1008.
67. Knopf, D., Park, M. J., & Muyle, T. P. (2008). The mental health of adolescents: A national profile, 2008. National Adolescent Health Information Center. Retrieved August 2008 from: <http://nahic.ucsf.edu/downloads/MentalHealthBrief.pdf>.
68. Kroger, J., Martinussen, M., & Marcia, J. E. (2010). Identity status change during adolescence and young adulthood: A meta-analysis. *Journal of Adolescence, 33*, 683–698.
69. Kunnen, E. S., Bosma, H. A., & VanGeert, P. L. C. (2001). A dynamic systems approach to identity formation: Theoretical background and methodological possibilities. In J. E. Nurmi (Ed.), *Navigating through adolescence: European perspectives* (pp. 251–278). New York: Routledge Falmer.
70. Larson, R., & Verma, S. (1999). How children and adolescents spend time across the world: Work, play and developmental opportunities. *Psychological Bulletin, 125*, 701–735.
71. Laursen, B., Coy, K. C., & Collins, W. A. (1998). Reconsidering changes in parent-child conflict across adolescence: A meta-analysis. *Child Development, 69*, 817–832.
72. Lenhart, M., & Madden, M. (2005). Teens and technology: Youth are leading the transition to a fully wired and mobile nation. Retrieved November 2008 from: <http://www.pewinternet.org/report_display.asp?r=162>.
73. Lenhart, M., Madden, M., Rankin-MacGill, A., et al. (2007). Teens and social media: The use of social media gains a greater foothold in teen life as they embrace the conversational nature of interactive online media. Retrieved November 2008 from: <http://www.pewinternet.org/PPF/r/230/report_display.asp>.
74. Levine, M. P., & Smolak, L. (2002). Body image development in adolescence. In T. F. Cash & T. Putzinsky (Eds.), *Body image* (pp. 74–82). New York: Guilford Press.
75. Magill-Evans, J., Darrah, J., Pain, K., et al. (2001). Are families with adolescents and young children with cerebral palsy the same as other families? *Developmental Medicine and Child Neurology, 43*, 466–472.
76. Marcia, J. E. (1991). Identity and self-development. In R. M. Lerner, A. C. Petersen, & T. Brooks-Gunn (Eds.), *Encyclopedia of adolescence* (Vol. 1, pp. 529–534). London: Garland Publishing.
77. Marsh, H. W., & Kleitman, S. (2002). Extracurricular school activities: The good, the bad and the nonlinear. *Harvard Educational Review, 72*, 465–515.
78. Martinez, G., Copen, C. E., & Abma, J. C. (2011). Teenagers in the United States: Sexual activity, contraceptive use, and childbearing, 2006–2010. National Survey of Family Growth. *Series, 23*(31). Retrieved from: <http://www.cdc.gov/nchs/data/series/sr_23/sr23_031.pdf>. Accessed June 23, 2014.
79. Mechanic, D. (1991). Adolescents at risk: New directions. *Journal of Adolescent Health, 12*, 638–643.
80. Meeropol, E. (1991). One of the gang: Sexual development of adolescents with physical disabilities. *Journal of Pediatric Nursing, 6*, 243–250.
81. Meeus, W. (2011). The study of adolescent identity formation 2000-2010: A review of longitudinal research. *Journal of Research on Adolescence, 21*, 75–94.
82. Miyahara, M., & Piek, J. (2006). Self-esteem of children and adolescents with physical disabilities: Quantitative evidence from meta-analysis. *Journal of Developmental and Physical Disabilities, 18*, 219–233.
83. Miyahara, M., & Register, C. (2000). Perceptions of three terms to describe physical awkwardness in children. *Research in Developmental Disabilities, 21*, 367–376.
84. Mpofu, E. (2003). Enhancing social acceptance of early adolescents with physical disabilities: Effect of role salience, peer interaction, and academic support interventions. *International Journal of Disability, Development, and Education, 50*, 435–454.
85. Murphy, K., Molnar, G., & Lankasky, K. (2000). Employment and social issues in adults with cerebral palsy. *Archives of Physical Medicine and Rehabilitation, 81*, 807–811.
86. Muyle, T. P., Park, M. J., Nelson, C. D., et al. (2009). Trends in adolescent and young adult health in the United States. *Journal of Adolescent Health, 45*, 8–24.
87. National Disability Authority. (2006). The WHO's ICF. Retrieved November 2008 from: <http://www.nda.ie/cntmgmtnew.nsf/0/6877A99815DA

544980257066005369D1?Open Document>.

88. Neinstein, L. S., & Kaufman, F. R. (2002). Normal physical growth and development. In L. S. Neistein (Ed.), *Adolescent health care: A practical guide* (4th ed., pp. 3–51). Philadelphia: Lippincott Williams & Wilkins.
89. Newacheck, P. W., & Halfon, N. (1998). Prevalence and impact of disabling chronic conditions in childhood. *American Journal of Public Health, 88,* 610–617.
90. National Institute of Occupational Safety and Health. (1997). Child labor research needs. Cincinnati, OH: NIOSH (NIOSH Publication No. 97-143).
91. Overton, W. F., & Byrnes, J. P. (1991). Cognitive development. In R. M. Lerner, A. C. Petersen, & T. Brooks-Gunn (Eds.), *Encyclopedia of adolescence, vol. 1* (pp. 151–156). London: Garland Publishing.
92. Palisano, R., Copeland, W., & Galuppi, B. (2007). Performance of physical activities by adolescents with cerebral palsy. *Physical Therapy, 8,* 77–87.
93. Parham, L. D., & Fazio, L. S. (2008). *Play in occupational therapy for children* (2nd ed.). St Louis: Mosby.
94. Passmore, A., & French, D. (2003). The nature of leisure in adolescence: A focus group. *British Journal of Occupational Therapy, 66,* 419–426.
95. Patchin, J., & Hinduja, S. (2013). Cyberbullying Research Center. <www.cyberbullying.us>. Accessed June 23, 2014.
96. Piaget, J. (1972). Intellectual evolution from adolescence to adulthood. *Human Development, 15,* 1–12.
97. Putzinsky, T., & Cash, T. F. (2002). Understanding body images: Historical and contemporary perspectives. In T. F. Cash & T. Putzinsky (Eds.), *Body image.* New York: Guilford Press.
98. Quint, E. (2008). Menstrual issues in adolescents with physical and developmental disabilities. *Annals of the New York Academy of Science, 1135,* 230–236.
99. Radzik, M., Sherer, S., & Neinstein, L. S. (2002). Psychosocial development in normal adolescents. In L. S. Neinstein (Ed.), *Adolescent health: A practical guide* (4th ed., pp. 52–58). Philadelphia: Lippincott Williams & Wilkins.
100. Rathus, S. A. (2008). *Child and adolescent development, voyages in development* (3rd ed.). Belmont, CA: Thomson Wadsworth.
101. Rojewski, J. W., Lee, I. H., Gregg, N., et al. (2012). Developmental patterns of occupational aspirations in adolescents with high incidence disabilities. *Exceptional Children, 78,* 157–179.
102. Rotherman-Borus, M. J., & Langabeer, K. A. (2001). Developmental trajectories of gay, lesbian, and bisexual youth. In A. R. D'Augelli & C. Patterson (Eds.), *Lesbian, gay, and bisexual identities among youth: Psychological perspectives* (pp. 97–128). New York: Oxford University Press.
103. Rubenstein, H., Sternabach, M. R., & Pollock, S. H. (1999). Protecting the health and safety of working teenagers. *American Family Physician, 60,* 575–587.
104. Safran, J. (2002). Supporting students with Asperger's syndrome in general education. *Teaching Exceptional Children, 34,* 60–66.
105. Sanford, C., Newman, L., Wagner, M., et al. (2011). *The post-high school outcomes of young adults with disabilities up to 6 years after high school: A report from the National Longitudinal Transition Study-2 (NLTS2) [NCSER 2009-30171].* Menlo Park, CA: SRT International. Retrieved from: <http://ies.ed.gov/ncser/pubs/20113004/pdf/20113004.pdf> Accessed June 23, 2014.
106. Santelli, J., Sandfort, T., & Orr, M. (2008). Transactional comparisons of adolescent contraceptive use: What can we learn from these comparisons? *Archives of Pediatrics and Adolescent Medicine, 162,* 92–94.
107. Santrock, J. W. (2012). *Adolescence* (14th ed.). New York: McGraw-Hill Higher Education.
108. Scales, P. C., & Leffert, N. (2004). *Developmental assets: A synthesis of the scientific research on adolescent development* (2nd ed.). Minneapolis, MN: Search Institute.
109. Schondel, C. K., & Boehm, K. E. (2000). Motivational needs of adolescent volunteers. *Adolescence, 35,* 335–344.
110. Schwartz, J., Engel, M., & Jensen, L. (1999). Pain in persons with cerebral palsy. *Archives of Physical Medicine and Rehabilitation, 80,* 1243–1246.
111. Schwartz, S. J., & Montgomery, M. J. (2002). Similarities or differences in identity development? The impact of acculturation and gender on identity process and outcome. *Journal of Youth and Adolescence, 31,* 359–372.
112. Skinner, H., Biscope, S., Poland, B., et al. (2003). Adolescents use technology for health information: Implications for health professionals from focus group studies. *Journal of Medical Internet Research, 5.* Retrieved October 2008 from: <http://www.jmir.org/2003/4/e25/HTML>.
113. Spencer, M. B., Dupree, D., & Hartman, T. (1997). A phenomenological variant of ecological systems theory (PVEST): A self-organization perspective of content. *Developmental and Psychopathology, 9,* 817–833.
114. Stainton, M. (2006). Raising a woman. *JAMA: The Journal of the American Medical Association, 296,* 1445–1446.
115. Stevens, S. E., Steele, C. A., Jutai, J. W., et al. (1996). Adolescents with physical disabilities: Some psychosocial aspects of health. *The Journal of Adolescent Health, 19,* 157–164.
116. Stewart, D. A., Law, M. C., Rosenbaum, P., et al. (2001). A qualitative study of the transition to adulthood for youth with physical disabilities. *Physical and Occupational Therapy in Pediatrics, 21,* 3–21.
117. Surgeon General. (1999). Surgeon General's Report on Mental Illness. Retrieved June 23, 2009 from: <http://www.surgeongeneral.gov/library/mentalhealth/home.html>.
118. Surís, J. C., Resnick, M., Cassuto, N., et al. (1996). Sexual behavior of adolescents with chronic disease and disability. *Journal of Adolescent Health, 19,* 124–131.
119. Tashie, C., Shapiro-Barnard, S., & Rossetti, Z. (2006). *See the charade: What we need to do and undo to make friendships happen.* Nottingham, UK: Inclusive Solutions Inc.
120. Tipton, L. A., Christensen, L., & Blacher, J. (2013). Friendship quality in adolescents with and without an intellectual disability. *Journal of Applied Research in Intellectual Disabilities, 26,* 522–532.
121. Van Cleave, J., & Davis, M. M. (2006). Bullying and peer victimization among children with special health care needs. *Pediatrics, 118,* e1212–e1219.
122. Vilhjalmsson, R., & Krisjansdottir, G. (2003). Gender difference in physical activity in older children and adolescents: The central role of organized sport. *Social Science and Medicine, 56,* 363–374.
123. Wagner, M., Newman, L., Cameto, R., et al. (2005). *After high school: A first look at the post-school experiences of youth with disabilities. A report from the National Longitudinal Transition Study-2 (NLTS2).* Menlo Park, CA: SRI International.
124. Wells, M., & Mitchell, K. J. (2013). Patterns of Internet use and risks of online victimization for youth with and without disabilities. *The Journal of Special Education,* 1–10.
125. U.S. Department of Education (2000). *Prohibited disability harassment: Reminder of responsibilities under Section 504 of the Rehabilitation Act of 1973 and Title II of the Americans with*

Disabilities Act. Washington, DC: Office for Civil Rights.
126. Williams, J., & Currie, C. (2000). Self-esteem and physical development in early adolescence: Pubertal timing and body image. *The Journal of Early Adolescence, 20,* 129–149.
127. Wolman, C., & Basco, D. (1994). Factors influencing self-esteem and self-consciousness in adolescents with spina bifida. *The Journal of Adolescent Health, 15,* 543–548.
128. Worley, G., Houlihan, C. M., Herman-Giddens, M. E., et al. (2002). Secondary sexual characteristics in children with cerebral palsy and moderate to severe motor impairment: A cross-sectional survey. *Pediatrics, 110,* 897–902.
129. Wynn, J. R. (2003). High school after school: Creating pathways to the future for adolescents. *New Directions for Youth Development, 97,* 59–74.
130. Ybarra, M. L., Mitchell, K. J., Wolak, J., et al. (2006). Examining characteristics and associated distress related to Internet harassment: Findings from the Second Youth Internet Safety survey. *Pediatrics, 118,* 1169–1177.
131. Yoder, A. (2000). Barriers to ego identity status formation: A contextual qualification of Marcia's identity status paradigm. *Journal of Adolescence, 23,* 95–106.
132. Youngblood, J., & Spencer, M. B. (2002). Integrating normative identity process and academic support requirements for special needs adolescents: The application of an identity focused cultural ecological (ICE) perspective. *Applied Developmental Science, 6,* 95–108.
133. Yurgelun-Todd, D. (2007). Emotional and cognitive changes in adolescence. *Current Opinion in Neurobiology, 17,* 251–257.
134. Zajicek-Faber, M. L. (1998). Promoting good health in adolescents with disabilities. *Health and Social Work, 23,* 203–214.
135. Zastrow, C. H., & Kirst-Ashman, K. K. (2004). *Understanding human behavior* (6th ed.). Belmont, CA: Brooks/Cole-Thomson Learning.

CHAPTER 5

Working with Families

Lynn Jaffe • Sharon Cosper

KEY TERMS

Families facing multiple challenges
Family adaptation and resilience
Family as a dynamic system
Family diversity
Family occupations: routines and rituals
Family-centered services
Functions of a family
Parent-professional partnership

GUIDING QUESTIONS

1. How does family systems theory describe the occupations and functions of families?
2. What is the family life cycle, and how do we identify times of potential stress for families of children with special needs?
3. How does having a child with special needs influence family function and the co-occupations of family members?
4. How do we learn about a family's culture and background, and why is knowledge of diversity important?
5. What are the roles of the occupational therapist when collaborating with families?
6. How does an occupational therapist establish and maintain partnership with a family?
7. How can families be empowered to facilitate their children's development?
8. What are the best strategies for supporting the strengths of families facing multiple challenges?

This chapter introduces a range of issues related to families, particularly families of children who have special developmental or health care needs. It considers how family members fulfill the functions of a family by collectively engaging in daily or weekly activities and by sharing special events. The chapter explores factors that contribute to the variety of families with whom occupational therapists may work in providing occupational therapy for children. After presenting this background on the occupations of families and family diversity, the chapter then discusses how the special needs of children bring opportunities and challenges to families. This discussion includes the ways in which having a child with disabilities can influence how family members organize their time, engage in activities, and interact with one another. Principles and strategies that follow a family-centered philosophy and research evidence are emphasized throughout the chapter.

Reasons to Study Families

"Why do I need to read a chapter on families? I was raised in a family, I know all about families. . . ."

Families are complex systems. Having a child with a disability or chronic health condition, which can happen in families anywhere on the socioeconomic spectrum, of any educational, ethnic, or genetic background, can add an appreciable degree of stress into this complex system. Families with low socioeconomic status, poor education, or minority status are more likely to have negative outcomes.[41] Occupational therapists encounter and must be prepared to work with every type of family. Children cannot be treated as isolated individuals; they are members of families, the social units that shape behavior and life experiences. Evidence has shown that child outcomes may be shaped by how well occupational therapists communicate with families and how well the partnership between them has been established.[28,57,82] Learning about family systems is important preparation for working in any practice setting.

The development of children's occupations cannot be understood without insight into what shapes their daily activities. All major health-related disciplines, including but not limited to psychology, sociology, and nursing practice, use the ecologic view of children and the family—that each is interconnected with the other and the environments that they experience. Although children's activities vary from one culture to the next, universally their families play the major role in guiding how children spend their time, influencing what they do, and helping them understand why the things they do are important.[70,125,149] The more completely occupational therapists understand these guiding factors, the better prepared they will be to support families in shaping their child's development.

Another reason to study families explicitly is to circumvent the inclination to reference one's own family experiences as a template for the way families operate. Walsh pointed out that when people speak of "the family," they suggest a socially constructed image of a "normal" family, giving the impression that an ideal family exists, in which optimal development occurs.[154] In reality, many different types of families are successfully raising children. In this chapter, two or more people who share an enduring emotional bond and a commitment to pool resources and carry out typical family functions can be seen as a family.[87,149,155] This chapter focuses on families raising children. One or more parents, grandparents, and stepparents, as well as adoptive or foster parents, can successfully bring up children. We refer to the caregiving adult as the "parent" of the child, and focus specifically on the "parent" only when it is germane to the discussion of family diversity (Box 5-1).

A third reason to study families is that the involvement of family members is central to the best practice of occupational therapy. In addition to organizing and enabling daily activities, the family provides the child's most enduring set of relationships throughout childhood, into early adulthood, and possibly beyond. During the course of his or her lifetime, a person with a disability may receive services from people working through health services, educational programs, and social agencies. These relationships exist because professionals bring the expertise required by the special needs of the young person. As the type of services needed changes, professionals enter and leave the young person's life. The family represents a source of continuity across this changing pattern of professional involvement. The family forms a unique emotional attachment to their child, and their continued involvement gives them special insight into the child's needs, abilities, and occupational interests. In light of the family's expertise, occupational therapists strive to collaborate with family members, follow their lead, and support their efforts in promoting the well-being and development of the child with special developmental or health care needs.[16,28,132] Case Study 5-1 on pp. 152–156, which describes the actual experiences of parents raising three children with special needs, provides additional insight into the essential nature of family relationships.

BOX 5-1 Therapists' Professional Responsibility in Light of Family Diversity

Family diversity is a social construct defined in the eyes of the beholder; families that appear atypical may have been defined as "just an average family" in another era or culture. It is not sufficient to strive to treat all families the same because each family has different needs and expectations for how professionals can support them.[152]

The therapist should strive to do the following:

- See each family in light of what makes it unique and also how similar it is to all other families raising children.
- Recognize differences among families by reflecting on one's own cultural model and associated beliefs and critically analyze how knowledge about families is constructed.[1,125]
- Gain an understanding of families with different backgrounds by reading the literature or finding other people who can share an insider's perspective because they have been parts of similar families.
- Initiate conversations that solicit a parent's explanation about family membership, family's cultural model, and activities valued for and by the child.
- Talk with parents about how they do things together during their daily and weekly routines and the meanings that they give these shared activities as a place to start.
- Design interventions that fit into daily routines and are compatible with family traditions.

Finally, including families in the process of providing services for children is not just best practice—it is the law. In recognizing the power of families, federal legislation requires service providers and educators to seek the input and permission of a parent or guardian in regard to any assessment, intervention plan, or placement decision. The importance of the family in the early part of the child's life (from birth to 3 years old) is reflected by the emphasis on family-centered services in Part C of the Individuals with Disabilities Education Improvement Act 2004 (IDEA; http://idea.ed.gov).[72] It requires providers to meet with parents and develop a family-directed, Individualized Family Service Plan (IFSP) regarding the resources that the family needs to promote the child's optimal development. Later, in the school system, parents are involved in developing the Individualized Educational Program (IEP), which guides special education and related services (see Chapters 22 and 23).

The Family: A Group of Occupational Beings

Family members, individually or together, engage in a variety of activities that are part of home management, caregiving, employed work, education, play, and leisure domains that help them feel connected to each other. A father fulfills one of his family roles by picking up groceries on his way home from work, or a child studies for a test because his or her parents expect good grades. Family occupations occur when daily activities or special events are shared among family members, such as a parent helping a son study for a test, the whole family going to a movie, or brothers shooting baskets. By engaging in occupations together, families with children fulfill the functions of the family unit expected of them by members of their community.

Societies first anticipate that families provide children with a cultural foundation for their development as occupational beings. Family members share and transmit a *cultural model,* a habitual framework for thinking about events, for determining which activities should be done and when, and for deciding on how to interact.[45] By providing a cultural foundation, families ensure that children learn how to approach, perform, and experience activities in a manner consistent with those in their cultural group (Box 5-2). Culture is passed from generation to

BOX 5-2 Outcomes of Family Occupations

Family occupations contribute to the following outcomes for children:

1. Establish a cultural foundation for learning occupations that enable children to participate in a variety of contexts
2. Help shape children's basic sense of identity and emotional well-being
3. Help children learn to master routines and habits that support physical health and well-being
4. Foster readiness to learn and participate in educational programs
5. Foster readiness to assume a place in the community and society

generation through rituals that include celebrations, traditions, and patterned interactions that give life meaning and construct family identity.[129]

Occupations have meaning because they convey a sense of self, connect us to other people, and link us to place.[59] Routine family occupations give order to life and structure the achievement of goals.[13] Routine family occupations and special events also form the basis for repeated interpersonal experiences that give family members a sense of support, identity, and emotional well-being.[134] The importance of family occupations is reflected by the fact that families create special activities for the specific purpose of spending time together.[128,147]

Families are expected to help their children develop fundamental routines and lifestyle habits that contribute to their physical health and well-being. In the context of receiving care and sharing in family activities, children acquire skills that lead to their independence in activities of daily living (ADLs) and learn habits that will influence their health across their life span. For example, in the context of sharing in family dinners and leisure activities after dinner, children establish habits that can reduce or increase future problems with obesity.

Families also prepare children for formal or informal educational activities and experiences that prepare young people to become productive adults.[125] Parents, in the context of their daily routines and through their encouragement, provide children with participation experiences that influence how they approach learning.[71] Families of children with disabilities must meet all these expectations.

Guided by their cultural models, special circumstances, and community opportunities for activities, families use their resources in different ways (Box 5-3). For example, one family may choose to pay (using financial resources) to have the yard work done so that time (another asset) on Saturday afternoons can be used for having a picnic together. Another family invests interpersonal energies (an emotional resource) to get everyone to help with the yard work on Saturday afternoon so that money will be available to pay for music lessons. Financial, human, and emotional resources, as well as time, are not limitless, and, in healthy families, members negotiate a give and take of their assets. Mothers of children with developmental coordination disorder (DCD) or attention-deficit/hyperactivity disorder (ADHD) may set aside extra time to help with their children's activities and rely on hired help or assistance from other family members to get household tasks done.[47,109] Typically, families with children have a hierarchical organization in which one or more family members (e.g., a parent) take(s) major responsibility for determining how the resources are distributed, enabling the family to engage in activities that fulfill family functions. Availability of resources varies for many reasons, within families and within their communities. Challenges for families and occupational therapists occur when families or the communities they live in have severely limited resources.[24,133]

BOX 5-3 Family Resources

Family resources: Properties family members use to engage in a balanced pattern of needed and desired activities in a way that enables them to fulfill the family functions

Financial: Remuneration from productive activities that enable the family to acquire material things such as a place to live, food, and clothing

This may also determine which types of community activities are available for family members.

Human: The knowledge and skills family members bring to activities

For example, a teenager who learns to use the Internet at school brings this skill home and can help his or her parent learn how to pay bills online.

Time: Minutes, hours, days to engage in activities that enable families to fulfill their functional roles

Emotional energy: Experiencing close interpersonal relationships during shared activities

System Perspective of Family Occupations

A family functions as a dynamic system in which its members, comprising subsystems, engage in occupations together to fulfill the functions of a family. As with any system, the activity of one person can influence the activities of other members. These *interdependent influences* define the dynamic relationship among the different parts, similar to the movement of a piece of a hanging mobile that causes movement of all the other parts. For example, a sixth grader may ask to stay after school with his friend, which means that he is not available to watch his sister that afternoon while his mother shops. Consequently, the mother brings her daughter to the grocery store. Shopping with the preschool daughter takes the mother longer than shopping alone. As a result, they do not get home as quickly, and dinner is started late. The interdependent nature of family members' activities is illustrated by the fact that the boy's choice of what he wanted to do in the afternoon altered the activities of his mother and sister and indirectly affected the family's mealtime routine that evening. Recognizing that a family functions as a whole, an occupational therapist who suggests an after-school horseback riding class for a child with cerebral palsy needs to appreciate that the recommendation must be weighed in light of the family resources and the implications of that activity for the entire family system. As a complex social system, family members have to coordinate what and when they do things to share in family routines and rituals (Box 5-4). They accomplish this within subsystems through their communications and family rules.[146]

BOX 5-4 Key Concepts of a Family System Model

1. A family system is composed of individuals who are interdependent and have reciprocal influences on each other's occupations.
2. Within the family, subsystems are defined, with their own patterns of interaction and shared occupations.
3. A family must be understood as a whole, and it is more than the sum of the abilities of each member.
4. The family system works to sustain predictable patterns in family occupations and be part of a larger community.
5. Change and evolution are inherent in a family.
6. A family, as an open system, is influenced by its environment.

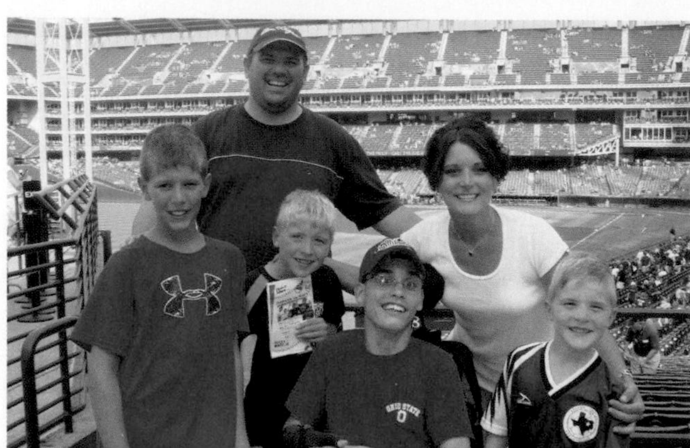

FIGURE 5-1 Matthew and his family enjoy a ball game. (Courtesy Jill and Mark McQuaid, Dublin, Ohio.)

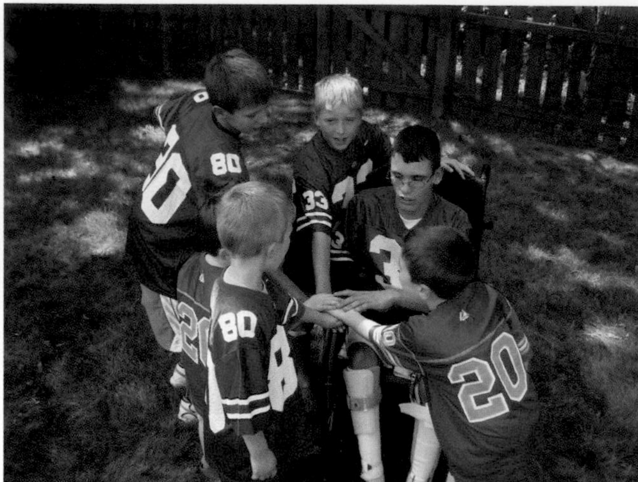

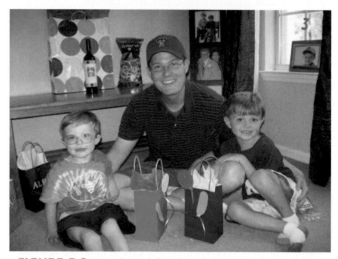

FIGURE 5-2 Matthew's brothers and friends play ball. (Courtesy Jill and Mark McQuaid, Dublin, Ohio.)

With all the activities a family does, and the different members who can carry out these tasks, it would become confusing and drain family resources if everyone had to negotiate daily who was going to do what, when, and in which way. An effective family system organizes itself into *predictable patterns* of daily and weekly activities and familiar ways with special events. Guided by their cultural models, and often organized through unspoken family rules, families settle into *daily routines* for various household activities.[29,48,134] These daily routines include interactive rituals that take on symbolic meaning and seem to be so habitual that people do not think of doing them any other way, and they resist changing them.[47,129,147] Bedtime routines for a child, for example, can have a set sequence of taking a bath, brushing teeth, and the parent reading a book. If routines are interrupted, even by a welcomed event, such as a grandparent coming to visit, family members invest extra family resources to reconfigure their daily routines under the changed circumstances. For example, time is spent making up a bed on the sofa rather than giving the daughter a bath, and emotional energy is expended to help the daughter fall asleep in the living room so that the grandparent can sleep in her bedroom. Families may experience the disruption of their daily routines as unsettling and taxing, and it is not uncommon to hear family members sigh in relief when they can return to predictable patterns—that is, when "things get back to normal."

In addition to routines for daily or weekly activities (Figure 5-1), families also establish predictable patterns for what they do during rituals, such as special events. *Family traditions,* such as cooking special food for birthday celebrations or sharing leisure activities on Sunday afternoons, help family members develop a sense of group cohesion and emotional well-being (Figure 5-2). Families may decide to maintain their traditions rather than address an individual member's needs because these customary activities fulfill family functions. For example, a family that traditionally vacations with grandparents for several weeks in the summer may value how special activities together reinforce their sense of being a family. Conflict with the occupational therapist could arise if the therapist assumes that the family will shorten their traditional vacation to attend some therapy sessions during the summer. When the occupational therapist offers a range of options and asks the family to set priorities, family members can consider all of their routines and traditions and determine how they want occupational therapy services to fit into their lives.

FIGURE 5-3 Noah and family celebrating Father's Day.

Celebrations are predictable patterns of doing activities, such as religious rituals, that are shared with members of the community. Therefore, what is done during family celebrations may be similar to what other families that share a similar background do for the same celebration. This link to others gives family members a sense of meaning associated with their special events that connects them to a community of families (Figure 5-3). Occupational therapists may be asked for assistance so that children can participate in celebrations. For example, a parent may want positioning suggestions so that her daughter with cerebral palsy will be comfortable during Christmas Eve services. The family of a boy with sensory processing problems may need ideas for coping that they can use while attending a Fourth of July fireworks display with the neighbors. By enabling these children's occupational engagement, the entire family participates in community celebrations and confirms their identity as a family, like every other family raising children. Needless to say, culturally aware occupational therapists are always respectful of families that choose to not engage in the celebrations thought to be typical in the larger society.

Among the researchers who have investigated family routines and practices, Fiese and colleagues[29,30,134] have examined the meaning of routines and related ritual interactions of families' daily activities and religious celebrations. Their studies show that families who reported finding more meaning and commitment to their routines and special activities experienced better health of family members and stronger interpersonal relationships. Occupational therapists who suggest home carryover of interventions must be sure that the activities will fit within the family's values and their existing routines; otherwise, the intervention may not be incorporated.[15,130,131]

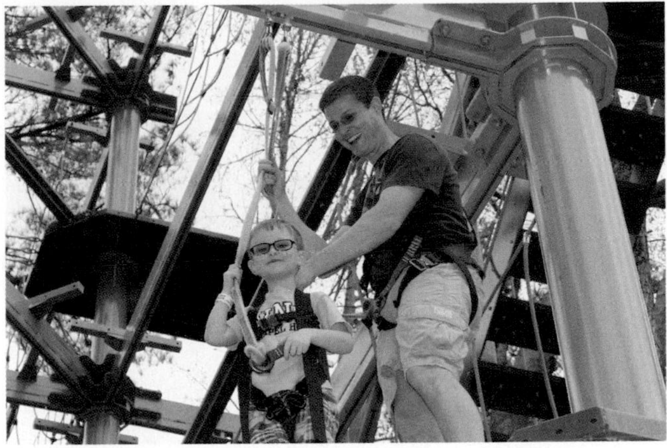

FIGURE 5-4 Noah doing a ropes course at the zoo with Dad's help.

Family Subsystems

Parents

Regardless of the type of family structure (e.g., birth, adoptive, partner, blended, foster), caregiving adults sharing parental duties need to coordinate their efforts. These adults form the *parent subsystem* of the family, which can be a positive force and can contribute to the child's ability to face developmental challenges. However, when stressed, it may be a negative influence on the child's development.[5] Parents may deal with childcare in a variety of forms, which may all be adaptive if they enable the system to operate and meet family functions.[79] Some studies note that the type and severity of a child's disability may necessitate additional time for caregiving co-occupations, such as in the mother-child subsystem.[33] Although some have found these time demands to be similar to those of typical children, the meaningfulness and enjoyment of the time and occupations may be different for parents of children with disabilities.[47]

All parents may experience increased levels of stress, especially when first taking on this role. Stresses may become even greater for parents of children with disabilities, although this is still equivocal.[12,17,34,35,139] Disabilities that seem to create more stress and caregiving effort for the family include autism, severe and multiple disabilities, behavior disorders, and medical problems that require frequent hospitalization and in-home medical care.[27,59,124] Although researchers had previously reported that mothers experience greater stress, currently, with the increase in the number of two-earner families and of fathers as primary caretakers, the stress level of both parents has been found to be more similar than earlier studies had suggested[33,79,134,143,150] (Figure 5-4). Often, the caregiving parent has the potential to be more isolated, yet is also the person who interacts with others about the child and may experience more support in that regard. The primary caregiving parent has the added burden of sharing information with his or her partner, which may also increase the level of stress. Professionals need to be sure to include both parents, as well as other caregivers, in their communications about a child to ensure that information is transmitted accurately and unburden the caregiving parent of the responsibility of transmitting all the information.

Children affect the relationship between husband and wife, in positive and negative ways. Although there is evidence that a child with disabilities can increase the stress on a marital relationship,[9] there is also evidence that marriages are strengthened when raising a child with a disability.[124] Differences in marital satisfaction between families of children with disabilities and those of typically developing children tend to be minimal.[24] Stress in dealing with the child may bring parents together for problem solving, and they may rely on each other for emotional support and coping. A strong relationship between husband and wife seems to buffer parenting stress. Teaching parents intervention techniques to use with behaviorally challenging children has also been shown to reduce stress levels.[14]

Siblings

Siblings are an important source of support to each other throughout life. Having a brother or sister with special needs may change the experiences of other children growing up in that family (Figure 5-5). In general, the relationships between children with disabilities and their siblings can be as strong and positive as those of typical siblings.[97] The research findings, however, are varied across types of disabilities, sibling place in the family (older or younger), and sibling genders. Conflict among siblings may be more prevalent when a child has a disability such as hyperactivity or behavioral problems. Conflict tends to be less prevalent when a child has Down syndrome or an intellectual disability.[66,83] Williams and colleagues[157] investigated factors that might influence behavioral problems or the self-esteem of children who had a sibling with a chronic illness (e.g., cancer, diabetes, cystic fibrosis) or developmental disability (e.g., autism, cerebral palsy). They found that the mental health of siblings of children with disabilities appeared more related to co-occurring risk factors, such as low socioeconomic status (SES) or single-parent household, than to the sibling relationship. These factors and the siblings' understanding of the disease or disability were related to whether the typically developing sibling had behavioral problems. When the siblings felt supported, their behavior, moods, and self-esteem were more positive than when they felt unsupported.[112]

Often, the roles of siblings are asymmetric, with the typically developing child dominating the child with the disability. Siblings without disability generally engage the child with a disability in play activities in which they can participate, such as rough and tumble play rather than symbolic play. Siblings may

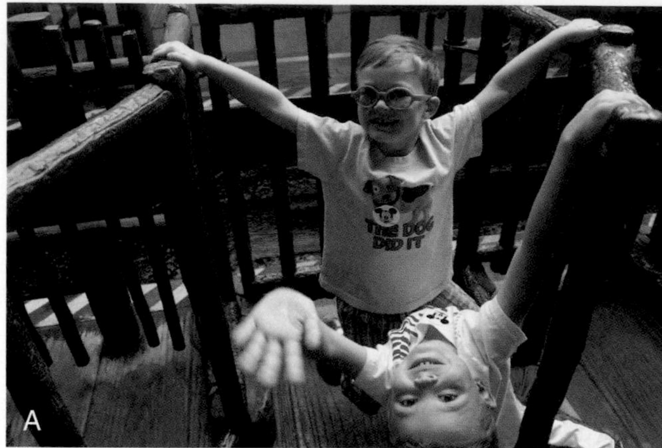

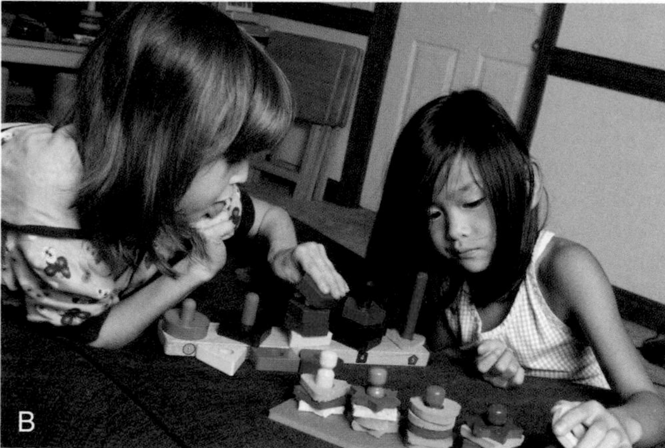

FIGURE 5-5 **A,** Two brothers enjoy playing together on the playground. **B,** Sisters play a sorting game together.

be asked to take on caregiving roles, and assuming caregiving roles can have positive and negative effects.[140] Siblings learn to relate and interact in the context of a family. Positive and solid marital systems seem to promote more positive sibling relationships, and marital stress has a deleterious effect on sibling relationships.[124]

Because occupational therapists promote engagement in a full range of activities as a way of helping a child participate in family life, the inclusion of siblings is an important step in occupation-centered practice. Siblings are likely to be the best playmates and can often elicit maximum effort from their brother or sister. In addition, sibling involvement gives the therapeutic activity additional meaning (play), and siblings can act as models for teaching new skills. Peer support groups for the typically developing siblings can also be occupation-centered. Occupational therapists can develop a recreational program for brothers and sisters of children with whom they work so that the siblings can meet one another and realize that their family is not the only one that faces challenging behaviors. These groups generally participate in structured activities and have open-ended discussions about what it means to have siblings with disabilities. One formalized support group for siblings is Sibshops, a recreational program that addresses needs and concerns through group activities.[108] Sibshops' primary goals for brothers and sisters of children with special needs are to meet their peers, discuss common joys and concerns, learn how others handle common experiences, and learn more about their siblings with special needs.

Extended Family

In the extended family, the experience of having a child with special needs depends on the meaning family members bring to their relationship with the child. Family members, such as grandparents, uncles, and aunts of the child, are especially important to fathers and mothers for emotional and practical assistance (Figure 5-6). When extended family members are not supportive, parents may experience frustration and hurt over their lack of contact.[38] For some grandparents, grandchildren represent a link to the future and an opportunity for vicarious achievement. Researchers have found that when children have disabilities, grandparents express positive and negative feelings and go through a series of adjustments similar to those of the parents.[99] Many of the negative feelings, such as anger and confusion, appear to decrease with time, although some may never completely disappear. Positive feelings, such as acceptance and a sense of usefulness, increase over time. A grandparent's educational level and sense of closeness to the child are positively associated with greater involvement with the child. Factors such as the grandparent's age and health and the distance the grandparent lives from the child do not appear to influence involvement. Grandparents learn information about their grandchild's condition primarily through the child's parents. However, some seek information from other sources, such as support groups for grandparents of children with special needs. Margetts et al.[99] found that grandparents of children with autism spectrum disorder felt strongly about the caring and support that they provided for their children and grandchildren. For professionals to be truly family-centered, they need to ask whether the parents want to include the grandparents in the initial assessment of the child.[99]

Family Life Cycle

Family systems undergo metamorphosis and adapt as family members change. Some transitions with developing children can be anticipated and seem to be tied to age more than ability. For example, *normative events* in children that require adjustments in families include the birth of a child, starting kindergarten, transitions between schools, leaving high school, and living outside the home. Other changes in the family are not anticipated. *Non-normative events* may include a grandparent coming to live with the family or a parent accepting a job in another city. Families that are cohesive and adaptable adjust interactive routines, reorganize daily activities, and return to a sense of "normal" family life. If interactive routines and role designation are set too rigidly, the family may not be able to operate effectively through periods of transition. This is especially true if the family experiences unanticipated, threatening events, such as a job loss or medical crisis. All families use coping strategies to accommodate periods of transition.

Occupational therapists must understand that all families are unique. Although life cycle models consist of predictable events, the individuality of each family must be acknowledged. The characteristics and issues at each life stage are highly variable, and each family moves through the stages at different

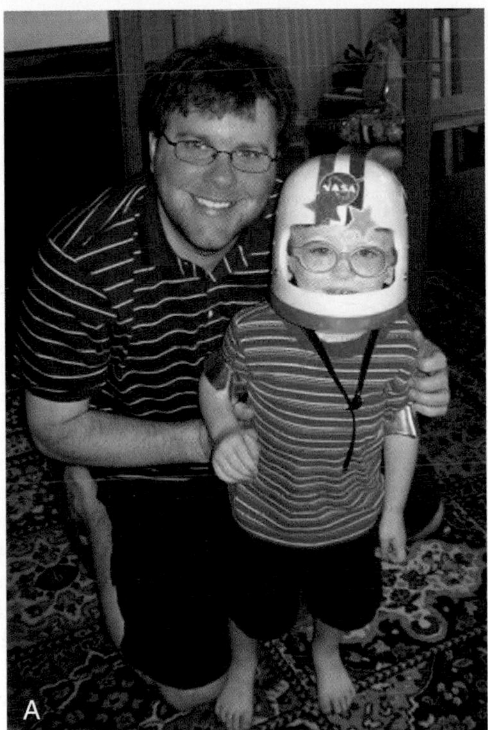

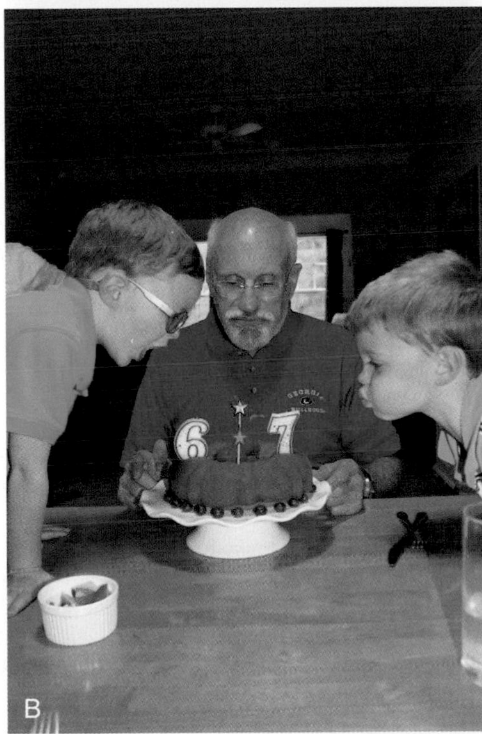

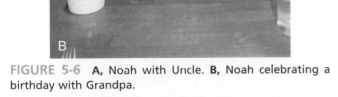

FIGURE 5-6 **A,** Noah with Uncle. **B,** Noah celebrating a birthday with Grandpa.

rates. Some family members may experience and resolve their feelings when they first learn about their child's diagnosis, or they may take months to "come to grips" with the information.[120] In addition, the family may experience additional cycles of sadness and acceptance, within and between life stages. Issues that the family seemed to resolve when the child was an infant may occur again when the child reaches school age and an educational diagnosis is made or a learning problem is identified. Other life stage–related events, such as the child's ability to develop friendships when first entering grade school, may become an issue again when the child enters high school. (Case Study 5-1 on pp. 152–156, provides examples of the issues that arise in each of the life stages.) Finally, different members of the family may be at different stages at the same time. Therefore, characteristics of the family members and child's phase of development must be considered. For example, in a skipped-generation family, grandparents frequently have to deal with changes associated with old age at the same time they are parenting their grandchildren. A young couple may have more energy and resources to cope with the birth of a child with special needs than an older couple with four other children participating in school activities.

Early Childhood

Identifying a child as being at risk for health or developmental problems is usually a complicated process. Unless the child is born with medical problems, congenital problems in a body structure, or features that suggest a syndrome, a child may be not diagnosed for months, and sometimes years. Families that describe their experiences in raising a child with a disability frequently recall their journey by looking back to a period when "something was not right."[42] Families of children with pervasive developmental delays recall a sense that they had to search for a diagnosis with repeated testing and visits to several clinics or evaluation centers. Even parents of a child with an unusual physical complaint, such as joint pain that occurs only at night, might have to persevere in finding the cause when professionals suggest that the child is only seeking attention. After receiving a diagnosis and ending a period of uncertainty, families hope for a period of stability, but, as one educated father commented, "No amount of professional or personal preparation trains you for the reality of chronic illness" (p. 243).[67] Parents' first questions often include accessing quality childcare, medication management, insurance issues, and available support systems.[69]

Parents whose first child has special needs do not have the same experiences to draw on as those of families with older children. Parents of young children may ask questions such as, "Do you think he can go into a regular classroom?" and "Do you think she will be able to live on her own some day?" Thoughtful responses to these questions recognize the parents' need for optimism and hope. However, the responses must be honest and realistic. Even occupational therapists with years of experience and extensive knowledge about disability and development cannot make definitive statements about the future. Long-range predictions about when the child will achieve a certain milestone or level of independence are always speculative. However, parents feel frustrated when they are told that the future cannot be predicted. Lawlor and Mattingly[91] found that families want to be exposed to anticipatory planning. Parents want to understand that they have reason to expect that their child, despite disabilities, will have a place in society and an opportunity to engage in socially valued occupations during adulthood. Occupational therapists can help parents understand the range of possibilities by telling them about the continuum of services for older children and young adults in the community. Talking with parents of older children with a similar condition or hearing the occupational therapist's story of a child with the same issues provides some insight into the future.[44,156] Even without knowing the child's developmental course, parents start to develop an understanding that services are in place, and they begin to create new stories about their child's future. Given information about the system, their rights, and the resources available to them in their communities, parents can solve problems and access needed services independently.

The caregiving routines of parents whose young child has a disability are not particularly different from those of all parents of young children. At this time in the child's life, the parent's work consists of managing the child's play environment and introducing new, developmentally appropriate objects and materials. The parent ensures the child's safety and may adjust or arrange the play environment so that an infant can access objects of interest. Feeding, diapering, bathing, and daily care are also natural parenting activities at this time. Only when infants and young children have serious medical conditions or behavioral problems are daily occupations significantly altered. When children are medically unstable, but still at home, a family may have home-based nursing for extended periods (i.e., months to several years). Murphy[110] has described the stress created by the constant presence of nurses and professional care providers in the home. Role ambiguity often results when parents think that they must take on unpaid nursing work and nurses take on a parenting role. Parents also report stress from a lack of privacy and the continual feeling that they are "on duty." Parents of medically fragile children must make tremendous accommodations, which must elicit high levels of sensitivity and responsiveness from professionals.[100] When parents have a medically unstable infant and 24-hour, in-home nursing care, services such as respite become a priority. When a child has life-threatening food allergies, the parent may need support sharing that information with personnel at the childcare center or preschool. Occupational therapists can be an essential support for families' interactions with the community (Research Note 5-1).

School Age

When a child enters school, all families are excited about the new opportunities for learning and the child's new demonstration of independence. However, school entry can be challenging for families of children with disabilities. Families who experienced early intervention services may be disappointed to find fewer family services and less family support offered by the school. Typically, parents are not encouraged to attend classes or school-based therapy sessions. Many parents view the transition to school as an opportunity to be less involved and a sign of their child's maturation, but some are distressed by the separation. To ease the transition from home to school, the parents of children with special needs should learn about the school's programs, schedules, rules, and policies (Figure 5-7).

For children with mild learning disabilities, entry into school may be the first time that the gap between a child's performance and teachers' expectations for performance is identified. Therefore, this may also be the first time that parents receive information that their child has special needs. When this is the case, parents can experience surprise, disbelief, or relief. School age is a time when children with disabilities may first discover that they have differences. How they make the adjustment to

RESEARCH NOTE 5-1

Khetani, M. A., Orsmond, G., Cohn, E., Law, M. C., & Coster, W. (2012). Correlates of community participation among families transitioning from part C early intervention services. OTJR: Occupation, Participation and Health, 32 *(3), 61–72.*

Abstract

Objective. This study examined factors that contributed to level (full or restricted) of community participation in order to guide practice.

Method. This was a secondary analysis of data from the National Early Intervention Longitudinal Study (NEILS) on data through computerized telephone interviews. This study used a subsample of 2003 families across 20 states. Classification and regression tree (CART) analysis was used to examine correlates of full and limited community participation.

Results. 1450 families were classified into the limited community participation group and 553 families into the full participation group. Families in the full participation group tended to have younger children, live in two-parent households with higher income, have more formal education, and have paid jobs.

Conclusion. Difficulty in managing the child's behavior is a significant barrier to community participation and is associated with the degree of social support.

Implications for Practice

Occupational therapists should ask caregivers about family's levels of participation in community events and whether that is satisfactory. They should also ask about their strategies to manage their child's behavior and their level of social supports.

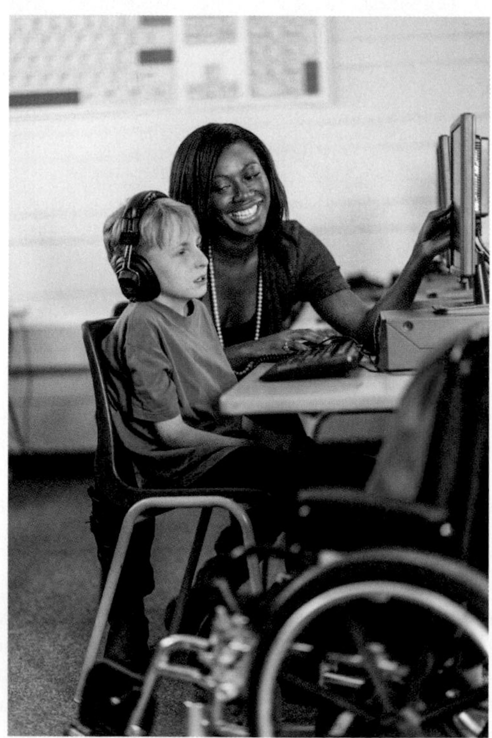

FIGURE 5-7 Child has an aide at school who supports his participation in both academic and nonacademic activities.

this information depends on the knowledge and sensitivity of the adults and children around them.

To the school-age child, making and keeping friends becomes critically important. Some parents report concern if their child appears lonely, isolated, and friendless. Children with behavioral problems frequently have no friends, leaving the parents with the additional responsibility of creating and supervising play opportunities with other children. Having peer friendships is associated with more positive school behaviors.[111] Teachers and occupational therapists can use different strategies to promote friendships in inclusive environments. Typically developing peers can take turns being a child's "special buddy," and they can offer assistance with projects or tutoring. In situations in which social stigma is an issue, peer relations can be promoted by explaining the disability to the other children and by designing classroom activities that promote cooperation and positive interaction.

Adolescence

Adolescence is a challenging and potentially stressful time for all families because the development of self-identity, sexuality, and expectations of emotional and economic autonomy herald the transition to adulthood. These issues may pose additional challenges in the lives of children with disabilities as they maneuver through adolescence. Parents need to prepare the young person to handle his or her growing social, financial, and sexual needs, as well as how to avoid substance abuse. (See the study of high-risk behaviors in adolescents with physical disabilities by Jones & Lollar.[75]) In certain cases, parents face decisions about their child's use of birth control and protection from sexually transmitted diseases.[51] With adolescence, new concerns about a son's or daughter's vulnerability increase as that child ventures further into the community and beyond. These decisions vary significantly depending on the nature of the disability—cognitive, physical, social, visible—and can be mediated by financial opportunities or constraints.

Although the child usually is well accepted by family members, the social stigma incurred from peers and others may increase during adolescence. The cute child with unusual behaviors may become a not so cute adolescent, with socially unacceptable behaviors. As one mother said, "The community accepts our children much more easily when they are small and cute. Babyish mannerisms are no longer acceptable. . . . [Our son] has had real problems with his social relationships. He simply does not know how to initiate a friendship. He has difficulty maintaining a sensible conversation with his peers. He doesn't handle teasing well, so he is teased unmercifully" (p. 90).[4]

Adolescence is the time when most parents must learn to let their children make their way in the world (Figure 5-8). For parents of children with disabilities, this time may require additional emotional support and financial resources. In addition, some parents experience difficulty caring for their child's growing physical needs. As the child reaches adulthood, parents who are reaching middle age may feel their strength and energy declining. As with all facets of the life cycle, this is a time for a sensitive, collaborative approach between families and service providers so that the right supports and resources are offered to each family. (See Chapters 4 and 12, on adolescent socialization, for more on this topic.)

Family Resources and the Child with Special Needs

Having a child with special needs does not eliminate any of the functions of a family. Families continue to provide a cultural and psychosocial foundation and guide their children's experiences in activities that will lead to optimal health and participation in the larger community. Understanding how families make choices in light of finite resources and their vision of a child's future puts some of the decisions families make about daily activities and what they want to work on in a different light. Sometimes, especially when a problem is recently diagnosed or when medical treatment is needed, family resources (e.g., time, money, emotional energy) may be directed primarily to the needs of the child.[106] For example, a mother who has a full-time job to help pay medical and therapy bills and spends 4 hours a day feeding her medically fragile child has limited time and emotional energy to devote to helping another child with homework or sharing in recreational activities. Over time, this allocation of resources may become more balanced or could have negative implications for family members.

Financial Resources

Having a child with special needs has implications for family economics. Parents with children who have disabilities have many hidden and ongoing expenses. When children are hospitalized, many expenses (e.g., days out of work, childcare for siblings, transportation, meals, motel rooms) are incurred, in addition to costs not covered by insurance.[117] Mothers on welfare have reported that they face multiple barriers. Although they wanted to become self-sufficient, they found that employment seemed like a distant dream as they struggled with transportation and finding childcare, particularly for older children.[94,153]

Many insurance plans have caps on the number of therapy visits allowed per year. Therefore, some parents must cut back on services or pay for sessions by finding a way to save somewhere else. Children who require extensive medical treatment can bring economic devastation to a family, especially when insurance coverage is inadequate.[117] Financial problems create added stress, and occupational therapists need to be aware of how costs associated with their own services and recommendations may affect the family and child whom they are serving. There might be times when a decision to cancel an appointment is made for financial reasons.[74]

Another challenge to financial resources occurs when a parent decides to remain unemployed so that he or she has time to provide extra caregiving. A number of studies have documented that a parent may need to work fewer hours, or not work at all, to care for the child.[49,121] With one spouse unable to take on paid employment, these households are at higher risk for problems associated with low income. Financial strain is increased in single-parent homes. Case-Smith[41] has found that mothers of children with medical conditions left employment because of the frequency of their children's illnesses. These children needed specialized medical care (e.g., nursing care) that prohibited them from attending community childcare centers. The need to stay home with a child who has multiple medical needs and frequent illnesses, coupled with lack

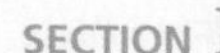

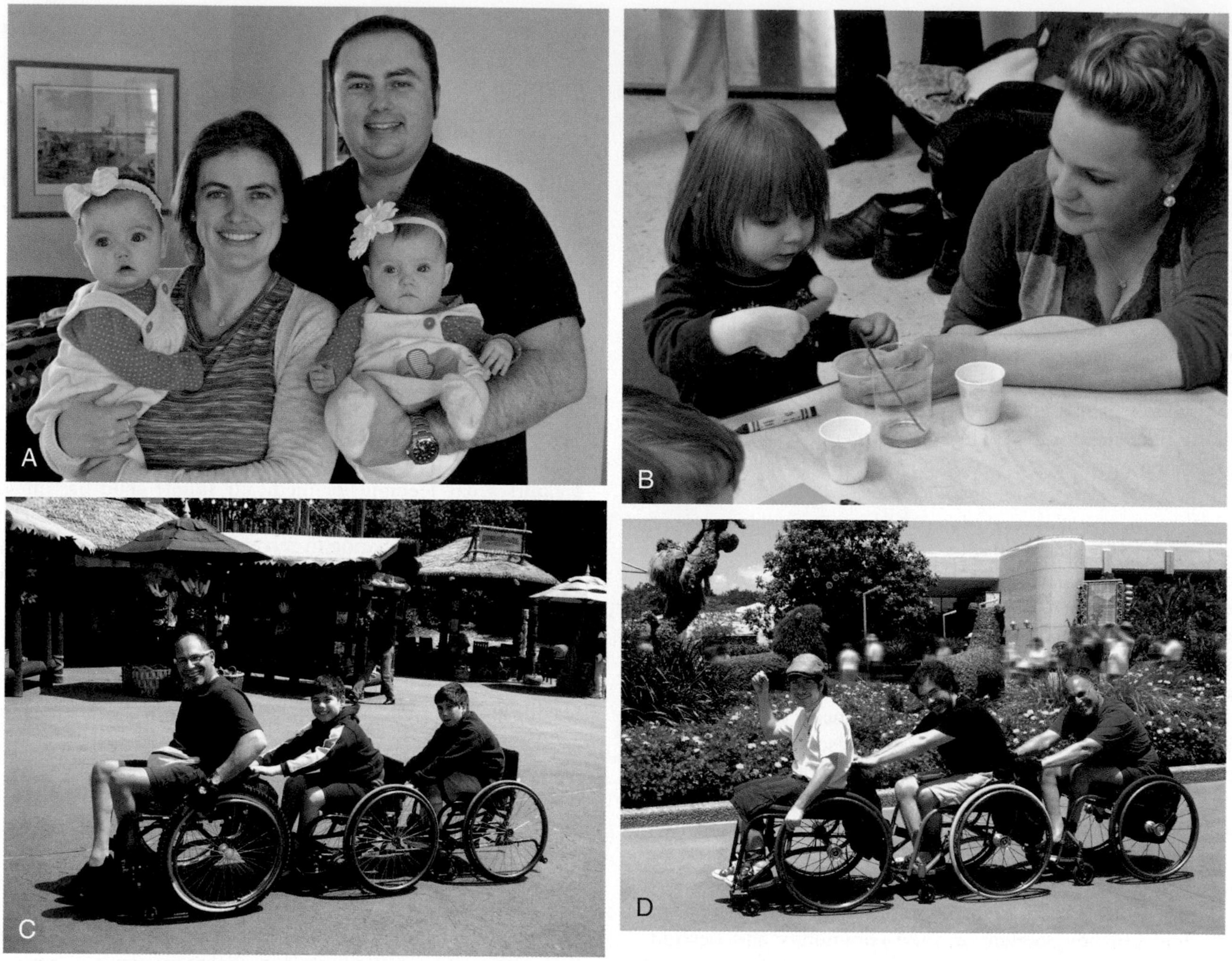

FIGURE 5-8 **Participation through the family life span. A,** Infant twins (Sadie and Madie) change the family dynamics as parents balance their new roles. **B,** School aged-children take on new roles (students) and associated responsibilities. **C,** Dad pulls his tired children through a theme park. **D,** Years later, young adult Keith helps his dad by taking his turn pulling through a theme park.

of community childcare for such a child, can become a particularly difficult situation for parents to manage. Part of the essence of family-centered care is addressing these needs in a family.[73]

Human Resources

The human resources important to a family raising children are education, practical knowledge, and problem-solving ability. Sometimes, the challenges of raising a child with disabilities are related to the sense of competence that the parent experiences.[30] An understanding of the basis of the child's problems and of possible adaptations is a powerful resource when helping families establish effective patterns of daily activities. A comprehensive parent-professional partnership should include ongoing sharing of information with parents. Initially, most parents want information about their children's conditions and about accessing services.[41] After that, they need information about potential complications and how to care for their child's physical and psychological needs on a daily basis.[69] The timing of parents' ability to use this knowledge and engage in home programs varies appreciably from the time of initial diagnosis of disability through adjustment to their situation. Qualitative studies have suggested that meeting the need for information is challenging because it is difficult to judge a family's priority needs and their readiness to assimilate information about managing their child's condition.[69,120] Occupational therapists need to keep their therapeutic listening and observation skills sharp and be flexible in their information sharing.

Families who are coping with stress have reported that "the ability to build on personal experience and expertise" (p. 261)[54] is an essential coping strategy. Parents can develop this knowledge through parent groups in which families can share strategies with other families who have had similar types of issues.[42,156] Occupational therapists, by listening to parents and individualizing the information, as well as connecting family members to other resources, help build the parents' personal resources. The CanChild Centre for Childhood Disability Research has developed a formal, individualized information package for parents, The KIT: Keeping It Together, which has been shown to increase parents' "perceptions of their ability and self-confidence in getting, giving and using information to assist their child with a disability" (p. 498).[138] Occupational therapists must remember that many parents are the experts on their own children and often have extensive information or stories to share about what works for them.[13]

Time Resources

Daily and weekly activities require time investment, and every family at some point experiences stress because there are too many things to be done and not enough time. Children with disabilities often depend on caregivers longer than typically developing children, and the extra daily care or supervision needed can extend for many years.[33,42,98,127] Much of the research on caregiving time has focused on mothers, although the distribution of caregiving between parents has changed in recent years, with a shift of some caregiving tasks to fathers.

Helitzer and colleagues[61] have found that mothers of children with disabilities reported that they used "structure, routine, and organized time management as a way to maintain a sense of control" (p. 28). However, their busy structured lives often were disrupted by crises, such as trips to the hospital or urgent care department, and, as a result, the mothers felt that they were "living on the edge" and that every disruption in their routine was experienced as a crisis. In a qualitative study of parents of children with chronic medical conditions and disabilities, parents reported that they had 24-hour responsibilities in administering medical procedures and performing caregiving tasks.[27] They described the challenges of "always being there" to care for their child's extraordinary medical needs and engage their very dependent child in developmentally appropriate activities. Children with feeding concerns also present a major challenge to managing time and tasks.[158]

Service providers need to consider the family's time and emotional resources when recommending home programs. Providers seeking to implement family-centered practice often expect parents to take on responsibility for implementing therapy.[93,96] These home assignments can become a source of guilt and marital difficulty as the family struggles to meet the demands of the provider or else be labeled as noncompliant. Less experienced occupational therapists, in their enthusiasm to help, often neglect to consider the family's time commitments when offering suggestions. Careful listening and asking about the degree of comfort that each caregiver has with aspects of intervention go a long way in building and maintaining good rapport and meeting the needs of the family. Exploring the possibilities of caregiving activities being shared between the parents, and possibly other family members, can make them more manageable and reduce the everyone's stress levels (Research Note 5-2).

RESEARCH NOTE 5-2

Fingerhut, P. E. (2013). Life Participation for Parents: A tool for family-centered occupational therapy. American Journal of Occupational Therapy, 67, *37–44.*

Abstract

Objective. This study describes the continued development of the Life Participation for Parents (LPP), an assessment to facilitate family-centered pediatric practice.

Method. A cohort of 162 parents of children with special needs receiving intervention at 15 pediatric private practice clinics completed LPP questionnaires. Instrument reliability and validity were examined.

Results. Good internal consistency and test-retest reliability were established. A construct validity was examined through an assessment of internal structure and comparison of the instrument to related variables. A principal components analysis resulted in a two-factor model accounting for 44% of the variance. As hypothesized, the LPP correlated only moderately with the Parenting Stress Index—Short Form. A child's diagnosis, age, and time in therapy did not predict parental responses.

Conclusion. The LPP is a reliable and valid instrument for measuring satisfaction with parental participation in life occupations.

Implications for Practice

The LPP can guide intervention by providing information on the caregiver's participation in life occupations.

Emotional Energy Resources

Families of children with disabilities may experience special forms of stress, social isolation, and less psychological well-being than families with typically developing children.[10,36,102] The idea that parents of children with disabilities experience recurrent grief is pervasive in the literature, but has been disputed.[43,149] Fox and colleagues[42] conducted a qualitative investigation to understand how children with developmental delays and behavioral problems influenced the family's lifestyle. The parents they studied reported that dealing with the child's 24-hour, 7-day-a week needs required emotional energy and often engendered frustration. Parents reported that individuals who offered "a shoulder to lean on" and professional assistance, encouragement, and information were particularly helpful.

There is evidence that parents of children with disabilities may experience anxiety and depression.[60,127] Mothers appear more vulnerable than fathers. Hastings,[60] investigating levels of stress, depression, and anxiety in a cohort of 18 couples with children with autism, found that mothers and fathers felt similar levels of stress; however, mothers were more anxious. It was suggested that mothers may feel more responsibility for the child and may take on a larger part of the extra care that a child with disabilities requires. Sawyer and colleagues[127] found that mothers who experienced increased time pressure to complete all their tasks had higher rates of mental health problems. When parents must administer medical support, beyond the typical parent-child activities of nurturance, caregiving, and play, they often find themselves exhausted and sleep-deprived, and appear to experience increased stress and anxiety.[62] In addition, they often do not have the time and resources to access energizing and relaxing activities, such as socializing or recreation.[10,127]

Stress level in families with children with chronic diseases or conditions has been found to have a strong relationship with family income and family function, with lower income associated with higher stress, especially as the children become adolescents.[10] Parents with limited resources, whether financial, educational, emotional, or a combination, are at higher risk of experiencing parental stress, which may lead to abusing or neglecting children with disabilities.[63,135]

Sources of Diversity in Families

Families with children who need occupational therapy services come from many different backgrounds and have a variety of forms. Occupational therapists working with these children have the rewarding opportunity to learn from these families, but must find a balance between focusing on the similarities and appreciating the differences among families. Because individuals are inclined to view the world through their own cultural model and use personal experiences as a point of reference, it takes professional commitment to become skilled at working with a variety of families.

Family researchers and service providers have focused on understanding how a family's culture and traditions affect child-rearing practices and how these might be adaptive, strengthening a family and bringing about positive developmental outcomes.[84] Families have patterns of different characteristics (e.g., family structure, family income, having a family member with a disability) and the ecology in which families' function varies (e.g., religious opportunity, crime rate in the neighborhood, period in history). Therefore, generalizations of research findings about diverse family groups may not be accurate, and sensitivity to the unique differences of each family is always needed.[32] The three sources of family diversity discussed next are the family's ethnic background, family structure, and socioeconomic status. A fourth section considers differences in parenting styles and practices.

Ethnic Background

Ethnicity is a term used to describe a common nationality or language shared by certain groups of families. It tends to be a broad concept, and heterogeneity among families within groups described as Hispanic, African American, Anglo American, or Asian is often anticipated. However, people may identify themselves as belonging to more than one ethnic group, making it harder to use this concept to guide how the occupational therapist works with families. Coll and Pachter[31] have offered two reasons for retaining ethnicity as an important variable when working with families raising children. First, families that are not part of the dominant ethnic group may experience a discontinuity between their cultural models and the majority culture, which shapes the social institutions. Thus, a cultural and language gap may exist among health systems, educational programs, and the families of minority ethnic groups.[2] In addition, as the proportion of ethnic groups grows in the United States, the sons and daughters of these groups will make up a larger proportion of the overall population of children in this country. Occupational therapists who serve children with special needs can anticipate working with an ever-growing, ethnically diverse group of families. The influence of ethnic background on how a family fulfills its functions and raises its children is a complex topic that is merely introduced here. Resources on the Evolve website provide further information.

Ethnic groups share cultural practices that can determine who has the authority to allocate family resources and a value system that sets priorities for family routines and special events. Families in an ethnic group may have similar daily activities, ways of interacting, and ways of thinking about events and may find similar meaning in their routines, traditions, and celebrations. Differences among ethnic groups are expressed in gender role expectations, child-rearing practices, and expectations at certain ages, as well as in definitions of health and views of disability. Cultural practices are not static traits but change when members of the group adapt to new situations.[58]

The recent influx of immigrants expands the diversity within ethnic groups that therapists encounter. Within a community, one family may have members who have been in a country for generations, and the family next door may have recently relocated to the country. Migration affects the family and how it functions at multiple levels.[40] Relocation to another country frequently includes a series of separations and reunions of children and family members, sometimes for 2 years or longer.[141] In some families, the tradition of having a child live with a grandparent or other relative may buffer the initial separation and help reduce the stress. When both parents emigrate ahead of their children, it is not unusual for the children subsequently brought into the country to have to adjust to living not only with their parents again, but also possibly with younger siblings born in the new country. Occupational therapists working with immigrant families need to be sensitive to the possibility of family friction, depression, and sense of uncertainty among family members.

For each immigrant family, the process of *acculturation* varies; this is the process of selectively blending their traditions of how things are done, which activities are important, and interactive styles with the cultural practices of the majority group.[40] Parenting practices might insulate children from exposure to the language, ways, and values of the majority culture until the children go to school. For example, some cultures may equate enrolling children in childcare programs with child abandonment. Those families may bring a grandparent with them as part of the immigration process to be the caregiver, so that both parents can find paid employment. These children may have had few experiences beyond their home environment before entering school. In school, surrounded by new peers, the children's acculturation process is accelerated, creating conflict among family members.[98] Unfortunately, feeling disconnected from home or discriminated against at school leads some youth, including youth with disabilities, to drop out of school as a way to ease the tension.[58]

Although every family wants its children to be successful members of the community, the family's vision of what this entails varies among different ethnic groups and influences the time use and expectations of children. Carlson and Harwood[26] observed Anglo American and Puerto Rican mothers in their daily routines and found that Puerto Rican mothers controlled their infants' behaviors more than the Anglo American mothers, who tolerated more off-task behaviors. Puerto Rican parents seemed to be guided by the anticipation that their children will join a Puerto Rican community that values respectful cooperation. The Anglo American willingness to follow the child's lead is compatible with valuing individual autonomy. Without insight into ethnic differences, an occupational therapist, observing a parent-child interaction, may mistakenly interpret a Puerto Rican mother's physical control and effort to divert a child's attention to the needs of others as intrusive and insensitive to the toddler's sense of self-efficacy. Occupational therapists avoid this type of error by understanding what a parent hopes to achieve before formulating an opinion about the appropriateness of a family's interactive routines.

Family Structure

Family features, such as the presence of children in the household, marital status, sexual orientation, and age or generation, are factors described as the *family structure*.[1] It is important to remember in working with families that acceptance of diversity within the family structure and family subsystems is necessary to be effective.

Family structure, in combination with its cultural model, influences how the family organizes itself to fulfill essential roles, such as caregiving of dependent family members or allocation of family resources. The idea that there is a best family structure in which children are raised is a myth.[8] For example, single-parent families have been portrayed as dysfunctional and as leaving children more vulnerable to having problems,[3] yet single parents, especially single fathers, have also been found to raise competent, well-adjusted children.[23] The Fragile Families and Child Wellbeing Study is an attempt to discard myths and replace them with evidence that will guide intervention and policy making to support low-resource families.[105] Some of their findings have demonstrated that "unwed parents are committed to each other and to their children at the time of birth.... Most unmarried mothers are healthy and bear healthy children" (p. 3).

Larson[88] sampled the activities and emotions of employed mothers in two-parent or single-parent homes of adolescents and found that the stereotype of the single-parent home was not necessarily the rule. Single mothers in his study had less stressed, more flexible routines after a day at work and friendlier relationships with their teenagers than their counterparts in two-parent homes. Mothers with a husband reported more hassles trying to make and serve dinner by a designated dinner time and experienced housework as more unpleasant. Larson[88] speculated that the negotiation of responsibilities and trying to live up to expectations of being a "wife" in a two-parent home contributed to these differences. Clearly, every family structure has advantages and risk factors.[11]

Many single-parent families are formed through divorce. This can cause disruption that alters household routines, traditions, and celebrations. Sometimes, the stress between marital partners leads to impaired occupational functioning of the children, and the divorce may come as a relief. Factors that contribute to positive developmental outcomes for children after couples break up include the parents' psychological well-being, economic resources, whether the family is part of a larger kinship network, and how parents navigate the separation and dissolution process. Greene, Anderson, Hetherington, Forgatch, and DeGarmo[55] reported contradictory findings regarding how well children adjust after their parents' divorce. Initially, parenting practices were erratic, and the parent-child relationship, especially between custodial mothers and young sons, could be stormy. Yet, 2 years after a divorce, many of the problems had diminished; therefore, some of the consequences of divorce depend on where in the adjustment process researchers conduct their study. The occupational therapist can be supportive by acknowledging that these parents face considerable challenges in raising children alone and by aiding the parent in identifying resources, such as friends, extended family, religious groups, and other single parents.

Gay, lesbian, and bisexual families reflect one variation of family structure that therapists encounter; parents who are not heterosexual comprise 1% to 12% of families.[136] Children may be the products of a parent's previous heterosexual relationship or may be born or adopted into families headed by adults who are gay, lesbian, or bisexual.[87,118] Studies comparing the psychological adjustment and school performance of children being raised by lesbian or gay parents with those of children with heterosexual parents have generally found no differences.[118]

When birth parents are unable or unavailable to care for children, ***kinship care*** is a way to preserve family ties that might be lost if children are placed in foster homes.[46] Households in which grandparents are raising their grandchildren are examples of those providing kinship care and are a growing source of differences between families. These families, primarily headed by middle-aged or older women, and disproportionately by women of color, are often formed after adverse events, such as child neglect or abandonment, maternal substance abuse, or incarceration or death of the parents.[46,86,123] Much of the research on grandparents raising their grandchildren has explored the issue of caregiver stress. Evidence from qualitative and quantitative studies has suggested that grandparents caring for their grandchildren (or great-grandchildren) find it rewarding and challenging.[46] Grandparents reported satisfaction in being able to "be there" for the child or children, and that they had to learn new parenting skills in response to the new generation. However, some also experienced parenting stress, which was exacerbated when they lacked social and/or financial resources or were in poor health.

During their childhood, many children experience changes in the family structure. Unwed mothers may marry, or parents in a family may divorce, and later one or both may remarry. A child may transition from a two- to three-generation family when an aging grandparent moves into the home. Therapists should talk with family members in an inclusive manner that does not suggest an assumed family structure. Asking a parent or child, "Can you tell me about your family?" does not suggest any expectations and helps family members openly express their definition of who is in their family.

Socioeconomic Status

The influence of the family's SES on children's occupations and development is complex.[66] SES reflects a composite of different factors, including the social prestige of family members, educational attainment of the parents, and family income. These factors influence each other, and have various implications for how a family fulfills its functions, by influencing the degree of access that families have to activities and experiences for their children. Parents who pursue higher or continued education may be more likely to incorporate new ideas about a healthy lifestyle and child development into their parenting practices. Factors that influence employment, such as a below-average education, inability to speak English, or disability of a family member, leave families more vulnerable as job opportunities come or go. When employment is found, the job may not pay enough to meet the family's needs, leaving the family with no resources if unexpected events occur.

Low income or limited education is associated with differences in the quality of parents' interactions with their children.[66,125] In these circumstances, parents may not be as responsive, addressing the child less often, providing fewer learning opportunities, and not engaging in an interactive teaching process. Factors associated with having children with disabilities, including the increased cost of raising such children and decreased ability of their mothers to be employed, increase the likelihood that families will live in poverty.[116] Suggestions for working with families with low SES are described later in this chapter.

Therapists need sensitivity and skill to work with families across the SES continuum. Having a higher SES clearly affords additional opportunities, time, and expectations of parents to advocate for those experiences that they desire for their children. The concept of "helicopter parents," who hover over every aspect of their child's life, also applies to parents of children with special needs. Therapists must draw on their many skills in assisting these parents to find balance between what can be done through direct service, what they can do themselves, and how to allow a child space in which to be a typical child and do for him- or herself.

Parenting Style and Practices

The individual interactive style and parenting practices of an adult raising a child are additional factors that must be considered to understand the diversity of families. Steinberg and Silk[137] have distinguished between *parenting style,* the emotional climate between parent and child, and *parenting practices,* goal-directed activities that parents do in raising their children. For example, two parents may believe that if they want their child to do well in school, it is their responsibility to spend time with the child reviewing the homework (a parenting practice). However, the interpersonal interactions while they engage in this shared activity (parenting style) can be distinctly different. One parent may discuss the work and help the child find solutions to problems, whereas the other parent may feel that she or he only has the emotional energy to point out errors. There is no test or license for parenting in this country. In the past, extended family members provided mentorship and modeling for parenting practices. In today's nuclear families, stresses run higher, and skills may be lacking.

A well-adapted child develops as a result of complex interactions between parenting style and practice. Regardless of ethnic background, socioeconomic status, or parenting practices, a parenting style that is warm, responsive, and positive, and that provides structure and learning opportunities, is associated with children who rank higher on many measures of social and cognitive development.[6,137]

The collaborative nature of the relationship between parents and occupational therapist may not be smooth if each holds different ideas about parenting style or parenting practices. This tension increases if the parents worry about the occupational therapist's disapproval.[39,93] The professional cannot assume to have more knowledge than the parent about what the child needs to be able to do or about the interactive style that best accompanies shared activities.[76] Occupational therapists can be supportive and empower parents by working with them so that family resources, such as time and emotional energy, are available when shared activities occur.

An Ecologic Perspective

As with any other open system, the social and physical features surrounding the family influence it. An ecologic and transactional perspective of development and parenting encourages occupational therapists to consider family resources and the adult's psychological background, personal history, and personality, which are in constant interaction with characteristics of the child being parented.[25,85,126] In addition, some occupations of families take place beyond the home. Many of the resources for family activities that enable families to function effectively are available in the neighborhood and larger community. Proximity to places of worship, stores, high-quality childcare, and friends is part of the family's ecology and influences how family members spend their time. It is important to take an ecologic perspective and investigate whether families can access a range of community activities that will enable them to fulfill their functions. At a slightly more removed level, family functions are supported when social institutions make services available (e.g., a health department that runs an immunization clinic, volunteer group that helps parents choose the best childcare centers, businesses that raise money for a school system). Occupational therapists who strive to enable children's occupations use a collaborative empowerment model in which families draw on their knowledge of their children's abilities and receive support from other families and professionals to make changes at the community level.[148] By joining with families in advocating for children's rights, occupational therapists contribute to a synergistic force that increases the family's access to resources outside their homes and helps them function as a family.

Supporting Participation in Family Life

Development of Independence in Self-Care and Health Maintenance Routines

Occupational therapists who understand the nature of family occupations can help parents manage and adapt daily living tasks with their children. The occupational therapist assists the parent in establishing goals about daily routines and tasks that the parent values, and then observes how they are being done. The occupational therapist may engage the parent in a discussion of alternative strategies or may model techniques that help the child perform daily living activities with greater skill and independence. With knowledge of the biomechanics of lifting and moving, the occupational therapist considers whether the task is performed in a way that conserves energy and avoids injury. This consideration is especially important when a physical impairment significantly limits mobility. Strategies to help a 5-year-old bathe, dress, and use the toilet may no longer be safe for the parent's back when the child becomes an adolescent. An occupational therapist's knowledge of adaptive solutions to self-care, such as Velcro fasteners or, if standing balance is too challenging, dressing while sitting, can be quite helpful to parents, especially first-time parents.[109] Any extra time that the therapist asks the parent to spend teaching new steps in self-care should be in response to a parent's identified need. In addition, the effort should be justified by evidence that the

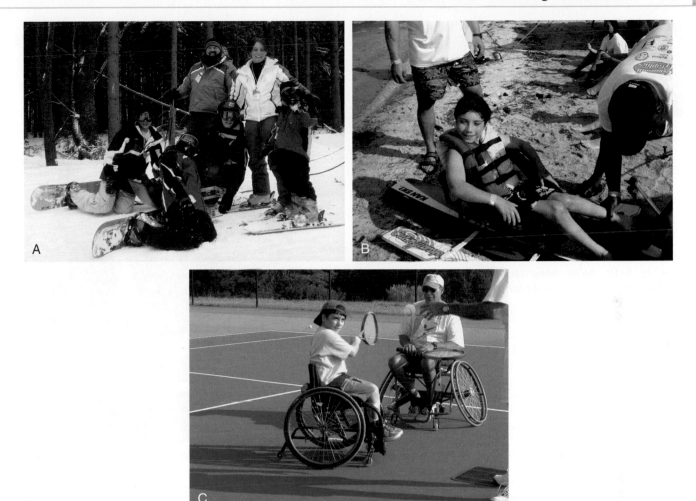

FIGURE 5-9 **A,** Recreational opportunities in the community provide an important family occupation. (Courtesy Jill and Mark McQuaid, Dublin, Ohio.) **B,** Wee Can Ski provides equipment for children with diverse abilities. **C,** Keith has a tennis lesson while Dad watches proudly.

altered routine has a good chance of bringing about an immediate change. Alternative suggestions should be made quickly when an adapted technique does not work. The goal of occupational therapy recommendations should be to benefit the entire family by increasing the child's independence at minimal cost in time and energy to the parents.[146]

Becoming independent in self-care occupations frequently requires repeated practice until performance becomes a habit. Occupational therapists can help parents reinforce a child's efforts at independence. Continuity in frequently repeated self-care occupations, such as using the toilet and eating with utensils, is increased when the occupational therapist initiates communication with teacher, parents, and others. A notebook that the child carries between school and home may serve this purpose.

Participation in Recreational and Leisure Activities

The family's ability to engage family members in recreational and leisure activities is the result of a multidimensional process that includes the community family and child with a disability[80,81] (Figure 5-9). One factor that can directly influence participation is the availability of an inclusive program, wherein peers and activity leaders support the child's ability to participate. Other factors, such as the extent to which the parents perceive acceptance from friends and neighbors and how parents view being active, indirectly shape whether families choose to participate in recreational activities in the community. Parents of children with developmental delays and behavioral problems sometimes limit taking their child into the community in response to negative reactions of other people.[21,43] Parents of children with a developmental coordination disorder may need to consider individual rather than team sports as options for their children[109] (Figure 5-10). Resources, such as money to purchase equipment and time to transport children, influence the extent to which a family can participate in recreational activities. Families that can afford vacations will find that many theme parks have become more accommodating to their needs.

Occupational therapists can communicate that they respect the value of recreation and leisure by including it in assessment and intervention plans. Occupational therapists can suggest

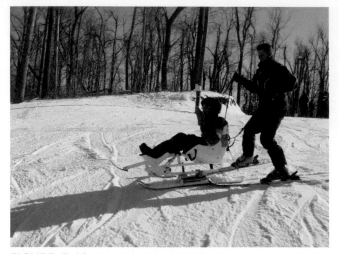

FIGURE 5-10 Most skiing facilities have equipment for children unable to stand independently.

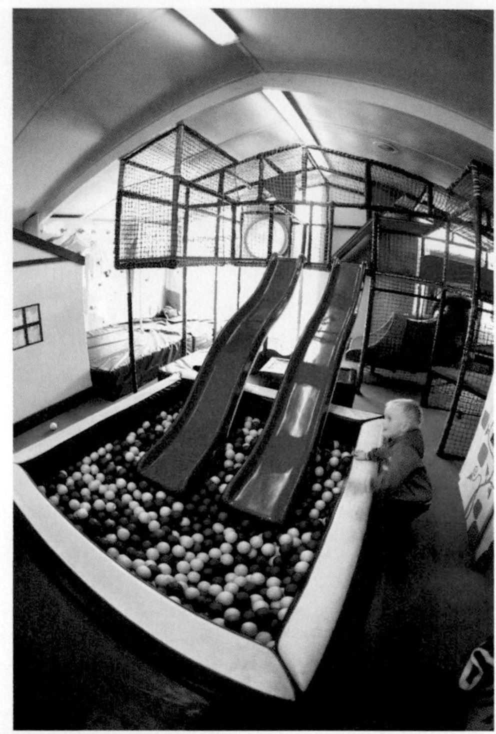

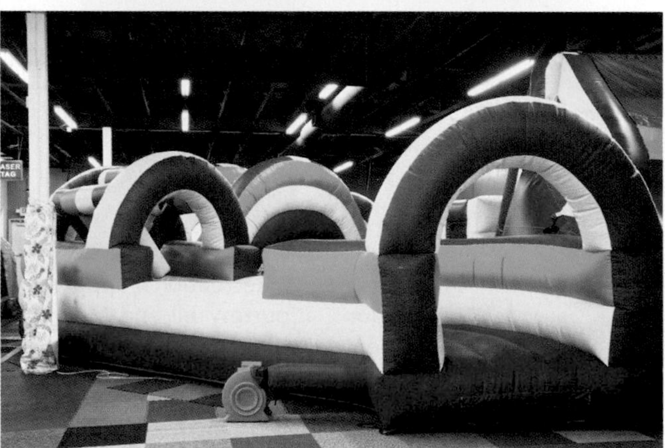

FIGURE 5-11 Activity centers with soft mats, bolsters, balls, and tunnels for tumbling offer safe and accessible environments for children with physical disabilities.

adapted equipment that the child can use to make recreational activities possible. With the passage of the Americans with Disabilities Act in 1990, more recreational opportunities became available to those with disabilities. Information about community recreational activities is often available in local newsletters or on websites. Occupational therapists can note which activities are accessible and appropriate for children with disabilities (Figure 5-11). They can also suggest strategies for making the family's outings more successful, such as providing headphones for a child with auditory sensitivity. Practitioners can also help parents accomplish caregiving tasks efficiently to make more time available for recreation. Scheduling therapy and education programs at times that allow families to engage in recreational activities can also support family function.

Socialization and Participation in Social Activities

Socialization not only is needed for health but is an important mechanism for preparing family members to enter their cultural group and participate in community activities. Most families of children with disabilities, particularly children with problem behaviors, report that far too few opportunities exist for participation in the community. Families perceive that they are the only socialization agents for their children because community social activities simply do not accommodate their children.[89] In addition, children with disabilities may interact more frequently with adults than with peers, particularly if they have classroom aides. Constant interaction with adults to the exclusion of peers may exacerbate feelings of social incompetence in interactions with peers. Educational and intervention programs should focus more attention on helping friendships develop and flourish.

A child's disability may also create barriers to the parents' opportunities to socialize. Families of children with special needs often feel that they have less time to spend participating in social activities.[33,89] Because childcare is typically difficult to arrange and must be set up in advance, taking advantage of spontaneous social opportunities is rarely possible.[7] Children who act out or demonstrate disruptive behaviors may be particularly difficult to manage in social situations.

Parents often find it helpful to develop friendships with other parents experiencing similar circumstances. A number of studies have found that increased social supports are associated with healthier family functioning and lower levels of stress.[20,150] Helitzer and colleagues[61] implemented a program for mothers of children with disabilities to address their concerns and difficulties in daily routines and coping. The mothers were encouraged to provide emotional support to one another and assist each other in resolving specific dilemmas in daily routines. They perceived that they had changed their self-image and coping strategies through participation in the group sessions. They placed great value on having "a supportive opportunity to discuss their feelings and thoughts in a setting that was nonjudgmental and comfortable" (p. 408).[150] Similar programs offer parents social supports and strategies to help in coping, as well as practical ideas that make everyday life easier, help them adapt to stress, and give them a more positive attitude toward their children.[156] These social supports appear to be of equal or greater importance to families than professional services.[24]

Fostering Readiness for Community Living

Families of children with disabilities express concerns about the future for their children, particularly once they leave school. They worry that their children will not have the life skills needed to live independently.[98] As children become adolescents and then young adults, parents need information on possible living arrangements in the community. Often, young adults are capable of leaving home but need support persons and arrangements for short- or long-term supervision and monitoring. These young adults may not have many options, and the options may be overly restrictive (to secure funding) or may not provide sufficient supervision. Parents of young adults with disabilities emphasize the need for information on housing, particularly innovative, supported, living arrangements. For these young adults to succeed in living in the community with support, families need assistance in finding roommates, other support persons, funding, and arrangements for supervision and monitoring.

Young adults with disabilities face many challenges in finding and maintaining employment; however, new models that support work performance and assisted community living have demonstrated success.[10,98,122] (See Case Study 5-1 for an example.) Families and professionals need to work together to advocate for changes in the community to create opportunities for young adults to become employed and productive members of society (see Chapters 12 and 25).

Family Adaptation, Resilience, and Accommodation

Despite the inclination of families to organize their activities into predictable patterns in the form of their routines, traditions, and celebrations, these are dynamic systems, and change is inherent in being a family. Pressures that can alter family activities include daily hassles, such as multiple demands on a parent's time or unpredictable transportation, as well as positive life transitions, such as the birth of a baby or an older son's leaving home to take a job, which alter household routines. Other events requiring that families adapt their routines and traditions may be unexpected, such as job loss, illness, or an event that affects the community (e.g., a natural disaster). When families experience new demands and stresses, they continue to function by creating meaning about the stressful event and by working as a system to adapt and continue their daily activities.

The process of ***adaptation*** starts when a family recognizes the state of affairs—an interruption in their activities or a loss of emotional well-being.[53,119] Families use a variety of strategies to make sense of what is happening.[154] They may tell stories about a similar situation or another generation that experienced a comparable event or redefine what seems like a catastrophic event by making a comparison with another family. Finding positive meaning in an adverse event is a way of changing how it is experienced. Regardless of the strategy used, by co-constructing their own definitions of events, families diminish the feeling of being out of control and, based on how they define the state of affairs, can allocate resources to manage the situation.

Families demonstrate resilience when they draw on resources to reconstruct their routines or create new ones that enable them to continue to fulfill family functions. McCubbin and colleagues[101] have identified factors that contributed to families' resilience and ability to manage when children were diagnosed with cancer. Based on their interviews of 42 parents, they found ***resiliency factors*** that made it easier for the family to construct new routines to deal with the situation. These families drew on their own resources, such as religious beliefs and emotional support of each other, and then reset their definition of how they would live or operate as a family. The parents rearranged their routines so that one parent could be with the child receiving inpatient medical treatment while the other stayed at home with the siblings. Parents reported that they also drew on resources in their community. For example, when neither parent had time to cook, members from their church brought in meals so that the family could share meals together. In a longitudinal study of families with a child with developmental delays, Bernheimer and Weisner[15] refer to these changes that maintain daily routines as ***accommodations***. They identified 10 accommodation domains (e.g., services, marital roles, social support) that varied in frequency of need over time. When the children were 3 years old, the highest frequency areas of accommodation were childcare tasks, sources of information, and support. They noted that family daily routines were strongly influenced by cultural and family values and goals.

The family members' ability to communicate with each other is important to co-construction of meaning and adaptation of daily routines. Families engage in affective and instrumental communication. In ***affective communication***, family members express their care for and support of each other. In ***instrumental communication***, members give each other role assignments, establish schedules, make decisions, and resolve conflicts. Clear, effective communication is important for establishing meaning for an event or problem and for planning resolution of the crisis. As Patterson[119] noted, "A family's belief in their inherent ability to discover solutions and new resources to manage challenges may be the cornerstone of building protective mechanisms and thereby being resilient" (p. 243).

A child with exceptional health or developmental needs creates new demands on a family system. Families with sufficient resources and flexibility respond by adapting their daily routines and special events so that they can fulfill their family functions. Occupational therapists who recognize the power of daily routines and family traditions are sensitive to the disruption of a family's pattern of activities and can assist parents in reestablishing or creating meaningful family routines. For example, the occupational therapist may suggest strategies that enable a child with a gastrostomy tube to participate in the family mealtime, such as explaining to the parents what foods the child can safely "taste" at the dinner table.

The fact that most families adjust successfully to children's disabilities should not lead occupational therapists to ignore the initial and ongoing challenges that families face. Times of coping and adaptation vary according to whether a family must adjust to an acute traumatic event leading to a disability or the family gains a gradual, unfolding understanding of the child's developmental differences. After the diagnostic period, when the child's problems are identified, the family goes about the process of living. During this period, the demands for adaptation and coping vary. The following sections describe how occupational therapists can offer support, intervention services, and education to families.

Partnering with Families

Parent-professional partnership grows from an appreciation that by working together, both the occupational therapist and parent can share important expertise and knowledge that will make a difference in the child's life. The sustained involvement and special insights that families bring were discussed earlier; this section goes into more specificity regarding the different ways occupational therapists work with families.

Family-centered services refers to a combination of beliefs and practices that define particular ways of working with families that are consumer-driven and competency-enhancing. These beliefs and practices are necessary if occupational therapists are to be successful in team development and implementation.[68,145] Definitions range from acting as service coordinators to addressing the needs of the family for financial and social resources as part of an intervention program to empowering family members as part of a team to make decisions about their child's program.[96] Three complementary models for family-centered services are family support, direct services, and family collaborative education.

Family support is designed to bolster a network of social support to enhance the family's natural strengths and family functions. DeGrace[36] has recommended being aware of how a disability affects family occupations in addition to addressing the child's issues. Social support, such as being able to talk with other parents, decreases the family members' feelings of isolation and stress.[31,102,156] Promoting a family's well-being through emotional support and practical suggestions allows families to engage in responsive interactions with their children. The occupational therapist's role in providing family support is to help the family secure needed resources and capitalize on its existing competencies and strengths.[52,56]

Direct services are provided when the occupational therapist engages a child in an activity with the goal of promoting the child's skill acquisition and minimizing the consequences of a disability. This is the traditional and, for the occupational therapist and most institutional facilities, the more reimbursable form of interaction. Family members should be present and participating in the therapeutic activity, but the occupational therapist's attention is on promoting the child's engagement in the activity. Unless handled with skill and sensitivity to the family, this type of service may fall outside family-centered practice.

Family collaborative education has a number of purposes and should be individualized to the families' interests, learning styles, and knowledge levels. In parent-mediated therapy, the caregiver is taught how to engage the child in an activity designed to achieve a parent-identified goal or outcome.[8] Interventionists then guide parents in using strategies that can be implemented within the natural flow of everyday activities.[77] Strong evidence indicates that the more parents know about development, the more responsive and supportive they are in interacting with their child and the better prepared they are to foster optimal development.[138,151]

When considering the father specifically, if he is the family's primary decision maker, it is critical that he receive complete information about the decisions that need to be made. Also, it has been reported that when teaching fathers an intervention that they then explain to their spouses, a resulting decrease in maternal stress levels was found.[14] Benefits to collaborative education are found beyond the scope of parental involvement and broaden to include grandparents and siblings.[99,144]

Sharing information with families is likely to be most effective when the child demonstrates interest in doing the activities that the team has targeted. At that point, the occupational therapist becomes a "coach" who facilitates an exchange of ideas that helps the parent discover ways of helping the child learn the activity.[57] This dialogue includes periods of observation and reflection. Coaches bring pragmatic understanding of the intervention strategy and serve as a resource.[52,77] Unlike in direct therapy, the family is the focus of the therapist's attention, and the parent or family member is the one interacting with the child (Research Note 5-3). Sharing with a family in

RESEARCH NOTE 5-3

Graham, F., Rodger, S., & Ziviani, J. (2013). Effectiveness of occupational performance coaching in improving children's and mothers' performance and mothers' self-competence. American Journal of Occupational Therapy, 67, *10–18.*

Abstract

Objective. This study examined the effectiveness of occupational performance coaching in improving children's and mothers' occupational performance and mothers' parenting self-competence.

Method. A one-group time-series design was used to evaluate changes in children's (n = 29) and mothers' (n = 8) occupational performance at four time points: (1) pre–wait list; (2) preintervention; (3) postintervention; and (4) follow-up.

Results. Significant improvements in occupational performance occurred postintervention for children and mothers that were maintained 6 weeks after intervention. Mothers' self-competence in parenting also improved.

Conclusion. These findings provide preliminary evidence supporting the effectiveness of occupational performance coaching in improving children's and mothers' occupational performance and mothers' parenting self-competence. Improvements were sustained and appeared to generalize to other areas of performance.

Implications for Practice

Family-centered care involves addressing the needs of the parents and child to foster the accomplishment of goals. Coaching caregivers may have more effect on children than direct service alone. Coaching in one area of performance may lead to generalized improvements in other areas.

this way requires a range of skills, including an understanding of development, well-grounded expertise in how to implement an intervention that has proved effective, and ability to communicate in an egalitarian way, which the family can choose to follow or not.[77,93] The therapist wants to empower the family, not engender dependence on a professional's expertise.[8,37,96]

Family education that focuses only on helping the parent minimize the child's disability and optimize developmental gains is too narrow. Furthermore, teaching must be a two-way process that will strengthen the family by recognizing the expertise of its members. Involving parents who are knowledgeable about community organizations and activities designed for children with special needs as educators in collaborative teams promotes their expertise. Parents can contribute information, resources, and strategies for caregiving for a child with special needs well beyond the professional's knowledge.[16]

Establishing a Partnership

The first interactions of the therapist with a family open the door to the establishment of a partnership. In a family-centered approach, the therapist demonstrates a family orientation that establishes trust and builds rapport through the use of open communication, mutual respect, shared decision making, and parental empowerment.[16] The therapist's initial interview reflects an interest not only in the child's behaviors but also in the family's concerns with managing those behaviors. These first interactions demonstrate that an equal partnership is desired, and encourage a give and take of information. At the same time, parents begin to understand that professionals are there to help them and can provide information and resources to support the child's development.[8,56,145]

Trust building is not easily defined; it is associated with nonverbal language, words, and mutual respect. Thinking the best of families is important to the development of this partnership. This may not always be easy, particularly when the family's lifestyle contradicts that of the professional. Being positive and maintaining a nonjudgmental position with a family can be challenging, but it is essential to establishing and building a trusting relationship. Parent participants in focus groups have defined respect as simple courtesies from professionals, such as being on time to meetings.[18] The professionals who were interviewed linked respect to being nonjudgmental and accepting of families. When professionals are disrespectful to families, parents may become reluctant to access services or may lose their sense of empowerment. Demonstrating respect for families becomes particularly important when they are of different racial, ethnic, cultural, and SES. Families from different cultures often have different perspectives on child rearing, health care, and disabilities. Table 5-1 lists cultural characteristics, examples, and possible consequences for intervention programs.

Qualitative studies have revealed snapshots of actual family experiences with service providers. Blue-Banning and colleagues[18] found that families emphasized that partnerships were built on equality and reciprocity. A sense of equality was created when professionals acknowledged the validity of the parents' points of view, and partnerships flourished when there were opportunities for each member to contribute. In contrast, Lea[92] found that teenage mothers perceived a lack of partnering on the part of the early intervention service providers and thought that their concerns were ignored. Professionals must reflect on their practices and determine whether they are truly valuing the families they are working with, and whether their expectations for intervention are aligned with the family's values and goals.[96]

Providing Helpful Information

Child-related information that may be of benefit to parents includes information about the child's development, disability, health, and assessment results.[90] To provide up-to-date information, occupational therapists must continually engage in reading and other professional development activities. Naturally, families want the most accurate and complete information, which places a responsibility on professionals to obtain current information and continually update their skills. The families in one qualitative study "admired providers who were willing to learn and keep up to date with the technology of their field. . . . [A] competent professional is someone who is not afraid to admit when he or she does not know something, but is willing to find out" (p. 178).[18]

Although parents express that they want information about their child and diagnosis, it must be given in a supportive manner. Describe what the child has accomplished using a criterion-referenced instrument, such as the Pediatric Evaluation of Disability Inventory, to help parents remain positive and encouraged. Use an occupation-centered approach by asking which self-care activities the child is attempting or which play skills are emerging. Articulate a therapeutic goal linked to an emerging skill that the parents have identified to reduce the use of professional jargon and help parents understand how the intervention plan relates to their child. Typically, parents hope to receive recommendations for activities that help the child play, toys that match the child's abilities, and strategies that lead to independence in self-care. They also look to the occupational therapist for help in managing motor impairments or differences in sensory processing that limit occupational performance.

Providing Flexible, Accessible, and Responsive Services

Because each family is different and has individualized needs, services must be flexible and adaptable. The occupational therapist should continually adapt the intervention activities as the family's interests and priorities change. Families value the commitment of professionals to their work and believe that it is important for professionals to view them as "more than a case."[18,57,103] Parents expressed appreciation when professionals exhibited "above and beyond" commitment by meeting with them outside the workday, remembering their child's birthday, or bringing them materials to use. See Box 5-5 for suggestions from parents.

Although occupational therapists are often flexible and responsive to the child's immediate needs and parent's concerns, the range of possible services is sometimes limited by the structure of the system. When a parent desires additional services, a change in location (e.g., home-based versus center-based care), or services to be provided at a different time, the occupational therapist may or may not be able to accommodate

TABLE 5-1 Cultural Considerations in Intervention Services

Cultural Considerations	Examples	May Determine:
Meaning of the disability	Disability in a family may be viewed as shameful and disgraceful or as a positive contribution to the family.	Level of acceptance of the disability and the need for services
Attitudes about professionals	Professionals may be viewed as persons of authority or as equals.	Level of family members' participation; may be only minimal if the partnership is based only on respect or fear
Attitudes about children	Children may be highly valued.	Willingness of the family to make many sacrifices on behalf of the child
Attitudes about seeking and receiving help	Problems in the family may be viewed as strictly a family affair or may be shared easily with others.	Level of denial; may work against acknowledging and talking about the problem
Family roles	Roles may be gender-specific and traditional or flexible. Age and gender hierarchies of authority may exist.	Family preference; may exist for the family member who takes the leadership role in the family-professional partnership
Family interactions	Boundaries between family subsystems may be strong and inflexible or relaxed and fluid.	Level of problem sharing or solving in families; family members may keep to themselves, deal with problems in isolation, or problem-solve as a unit
Time orientation	Family may be present or future-oriented.	Family's willingness to consider future goals and future planning
Role of the extended family	Extended family members may be close or distant, physically and emotionally.	Who is involved in the family-professional partnership
Support networks	Family may rely solely on nuclear family members, on extended family members, or on unrelated persons (e.g., godparents).	Who can be called on in time of need
Attitude toward achievement	Family may have a relaxed attitude or high expectations for achievement.	Goals and expectations of the family for the member with the disability
Religion	Religion and the religious community may be strong or neutral factors in some aspects of family life.	Family's values, beliefs, and traditions as sources of comfort
Language	Family may be non–English-speaking, bilingual, or English-speaking.	Need for translators
Number of generations removed from country of origin	Family may have just emigrated or may be several generations removed from the country of origin.	Strength and importance of cultural ties
Reasons for leaving country of origin	Family may be immigrants from countries at war.	Family's readiness for involvement with external world

From Turnbull, A. P., & Turnbull, H. R. (1990). *Families, professions and exceptionality: A special partnership* (pp. 156–157). Columbus, OH: Merrill.

BOX 5-5 Suggestions for Therapists from Parents on Providing Flexible and Responsive Services

1. Listen with empathy to understand family concerns and needs.
2. Verbally acknowledge family priorities.
3. Make adaptations to services based on parent input.
4. Explain the constraints of the system when the parents' requests cannot be met.
5. Suggest alternative resources to parents when their requests cannot be met within the system.
6. Discuss parents' suggestions and requests with administrators to increase the possibilities that policies and agency structure can change to benefit families.

From Turnbull, A. P., & Turnbull, H. R. (1990). *Families, professions and exceptionality: A special partnership* (pp. 156–157). Columbus, OH: Merrill.

the request because of his or her schedule. Often, the agency or school system enforces policies regarding the occupational therapist's caseloads and scope of services. Practitioners are caught in the middle—between the system's structure and individualized family needs. A ready solution does not always exist for the occupational therapist who is constrained by time limitations, demands of a large caseload, or institutional policies.

Much of the time, the occupational therapist recognizes that he or she cannot change the structure of the system and must work as efficiently as possible within it. At the same time, the occupational therapist should inform the family of the program's rules and policies so that family members are aware of the constraints of the system. The occupational therapist can also take the initiative to work toward changing the system to allow more flexibility in meeting family needs. It is necessary for occupational therapists to have a voice in policy issues.

Respecting Family Roles in Decision Making

Parents who share in decision making regarding intervention for their child are more satisfied with services.[50,107] Although professionals readily tend to acknowledge the role of parents as decision makers, they do not always give parents choices or explain options in ways that enable parents to make good decisions. Too often, plans that should be family-centered are written in professional jargon and do not always address family concerns.[39] Parents are involved in decision making about their child in the following ways:

1. Parents can defer to the therapist in decision making. Deferring to the therapist may reflect confidence in the therapist's judgment and may be an easy way for parents to make a decision about an issue that they do not completely understand.
2. Parents have veto power. It is important that parents know that they have the power to veto any decision made or goal chosen by the team. Awareness of the legitimacy of this role gives parents assurance that they have an important voice on the team and can make changes, should they desire them.
3. Parents share in decision making. As described earlier, when parent-professional partnerships have been established, the parents fully participate in team discussions that lead to decisions about the intervention plan. Service options and alternatives are made clear, and parents have the information needed to make final decisions. Requests of parents are honored (within the limitations of the program).

Families cannot always be given a wide range of choices about who will provide services and when and where these services will be provided. However, their role in decision making should still be emphasized; otherwise, family-centered practice is not being implemented.[15,39,93,96] Families who are empowered to make decisions early in the intervention process will be better prepared for that role throughout the course of the child's development. In most cases, assessment of choices and good decision-making are skills that parents promote in their children as they approach adulthood.

Communication Strategies

Effective communication is built on trust and respect; it requires honesty and sensitivity to what the parent needs to know at the moment. Therapists have tremendous amounts of information to impart to parents. Effective helping is most likely to occur when the information given is requested or sought by the parent.

Occupational therapists communicate with parents using a variety of methods formal and informal, written, verbal, and nonverbal. Table 5-2 describes communication strategies consistent with the principles described earlier. These strategies are based primarily on feedback from parents regarding what they have found to be effective help from occupational therapists.[57,64]

Home Programs: Blending Therapy into Routines

Throughout this text, recommendations are given for ways to integrate therapeutic strategies into the daily occupations of children, with the clear recognition that learning occurs best in the child's natural environment. Skills demonstrated in therapy translate into meaningful functional change only when the child can generalize the skill to other settings and demonstrate the skill in his or her daily routine. Occupational therapists often recommend home activities for parents to implement with their child, so that he or she can apply new skills at home. However, before making recommendations, the occupational therapist should ask the parents about daily routines and the typical flow of family activities during the week. Home programs are most effective when the child responds well to the procedures and the demands on the parent are reasonable.[113,130,143] Understanding which routines and traditions hold special meaning for the family will help occupational therapists focus.[95] The result of this close examination of the typical week enables the occupational therapist and parents to embed goals and activities in interactive routines, in which the therapeutic process does not diminish the value and pleasure.

Working with Families Facing Multiple Challenges

Challenges to a family's ability to fulfill its functions (e.g., living in poverty, acute onset of a disability in the parent) increase the vulnerability of children with special needs and add unique challenges to family functions. Parents with their own chronic illnesses may require extra physical or emotional support.[115] By identifying protective factors that bolster the child's resilience, the occupational therapist can approach issues from a positive perspective to support strengths, capitalize on family assets, and work to make maximum use of community resources.

The occupational therapist grounded in family systems' perspective and committed to empowering families works effectively with a whole-family system, regardless of the type of disability of one or more family members. Understanding and valuing how the family system orchestrates members' occupations to fulfill family function allows the occupational therapist to take a holistic view of the family's needs and priorities. Although parents advocate a positive view, it is important to recognize when an unusual parental behavior reflects family dysfunction (e.g., child abuse, child neglect). When family dysfunction is pervasive, most occupational therapists need input from colleagues with expertise in counseling and family systems. Services for the child with special needs continue, but the occupational therapist considers ecologic and family systems factors in collaborating with the team to set priorities and provide services.

Families in Chronic Poverty

Chronic poverty has a pervasive effect on family and child experiences. Poverty has any number of causes. Most families receiving public assistance are children and mothers with poor educational backgrounds, an inconsistent work history, and

TABLE 5-2 Communication Methods between Parents and Professionals

Type of Communication Method	Purpose	Role of Professional
Formal team meeting with the family to develop an IFSP or IEP	To increase the parents' participation and comfort level	Provide parents with specific information about the purpose, structure, and logistics of the meeting. Information about parental rights must be explained to parents before and during the meeting. Decipher legal terms so that parents have practical knowledge regarding IDEA safeguards. Before meeting, parents should be informed of the questions that the team members may ask (e.g., "What are your visions for your child?") so that they can formulate thoughtful responses. Parents should receive assessment results before the meeting so they have an opportunity to think about the assessment and be prepared to discuss their goals for the child in the team meeting. A telephone call before the meeting also gives the therapist an opportunity to ask about the parents' concerns and prepare options for meeting those concerns in the child's educational program or intervention plan. Encourage parents to ask questions, express opinions, or take notes. Use jargon-free language, avoiding technical terms. Plans should be specific and should include dates, tasks, and the names of those who are responsible for the plans.
Informal meetings during or after the child's therapy		The therapist needs to be organized and prepared for parent encounters. Casual or general responses are not adequate. The therapist should give specific examples of recent performance or state when reevaluation will occur and how those results will be reported. Listen to and acknowledge the parent's concerns. Indicate preference to respond after reviewing daily notes and charts on the child. The therapist can later make a telephone call to the parent with the child's chart in hand to avoid giving the parent erroneous or misleading information.
Written and electronic communication	If parents are not physically present, regular communication with family members relies on written strategies or phone calls.	*Notebooks* shared between therapists and parents are a highly valued way to have a regular reliable method for expressing concerns. Team members may describe a new skill that the child demonstrated that day, an action by the child that delighted the class, an upcoming school event, materials requested from the parent, snack information, or the current strategy for working on self-feeding. The parents can share their perceptions of the child's feelings, new accomplishments at home, new concerns, or reminders of appointments that will keep a child out of school. Home-based therapists may initiate a notebook for the parent to record significant child behaviors and for the therapist to make weekly suggestions for activities. In the neonatal intensive care unit, notebooks are sometimes kept at the infant's bedside to provide a method for parents and therapists to communicate with the nursing staff on successful strategies for feeding and handling the infant. *Handouts* should be individualized and applicable to the family's daily routine. Handouts copied from books and manuals are appropriate if they are individualized. Many parents prefer pictures and diagrams. Other parents have remarked that triplicate forms that could be shared among the therapist, parent, and preschool were very useful.[57] Parents' perceptions of their ability, confidence, and satisfaction significantly improved after using the Keeping It Together information organizer (see earlier).[138] Photographs are also helpful to serve as a reminder to parents and staff on ways to improve postural alignment.
E-mail and other methods of communication		E-mail has become an easy, end-of-the-day method for noting any particular daily occurrences that would be of interest to the parents. A blog or even a wiki may be a viable method for regular communication with technology-proficient partners. Regular progress reports are important to parents and are required in most school systems. A simple report covering a few areas of performance may be more meaningful to the parents than a lengthy, complicated report. A child's quotes and reports of specific performance send the message that the child is receiving individualized attention. Camcorders with software for sharing have become less expensive and the videos could be uploaded to the Internet or recorded to videocassettes or DVDs. Videos can convey information about handling, feeding, and positioning methods. Keep in mind that parents must invest time in watching the tape; short clips of direct relevance to current goals are most efficient. Written materials (and videotapes and DVDs) are helpful because parents were "not always ready to hear, understand, or accept some information, but . . . it could be available for later use" (p. 91).[142]

low-wage jobs. The process of "qualifying" for services can be frustrating, depersonalizing, and degrading. Once a family qualifies for help, resources are not always enough to make ends meet. Sometimes, the family needs to forgo health care because of the pressure of other bills to pay.[74] Single parents are particularly vulnerable[105]; without family members to help, these mothers lack control over the events in their lives. Unexpected events, such as a car breaking down or special meetings at school about a child, can cause the parent to miss hours at a job and increase financial strain. Poverty represents a multidimensional issue, and occupational therapists cannot make assumptions about why a family lives in poverty.

Recognizing that poverty creates a unique cultural worldview enables occupational therapists to consider what it means to provide family-centered services.[74,92] For example, time may be perceived in the here and now, making it harder to schedule or keep appointments. Families with low SES may have difficulty following through with their plans. Therefore, planning for the future has little meaning, and participating in the setting of annual goals at IFSP or IEP meetings may not be considered important.

It is necessary to look beyond simple associations between poverty and parenting because some parents do better than others, despite a low SES.[147] Some parents living in poverty adapt and raise children successfully. Single parents who have strict disciplinary standards may seem harsh; however, their parenting practices may be grounded in an anticipation that their children will grow into a world in which obedience to those in authority is important for keeping a job. Other parents who restrict their children's community activities may be effective in monitoring who they are with, minimizing the negative influences of poor neighborhoods. When a therapist is sensitive to and deeply understands a family, she or he can make recommendations that help the child with special needs while supporting the family in its precarious position.

Parents with Special Needs

Parents themselves may have special needs that require an emphasis on supportive services. Parents who face physical or sensory challenges may need help in solving problems, such as monitoring the activity of an active child or being alerted to the cry of an infant. Occupational therapists, from their extensive knowledge of activity analysis, can assist the parent in the modification of tasks. For example, adapting the location of routines, such as diaper changing and infant bathing, can enable parents with physical limitations to participate in caregiving and simple routines that build affection between the parent and child. Occupational therapists can explore the use of adaptive equipment, such as motion detectors or sound-activated alarm systems, to compensate for the parents' sensory deficits and ensure responsiveness to their child's cues. Most parents who have had long-term experiences with a physical limitation independently develop creative solutions for providing care for their children, and they only occasionally seek an occupational therapist's assistance for determining how to perform specific caregiving tasks.

Parents who struggle with drug addiction or mental health conditions may worry whether they are up to caregiving responsibilities.[104] They often require counseling, mental health services, and opportunities to participate in support groups.[114] When parents have special needs that strongly influence their caregiving abilities, their needs often become the first emphasis of intervention. Professionals helping parents with intellectual or mental health impairments may need to address self-esteem and confidence issues, as well as build problem-solving skills. Everyday care for children requires constant problem solving. Therapists can help empower parents to make their own decisions, thereby increasing their sense of self-control. Often, professionals give advice or recommendations without encouraging the parents to solve the problem independently or try their own actions first. When others direct parents, they become more dependent. However, when parents successfully solve a problem, they become empowered to act independently in daily decision making. Problem solving can be taught and modeled.

Parents with intellectual disabilities, mental health issues, or drug addiction are at risk for having children with developmental disabilities. Professionals have questioned the competency of parents with intellectual delays, and courts have removed their children in disproportionate numbers.[19] However, with support systems in place, these parents can be surprisingly successful. Parents at risk because of intellectual or mental health impairments appear to be most successful in caring for young children when they are married, have few children, have adequate financial support, and have multiple sources of support, attributes similar to those needed by most parents.[78,89,102]

When occupational therapists work with parents with intellectual or mental health impairments, it becomes essential to know the parents' learning styles and abilities. Often, instructions need to be repeated and reinforced. Occupational therapists must use good judgment about which techniques are taught to these parents, with an emphasis on safe and simple methods. The occupational therapist should also recognize the need for additional support to help parents with intellectual delays access those needed services. Regular visits in the home by aides, nurses, or teaching assistants can meet the level of support needed. If the occupational therapist communicates his or her goals and strategies to the visiting aide, therapy activities are more likely to be implemented by the parents and other professionals working with the family.

Working with parents with intellectual or mental health impairments can be frustrating when appointments are missed or requests are not followed. Therefore, an understanding of the parents' needs is essential. The development of simple repetitive routines and systems that the parents can learn and follow enables them to become competent caregivers. With support, they can offer a child a positive and loving environment that fosters health and development.

Professionals use a variety of strategies when providing services to families with multiple challenges. When families have continual stress and problems, it is important for therapists to begin to build trust slowly, share observations and concerns, and accept parents' choices.[22] Professionals can attempt to establish rapport by using concrete, simple terms, by providing graphic and oral information, and by providing ideas that would immediately help the child. Focusing on the child's strengths and developing trust and responsiveness are also important when parents are coping with their own challenges.

Text continued on p. 157

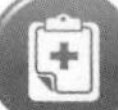

CASE STUDY 5-1 A Parent's Perspective

Beth Ball

When I was first asked to contribute to this chapter, I reflected on the myriad experiences and feelings that have emerged as a result of having children with disabilities. This seemed too vast a topic to be captured in a few typed pages. The following is a brief glimpse into my thoughts and feelings about life with my three children. There is much more than facts or history about our lives. There is, of course, emotion—deep and undeniable—and there is poetry. There is the first shed tear of realization that my child will have a life that is more difficult than most. There is the happy smile of childhood shared with supportive therapists and teachers. There is the frustrated panic of adolescence when social situations are hard and troublesome and the phone does not ring on Saturday night.

Initial Response

Learning about the disabilities of each of my children came at different times in their lives. The impact varied because of the timing of the news and disability of each child. Benjamin was born on a warm June day in 1971. On the delivery table, the nurse turned the mirror away, and I didn't understand why I couldn't see the baby. Everything seemed to happen in slow motion. The physician held him up and announced that he was a boy, but there was a small problem. His right arm tapered from the elbow to a thumblike digit for a right hand, and his left arm ended in a modified claw hand, having a center cleft halfway into his palm and syndactyly webbing between the other fingers.

The nurse placed him on my tummy, and he peed a fountain all over the sterile drapes. She said, "That works," which was comforting, but scary, because I considered that other anomalies could exist. It was not until that night in the privacy of my room that I felt the bifid femur of his right leg; the block at his knee that refused to let it extend; the very thin lower leg, which turned out to be missing the tibia; and the clubfoot. I discovered these problems one at a time. The sick feeling in my stomach was guilt. There must have been something that I had done wrong that had caused this. Even though I had followed all the doctor's instructions, I must have missed something. What would everyone think? I thought or rather felt that I must not be good enough to have a child.

Mick, my husband, and I were lucky to have a wonderful pediatrician whose first advice was exactly what we needed to hear. He told us not to withdraw from our family and friends (alluding to the feelings of shame and guilt that we had not overtly expressed). He told us to allow them to give us support—they would only want to help. The unspoken message that they would not judge us was very important to us.

And so we started on our journey of new experiences with orthopedic surgeons, prosthetists, genetic counselors, neurologists, urologists, internists, and pediatricians. Later came more professionals, occupational therapists, physical therapists, ENT specialists, vision therapists, special education teachers, and psychologists. We searched for answers to "Why?" We searched for options to deal with the issues of discrepancies in leg length and hand function. We searched for resolution to our own feelings. But we were fortunate because, as husband and wife, we never blamed each other.

Mick and I started the journey together, and we have always turned to each other for support. Sometimes it was an "us against the world" attitude and a fierce, protective response that got us through the hard times. When joyous times came, they did so with the realization that it had taken all our efforts to get there. The reason that we have been able to deal with the problems and come out on top is that we have a commitment to each other and a deep faith in God. This statement is much too simplistic for the deep feelings of need, grace, and oneness that we have. This oneness has allowed us to go forward to meet challenges as they have come.

Another reason we have been able to go forward is that we see each of our children as a gift. They are grace without gracefulness. They are charm without all the social skills. They are fun with a sometimes struggling sense of humor. They are individuals who have enriched our lives and given us humility, wonder, and awe at their commitment to living, loving, and succeeding.

Accessing Services and Resources

Gaining services and resources for our children has not come without pain, questioning, depression, and anger. It has been a struggle that has required persistence and patience. We faced the first barrier when we attempted to find the money to cover the costs of prosthetics for our son. When we were told that it would be better to amputate Benjy's leg above the knee than to try to keep it and work through the lack of joints and musculature, we were also told about the costs of prosthetics. One of the first things our orthopedic surgeon told us was that we needed to find a source of funding beyond our insurance, because prosthetics would cost more than a small house by the time Benjy was 16. I will not go into all the details, but parents have to be persistent if they do not know where to turn to find funds. The doctors have a few ideas, but they are not the best source of information in this area. Agencies and hospitals may have more information, but getting connected to the right person to gain the information is not an easy task. Even now with SSI and waivers and additional funding available, funding for disabilities comes with reams of paperwork, confusion about agency services and a maze of providers, each with a different set of rules and information.

In the search for money to cover the costs of prosthetics, we approached a well-known agency that worked with individuals who had physical disabilities. This agency had fundraising campaigns that were earmarked for this purpose. After being told that providing prosthetics was not among its services, and because this was the third or fourth rejection that we had encountered, Mick broke down and joined me in some tears. We were then informed by the agency director that we had better pull ourselves together. This was *our* child and *our* responsibility, and we had better "face it." Shame turned to anger as we left. I felt judged, and included in the

CASE STUDY 5-1 A Parent's Perspective—cont'd

anger was the fear that we would not be able to provide for Benjy. How could this man judge us? Why didn't this administrator of an agency that provides services to children with disabilities and parents have more empathy for our situation? If he didn't help, then to whom could we turn?

This experience made us even more leery of asking for assistance. Luckily, the Shriners accepted our application, and they provided most of the funds for Benjy's prosthetics until he turned 18. I do not want to think of what might have happened if we had not had their help. Dealing with financial issues created a new level of trauma that was added to our earlier pain. Because the Shriners helped with the finances for the prosthetics, we could focus our energy on education plans and homework and hope.

One of the things we discovered from this process was the necessary and valuable aspect of networking. It was through work, friends, and family that we made contact with the Shriners. It was through people at school that we were put in touch with the local Special Education Regional Resource Center and became a part of the Parent Advisory Council. It was through many of the parents that we met in these places that we learned about the Ohio Coalition for the Education of Children with Disabilities. It has always been invaluable to us to be able to share with other parents who have similar feelings, frustrations, and breakthroughs. If it had not been for these people and these agencies, we would not have received the valuable personal, educational, and emotional support that we needed. Parents are invaluable sources of information.

Whose Distress, Whose Struggle?

When my children were small, the feelings about their disabilities could be set aside for the new dream of having the brightest, cutest, most wonderful child with special needs. I dreamed of the well-spoken poster child. These dreams might have also been called denial and led others to believe that I was unaware of the true impact of my children's problems. In truth, that may have been, but I chose to live with faith and hope.

Most feelings do not come from the big picture of the disability. They come from all the little incidents. For example, when Benjy was 12 or 13 months old, I took him out of a nice, warm tub of sudsy water and stood his chubby, slippery little nude body next to the tub so that he could hold on while I toweled him dry. He stood straight and tall on his left leg, but as I watched, he tried to bear weight on his useless, dangling right leg. He bent his left leg so that his right toes touched the floor, and then he leaned to see why he could not reach the floor with his right foot. It was a moment of revelation for me. Until that moment, I think that all the focus had been on me: my inadequacy, my problem, my pain. This was a breathless revelation; it was too deep even for tears. We had been struggling with the decision of whether or not to move forward with the amputation of the malformed leg so he could be fitted with a functional prosthetic leg. We had chosen to avoid the decision; to buy time; hoping that a better solution—something less painful for us—would appear. Yet this was Benjy's life, *his* surgeries, *his* pain, and *his* inability to run swiftly through life. Seeing him search for the leg intended to support him changed my perspective. My role was and is to help and support him. Of course, every now and then, I have my own private pity party. However, it is not my pain that is the issue; it is each child's. Somehow, there is a deeper pain in watching someone I love struggle than the pain I feel when struggling myself.

In our minds, Jessica, our second child, had no disabilities through her first 5 years of life. My dream was of a baby ballerina with grace and coordination. She did have four eye surgeries by age 5 (because of crossed eyes, muscle imbalance, and rotary nystagmus). She attended a church-related preschool. At parent conference times, when the teacher would indicate problems or ask pointed questions about behaviors at home, I would justify Jessica's performance by telling myself, or Mick, that every surgery sets a child back about 3 months. She would "catch up."

When Jessica was old enough to go to kindergarten, we were called into a special conference in which we were carefully told that she was not ready to do so. I did not hear anything else that conference that day. The impact of that statement and the carefully worded explanation was like an icy shower. It was almost as if I had awakened from a dream with a clear vision of how disabled and delayed my daughter really was. I felt guilty and ashamed. I am an occupational therapist, and I know developmental milestones. I had let my doctor and others calm my fears about delays in walking, ataxia, and fine motor challenges because I did not want to believe that this second child of mine could have more than visual impairments. I was in denial for 5 years, helped by well-meaning people who did not want to hurt me.

The night after Jessica's conference, I received an answer to my prayer of "Where do I go from here?" I attended a presentation by Ken Moses, a psychologist and counselor who writes and speaks about parenting children with disabilities. I then experienced a new step on my journey. He spoke about the grief cycle and how we are grieving not for a lost child but for a lost dream. His discussion supported what I had been feeling and experiencing. The most important factor to me was the permission he gave me to feel the way I did. He emphasized how important denial is in helping us to deal with life-affecting decisions. He pointed out that denial buys us the time to gather our resources so that we can deal head on with problems.

Ken Moses also spoke about the importance of recognizing that anger gives us the energy to take action. Many times, my children's disabilities required so many appointments, surgeries, exercises, prescriptions, Individualized Education Program (IEP) meetings, and other details that I was left with only enough energy to put one foot in front of the other. I ignored, or put on hold, things or decisions that I should have taken care of immediately. Often, it was anger that got me energized and sparked my determination to get things done. I learned that anger can actually help as long as it is not turned inward or unleashed on others. I came away from this talk with a sense of relief. To have these feelings was normal, and I was not a bad person, mom, or therapist.

Some professionals and parents believe that the word *denial* should not be used to describe parents' reactions to their children's disabilities. Instead they assert that parents'

Continued

CASE STUDY 5-1 A Parent's Perspective—cont'd

reactions are *hope*. *Denial* has been a word that has allowed professionals to make judgments about parental actions. They have used the word *denial* when parents are not following through on something recommended or are having difficulty accepting decisions about education or diagnoses. Having been on both sides of the table, I understand the issues. I have what I think is a realistic view that the word *denial* is not going to go away. Also, the anticipation and hope for each of my children's futures cannot be erased by a word called *denial.* My hopes are real and if I choose to live with them, I don't mind if someone calls them *denial.* I embrace my whole journey and all aspects of my children. I can wallow with the best of them, dig in my heels, and go in the direction that I believe is right—no matter whether someone thinks I am denying reality. I believe that parents "in denial" need to hold onto their hope and/or don't yet have the resources they need to deal with their child's disability. So, dear OTs, give them some!

I have also recently come to believe that parent's reactions come from fear as well as hope. I have been afraid that I would not do the "right" things for my children. I wanted so much to allow them to be and do their best. I wanted for them to have the "right" experiences. I wanted them to experience the "right" education. I wanted them to be in the "right" situations. I wanted them to see the "right" doctors.

Mick says that he believes, regardless of the words, parents' behaviors and attitudes are justified: "If the judgment word is denial, parents are just buying time to accumulate resources. If the word is hope, they are focusing on being buoyed up out of some of the harsh realities. Empowerment of parents in impossible situations is a noble mission. As parents, we want to be powerful advocates and capable guardians. To do that, we need to be emotionally healthy and grounded in reality. We arrive at that point by working though the emotions associated with our disillusionment, our fear, our anger, to ultimately be at peace *each* time we encounter another in the endless series of emotion-filled transitions of life."

Where Do We Go From Here?

Decisions are forced on parents. There are medical decisions, therapy decisions, educational decisions, second opinion decisions, and decisions made in the middle of the night and in the emergency room. Decision making starts immediately with a diagnosis or with the search for a diagnosis. Which doctor should we use? Which hospital? What about insurance? How much intervention do we need? How much do we want? What will *they* think if we say no to this thing that they think is important for our family? Is it important?

When Jessica was in elementary school, we would wait for the bus together. Each morning while sitting on our staircase landing, Jessica and I spent 20 minutes practicing eye exercises. Some days it was easy; other days Jessica would complain, resist, and attempt to divert my attention from the task. One day, when she was 7 or 8 years old, we were doing her exercises and discussing her braces, her eye surgery, and her occupational therapy session scheduled for that afternoon. She wanted to know for the thousandth time why we had to do these things. I explained that we were trying to fix things so she would have an easier time of it. She suddenly looked up at me and asked, "Is there anything about me that you don't have to fix?" I quickly named all of her gifts and attributes that I treasured. Later, as Jessica's bus turned the corner, I was left sitting on the steps with emptiness and guilt. I also had a new insight into the impact on her confidence from countless therapy sessions, surgeries, and home programs.

This incident also made me face another aspect of parenting. There is an unavoidable fact that there are some aspects of disabilities that cannot be fixed. I became an occupational therapist so that I could help people and make things better for them. I truly believed (and believe) that I could help eliminate some problems, that I could help heal hurts, and that I could provide training so that people could be more independent. Once I saw Jessica's problems, I was off and running. I wanted to make up for lost time. Fear drove me to leave no stone unturned if I thought that it would help Jessica get better. As a result of Jessica's question I began to understand that all needs do not require "fixing." I stopped doing many of the recommended home programs. I found out that I needed to be "Mom" and others could be therapists. When professionals criticize parents for not following through on recommendations, I tell them that each family has its own story and now may be the time for re-grouping and just being the mom instead of the scheduler, therapist, taxi driver, MD, or counselor.

School

Other than their child's medical issues, qualifying for special education is one of the greatest traumas parents of a special needs child will encounter. It was obvious that Benjy had an orthopedic handicap. However, to qualify for special education, we had to go through an intake process. Benjy had to be tested, and we waited with bated breath to see if he would receive educational services. He did qualify, and Benjy attended kindergarten through third grade in a school that had an orthopedic handicap program. He was in a self-contained classroom for disabled children until third grade.

When attention turned to education instead of surgeries and therapies, we found that physical disabilities are more apparent than learning disabilities. Soon our priorities switched to cognition and classroom skill building. During that time, Benjy was retained in first grade because the teachers had decided that he should be assessed for a learning disability. This evaluation provided another chance for the ever-present grief cycle to jump up and bite us. Acceptance of the physical part of the disability was almost in place. However, this new evaluation crushed my new dream of having the brightest, most socially adept physically disabled child. Even though he was adorable and happy, I went through an equally bitter (if not more so) period of guilt. Once again, I also feared for his success.

When Jessica was tested, *we* requested the testing because the preschool had prepared us for the possibility that she would have trouble learning. The school said that it was too early to find a discrepancy, but we pursued it, and one was found. She qualified for the learning disabled program. For each of the next 5 years, Jessica's resource room moved from one school to another. This meant that each year, she had to adjust to a *new* building, *new* teachers, and *new* classmates. When Jessica was in fourth grade, we were told to take her to counseling because she was withdrawn and had no friends

CASE STUDY 5-1 A Parent's Perspective—cont'd

on the playground. Guess what contributed to this. I can still see her sitting on the edge of the playground playing with her imaginary "little people" in the dirt. When Jessica was in sixth grade, we moved to another district because it had neighborhood schools with special education resources in each building. There, too, the resource room for her particular grade level had been moved from the neighborhood school. She couldn't win. She still struggles with feelings of not belonging.

When Benjy was in the third grade, Mick and I decided that he would benefit from being in the regular classroom for most of his instruction. We were a little ahead of the curve regarding inclusion, and our request received quite a response! In 1980, Benjy was a pioneer. That year was difficult for us because we decided to change priorities to allow the learning disabled program to meet his needs instead of the orthopedic handicapped program. One of the most intimidating places in the world is a room full of educators, including heads of programs, psychologists, teachers, occupational therapists, and physical therapists, and the only people who believe that you are doing the right thing for your child seem to be you and your spouse. Allowing the school's LD program to meet our son's needs turned out to be the right decision, but I still get uneasy when it is time for an IEP meeting (even an IEP meeting in which I am the occupational therapist). We worked very hard to get services to follow the student rather than placing the student into an existing special education program. This is becoming more the norm.

Mick and I always helped our children with their homework and school projects. I rationalized that their success with their schoolwork would help them achieve in life. Their work ethic for school was high. Unfortunately, because we provided continual support in completing their homework, they never had the opportunity to fail. It is now very clear to me that children have to learn responsibility for themselves and that failure is a vital part of the learning process. Otherwise they can become too dependent. I wanted to cushion my children's self-esteem by ensuring that they were successful in school. However, with the complex pattern of learning and growth, there is no clear path for children who have more challenges than most. Children with disabilities do need more help with schoolwork, but how much is too much? Lessons learned later are just as valuable, but they are more challenging because there is more at stake. There is a fine line also between teaching our children to ask for help and not feel guilty that they need it but not to assume that they *deserve* more help than others.

When we find ourselves making judgments about families, a red flag needs to go up. As was pointed out earlier in this chapter, each family has a different structure and different values. Decision making in each family is complicated and sacred. I know many people thought we were crazy when we decided to have a third child. Some were even brave enough to tell us so to our faces. Service providers held their breath, and educators looked for another Ball child in their classrooms. Having another child was a decision about which Mick and I prayed. This time in our lives was like a pause in a heartbeat, filled with hope and fear but also with the knowledge that we were in it together.

Alexander was born on a cold day in February of 1981. He had no physical problems, but he was just as colicky as the other two children. He walked at 9 months and never stopped after that. He was *very busy*. In preschool meetings, *I* was the one to point out discrepancies in Alexander's progress. The teacher complimented me on being accepting, and I carefully informed her that I had been through this twice before and had not been as accepting then. I told her that that was okay, too. My children did not lose everything because it took time for me to face their delays. They were doing just fine, and parents need to be allowed to feel the way they do. However, that does not mean that professionals should not be honest with them!

Receiving sympathetic and respectful honesty from professionals is the only way to know I have all the facts before I make a decision. Honesty is a gift that you, as a therapist, give parents. It does not mean that parents will hear you, follow your suggestions, or even believe that you are right. But your honest appraisal of the situation gives parents a piece of the picture and the truth that they need to help their child succeed. It helps if you take the time to listen to the parents' dreams or if you help them put words to those dreams.

Alexander turned out to be gifted, charming, and learning disabled, with attention-deficit disorder and dyslexia. Auditory and visual processing problems and sensory defensiveness completed the picture. His disabilities were identified between kindergarten and first grade, again at our insistence. Alexander continues to reverse letters as he reads and writes. He often reads the end of words first. At age 9, he wrote out, in bold letters on a T-shirt, a commitment to avoid drugs: "Lust say on!" Classic notes left for me on the kitchen counter often told me that his "homework is bone" or the "bog ben out."

Alexander's disability diagnosis was also difficult for me and my husband. The feelings of loss and sadness that accompanied identification again resurfaced. Again I had to be persistent to get the correct services. I also had to watch him struggle through years of extra tutoring, vision therapy, and occupational therapy just to begin to decode words. Alexander has borne the burden of being the articulate, social child in the family. He has struggled with feelings of guilt that his disabilities are not as great as those of his siblings. He received counseling to help him deal with these feelings as well as feelings of his own inadequacy.

However, part of Alexander's disability was a gift for me. He always needed books read to him for school. When he could not get a particular recorded book or he needed to complete one in a hurry, I spent time reading with him. We have shared insights on comparisons of religions, how Native Americans smoke peace pipes, and how to save yourself if you become lost in the middle of a forest. It has been cherished time that would not have occurred if he had the ability to read on his own.

Gifts and Dreams

Recently I heard that old saying, "I'm playing the hand I've been dealt." I think that applies to all of us. It seems to me that *everyone* has many sources of distress in their lives. We, as the parents of children with disabilities, often focus on the delays and the fears. We should be allowed to feel the feelings

Continued

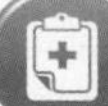

CASE STUDY 5-1 A Parent's Perspective—cont'd

that are associated with this situation. However, I think you'll find that we are proud of our children's small accomplishments: learning to put on a prosthesis independently, learning to turn a somersault, or hitting the right key on the keyboard to match the computer screen. We are happy and want to spend time with these individuals with unique perspectives on life.

There are some things our children will never be able to do, activities they choose not to attempt. These things would be next to impossible for them, but I never told them they couldn't do them. Parents are always in the position of encouraging the impossible. However, the reality is that it is the child who will ultimately determine what he or she can or cannot do. We have made and will make many mistakes parenting our children with disabilities, but we refuse to let their disabilities limit the possibilities.

I remember crying over *The Velveteen Rabbit* when I read it to the kids. It seemed that the problems of my children kept them from being "real" too. I knew that all the love I was showering on them could not change their physical makeup; however, I also knew that the love I was showering on them might help them cope with their "realness." Benjy has told me that he will run in heaven, and I believe that. I also know that all three of them run in their hearts every day here, and that others seeing them are challenged to be more.

As part of my job, I was asked to evaluate a student who had hands similar to Benjy's "claw" hand. He had a hearing impairment, and the special education team met to determine how best to serve him in the school setting. When we sat down in the meeting, one of my colleagues made a comment about his hands. She said she couldn't understand why his parents didn't have his hands "fixed"—they looked so strange. I sucked in a breath and my heart pounded. I could not respond. I felt immobilized in my chair, without a voice. How did my colleague have the right to judge that the boy's hands needed fixing? My pounding heart was accompanied by the resounding thought, "He has a right to those hands, his hands. He has a right to be different." In part I had these feelings because I had evaluated his hand skills and knew that despite how different his hands appeared, he was able to use them skillfully. Only after the meeting was I able to express what I thought and felt. I realized that this person had made the comment because she thought that "fixing" his hands would take away the staring and teasing that always accompany looking different.

To express my feelings, I wrote my colleague a letter. In it I explained that my husband and I had made the decision to increase function in Benjy's left hand when he was 7 months old, wishing it would look more like everyone else's. It was hard to admit that I had those feelings. I told her that Benjy's right arm, which we affectionately call "Super Pinky," will never look like everyone else's. I told her about the scars on his hand and the scars on his wrist from the site where the graft skin was taken. I talked about Benjy's surgery allowing for a little stronger grasp but not full extension or flexion. I told her that the young man about whom she had commented had an adapted grasp for scissors and functional cutting skills.

My letter also explained that this is a bigger issue than hands; it is about attitudes. I see our roles as professionals who work with children who are different as teaching not only the children but also everyone else. The message about our kids needs to be that *different is not worse, just different.* I know that people have the capacity to be open to difference. If we lived in a perfect world, all differences would be okay, and we would not feel that we have to fix them. However, we live in the ever-present face lift, nose fix, and "Extreme Makeover" society. People are judged on their appearance. Part of our role as professionals is to learn to accept differences, particularly in appearance, and not to try to fix everything. Our job is to help others understand that different is not wrong. This is a very simplistic view of a complex problem.

When I told Benjy about the incident, he said, "That person is not cold. She just doesn't know all the facts. If God wanted everyone to look like everyone else, He wouldn't have made handicapped people. There have been times when I wanted to look like everyone else. True people are the ones who remember you for more than your physical side, and that's what really matters. True people are able to look at you and not think you are different, but that you are unique."

Benjy is living independently and working as a cashier at a grocery. He has a new diagnosis of spinal muscle atrophy. He is gradually losing function in his remaining leg and has been using a wheelchair for a couple of years. Jessica is on disability, living independently. Her diagnoses increased to include celiac disease, chronic anxiety, and also an unknown neurologic degenerative disease causing footdrop, scissor gait and falling. She has published two poetry books. Alexander is married to a wonderful young lady, and has a beautiful daughter and son. His word-decoding skills have improved. He says this is a result of helping his children learn to read. As parents of children with disabilities, we continue to be very involved in our children's lives beyond the usual time. My prayers and dreams for them remain the same as when they were small: that they will be happy, that they will be as independent as they can be, and that they will always have someone who loves them. As the kids have grown into adults, we have had to practice involvement and support—without control. We also continue to deal with emotions, because the disabilities our children have are for life.

In all stages and at all ages, families of people with disabilities value support and resources. If you take the time to hear a parent's dream, you may hear the sound of laughter and tears. You may hear the strong heartbeat of anger or the resistance to a life that is less than it could be. As a therapist, you are a gift to the parents whose lives you touch. You have a solution to some of their frustrations. You can help uncover the hope. You have the opportunity to be as honest as you can be and provide them with the information they need to make decisions. You have the answer to some parent's question.

Thank you.

Beth Ball is the mother of three children with disabilities. She is also an occupational therapist and has worked in the public school system for a number of years.

Summary

Working with families is one of the most challenging and rewarding aspects of pediatric occupational therapy. The family's participation in intervention is of critical importance in determining how much the child can benefit. Therapy goals and activities that reflect the family's priorities often result in meaningful outcomes. The following summarizes the main points of this chapter.

Summary Points

- Family systems theory describes families as unique subsystems (parent, child, extended family) whose interactive patterns affect the behaviors and physical and mental health of each member as the family works to enable children to become participating members of society.
- The family life cycle defines life stages and the ecologic influences at each stage. Raising a child with special needs influences the co-occupations of family members by influencing time use, stress levels, satisfaction with life, and the meaning found in daily occupations.
- Families' cultures and backgrounds influence their unique perceptions of the world and what they want their children to do. For intervention to be effective, occupational therapists must listen carefully and respond to what is important to each family.
- When collaborating with families, occupational therapists focus on family priorities, partner in decision making, may coach caregivers to apply specific strategies, and support caregivers in becoming advocates for their child.
- Occupational therapists establish and maintain partnership with families through respectful interaction, honest and consistent communication, and supportive attitudes.
- Families can be empowered to facilitate their children's development through effective information sharing, full inclusion in team decision making, and provision of adequate support.
- Strategies for supporting the strengths of families facing multiple challenges are similar to those for supporting all families—using clear communication, adapting tasks and routines if modification will ensure a better result, and attending to the specific needs of those caregivers so that they feel competent to fulfill their roles.

REFERENCES

1. Allen, K. R., Fine, M. A., & Demo, D. H. (2000). An overview of family diversity: Controversies, questions and values. In D. H. Demo, K. R. Allen, & M. A. Fine (Eds.), *Handbook of family diversity.* New York: Oxford University Press.
2. Alvarado, M. I. (2004). Mucho camino: The experiences of two undocumented Mexican mothers participating in their child's early intervention program. *American Journal of Occupational Therapy, 58*, 521–530.
3. Amato, P. R. (2000). Diversity within single-parent families. In D. H. Demo, K. R. Allen, & M. A. Fine (Eds.), *Handbook of family diversity* (pp. 149–172). New York: Oxford University Press.
4. Anderson, C. (2003). The diversity, strengths and challenges of single-parent households. In F. Walsh (Ed.), *Normal family processes: Growing diversity and complexity* (3rd ed.). New York: Guilford Press.
5. Anthony, L. G., Anthony, B. J., Glanville, D. N., et al. (2005). The relationships between parenting stress, parenting behavior and preschoolers' social competence and behavior problems in the classroom. *Infant and Child Development, 14*, 133–154.
6. Aran, A., Shalev, R. S., Biran, G., et al. (2007). Parenting style impacts on quality of life in children with cerebral palsy. *Journal of Pediatrics, 151*, 56–60.
7. Bagby, M. S., Dickie, V. A., & Baranek, G. T. (2012). How sensory experiences of children with and without autism affect family occupations. *American Journal of Occupational Therapy, 66*, 78–86.
8. Bailey, D. B., Bruder, M. B., Hebbeler, K., et al. (2006). Recommended outcomes for families of young children with disabilities. *Journal of Early Intervention*, 227–251.
9. Baker, B. L., McIntyre, L. L., Blacher, J., et al. (2003). Pre-school children with and without developmental delay: behaviour problems and parenting stress over time. *Journal of Intellectual Disability Research, 47*, 217–230.
10. Barakat, L. P., Patterson, C. A., Tarazi, R. A., et al. (2007). Disease-related parenting stress in two sickle cell disease caregiver samples: Preschool and adolescent. *Families, Systems, & Health, 25*, 147–161.
11. Barrett, A. E., & Turner, R. J. (2005). Family structure and mental health: The mediating effects of socioeconomic status, family process, and social stress. *Journal of Health and Social Behavior, 46*, 156–169.
12. Bayat, M. (2007). Evidence of resilience in families of children with autism. *Journal of Intellectual Disability Research, 51*, 702–714.
13. Bedell, G. M., Cohn, E. S., & Dumas, H. M. (2005). Exploring parents' use of strategies to promote social participation of school-age children with acquired brain injuries. *American Journal of Occupational Therapy, 59*, 273–284.
14. Bendixen, R. M., Elder, J. H., Donaldson, S., et al. (2011). Effects of a father-based in-home intervention on perceived stress and family dynamics in parents of children with autism. *American Journal of Occupational Therapy, 65*, 679–687.
15. Bernheimer, L. P., & Weisner, T. S. (2007). "Let me just tell you what I do all day. . . .": The family story at the center of intervention research and practice. *Infants & Young Children, 20*(3), 192–201.
16. Betz, C. L. (2006). Parent-professional partnerships: Bridging the disparate worlds of children, families, and professionals [Editorial]. *Journal of Pediatric Nursing: Nursing Care of Children & Families, 21*(5), 333–335.
17. Blacher, J., Begun, G. F., Marcoulides, G. A., et al. (2013). Longitudinal perspectives of child positive impact on families: Relationship to disability and culture. *American Journal on Intellectual and*

Developmental Disabilities, 118, 141–155.
18. Blue-Banning, M., Summers, J. A., Frankland, H. C., et al. (2004). Dimensions of family and professional partnerships: Constructive guidelines for collaboration. *Exceptional Children, 70*(2), 167–184.
19. Booth, T., & Booth, W. (2004). Brief research report: Findings from a court study of care proceedings involving parents with intellectual disabilities. *Journal of Policy and Practice in Intellectual Disabilities, 1*, 179–181.
20. Bourke, J., Ricciardo, B., Bebbington, A., et al. (2008). Physical and mental health in mothers of children with Down syndrome. *Journal of Pediatrics, 153*, 320–326.
21. Bourke-Taylor, H., Howie, L., & Law, M. (2010). Impact of caring for a school-aged child with a disability: Understanding mothers' perspectives. *Australian Occupational Therapy Journal, 57*, 127–136.
22. Bourke-Taylor, H., Pallant, J. F., Law, M., et al. (2012). Predicting mental health among mothers of school-aged children with developmental disabilities: The relative contribution of child, maternal and environmental factors. *Research in Developmental Disabilities, 33*, 1732–1740.
23. Bramlett, M. D., & Blumberg, S. J. (2007). Family structure and children's physical and mental health. *Health Affairs, 26*, 549–558.
24. Britner, P. A., Morog, M. C., Pianta, R. C., et al. (2003). Stress and coping: A comparison of self-report measures of functioning in families of young children with cerebral palsy or no medical diagnosis. *Journal of Child and Family Studies, 12*, 335–348.
25. Bronfenbrenner, U. (1990). Discovering what families do. In D. Blankenhorn, S. Bayme, & J. B. Elshtain (Eds.), *Rebuilding the nest.* Milwaukee: Family Service America.
26. Carlson, V. J., & Harwood, R. L. (2003). Attachment, culture, and the caregiving system: The cultural patterning of everyday experiences among Anglo and Puerto Rican mother-infant pairs. *Infant Mental Health Journal, 24*, 53–73.
27. Case-Smith, J. (2004). Parenting a child with a chronic medical condition. *American Journal of Occupational Therapy, 58*, 551–560.
28. Case-Smith, J., Sainato, D., McQuaid, J., et al. (2007). IMPACTS project: Preparing therapists to provide best practice early intervention services. *Physical & Occupational Therapy in Pediatrics, 27*(3), 73–90.
29. Christian, L. G. (2006). Understanding families: Applying family systems theory to early childhood practice. *Journal of the National Association for the Education of Young Children, 61*, 12–20.
30. Cohn, E., May-Benson, T. A., & Teasdale, A. (2011). The relationship between behaviors associated with sensory processing and parental sense of competence. *OTJR: Occupation, Participation and Health, 31*(4), 172–181.
31. Coll, C. G., & Pachter, L. M. (2002). Ethnic and minority parenting. In M. H. Bornstein (Ed.), *Handbook of parenting* (2nd ed., Vol. 4). Mahwah, NJ: Lawrence Erlbaum.
32. Croot, E. (2012). The care needs of Pakistani families caring for disabled children: How relevant is cultural competence? *Physiotherapy, 98*, 351–356.
33. Crowe, T. K., & Florez, S. I. (2006). Time use of mothers with school-age children: A continuing impact of a child's disability. *American Journal of Occupational Therapy, 60*, 194–203.
34. Dabrowska, A., & Pisula, E. (2010). Parenting stress and coping styles in mothers and fathers of pre-school children with autism and Down syndrome. *Journal of Intellectual Disability Research, 54*, 266–280.
35. Deater-Deckard, K., Smith, J., Ivy, L., et al. (2005). Differential perceptions of and feelings about sibling children: Implications for research on parenting stress. *Infant and Child Development, 14*, 211–225.
36. DeGrace, B. W. (2004). The everyday occupation of families with children with autism. *American Journal of Occupational Therapy, 58*, 543–550.
37. Dolev, R., & Zeedyk, M. S. (2006). How to be a good parent in bad times: Constructing parenting advice about terrorism. *Child: Care, Health and Development, 32*(4), 467–476.
38. Dyson, L. (2010). Unanticipated effects of children with learning disabilities on their families. *Learning Disability Quarterly, 33*, 43–55.
39. Egilson, S. T. (2011). Parent perspectives of therapy services for their children with physical disabilities. *Scandinavian Journal of Caring Sciences, 25*, 277–284.
40. Falicov, C. J. (2003). Immigrant family processes. In F. Walsh (Ed.), *Normal family processes: Growing diversity and complexity* (3rd ed.). New York: Guilford Press.
41. Fernandez, E. (2007). Supporting children and responding to their families: Capturing the evidence on family support. *Children and Youth Services Review, 29*, 1368–1394.
42. Fox, L., Vaughn, B. J., Wyatte, M. I., et al. (2002). "We can't expect other people to understand": Family perspectives on problem behaviors. *Exceptional Children, 68*, 437–450.
43. Gallagher, P. A., Fialka, J., Rhodes, C., et al. (2001). Working with families: Rethinking denial. *Young Exceptional Children, 5*(2), 11–17.
44. Gallagher, P. A., Rhodes, C. A., & Darling, S. M. (2004). Parents as professionals in early intervention: A parent educator model. *Topics in Early Childhood Special Education, 24*(1), 5–13.
45. Gallimore, R., & Lopez, E. M. (2002). Everyday routines, human agency and ecocultural context: Construction and maintenance of individual habits. *Occupational Therapy Journal of Research, 22*, 70–77.
46. Geen, R. (2004). The evolution of kinship care policy and practice. *The Future of Children, 14*, 130–149.
47. Gevir, D., Goldstand, S., Weintraub, N., et al. (2006). A comparison of time use between mothers of children with and without disabilities. *OTJR: Occupation, Participation and Health, 26*(3), 117–127.
48. Gillett, K. S., Harper, J. M., Larson, J. H., et al. (2009). Implicit family process rules in eating-disordered and non-eating-disordered families. *Journal of Marital and Family Therapy, 35*(2), 159–174.
49. Glasscock, R. (2000). A phenomenological study of the experience of being a mother of a child with cerebral palsy. *Pediatric Nursing, 26*, 407–410.
50. Golnik, A., Maccabee-Ryaboy, N., Scal, P., et al. (2012). Shared decision making: Improving care for children with autism. *Intellectual and Developmental Disabilities, 50*, 322–331.
51. Gordon, P. A., Tschopp, M. K., & Feldman, D. (2004). Addressing issues of sexuality with adolescents with disabilities. *Child and Adolescent Social Work Journal, 21*(5), 513–527.
52. Graham, F., Rodger, S., & Ziviani, J. (2013). Effectiveness of occupational performance coaching in improving children's and mothers' performance and mothers' self-competence.

American Journal of Occupational Therapy, 67, 10–18.
53. Grant, G., Ramcharan, P., & Goward, P. (2003). Resilience, family care and people with intellectual disabilities. *International Review of Research in Mental Retardation, 26*, 135–173.
54. Grant, G., & Whittell, B. (2000). Differentiated coping strategies in families with children or adults with intellectual disabilities: The relevance of gender, family composition and the life span. *Journal of Applied Research in Intellectual Disabilities, 13*, 256–275.
55. Greene, S. M., Anderson, E. R., Hetherington, E. H., et al. (2003). Risk and resilience after divorce. In F. Walsh (Ed.), *Normal family processes: Growing diversity and complexity* (3rd ed.). New York: Guilford Press.
56. Hanft, B. E., Rush, D. D., & Shelden, M. L. (2004). *Coaching families and colleagues in early childhood.* Baltimore: Paul H. Brookes.
57. Harrison, C., Romer, T., Simon, M. C., et al. (2007). Factors influencing mothers' learning from paediatric therapists: A qualitative study. *Physical & Occupational Therapy in Pediatrics, 27*, 77–96.
58. Harwood, R. L., Leyendecker, B., Carlson, J., et al. (2002). Parenting among Latino families in the U.S. In M. H. Bornstein (Ed.), *Handbook of parenting: Social conditions and applied parenting* (2nd ed.). Mahwah, NJ: Lawrence Erlbaum.
59. Hasselkus, B. R. (2002). *The meaning of everyday occupation.* Thorofare, NJ: Slack.
60. Hastings, R. P. (2003). Child behavior problems and partner mental health as correlates of stress in mothers and fathers of children with autism. *Journal of Intellectual Disability Research, 47*, 231–237.
61. Helitzer, D. L., Cunningham-Sabo, L. D., VanLeit, B., et al. (2002). Perceived changes in self-image and coping strategies of mothers of children with disabilities. *Occupational Therapy Journal of Research, 22*(1), 25–33.
62. Hemmingsson, H., Stenhammar, A. M., & Paulsson, K. (2008). Sleep problems and the need for parental night-time attention in children with physical disabilities. *Child: Care, Health and Development, 35*, 89–95.
63. Hibbard, R. A., Desch, L. W., & Committee on Child Abuse and Neglect, and Council on Children with Disabilities. (2007). Maltreatment of children with disabilities. *Pediatrics, 119*(5), 1018–1025.
64. Hinojosa, J., Sproat, C. T., Mankhetwit, S., et al. (2002). Shifts in parent-therapist partnerships: Twelve years of change. *American Journal of Occupational Therapy, 56*, 556–563.
65. Hodapp, R. M. (2007). Families of persons with Down syndrome: New perspectives, findings, and research and service needs. *Mental Retardation and Developmental Disabilities Research Reviews, 13*, 279–287.
66. Hoff, E., Laursen, B., & Tardif, T. (2002). Socioeconomic status and parenting. In M. H. Bornstein (Ed.), *Handbook of parenting* (2nd ed., Vol. 2). Mahwah, NJ: Lawrence Erlbaum.
67. Holloway, R. L. (2007). Families and chronic illness: Introduction to the special section for *Families, Systems, and Health. Families, Systems, & Health, 25*, 243–245.
68. Hornberger, S., & Smith, S. L. (2011). Family involvement in adolescent substance abuse treatment and recovery: What do we know? What lies ahead? *Children and Youth Services Review, 33*, 570–576.
69. Hummelinck, A., & Pollock, K. (2006). Parents' information needs about the treatment of their chronically ill child: A qualitative study. *Patient Education and Counseling, 62*, 228–234.
70. Humphry, R. (2002). Young children's occupations: Explicating the dynamics of developmental processes. *American Journal of Occupational Therapy, 56*, 171–179.
71. Humphry, R., & Wakeford, L. (2008). Development of everyday activities: A model for occupation-centered therapy. *Infants & Young Children, 21*(3), 230–240.
72. Individuals with Disabilities Education Act of 2004 (IDEA). (P.L. 108-446.) Retrieved from: <http://idea.ed.gov/>.
73. Johnson, C. P., Kastner, T. A., & American Academy of Pediatrics Committee/Section on Children With Disabilities. (2005). Helping families raise children with special health care needs at home. *Pediatrics, 115*(2), 507–511.
74. Jones, K., & Flores, G. (2009). The potential impact of Medicaid reform on the health care–seeking behavior of Medicaid-covered children: A qualitative analysis of parental perspectives. *Journal of the National Medical Association, 101*, 213–222.
75. Jones, S. E., & Lollar, D. J. (2008). Relationship between physical disabilities or long-term health problems and health risk behaviors or conditions among US high school students. *Journal of School Health, 78*, 252–300.
76. Kadlec, M. B., Coster, W., Tickle-Degnen, L., & et al. (2005). Qualities of caregiver-child interaction during daily activities of children born very low birth weight with and without white matter disorder. *American Journal of Occupational Therapy, 59*, 57–66.
77. Kaiser, A. P., & Hancock, T. B. (2003). Teaching parents new skills to support their young children's development. *Infants and Young Children, 16*, 9–22.
78. Karst, J. S., & Van Hecke, A. V. (2012). Parent and family impact of autism spectrum disorders: A review and proposed model for intervention evaluation. *Clinical Child and Family Psychology Review, 15*, 247–277.
79. Keller, D., & Honig, A. S. (2004). Maternal and paternal stress in families with school-aged children with disabilities. *American Journal of Orthopsychiatry, 74*(3), 337–348.
80. King, G., Law, M., Hanna, S., et al. (2006). Predictors of the leisure and recreation participation of children with physical disabilities: A structural equation modeling analysis. *Children's Health Care, 35*(3), 209–234.
81. King, G., Law, M., King, S., et al. (2003). A conceptual model of factors affecting the recreation and leisure participation of children with disabilities. *Physical and Occupational Therapy in Pediatrics, 23*, 63–89.
82. King, G., Tucker, M. A., Baldwin, P., et al. (2002). A life needs model of pediatric service delivery: Services to support community participation and quality of life for children and youth with disabilities. *Physical & Occupational Therapy in Pediatrics, 22*(2), 53–77.
83. Knott, F., Lewis, C., & Williams, T. (2007). Sibling interaction of children with autism: Development over 12 months. *Journal of Autism and Developmental Disorders, 37*, 1987–1995.
84. Koramoa, J., Lynch, M. A., & Kinnair, D. (2002). A continuum of child-rearing: Responding to traditional practices. *Child Abuse Review, 11*, 415–421.
85. Kotchick, B. A., & Forehand, R. (2002). Putting parenting in perspective: A discussion of the contextual factors that shape parenting practices. *Journal of Child and Family Studies, 11*, 255–269.
86. Kroll, B. (2007). A family affair? Kinship care and parental substance

misuse: Some dilemmas explored. *Child and Family Social Work, 12*, 84–93.

87. Laird, J. (2003). Lesbian and gay families. In F. Walsh (Ed.), *Normal family processes: Growing diversity and complexity* (3rd ed.). New York: Guilford Press.
88. Larson, R. (2001). Mothers' time in two-parent and one-parent families: The daily organization of work, time for oneself, and parenting of adolescents. In *Minding the time in family experiences: Emerging perspectives and issues* (Vol. 3). New York: Elsevier Science.
89. LaVesser, P., & Berg, C. (2011). Participation patterns in preschool children with an autism spectrum disorder. *OTJR: Occupation, Participation and Health, 31*, 33–39.
90. Law, M., Teplicky, R., King, S., et al. (2005). Family-centered service: Moving ideas into practice. *Child: Care, Health and Development, 31*, 633–642.
91. Lawlor, M. C., & Mattingly, C. F. (1998). The complexities embedded in family-centered care. *American Journal of Occupational Therapy, 52*, 2059–2067.
92. Lea, D. (2006). You don't know me like that: Patterns of disconnect between adolescent mothers of children with disabilities and their early interventionists. *Journal of Early Intervention, 28*(4), 264–282.
93. Leiter, V. (2004). Dilemmas in sharing care: Maternal provision of professionally driven therapy for children with disabilities. *Social Science & Medicine, 58*, 837–849.
94. LeRoy, B. W. (2004). Mothering children with disabilities in the context of welfare reform. In S. A. Escaile & J. A. Olson (Eds.), *Mothering occupations: Challenge, agency, and participation*. Philadelphia: F. A. Davis.
95. Lietz, C. A. (2009). Examining families' perceptions of intensive in-home services: A mixed methods study. *Children and Youth Services Review, 31*, 1337–1345.
96. MacKean, G. L., Thurston, W. E., & Scott, C. M. (2005). Bridging the divide between families and health professionals' perspectives on family-centred care. *Health Expectations, 8*, 74–85.
97. Macks, R. J., & Reeve, R. E. (2007). The adjustment of non-disabled siblings of children with autism. *Journal of Autism and Developmental Disorders, 37*, 1060–1067.
98. Magill-Evans, J., Wiart, L., Darrah, J., et al. (2005). Beginning the transition to adulthood: The experiences of six families with youths with cerebral palsy. *Physical & Occupational Therapy in Pediatrics, 25*(3), 19–36.
99. Margetts, J. K., Le Couteur, A., & Croom, S. (2006). Families in a state of flux: The experiences of grandparents in autism spectrum disorder. *Child: Care, Health and Development, 32*, 565–574.
100. McBride, C., McBride-Henry, K., & van Wissen, K. (2010). Parenting a child with medically diagnosed severe food allergies in New Zealand: The experience of being unsupported in keeping their children healthy and safe. *Contemporary Nurse, 35*, 77–87.
101. McCubbin, M., Balling, K., Possin, P., et al. (2002). Family resiliency in childhood cancer. *Family Relations, 51*, 103–111.
102. McGuire, B. K., Crowe, T. K., Law, M., et al. (2004). Mothers of children with disabilities: Occupational concerns and solutions. *OTJR: Occupation, Participation and Health, 24*, 54–63.
103. McIntosh, J., Runciman, P. (2008). Exploring the role of partnership in the home care of children with special health needs: Qualitative findings from two service evaluations. *International Journal of Nursing Studies, 45*, 714–726.
104. McKay, E. A. (2004). Mothers with mental illness: An occupation interrupted. In S. A. Escaile & J. A. Olson (Eds.), *Mothering occupations: Challenge, agency, and participation*. Philadelphia: F. A. Davis.
105. McLanahan, S., Garfinkel, I., Reichman, N., et al. (2003). *The fragile families and child wellbeing study: Baseline national report*. Retrieved from: <http://www.fragilefamilies.princeton.edu/publications.asp>.
106. Melamed, B. G. (2002). Parenting the ill child. In M. H. Bornstein (Ed.), *Handbook of parenting* (2nd ed., Vol. 5). Mahwah, NJ: Lawrence Erlbaum.
107. Merenstein, D., Diener-West, M., Krist, A., et al. (2005). An assessment of the shared-decision model in parents of children with acute otitis media. *Pediatrics, 116*, 1267–1275.
108. Meyer, D. J., & Vadasy, P. F. (2007). *Sibshops: Workshops for siblings of children with special needs* (revised edition). Baltimore: Paul H. Brookes.
109. Missiuna, C., Moll, S., King, S., et al. (2007). A trajectory of troubles: Parents' impressions of the impact of developmental coordination disorder. *Physical & Occupational Therapy in Pediatrics, 27*(1), 81–101.
110. Murphy, K. E. (1997). Parenting a technology-assisted infant: Coping with occupational stress. *Social Work in Health Care, 24*(3/4), 113–126.
111. Murray, C., & Greenberg, M. T. (2006). Examining the importance of social relationships and social contexts in the lives of children with high-incidence disabilities. *Journal of Special Education, 39*, 4220–4233.
112. Neely-Barnes, S., Graff, S. L., & Carolyn, J. (2011). Are there adverse consequences to being a sibling of a person with a disability? A propensity score analysis. *Family Relations, 60*, 331–341.
113. Novak, I., Cusick, A., & Lannin, N. (2009). Occupational therapy home programs for cerebral palsy: Double-blind, randomized, controlled trial. *Pediatrics, 124*, 606–614.
114. O'Keefe, N., & O'Hara, J. (2008). Mental health needs of parents with intellectual disabilities. *Current Opinion in Psychiatry, 21*(5), 463–468.
115. Opacich, K., & Savage, T. A. (2004). Mothers with chronic illness: Reconstructing occupation. In S. A. Escaile & J. A. Olson (Eds.), *Mothering occupations: Challenge, agency, and participation*. Philadelphia: F. A. Davis.
116. Parish, S. L., & Cloud, J. M. (2006a). Child care for low-income school-age children: Disability and family structure effects in a national sample. *Children and Youth Services Review, 28*, 927–940.
117. Parish, S. L., & Cloud, J. M. (2006b). Financial well-being of young children with disabilities and their families. *Social Work, 51*(3), 223–232.
118. Patterson, C. J. (2002). Lesbian and gay parenthood. In M. H. Bornstein (Ed.), *Handbook of parenting* (2nd ed.). Mahwah, NJ: Lawrence Erlbaum Associates.
119. Patterson, J. M. (2002). Integrating family resilience and family stress theory. *Journal of Marriage and Family, 64*, 349–360.
120. Piggot, J., Hocking, C., & Paterson, J. (2003). Parental adjustment to having a child with cerebral palsy and participation in home therapy programs. *Physical & Occupational Therapy in Pediatrics, 23*(4), 5–29.
121. Porterfield, S. L. (2002). Work choices of mothers in families with children with disabilities. *Journal of Marriage and Family, 64*, 972–981.
122. Powers, K., Hogansen, J., Geenen, S., et al. (2008). Gender matters in

transition to adulthood: A survey study of adolescents with disabilities and their families. *Psychology in the Schools, 45*(4), 349–364.

123. Raphel, S. (2008). Kinship care and the situation for grandparents. *Journal of Child and Adolescent Psychiatric Nursing, 21*, 118–120.
124. Rivers, J. W., & Stoneman, Z. (2003). Sibling relationships when a child has autism: Marital stress and support coping. *Journal of Autism and Developmental Disorders, 33*(4), 383–394.
125. Rogoff, B. (2003). *The cultural nature of human development.* New York: Oxford University Press.
126. Sameroff, A. J., & Fiese, B. H. (2000). Transactional regulation: The developmental ecology of early intervention. In J. P. Shonkoff & S. J. Meisels (Eds.), *Handbook of early childhood intervention* (2nd ed.). New York: Cambridge University Press.
127. Sawyer, M. G., Bittman, M., La Greca, A. M., et al. (2010). Time demands of caring for children with autism: What are the implications for maternal mental health? *Journal of Autism and Developmental Disorders, 40*, 620–628.
128. Schultz-Krohn, W. (2004). Meaningful family routines in a homeless shelter. *American Journal of Occupational Therapy, 58*(5), 531–542.
129. Segal, R. (2004). Family routines and rituals: A context for occupational therapy interventions. *American Journal of Occupational Therapy, 58*(5), 499–508.
130. Segal, R., & Beyer, C. (2006). Integration and application of a home treatment program: A study of parents and occupational therapists. *American Journal of Occupational Therapy, 60*(5), 500–510.
131. Segal, R., & Hinojosa, J. (2006). The activity setting of homework: An analysis of three cases and implications for occupational therapy. *American Journal of Occupational Therapy, 60*(1), 50–59.
132. Shonkoff, J. P., & Phillips, D. A. (2000). *From neurons to neighborhoods: The science of early childhood development.* Washington, DC: National Academy Press.
133. Skogrand, L., & Shirer, K. (2007). *Working with low-resource and culturally diverse audiences.* Retrieved from: <https://www.childwelfare.gov/systemwide/cultural/families/>.
134. Spagnola, M., & Fiese, B. H. (2007). Family routines and rituals: A context for development in the lives of young children. *Infants & Young Children, 20*(4), 284–299.
135. Spratt, E. G., Saylor, C. F., & Macias, M. M. (2007). Assessing parenting stress in multiple samples of children with special needs (CSN). *Families, Systems, & Health, 25*(4), 435–449.
136. Stacey, J., & Biblarz, T. J. (2001). How does the sexual orientation of parents matter? *American Sociological Review, 66*, 159–183.
137. Steinberg, L., & Silk, J. S. (2002). Parenting adolescents. In M. H. Bornstein (Ed.), *Handbook of parenting* (2nd ed., Vol. 1). Mahwah, NJ: Lawrence Erlbaum.
138. Stewart, D., Law, M., Burke-Gaffney, J., et al. (2006). Keeping It Together: An information KIT for parents of children and youth with special needs. *Child: Care, Health and Development, 32*, 493–500.
139. Stokes, R. H., & Holsti, L. (2010). Paediatric occupational therapy: Addressing parental stress with the sense of coherence. *Canadian Journal of Occupational Therapy, 77*(1), 30–37.
140. Stoneman, Z. (2001). Supporting positive sibling relationships during childhood. *Mental Retardation and Developmental Disabilities Research Reviews, 7*, 134–142.
141. Suarez-Orozco, C., Todorova, L. G., & Louie, J. (2002). Making up for lost time: The experiences of separation and reunification among immigrant families. *Family Process, 41*, 625–643.
142. Summers, J. A., Dell'Oliver, C., Turnbull, A. P., et al. (1990). Examining the individualized family service plan process: What are family and practitioner preferences? *Topics in Early Childhood Special Education, 10*(2), 78–99.
143. Tetreault, S., Parrot, A., & Trahan, J. (2003). Home activity programs in families with children presenting with global developmental delays: Evaluation and parental perceptions. *International Journal of Rehabilitation Research, 26*, 165–173.
144. Trent-Stainbrook, A., Kaiser, A. P., & Frey, J. R. (2007). Older siblings' use of responsive interaction strategies and effects on their younger siblings with Down syndrome. *Journal of Early Intervention, 29*(4), 273–286.
145. Trivette, C. M., & Dunst, C. J. (2005). DEC recommended practices: Family-based practices. In S. Sandall, M. L. Hemmeter, B. J. Smith, & M. E. McLean (Eds.), *DEC recommended practices: A comprehensive guide for practical application in early intervention/early childhood special education.* Missoula, MT: Division for Early Childhood.
146. Trivette, C. M., Dunst, C. J., & Hamby, D. W. (2010). Influences of family-systems intervention practices on parent-child interactions and child development. *Topics in Early Childhood Special Education, 30*(1), 3–19.
147. Tubbs, C. Y., Roy, K. M., & Burton, L. M. (2005). Family ties: Constructing family time in low-income families. *Family Process, 44*(1), 77–91.
148. Turnbull, A. P., Turbiville, V., & Turnbull, H. R. (2002). Evolution of family-professional partnerships: Collective empowerment as the model for the early twenty-first century. In J. P. Shonkoff & S. J. Meisels (Eds.), *Handbook of early childhood intervention* (2nd ed.). New York: Cambridge University Press.
149. Turnbull, A., Turnbull, R., Erwin, E. J., et al. (2006). *Families, professionals, and exceptionality: Positive outcomes through partnerships and trust* (5th ed.). Columbus, OH: Merrill.
150. VanLeit, B., & Crowe, T. K. (2002). Outcomes of an occupational therapy program for mothers of children with disabilities: Impact on satisfaction with time use and occupational performance. *American Journal of Occupational Therapy, 56*, 402–410.
151. Wacharasin, C., Barnard, K. E., & Spieker, S. J. (2003). Factors affecting toddler cognitive development in low-income families: Implications for practitioners. *Infants and Young Children, 16*, 175–187.
152. Walker, S. (2002). Culturally competent protection of children's mental health. *Child Abuse Review, 11*, 380–393.
153. Wall, S., Kisker, E. E., Peterson, C. A., et al. (2006). Child care for low-income children with disabilities: Access, quality, and parental satisfaction. *Journal of Early Intervention, 28*(4), 283–298.
154. Walsh, F. (2002). A family resilience framework: Innovative practice applications. *Family Relations, 51*, 130–137.
155. Walsh, F. (2003). *Normal family processes: Growing diversity and complexity* (3rd ed.). New York: Guilford Press.
156. Williams, L. (2007). The many roles of families in family-centered care—Part III. *Pediatric Nursing, 33*(2), 144–146.

157. Williams, P. D., Williams, A. R., Graff, J. C., et al. (2002). Interrelationships among variables affecting well siblings and mothers in families of children with chronic illness or disability. *Journal of Behavioral Medicine*, *25*, 411–424.
158. Winston, K. A., Dunbar, S. B., Reed, C. N., et al. (2010). Mothering occupations when parenting children with feeding concerns: A mixed methods study. *Canadian Journal of Occupational Therapy*, *77*(3), 181–189.

CHAPTER 6

Use of Standardized Tests in Pediatric Practice

Pamela K. Richardson

KEY TERMS

Standardized test
Performance-based test
Self-report test
Reliability
Norm-referenced test
Criterion-referenced test
Normative sample
Measures of central tendency
Measures of variability
Standard score
Correlation coefficient
Validity
Ethics in testing

GUIDING QUESTIONS

1. What are the characteristics of commonly used standardized pediatric tests?
2. What are the differences between norm- and criterion-referenced tests and the purpose of each?
3. How do performance- and observation-based tests differ?
4. What descriptive statistics are used in standardized pediatric tests?
5. What do standard scores used in standardized pediatric tests mean?
6. How do reliability and validity relate to a test's integrity?
7. How do occupational therapists demonstrate competency in and ethical use of standardized tests?

What are standardized tests, and why are they important to occupational therapists? A test that has been standardized has uniform procedures for administration and scoring.[63] This means that examiners must use the same instructions, materials, and procedures each time they administer the test, and they must score the test using criteria specified in the test manual. A number of standardized tests are in common use. Most schoolchildren have taken standardized achievement tests that assess how well they have learned the required grade-level material. College students are familiar with the Scholastic Aptitude Test (SAT), the results of which can affect decisions on admission at many colleges and universities. Intelligence tests, interest tests, and aptitude tests are other examples of standardized tests frequently used with the general public.

Pediatric occupational therapists use standardized tests to help determine the eligibility of children for therapy services, monitor their progress in therapy, and make decisions on the type of intervention that would be most appropriate and effective for them. Standardized tests provide measurements of a child's performance in specific areas, and this performance is described as a standard score. The standard score can be used and understood by other occupational therapists and child development professionals familiar with standardized testing procedures.

Using anthropometric measurements and psychophysical testing to measure intelligence, Galton and Cattell developed the initial concept of standardized assessments of human performance late in the nineteenth century. The first widespread use of human performance testing was initiated in 1904, when the minister of public education in Paris formed a commission to create tests that would help to identify "mentally defective children," with the goal of providing them with an appropriate education. Binet and Simon developed the first intelligence test for this purpose. Terman and Merrill incorporated many of Binet and Simon's ideas into the construction of the Stanford-Binet Intelligence Scale,[60] which remains widely used today.[57] Although intelligence was the first human attribute to be tested in a standardized manner, tests have been developed over the past several decades that assess children's developmental status, cognition, gross and fine motor skills, language and communication skills, school readiness, school achievement, visual-motor skills, visual-perceptual skills, social skills, and other behavioral domains. Although the number and types of tests have changed radically since the time of Simon and Binet, the basic reason for using standardized tests remains the same: to identify children who may need specialized intervention or environmental adaptations because their performance in a given area is outside the norm, or average, for their particular age.

The use of standardized tests requires a high level of responsibility on the part of the tester. The occupational therapist who uses a standardized test must be knowledgeable about scoring and interpreting the test, must know for whom the test is and is not appropriate, and must understand how to report and discuss a child's scores on the test. The tester must also be aware of the limitations of standardized tests in providing information about a child's performance or participation. This, in turn, requires a working knowledge of standardized testing concepts and procedures, familiarity with the factors that can affect performance on standardized tests, and awareness of the ethics and responsibilities of testers when using standardized tests.

This chapter introduces pediatric standardized testing used by occupational therapists. The purposes and characteristics of standardized tests are discussed, technical information about standardized tests is presented, practical tips to help the student become a competent user of standardized assessments are given, and ethical considerations are explained. The chapter concludes with a summary of the advantages and disadvantages of standardized tests and a case study that incorporates the concepts presented in the chapter into a "real-life" testing scenario. Throughout the chapter, several standardized assessments commonly used by pediatric occupational therapists are highlighted to illustrate the concepts of test administration, scoring, and interpretation.

Influences on Standardized Testing in Pediatric Occupational Therapy

When standardized tests became widely used in pediatric practice in the 1970s and 1980s, the tests available for occupational therapists focused primarily on the developmental domains of gross motor skills, fine motor skills, and visual-motor/visual-perceptual skills. These early tests were developed by educators and psychologists. The first pediatric standardized test developed by an occupational therapist was the Southern California Sensory Integration Test (SCSIT), published by A. Jean Ayres in 1972. The SCSIT assessed sensory integration and praxis, domains that were of specific interest to occupational therapists, and was instrumental in defining the measurement standards in these areas.

In the ensuing years, the number of standardized tests created by and for pediatric occupational therapists has increased dramatically, and the number of behavioral and performance domains assessed has expanded. This evolution in standardized testing in occupational therapy has been influenced by developments both inside and outside the profession. Some key developments are briefly summarized next.

The Individuals with Disabilities Education Act (IDEA) Part B defined the role of occupational therapy as a related service in school-based settings for children age 3-21 years. In this setting, standardized tests provide information that is used to determine children's eligibility for services, measure progress, and develop individualized education programs (IEPs).

The IDEA Part C created federal support for family-centered services for children age 0-3 and their families. Occupational therapy is a supportive service that participates in multidisciplinary evaluations to determine eligibility for services, assessment of family needs, resources, and priorities to support development of an individualized family service plan (IFSP) and periodic review of progress. Standardized tests of children's developmental status, caregiver-child interactions, and the home environment are an important part of this process.

The development of occupational therapy frameworks that consider environmental characteristics and the performance of activities within daily contexts expanded evaluation to include information about how individuals engage with their environment and how environments may support or inhibit participation in daily life. This new focus required the development of evaluation procedures that assessed characteristics of the environment and the quality of children's interactions within the environment. Strategic frameworks that define this person-environment interaction include the model of human occupation,[38] the ecology of human performance,[19] and the person-environment-occupation model.[42]

The development of client-centered models of practice that advocated involvement of the client and family in the evaluation and intervention planning process required the development of evaluation methods that collected information from clients about their needs, priorities, and satisfaction with their performance. The Canadian Occupational Performance Measure (COPM) is frequently used for this purpose.[41] In pediatric practice this information is generally collected from parents/caregivers and teachers. Increasingly, however, the importance of obtaining information directly from children is being acknowledged, and evaluation methods to obtain this information have been developed.[37,39,43]

Recognition of the limitations of collecting evaluation data focused on sensorimotor skills and the need to address multiple aspects of children's occupational performance created a call for a "top down" evaluation process[13] whereby initial focus of the evaluation shifted to the quality and quantity of children's engagement in daily occupations. Assessments such as the School Function Assessment (SFA)[14] and the Pediatric Evaluation of Disability Inventory (PEDI)[32] incorporate this approach to assessment.

The International Classification of Functioning, Disability, and Health (ICF) identified three levels of focus for interventions: body structure or function (impairment), whole body movements or activities (activity limitations), and involvement in life situations (participation restrictions).[66] The ICF for Children and Youth (ICF-CY) added characteristics associated with growth and development in children and youth, facilitating the inclusion of the school and other learning environments in intervention programs. Incorporation of participation restrictions as an area of intervention created a new focus on the effect of impairments or activity limitations on children's abilities to participate in all aspects of daily life. As a result, methods to assess children's participation have been developed. Participation measures are incorporated into some standardized pediatric assessments such as the SFA[14] and the Miller Function & Participation Scales (M-FUN).[45] Assessments that focus on children's participation include the Children's Assessment of Participation and Enjoyment (CAPE), the Preferences for Activities of Children (PAC),[39] the Child and Adolescent Scale of Participation (CASP),[9] and the Pediatric Evaluation of Disability Inventory Computer Adaptive Test (PEDI-CAT).[32]

The preceding discussion illustrates how evolution of the occupational therapy profession has contributed to the ongoing development of standardized testing practices. One of the most significant changes in standardized testing over the past 30 years involves the inclusion of multiple information sources in the standardized testing process. Pediatric occupational therapists no longer draw conclusions about a child's abilities and needs based only on the child's performance on test items administered in a highly structured setting. Self-report and parent-report assessments allow therapists to obtain information about children's performance and participation in a variety of daily contexts based on information provided by adults who are familiar with the child and in some cases from the children themselves. These multiple sources of information provide a well-rounded picture of how personal and environmental factors interact to influence children's ability to engage productively in age-appropriate occupations. Table 6-1 lists some of the most commonly used pediatric standardized assessments.

TABLE 6-1 Summary of Selected Pediatric Standardized Tests

Test	Age Range	Domains Tested	Sources of Information	Standard Scores Used	Duration of Test
Bayley Scales of Infant & Toddler Development Motor Scale (3rd ed.) (BSID-III)	1-42 mo	Fine Motor Subtest: Prehension, perceptual-motor integration, motor planning, motor speed Gross Motor Subtest: Static positioning, locomotion and coordination, balance, motor planning	Performance-based	Scaled scores Composite scores Percentile ranks Confidence intervals Growth scores Developmental age equivalent	15-20 min
Peabody Developmental Motor Scales (2nd ed.) (PDMS-2)	1-84 mo	Fine Motor Scale: Grasping, hand use, eye-hand coordination, manual dexterity Gross Motor Scale: Reflexes, balance, locomotor, nonlocomotor, receipt and propulsion	Performance-based	Z-scores T-scores Scaled scores Age-equivalent scores Developmental motor quotient scores	45-60 min for total test, 20-30 min for each scale
Miller Function & Participation Scale (M-FUN)	2 yr 6 mo-7 yr 11 mo	Fine Motor, Visual Motor, and Gross Motor subtests each assess aspects of four neurologic foundations: hand function, postural abilities, executive function and participation, nonmotor visual perception Test Observations: Examiner rating of child's behavior during testing session Home Observations: Caregiver rating of child's participation in activities of daily living (ADLs) and leisure activities at home Classroom Observations: Teacher or examiner rating of participation in classroom activities	Performance-based Context-based: examiner, caregiver, and teacher ratings	Scaled scores Confidence intervals Percentile scores Age equivalents Progress scores Criterion-referenced participation scores	40-60 min for performance activities 5-10 min for participation checklists
Bruininks-Oseretsky Test of Motor Proficiency (2nd ed.) (BOT-2)	4 yr 0 mo-21 yr 11 mo	Fine Manual Control: Motor skills for drawing and writing Manual Coordination: Motor skills for reaching, grasping, and manipulating objects; emphasis on speed, dexterity, and coordination Body Coordination: Motor skills involved in balance and coordination of upper and lower extremities Strength and Agility: Large muscle strength, motor speed, motor skills for maintaining body position for walking and running	Performance-based	Scale scores Composite standard scores Percentile ranks Total motor composite Age-equivalent scores Descriptive categories Confidence intervals	40-60 min for complete form; individual subtests can also be administered
Pediatric Evaluation of Disability Inventory Computer Adaptive Test (PEDI-CAT)	6 mo-7 yr	Social Function, Self-Care, and Mobility scales: Each scale is scored according to functional skills, amount of caregiver assistance, and modifications	Self-report: caregiver and/or therapist/professional ratings; can be completed by one or more respondents	Normative standard score Scaled score	40-60 min when scoring by caregiver report
School Function Assessment (SFA)	Grades K-6	Participation in nonacademic school tasks Task Supports: Five assistance and five adaptation scales Activity Performance: Physical tasks and cognitive-behavioral tasks	Self-report: teachers and other school staff ratings. Can be completed by one or more respondents	Criterion scores for each scale Cutoff scores for each scale for grades K-3 and grades 4-6	Total time 1.5-2 hr; 5-10 min per scale

Continued

TABLE 6-1 Summary of Selected Pediatric Standardized Tests—cont'd

Test	Age Range	Domains Tested	Sources of Information	Standard Scores Used	Duration of Test
Sensory Profile (SP)	3-10 yr	Sensory Processing: Auditory, visual, vestibular, touch, multisensory, and oral sensory processing Modulation: Sensory Processing Related to Endurance/Tone, Modulation Related to Body Position and Movement, Modulation of Movement Affecting Activity Level, Modulation of Sensory Input Affecting Emotional Responses Behavioral and Emotional Responses: Emotional/Social Responses, Behavioral Outcomes of Sensory Processing, Thresholds for Response	Self-Report: completed by caregiver	Cut score and classification system based on normative information: typical performance, probable difference, definite difference	20-30 min
Adolescent/Adult Sensory Profile (AASP)	11 yr and up	Sensory processing categories—Taste/Smell, Movement (vestibular/proprioceptive), Visual, Touch, Activity Level, and Auditory—are evaluated for each quadrant: Low Registration, Sensation Seeking, Sensory Sensitivity, and Sensation Avoiding, on a neurologic threshold continuum and behavioral response/self-regulation continuum	Context-based self-report	Cut score and classification system based on normative information: Quadrant grid Quadrant summary Quadrant profile	10-15 min
Sensory Processing Measure (SPM)	5-12 yr (Grades K-6)	Social participation Vision Hearing Touch Body awareness Balance and motion Planning and ideas Total sensory systems	Self-Report: completed by caregiver (Home Form), teacher (Main Classroom Form), teacher and other school staff (School Environments Form)	Standard scores, T-score, percentile score (Home and Main Classroom Forms) Cutoff scores (School Environments Form)	15-20 min for Home and Main Classroom Forms 5 min for each of six rating sheets for School Environments Form
Assessment of Motor and Process Skills (AMPS)	3 yr and up	Motor and process skills in performance of basic and instrumental activities of daily living (IADLs)	Performance-based	ADL ability measure Logit scores for motor and process scales	30-40 min
School Assessment of Motor and Process Skills (School AMPS)	3-11 yr	Occupational performance in school motor and process skills in five classroom tasks: pen/pencil writing, drawing and coloring, cutting and pasting, computer writing, manipulatives	Performance-based	Logit scores for motor and process scales	30-40 min
Goal-Oriented Assessment of Life Skills (GOAL)	7-17 yr	Functional motor skills needed for activities of daily living	Seven gross and fine motor activities composed of 54 steps—small units of easily observed behavior based on childhood occupations: Gross Motor and Fine Motor Standard Scores and Progress Scores	Performance-based	45-60 min

TABLE 6-2 Developmental Domains Assessed in Four Screening Tools

Screening Tool	Age Range	Domains Assessed
Ages and Stages Questionnaire (3rd ed.)	1-66 mo	Communication, gross motor, fine motor, problem-solving, personal-social
Denver Developmental Screening Test (Revised)	1 mo-6 yr	Personal-social, fine motor adaptive, language, gross motor
Developmental Indicators for Assessment of Learning (3rd ed.)	2.5-6 yr	Motor, language, concepts
FirstSTEP: Screening Test for Evaluating Preschoolers	2 yr 9 mo-6 yr 2 mo	Cognition, communication, physical, social, and emotional, adaptive functioning

Purposes of Standardized Tests

Standardized tests are used for several reasons. For example, a standardized test can be used as a screening tool to assess large numbers of children quickly and briefly and identify those who may have delays and are in need of more in-depth testing. Examples of screening tests frequently used by occupational therapists include the revised Denver Developmental Screening Test (Denver-II),[25] Ages and Stages Questionnaire–2nd (ASQ), and the FirstSTEP (Screening Test for Evaluating Preschoolers).[44]

Screening tests typically assess several developmental domains, and each domain is represented by a small number of items (Table 6-2). Screening tests generally take 20 to 30 minutes and can be administered by professionals or by paraprofessionals such as classroom aides, nurse's aides, or teaching assistants. Therapists who work in settings that primarily serve typically developing children (e.g., a public school system or Head Start program) may become involved in developmental screening activities. In addition, occupational therapists frequently use assessment tools to evaluate children with specific developmental problems. Therefore it is important for all therapists to be aware of the strengths and weaknesses of specific tests used in their settings. Although the screening tools mentioned are not discussed in greater depth, the concepts of developing, administering, scoring, and interpreting standardized tests (discussed later in this chapter) should also be considered when using screening tools.

Occupational therapists most frequently use standardized tests as in-depth assessments of various areas of occupation and performance skills. Standardized tests are used for five main purposes:

1. To assist in the determination of a medical or educational diagnosis
2. To document a child's developmental, functional, and participation status
3. To aid the planning of an intervention program
4. To measure outcomes of programs
5. To measure variables in research studies

Determination of Medical or Educational Diagnoses

A primary purpose of standardized tests is to assist in the determination of a diagnosis through use of normative scores that compare the child's performance with that of an age-matched sample of children. Standardized tests are frequently used to determine if a child has developmental delays or functional deficits significant enough to qualify the child for remedial services such as occupational therapy. Many funding agencies and insurance providers use the results of standardized testing as one criterion in deciding whether a child will receive occupational therapy intervention. In school-based practice, standard scores are helpful for identifying specific student problems that may indicate that the involvement of an occupational therapist is appropriate. Funding approval for special services generally depends on documentation of a predetermined degree of delay or deficit in one or more developmental or academic domains, and standardized test results are an important component of this documentation. The results of standardized testing performed by occupational therapists, when used in conjunction with testing done by other professionals, can help physicians or psychologists arrive at a medical or educational diagnosis.

Documentation of Developmental, Functional, and Participation Status

Another purpose of standardized testing is to document a child's status. This can include developmental levels, functional skills, and the child's level of participation in home, school, and community activities. Many funding and service agencies require periodic reassessment to provide a record of a child's progress and to determine if the child continues to qualify for services. Standardized testing is often a preferred way of documenting progress because the results of the most current assessment can be compared with those of earlier ones. Periodic formal reassessment can also provide valuable information to the therapist working with the child. Careful scrutiny of a child's test results can help identify areas of greatest and least progress. This can assist the therapist in prioritizing intervention goals. Many parents are also interested in seeing the results of their child's periodic assessments. Standardized tests used in periodic assessments must be chosen carefully so that areas of occupation or performance skills addressed in the intervention plan are also the focus of the standardized testing.

A discussion about the child's progress in areas that may not be measured by standardized testing should accompany the discussion of test performance. Structured or unstructured observations of the child's play, academic, social, and/or self-care performance; interviews with the caretaker or teacher about the child's home or school routine; the developmental, educational, and medical histories; and a review of pertinent medical or educational records are equally important components of the assessment process.

Planning Intervention Programs

A third purpose of standardized testing is program planning. Standardized tests provide information about a child's level of function, and they help therapists determine the appropriate starting point for therapy intervention. Most commonly, criterion-referenced standardized tests are used as the basis for developing goals and objectives for individual children and measuring progress and change over time. Criterion-referenced tests are used extensively in educational settings and include tools such as the Hawaii Early Learning Profile (HELP)[50]; the Assessment, Evaluation, and Programming System for Infants and Children[10]; and the SFA.[14] Criterion-referenced tests are described in more detail in the following section.

Measuring Program Outcomes

Occupational therapists are increasingly being required to document efficacy of their interventions, not only individually but at the program level. When a number of children participate in a similar intervention program and standardized instruments are used to evaluate change of status, the data can be combined and analyzed to provide outcome data about the program.[48] These data can be used for program development and modification and to support allocation of necessary resources to continue the program.

Measurement Instruments for Research Studies

Because of the psychometric properties of standardized tests, standard scores obtained from these tests can be statistically manipulated and analyzed. This allows test scores to be used for both descriptive and experimental research. Standardized tests can be used to obtain descriptive data about particular populations or groups. Experimental studies compare scores obtained before and after interventions or compare the outcome scores for two different interventions. Data obtained through descriptive and experimental studies enhance our knowledge about client groups and provide evidence regarding the efficacy of occupational therapy interventions.

Characteristics

As stated, standardized tests have uniform procedures for administration and scoring. These standard procedures permit the results of a child's tests to be compared either with the child's performance on a previous administration of the test or with the test norms developed by administration of the test to a large number of children.

Standardized tests characteristically include a test manual that describes the purpose of the test (i.e., what the test is intended to measure). The manual should also describe the intended population for the test. For pediatric assessments, this generally refers to the age range of children for whom the test was intended, but it may also refer to specific diagnoses or types of functional impairments. Test manuals also contain technical information about the test, such as a description of the test development and standardization process, characteristics of the normative sample, and studies done during the test development process to establish reliability and validity data. Finally, test manuals contain detailed information about the administration, scoring, and interpretation of the test scores.

Another characteristic of standardized tests is that they are composed of a fixed number of items. Items may not be added or subtracted without affecting the standard procedure for test administration. Most tests have specific rules about the number of items that should be administered to ensure a standardized test administration. These rules may differ significantly from test to test. For instance, the Bruininks-Oseretsky Test of Motor Proficiency (2nd ed.) (BOT-2) specifies that within each subtest the entire item set be administered regardless of the child's age.[11,67] In contrast, the Bayley Scales of Infant and Toddler Development (3rd ed.) (BSID-III) has 17 start points for the test.[7] Examiners are instructed to begin testing at the start point corresponding to the child's chronologic age (or corrected age, if the child was born prematurely) and move to easier or more difficult items, depending on the child's performance. Box 6-1 explains how to compute ages corrected for prematurity.

A third characteristic of standardized tests is fixed protocol for administration. The term *fixed protocol for administration* refers to the way each item is administered and the number of items administered. Generally, the protocol for administration specifies the verbal instruction or demonstration to be provided, the number of times the instructions can be repeated, and the number of attempts the child is allowed on the item. For some tests, instructions for each item are printed in the manual, and the tester is expected to read the instructions verbatim to the child without deviating from the text. However, other tests allow for more freedom of instruction, especially when the test involves a physical activity (Figure 6-1).

Standardized tests also have a fixed guideline for scoring. Scoring guidelines usually accompany the administration guidelines and specify what the child's performance must look like to receive a passing score on the item. Depending on the nature of the item, passing performance may be described using text, a picture, or a diagram. The administration and scoring guidelines for a test item from the BOT-2 are shown in Figure 6-2. In this example, the instructions to be given to the child are printed in bold type. Also included are the criteria for a passing score on the item, examples of incorrect responses, the number of trials, and the time allowed for completion of the item. This example (see Figure 6-2) describes how to present the item and what constitutes a passing score and includes a diagram of what a passing performance looks like.

Types of Standardized Tests

The two main types of standardized tests are norm-referenced tests and criterion-referenced tests. Many pediatric occupational therapists use both types in their practices. Each type has a specific purpose, and it is important for testers to be aware of the purpose of the test they are using.

A norm-referenced test is developed by giving the test in question to a large number of children, usually several hundred or more. This group is called the normative sample, and norms,

BOX 6-1 Calculating the Chronologic Age and Corrected Age

Many standardized tests require that the examiner calculate the child's exact age on the date of testing. The method for calculating both the chronologic and the corrected age is presented in the following.

Calculating the Chronologic Age

First, the date of testing and the child's birth date are recorded in the following order:

	Year	Month	Day
Date of testing	99	6	15
Birth date	95	3	10
Chronologic age	4	3	5

Beginning on the right (the Day category), the day, month, and year of the child's birth date are subtracted from the date of testing. In the above example, the child's chronologic age is 4 years, 3 months, 5 days at the time of testing.

The convention in calculating age is that if the number of days in the chronologic age is 15 or less, the month is rounded down. Therefore in the above example, the child's age would be stated as 4 years, 3 months, or 4-3. If the number of days in the chronologic age is between 16 and 30, the month is rounded up. If the above child's chronologic age had been 4 years, 3 months, 16 days, the chronologic age would be expressed as 4 years, 4 months, or 4-4.

Sometimes, "borrowing" is necessary to subtract the birth date from the date of testing correctly:

	Year	Month	Day
Date of testing	99	6	15
Birth date	95	10	22
Chronologic age	3	7	23

Begin with the Day category. Twenty-two cannot be subtracted from 15 without borrowing from the Month category. One month must be borrowed and placed in the Day category. One month equals 30 days; 30 is added to the 15 days in the Date of testing, giving a total of 45. Twenty-two is subtracted from 45, leaving 23 days. Moving to the Month category, 1 month has been borrowed by the Day category, leaving 5 months. Because 10 cannot be subtracted from 5, 1 year must be borrowed from the Year category. One year equals 12 months; therefore 12 will be added to the 5 in the Month category for Date of testing, totaling 17. Ten is subtracted from 17, leaving 7 months. Moving to the Year category, 1 year has been borrowed by the Month category, leaving 98. Ninety-five can be subtracted from 98, leaving 3 years. Therefore this child's chronologic age is 3 years, 7 months, 23 days. Using the rounding convention as discussed, the month is rounded up, giving a chronologic age of 3 years, 8 months.

Calculating the Corrected Age

Corrected age is used for children who were born prematurely to "correct" for the number of weeks they were born before the due date. Generally, the age is corrected until the child turns 2 years of age, although this convention can vary. Given 40 weeks' gestation as full term, the amount of correction is the difference between the actual gestational age at birth and the 40 weeks' full-term gestational age. Therefore a child born at 30 weeks' gestation is 10 weeks premature. Many practitioners consider 36 or 37 weeks or above to be full-term gestation; therefore children with a gestational age of 36 weeks or above do not receive a corrected age. Because there is some variation in how and when corrected age is used, it is wise for the therapist to learn the procedures of his or her facility and to adhere to them when calculating corrected age.

If the expected due date and birth date are both known, subtracting the birth date from the due date yields an exact measurement of prematurity.

	Year	Month	Day
Due date	98	9	20
Birth date	98	6	12
	—	3	8

This child is 3 months, 8 days premature. To calculate corrected age, subtract the prematurity value from the chronologic age:

	Year	Month	Day
Chronologic age	1	1	25
Prematurity	—	3	8
	—	10	17

The child's corrected age is 10 months, 17 days, or, when rounded, 11 months.

or average scores, are derived from this sample. When a norm-referenced test is administered, the performance of the child being tested is compared with that of the normative sample. The purpose of norm-referenced testing, then, is to determine how a child performs in relation to the average performance of the normative sample.

Test developers generally attempt to include children from a variety of geographic locations, ethnic and racial backgrounds, and socioeconomic levels so that the normative sample is representative of the population of the United States, based on the most recent U.S. census data. Generally, the normative sample is composed of children who have no developmental delays or conditions, although many tests include data from subsamples of clinical populations as a means of determining whether the test discriminates between children whose development is proceeding normally and those who have known developmental delays.

Norm-referenced tests address one or more areas of behavior. If the test evaluates more than one area, each area typically has one or more subtests. For instance the BOT-2 assesses performance in four motor-area composites: fine manual control, manual coordination, body coordination, and strength and agility. Items are chosen to represent a broad range of skills within these composite areas. Additionally, items are chosen to

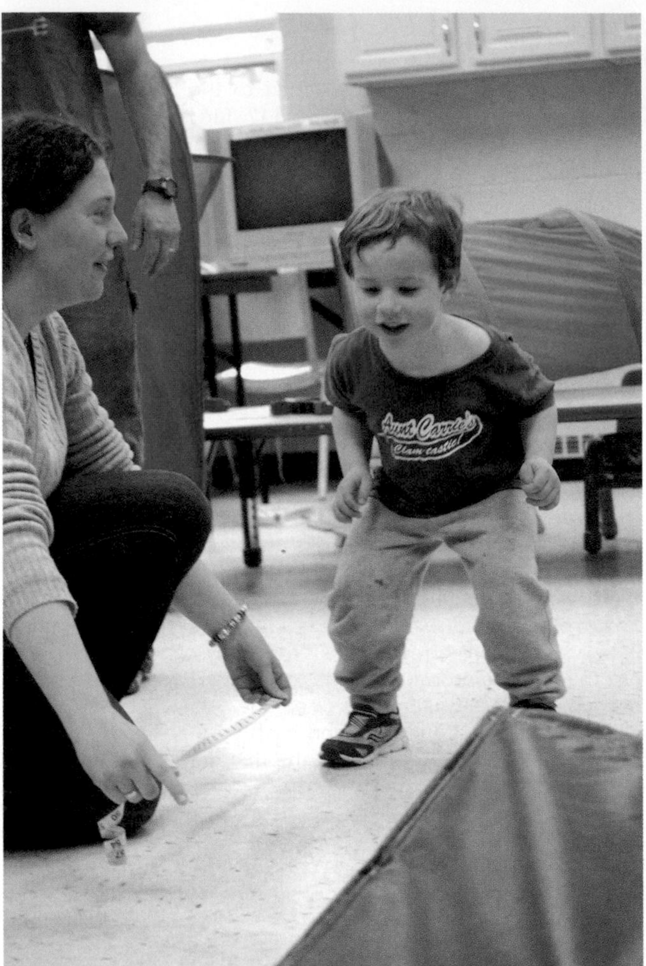

FIGURE 6-1 A therapist prepares to test a child on the broad jump item from the Bruininks-Oseretsky Test of Motor Proficiency 2.

incorporate materials and activities that are reasonably familiar and typical for children of the age group being tested. A child's performance on an individual test item is not as important as the overall subtest or area score. However, it is important for the therapist to observe the quality and characteristics of a child's performance on each item, as these qualitative observations provide important information to complement the obtained standard scores.

Norm-referenced tests have standardized protocols for administration and scoring. The tester must adhere to these protocols so that each test administration is as similar as possible to that of the normative sample. This is necessary to compare any child's performance fairly with that of the normative sample.

Sometimes the examiner must deviate from the standard protocol because of special needs of the child being tested. For instance, a child with visual impairments may need manual guidance to cut with scissors, or a child with cerebral palsy may need assistance stabilizing the shoulder and upper arm to reach and grasp a crayon. If changes are made in the standardized procedures, the examiner must indicate this in the summary of assessment, and standard scores cannot be used to describe that child's performance in comparison with the normative sample.

Norm-referenced tests have specific psychometric properties. They have been analyzed by statisticians to obtain score distributions, mean or average scores, and standard scores. This is done to achieve the primary objective of norm-referenced tests: comparability of scores with the normative sample. A test under development initially has a much larger number of items than the final version of the test. Through pilot testing, items are chosen or rejected based partly on how well they statistically discriminate between children of different ages and/or abilities. Items are not chosen primarily for their relevance to functional skills. Consequently, some norm-referenced tests are not intended to link test performance with specific objectives or goals for intervention. Other norm-referenced tests, such as the Sensory Profile, are designed to specifically evaluate the effect of sensory processes on functional performance in daily life and, when combined with other evaluation and observation data, to allow therapists to develop intervention goals. A portion of the Sensory Profile questionnaire is presented in Figure 6-3.

A criterion-referenced test, by contrast, is designed to provide information on how children perform on specific tasks. The term *criterion-referenced* refers to the fact that a child's performance is compared with a particular criterion, or level of performance of a particular skill. The goal of a criterion-referenced test is to determine which skills a child can and cannot accomplish, thereby providing a focus for intervention. In general the content of a criterion-referenced test is detailed and in some cases may relate to specific behavioral or functional objectives. The intent of a criterion-referenced test is to measure a child's performance on specific tasks rather than to compare the child's performance with that of his or her peers.

Many developmental checklists have been field tested and then published as criterion-referenced tests. The HELP is a good example of a developmental checklist designed to be used with children from birth to 3 years of age, and from 3 to 6 years of age.[59] It contains a large number of items in each of the domains of gross motor, fine motor, language, cognitive, social-emotional, and self-help skills. Each item correlates with specific intervention objectives. For instance, if a child is not able to pass Fine Motor item 4.81, Snips with Scissors, a list of intervention ideas is presented in the HELP activity guide.[28] The activity guide provides ideas for developmentally appropriate activities that link to the assessment items. The administration protocol for this item and the associated intervention activities are presented in Boxes 6-2 and 6-3.

Administration and scoring procedures may or may not be standardized on a criterion-referenced test. The HELP has standard procedures for administering and scoring each item. In contrast, the SFA is a judgment-based questionnaire completed by one or more school professionals familiar with the child's performance at school.[14] Criteria for rating the child's performance on each item are provided. School professionals are encouraged to collaborate in determining ratings and to use these ratings as a basis for designing an intervention plan. Figure 6-4 shows a category of activity performance with the associated rating scale. Many other criterion-referenced tests take the form of checklists, in which the specific performance needed to receive credit on an item is not indicated. Many therapist-designed tests for use in a particular facility or setting are non-standardized, criterion-referenced tests.

Criterion-referenced tests are not subjected to the statistical analyses performed on norm-referenced tests. No mean score

Item 8: **Standing Heel-to-Toe on a Balance Beam**

Number of Trials	Maximum Raw Score
2	10 seconds

Equipment
Balance Beam
Target
stopwatch

Procedure

- The examinee stands with preferred foot on the balance beam and non-preferred foot on the floor.
- The examinee places hands on hips.
- The examinee takes one step forward, placing non-preferred foot on the balance beam and touching heel of front foot to toe of back foot, and looks at the target.
- Conduct the second trial *only if* the examinee does not earn the maximum score of 10 seconds on the first trial.

Scoring

- Record the number of seconds, to the nearest tenth of a second, that the examinee maintains proper form, up to 10 seconds.
- Stop the trial after 10 seconds or if the examinee fails to keep feet heel-to-toe, fails to keep hands on hips, or steps or falls off the beam.

Administration

Teach the task to the examinee. Then, say,

Stand heel-to-toe on the beam until I tell you to stop. Ready? Begin.

Begin timing *when the examinee attains proper form.* After 10 seconds or when the examinee breaks proper form, say,

Stop.

If the examinee does not earn the maximum score of 10 seconds, conduct the second trial. If necessary, reteach the task after you say,

Let's try it again.

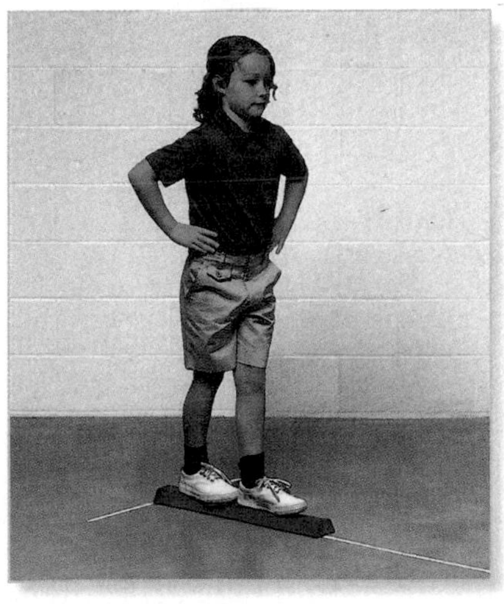

Subtest 5: **Balance** 71

FIGURE 6-2 Administration and scoring protocol for Bruininks-Oseretsky Test of Motor Proficiency 2, subtest 5, item 8. (From Bruininks, R. H., & Bruininks, B. [2005]. *Bruininks-Oseretsky Test of Motor Proficiency 2*. Circle Pines, MN: American Guidance Service.)

Sensory Processing

Item			A. Auditory Processing	ALWAYS	FREQUENTLY	OCCASIONALLY	SELDOM	NEVER
👂	L	1	Responds negatively to unexpected or loud noises (for example, cries or hides at noise from vacuum cleaner, dog barking, hair dryer)					
👂	L	2	Holds hands over ears to protect ears from sound					
👂	L	3	Has trouble completing tasks when the radio is on					
👂	L	4	Is distracted or has trouble functioning if there is a lot of noise around					
👂	L	5	Can't work with background noise (for example, fan, refrigerator)					
👂	H	6	Appears to not hear what you say (for example, does not "tune-in" to what you say, appears to ignore you)					
👂	H	7	Doesn't respond when name is called but you know the child's hearing is OK					
👂	H	8	Enjoys strange noises/seeks to make noise for noise's sake					
			Section Raw Score Total					

Comments

FIGURE 6-3 A portion of the caregiver questionnaire for the Sensory Profile. (From Dunn, W. [1999]. *Sensory Profile user's manual.* San Antonio, TX: Psychological Corp.)

BOX 6-2 Administration and Assessment Procedures and Processes for Hawaii Early Learning Profile: Item 4.81—Snips with Scissors (23-25 Months)

- Definition: The child cuts a paper edge randomly, one snip at a time, rather than using a continuous cutting motion.
- Example observation opportunities: Incidental—May observe while the child is preparing for a tea party with stuffed animals or dolls. Demonstrate making fringe on paper placemats and invite the child to help. Structured—Using a half piece of sturdy paper and blunt scissors, make three snips in separate places along the edge of the paper while the child is watching. Exaggerate the opening and closing motions of your hand. Offer the child the scissors and invite him or her to make a cut. Let the child explore the scissors (if interested), helping him or her position the scissors in his or her hand as needed.
- Credit: Snips paper in one place, holding the paper in one hand and scissors in the other (see also Credit Notes in this strand's preface).

From Parks, S. (2006). *Inside HELP: Administration and reference manual for the Hawaii Early Learning Profile.* Palo Alto, CA: VORT.

BOX 6-3 Administration and Assessment Procedures and Processes for Hawaii Early Learning Profile Item 4.81—Snips with Scissors: Activity Guide Suggestions

The child cuts with the scissors, taking one snip at a time rather than doing continuous cutting.

1. Let the child use small kitchen tongs to pick up objects and to practice opening and closing motions.
2. Let the child use child-sized scissors with rounded tips.
3. Demonstrate by placing your finger and thumb through the handles.
4. Position the scissors with the finger holes one above the other. Position the child's forearm in mid-supination (i.e., thumb up). Let the child place his or her thumb through the top hole and the middle finger through the bottom hole. If the child's fingers are small, place the index and middle fingers in the bottom hole. The child will adjust his or her fingers as experience is gained.
5. Let the child open and close the scissors. Assist as necessary by placing your hand over the child's hand.
6. Let the child snip narrow strips of paper and use it for fringe in art work.
7. The different types of scissors available for children are a scissors with reinforced rubber coating on the handle grips; a scissors with double handle grips for your hand and the child's hand; a left-handed scissors; and a scissors for a prosthetic hook. Use the different types of child's scissors appropriately as required.

From Furuno, S., O'Reilly, K. A., Hosaka, C. M., Zeisloft, B., & Allman, T. (2005). *HELP activity guide.* Palo Alto, CA: VORT.

or normal distribution is calculated; a child may pass all items or fail all items on a particular test without adversely affecting the validity of the test results. The purpose of the test is to learn exactly what a child can accomplish, not to compare the child's performance with that of the peer group. This goal is also reflected in the test development process for criterion-referenced tests. Items are generally chosen based on a process of task analysis or identification of important developmental milestones rather than for their statistical validity. Therefore the specific items on a criterion-referenced test have a direct relationship with functional skills and can be used as a starting point for generating appropriate goals and objectives for therapy intervention.

The characteristics of norm- and criterion-referenced tests are compared in Table 6-3. As is shown in the table, some tests are both norm- and criterion-referenced. This means that although the items have been analyzed for their ability to perform statistically, they also reflect functional or developmental skills that are appropriate for intervention. These tests permit the therapist to compare a child's performance with that of peers in the normative sample, and they also provide information about specific skills that may be appropriate for remediation.

The Peabody Developmental Motor Scales (2nd ed.; PDMS-2) is an example of both a norm- and criterion-referenced test. Although the PDMS-2 has been subjected to the statistical analyses used in norm-referenced tests, many individual items in the test also represent developmental milestones that can be targeted as specific intervention goals. The SFA, although primarily a criterion-referenced test, provides a criterion score and standard error for each raw score based on a national standardization sample.

Standardized tests can also be categorized as performance-based or self-report. Self-report tests collect data on the child's performance, behavior, or participation in daily activities and natural environments from adults such as parents, caregivers, teachers, or therapists who interact regularly with the child or from the child himself or herself. The advantage of self-report tests is that the score represents typical or usual behavior, performance, or participation based on multiple observations of the child in different times and places. The disadvantage of self-report tests is that respondents may not carefully read or understand the test instructions or may answer according to what they believe the evaluator wants to hear. Clarity of questions and criteria for respondent ratings is crucial to the quality of a self-report test. Test development procedures include data collection from potential respondents so that they can provide input to ensure that the test content is meaningful and the items and procedures are easily understandable.[40] Careful instruction of respondents at the time of the evaluation can also facilitate accuracy of responses. Self-report tests have been developed for developmental screening—the Ages and Stages Questionnaire,

Behavior Regulation

1. Displays appropriate restraint regarding self-stimulation (e.g., refrains from head banging, hand flapping).	1 2 3 4
2. Accepts unexpected changes in routine.	1 2 3 4
3. Refrains from provoking others.	1 2 3 4
4. Uses nonaggressive words and actions.	1 2 3 4
5. Maintains behavioral control in large groups of students (e.g., cafeteria, assemblies).	1 2 3 4
6. Hears constructive criticism without losing temper.	1 2 3 4
7. Uses words rather than physical actions to respond when provoked or angry at others.	1 2 3 4
8. Seeks adult assistance, if necessary, when experiencing peer conflict, especially conflicts involving violence.	1 2 3 4
9. Responds to/handles teasing in a constructive way.	1 2 3 4
10. Handles frustration when experiencing difficulties with school tasks/activities.	1 2 3 4
11. Shows common sense in words and actions around bullies, gangs, or strangers.	1 2 3 4
12. Resolves ordinary peer conflicts or problems adequately on his/her own without requesting teacher assistance.	1 2 3 4
Respondent's Initials — **Behavior Regulation Raw Score**	

Ratings Key for Activity Performance

1: Does not perform **2:** Partial performance **3:** Inconsistent performance **4:** Consistent performance

FIGURE 6-4 One category of activity performance and corresponding rating scale for the School Function Assessment (SFA). (From Coster, W., Deeney, T., Haltiwanger, J., & Haley, S. [1998]. *School Function Assessment.* San Antonio, TX: Psychological Corp.)

TABLE 6-3 Comparison of Norm-Referenced and Criterion-Referenced Tests

Characteristic	Norm-Referenced Test	Criterion-Referenced Test
Purpose	Comparison of child's performance with normative sample	Comparison of child's performance with a defined list of skills
Content	General; usually covers a wide variety of skills	Detailed; may cover specific objectives or developmental milestones
Administration and scoring	Always standardized	May be standardized or non-standardized
Psychometric properties	Normal distribution of scores; means, standard deviations, and standard scores computed	No score distribution needed; a child may pass or fail all items
Item selection	Items chosen for statistical performance; may not relate to functional skills or therapy objectives	Items chosen for functional and developmental importance; provides necessary information for developing therapy objectives
Examples	BSID-III; PDMS-2; BOT-2; PEDI-CAT	PDMS-2, PEDI-CAT, HELP, Gross-Motor Function Measure, SFA

BOT-2, Bruininks-Oseretsky Test of Motor Proficiency (2nd ed.); BSID-III, Bayley Scales of Infant and Toddler Development (3rd ed.); HELP, Hawaii Early Learning Profile; PDMS, Peabody Developmental Motor Scales; PEDI-CAT, Pediatric Evaluation of Disability Inventory Computer Adaptive Test; SFA, School Function Assessment.

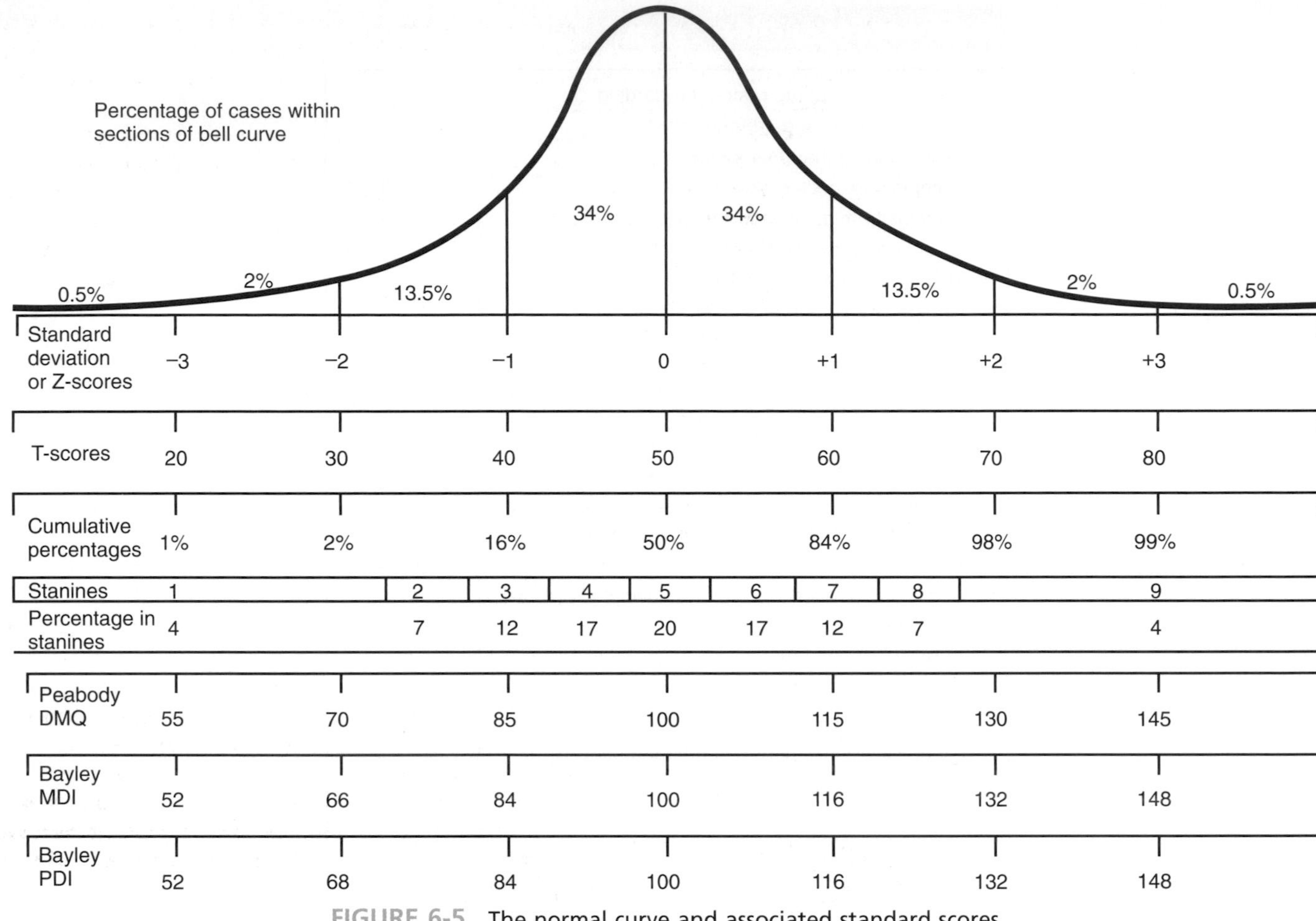

FIGURE 6-5 The normal curve and associated standard scores.

3rd ed.[56]—and for assessing aspects of participation and function—SFA,[14] CAPE, PAC,[39] CASP,[9] and PEDI-CAT.[32,34]

Technical Aspects

The following discussion of the technical aspects of standardized tests focuses on the statistics and test development procedures used for norm-referenced tests. Information on how standard scores are obtained and reported is included, as well as on how the reliability and validity of a test are evaluated. It is the responsibility of the test author to provide initial data on test reliability and validity. However, these test characteristics are never definitively determined, and ongoing evaluation of validity and reliability is necessary. Occupational therapists must comprehend the technical aspects of standardized tests to be able:

1. To analyze and select standardized tests appropriately, according to the child's age and functional level and the purpose of testing.
2. To interpret and report scores from standardized tests accurately.
3. To explain test results to caregivers and other professionals working with the child in a clear, understandable manner.

Presented next is information on (1) descriptive statistics, (2) standard scores, (3) correlation coefficients, (4) reliability, and (5) validity.

Descriptive Statistics

Descriptive statistics provide information about the characteristics of a particular group. Many human characteristics, such as height, weight, head size, and intelligence, are represented by a distribution called the normal curve (or bell-shaped curve) (Figure 6-5). The pattern of performance on most norm-referenced tests also follows this curve. The greatest number of people receive a score in the middle part of the distribution, with progressively smaller numbers receiving scores at either the high or the low end. Descriptive statistics also provide information about where members of a group are located on the normal curve. The two types of descriptive statistics are the measure of central tendency and the measure of variability.

The measure of central tendency indicates the middle point of the distribution for a particular group, or sample, of children. The most frequently used measure of central tendency is the mean, which is the sum of all the scores for a particular sample divided by the number of scores. It is computed mathematically using a simple formula:

$$\bar{X} = \frac{\sum X}{n}$$

where Σ means to sum, X is each individual score, and n is the number of scores in the sample. (The mean is also often called the *average score*.)

Another measure of central tendency is the median, which is simply the middle score of a distribution. Half the scores lie below the median and half above it. The median is the preferred measure of central tendency when outlying or extreme scores are present in the distribution. The following distribution of scores is an example:

2 3 13 14 17 17 18

The mean score is 12 [i.e., (2 + 3 + 13 + 14 + 17 + 17 + 18) ÷ 7]. The median, or middle score, is 14. In this case the score of 14 is a more accurate representation of the middle point of these scores than is the score of 12 because the two low scores, or outliers, in the distribution pulled down the value of the mean.

The measure of variability determines how much the performance of the group as a whole deviates from the mean. Measures of variability are used to compute the standard scores used in standardized tests. As with measures of central tendency, measures of variability are derived from the normal curve. The two measures of variability discussed are the variance and the standard deviation.

The variance is the average of the squared deviations of the scores from the mean. In other words, it is a measure of how far the score of an average individual in a sample deviates from the group mean. The variance is computed using the following formula:

$$S^2 = \frac{\sum(X-\bar{X})^2}{n}$$

where S^2 is the variance, $\sum(X-\bar{X})^2$ is the sum of each individual score minus the mean score, and n is the total number of scores in the group. The standard deviation is simply the square root of the variance. To illustrate, calculations are provided for the mean, the variance, and the standard deviation for the following set of scores from a hypothetical test:

17 19 21 25 28

To calculate the mean, the following equation is used:

$$\frac{(17+19+21+25+28)}{5} = 22$$

To calculate the variance, the mean must be subtracted from each score, and that value then must be squared:

$$17-22=(-5)^2=25$$
$$19-22=(-3)^2=9$$
$$21-22=(-1)^2=1$$
$$25-22=(3)^2=9$$
$$28-22=(6)^2=36$$

The squared values are summed and then divided by the total number of scores:

$$25+9+1+9+36=80$$
$$80 \div 5 = 16$$

The variance of this score distribution is 16. The standard deviation is simply the square root of the variance, or 4.

The standard deviation (SD) is an important number because it is the basis for computing many standard scores. In a normal distribution (see Figure 6-5), 68% of the people in the distribution score within 1 SD of the mean (±1 SD); 95% score within 2 SD of the mean (±2 SD); and 99.7% score within 3 SD of the mean (±3 SD). In the score distribution with a mean of 22 and a standard deviation of 4, three of the five scores were within 1 SD of the mean (22 ± 4; a score range of 18-26), and all five scores were within 2 SD of the mean (22 ± 8; a score range of 14-30). The standard deviation, then, determines the placement of scores on the normal curve. By showing the degree of variability in the sample, the standard deviation reveals how far the scores can be expected to range from the mean value.

Standard Scores

Standardized tests are scored in several different ways. Scoring methods include Z-scores, T-scores, deviation intelligence quotient (IQ) scores, developmental index scores, percentile scores, and age-equivalent scores.

The Z-score is computed by subtracting the mean for the test from the individual's score and dividing it by the standard deviation, using the following equation:

$$Z = \frac{X-\bar{X}}{SD}$$

For the score distribution above (i.e., 17 19 21 25 28), the person receiving the score of 17 would have a Z-score of (17 − 22) ÷ 4 = −1.25. The person receiving the score of 28 would have a Z-score of (28 − 22) ÷ 4 = 1.5. The negative value of the first score indicates that the Z-score value is below the mean for the test, and the positive value of the second score indicates that the Z-score value is above the mean. Generally, a Z-score value of −1.5 or less is considered indicative of delay or deficit in the area measured, although this can vary, depending on the particular test.

The T-score is derived from the Z-score. In a T-score distribution, the mean is 50 and the standard deviation is 10. The T-score is computed using the following equation:

$$T = 10(Z) + 50$$

For the two Z-scores computed in the preceding, the T-score values are as follows: for the first Z-score of −1.25, the T-score is 10(−1.25) + 50 = 37.50. For the second Z-score of 1.5, the T-score is 10(1.5) + 50 = 65. Note that all T-scores have positive values, but because the mean of a T-score distribution is 50, any number less than 50 indicates a score below the mean. Because the standard deviation of the T distribution is 10, the first score of 37.50 is slightly more than 1 SD below the mean. The second score of 65 is 15 points, or 1.5 SD, above the mean.

Two other standard scores that are frequently seen in standardized tests are the deviation IQ score and the developmental index score. Deviation IQ scores have a mean of 100 and a standard deviation of either 15 or 16. These are the IQ scores obtained from such tests as the Stanford-Binet[61] or the Wechsler Intelligence Scale for Children (WISC).[65] On these tests, individuals with IQ scores 2 SD below the mean (IQs of 70 and 68, respectively) are considered to have an intellectual disability. Individuals with IQ scores 2 SD above the mean (IQs of 130 and 132, respectively) are considered gifted. Developmental index scores are used in developmental tests such as the

PDMS-2 and the BSID-III. Like the deviation IQ scores, they have a mean of 100 and a standard deviation of 15 or 16. Children who receive a developmental index score of 2 SD below the mean (index score of 68 or 70) in one or more skill areas are considered to be in need of remedial services. In many cases children who receive developmental index scores lower than −1.5 SD (index score of 85) may also be recommended for occupational therapy services.

Two other types of scores (i.e., percentile scores and age-equivalent scores) are frequently used in standardized tests. These are not standard scores in the strictest sense, because they are computed directly from raw scores rather than through the statistically derived measures of central tendency and variability. However, they give an indication of a child's performance relative to that of the normative sample.

The percentile score is the percentage of people in a standardization sample whose score is at or below a particular raw score. A percentile score of 60, for instance, indicates that 60% of the people in the standardization sample received a score that was at or below the raw score corresponding to the 60th percentile. Tests that use percentile scores generally include a table in the manual by which raw scores can be converted to percentile scores. These tables usually indicate at what percentile rank performance is considered deficient. Raw scores can be converted to percentile rank (PR) scores by a simple formula:

$$PR = \frac{(\text{Number of people below score} + \text{One half of people at score}) \times 100}{\text{Total number of scores}}$$

Using the previous sample data (i.e., 17 19 21 25 28), percentile ranks for the highest and lowest scores can be computed. The raw score of 17 is the lowest score in the distribution and is the only score of 17. Therefore the equation is as follows:

$$\frac{(0+0.5)}{5} \times 100 = \frac{0.5}{5} \times 100 = 10$$

The highest score in the distribution is 28; therefore four people have lower scores and one person received a score of 28. The equation is as follows:

$$\frac{(4+0.5)}{5} \times 100 = \frac{4.5}{5} \times 100 = 90$$

In this distribution, then, the lowest score is at the 10th percentile and the highest score is at the 90th percentile.

Although PR scores can be easily calculated and understood, they have a significant disadvantage: The percentile ranks are not equal in size across the score distribution. Distances between percentile ranks are much smaller in the middle of the distribution than at the ends; consequently, improving a score from the 50th to the 55th percentile requires much less effort than improving a score from the 5th to the 10th percentile (see Figure 6-5). As a result, an improvement in performance by a child functioning at the lower end of the score range may not be reflected in the PR score the child achieves. Other standard scores are more sensitive at measuring changes in the performance of children who fall at the extreme ends of the score distribution.

The age-equivalent score is the age at which the raw score is at the 50th percentile. The age-equivalent score generally is expressed in years and months, e.g., 4-3 (i.e., 4 years 3 months). It is a score that is easily understood by parents and caregivers who may not be familiar with testing concepts or terminology. However, age-equivalent scores have significant disadvantages. Although they may provide a general idea of a child's overall developmental level, it may be misleading to say, for example, that a 4-year-old is functioning at the 2.5-year level. The age-equivalent score may be more or less an average of several developmental domains, some of which may be at the 4.5-year level and some at the 1.5-year level. Therefore the child's performance may be highly variable and may not reflect that of a typical 2.5-year-old. In addition, because the age-equivalent score represents only the score that a child of a particular age who is performing at the 50th percentile would receive, a child who is performing within normal limits for his or her age but whose score is below the 50th percentile would receive an age-equivalent score below his or her chronologic age. This can cause parents or caregivers to conclude incorrectly that the child has delays. Age equivalents, then, are a type of standard score that can contribute to an understanding of a child's performance, but they are the least psychometrically sound, can be misleading, and should be used only with caution.

Reliability

The reliability of a test describes the consistency or stability of scores obtained by one individual when tested on two different occasions with different sets of items or under other variable examining conditions.[63] For instance, if a child is given a test and receives a score of 50 and 2 days later is given the same test and receives a score of 75, the reliability of the test is questionable. The difference between the two scores is called the error variance of the test, which is a result of random fluctuations in performance between the two testing sessions. Some amount of random error variance is expected in any test situation because of variations in such things as mood, fatigue, or motivation. Error variance can also be caused by environmental characteristics such as light, temperature, or noise. However, it is important that error variance caused by variations in examiners or by the characteristics of the test itself be minimal. Confidence in the scores obtained requires that the test have adequate reliability over a number of administrations and have low error variance.

Most standardized tests evaluate two or three forms of reliability. The three forms of reliability most commonly used in pediatric standardized tests are (1) test-retest reliability, (2) inter-rater reliability, and (3) standard error of measurement (SEM).

Test-Retest Reliability

Test-retest reliability is a measurement of the stability of a test over time. It is obtained by giving the test to the same individual on two different occasions. In the evaluation of test-retest reliability for a pediatric test, the time span between test administrations must be short to minimize the possibility of developmental changes occurring between the two test sessions. However, the time span between tests should not be so short that the child may recall items administered during the first test session, thereby improving his or her performance on the second test session (this is called the learning, or practice, effect).

During the process of test development, test-retest reliability is evaluated on a subgroup of the normative sample. The size and composition of the subgroup should be specified in the manual. The correlation coefficient between the scores of the two test sessions is the measure of the test-retest reliability. A test that has a high test-retest reliability coefficient is more likely to yield relatively stable scores over time. That is, it is affected less by random error variance than is a test with a low test-retest reliability coefficient. When administering a test with a low test-retest reliability coefficient, the examiner has less confidence that the score obtained is a true reflection of the child's abilities. If the child were tested at a different time of day or in a different setting entirely, different results might be obtained.

A sample of 197 children was evaluated twice within 2 weeks (mean retest interval of 6 days) to assess the test-retest reliability (stability) of the BSID-III Motor Scale.[7] Overall stability coefficients were 0.80 for the Fine Motor Scale, 0.82 for the Gross Motor Scale, and 0.83 for the Motor Composite. Test-retest stability was slightly higher for the older age groups. The performance of a young child often varies within short periods because he or she is highly influenced by variables such as mood, hunger, sleepiness, and irritability. The test-retest reliability coefficients for 50 children tested twice within 1 week with the PDMS-2 ranged from 0.73 for the Fine Motor Quotient and 0.84 for the Gross Motor Quotient for 2- to 11-month-old children to 0.94 for the Fine Motor Quotient and 0.93 for the Gross Motor Quotient for 12- to 17-month-old children.[24]

To evaluate test-retest reliability of the Sensory Processing Measure (SPM),[49] a rating scale of sensory processing, praxis, and social participation in home and school environments for children age 5-12, caregivers and teachers of 77 typically developing children completed the rating scale two times within a 2-week interval. Correlation coefficients for the scales ranged from 0.94 to 0.98. These three examples of good to excellent test-retest reliability are typical examples of scales that measure children's sensory processing and motor performance. The rapid and variable development of young children and the practice effect are two factors that negatively influence a test's stability over time. The test-retest reliability of a test is critical to its use as a measure of the child's progress or of intervention efficacy.

Inter-rater Reliability

Inter-rater reliability refers to the ability of two independent raters to obtain the same scores when scoring the same child simultaneously. Inter-rater reliability is generally measured on a subset of the normative sample during the test development process. This is often accomplished by having one rater administer and score the test while another rater observes and scores at the same time. The correlation coefficient calculated from the two raters' scores is the inter-rater reliability coefficient of the test. It is particularly important to measure inter-rater reliability on tests for which the scoring may require some judgment on the part of the examiner.

Although the scoring criteria for many test items are specific on most tests, scoring depends to a certain extent on individual judgment, and scoring differences can arise among different examiners. A test that has a low inter-rater reliability coefficient is especially susceptible to differences in scoring by different raters. This may mean that the administration and scoring criteria are not stated explicitly enough, requiring examiners to make judgment calls on a number of items. Alternatively, it can mean that the items on the test call for responses that are too broad or vague to permit precise scoring.

The inter-rater reliability of the M-FUN52 was evaluated by having pairs of examiners score the performance of 29 children on the M-FUN using the scoring rubrics developed for the standardization edition of the test. One examiner administered and scored while the second examiner observed and scored independently. Correlation coefficients were 0.91 for Visual Motor, 0.93 for Fine Motor, and 0.91 for Gross Motor. A second aspect of inter-rater reliability, decision agreement, was also evaluated. Decision agreement is the degree to which examiners' scores agree in the identification of a child as performing in the average range or below average range. Because standardized tests are used frequently to qualify children for services, it is important to know whether different examiners can consistently identify whether or not a child has impairments. On the M-FUN, decision agreement was 96% for Visual Motor, 97% for Fine Motor, and 93% for Gross Motor. The results of the inter-rater reliability studies on the M-FUN suggest that examiners can reliably score children's performance, and based on the obtained scores can make reliable determinations about the presence of impairment.

Inter-rater reliability for the PDMS-2 was evaluated using a slightly different method. Sixty completed test protocols were randomly selected from the normative sample and were independently scored by two examiners. The resulting correlation coefficients were 0.97 for the Gross Motor Composite and 0.98 for the Fine Motor Composite.[24] It should be noted that this method of determining reliability is not based on two independent observations of the child's performance but on review of completed scoring protocols. Hence, potential error related to the way examiners interpreted and applied the scoring criteria to determine scores on individual items was not addressed. This could result in spuriously high inter-rater reliability coefficients. In a test such as the DTVP-II, in which scores are based on a written record of the child's response, inter-rater reliability is excellent. When two individuals scored 88 completed DTVP-II protocols, the inter-scorer reliability was 0.98.[33]

Examiners can exert some control over the inter-rater reliability of tests they use frequently. It is good practice for examiners to check inter-rater reliability with more experienced colleagues when learning a new standardized test before beginning to administer the test to children in the clinical setting. Also, periodic checking of inter-rater reliability with colleagues who are administering the same standardized tests is a good practice. Some simple methods for assessing inter-rater reliability are discussed in more detail later in the chapter.

For self-report tests, inter-rater reliability is generally not a meaningful indicator of the psychometric integrity of the test, because each individual who contributes information to the test does so based on knowledge of the child in a specific environment with unique demands. However, because different raters may be evaluating the child on similar constructs, some agreement between ratings should be expected. This is known as cross-rater concordance, and is a measure of the validity of the instrument rather than reliability. For instance, on the SPM, concordance between caregiver (home) and teacher (school) ratings ranged from a coefficient of 0.31 for balance and motion to 0.55 for planning and ideas. These represent moderate to high correlations, but are lower than minimum inter-rater reliability standards for performance-based tests. These results are acceptable for a context-based instrument and reflect the importance of gathering data on a child's ability to engage in daily life tasks, activities, and occupations based on observations of the child over time in daily environments.

Acceptable Reliability

No universal agreement has been reached regarding the minimum acceptable coefficient for test-retest and inter-rater reliability. The context of the reliability measurement, the type of test, and the distribution of scores are some of the variables that can be taken into account when determining an acceptable reliability coefficient. One standard suggested by Urbina and used by a number of examiners is 0.80.[63]

Not all tests have test-retest or inter-rater reliability coefficients that reach the 0.80 level. Lower coefficients indicate greater variability in scores. When examiners use a test that has a reliability coefficient below 0.80, scores must be interpreted with great caution. For example, if one subtest of a test of motor development has test-retest reliability of 0.60, the examiner who uses it to measure change over time must acknowledge that a portion of the apparent change between the first and second test administration is a result of the error variance of the test.

When individual subtests of a comprehensive test have a low reliability coefficient, it is generally not recommended that the standard scores from the subtests be reported. Often the reliability coefficient of the entire test is much higher than that of the individual subtests. One reason for this is that reliability increases with the number of items on a test. Because subtests have fewer items than the entire test, they are more sensitive to fluctuations in the performance or scoring of individual items. When this occurs, it is best to describe subtest performance qualitatively, without reporting standard scores.

Standard scores can be reported for the total, or comprehensive, test score. Examiners should consult the reliability information in the test manual before deciding how to report test scores for individual subtests and for the test as a whole. The test-retest and inter-rater reliability coefficients reported in the manual are estimates based on the context and conditions used during test development and may vary when children are tested in different contexts or when examiners have differing levels of training and experience.

Standard Error of Measurement

The standard error of measurement (SEM) is a statistic used to calculate the expected range of error for the test score of an individual. It is based on the range of scores an individual might obtain if the same test were administered a number of times simultaneously, with no practice or fatigue effects. Obviously, this is impossible; the SEM, therefore, is a theoretical construct. However, it is an indicator of the possible error variance in individual scores.

The SEM creates a normal curve for the individual's test scores, with the obtained score in the middle of the distribution. The child has a higher probability of receiving scores in the middle of the distribution than at the extreme ends. The SEM is based on the standard deviation of the test and the test's reliability (usually the test-retest reliability). The SEM can be calculated using the following formula:

$$\text{SEM} = \text{SD}\sqrt{(1-r)}$$

where SEM is the standard error of measurement, SD is the standard deviation, and r is the reliability coefficient for the test (test-test reliability coefficients are the ones most commonly used). Once the SEM has been calculated for a test, that value is added to and subtracted from the child's obtained score. This gives the range of expected scores for that child, a range known as the confidence interval. The SEM corresponds to the standard deviation for the normal curve: 68% of the scores in a normal distribution fall within 1 SD on either side of the mean, 95% of the scores fall within 2 SD on either side of the mean, and 99.7% of the scores fall within 3 SD on either side of the mean. Similarly, a child receives a score within 1 SEM on either side of his or her obtained score 68% of the time; a score within 2 SEM of the obtained score 95% of the time; and a score within 3 SEM of the obtained score 99.7% of the time.

Generally, test manuals report the 95% confidence interval. As can be seen by the preceding equation, when the SD of the test is high or the reliability is low, the SEM increases. A larger SEM means that the range of possible scores for an individual child is much greater (i.e., a larger confidence interval) and consequently the degree of possible error is greater. This means that the examiner is less confident that any score obtained for a child on that test represents the child's true score.

An example may help to illustrate this point. Two tests are given, both consisting of 50 items and both testing the same skill area. One test has an SD of 1.0 and a test-retest reliability coefficient of 0.90. The SEM for that test is calculated as follows:

$$\text{SEM} = \sqrt{(1-0.90)}$$
$$\text{SEM} = 0.32$$

The second test has an SD of 5.0 and a test-retest reliability coefficient of 0.75. The SEM for that test would be calculated as follows:

$$\text{SEM} = 5\sqrt{(1-0.75)}$$
$$\text{SEM} = 2.5$$

Using the SEM, a 95% confidence interval can be calculated for each test. A 95% confidence interval is 2 SEM; therefore, test 1 has a confidence interval of ±0.64 points from the obtained score, or a total of 1.28 points. Test 2 has a confidence interval of ±5 points, or a total of 10 points. If both tests were available for a particular client, an examiner could use test 1 with much more confidence that the obtained score is truly representative of that individual's abilities and is not caused by random error variance of the test.

Occupational therapists who use standardized tests should be aware of how much measurement error a test contains so that the potential range of performance can be estimated for each individual. Currently, the trend is to report standardized test results as confidence intervals rather than as individual scores.[16,30] Several tests, such as the BSID-III, the M-FUN, and the BOT-2, include confidence intervals for subtest or scaled scores so that examiners can determine the potential score range for each child. According to Bayley, "Confidence intervals also serve as a reminder that measurement error is inherent in all test scores and that the observed test score is only an estimate of true ability" (p. 104).[7]

Consideration of the SEM is especially important when the differences between two scores are evaluated (e.g., when the progress a child has made with therapy over time is evaluated).[63] If the confidence intervals of the two test scores overlap, it may be incorrect to conclude that any change has occurred. For instance, a child is tested in September and receives a raw score of 60. The child is tested again in June with the same test and receives a raw score of 75. Comparison of the two raw scores would seem to indicate that the child has made substantial progress. However, the scores should be considered in light of an SEM of 5.0. Using a 95% confidence interval (the 95% confidence interval is 2 SEM on either side of the obtained score), the confidence interval for the first score is 50-70, and the confidence interval of the second score is 65-85.

Based on the two test scores, it cannot be conclusively stated that the child has made progress because the confidence intervals overlap. It is conceivable that a substantial amount of the difference between the first and second scores is a result of error variance rather than actual change in the child's abilities. Therefore the SEM is a tool to aid in determining whether changes in test scores over time are statistically significant.[46] This statistically significant difference is sometimes called the minimum detectable change (MDC). Because the MDC is a statistical measure, some authors discuss the need to also calculate the minimal clinically important difference (MCID), which is an observable difference in the individual's performance or perceived quality of life.[27] To determine the MCID, therapists can use additional methods of obtaining data on satisfaction, perceived quality of life, or perceived improvement in conjunction with the standardized test. Assessment of clinically important difference is also consistent with recommended practice of evaluating all relevant aspects of occupational performance, including client, context, and activity.[1]

Validity

Validity is the extent to which a test measures what it claims it measures.[63] For example, it is important for testers to know that a test of fine motor development actually measures fine motor skills and not gross motor or perceptual skills. The validity of a test must be established with reference to the particular use for which the test is being considered.[63] For instance, a test of fine motor development is probably highly valid as a measure of fine motor skills. It is less valid as a measure of visual motor skills and has low validity as a measure of gross motor skills.

The information on validity reported in test manuals has been obtained during the test development process. In addition, after a test becomes available commercially, clinicians and researchers continue to evaluate validity and to publish the results of their validation studies. This information about test validity can help examiners make decisions about appropriate uses of standardized tests. The four categories of validity are construct-related validity, content-related validity, criterion-related validity, and Rasch analysis.

Construct-Related Validity

Construct-related validity is the extent to which a test measures a particular theoretical construct. Some constructs frequently measured by pediatric occupational therapists include fine motor skills, visual-perceptual skills, self-care skills, gross motor skills, and functional performance at home or school. This chapter discusses a few of the many ways to determine construct validity.

One method of establishing construct validity involves investigating how well a test discriminates among different groups of individuals. For instance, a developmental test (e.g., BSID-III, PDMS-2, BOT-2) is expected to differentiate between the performance of older and younger children. Older children should receive higher scores than younger children, providing clear evidence of developmental progression with advancing age. Because these tests are also intended to discriminate typically developing children from children with developmental delays, children in specific diagnostic categories should receive lower scores than children with no documented deficits. This type of construct validity analysis is termed the ***known groups*** method.[52]

For example, during development of the Sensory Profile,[17] the sensory processing patterns of children in the following clinical groups were evaluated: attention deficit hyperactivity disorder, autism/pervasive developmental disorder, fragile X disorder, sensory modulation disorder, and other disabilities. The scores for children in each of these groups differed from that of the standardization sample, with the score ranges for all factors generally lower than those for the standardization sample. Therefore the Sensory Profile is able to differentiate children with typical sensory processing from those who have sensory processing differences. In addition, score patterns for various clinical groups were identified, allowing therapists to compare client scores with those of the corresponding clinical group. Subsequent research using the Sensory Profile has identified specific differences in sensory processing scores and sensory processing profiles for children with autism spectrum disorder, fragile X disorder, and fetal alcohol syndrome.[19,26,53,62,64]

Factor analysis can be used as another method of establishing construct-related validity. Factor analysis is a statistical procedure for determining relationships between test items. In a test of motor skills that includes gross motor items and fine motor items, factor analysis is expected to identify two factors on which items showed the strongest correlation, one composed mostly of gross motor items and one composed mostly of fine motor items. Factor analysis of the Sensory Integration and Praxis Tests (SIPT)[4] resulted in identification of four primary factors. The constructs measured were visual-perceptual skills (related to praxis), somatosensory-praxis skills, bilateral integration and sequencing of movements, and praxis on verbal command.[5] Factor analysis helped establish the functions that are measured by the SIPT and that can be used to interpret the results of testing individual children.

The third method of establishing construct-related validity requires repeated administration of a test before and after a period of intervention. For example, a group of children are given a test of visual-perceptual skills and subsequently receive intervention focused on improving those skills. They are then retested with the same test and the difference in scores is analyzed. A rise in test scores supports the assertion that the test measured visual-perceptual skills and provides evidence of construct-related validity.

TABLE 6-4 Correlations Between the Sensory Profile and the School Function Assessment

	School Function Assessment			
	Behavioral Regulation		Positive Interaction	
Sensory Profile	*Adaptations*	*Assistance*	*Adaptations*	*Assistance*
1 Sensory Seeking	−0.434	−0.436	−0.095	−0.328
2 Emotionally Reactive	−0.372	−0.360	−0.245	−0.282
3 Low Endurance/Tone	−0.584*	−0.721*	−0.584*	−0.716*
4 Oral Sensory Sensitivity	−0.199	−0.320	0.007	−0.300
5 Inattention/Distractibility	−0.582*	−0.584*	−0.495	−0.373
6 Poor Registration	−0.615*	−0.340	−0.348	−0.388
7 Sensory Sensitivity	−0.452	−0.478	−0.546*	−0.388
8 Sedentary	−0.551*	−0.554*	−0.545*	−0.368
9 Fine Motor/Perceptual	−0.502	−0.720†	−0.703†	−0.681†

*Correlation is significant at the 0.05 level (two-tailed).
†Correlation is significant at the 0.01 level (two-tailed).
Modified from Dunn, W. (1999). *Sensory Profile user's manual* (p. 54). San Antonio, TX: Psychological Corporation.

Content-Related Validity

Content-related validity is the extent to which the items on a test accurately sample a particular behavior domain. For instance, to test self-care skills, it is impractical to ask a child to perform every conceivable self-care activity. A sample of self-care activities must be chosen for inclusion on the test, and conclusions can be drawn about the child's abilities on the basis of the selected items. Examiners must have confidence that self-care skills are adequately represented so that accurate conclusions regarding the child's self-care skills can be made. Test manuals should show evidence that the authors have systematically analyzed the domain being tested. Content validity is established by review of the test content by experts in the field, who reach some agreement that the content is, in fact, representative of the behavioral domain to be measured.

Criterion-Related Validity

Criterion-related validity is the ability of a test to predict how an individual performs on other measurements or activities. To establish criterion-related validity, the test score is checked against a criterion, an independent measure of what the test is designed to predict. The two forms of criterion-related validity are concurrent validity and predictive validity.

Concurrent validity describes how well test scores reflect current performance. The degree of relationship between the test and the criterion is described with a correlation coefficient. Most validity correlation coefficients range from 0.40 to 0.80; a coefficient of 0.70 or above indicates that performance on one test can predict performance on a second test.

Concurrent validity is examined in the test development process to determine the relationship between a new test and existing tests that measure a similar construct. For instance, during the development of the Sensory Profile, children were scored with both the Sensory Profile and the SFA. The SFA was chosen because some aspects of children's performance at school depend on sensory processing and modulation.[17] High correlations between SFA performance items and the Fine Motor/Perceptual factor on the Sensory Profile were expected, because both tests address hand use. In addition, the SFA socialization and behavior interaction sections were expected to correlate highly with the modulation sections and factors on the Sensory Profile, because problems with regulating sensory input could result in problems with generating appropriate responses. The scores on the two tests were compared for a random sample of 16 children enrolled in special education programs. Portions of the correlational data are presented in Table 6-4. The correlations are negative because of the different scoring systems on the two tests; lower scores are desirable on the SFA but undesirable on the Sensory Profile.

As Table 6-4 shows, the two tests share areas of moderate to high correlation and areas of low correlation. Factor 9, which consists of items describing product-oriented behaviors, correlated strongly with three sections of the SFA. Factors 3, 6, and 8 on the Sensory Profile contain items that indicate low responsiveness, whereas Factor 5 contains items indicating over-responsiveness. These four factors correlated moderately with the Behavioral Regulation and Positive Interaction sections of the SFA, suggesting relationships between sensory processing and modulation, and children's social/behavioral repertoires.[17] This pattern of correlation coefficients supports the research hypotheses about relationships between the constructs measured by the two tests and also supports the validity of the Sensory Profile as a measure of sensory processing and modulation.

In contrast with concurrent validity, predictive validity identifies the relationship between a test given in the present and some measure of performance in the future. Establishing predictive validity is a much lengthier process than establishing other forms of validity because often several years must elapse between the first and second testing sessions. The predictive validity of a test often is not well documented until it has been in use for several years. Barbosa, Campbell, and Berbaum studied the predictive validity of the Test of Infant Motor Performance (TIMP).[6] These researchers examined how well the TIMP, when administered shortly after birth, predicted the infant's outcome at 12 months. Using a sample of 96 at-risk infants recruited from special care nurseries, the infants were categorized as developmentally delayed, cerebral palsy, or typical at 12 months on the basis of their scores on the Alberta

Infant Motor Scale and physician's clinical judgment. The TIMP scores at 13 weeks correctly classified all of the infants at 12 months. Two items, hand-to-mouth and fingering objects, were identified as highly accurate predictors of cerebral palsy (i.e., children with cerebral palsy did not exhibit fingering or hand-to-mouth movements).

One final point about criterion-related validity: The meaningfulness of the comparison between a test and its criterion measure depends on both the quality of the test and the quality of the criterion. Because no single measure of criterion-related validity provides conclusive evidence of the test's validity, multiple investigations should be undertaken. Important standardized assessments undergo extensive evaluation of validity after publication. The resulting information helps the test user decide when and with whom the test results are most valid.

In summary, validity is an important but sometimes elusive concept that rests on a number of judgments by authors of the tests, users of the tests, and experts in the field. It is important to remember that validity is not an absolute and that a test that is valid in one setting or with one group of children may not be valid for other uses. Test users must not assume that because a test has been developed and published for commercial distribution, it is universally useful and appropriate. An examiner must apply his or her clinical knowledge and experience, knowledge of normal and abnormal development, and understanding of an individual child's situation when deciding whether test findings are a valid measure of the child's abilities.

Rasch Models of Measurement

The Rasch models of measurement[2] have been used to develop item scaling for several tests in the field of occupational therapy. The SFA, the PEDI-CAT, and the Assessment of Motor and Process Skills (AMPS)[21,22] have used Rasch methodology in the test development process. Rasch methodology has also been used to develop a school version of the AMPS (School AMPS).[3,23]

A test instrument developed using Rasch methodology must meet several assumptions.[14] The construct being measured (e.g., activities of daily living) can be represented as a continuous function with measurement covering the full range of possible performance from dependent to independent. The instrument (or individual scale of the instrument) measures one characteristic (or construct) of performance, and each item represents a sample of the characteristics measured. The scale provides estimates of item difficulty that are independent of the sample of persons tested, and an individual's ability estimate is independent of the specific items tested.

The Rasch model generates a hierarchic ranking of items on the test from easiest to most difficult, creating a linear scale of items from ordinal observations. With the items ranked along the continuum within each skill area, an individual's performance can be assessed in light of an item's difficulty rather than against a normative sample. The ranking of items creates an expected pattern of mastery of items; the model predicts that more difficult items on the continuum are mastered only after easier items have been learned. Therefore therapists who administer an assessment tool developed using Rasch methodology generally can assume that the most appropriate goals for intervention will be the items and/or skills immediately above the items successfully passed by the client.

Occupational therapy tests developed using Rasch methodology emerge from a different philosophic base than traditional standardized tests. The two main methods of data collection are naturalistic observation and parent/teacher/caregiver report. The tasks observed are the ones the child engages in daily (e.g., schoolwork, self-care, social participation, mobility) rather than items administered in a controlled testing situation. Intervention recommendations can be generated directly from the child's observed and/or reported performance and participation.

Tests developed using the Rasch model are generally not considered norm-referenced tests because individual performance is not compared against that of a normative sample. However, some of these tests provide options to calculate standard scores. For instance, PEDI-CAT scores can be converted to T-scores.[32] The Rasch model provides an objective measure of performance that can be linked directly to desired occupational performance outcomes. The Rasch model has been applied to a variety of rating scales and traditional measurement instruments to assess disablement and functional status.[31,54] It is a model that can be used alone or in conjunction with traditional test development and measurement theory to produce measurement tools that provide a clearer connection between the assessment process and intervention planning.

Becoming a Competent Test User

The amount of technical information presented here might make the prospect of learning to administer a standardized test seem daunting. However, potential examiners can take a number of specific steps to ensure that they administer and score a test reliably. These steps also help examiners interpret test results accurately so that they provide a valid representation of each child's abilities. This section discusses the process of learning to administer and interpret any standardized test, be it a screening tool or a comprehensive assessment.

Choosing the Appropriate Test

The therapist's first step is to decide which test, or tests, to learn. A number of standardized tests used by pediatric occupational therapists address a wide age span and a number of different performance skills and areas of occupation. The examiner must decide which tests are most likely to meet the assessment needs of his or her particular work setting and the children served in that setting. For instance, an occupational therapist working in an early intervention setting might use the BSID-III or the PEDI-CAT.[32] A therapist working in preschools might use the M-FUN or the PDMS-2. A therapist working in a school-based setting might use the SFA, the School AMPS, or BOT-2. Instruments such as the PEDI-CAT or the AMPS can be used in a variety of settings.[34]

A number of other standardized tests are available that assess more specialized areas of function, such as the SIPT, the Developmental Test of Visual-Motor Integration,[8] the Sensory Profile, or the DTVP-II. Examiners should consult with other therapists working in their practice settings to determine which tests are most commonly used. In addition, they should examine the characteristics of the children referred to them for assessment to determine which tests are most appropriate.

Some children may not be able to comply with standardized testing procedures. Occupational therapists evaluating children whose behavior, cognition, motor skills, or attention limit their ability to follow standardized testing procedures often make adjustments in the standardized testing procedures or use parent-report assessments.[58]

Some standardized tests provide specific instructions, guidelines, or norms to be used with children who have a variety of disabilities. For example, the PDMS-2 provides case illustrations of how the test can be adapted for children with vision impairment and cerebral palsy. The BSID-III and the Sensory Profile provide normative data for several clinical groups. Piper and Darrah, in developing the AIMS, used infants who were preterm or born with congenital anomalies, as well as those who were full term and those who did not have an unusual diagnosis.[51] The PEDI-CAT, the Gross Motor Function Measure (GMFM),[55] and the SFA are examples of tests that evaluate function and participation of children with identified disabilities. The PEDI-CAT measures the level of caregiver assistance and environmental modifications required for children to perform specific functional tasks. The PEDI-CAT assesses the level of independence and the quality of performance of children whose disabilities may prevent them from executing a particular task in a typical way. The GMFM is a criterion-referenced test that measures the components of a gross motor activity accomplished by children with cerebral palsy. It provides information necessary for designing intervention programs and measuring small increments of change. The SFA evaluates the child's performance of functional tasks that support participation in the academic and social aspects of an elementary school program.

It may also be appropriate to consult other sources for information about a test. The Seventeenth Mental Measurements Yearbook[29] and Tests in Print VII[47] publish descriptions and critical reviews of commercially available standardized tests written by testing experts. These resources can also be accessed online through most university library systems. In addition, published studies of the validity or reliability of tests relevant to pediatric occupational therapists appear throughout the occupational therapy literature. See Table 6-1 for a list of selected standardized tests arranged by information source.

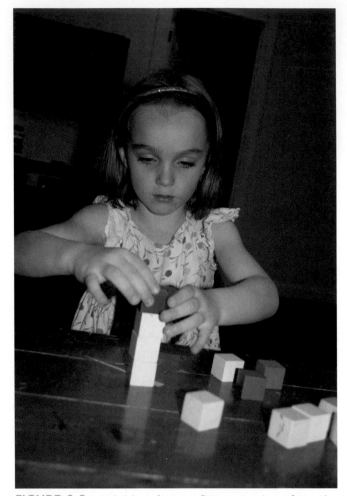

FIGURE 6-6 A child performs a fine motor item from the PDMS-2.

Learning the Test

Once a decision has been made about which test to learn, the therapist should read the test manual carefully. In addition to administration and scoring techniques, the technical attributes of the test should be studied. Particular attention should be paid to the size and composition of the normative sample, the reliability coefficients, the validation data, and the intended population for the test. The examiner should determine the standardized administration procedures and whether they can be altered for children with special needs. He or she should also understand how the scores should be reported and interpreted if the standardized procedure is changed.

The next step in learning a test is to observe it being administered by an experienced examiner. If possible, the therapist should also discuss administration, scoring, and interpretation of the test results. One observation may suffice; however, it may be helpful to watch several administrations of the test to children of different ages and abilities. Observation is an excellent way to learn how other examiners deal with the practical aspects of testing (e.g., arranging test materials, sequencing test items, handling unexpected occurrences, managing behavior). A discussion with the examiner about the interpretation of a child's performance can also be extremely helpful for acquiring an understanding of how observed behaviors are translated into conclusions and recommendations.

Once these preparatory activities have been completed, the learner should practice administering the test. Neighborhood children, friends, or relatives can be recruited to be "pilot subjects." It is a good idea to test several children whose ages are similar to those for whom the test is intended. Testing children, rather than adults, provides the realism of the mechanical, behavioral, and management issues that arise with a clinical population (Figure 6-6).

Checking Inter-rater Reliability

When possible, an experienced examiner should observe the testing and simultaneously score the items as a check of inter-rater reliability (Research Note 6-1). A simple way to assess inter-rater agreement is to use point-by-point agreement.[36] With this technique, one examiner administers and scores the test, while the other observes and scores (Figure 6-7). The two

RESEARCH NOTE 6-1

Eldred, K., & Darrah, J. (2010). Using cluster analysis to interpret the variability of gross motor scores of children with typical development. Physical Therapy, 90, *1510–1518.*

Abstract

This descriptive study explored the utility of cluster analysis as a method to organize gross motor scoring patterns of children with typical development into clinically relevant groups using data from 66 typically developing children from two longitudinal studies. The children were assessed on the gross motor subscale of the Peabody Developmental Motor Scales at 9, 11, 13, 16, and 21 months of age and on the gross motor subscale of the Peabody Developmental Motor Scales, 2nd ed., at 4, 4.5, 5, and 5.5 years of age. Parents were interviewed when the children were 8 years of age. Cluster analysis was conducted. Four distinct and clinically relevant clusters were identified, designated as "robust scores," "decreasing scores," "increasing scores," and "low scores." The clusters illustrate that among typically developing children there are different patterns of motor development.

Implications for Practice

Aggregation of scores of children in the "low score" cluster later identified as having motor concerns suggests that children with motor problems can be identified by a consistently low scoring profile.

Children whose performance fell into the "increasing scores" cluster demonstrate that improvements in motor assessment scores can occur spontaneously without intervention.

Children whose scores decreased over time did not have a diagnosis or motor intervention by the age of 8, suggesting that decreasing scores alone are not a cause for concern.

The results reinforce the variability of skill development in typically developing children and the need to assess qualitative and functional aspects of motor performance.

The study supports the practice of developmental surveillance as a screening strategy.

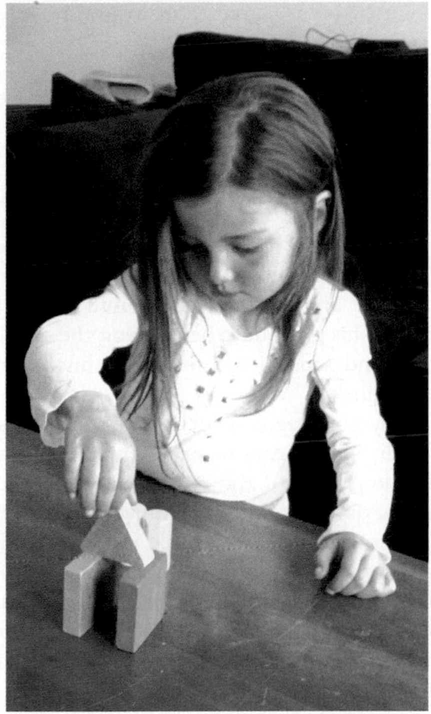

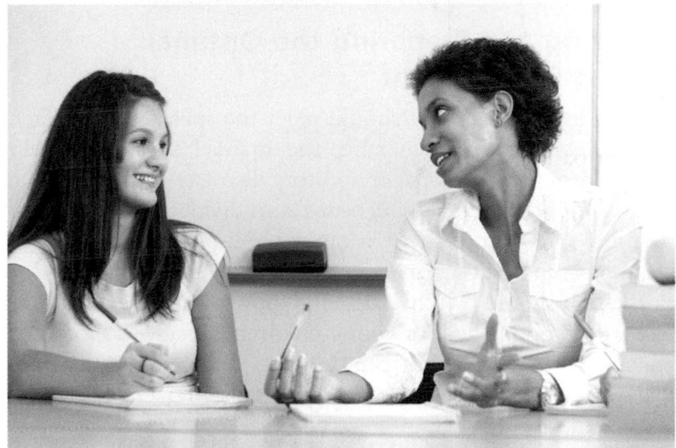

FIGURE 6-7 Two therapists check their inter-rater reliability by scoring the same testing session of this child. (Bottom photo © istock.com.)

examiners then compare their scores on each item. The number of items on which the examiners assigned the same score is then added.

Inter-rater agreement then is computed using this formula:

$$\text{Point-by-point agreement} = \frac{A}{A + D} \times 100$$

where A equals the number of items on which there was agreement and D equals the number of items on which there was disagreement.

The following example illustrates point-by-point agreement.

Two examiners score a test of 10 items. The child receives either a pass (+) or fail (−) for each item. The scores for each examiner are shown in Table 6-5. According to the data, the raters agreed on 7 of the 10 items. They disagreed on items 2, 7, and 9.

TABLE 6-5 Raters' Scores for Point-by-Point Agreement

Item	Rater 1	Rater 2
1	+	+
2	+	−
3	+	+
4	−	−
5	−	−
6	+	+
7	−	+
8	−	−
9	−	+
10	+	+

Their point-by-point agreement would be calculated as follows:

$$\frac{7}{7+3} = 0.70 \times 100 = 70\% \text{ Point-by-point agreement}$$

This means that the examiners agreed on the scores for 70% of the items. To benefit from this exercise, the two examiners should discuss the items on which they disagreed and their reasons for giving the scores they did. A new examiner may not understand the scoring criteria and may be making scoring errors as a result. The experienced examiner can help clarify scoring criteria. This procedure helps bring the new examiner's administration and scoring techniques in line with the standardized procedures.

The point-by-point agreement technique can also be used for periodic reliability checks by experienced examiners, and it is particularly important if the examiners may be testing the same children at different times. No universally agreed-on standard exists for a minimum acceptable level for point-by-point agreement. However, 80% is probably a good guideline. Examiners would be well advised to aim for agreement in the range of 90% if possible. Organization of the testing environment and materials can improve reliability by creating a standard structured environment.

Selecting and Preparing the Optimal Testing Environment

The testing environment should meet the specifications stated in the test manual. Generally, the manual specifies a well-lighted room free of visual or auditory distractions. If a separate room is not available, a screen or room divider can be used to partition off a corner of the room. An example of an appropriate test setup is shown in Figure 6-8.

Testing should be scheduled at a time when the child is able to perform optimally. For young children, caregivers should be consulted about the best time of day for testing so that the test session does not interfere with naps or feedings. Older children's school or other activities should be considered in the scheduling of assessments. For instance, a child who has just come from recess or a vigorous physical education session may have decreased endurance for gross motor activities.

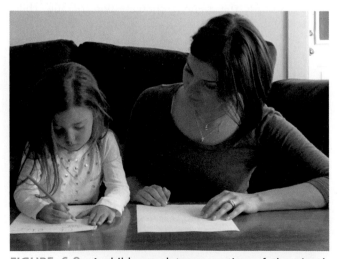

FIGURE 6-8 A child completes a portion of the visual-motor subtest of the Bruininks-Oseretsky Test of Motor Proficiency 2.

The test environment should be ready before the child arrives. Furniture should be appropriately sized so that children sitting at a table can rest their feet flat on the floor and can comfortably reach items on the table. If a child uses a wheelchair or other adaptive seating, he or she should be allowed to sit in the equipment during testing. Infants or young children generally are best seated on the caregiver's lap unless particular items on the test specify otherwise. The examiner should place the test kit where he or she can easily access the items but not where the child can see or reach the kit. Often a low chair placed next to the examiner's chair is a good place to put a test kit.

Each examiner should consider what adaptations are necessary to administer the test efficiently. In many cases a test manual is too large and unwieldy to have at hand during testing, and the score sheet does not provide enough information about administration and scoring criteria. Examiners have developed many ways to meet this need. A common method is preparation of a cue card on which the examiner records specific criteria for administration and scoring, including the instructions to be read to the child. This can be accomplished by making a series of note cards, putting color codes on a score sheet, or developing a score sheet with administration information.

Administering Test Items

Most important, the examiner must be so familiar with the test that his or her attention can be focused on the child's behavior and not on the mechanics of administering the test. This is a critical part of preparation, because much valuable information can be lost if the examiner is unable to observe carefully the quality of the child's responses because he or she instead must devote energy to finding test materials or looking through the test manual. In addition, young children's attention spans can be short, and the examiner must be able to take full advantage of the limited time the child is able to attend to the activities.

Familiarity with the test also allows the examiner to change the pace of activities if necessary. The child can be given a brief break to play, have a snack, or use the bathroom while the examiner interviews the caregiver or jots down notes. Most standardized tests have some flexibility about the order or arrangement of item sets, and an examiner who knows the test can use this to his or her advantage. Sometimes, because of the child's fatigue or behavior or because of time constraints, a test cannot be administered completely in one session. Most tests provide guidelines for administering the test in two sessions, and examiners should be familiar with these guidelines before starting to test.

Interpreting the Test

Before administering the test, the examiner should read the test interpretation section of the examiner's manual and discussion interpretation of the test with experienced examiners. It is essential for examiners to understand which conclusions can and cannot be drawn about a child's performance based on the items administered and standard scores obtained. In addition to the guidelines and interpretation standards specified in the test manual, the examiner must take into account a number of other factors when interpreting an individual child's test score. The following questions should be asked when interpreting test results: How representative or typical was the child's response to the testing situation? If the child did not appear to perform optimally during testing, what influenced the child's performance? When the parent observes the testing, the examiner should ask the parent if the child's performance was typical. The parent's judgment of the child's performance during testing can be included in the report of findings.

How closely do the test scores obtained by the occupational therapist concur with standardized or non-standardized test results of other professionals or from previous testing? Are the scores congruent with observations or reports by caregivers, teachers, or other professionals? Possible reasons for discrepancies can include different performance demands or expectations in various environments, differences in characteristics and environmental supports provided to the child, differing levels of tolerance for children's behavior, or discrepant ability in different developmental or performance domains (which may be identified when several disciplines are evaluating a child).

Which strategies used during the testing were either particularly effective or ineffective in organizing, motivating, or facilitating the child's best performance? Evaluating and discussing the efficacy of management strategies can provide important information to augment test results and recommendations.

Did the tests administered provide a complete picture of the child's occupational performance and participation or is additional testing, observation, or interview required?

Evaluating the Clinical Usefulness of the Test

The final area of preparation is to evaluate the clinical usefulness of the test. The learner should discuss the test with colleagues: What are its strengths and weaknesses? What important information does it give? What information needs to be collected through other techniques? For which children does it seem to work especially well and for which is it an especially poor choice? Can it be adapted for children with special needs? Does it measure what it claims it measures? Do other tests do a better job of measuring the same behavioral domain? Is it helpful for program planning or program evaluation? An ongoing dialog is an important way to ensure that the process of standardized testing meets the needs of the children, families, therapists, and service agencies that use the tests. The steps to becoming a competent user of standardized tests are summarized in Box 6-4.

BOX 6-4 Steps to Becoming a Competent Test User

1. Study the test manual.
2. Observe experienced examiners; discuss your observations.
3. Practice using the test.
4. Check inter-rater agreement with an experienced examiner.
5. Prepare administration and scoring cue sheets.
6. Prepare the testing environment.
7. Consult with experienced examiners about test interpretation.
8. Periodically recheck inter-rater agreement.

Ethical Considerations in Testing

All pediatric occupational therapists who use standardized tests in their practice must be aware of their responsibilities to the children they evaluate and to their families. Urbina has discussed several ethical issues relevant to standardized testing, including (1) examiner competency, (2) client privacy, (3) communication of test results, and (4) cultural bias.[63]

Examiner Competency

Examiner competency was discussed in detail in the previous section. However, it is important to re-emphasize here that examiners must achieve a minimal level of competency with a test before using it in practice. Along with knowing how to administer and score a test, a competent examiner should know for whom the test is intended and for what purpose. This also means knowing when it is not appropriate to use a particular standardized instrument. The examiner should be able to evaluate the technical merits of the test and should know how these characteristics may affect its administration and interpretation. The examiner also should be aware of the many things that can affect a child's performance on a test, such as hunger, fatigue, illness, or distractions, as well as sources of test or examiner error.

The competent examiner draws conclusions about a child's performance on a standardized test only after considering all available information about the child. Such information can include the results of non-standardized tests, informal observations, caregiver interviews, and reviews of documentation from other professionals. It is extremely important to put a child's observed performance on standardized testing in the context of all sources of information about the child; this ensures a more accurate and meaningful interpretation of standard scores.

Client Privacy

The Privacy Rule of the Health Insurance Portability and Accountability Act (HIPAA) mandates that all recipients of health care services be notified of their privacy rights; that they have access to their medical information, including provision of copies at their request; and that they be notified of any disclosure of medical information for purposes other than treatment or billing. For minor children, the parent or legal guardian must provide consent before initiation of any evaluation or intervention procedures. Agencies have different forms and processes for obtaining consent, and examiners must be aware of the procedures for their particular institution. Informed consent generally is obtained in writing and consists of an explanation of the reasons for testing, the types of tests to be used, the intended use of the tests and their consequences (i.e., program placement or qualification for remedial services), and the testing information that will be released and to whom it will be released. Parents/guardians should be given a copy of the summary report and should be informed about who will receive the additional copies. If test scores or other information will be used for research purposes, additional consent procedures must be followed.

Verbal exchanges about the child should be limited. Although it is often necessary to discuss a case with a colleague for the purposes of information sharing and consultation, it is not acceptable to have a casual conversation about a particular child in the elevator, lunchroom, or hallway. If others overhear the conversation, a violation of confidentiality could result.

Communication of Test Results

Evaluation reports should be written in language that is understandable to a nonprofessional, with a minimum of jargon. Each report should be objective in tone, and the conclusions and recommendations should be clearly stated. When the results of tests are discussed, the characteristics of the person receiving the information should be taken into account.

Speaking with other professionals and speaking with family members require different communication techniques. When sharing assessment results with family members, the examiner should be aware of the general level of education and, in the case of bilingual families, the level of proficiency with English. Even if family members have a reasonable capability in the English language, it may be a good idea to have an interpreter available. Often the family members most skilled in English act as interpreters. However, this may not be the optimal arrangement for sessions in which test results are discussed because of the technical nature of some of the information. The ideal interpreter is one who is familiar with the agency and the kinds of testing and services it offers and who has developed techniques for helping examiners offer information in an understandable and culturally meaningful way.

When presenting information to family members, examiners must also consider the anticipated emotional response. A parent who hears that his young child has developmental delays may be emotionally devastated. Therefore the information should be communicated sensitively. Every child has strengths and attributes that can be highlighted in the discussion of his or her overall performance. The examiner should also avoid any appearance of placing blame on the parent for the child's difficulties, because many parents are quick to blame themselves for their child's problems. The examiner also gives opportunities for the caregivers to ask questions about the assessment and the findings. The tone of any discussion should be objective, yet positive, with the emphasis placed on sharing information and making joint decisions about a plan of action.

Cultural Considerations When Testing

Tests developed primarily on a white, middle-class population may not be valid when used with children from diverse cultural backgrounds. It is important for examiners to be aware of the factors that may influence how children from diverse cultures perform on standardized tests.

Children who have not had any experience with testing may not understand the unspoken rules about test taking. They may not understand the importance of doing a task within a time limit or of following the examiner's instructions. They may not be motivated to perform well on tasks because the task itself has no intrinsic meaning to them. The materials or activities may be seen as irrelevant, or the child, having had no experience with the kinds of materials used in the tests, may not know how to interact with them. Establishing a rapport may be difficult either because of language barriers or because of a cultural mismatch between the child's social interaction patterns and those of the examiner. If the examiner is aware of these potential problems, steps can be taken to minimize possible difficulties.

For example, the caregiver or an interpreter can be present to help put the child more at ease. The caregiver can be questioned about the child's familiarity with the various test materials; this information can help the examiner determine whether the child's failure to perform individual items is the result of unfamiliarity with the materials or of inability to complete the task. The caregiver can also be shown how to administer some items, particularly those involving physical contact or proximity to the child. This may make the situation less threatening for the child. However, if these adjustments are made, standard procedure may have been violated, and it may be inappropriate to compute a standard score. Even so, the test can provide a wealth of descriptive information about the child's abilities.

Standardized tests should be used cautiously with children from diverse cultures. Occupational therapists who find themselves frequently evaluating children from cultural or ethnic groups that are underrepresented in the normative samples of most standardized tests may want to consider developing "local norms" on frequently used instruments that reflect the typical patterns of performance among children of that culture. This information can help provide a more realistic appraisal of children's strengths and needs. Several studies have evaluated the performance of children from different countries and/or different cultural groups on pediatric standardized tests developed in the United States and identified differences in test outcomes.[11,12,15,20,35] In addition, observation of the child in a variety of contexts and communication with the family, caregivers, and others familiar with the child are essential to the assessment process.

Clearly, professional communication skills are essential when administering tests and reporting information. Awareness of family and cultural values helps put the child's performance in a contextual framework. An understanding of the professional and ethical responsibilities involved in dealing with sensitive and confidential information is also extremely important. A competent examiner brings all of these skills into play when administering, scoring, interpreting, and reporting the results of standardized tests.

Advantages and Disadvantages of Standardized Testing

Standardized tests have allowed occupational therapists and other professionals to develop a more scientific approach to assessment, and the use of tests that give statistically valid numeric scores has helped give the assessment process more credibility. However, standardized tests are not without their drawbacks. This section discusses the advantages and disadvantages of using standardized tests and presents suggestions on how to make test results more accurate and meaningful.

Advantages

Standardized tests have several characteristics that make them a unique part of the assessment inventory of pediatric occupational therapists. For example, they are tests that in general are well known and commercially available. This means that a child's scores on a particular test can be interpreted and understood by therapists in other practice settings or geographic locations.

Standard scores generated by standardized tests allow testers from a variety of professional disciplines to "speak the same language" when it comes to discussing test scores. For example, a child may be tested by an occupational therapist for fine motor skills, by a physical therapist for gross motor skills, and by a speech pathologist for language skills. All three tests express scores as T-scores. An average T-score is 50. The child receives a fine motor T-score of 30, a gross motor T-score of 25, and a language T-score of 60. It is apparent that although this child is below average in both gross and fine motor skills, language skills are an area of strength; in fact, they are above average. These scores can be compared and discussed by the assessment team, and they can be used to identify areas requiring intervention and areas in which the child has particular strengths.

Standardized tests can be used to monitor developmental progress. Because they are norm-referenced according to age, the progress of a child with developmental delays can be measured against expected developmental progress compared with the normative sample. In this way, occupational therapists can determine if children receiving therapy are accelerating their rate of development because of intervention. Similarly, children who are monitored after discharge from therapy can be assessed periodically to determine whether they are maintaining the expected rate of developmental progress or are beginning to fall behind their peers without the assistance of intervention.

Standardized tests can be used for program evaluation to determine response to intervention across a large number of clients. Standard test scores can be subjected to statistical analysis to evaluate efficacy of interventions. These data can contribute to evidence-based practice and provide information about areas of strength and weakness in the intervention program that can be addressed through quality improvement processes.

Disadvantages

A standardized test cannot stand alone as a measure of a child's abilities. Clinical judgment, informal or unstructured observation, caregiver interviews, and data gathering from other informants are all essential parts of the assessment process. These less structured evaluation procedures are needed to provide meaning and interpretation for the numeric scores obtained by standardized testing.

Several other considerations must be taken into account when performance-based standardized tests are used. For example, a test session provides only a brief "snapshot" of a child's behavior and abilities. The performance a therapist sees in a 1-hour assessment in a clinic setting may be different from that seen daily at home or at school. Illness, fatigue, or anxiety or lack of familiarity with the test materials, the room, or the tester can adversely affect a child's performance. The tester must be sensitive to the possible impact of these factors on the child's performance.

A competent tester can do a great deal to alleviate a child's anxiety about testing and ensure that the experience is not an unpleasant one. However, any test situation is artificial and usually does not provide an accurate indication of how the child performs on a daily basis. Therefore it is important for the therapist to speak to the child's parent, caregiver, or teacher at the time of testing to determine whether the observed behavior is truly representative of the child's typical performance, and the representativeness of the behavior must be taken into account when the child's test scores are interpreted and reported.

Another concern about standardized tests is the rigidity of the testing procedures themselves. Standardized tests specify both particular ways of administering test items and, in many cases, exactly what instructions the tester must give. In view of these administration requirements, children who have difficulty understanding verbal instruction (e.g., with autism, hearing impairment, or attention deficit) or lack control of movement (e.g., with muscle weakness or lack of coordination) may be disadvantaged on performance-based tests. Although this issue is not addressed by all standardized tests, some provide guidelines for administering the test under nonstandard conditions, and some are specifically designed to evaluate functional performance and participation of children with disabilities using performance- and observation-based formats.

It is important to reiterate that although it is permissible to alter the administration procedures of most performance-based tests to accommodate children's individual needs, the child's performance cannot be expressed as a standard score. Rather, the purpose of the testing is to provide a structured format for describing the child's performance (Case Study 6-1). The test manual should always be consulted for guidelines on alterations in test procedures.

CASE STUDY 6-1 Caitlin

Caitlin is a 5.5-year-old kindergarten student referred for occupational therapy assessment by her teacher, Mrs. Clark, who notes that Caitlin is having difficulty learning to write; she holds her pencil awkwardly and exerts too much pressure on the paper. On the playground she has difficulty keeping up with her peers, falls frequently, appears uncoordinated, and has difficulty learning new motor skills. Her energy level is low. She is easily overwhelmed by typical classroom activity and often has emotional outbursts, which affect her ability to complete her work and interact with classmates.

The occupational therapist, Debra, spoke to Caitlin's parents and discovered that Caitlin received physical therapy as an infant because of low muscle tone and slow achievement of developmental milestones. Her parents were worried

Continued

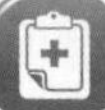

CASE STUDY 6-1 Caitlin—cont'd

about her ability to cope with the increase in writing assignments in first grade and her social acceptance by other children.

Debra considered Caitlin's age (5.5 years) and the areas of concern (gross and fine motor skills and social adjustment) in choosing which standardized tests to use. She decided to administer the PDMS-2, along with clinical observations of Caitlin's posture, muscle tone, strength, balance, motor planning, hand use and hand preference, attention, problem-solving skills, and visual skills. She asked Caitlin's teacher to complete the SFA to provide information on Caitlin's performance of functional school-related behaviors. In addition, she had the teacher complete the Sensory Profile School Companion (SPSC) to determine whether sensory processing problems were contributing to Caitlin's motor delays.

Test Results

Caitlin's testing session was scheduled at midmorning to avoid possible effects of fatigue or hunger. She attended well, although she needed encouragement for the more challenging items. By the end of the session she complained of fatigue, but Debra believed she was able to get a representative sample of Caitlin's motor skills and that the scores obtained were reliable.

On the PDMS-2 Caitlin received a gross motor quotient of 81, placing her at the 10th percentile for her age. Her fine motor quotient was 76, placing her at the 5th percentile. In the gross motor area, ball skills were an area of relative strength, but she had difficulty with balance activities and activities involving hopping, skipping, and jumping. In the fine motor area, Caitlin used a static tripod grasp on the pencil, frequently shifting into a fisted grasp if the writing task was challenging. Based on the small number of visual-motor items on this test, visual-perceptual skills appeared to be an area of strength, whereas tasks involving speed and dexterity were difficult.

Debra found that Caitlin had low muscle tone overall, particularly in the shoulder girdle and hands, and strength was somewhat decreased overall. Caitlin's endurance was poor. Motor planning difficulties were evident in the way she handled test materials and moved about the environment. She had difficulty devising alternate ways to accomplish tasks that were challenging for her and required manual guidance to complete some tasks.

Debra obtained a functional profile on the SFA based on Mrs. Clark's responses to the items on the test. On the scales of recreational movement, using materials, clothing management, written work, and task behavior and/or completion, Caitlin received scores below the cutoff for her grade level. Other scales were within grade-level expectations, with strengths in the scales of memory and understanding, following social conventions, and personal care awareness.

On the SPSC, scores indicated that Caitlin had definite differences in Environmental Sensations–Auditory and Body Sensations–Movement. She also received definite difference scores in School Factor 1, indicating a need for external support for sensory input, and School Factor 3, a low tolerance for sensory input. The scale confirmed that she could easily become overloaded by environmental stimuli.

Observations and Recommendations

According to her scores on the PDMS-2, Caitlin had mild delays in her gross motor skills and mild to moderate delays in her fine motor skills. Although Debra believed that the PDMS-2 gave a good indication of what Caitlin could do under optimal circumstances (i.e., a nondistracting environment, individual attention and encouragement, and structuring of tasks to maximize success and minimize frustration), she also thought it did not represent the level of performance that would be seen over the course of a typical day.

In the classroom Debra observed that Caitlin avoided motor activities and completed writing and drawing activities rapidly, resulting in poor quality of the end product. Her materials were disorganized, she required multiple reminders to complete tasks, and she became upset when unable to finish on time. Her SFA results indicated that her performance of tasks involving fine and gross motor coordination and task organization was below grade-level expectations.

Debra met with the teacher, psychologist, principal, and Caitlin's parents to determine a plan of action. The SFA was used to facilitate collaborative problem solving by helping to identify which specific areas of school function could be targeted in the classroom and which skills should be identified as functional outcomes. Based on the collaborative problem solving process, the team developed the following 6-month outcomes for Caitlin:

- Given appropriate seating support, Caitlin will complete written assignments within the time allotted, 75% of the time, no verbal cues required.
- Given appropriate seating support, Caitlin will produce written work of 85% letter legibility, 80% of the time.
- Given verbal reminders, Caitlin will maintain an orderly workspace (desktop clear of extraneous items and supplies stored neatly within the desk), 90% of the school day.
- Caitlin will participate in age-appropriate playground activities with peers for a 20-minute recess period without falling or requiring a rest break, 80% of the time.

The team determined that Debra would provide recommendations to Mrs. Clark about classroom modifications and activities that would increase Caitlin's success and build her motor skills. The team members also collaborated to design strategies and routines that could be used at school and at home to improve Caitlin's on-task behavior, sensory responsiveness, organization, and ability to manage daily tasks at school.

Debra provided a chair that better fit Caitlin and allowed optimal positioning for writing. She provided Mrs. Clark with ideas for appropriate activities and ways of teaching Caitlin new motor skills and addressing her sensory needs. Debra provided Caitlin's parents with suggestions for family activities that would improve general strength and endurance (e.g., bicycle riding and swimming) and provided specific ideas for ways they could build Caitlin's fine motor skills at home. She also agreed to be available to Mrs. Clark for periodic informal

CASE STUDY 6-1 Caitlin—cont'd

consultation. It was agreed that a reassessment would be scheduled at the end of the school year so that the team could make a decision about further intervention and program planning for the next school year.

Summary

Standardized testing, specifically the PDMS-2, SFA, and SPSC, provided a helpful framework for Debra's assessment of Caitlin and gave specific information about areas of strength and difficulty. Debra made use of her clinical observations and information gathering from a variety of sources to recommend interventions she felt would be beneficial, efficient, and relatively easy to implement. The standardized scores helped her identify Caitlin's problems in fine and gross motor skills, and the test items provided activities that revealed the challenges Caitlin faced when performing motor tasks. However, if Debra had simply relied on the standardized test scores, she would not have acquired the breadth of knowledge that led to her decision-making process for developing intervention options. This example illustrates the important roles of both standardized testing and other methods of data collection in arriving at meaningful and realistic conclusions about children's intervention needs and modes of service delivery.

Summary

- Standardized tests are used by pediatric occupational therapists to assist in the determination of a medical or educational diagnosis, document a child's developmental, functional, and participation status, aid the planning of an intervention program, measure outcomes of programs, and measure variables in research studies.
- Standardized tests have a uniform procedure or protocol for administration, scoring, and interpretation of scores.
- Standardized tests have undergone test development procedures that result in computation of standard scores so that findings can be compared over time and among different domains of function.
- Competency in standardized test administration requires that the user understands basic measurement concepts and is familiar with the test before using it in practice.
- Users evaluate the validity (appropriateness) of a standardized test for specific children and practice contexts.
- Ethical testing procedures include that the examiner considers the purpose of the assessment; adapts procedures to match child and family culture, characteristics, and values adjusts for the testing context; and is knowledgeable about the test instrument.
- Standardized tests should be administered in conjunction with other methods of data gathering, such as observation and interview.

REFERENCES

1. American Occupational Therapy Association. (2008). Occupational therapy practice framework: Domain and process. (2nd ed.). *American Journal of Occupational Therapy, 62*, 625–683.
2. Andrich, D. (1988). *Rasch models for measurement.* Beverly Hills, CA: Sage.
3. Atchison, B. T., Fisher, A. B., & Bryze, K. (1998). Rater reliability and internal scale and person response validity of the School Assessment of Motor and Process Skills. *American Journal of Occupational Therapy, 52*, 843–850.
4. Ayres, A. J. (1989). *Sensory integration and praxis test manual.* Los Angeles: Western Psychological Corporation.
5. Ayres, A. J., & Marr, D. (1991). Sensory integration and praxis tests. In A. Fisher, E. Murray, & A. Bundy (Eds.), *Sensory integration: Theory and practice* (pp. 201–233). Philadelphia: F. A. Davis.
6. Barbosa, V. M., Campbell, S., & Berbaum, M. (2007). Discriminating infants from different developmental outcome groups using the Test of Infant Motor Performance (TIMP) Item Responses. *Pediatric Physical Therapy, 19*, 28–39.
7. Bayley, N. (2006). *Bayley Scales of Infant and Toddler Development, Motor Scale* (3rd ed.). San Antonio, TX: Psychological Corporation.
8. Beery, K. E., Buktenica, N. A., & Beery, N. A. (2004). *Developmental Test of Visual-Motor Integration* (5th ed.). Los Angeles: Western Psychological Services.
9. Bedell, G. (2009). Further validation of the Child and Adolescent Scale of Participation (CASP). *Developmental Neurorehabilitation, 12*(5), 342–351.
10. Bricker, D. (2002). *Assessment, evaluation, and programming system for infants and children* (2nd ed.). Baltimore: Brookes.
11. Bruininks, R. H., & Bruininks, B. D. (2005). *Bruininks-Oseretsky Test of Motor Proficiency* (2nd ed.). Circle Pines, MN: AGS Publishing.
12. Chow, S. M. K., Henderson, S. E., & Barnett, A. L. (2001). The Movement Assessment Battery for Children: A comparison of 4-year-old to 6-year-old children from Hong Kong and the United States. *American Journal of Occupational Therapy, 55*, 55–61.
13. Coster, W. (1998). Occupation-centered assessment of children. *American Journal of Occupational Therapy, 52*, 337–344.
14. Coster, W., Deeney, T., Haltiwanger, J., et al. (1998). *School Function Assessment.* San Antonio, TX: Psychological Corporation.
15. Crowe, T. K., McClain, C., & Provost, B. (1999). Motor development of Native American children on the Peabody Developmental Motor Scales. *American Journal of Occupational Therapy, 53*, 514–518.
16. Deitz, J. C. (1989). Reliability. *Physical and Occupational Therapy in Pediatrics, 9*(1), 125–147.
17. Dunn, W. (1999). *Sensory profile user's manual.* San Antonio, TX: Psychological Corporation.
18. Dunn, W., Brown, C., & McGuigan, A. (1994). The ecology of human

performance: A framework for considering the effect of context. *American Journal of Occupational Therapy, 48*, 595–607.

19. Dunn, W., Myles, B. S., & Orr, S. (2002). Sensory processing issues associated with Asperger syndrome: A preliminary investigation. *American Journal of Occupational Therapy, 56*, 97–102.
20. Egilson, S. T., & Coster, W. J. (2004). School Function Assessment: Performance of Icelandic students with special needs. *Scandinavian Journal of Occupational Therapy, 11*, 163–170.
21. Fisher, A. G. (2003). *Assessment of motor and process skills. Vol. 1: Development, standardization, and administration manual* (5th ed.). Fort Collins, CO: Three Star Press.
22. Fisher, A. G. (2003). *Assessment of motor and process skills. Vol. 2: User manual* (5th ed.). Fort Collins, CO: Three Star Press.
23. Fisher, A. G., Bryze, K., & Atchison, B. T. (2000). Naturalistic assessment of functional performance in school settings: Reliability and validity of the School AMPS scales. *Journal of Outcome Measurement, 4*, 504–522.
24. Folio, M. R., & Fewell, R. R. (2000). *Peabody Developmental Motor Scales* (2nd ed.). Austin, TX: Pro-Ed.
25. Frankenburg, W. K., & Dodds, J. B. (1990). *Denver II Developmental Screening Test.* Denver: Denver Developmental Materials.
26. Franklin, L., Deitz, J., Jirikowic, T., et al. (2008). Children with fetal alcohol spectrum disorders: Problem behaviors and sensory processing. *American Journal of Occupational Therapy, 62*, 265–273.
27. Fritz, S. L., Blanton, S., Uswatte, G., et al. (2009). Minimal detectable change scores for the Wolf Motor Function Test. *Neurorehabilitation and Neural Repair, 23*, 662–667.
28. Furuno, S., O'Reilly, K. A., Hosaka, C. M., et al. (2005). *HELP activity guide (0-3).* Palo Alto, CA: Vort.
29. Geiger, K. F., Spies, R. A., Carlson, J. F., et al. (2007). *Seventeenth mental measurements yearbook.* Lincoln, NE: Buros Institute of Mental Measurements.
30. Gregory, R. J. (2000). *Psychological testing: History, principles and applications* (3rd ed.). Needham Heights, MA: Allyn & Bacon.
31. Grimby, G., Andren, E., Holmgren, E., et al. (1996). Structure of a combination of functional independence measure and instrumental activity measure items in community-living persons: A study of individuals with cerebral palsy and spina bifida. *Archives of Physical Medicine and Rehabilitation, 77*, 1109–1114.
32. Haley, S. M., Coster, W. J., Dumas, H. M., et al. (PEDI-CAT Version 1.3.6 Development, standardization and administration manual. (2012). Retrieved from <http://pedicat.com>.
33. Hammill, D. D., Pearson, N. A., & Voress, J. K. (1993). *Developmental test of visual perception* (2nd ed.). Austin, TX: Pro-Ed.
34. Kao, Y.-C., Kramer, J. M., Liljenquist, K., et al. (2012). Comparing the functional performance of children and youths with autism, developmental disabilities, and no disability using the Revised Pediatric Evaluation of Disability Inventory Item Banks. *American Journal of Occupational Therapy, 66*, 607–616.
35. Katz, N., Kizony, R., & Parush, S. (2002). Visuomotor organization and thinking operations of school-age Ethiopian, Bedouin, and mainstream Israeli children. *Occupational Therapy Journal of Research, 22*, 34–43.
36. Kazdin, A. E. (2010). *Single-case research designs: Methods for clinical and applied settings* (2nd ed.). New York: Oxford University Press.
37. Keller, J., Kafkes, A., & Kielhofner, G. (2005). Psychometric characteristics of the Child Occupational Self-Assessment (COSA), Part One: An initial examination of psychometric properties. *Scandinavian Journal of Occupational Therapy, 12*, 118–127.
38. Kielhofner, G. (2007). *Model of human occupation: Theory and application* (4th ed.). Philadelphia: Lippincott Williams & Wilkins.
39. King, G., Law, M., King, S., et al. (2004). *Children's Assessment of Participation and Enjoyment (CAPE) and Preferences for Activities of Children (PAC).* San Antonio, TX: Harcourt Assessment.
40. Kramer, J. M., Coster, W. J., Kao, Y.-C., et al. (2012). A new approach to the measurement of adaptive behavior: Development of the PEDI-CAT for children and youth with autism spectrum disorders. *Physical & Occupational Therapy in Pediatrics, 32*, 34–47.
41. Law, M., Baptiste, S., Carswell, A., et al. (1998). *Canadian Occupational Performance Measure* (3rd ed.). Ottawa: CAOT Publications.
42. Law, M., Cooper, B., Strong, S., et al. (1996). Person-environment-occupation model: A transactive approach to occupational performance. *Canadian Journal of Occupational Therapy, 63*, 9–23.
43. McDougall, J., Bedell, G., & Wright, V. (2013). The youth report version of the Child and Adolescent Scale of Participation (CASP): Assessment of psychometric properties and comparison with parent report. *Child: Care, Health and Development, 39*(4), 512–522.
44. Miller, L. J. (1990). *First STEP screening tool.* San Antonio, TX: Psychological Corporation.
45. Miller, L. J. (2006). *Miller function and participation scales examiner's manual.* San Antonio, TX: Psychological Corporation.
46. Munkholm, M., Lofgren, B., & Fisher, A. (2012). Reliability of the School AMPS measures. *Scandinavian Journal of Occupational Therapy, 19*, 2–8.
47. Murphy, L. L., Spies, R. A., & Plake, B. S. (Eds.), (2006). *Tests in print VII.* Lincoln, NE: Buros Institute of Mental Measurements.
48. Ohl, M., Graze, H., Weber, K., et al. (2013). Effectiveness of a 10-week Tier-1 Response to Intervention program in improving fine motor and visual-motor skills in general education kindergarten students. *American Journal of Occupational Therapy, 67*, 507–514.
49. Parham, L. D., Ecker, C., Kuhaneck, H. M., et al. (2007). *Sensory processing measure manual.* Los Angeles: Western Psychological Services.
50. Parks, S. (2006). *Inside HELP: Administration manual (0-3).* Palo Alto, CA: Vort.
51. Piper, M. C., & Darrah, J. (1994). *Motor assessment of the developing infant.* London: Saunders.
52. Portney, L. G., & Watkins, M. P. (2006). *Foundations of clinical research: Applications to practice.* Upper Saddle River, NJ: Prentice Hall Health.
53. Rogers, S. J., Hepburn, S., & Wehner, E. (2003). Parent reports of sensory symptoms in toddlers with autism and those with other developmental disorders. *Journal of Autism and Developmental Disorders, 25*, 61–70.
54. Roth, E. J., Heinemann, A. W., Lovell, L. L., et al. (1998). Impairment and disability: Their relation during stroke rehabilitation. *Archives of Physical Medicine and Rehabilitation, 79*, 329–335.
55. Russell, D., Rosenbaum, P., Avery, L. M., et al. (2002). *Gross Motor Function Measure.* Cambridge: Cambridge University Press.
56. Squires, J., Twombly, E., Bricker, D., et al. (2009). *Ages and Stages Questionnaire* (3rd ed.). Baltimore: Paul H. Brookes.
57. Sternberg, R. J. (1990). *Metaphors of mind: Conceptions of the nature of intelligence.* Cambridge: Cambridge University Press.
58. Stuhec, V., & Gisel, E. G. (2003). Compliance with administration procedures of tests for children with pervasive developmental disorder: Does it

exist? *Canadian Journal of Occupational Therapy, 70*, 33–41.

59. Teaford, P., et al. (2010). *HELP 3-6 assessment manual* (2nd ed.). Palo Alto, CA: Vort.
60. Terman, L. M., & Merrill, M. A. (1937). *Measuring intelligence*. Boston: Houghton Mifflin.
61. Thorndike, R. L., Hagen, E. P., & Sattler, J. M. (1986). *Technical manual, Stanford-Binet Intelligence Scale* (4th ed.). Chicago: Riverside.
62. Tomchek, S. D., & Dunn, W. (2007). Sensory processing in children with and without autism: A comparative study using the Short Sensory Profile. *American Journal of Occupational Therapy, 61*, 190–200.
63. Urbina, S. (2004). *Essentials of psychological testing*. Hoboken, NJ: Wiley.
64. Watling, R. L., Deitz, J., & White, O. (2001). Comparison of sensory profile scores of young children with and without autism spectrum disorders. *American Journal of Occupational Therapy, 55*, 416–423.
65. Wechsler, D. (1991). *Wechsler Intelligence Scale for Children*. San Antonio, TX: Harcourt.
66. World Health Organization (2007). *International classification of functioning, disability, and health—children and youth version (ICF-CY)*. Geneva: WHO.
67. Wuang, Y.-P., & Su, C.-Y. (2009). Reliability and responsiveness of the Bruininks-Oseretsky Test of Motor Proficiency-second edition, in children with intellectual disability. *Research in Developmental Disabilities, 30*, 847–855.

CHAPTER 7

Application of Motor Control/Motor Learning to Practice

Jane O'Brien

KEY TERMS

- Dynamic systems
- Degrees of freedom
- Attractor state
- Perturbation
- Postural control
- Motor control
- Motor learning
- Feedback
- Transfer of learning
- Mental rehearsal
- Skill acquisition

GUIDING QUESTIONS

1. What are the key concepts of motor control and motor learning theories?
2. What are the principles and strategies of contemporary motor control interventions?
3. How do practitioners develop evidence-based interventions for children with motor control deficits?
4. Which child, task, and environmental factors influence motor skill acquisition and occupational performance?
5. How do practitioners apply motor learning concepts to promote children's occupational performance?
6. How are transfer of learning, feedback, practice, sequencing and adapting tasks, modeling or demonstration, and mental rehearsal used to promote children's motor performance?

Typically developing children move into and out of positions fluidly and with ease, exploring their worlds, learning about their bodies, and developing motor, cognitive, sensory, and social skills. They use their hands for feeding, dressing, bathing, play, and academics (Figures 7-1 and 7-2). They practice sitting, walking, jumping, and crawling. They play in a variety of positions and show variability in their movements. Conversely, children who have difficulties with motor control may not have the same opportunities to explore their surroundings; they may take longer and often do not master movements. Because motor control is central to participation, occupational therapists provide interventions to improve children's motor control and ability to engage in occupations.

This chapter delineates the principles of motor control and motor learning related to occupational therapy practice, beginning with a definition of motor control. A description of contemporary dynamic systems theory is provided, including research evidence to support its use in practice. The author examines the importance of examining the child (e.g., motivation, goals), task (e.g., nature, object properties, goals, and rules), and environment (e.g., setting, terrain) when evaluating movement. A review of motor learning concepts, including practice, feedback, modeling or demonstration, and mental rehearsal, is provided. The author reviews the evidence, principles, and strategies for motor control approaches and provides evidence for current motor control theory as it relates to intervention. Case examples are used to illustrate the application of motor control and motor learning in occupational therapy practice. *Examples of motor control deficits:*

- Teagan is a 4-year-old boy with Down syndrome who loves to play tee-ball. His gross motor skills are awkward and he must take breaks when running around the bases. (See the Evolve website for accompanying video.) Teagan has low muscle tone throughout. He runs with a wide-based gait and holds his arms close to his body for balance. His posture is asymmetric (he elevates his shoulders and leans) when he runs. He holds objects in a palmar grasp and exhibits delayed visual-perceptual skills interfering with his fine-motor performance. Teagan engages in parallel play with other children at the day care center. When he does interact with his peers, he engages at a much younger level and frequently interferes in their play.
- Georgia is a 2-year-old girl who has difficulty playing on the playground. She is diagnosed with cerebral palsy, right hemiplegia. She walks but her movements are awkward and slow. She leans to the left and drags her right toe on the ground. Her right leg is positioned in the "typical" hemiplegic pattern (internally rotated, foot pronated, ankle extended). She does not use her right hand when playing with her toys and has difficulty manipulating objects. The other children run quickly past her. Georgia falls frequently. She looks frustrated at times that her body will not cooperate with her intentions.
- Devin is a 10-year-old boy who has difficulty with fine-motor tasks, such as tying his shoes, buttoning, and writing. He takes longer than his peers to get ready for recess. Devin is awkward in his movements, falls frequently, and experiences difficulty with balance and coordination skills. He cannot skip, hop, or ride a bicycle. Eye-hand coordination is poor as shown in his inability to catch a ball or play games

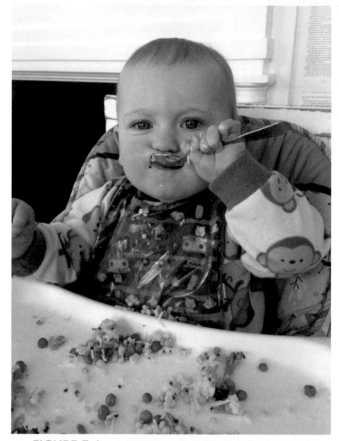

FIGURE 7-1 Children use their hands for feeding.

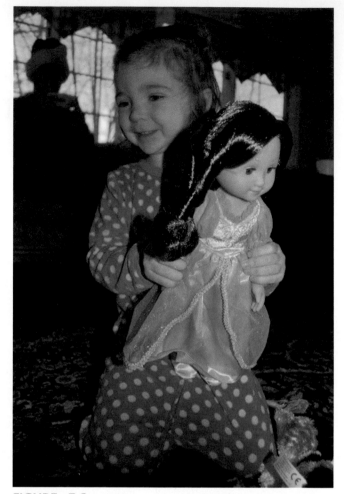

FIGURE 7-2 Children move in many positions when playing.

BOX 7-1 Description of Developmental Coordination Disorder

Developmental coordination disorder (DCD) refers to children whose acquisition and execution of motor skills is substantially below that expected for their chronologic age and opportunity for skill learning and use. Difficulties are manifested as clumsiness, slowness, and inaccuracy of performance of motor skills. The motor skill deficits must significantly and persistently interfere with activities of daily living and impact academic/school productivity, prevocational and vocational activities, leisure, and play. The motor skills deficits are not explained by intellectual disability, visual impairment, or neurologic conditions affecting movement.

Adapted from American Psychiatric Association. (2013). *Diagnostic and statistical manual of mental disorders* (5th ed., pp. 74–77). Arlington, VA: American Psychiatric Publishing.

such as baseball or Frisbee. Devin has been diagnosed with developmental coordination disorder (DCD) (Box 7-1). He has above average intelligence and enjoys playing with other children, although he tends to stay on the "fringes" of the activity.

These three examples illustrate the diversity of motor control challenges found in children. Motor control is important for occupational performance in activities of daily living, self-care, social participation, play, and academics. Occupational therapists help children develop the motor performance required to engage in daily activities. Practitioners develop strategies and interventions to remediate a variety of motor control deficits and therefore therapists must fully understand theories of motor control and the underlying components and mechanisms essential to movement.

Motor Control: Overview and Definition

Motor control is defined as the "ability to regulate or direct the mechanisms essential to movement" (p. 4).[93] Motor control refers to how the central nervous system organizes movement, how we quantify movement, and the nature of movement. Practitioners and researchers interested in motor control examine the mechanisms, strategies, and development of movement, as well as causes of motor dysfunction.[54,70,73,95] Occupational therapy practitioners use this knowledge to design effective intervention so that children with motor control deficits may participate in their desired occupations.

Movement deficits occur in numerous conditions including cerebral palsy, DCD, autism spectrum disorder, Down syndrome, sensory integration disorders, and acquired brain injury.

Motor problems may present as poor coordination, timing, sequencing, bimanual control, force production, balance, sensory processing, and motor planning. These issues interfere with the child's ability to engage in activities of daily living, play, academics, and social events at home, at school, and in the community.

Children with a variety of diagnoses manifest motor problems. Children with cerebral palsy exhibit difficulty with postural control because of neuromuscular and sensory impairments, which leads to motor deficits.[88] Abnormal muscle tone and spasticity interfere with voluntary muscle control, and children with cerebral palsy exhibit sensory impairments that may result in poor motor planning and body awareness.[88] Children with Down syndrome experience poor timing, decreased strength, and decreased postural control.[110] Given the importance of motor skills to young children's play, early intervention aimed at skill acquisition is recommended to maximize their motor control.[46,54] A systematic review of the literature showed that the motor deficits of children with autism spectrum disorder fall into two areas: poor integration of information for motor planning and increased variability in sensory inputs and motor output.[36] Children with DCD experienced slower reaction times, less accuracy in bimanual tasks, and timing and sequencing problems.[60,76] In a meta-analysis of studies examining the performance deficits associated with DCD, Wilson et al.[117] found that children with DCD experience difficulty with anticipatory movement, rhythmic coordination, executive function (e.g., set shifting, attention, flexibility), gait and postural control, catching and interceptive action, and aspects of sensory-perceptual function (e.g., visuosensory processing, tactile perception, kinesthesia, processing speed). Raynor[87] found that children with DCD experienced strength and power deficits as compared with matched controls in knee extension and flexion tasks. Children with sensory integration deficits experience a host of motor problems including disorders of the vestibular system, body perception and motor planning, and sensory processing and modulation difficulties.[4,5]

Historically, intervention strategies used by practitioners varied according to the etiology and nature of motor impairments.[61,93] Therapists used bottom-up approaches, hypothesizing that if they treated the underlying causes of motor dysfunction, the child's function would improve. Therefore, the goals of intervention included normalizing muscle tone, remediating sensory dysfunction, and improving dyspraxia. Bottom-up approaches include sensory integration, neurodevelopmental treatment, reflex integration therapy, and strength training. Table 7-1 describes selected motor control approaches. These interventions focus on addressing the underlying deficit to improve performance.[3,16,17] These bottom-up frames of reference are based on a hierarchic development model based on neuroscience understandings of the 1970s and 1980s.

Overall, bottom-up approaches appear to have limited effectiveness in improving the occupations of children.[16,17,25,57,67,75,82,97] Because bottom-up approaches have minimal evidence, they should be used in combination with other approaches, carefully evaluated when used, and continuously monitored to document the child's progress. In contrast, dynamic systems theory describes how systems interact and how these interactions are responsible for motor performance.[3,17,24,93,102,103]

Dynamic Systems Theory

Dynamic systems theorists propose that movement derives from a variety of sources and takes place within a variety of natural and meaningful contexts.[93,102,103] This evolving and contemporary theory can be applied to motor control to assist practitioners in framing evaluation and subsequent intervention to facilitate movement in children and youth. Dynamic systems theory suggests that motor control is dependent on nonlinear and transactive person factors (i.e., cognitive, musculoskeletal, neurologic, sensory, perceptual, social-emotional), task characteristics (i.e., goals, rules, object properties) and environmental systems (i.e., contexts).[102,103] See Figure 7-3.

The principles of dynamic systems theory include:

- The interaction among systems is essential to adaptive control of movement.
- Motor performance results from an interaction between adaptable and flexible systems.
- Dysfunction occurs when movement patterns lack sufficient adaptability to accommodate task demands and environmental constraints.
- Because task characteristics influence motor requirements, practitioners modify and adapt the requirements and affordances of tasks to help children succeed.

According to dynamic systems theory, multiple systems of the person, task, and environment transact for predictive and adaptive control of movement.[93,102,103] The person factors include the child's cognitive (e.g., attention, motivation, and self-efficacy), musculoskeletal, neuromotor, sensory, perceptual, and social-emotional factors.

Person

Occupational therapy practitioners examine personal factors using knowledge of biomechanics, neurology, and kinesiology to identify areas that may be interfering with motor performance. Practitioners develop goals based on quantitative and qualitative data. Assessments or evaluation tools may provide objective measurements of the child's current level of functioning for purposes of planning intervention and evaluating progress (see Chapter 6). A thorough evaluation of the person factors that influence motor performance includes many of the components described in the following paragraphs.

Cognition

Cognitive factors include a child's attention, motivation, and self-efficacy. Attention is required to explore the environment and move around objects and through space. Children must attend to activity to explore and learn. Typical infants and children are innately motivated to move through the environment; they exhibit interest in activities and enjoy movement. Understanding a child's motivation or interests helps the practitioner design fun and inviting activities to promote effective motor performance. Self-efficacy refers to one's belief in his or her abilities.[49] Children who feel they will be successful are more apt to attempt new actions leading to improved neural plasticity. They engage in habits and routines that allow them to develop new skills.[49,52] They may move more confidently and try out new activities freely.

TABLE 7-1 Selected Motor Control Approaches

Approach	Brief Description	Principles	Strategies
Activity-focused motor intervention[107]	Activity-focused motor intervention emphasizes the need for practice and repetition of purposeful motor actions. Provides movement experiences that promote motor learning within the context of the daily routines of the family.	Motor learning principles are a natural fit for therapy if they are complemented by a methodology to address impairments in body function and structure that affect motor learning. Neurologic impairments that affect motor learning can be addressed by: 1. Adapting motor learning guidelines to meet individual needs 2. Integrating activity-focused and impairment-focused intervention	1. Develop activity-related goals with the child and family. 2. Plan activity-focused interventions by adapting knowledge of motor leaning to the child's learning strengths and needs. 3. Integrate impairment-focused intervention with activity-focused intervention.
Neurodevelopmental treatment (NDT)	Children who have a brain lesion benefit from "feeling" typical movement patterns. Children with brain lesions (cerebral palsy) experience abnormal muscle tone that interferes with movement, which can be addressed through handling techniques.	The therapist's role is to facilitate normal movement patterns to help children acquire more normal movement. The goal is to provide input to the child to help "normalize" muscle tone. NDT theorists suggest that normalizing muscle tone may improve movement. Although movement is often guided by subcortical brain centers, the role of higher level brain function in guiding movement is acknowledged (e.g., the role of cognition in guiding movement).	The therapist begins by inhibiting or facilitating muscle tone. A variety of strategies is used to inhibit or facilitate muscle tone in children. The therapist uses *key points of control* and *handling techniques* to facilitate movement. NDT intervention also considers symmetrical alignment of the body, movement with full range of motion, base of support and weight-bearing, muscle strength, and postural control.[7]
Reflex integration therapy	Reflex integration therapy is based on the premise that reflexes that are not integrated in the sequence and rate of typical development interfere with the acquisition of normal movement.	The principles of this approach are based on dated neuroscientific and hierarchical models for motor development.	Provide intervention strategies to integrate reflexes.
Sensory integration	Sensory integration addresses the underlying components of movements by engaging children in intervention in enriched, simulated environments to which they adapt and respond to sensory stimuli (vestibular, tactile, proprioceptive). The practitioner helps the child to engage in activities that provide the "just-right" challenge.	When children complete adaptive responses, change occurs at the neuronal level (brain plasticity).	Provide child-directed vestibular, proprioceptive, tactile activities designed to facilitate the "just-right" challenge so the child makes an adaptive response. The use of suspended equipment is required.
Strength training	Strength training uses progressively more challenging resistance to muscular contraction to build muscle strength and endurance.[75]	Strength training programs develop a child's muscle strength to improve quality of movement or performance.	Increase weight of objects or increase repetition of movements to build strength.
Task-specific training	Task-specific training involves practicing the specific actions or activity (task) while considering the concepts of motor learning. Clients "practice context-specific motor tasks and receive some form of feedback" (p. 576).[101]	The focus of task-specific training is on the functional task, rather than the impairment. Task-specific training resonates with occupational therapy principles.	1. Training is relevant to the client and context. 2. Practice sequences are randomly ordered. 3. Training is repetitive. 4. The goal is for the client to complete the whole task (occupation). 5. The client should be positively reinforced.

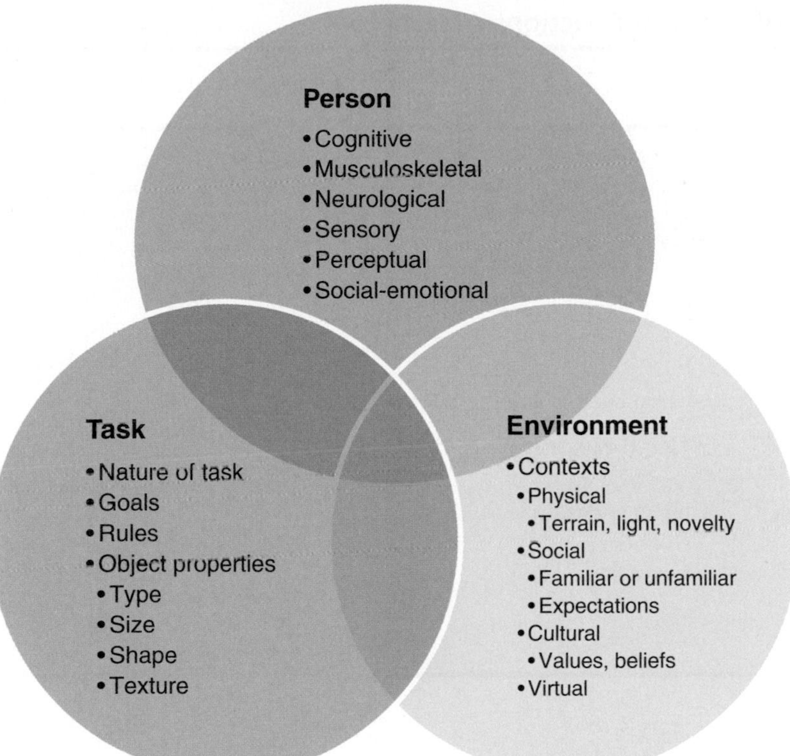

FIGURE 7-3 Dynamic systems theory. (Adapted from Shumway-Cook, A., & Woollacott, M. H. (2007). *Motor control: Translating research into clinical practice* (3rd ed.). Philadelphia: Lippincott Williams & Wilkins.)

Musculoskeletal

Observation of a child's physical appearance provides the practitioner with an overview of musculoskeletal structures required for movement. Physical appearance includes symmetry between the right and left sides of the body, muscular structures, and physical stature. Range of motion of joints allows for effective and full movement.

Muscle tone is defined as the resting state of the muscle.[63] Typical muscle tone allows movement into and out of positions with ease, fluidity of movement, and variety in movement. Children with hypertonicity exhibit increased muscle tone, resulting in limited movements; those with hypotonicity exhibit low muscle tone, which results in excessive range of movement and limited control over movement. Some children may experience fluctuating muscle tone, which interferes with quality of motor control. The goal of occupational therapy intervention is not to change the muscle tone but rather to improve the child's ability to perform occupations.

Strength is defined as the voluntary recruitment of muscle fibers. Strength is needed to perform movements against gravity or to pick up objects of varying weights. A degree of trunk strength is required to maintain posture. In strength training programs, the child repeats movements, often with added resistance or weight.

Posture refers to one's core stability and involves the trunk and neck musculature. To demonstrate postural control, a person maintains the center of mass over the base of support.[43,44,111] Postural control is required for functional movement and involves an interplay between sensory, motor, and musculoskeletal systems.[37,111] Children stabilize the head and trunk and remain upright for reaching, feeding, dressing, and play. A stable posture is essential for refined movement and mobility.[37,111]

Children with cerebral palsy, developmental coordination disorder, or other movement difficulties may have difficulty with postural control and exhibit awkward movements or inadequate balance.[19,20,88,93] Children with cerebral palsy may not be able to stabilize the shoulder for arm and hand movement; they may walk with a wide or inefficient gait. They may slouch in their seats at school, interfering with writing and academic tasks. Postural stability provides the foundation for simple and complex movements. Core strengthening activities may help children with postural challenges.[47] Meaningful engagement in a variety of activities can help develop posture and core muscle control for coordinated movement.

Neuromotor Development

The neurologic system (i.e., the peripheral and central nervous systems) is primary in controlling movement. Examining how a child responds to movement helps practitioners better understand the child's neurologic functioning. Infants are born with reflexes that integrate over time and are believed to be the building blocks for functional movement.[120] Reflexes may remain obligatory for some children who have neurologic deficits. When a primitive reflex remains obligatory over time, it interferes with voluntary movement. For example, an 8-year-old child who is still bound by the Moro reflex or asymmetric

TABLE 7-2 Age of Postural Reactions Acquisition

			Immature (Months)	Mature (Months)
Righting Reactions				
	Neck on body		Birth	4-5
	Body on body		Birth	4-5
	Body on head			
		Prone	1-2	4-5
		Supine	2-4	5-6
	Landau			
		Flexion	3-4	6-7
		Vertical	2	6
Protective Extension	Emerge and continue throughout lifespan			
		Forward		6-7
		Lateral		6-11
		Backward		9-12
Equilibrium Reactions	Emerge and continue throughout lifespan			
		Prone		5-6
		Supine		7-8
		Sitting		7-10
		Quadruped		9-12
		Standing		12-21

tonic neck reflex will experience difficulty with voluntary or functional movement. Although some reflexes emerge under stressful situations (e.g., associated movements), they are not obligatory and consistent.

Children tend to develop postural reflexes in a predictable sequence: prone and supine positions to quadruped to standing. There are three major categories of postural reflexes: primitive, righting, and equilibrium and protective reflexes (Table 7-2 provides an overview of postural reactions.)

Primitive reflexes appear within the first year and are thought to serve a survival function. For example, the rooting reflex allows the infant to orient to a food source; the suck reflex enables the infant to receive nutrients. Most primitive reflexes are suppressed early in infancy but may reappear after injury or trauma to the brain.[39,120]

Righting reflexes are typically observed at about 3 months of age and persist to 6 months of age and are designed to align the head with the body (limbs) and the upper body with lower body. When rotation is imposed on the body, the righting reflexes realign the segments of the body and bring the body into appropriate alignment. They align the head with gravity (keep the child's head upright) and include optical righting, labyrinthine righting reflexes, and Landau. These reflexes realign the head vertically when the body is displaced and are mediated, respectively, by the visual and vestibular systems.

Equilibrium and protective reflexes, the third category, are present at about 6 months of age and persist throughout life to help the child remain upright. Equilibrium and protective reflexes are whole-body responses to postural instability. Protective extension responses are elicited by sudden shoves or pushes to the body. Protective extension helps the child protect the body from injury during loss of balance. For example, in sitting, a toddler extends his or her arm and hand to prevent falling to the side when pushed. Equilibrium responses are elicited when one's center of gravity shifts (e.g., by slowly tilting surfaces on which the child is standing or sitting). If some instability occurs, the child adjusts by extending limbs or changing muscle tone to remain in position. Children develop equilibrium reactions in supine and prone positions between 5 and 8 months of age and continue to develop equilibrium in more upright positions throughout early childhood.

Equilibrium responses are required to maintain one's upright position or balance. Balance is essential to functional movement. To balance, a child must sense changes in position and respond via movement or muscle tone. These subtle adjustments (equilibrium responses) enable the child to continue a movement and aid in the quality of that movement. Children with motor control deficits may experience balance difficulties.

Soft neurologic signs are often associated with motor control difficulties and provide indicators of brain dysfunction.[18,38,120] Practitioners can evaluate the presence of the following soft neurologic signs:

- Mild dysfunction in muscle tone
- Dysdiadokokinesis—impairment of the ability to make movements exhibiting a rapid change of motion that is caused by cerebellar dysfunction[112]
- Intention tremor—a slow tremor of the extremities that increases on attempted voluntary movement and is observed in certain diseases of the nervous system[74,112]
- Dysmetria—impaired ability to estimate distance in muscular activity[74]
- Limited force control—limited strength or energy
- Poor bilateral motor coordination—inability to perform movements using both sides of the body (e.g., alternating jumps)
- Difficulty with coordination (fine and gross motor)—inability to complete movements in a smooth manner (e.g., walk on heels, finger opposition)
- Difficulty with balance—inability to maintain one's center of gravity (e.g., stand on one foot)

- Associated reactions (synkinesis)—involuntary movement in one part when another part is moved: an associated movement[112]

Children with DCD, acquired brain injury, or mild intellectual disability may exhibit soft neurologic signs.[18,38] Lundy-Ekman et al.[60] sought to identify the neurologic systems responsible for soft neurologic signs to shed light on why some children are clumsy or exhibit motor control difficulties.[60] They found that children with basal ganglia deficits showed difficulty controlling force as compared with matched controls. The children with cerebellum dysfunction were more variable than controls with timing tasks (tapping) and produced less force.[60]

Sensory

The sensory systems that relate to motor control include visual, auditory, vestibular, kinesthesia, proprioception, and tactile. Auditory input may motivate children to respond and explore the environment by turning and locating the source of the noise. Vestibular processing allows the child to sense changes in movement or position that allow the body to respond. Children who under- or overrespond to vestibular sensations may demonstrate ill-timed or awkward responses to position changes. Kinesthesia refers to the sense and direction that one is moving. Children with poor kinesthetic awareness may not realize how their body is performing. Kinesthetic awareness allows children to sense that the body is in motion (e.g., the hand is moving), whereas proprioception provides a sense of the position of one's muscles and joints. Without proprioceptive sense, children are unsure of where they are in space or how the body is positioned. For example, a child may not realize how his or her feet are moving or if his or her feet are positioned on the ground when not looking at the feet. Therefore, poor kinesthetic or proprioceptive perception can result in poor quality of movement and inefficient motor control. Tactile processing provides children with information about the environment through direct body contact. Children first learn about their environment through tactile sensations. They explore objects and their bodies by putting toys and their hands in their mouths.

Perceptual

Perception refers to the ability to make sense of sensory stimuli and involves cognition and sensory awareness. Visual perception, for example, refers to understanding letter formations (visual closure, figure-ground) and identifying letters (shape recognition). Depth perception refers to an understanding of how far apart things are.

The development of the concept of the physical self involves at least three major components: body schema, body image, and body awareness. Figure 7-4 shows a schematic of the components of the concept of the physical self and the behavioral components specific to body awareness. Body schema is the neural substrate for body awareness. It is present at birth, and as children grow and develop, this so-called diagram of the body (homunculus) in the sensory and motor areas of the brain is modified, in part, through sensory motor experiences and feedback received. Body image refers to the image one has of oneself as a physical entity; it includes the perception that one has of the body's physical or structural characteristics (e.g., "Am I short, tall, heavy, or lean?") and of one's physical performance abilities. Body awareness is defined as the ability to visually discriminate, recognize, and identify labels for various aspects of the body's physical and motor dimensions. Internal aspects of body awareness tend to develop slightly in advance of external components.[10,13,69,113] External aspects are associated with development and awareness of the relationship of the body to the environment. Understanding one's physical self allows a child to move in many ways through a variety of environments.

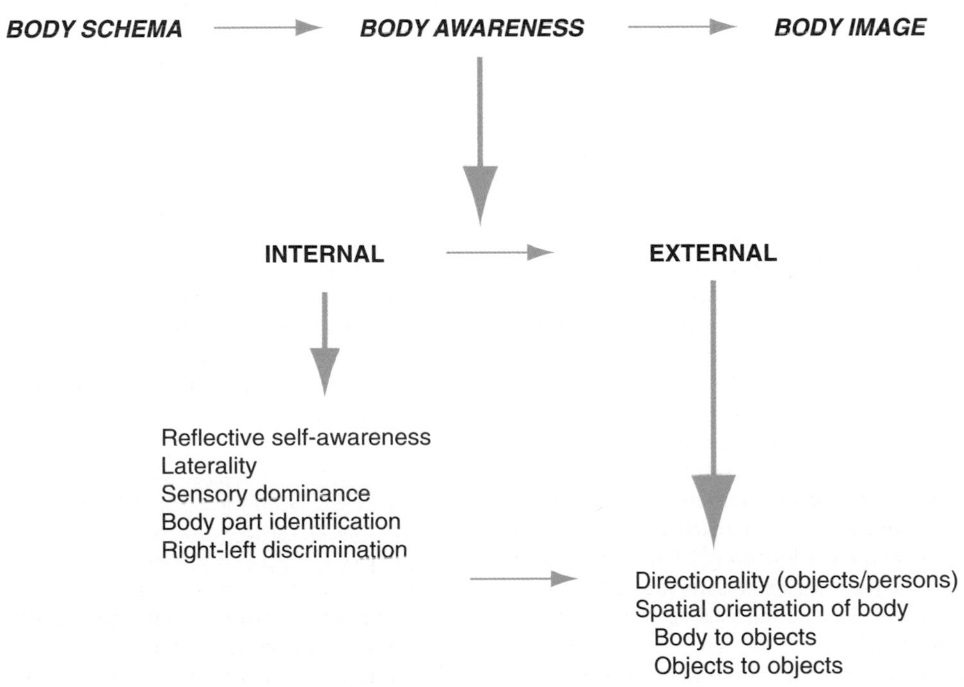

FIGURE 7-4 **Body Concepts.**

Children with poor body awareness may bump into objects; they do not have an internal representation of their body in space. Being unaware of body position, they may stand closer to people. They may not perceive left and right.

Social-Emotional Factors

Emotion is a psychological state that may affect motor performance. Individuals are able to achieve motor challenges for which they attribute positive feelings.[71,78,86] For example, athletes use the "power of positive thinking" to visualize achievement and subsequently exhibit improved motor performance as a result.[71] Conversely, children may have difficulty performing at their best when they are experiencing negative emotions (such as anxiety or fear). Children may perform less effectively if they are feeling pushed or judged; they may be afraid of failure. Children may want to perform an activity or skill and feel frustrated when they cannot. Watching the child's expressions during motor performance can provide cues to therapists about the child's emotions and perceived task difficulty.

When a child is overly stressed or afraid, the sympathetic system is activated, making it difficult for the child to problem solve or learn a new motor skill. Children learn movement best when they are challenged at a level in which success is achievable and they are emotionally ready to engage in problem solving.

Task

Task characteristics refer to the nature, object properties, goals, and rules. The nature of the task may be defined as simple or complex. Generally speaking, simple tasks require minimal attention and brief motor responses. Complex motor tasks require a high degree of attention and are generally more engaging.[70] Tasks that require precision are often defined as complex and may be more difficult for children (such as handwriting as compared with scribbling). Practice of complex motor tasks results in greater neuroplastic changes than practice of a simple motor task.[70] When compared with simple motor tasks, adults show greater increase of neural activity during and after practice of a complex task.[70] Interestingly, these findings are reported after a single practice session. These findings suggest that practice of a more complex task results in greater neuroplastic changes than practice of a simple motor task.[70]

The nature of the task determines the speed, smoothness, force, and accuracy of movement required.[93,119] Open tasks involve supporting surfaces, objects, or people in the environment that are in motion. Closed tasks involve objects, people, and terrain that are stationary; the learner decides the start and finish.

The properties of the objects (size, shape, weight, texture, sensory aspects) and the ascribed meaning of task (goals, rules) influence motor requirements. Children respond differently when reaching for large as compared with small objects. They orient the hand at the beginning of a reach and adjust the fingers at the end to grasp the small object.[30] The shape of the object determines how a person prepares to grasp. Children with motor challenges such as cerebral palsy experience difficulty with these adjustments.[118]

Object affordance along with the rules and goals associated with the objects help to cue children regarding the expected movement. Object affordance is a property of an object or an environment that allows an individual to perform an action.[112] For example, providing a child with a spoon and food presents a cue of how to use the object and consequently the motor performance required. Research suggests that practitioners should pay attention to several object features: the number of objects required for action, the information conveyed by objects, and the goals.[42,119] Overall, using the number of objects required for the task along with the actual objects enhances motor responses (as measured by movement time, grasp pattern, and motor performance). Making a clear relationship between the goal and the object(s) enhances motor performance.[42]

Environmental Contexts

Practitioners evaluate the physical, social, cultural, temporal, virtual, and personal contexts in which movement and occupational performance occur. For example, children may move successfully in a structured clinical setting but have difficulty navigating the uneven terrain outdoors. The light, terrain, setting, gravity, and novelty of the setting may influence a child's performance.[56] For example, children were more playful and moved more (as measured by Actiograph measures) at recess when novel objects (e.g., hay bales, tires) were introduced.[15]

The social environment can place additional motor requirements on activities. For example, a child may perform "dance moves" in front of his family but show poor quality when in front of classmates at school. The social pressure of "performing" influences the movement. Cultural expectations may influence motor actions. Some family cultures accept less than quality movement, whereas others expect fine and precise movements. Temporal aspects include the developmental stage of the child. Younger children are allowed to be "silly" in their movements, whereas an adolescent may need to control movements more carefully for success. Virtual contexts include motor interactions with a computer screen. Playing video games may help children develop motor skills in a controlled setting. Personal contexts include the features of the child that promote or inhibit movement.

The skilled practitioner considers all these contexts when analyzing a child's motor performance. Careful analysis of the child's motor functioning in a variety of contexts allows the practitioner to establish the child's strengths and weaknesses.[24] The Test of Environmental Supportiveness[14,94] measures the influence of the environment on play and can provide practitioners with a structure when analyzing the play environment. Most often therapists informally assess the environment, with a focus on identifying the factors that seem to most influence the child's occupational performance.

Motor Performance Results from an Interaction Between Adaptable and Flexible Systems

Movement arises from interactions among many systems. The complexity of movement can be illustrated by examining the system requirements for the complex motor task of handwriting. (Chapter 9 provides more information on handwriting.)

Handwriting involves fine motor skills, visual-motor coordination, motor planning, proprioception, sustained attention, perceptual skills, and tactile and kinesthetic sensitivities; children must hold the pencil and maintain posture, requiring an intact neuromuscular system.[6,32] Children sit upright (postural control), coordinate fine motor movement, and plan how to move the pencil in relationship to the paper (visual-motor and perception). They feel the object (pencil) in their hand (stereognosis) and detect how it is moving (kinesthesia). As they fluidly draw on the paper, children experience subtle changes in the center of gravity (equilibrium), which they must process and make subtle tone changes in response to (to remain in an upright position). They stabilize the trunk and shoulder muscles to control elbow, wrist, and fingers for writing. They exert pressure (force) on the pencil and paper and use timing and sequencing to form letters in order. They attend to the task along with environmental influences (e.g., teacher or children talking). Cognitive and motivational factors may influence handwriting, as well as feelings of self-efficacy. Handwriting provides an example of the complexity of a motor task and how multiple systems influence movements (Figure 7-5).

Dynamic systems theorists acknowledge the interactions among the systems. The personal aspects such as the child's age, body stature, and neuromotor status interact with the task (e.g., handwriting versus printing) and environment (e.g., classroom with child-sized tables and chairs). Instead of focusing on one component (e.g., hand strength), they propose that practitioners consider multiple systems when designing intervention.

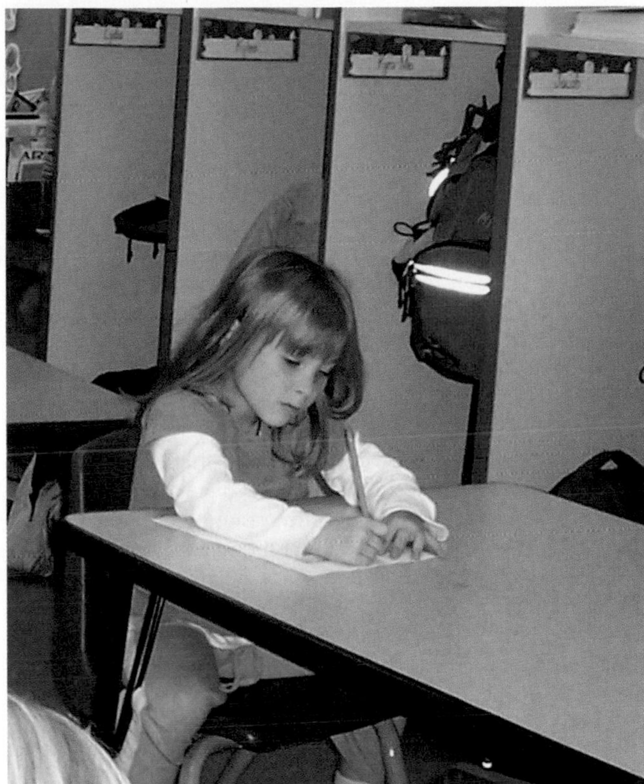

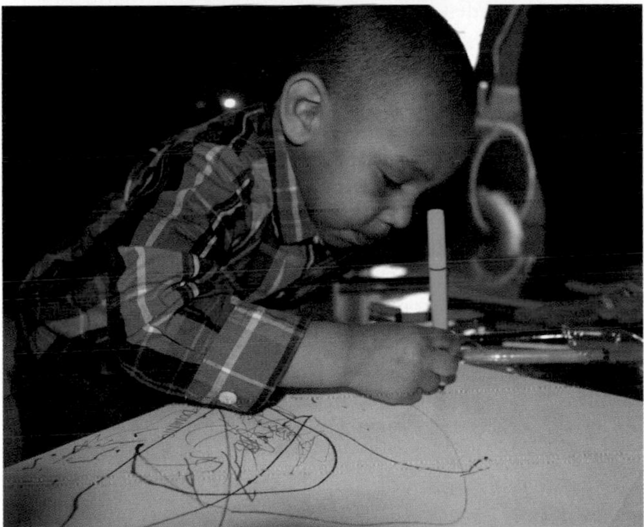

FIGURE 7-5 Children working on academics.

Dysfunction Occurs When Movement Lacks Sufficient Adaptability to Accommodate Task Demands and Environmental Constraints

Performance is affected when components of one or more systems are rigid, impaired, or inflexible. Children with motor deficits who experience difficulty with flexible movements may exhibit timing and sequencing deficits, poor postural control, slow reaction time responses, and/or difficulty with sensory-perceptual function (e.g., tactile perception, visuosensory processing, kinesthesia).[60,77] Delayed reactions and processing interfere with the accuracy and quality of the movements. Consequently, their movements are not smooth, coordinated, or timely.

Children with motor or processing deficits often lack adaptability and variety in their movements. They move in the same manner and exhibit difficulty maneuvering in unfamiliar ways, such as when navigating an obstacle course. Children with motor impairments frequently move in limited or stereotypical ways and exhibit a small repertoire of movements. For example, a 3-year-old girl who experienced motor planning deficits had only one motor pattern for climbing onto a tricycle and could not get on the tricycle when it was turned at a different angle. This toddler's praxis (ability to process, plan, and execute a movement) was impaired.

Typical children move in a variety of ways so that they can easily navigate through the environment. They process sensory information quickly and correctly, allowing them to move smoothly. They problem solve new movements to address motor challenges. Variability is a hallmark of efficient movement, therefore occupational therapists work to help children develop a variety of movements they can use in multiple contexts.

Therapists Modify and Adapt the Requirements and Affordances of Tasks to Help Children Succeed

According to dynamic systems theory, the difficulty of planning and executing movement may be changed by altering the degrees of freedom required to accomplish a movement.[9,51,102,103]

Bernstein[9] suggested that an essential central nervous system (CNS) function is to control redundancy by minimizing the degrees of freedom for a movement. Degrees of freedom are defined as possible planes of motion in the joints controlled by the musculoskeletal and central nervous systems.[9,59,93] When multiple systems interact there are many options (degrees of freedom) available to perform the given action.[9,51,102,103] Therefore, the practitioner can control or limit some of the options to help the child be successful. For example, providing an alternative position (supported sitting, prone) limits the need for the child to control posture, which may allow him or her more success with hand skills.

Decreasing the degrees of freedom required for movement may result in more functional movement.[59] A child with cerebral palsy may use his hand more effectively if the wrist or thumb is stabilized with a splint. The splint decreases the degrees of freedom the child must control and allows for more accuracy in movements. In a study examining violin playing, Konczak and colleagues (2009) found that expert child or adult violinists decreased the degrees of freedom of movement through practice (e.g., stabilized shoulder flexion-extension), which resulted in greater accuracy and movement at the elbow and shoulder (abduction-adduction).[51] The findings imply that restricting degrees of freedom while leaving other degrees of freedom unconstrained may be an effective strategy for learning complex, precise motor patterns in children and adults.[51]

Dynamic systems theorists use the term *attractor state* to describe the tendency to stay in the patterns of the status quo, preferred state, or the state requiring the fewest degrees of freedom to maintain.[102,103] For example, a child may have a tendency to sit in a posterior pelvic tilt. This pattern may not be most efficient and may even prevent the child from achieving other milestones (e.g., such as reaching with ease). The therapist's role is to identify the attractor state, and when it limits function, facilitate movement away from this state to promote engagement in occupation. Facilitating a child away from an attractor state is often referred to as a *perturbation*—a force that alters the movement pattern. Perturbations can be used to help children move in different ways. They may be psychological (e.g., motivating the child to move to change the task or environment) or physical (e.g., body feels misaligned and therefore the child must right him- or herself).

Functional goals in addition to environmental and task constraints play a major role in determining movement.[44,81,102] When following a dynamic systems approach, practitioners analyze the task requirements in relation to child and environmental factors so they can adapt the task to help the child successfully perform.[81] Understanding and manipulating task characteristics is an essential feature of occupational therapy intervention planning.

Practice Models That Use Dynamic Systems Theory

Occupational therapy models (e.g., Canadian Occupational Performance[55]; Person, Environment, Occupation, Performance Capacity[21]; Model of Human Occupation[49]) can guide one's thinking and help practitioners develop intervention based on the principles of dynamic systems theory. Each of these models places the client and family at the center while considering multiple systems. A variety of motor control approaches have been developed to apply dynamic systems theory to practice.

Task-specific training involves practicing the specific actions or activity (task) while considering the concepts of motor learning. Clients "practice context-specific motor tasks and receive some form of feedback" (p. 576).[90,101] The focus of task-specific training is on the functional task, rather than the impairment. Task-specific training resonates with occupational therapy principles. According to Hubbard et al.,[45] practitioners using task-specific training follow these guidelines:

1. Training is relevant to the client and context.
2. Practice sequences are randomly ordered.
3. Training is repetitive.
4. The goal is for the client to complete the whole task (occupation).
5. Client should be positively reinforced.

Activity-focused motor intervention emphasizes the need for practice and repetition of purposeful motor actions.[106,107] The practitioner develops goals with the family and engages the child in repetition of actions in functional movement within the environment. This approach is consistent with current motor control theory, supporting the idea that coordination and motor control emerge in the context of functional activity.[39,93] Practitioners using the activity-focused approach provide movement experiences that promote motor learning within the context of the daily routines of the family.[107]

Framework for Occupational Gradation[85] provides a systematic process for treating persons with CNS impairments that aligns with dynamic systems theory. The authors suggest ways to manipulate the person, task, or object properties and the environment as ways to decrease the degrees of freedom. The authors base this approach on strength training and practice of meaningful occupations and provide an outline of how to analyze and grade occupations by altering the task, person, and environment.[85] This framework illustrates how a practitioner may successfully combine strength training with dynamic systems approach.

Case Study 7-1 provides a sample description using the Model of Human Occupation[49] and a dynamic systems approach to plan occupational therapy intervention.

Translating Dynamic Systems Theory Principles to Occupational Therapy

Dynamic systems theory integrates well with occupational therapy principles. Specifically, a child learns movement more easily and effectively if: (1) The movement is taught as a whole (versus part); (2) the movement is performed in variable situations; (3) the child is allowed to actively problem solve the actions required; and (4) the activity is meaningful to the child.

These principles are described and illustrated in the following sections.

Whole Learning

According to dynamic systems theory, many systems are involved and interact with each other to plan and execute movement.[93] Therefore, engaging in a whole activity

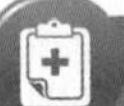

CASE STUDY 7-1 Intervention Plan

See accompanying video clip on the Evolve website.

Occupational Profile

Teagan is a 4-year-old boy who lives with his mothers and 7-year-old brother in a rural town. Both mothers are employed; one is a teacher and the other is a business manager. Teagan has Down syndrome and had cardiac surgery at 7 months. He has not experienced any other health issues. He receives physical therapy and occupational therapy at preschool.

Volition

Teagan loves to play tee-ball and play outside with his brother. He follows his brother, imitates his play, and indicates what he would like to do. Teagan enjoys being outside at preschool and watches his peers but does not interact with them. They run quickly by him. His parents state that he is an active boy. They are concerned that he does not play with his peers.

Habituation

Teagan attends a preschool for 4-year-olds. Teagan needs help getting dressed and he is not toilet trained. He washes his face and hands. He feeds himself with a spoon (with spillage) and uses a sippy cup to drink. He participates in recreational tee-ball. Teagan's parents report that he goes to bed at a reasonable hour (9 pm) during school days and awakes at 8 am. Teagan has chores to do each day, including picking up his plates after meals, putting his dirty clothes in the hamper, and walking the dog. He takes a 2-hour nap daily.

Performance Capacity

Teagan's gross motor skills are awkward and he must take breaks when running around the bases. He has low muscle tone throughout. He runs with a wide-based gait and holds his arms close to his body for balance. His posture is asymmetric (he elevates his shoulders and leans) when he runs. He falls frequently and shows difficulty moving around obstacles. His movements are slow and he watches his peers play instead of engaging. Teagan climbs up the slide, but does not slide down. Rather, he sits at the top of the slide, frustrating his peers. Teagan engages in some parallel play with other children at day care. When he does interact with his peers, he plays at a much younger level and frequently interferes in their play.

Environment

The preschool is a playful environment with a large fenced-in playground with a large slide, swings, and grassy play area. The inside rooms are full of toys and child-friendly decorations, small tables, and child-sized chairs.

Strengths

Teagan is a physically active 4-year-old who imitates his older brother's play. He enjoys rough play with his brother, playing tee-ball, and water play.

Weaknesses

Teagan does not play with his peers, but rather watches them or interferes in their play (i.e., sits at the top of the slide). He spends outdoor playtime at preschool playing alone.

Assessment

Teagan's motor difficulties are interfering with his ability to engage in play with his peers. He has difficulty initiating movement, as observed by his not moving down the slide. He falls frequently and has poor timing and sequencing of movements. Helping Teagan become more proficient in motor skills may improve his ability to keep up with peers on the playground.

Intervention Plan

Goals: To improve initiation, timing, and sequencing of motor skills for play.

1. At preschool, Teagan will initiate movement by climbing up and sliding down the slide five times consecutively (without stopping at the top for more than 10 seconds) within a 30-minute play session. [initiation]
2. Teagan will complete a 4-step obstacle course (walk on balance board for 5 feet, reach and throw object in container × 3, crawl through tunnel for 5 feet, and run 10 feet) within 10 minutes without falling or requiring verbal cues. [timing and sequencing]

The practitioner used the Model of Human Occupation (MOHO) to understand Teagan's occupational needs. The model fit well with dynamic systems theory because MOHO provides a framework to examine multiple systems, allowing the therapist to design intervention using motor control/motor learning principles. When developing client-centered goals the occupational therapy practitioner considered Teagan's preference for playing outside and the parents' goal for Teagan to play with his peers. These goals helped Teagan establish positive habits and routines at preschool and provided him with confidence in his ability to play with peers (self-efficacy). The practitioner engaged Teagan in activity in his environment and was able to train the teacher and caregivers through modeling and instruction. The practitioner designed interventions to specifically improve his performance capacity, to allow for occupational engagement by focusing on initiation of movement, sequencing, and timing of motor actions for play.

The practitioner focused on activities in which Teagan would be successful to improve his belief in his skills and abilities (self-efficacy) so that he would engage in play with peers. See Table 7-3 for examples of how a practitioner may consider the child, task, and environment when designing intervention activities.

Therapy sessions were fun and included a variety of games (e.g., follow the leader, obstacle course parades in ride-on cars) where other children could participate. The practitioner determined that person factors (e.g., limited initiation, inadequate timing, and difficulty sequencing) interfered with Teagan's movement for play. Teagan's low muscle tone may

Continued

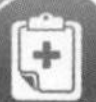

CASE STUDY 7-1 Intervention Plan—cont'd

result in poor postural control and subsequent difficulty with gross motor activities. Because Teagan engaged in rough play with his older brother at home, the practitioner hypothesized that the social environment at preschool was causing him to be "nervous" or "anxious" because the children ran quickly around him, seldom paying attention to him. The practitioner conducted a task analysis and concluded that activities involving complex motor tasks and multiple children were very difficult for him. The practitioner graded activities to allow Teagan to practice new motor actions in a safe and fun setting. During these sessions, the therapist adapted the course (environment), task (a car that was easier to move), or child requirements (allowing Teagan to perform a task differently) to help him be successful. Engaging Teagan in play activities that involved other children provided him with opportunities to socialize in nonthreatening and successful ways. For example, the practitioner allowed him to be the leader of the course, allowing him to practice prior to inviting other children. Teagan was proud that he could provide "tips" and directions for his peers. This helped develop his motivation for motor activities, further reinforcing practice and socialization.

TABLE 7-3 Sample Intervention Activities

	Child	Task	Environment
Ride-on-car obstacle course	Require the child to challenge motor skills or perform for longer period of time. Require the child to perform a less challenging motor task but a more challenging social task.	Change the type of "ride-on-car" so that it is easier or more difficult to operate. The car could be operated by pedaling, pushing, or walking or even be motorized. These different cars change the task requirements.	Change the course so that it is a flat or hilly course or a grass-covered or tarred surface.
Follow the leader	Provide a one-on-one assistant to help the child complete the tasks. Provide pictures or cues to the child and vary the time required to follow.	Change the motor movements required when imitating the leader. The leader could walk slowly or hop on one foot. The leader could do bilateral activities or unimanual activities.	Perform game in a structured setting with few distractions. Vary the type of terrain or area that the children must "follow."
Safari trip	Provide hand-over-hand assistance or modify the tasks so the child can achieve the motor task.	Change the requirements for each stage of the trip. The child may have to reach, pull, throw, or push objects.	Perform the trip in a variety of settings (e.g., ball pit, trampoline, outside, inside).

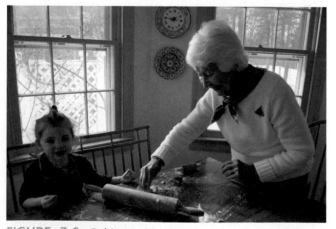

FIGURE 7-6 Baking with Grandma is meaningful and allows the child to engage in a variety of motor actions.

(occupation) facilitates multiple systems and the interactions required for effective movement (Figure 7-6). Overall, learning the whole motor task is more effective and motivating than learning only a part of the movement.[62,64,93,108]

Children perform whole tasks more efficiently and with better coordination than when they are asked to perform only a part or component of the movement.[31,62] Van der Weel and colleagues found that children with cerebral palsy used more supination when banging a drum than when simply exercising.[108] Not only did children perform the task more efficiently, but they also engaged in the task for longer periods of time and activated more areas of the brain during the activity. In addition, functional magnetic resonance imaging studies indicate that more areas of the brain are activated when subjects engage in meaningful whole tasks versus parts of the tasks.[50] Van de Winckel and colleagues found significantly more brain activation for both children with cerebral palsy and typically developing children when they were engaged in active movement (grasp and release of an object) compared with passive movements (robot moved finger up and down) and tactile stimulation (stroking back of hand with sponge cotton cloth).[109] The findings suggest engaging children in active tasks results in more brain activation for both typical children and children with cerebral palsy.[58,109]

Engaging in the whole activity or occupation requires children to process stimuli and respond to changes within and between systems. The ability to respond in variable ways is a hallmark of functional movement. Typically developing children, for example, use multiple strategies when moving, as opposed to children with DCD, who have been found to exhibit limited variability and adaptability in their movement.[61,91,100] Therefore, one goal of occupational therapy intervention is to promote variability and flexibility in movements.

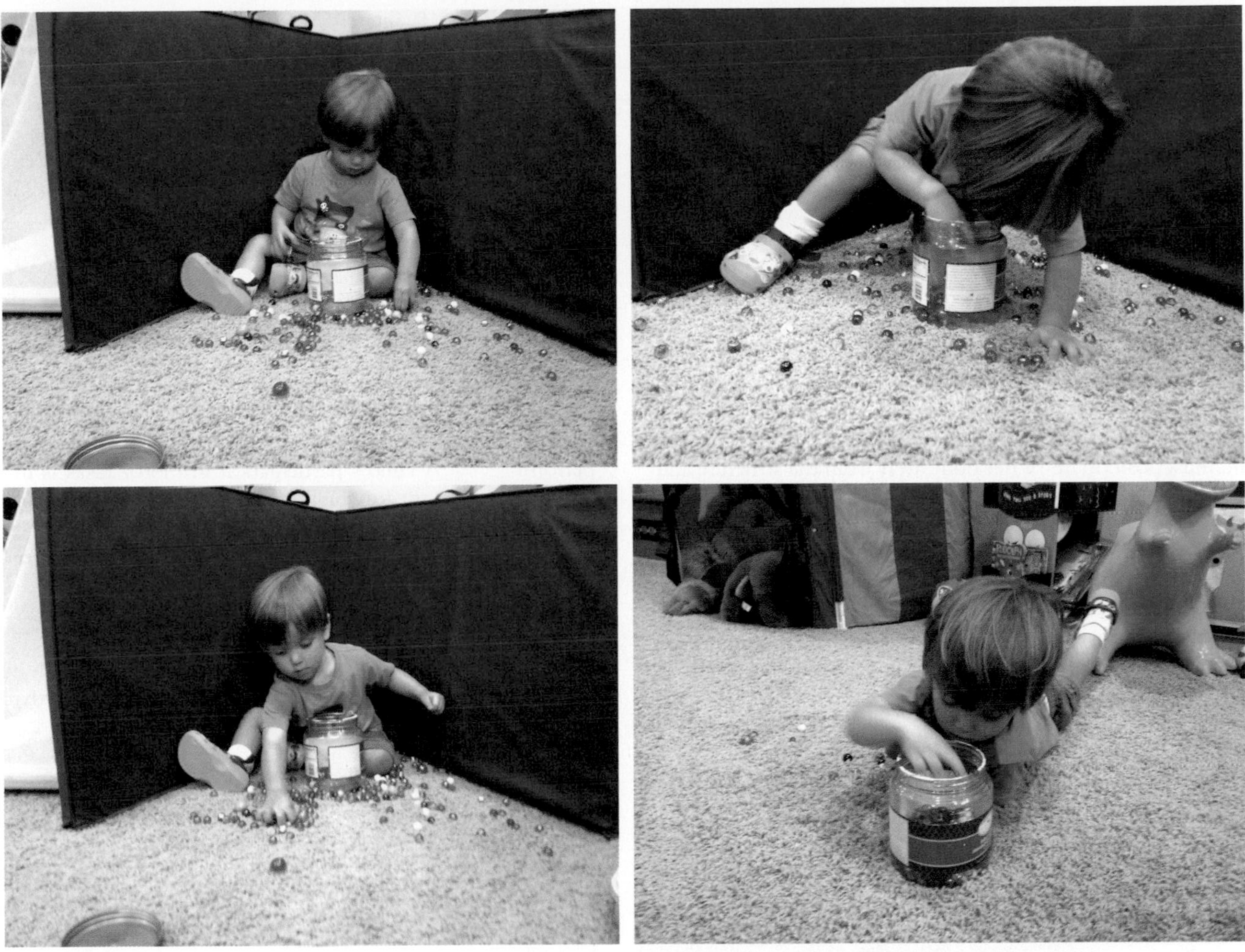

FIGURE 7-7 The child enjoys playing with marbles in a variety of positions. This activity requires he use a variety of movements.

Variability

Dynamic systems theorists propose that movement requires an ability to adapt to changes within and between systems; in other words, variability is central to functional movement.[98,102,103] Variability is inherent in activity (e.g., reaching for different objects, environmental stimuli) as well as within and between systems (e.g., interactions between visual and sensory systems).

Movement occurs in a variety of contexts and requires that children adapt to environmental changes (using visual and auditory systems) or internal changes (perceived through vestibular and proprioceptive systems). For example, children may need to adjust movements in response to interpretations of visual input (e.g., the ball is coming quickly versus slowly); children may experience physiologic changes (e.g., low energy) affecting movement patterns. The environment may pose changes (e.g., weather, terrain, peers). Functional movement, the goal of motor control intervention, requires that children possess a variety of motor skills.

Because variability is essential to functional movement, occupational therapists encourage children to move in variable ways while engaging in occupations. Thus the expectation of intervention is that the child performs movements in a variety of ways versus repeating and learning one pattern of movement. For example, requesting a child who is sitting in a corner seat to repeatedly pick up a block and drop it into a stationary container requires minimal adaptability on the child's part. A better intervention session would include combining the whole task with variability such as engaging the child in playing with marbles scattered on the floor (Figure 7-7).

In certain children, variability of performance is too great and the practitioner's goal is to establish consistency in movements. Variability in movements can be measured by intra-individual variability. In a simple reaction time task to examine intra-individual variability, children with attention-deficit/hyperactivity disorder (ADHD) or dyslexia did not differ from each other but were more variable than typically developing children.[11] Children with ADHD produced fewer writing sequences than did the children with dyslexia (controls were not significantly different from children with dyslexia). Excessive variability found in the children with ADHD and those with dyslexia interfered with consistency in handwriting performance. These findings support the need to encourage more accuracy in movements while allowing for variability for functional performance. Understanding the range of typical development and factors influencing movement is essential to designing effective intervention. Performing movements in multiple ways requires that children problem solve and self-correct. All children use problem solving to develop and refine movement; therefore, problem solving is an important part of motor control.

Problem Solving

Improved retention of motor skills occurs when children problem solve and self-correct for motor errors.[12,65,68,83] Children learn and retain motor skills better from intrinsically problem solving than they do from receiving external feedback during an action (such as hand-over-hand assistance). For example, to learn to build a sand castle, the child problem solves his or her position in the sand and how to scoop and place the sand (Figure 7-8). The child is more likely to learn a new motor task in a meaningful, socially engaging activity. The child must position his or her body away from the structure and use adequate timing and force to make the castle of choice. Self-correcting enables children to rely on internal cues that indicate the effectiveness of movement and thereby help them adapt and modify movements in a variety of contexts.[34,41]

Therefore, therapists working to improve a child's motor performance provide many opportunities for the child to actively solve motor problems by doing, rather than repetitive practicing of a part of the movement. Setting up the environment to facilitate physical, social, and cognitive tasks encourages the child to discover how to move, explore options, and self-correct movement errors beneficial to motor learning. Not only do children benefit from problem solving how to move, they also benefit from engaging in activities that they find meaningful. Participation in meaningful activities is central to occupational therapy practice and also improves the child's motor control.

Meaning

Dynamic systems theory proposes that the interactions between systems (including the emotional system) influence movements. Occupational therapists have historically viewed the meaningfulness of activities as essential to practice and acknowledge the benefits of purposeful activity in motivating clients to perform.[33,49,105] A child's participation in motor tasks is influenced by the extent to which he or she can identify his or her own interests and goals and believes he or she will be effective in those motor tasks (Figure 7-9, *A-C*). Children are more motivated to engage in difficult motor skills if they find the activity important and fun and if they believe they can be successful.[49,52]

In addition, children and youth participate for longer periods of time and perform more repetitions when activities

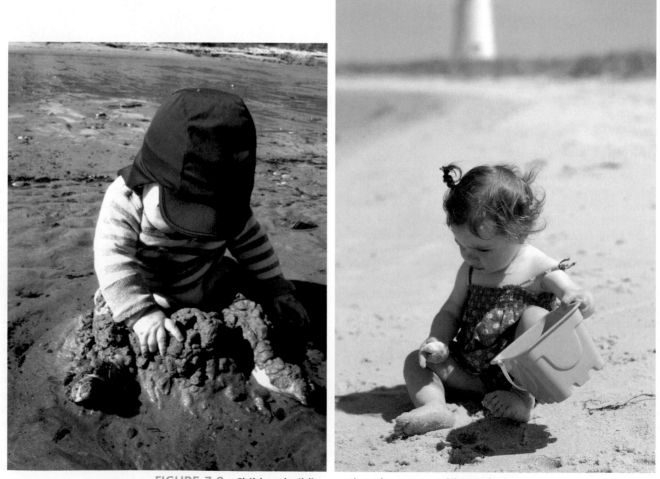

FIGURE 7-8 Children building sand castles must problem solve.

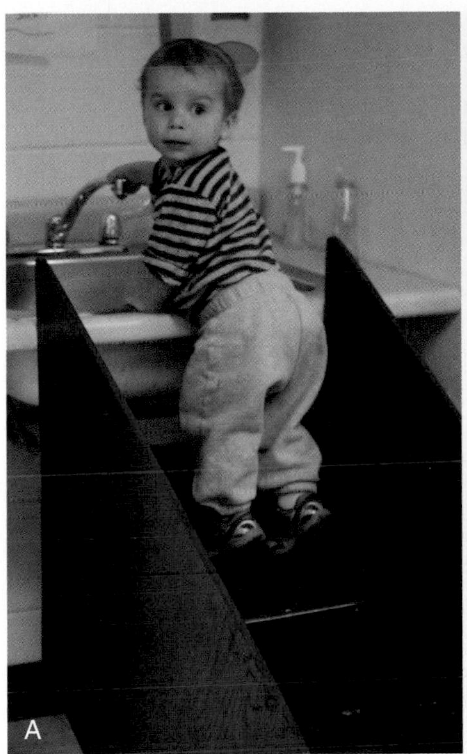
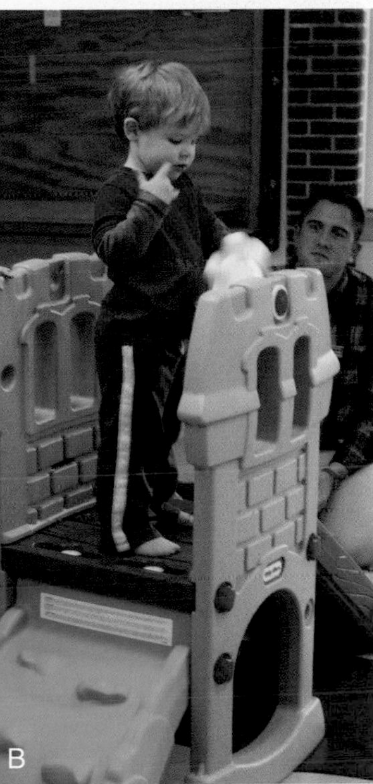
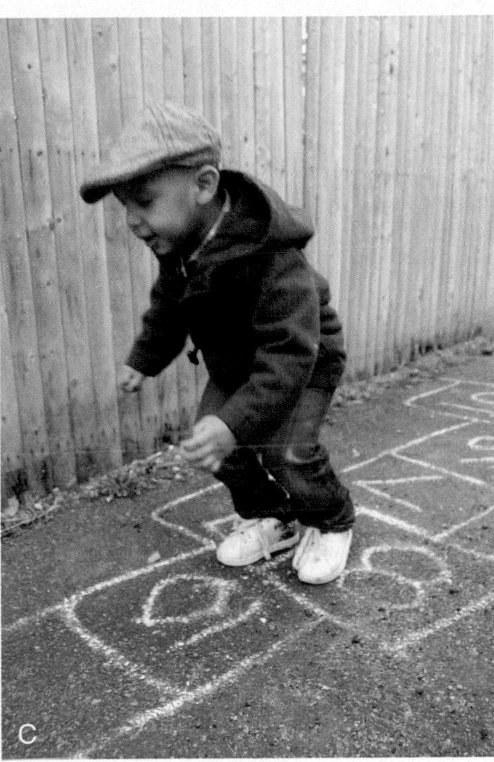

FIGURE 7-9 **A,** Sometimes children look very serious while playing as they try to problem solve how to motor plan. **B,** Children are more likely to engage in a difficult task if they find it meaningful. **C,** Hopscotch requires motor planning, coordination, timing, and sequencing.

are meaningful.[118] Not only do they perform longer, but, in addition, the quality of movement improves when the activity has meaning to the child.[35] Meaning may be determined by asking children directly using semistructured interviews. Cohn, Miller, and Tickle-Degnen[22] and O'Brien et al.[76] found that children with motor deficits wanted to participate in "regular" activities with friends. These expressed interests suggest that practitioners promote meaningful physical activity (such as skiing, swimming, cycling, running, and skating) for children who have motor impairments.

Hetu and Mercier[42] examined the influence of purposeful activity by reviewing 35 articles. They suggest that clinicians use tasks with high object affordance to promote optimal motor performance. They defined object affordance tasks as those in which the objects used conveyed functional information, included functional goals, and consisted of the correct number of actual objects required for the task. The affordance refers to the purposefulness of the object. For example, the object is meaningful to the person (i.e., child's favorite toy) and the object suggests a specific motor action (e.g., flying a toy helicopter).

Practitioners may also observe children to better understand meaning. The Pediatric Volitional Questionnaire[8] and the Test of Playfulness[94] provide observational assessments to measure interest, motivation, and approach toward activity (play). To design effective motor control intervention, occupational therapists acknowledge the meaning a child attaches to the activity by learning the child's goals and desires.[1,49,61] Meaning is derived from an individual's experience and viewpoint; thus therapists involve the child in selecting and designing the activity. The Child Occupational Self-Assessment (COSA)[48] provides a measure to help the child identify activities in which he or she would like to engage. The authors suggest that practitioners interviewing children set up a comfortable environment, engage in informal discussion, begin with open-ended questions and follow up with probing questions, pay attention to nonverbal cues, and be aware of how the child perceives the interview. The assessment may be given in multiple sessions and practitioners can adapt or modify the approach to meet the child's needs. The intent of the COSA is to gain information about the child. In focus group discussions, practitioners using the COSA felt it helped them engage in important discussions with children while providing information on the child's interests and belief in abilities.[53]

Therapists use the Cognitive Orientation to daily Occupational Performance (CO-OP) model to engage children in goal setting and problem solving.[83] This model is congruent with dynamic systems theory and has been found to be effective for improving movement for children with DCD.[66,68,116,117] By including children in the process, the therapist empowers the child to make decisions and actively engage. The CO-OP model is explained in Chapter 10. See Box 7-2 for tips to design intervention using motor control concepts.

Development of Motor Control

The development of motor skills occurs in three stages—cognitive, associative, and autonomous—and involves an interaction among three processes (i.e., cognition, perception, and

BOX 7-2 Tips for Designing Intervention Using Motor Control Concepts

Whole Learning
- Play activities (e.g., crafts, dress-up, cooking, dance moves)
- Games
- Themed activities

Variability
- Develop occupations as goals (e.g., play with peers)
- Provide variety of activities or different ways to do tasks
- Same motor movement in different forms
- Vary the objects or placement
- Vary the requirements of the task
- Consider the social nature of the task
- Vary the environmental context (e.g., clinic versus playground)

Problem Solving
- Set up activities with different degrees of difficulty
- Repeat movements so child must figure it out
- Wait for child to figure it out

BOX 7-3 Strategies for Each Stage of Motor Control

Stage	Strategies
Cognitive	Use simple statements and verbal cues. Use catchy words or pneumonics. Repeat skills. Provide time for problem solving. Allow child to review progress.
Associative	Relate new tasks to past activities. Use the same words or cues for similar tasks. Help child see links to previous successful activity. Allow child to review progress by relating to other activity.
Autonomous	Set up an environment in which the child can be successful. Allow the child to self-reflect. Provide few if any cues. Do not correct or address quality—allow the child to self-evaluate.

action).[93] These stages and processes are considered dynamic in that they are constantly changing and interacting with each other in relation to the motor skill or task requirements. Practitioners may change intervention strategies based on the stage of development in which the child is performing. See Box 7-3 for sample strategies as related to stage of development.

The cognitive stage refers to the skill acquisition stage. In this stage the learner practices new movements, errors are common, and movements are inefficient and inconsistent. During this stage, learners need frequent repetition and feedback. Children learning to hold a spoon, for example, may need reminders to take little scoops of food and to move the spoon to the mouth slowly.

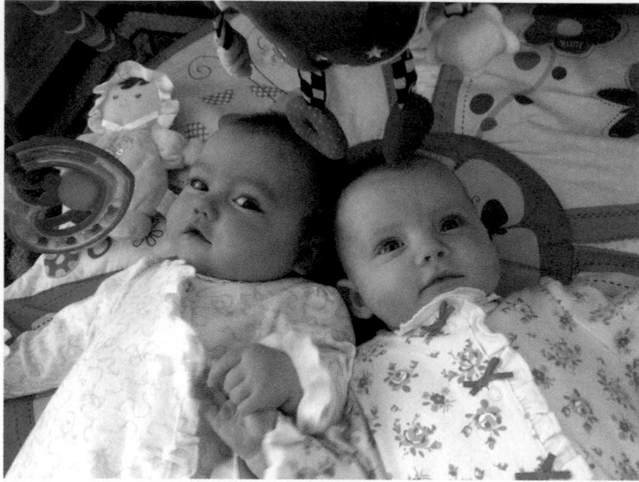

FIGURE 7-10 Infants enjoy sensory motor play as they look around and feel things to learn about their environment and movements.

The associative stage involves skill refinement, increased performance, decreased errors, and increased consistency and efficiency. During this stage the learner relates past experiences to the present, thereby "associating" movements (e.g., the child may realize that the last time she moved her hand too quickly, the food dropped off the spoon, so she reminds herself to slow down).

During the autonomous stage, the learner retains the skills and can perform the movement functionally. During this stage, skills are transferred easily to different settings and are refined. For example, during this stage a child can feed himself or herself a variety of foods using a spoon and simultaneously carry on a conversation at the table. At this stage the motor skill has been learned and requires little attention, which supports evidence suggesting that less brain activation is required.[84]

Each stage of movement involves interactions among the processes of cognition, perception, and action[93] (Figure 7-10). Cognition refers to intent or the child's motivation to move and also to the ability to plan the movement. Cognitive processes are used in decisions about how to use an object (e.g., throw versus catch).

Perception refers to how the individual receives and makes sense of a stimulus (visual, auditory, tactile, kinesthetic, vestibular, or olfactory). Perception involves attributing meaning to sensory input. Perception refers to both peripheral sensory mechanisms and higher level processing that interprets the meaning of stimuli.[93] For example, the child must be able to identify the object coming toward him or her or "feel" balance.

The process of action includes muscle contractions, patterns, precision, and nature of the movement (dynamic versus static). Research devoted to the action stage explores how factors such as strength, ability to co-activate muscle groups, reaction time, and timing and sequencing contribute to movement.[77,80,87]

When looking at skill acquisition, practitioners help clients demonstrate consistency, flexibility, and efficiency in movements. Consistency refers to ability of the child to perform a task consistently over time. Flexibility refers to the ability to adapt and modify the task performance based on changing environments or conditions.[72] Efficiency pertains to the cardiovascular and musculoskeletal systems (e.g., Can the child perform the task without tiring?).

Motor Learning

Motor learning refers to the acquisition or modification of motor skills. Motor learning literature explores transfer of learning, sequencing, and adapting tasks, type and amount of practice, error-based learning, timing, type of feedback, and mental rehearsal. These concepts provide useful information on techniques involved in the teaching-learning process of movement. Being knowledgeable and aware of the teaching-learning process enables therapists to incorporate motor learning principles into practice so that children learn and retain motor function for their daily lives. Williams (Box 7-4) provides an overview of motor learning strategies shown to increase motor control. Occupational therapy practitioners are encouraged to use these techniques to promote motor learning. These motor learning strategies can easily be integrated into occupational therapy practice.

Niemeijer and colleagues[74] examined the outcomes of physical therapy sessions when the practitioners used teaching principles during neuromotor task training. The authors provided 11 practitioners with a taxonomy of principles aimed at improving motor learning for children with DCD. Twenty teaching-learning principles were organized into three categories: giving instructions, sharing knowledge, and providing or asking for feedback. The data revealed that four principles were associated with improved performance as measured by the Test of Gross Motor Development: giving clues, explaining why, providing rhythm, and asking about understanding. Two principles were associated with improved performance on the M-ABC (adjusting body position and explaining why).[74]

Transfer of Learning

Transfer of learning, or generalization, refers to applying learning to new situations. The goal of occupational therapy intervention is that the child transfer learning performed in the clinic or intervention setting to a natural context. For example, after working on maneuvering a new wheelchair through an obstacle course at the clinic with ease, the therapist hopes the child will be able to maneuver the wheelchair through the school hallway.

Children are best able to transfer motor skills when they have practiced the motor skill within the natural context or in the "real world" situation. Therefore, the best way to help the child successfully maneuver his wheelchair through the school hallway is to practice in that setting. The occupational therapist may initially teach basic wheelchair skills to the child, then practice in the hallway after school hours (to decrease obstacles), and finally work up to maneuvering the wheelchair during class change. Research suggests that children transfer the task more quickly with this intervention strategy than with practicing in a clinic setting only.[23,99]

In addition, transfer of learning occurs more easily when the motor task is performed during a functional activity or actual occupation.[23,31,35,79] When selecting activities to practice, the practitioner recognizes that motor skills with similar components are more likely to transfer. For example, a child who has just successfully learned to throw a ball would more easily learn to throw a bean bag at a target.

Sequencing and Adapting Tasks

Grading and adapting motor tasks so that children are successful constitute part of the occupational therapy process (Table 7-4). Generally, discrete tasks are easier to accomplish than continuous tasks. Discrete tasks are those with a definite beginning and end (e.g., picking up an object), whereas continuous task are ongoing (e.g., walking, running). Tasks involving unimanual movements are often learned or mastered before bimanual movements.[114] Skills manipulating stationary objects develop before skills with moving objects.

"Closed tasks are those in which the environment is stationary during task performance" (p. 407),[93] whereas open tasks are ones in which the environment is changing or in motion and involve some intertrial variability. Closed tasks are generally simpler for most children to accomplish.

Therapists also consider the cognitive demands of activities; children more easily complete simple motor tasks that have fewer cognitive requirements. Tasks with fewer steps are accomplished more readily than those with multiple steps (e.g., throwing at a target is easier than picking up a ball from the container, moving to the starting line, and then throwing at a target). Children acquire tasks that require less precision (e.g., scribbling will be easier than coloring within the lines) more easily than those that require more precision. When sequencing and adapting activities for children, therapists consider the amount of direction required; movement requiring less direction is easier to learn than that requiring multiple directions.

The structure of the environment plays an important role in the nature and complexity of the demands of the activity. For example, environments with variability and extraneous stimuli (e.g., other children) are more challenging and thus more

TABLE 7-4 Grading and Adapting Activity

Uncomplicated	Example	More Difficult	Example
Discrete	Jump over rope × 1	Continuous	Jumping rope
Unimanual	Grasp toy in one hand	Bimanual	Grasping toy with two hands
Stationary	Hold toy	Dynamic	Catching a moving ball
Closed	Scribble on paper	Open	Following with pen moving target on computer
One-step	Write name	Multistep	Writing name and drawing picture
Simple	Place ball in container	Complex	Playing a game of mini-golf

BOX 7-4 Williams' Motor Learning Principles

Transfer of Learning

- Skill experiences are presented in logical progression.
- Simple, foundational skills are practiced before more complex skills.
- Skill practice includes "real life" and simulated settings.
- Skills with similar components are more likely to show transfer effect.
- Practice in natural context with actual objects is most effective

Feedback

Modeling or demonstration

- Demonstration is best if it is given to the individual before practicing the skill and in the early stages of skill acquisition.
- Demonstration should be given throughout practice and as frequently as deemed helpful.
- Demonstrations should not be accompanied by verbal commentary because this can reduce attention paid to important aspects of the skill being demonstrated.
- It is important to direct the individual's attention to the critical cues immediately before the skill is demonstrated.
- Allow child time to "figure it out."

Verbal Instructions

- Verbal cues should be brief, to the point, and use one to three words.
- Verbal cues should be limited in terms of numbers of cues given during or after performance.
- Only the major aspect of the skill that is being concentrated on should be cued.
- Verbal cues should be carefully timed so they do not interfere with performance.
- Verbal cues can and should be initially repeated by the performer.
- Verbal cues should emphasize key aspects of movement

Knowledge of Results (KR) and Knowledge of Performance (KP)

- A variety of different combinations of both KR and KP typically helps to facilitate learning.
- KP error information may help the performer change important performance characteristics and thus may help facilitate skill acquisition.
- Information about "appropriate" or "correct" aspects of performance helps to motivate the child to continue practicing.
- It is important to balance between feedback that is error-based and that which is based on "appropriate" or "correct" characteristics of the performance.
- KP feedback can also be descriptive or prescriptive; prescriptive KP is more helpful than just descriptive KP in the early or beginning stages of learning.
- KP and KR should be given close in time to but after completion of the task.
- KP and KR typically should not necessarily be given 100% of the time.
- Learning is enhanced if KR/KP is given at least 50% of the time.
- A frequently used procedure for given KR/KP is to practice a skill several times and then provide the appropriate feedback.

Distribution and Variability of Skill Practice

- Shorter, more frequent practice sessions are preferable to longer, less frequent practice.
- If a skill or task is complex and/or requires a relatively long time to perform or if it requires repetitive movements, relatively short practice trials/sessions with frequent rest periods are preferable.
- If the skill is relatively simple and takes only a brief time to complete, longer practice trials/sessions with less frequent rest periods are preferable.
- It can enhance skill acquisition to practice several tasks in the same session.
- If several tasks are to be practiced, divide the time spent on each and either randomly repeat practice on each or use a sequence that aids the overall practice.
- Providing a number of different environmental contexts in which the skill is practiced appears to facilitate learning.
- With regard to the "amount" of practice, more is not necessarily always better.
- Clinical judgment should be used to recognize when practice is no longer producing changes; at this time, a new or different task could and probably should be introduced.

Whole Versus Part Practice

- Whole practice is better when the skill or task to be performed is simple.
- Part practice may be preferable when the skill is more complex.
- If part practice is used, be sure that the parts practiced are "natural units"—that they go together.
- To simplify a task, reduce the nature and/or complexity of the objects to be manipulated—for example, use a balloon for catching instead of a ball.
- To simplify a task, provide assistance to the learner that helps to reduce attention demands—for example, provide trunk support during practice of different eye-hand coordination tasks.
- To simplify a task, provide auditory or rhythmic accompaniment; this may help to facilitate learning through assisting the learner in getting the appropriate "rhythm" of the movement.

Mental Practice

- Mental practice can help to facilitate acquisition of new skills as well as the relearning of old skills.
- Mental practice can help the child to prepare to perform a task.
- Mental practice combined with physical practice works best.
- For mental practice to be effective, the individual should have some basic imagery ability.
- Mental practice should be relatively short, not prolonged.

Adapted from Williams, H. (2006). Motor control. In J. Solomon & J. O'Brien (Eds.), *Pediatric skills for occupational therapy assistants* (2nd ed., pp. 474–480). St. Louis: Mosby.

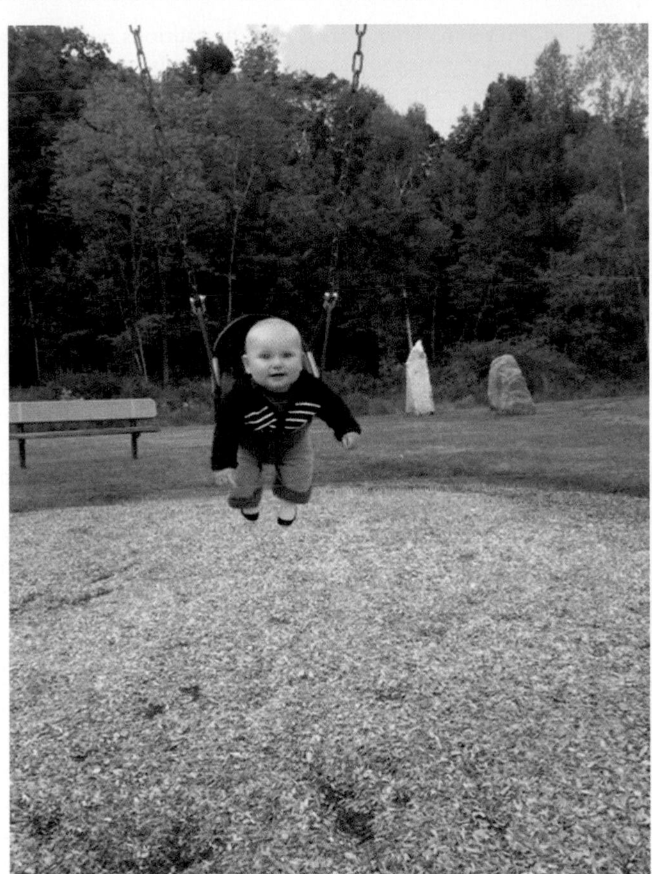
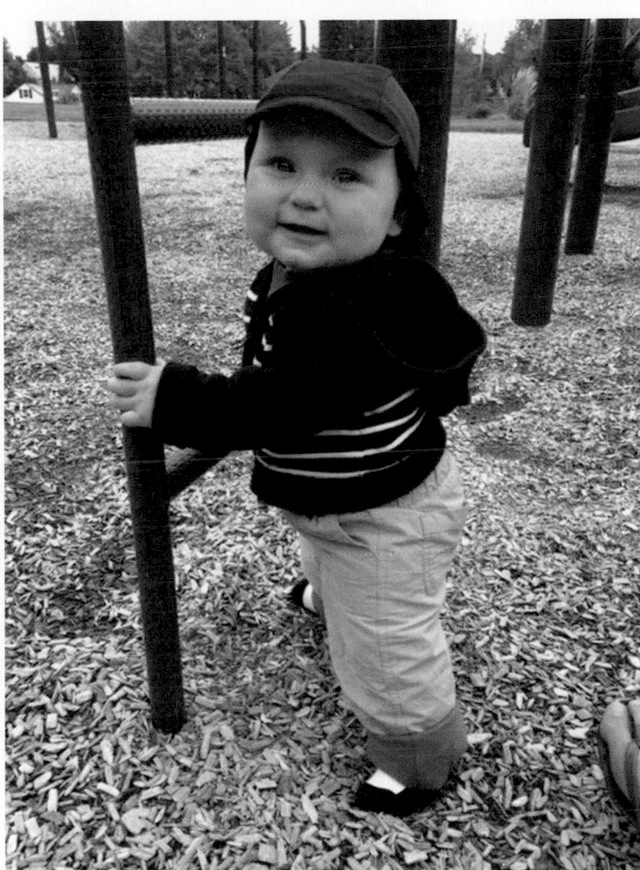

FIGURE 7-11 **Distributed Practice.** Taking breaks between swinging is an example of distributed practice.

difficult for children because they must continually adapt and adjust. Occupational therapy practitioners consider how to sequence activities and adapt them accordingly to promote a child's success. Recent research suggests that children with cerebral palsy may have less ability to adapt or vary their movement patterns given different contexts.[104] For example, children with cerebral palsy within the same Gross Motor Function Classification System[89] exhibited varying degrees of independence depending on the setting and terrain.[104] They performed higher at home and lowest in the outdoors or community. Thus, therapists are encouraged to consider the contextual features that can promote skills when planning interventions.

Practice Levels and Types

Practice is an essential feature of occupational therapy intervention. A considerable amount of research has been conducted on the use of practice to improve or develop motor skills.[79,99]

Massed practice (also known as blocked) is defined as practice in which the period performing the movement is greater than the rest period. This type of practice works best during the cognitive stage, as the subject is just beginning to learn the movements. An example of blocked practice may include working on grasp pattern and release by asking a child to pick up 10 blocks and put them all in a container before taking a break and then repeating the game again.

Distributed practice is defined as practice in which rest between trials is greater than the time of the trial and is most useful during the associative stage (Figure 7-11). A clinical example of distributed practice includes asking the child to pick up bean bags placed on the floor while engaged in a game of swinging. In this scenario, the child is still practicing grasp and release, but the child is also working on postural control and processing vestibular input. Therefore, the child grasps and releases a few bean bags, has a rest while swinging in which he must work on other aspects of skill, and then returns to grasp and release.

Variable or random practice is most effective during the autonomous stage. Variable practice requires that learners repeat the same patterns but make small changes as necessary (Figure 7-12). This type of practice increases the ability to adapt and generalize learning. In general, short frequent practice is better than longer, less frequent practice because it decreases fatigue and increases reinforcement.[114] Persons with Down syndrome showed improvement in a simple reach (to a target) with variable practice.[46] An example of random practice includes intervention working on grasp and release while the child is engaged in a variety of play activities. This type of practice is most closely related to the actual occupation. The child must pick up and release toys during the play session. The child picks up a variety of objects: small blocks, large balls, light toys, and heavy scooter boards.

Mental practice includes performing the skill in one's imagination, without any action involved. It consists of role playing, watching a video, or imagining. Mental practice is effective in teaching motor skills and retraining the timing and

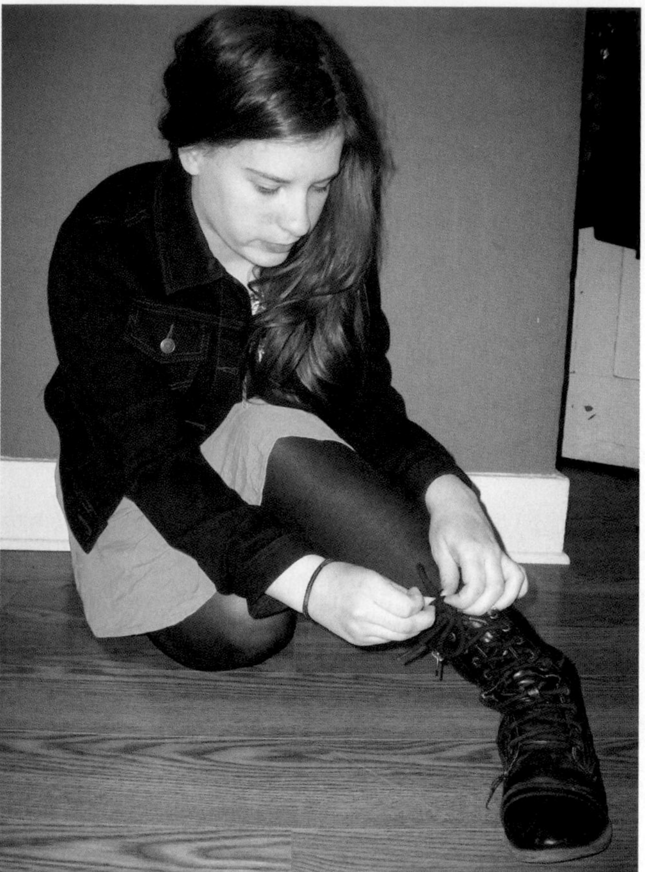

FIGURE 7-12 Variable Practice. The child ties her shoes right before she goes outside to play. She is able to tie different sneakers and often she sits on the floor to complete the task.

coordination of muscle group activity.[26-29,40,78] It is most effective at the early and later stages of learning and may be task-specific. Much of the research on mental practice is conducted on athletes trying to maximize their performance.[71,78] However, the techniques used may be beneficial to children with motor difficulties.[91,96,115] For middle school children with mild mental disabilities, mental imagery enhanced their motor performance on a peg board and pursuit rotor task.[91] Some positive results regarding motor performance were reported for children with attention deficit disorder and developmental coordination disorder.[115] Taktek and colleagues found performance (in throwing a ball) resulting from mental imagery combined with physical practice was equal during the retention phase, but superior during the transfer of learning phase.[100] The researchers examined visual and kinesthetic imagery in young children and found that they were both effective for children as young as 8 years. Many theorists suggest imagery is effective because it requires cognitive processes and helps children problem solve motor solutions.[29,40]

Driskell and colleagues suggest that practitioners using mental practice consider the type of task, duration of mental practice, and time between practice and performance for retention.[29] Tasks in which the child has experience may be easier to imagine. However, the child may be able to imagine movements after observing them on a video or observing someone else perform them. Therapists should be cautious not to incorporate a too-long mental practice because this may be difficult for children and result in a lack of motivation. Finally, therapists should incorporate actual performance shortly after the mental practice for the best retention. Techniques of watching a video, pointing out components of the movement, or simply reviewing mentally how the movement will look in combination with physical practice may provide improved motor learning.

In a descriptive study, researchers compared EEG topographic maps in four typically developing children and four children with cerebral palsy while they were engaged in motor execution and motor imagery tasks.[92] The researchers asked the children to reach and grasp a small ball with their dominant hand, imagine hand movement needed to reach and grasp the ball, observe an animated reaching and grasping movement on the monitor, visualize the right-handed reaching and grasping movement, and create a "mental video" of the virtual hand movement. The authors found that different areas of the brain were activated during the imagery tasks for typical children and those with cerebral palsy.[92]

Error-Based Learning

Children learn movement by making errors or mistakes and self-correcting.[6,99] Therefore, clinicians sometimes allow the challenge to exceed the capacity of the child, to give him or her the opportunity to make errors, correct them (if possible), and learn from the experience. Children with disabilities must learn to adapt to new, different, or unexpected situations. In the past, therapists typically have been hesitant to allow children to learn through making errors. However, making errors in controlled settings allows children to resolve problems and is important for facilitating motor skill learning. Encouraging children to explore, adjust movements, and evaluate their responses and reactions helps them learn and refine motor skills.

Feedback

Intrinsic feedback, which allows the child to self-correct, is most effective for sustaining motor performance and should be the goal of intervention sessions. Intrinsic feedback may be elicited through discovery, a situation in which the therapist sets up the environment and the child is allowed to explore and discover, make errors, and consequently learn new ways of moving.

Children may require extrinsic feedback in the early stages of motor skill development. Extrinsic feedback consists of providing verbal cueing or physical guidance. Demonstrative feedback refers to modeling or imitating movements. Demonstrative feedback is best if it is provided before the child actually practices the movement, as well as throughout early stages of skill acquisition. The practitioner provides modeling without verbal commentary, because simultaneous verbal cues can decrease the child's attention to the movement.[23,99]

Knowledge of Performance

Feedback to improve movement is most helpful when it is specific and clear. Knowledge of performance helps children understand how they performed the desired movement. Knowledge of performance is helpful in refining and adjusting motor skills and therefore is useful after the child has established basic skills. Therapists may provide descriptive feedback to the child about performance of a specific task (i.e., writing), such as "You held the pencil between thumb and fingers and pressed lightly" or therapists may provide prescriptive feedback, such as "Next time, press a little more."

Knowledge of Results

Feedback related to the desired outcome helps children understand movement. Providing this knowledge is most effective when specific information on the movement's goal is stated. Thus, saying "Each button is lined up with its buttonhole" is preferred over "Good job." Knowledge of results is motivating and encourages children to continue; it is most helpful when learning new motor tasks.

Verbal Feedback

Verbal praise and reinforcement are useful in motivating clients and changing behaviors but may be overused in clinical settings. Allowing children to make their own assessments of their performance is beneficial and will increase their sense of efficacy.[99] Verbal feedback is best if provided immediately after completion of the task. Using one to three brief cue words that can be repeated easily by the performer is best. Knowledge of correct performance motivates a child to continue practicing, so such reinforcement may be used frequently. Positive feedback with specific cues improves performance, such as saying "You pressed firmly with the pencil!"

Application of Motor Control/Learning Theory in Occupational Therapy Practice

Case Study 7-2 illustrates how therapists may apply current motor control/motor learning principles to practice. Specifically, this example applies dynamic systems theory from an occupational therapy perspective to intervention of a child's motor deficits. The practitioner uses concepts from dynamic systems theory with motor learning strategies as outlined by Williams (see Box 7-4).

Case Study 7-2 shows how a practitioner works within the multiple systems involved in movement to evaluate and design intervention. The therapist used principles of variability, meaning, occupation, and natural context when designing intervention. The therapist incorporated motor learning principles of feedback, demonstration, practice, and sequencing and adapting tasks. All activities were playful and fun for the child so that he would optimally engage in them.

CASE STUDY 7-2 Occupational Profile

Paul is a 7-year-old boy referred to occupational therapy after his mother expressed concern that he has difficulty using his hands, completing school work, and playing on the playground. Paul's mother states that "he has trouble coloring, doing anything with his hands, and can't climb up the slide or get on the swing." She noted that Paul has stomachaches in the mornings and does not want to go to school. She reported that Paul enjoys playing with trucks on the floor in the living room with his friend.

Paul is in the first grade. His teacher is concerned that Paul is not "picking up things" as quickly as his peers and noted he has trouble with handwriting and reading. She acknowledged that Paul verbally contributes in class.

Occupational Performance

Living Situation

Paul lives with his parents and 2-year-old sister in a neighborhood with many children who frequently play together outside. Paul stated he has "one good friend" with whom he plays in the afternoons and sees at school. Paul participates in recreational soccer (although he says, "I'm not very good").

Gross Motor

Paul presented as a thin, small 7-year-old boy, who stood with his shoulders depressed. Range of motion is within normal limits. His muscle tone throughout was slightly low, especially in the trunk. He sat with a rounded back and could not maintain balance with eyes closed. Paul ran with his feet apart and his arms did not swing consistently or in rhythm. He had difficulty changing positions as observed by stopping and reorienting himself as his friend ran around him. Paul showed poor sequencing and timing of movements—he could not jump with both feet together and or catch a ball. He fell three times on the tires when he tried to balance on them during recess.

Handwriting

Paul held a pencil in a tight pronated grasp and made dark marks on the paper. He did not draw a straight line (3 inches) within the ¼-inch markings—his line went over in more than five places. He printed his name slowly; spacing was inconsistent between letters; the letters were of uneven size; and he did not stay within the large ruled lines. When writing, he sat with his feet on the floor, his back was rounded, and his face was close to the paper. He showed some associated reactions (e.g., facial movements) when writing. He was not able to perform alternating hand movements.

Self-Care

Paul independently donned his coat and hat. He had difficulty with buttoning, and required several minutes to accomplish. He demonstrated beginning skills in tying his shoes, making multiple knots instead. He feeds himself but has difficulty with opening cartons and tearing packages. He washes his face and hands.

Play

Paul was the last child to go outside for recess. He played with his friend and watched others. His friend waited for him and frequently repeated, "Hurry up, Paul." Paul watched others on the swings and slides, but did not try to interact with others. He played on the tires by himself.

Continued

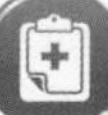

CASE STUDY 7-2 Occupational Profile—cont'd

Systems Contributing to Performance

Environment

Paul lives in a three-bedroom home. He has access to toys inside and outside. His home is child-friendly. The backyard is fenced in and includes a swing set, slide, and sandbox. He does not ride a bike, swing, or go down the slide. He prefers to play indoors. If he must play outside, he likes to play with his trucks on the deck.

School

Paul attends a local elementary school; there are 15 students in his class. The teacher provides structure and is consistent. She expressed concern that Paul is falling behind his classmates and notes difficulty with handwriting, paying attention, and getting things done in a timely manner. She commented that Paul is always the last one out the door, forgets things in the classroom, and seems frustrated at times. However, she revealed that Paul is verbal, answers questions readily, behaves well, and is polite.

Neuromotor

Paul's low muscle tone, poor postural control, and difficulty with timing and sequencing are interfering with his ability to move in a coordinated fashion. Paul shows some soft neurologic signs, such as associated reactions. He demonstrates poor standing balance with his eyes closed and poor dynamic balance. He fell three times on playground tires within a 30-minute recess.

Sensory

Paul's poor balance and motor planning are interfering with his movement. Paul's body awareness is somewhat affected because he struggles to identify right-left, a skill expected at his age. His internal body awareness is not quite developed.

Assessment

Paul exhibits developmental coordination disorder (DCD), as his motor abilities are interfering with his daily activities of play, self-care, and academics. He is aware of his difficulties and experiencing frustration with an inability to keep up with his peers. He has changed his activity preferences (to indoor activities) and is beginning to resist going to school.

Goals

1. *Academic performance*: Paul will improve fine motor skills for academics.
   a. Paul will write his first name in a 2 inch by 3 inch rectangle on the upper right hand corner of his paper with 90% legibility.
   b. Given a verbal prompt, Paul will complete a short writing assignment (three lines) in 15 minutes with 80% legibility.
2. *Play*: Paul will improve motor skills to engage in play on playground with peers.
   a. Paul will show improved timing and sequencing by pumping a swing consecutively for 5 minutes on the school playground.
   b. Paul will demonstrate posture and balance for play as evidenced by remaining upright while climbing on at least 10 tires (on the playground tire hill) within a 30-minute play session.

Analysis of Intervention Planning

The occupational therapist, Cora, a school-based practitioner, developed an intervention plan to help Paul play with his peers and perform in the classroom. These goals address the parents' concern that Paul is having "difficulty playing on the playground and doing anything with his hands." Cora hypothesized that helping Paul gain postural control, balance, timing, and sequencing through playground activities would provide a foundation for hand skills. Improving the quality, speed, and timing of his motor performance allows him to keep up with his peers. Engaging in successful activities contributes to his sense of competency and leads to a positive view of school. Because children spend so much of their day writing, Cora felt targeting handwriting would significantly effect his occupational performance in school.

Keeping in mind that children learn best when they are presented with the whole versus a part of the activity that is meaningful and carried out in natural contexts, Cora designed a variety of fun gross motor games for the playground. The intervention was designed to help Paul develop postural control, balance, timing, and sequencing while completing fun games with peers and helping him feel better about his abilities. Providing Paul with the opportunity to develop some basic skills will help him succeed on the playground. The therapist graded and adapted activities to promote his success in this context.

Cora spent the first session recording baseline measurements directly related to the established goals. She recorded the time and legibility of Paul's performance of writing his name on his paper and writing three sentences after being given a verbal prompt ("Tell me about your favorite animal."). She also measured how many consecutive swings (back and forth) Paul could complete on the swing in 5 minutes and how many times he fell on the tires. Cora videotaped the baseline measurements, recorded the results, and documented her observations of the quality of his motor performance. This data provided her with solid measurements to determine the effectiveness of occupational therapy intervention.

During the subsequent sessions, Cora designed fun activities to target postural control, balance, timing, and sequencing play by setting up a five-step obstacle course on the playground, which included that Paul:

1. Climb over three tires (lined up on flat surface)
2. Run to the slide (10 feet)
3. Pick up an object sitting on the fourth rung of the slide
4. Swing back and forth two times on the swing
5. Stand in the center of the hula hoop

Cora used motor learning principles by demonstrating the movement for each step before asking Paul to perform. Once she reviewed each step, she asked him to complete them in order. Paul made many mistakes but started to problem solve how to better perform toward the end of the course. On

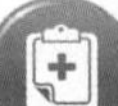

CASE STUDY 7-2 Occupational Profile—cont'd

completion, he said, "Let me try it again and see if I can go faster." Cora provided some key points about the part of the course with which he had trouble (e.g., swinging). She cued him using one to three key words to "Pump back and forth." Providing one to three key words as verbal feedback after the child has performed is recommended for motor learning. Furthermore, allowing Paul to make and learn from his own motor mistakes allowed him to internalize the motor learning. This technique has been found to improve generalization. The therapist periodically changed the format, allowing Paul to make some revisions in the course, to ensure that the course was meaningful. For example, Paul added more tires to the course and requested that the toy be placed higher on the ladder.

Cora was fortunate to be able to provide intervention in the natural context, which provides cues to the child and allows for transfer of learning. Cora waited to invite peers to join Paul so that he could develop competence in skills before the added social "pressure" and stimuli.

Cora continued the session in her classroom space by talking to Paul about his writing and discussing strategies that might help make it easier for him in terms of motor functioning. Paul decided his writing would improve if he held the paper down with his left thumb; he liked the idea of using a mechanical pencil with a new pencil grip. Research suggest that discussing handwriting performance may help children improve motor performance.[6] For example, Banks and colleagues found that discussing strategies (so the children come up with the solutions) helped four children with developmental coordination disorder to improve handwriting performance more than physical practice alone.[6] Problem solving with the child may not work with all groups of children and requires an adequate level of cognition. Using mental practice strategies, Cora asked Paul to visualize how he would complete his writing tasks in school. She suggested that he visualize his handwriting immediately before beginning the writing task.

In the therapy session, they played with a spirograph, using it to help Paul improve his handwriting grasp. The spirograph requires repetitive movement and is fun for children. It improves sequencing and allows the child to work on grip strength. This proved to be a nice activity to work on the mechanics of writing. Later in the intervention sessions, Cora purchased a set of colored pencils, an art book, and some stencils that Paul found interesting. Paul brought his "art portfolio" to class and home, which allowed him practice time.

Cora provided Paul with a variety of activities to promote postural control, coordination, timing and sequencing, and handwriting that were meaningful and fun for him. Periodically, she stopped the spirograph activity and reviewed how to hold the pencil or reinforced correct posture. On the playground she spent time explaining pumping and working on songs to improve timing and rhythm. Cora paid close attention to the nonverbal and verbal cues Paul gave her. If activities were too challenging, she adapted them almost effortlessly. She used humor and paid attention to therapeutic use of self so she could optimize the session. Cora was attentive to Paul, provided positive facial expressions, and encouraged gently.

She used a block practice schedule to teach the new skills, such as climbing to the top of the slide alternating one's feet and hands (bilaterally). As Paul became more competent, she used a distributed practice schedule and later a random or variable schedule. She focused on her goal to enable Paul to participate in play on the playground with peers and complete handwriting assignments with better quality and speed.

By capturing the child's interest in playing with friends and the parent's goal of helping him play with his peers and school, the therapist targeted intervention to help the child improve occupational performance in a meaningful way. The practitioner addressed his fine motor skills for handwriting. This approach promotes practice and learning by empowering children to meet their own occupational goals.

Summary

- Motor control refers to the "ability to regulate or direct mechanisms essential to movement" (p. 4).[93] It includes examination of the mechanisms, strategies, development of movement, and causes of motor dysfunction. Motor learning refers to how people learn and retain motor skills. It helps practitioners understand how to instruct and teach children to perform movements.
- Contemporary motor control interventions support a dynamic systems approach that movement derives from an interaction of person factors, task characteristics, and environmental systems. The principles of dynamic systems theory include:
  - The interaction among systems is essential to adaptive control of movement.
  - Motor performance results from an interaction between adaptable and flexible systems.
  - Dysfunction occurs when movement patterns lack sufficient adaptability to accommodate task demands and environmental constraints.
  - Because task characteristics influence motor requirements, practitioners modify and adapt task requirements and affordances to help children succeed.
- The research evidence supports a dynamic systems approach to motor control intervention by considering the multiple systems in which the child moves. Using an occupation-based model of practice can frame the occupational therapist's use of a dynamic systems approach. Interventions that allow the child to perform meaningful whole activities using real objects in the natural setting promote motor performance.
- An understanding of the stages of motor control (cognitive, associative and automatic) helps guide practitioners when developing intervention. The practitioner analyzes child, task, and environmental systems to determine how the components and systems interact for purposeful movement.

Child factors include cognitive, musculoskeletal, neuromotor, perceptual, and social-emotional influences. Task characteristics consider nature of task, object properties, goals, and rules. Environmental systems include physical, social, cultural, virtual, and personal contexts.
- Practitioners use knowledge of motor learning concepts during intervention to teach children motor actions.
- Motor learning strategies (such as transfer of learning, feedback, practice, sequencing and adapting tasks, modeling or demonstration, and mental rehearsal) are techniques to promote motor acquisition and motor control. Motor learning strategies help practitioners decide how and when to provide feedback and how to promote generalization of skills (transfer of learning). Practice information helps define which type of practice to provide at each stage of learning. Practitioners are encouraged to use evidence-based motor learning strategies to enhance a child's occupational performance.

REFERENCES

1. American Occupational Therapy Association. (2008). *Occupational therapy practice framework: Domain and process.* Bethesda, MD: AOTA, Inc.
2. American Psychiatric Association. (2013). *Diagnostic and statistical manual of mental disorders* (5th ed.). Arlington, VA: American Psychiatric Publishing.
3. Armstrong, D. (2012). Examining the evidence for interventions with children with developmental coordination disorder. *British Journal of Occupational Therapy, 75*(12), 532–540.
4. Ayres, A. J. (1972). *Sensory integration and learning disorders.* Los Angeles: Western Psychological Services.
5. Ayres, A. J. (2005). *Sensory integrations and the child: Understanding hidden sensory challenges.* Revised and updated by the Pediatric Therapy Network. Los Angeles: Western Psychological Services.
6. Banks, R., Rodger, S., & Polatajko, H. (2008). Mastering handwriting: How children with developmental coordination disorder succeed with CO-OP. *OTJR: Occupation, Participation and Health, 28*(3), 100–109.
7. Barthel, K. A. (2010). A frame of reference for neuro-developmental treatment. In P. Kramer & J. Hinojosa (Eds.), *Pediatric occupational therapy* (3rd ed., pp. 187–233). Baltimore: Lippincott, Williams & Wilkins.
8. Basu, S., Kafkes, A., Geist, R., et al. (2002). *Pediatric volitional questionnaire.* Chicago: Model of Human Occupation Clearinghouse.
9. Bernstein, N. (1967). *The coordination and regulation of movements.* London: Pergamon.
10. Bertoldi, A. L. S., Ladewig, E., & Israel, V. L. (2007). Influence of selectivity of attention on the development of body awareness in children with motor deficiencies. *Revista Brasileira de Fisioterapia, 11*, 319–324.
11. Borella, E., Chicherio, C., Re, A. M., et al. (2011). Increased intraindividual variability is a marker of ADHD but also of dyslexia: A study on handwriting. *Brain and Cognition, 77*, 33–39.
12. Bouffard, M., & Wall, A. E. (1990). A problem-solving approach to movement skill acquisition: Implications for special populations. In G. Reid (Ed.), *Problems in movement control* (pp. 107–131). Amsterdam: Elsevier Science.
13. Brownwell, C., & Zerwas, S. (2007). "So big": The development of body self-awareness in toddlers. *Child Development, 78*, 1426–1440.
14. Bundy, A. C. (1999). *Test of environmental supportiveness (TOES).* Fort Collins, CO: Colorado State University.
15. Bundy, A., Luckett, T., Naughton, G., et al. (2008). Playful interaction: Occupational therapy for all children on the school playground. *American Journal of Occupational Therapy, 62*(5), 522–528.
16. Case-Smith, J., Clark, J., & Schlabach, T. L. (2013). Systematic review of interventions used in occupational therapy to promote motor performance for children ages birth-5 years. *American Journal of Occupational Therapy, 67*(4), 413–424.
17. Casillas, D., Davis, N., Loukas, K., et al. (2008). The nonlinear dynamics of occupation: A comparative analysis of nonlinear dynamics and sensory integration. *Journal of Occupational Therapy, Schools & Early Intervention, 1*, 123–141.
18. Chan, R. C. K., McAlonan, G. M., Yang, B., et al. (2010). Prevalence of neurological soft signs and their neuropsychological correlates in typically developing Chinese children and Chinese children with ADHD. *Developmental Neuropscyhology, 35*(6), 698–711.
19. Chen, C. L., Chen, C. Y., Chen, H. C., et al. (2013). Potential predictors in changes in gross motor function during various tasks for children with cerebral palsy: A follow-up study. *Research in Developmental Disabilities, 34*, 721–728.
20. Chen, Y., & Yang, T. (2007). Effect of task goals on the reaching patterns of children with cerebral palsy. *Journal of Motor Behavior, 39*, 317–324.
21. Christiansen, C., Baum, C. M., & Bass, J. (2011). The person-environment-occupational performance model. In E. A. S. Duncan (Ed.), *Foundations for practice in occupational therapy* (5th ed., pp. 93–104). London: Elsevier.
22. Cohn, E., Miller, L. J., & Tickle-Degnen, L. (2000). Parental hopes for therapy outcomes: Children with sensory modulation disorders. *American Journal of Occupational Therapy, 54*, 36–43.
23. Correa, V., Poulson, C., & Salzberg, C. (1984). Training and generalization of reach-grasp behavior in blind, retarded young children. *Journal of Applied Behavior Analysis, 17*, 57–69.
24. Darrah, J., Law, M., Pollock, N., et al. (2011). Context therapy: A new intervention approach for children with cerebral palsy. *Developmental Medicine & Child Neurology, 53*(7), 615–620.
25. Davidson, T., & Williams, B. (2000). Occupational therapy for children with developmental coordination disorder: A study of the effectiveness of a combined sensory integration and perceptual-motor intervention. *British Journal of Occupational Therapy, 63*, 495–499.
26. Deecke, L. (1996). Planning, preparation, execution, and imagery of volitional action. *Cognitive Brain Research, 3*, 59–64.
27. Denis, M. (1985). Visual imagery and the use of mental practice in the development of motor skills. *Canadian Journal of Applied Sport Sciences, 10*(4), 4S–16S.
28. Doussoulin, S., & Rehbein, L. (2011). Motor imagery as a tool for motor skill training in children. *Motricidade, 7*(3), 37–43.
29. Driskell, J. E., Cooper, C., & Moran, A. (1994). Does imagery practice enhance

performance? *Journal of Applied Psychology*, *79*, 481–492.

30. Elliasson, A. C., & Gordon, A. M. (2000). Impaired force coordination during object release in children with hemiplegic cerebral palsy. *Developmental Medicine & Child Neurology*, *42*, 228–234.
31. Emanuel, M., Jarus, T., & Bart, O. (2008). Effect of focus of attention and age on motor acquisition, retention, and transfer: A randomized trial. *Physical Therapy*, *88*, 251–260.
32. Feder, K., & Majnemer, A. (2007). Handwriting development, competency, and intervention. *Developmental Medicine & Child Neurology*, *49*, 312–317.
33. Fisher, A. G. (1998). Uniting practice and theory in an occupational framework. *American Journal of Occupational Therapy*, *52*, 509–521.
34. Goodgold-Edwards, S. A., & Cermak, S. A. (1990). Integrating motor control and motor leaning concepts with neuropsychological perspectives on apraxia and developmental dyspraxia. *American Journal of Occupational Therapy*, *44*, 431–439.
35. Gordon, A., Schneider, J., Chinnan, A., et al. (2007). Efficacy of a hand-arm bimanual intensive therapy (HABIT) in children with hemiplegic cerebral palsy: A randomized control trial. *Developmental Medicine and Child Neurology*, *49*, 830–839.
36. Gowen, E., & Hamilton, A. (2012). Motor abilities in autism: A review using a computational context. *Journal of Autism Developmental Disorders*, *43*, 323–344.
37. Grove, C. R., & Lazarus, J. A. (2007). Impaired re-weighting of sensory feedback for maintenance of postural control in children with developmental coordination disorder. *Human Movement Science*, *26*, 457–476.
38. Gustafsson, P., Svedin, C. G., Ericsson, I., et al. (2009). Reliability and validity of the assessment of neurological soft-signs in children with and without attention-deficit-hyperactivity disorder. *Developmental Medicine & Child Neurology*, *52*, 364–370.
39. Hadders-Algra, M., Brogren, E., & Forssberg, H. (1996). Ontogeny of postural adjustments during sitting in infancy: Variation, selection, and modulation. *Journal of Physiology*, *493*, 273–288.
40. Hall, C. R. (1985). Individual differences in mental practice and imagery of motor skill performance. *Canadian Journal of Applied Science*, *10*, 17S–21S.
41. Hay, J., & Missiuna, C. (1998). Motor proficiency in children reporting low levels of participation in physical activity. *Canadian Journal of Occupational Therapy*, *65*, 64–71.
42. Hetu, S., & Mercier, C. (2012). Using purposeful tasks to improve motor performance: Does object affordance matter? *British Journal of Occupational Therapy*, *75*(8), 367–376.
43. Horak, F., Diener, H., & Nashner, L. (1990). Postural strategies associated with somatosensory and vestibular loss. *Experimental Brain Research*, *82*, 167–177.
44. Horak, F., Jones-Rycewicz, C., Black, F., et al. (1992). Effects of vestibular rehabilitation on dizziness and imbalance. *Otolaryngology Head and Neck Surgery*, *106*, 175–180.
45. Hubbard, I. J., Parsons, M. W., Neilson, C., et al. (2009). Task-specific training: Evidence and translation to clinical practice. *Occupational Therapy International*, *16*(3–4), 175–189.
46. Jaric, S., Corcos, D. M., Agarwal, G. C., et al. (1993). Principles of learning single joint movements. II. Generalizing a learned behavior. *Experimental Brain Research*, *94*, 514–521.
47. Kaufman, L. B., & Schilling, D. L. (2007). Implementation of a strength training program for a 5-year-old child with poor body awareness and developmental coordination disorder. *Physical Therapy*, *87*, 455–467.
48. Keller, J., Kafkes, A., Basu, S., et al. (2005). *The child occupational self-assessment (COSA) (version 2.1)*. Chicago: MOHO Clearinghouse, Department of Occupational Therapy, College of Applied Health Sciences, University of Illinois at Chicago.
49. Kielhofner, G. (2008). *Model of human occupation: Theory and application* (4th ed.). Philadelphia: F. A. Davis.
50. Klingberg, T., Forssberg, H., & Westerberg, H. (2002). Increased brain activity in frontal and parietal cortex underlies the development of visuospatial working memory capacity during childhood. *Journal of Cognitive Neuroscience*, *14*, 1–10.
51. Konczak, J., vander Velden, H., & Jaeger, L. (2009). Learning to play the violin: Motor control by freezing, not freeing degrees of freedom. *Journal of Motor Behavior*, *41*(3), 243–252.
52. Kramer, J. M. (2007). Using a participatory action approach to identify habits and routines to support self-advocacy. *OTJR: Occupation, Participation and Health*, *27*, 84S–85S.
53. Kramer, J., Walker, R., Cohn, E., et al. (2012). Striving for shared understandings: Therapists' perspectives of the benefits and dilemmas of using a child self-assessment. *OTJR: Occupation, Participation & Health*, *32*, S48–S58.
54. Latash, M. L. (2007). Learning motor synergies by person with Down syndrome. *Journal of Intellectual Disability Research*, *51*(12), 962–971.
55. Law, M., Baptiste, S., Carswell, A., et al. (1991). *Canadian occupational performance measure*. Ottawa: CAOT Publications ACE.
56. Law, M., Darrah, J., Pollock, N., et al. (2011). Focus on function: A cluster, randomized controlled trial comparing child- versus context-focused intervention for young children with cerebral palsy. *Developmental Medicine & Child Neurology*, *53*(7), 621–629.
57. Law, M., Russell, D., Pollock, N., et al. (1997). A comparison of intensive neurodevelopmental therapy plus casting and a regular occupational therapy program for children with cerebral palsy. *Developmental Medicine & Child Neurology*, *39*, 664–670.
58. Lee, J. J., Lee, D. R., Shin, Y. K., et al. (2013). Comparative neuroimaging in children with cerebral palsy using fMRI and a novel EEG-based brain maping during a motor task—A preliminary investigation. *Neurorehabilitation*, *32*, 279–285.
59. Li, K. (2012). Examining contemporary motor control theories from the perspective of degrees of freedom. *Australian Occupational Therapy Journal*, *60*, 138–143.
60. Lundy-Ekman, L., Ivry, R., Keele, S., et al. (1991). Timing and force control deficits in clumsy children. *Journal of Cognitive Science*, *3*(4), 367–376.
61. Mandich, A. D., Polatajko, H. J., Macnab, J. J., et al. (2001). Treatment of children with developmental coordination disorder: What is the evidence? *Physical and Occupational Therapy in Pediatrics*, *20*, 51–58.
62. Mathiowetz, V., & Bass-Haugen, J. (1994). Motor behavior research: Implications for therapeutic approaches to central nervous system dysfunction. *American Journal of Occupational Therapy*, *48*, 733–745.
63. Merriam Webster online medical dictionary. Retrieved February 14, 2014 from: <http://www.merriam-webster.com/medlineplus/dysmetria>.
64. Miller, L., & Nelson, D. L. (1987). Dual-purpose activity versus single-purpose activity in terms of duration on task, exertion level, and affect. *Occupational Therapy in Mental Health*, *7*, 55–67.
65. Missiuna, C., & Mandich, A. (2002). Integrating motor learning theories into practice. In S. Cermak & D. Larkin (Eds.), *Developmental coordination disorder* (pp. 221–233). Albany, NY: Delmar Thomson Learning.

66. Miyahara, M. (2013). Meta review of systematic and meta analytic reviews on movement differences, effect of movement based interventions, and the underlying neural mechanisms in autism spectrum disorder. *Frontiers in Integrative Neuroscience*, *7*, 16.
67. Miyahara, M. (1996). A meta-analysis of intervention studies on children with developmental coordination disorder. *Corpus, Psyche & Societas*, *3*, 11–18.
68. Miyahara, M., & Wafer, A. (2004). Clinical intervention for children with developmental coordination disorder: A multiple case study. *Adapted Physical Activity Quarterly*, *21*, 281–300.
69. Moore, C., Mealiea, J., Garon, N., et al. (2007). The development of body self-awareness. *Infancy*, *11*, 157–174.
70. Muir, A. L., Jones, L. M., & Signal, N. E. J. (2009). Is neuroplasticity promoted by task complexity? *New Zealand Journal of Physiotherapy*, *37*(3), 136–146.
71. Murphy, S. M. (1994). Imagery interventions in sport. *Medicine and Science in Sports and Exercise*, *26*, 486–494.
72. Muratori, L. M., Lamberg, E. M., Quinn, L., et al. (2013). Applying principles of motor learning and control to upper extremity rehabilitation. *Journal of Hand Therapy*, *26*, 94–103.
73. Nagel, M. J., & Rice, M. S. (2000). Cross-transfer effects in the upper extremity during an occupationally embedded exercise. *American Journal of Occupational Therapy*, *55*(3), 317–323.
74. Niemeijer, A. S., Schoemaker, M. M., & Smits-Engelsman, B. (2006). Are teaching principles associated with improved motor performance in children with developmental coordination disorder? A pilot study. *Physical Therapy*, *86*(9), 1221–1231.
75. Novak, I., McIntyre, S., Morgan, C., et al. (2013). A systematic review of interventions for children with cerebral palsy: State of the evidence. *Developmental Medicine & Child Neurology*, *55*, 885–910.
76. O'Brien, J., Bergeron, A., Duprey, H., et al. (2009). Children with disabilities and their parents' views of occupational participation needs. *Occupational Therapy in Health Care*, *25*, 1–17.
77. O'Brien, J., Williams, H., Bundy, A., et al. (2008). Mechanisms that underlie coordination in children with developmental coordination disorder. *Journal of Motor Behavior*, *40*, 43–61.
78. Page, S., Sime, W., & Nordell, K. (1999). The effects of imagery on female college swimmers' perceptions of anxiety. *The Sport Psychologist*, *13*, 458–469.
79. Painter, M., Inman, K., & Vincent, W. (1994). Contextual interference effects: I. The acquisition and retention of motor tasks by individuals with mild mental handicaps. *Adapted Physical Activity Quarterly*, *11*, 383–395.
80. Piek, J., & Skinner, R. (1999). Timing and force control during a sequential tapping task in children with and without motor coordination problems. *Journal of International Neuropsychological Society*, *5*, 320–329.
81. Pless, M., & Carlsson, M. (2000). Effects of motor skill intervention on developmental coordination disorder: A meta-analysis. *Adapted Physical Activity Quarterly*, *17*(4), 381–401.
82. Polatajko, H. J., Kaplan, B. J., & Wilson, B. N. (1992). Sensory integration treatment for children with learning disabilities: Its status 20 years later. *Occupational Therapy Journal of Research*, *12*, 323–341.
83. Polatajko, H., Mandich, A., Miller, L., et al. (2001). Cognitive orientation to daily occupational performance (CO-OP): Part II—the evidence. *Physical & Occupational Therapy in Pediatrics*, *20*, 83–106.
84. Poldrack, R. A. (2010). Mapping mental function to brain structure: How can cognitive neuroimaging succeed? *Perspectives on Psychological Science*, *5*(6), 753–761.
85. Poole, J. L., Burtner, P. A., & Stockman, G. (2009). The framework of occupational gradation (FOG) to treat upper extremity impairments in persons with central nervous system impairments. *Occupational Therapy in Health Care*, *23*(1), 40–59.
86. Rathunde, K. (2001). Toward a psychology of optimal human functioning: What positive psychology can learn from the "experiential turns" of James, Dewey, and Maslow. *The Journal of Humanistic Psychology*, *41*, 135–153.
87. Raynor, A. J. (2001). Strength, power, and coactivation in children with developmental coordination disorder. *Developmental Medicine and Child Neurology*, *43*, 676–684.
88. Rose, J., Wolff, D. R., Jones, V. K., et al. (2002). Postural balance in children with cerebral palsy. *Developmental Medicine and Child Neurology*, *44*, 58–63.
89. Russell, D. J., Avery, I. M., Rosenbaum, P. L., et al. (2000). Improved scaling of the Gross Motor Function Measure for children with cerebral palsy: Evidence of reliability and validity. *Physical Therapy*, *80*, 873–885.
90. Schoemaker, M. M., Niemeijer, A. S., Reynders, K., et al. (2003). Effectiveness of neuromotor task training for children with developmental coordination disorder: A pilot study. *Neural Plasticity*, *10*, 153–163.
91. Screws, D. P., & Surburg, P. R. (1997). Motor performance of children with mild mental disabilities after using mental imagery. *Adapted Physical Activity Quarterly*, *14*, 119–130.
92. Shin, Y. K., Lee, D. R., Hwang, H. J., et al. (2012). A novel EEG-based brain mapping to determine cortical activation patterns in normal children and children with cerebral palsy during motor imagery tasks. *Neurorehabilitation*, *31*, 349–355.
93. Shumway-Cook, A., & Woollacott, M. (2007). *Motor control: Theory and practical applications* (3rd ed.). Philadelphia: Lippincott Williams & Wilkins.
94. Skard, G., & Bundy, A. (2008). The test of playfulness. In L. D. Parham & L. S. Fazio (Eds.), *Play in occupational therapy for children* (2nd ed., pp. 71–94). St. Louis: Mosby.
95. Smyth, C., Summers, J. J., & Garry, M. (2010). Differences in motor learning success are associated with M1 excitability. *Human Movement Science*, *29*, 618–630.
96. Steenbergen, B., Jongblod-pereboom, M., Spruijt, S., et al. (2013). Impaired motor planning and motor imagery in children with unilateral spastic cerebral palsy: Challenges for the future of pediatric rehabilitation. *Developmental Medicine & Child Neurology*, *55*, 43–46.
97. Steultjens, E. M. J., Dekker, J., Bouter, L. M., et al. (2005). Evidence of the efficacy of occupation therapy in different conditions: An overview of systematic reviews. *Clinical Rehabilitation*, *19*, 247–254.
98. Sugden, D., & Dunford, C. (2007). Intervention and the role of theory, empiricism and experience in children with motor impairment. *Disability & Rehabilitation*, *29*, 3–11.
99. Sullivan, K., Kantuk, S., & Burtner, P. (2008). Motor learning in children: Feedback effects on skill acquisition. *Physical Therapy*, *88*, 720–732.
100. Taktek, K., Zinsser, N., & St.-John, B. (2008). Visual versus kinesthetic mental imagery: Efficacy for the retention and transfer of a closed motor skill in young children. *Canadian Journal of Experimental Psychology*, *62*, 174–187.
101. Teasell, R. W., Foley, N. C., Salter, K. L., et al. (2008). A blueprint for transforming stroke rehabilitation care in Canada: the case for change. *Archives of Physical Medicine and Rehabilitation*, *89*, 575–578.
102. Thelen, E. (2000). Motor development as foundation and future of developmental psychology.

International Journal of Behavioral Development, *24*(4), 385–397.

103. Thelen, E., Kelso, J., Kelso, J. S., et al. (1987). Self-organizing systems and infant motor development. *Developmental Review*, *7*, 39–65.

104. Tieman, B., Palisano, R. J., Gracely, E. J., et al. (2007). Variability in mobility of children with cerebral palsy. *Pediatric Physical Therapy*, *19*(3), 180–187.

105. Trombly, C. A. (1995). Occupation: Purposefulness and meaningfulness as therapeutic mechanisms. 1995 Eleanor Clarke Slagle Lecture. *American Journal of Occupational Therapy*, *49*, 960–972.

106. Valvano, J. (2004). Activity-focused motor interventions for children with neurological conditions. *Physical & Occupational Therapy in Pediatrics*, *24*(1/2), 79–107.

107. Valvano, J., & Rapport, M. J. (2006). Activity-focused motor interventions for infants and young children with neurological conditions. *Infants & Young Children*, *4*, 292–307.

108. Van der Weel, F. R., Van der Meer, A. L., & Lee, D. N. (1991). Effect of task on movement control in cerebral palsy: Implications for assessment and therapy. *Developmental Medicine & Child Neurology*, *33*, 419–426.

109. Van de Winckel, A., Klingels, K., Bruyninckx, F., et al. (2013). How does brain activation differ in children with unilateral cerebral palsy compared to typically developing children, during active and passive movements, and tactile stimulation? An fMRI study. *Research in Developmental Disabilities*, *34*, 183–197.

110. Wang, H. Y., Long, I. M., & Liu, M. F. (2012). Relationships between task-oriented postural control and motor ability in children and adolescents with Down syndrome. *Research in Developmental Disabilities*, *22*, 1792–1798.

111. Westcott, S. L., & Burtner, P. (2004). Postural control in children: Implications for pediatric practice. *Physical and Occupational Therapy in Pediatrics*, *24*(1/2), 5–55.

112. Wikipedia: The Free Encyclopedia. Retrieved February 22, 2014 from: <https://en.wikipedia.org/wiki/Diadochokinesia>.

113. Williams, H. (2002). Motor control in children with developmental coordination disorder. In S. A. Cermak & D. Larkin (Eds.), *Developmental coordination disorder* (pp. 117–137). Albany, NY: Delmar Thomson Learning.

114. Williams, H. (2006). Motor control. In J. Solomon & J. O'Brien (Eds.), *Pediatric skills for occupational therapy assistants* (2nd ed., pp. 461–480). St. Louis: Mosby.

115. Williams, J., Omizzolo, C., Galea, M. P., et al. (2013). Motor imagery skills of children with attention deficit hyperactivity disorder and developmental coordination disorder. *Human Movement Science*, *32*, 121–135.

116. Wilson, P. H. (2005). Practitioner review: Approaches to assessment and treatment of children with DCD: An evaluative review. *Journal of Child Psychology and Psychiatry*, *46*(8), 806–823.

117. Wilson, P. H., Ruddock, S., Smits-Engelsman, B., et al. (2012). Understanding performance deficits in developmental coordination disorder: A meta-analysis of recent research. *Developmental Medicine & Child Neurology*, *55*, 217–228.

118. Wright, M. G., Hunt, L. P., & Stanley, O. H. (2005). Object/wrist movements during manipulation in children with cerebral palsy. *Pediatric Rehabilitation*, *8*(4), 263–271.

119. Wu, C., Trombly, C. A., Lin, K., et al. (1998). Effects of object affordances on movement performances: a meta-analysis. *Scandinavian Journal of Occupational Therapy*, *5*(20), 83–92.

120. Zafeiriou, D. I. (2004). Primitive reflexes and postural reactions in the neurodevelopmental examination. *Pediatric Neurology*, *31*(1), 1–8.

CHAPTER

8 Hand Function Evaluation and Intervention

Jane Case-Smith • Charlotte E. Exner

KEY TERMS

Hand function
Reach and carry
Grasping patterns
In-hand manipulation
Bimanual skills
Biomechanical approaches
Neurodevelopmental therapy
Motor learning
Constraint induced movement therapy
Adaptation and assistive technology

GUIDING QUESTIONS

1. What is the sequence of hand function development in infants and children?
2. Which factors contribute to development of hand function?
3. How do hand function problems affect children's occupational performance?
4. Which assessment tools and methods are useful in evaluating children's hand skills?
5. How are intervention practice models and principles used by occupational therapists to promote hand function?
6. Given a range of diagnoses, how do occupational therapists use specific intervention strategies to improve hand function?
7. How do assistive technologies and adapted techniques improve children's hand function and increase participation in play, school, and activities of daily living?
8. How does research support occupational therapy practice models for hand function interventions?

Hand function is critical to children and youth's interaction with objects (e.g., tools), materials, and other persons within everyday environments. Hands are the dynamic "tools" most often used to accomplish activities of daily living (ADLs), school, work, and play activities. The child who has a disability affecting hand function has less opportunity to interact with, explore, and act on the environment.

Components of Hand Skills

Effective use of the hands to engage in a variety of occupations depends on a complex interaction of hand functions, postural mechanisms, cognition, social-emotional function, and visual perception. The term *visual-motor integration* refers to the interaction of visual skills, visual-perceptual skills, and motor skills. The term *hand function* is used interchangeably with the terms *fine motor coordination, fine motor skills,* and *hand skills,* and this chapter uses the term hand function to refer to all of these skills.

Although a child's development of hand functions depends on adequate postural functions and sufficient visual-perceptual and cognitive development, these areas are described in other chapters and not in detail in this chapter. Patterns of hand function include reach, grasp, carry, and voluntary release, as well as the more complex skills of in-hand manipulation and bimanual skills. These terms are briefly defined:

- Reach: extension away from the body and movement of the arm for grasping or placing objects
- Grasp: attainment of an object with the hand; holding within the hand
- Carry: transportation of a hand-held object from one place to another
- Voluntary release: finger extension allowing intentional release of a hand-held object at a specific time and place
- In-hand manipulation: adjustment or movement of an object within the hand
- Bimanual skills: coordinated use of two hands together sequentially or simultaneously to accomplish an activity

Factors That Contribute to the Development of Hand Function

Occupational therapists often use occupation-based models and dynamic systems theory to understand development of inter-related performance areas. Through the lens of these conceptual models, a child's performance reflects his or her innate developmental abilities and the contextual opportunities and barriers that affect performance. As described in Chapters 2 and 8, performance is dynamically influenced by intrinsic variables, including motivation, cognition, and social-emotional function as well as extrinsic variables, including the social, physical, and cultural context. These models are used to guide analysis of hand function by identifying potential factors associated with a child's delay or impairment in hand function. Using a top-down approach, this section describes factors that influence the development of hand function, recognizing that as a child develops, the factors associated with efficient hand use and skilled manipulation of objects have greater or lesser influence.

Social and Cultural Factors

Knowledge of contextual factors is critical for understanding, evaluating, and providing interventions to enhance hand functions. Social and cultural factors, in particular, are likely to play important roles in the acquisition and use of various hand skills. Social factors that can affect the development of hand functions include socioeconomic status, gender, and role expectations. These cultural and social factors may not influence the development of basic hand skills but can influence the development of complex manipulation of objects and tool use. For example, children who live in conditions of poverty may not have access to writing utensils, scissors, and other materials common to children from middle-class environments.

The objects that are important to the child's cultural group influence the development of object manipulation. Because tools that are important in one culture may not be available in another, children may not have the opportunity to develop some tool-specific skills. For example, eating utensils vary from chopsticks to forks and spoons. Scissors use may be important for school performance in some cultures but not in others. As explained by Flynn and Whiten,[53] children's pattern of tool use is influenced by observing the actions of familiar individuals using tools over time, thereby reinforcing the significance of that action to the child. Children learn to use tools through repeated observation of adults and their peers, suggesting that tool use may be delayed when models are not available and most often reflect patterns within their immediate environments.

In addition, the age at which children are expected to achieve skills in object manipulation can vary. Safety concerns influence parents in some cultural groups to delay introduction of a knife to a child, whereas parents in other cultural groups encourage early independence in knife use.[109] Some cultures introduce children to the use of writing materials before 1 year of age. Parents from other cultures and socioeconomic groups do not provide children with these materials until they can be expected to adhere to requirements such as using them only on paper (rather than on the wall or on clothing).

Culture also influences the perception of children's need for manipulative materials and the cultural group's view of the importance of play. Play materials that provide opportunities for the development of manipulative skills (e.g., building sets, beads, puzzles, table games) are highly valued in some cultural groups, whereas in other groups, play with gross motor objects (e.g., balls, riding toys) or play with animals is more valued. Some cultural groups do not view children's play as important; therefore few play materials of any type are available.[6]

Although the types of activities encouraged can promote the development of specific skills, acquisition of the basic hand functions of reach, grasp, release, and manipulation does not rely on the availability of any particular materials; rather, it relies on reasonable exposure to a variety of materials with the opportunity to handle them. In a comparative study of children in Hong Kong and those in the United States, children in Hong Kong demonstrated higher level manual dexterity and, at earlier ages, more proficient writing.[23] Hong Kong children's proficient hand skills at early ages may relate to using chop sticks to eat, having less access to gross motor activities, or attending early childhood programs that emphasize writing. Although dexterity of children in Eastern cultures may be higher than that of American children, hand strength may be lower. Studies have found that on average, children from Eastern cultures, such as Korea, demonstrate lower hand strength than children of Western cultures.[131]

Although contextual variables influence a child's development of hand function, intrinsic variables, including the child's somatosensory functions, visual perception, and cognition, have strong, direct association with the child's rate of development, level of performance, and proficiency across tasks. Musculoskeletal integrity also influences patterns of hand function, coordination, and dexterity. As hand functions mature beyond grasp and release patterns, children learn to coordinate visual skills with hand skills, develop praxis and dexterity, and later, coordinate visual-perceptual and motor planning skills.[37,98]

Somatosensory Functions

The role of somatosensory information and feedback is critical in the development of hand functions, particularly those involving isolated movements of the fingers and thumb. Practitioners acknowledge that intact somatosensory functioning is required for development of precise and dexterous hand and finger movements. Haptic perception is the child's interpretation of somatosensory information (through active touch) for purposes of understanding object properties and characteristics. Although haptic perception emerges by 6 months when grasping patterns are immature, full haptic perception (perception of object texture, shape, and hardness through active touch) does not mature until 5 or 6 years when the child can manipulate objects within the hand.[13] As a more direct sense than vision, haptic perception allows for immediate feedback on the child's use of force, accuracy of movement, and precision of movement.[111] A 6-year-old can identify three-dimensional common objects and all aspects of objects' characteristics by active touch alone.[21]

The fingertips gather precise information about many types of object qualities. Children with impaired control of finger movement have limited access to somatosensory information, and/or the impaired control of finger movement may reflect their difficulties in perceiving and using sensory information. Initiating and sustaining grasp force requires tactile and proprioceptive input and integration, and the ability to hold objects in the hand (i.e., without dropping them) is related primarily to intact somatosensory functioning.[55,58,59] Hand functions and accurate use of force clearly relate to tactile sensibility; for example, in children with cerebral palsy, tactile information was found to be critical for anticipating the amount of force needed to grasp and lift an object.[56]

Somatosensory functioning is difficult to assess in children, particularly in young children (e.g., less than 4 years) and those with disabilities. When testing haptic perception (e.g., using stereognosis) or tactile sensitivity (e.g., using two-point discrimination), a child's performance often varies within a session or from one session to another. Although formal testing may be unreliable, therapists informally evaluate somatosensory functioning to understand delays or impairment in hand function. For example, a child with poor somatosensory registration may engage in few activities involving active manipulation. A child with tactile hypersensitivity may avoid contact with certain materials, thus limiting exposure to various objects. Limitations in somatosensory function are associated with poor coordination, problems in timing and speed of response, and clumsiness, including dropping objects or use of excessive force.[57] In particular, children with cerebral palsy[35,56] and developmental coordination disorder (DCD)[78] often demonstrate these somatosensory perception difficulties and associated impaired hand function.

Visual Perception and Cognition

Visual perceptual and visual-motor development has a major role in the development of hand function.[9,21,71] Vision is particularly important for learning new motor skills. The 4-month-old infant uses vision as a dominant sense to guide arm and hand movements in reaching for objects and making differentiated finger movements. The visual-motor development required for accurate reach matures by approximately 6 months of age. During the first 6 months, the infant demonstrates emerging skills in using visual and tactile perception to guide reach, object carry, and object placement.[110] The infant's visual-motor coordination continues to refine, and by 9 months of age the infant guides his or her hand movements using visual-somatosensory integration (i.e., these sensory inputs are combined and compared as the infant anticipates and plans arm and hand movements).

Because the child acquires knowledge about objects through object manipulation, hand use and cognitive development seem to be particularly linked in infancy and very early childhood.[50] Early manual exploratory behavior plays an important role in the development of visual-spatial skills and learning about the environment.[96,112] Object manipulation in infants between 6 and 12 months of age leads to learning about object characteristics and understanding of spatial relationships. For example, by 9 to 10 months of age, infants adapt their arm positions to horizontal versus vertical object presentations and shape their hands appropriately for convex and concave objects.[110]

During the second year, infants learn to relate objects to one another with more accuracy and purpose. Before 18 months of age, infants modify their movement approach in anticipation of the weight of the object.[13,27] As eye-hand coordination continues to develop, the toddler learns movements that require precise guidance by vision (e.g., stringing small beads or putting together a puzzle). For example, in the second half of the first year the infant adjusts the actions of the hand in response to object characteristics, such as size, shape, and surface qualities.[27] By preschool age, the development of hand function allows for more complex interaction with objects, and the child uses well-developed visual-perceptual skills to guide manipulation of objects in the course of play and social interaction.

Like visual-perceptual skills, cognitive skills are associated with the development of hand function in the young child.[82] Changes in attentional control and the development of problem-solving strategies are seen in the infants' gradual improvement in handling two objects simultaneously. The infant attends to two objects simultaneously when, at 10 months, he or she bangs two objects together and, at 15 months, he or she stabilizes an object with one hand while manipulating with the other. With further cognitive development, the toddler, at 18 to 20 months, manipulates two or more objects simultaneously. As attention and planning skills increase, the child develops facility in using two hands together to manipulate objects.[17,27]

Musculoskeletal Integrity

The integrity of the hand's joint and bone structures is an important consideration in hand function. Children with congenital hand anomalies may be missing one or more digits, a condition that significantly affects the variety of possible prehension patterns. Refined finger movements and in-hand manipulation skills may also be limited or absent. Congenital anomalies in which the thumb is missing or contracted significantly affect grasp. Children with congenital anomalies affecting hand structures often undergo orthopedic surgeries to optimize grasp and hand function.

Limitations in joint range of motion (ROM) can occur as a result of abnormal joint structure, muscle weakness, abnormal muscle tone, or joint inflammation. These limitations can affect the child's range of reach and carry, active supination for tool uses, and hand and finger mobility. Effective hand function depends on adequate mobilization of distal muscle groups that control palmar arches. ROM limitations or hand contractures affect a child's ability to grasp small or large objects, use dynamic grasp and release patterns, and move objects within the hand.

Aspects of muscle functions include muscle power (strength), muscle tone, and muscle endurance. Sufficient strength is necessary to initiate all types of grasp patterns and to maintain these patterns during lifting and carrying. Children's grasp strength gradually increases through the preschool years,[80] the elementary school years,[131] and adolescence.[25] This increase allows them to engage in activities with objects of increasing weight and to use greater resistance.

Children with poor strength may be unable to initiate the finger extension or the thumb opposition pattern necessary before grasp. They also may not have the flexor control to hold a grasp pattern. Many children with diminished strength are unable to use patterns that rely on the intrinsic muscles for control and therefore are unable to use thumb opposition or metacarpophalangeal (MCP) joint flexion with interphalangeal (IP) joint extension. Children with fair strength may be able to initiate a grasp pattern but may be unable to lift an object against gravity while maintaining the grasp. Children with mildly diminished strength may demonstrate limited activity endurance, particularly in situations in which they must use a sustained grasp pattern or hold an object against resistance (e.g., during eating with utensils, coloring, handwriting, and scissors activities).

When children with cerebral palsy demonstrate increased or decreased muscle tone in the upper extremity, arm and hand movements tend to be unstable and motor control is diminished. Finger and hand movements are often limited or missing. Children with spasticity or hypertonicity frequently demonstrate limited ROM, poor control, and decreased movement efficiency. Children with hypotonia or low muscle tone often exhibit exaggerated joint ROM and decreased stability. With fluctuating tone, a child may have full ROM but attains joint stability only at the extreme end of a joint position (full flexion or full extension). With fluctuating tone, movements are less controlled and appear to be random or unrelated to the child's goal.

Although intrinsic and extrinsic factors influence the development of hand function, the sequence of hand skill development is remarkably similar in typical children. The sequence of development guides the occupational therapist in evaluating hand function and fine motor skills, establishing goals that reflect the next developmental steps, and selecting developmentally appropriate activities as the context for intervention.

Development of Hand Skills

Developmental theories and principles are used in conjunction with other practice models to select appropriate goals, design intervention activities, and assess the child's progress. The occupational therapist uses comprehensive knowledge of hand function development to select tasks that challenge the child's emerging skills and provide or fade out supports that enable the child to reach the next developmental level. Hand functions develop through childhood, continuing into the adolescent years.[4,46] This long course of development mirrors other aspects of development and reflects the complexity of hand skills as humans interact with objects and their environments. Developmental theories are further described in Chapter 3; this section describes the sequence of hand function development by considering its components.

Reach and Carry

An important sequence in the development of motor control is the use of linear movement patterns before the emergence of controlled rotation patterns. As illustrated in the development of reach and carry, the infant first develops controlled stability and mobility in basic flexion and extension of the shoulder, elbow, and wrist. Within the first year, control of internal and external rotation of the shoulder and pronation and supination of the forearm emerges and these rotational arm movements characterize the reaching patterns required in functional tasks (e.g., reach to be picked up, reach for a bottle or cup). The goal of reach is to transport the hand to the target, with precision in both time and space,[110,117] and therefore requires control of the hand's movement toward the object and the preparation of the hand for grasp.

Within the first several days of life the neonate shows visual regard of objects close to him or her and activation of the arms in response to objects.[126] Over the next few months of life the arms become more active and the infant swipes or bats at objects with the arm abducted at the shoulder. Reach with an extended arm to contact an object with the hand is likely to occur between approximately 12 and 22 weeks of age.[126,127] Objects are rarely grasped and then only by accident. If grasped, they are released at random, generally in association with arm movements.

By 3 to 4 months a midline orientation of the hands develops. Initially the hands are held close to the body. Soon, with an increased desire for visual regard of the hands and greater proximal arm stability, the 4- to 5-month-old infant holds the hands further away to view them. This pattern precedes the onset of symmetric bilateral reaching, which usually occurs first in the supine and then in the sitting position. At this stage the infant initiates reach with humeral abduction, partial shoulder internal rotation, forearm pronation, and full finger extension.[110]

As the infant shows increasing dissociation of the two body sides during movement, unilateral reaching begins. Abduction and internal rotation of the shoulder are less prominent in reach. The hand opens in preparation for grasping the object and is usually more open than necessary for the size of the object.[128]

As scapular control and trunk stability mature, the infant begins to use shoulder flexion, slight external rotation, full elbow extension, forearm supination, and slight wrist extension during reaching. Active supination of the forearm requires some external rotation of the shoulder to stabilize the humerus. In addition, well-controlled elbow extension evolves as control of shoulder rotation develops. Mature reach is usually seen with sustained trunk extension and a slight rotation of the trunk toward the object of interest. Over the next few years the child refines this unilateral reaching pattern, increasing the accuracy of arm placement and the grading of finger extension as appropriate to the size of the object (Figure 8-1), as well as the timing of the various movement elements. With increasing age, reaching patterns become direct, highly accurate, and highly consistent. The quality of reach with grasp continues to mature until approximately 12 years of age, at which time the child prepares the hand with the optimal hand opening for the object size at the initiation of reach.[75]

Carrying (moving and lifting) involves a smooth combination of body movements accompanied by stabilization of an object in the hand. When carrying objects to perform a task, small ranges of movements are used and adjusted in accordance with the demands of the activity. The child carries an object by maintaining co-contraction of the forearm, wrist, and hand and may modify the forearm and wrist positions to correctly orient the object. Similarly, the child uses shoulder rotation movements with shoulder flexion and abduction to orient the object during carry.

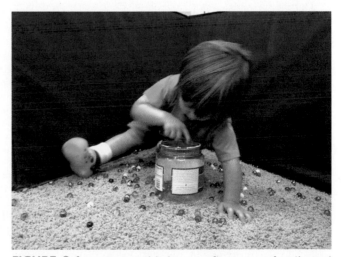

FIGURE 8-1 A 2-year-old shows refinement of unilateral reach with graded finger extension.

Grasp Patterns

Broadly, grasp patterns are determined by whether a person needs to perform with precision or power to accomplish an activity. Precision grasps involve opposition of the thumb to fingertips. Power grasps involve the use of the entire hand. In a power grasp, the thumb is held flexed or abducted to other fingers, depending on control requirements. In most cases the activity and the object's characteristics determine the grasp pattern used. Small objects are generally held in a precision grasp, using the extensive sensory feedback available through the fingertips and the fine control of intrinsic muscles. Medium objects can be held with either pattern, and large objects are generally held with a power grasp. The child uses interplay between precision and power handling of objects based on the activity demands.[17,98] Specific grasp patterns are described in Table 8-1.

Sequential Development of Grasp Patterns

The sequences of grasp pattern development reflect three types of progression: (1) Ulnar fingers show activation before radial fingers and thumb; (2) palmar grasp (proximal) patterns precede finger grasp (distal) patterns; and (3) extrinsic muscle activation dominates before intrinsic muscle activation. These progressions interact and overlap as the infant develops. The infant's growing interest in objects and desire to attain and explore them and relate them to other objects interact with motor and sensory development to influence the grasp patterns. Haptic development and visual-perceptual development contribute to the infant's ability to shape the hand to the object's form and to approach the object with optimal orientation of the arm and hand.

Another aspect of motor development that contributes to the infant's use of increasingly mature and more varied patterns is the arm's internal stability to hold a position of forearm supination and wrist extension. Stability of wrist and forearm allow controlled thumb opposition and isolated finger movements for precision grasp patterns. The ability to stabilize the wrist in a slightly extended position is important for grasp patterns that use distal (fingertip) control. Slight forearm supination positions the hand so that the thumb and radial fingers are free for active object exploration and allows the infant to view fingers and thumb during grasp.[17]

The typical sequence of grasp development begins with the neonate appearing to have no voluntary hand use. A newborn infant's hands alternately open and close in response to sensory input. Within the first 3 months the automatic traction response and grasp reflex decrease, and a voluntary palmar grasp emerges (Figure 8-2). By approximately 6 months the infant exhibits a radial palmar grasp when prehending objects.

The second 6 months is a significant period for the development of hand skills. The ability to grasp a variety of objects

TABLE 8-1 Mature Grasping Patterns Used in Functional Activities

Grasp Pattern	Functionality	Description
Power grasp	Used to control tools or other objects. Used with hand strength is required in activity	The object is held obliquely in the hand; ulnar fingers are flexed; radial fingers are less flexed. Thumb is in extension and adduction. The child stabilizes the object with the ulnar side of the hand and controls the object using the radial side of the hand.
Hook grasp	Used to carry objects such as a purse or briefcase	The transverse metacarpal arch is flat; the fingers are adducted with flexion at the interphalangeal (IP) joints. The metacarpophalangeal (MCP) joints may be flexed or extended.
Spherical grasp	Used to hold a small ball	The wrist is extended, fingers abducted, with some flexion at the MCP and IP joints. Stability of the longitudinal arch is needed to use this pattern to grasp a larger ball. The hypothenar eminence assists in cupping the hand for control of the object.
Cylindrical grasp	Used to hold a glass, cup, or can with hand around the object	The transverse arch is flattened to allow the fingers to hold against the object. The fingers are only slightly abducted, and IP and MCP joint flexion is graded according to the size of the object. When additional force is required, more of the palmar surface of the hand contacts the object.
Disk grasp	Used to hold a disk such as a jar lid	The fingers hold the disk with extension of the MCP joints and flexion of the IP joints. The wrist flexes and thumb extends when objects are larger, and only the pads of the fingers contact the object. This pattern involves dissociation of flexion and extension movements and use of a combination of wrist flexion with MCP extension and IP flexion.
Lateral pinch	Used to exert power on or with a small object	The index finger is slightly flexed and the thumb is flexed and adducted. The pad of the thumb is placed against the radial side of the index finger at or near the distal interphalangeal (DIP) joint.
Pincer grasp	Used to hold and handle small objects and precision tools (e.g., a pencil)	The thumb is opposed to the index finger pad and the object is held within the finger pads. The ulnar fingers are often flexed.
Three-jaw chuck or tripod grasp	Used to hold and manipulate a writing utensil or eating utensil	The thumb is simultaneously opposed to the index and middle finger pads. These fingers provide stability for prehension of a tool. The thumb forms an oval or a modified oval shape with the fingers. When using a tripod grasp on a tool, the forearm is slightly supinated.
Tip pinch	Used to prehend and hold tiny objects	The thumb is opposed with thumb tip meeting index finger tip, forming a circle. All joints of the index finger and thumb are partly flexed.

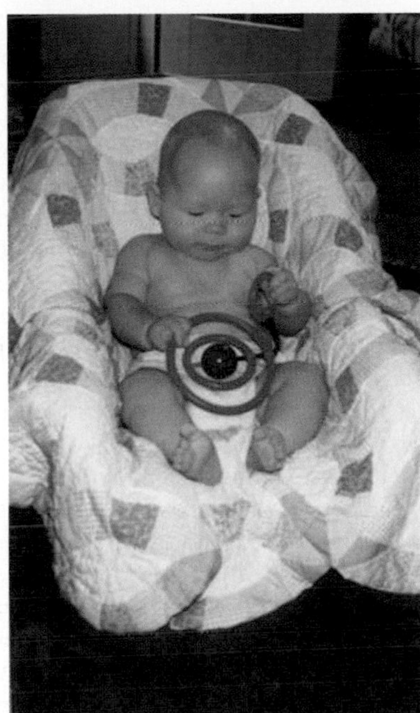

FIGURE 8-2 A 4-month-old exhibits voluntary palmer grasp. (From Case-Smith, J. (2013). Applying occupation and motor learning principles in pediatric CIMT: Theoretical foundations and conceptual framework. In S. L. Ramey, P. Coker-Bold, & S. C. DeLuca (Eds.). *Handbook of pediatric constraint-induced movement therapy (CIMT)* (pp. 41–54). Bethesda, MD: AOTA Press.)

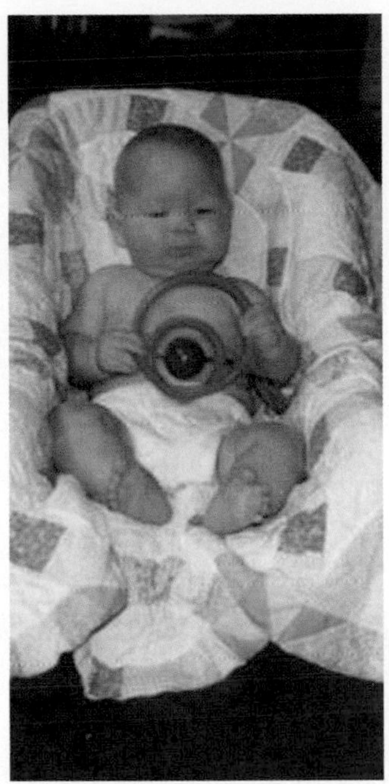

FIGURE 8-3 This child uses a radial-digital grasp to hold a rattle. (From Case-Smith, J. (2013). Applying occupation and motor learning principles in pediatric CIMT: Theoretical foundations and conceptual framework. In S. L. Ramey, P. Coker-Bold, & S. C. DeLuca (Eds.), *Handbook of pediatric constraint-induced movement therapy (CIMT)* (pp. 41–54). Bethesda, MD: AOTA Press.)

increases significantly between 6 and 9 months of age. During this time grasp patterns with active thumb use emerge. Crude raking of a tiny object is present by about 7 months of age, and by 9 months of age the infant holds a tiny object between the finger surface and the thumb. By 8 to 9 months of age the infant grasps a larger object between the thumb and the radial fingers (Figure 8-3) and readily varies the grasping pattern according to the shape of the object. However, intrinsic muscle control is not yet effective because the infant does not use grasp with MCP flexion and IP extension. Between 9 and 12 months of age, refinement occurs in the ability to use thumb and finger pad control for tiny and small objects. More precise preparation of the fingers before initiation of grasp, more inhibition of the ulnar fingers, and slight wrist extension and forearm supination are characteristics of this refinement.

After 1 year of age the infant further refines grasp patterns and more sophisticated patterns emerge. By 15 months the infant can hold crackers, cookies, and other flat objects, signifying increasing control of the intrinsic muscles. Between 18 months and 3 years of age most children with typical development acquire the ability to use a disk grasp, a cylindrical grasp, and a spherical grasp with control (see Table 8-1). Control of a power grasp continues to develop through the preschool years. The pattern for a lateral pinch may be present by 3 years of age, but children generally do not use this pattern with power until later in the preschool years. Overall grasp patterns for a variety of objects are well developed by 5 years of age, but those involving tools may continue to mature into the early school years.[88,98]

In addition to refinement of grasp patterns, strength of grasp increases throughout childhood. Strength for palmar grip, key (lateral) pinch, and tripod (three-point) pinch significantly increase in children between 3 and 5 years of age.[81] Strength appears to continue to increase in grip, lateral pinch, palmar pinch, and tip pinch until children reach 12 years, with differences in grip strength between boys and girls common.[86] Isometric force gradually increases during the 5- to 10-year-old age span, reflecting corticospinal system maturation.[119,120] Compared with 10- to 12-year-olds, adults exhibit greater isometric strength and use alternative strategies for selecting and monitoring the hand strength needed during a task.[51]

In-Hand Manipulation Skills

In-hand manipulation includes five basic types of patterns: finger-to-palm translation, palm-to-finger translation, shift, simple rotation, and complex rotation.[44] All skills require the ability to control the arches of the palm (Figure 8-4, *A* and *B*). In finger-to-palm translation, the child grasps the object with the pads of the fingers and thumb and moves it into the palm.[44] The finger pad grasp is released so that the object rests in the palm of the open hand or is held in a palmar grasp. The child moves the object in a linear direction within the hand, and the fingers move from an extended to flexed position during the translation. An example of this skill is picking up a coin with the fingers and thumb and moving it into the palm of the hand.

Palm-to-finger translation is the reverse of finger-to-palm translation and requires isolated control of the thumb.[43,99] In palm-to-finger translation, the child begins with finger flexion and moves to finger extension (see Figure 8-4, *B*). This pattern is more difficult for the child to execute than finger-to-palm translation. An example of this skill is moving a coin from the

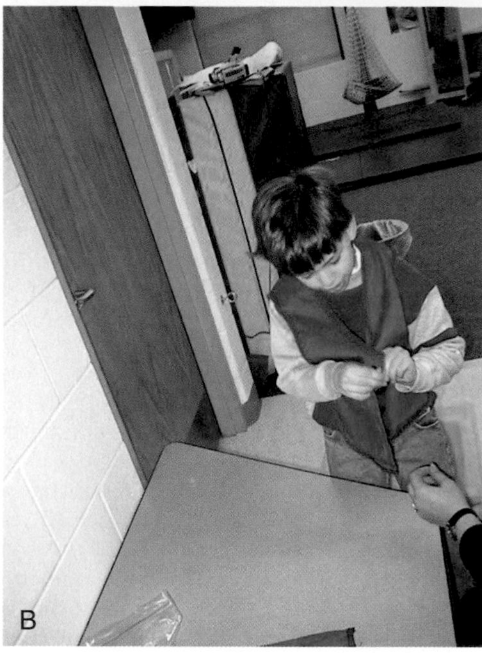

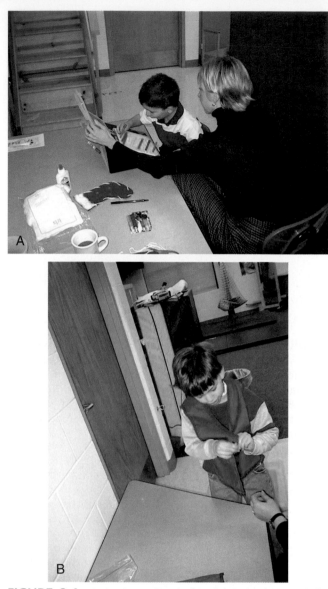

FIGURE 8-4 **A,** In emerging in-hand manipulation skills, child demonstrates increasing control of isolated finger movements. **B,** In buttoning, child uses palm-to-finger translation.

palm of the hand to the finger pads before placing the coin in a vending machine.

Shift involves linear movement of the object on the finger surface to allow for repositioning of the object on the pads of the fingers.[44,98] In this pattern the fingers move just slightly at the MCP and IP joints, and the thumb typically remains opposed or adducted with MCP and IP extension throughout the shift. The object usually is held solely on the radial side of the hand. Examples of this skill are separating two pieces of paper, moving a coin from a position against the volar aspect of the DIP joints to a position closer to the fingertips (e.g., to insert a coin into the slot of a vending machine), and adjusting a pen or pencil after grasp so that the fingers are positioned close to the writing end of the tool. This skill is used frequently in dressing tasks such as buttoning, fastening snaps, lacing shoes, and putting a belt through belt loops.

The two patterns of rotation are simple rotation and complex rotation. In simple rotation the child turns or rolls an object held at the finger pads approximately 90 degrees or less.[44] The fingers act as a unit, without differentiation of action, and the thumb is in an opposed position. Examples of simple rotation are unscrewing a small bottle cap, reorienting a puzzle piece in the hand by turning it slightly before placing it in the puzzle, and picking up a small peg and rotating it from a horizontal to a vertical position for insertion into a pegboard.

In complex rotation, the child rotates a small object 180 to 360 degrees once or repetitively.[44,100] During complex rotation the fingers and thumb alternate in producing the movement, and the fingers typically move independently of one another. An object may be moved end over end, such as in turning a coin or a peg over or in turning a pencil over to use the eraser.

In-hand manipulation skills also are used when a child has two or more pieces of cereal in his or her hand and moves one piece to the finger pads before placing it in the mouth. The term *with stabilization* refers to the use of an in-hand manipulation skill while other objects are stabilized in the hand. In-hand manipulation skills with stabilization are generally more difficult to perform than the same skill without the simultaneous stabilization of other objects in the hand.

Developmental Considerations

Postural and motor skill prerequisites for in-hand manipulation and dynamic grasping patterns include that the child demonstrates:

- Active forearm supination with stability when moving hand and fingers
- Wrist extension with stability
- Controlled and dynamic thumb opposition
- Fingertip prehension of objects with control of fingertip forces
- Isolated thumb and radial finger movement
- Stability with mobility of the transverse MCP arch
- Dissociation of the radial and ulnar sides of the hand[44]

Children with delayed or limited in-hand manipulation skills are likely to substitute other patterns. Typical patterns that compensate for limited in-hand manipulation include (1) changing hands, (2) transferring from hand to hand, or (3) stabilizing the object on a table surface to reorient its position. The child uses these patterns after the initial grasp when he or she realizes that the object needs to be repositioned for use. For example, a child picks up a crayon with the right hand but is unable to shift it to place the fingers near the writing end; therefore, he or she grasps the object with the left hand and then transfers it back to the right hand. Some children preplan for this by picking up the crayon with the non-preferred hand and changing it to the preferred hand. Children commonly use two hands to compensate for limited shift and complex rotation.

In-hand manipulation skills develop after primary grasp and release skills have matured. By approximately 12 to 15 months of age, infants use finger-to-palm translation to pick up and "hide" small pieces of food in their hands. By 2 to 2.5 years of age, children use palm-to-finger translation and simple rotation with some objects.[99] Complex rotation skills are observed in children at 2.5 to 3 years of age, although children of this age group often have difficulty with them. By 4 years of age, children consistently use complex rotation without using an external support.[100] Children between 3.5 and 5.5 years of age develop skills in rotating a marker (regardless of its initial orientation) and shifting it into optimal position for coloring and writing.[69] Children 3 and 3.5 years old demonstrate shift, although use is inconsistent.[43]

After 3 years of age, a child's in-hand manipulation skills become more proficient and consistent. For example, objects are seldom dropped during in-hand manipulation tasks.[98] In-hand manipulation speed and accuracy continue to improve during the preschool years. By 6 years of age children develop the ability to use a variety of in-hand manipulation skills with stabilization.[97] Between 6 and 7 years of age, children more consistently use combinations of in-hand manipulation skills in complex fine motor activities (e.g., palm-to-finger translation with stabilization followed by complex rotation with stabilization). These skills continue to refine and speed improves through 12 years of age, at which time skills are similar to those of adults.[55]

Object characteristics influence the in-hand manipulation pattern used. In general, medium-sized objects (e.g., standard crayons) are easier for children to manipulate than slightly larger objects (e.g., larger-diameter crayons) or tiny objects. Tiny objects require precise fingertip control, whereas medium-sized and larger objects require control with more fingers. Other factors that contribute to a child's use of in-hand manipulation skills include the cognitive-perceptual demands of the activity and the objects' shape and texture. The child's motor-planning skills, strength, and tactile sensibility can influence development of in-hand manipulation skills.

Voluntary Release

Voluntary release, like grasp, depends on control of arm and finger movements. To place an object for release, the arm must move into position accurately and then stabilize as the fingers and thumb extend. Object release requires precise coordination of fingertip forces and timing for predicting accurate object placement (e.g., on a surface).[60]

Initially the infant does not voluntarily release an object; objects either drop involuntarily from the hand or must be forcibly removed from the hand. As the infant's tactile and proprioceptive perception, eye-hand coordination, and cognitive development improve, volitional control of release emerges. The infant first demonstrates object release when transferring objects from one hand to another. Initially the child stabilizes the object in the mouth during transfers or pulls it out of one hand with the other. By 5 to 6 months the infant transfers the object from one hand to the other by fully opening the releasing hand.

By 9 months of age the infant begins to release objects without stabilizing them with the other hand. Typically, the arm (i.e., elbow and wrist) extends during release. The infant exhibits increasing shoulder control as he or she moves the arm to drop objects in different locations. With the development of dissociation of arm and hand and increasing elbow stability, the infant begins to release with the elbow in mid ranges (i.e., with some degree of flexion). To control release, the child may stabilize the arm or hand on the surface during release. At about 1 year of age, the child can release objects with shoulder, elbow, and wrist stability; however, the MCP joints remain unstable during this pattern, therefore the infant continues to show excess finger extension (Figure 8-5). Gradually the child

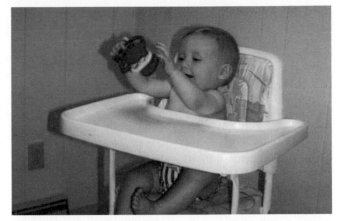

FIGURE 8-5 A 10-month-old infant exhibits object release with full finger extension.

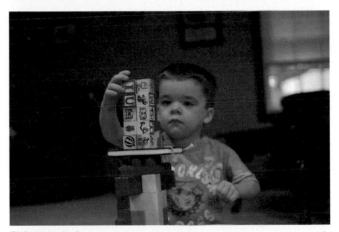

FIGURE 8-6 A 2-year-old exhibits precision release with partial finger extension.

develops the ability to release objects into smaller containers and to stack blocks. The release pattern is refined over the next few years until the child can release small objects with graded extension of the fingers, indicating control over the intrinsic hand muscles (Figure 8-6). Between 7 and 13 years of age, children acquire effective modulation of fingertip force when grasping lighter and heavier objects to accurately time their release and placement.[39,97] Development of precision release, similar to precision grasp, illustrates the integration of perceptual, motor, cognitive, and sensory functions.

Bimanual Skills

In typical development the infant gradually learns to use both sides of the body together in effective ways and to use each side of the body independently of the other. Initially the newborn moves his or her arms in asymmetrical patterns that are not coordinated. Movements of one arm often elicit reflexive, nonpurposeful reactions in the other arm. Gradually the infant develops the ability to move the two arms together in the same pattern. As skilled use of symmetrical hand and arm patterns is refined, the infant begins to use the two arms independently of one another to perform different roles in an activity.[27,47,48] For example, one hand stabilizes an object while the other hand manipulates it. Overflow and associated movements gradually decrease to allow separate but coordinated action of the two hands.

As discussed previously, infants progress from asymmetry to symmetry to differentiated asymmetrical movements for bilateral hand activities. Asymmetry is a characteristic of movement patterns until almost 3 months of age. Symmetric patterns predominate between 3 and 10 months of age, when bilateral reach, grasp, and mouthing of the hands and objects are primary activities. Control of these movements originates proximally at the shoulders, allowing the hands to engage at midline. By 9 to 10 months of age the infant can hold one object in each hand and bang them together. This ability to hold an object in each hand at the same time is critical for further bimanual skill development. By 10 months of age bimanual action is well differentiated, with one hand grasping the object and the other exploring parts of it (Figure 8-7).[48,49]

Differentiated bimanual action, first as reciprocal or alternating hand movements, then as simultaneous hand movements, allows the child to engage in ADLs and object interactions of increasing complexity. By 17 to 18 months of age, infants frequently use role-differentiated strategies (i.e., one hand stabilizes or holds the materials and the other manipulates or activates them).[17] For these skills to emerge, the infant must be able to dissociate the two sides of the body and begin to use the two hands simultaneously for different functions (see Figure 8-7). Effective stabilization of materials also depends on adequate shoulder, elbow, and wrist stability.

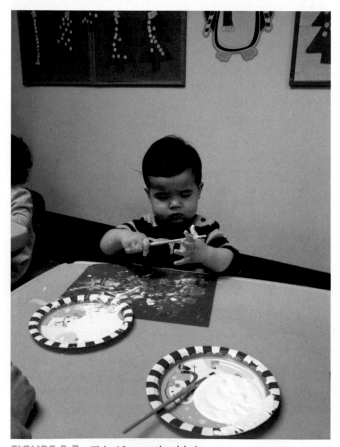

FIGURE 8-7 This 10-month-old shows emerging bimanual skills with one hand holding the object and the other manipulating it.

Between 18 and 24 months of age, the child begins to develop skills that are precursors to simultaneous manipulation. Continuing development of reach, grasp, release, and in-hand manipulation skills complements bimanual skill refinement. Skills in visual-perceptual, cognitive, and motor areas become more integrated, leading to the child's effective use of motor planning for task performance. Simultaneous manipulation using both hands together—that is, opposing hand and arm movements for highly differentiated activities (e.g., cutting with scissors)—emerges at about 2.5 years of age.[27,47] This mature pattern is refined, including increases in speed and efficiency, as the school-age child engages in increasingly complex manipulation tasks.

Ball-Throwing Skills

Ball-throwing skills reflect the child's ability to use shoulder strength and control with release skills. In throwing a small ball, the child must sequence and time movements throughout the entire upper extremity. The child brings the arm into a starting position, then prepares for projection of the ball into space by moving the trunk with the scapulohumeral joint, stabilizing the shoulder while beginning to extend the elbow, stabilizing the elbow while moving the wrist from extension to a neutral position, and simultaneously forcefully extending the fingers and thumb.

Children progress through a series of skill levels before they can smoothly sequence these movements and project the ball to the desired location. Research on the development of ball-throwing skills is quite limited and has primarily been identified in the context of standardized test development.[12,54] By 2 years of age the child can throw a ball forward and maintain balance so that his or her body does not also move forward. At this age the child uses arm extension without sustained shoulder flexion to fling the ball.[54] The child dissociates trunk and arm movement but does not completely dissociate humeral and forearm movements. By 2.5 to 3 years of age, the child projects the ball approximately 3 feet forward toward a target. This ability to control the direction of the ball to some degree implies that the child can control the humerus so that the elbow is in front of the shoulder when the ball is released. Thus the shoulder has sufficient stability to support controlled elbow and finger movement. By 3.5 years of age, the child throws a ball 5 to 7 feet toward a target with little deviation from a straight line.[54] To accomplish this level of throwing accuracy, the child positions his or her elbow in front of the shoulder before releasing the ball.

Further refinement of ball-throwing skills continues over the next few years. Distance and accuracy improve as the child gains scapulohumeral control, the ability to sustain the humerus above the shoulder, and the ability to control the timing of elbow, wrist, and finger extension. Thus at approximately 5 years of age, the child uses an overhand throw to consistently hit a target at 5 feet. Children between 6 and 7 years of age can hit a target 12 feet away using an overhand throw.[54] Children 5 years of age or older also use underhand throws to contact a target. Underhand throwing requires the ability to move the humerus into flexion while sustaining full external rotation.

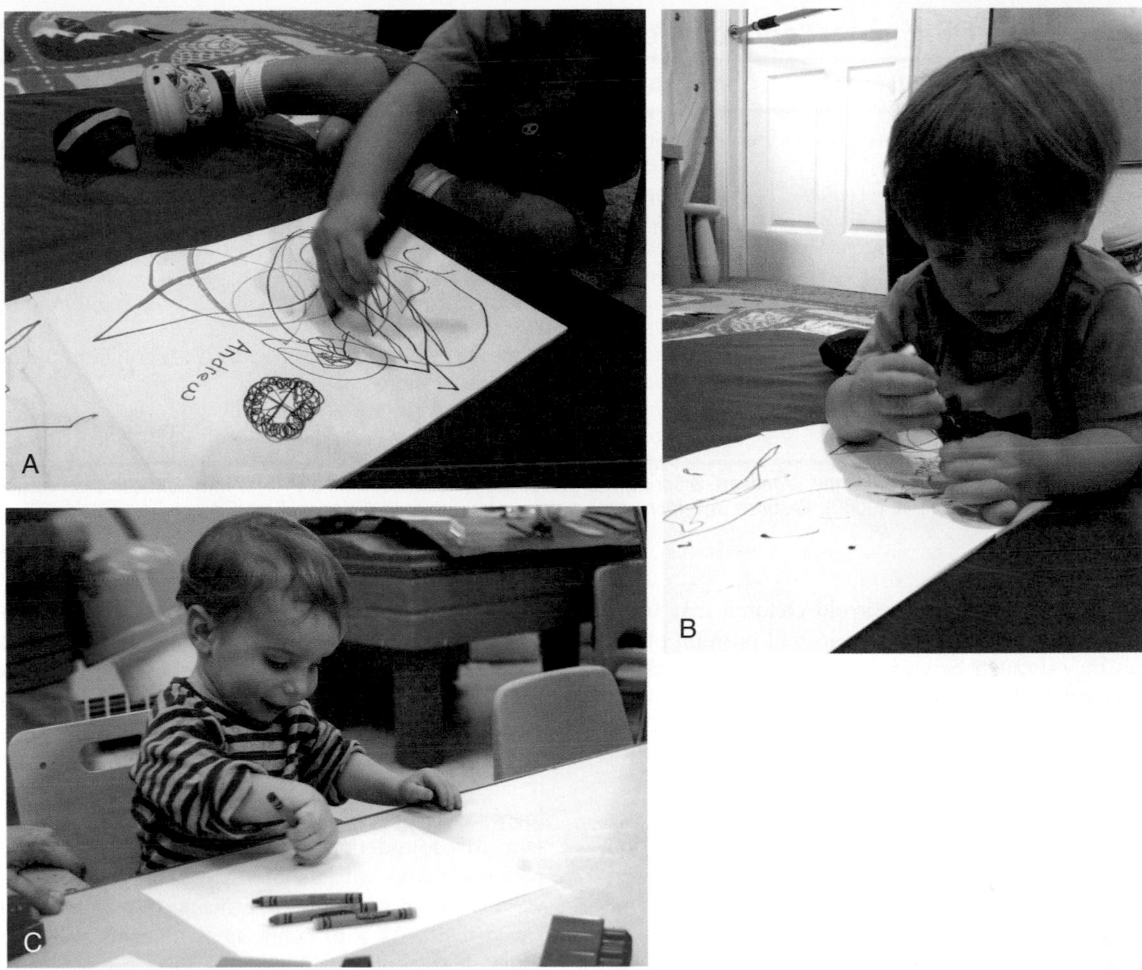

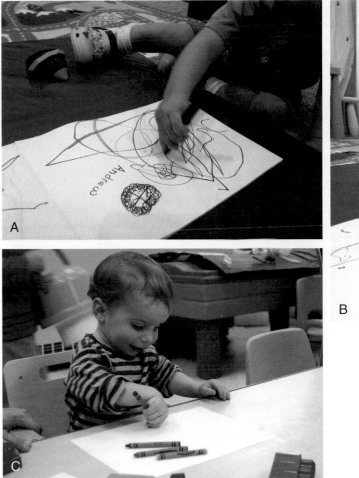

FIGURE 8-8 A 2-year-old experiments with using a marker (**A** and **B**) and a crayon (**C**), exhibiting a variety of transitional grasping patterns.

Tool Use

Tool use is part of everyday life and is an essential method for children and adults to interact with their environment. It involves purposeful, goal-directed manipulation of a tool to interact with other objects or materials.[26,105] Proficient tool use is essential to participation in a variety of self-care, play and leisure, and school and work tasks. Tool use competence for eating and play typically emerges during the second year, after the child has mastered the basic skills of reach, grasp, and release.[27] These skills emerge concurrently with in-hand manipulation skills that allow the tool to be dynamically held with fingers adjusting it within the hand.

A child's acquisition of tool-use skills highly relates to cognitive development. In proficient tool use, an individual understands the goal of the task (the intentional aspect of the task) and knows how to accomplish it (the operational aspect of the task).[82,105] Acquisition of tool use follows the stages of motor learning (later defined in the motor learning section). Initially, the child experiments with a tool (e.g., a marker) by trying a wide variety of actions (e.g., holding in either hand, with fist or fingers, at top or base of marker). Experimenting with a tool is an important stage in the skill-acquisition process. As skill acquisition progresses, practice allows the skill to progress from the child demonstrating a high level of attention to his or her action to performing at a more automatic level. With practice, performance becomes faster, more accurate, and smoother (i.e., more automatic), resulting in proficient tool use for daily life tasks (Figure 8-8, *A* to *C*).

The first tools that a child learns to use with proficiency are those required for eating. A toddler uses a spoon by 18 months of age, a fork by 2.5 years of age, and a knife by 6 years of age.[65] In a longitudinal study on development of spoon use skills in infants between 11 and 23 months of age, 17- to 23-month-old toddlers showed a clear hand and grasping pattern[26] preference for eating. Between these ages, children used 10 different grasp patterns, none of which was typical of an adult pattern. The most commonly used pattern was a transverse palmar grasp with all four fingers flexed around the handle of the spoon. By 17 months toddlers held the spoon primarily in their fingers and used some degree of finger extension to hold and orient the spoon. This pattern, which continues to refine through the second year, improves eating efficiency.

Another example of tool use that emerges in young children is cutting with scissors.[54] Early cutting is actually snipping, a process of closing the scissors on the paper with no movement of the paper and with no ability to repetitively open and close the scissors while flexing the shoulder and extending the elbow

TABLE 8-2 Developmental Sequence for Scissors Skills

Age (years)	Scissors Skill	Arm Actions
2	Snips with scissors	Hand holding paper is minimally involved; may hold paper awkwardly or with lateral pincer; hand with scissors often pronated.
2.5	Cuts across a 6-inch piece of paper	Hand holding paper in active supination; holds paper with stability; hand with scissors supinated.
3 to 3.5	Cuts on a line 6 inches long	Hand holding paper with stability, forearm in partial supination; hand holding scissors supinates to 90 degrees.
3.5 to 4	Cuts out a circle*	Hand holding paper moves it in coordination with cutting; hand holding scissors is supinated 90 degrees or more.
4 to 5	Cuts out a square	Hand holding paper moves it in coordination with cutting; hand holding scissors is supinated 90 degrees or more.
6 to 7	Cuts a variety of shapes	Both hands cooperate in synchronous and reciprocal interaction during cutting actions.

*The research of Rodger, Ziviani, Watter, Ozanne, Woodyatt, & Springfield (2003) suggests that cutting a circle is more difficult than cutting a square.
Adapted from Folio, R. M., & Fewell, R. (2000). *Peabody developmental motor scales—revised.* Chicago: Riverside.

to move across the paper. Three-year-old children may use a pronated forearm position or a forearm-in-mid-position placement, or they may alternate between the two forearm positions. By 4 years of age children typically hold both forearms in mid position for the cutting activity.[92] Table 8-2 describes the typical sequence for the development of scissors skills.

The child's grasp on the scissors changes over time. The thumb position in one hole remains consistent, but the finger positions change according to the child's level of maturation and the type of scissors used. Although grasp pattern is determined by the type of scissors, by 6 years of age a child demonstrates a mature grasp with the ulnar two fingers flexed (inside or outside the lower hole, depending on its size) and the radial fingers within the top scissor hole to provide the cutting action.

One component of tool use is the role of the assisting hand. For example, in using scissors and eating, the assisting hand has an active role, while in writing and drawing, the assisting hand primarily stabilizes the paper. In cutting, the assisting hand holds the paper and orients it using rotational movements in the same or the opposite direction as the hand with the scissors. In eating, the child's assisting hand may be involved in a variety of activities, depending on the child's age and the utensils used. Infants between 18 and 23 months of age appear to have significantly more involvement of the assisting hand in stabilizing a dish during spoon feeding than do infants between 12 and 17 months of age.[26]

Hand Preference

Hand preference, sometimes termed ***hand dominance,*** is a complex concept. In typical children hand preference evolves over a long period of time and gradually becomes more consistent, as do other expressions of motor functioning. In children 6 to 24 months of age, use of a preferred hand is inconsistent in about 60% of the children performing a simple grasp task. When one hand is used as a stabilizer and one as a manipulator, 65% or more of the children over 18 months use the right hand as the manipulator. Inconsistency of preferred hand was noted in some children in the 2.5- to 3-year-old group but not in the 4-year-old group. Handedness is highly influenced by the task demands; for example, 18- to 36-month-old infants show a preferred hand in bimanual manipulation tasks that mandate a dominant hand but not in simple grasping tasks. When exploring objects, infants tend to use both hands and not demonstrate a preferred hand.[49]

Hand preference continues to develop until at least 8 years of age, as illustrated in a study of a reaching activity that involved crossing the midline of the body. Carlier, Doyen, and Lamard[15] found that with increasing age, children used the preferred hand with greater frequency to pick up cards in various locations, including crossing the midline with the preferred hand. As with other areas of hand skill development, some degree of variability and inconsistency is the typical pattern for young children. It is worrisome and atypical when infants (less than 7 months) consistently use one hand, and these infants should be further evaluated for possible neurologic impairment.

Relationship of Hand Skills to Children's Occupations

Hand skills are vital to the child's interaction with the environment. Engagement in most occupations requires object and material handling with one's hands.

Play

Although infants engage with people and objects through their visual and auditory senses, these are distant senses and do not readily bring the infant essential information that can be gained only through touch. In early exploratory play with objects, an infant learns object properties through manipulating them.[17,117] The interaction of touching, grasping, and manipulating, while visually inspecting, allows the infant to integrate sensory information and to learn that objects remain the same regardless of visual orientation.

With increasing age, until at least the early school years, participation in play depends on hand function and fine motor skill competence. These skills are reflected in the child's interest in activities such as cutting with scissors, dressing and undressing dolls, putting puzzles together, constructing with various types of building materials and model sets, participating in sand and water play, completing craft projects, and engaging in imaginary play with objects. Playing video games and using computers also require fine motor control. Dramatic play with dolls or figurines in doll houses and vehicles involves precision hand movement including in-hand and bimanual manipulation.

Activities of Daily Living

Activities of daily living (ADLs) often entail a sequence of steps using a variety of hand functions. Specific hand functions needed for ADLs include (1) precision and power grasps of objects and materials; (2) complementary and reciprocal bimanual skills; (3) hand movements, including in-hand manipulation, with and without vision; (4) complex action sequences; and (5) development of automaticity.[65] In-hand manipulation speed, grasp strength, motor accuracy, and tool handling are correlated with self-care skill development.[16]

Dressing skills (i.e., donning shirts, pants, socks, and shoes) involve complex grasping patterns and in-hand manipulation skills to fasten and a variety of bimanual skills to manipulate the clothing. Donning jewelry requires the ability to use delicate grasp patterns and in-hand manipulation. Bathing, showering, and other personal hygiene skills depend on the child's increasing control of dynamic grasping patterns to handle slippery objects (e.g., soap). In addition, these skills are likely to be needed when an individual is in a standing position, such as when putting toothpaste on a toothbrush, brushing the teeth, shaving, or applying makeup. Youth need high competency in precision grasp, in-hand manipulation, and dynamic tool use to perform complex hygiene activities such as shaving, applying makeup, using tweezers, cutting nails, and styling hair (applying barrettes or rubber bands and using a curling iron, a brush, and a hair dryer).

Eating skills require refinement of the ability to use forearm control with a variety of grasp patterns and tools. The ability to use both hands together effectively is necessary for spreading and cutting with a knife, opening all types of containers, pouring liquids, and preparing food. In-hand manipulation skills are used to adjust eating utensils and finger foods within the hand, to handle a napkin, and to manipulate the opening of packaged food and utensils.

Typically developing children 8 years of age and older are independent in self-care skills and the manipulation skills required to perform eating, dressing, and hygiene tasks. In contrast, children with DCD and poor coordination are frequently delayed in development of dressing, personal hygiene, toileting, and independent eating skills.[91,108] Older children with DCD perform similarly to younger typical children. Because older children with DCD demonstrate delays in self-care, parents continue to support their self-care participation by providing cues, assistance, and substitutions.[108]

School Functions

Independent functioning in the school environment requires effective hand function and competence in fine motor skills. In preschool classrooms, children engage in a variety of manipulative activities, for example, using crayons, scissors, small building materials, and puzzles, and participate in simple cooking and art projects. During kindergarten and the early elementary school years, children use fine motor skills most of the school day. McHale and Cermak[89] found that first and second grade children spend 45% to 55% of the school day engaged in fine motor activities. Fourth grade children spend approximately 30% of their school day participating in fine motor activities, primarily paper-pencil tasks. Writing activities include preparing one's paper, obtaining a writing tool, and using an eraser. Other typical fine motor activities in children's classrooms include cutting with scissors, folding paper, using paste and tape, carrying out simple science projects, assuming responsibility for managing one's own snack and lunch items, and organizing and maintaining one's desk.[28] Elementary school children also need computer and keyboarding skills to function in the classroom.

Older children and adolescents use high-level fine motor skills for science projects, vocational courses (e.g., woodworking, metal shop, and home economics), art classes, music classes (other than vocal music), managing a high volume of written work and notebooks, keyboarding, and maintaining a locker. Greater speed (e.g., in writing and keyboarding) and greater strength (e.g., for physical education and vocational courses) are required. As demands in high school increase, proficiency and speed in using keyboards, calculators, and writing utensils is expected. Children and adolescents with hand function difficulties often demonstrate limited productivity and require accommodations for written communication tasks, managing school-related materials, and manipulating learning materials.[7]

Evaluation of Hand Skills in Children

The developmental sequence provides a backdrop for evaluation of hand function. The occupational therapist evaluates a child's hand skills in the context of play, self-care, and school occupations when the evidence suggests that problems with performance are associated with delays or impairment in hand function. Based on the evaluation purpose, a variety of standardized and non-standardized assessments can be used (see Chapter 6). Parents, teachers, and the child often are the best sources of information about difficulties with participation at home and in the community; this information is obtained through the development of an occupational profile.

When a problem with occupational performance that implies hand function delays has been identified, the occupational therapist plans a full evaluation of fine motor, visual-motor, and hand function performance. To fully analyze hand function and potential reasons for difficulties, related performance areas may need to be screened and/or assessed using standardized methods. Postural alignment and stability, gross motor skills, cognitive and perceptual skills, sensory processing, social skills, and emotional functioning are associated performance areas that can contribute to hand function.

Analysis of the identified hand function problems follows administration of specific assessments or scales that define the basis of the problem and the extent of the impairment. A sample analysis of an occupational performance problem in the area of constructive play associated with delayed and impaired hand function is presented in Box 8-1. The occupational

BOX 8-1 Analysis of Performance Components Potentially Associated with Delays or Impairment in Constructive Play

Occupational therapists apply clinical reasoning to analyze potential reasons for a child's delay or limitation in constructive play activities. Constructive activities vary by the child's age and may include completing puzzles, building with blocks and Legos, stacking toys, and participating in games that involve moving and combining small objects. When the basis for a child's performance delay is identified, these components can be targeted in designing play activities for intervention.

1. Delayed or limited in-hand manipulative skills may be associated with:
   a. Unstable wrist in neutral position or extension, uses wrist flexion
      (1) Decreased tone in wrist extensors
      (2) Increased tone in wrist flexors
   b. Unstable metacarpophalangeal (MCP) joints and limited stability of finger joints
      (1) Increased tightness of extensor digitorum muscles
   c. Inability to identify finger being touched; decreased tactile discrimination
   d. Lack of midrange movements of finger joints
      (1) Poor co-contraction of MCP and interphalangeal (IP) flexors and extensors
      (2) Tightness in intrinsic muscles and long finger flexors
2. Breaking materials, often by dropping and crushing them, may be associated with:
   a. Inability to sustain finger pad grasp; may be associated with:
      (1) Poor tactile or proprioceptive awareness
      (2) Poor co-contraction of muscle groups
   b. Excessive finger flexion in grasp may be associated with:
      (1) Poor proprioceptive awareness of size and weight of object
      (2) Increased finger flexor tone
      (3) Associated reactions
      (4) Inactivity in intrinsic muscles
3. Ineffective bilateral handling may be associated with:
   a. Weakness and limited control of movement in one arm and hand
      (1) Unstable grasp because of poor wrist extension caused by increased flexor tone
      (2) Learned nonuse of one hand
   b. Delays in bimanual coordination, reciprocal and simultaneous use of two hands together
      (1) Difficulty in motor planning of sequential, coordinated movements
      (2) Limited or inaccurate tactile and kinesthetic feedback from arm and hand movement.
      (3) Delays in performance of cooperative, precise hand and finger movements, possibly related to delayed somatosensory or visual motor integration.

therapist analyzes potential sensory, musculoskeletal, and neuromotor functions that may contribute to a child's difficulties in construction activities. To support analysis of the child's performance in specific tasks and interpret which sensory, motor, perceptual, and cognitive factors influence performance, therapists administer a combination of standardized assessments. Examples of measures used in comprehensive evaluation of hand function are listed in Table 8-3.

Intervention Models, Principles, and Strategies

Occupational therapists use a variety of evidence-based practice models to guide interventions to improve a child's hand function. The child's diagnosis (e.g., cerebral palsy, developmental coordination disorder), severity of involvement (e.g., mild, moderate, severe), context for intervention (e.g., clinic, home, school), service delivery model (e.g., direct, consultation), and phase of intervention (e.g., preparation, practice, generalization) influence which practice approach is used. Practice models used by occupational therapists to improve children's hand function can be categorized as biomechanical/neurodevelopmental, occupation-based, and adaptation/ecologic and are described in the following sections. These practice models, with their corresponding principles and strategies, are generally used in combination or sequentially throughout a course of interventions to improve a child's hand function.

Biomechanical and Neurodevelopmental Approaches

Practice models that focus on the child's musculoskeletal and neuromotor systems are considered to be bottom-up approaches because they focus on enhancing specific components of performance. The approaches are based on an understanding of normal movement patterns and body alignment and incorporate handling and positioning of the child to inhibit and facilitate posture and movement. The occupational therapist embeds these techniques in specific activities that promote strengthening and motor control of targeted movements. These approaches require careful, in-depth analysis of performance to identify missing, atypical, or delayed body functions that are the basis for hand function problems. Biomechanical approaches focus on the musculoskeletal system, including spinal alignment, joint alignment throughout the body, muscle tone, and muscle strength as foundational elements of a child's motor skill. In neurodevelopmental therapy, therapists use facilitation and inhibition handling techniques within activities designed to enhance the child's motor control.

Biomechanical Practice Model

The biomechanical approach or practice model is used primarily to assess and provide intervention activities that improve a child's ROM, strength, or endurance. Biomechanical approaches focus on postural alignment, joint stability and relationships, and musculoskeletal problems. For example, biomechanical principles explain the basis for tenodesis grasp (i.e., automatic finger flexion when the wrist is extended) and the relationship of intrinsic and extrinsic muscle control for grasp and in-hand manipulation patterns.

Types of Children Who Benefit from Biomechanical Approaches

Children with musculoskeletal and neuromotor disorders associated with prenatal or perinatal central nervous system lesions or anomalies often receive interventions that use biomechanical

TABLE 8-3 Comprehensive Hand Function Evaluation

Evaluation Objective	Examples of Tools
Measurement of active and passive range of motion (ROM)	Goniometer Observation of ADL tasks
Evaluation of strength	Muscle testing (modified for children) Grip and pinch strength testing Observation of strength and endurance across motor tasks
Evaluation of tactile perception/sensibility	Two-point discrimination[40] Finger identification with vision occluded
Stereognosis	Identification of common objects with vision occluded Matching of object in hand (with hand behind barrier) to one visualized
Postural alignment and postural stability	Observation of posture when trunk is unsupported. Postural tilt with observation of equilibrium responses.
Classification of hand function to document outcomes	Manual Abilities Classification System (MACS)[41]
Assessment of developmental hand skills in young children	Bayley Scales of Infant and Toddler Development (3rd ed.): Motor Scale[5] Peabody Developmental Motor Scales (2nd ed): Fine Motor[54] Hawaii Early Learning Profile: Fine Motor[97]
Assessment of fine motor coordination in older children and adolescents	Bruininks-Oseretsky Test of Motor Proficiency (BOT-2)[12] Purdue Pegboard Test Box & Block Test of Manual Dexterity[85] Test of In-Hand Manipulation[101]
Assessment of quality of movement and dissociated movement patterns (for children with cerebral palsy)	Quality of Upper Extremity Skills Test (QUEST)[32,33]
Assessment of visual motor integration	Developmental Test of Visual Motor Integration (5th ed.) (VMI)[8] Developmental Test of Visual Perception (DTVP-3)[64]
Assessment of bimanual hand function	Assisting Hand Assessment[74] Melbourne Assessment of Unilateral Upper Limb Function[104]
Assessment of hand function for prevocational or work tasks	Job task simulations

approaches. Primary features of neuromotor disorders such as cerebral palsy are abnormal muscle tone, muscle weakness, and sensory loss. Muscle tone may be lower or higher than the normal muscle tension (e.g., hypotonia or spasticity) and is associated with shortening and tightness of muscle groups and malalignment or contracture of joints. With imbalance of muscle groups around joint structures, upper extremity joints can tighten into a position of flexion or extension that counters full hand function.

The biomechanical problems associated with hypotonia include poor postural stability that affects hand function in a seated or standing position and poor control of arms in space (i.e., when posture is unsupported). Therefore, children with hypotonia may need seating supports such as a high chair back, lateral supports, firm seating, and strapping to maintain a midline, upright posture when sitting in a chair or wheelchair to effectively use their arms and hands. When children with cerebral palsy have spasticity, they exhibit limited ROM, stiffness that restricts movements, asymmetrical postures and movements, and difficulty maintaining upright postures. Arm and hand function is often limited to small ranges of movement with reduced isolated thumb and finger movements and limited control of their arms when not stabilized on a surface. Children with spastic quadriparesis may exhibit primitive reflexes, such as the asymmetrical tonic neck reflex, and stereotypical patterns of movement (e.g., a pattern of pronation, elbow, wrist, and finger flexion when bringing hands to mouth). Patterns of hip adduction and internal rotation may dominate in the low extremities. These movement problems are associated with poor postural alignment and significantly delayed motor skill development.

Biomechanical Model Principles and Strategies

Biomechanical approaches consider postural alignment, postural stability, the level of motor skill performance, effects of gravity, effects of the supporting surface, and the most efficient postures for functional performance. Biomechanical approaches for children with cerebral palsy and neuromotor disorders as described previously often focus on minimizing spinal asymmetries and optimizing support of posture. Box 8-2 defines key concepts of the biomechanical approach. The occupational therapist often implements biomechanical techniques that support optimal function before making activity demands on the child or before need for performance. Principles and examples for the biomechanical model are listed in Table 8-4.

In selecting the positioning of the child for hand function interventions, the occupational therapist must consider the optimal position for eliciting the particular skills desired, given activity demands and environmental contexts. Positions are carefully selected and optimally supported to promote the child's alignment, postural stability, and control of arm and hand movements. Supported side-lying, prone, sitting, or standing may be optimal positions to elicit and practice fine motor skills. For example, a child with significant weakness or spasticity may achieve hands-to-midline or reach only in the side-lying position. The side-lying position may reduce the effects of gravity on overall body posture and may make it

BOX 8-2 Biomechanical Model Concepts

Range of Motion (ROM)
ROM requires joint movement and flexibility. Strength and coordination of arm movement relates to ROM, and optimal position for function is usually midrange of the joint. Joints may be limited in ROM because of muscle tightness, soft tissue contracture, or fascial restrictions.

Base of Support
The body's base of support includes the areas of the body that are in contact with the supporting surface. The center of pressure in standing or sitting depends on the characteristics of the base of support. Postural activity is initiated at the base of support (e.g., when sitting, pelvic movement allows the trunk to shift forward or laterally for reach).

Changes in the base of support influence alignment of the spine and limbs.

Alignment of the Body
The alignment of shoulders, pelvis, and feet is influenced by gravity. Body alignment reflects the interaction of gravity, postural tone, position, and supporting surfaces. Alignment of the trunk influences the possible ROM and control of head, arms, and legs.

Muscle Strength and Postural Control
The musculoskeletal system maintains posture and movement through muscle force (muscle fiber activation). Postural control requires spinal alignment, muscle tone (active muscle tension), and muscle strength.

Mobility
Movement of the body through space requires postural control, muscle strength, and muscle control.

Adapted from Adolph, K.E., Vereijken, B., & Shrout, P. E. (2003). What changes in infant walking and why? *Child Development, 74*(2), 475–497.

TABLE 8-4 Biomechanical Model Principles and Examples

Principles	Description and Examples
Optimal positioning of the child includes natural spinal alignment with trunk stable or well supported.	The child's head is aligned over the pelvis. When the child is in a prone stander, head and pelvis are aligned over the feet. A straight line can be drawn from head to feet.
Central control at shoulders and pelvis is prerequisite to control of arm and hand movement in space.	The pelvis anchors the trunk and provides a base of support for shoulder and arm movement. The shoulder and scapula complex anchor the arms' movement in space and allows for rotational movement in reach and carry.
Postural control is influenced by the child's postural tone, spinal alignment, and gravity and supporting surfaces.	When sitting square on buttocks on a firm surface, postural tone is likely to be neutral with extension against gravity dominating.
Midline position of the head, arms, and hands is optimal for most functional tasks.	Many positioning devices facilitate midline position of head and arms. Lateral supports on a wheelchair or feeder chair can guide arms to midline.
Equipment to support a child's alignment and trunk control should be firm, stable, and solid.	A firm seat such as that of a Rifton chair or wheelchair allows the child to sit in a neutral pelvic position (i.e., square on buttocks). A firm seat can prevent adduction of hips and reduce posterior pelvic tilt.
For optimal function, a child should feel stable, able to move against gravity, able to shift weight, and able to flexibly adjust his or her position when needed.	Strapping on a wheelchair should allow weight shift, movement of arms, and reach in all directions. For optimal function, the child sits with dynamic stability and can move his or her arms overhead and across the midline.
For optimal function, the child's postural tone should be relaxed, allowing him or her to actively maintain upright posture and flexibly maintain functional postural alignment.	A child's postural tone may be optimal when sitting on a firm surface, when feet are well supported, and when a midline position is facilitated. See Chapter 20 for additional information on seating and positioning.

possible for the child to more easily open his or her hands. However, side-lying positions tend to limit most hand functions, and in general children exhibit more varied and skillful hand function in supported sitting positions.

The occupational therapist can use certain body positions to elicit specific hand skills. The supine position is effective for working with infants on initial control of arm movements with visual regard of the hands during movement. Supine positioning can be used to reinforce midline movements of hands and reach against gravity; however, a supine position is not functional for most activities and is most appropriate for infants (less than 12 months). A prone position with weight bearing on the forearms can elicit and reinforce shoulder stability and co-contraction, dissociation of the two sides of the body during weight bearing on one arm while manipulating with the other, bilateral manipulation of objects, and visual regard of the hands. By placing a child prone on a wedge, the effect of gravity is reduced, allowing for more trunk and next extension. Prone positioning can be an advantageous position for the child to visualize his hands but limits the child's viewing of the environment. Use of prone positioning for play activities is always fatiguing and should be used only for brief periods with the occupational therapist or caregiver present to support the child's actions.

Through assessment of the child's alignment, postural control, and arm/hand control, the occupational therapist identifies and recommends positioning and seating that offer sufficient stability and mobility for optimal hand function across a range of home and school activities. For optimal hand use in sitting, the child needs a chair that provides appropriate shoulder, pelvis, leg, and foot support.[24,113] Even young children without motor disabilities benefit from sitting in furniture that fits appropriately. Children demonstrate higher level manipulation skills when seated in chairs and at a table fitted to them than when seated in chairs and at a table that do not fit. Appropriately fitted furniture may enhance hand function by supporting proximal stability, thereby allowing the child to focus more on the manipulative tasks and less on postural readjustments.[129]

To promote optimal alignment and control of hand function for children with disabilities, adapted seating and positioning may be needed. When in a seated position, the child should be able to shift weight in the anterior-posterior and lateral directions; his or her trunk should be aligned over the pelvis or leaning slightly forward; and the pelvis and shoulders should be stable. Spinal alignment with trunk stability and mobility is important to functional movement of the head and arms. Examples of adaptations for sitting, such as lateral supports, pelvic straps, pelvic stabilizers, and chest harnesses, can provide the just-right support for a child to competently perform fine motor activities.[113] In a systematic review of the effect of positioning on upper extremity function, Stavness[121] found that upper extremity function was optimal when the child was in a functional sitting position with slight (0 to 15 degrees) forward orientation, a pelvic strap, footrests, and a cutout tray. Caregivers of children with cerebral palsy report that adapted seating is useful to their families and enables the child's participation in important everyday activities.[107] Rigby and colleagues[107] found that adaptive seating was particularly important to the child's ability to participate in eating, self-care, play, and recreational activities. Case Study 8-1 illustrates use of the biomechanical approach to improve hand function in a child with spastic cerebral palsy (Figure 8-9).

In addition to supportive and functional seating, children with neuromotor disabilities may benefit from a wheelchair tray in supporting the upper extremity during fine motor activities. For optimal support, the tray or table surface should be only slightly above elbow height, because a lower table may cause trunk flexion and a higher surface can cause abduction and internal rotation of the arms. The tray's height can be adjusted to meet specific goals; for example, children with muscle weakness more effectively reach and carry objects when the table or tray surface is at or slightly above elbow height. With this biomechanical advantage, the child's control in manipulating

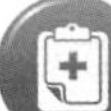

CASE STUDY 8-1 Biomechanical Model for Child with Cerebral Palsy

Zeza with Spastic Quadriparesis

Zeza was 3 years old and had severe spastic quadriparesis. She received occupational therapy each week through an outpatient clinic; she also received occupational therapy in her early childhood program. She was dependent in all of her self-care skills. Her parents fed her most meals, although she independently self-fed finger foods. She also drank from a sippy cup with handles with minimal assistance. She did not sit independently but she sat with minimal assistance when provided full back support. She used a Rifton chair in the early childhood program and is transported in an umbrella stroller. Her occupational therapist discussed with the family the purchase of a manual wheelchair that would offer her more support. Recognizing that a wheelchair, if well-fitting and adapted to her postural needs, could become a more functional sitting device at home and school, the family agree to purchase a wheelchair that would replace the stroller.

The occupational therapist with the family selected a manual wheelchair that offered features to support her posture and enhance hand function. The therapist and family selected a new chair that would facilitate Zeza's achievement of the following Individual Education Program goals:

1. Eat yogurt and other thickened foods using a spoon with enlarged handle and suction bowl with minimal support in grasping the spoon.
2. Successfully activate her iPod or CD player using a button switch on her wheelchair tray.
3. Participate in circle time songs and activities by imitating the teacher's gestures with arms and hands, turning to greet her peers, and vocalizing when appropriate.

The manual chair that the occupational therapist and family selected had the following features:

1. The back extended to the top of her head to support her head in neutral and midline.
2. A neck support helped to align her head in midline but did not prevent full head turning and neck ROM.
3. Shoulder straps that gently maintained neutral, upright trunk.
4. A pelvic strap held her buttocks against the back of the chair and maintained neutral pelvis.
5. Lateral supports helped to maintain her trunk in neutral.
6. Arm rests that supported her arms in neutral forearm and wrist positions; the arm rests also supported a tray.
7. A tray supported her arms and gave her a surface to stabilize her hand in fine motor activities.
8. A foot rest fully supported her feet with hips, knees, and ankles at 90 degrees.

The new wheelchair offered positioning that increased her function in hand function activities, including eating and use of switches. The wheelchair enabled Zeza to achieve the established objectives. In her new chair, she more fully participated in the early childhood program including circle time, story time, art, and snack. Although she did not sit in her new wheelchair all day, it was her optimal seating device for activities that required her highest level hand function. Often a child's well-fitting wheelchair, because it has adapted features that support postural alignment, gives the child a biomechanical advantage and is an optimal seating device for hand function and fine motor activities.

See Figure 8-9 for an example of manual wheelchair.

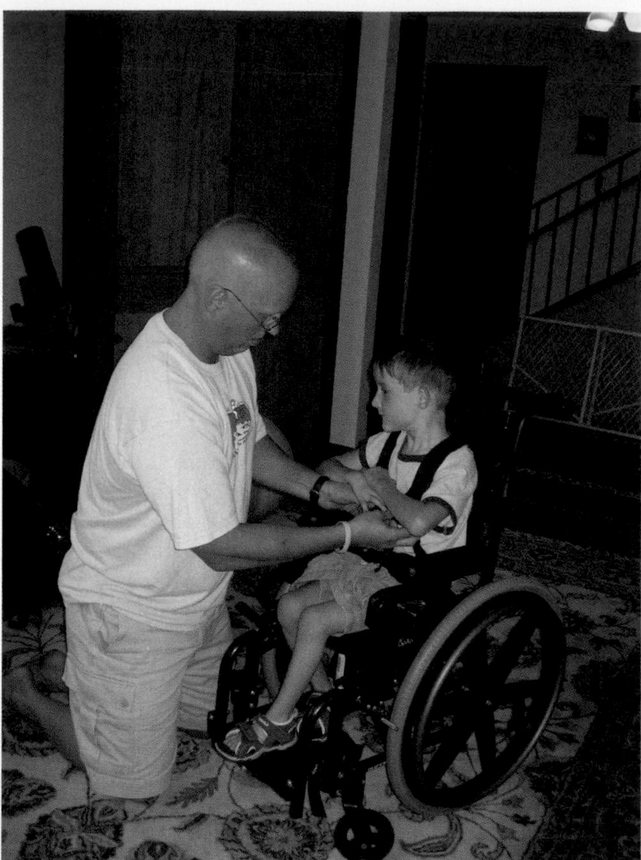

FIGURE 8-9 This manual wheelchair provides optimal supports for a child with spastic quadruparesis to effectively participate in visual-motor and fine motor activities.

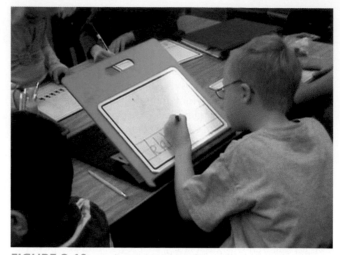

FIGURE 8-10 A slanted surface for writing promotes wrist extension and active grasping patterns.

objects can increase. Another biomechanical advantage that supports hand postures for effective tool use and other hand functions (e.g., for writing or fine motor activities) is use of an elevated or slanted table or tray surface. An elevated surface, such as a slant board positioned at an angle of 20 to 30 degrees, can facilitate a hand position of wrist extension, increasing the child's control of finger flexion for grasping activities[92] (Figure 8-10). Table 8-5 presents characteristics of optimal postural support for fine motor tasks when sitting.

For children with mild to moderate motor involvement, standing may be an appropriate position for practice of fine motor activities. Standing facilitates extension through the trunk and neck and may promote more active postural tone when compared with sitting. Many daily living skills that rely on hand skills, such as brushing the teeth, zipping and buttoning clothing, shaving, applying makeup, and cooking, are most commonly done while standing. For children who have substantial difficulties with standing, the occupational therapist should use this position only after the child has mastered the skills in a sitting position.

Neurodevelopmental Therapy

Neurodevelopmental therapy (NDT) uses biomechanical principles in addition to a range of handling and positioning techniques that promote motor function in children with cerebral palsy. Originally termed neurodevelopment treatment, NDT was proposed by the Bobaths in the 1960s and has been widely used by occupational and physical therapists since that time. The Bobaths were innovative in their understanding of cerebral palsy and the effects of abnormal muscle tone (e.g., spasticity) on postural control and movement. They recognized that spasticity interfered with normal movement patterns and that inhibition of spasticity was important to improving a child's movement patterns. They also believed that through sensory feedback, a child with atypical muscle tone and movement patterns could learn normal movement patterns. The goals of therapeutic handling are to inhibit spasticity, facilitate more normal muscle tone, and guide the child with cerebral palsy in using more normal movement patterns.[66]

Types of Children for Whom Neurodevelopmental Therapy Principles and Techniques Are Appropriate

The NDT practice model was specifically designed for children with cerebral palsy who have abnormal muscle tone. The Bobaths characterized spasticity as tonic reflexes, muscle co-contraction, and stereotypic movement patterns and specified that an important goal of therapy was to reduce spasticity and its associated abnormal movement patterns. NDT theories and postulates have enabled occupational therapists to understand how abnormal muscle tone, primitive reflexes, abnormal movement patterns, loss of strength, and impaired muscle synergies interfere with motor control.[66,125] By analyzing these components of posture and movement in children with cerebral palsy, occupational therapists have conceptualized new methods to improve these elements of the child's motor function.

When a child has cerebral palsy, control of arms in reach and carry; development of precise hand and finger movements; bimanual coordination; and sequential, reciprocal, fluid movement patterns are delayed, limited, or missing. Gordon and Duff[35,57,58] described the characteristics of hand function in children with cerebral palsy, explaining that they have difficulty grading force and sustaining force during grasping, holding, and carrying objects. Children with cerebral palsy also have difficulty releasing objects with control and grading hand movements.[60] The characteristics associated with cerebral palsy and related effects on hand function are described in Table 8-6.

TABLE 8-5 Characteristics of Sitting Supports for Optimal Hand Function in Children with Cerebral Palsy, Spastic Quadriparesis

Characteristic	Rationale	Example
The pelvis is supported on a solid surface.	Solid support promotes trunk symmetry and trunk extension	Chair seat is a firm cushion or wooden surface.
The back support ends at the scapula unless shoulder and head support is needed.	Support through the scapula area can enhance shoulder stability for distal (hand) function.	Most wheelchair backs end at the scapula, although chair backs can extend to include head support.
A pelvic strap holds the pelvis in place. The pelvis is in a neutral position and the hips are at 90 degrees.	With hips at 90 degrees, the pelvis is upright or in a neutral position (without anterior or posterior tilt). A neutral pelvis supports an upright trunk.	The strap holds hips at 90 degrees with a 45 degree angle across the hips.
The chair promotes symmetric weight bearing on thighs.	Symmetric weight bearing results in symmetric posture, facilitating midline movement of arms and hand.	Chair may include hip guides. A firm seat also promotes symmetrical weight bearing.
Knees and ankles are positioned at 90-degree angles.	Solid foot support anchors the lower extremity, giving the trunk, head, and hands a firm base of support. When knees and ankles are at 90 degrees, muscle tone tends to be neutral; tension on the hamstrings is optimal; and a stable, neutral pelvis can be maintained.	Foot supports on wheelchair or other chair that angle at 90 degrees. A well-fitting chair seat that does not extend beyond knee angle.
Lateral trunk supports can provide lateral stability and increase midline alignment of trunk.	Lateral support guides the trunk but do not support or hold the trunk. Lateral supports can promote symmetry and midline.	Lateral supports on wheelchair. Lateral supports on floor sitter or other chair.
A lap tray can improve shoulder and trunk position.	A lap tray can provide a surface to support arms and hands.	Wheelchair tray.
A harness may be needed to promote an upright trunk and to guide child's weight shift when moving arms.	A harness helps the child maintain an upright and symmetric posture. When using a harness, the child should be dynamically stable (stable with mobility to move arms and hands).	When fitting appropriately, most harnesses firmly support the chest and pelvis while allowing the child to shift weight and reach.

TABLE 8-6 Characteristics of Cerebral Palsy and Associated Hand Function Limitations

Characteristic of Cerebral Palsy	Associated Hand Function Limitations
Muscle tone characterized by hyper- or hypotonicity	Limited ROM at wrist, forearm, and fingers. In hypertonicity, the finger flexors may be tight; the child cannot fully extend fingers. In hypotonicity, the joints may be hypermobile and the hand lacks stability. Over time, joints stiffen owing to limited or minimal joint movement.
Excessive co-contraction at joints (with spasticity)	Wrist, forearm, and metacarpals are stiff; wrist and finger joint movements are limited. Hand may tighten when child attempts to move fingers. Excessive thumb adduction.
Muscle synergies are inefficient and stereotypical	Flexor synergies may dominate upper extremity movement. These include shoulder internal rotation with elbow flexion, forearm pronation, and wrist flexion.
Muscle weakness	The hand may not have sufficient force to hold or move heavy objects. The hand may not generate appropriate forces to hold and use writing utensils, scissors, eating utensils.
Limited dissociated movement	Fingers move together in full flexion or extension; child has difficulty moving isolated fingers with control. Reciprocal, precise finger movements are limited. Inability to initiate or sustain thumb opposition. Intrinsic muscle action is limited.
Impaired sensory feedback	Tactile, kinesthetic, and proprioceptive feedback is limited; sensory feedback is not available to guide precise hand and finger movements

From Vogtle, L. K. (2006). Upper extremity intervention in cerebral palsy: A neurodevelopmental approach. In A. Henderson & C. Pehoski (Eds.). *Hand funciton in the child: Foundations for remediation* (2nd ed., pp. 345–368). St. Louis: Mosby/Elsevier.

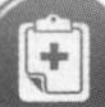

CASE STUDY 8-2 Use of Neurodevelopmental Therapy Techniques to Promote Hand Function in a Young Child with Cerebral Palsy

Susan, 5-Year-Old with Spastic Quadriparesis

Susan was currently in regular kindergarten where she received special education, occupational therapy, and physical therapy. She had a power wheelchair that gives her mobility in the classroom and school. Susan spent 20 to 30 minutes each day in her prone stander and 30 minutes twice a day in her Rifton chair. Most of the day she stayed in her power chair using the tray that supports her fine motor activities.

The occupational therapist and physical therapist often worked together to provide NDT techniques in their clinic space. The occupational therapy goals were:

1. Given minimal physical assist at her shoulder, Susan will use a spoon with enlarged handle and scoop bowl on her wheelchair to feed herself applesauce.
2. Given preparation using upper extremity weight bearing, Susan will demonstrate hand opening sufficient to turn pages of her book.
3. Given preparation using upper extremity weight bearing and trunk rotation, Susan will use her open hand to consistently activate a button switch.

Each session began with Susan lying on the mat, stretching and practicing trunk rotation. This trunk rotation was followed by weight bearing on her hands while kneeling beside a bench. She moved from tall kneeling to trunk rotation in side sitting. She moved into side sitting to the right and left to reinforce the trunk rotation patterns. Frequently the occupational therapists placed her in a prone position over a therapy ball and rolled the ball forward to allow her to place her hands on the floor. This activity helped her develop full shoulder flexion range, equilibrium reactions in prone, and weight bearing on her hands.

After these preparatory activities, often Susan elected to sit in her Rifton chair with a tray. She practiced prehending and manipulating puzzle pieces to complete a puzzle with assistance from the occupational therapist supporting her shoulder, and she practiced using different switches to active her favorite toys. The occupational therapist gave her graded support, that is, the just-right support that she needed to accomplish the isolated (dissociated) arm and hand movements. Although she held her hand in a more open position, she continued to demonstrate difficulty in isolating and controlling finger movements.

After the occupational therapy and physical therapy session, the occupational therapists discussed with the teacher Susan's successes in completing the puzzles and in activating the switches, noting the level of support and the position in her chair that were optimal for achieving these activities. They recommended that she continue to practice in the classroom.

Principles of Neurodevelopmental Therapy Used to Promote Hand Function

Principles of the neurodevelopmental approach have evolved since the Bobaths originated the intervention concepts. At its inception and as practiced through the 1970s and 1980s, NDT involved extensive handling by a trained occupational therapist.[66] More recently, NDT-trained occupational therapists have adopted motor learning principles and dynamic systems theories.[66] Many of the principles have been integrated into other practice models and approaches; for example, Howle[67] defines how the goals and principles of NDT and motor learning are integrated in current practice. Child goals include:

- Postural alignment and postural tone that allows fluid transitional movements through a variety of positions
- Improved foundational postural stability to support optimal hand function
- Efficient weight shift and equilibrium responses in upright positions
- Improved control of isolated and dissociated extremity movements
- Enhanced mobility and dynamic stability within and between body positions

Occupational therapists implement NDT techniques to inhibit spasticity and primitive reflexes and facilitate normal movement patterns. Specifically, the occupational therapist uses sensory input such as deep pressure and upper extremity weight bearing with the spine and body in good alignment. These techniques facilitate postural tone to increase dynamic stability, that is, postural tone that supports movements through different planes (e.g., lateral weight shifts when sitting or rotational movements in a quadruped position). Specialized handling of children with cerebral palsy is believed to allow the development of new patterns of more normal movement and provide the basis for ongoing motor skill development. Case Study 8-2 explains how the NDT approach can be applied to improve a child's development of hand function.

Postural stability is important to hand function, and a child's ability to control isolated movements of fingers, thumb, and hand arches requires a stable base of support that allows these precise and coordinated movements. Stability of all proximal structures—the pelvis, trunk, shoulders, elbow, forearm, and wrist—allows these fine hand movements. Occupational therapists facilitate postural tone through therapeutic handling at key points (most often, the shoulders and pelvis). By handling in a play activity, the occupational therapist guides the child through small weight shifts and movements in different planes that specifically activate or modulate postural tone. When a child learns to control weight shifts and equilibrium responses, he or she may gain improved control of arm movement for reach and bimanual tasks. The occupational therapist primarily facilitates rotational patterns of movement as the basis for normal movement patterns. For example, the occupational therapist can facilitate slow rotary movements in small ranges of motion in shoulder rotation and forearm pronation and supination to inhibit the child's arm tone before implementing a fine motor activity.

Weight bearing on hands during intervention activities is particularly useful for improving postural control and improving stability in the scapulohumeral area (Figure 8-11). The occupational therapist can also use upper extremity weight bearing to encourage the child to maintain elbow co-contraction

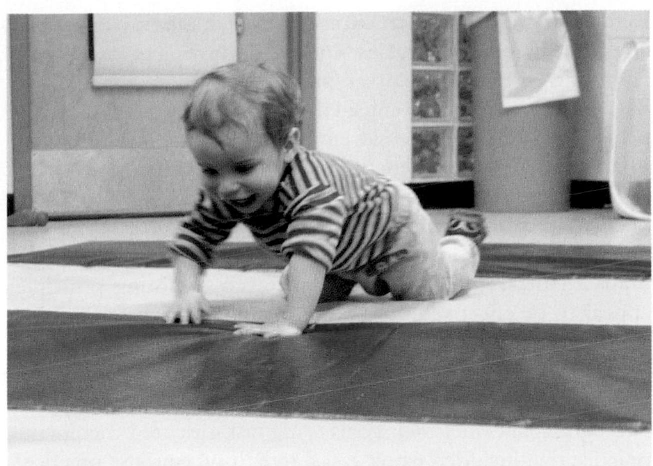

FIGURE 8-11 Weight bearing on hands improves shoulder and arm stability. It also promotes wrist extension and, for certain children, finger extension.

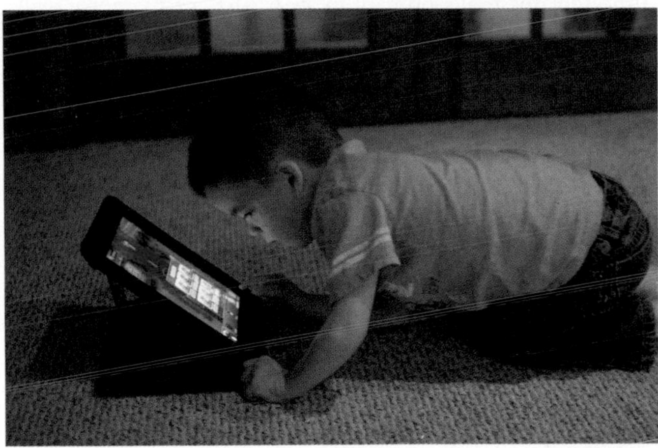

FIGURE 8-12 Weight bearing on forearms or hands can be practiced using functional activities. This child maintains an upper extremity weight-bearing position on his affected arm while engaged in a computer tablet activity.

and wrist extension.[10] Depending on the child's skill level, the occupational therapist can carry out weight-bearing activities with the child in a prone position on forearms, a prone position on extended arms, or a side-sitting position (Figure 8-12).

For the child who has tightness in wrist flexion, a position of upper extremity weight bearing on hands with the arms extended may be difficult, if not impossible, to achieve. The most appropriate positions for children with wrist tightness to use for weight bearing include prone on the forearms and side-lying. If the child's thumb is tightly adducted and flexed, the occupational therapist can apply firm pressure over the first MCP joint and use slow, small, rotary movements to relax the child's hand before this activity.

Important functional outcomes of NDT include improved control of isolated arm, hand, and finger movements required in manipulation and bimanual activities.[125] For example, often children with cerebral palsy lack control of supination and forearm muscles can be spastic. Active supination is easiest to perform in an elbow flexed position, and the child can first practice active supination in activities that position the elbow in greater than 90 degrees of flexion (e.g., eating finger foods, donning dress-up hats, and putting lotion on the face). Supination of 90 degrees or more is needed to accomplish functional activities such as drinking, eating with utensils, or turning a doorknob.

As noted above, manipulation is often optimal when the child is positioned with good postural stability and support, including support of shoulder stability and a working surface that fully supports forearm and hand. The MCP joints (i.e., the palmar arch) can be key points of control to promote isolated fingers movements. The occupational therapist may offer support of palm at the MCP joints as the child practices activities that specifically require isolated movements in a supportive surface.[125] Games that include grasping chips, marbles, small boxes, or pick-up sticks provide practice of isolated finger movement. The occupational therapist may handle the child during these activities by supporting the shoulder, guiding the wrist into extension, supporting the palmar arch, or guiding the forearm into supination.

Research of Neurodevelopmental Therapy Related to Hand Function Interventions

Although understanding of cerebral palsy and diagnoses in which muscle tone and function are impaired has increased because of Bobath's work and that of NDT-trained therapists, the trials of NDT principles and handling techniques have not demonstrated strong efficacy. NDT handling techniques by occupational therapists were examined in two randomized trials by Law and colleagues in the 1990s. Neither study found support for NDT in improving the hand function of children with cerebral palsy more than regular (usual care) intervention. In the second trial the preschool children received more NDT sessions than regular occupational therapy but did not differ in hand function or quality of movement after the interventions.[79] Both groups made significant gains in hand function. Three systematic reviews[11,20,94] synthesized the research evidence for NDT and concluded that NDT does not appear to result in positive benefit and functional improvement in children with cerebral palsy. Of 15 studies, Novak found only three that demonstrated benefit from NDT and concluded that the evidence does not support NDT for improving contractures, muscle tone, or functional outcomes. These studies suggest that the specific handling techniques used in NDT may not result in significant improvement in motor function, and use of NDT techniques in occupational therapy should be carefully monitored and evaluated to determine if the child is benefitting and making expected progress.

Despite lack of evidence, the principles introduced by the Bobaths have deepened therapists' understanding of cerebral palsy and disorders that include muscle tone impairments. As explained by Howle,[67] certain NDT practices translate to other practice models and have validity through clinical practices with children with cerebral palsy. Therapists recognize the importance of enhancing postural stability as the child's base of support for control of hand function. The occupational therapist can provide activities and handling that inhibit stereotypic movement patterns or reduce joint stiffness. The goals that were originally identified within the NDT practice model are often achieved in current practices through positioning and seating, Botox or baclofen treatments, electrical stimulation, practice opportunities, and motor learning techniques.

More recently developed practice models are based on learning and behavioral theories. These models have emerging evidence of effectiveness and translate well into occupation-based interventions. Efficacious practice models, such as motor learning, that use occupation-based theories are described in the following section.

Occupation-Based Approaches

Occupation-based approaches emphasize the interaction of person, environment, and occupation and use holistic methods to support the child's skill development. Using this approach, an occupational therapist selects and creates activities that facilitate the child's functional performance by considering (1) the child's motivation and interests; (2) the context of performance, including activity demands, constraints, and natural supports; and (3) the child's performance strengths and limitations. The interaction of child, environment, and occupation determines how well and at which developmental level the child participates in play, mobility, social relationships, and ADLs. Interventions may focus on any or all of these variables, and in typical practice the focus shifts among them. Occupation-based models are congruent with dynamic systems theories (see Chapters 2 and 7) in understanding the multiple child-related and context-specific variables that influence performance. Key to these approaches is appreciation of meaningful and preferred play occupations, particularly social play, as the context for intervention and the context for much of the child's learning and development. Two practice models that reflect occupation-based approaches to improve children's hand function are (1) motor learning and (2) pediatric-constraint induced movement therapy. Two other occupation-based models are frequently used to promote children's hand function: Cognitive Orientation to daily Occupational Performance (CO-OP) and occupational therapy using sensory integration (OT-SI). CO-OP is described in Chapter 10 and OT-SI is explained in Chapter 9; therefore these practice models and associated strategies are not described in this chapter.

Motor Learning Practice Model

Motor learning is an occupation-based approach that helps the child achieve motor goals using problem solving, practice with reinforcement, whole task activities, and refinement of skill in everyday activities.[18] Using motor learning principles, the occupational therapist assists the child in acquiring motor skills through structured activities, practice of targeted skills, and specific types of feedback. The occupational therapist selects the type of practice and feedback based on the child's level of performance and response to intervention. Using the child's interest to guide activity selection, the child is engaged in meaningful whole tasks that have embedded targeted movement patterns. Through practice of these activities with reinforcement that specifically guides the child's learning, the child masters new skills.

Types of Children Who Benefit from Motor Learning Approaches

Because motor learning approaches are based on general learning theories, many types of children can participate in and benefit from this practice model. Children who have aptitude to follow a model or instructions, engage in repetitive practice, and understand specific, descriptive reinforcement can benefit from motor learning interventions. Although infants may have difficulty staying engaged and repeating action, most preschoolers and older children are easily motivated to engage in activities with high repetition and some challenge.

Application of motor learning approaches and principles has been examined in children with developmental coordination disorder,[90] children with cerebral palsy,[73] and adults with brain injury.[87] Interventions that explicitly access learning principles appear to be effective in promoting hand function for children with developmental coordination disorder.[90] Mastos and colleagues[87] studied the effects of goal-directed therapy using motor learning principles on individuals post brain injury. The two participants met their goals using task-oriented therapeutic practice that included whole tasks, repetition (intense practice), and structured feedback. In a randomized controlled trial, children with cerebral palsy, including those with hemiparesis, diplegia, and quadriplegia, made gains in functional performance following 6 months of physical therapy using a functional program that included motor learning principles.[73] Although this trial's primary focus was on gross motor skills, the children, most of whom had upper extremity impairments, improved in self-care, suggesting improvement in hand function. Using case reports, Eliasson[36] explained how the complexity of hand function in children with cerebral palsy warrants holistic approaches such as occupation-based and motor learning models. These models incorporate the multiple variables that she identified influence hand function, that is, self-efficacy, attention, cognition, motivation, sensorimotor systems, perception, and musculoskeletal/biomechanical structures. The case reports[36,73] and small trials suggest that motor learning models can have positive effects on hand function in children and youth with a variety of diagnoses.

Motor Learning Principles and Techniques

Motor learning theories posit how children develop motor skills in the course of daily activity[132] and include both foundational theories that explain how children learn movement and transformational principles that form the basis for intervention principles and strategies. For our purposes, foundational motor learning theories are (1) schema theory, (2) dynamic systems theory, and (3) stages of learning. These basic concepts about motor development and learning provide a context for designing interventions and are briefly described below. They are further explained in this chapter and in Chapter 2. Schema theory defines how a child learns movement patterns by building new movements on established motor patterns.[116,132] To improve efficiency of learning and to allow automatic movements, humans use similar movement patterns repeatedly, albeit with variation and flexibility, to accomplish everyday tasks. For example, similar movement patterns are used to brush teeth, comb hair, and wash the face. Dynamic systems theory and occupation-based theories recognize how multiple variables in the child, the activity, and the environment influence performance. When interventions use motor learning theories, constraints and resources of environment, activity demands, and child strengths and limitations are considered and purposely manipulated to promote new learning and skill development.

The child's stage of learning (i.e., cognitive, associative, or automatic) also provides a foundation for selecting an appropriate intervention activity and planning how to elicit and support

TABLE 8-7 Principles and Examples of Motor Learning Theory

Principle	Application
Learning a whole motor task is more effective and motivating than learning part of a movement.	Whole motor tasks can provide the child with a meaningful goal, sustain his or her attention, and become the context for repetition.
A meaningful, preferred activity is selected.	When a preferred activity is selected, the child is more likely to remain engaged.[61]
Frequent, repetitive practice is required to learn new motor skills.	Children must practice motor actions repeatedly to reach the automatic stage of learning. Generally, the number of repetitions required is underestimated. For example, children take thousands of steps with supports before they achieve independent ambulation[3] (Adolf, Vereijken, & Shrout, 2003). Practice is equally important for learning hand functions.
Practice should include variability and should be distributed across time	Children retain more when motor practice is varied within the context of the activity. This generally happens naturally when building a structure, playing a game, or performing ADLs.
The occupational therapist provides structured reinforcement that includes specific feedback about performance.	Specific feedback reinforcement learning by increasing the child's understanding of his or her performance. "You reached higher that time!" "You made a perfect letter B."
Feedback or reinforcement is provided frequently and consistently.	Children appear to perform best when they receive consistent reinforcement.[122]
Specific activities are structured to support transfer of learning to a variety of natural environments.	Learning of specific motor skills in a therapy session may not generalize to natural environment and varied contexts. Therapists encourage practice of new skills in a variety of environments with supports as needed. Caregivers and teachers reinforce the child attempting new motor skills in a variety of environments.

practice of the child's highest level skills. Understanding these stages helps the occupational therapist identify the next step in the child's learning and select appropriate challenges and supports for each stage.[18,52] In the cognitive stage of learning the child is highly attentive to the activity, learning how to approach it, often using trial-and-error to develop a strategy for accomplishing the activity goal (e.g., creating a bridge out of Legos). In the associative stage of learning, movements are less variable and the child refines the movements that accomplish the goal. In the automatic stage, the child practices his or her skills with less cognitive effort and less attention required. Performance that is automatic (e.g., putting on a coat, opening a jar) allows people to perform efficiently and attend to meaningful goals. The stages of learning also suggest that learning processes extend over time, requiring repeated practice in varied environments.

The transformation principles used to design motor learning interventions are listed in Table 8-7 with examples. These principles define how to select intervention activities, structure practice and reinforcement, and help the child generalize new motor skills. To apply motor learning principles to occupational therapy intervention, first the occupational therapist selects a meaningful goal-directed activity that is preferred by the child. The activity selected allows practice of movements that are missing, delayed, or difficult for the child and a just-right challenge for his or her emerging hand functions. For example, a therapist may select building a train track with a 4-year-old child who has unilateral cerebral palsy. Fitting together train track pieces requires two hands working together with precision grasp, stable wrists, and forearm supination. Pressing the train track pieces together using weight bearing on hands requires shoulder strength and bimanual coordination (Figure 8-13). The child selected this activity because he loves trains and wanted to build an entire track to show his father. Building the track required 22 repetitions of placing pieces together, naturally requiring repetition. Therefore this activity exemplifies a good choice using motor learning principles. Case Study 8-3 illustrates use of motor learning principles with a child with cerebral palsy.

Repetition and practice are important to establishing and retaining new motor skills and hand functions.[36] Therefore, eating activities and toys and games with many pieces can be particularly useful and enjoyable for developing precision grasping skills (Figures 8-14). Eating is often motivating and if designed to provide the just-right challenge, for example, using a spoon with a new food (such as blueberries) that is challenging to scoop, the child will engage in the challenging activity repeatedly. The occupational therapist reinforces the child's actions and praises how she is holding the spoon and scooping blueberries onto the spoon.

Although children with cerebral palsy can acquire new hand function, including more precise grasp and release, they require more practice than do typically developing children.[57] Research has demonstrated that as children with cerebral palsy learn new skills, each stage of learning (i.e., cognitive, associative, and automatic) takes longer and requires more practice than these learning stages require for typical children.[36,37]

For children with autism spectrum disorder (ASD) or DCD, hand function goals may include managing fasteners to dress independently each morning or legible handwriting for school assignments. Because children with ASD or DCD often struggle with higher level hand function, such as in-hand manipulation and bimanual coordination, one component emphasized in designing intervention activities are tasks that facilitate in-hand manipulation skills. Box 8-3 lists examples of specific activities that can be incorporated in games, ADLs, and play to

 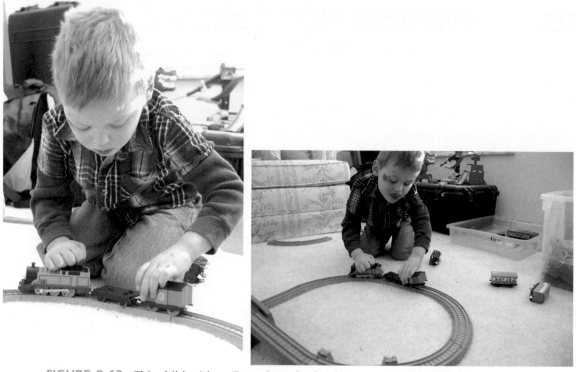

FIGURE 8-13 This child with unilateral cerebral palsy puts together the train cars and places them on the track. This activity inherently has repetition and requires bimanual skill.

CASE STUDY 8-3 Use of Motor Learning Principles to Improve Hand Function

Simon: Use of Motor Learning Principles with Child with Hemiparesis

Simon was 4 years old and had right hemiparesis cerebral palsy following preterm birth and a grade III intraventricular hemorrhage. He was bright and cooperative, although he struggled to use his right hand and typically performed activities using only his left hand. Simon's father was an airplane pilot, and Simon loves airplanes and airports.

Simon's occupational therapist provided services in the home. In this session Simon and the occupational therapist decided to build an air control tower that included a garage for airplanes to trolley through and park for repairs. They used medium-sized Legos that required firm fingertip grasp with stable wrist and arm to fit the pieces together. The occupational therapist assisted Simon intermittently in fitting pieces together and allowed him to sometimes press them together using one hand with the Lego stabilized on the floor surface. The tower required that 40 Legos be pressed together; it required 30 minutes to complete the tower with the occupational therapist providing some assistance with stabilizing the Legos and giving frequent reinforcement and encouragement. As the tower became taller, Simon did not have a supporting surface and was challenged to hold both arms in space. The occupational therapist suggested ways to place the Legos to make the task easier when he observed that Simon was fatiguing and to make the task more challenging when he wanted to push Simon to the next skill level.

The 30-minute activity was fatiguing but Simon remained engaged because the occupational therapist was encouraging and airports were a favorite activity. He knew that when the air control tower was completed, he could play with his airplane, driving through the port at the base and flying by it.

When the air control tower was completed, the occupational therapist discussed with Simon's father how to use Lego activities to encourage bimanual hand skills. The father planned to build another tower with Simon that weekend, to continue his practice and to generalize his skills to play with partners who would offer different levels and types of reinforcement. See Figure 8-11.

promote in-hand manipulation. The occupational therapist can guide and support repeated practice of dressing skills in pretend dress-up play, doll dress-up, or morning dressing. Because dressing most often occurs with caregivers, the occupational therapist recommends to parents how to arrange dressing tasks to promote success and how to motivate the child to practice the tasks (e.g., fastening) that are most difficult.

Handwriting is also a frequent goal for children with ASD or DCD. Denton et al.[34] found that intensive handwriting practice was more effective in promoting handwriting legibility

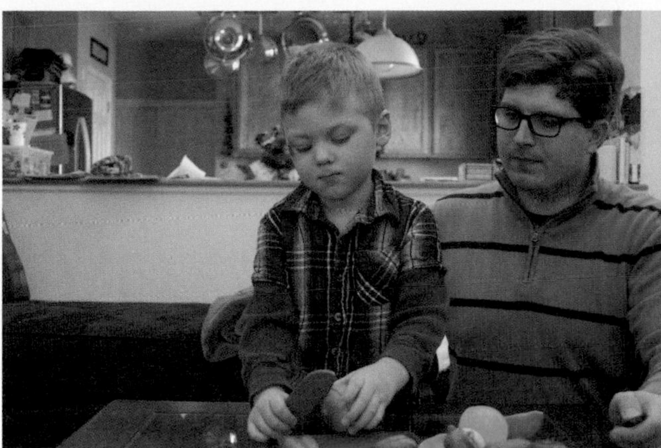
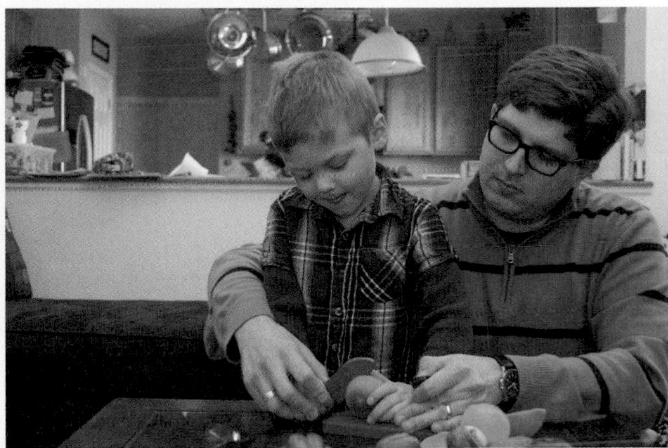
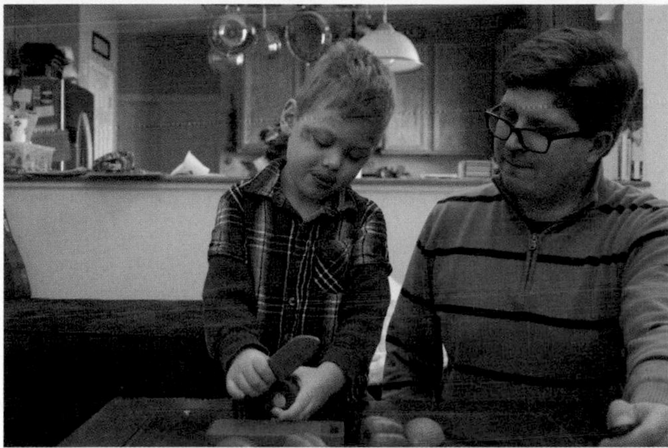

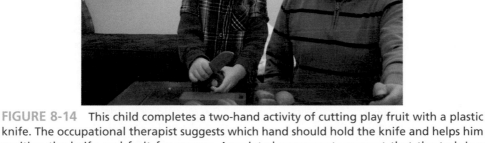

FIGURE 8-14 This child completes a two-hand activity of cutting play fruit with a plastic knife. The occupational therapist suggests which hand should hold the knife and helps him position the knife and fruit for success. Associated movements suggest that the task is a challenge for this boy.

than practice of sensorimotor performance components. Case-Smith et al.[19] also used motor learning principles to enhance handwriting legibility in first grade students. They incorporated handwriting practice into meaningful activities (e.g., small group activities with playful, social elements) and encouraged peer supports. The occupational therapist and teacher team structured handwriting practice, provided immediate reinforcement, solicited peer feedback, and guided transfer of handwriting skills to writing tasks. These learning strategies resulted in significant improvement in handwriting legibility when compared with traditional handwriting instruction.[19]

For children with mild delays in hand function who have limited in-hand manipulation, games and crafts with small objects and dynamic use of tools (e.g., scissors) can be used to practice, reinforce, and gain control of isolated finger movements. The occupational therapist selects manipulative tasks that require practice of dissociated movements, translation of small game pieces in and out of the hand, and rotation of small objects within the hand.[44] Games with marbles, pick-up sticks, or chips require that children practice and repeat in-hand manipulation. Children often experience more success when their hand is stabilized on a surface. As skills progress they should be encouraged to manipulate objects without the forearm and wrist supported. Table 8-8 lists games and activities that can be practiced to develop dynamic grasping patterns and in-hand manipulation skills for children with developmental coordination disorder or mild delays in hand function.

Motor Learning Research

Motor learning interventions have been researched in adults[86]; however, few studies of motor learning interventions for children have been published. In a descriptive study, Eliasson[36] explains how to design interventions that incorporate motor learning principles, using examples of tasks for children with cerebral palsy. Using case reports, she explains how to structure meaningful, child-selected tasks, elicit distributed practice, and provide reinforcement. Each case demonstrated qualitative improvement in hand function.

Several group comparative studies of motor learning principles have been completed. In a study of "neuromotor task training" in which motor learning principles were applied to children with DCD, therapists were trained to teach children whole motor tasks by giving explicit instruction, sharing specific information about the child's performance, and providing feedback when the task was completed.[93] The children who received this intervention improved more in motor coordination and gross motor function than children who received no intervention. In a second study of children with DCD who received a task-oriented treatment program using motor learning principles, the intervention group improved more in

BOX 8-3 In-Hand Manipulation Activities That Can Be Embedded When Using Motor Learning Principles

Preparation Activities

1. Activities involving general tactile awareness (easily repeated, generally not a skill challenge)
   - Using Crazy Foam
   - Using shaving cream
   - Applying hand lotion
   - Finger painting
2. Activities involving proprioceptive input (increases cocontraction, strength, endurance; easily repeated)
   - Weight bearing (e.g., wheelbarrow, activities on a small ball)
   - Pushing heavy objects (e.g., boxes, chairs, benches)
   - Pulling (e.g., tug-of-war)
   - Pressing different parts of the hand into clay
   - Pushing fingers into clay or therapy putty
   - Pushing shapes out of perforated cardboard
   - Tearing open packages or boxes
3. Activities involving regulation of pressure
   - Rolling clay into a ball
   - Squeezing water out of a sponge or washcloth
   - Pushing snaps together
4. Activities involving tactile discrimination
   - Playing finger games and singing songs
   - Playing finger identification games
   - Discriminating among objects or textures by manipulating with vision occluded

Specific In-Hand Manipulation Activities

1. Translation (fingers to palm)
   - Prehending coins from a container
   - Hiding pennies in the hand (magic trick)
   - Crumpling paper
   - Picking up small pieces of food
   - Taking chips attached to a magnetic wand
   - Picking up pegs or paper clips for use in a game or craft
   - Picking up several utensils one at a time
2. Translation (palm to fingers)
   - Moving pennies from the palm to the fingers
   - Moving game pieces to place onto a game board
   - Moving small food items into the mouth
   - Holding several chips to put on a wand
   - Handling money to put it into a coin bank
3. Shift
   - Turning pages in a book
   - Picking up sheets of paper, tissue paper, or dollar bills
   - Separating playing cards
   - Stringing beads (shifting string and bead as string goes through the bead)
   - Shifting a crayon, pencil, or pen for coloring or writing
   - Shifting paper in the nonpreferred hand while cutting
   - Playing with Tinker Toys (long, thin pieces) or pick-up sticks
   - Adjusting a spoon, fork, or knife for appropriate use
   - Holding a pen and pushing the cap off with the same hand
   - Holding chips while flipping one out of the fingers
   - Holding fabric in the hand while attempting to button or snap
4. Simple or complex rotation (depending on object orientation)
   - Removing or putting on a small jar lid
   - Putting on or removing bolts from nuts
   - Rotating a crayon or pencil
   - Removing crayons from the box and preparing for coloring
   - Rotating a pen or marker to put the top on it
   - Rotating toy people to put them in chairs, a bus, or a boat
   - Rotating a puzzle piece for placement in the puzzle
   - Feeling objects or shapes to identify them
   - Handling construction toy pieces
   - Turning cubes that have pictures on all six sides
   - Constructing twisted shapes with pipe cleaners
   - Handling parts of a small-shape container while rotating the shape to put it into the container
   - Holding a key ring with keys, rotating the correct one for placement in a lock

TABLE 8-8 Examples of Activities That Promote Hand Function in Children 3 to 8 Years Old

Activity	Child Goal	Specific Hand Functions Targeted
Basket weaving Repetition of pulling yarns through basket frame	Make a basket for mother; share yarn colors with friends	In-hand manipulation simple rotation as child moves basket while pulling through yarn
Sponge painting	Create colorful painting using small sponges, making favorite animals	Precision grasp of sponge, carry of sponge; translation when prehending sponge
Nuts and bolts	Make box with nuts and bolts around top; make design with nuts and bolts	Rotation and translation
Eye dropper painting	Make multicolor painting for parents or for holiday	Precision grasp, precision release
Cleaning the white board with water spray	Helping the teacher with classroom cleanup	Isolated finger strength and coordination to operate spray bottle
Perfection game	Play with peers; social elements promote motivation and effort	Translation to move piece in and out of hand; precision placement; precision release, repetition
Tissue paper mural	Create a mural for classroom with peers, tearing small pieces of tissue paper and pasting to a large piece of paper	Precision grasp; hand strength, bimanual hand skills

handwriting, dexterity, and ball skills performance when compared with a control group.[118]

In a study of typical children, Sullivan, Kantak, and Burtner[122] provided different frequencies of feedback as children learned a task involving arm movements. Compared with adults who perform optimally with intermittent feedback, the children performed optimally with continuous feedback and required longer periods of practice. This emerging but promising research evidence supports the use of motor learning principles to improve hand function in children with a variety of diagnoses.[132]

Pediatric Constraint-Induced Movement Therapy

Pediatric constraint-induced movement therapy (P-CIMT) is a well-researched, widely used intervention for children with hemiparesis cerebral palsy (i.e., unilateral cerebral palsy). P-CIMT evolved from constraint-induced movement therapy for adults post stroke, which was originally developed and researched in the 1980s.[95,130] Research applying CIMT to young children with cerebral palsy emerged after 2000 with studies in New York, Alabama, and Sweden.[22,29,42] Currently many variations of P-CIMT have been studied, and virtually all studies have produced positive effects on hand function in children with unilateral cerebral palsy. The core elements of P-CIMT are (1) constraint of the child's less impaired upper extremity, (2) selection of activities and techniques to elicit specific movements of the more impaired arm and hand, (3) high intensity intervention with repetition of targeted movements, (4) sessions in the child's natural environment (note: sessions are sometimes held in clinics, hospitals, or schools), (5) systematic reinforcement that directs the child to attempt higher level skills or demonstrate increased strength and endurance, and (6) transfer of the intervention program to caregivers and the child's daily routines. Although constraint is an essential part of P-CIMT, virtually all programs include sessions without constraint (most often in the final weeks or days of the intervention) that emphasize integration of bimanual skills. The variations of these essential components are explained in the following sections.

Types of Children Who Benefit from P-CIMT

P-CIMT was originally developed for children with hemiparetic cerebral palsy and hemiparesis caused by acquired brain injury.[72] Research findings suggest that P-CIMT is successful with children across age groups (15 months to 20 years).[66,103] Eliasson et al. found that older children improved more with P-CIMT than younger, but this finding has been inconsistent across studies, with most showing no difference in improvement based on age. Recent studies have shown benefits for infants with unilateral cerebral palsy.[83] Although practitioners recognize that neuroplasticity is greatest in infancy, certain scholars are concerned about use of constraint at early stages of bimanual development; therefore, careful monitoring for potential negative effects is warranted when applying P-CIMT to infants less than 12 months.

One rationale for using P-CIMT with infants is the potential to prevent the phenomenon of "developmental disregard." Developmental disregard refers to a pattern observed in children with congenital hemiparesis in which they neglect their affected arm and hand.[31,103] This pattern seems to evolve from repeated experiences when the child attempts to use the hemiparetic hand and fails to achieve his or her goal. Therefore, early on in development the child learns adapted techniques for accomplishing his goals by using only the skillful or unaffected arm and hand. Intervention such as P-CIMT that can promote and help integrate bimanual skills during infancy may prevent this pattern of disregard.

P-CIMT has been used with children with a wide range of impairment (i.e., severe to moderate) with equivalent benefit across level of involvement. Citing one exception, DeLuca et al.[30] found that children with dystonia did not improve with P-CIMT and suggested that children with dystonia may not benefit from P-CIMT. Because a child with dystonia has very poor control of extremity movement with fluctuating tone, gains with intervention may be limited, and such a child may benefit most from adapted techniques and assistive technology.

In recent examples, occupational therapists have implemented P-CIMT with children recovering from brachial plexus injuries. In two case reports, P-CIMT was applied to children with Erb-Duchenne palsy (brachial plexus injury with impairment to spinal nerves C5 and C6 resulting in paralysis of shoulder muscles, elbow flexors, and forearm supinators).[115,124] In Santamato et al.[115] the children (age 6 and 7 years) had contractures and were treated with botulinum toxin injections before the P-CIMT program. Both studies reported significant improvement in arm movement and hand function with P-CIMT, suggesting potential benefit for children with brachial plexus injuries.[106]

P-CIMT Principles and Strategies

As noted, a feature of P-CIMT is use of constraint of the child's less affected or unaffected upper extremity. Researchers and practitioners have used different types of constraints, including mitts,[22] splints inserted into gloves, slings,[1] and full arm casts.[19] Although the effects of constraints cannot be compared across studies, the principles supporting type of constraint are distinctly different. When splints and mitts are used, the child wears these forms of constraint only during the intervention sessions. In P-CIMT using full-arm casts, the child wears the cast continually (i.e., full time), "forcing" him or her to primarily use the affected arm and hand throughout the day and beyond the intervention session (Figure 8-15).

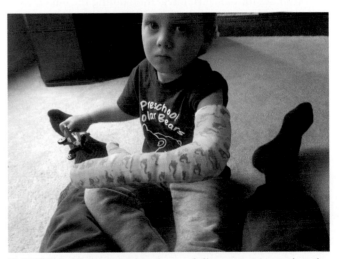

FIGURE 8-15 In P-CIMT often a full arm cast is used as the constraint. The child wears a typical CIMT full-arm cast.

TABLE 8-9 Pediatric Constraint-Induced Movement Therapy (P-CIMT) Principles and Strategies

Principle	Explanation and Examples
Intervention takes place in the child's natural environment.	The child's home is a comfortable environment for intensive practice of skills, allows selection of meaningful and preferred activities, and allows easy engagement of the caregiver in the intervention sessions.
The child's less-affected arm and hand are constrained.	Constraints include mitts, splints, slings, gloves, or casts. A full-arm cast limits sensorimotor input to the less affected arm, potentially inhibiting brain activity in the nonimpaired hemisphere.
The occupational therapist guides intensive practice or targeted movements in whole tasks.	The occupational therapist encourages the child to repeat specific, targeted movement patterns in meaningful (fun) play activities and family-selected self-care activities.
The occupational therapist encourages the child to master emerging skills or the just-right challenge.	Using a process termed "shaping," the occupational therapist encourages the child to attempt challenging skills, reinforces the child's efforts, reinforces repetition, monitors performance, and guides activity to refine movement patterns.
The occupational therapist uses reinforcement that is specific and positive and supports the child's learning about performance.	The occupational therapist uses immediate reinforcement (i.e., praise) that encourages sustained performance, guides higher level performance, and results in skills refinement.
The occupational therapist collaborates with the parents in establishing goals, assessing and monitoring the child's progress.	The occupational therapist establishes goals with the caregiver at the initiation of the P-CIMT program. The goals are assessed and monitored routinely (e.g., each week). Formal communication methods are established to communicate the child's performance during therapy sessions and at home after therapy sessions.
The occupational therapist transfers the intervention program to the caregiver.	At the conclusion of the P-CIMT session, the occupational therapist develops a home program that extends the original goals and suggests activities that encourage the child's practice of bimanual skills and the next developmental steps.

Emerging evidence suggests that by inhibiting sensorimotor functions of the less affected arm and hand for an extended period (e.g., 3 weeks), the brain may reorganize. A neuroimaging study found that inhibiting the unaffected hemisphere was associated with activation in the impaired hemisphere.[123] The slowing of neural input to the unimpaired hemisphere may allow the development of new pathways within the impaired hemisphere.[18] Although emerging evidence from imaging studies suggests benefit[123] and the full-time full arm cast results in more practice with the affected arm and hand, it may reduce opportunities for bimanual integration during the intervention period. Some researchers believe that intensive, highly structured bimanual interventions in which the child is not constrained better align with the goal of increasing bimanual function. Intensive bimanual interventions,[61] when provided with high structure, appear to be as effective as P-CIMT.[62]

Most often P-CIMT is provided in an intensive (3-6 hour) daily program of 2 to 4 weeks.[103] Short-term, intensive occupational therapy services allow the child and family to focus on specific functional goals, engage in daily goal-directed practice, and assess intervention outcomes. Pediatric hospitals and clinics across the United States are implementing short-term intensive occupational and physical therapy services as a service delivery model that may be more effective, more accountable, and more family-friendly than continuous (year round) weekly therapy services. Short-term, intensive P-CIMT has resulted in significantly improved hand function and bimanual hand use with sustained outcomes at follow-up.[19]

The occupational therapist incorporates both motor learning and shaping techniques in the P-CIMT sessions. These principles that guide intervention with example strategies are presented in Table 8-9. After analysis of the missing or impaired components of arm and hand movements, the occupational therapist designs play and social activities that elicit and provide a context for practice of specific hand functions. With sessions of 2 to 3 hours, the occupational therapist can select meaningful activities that may require many steps to complete (e.g., making muffins, building a castle of Legos, a morning dressing and bathing routine). The child repeats targeted movements within the play or self-care activity that are reinforced by the occupational therapist's praise, descriptive feedback, and encouragement. The occupational therapist prompts and cues the child to attempt movements that are higher level (e.g., to reach higher, supinate more, grasp multiple pieces). Using continual activity analysis, the occupational therapist judges when the child needs supports or encouragement and when the child can be further challenged. The intervention sessions provide continuous cycles of (1) selecting an activity that presents a motor challenge (elicits the targeted movement), (2) observing the child's performance, (3) reinforcing the child's performance, (4) encouraging the child to repeat the action, and (5) monitoring how the child refines the movement pattern.[30] For example, during the bimanual intervention phase the occupational therapist designs a folding, cutting, and pasting activity that includes easy shapes and more difficult shapes to cut with scissors. The occupational therapist initially helps the child stabilize the paper, then encourages the child to stabilize it. The child is positioned at a table for the activity; however, the occupational therapist encourages the child to cut without using the table as a support, facilitates movement of

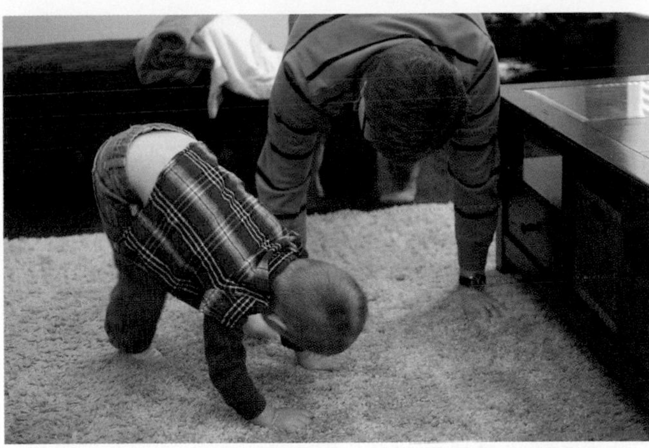

FIGURE 8-16 Bear crawling on carpet allows more weight bearing on hands than does the quadruped position. The occupational therapist demonstrates and joins in the race.

the affected arm into different planes, and encourages active supination. The occupational therapist increases or fades out supports depending on the complexity and challenges inherent in each cutting and folding task.

For young children, scooping and eating with a spoon can be challenging and is naturally repetitive. Eating can be a motivating activity with multiple steps that the occupational therapist can grade to challenge the child's current skill level. Crawling through the living room over carpet and pillows elicits wrist extension, open hand (finger extension), and shoulder external rotation (Figure 8-16). Sustained crawling requires upper extremity stability and strength. The carpet texture may be beneficial to children whose hands are hypersensitive to touch. Crawling games can include siblings, can be extended by playing hide and seek, can provide a break from intensive practice of grasp in fine motor activities, and are appropriate across age groups.

Although P-CIMT is provided in clinics and outpatient hospital settings, Ramey et al.[103] recommend that therapists provide the sessions in the child's home and other natural environments. Services in the home with parents present during some or most of the sessions promote easier transfer of learning. Using the child's own toys and objects ensures that he or she can continue to practice new skills after the intervention session. The occupational therapist can model techniques that elicit the child's highest level skills (Figure 8-17). Parent education is an essential element of P-CIMT. Parent education is most likely to result in behavioral change when (1) the occupational therapist first develops a positive relationship with the family; (2) the parents' learning styles and motivation are considered; (3) the family's routine and time demands are considered; and (4) the occupational therapist is responsive and sensitive to the family's needs and priorities. When services are provided in the home, the occupational therapist can model for the parent, interact on a regular basis, discuss the child's progress, and provide education about the intervention according the pace that is most comfortable for the parent. Case Study 8-4 describes P-CIMT for a child with unilateral cerebral palsy.

P-CIMT Research

Since 2000, more than 50 studies of P-CIMT have been published. Research has been completed in more than 10 countries, suggesting that this intervention has been broadly adopted. Although almost all studies have shown that P-CIMT has positive effects on hand function for children with unilateral cerebral palsy, the studies have been criticized for lack of follow-up measures and differences in intensity between the intervention and control groups that may account for differences in

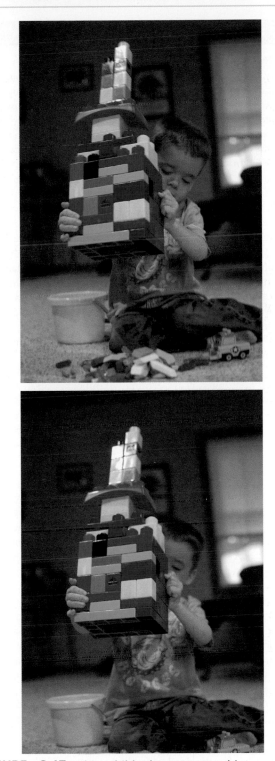

FIGURE 8-17 This child demonstrates his emerging strength and highest level skill using two hands to lift his Lego construction.

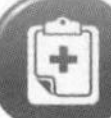

CASE STUDY 8-4 P-CIMT for a Child with Unilateral Hemiparesis

P-CIMT Camp

Many hospitals and clinics offer P-CIMT during the summer using a camp model with groups of children with hemiparesis cerebral palsy participating. Examples of camps are those with specific themes, such as a rock 'n' roll P-CIMT camp or one that is held outdoors and includes many adapted outdoor activities (e.g., scavenger hunts, boating, animal exploration, obstacle courses).

Camps offer many positive social elements, making it easy to create fun activities while promoting shaping and repetitive practice. Once an age range is selected, the types of activities can be selected. Most camps offer all-day activities that include eating, social activities, fun yet challenging activities, and housekeeping activities. For example, using a rock 'n' roll theme with children 8 to 12 years, the camp provides dancing, singing, playing musical instruments, making collages of rock 'n' roll images, and performing for families. These fun activities are scheduled before and after preparing and eating lunch with cleanup.

A preschool camp may include a Disney theme with pretend play activities focused on Disney characters, singing and dancing, Disney arts and crafts, and gross motor play.

Aarts, Jongerius, Geerdink, Limbeek, and Geurts[1] described a group intervention for children with unilateral cerebral palsy (ages 2.5-8 years) that included 6 weeks of constraint and 2 weeks of bimanual task-specific training. The theme of their intervention program was "Pirates," and it took place in the Netherlands. The children attended the camp for 3-hour sessions, 3 days per week, and daily activities included the following:

- As a group they dressed in pirate costumes that included a sling for their less affected arm (during the constraint weeks).
- They practiced targeted movement with a plastic sword while singing pirate songs.
- Each then had an individualized session to target specific tasks.
- As a group they participated in eating and drinking, reinforcing use of their more affected arm and hand.
- In small groups they participated in board games, card games, puzzles, and arts and crafts according to their developmental level and targeted goals.
- At the conclusion they changed into their own clothes to prepare to go home.

The pirate group intervention resulted in significant positive effects on individualized goals as measured by Goal Attainment Scaling and standardized measures (the Assisting Hand Assessment and the ABILHAND-Kids).

Aarts et al. concluded that "the Pirate group provided a meaningful and challenging environment for the children, who enjoyed the playlike treatment and the provocative activities with peers."

outcomes. As noted earlier, researchers have used widely varied forms of constraint (mitt, sling, splint, cast) and different intensities (2-6 hours/day over 2 to 4 weeks). Because studies have used different measures and study samples have different characteristics, comparison of these important variables across studies is not possible.[100]

Four systematic reviews that included P-CIMT have been published since 2007.[18,66-68,114] Each review included three randomized controlled trials and concluded that although most studies reported positive evidence, the trials remained small and differences in procedures prevented comparability across studies. Among the recent studies, Aarts et al.[1] examined the effects of a group intervention that combined constraint and bimanual interventions with usual care. The children in the CIMT/bimanual groups demonstrated improved function in the affected hand (including improved effectiveness as an assisting hand and increased bimanual performance during self-care and leisure activities) but did not improve in strength and automaticity.[2] In a randomized controlled trial reported by DeLuca et al.[30] and Case-Smith et al.,[19] the effects of 3 hours per day P-CIMT was compared with 6 hours per day P-CIMT for a sample of preschool children. This team used continuous full-arm casting, home-based services, and shaping/motor learning principles in the intervention sessions. The children who received P-CIMT 3 hours per day, when compared with those who received 6 hours per day, made comparable improvements in affected hand function and bimanual hand skills at 1 and 6 months post intervention. Effect sizes on hand function measures for both groups were large. This small study concluded that a program of 3 hours per day may yield as many benefits to a child's hand function as a program of 6 hours per day.

A recent large randomized trial completed in Italy[45] compared three groups of children with hemiplegic cerebral palsy (N = 105): P-CIMT, bimanual training, and standard treatment. The children in the P-CIMT group wore a glove with a splint 3 hours per day for 10 weeks. The P-CIMT and bimanual interventions were provided in a clinic, 3 days per week for 3 hours a day over 10 weeks, and the parents were instructed to provide 3 hours per day on the other 4 days. Standard treatment occurred once or twice a week. The two intensive interventions resulted in significant effects on isolated arm and hand movements, grasp, and bilateral manipulation. ADLs improved for the younger (2- to 6-year-old) but not older (7- to 8-year-old) children. With positive results for most P-CIMT studies, occupational therapists should prioritize translation of this intervention to clinic and program. Although major pediatric hospitals and some clinics provide CIMT using intensive schedules, modified intervention models that obtain similar results are needed. Further study of P-CIMT models, including those that vary by types of constraint, dosage, individual or group, and types of children who benefit, is needed.

A barrier to broad use of CIMT is the intensive therapy schedule that translates into commitment of therapist resources and family time. Clinics have begun to provide group P-CIMT to maximize therapist resources.[38] Home-based models are family-friendly models; however, they are most costly for therapy resources. With positive outcomes, expansion of P-CIMT is anticipated.

Adaptation Models

In many cases, children with neuromotor or musculoskeletal disorders experience hand function impairments that remain limiting despite interventions focused on remediation. Children with congenital orthopedic disorders (e.g., arthrogryposis), trauma resulting in permanent hand impairments (e.g., spinal cord injury or amputation), or severe neuromotor disorders (e.g., spastic quadriparesis cerebral palsy), may benefit from adapted techniques or assistive technology to increase their participation in hand function activities. Adaptation models reflect ecologic practice models in which contextual features of the environment and activity are modified to increase the child's participation in play, school functions, social interaction, and ADLs. When a child has impaired hand function of anticipated long duration, occupational therapists recommend, select, and implement adapted techniques, adapted equipment, and assistive technology to improve the child's participation in everyday activities.

To select appropriate adapted equipment or assistive technology, the occupational therapist analyzes the child's performance and the activity demands and, using this information, identifies potential devices or technology that can compensate for the gap between the child's performance and activity demands. Application of assistive technology to support a child's hand function and participation also includes the occupational therapist's involvement in purchasing, fitting, problem solving or troubleshooting, adjusting, and training to successfully use equipment or technology. Following analysis of performance and desired activities, the occupational therapist identifies available technology and assesses its potential usefulness, fit to the environment, cost, durability, and usability for a particular child's hand function limitations and routine activity demands. Once the family (or school), based on the occupational therapist's recommendations, decides to purchase a specialized device, the occupational therapist adjusts or fits the device; explains how it is used; models and instructs the child in how to use it; trains the family, teachers or other caregivers; and assesses its functionality. These roles in selecting, training, and assessment may be minimal or extensive depending on whether the technology is simple or complex (see Chapter 20). This section describes the adaptation practice model, including use of adapted equipment and assistive technology, to support and improve hand function.

Types of Children Who Benefit from Activity Adaptation

For children with significant loss of hand function, therapists and families select adapted techniques and assistive technology to increase their participation in play, self-care, and school activities. Although technology is used to support hand function for children with a broad range of disabilities, to illustrate how technologies can support play, self-care, and school occupations, this section focuses on three types of children. Children and youth with (1) orthopedic conditions that restrict upper extremity function, (2) neuromuscular disorders with significant weakness or loss of movement, and (3) cerebral palsy with severe spasticity and limited ROM often benefit from adapted techniques and assistive technology.

Children born with congenital orthopedic disorders, such as arthrogryposis, may have significant limitations in hand function beginning at birth with limited increase in function over the course of development. Arthrogryposis multiplex congenital is characterized by abnormal fibrosis of muscle tissue, causing contracture of upper and lower extremity joints.[63] Often the child's elbow is locked in extension with forearm pronated, creating difficulty in eating and activities that require bringing hands to face. Because children with arthrogryposis experience limited ROM from birth, they often learn adapted methods for accomplishing their goals and tend to be good problem solvers.

Congenital limb deficiencies can also affect hand function. Conditions such as polydactyly (more than 5 fingers [including an extra finger with bone but no joints]), syndactyly (webbed or fused fingers) or amelia (missing fingers or limbs) can result in participation limitations for activities involving hand and finger function. Children with congenital anomalies such as polydactyly or syndactyly generally undergo reconstructive surgeries to increase hand function (see Chapter 29). Depending on the extent of involvement and success of the surgery, these children may benefit from adapted techniques and equipment. Often children who are missing hands or parts of the hand learn to perform ADLs and school activities with other body parts, rather than learn to use prostheses. When a child determines that use of other body parts is more efficient than use of a prosthesis, these adapted methods need to be respected.

When a child or youth experiences a spinal cord injury that results in quadriparesis, hand function can be permanently impaired. When high-level injuries resulting in minimal arm and hand movement (e.g., at cervical vertebrae C3 or C4) occur, children benefit from assistive technologies such a joy sticks, switches, or mobile arm supports. When the spinal cord injury is lower and the child retains wrist movement and partial hand function (e.g., at C6 or C7), adapted equipment, such as universal cuffs, built up handles, or handles on cups, allows independence in specific ADLs. Children and youth with spinal cord injury with quadriplegia can benefit from both low technology, such as adapted spoons and writing utensils, and high technology, such as computer tablets, adapted computers, and electronic aids for daily living.

Children with quadriparesis spastic cerebral palsy whose movement is restricted or poorly controlled may benefit from use of assistive technologies such as switches and electronic devices. When severe muscle tone and muscle weakness limit range of reach and motor control is minimal, adapted equipment and technology become important to the child's participation in play and ADLs. Children with severe athetoid cerebral palsy and minimal control of extremity movements, particularly in midranges, often need switches or adapted interfaces to access computers, tablets, and other devices.[84] Examples of assistive technology for children with severe cerebral palsy and limited hand function are described in the following sections.

Assistive Technology to Enhance Children's Participation in Play Activities

Children with severely limited upper extremity ROM or hand function can increase their participation in play activities with application of assistive technology.[77] Lane and Mistrett[77] recommend the family access lending libraries to explore different options in adapted toys and play activities. Toy adaptations

TABLE 8-10 Switches and Computer Devices for Children with Limited Hand Function

Switch or Device	Examples of Use	Functionality Required to Operate
Button switch	Operates a battery powered toy; can interface with a computer; can be used with online scanning	The child presses down with hand or arm. Releases by lifting hand and arm Can operate with fist or open hand
Grasp switch	Turns devices on and off, can interface with computer and operate online scanning; operates a battery-powered toy	The child squeezes the switch using palmar grasp. Must be able to release the grip to prevent switch latching
Ribbon or leaf switch	Turns devices on and off; operates a battery-powered toy	The child activates by swiping against the switch and bending it. A child who reaches and swipes with fair accuracy can operate this switch.
Plate switch	Turns on and off other devices; operates a battery-powered toys	The child activates with very light touch. A child with poor strength and minimal hand movement can activate this switch.
Joystick	Turns devices on and off; can be used as the computer's mouse; because it has directionality can be used to operate a power wheelchair	The child can operate without full grasp if positioned in thumb web space. Usually the full arm is used to push the joystick forward and backward. Backward pull requires grasp, but child with minimal strength can operate a joystick. Child must have directionality sense. Sensitivity of joystick can be adjusted for a child with poor control of arm movements.
Head proximity switches, mouth-activated switches (e.g., pneumatic)	Turns devices on and off; can include activate computer	For a child with no hand movement or extremely poor control of arm and hand movement, the head or mouth can be used to activate a switch.
Adapted mouse: joystick	Provides mouse functions	For a child with poor control of arm movement or limited grasp. Child controls the mouse movement by moving joystick in different directions. Joystick can be calibrated to become more or less responsive to child's movements.
Adapted mouse: trackball	Provides mouse functions	For a child with limited hand strength and movement, or a child with limited arm control. Computer's cursor moves with minimal movement of hand on trackball.
BigKeys keyboard	Provides large, easily visible keys to access the computer's keyboard	For a child with limited fine motor control who needs a bigger key target. Child with poor hand coordination or ataxia is more accurate with BigKeys.
Membrane keyboard	Provides alternative keyboard for computer access and word processing	For a child with poor strength and limited arm and hand movement

See Ablenet at http://www.ablenetinc.com.

include easy-to-grasp handle extensions or handles on puzzle pieces, methods to stabilize the toy by placing on a nonslip material or materials, and attaching toys to the hand using Velcro or a strap. Campbell et al.[14] summarized 12 studies that examined young children's use of switches to activate toys or a computer. These studies demonstrated that young children with a variety of disabilities can learn to use a switch and that switch-activated toys are motivating and reinforcing. Children with minimal arm and hand function can activate switches using an arm swipe, full hand grasp, or pressing motion with hand open. Once a reliable and controlled arm or hand movement is identified, an appropriate switch is selected and placed optimally for the child to activate. When a child can consistently activate a switch, it can be used to operate different battery-operated toys and computer play activities. For children with limited reach and minimal manipulation, switch-activated toys can offer an engaging and meaningful play activity that reinforces the child's motivation and self-initiation. Table 8-10 lists different types of switches and the arm and hand function required to activate them.

Adapted Equipment for Activities of Daily Living

For children with limited reach, grasp, and manipulation, use of adapted equipment and simple devices can significantly increase their independence in ADLs. When selecting adapted equipment to improve the child's participation in ADLs, the occupational therapist selects and recommends devices that the child can (1) easily use to achieve the ADL goal with minimal caregiver supports, (2) independently don and doff, (3) learn to use without extensive training, and (4) use in different circumstances and environments. The device or adapted materials need to easily fit into the family daily life and should be durable and reliable. Examples of adapted equipment that can support a child eating independently include Dycem underneath the plate to stabilize it, a scoop bowl that allows easy scooping with a spoon, a spoon or fork with built-up handle, bent spoon or fork, a cup with handles and lid, or a long straw to a stabilized cup.

Adapted equipment helpful for dressing includes reachers, hooks to pull up pants, button hooks, and long-handled shoe horns. Choice of clothing can also make dressing tasks easier. Although family and child preference in clothing must always be considered, therapists often recommend pants with elastic waistbands, looser fitting clothing, shirts with large open necklines, large zipper pulls, Velcro closures, and stretchy materials. Adapted equipment for hygiene includes bath mitts, liquid soap instead of a soap bar, easy grip handles for the toothbrush, and easy-to-dispense toothpaste.

Assistive Technology for School Functions

School-based occupational therapists frequently consider and, when appropriate, recommend technology and device solutions for children with limited hand function. The Individuals with Disabilities Education Act requires that schools provide assistive technology devices and services to students who can benefit from these services, and in the past 20 years assistive technologies have become an important resource for students with disabilities. Fifty percent of students who use assistive technology receive occupational therapy services to support that use,[102] and occupational therapists are frequently part of a school's interdisciplinary assistive technology team. These teams assess the student's functional performance relative to environmental and activity demands, decide as a team which technology is needed, and work with the school and family to obtain the technology.[76] These teams also fit or adjust the technology, troubleshoot when needed, and train school personnel in its use.

Among school functions, children with limited hand skills often need assistive technology to support writing tasks. Adapted pencils or pens with larger grasping surfaces can be used with a supportive writing surface (e.g., correct height, supporting the forearm and wrist). Children with a tight or fisted grasp on the pencil may benefit from a pencil grip to encourage a tripod grasp.

Children and youth with severely limited hand function often abandon handwriting and transition to word processing using a computer. Adapted computers and tablets may be recommended to optimize the student's function in classroom tasks. When accessing a keyboard, a child with poor arm and hand control may benefit from using a keyguard or forearm stabilizer. The keyguard is a clear plastic cover for the keyboard with key holes over the letters; therefore, it offers a surface for stabilizing the hand when using isolated finger movements to access the keys. For a student with limited control and some isolated finger movement, a larger keyboard, such as Intellikeys or BigKeys, may improve accuracy. Use of a typing stick may improve the child's accuracy on the keyboard. In addition, the responsiveness of the mouse and keyboard can be slowed to accommodate a child whose performance is slower or error-prone. Using an adapted mouse can be helpful to children with weak hands or poor control of hand function. A large track ball may be easier to use than a regular mouse, or a joystick can replace the mouse (see Table 8-10). For students with minimal arm and hand control, a switch can be used to access an online keyboard. A rocker or button switch can be optimal for scanning to a word processor (Case Study 8-5). Chapter 20 describes for examples of computer programs to support school functions.

Students also use assistive technology and adapted equipment to manage materials, (e.g., math cubes, rulers, books). Occupational therapists may recommend or obtain dividers or containers that are easy to open and stable when handling. Placement of enlarged handles, large zipper pulls, and Velcro fasteners can help the student manage his or her materials with less support from caregivers and aides.

Assistive Technology Research

Because the types of technology vary according to the activity and the hand performance problem, few studies of assistive technology use have been completed. In pre- to post-test, repeated-measures study of students who received assistive technology services in school, their individualized education program goals and objectives improved.[128] Frequently applied technology to support limited hand function included adapted devices for computer access (e.g., Intellikeys) and adapted keyboards for word processing (e.g., AlphaSmart word processors).[128]

Isabelle and colleagues[70] explained that because children mature quickly, their need for assistive technology changes quickly, therefore limiting opportunities to collect outcomes data on assistive technology use. Assistive technology application appears to be very fluid with children, and often devices are used to help them reach the next developmental level and then are no longer needed. Therefore, one indicator of assistive technology success may be that the device is not used and is replaced with a simpler device or no device. Although research on the effectiveness of assistive technology to augment and increase hand function is limited, the tools presented in this section are widely used in practice. Occupational therapists who combine adapted techniques and assistive technology with interventions to improve performance can optimize children's participation in school and home activities.

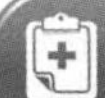

CASE STUDY 8-5 The Use of Assistive Technology

Suzanne, at 8 years old, had infantile spinal muscular atrophy. Spinal muscular atrophy is a genetic disorder that affects neuronal cells in the anterior horn of the spinal cord, causing atrophy of motor neurons. Spinal muscular atrophy progresses from birth, and often children die in infancy. Generally, lower extremity muscles are first affected, then upper extremities, trunk, and neck; the disease progresses from proximal to distal muscle. Although Suzanne was diagnosed in the first months of life, at 8 she continued to be healthy despite profound weakness throughout her body. She was on a respirator and had limited head movement, no functional movement in her trunk and legs, and minimal movement of her right arm and

Continued

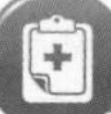

CASE STUDY 8-5 The Use of Assistive Technology—cont'd

hand, with some active range in supination, wrist extension, finger flexion, and extension. Suzanne operated her power chair with an adapted joy stick calibrated to require minimal movement to activate the chair's movement.

Suzanne was very bright and social. She did well in her academic work and in particular enjoyed drawing and art. The following adaptations were made to enable her mobility in school, her participation in art, and her participation in second grade academic work. The second grade curriculum was adapted for her with significant reduction in written work, emphasis on reading/literacy, and emphasis on adapting leisure activities. Suzanne's attendance in school was intermittent because the family was very cautious about maintaining her health. She spent most of her day in her wheelchair because it offered full pelvic, trunk, head, and foot support and had a tray to support her arms. The wheelchair tray was also used to support her computer, computer tablet, switches, and other materials. She received occupational therapy at home and at school.

Goals for Suzanne included:

1. With supervision and an obstacle-free environment, she will operate her power chair for short distances at home and school.
2. With minimal assistance and setup, she will operate painting programs on her computer and her computer tablet using a touch mouse and an adapted joystick.
3. With setup of the book on her book stand, she will turn pages using a mouth stick.

Power Mobility

Suzanne was fitted for an adapted joystick on her power wheelchair's right arm rest (she is stronger on the right). Although Suzanne could not raise her arm at this time, she moved her arm forward when it was resting on the arm rest and she cupped her hands on the joy stick to move it to the right and left. This adapted joystick responded to very subtle movements, and although Suzanne was profoundly weak, she had precise control of her arm movements within a limited range. At times the occupational therapist or parents needed to readjust her arm on the joystick and a small platform was placed over her arm rest to give her a larger surface for sliding her arm (and to keep her arm from falling). Although Suzanne traveled short distances in her chair, she had limited neck ROM and therefore needed adult guidance when turning or when she needed to avoid obstacles in her environment.

Computer Painting

Suzanne received great pleasure from painting using computer and tablet programs. These programs allowed her to select different colors and make designs on the computer screen with movements of her hand over the touch pad or with the adapted joystick. She loved to select different colors. The touchpad was mounted on a gooseneck mount on her wheelchair to position it for her right hand in the range where she had the most control of her movement (to the right of midline and near her body). She rested her hand on the pad and used the movement of second and third fingers, where she had the greatest active range. She required assistance to print her paintings. Family and staff were most pleased when Suzanne shared her artwork with them.

Turning Pages of a Book

The occupational therapist had to problem solve where to place Suzanne's book stand for her to easily visualize the page and to use her hand to turn pages. He originally set up computer books for Suzanne to use on the computer and to turn pages by lightly hitting a switch. Although computer books worked well, not all of Suzanne's required reading was available on the computer with page-turning capacity, and therefore a set up for paper books was needed. Using a mounting system on her wheelchair tray, the books were placed to the right at the height of her arm rest. She was fitted with a pointer with rubber end on a U-shaped universal cuff. The point angled from her palm and she used a rocking motion of her hand and a sliding motion of her arm (across the tray) to turn the pages. With this system Suzanne sometimes required multiple tries, but she was successful 90% of the time. The book holder had a small bar that holds down the page once it was turned.

Although these adapted activities required teacher or therapist support, they gave Suzanne great pleasure, enabled social and academic participation, and promoted her overall quality of life.

Summary

Occupational therapists are experts in children's hand function and often take the lead in providing interventions to improve hand function. The typical sequences of development for basic skills of reach, carry, grasp, and release, as well as advanced functions of in-hand manipulation and bilateral hand use, were reviewed. A deep understanding of hand skill development and the factors associated with hand function enable occupational therapists (1) to analyze performance in play, social, school, and ADLs; (2) to determine the variables associated with performance, including contextual factors; and (3) to prioritize and plan interventions. The chapter includes description of intervention principles and strategies, based on primary occupational therapy practice models, and research that supports these practice models.

- Children rapidly develop basic hand functions of reach, carry, grasp, release, and bimanual skills in the first 2 years of life. They continue to refine these hand functions, with emphasis on increasing strength and coordination, development of in-hand manipulation and dynamic grasping patterns, and increasing competency of bimanual skills through elementary school ages.
- Factors that contribute to hand function development include musculoskeletal systems, somatosensory function, visual perception, and cognition. Social cultural context also influences hand function development.

- The child's proficiency in tool use, ADLs and school functions is highly influenced by competency in bimanual skills, dynamic grasping patterns including precision grasp and release, and in-hand manipulation.
- Biomechanical and neurodevelopmental therapy practice models are used with children with cerebral palsy and neuromotor disorders. These approaches emphasize body alignment, ROM techniques that influence muscle tone, facilitation of postural stability and equilibrium, and techniques that facilitat e normal patterns of posture and movement.
- Motor learning principles and strategies include (1) engaging the child in a meaningful, preferred activity; (2) using frequent, repetitive practice; (3) systematically varying the practice; (4) providing a just-right challenge to elicit emerging skills; (5) providing structured reinforcement that includes specific feedback about performance; and (6) structuring activities to facilitate the transfer of newly learned skills to the natural environment.
- Pediatric constraint-induced movement therapy (P-CIMT) is the most extensively researched intervention for children with unilateral cerebral palsy. In P-CIMT, occupational therapists provide (1) systematic constraint of the child's less-affected arm and hand either continuously throughout the intervention program or during intervention sessions, (2) high-intensity intervention that engages the child in activities to improve function of the more involved arm and hand, (3) systematic repetition and reinforcement based on motor learning principles, (4) activities that challenge the child's skills and elicit emerging skills, and (5) transfer of intervention program (generally at 2 to 4 weeks) to the caregivers.
- Children with significant hand function impairments may benefit from acquiring and using adapted equipment and assistive technology. A range of assistive technologies can increase the child's participation in play, ADLs and school functions.

REFERENCES

1. Aarts, P. B., Jongerius, P. H., Geerdink, Y. A., et al. (2010). Effectiveness of modified constraint-induced therapy in children with unilateral spastic cerebral palsy: A randomized controlled trial. *Neurorehabilitation and Neural Repair, 24*, 509–518.
2. Aarts, P. B., Jongerius, P. H., Geerdink, Y. A., et al. (2011). Modified constraint-induced movement therapy combined with bimanual training (CIMT-CiT) in children with unilateral spastic cerebral palsy: How are improvements in arm-hand use established? *Research in Developmental Disabilities, 32*, 271–279.
3. Adolph, K. E., Vereijken, B., & Shrout, P. E. (2003). What changes in infant walking and why? *Child Development, 74*(2), 475–497.
4. Bard, C., Fleury, M., & Gagnon, M. (1990). Coincidence anticipation timing: An age-related perspective. In C. Bard, M. Fleury, & L. Hay (Eds.), *Development of eye-hand coordination across the life span*. Columbia, SC: University of South Carolina Press.
5. Bayley, N. (2005). *Bayley scales of infant and toddler development* (3rd ed.). San Antonio, TX: Psychological Corp.
6. Bazyk, S., Stalnaker, D., Llerena, M., et al. (2003). Play in Mayan children. *American Journal of Occupational Therapy, 57*, 273–283.
7. Bayona, C. L., McDougall, J., Tucker, M., et al. (2006). School-based occupational therapy for children with fine motor difficulties: Evaluating functional outcomes and fidelity of services. *Physical & Occupational Therapy in Pediatrics, 26*(3), 90–110.
8. Beery, K. E., Buktenica, N. A., & Beery, N. A. (2004). *Developmental test of visual-motor integration* (5th ed.). Los Angeles: Western Psychological Services.
9. Bertenthal, B., & Von Hofsten, C. (1998). Eye, head and trunk control: The foundation for manual development. *Neuroscience and Biobehavioral Reviews, 22*, 515–520.
10. Boehme, R. H. (1988). *Improving upper body control: An approach to assessment and treatment of tonal dysfunctioni*. Tucson, AZ: Therapy Skill Builders.
11. Brown, T., & Burns, S. (2001). The efficacy of neurodevelopmental treatment in paediatrics: A systematic review. *British Journal of Occupational Therapy, 54*, 235 244.
12. Bruininks, R. H., & Bruininks, B. D. (2005). *Bruininks-Oseretsky test of motor proficiency* (2nd ed.). Manual Circle Pines, MN: AGS Publishing.
13. Bushnell, E. W., & Boudreau, J. P. (1999). Exploring and exploiting objects with the hands during infancy. In K. J. Connolly (Ed.), *The psychobiology of the hand* (pp. 144–161). London: Cambridge University Press.
14. Campbell, P., Milbourne, S., Dugan, L., et al. (2006). A review of evidence on practices for teaching young children to use assistive technology devices. *Topics in Early Childhood Special Education, 26*(1), 3–13.
15. Carlier, M., Doyen, A.-L., & Lamard, C. (2006). Midline crossing: Developmental trend from 3 to 10 years of age in a preferential card-reaching task. *Brain and Cognition, 61*(3), 255–261.
16. Case-Smith, J. (1996). Fine motor outcomes in preschool children who receive occupational therapy services. *American Journal of Occupational Therapy, 50*, 52–61.
17. Case-Smith, J. (2006). Hand skill development in the context of infants' play: Birth to 2 years. In A. Henderson & C. Pehoski (Eds.), *Hand function in the child: Foundations for remediation* (pp. 117–142). St. Louis: Mosby.
18. Case-Smith, J. (2013). Applying occupation and motor learning principles in pediatric CIMT: Theoretical foundations and conceptual framework. In S. L. Ramey, P. Coker-Bolt, & S. C. DeLuca (Eds.), *Handbook of pediatric constraint-induced movement therapy (CIMT)* (pp. 41–54). Bethesda, MD: AOTA Press.
19. Case-Smith, J., DeLuca, S. C., Stevenson, R., et al. (2012). Multicenter randomized controlled trail of pediatric constraint-induced movement therapy: 6-month follow-up. *American Journal of Occupational Therapy, 66*, 15–23.
20. Case-Smith, J., Frolek Clark, G. J., & Schlabach, T. L. (2013). Systematic review of interventions used in occupational therapy to promote motor performance for children ages birth-5 years. *American Journal of Occupational Therapy, 67*, 413–424.
21. Cermak, S. (2006). Perceptual functions of the hand. In A. Henderson & C. Pehoski (Eds.), *Hand function in the*

child: Foundations for remediation (pp. 63–88). St. Louis: Mosby.
22. Charles, J. R., Wolf, S. L., Schneider, J. A., et al. (2006). Efficacy of a child-friendly form of constraint-induced movement therapy in hemiplegic cerebral palsy: A randomized control trial. *Developmental Medicine and Child Neurology, 48*, 635–642.
23. Chow, S., Henderson, S., & Barnett, A. (2001). The movement assessment battery for children: A comparison of 4-year-old to 6-year-old children from Hong Kong and the United States. *American Journal of occupational Therapy, 55*, 55–61.
24. Chung, J., Evans, J., Lee, C., et al. (2008). Effectiveness of adaptive seating on sitting posture and postural control in children with cerebral palsy. *Pediatric Physical Therapy, 20*, 303–317.
25. Cohen, D., Voss, C., Taylor, M., et al. (2009). Handgrip strength in English schoolchildren. *Acta Paediatrica, 99*, 1065–1072.
26. Connolly, K., & Dalgleish, M. (1989). The emergence of a tool-using skill in infancy. *Developmental Psychology, 25*, 894–912.
27. Corbetta, D., & Mounoud, P. (1990). Early development of grasping and manipulation. In C. Bard, M. Fleury, & L. Hay (Eds.), *Development of eye-hand coordination across the life span* (pp. 188–213). Columbia, SC: University of South Carolina Press.
28. Coster, W., Deeney, T., Haltiwanger, J., et al. (1998). *School function assessment*. San Antonio, TX: Psychological Corp.
29. DeLuca, S. C., Echols, K., Law, C. R., et al. (2006). Intensive pediatric constraint-induced therapy for children with cerebral palsy. *Journal of Child Neurology, 21*, 931–938.
30. DeLuca, S. C., Case-Smith, J., Stevenson, R., et al. (2012). Constraint-induced movement therapy (CIMT) for young children with cerebral palsy: Effects of therapeutic dosage. *Journal of Pediatric Rehabilitation Medicine, 5*, 133–142.
31. DeLuca, S. C., Ramey, S. L., Trucks, M. R., et al. (2013). The ACQUIREc protocol: What we have learned from a decade of delivering a signature form of pediatric CIMT. In S. L. Ramey, P. Coker-Bolt, & S. C. DeLuca (Eds.), *Handbook of pediatric constraint-induced movement therapy (CIMT)* (pp. 129–148). Bethesda, MD: AOTA Press.
32. DeMatteo, C., Law, M., Russell, D., et al. (1992). *QUEST: Quality of Upper Extremity Skills Test manual*. Hamilton, OH: Neurodevelopment Research Unit, Chedoke Campus, Chedoke-McMasters Hospital.
33. DeMatteo, C., Law, M. C., Russell, D. J., et al. (1993). The reliability and validity of the Quality of Upper Extremity Skills Test. *Physical and Occupational Therapy in Pediatrics, 13*, 1–18.
34. Denton, P., Cope, S., & Moser, C. (2006). Effects of sensorimotor-based intervention versus therapeutic practice on improving handwriting performance in 6- to 11-year-old children. *American Journal of Occupational Therapy, 60*, 16–27.
35. Duff, S. V., & Gordon, A. M. (2003). Learning of grasp control in children with hemiplegic cerebral palsy. *Developmental Medicine and Child Neurology, 5*, 746–757.
36. Eliasson, A. C. (2005). Improving the use of hands in daily activities aspects of the treatment of children with cerebral palsy. *Physical and Occupational Therapy in Pediatrics, 25*(3), 37–60.
37. Eliasson, A. C. (2005). Normal and impaired development of force control in precision grip. In A. Henderson & C. Pehoski (Eds.), *Hand function in the child* (pp. 45–62). St. Louis: Mosby.
38. Eliasson, A., & Coker-Bolt, P. (2013). Group-based models of pediatric CIMT: Special camps, school-based treatment and home environment models. In S. L. Ramey, P. Coker-Bolt, & S. C. DeLuca (Eds.), *Handbook of pediatric constraint-induced movement therapy (CIMT)* (pp. 161–180). Bethesda, MD: AOTA Press.
39. Eliasson, A. C., & Gordon, A. M. (2000). Impaired force coordination during object release in children with hemiplegic cerebral palsy. *Developmental Medicine and Child Neurology, 42*, 228–234.
40. Eliasson, A. C., Gordon, A. M., & Forssberg, H. (1995). Tactile control of isometric finger forces during grasping in children with cerebral palsy. *Developmental Medicine and Child Neurology, 37*, 216–255.
41. Eliasson, A. C., Krumlinde-Sundholm, L., Rosblad, B., et al. (2006). The Manual Ability Classification System (MACS) for children with cerebral palsy: Scale development and evidence of validity and reliability. *Developmental Medicine and Child Neurology, 48*, 549–554.
42. Eliasson, A. C., Krumlinde-Sundholm, L., Shaw, K., et al. (2005). Effects of constraint-induced movement therapy in young children with hemiplegic cerebral palsy: An adapted model. *Developmental Medicine and Child Neurology, 47*, 266–275.
43. Exner, C. E. (1990). The zone of proximal development in in-hand manipulation skills of nondysfunctional 3- and 4-year-old children. *American Journal of Occupational Therapy, 44*, 884–891.
44. Exner, C. E. (2006). Intervention for children with hand skill problems. In A. Henderson & C. Pehoski (Eds.), *Hand function in the child* (pp. 239–266). St. Louis: Mosby.
45. Facchin, P., Rosa-Rizzotto, M., Pozza, L. V., et al. (2011). Multisite trial comparing the efficacy of constraint-induced movement therapy with that of bimanual intensive training in children with hemiplegic cerebral palsy. *American Journal of Physical Medicine and Rehabilitation, 90*, 539–553.
46. Fagard, I. (1990). The development of bimanual coordination. In C. Bard, M. Fleury, & L. Hay (Eds.), *Development of eye-hand coordination across the life span*. Columbia, SC: University of South Carolina Press.
47. Fagard, J. (1993). Manual strategies and interlimb coordination during reaching, grasping and manipulating throughout the first year of life. In S. Swinen, J. Massion, J. Heuer, & P. Caeser (Eds.), *Interlimb coordination: Neural, dynamical and cognitive constraints* (pp. 438–460). San Diego: Academic Press.
48. Fagard, J., & Jacquet, A. Y. (1989). Onset of bimanual coordination and symmetry versus asymmetry of movement. *Infant Behavior and Development, 12*, 229–236.
49. Fagard, J., & Lockman, J. J. (2005). The effect of task constraints on infants' (bi)manual strategy for grasping and exploring objects. *Infant Behavior & Development, 28*, 305–315.
50. Fagard, J., & Lockman, J. J. (2010). Change in imitation for object manipulation between 10 and 12 months of age. *Developmental Psychobiology, 52*, 90–99.
51. Falk, B., Usselman, C., Dotan, R., et al. (2009). Child-adult differences in muscle strength and activation pattern during isometric elbow flexion and extension. *Applied Physiology Nutrition & Metabolism, 34*, 609–615.
52. Fitts, P. M., & Posner, M. I. (1967). *Human performance*. Belmont, CA: Brooks/Cole.
53. Flynn, E., & Whiten, A. (2008). Cultural transmission of tool use in young children: A diffusion chain study. *Social Development, 17*(3), 699–718.
54. Folio, R. M., & Fewell, R. (2000). *Peabody developmental motor scales—revised*. Chicago: Riverside.
55. Garvey, M. A., Ziemann, U., Bartko, J., et al. (2003). Cortical correlates of neuromotor development in healthy children. *Clinical Neurophysiology, 114*, 1662–1670.

56. Gordon, A. W., & Duff, S. V. (1999). Relation between clinical measures and fine manipulative control in children with hemiplegic cerebral palsy. *Developmental Medicine and Child Neurology, 41*, 586–591.
57. Gordon, A. M., & Duff, S. V. (1999). Fingertip forces in children with hemiplegic cerebral palsy. I: Anticipatory scaling. *Developemntal Medicine & Child Neurology, 41*, 166–175.
58. Gordon, A. M., & Duff, S. V. (1999). Relationship between clinical measures and fine manipulative control in children with hemiplegic cerebral palsy. *Developmental Medicine & Child Neurology, 41*, 586–591.
59. Gordon, A. M., Charles, J., & Steenbergen, B. (2006). Fingertip force planning during grasp is disrupted by impaired sensorimotor integration in children with hemiplegic cerebral palsy. *Pediatric Research, 60*, 587–591.
60. Gordon, A. M., Lewis, S. R., Eliasson, A. C., et al. (2003). Object release under varying task constraints in children with hemiplegic cerebral palsy. *Developmental Medicine and Child Neurology, 45*, 240–248.
61. Gordon, A. M., Schneider, J. A., Chinnan, A., et al. (2007). Efficacy of a hand-arm bimanual intensive therapy (HABIT) in children with hemiplegic cerebral palsy: A randomized control trial. *Developmental Medicine and Child Neurology, 49*, 830–838.
62. Gordon, A. M., Hung, Y.-C., Brandao, M., et al. (2011). Bimanual training and constraint-induced movement therapy in children with hemiplegic cerebral palsy: A randomized trial. *Neurorehabilitation & Neural Repair, 25*, 692–702.
63. Hall, J. G. (1997). Arthrogryposis multiplex congenital: Etiology, genetics, classification, diagnostic approach, and general aspects. *Journal of Pediatric Orthopedics, 6*, 159–166.
64. Hammill, D. D., Pearson, N. A., & Voress, J. K. (2014). *Developmental test of visual perception* (3rd ed.). Austin, TX: Pro-Ed.
65. Henderson, A. (2006). Self-care and hand skill. In A. Henderson & C. Pehoski (Eds.), *Hand function in the child* (pp. 193–216). St. Louis: Mosby.
66. Hoare, B., Imms, C., Carey, L., et al. (2007). Constraint-induced movement therapy in the treatment of the upper limb in children with hemiplegic cerebral palsy: A Cochrane systematic review. *Clinical Rehabilitation, 21*(8), 675–685.
67. Howle, J. M. (2002). *Neuro-developmental treatment approach: Theoretical foundations and principles of clinical practice.* Laguna Beach, CA: Neuro-Developmental Treatment Association.
68. Huang, H. H., Fetters, L., Hale, J., et al. (2009). Bound for success: A systematic review of constraint-induced movement therapy in children with cerebral palsy supports improved arm and hand use. *Physical Therapy, 89*, 1126–1141.
69. Humphry, R., Jewell, K., & Rosenberger, R. C. (1995). Development of in-hand manipulation and relationship with activities. *American Journal of Occupational Therapy, 49*, 763–774.
70. Isabell, S., Bessey, S. F., Dragas, K. L., et al. (2002). Assistive technology for children with disabilities. *Occupational Therapy in Health Care, 16*, 29–52.
71. Jeannerod, M. (1994). The hand and the object: The role of posterior parietal cortex in forming motor representations. *Canadian Journal of Physiology and Pharmacology, 72*, 535–541.
72. Karman, N., Maryles, J., Baker, R. W., et al. (2003). Constraint-induced movement therapy for hemiplegic children with acquired brain injuries. *Journal of Head Trauma Rehabilitation, 18*, 259–267.
73. Ketelaar, M., Vermeer, A., Hart, H., et al. (2001). Effects of a functional therapy program on motor abilities of children with cerebral palsy. *Physical Therapy, 81*, 1524–1545.
74. Krumlinde-Sundholm, L., Holmefur, M., Kottorp, A., et al. (2007). The Assisting Hand Assessment: Current evidence of validity, reliability, and responsiveness to change. *Development Medicine and Child Neurology, 49*, 259–264.
75. Kuhtz-Buschbeck, J. P., Stolze, H., Johnk, K., et al. (1998). Development of prehension movements in children: A kinematic study. *Experimental Brain Research, 122*, 424–432.
76. Lahm, E. A., & Sizemore, L. (2002). Factors that influence assistive technology decision making. *Journal of Special Education Technology, 27*, 15–26.
77. Lane, S. J., & Mistrett, S. (2002). Let's play! Assistive technology interventions for play. *Young Exceptional Children, 5*, 19–27.
78. Law, S.-H., Lo, S. K., Chow, S., et al. (2011). Grip force control is dependent on task constraints in children with and without developmental coordination disorder. *International Journal of Rehabilitation Research, 34*, 93–99.
79. Law, M., Russell, D., Pollock, N., et al. (1997). A comparison of intensive neurodevelopmental therapy plus casting and a regular occupational therapy program for children with cerebral palsy. *Developmental Medicine and Child Neurology, 39*, 664–670.
80. Lee-Valkov, P. M., Aaron, D. H., Eladoumikdachi, F., et al. (2003). Measuring normal hand dexterity values in normal 3-, 4-, and 5-year-old children and their relationship with grip and pinch strength. *Journal of Hand Therapy, 16*, 22–28.
81. Link, L., Lukens, S., & Bush, M. A. (1995). Spherical grip strength in children 3 to 6 years of age. *American Journal of Occupational Therapy, 49*, 318–326.
82. Lockman, J. J. (2000). A perception–action perspective on tool use development. *Child Development, 71*(1), 137–144.
83. Lowes, L., Mayhan, M., Orr, T., et al. (2014). Pilot study of the efficacy of constraint-induced movement therapy for infants and toddlers with cerebral palsy. *Physical and Occupational Therapy in Pediatrics, 34*, 4–21.
84. Man, D. W., & Wong, M-S. L. (2007). Evaluation of computer-access solutions for students with quadriplegic athetoid cerebral palsy. *American Journal of Occupational Therapy, 61*, 355–364.
85. Mathiowetz, V., Federman, S., & Wiemer, D. (1985). Box and Block Test of manual dexterity: Norms for 6-19 year olds. *Canadian Journal of Occupational Therapy, 52*, 241–245.
86. Mathiowetz, V., Weimer, D. M., & Federman, S. M. (1986). Grip and pinch strength: Norms for 6- to 19-year-olds. *American Journal of Occupational Therapy, 40*, 705–711.
87. Mastos, M., Miller, K., Eliasson, A. C., et al. (2007). Goal-directed training: Linking theories of treatment to clinical practice for improved functional activities in daily life. *Clinical Rehabilitation, 21*, 47–55.
88. McCarty, M. E., Clifton, R. K., & Collard, R. R. (2001). The beginnings of tool use by infants and toddlers. *Infancy, 2*, 233–256.
89. McHale, K., & Cermak, S. A. (1992). Fine motor activities in elementary school. Preliminary findings and provisional implications for children with fine motor problems. *American Journal of Occupational Therapy, 46*, 898–903.
90. Missiuna, C., Mandich, A. D., Polatajko, H., et al. (2001). Cognitive Orientation to daily Occupational Performance (CO-OP): Part I—Theoretical foundations. *Physical and Occupational Therapy in Pediatrics, 20*, 69–81.
91. Missiuna, C., Mole, S., King, S., et al. (2007). A trajectory of troubles: Parents' impressions of the impact of developmental coordination disorder.

Physical and Occupational Therapy in Pediatrics, 27(1), 81–101.

92. Myers, C. A. (2006). A fine motor program for preschoolers. In A. Henderson & C. Pehoski (Eds.), *Hand function in the child: Foundations for remediation* (2nd ed., pp. 267–292). St. Louis: Mosby.
93. Niemeijer, A. S., Smits-Engelman, B. C., & Schoemaker, M. M. (2007). Neuromotor task training for children with developmental coordination disorder: A controlled trial. *Developmental Medicine and Child Neurology, 49*, 406–522.
94. Novak, I., McIntyre, S., Morgan, C., et al. (2013). A systematic review of interventions for children with cerebral palsy: State of the evidence. *Developmental Medicine & Child Neurology, 55*, 885–910.
95. Ostendorf, C. G., & Wolf, S. L. (1981). Effect of forced use of the upper extremity of a hemiplegic patient on changes in function. *Physical Therapy, 61*, 1022–1028.
96. Palmer, C. F. (1989). The discriminating nature of infants: Exploratory actions. *Developmental Psychology, 25*, 885–893.
97. Parks Warshaw, S. (2006). *Inside HELP: Hawaii Early Learning Profile.* Palo Alto, CA: VORT.
98. Pehoski, C. (2006). Object manipulation in infants and children. In A. Henderson & C. Pehoski (Eds.), *Hand function in the child: Foundations for remediation* (pp. 143–160). St. Louis: Mosby.
99. Pehoski, C., Henderson, A., & Tickle-Degnen, L. (1997). In-hand manipulation in young children: Rotation of an object in the fingers. *American Journal of Occupational Therapy, 51*, 544–552.
100. Pehoski, C., Henderson, A., & Tickle-Degnen, L. (1997). In-hand manipulation in young children: Translation movements. *American Journal of Occupational Therapy, 51*, 719–728.
101. Pont, K., Wallen, M., Bundy, A., et al. (2008). Reliability and validity of the Test of In-Hand Manipulation in children ages 5 to 6 years. *The American Journal of Occupational Therapy, 62*, 384–392.
102. Quinn, B. S., Behrmann, M., Mastropieri, S., et al. (2009). Who is using assistive technology in schools? *Journal of Special Education Technology, 24*, 1–11.
103. Ramey, S. L., & DeLuca, S. C. (2013). Pediatric CIMT: History and definition. In S. L. Ramey, P. Coker-Bolt, & S. C. DeLuca (Eds.), *Handbook of pediatric constraint-induced movement therapy (CIMT)* (pp. 19–40). Bethesda, MD: AOTA Press.
104. Randall, M., Johnson, I., & Reddihough, D. (1999). *The Melbourne Assessment of Unilateral Upper Limb Function: Test administration manual.* Melbourne, Australia: Royal Children's Hospital.
105. Rat-Fischer, L., O-Regan, J. K., & Fagard, J. (2012). The emergence of tool use during the second year of life. *Journal of Experimental Child Psychology, 113*, 440–446.
106. Reidy, T. G., Coker-Bolt, P., & Wallace, D. A. (2013). Adapting pediatric CIMT for children with brachial plexus injuries, traumatic brain injury and hemispherectomy and other surgical intervention. In S. L. Ramey, P. Coker-Bolt, & S. C. DeLuca (Eds.), *Handbook of pediatric constraint-induced movement therapy (CIMT)* (pp. 149–160). Bethesda, MD: AOTA Press.
107. Rigby, P. J., Ryan, S. E., & Campbell, K. A. (2009). Effect of adaptive seating devices on the activity performance of children with cerebral palsy. *Archives of Physical Medicine and Rehabilitation, 90*, 1389–1396.
108. Rodger, S., Ziviani, J., Watter, P., et al. (2003). Motor and functional skills of children with developmental coordination disorder: A pilot investigation of measurement issues. *Human Movement Science, 22*, 461–478.
109. Rogoff, B., Mosier, C., Mistry, J., et al. (1993). Toddlers' guided participation in cultural activity. *Cultural dynamics, 2*, 209–237.
110. Rosblad, B. (2006). Reaching and eye-hand coordination. In A. Henderson & C. Pehoski (Eds.), *Hand function in the child* (pp. 89–100). St. Louis: Mosby.
111. Ruff, H. A. (1980). The development of the perception and recognition of objects. *Child Development, 51*, 981–992.
112. Ruff, H. A. (1989). The infant's use of visual and haptic information in the perception and recognition of objects. *Canadian Journal of Psychology, 43*, 302–319.
113. Ryan, S. E. (2012). An overview of systematic reviews of adaptive seating interventions for children with cerebral palsy: Where do we go from here? *Disability and Rehabilitation: Assistive Technology, 7*, 103–111.
114. Sakzewski, L., Ziviani, J., & Boyd, R. (2009). Systematic review and meta-analysis of therapeutic management of upper limb dysfunction in children with congenital hemiplegia. *Pediatrics, 123*, e1111–e1122.
115. Santamato, A., Panza, F., Ranieri, M., et al. (2011). Effect of botulinum toxin type A and modified constraint-induced movement therapy on motor function of upper limb in children with obstetrical brachial plexus palsy. *Children's Nervous System, 27*, 2187–2192.
116. Smits-Engelsman, B. C., Westenberg, Y., & Duysens, J. (2003). Development of isometric force and force control in children. *Cognitive Brain Research, 17*, 68–74.
117. Schneiberg, S., Sveistrup, H., McFadyen, B., et al. (2002). The development of coordination for reach-to-grasp movements in children. *Experimental Brain Research, 146*(2), 142–154.
118. Schoemaker, M. M., Niemeijer, A. S., Reynder, K., et al. (2003). Effectiveness of neuromotor task training for children with developmental coordination disorder: A pilot study. *Neural Plasticity, 10*, 155–163.
119. Smits-Engelsman, B. C., Westenberg, Y., & Duysens, J. (2003). Development of isometric force and force control in children. *Cognitive Brain Research, 17*, 68–74.
120. Smits-Engelsman, B. C., Wilson, P. H., Westenberg, Y., et al. (2003). Fine motor deficiencies in children with developmental coordination disorder and learning disabilities: An underlying open-loop control deficit. *Human Movement Science, 22*, 495–513.
121. Stavness, C. (2006). The effect of positioning for children with cerebral palsy on upper-extremity function: A review of the evidence. *Physical and Occupational Therapy in Pediatric, 26*, 39–53.
122. Sullivan, K., Kantak, S. S., & Burtner, P. A. (2008). Motor learning in children: Feedback effects on skill acquisition. *Physical Therapy, 88*(6), 720–732.
123. Sutcliffe, T. L., Gaetz, W. C., Logan, W. J., et al. (2007). Cortical reorganization after modified constraint-induced movement therapy in pediatric hemiplegic cerebral palsy. *Journal of Child Neurology, 22*, 1281–1287.
124. Vaz, D. V., Mancini, M. C., do Amaral, M. F., et al. (2010). Clinical changes during an intervention based on constraint-induced movement therapy principles on the affected arm of a child with obstetric brachial plexus injury: A case report. *Occupational Therapy International, 17*, 159–167.
125. Vogtle, L. K. (2006). Upper extremity intervention in cerebral palsy: A neurodevelopmental approach. In A. Henderson & C. Pehoski (Eds.),

Hand function in the child: Foundations for remediation (2nd ed., pp. 345–368). St. Louis: Mosby/Elsevier.

126. Von Hofsten, C. (1982). Eye-hand coordination in the newborn. *Developmental Psychology, 18*(3), 450–461.
127. Von Hofsten, C. (1991). Structuring of early reaching movements: A longitudinal study. *Journal of Motor Behavior, 23*(4), 280–292.
128. Watson, A. H., Ito, M., Smith, R. O., et al. (2010). Effect of assistive technology in a public school setting. *American Journal of Occupational Therapy, 64*, 18–29.
129. Wingrat, J., & Exner, C. E. (2005). The impact of school furniture on fourth grade children's on-task and sitting behavior in the classroom: A pilot study. *Work (Reading, Mass.), 25*, 263–272.
130. Wolf, S. L., Winstein, C. J., Miller, J. P., et al.; EXITE Investigators. (2006). Effect of constraint-induced movement therapy on upper extremity function 3 to 9 months after stroke: The EXCITE randomized clinical trial. *JAMA: The Journal of the American Medical Association, 296*, 2095–2104.
131. Yim, S. Y., Cho, J. R., & Lee, I. Y. (2003). Normative data developmental characteristics of hand function for elementary school children in Suwon area of Korea: Grip, pinch, and dexterity study. *Journal of Korean Medical Science, 18*, 552–558.
132. Zwicker, J. F., & Harris, S. R. (2009). A reflection on motor learning theory in pediatric occupational therapy practice. *Canadian Journal of Occupational Therapy, 76*(1), 29–37.

CHAPTER

9

Sensory Integration

L. Diane Parham • Zoe Mailloux

KEY TERMS

Ayres Sensory Integration (ASI)
Adaptive response
Neural plasticity
Sensory integration
Sensory modulation
Under-responsiveness
Sensory registration
Over-responsiveness
Perception
Sensory discrimination
Praxis
Dyspraxia
Ideation
Motor planning
Sensory seeking
Intervention fidelity

GUIDING QUESTIONS

1. What does the term "sensory integration" mean, as a term referring to neurobiologic processes and as a frame of reference in occupational therapy practice?
2. Which sensory systems are emphasized in Ayres Sensory Integration (ASI), and why are they considered important?
3. How do sensory experiences support brain functions, and what are the conditions under which they optimally influence neuroplastic changes?
4. What are the key hallmarks of development in the tactile, proprioceptive, and vestibular systems, and how does each developmental achievement in each system contribute to mastery of occupations from early infancy through childhood?
5. Does evidence exist for the different types of sensory integration problems in childhood, and if so, what type of evidence is available and where can this evidence be found?
6. What are the key indicators of problems in sensory modulation, perception, vestibular-bilateral functions, and praxis, and how does each of these areas affect child behavior?
7. What are the primary methods and specific instruments used to assess sensory integration?
8. How are assessment data from different sources and contexts organized to make recommendations that will benefit the child and family?
9. What are the active ingredients of occupational therapy applying a sensory integration approach (OT-SI), and what are the benefits and drawbacks of this intervention approach?
10. What is the purpose of the Fidelity Measure for Ayres Sensory Integration Intervention?
11. Which children are appropriate for OT-SI, and what are the expected outcomes of OT-SI?
12. Does evidence exist for effectiveness of OT-SI intervention, and if so, what type of evidence exists and where can it be found?
13. What are alternative interventions that may be used in conjunction with or instead of OT-SI intervention to help children with sensory integration problems, what are the benefits and limitations of each, and what evidence exists for each?

The term *sensory integration* has held significance for occupational therapists for more than 50 years. Recognized as a way of viewing the neural organization of sensory information for functional behavior, this term also refers to a clinical frame of reference that includes theoretic tenets, assessment methods, and intervention principles and strategies. Both the biobehavioral and the clinical meanings of this term originated in the work of A. Jean Ayres, an occupational therapist and psychologist whose brilliant clinical insights and original research revolutionized occupational therapy practice with children and in many ways led the way for theory development and evidence-based practice for the profession as a whole.

The ideas developed by Ayres ushered in a new way of looking at children and understanding many of the developmental, learning, and emotional problems that arise during childhood. When introduced in the late 1960s and 1970s, her innovative practice and groundbreaking research met some resistance from within the profession, as well as from outside fields. The intervention methods that she pioneered continue to be questioned and investigated today. However, the substantial and evolving body of research and practice applications that have emanated from her work leave little doubt that the Ayres' perspective has had a profound influence on occupational therapy. The presence of sensory integration concepts in many of the chapters of this book attests to the extent to which these ideas have affected the thinking of pediatric occupational therapists. Even more broadly, the research base of the sensory integration approach has elevated many aspects of assessment, intervention planning, and outcome monitoring in the profession of occupational therapy.

The practice approach that occupational therapists call *sensory integration* is now trademarked through the Franklin B. Baker/A. Jean Ayres Baker Trust as *Ayres Sensory Integration* (ASI).[209] According to the trademark document, ASI encompasses the theory, assessment methods, patterns of sensory integration and praxis problems, and intervention concepts, principles, and techniques developed by Ayres.[208] This chapter uses the abbreviation OT-SI (occupational therapy using a sensory integration approach) when discussing the clinical methods developed by Ayres, to emphasize that this kind of intervention generally is provided within the context of occupational therapy.

This chapter provides an in-depth orientation to this fascinating and important aspect of occupational therapy practice for children. The reader will gain a general sense of how sensory integration as a brain function is related to everyday occupations, how sensory integration is manifested in typically developing children, and how some children experience difficulties with sensory integration that may lead to daily life problems. Research on sensory integration problems is reviewed to give the reader a perspective on the evolving research base of this field and how we currently classify patterns of sensory integration problems. We discuss OT-SI practice with respect to methods of clinical assessment, key principles of individual intervention, and other interventions that may be used in conjunction with or in place of individual OT-SI intervention. Effectiveness research on individual OT-SI intervention is reviewed, and case examples of children who have been helped by occupational therapists using an OT-SI approach are provided.

Introduction to Sensory Integration Theory

Ayres understood that brain function is a critical factor in human behavior.[14] She reasoned, therefore, that knowledge of brain functioning would give her insight into the ways children develop, learn, and interact in the world. However, Ayres also had a pragmatic orientation that sprang from her professional background as an occupational therapist. She was concerned particularly with how brain functions affected the child's ability to participate successfully in daily occupations. Consequently, her work represents a fusion of neurobiologic insights with the practical, everyday concerns of human beings, particularly children and their families.

As Ayres developed her ideas about sensory integration, she used terms such as *sensory integration, adaptive response,* and *praxis* in ways that reflected her concern with child occupations. Ayres coined some of these terms, whereas others were drawn from the literature of a variety of fields of study. When Ayres borrowed a term from another field, however, she imparted a particular meaning to it. For example, Ayres did not use the term *sensory integration* to refer solely to intricate synaptic connections within the brain, as neuroscientists typically do. Rather, she applied it to neural processes as they relate to functional behavior. Hence, her definition of sensory integration is the "organization of sensation for use" (p. 5).[20] It is the inclusion of the final clause "for use" that is Ayres' hallmark, because it ties sensory processing to the person's occupation.

Ayres introduced a new vocabulary of sensory integration theory and synthesized important concepts from the neuroscience literature to organize her views of child development, as well as the types of difficulties she observed in children. Many of these ideas were first published in her seminal book, *Sensory Integration and Learning Disorders.*[14] Later she wrote a book for parents, *Sensory Integration and the Child,*[20,23] which identified the ways in which sensory integration develops as well as the ways in which inefficient sensory integration affects behavior, learning, and participation. Major points made in these books regarding neurobiological concepts in relationship to child development and the ontogeny of sensory integration are presented in the following sections.

Neurobiologically Based Concepts

Role of Sensory Experiences in Development and Brain Function

Sensory input is necessary for optimal brain function. The brain is designed to constantly take in sensory information, and it malfunctions if deprived of it. The classic sensory deprivation experiments conducted in the 1950s and 1960s made it clear that without an adequate inflow of sensation, the brain generates its own input in the form of hallucinations and subsequently distorts incoming sensory stimuli.[231] If adequate sensory experiences are not available at critical periods in development, neuronal and brain connectivity abnormalities emerge that influence behavior, limiting the ability to function.[90,116,126,242] It is now well established that persistent, serious impairments in cognitive, social, and emotional functioning often result when infants and young children are institutionalized in environments that are impoverished with respect to availability of a wide range of sensory experiences, the presence of a nurturing caregiver, and opportunities for sensorimotor exploration.[38,40,75]

Ayres considered sensory input to be *sensory nourishment* for the brain, just as food is nourishment for the body.[20] Wilbarger, a colleague of Ayres, built on this concept with the term *sensory diet*, an intervention program that involves provision of individualized sensory experiences and activities throughout the day to support optimal functioning of the child with sensory integration challenges.[244] The therapeutic sensory diet provides an optimal combination of sensory-based activities at the appropriate intensities for the specific child. For most typically developing children, the naturally occurring sensory diet does not require conscious monitoring by caregivers. The environment continuously "feeds" the child a variety of nourishing sensations in the flow of everyday life.

As critical as input is to the developing brain, the mere provision of sensory stimulation is limited in value. Too much stimulation can generate stress that is detrimental to brain development and may reduce the person's subsequent ability to cope with stress.[105] To have an optimal effect on development, learning, and behavior, the sensory input must be actively organized and *used* by the child to act on and respond to the environment.

Sensory Integration and Adaptive Responses

A child does not passively absorb whatever sensations come along. The child actively selects the sensations most useful at the time and organizes them in a fashion that facilitates accomplishing goals. This involves brain processes of *sensory integration*, "the organization of sensation for use" (p. 5).[20] When these processes are going well, the child also organizes a successful, goal-directed action on the environment, which is called an *adaptive response*. When a child makes an adaptive

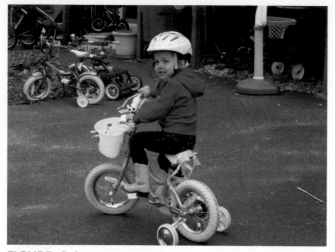

FIGURE 9-1 Adaptive responses help the child acquire skills such as riding a bicycle. Amelia's nervous system must integrate vestibular, proprioceptive, and visual information adequately for her to successfully steer the bicycle while it is moving.

response, he or she successfully meets some challenge presented in the environment. The adaptive response is possible because the brain has been able to efficiently organize incoming sensory information, which then provides a basis for action (Figure 9-1). Adaptive responses are powerful forces that drive development forward. When a child makes an adaptive response that is more complex than any previously accomplished response, Ayres hypothesized that the brain attains a more organized state, and its capacity for further sensory integration is enhanced. Thus, sensory integration leads to adaptive responses, which in turn result in more efficient sensory integration.

Ayres provides the example of learning to ride a bicycle to illustrate this process.[20] The child must integrate sensations, particularly from the vestibular and proprioceptive systems, to learn how to balance on the bicycle. The vestibular, proprioceptive, and visual senses must accurately and quickly detect when the child begins to fall, and then must be rapidly integrated with each other to produce motor reactions that counteract the direction of the fall. Eventually, often after many trials of falling, the child integrates sensory information efficiently enough to make the appropriate weight shifts over the bicycle to maintain balance. This adaptive response, and those that follow, enable the child to balance effectively to ride the bike. The child's nervous system has changed in how it integrates multisensory information to produce refined, dynamic balancing, so the child is now more adept at bicycle riding.

In making adaptive responses, the child is an active doer, not a passive recipient. Adaptive responses come from within the child. No one can force a child to respond adaptively, although a situation may be set up that is likely to elicit adaptive responses from the child. Typically developing children and most children with disabilities have an innate drive to develop sensory integration through adaptive responses. Ayres called this *inner drive* and speculated that it is generated primarily by the limbic system of the brain, a network of neural structures known to be critical in both motivation and memory.[20] Ayres designed therapeutic activities and environments to engage the child's inner drive (to elicit adaptive responses) and, in so doing, advance sensory integrative development and the child's occupational competence.

Neural Plasticity

It is thought that when a child makes an adaptive response, change occurs in neural synapses and circuits. This change is a function of the brain's neural plasticity. *Plasticity* is the ability of a structure and concomitant function to be changed gradually by its own ongoing activity.[14] The term *neuroplasticity* is used to refer to specific changes in neuron structure and function that last longer than a few seconds and are not simply part of a periodic cycle. The processes of habituation, experience-dependent learning and memory, and cellular recovery after injury all provide examples of types of neuroplasticity.[225] It is well established in the neurobehavioral literature that when organisms are permitted to explore interesting environments, significant increases in dendritic branching, synaptic connections, synaptic efficiency, and size of brain tissue result.[126] These changes are most dramatic in a young animal and probably represent a major mechanism of brain development,[116] although it is clear that such manifestations of plasticity are characteristic of optimal brain functioning throughout the life span.[28,74,143]

Studies of the effects of enriched environments on animals indicate that the essential ingredient for positive brain changes is that the organism actively interacts with a meaningful and challenging environment.[43,126] Passive exposure to sensory stimulation does not produce these same positive changes.[74,79] Recent research suggests that neural circuit reorganization is more extensive and optimal when an animal actively engages in goal-directed activity rather than being passive, for example, when an owl is allowed to hunt instead of being fed.[212] It can be hypothesized from this body of research that adaptive responses activate the brain's neuroplastic capabilities. Furthermore, the brain's plasticity makes it possible for an adaptive response to increase the efficiency of sensory integration at a neuronal level.

Central Nervous System Organization

Ayres looked to the organization of the central nervous system (CNS) for clues to how children use sensory information and how sensory integration develops over time.[14] Her postdoctoral studies in neuroscience led her to hypothesize that critical aspects of sensory integration are seated in parts of the brain that are phylogenetically older and more primitive than the neocortex.[14] For example, most of the CNS processing of vestibular information occurs in the brainstem, and a great deal of somatosensory processing takes place in the thalamus. One of the basic propositions of Ayres' theory is that, because older parts of the brain integrate and filter information before it is relayed to the cortex, increased efficiency in structures such as the brainstem and thalamus enhance[5] higher-order functioning.[14] This view differs from traditional neuropsychology and education models, which have tended to emphasize the direct study and remediation of high-level, cortically directed skills such as reading and writing, without attention to more basic modes of processing information.

Ayres also assumed that the more primitive parts of the CNS develop before maturation of higher brain centers.[14] At the time that Ayres was developing her theory, this was somewhat speculative, although generally accepted by neuroscientists. In later research, the use of positron electron tomography (PET) scans with infants provided direct support for the notion that postnatal brain development proceeds in a bottom-to-top direction.[65]

Her view of the interdependence between the more primitive and more refined processing centers of the brain led Ayres to emphasize the more primitive vestibular and somatosensory systems in her work with young children. These systems mature early and are seated in the lower CNS centers (particularly the brainstem, cerebellum, and thalamus).[14,149] Ayres reasoned that the refinement of primitive functions, such as postural control, balance, and tactile perception, provides a sensorimotor foundation for higher-order functions, such as academic ability, behavioral self-regulation, and complex motor skills (e.g., those required in sports). Thus, she viewed the developmental process as one in which the more primal body-centered functions serve as building blocks upon which complex cognitive and social skills can be scaffolded. This view undergirds a basic premise of the therapy approach that she developed: enhancing lower-level functions related to the proximal senses might have a positive influence on higher-level cortical functions. In many ways, Ayres was ahead of her time in suggesting that the brain operates in a holistic manner.

Sensory Integrative Development and Childhood Occupations

One of the most distinctive contributions that Ayres made to understanding child development was her focus on the role of primary sensory motor experiences in early childhood, with a unique and original view of the proximal senses (vestibular, tactile, and proprioceptive). From the sensory integration viewpoint, these senses are emphasized because of their importance in shaping a child's interactions with the world early in life. The distal senses of vision and hearing are also critical and become increasingly more dominant as the child matures. Ayres believed, however, that the body-centered senses provide a foundation on which complex occupations are scaffolded. Furthermore, when Ayres began her work, consideration of the vestibular, tactile, and proprioceptive senses was virtually absent in the literature on child development. She devoted her career to studying the roles played by these overlooked senses in development and the genesis of developmental problems of children.

Ayres believed that the first decade of life is a period of rapid development in sensory integration.[20] She drew this conclusion not only from her many years of observing children, but also from research in which she gathered normative data on tests of sensory integration.[22] By the time most children reach 7 or 8 years of age, their scores on standardized tests of sensory integrative capabilities reflect almost as much maturity as an adult's.

Development, from a sensory integrative standpoint, occurs as the brain organizes sensory information and the child forms adaptive responses with increasing degrees of complexity in order to respond to and interact with early sensory experiences. Sensory integration, of course, enables adaptive responses to occur, which in turn promote the *development of sensory integration* and the emergence of occupational engagement and social participation.[184,232] As this process unfolds in infancy, the developing child begins to attach meaning to the stream of sensations experienced. The child becomes increasingly adept at shifting attention to what he or she perceives as intriguing and essential, tuning out that which is irrelevant to current needs and interests. As a result, the child can organize play behavior for increasing lengths of time and gains control in the regulation of emotions.

Inner drive leads children to search for opportunities in the environment that offer "just-right" challenges to their emerging abilities and are aligned with their temperament and interests. These are challenges that are not so complex that they overwhelm or induce failure nor so simple that they are routine or uninteresting. The just-right challenge is one that requires effort but is accomplishable and satisfying. Because there is an element of challenge, a successful adaptive response engenders feelings of mastery and a sense of oneself as a competent being.

It is fascinating to watch this process unfold. Most children require no adult guidance or teaching to acquire basic developmental skills such as manipulating objects, sitting, walking, and climbing. Children need little, if any, step-by-step instruction to learn daily occupations, such as playing on playground equipment, dressing and feeding oneself, drawing and painting, and constructing with blocks. These achievements seem to just happen. They are the product of an active nervous system busily organizing sensory information and searching for challenges that bring forth more complex behaviors, all shaped within the context of a world saturated with sociocultural expectations and meanings.[184]

In this section, developmental hallmarks of sensory integration are identified and connected to the occupations attained during childhood. The proximal senses dominate early infancy and continue to exert their influence in critical ways, as the visual and auditory systems gain ascendancy. Although there is some variability across children in the sequence in which developmental achievements unfold during the first year of life, this variability becomes increasingly apparent after this first year. By kindergarten age, skills vary tremendously among children because of differences in environmental opportunities, familial and cultural influences, personal experiences, and genetic makeup. It is important to keep in mind that, throughout development, sensory integrative processes contribute to children's construction of their identities, but many other influences are powerful as well—the family and cultures that shape occupational routines, the interpretations given to behaviors by others, individual talents and abilities, and even chance events that carry special meaning for children and families.[184]

Prenatal Period

The first known responses to sensory stimuli occur early in life, at approximately 5.5 weeks after conception.[125] These first responses are to tactile stimuli. Specifically, they involve reflexive avoidance reactions to a perioral stimulus (e.g., the embryo bends its head and upper trunk away from a light touch stimulus around the mouth). This is a primitive protective reaction. It is not until a gestational age of about 9 weeks that an approach response (moving of the head toward the chest) occurs,[125] probably as a function of emerging proprioception.

The first known responses to vestibular input in the form of the Moro reflex also appear at about 9 weeks after conception. The fetus continues to develop a repertoire of reflexes such as rooting, sucking, Babkin, grasp, flexor withdrawal, Galant, neck righting, Moro, and positive supporting in utero that are fairly well established by the time of birth. Thus, when the time comes to leave the uterus, the newborn is well equipped with the capacity to form a strong bond with a caregiver and to actively participate in the critical occupation of nursing. These innate capacities require rudimentary aspects of sensory integration that are built into the nervous system. However, even in this earliest period of development, environmental influences, such as maternal stress, can have a significant impact on the quality of sensory integrative development. For example, Schneider and her colleagues found that infant rhesus monkeys born to mothers who had experienced stress in early pregnancy had signs of diminished responses to vestibular input, such as impaired righting responses, weak muscle tone, and attenuated postrotary nystagmus (i.e., normal reflexive back-and-forth movements of the eyes that occur following rotary movement and reflect central vestibular function).[220,221]

Neonatal Period

Touch, smell, and movement sensations are particularly important to the newborn infant, who uses these to maintain contact with a caregiver through nursing, nuzzling, and cuddling. Tactile sensations, especially, are critical in establishing a primary attachment relationship with a caregiver and fostering feelings of security in the infant. This is just the beginning of the important role that the tactile system plays in a person's emotional life because it is directly involved in making physical contact with others (Figure 9-2). Proprioception is also critical in the mother-infant relationship, enabling the infant to mold to the adult caregiver's body in a cuddly manner. The phasic movements of the infant's limbs generate additional proprioceptive inputs. Together, all of these tactile and proprioceptive inputs set the stage for the eventual development of body scheme (the brain's map of the body and how its parts interrelate).

The vestibular system is fully functional at birth, although refinement of its sensory integrative functions, particularly its integration with visual and proprioceptive systems, continues through childhood.[158] Most caregivers who use rocking and carrying to soothe and calm the infant instinctively appreciate the influence of vestibular stimuli on the infant's arousal level. Ayres pointed out that sensations such as these, which make a child contented and organized, tend to be integrating for the child's nervous system.[20]

Experiences that activate the vestibular sense have other integrating effects on the infant as well. Being lifted into an upright position against the caregiver's shoulder is known to increase alertness and visual pursuit.[103] While being held in such a position, the young infant's vestibular system detects the pull of gravity and begins to stimulate the neck muscles to raise the head off the caregiver's shoulder. This adaptive response reaches full maturation within 6 months. In the first month of life, head righting may be minimal and intermittent with much wobbling, but it will gradually stabilize and become firmly established as the baby assumes different positions (first when the baby lies in a prone position and later in the supine position).

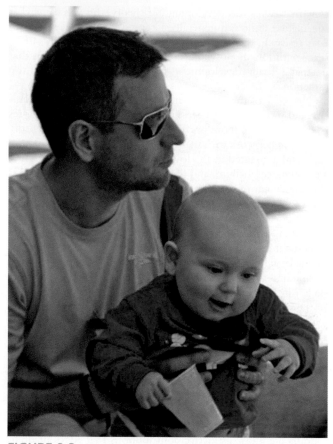

FIGURE 9-2 Tactile sensations play a critical role in generating feelings of security and comfort in the infant and are influential in emotional development and social relationships throughout the life span.

The visual and auditory systems of the newborn are immature. The newborn orients to some visual and auditory inputs and is particularly interested in human faces and voices, although meaning is not yet attached to these sensations. Visually the infant is attracted to high-contrast stimuli, such as black-and-white designs, and the range of visual acuity for most stimuli is limited to approximately 10 inches. The infant's visual acuity and responsiveness to visual patterns expand dramatically over the first few months of life.[158] During this time the infant begins to sustain eye contact with the caregiver, further strengthening the bond between them.

Stimulation in each of the sensory systems potentially affects the infant's state of arousal. The infant's capacity to behaviorally adapt to changing sensations is another important aspect of sensory integrative development—the development of self-regulation. It is relatively easy to overstimulate young infants, for example, with changes in water temperature, changes in body position, or an increase in auditory or visual stimuli.[213] However, as sensory integration develops, the older child is better able to self-regulate his or her responses to changing stimuli by initiating behaviors that facilitate calming and soothing (e.g., thumb sucking or cuddling with a favorite blanket) or exciting and energizing (e.g., jumping or singing).[195] This process of self-regulation begins in the neonatal period and develops throughout early childhood.

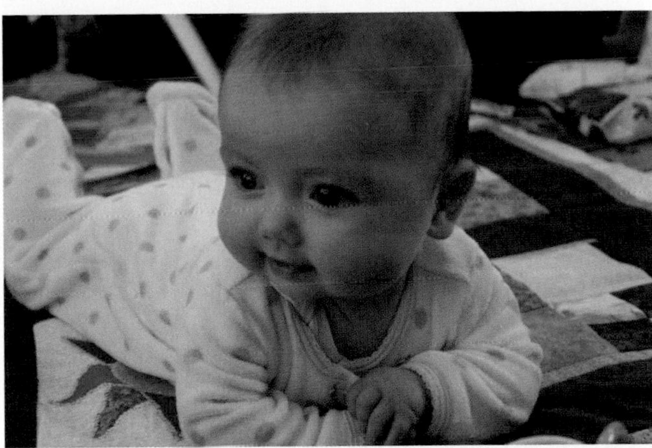

FIGURE 9-3 Strong inner drive to master gravity is evident in this infant's efforts to lift her head and shoulders off the floor. This is an early form of the prone extension posture.

First Six Months

By 4 to 6 months of age, a shift occurs in the infant's behavioral organization. The sensory systems have matured to the extent that the baby has much greater awareness and interest in the world, and developing vestibular-proprioceptive-visual connections provide the beginnings of postural control. During the first half of the first year, the infant begins to show a strong inner drive to rise up against gravity (Figure 9-3), and this drive is evident in much of the baby's spontaneous play. Body positions during the first 6 months characteristically involve the prone position, with gradually increasing extension from the neck down through the trunk as the arms gradually bear more weight to help push the chest off the floor. By 6 months of age, many infants spend much of waking playtime in the prone position with full active trunk extension, and most are able to sit independently, at least if propped with their own hands. These body positions usually are the infant's preferred positions for play and reflect the maturing of the lateral vestibulospinal tract. Head control is well established by 6 months of age and provides a stable base for control of eye muscles. The development of head control reflects the growing integration of vestibular, proprioceptive, and visual systems, which becomes increasingly important in providing a stable visual field as the baby becomes mobile.

Somatosensory maturation at this time is particularly evident in the infant's hands. The infant uses tactile and proprioceptive sensations to grasp objects, albeit with primitive grasps. Touch and visual information are integrated as the baby begins to reach for and wave or bang objects. The infant has a strong inner drive to play with the hands by bringing them to midline while watching and touching them. Connections between the tactile and visual systems pave the way for later hand-eye coordination skills. Midline hand play is a significant milestone in the integration of sensations from the two sides of the body.

By now, neonatal reflexes no longer dominate behavior; the baby is beginning to exercise voluntary control over movements during play. The earliest evidence of motor planning is observed as the infant produces simple novel actions, that is, handling objects and initiating transitions from one body position to another. Although reflexes play a role in such actions (e.g., grasp and neck righting reflexes), the infant's actions have a goal-directed, volitional quality and are not stereotypically reflex-bound. The emergence of intentionality is a marker of the beginning of occupational engagement.

Six to Twelve Months

Another major transition occurs during the latter half of the first year. Infants become mobile in their environments, and by the first birthday they can willfully move from one place to another, many walking while others creep or crawl. These locomotor skills are the product of the many adaptive responses in prior months, resulting in increasingly more sophisticated integration of somatosensory, vestibular, and visual inputs.

As the infant explores the environment, greater opportunities are generated for integrating a variety of complex sensations, particularly those responsible for developing body scheme and spatial perception. The child learns about environmental space and about the body's relationship to external space through sensorimotor experiences.

During the second 6 months after birth, tactile perception becomes further refined and plays a critical role in the child's developing hand skills. The infant relies on precise tactile feedback in developing a fine pincer grasp, which is used to pick up small objects. Proprioceptive information is also an important influence in developing manipulative skills, and now the baby experiments with objects using a variety of actions. These somatosensory-based adaptive responses contribute to development of motor planning ability. Growing evidence indicates that these early sensory motor experiences not only inform children about their own actions, but also the actions of others.[252] Further development of midline skills is also apparent as the baby easily transfers objects from one hand to the other and may occasionally cross the midline while holding an object.

Through the first year, auditory processing plays a significant role in the infant's awareness of environment, especially the social environment. Auditory information is integrated with tactile and proprioceptive sensations in and around the mouth as the infant vocalizes. The fruits of this process begin to blossom in the latter half of this first year, when the infant experiments with creating the sounds of the language used by caregivers. Vocalizations such as consonant-vowel repetitions ("baba" and "mamama") are common. Parents often attach meaning to these infant vocalizations and strongly encourage them, thus leading the infant also to attach meaning to these sounds. By their first birthday, many infants have a small vocabulary of words or wordlike sounds that they use meaningfully to communicate desires to caregivers.

Another major landmark toward the end of the first year is beginning independence in self-feeding. This complex achievement requires refined somatosensory processing of information from the lips, the jaw, and inside the mouth to guide oral movements in the chewing and swallowing of food. Taste and smell sensations are also integral to this process, but self-feeding involves more than the mouth. All of the acquired sensory integrative milestones involving hand-eye coordination are important to self-feeding. The infant at this period of life uses the fingers directly to feed him- or herself and to explore the textures of foods. At this stage, use of a spoon is not very functional and is messy because motor planning skills have not progressed to the point that the child can manipulate it successfully. However, many infants begin to demonstrate a drive

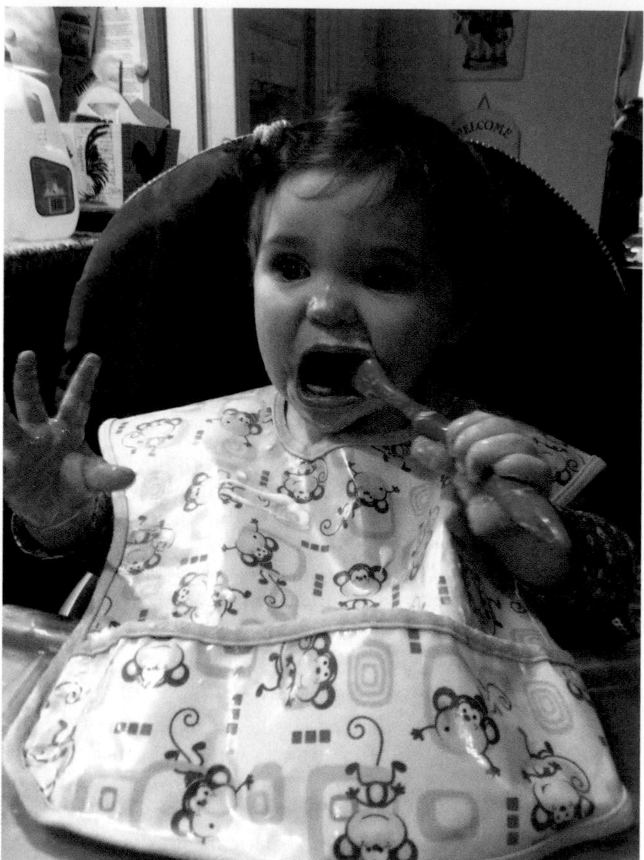

FIGURE 9-4 Because somatosensory processing and visual motor coordination strongly influence self-feeding skills, sensory integration is an important contributor to the development of dining, a fundamental occupation.

to use the spoon in self-feeding by the end of the first year. For many contemporary U.S. infants, use of a spoon is the first experience in using a tool (Figure 9-4).

The occupation of eating, then, begins to emerge in infancy as sensory integrative abilities mature, allowing the child to engage in self-feeding. As an occupation, eating in its fullest sense goes far beyond the physical, sensorimotor act. Mealtime usually takes place within a social context, whether at a family dinner at home or in a formal restaurant, so social standards for acceptable behavior and etiquette become increasingly important as the child develops. Partaking in a meal and sharing certain types of food gradually come to take on powerful symbolic meanings. The sensory integrative underpinnings of the eating experience influence how the child experiences mealtimes and how others view the child as a dining partner, thus playing a role in shaping the social and symbolic aspects of this vitally important occupation.

Second Year

As the child moves into the second year, the basic vestibular-proprioceptive-visual connections that were laid down earlier continue to refine, resulting in growing finesse in balance and fluidity of dynamic postural control. Discrimination and localization of tactile sensations also become much more precise, allowing for further refinement of fine motor skills.

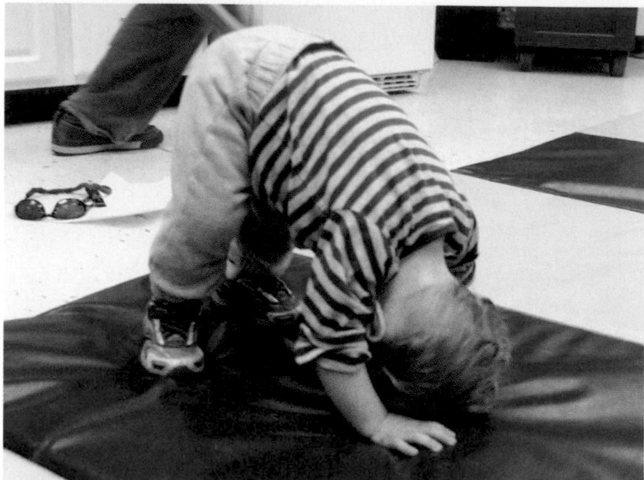

FIGURE 9-5 As motor planning develops during the second year of life, the infant experiments with a variety of body movements and learns how to transition easily from one position to another. These experiences are thought to reflect the development of body scheme.

Increasingly complex somatosensory processing contributes to the continuing development of body scheme. Ayres hypothesized that as body scheme becomes more sophisticated, so does motor planning ability.[14] The child draws on knowledge of how the body works to program novel actions (Figure 9-5). Throughout the second year, the typically developing toddler experiments with many variations in body movements. Imitation of the actions of others contributes further to the child's movement repertoire. In experiencing new actions, the child generates new sensory experiences, thus building an elaborate base of information from which to plan future actions.

Although motor planning ability becomes increasingly more complex in the second year, another aspect of praxis, ideation, begins to emerge. Ideation is the ability to conceptualize what to do in a given situation. Ideation is made possible by the cognitive ability to use symbols, first expressed gesturally and then vocally during the second year of life.[49] Symbolic functioning enables the child to engage in pretend actions and to imagine doing actions, even actions that the child has never before done. By the end of the second year, the toddler can connect several pretend actions in a play sequence.[165] Furthermore, the 2-year-old child demonstrates that he or she has a plan before performing an action sequence, either through a verbal announcement or through a search for a needed object.[165] Thus, a surge in practic development occurs in the second year as the child generates many new ideas for actions and begins to plan actions in a systematic sequence.

The burgeoning of praxis abilities plays an important role in the development of self-concept. Infant psychiatrist Daniel Stern suggests that the sense of an integrated core self begins in infancy as an outcome of the volition and the proprioceptive feedback involved in motor planning.[233] The consequences of the child's voluntary, planned actions add to the developing sense of self as an active agent in the world. Because praxis takes giant leaps during the second year, so does this sense of self as an agent of power. The child feels in command of his or her own life when sensory integration allows the child to move freely and effectively through the world.[20]

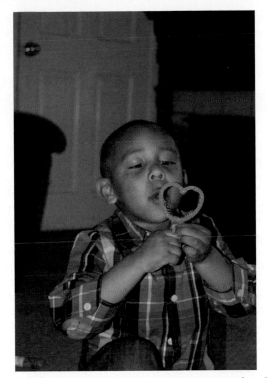

FIGURE 9-6 Blowing bubbles requires motor planning of oral movements to blow with the right amount of force, in coordination with upper extremity actions to manage the object.

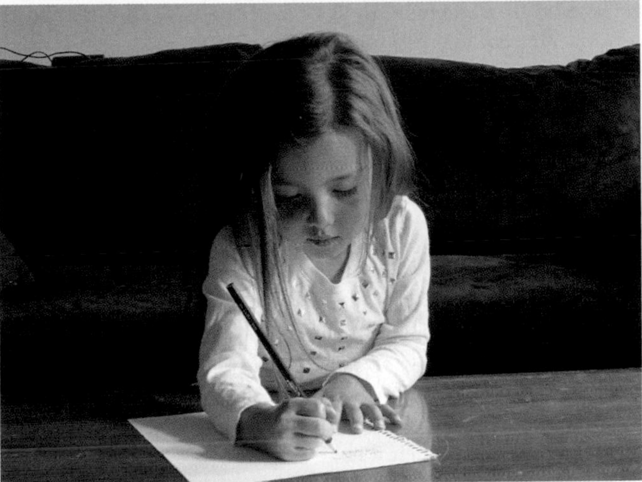

FIGURE 9-7 By the time a child reaches school age, sensory integrative capacities are almost mature. The child now can devote full attention to the demands of academic tasks because basic sensorimotor functions, such as maintaining an upright posture and guiding hand movements while holding a tool, have become automatic.

Third Through Seventh Years

The child's competencies in the sensorimotor realm mature in the third through seventh years of life, which Ayres considered a crucial period for sensory integration because of the brain's receptiveness to sensations and its capacity for organizing them at this time.[20] This is the period when sensorimotor functions become consolidated as a foundation for higher intellectual abilities. Although further sensory integrative development occurs beyond the eighth birthday, changes are fewer and less dramatic than in infancy and early childhood.

In the third through seventh years, children have strong inner drives to produce adaptive responses that not only meet complicated sensorimotor demands but also sometimes require interfacing with peers. The challenges posed by children's games and play activities attest to this complexity. In the visual-motor realm, sophistication develops through involvement in crafts, drawing and painting, constructional play with blocks and other building toys, and video games (Figure 9-6). Children are driven to explore playground equipment by swinging, sliding, climbing, jumping, riding, pushing, pulling, and pumping. Toward the end of this period they enthusiastically grapple with the motor-planning challenges posed by games such as jump rope, jacks, marbles, and hopscotch. It is also during this period that children become expert with cultural tools such as scissors, pencils, zippers, buttons, forks and knives, pails, shovels, brooms, and rakes (Figure 9-7). Many children begin to participate in occupations that present sensorimotor challenges for years to come, such as soccer, softball, karate, gymnastics, playing a musical instrument, and ballet. Furthermore, children develop the ability to organize their behavior into more complex sequences over longer time frames. This makes it possible for them to become more autonomous in orchestrating daily routines, such as getting ready for school in the morning, completing homework and other school projects, and performing household chores.

As children participate in these occupations, they must frequently anticipate how to move in relation to changing environmental events by accurately timing and sequencing their actions.[53] This is particularly challenging in sports when peers, with their often unpredictable moves, are involved. Their bodies are challenged to maintain balance through dynamic changes in body position. In fine motor tasks, children must efficiently coordinate visual with somatosensory information to guide eye and hand movements with accuracy and precision while maintaining a stable postural base.

Children meet these challenges with varying degrees of success. Some are more talented than others with respect to sensory integrative abilities, but most children eventually achieve a degree of competency that allows them to fully participate in the daily occupations that they are expected to do and wish to do at home, in school, and in the community. Furthermore, most children experience feelings of satisfaction and self-efficacy as they master occupations that depend heavily on sensory integration.

When Problems in Sensory Integration Occur

Not every child develops sensory integration in the same way, and for some children, differences in sensory integrative functions create challenges in daily life. When some aspect of sensory integration does not work well, the child may experience difficulties in the course of everyday occupations because processes that should be automatic or accurate are not. It may be stressful, for example, to get dressed in the morning before school, attempt to play jump rope, or eat lunch in a socially acceptable manner. The child may be aware of these difficulties and become frustrated by frequent failure when confronted with ordinary tasks that come easily for other children. Many children with sensory integrative problems develop a tendency to avoid or reject simple sensory or motor challenges, responding with refusals or tantrums when pushed to perform. If this becomes a long-term pattern of behavior, the child may miss important experiences, such as playing games with peers, which are critical in building feelings of competency, mastering a wide repertoire of useful skills, and developing flexible social strategies. Thus, the capacity to participate fully in the occupations that the child wants and needs to do is compromised.

Often behavioral, social, academic, or motor coordination concerns are cited when a child with sensory integrative challenges is referred for occupational therapy. The occupational therapist evaluates whether a sensory integration problem may underlie these concerns. The therapist then must decide on a course of action to help the child move toward the goal of greater success and satisfaction in engaging in meaningful occupations. These challenges to the occupational therapist—to identify a problem that may be hidden and decipher how to best help the child—were the challenges to which Ayres devoted most of her career.

Beginning in the 1960s, Ayres[6] conducted research over several decades to develop her theory of sensory integration and evaluate the assessment and intervention methods that she created to help children who have difficulty processing sensory information. She also mentored many occupational therapists who used her theory in practice and conducted research to evaluate, expand on, or modify her theory. While conducting her research, she maintained a private practice; thus, she had many years of firsthand clinical experience on which to ground her theoretical work.

As a step toward better understanding the difficulties of children with learning and behavior problems, Ayres developed standardized tests[12,22] that measured visual, tactile, and kinesthetic perception, as well as central vestibular processing, motor planning, and other sensorimotor abilities. She statistically analyzed test scores and behavior observations to identify different patterns of sensory integration functioning among children with a variety of learning and behavior difficulties.

Ayres found similar patterns of sensory integration functions as well as problems across multiple studies involving diverse samples of children. The key factors discovered by Ayres were replicated by Mulligan in a confirmatory factor analytic study of more than 10,000 children across the United States who had been clinically referred to occupational therapists.[179] Mailloux et al.[155] also replicated most of the factors identified by Ayres and Mulligan. Tables 9-1e and 9-2e in Evolve summarize these studies and other studies of sensory integration patterns. The robustness of patterns across many studies strengthens the hypothesis that these patterns are generalizable and relevant to a child's ability to be successful in everyday life. Evidence-based practice in sensory integration assessment, therefore, includes a comprehensive effort to evaluate these patterns. Knowledge of these patterns provides the therapist with critical information to accurately interpret assessment data and develop individualized intervention that addresses the child's specific strengths and limitations in the various patterns of sensory integration functions and problems. In the following sections, the general categories of sensory integrative problems that concern clinicians today, based on research findings and clinical experience, are discussed.

Types of Sensory Integration Problems

The results of research, combined with the experiences of practitioners and the ongoing work of scholars in the field, have led to the identification of patterns of individual differences in sensory integration. The terms *sensory integrative problems*, *sensory integrative disorder*, *sensory integrative dysfunction*, and *sensory processing disorder* do not refer to one specific type of difficulty but to a heterogeneous group of patterns that emerge developmentally (i.e., not owing to trauma) and are thought to reflect subtle neural processing differences involving sensory and motor systems. This chapter uses words such as *dysfunction* or *disorder* primarily when referring to particular work in the field that has used these terms. In general, however, we use the terms *sensory integrative patterns*, *problems*, *differences*, or *difficulties*, instead of *disorders* or *dysfunction*, to emphasize our view that differences in sensory integration are part of being human, rather than pathologies. All of us encounter problems or difficulties in life, and for those of us who have difficulty with sensory integration, the problems often fall into predictable patterns. Familiarity with these patterns, and with the related research, assists the occupational therapist in determining how sensory integration problems should be addressed when planning intervention for a particular child.

Most discussions of sensory integrative problems assume normal sensory receptor function. In other words, sensory integrative differences involve central, rather than peripheral, sensory functions. This assumption has been supported in several well-designed studies. For instance, Parush and her colleagues found that the somatosensory-evoked potentials of children with attention deficit hyperactivity disorder (ADHD) differ from those of typically developing children with respect to indicators of central tactile processing but not peripheral receptor responses.[189] Many of the children with ADHD in this study were also identified as having tactile defensiveness, a sensory integrative problem. In another study, researchers found that children with learning disabilities, compared with nondisabled children, had impaired postural responses involving central integration of vestibular, proprioceptive, and visual inputs, whereas measures of peripheral receptor functions were normal.[223] Thus, when sensory integrative problems involving the vestibular system are discussed, these problems are generally thought to be based within CNS structures and pathways (i.e., the vestibular nuclei and its connections) rather than the vestibular receptors (i.e., the semicircular canals, utricle, or saccule).[251] In this chapter, the discussions of sensory integrative problems assume that peripheral receptor function is normal.

As noted, different conceptualizations of sensory integrative problems have been generated over the years. Although perfect consensus on how to categorize these problems does not exist, clearly there are recurring themes across authors. Distinct but overlapping taxonomies and models of sensory integrative problems include, for example, those of Bundy and Murray[53] and Kimball.[130] Bundy and Murray presented a taxonomic model that depicts sensory integrative dysfunction as manifested in two major ways: poor sensory modulation and poor praxis.[53] Miller, Anzalone, Lane, Cermak, and Osten[169] proposed use of the term *sensory processing disorder* to include three main types of problems: sensory modulation disorder (i.e., over-responsiveness, under-responsiveness, and sensory seeking), sensory-based motor disorder (incorporating the postural-bilateral and dyspraxia patterns identified by Ayres),[21] and sensory discrimination disorder (perceptual problems identified by Ayres). Some models specifically focus on sensory modulation. For example, Cermak[60] and Royeen[211] hypothesized that sensory responsiveness follows a continuum, with hypo-responsiveness at one end and hyper-responsiveness at the other. Dunn later presented a quadrant model that takes into account the potential roles of various neural processes in generating patterns of under-responsiveness and over-responsiveness.[80,82]

For the purposes of this chapter, four general categories of sensory integration problems are discussed:

1. Sensory modulation problems
2. Sensory discrimination and perception problems
3. Vestibular-bilateral functional problems
4. Praxis problems

These four categories are used here because they are consistent with research that has accumulated from the 1960s to the present. Although variations were reported across studies, these patterns of sensory integration problems emerged in research on different samples of children over many decades. This research indicated that the patterns are interrelated and often coexist in individual children. When planning intervention, occupational therapists need to carefully analyze assessment data to discern whether one or more specific patterns of sensory integration problems seem to be affecting an individual child's participation in activities.

Sensory-seeking behavior is often seen in conjunction with these four main types of sensory integration problems. Although sensory seeking sometimes is addressed as a type of sensory integration problem, this chapter discusses it as a set of diverse behaviors that often co-occur with the four main types of SI problems. Sensory seeking may serve a variety of adaptive purposes for a child who is struggling with some aspect of sensory integration. When planning intervention for children whose sensory-seeking behavior is a concern, the therapist must carefully analyze why the behavior may be occurring, in light of assessment data on SI functioning as well as other factors such as temperament and events in the child's life. In the next section of this chapter, we discuss each of the four main categories of sensory integration problems. This is followed by a discussion of sensory-seeking behaviors and some of the diverse reasons why these behaviors may occur.

Sensory Modulation Problems

Modulation refers to CNS regulation of its own activity.[20] The term *sensory modulation* refers to the tendency to generate responses that are appropriately graded in relation to incoming sensory stimuli, rather than under-responding or over-responding to them.

Sensory modulation has been widely studied in the past decade. Most studies of the sensory characteristics of children use sensory questionnaires completed by adults, which are valuable instruments but rely on the reports of parents and teachers. Sensory questionnaires tend to focus on over-responsiveness (one type of modulation problem that involves strong reactions to ordinary stimuli), because the child behaviors associated with this condition are easily noticed and relatively easy to report in a reliable manner. Consequently, it has become commonplace for many professionals outside occupational therapy (and some inside the profession) to think of sensory modulation problems, and over-responsiveness in particular, when they hear the terms *sensory processing* or *sensory integration*. Prevalence of sensory modulation problems among 4- to 6-year-old children in the general population, as determined through parent questionnaire data, is estimated to be about 5%.[1] No large epidemiological studies have been conducted for children with developmental challenges, but prevalence estimates based on smaller studies consistently indicate a relatively high incidence of modulation problems. It may be greater than 80% among children with autism.[34,144]

Research on patterns of sensory modulation and their manifestations in everyday activities is an area of focused investigation in occupational therapy[32,86,172] and in interdisciplinary research on children with diagnoses such as autism[42,139,140,148] and attention deficit disorder.[85,253] Many children (e.g., children with autism spectrum disorder [ASD]) demonstrate behavioral characteristics of both under-responding and over-responding, often within the same sensory system.[33,41,138,235] In addition, the relationship between physiologic measures and patterns of behavior that characterize sensory modulation problems continues to be explored through studies of brain electrical activity[76] and autonomic responses[64,170,214,215,222] to sensory input.

Although much remains to be learned about sensory modulation, a general consensus exists among sensory integration experts regarding the behaviors that characterize different kinds of sensory modulation difficulties. These behaviors are described in the following sections.

Under-responsiveness and Sensory Registration Problems

As noted previously, sensory integration is the "organization of sensory input for use" (p. 184).[20] However, for sensory information to be used functionally, it must first be registered within the CNS. When the CNS is working well, it knows when to "pay attention" to a stimulus and when to "ignore" it. Most of the time, this process occurs automatically and efficiently. For example, a student may not be aware of the noise of traffic outside the window of a classroom while listening to a lecture, instead focusing attention on the sound of the lecturer's words. In this situation, the student registers the auditory stimuli generated by the lecturer but not the stimuli generated by the traffic. The process of sensory registration is critical in enabling efficient function so that people pay attention to stimuli that enable them to accomplish desired goals. Simultaneously, if the process is working well, energy is not wasted attending to irrelevant sensory information.

Traditionally, occupational therapists, beginning with Ayres,[20,27] have used the term *sensory registration* problem to refer to the difficulties of the person who frequently does not notice or "register" relevant environmental stimuli. This kind of problem is considered to be a form of modulation difficulty involving under-responsiveness (also called *hypo-responsiveness*). It is often seen in individuals with autism[33,42,204] but may also be seen in other individuals. Under-responsiveness appears to be one of the earliest developing features of autism, particularly lack of response to social signals from others, such as the sound of a caregiver calling the child's name.[31,98] When a pervasive sensory registration problem is present, the child often seems oblivious to touch, pain, movement, taste, smells, sights, or sounds. The key point is that the child is not aware that the stimulus is present. Usually more than one sensory system is involved, but for some children one system may be particularly affected. Among children with ASD, a common finding is that the child does not register socially relevant stimuli but is over-focused on irrelevant stimuli. Children with developmental problems, including ASD, may lack sensory registration in some situations but react with extreme sensory over-responsiveness in other situations.[33,101]

Safety concerns are frequently an important issue among children with sensory registration problems. For example, the child who does not register pain sensations may not have learned that certain actions naturally lead to the negative consequence of pain, and therefore may not withdraw adequately from dangerous situations. Instead of avoiding situations likely to result in pain, the child may repeatedly engage in activities that may be injurious, such as jumping from a dangerous height onto a hard surface or walking over toys with sharp edges. Other children with sensory registration problems may not register noxious tastes and smells that warn of hazards. Similarly, sights and sounds such as sirens, flashing lights, firm voice commands, and hand signals or signs that are meant to warn of perils go unheeded if not registered. This can be a life-endangering problem in some circumstances (e.g., when a child is at risk for stepping into traffic).

When a child appears to not notice or respond to certain stimuli, it is important to consider whether the underlying problem is a perceptual or cognitive difficulty, rather than a lack of registration. For example, a child who has a tactile perception problem may register the sensation of a tactile stimulus in the hand, but have so much difficulty with stereognosis (a form of tactile perception) that she does not actively manipulate objects. She is unable to interpret the complex, changing three-dimensional tactile sensations that occur when an object moves in her hand, so she has not learned to use object manipulation to gain tactile information as a guide to movement. To the novice therapist, it may appear that this child does not notice the stimulus and therefore is under-responsive, when actually the child may be aware that the stimulus is present but is not able to accurately perceive the complex three-dimensional tactile information provided by the object. In this example, the child's lack of active object manipulation is caused by tactile perception or cognitive limitations rather than under-responsiveness (i.e., a registration problem).

A sensory registration problem interferes with the child's ability to attach meaning to an activity or situation because critical information is not being noticed. Consequently, in severe cases, the child lacks the inner drive that compels most children to master ordinary childhood occupations (e.g., the child who is generally unmotivated to engage in play activities or to practice skills). Symbolic play and language development may be impeded, particularly if auditory and visual stimuli related to social meanings and messages are not registered.[241] Therefore the long-term effects on the child's development can be profound.

Over-responsiveness

At the opposite end of the sensory modulation continuum are problems associated with over-responsiveness, sometimes called *hyper-responsiveness* or *sensory defensiveness.* The term *sensory defensiveness* was first introduced by Knickerbocker[132] and later used by Wilbarger and Wilbarger[153] to describe sensory modulation difficulties involving over-responsiveness in multiple sensory systems, such as over-reactions to touch, movement, sounds, odors, and tastes, that are often associated with discomfort, avoidance, distractibility, and anxiety. The child who is over-responsive is overwhelmed by ordinary sensory input and reacts defensively to it, often with strong anxiety[192] and activation of the sympathetic nervous system.[64] This condition may occur as a general response to all types of sensory input, or it may be specific to one or a few sensory systems.

A large study of tactile and auditory over-responsiveness in randomly selected elementary school-aged children with no disabilities produced a prevalence estimate of about 17%.[42] In this study, most of the children who were scored as over-responsive demonstrated difficulty specifically with tactile sensations but not auditory. Similarly, a large study of twin toddlers found that tactile and auditory over-responsiveness appear to be distinct conditions, with tactile over-responsiveness particularly likely to have a genetic influence.[100] However, sociodemographic factors such as poverty, minority ethnicity, low birthweight, and exposure to environmental toxins may also play a significant role in the prevalence of over-responsiveness.[42,200,210]

Anxiety is so common among children with sensory over-responsiveness that the relationship between these two conditions has been given increasing scrutiny in recent years. Unusually high rates of coexisting sensory over-responsiveness and anxiety disorders have been documented for children with attention deficit disorders,[141,198] children with autism,[102] and children and adults with obsessive-compulsive disorder.[201] Both anxiety and sensory over-responsiveness involve states of over-arousal in response to stimuli, perhaps because of neurophysiologic mechanisms such as abnormal amygdala activity.[102,192] Green and Ben-Sasson[102] proposed three possible theories that could explain the association between sensory over-responsiveness and anxiety disorders: (1) anxiety causes sensory over-responsiveness, (2) sensory over-responsiveness causes anxiety, or (3) these two conditions are associated through a common risk factor, such as abnormal amygdala activity. Because an understanding of the underlying causal mechanisms for these conditions will inform decisions regarding appropriate interventions, ongoing research on this issue is imperative.

Over-responsiveness to particular sensory stimuli is very common among children with autism and, as noted earlier, often coexists with under-responsiveness.[33,42,204] In other words, a child may be unusually over-responsive to certain types of stimuli, but does not register other types of stimuli that peers notice. Over-responsiveness in autism is very often manifested as tactile defensiveness, for example, avoidance of certain textures of clothing or food, or as auditory defensiveness, as in showing distress or holding hands over the ears in reaction to certain sounds.

Tactile Defensiveness

Tactile defensiveness involves a tendency to over-react to ordinary touch sensations.[7,14,20] It is one of the most commonly observed sensory modulation problems. Individuals with tactile defensiveness experience irritation and discomfort from sensations that most people do not find bothersome. Light touch sensations are especially likely to be disturbing. Common irritants include certain textures of clothing, grass or sand against bare skin, glue or paint on the skin, the light brush of another person passing by, the sensations generated when having one's hair or teeth brushed, and certain textures of food. Common responses to such irritants include anxiety, distractibility, restlessness, anger, throwing a tantrum, aggression, fear, and emotional distress.

Common self-care activities such as dressing, bathing, grooming, and eating are often affected by tactile defensiveness. Classroom activities such as finger painting, sand and water play, and crafts may be avoided. Social situations involving close proximity to others, such as playing near other children or standing in line, tend to be uncomfortable and may be disturbing enough to lead to emotional outbursts. Thus, ordinary daily routines can become traumatic for children with tactile defensiveness and for their parents. Individuals with tactile defensiveness can be stressed when they realize that others do not share their discomforts and may actually enjoy situations that they find so upsetting. Teachers and friends are likely to misinterpret the child with tactile defensiveness as being rejecting, aggressive, or simply negative.

An occupational therapist working with a child who is tactually defensive must become aware of the specific kinds of tactile input that are aversive and the kinds that are tolerated by that particular child. Usually, light touch stimuli are aversive, especially when they occur in the most sensitive body areas such as the face, abdomen, and palmar surfaces of the upper and lower extremities. Generally, tactile stimuli that are actively self-applied by the child are tolerated much more easily than stimuli that are passively received, as when being touched by another person. Tactile stimuli may be especially threatening if the child cannot see the source of the touch. Most individuals with tactile defensiveness feel comfortable with deep touch stimuli and may experience relief from irritating stimuli when deep pressure is applied.

Knowledge of these characteristics of tactile defensiveness helps the occupational therapist identify strategies that help the child and others who interact with the child to cope with this condition. For example, the occupational therapist may recommend to the teacher that if the child needs to be touched, it should be done with firm pressure in the child's view, rather than with a light touch from behind the child. Helping a child prepare for sensory experiences in advance can lower stress and anxiety for many children. For example, showing pictures of children getting haircuts may make the situation less anxiety-provoking for some children, as it may help them to know what to expect. Using other forms of sensory feedback, such as a mirror for teeth brushing or hair washing, may also reduce the aversion felt by some children in these tasks. Deep touch pressure is a naturally calming and overriding sensation (e.g., when we rub a place on the body that hurts). Helping a child by rubbing away ticklish or irritating sensory input with soothing words that Dr. Ayres used, such as, "Sometimes rubbing will make that bothersome feeling go away," are still useful today.

Gravitational Insecurity

Gravitational insecurity is a form of over-responsiveness to vestibular sensations involving linear movement, particularly sensations from the pull of gravity and from vertical movement through space.[20] Children with this problem have an insecure relationship to gravity characterized by excessive fear during ordinary movement activities. The gravitationally insecure child is overwhelmed by changes in head position and movement, especially when moving backward or upward through space. Fear of heights, even those involving only slight distances from the ground, is a common problem associated with this condition. Research evidence suggests that some children with autism have this distinct type of over-responsiveness to movement.[139,140]

Children with gravitational insecurity often display signs of inordinate fear, anxiety, or avoidance in relation to stairs, escalators or elevators, stepstools or ladders, playground equipment that moves, and uneven or unpredictable surfaces. Some children are so insecure that only a small change from one surface to another, as when stepping off the curb or from the sidewalk to the grass, is enough to send them into a state of high anxiety or panic.

Common reactions of children with gravitational insecurity include extreme fearfulness during low-intensity linear movement or when anticipating movement, and avoidance of tilting the head in different planes (especially backward). They tend to move slowly and carefully, and they may refuse to participate in many gross motor activities. When they do engage in movement activities such as swinging, many of these children resist lifting their feet off the ground. When threatened by simple motor activities, they may try to gain as much contact with the ground as possible or they may tightly clutch a nearby adult for security. These children often have signs of poor proprioception in addition to the vestibular over-responsiveness. May-Benson and Koomar developed a Gravitational Insecurity (GI) Assessment (see Evolve website) and found that scores on this standardized tool, which involves activities such as performing a backward roll and stepping off a chair with eyes closed, significantly discriminated between children with gravitational insecurity and typical children.[161]

Playground and park activities are often difficult for children with gravitational insecurity, as are other common childhood activities such as bicycle riding, ice skating, roller skating, skateboarding, skiing, and hiking. The ability to play with peers and explore the environment is therefore significantly affected. Functioning in the community may also be affected when the child needs to use escalators, stairs, and elevators.

A distinction may be made between gravitational insecurity and a similar condition called *postural insecurity*. Postural insecurity refers to fearfulness of full body movement resulting from limited postural stability or motor control. The fears of children with postural insecurity result from a learned, realistic appraisal of their motor limitations, not a modulation problem per se. Often it is difficult to discern whether a child's anxiety during movement activities is primarily sensory, that is, caused by vestibular over-responsiveness, or primarily resulting from limited motor control, because these two conditions can coexist in the same child. Sometimes, however, the distinction is clear. Children with mild spastic diplegia, for example, commonly have postural but not gravitational insecurity. These children typically (and appropriately) react with anxiety when faced with a minimal climbing task because they are aware that they lack the refined motor control needed to safely climb. However, these same children may show pleasure at receiving vestibular stimulation, including movement of the head in different planes, as long as they are securely held and do not have to rely on their own motor skills to maintain a safe position.

Over-responsiveness in Other Sensory Modalities

Over-responsiveness in other sensory systems can also have a significant influence on a person's life. For example, most people interpret the raucous sounds found at birthday parties, parades, playgrounds, and carnivals as happy sounds, but these can be overwhelming and distressing to a child with auditory defensiveness. Similarly, a visually busy and unfamiliar environment may evoke an unusual degree of anxiety in a child with visual defensiveness. The variety of tastes and odors encountered in some environments may be disturbing to a child with over-responsiveness in these systems.

Auditory defensiveness is very common among children with autism or other developmental disabilities[32] and probably contributes greatly to difficulties with social participation. Lane and colleagues have documented that a subgroup of children with autism have extreme taste and smell sensitivities.[139,140] These types of problems, like over-responsiveness to touch and movement, may create discomfort, avoidance, distractibility, and anxiety.

Sensory Discrimination and Perception Problems

Sensory discrimination and perception allow for refined organization and interpretation of sensory stimuli. *Discrimination* refers to the brain's ability to distinguish between different sensory stimuli, such as two points touched on the skin simultaneously. *Perception* is the brain's process of giving meaning to sensory information, as when the complex visual stimuli from a person's face are integrated and interpreted as a particular facial expression of emotion. Some types of sensory integrative disorders involve inefficient or inaccurate organization of sensory information (e.g., difficulty differentiating one stimulus from another or difficulty perceiving the spatial or temporal relationships among stimuli). A classic example involving the visual system is that of the older child with a learning disability who persists in confusing a *b* with a *d*. A child with an auditory discrimination problem may be unable to distinguish between the sounds of the words *doll* and *tall*. A child with a tactile perception problem may not be able to distinguish between a square block and a hexagonal block using touch only, without visual cues.

Some children with perceptual problems have no difficulty with sensory modulation. However, modulation problems often coexist with perceptual problems. It is reasonable to expect that these two types of problems are associated, because a child who has registration problems may have limited perceptual skills owing to a lack of experience interacting with sensory information. The child who has sensory defensiveness may exert energy trying to avoid certain sensory experiences. Defensive reactions may make it difficult to attend to the detailed features of a stimulus and thereby may impede perception.

Discrimination or perception problems can occur in any sensory system. They are best detected by standardized tests, except in the case of proprioception, which is difficult to measure in a standardized manner. Although most factor analytic studies of the Sensory Integration and Praxis Tests (SIPT) scores revealed patterns that linked perception with motor functions, certain patterns reflected perception factors that were specific to a particular sensory system (e.g., a visual form and space perception factor or a tactile perception factor as well as a somatosensory perception factor). Professionals in many fields, such as clinical psychology, special education, and speech language pathology, are trained to evaluate perceptual problems, and their focus usually is on the visual and auditory systems. Most of the clinical assessment tools in visual and auditory perception focus on literacy-related perceptual functions, such as visual discrimination of two-dimensional diagrams or letters and auditory discrimination of phonemes. In contrast, occupational therapists have expertise in the functional aspects of lesser known areas of perception such as tactile, proprioceptive, and vestibular processing.

Tactile Discrimination and Perception Problems

Poor tactile perception is a common sensory integrative problem. Children with this disorder have difficulty interpreting tactile stimuli in a precise and efficient manner. For example, they may have difficulty localizing precisely where an object has brushed against them or using stereognosis to manipulate an object that is out of sight. Fine motor skills are likely to be affected when a tactile perception problem is present, especially if tactile defensiveness is also present.[58]

As discussed, the tactile system is a critical modality for learning during infancy and early childhood. Tactile exploration using the hands and mouth is particularly important. If tactile perception is vague or inaccurate, the child is at a disadvantage in learning about the different properties of objects and substances. It may be difficult for a child with such problems to develop the manipulative skills needed to efficiently perform tasks such as connecting pieces of constructional toys, fastening buttons or snaps, braiding hair, or playing marbles. Inadequate tactile perception also interferes with the feedback that is normally used to precisely guide movement during activities such as writing with a pencil, manipulating a spoon, or holding a piece of paper with one hand while cutting with the other.

Tactile perception is associated with visual perception[25]; thus, it is fairly common to see children with problems in both of these sensory systems. Not surprisingly, these children tend to have concomitant problems with hand-eye coordination. A discrete somatosensory perception factor emerged as a pattern in analyses of the SIPT,[22] but a more striking finding in the factor analytic studies of sensory integration tests over many decades was the link between tactile perception and motor planning, which recurred in many different studies.[8-10,12,13,18,25,179] These findings led Ayres to hypothesize that tactile perception is an important contributor to the ability to plan actions. She speculated that the tactile system is responsible for the development of body scheme, which then becomes an important foundation for praxis.

Ordinarily, tactile perception operates at such an automatic level that, when it is not working well, compensation strategies take a great deal of energy. For example, a child who cannot make the subtle manipulations to fasten a button needs to use compensatory visual guidance; as a result, the task of buttoning, usually performed rapidly and automatically, becomes tedious, tiring, and frustrating. The necessity of using such compensatory strategies throughout the day tends to interrupt the child's ability to focus on the more complex conceptual and social elements of tasks and situations.

Proprioception Problems

Another type of perceptual problem involves proprioception, wherein the muscles and joints inform the brain about the position of body parts. Research on this sensory system is limited because specific measures of proprioception with adequate normative data are not available. However, the experiences of master clinicians suggest that many children have serious difficulties interpreting proprioceptive information.

Children who do not receive reliable information about body position often appear clumsy and awkward. Children with inadequate feedback about body position must often rely on visual cues or other cognitive strategies (e.g., use of verbalizations) to perform simple aspects of tasks, such as staying in a chair or using a fork correctly. Other common attributes of children with poor proprioception include using too much or too little force in activities such as writing, clapping, marching, or keyboarding. Breaking toys, bumping into others, and misjudging personal space are other consequences of poor proprioception that have strong social implications.

Many children thought to have proprioception problems seek firm pressure to their skin or joint compression and traction. These sensation-seeking behaviors may be an attempt to gain additional feedback about body position, or they may reflect a concomitant hypo-responsiveness to tactile and proprioceptive sensations. In any case, if these behaviors are done in socially inappropriate ways or at inopportune times, such as leaning on another child during circle time or hanging from a doorway at school, the child's behavior may be misinterpreted as being willfully disruptive.

For many years, occupational therapists have hypothesized that children with autism have difficulty with proprioception.[48] A recent study of adolescents with autism found no deficits in simple proprioception of isolated limb position.[99] This finding indicates that peripheral proprioceptors probably function normally in autism. However, it is plausible that the proprioceptive problems of concern to occupational therapists are related to integration of proprioceptive information from the entire body to guide complex action. Praxis difficulties in ASD may relate to proprioceptive inefficiencies and are discussed later in this chapter.

Visual Perception Problems

Visual perception is an important factor in the competent performance of many constructional play activities and fine motor tasks. Early factor analyses of sensory integration test scores revealed a form and space perception factor. Tests are available to measure figure-ground perception, spatial orientation, depth perception, and visual closure, to name just a few of the many aspects of visual perception that have been of concern to professionals in many disciplines.

Problems with visual perception are commonly seen in children with sensory integrative difficulties, particularly when poor tactile perception or dyspraxia is present.[22,25] Whereas some children have only a specific visual perception problem without any other sign of sensory integrative difficulty, many others who have visual perception problems also have broader sensory integration difficulties. Henderson, Pehoski, and Murray point out the many relationships between visual spatial abilities and functions such as grasp, balance, locomotion, construction, and cognition.[109] As these authors note, low scores on tests of visual perception can occur for a variety of reasons and in some cases will represent a problem that therapists would not view as reflective of a sensory integrative issue.

A sensory integrative intervention approach, as described later in this chapter, may be appropriate for the child who demonstrates visual perception problems along with other indicators of sensory integrative difficulties, such as poor tactile perception or praxis. However, if the child has a discrete problem with visual perception, an alternative intervention may be more helpful. When other sensory integration issues are not present or have been resolved with intervention, the occupational therapist may choose to work with the child using another approach, such as visual perception training, use of compensatory strategies, or skill training in specific activities.

Many children with autism have strengths in visual perception, especially in regard to ability to perceive visual details.[34,177] However, children with these talents may also have difficulty with more global, gestalt-type visual perception as well as decreased perception of moving visual stimuli.

Other Perceptual Problems

Many other dimensions of perception and sensory discrimination exist. For example, perception of movement through space involves the integration of vestibular, proprioceptive, and visual sensations and may be affected in children with vestibular-proprioceptive problems. Auditory perception is an important function that may, when impaired, contribute to sensory integrative disorders in some children. The field of speech pathology has introduced the term *central auditory processing disorders* in reference to problems with auditory perception and modulation, and some authors have suggested that more attention should be given to the role of the auditory system in the sensory integration literature.[56] However, because so much of the function of the auditory system is related to the functions of hearing, speech, and language, this area of study in sensory integration may be most appropriately pursued in collaboration with speech-language pathologists and audiologists. Although auditory perception problems are not usually considered to be a type of sensory integrative condition when seen in isolation, difficulties with auditory perception and language development often coexist with signs of sensory integrative difficulties. The relationship between these processes warrants further research.

Vestibular-Bilateral Problems

A type of sensory integration problem that was identified early in Ayres' research involves difficulty with functions that are closely associated with the vestibular system. As research emerged using different measures across several decades, different terms were used to refer to this type of problem, including *postural and bilateral integration* disorder,[14] *vestibular-bilateral integration* (VBI) disorder, [19] *bilateral integration and sequencing* (BIS) pattern,[22] and *vestibular bilateral integration and sequencing* (VBIS) pattern. These terms refer to the same general constellation of clinical signs and test scores that involve motor outcomes of vestibular processing. This chapter uses the term *vestibular-bilateral problems* to refer to this type of sensory integration pattern.

Vestibular-bilateral functions are assessed primarily using informal and formal clinical observations, as well as standardized tests. Observations of head and trunk control, balance and bilateral coordination, and vestibular-ocular functions during spontaneous, naturally occurring activities are informative. Clinical observations such as the ability to assume and maintain a prone extension ("superman") body position are valuable as well. Relevant SIPT tests include Standing and Walking Balance, Bilateral Motor Coordination, and Postrotary Nystagmus (PRN). Postrotary nystagmus, a normal reflexive back-and-forth movement pattern of the eyes following rotary vestibular stimulation, may be shorter than average in duration. Shortened duration of postrotary nystagmus is associated with other signs of vestibular processing difficulty, including limitations in smooth sequencing of bilateral movements.[22,95,155] A recent study indicated that the PRN test is feasible to administer to infants and toddlers when they are seated on an adult's lap and that PRN scores for these young children are comparable to those of typical 5-year-olds. These findings suggest that the PRN test may be valid to use in assessment of infants and toddlers.[156]

Inefficient balance and equilibrium reactions, as well as poor bilateral coordination, are likely to affect competence in performing activities such as bicycle riding, roller-skating, skiing, and playing games like hopscotch. In addition, difficulty with bilateral coordination may make activities such as cutting with scissors, buttoning a shirt, or doing jumping jacks especially challenging. Bilateral motor difficulties are sometimes associated with delays in body midline skill development, such as hand preference, spontaneous crossing of the body midline, and right-left discrimination.

Children with vestibular-bilateral signs, and no other sensory integration problems, typically do not appear to have a disability so they are seldom referred to a health professional for assessment. When they are referred, the reasons for referral usually include clumsiness or incoordination, difficulty with team sports, slumping or slouching when sitting and doing academic tasks, and attention difficulties.

Although some children with vestibular-bilateral problems have no other sensory integration difficulties, research has shown that vestibular functions such as postural control may be impaired in children with sensory modulation difficulties.[234] The limited research that has examined vestibular functions of children with ASD suggests that postural control in these children may be underdeveloped.[176] A prospective study of infants who were siblings of children with autism, and therefore at high risk for autism, showed that delayed head lag (a measure of emerging head control and postural stability) was a predictor of diagnosis of autism at age 36 months.[96]

Praxis Problems

Praxis is the ability to conceptualize, plan, and execute a nonhabitual motor act.[20] Problems with praxis are often referred to as *dyspraxia* or *problems in motor planning*. When the term *dyspraxia* is used in regard to children, it usually refers to a condition characterized by difficulty with motor planning that emerges in early childhood and cannot be explained by a medical diagnosis, developmental disability, or environmental constraint.

Ayres was struck with the relationship between tactile perception and praxis that emerged in her studies. She hypothesized that tactile perception contributes to development of an accurate and precise body scheme, which is necessary for planning new actions. Ayres introduced the idea that praxis problems may be manifested in different forms, not all of which are sensory integrative in nature.[22] She coined the term *somatopraxis* to refer to the aspect of praxis that is sensory integrative in origin and grounded in somatosensory processing. At the same time she introduced the term *somatodyspraxia* to refer to a sensory integrative deficit that involves poor praxis and impaired tactile and proprioceptive processing. By definition, somatodyspraxia involves poor tactile perception in conjunction with signs of poor motor planning.[61] This pattern of sensory integrative dysfunction was identified by Ayres and replicated in recent factor analytic studies.[155,179]

The child with somatodyspraxia typically appears clumsy and awkward. Novel motor activities are performed with great difficulty and often result in frustration. Transitioning from one body position to another or sequencing and timing the actions involved in a motor task may pose a great challenge. These children typically have difficulty relating their bodies to physical objects in environmental space. They often have difficulty accurately imitating actions of others. Precision of movement may be poor, resulting in unintentional knocking down of toys or inefficient placement of materials and objects. Many of these children have difficulties with oral praxis, which may affect eating skills or speech articulation.

Ayres also demonstrated the relationship between visual perception and visually directed praxis in numerous studies. She used the term *visuopraxis* to describe this relationship and the term *visuodyspraxia* for patterns in which these functions were paired as areas of difficulty. In both the studies conducted by Ayres as well as subsequent research, visuodyspraxia was shown to sometimes occur in conjunction with somatodyspraxia.[25] Some children with dyspraxia have problems with *ideation* (i.e., they have difficulty generating ideas of what to do in a novel situation or conceiving play possibilities when presented with unfamiliar toys or objects). When asked to simply play, without being given specific directions, these children may not initiate any activity or they may initiate activity that is habitual and limited or seems to lack a goal. Typical responses may include wandering aimlessly; performing simple repetitive actions such as patting or pushing objects around; randomly piling up objects with no apparent plan; or, for the more sophisticated child, waiting to observe others doing an activity and then imitating them rather than initiating a new activity independently. The work of May-Benson highlighted the role of language and the social environment in the development of ideation as an aspect of praxis.[159]

For children with dyspraxia, skills that most children attain rather easily can be excessively challenging (e.g., donning a sweater, feeding oneself with utensils, writing the alphabet, jumping rope, completing a puzzle). These skills may be mastered only with high motivation on the part of the child, coupled with a great deal of practice, far more than most children require. Participation in sports is often embarrassing and frustrating, and organization of schoolwork may be a problem of particular concern. Children who have somatodyspraxia and are aware of their deficits often avoid difficult motor challenges and may attempt to gain control over such situations by assuming a directing or controlling role over others.

Praxis may be a significant area of concern for children with autism. Ideation may be affected[146] and could be related to the repetitive, stereotyped behaviors that comprise one of the defining characteristics of this diagnosis. Motor planning difficulties are well documented in this population. For example, many studies have demonstrated that children with autism have difficulty imitating gestures.[88,107,203] In one recent study, children with autism were shown to have worse praxis than typical controls, after accounting for age, IQ, and basic motor skills.[78] In another study, children with Asperger's syndrome who were tested with the SIPT demonstrated evidence of poor proprioceptive and vestibular processing, as well as motor planning impairment, leading the investigators to suggest that these sensorimotor impairments exacerbate the limited social participation of individuals with Asperger's.[224]

Praxis in children is best evaluated using the SIPT, which is very sensitive to detecting differences in several aspects of praxis. Five standardized tests on the SIPT—Oral Praxis, Sequencing Praxis, Postural Praxis, Constructional Praxis, and Design Copying—measure motor planning aspects of somatopraxis and visuopraxis. However, parent interview, questionnaires, and informal observations also provide critical information in the assessment process, particularly in the assessment of the ideational aspects of praxis, which are difficult to appraise using conventional standardized tests. A recently developed instrument, the Test of Ideational Praxis, is promising as a standardized, objective means for assessing ideation.[160] In addition, emerging work on assessments of praxis for younger children will hopefully contribute valuable new options in the future for assessment of praxis.[237]

Sensory-Seeking Behavior

Some children seek intense stimulation in particular sensory modalities. For example, a child may jump excessively, make sounds frequently, or want to swing or spin his body more often and more intensely compared with most children. Traditionally, in the field of sensory integration, sensory seeking often has been considered to be a sign of under- or over-responsiveness, and accordingly, previous editions of this textbook discussed it as a modulation disorder. However, as new research emerges and more in-depth case examples become available (e.g., personal reflections by individuals with autism),[63] it is becoming clear that sensory-seeking behaviors probably occur for diverse reasons. This section reviews the plausible explanations for behaviors that are generally considered to reflect sensation seeking. These potential explanations for what we call *sensory-seeking behaviors* are that they: (1) generate additional sensory input to compensate for weak processing in a particular sensory system, (2) regulate general arousal level, (3) modulate over- or under-responsiveness in other sensory systems, (4) are part of a multifaceted modulation disturbance, (5) reflect limited praxis and are not really sensory-seeking behaviors, and (6) are an expression of temperament and not related to sensory integration problems. These proposed reasons currently serve as tentative explanations that should be examined in future research. Underlying many of these potential explanations is the hypothesis that sensory-seeking behavior may serve an adaptive function for particular sensory integration difficulties.

One kind of adaptive function that sensory-seeking behaviors may serve is generating additional sensory input to compensate for weak processing in a particular sensory system. For example, some children seek very strong proprioceptive input in the form of active resistance to muscles, deep touch pressure stimulation, or strong joint compression and traction (e.g., by stomping instead of walking, jumping forcefully, intentionally falling or bumping into objects and people, pushing against large objects, or pushing and throwing objects with excessive force). In such cases, the occupational therapist might hypothesize that the child is not aware of the positions of body parts without intense proprioceptive stimulation. For example, when assessment data indicate that the child has tactile perception and proprioceptive difficulties, demonstrates signs of poor body awareness, and frequently initiates jumping and throwing movements with excessive force, the practitioner might interpret the sensory-seeking behaviors as strategies for obtaining additional touch pressure and proprioceptive sensations to compensate for inefficient processing in these sensory systems. The forceful movements can be viewed as proprioceptive-seeking behaviors, which may serve to provide enhanced feedback about dynamic changes in body position during action.

Similarly, some children who have signs of poor tactile perception are observed to touch things and people excessively. This tactile seeking behavior might be a way to compensate for inadequate tactile information by increasing the flow of tactile sensations into the central nervous system, to enhance interpretation of touch sensations during object manipulation and social contacts. Vestibular sensation seeking may also serve a similar function. For example, some children who have difficulty processing vestibular sensations seek large quantities of intense stimulation by swinging or spinning on suspended equipment in a therapy setting, but do not easily become dizzy or show the expected autonomic responses demonstrated by most peers. This intense vestibular seeking behavior may serve the adaptive function of increasing the intensity of vestibular input to adequately activate responses such as maintaining head and trunk stability during movement.

Sensory seeking may also serve the purpose of regulating arousal level. For example, intense vestibular sensation seeking may serve to increase the arousal level of a nervous system that is generally under-aroused. It is well documented in research that vestibular stimulation involving fast changes in head position or movement through space has a generally arousing effect.[151,194,230] So again, sensory seeking may be playing an adaptive role. That is, children with low baseline arousal may be engaging in vestibular seeking behaviors to reach levels of alertness that help them to perform more optimally.

Another potential reason for sensory seeking is that it may serve to help dampen or override over-responsivity in a particular sensory system. Children who seek intense proprioceptive input sometimes demonstrate concomitant signs of tactile defensiveness or gravitational insecurity. Because animal research as well as clinical experience indicates that proprioceptive and deep touch pressure sensations have an inhibitory effect on light touch[166] and vestibular[97] sensations, these children may be seeking increased proprioceptive input to help themselves modulate the overwhelming touch and movement sensations that they often experience.

Sensory-seeking behavior is prevalent among children with autism. In their recent review of sensory characteristics in autism, Baranek and her colleagues separate sensory seeking from hypo-responsiveness (which they treat as low sensory registration).[34] These authors categorize sensory features in autism as falling into four main categories: (1) hypo-responsiveness; (2) hyper-responsiveness; (3) sensory interests, repetitions, and seeking; and (4) enhanced perception. Examples of "sensory interests, repetitions, and seeking" in autism often involve visual, tactile, and auditory-seeking behaviors such as fascination with flickering lights, repeatedly rubbing textures, or wanting to listen to the same sound over and over. Proprioception seeking is also very common in this population.[142] Because sensory-seeking behaviors are associated with under- and over-responsiveness in children with autism, it is plausible that sensory-seeking behaviors in this population serve arousal modulation functions.[34,80,148] For example, a child who is over-responsive to environmental sounds may find that staring at flickering lights helps to block out the disturbing stimuli by focusing attention on the light stimuli. In this example, the visual sensory seeking may be viewed as a strategy for modulating disturbing auditory stimuli or as a direct reflection of a sensory modulation disturbance.

Children who have difficulty with praxis may also appear to have sensory-seeking behavior. Those who struggle with ideation, imitation, sequencing, timing, and multistep planning tend to use play equipment in very simple, repetitive ways because they lack the ability to conceptualize and plan novel and complex actions. These children typically perform familiar actions excessively, such as swinging, jumping, throwing, hitting, or splashing. When these behaviors occur in a child with signs of poor praxis, the possibility exists that these are the only movement strategies available to the child, given the limited repertoire of play skills.

The behaviors generated by sensation-seeking children may be disruptive or inappropriate in social situations. Safety issues frequently are of paramount concern, and often these children are labeled as having social or behavioral problems. A challenge for the occupational therapist working with these children is to identify strategies by which they can receive the high levels of stimulation they seem to need without being socially disruptive, inappropriate, or dangerous to themselves or others.

Finally, occupational therapists should bear in mind that people of all ages (including children) have natural, individual proclivities for certain sensory experiences. Although some children inherently love the thrill of fast rides and high vistas, others prefer slow movements and do not find pleasure in speedy movement or ascending to high places. If no other indicators of a sensory integration difficulty are present, then the sensation-seeking behavior probably is an expression of temperament, and not a manifestation of a sensory integration problem, so a sensory integration approach to intervention would not be appropriate. However, if occupational therapy is indicated to support self-care, play, school, or work skills, the child's inclination toward sensory seeking should be addressed when considering daily activity routines to ensure that the child's preferences for intense sensations are met in ways that are safe and socially acceptable.

Impact on Participation

Research tells us that sensory integration difficulties may limit the quality of children's participation in occupations that they want or need to do as a member of a family, classroom, or community. A systematic review of research on the occupational performance challenges of children with sensory integration difficulties identified 35 studies that addressed difficulties in the areas of play, leisure, and social participation; activities of daily living and instrumental activities of daily living; rest and sleep; and education and work.[134] Results indicated that sensory problems were related to occupational performance difficulties in all of these areas.

The severity of the sensory difficulties and the presence of other disabilities very likely have an impact on the degree to which participation is affected and the aspects of participation that are impacted. Research has shown that Sensory Profile scores of high functioning children with autism are significantly correlated with scores on a social competence measure, indicating that more extreme sensory differences—especially those involving over-responsiveness—are related to more severe social problems.[118] For children with sensory processing problems but no identified disability, the social impact may be milder. For example, a study of these children compared with closely matched typical peers found that, in many ways, these children were very similar to peers in activity preferences and participation. However, they were less involved with team sports, reported less enjoyment and intensity of involvement in general, and had more limited social networks.[71] Qualitative research suggests that sensory experiences of children with autism have a powerful effect on family occupations and daily routines.[30] Tactile defensiveness, in particular, seems to strongly affect family routines and self-care activities, even in children with no medical, developmental, or learning disabilities.[197] For example, sensory processing problems can be a significant source of child-related parenting stress.[127]

How others, especially parents, respond to a child's struggles with sensory integration challenges may have a powerful effect on the child's developing competence and self-image. First-hand parent accounts provide vivid illustrations of the challenges involved in raising a child with significant sensory issues.[181] Sensory integrative difficulties can be both "invisible" (i.e., their presence or origin may not be obvious, especially for children who have no medical or developmental diagnosis) and fluctuating (i.e., their presentation may vary from one time and situation to another). These features often lead parents, teachers, neighbors, and even strangers to assume that the child is capable of performing or behaving better and more consistently and is willfully refusing to do so. Consequently, the child may be punished or responded to inappropriately for behavior not under voluntary control, which may lead to chronic feelings of hopelessness. Moreover, the variability of the sensory integrative problems across time, events, and environments makes it difficult to predict which situations cause problems for a particular child, how much discomfort results, and when distress is likely to occur. Parents and teachers of children with these disorders often find the unpredictability of the child's behavior to be frustrating and difficult to understand.

Sensory integration difficulties can also have a negative influence on skill development, secondary to limited participation in the typical childhood occupations that afford children with opportunities for practice and exposure to challenges. The child who avoids finger painting because of tactile defensiveness or who rarely attempts climbing on the jungle gym because of poor praxis not only misses these singular experiences, but also misses opportunities to hone underlying functions such as tactile discrimination, hand strength and dexterity, shoulder stability, balance and equilibrium, hand-eye coordination, bilateral coordination, ideation, and motor planning. If the child misses a substantial number of such experiences over time, the gap between the child's sensorimotor skills and the skills of peers may grow.

In addition, typical interactions that occur in the context of sensorimotor play and are important to the development of communication and social skills may be limited. Thus, some children with sensory integrative problems may lack the ability to play successfully with peers partly because they have not participated fully in the childhood occupations in which sensory, motor, cognitive, and social skills typically emerge and develop. The fear, anxiety, or discomfort that accompanies many everyday situations is also likely to work against the expression of the child's inner drive toward growth-inducing experiences. Therefore, lack of experience and diminished drive to participate can compound the direct effects of a sensory integrative disorder. A qualitative case study of "Jake," a young man with praxis difficulties and sensory modulation problems, illustrates how sensory integration challenges can strongly influence activity and lifestyle choices from childhood into adulthood.[191]

Sensory integrative problems can also undermine self-esteem and self-confidence over time. Autobiographical accounts by people with sensory integration difficulties provide concrete examples of how this negative cycle may unfold.[101,164] Children with sensory integrative problems are often aware of their struggles with commonplace tasks, so it is natural for them to react with frustration. Chronic frustration, compounded by fear of failure and humiliation, can negatively affect the child's feelings of self-efficacy. Instead, the child may develop feelings of helplessness. This leads to further limitations in the child's experiences because the child becomes less likely to attempt challenging activities.

These obstacles to participation may actually have a more powerful impact on the child's life outcomes than the original sensory integration difficulty. In some cases, minor sensory integration difficulties can become magnified by losses in self-efficacy and limitations in social relationships, ultimately leading to significant barriers to life satisfaction.

This kind of negative cycle is not inevitable. Children's resilience and capacity to grapple and cope with challenging experiences will influence their occupational lives over the years.[184] Resilient families and children find successful strategies on their own. For many others, however, professional support may provide critical experiences that alter the child's life trajectory in a positive direction. How occupational therapists may help through assessment, intervention, and other supportive approaches is the next topic in this chapter.

Assessment of Sensory Integrative Functions

Assessment of sensory integration, like all other areas addressed in occupational therapy, requires a multifaceted approach because of the need to understand the child's presenting problems in relation to the family and environments in which that child participates. Assessment by the occupational therapist begins with a general exploration of the occupations of the child and family, focusing on their concerns and hopes in relation to the child's strengths and challenges. A variety of tools is needed to help the occupational therapist discern whether problems in sensory integration are relevant to the child's life situation, to understand the nature and scope of these difficulties, to consider how the difficulties may be offset by the child's talents and strengths, and to decide whether intervention should be recommended. Assessment tools employed by occupational therapists using a sensory integration perspective include interviews and questionnaires, informal and formal observations, standardized tests, and consideration of services and resources available to and appropriate for the family. Smith Roley[172] explained how this process of assessment is consistent with the Occupational Therapy Practice Framework.[4]

Interviews and Questionnaires

The need for an occupational therapy assessment of sensory integration usually arises when a parent, teacher, physician, or other person who knows the child notices difficulties that are not easily explained by some known condition or circumstance. The referral source, family members, and others who work with the child may all be valuable sources of information through interviews or questionnaires (Figure 9-8). This initial phase of evaluation identifies the main concerns about the child and begins the process of determining if examination of sensory integration functions might help to explain some of the child's challenges.

The initial interview with the parent, teacher, or other referral source provides an opportunity for the therapist to gather important information about sensory integration problems that may be present. For example, the teacher may report that the child seems to frequently become agitated while standing in line and cannot seem to stay seated during reading circle time. Further questioning may reveal signs of tactile defensiveness

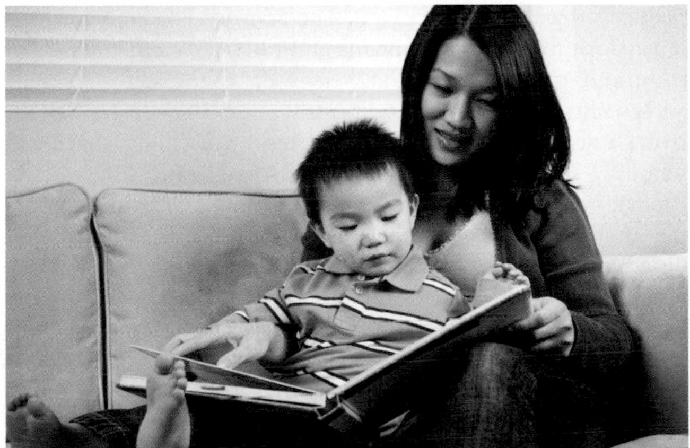

FIGURE 9-8 Because parents know their child better than anyone else, they are invaluable sources of information to the therapist, especially in beginning phases of the assessment process. (Photo © istock.com.)

that explain the child's behavior, but may not have been considered by a teacher unfamiliar with this condition. A parent may provide critical information about the child's development, which may be helpful in identifying early signs of sensory integrative difficulties. For instance, parents may have noticed that specific tasks, such as cutting with scissors or pedaling a tricycle, were especially difficult for the child. Because difficulty coordinating the two sides of the body is common when vestibular processing difficulties are present, this type of information can inform the therapist about additional observations and tests that are needed to determine whether this is the case. Another important role of the interview is to uncover alternative explanations of the child's difficulties that may rule out sensory integration problems, such as when a recent emotional crisis (e.g., a divorce or death) coincides with the onset of problems.[173]

Cohn[68] identified the themes of child abilities, activities, and re-establishment of self-worth as important priorities for parents seeking intervention for their children with sensory integration challenges. These themes may be strategic areas to address in initial parent interview questions or conversations with the child. Discussion of these topics goes beyond identification of sensory integration problems and lays the groundwork for intervention planning. When possible, it is also useful to talk with the child directly. Children with sufficient verbal skills to discuss their own abilities, perceptions, and difficulties can sometimes provide invaluable insight into their sensory experiences, challenges, skills, and interests.

Questionnaires, checklists, and histories given by caregivers and other adults who know the child well are other means for gathering information that aids in identifying presenting problems and strengths, and in clarifying the priorities of the family. One such instrument is a sensory history or similar questionnaire. Originally developed by Ayres as an unpublished questionnaire, this type of instrument asks parents questions regarding specific child behaviors indicative of sensory integrative problems, and parents respond by rating the child using a Likert-style scale. These types of questionnaires were subsequently developed using normative samples to produce reliable and valid scores.

The Sensory Profile[81] and the Sensory Processing Measure (SPM)[187] are two sensory questionnaires used extensively in pediatric occupational therapy. The Sensory Profile is normed in versions for parents of infants and toddlers[83] and children in early and middle childhood,[81] as well as for self-reports of adolescents and adults.[50] Additionally, a Sensory Profile School Companion is available for teacher report of child behavior at school.[84] The SPM has two forms, Home[115] and Main Classroom,[175] that are normed on the same sample of 5- to 12-year-old children and can furnish a score that aids the therapist in discerning whether a child's sensory issues are manifested differently in the contexts of home versus school. In addition, the SPM contains separate rating scales for school personnel other than the main teacher, such as art teacher, music teacher, or bus driver. The SPM-Preschool (SPM-P)[174] is normed for ages 2 to 5 years old, and is structured similarly, with separate Home and School forms for parents and day care providers or preschool teachers, respectively. Normative data for 2-year-olds are separate from that of 3- to 5-year-olds, because this instrument is sensitive to developmental changes in sensory processing of young preschoolers.

The information garnered through the initial interview process and, when available, through review of the educational or medical records is used to decide whether further assessment is warranted and, if so, which evaluation procedures are most appropriate. This information is also critical in interpreting the final pool of information gathered through assessment and in prioritizing goals for the child in light of the main concerns and wishes of the family and child.

Direct Observations

Direct observation of the child is essential to the evaluation of sensory integration. Both unstructured observations within natural environments as well as more structured clinical observations are essential for a comprehensive assessment and a full understanding of the child's strengths and challenges.

Naturalistic Observations

When feasible, informal observation of the child during familiar routines in natural settings, such as a classroom, playground, or home, is informative and helpful. Informal observation influences the conclusion as to whether sensory integrative challenges are present and, if so, helps to clarify how the child's difficulties, as well as capabilities, are affecting the child's participation in daily occupations. For example, an experienced therapist can often detect signs of poor proprioceptive body awareness by observing the child at school. Such signs may include exerting too much pressure on a pencil, standing too close to classmates in line, using poor foot placement when climbing on a jungle gym, or sitting in an ineffective position in a chair while completing class assignments. Teachers may not report these behaviors to the therapist if they perceive them as signs of inattentiveness or clumsiness.

Observation of the child in the clinical setting can also be useful for discovering how the child responds to situations that are novel or unpredictable. A child with praxis problems may struggle to mount an unfamiliar climbing structure in a therapeutic setting, even though performance is adequate on play equipment at home or in school, on which the child has practiced familiar actions. The novelty of the specialized therapy room elicits responses from children that may be diagnostically relevant. For children with good ideation and sensory processing abilities, the endless opportunities afforded by sensory integration equipment in the clinic can be exhilarating. For the child who experiences difficulty with praxis or bilateral integration, the same environment may be confusing, puzzling, or frustrating. A child with gravitational insecurity may be terrified by the prospect of equipment that moves, whereas a child with autism may be distressed by the clinic environment because of its unpredictability and discrepancy from familiar settings. Parham has provided some guidelines for organizing informal observations in a therapeutic setting, with special attention to issues related to praxis.[183] Although focused on the assessment of preschoolers, these suggestions can also be applied to older children and may be particularly helpful in evaluating children who are unable to cooperate with standardized testing. Roley[207] and Windsor, Roley, and Szklut[250] provide additional guidelines for assessing praxis through informal observations. May-Benson and Cermak[160] offer guidance for specifically assessing ideational aspects of motor planning.

BOX 9-1 Examples of Commonly Used Clinical Observations

- *Crossing body midline:* Intentional movement of a body part (usually the hand) to reach for or manipulate an object in contralateral space. This capacity typically emerges during toddlerhood and early childhood and is related to the development of hand preference. Delays in midline crossing may be related to inadequate hand preference and bilateral integration.
- *Equilibrium reactions:* Automatic postural and limb adjustments that occur when the body's center of gravity is displaced enough to cause potential loss of balance. These adjustments serve to restore the body's center of gravity over its base of support so that balance is maintained or restored. Difficulties with equilibrium reactions are associated with vestibular processing problems.
- *Muscle tone:* The readiness of a muscle to contract. Force with which a muscle resists being lengthened.
- *Prone extension:* Ability to assume and hold an "airplane" position (neck, upper body, and hips extended to lift head, arms, and legs off the floor) while lying prone. Difficulty maintaining this position for 30 seconds is related to inefficient vestibular processing in children 6 years of age and older.
- *Supine flexion:* Ability to assume and hold a curled position (neck, upper body, hips, and knees flexed so that knees are drawn close to the face) while lying supine. Difficulty maintaining this position for 30 seconds is related to poor praxis in children 6 years of age and older.

Structured Clinical Observations

Formal observations that are highly structured and similar to test items are often used in an occupational therapy assessment of sensory integration. Usually referred to as *clinical observations*, these typically involve a set of specific procedures that allow the therapist to observe signs of neurologic system integrity that are associated with sensory integrative functioning. Ayres developed a set of clinical observations that she used in clinical practice. These unpublished, non-standardized evaluation tools were intended to supplement standardized test scores and subsequently were revised, expanded on, and studied by many other therapists over the years.[46,52,249] Examples of some of the most commonly used clinical observations are presented in Box 9-1. Recently, Blanche and colleagues reported on a developing scale, the Comprehensive Observations of Proprioception (COP), specifically for assessment of proprioceptive functions in children.[48]

Because these types of clinical observations usually involve administration and scoring criteria that are not rigorously standardized, different procedures are often applied from one clinician to another. Furthermore, most of these observations lack normative data to aid in interpretation of the scores, although some clinical observations are supported by research using standardized administration and data on typically developing children.[48,104,150,160,161,250] In light of the limited information available regarding expected performance across age, gender, and other demographic characteristics, clinical observations are generally considered supplemental rather than stand-alone information within a comprehensive assessment.

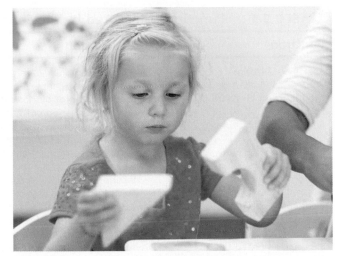

FIGURE 9-9 Constructional praxis is the ability to motor plan actions in order to create a 2- or 3-dimensional design or structure, as when drawing or building with blocks. This ability is used when children engage in constructional play. It is evaluated by the Constructional Praxis Test of the Sensory Integration and Praxis Tests (SIPT).

Standardized Testing

Occupational therapists frequently use standardized tests to evaluate sensory integration. Although several tests are available that contribute incidental information regarding sensory integrative functions, the Sensory Integration and Praxis Tests (SIPT) comprise the gold standard for comprehensive, in-depth evaluation of sensory integration. The SIPT evolved from a series of tests that Ayres developed in the 1960s[6,7,9,10,20] and later published as the SCSIT[15] and the SCPNT.[17] The standardization process used in the development of the SIPT was rigorous, involving normative data on approximately 2000 children in North America and extensive reliability and validity studies.[22] Its 17 tests measure tactile, vestibular, and proprioceptive sensory processing; form and space perception and visuomotor coordination; bilateral integration and sequencing abilities; and praxis.[26] A list of the 17 tests and the functions measured by each is presented in Table 9-1.

Administration of the SIPT by an experienced examiner requires about 1.5 to 2 hours with an additional 30 to 45 minutes for scoring (Figure 9-9). Raw scores are translated into standard scores through a computerized scoring program available from the test publisher. After standard scores are obtained for both the major and subtests of the SIPT, the therapist critically reviews them, keeping in mind the patterns of sensory integration problems that were identified in research. The SIPT scores are integrated with observations of the child's behavior during testing, as well as all other sources of assessment information, so as to reach a conclusion regarding the status of the child's sensory integrative functioning.

Other pediatric tests include items or subtests from which inferences regarding sensory integration may be drawn. For example, the Miller Function & Participation Scales include tests that challenge praxis, visual-motor integration, figure-ground perception, and some vestibular functions.[168] The

TABLE 9-1 Functions Measured by the Sensory Integration and Praxis Tests

Function	Description
Space visualization	Motor-free visual space perception; mental manipulation of objects
Figure-ground perception	Motor-free visual perception of figures on a rival background
Manual form perception	Identification of block held in hand with visual counterpart or with block held in other hand
Kinesthesia	Somatic perception of hand and arm position and movement
Finger identification	Tactile perception of individual fingers
Graphesthesia	Tactile perception and practice replication of designs
Localization of tactile stimuli	Tactile perception of specific stimulus applied to arm or hand
Praxis on verbal command	Ability to motor-plan body postures on the basis of verbal directions without visual cues
Design copying	Visuopractic ability to copy simple and complex two-dimensional designs, and the manner or approach one uses to copy designs
Constructional praxis	Ability to relate objects to each other in three-dimensional space
Postural praxis	Ability to plan and execute body movements and positions
Oral praxis	Ability to plan and execute lip, tongue, and jaw movements
Sequencing praxis	Ability to repeat a series of hand and finger movements
Bilateral motor coordination	Ability to move both hands and both feet in a smooth and integrated pattern
Standing and walking balance	Static and dynamic balance on one or both feet with eyes opened and closed
Motor accuracy	Hand-eye coordination and control of movement
Postrotary nystagmus	Central nervous system processing of vestibular input assessed through observation of the duration and integrity of a vestibular-ocular reflex

From Mailloux, Z. (1990). An overview of the sensory integration and praxis tests. *American Journal of Occupational Therapy, 44*, 589–594.

Bruininks-Oseretsky Test of Motor Proficiency (BOT-2)[51] measures aspects of fine and gross motor skills (such as bilateral coordination) that are related to sensory integrative functions. Other tests, such as the Developmental Test of Visual Motor Integration,[39] provide specific information related to visual-perceptual and perceptual-motor skills.

Some instruments geared toward the broader evaluation of occupation can provide critical information, such as the School Function Assessment (SFA),[72] the Goal-Oriented Assessment of Lifeskills (GOAL),[171] or the Social Participation Scale of the SPM.[187] These tools are useful for identifying the extent to which sensory integrative difficulties may be affecting the child's participation in occupations within specific settings. For the child with suspected sensory integrative problems, tests such as these are most effectively used along with specific measures of sensory integration. When combined, these tests assist the therapist in identifying the child's functional strengths and challenges, as well as the underlying reasons for the child's difficulties and accomplishments, to target in intervention.

Interpreting Data and Making Recommendations

Once the information from interviews, questionnaires, informal and formal observations, and standardized tests has been collected, the occupational therapist must integrate and interpret these data to reach meaningful conclusions and appropriate recommendations for the individual child. Conclusions and recommendations are framed with an overriding consideration of the presenting problems and concerns from the family and other professionals (such as teachers), the occupations of the child and family, and the contexts that influence occupational engagement.[4,206] Burke, Schaaf, and Hall advocate the strategy of creating a narrative, or story, to form an integrated understanding of the child and family to focus assessment and intervention planning on issues that are most meaningful and important to them.[55] In using such a future-oriented outlook, the therapist not only generates a picture of the child and family in the present, but also imagines how changes might unfold over the next few years.[184] Occupational therapists use research as well as training and experience to formulate conclusions and recommendations.

One of the important steps in interpretation of assessment findings is to evaluate whether a sensory integrative problem may contribute to the occupational challenges of the child. To do this, data are classified into categories that either support or refute the presence of particular types of sensory integrative problems. After a detailed analysis of the constellation of assessment findings, a hypothesis is generated as to whether any sensory integrative issues appear to affect the child's daily functioning, and if so, what kinds of difficulties appear to be present. For example, a child may present as having difficulties in the classroom with sitting still, staying upright at his or her desk, and losing his or her place when copying from distances. If the interviews, observations, questionnaires, and standardized assessments reveal signs of a vestibular bilateral integration problem (e.g., depressed postrotary nystagmus, poor extensor muscle tone, inefficient postural and ocular control, low scores on balance and bilateral coordination tests), then the therapist forms a hypothesis that this child's classroom struggles relate to vestibular bilateral difficulties. This type of analysis requires both advanced knowledge and skills about these complex sensory integrative functions and patterns, as well as the ability to translate the relationship of these functions to everyday childhood activities.

As the preceding example illustrates, the relationships between sensory integrative functions and daily occupations can be difficult to understand without advanced training. As in any aspect of occupational therapy, it is critical to relate the assessment findings to the presenting problems and initial concerns of the family or referral source, and when applying the sensory integrative framework, therapists will often find that they need to take some extra steps to make the connections understandable and meaningful.[153] For example, an assessment may uncover signs of tactile defensiveness in a child described by the parents as destructive and impulsive. It may not have occurred to the parents that difficulty responding to touch input has any relationship to the child's behavior. The evaluating therapist will likely not only need to explain the concept of tactile defensiveness, but also to present a description of how and why tactile defensiveness may be related to the child's behavior problems. An interpretation of how the assessment findings are linked to the daily life experiences and occupations of the child and family also lays the foundation for intervention recommendations.

In addition to the information that is gathered about the child, an occupational therapy assessment of sensory integration takes into consideration the services and resources that are available to the child and family. Information regarding the types of services that the child is currently receiving, how he or she is responding to these services, and which services, programs, and resources are available to the child need careful consideration in light of the purpose and findings of the evaluation before recommendations can be formulated. For example, a child who lives in an area where no occupational therapists are qualified to provide sensory integration intervention needs a program recommendation different from one for a child who has easy access to this type of service. Understanding family aspirations and values, caregivers' concerns, child interests and talents, and resources such as funding, transportation, and time are also critical in identifying the types of services that will be most helpful to the child and family. These issues are as important to the assessment process as the child factors that are addressed in a sensory integration evaluation.

If an assessment leads to a recommendation for occupational therapy intervention, it generally includes an estimate of the duration of time that the child should receive therapy, some indication of prognosis, and a statement regarding expected areas of change. The anticipated gains can be further clarified through the establishment of specific goals and objectives. Writing and explaining goals will provide the occupational therapist with an opportunity to illuminate the ways in which the identified sensory integration issues relate to the presenting problems and desired functional outcomes.[153] The format in which goals are specified is often a function of the setting in which therapy is delivered. For example, a school district may mandate a particular format for goals in an individualized education plan, whereas a hospital setting may require medically related outcomes. Goal attainment scaling may be useful in many settings.[154] Regardless of the types of goals that are written, goals are established in a manner that is culturally relevant for the family and considers the needs, wishes, talents, and interests of the individual child.

Interventions for Children with Sensory Integrative Problems

Planning an occupational therapy program around a child's strengths and sensory integrative challenges requires the same careful analysis that is used in applying any theoretical framework in therapeutic practice. As for any occupational therapy practice, the aim of sensory integration intervention is "supporting health and participation in life through engagement in occupation."[4] When a sensory integration approach is used in occupational therapy, intervention decisions are based on an understanding of the unique ways in which sensory integrative problems affect the engagement and participation of children and their families.[206] Intervention is continually planned and evaluated in relation to the occupations that the child wants and needs to do in the contexts of home, school, and community.

The comprehensive assessment process, combined with knowledge of available evidence, helps the therapist to evaluate whether intervention is indicated and, if so, which kinds of approaches are likely to be of the most benefit to the child and family. Regardless of the form in which intervention is delivered, theory-based reasoning regarding the nature of sensory integration should be applied in services to children with sensory integrative difficulties. Therapists who plan interventions for children with sensory integrative problems are responsible for developing their professional expertise through advanced training, mentorship, and ongoing review of evidence. The field of sensory integration is a complex, specialized area of occupational therapy practice that demands that the occupational therapist synthesize information from many sources. Because it is a dynamically changing field, it is important that the therapist stay abreast of research evidence, as well as new developments in sensory integration theory and practice, to guide practice decisions.

The remainder of this chapter provides a description of Ayres sensory integration intervention (OT-SI), including intervention principles, effectiveness research, methods for measuring outcomes, and expected child outcomes. In addition, we discuss several other types of intervention approaches that are often used along with OT-SI or as alternatives to OT-SI: specific sensory strategies and regimes, individual skill development training, group skill development interventions, and consultation, including individualized coaching and modification of everyday activities, routines, and environments.

Ayres Sensory Integration Intervention

The term *Ayres Sensory Integration* (ASI) intervention refers to the individualized occupational therapy practice approach that Ayres developed specifically to remediate sensory integrative problems of children.[209] ASI intervention is also called OT-SI to emphasize that it is occupational therapy. In this intervention, the occupational therapist presents activity challenges that are individually tailored to improve sensory integration capacities of the child. Ultimately, this intervention is designed to help a child gain competencies and confidence in performing everyday occupations at home, in play, at school, or in the community (Case Study 9-1). Although Ayres originally designed this therapy for children with learning disabilities who presented signs of sensory integration difficulties,[14] she and many other expert practitioners have used this kind of intervention, alongside other compatible occupational therapy intervention frameworks, to help children with other disabilities, including autism.[152,157]

In designing this specialized form of occupational therapy, Ayres was influenced by the neuroscience literature, which shows that the nervous system has plasticity or changeability, particularly when the organism has opportunities to explore

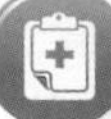

CASE STUDY 9-1 Karen

History

Karen was born after a full-term pregnancy complicated by gestational diabetes. Labor, which was induced at 40 weeks, was prolonged, and it was believed that Karen broke her right collarbone during delivery. Karen achieved her early motor and language milestones within average age ranges. However, she was described as an irritable baby who had difficulty breastfeeding, startled easily, and could be calmed only by swinging. Karen attended a parent cooperative child development program as a toddler, and at 4 years of age she was eligible for a special education preschool program through her school district. She has not been given any specific medical or educational diagnosis.

Reason for Referral

Karen's mother expressed concern about Karen's fine and gross motor skills to a neurologist, who referred Karen for an occupational therapy assessment when she was 4 years of age. When asked why she was seeking an evaluation for Karen, her mother wrote, "Up until recently I had been very patiently waiting for normal development to occur (for example, handedness, fine motor). The school psychologist feels that this still may occur, but I am convinced that something isn't right. Karen's increasing frustration and decreasing belief in herself prompted me to seek evaluations. While a part of me wishes to have a 'normal child,' the other part will be relieved to find that the child I have had so many doubts about since infancy does indeed have some behaviors and actions that are unusual."

Evaluation Procedure

The Sensory Integration and Praxis Tests (SIPT) were administered in one testing session. Karen was also observed in a clinical therapy setting and at home. In addition, Karen's mother was interviewed, and she completed a developmental and sensory history on which she provided detailed accounts of Karen's early and current sensorimotor, language, cognitive, social, and self-care development.

Evaluation Results

On the SIPT, Karen scored below average for age expectations on 7 of 17 tests. This profile was generated through computer scoring by the test publisher. The unit of measure represented by the scores is a statistical measure called a *standard deviation*, which represents how different the child's score is from that of an average child of the same age. The closer a child's score is to 0 on the horizontal axis, the closer to average is the child's performance on that test. Karen's scores are plotted as solid squares that are connected by a dark line on the computer-generated profile. Scores falling below −1.0 on the horizontal axis are considered to be possibly indicative of dysfunction.

One of Karen's scores was low on a motor-free visual perception test (space visualization), and it was noted that she had difficulty fitting a geometric form into a puzzle board during this test. Her mother reported that Karen knew colors at 18 months of age but had trouble learning shapes. However, she was reported to have a strong visual memory for roads, signs, and faces. These findings suggested difficulty with spatial orientation of objects but relative strengths in visual memory.

Karen had several low scores and showed signs of difficulty performing on several of the tests of somatosensory and vestibular processing. A low score on finger identification suggested inefficient tactile feedback involving the hands. This was corroborated by observations of poor manipulative skills during activities such as buttoning and using utensils. She was also observed to have signs of tactile defensiveness, also corroborated by her mother's report. Her low score on Kinesthesia, as well as her difficulty in exerting the appropriate amount of pressure on a pencil and in positioning her body for dressing, suggested problems with proprioceptive feedback. Karen's lowest score on the SIPT was on the Postrotary Nystagmus test (−2.2 standard deviations). This low score, as well as below-average scores on Standing and Walking Balance, observations of poor functional balance in dressing and playground activities, a tendency not to cross her body midline, poor bilateral coordination in activities such as cutting, and reports that she never appeared to get dizzy, pointed to the probability of vestibular processing problems.

Karen showed above-average performance on a praxis test on which she could rely on verbal directions. However, tests of motor planning that were more somatosensory dependent (Oral Praxis and Postural Praxis) were substantially more difficult for her. Karen was unable to ride a tricycle, pump a swing, or skip. She had extreme difficulty planning her movements to dress herself or even letting someone else dress her. She also had a great deal of difficulty using utensils during eating and often choked on food and drinks. Writing skills were particularly difficult for Karen, and her lack of hand preference, immature grasp, and hesitancy to cross her midline hampered her attempts at drawing or writing.

Karen was reported to be a social child who was liked by adults and younger peers. However, her mother worried that she did not seem able to "pick up on the hints and unwritten rules of her peers" and was "definitely starting to march to her own beat." She noticed increasing signs of frustration that she thought were beginning to impinge on Karen's willingness to participate with peers.

Overall, the evaluation results suggested problems in sensory processing of some aspects of visual, tactile, proprioceptive, and vestibular sensory information. These difficulties were seen as related to somatodyspraxia, poor balance and bilateral integration, difficulties with specific gross and fine motor skills, and emerging concerns around socialization. Karen's strengths included age-appropriate cognitive and language skills, good ability to motor plan actions using verbal directions, and an exceptionally supportive and involved family.

Recommendation

Based on the evaluation results and a meeting of Karen's IEP team, who met shortly after the assessment, it was

CASE STUDY 9-1 Karen—cont'd

recommended that Karen receive individual occupational therapy using a sensory integration approach to enhance foundational sensory and motor processes. Because of her significant sensory integrative problems and need for a specialized approach, the therapy was recommended to initially occur in a setting equipped for Ayres Sensory Integration (ASI) intervention.

Occupational Therapy Program

In the first 6 months of individual occupational therapy, an ASI approach was used that included individualized, carefully selected therapeutic activities aimed at enhancing visual, tactile, proprioceptive, and vestibular sensory processing. As part of her intervention program, Karen's occupational therapist provided her with graded challenges to praxis, bilateral coordination, and balance.

After 6 months of therapy, Karen has shown decreasing tactile defensiveness, a reduced tendency to choke on food, acquisition of the ability to ride a tricycle, and an improved ability to plan new or unusual motor actions. Although these are significant gains for Karen, she continues to exhibit substantial difficulties with many aspects of sensory processing, general motor planning ability, and many age-appropriate fine and gross motor skills. If she continues to respond to occupational therapy using an ASI approach, it is expected that by the beginning of the next school year (in about 6 months), she will have improved in basic sensory and motor functions to the extent that some specific skill training will become more appropriate. It is likely that at that time some therapy will occur at school with the introduction of a consultation program for her teacher. Her parents have already begun a home program, which appears to support the gains she is making through direct services. Karen's young age and initial positive response to therapy make her an optimal candidate for application of the sensory integration approach, and her long-term outlook is excellent.

and engage in activities within an enriched environment. Plasticity is particularly characteristic of the developing young child. This led Ayres to hypothesize that neural system functions can be improved with active engagement in an enriched environment that presents activity challenges, especially for the young child. Accordingly, she set out to design therapy that capitalized on the plasticity of the nervous system to improve sensory integrative functioning. This is *not* to say that OT-SI cures conditions such as learning disability, autism, or developmental delays. Rather, the intent is to improve the efficiency with which the nervous system interprets and uses sensory information for functional use. Therefore OT-SI promotes underlying capabilities to the greatest degree possible. Recently, Reynolds, Lane, and Richards reviewed five decades of animal studies on the effects of enriched environments on brain structure and function and concluded that essential features of enriched environments historically have been incorporated into OT-SI and should continue to do so.[199] These essential features are multiple sensory experiences, novelty in the environment, and active engagement in challenging cognitive, sensory, and motor tasks. Thus, the basic science research on effects of enriched environments studies provides empirical support for the underlying assumptions and strategic intervention strategies of OT-SI intervention.

Some basic assumptions underlying the OT-SI approach are summarized in Box 9-2, drawn from the classic work of Ayres.[14,20] The principal ideas behind these assumptions were introduced previously in this chapter in the sections on neurobiologically based concepts, sensory integrative development, and types of problems.

OT-SI is applied on an *individual* basis because the therapist must adjust therapeutic activities moment by moment in relation to the individual child's interest in the activity or response to a specific challenge or sensory experience.[66,130,136] This requires the occupational therapist to continually focus attention on the child while being mindful of opportunities in the environment for eliciting adaptive responses. Of particular importance is the delicate interplay between the potential therapeutic value of an activity and the child's motivation to engage in it. Therefore, the occupational therapist's session plan is fluid, changing according to the child's behaviors. The occupational therapist establishes a relationship with the child that fosters the child's inner drive to actively explore the environment and to master challenges posed by the environment. Because of the high degree of personal attention continuously given to the child during the therapy session, a fine gradient of complexity can be built into therapeutic activities while simultaneously ensuring that the child's interests are prioritized and the child experiences success and a growing sense of "I can do it!"

The occupational therapist's job is to create an environment that evokes increasingly complex adaptive responses from the child. To accomplish this, the occupational therapist respects the child's needs and interests while structuring opportunities to help the child successfully meet a challenge. An example is a child who needs to develop more efficient righting and equilibrium reactions and chooses to sit and swing on a platform swing. The occupational therapist may allow the child to swing

BOX 9-2 Basic Assumptions Underlying Ayres Sensory Integration Intervention

1. Sensory input can be used systematically to elicit an adaptive response.
2. Registration of meaningful sensory input is necessary before an adaptive response can be made.
3. An adaptive response contributes to the development of sensory integration.
4. Better organization of adaptive responses enhances the child's general behavioral organization.
5. More mature and complex patterns of behavior emerge from consolidation of simpler behaviors.
6. The more inner-directed a child's activities are, the greater the potential for the activities to improve neural organization.

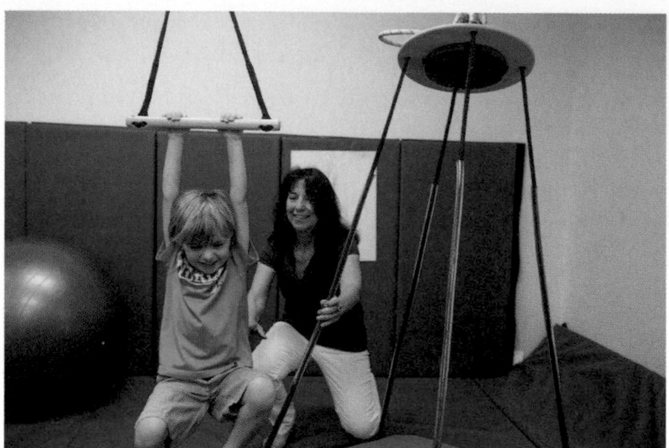

FIGURE 9-10 Individual OT-SI intervention requires the therapist to attend closely to the child on a moment-by-moment basis to ensure that therapeutic activities are individually tailored to changing needs and interests of the child.

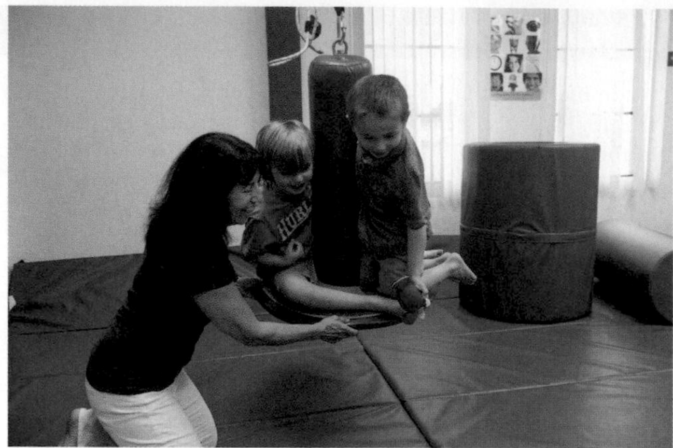

FIGURE 9-11 Rather than passively imposing vestibular input on the child, classic sensory integration treatment emphasizes active participation and self-direction of the child.

awhile to become accustomed to the vestibular sensations. Once the child seems comfortable, the occupational therapist steps in to jiggle the swing to stimulate the desired responses. However, if the child responds to this challenge with signs of anxiety or fear, the occupational therapist needs to intervene quickly to help the child feel safer. For example, the occupational therapist might set an inner tube on the swing to provide a base to stabilize the lower part of the child's body and increase feelings of security while the child's upper body is free to make the required righting reactions. Therapeutic activities thus emerge from the interaction between the occupational therapist and the child. Such individualized treatment can be fully realized only with one-to-one interaction between the occupational therapist and the child (Figure 9-10).

Occupational therapy using a sensory integration approach intervention capitalizes on the *inner drive* of the child during intervention.[14,20,66,136] Self-direction on the part of the child is encouraged because therapeutic gains are maximized if the child is fully invested as an active participant. This is not the same as permitting the child to engage in free play with no adult guidance. The optimal therapy situation is one in which a balance is struck between the structure provided by the occupational therapist and freedom of choice on the part of the child.[14,20] Drawing on the child's interests and imagination is often key to encouraging greater effort on a difficult task or staying with a challenging activity for a longer time. However, because children with sensory integrative problems do not always demonstrate inner drive toward growth-inducing activities, it may be necessary to modify activities and find ways to entice such children toward interaction. When facilitating engagement in children with autism or other children whose inner drive is limited, the occupational therapist may need to frequently initiate activities and guide the child on how to perform them. Occasionally an occupational therapist may use a greater degree of directedness within the context of a particular activity to show a child that the challenging activity is possible not only to achieve, but also to enjoy. In situations in which the occupational therapist intervenes by directing the child, the occupational therapist always looks for opportunities in which the child can increase his or her active engagement and control of the activity, including supporting the child's initiation of a new activity.

Active participation is also emphasized because the brain responds differently and learns more effectively when an individual is actively involved in a task, rather than merely receiving passive stimulation. Therefore, in OT-SI intervention, the occupational therapist actively engages the child to the greatest degree possible. For example, sensory integration theory posits that a child experiences a greater degree of integration from pumping a swing or pulling on a rope to make it go than from being swung passively.

Maximal active involvement generally takes place when therapeutic activities are at just the right level of complexity, at which the child not only feels comfortable and non-threatened but also experiences some challenge that requires effort. The course of therapy usually begins with activities with which the child feels comfortable and competent and then moves toward increasing challenges. For example, for children with gravitational insecurity, therapy usually begins with activities close to the ground and with close physical support from the therapist to help the child feel secure. Gradually, over weeks of therapy, activities that require higher level surfaces and moving away from the floor are introduced as the therapist subtly withdraws physical support. Introducing the "just right" level of challenge, while respecting the child's need to feel secure and allowing the child to have degree of control, is a key to maximizing the child's active involvement in therapy (Figure 9-11).

At times, sensory experiences may be initiated and provided by the occupational therapist to help prepare a child for more complex or challenging activities that he or she may later perform. For example, a child with autism may show improved awareness of and interest in movement activities after receiving passive vestibular sensation on a swing that the occupational therapist has moved in a linear or rotary fashion.[230] The improved awareness of the joys and affordances of movement will also likely mean that the child has greater awareness of the environment. In this way, therapist-initiated sensory experiences can be a stepping stone toward active involvement in an activity. Another example is the use of carefully introduced tactile activities as a means for reducing tactile defensiveness and improve the child's comfort in situations and activities that involve frequent tactile contact with objects and people.[14] Overall, therapist-directed or induced sensory experiences are a limited component of a sensory integrative treatment program and are used only as a step toward facilitating more active participation.

The setting in which OT-SI takes place, including the availability of specialized therapeutic equipment, is another important aspect of this type of intervention.[163,229,239] Consistent with research that shows that brain structure and function are enhanced when animals are permitted to actively explore an interesting environment,[126,199] a sensory-enriched environment is designed to evoke active exploration on the part of the child. A therapy room that is designed for OT-SI contains large activity areas with an array of specialized equipment.[163] The availability of suspended equipment is a hallmark of this treatment approach.[66,136] Suspended equipment provides rich opportunities for engaging and challenging the vestibular system. In addition, equipment and materials are available that provide a variety of somatosensory activities, including tactile, vibratory, and proprioceptive input. Mats and large pillows are used for safety. Overall, this special environment provides the child with a safe and interesting place in which to explore his or her capabilities. At the same time the equipment and setting provide the occupational therapist with a tool kit and workshop for creating sensory experiences that are enticing to the child and for gently guiding the child toward activities that challenge perception, dynamic postural control, and motor planning (Figure 9-12).

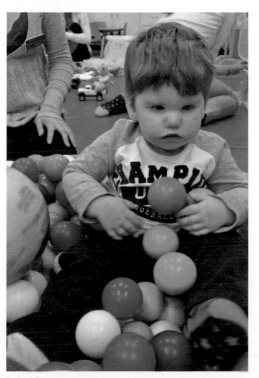

FIGURE 9-12 The setting in which OT-SI intervention takes place provides a variety of sensory experiences. Immersion in a pool of balls presents challenges to sensory modulation.

A few cautionary words are in order regarding responsible use of vestibular and tactile stimulation as therapeutic tools. These are powerful tools that can have profound effects on the physiologic state. For example, activation of the vestibular system, usually in the form of linear movement, is commonly introduced early in the course of treatment for many children because it is believed to have an organizing effect on other sensory systems.[14,20] However, it can have a disturbing and disorganizing effect on the child if used without careful monitoring of the child's response. Vestibular system activation may produce strong autonomic responses, manifested as blanching and nausea. It directly influences arousal level and, if not regulated carefully, may produce hyperactive, distractible states or lethargic, drowsy states. Because OT-SI intervention emphasizes active participation on the part of the child, vestibular stimulation is rarely passively imposed on the child. Whenever vestibular stimulation is used, the occupational therapist constantly monitors the child's responses and frequently adjusts the activity in response to the child's state. For example, if a child is actively rotating while sitting in a tire swing and begins to exhibit mild signs of autonomic activation, the occupational therapist might intervene by acting to reduce the intensity of the swinging, guide the child to shift to slow linear swinging, or increase proprioceptive input by offering the child a trapeze to pull. This latter strategy (increasing proprioceptive input) is derived from animal research showing that proprioceptive input has an inhibitory effect on vestibular activation.[97] Therefore, knowledge of the effects of vestibular stimulation and its interactions with other sensory systems is critical in this treatment approach.

Similarly, tactile stimulation during OT-SI is informed by knowledge about this sensory system and how it interacts with arousal processes as well as other sensory systems. Passive tactile stimulation is not often used. Imposing tactile stimulation on a child who is tactile defensive may lead to a state of sensitization, in which the child becomes increasingly more defensive instead of habituating to the sensation. Instead of using passive tactile stimulation, tactile stimuli are usually incorporated into the materials and surfaces that the child contacts while engaging in activities under his or her active control, for example, through manipulation of objects with varying shapes and textures or through contact with surfaces that have diverse textures.

To summarize the critical features of OT-SI intervention, therapeutic activities are neither predetermined nor are they simply free play. The flow of the treatment session involves collaboration between the occupational therapist and child in which the therapist encourages and supports the child in a way that moves the child toward therapeutic goals. This all takes place within a special environment that is safe yet challenging. To determine if a child can benefit from OT-SI intervention, a comprehensive occupational therapy assessment, including in-depth evaluation of sensory integration, must be conducted. Assessment findings are used to determine whether OT-SI is appropriate and desirable for the individual child. If so, assessment findings guide treatment planning.[217] Because challenges in sensory integration are often identified early in life and can affect occupational performance over many phases of development, OT-SI intervention may be appropriate for extended or intermittent periods across childhood.

After Ayres developed OT-SI intervention,[14,20] her colleagues and students continued to further develop and expand on her intervention concepts. Koomar and Bundy provided a particularly thorough description of the application of sensory integration procedures for specific types of sensory integrative disorders.[136] Holloway imported OT-SI concepts into the neonatal intensive care unit (NICU), where the treatment principles are used to help young infants when their developing nervous systems are most plastic.[121] Others have adapted OT-SI intervention to address the needs of infants and toddlers who are developmentally at risk,[213] as well as the needs of children with visual impairments,[205] cerebral palsy,[47] environmental deprivation,[75] and fragile X syndrome.[117]

Application of the OT-SI approach requires special training beyond the entry level of practice in occupational therapy.[240] Koomar and Bundy advocated a mentorship process as the best preparation for learning how to clinically apply sensory integration principles.[136] Ayres also advocated this and established a 4-month course in which therapists receive both didactic instruction and intensive hands-on experience treating children under close supervision. Ayres believed that this level of intensity was required to master the sensory integration approach. Because of the highly specialized and complex nature of the OT-SI approach, it is important that occupational therapists gain post-professional education and mentored experience in this area before independently engaging in this form of practice. Self-study of professional and scholarly resources relevant to this area of practice is also important in developing professional competencies. A list of these resources is available on the Evolve website.

In addition, ongoing personal study and discussion with peers are highly recommended after acquiring advanced training, to hone clinical expertise and explore emerging evidence in the field. Although OT-SI intervention often occurs within specialized therapy centers, many of the concepts can be applied in other settings as well. School-based occupational therapists have found ways to incorporate the central principles of OT-SI into the educational setting, including bringing specialized equipment into classrooms, therapy rooms, and playgrounds in ways that help to organize and prepare a child for learning. Successful therapy programs frequently involve helping families to understand and use the sensory integration concepts that support and facilitate their children's success by developing activities at home and identifying resources within the community that reinforce the experiences emphasized during therapy.[190]

Evidence of Effectiveness of Ayres Sensory Integration Intervention

Occupational therapists who wish to use an OT-SI approach in practice need to keep up-to-date on research in this field to ensure that intervention is informed by the growing knowledge base. Research on the effectiveness of OT-SI is particularly critical to evidence-based practice in this specialty area. May-Benson and Koomar[162] conducted a systematic review of 27 effectiveness studies that were published in peer-reviewed journals over a span of 37 years. Two meta-analyses were included: an early one that found a large, significant, positive treatment effect for motor outcomes in children with learning and intellectual disabilities[182] and a later one that found moderate motor and psychoeducational benefits across different populations but no significant difference from interventions that used other approaches.[238] These findings, taken together with the results of other studies, led these authors to conclude that sensory integration intervention leads to positive results, especially compared with no intervention.[162]

However, these encouraging findings must be interpreted with caution because of a variety of methodologic limitations that are common in research on interventions for children with developmental, learning, and behavioral challenges.[162,167,180] For example, a common limitation in outcomes studies of OT-SI is that children may have been provided this intervention without confirming whether they actually have any problems with sensory integration. Another common limitation is that the intervention provided in a study may have been called sensory integration but was not actually provided in a manner that matches the defining characteristics of OT-SI.[185] This type of limitation is called a fidelity problem. In intervention research, fidelity refers to the extent to which the intervention provided in a study is faithful to the key elements of the intervention approach.

A reliable and valid fidelity instrument, the Fidelity Measure for ASI Intervention, was developed recently to provide researchers with a systematic method for ensuring fidelity of OT-SI intervention[163,188] (Box 9-3). Table 9-2 presents evidence from group design studies that used the Fidelity Measure for ASI Intervention or a similar fidelity instrument to document that the intervention provided in the study was delivered in a manner that reflects OT-SI principles. As shown in Table 9-2, several studies examining the effectiveness of OT-SI have demonstrated positive outcomes of this approach for children with autism. In a randomized controlled trial (RCT) comparing fine motor intervention with OT-SI, Pfeiffer et al.[193] reported that children with ASD had greater gains in individual goals using Goals Attainment Scaling (GAS) as well as a significant decrease in autistic mannerisms. Similarly, Schaaf et al.[216] conducted an exceptionally well-designed RCT involving 32 children with ASD. The group who received OT-SI for 10 weeks, three times per week, showed statistically significant improvements in primary outcome measures using GAS, as well as improved performance in self-care and social activities and decreased caregiver assistance, which were secondary outcome measures. Both the Pfeiffer et al. and Schaaf et al. studies used the Fidelity Measure for ASI Intervention throughout the study to ensure adherence to the intended intervention.

An important issue in intervention trials is the maintenance of long-term gains after completion of a period of OT-SI intervention. An encouraging finding reported by Wilson and Kaplan[247] suggests that children who receive sensory integration intervention may obtain long-term benefits that are not obtained by children who receive other interventions. Although this study was published before development of the Fidelity Measure for ASI Intervention, a systematic review of fidelity in sensory integration research found that the intervention in this study included most of the key fidelity elements of OT-SI identified by Parham et al.[185] Although no significant differences in outcomes were found between the two intervention groups in the original study (i.e., both the OT-SI and tutoring groups made significant gains),[248] at follow-up 2 years later only the children who had received OT-SI maintained the gains that they had made after intervention. Maintenance of intervention gains is a critical issue that is relevant to cost-effectiveness of

TABLE 9-2 Effectiveness Studies Using Group Comparison and Fidelity Measure to Verify Occupational Therapy Using a Sensory Integration Approach Intervention

Author/Year	Purpose	Study Design and Subjects	Intervention and Outcome Measures	Results and Limitations	Conclusions
Iwanaga, Honda, Nakane, Tanaka, Toeda, & Tanaka[123]	Investigate the effectiveness of OT-SI for high-functioning children with ASD	Level III—Cohort study of two groups *Subjects*: 20 children with ASD (IQ > 70), ages 2-6 yr. Children received individual OT-SI (N = 8) if standard group therapy (GT) (N = 12) was not available. Groups were similar for gender and age.	*Intervention*: All participants received 8-10 mo of intervention, 1 session per week. GT focused on social skills. OT-SI included all elements in Fidelity Measure for ASI. *Measures*: JMAP before and after intervention.	OT-SI group made treatment gains in JMAP Total and 4 subscale scores. GT group made gains only on total score. Group differences in changes found for Total and 3 subscale scores, with OT-SI group benefitting more. Results may be biased by non-blinded ratings.	High-functioning young children with ASD may benefit from OT-SI in motor, nonverbal cognitive, and complex perceptual-motor functions.
Miller, Coll, & Schoen[170]	Determine whether OT-SI is more effective than a placebo treatment or no treatment	Level II—Small RCT *Subjects*: 24 children with SMD. N = 7 in OT-SI group, 10 in placebo group, and 7 no treatment. Groups equivalent for gender, ethnicity, parent education, & age. Mean age 6 yr in each group.	*Intervention*: Individual OT-SI twice per week for 10 weeks. Placebo was child-selected tabletop play activities in 1:1 sessions. Structured assessment to monitor fidelity. *Measures*: Leiter Parent Rating Scales, SSP, VABS, CBC, GAS, electrodermal reactivity.	OT-SI group made significantly greater gains than other groups on GAS and Leiter scales. Very large effect size found in OT-SI group for GAS. Parent involvement in OT-SI sessions may have biased results.	Children with sensory modulation problems may benefit from OT-SI. GAS outcomes may be especially sensitive to gains owing to OT-SI.
Pfeiffer, Koenig, Kinnealey, Sheppard, & Henderson[193]	Establish model RCT, identify appropriate outcome measures, and examine effectiveness of OT-SI for children with ASD	Level II—Small RCT *Subjects:* 32 boys and 5 girls with ASD, age 6-12 (mean = 8.8 yr) attending therapeutic activities program; 21 with autism and 16 with PDD-NOS. All scored ≥ 60 on the SPM. 20 received OT-SI & 17 received OT individualized fine motor (FM) intervention.	*Intervention*: Individual 45-min sessions for 18 days over a 6-week period. Fidelity Measure for ASI and a fidelity measure for FM group were used to monitor and manualize interventions. *Measures:* SPM, SRS, QNST-II, GAS, VABS-II. All evaluators blinded to group assignment.	SI group had more gains than FM group in GAS goals rated by parents and teachers. No differences found for SPM or QNST-II scores. Sample heterogeneity and short intervention period may have limited outcomes.	Short-term intensive OT-SI (3 × per week for 6 weeks) is more effective for children with ASD than fine motor intervention for attaining GAS goals. SPM and QNST may not be sensitive to short-term OT-SI gains.
Schaaf et al.[216]	Evaluate the efficacy of OT-SI for children with autism	Level II—Small RCT *Subjects*: 32 children randomly assigned to OT-SI (N = 17) + usual care or usual care control group (N = 15). All had confirmed diagnosis of ASD, ages 4-7 yr, IQ > 65, and assessment indicating SI problems. Groups similar for gender, race, parent education, age, autism severity, cognition, and non–study related services.	*Intervention*: Individual 1-hr OT-SI, 3 times per week for 10 weeks, provided by SI-certified OTs. Fidelity Measure for ASI used to monitor manualized OT-SI intervention. *Measures*: Primary measure was GAS. Goals set by independent evaluators using standard questions for parents. Secondary measures were PEDI, PDDBI, and VABS-II. All evaluators blinded to group assignment.	OT-SI group made significantly greater gains than control group on GAS and PEDI scores for Self-Care Caregiver Assistance and Social Function Caregiver Assistance.	Children with ASD + SI problems, and mild or no intellectual disability, are likely to benefit from OT-SI. Benefits include gains in daily life functioning and decreased need for caregiver assistance during self-care and social activities.

Note: Levels of evidence are rated using the AACPDM[2] Methodology for quantitative group designs (AACPDM, 2008) or for single-subject research designs (Logan, Hickman, Harris, & Heriza, 2008). ASD, autism spectrum disorder; CBC, Child Behavior Checklist; GAS, goal attainment scaling; JMAP, Japanese version of Miller Assessment for Preschoolers; OT-SI, occupational therapy using Ayres Sensory Integration (ASI) intervention; PDDBI, Pervasive Developmental Disorders Behavior Inventory; PDDNOS, pervasive developmental disorder not otherwise specified; PEDI, Pediatric Evaluation of Disability Inventory; QNST-II, Quick Neurological Screening Test (2nd ed.); RCT, randomized controlled clinical trial; SMD, sensory modulation disorder; SPM, Sensory Processing Measure; SRS, Social Responsiveness Scale; SSP, Short Sensory Profile; VABS, Vineland Adaptive Behavior Scales (VABS-II = 2nd ed.).

BOX 9-3 Fidelity Process Elements of Occupational Therapy Using Ayres Sensory Integration Intervention

OT-SI intervention is implemented with moment by moment adjustments that are made based on the child's responses and choices in concert with the occupational therapist's clinical reasoning. The fidelity elements listed here describe the process of therapy, that is, what the therapist is responsible for doing throughout OT-SI therapy sessions.[188] In action, these elements occur simultaneously and interactively. Additionally, structural elements are required for the appropriate implementation of OT-SI.[163,188] These include specified therapist qualifications and training, space and equipment requirements, safety monitoring measures, and assessment and documentation procedures.

1. *Ensures physical safety:* The physical space arrangement and materials in the therapy room, as well as the occupational therapist's actions, ensure the child's physical safety.
2. *Presents sensory opportunities:* Using therapeutic equipment, materials, and activities, the occupational therapist provides the child with sensory-rich activities, particularly those that involve body-centered (tactile, proprioceptive, and vestibular) sensory experiences
3. *Supports sensory modulation for attaining and maintaining a regulated state:* The occupational therapist modifies sensory conditions and activity challenges to help the child attain optimal arousal, alertness, and affect for engagement in activities.
4. *Challenges postural, ocular, oral, and/or bilateral motor control:* Using assessment data regarding areas of need, the occupational therapist introduces, supports, or modifies activities to provide challenges to these areas of motor control.
5. *Challenges praxis and organization of behavior:* Using assessment data regarding areas of need, the occupational therapist introduces, supports, or modifies activities to challenge the child's motor planning, ideation, and/or ability to plan and engage in organized activities.
6. *Collaborates in activity choice:* The occupational therapist strives to shares control with the child in choosing, modifying, or changing activities; ultimately the goal is that activities are chosen collaboratively by the occupational therapist and child.
7. *Tailors activity to present just-right challenge:* To ensure the child's optimal engagement, the occupational therapist tailors activities so that they are at the "just-right" level of challenge, by suggesting or supporting an increase or decrease in task complexity so that the activity is not too difficult or too easy for the child to do independently or with therapist support.
8. *Ensures that activities are successful:* The occupational therapist strives to provide challenges in which the child will experience feelings of success.
9. *Supports child's intrinsic motivation to play:* The child's intrinsic motivation to play is prioritized in the OT-SI approach, so the occupational therapist creates a setting that supports play as a way to fully engage the child in the intervention.
10. *Establishes a therapeutic alliance with the child:* In OT-SI, a strong positive relationship between the child and occupational therapist is essential; therefore, the occupational therapist establishes an interpersonal connection with the child, forming a therapeutic alliance that entails working together in a mutually enjoyable partnership.

From Parham, L. D., Roley, S. S., May-Benson, T., et al. (2011). Development of a fidelity measure for Research on Ayres Sensory Integration. *American Journal of Occupational Therapy, 65,* 133–142.

intervention. Additional studies are needed to measure long-term outcomes of OT-SI.

Although randomized clinical trials are considered to be the gold standard of effectiveness studies, other research designs examining intervention outcomes also make valuable contributions to understanding the potential effects of sensory integration intervention. In research using single-subject designs, a child serves as his or her own control and is monitored repeatedly before intervention (the baseline phase) and during intervention. An advantage to this approach is that behavioral outcomes can be highly individualized and tracked over time to provide an understanding of each child's response to intervention. For example, Linderman and Stewart measured three behavioral outcomes of OT-SI for two preschool children with pervasive developmental disorders.[147] Each outcome was observed in the child's home and was tailored to address functional issues for each child (e.g., response to holding and hugging for one child and functional communication during mealtime for the other). Results indicated significant improvements between baseline and intervention phases for five of the six outcomes measured. These results are encouraging, but should be considered tentative because of the small number of participants and the absence of a fidelity measure.

Future studies can build on current research to explore new questions regarding who is a good candidate for OT-SI intervention and what kinds of outcomes can be expected. For example, it would be reasonable to expect different intervention outcomes for children with different kinds or different levels of severity of sensory integration difficulties, yet this has not been systematically studied since Ayres' early work.[13,19,24,27] Research addressing this issue could help practitioners predict who will best respond to individual OT-SI intervention and who may be better served by other intervention approaches. The effectiveness of systematically combining individual OT-SI intervention with other interventions, such as sensory strategies at home or in the classroom, specific skill training, group programs, or consultation, also needs further research. Finally, long-term maintenance of gains, particularly those related to social participation outcomes, is an important question that should be addressed in future research.

Expected Outcomes of Ayres Sensory Integration Intervention

Occupational therapy aims to improve a child's health and quality of life through engagement in meaningful and important occupations or activities. To accomplish this with a young child who has sensory integrative problems, the occupational therapist usually first aims to improve sensory integrative functions through direct OT-SI intervention. Based on the premise of neuroplasticity in the young and developing brain, sensory integration theory holds that many of the child's sensory integration functions improve with individually tailored therapeutic activities that provide opportunities for exploration and challenge. In addition to addressing the underlying sensory integration problems, occupational therapists also often help the child to develop specific skills and strategies, to minimize the effects of the problems the child is experiencing and help the child to cope with the current day-to-day demands. Finally, consulting with parents and teachers to allow for carry-over of direct intervention and to plan modifications of activities, routines, and environments is an important component of any intervention program involving children. Often direct intervention, specific skill training, and consultation are thoughtfully combined in a treatment plan that is designed to meet the particular needs of the child and family.

The child's goals and objectives target specific occupations, such as eating, play, rest, work, and self-care, in which positive changes are expected. For example, a toddler who tends to be overstimulated much of the time because of severe sensory modulation problems may consequently have difficulty falling and staying asleep. Sleep deprivation can aggravate over-responsiveness and behavior problems for the child and can also disrupt occupational performance of other family members. A goal may be for the child to acquire more predictable sleep patterns with adequate amounts of sleep. A related objective might be that the child will tolerate unpredictable sensations such as household sounds, change in room temperature, or the texture of sheets and blankets in order to successfully nap without interruption for at least 1 hour for 3 days per week. The intervention could involve direct remediation to reduce the sensory defensiveness, as well as parent consultation on strategies such as calming activities, a predictable activity schedule including a specific rest time ritual, and creation of an arousal-reducing environment after lunch (e.g., lights dimmed and noise reduced and screened with rhythmic sounds or "white noise").

Sometimes specific objectives that address performance skills are appropriate as a way to monitor progress toward the desired changes in daily occupations. Expected outcomes are summarized in Box 9-4; more detailed descriptions of each category follow.

Increase in the Frequency or Duration of Adaptive Responses

As discussed in the introduction of this chapter, adaptive responses occur when an individual responds to environmental challenges with success. A priority for an occupational therapist applying OT-SI principles is to create opportunities for the child to make adaptive responses. Ensuring that the sensory experiences inherent in activities are organizing rather than disorganizing and integrating rather than overwhelming requires careful monitoring on the part of the occupational therapist, who must be sensitive to the child's response to each aspect of an activity and to each type of sensory input involved. The OT-SI intervention approach intensively focuses on the child's acquisition of higher level adaptive responses.

Increasing the duration and frequency of adaptive responses is an important outcome of sensory integration because functional behavior and skills are developed by mastering simple adaptive responses. For example, a child who has difficulty staying with an activity for more than a few seconds tends to shift from one activity to another, thus never having the chance to fully process the sensation and develop purposeful actions in response to it. A desirable outcome for that child might be to remain involved in a simple activity, such as swinging, for longer periods of time. The specific goal might be worded as, "The child will sustain engagement for two minutes in a simple movement activity, such as remaining seated in a swing while holding onto the side ropes as it moves, with therapist providing verbal and physical cues for support." Achievement of this simple adaptive response can lead to increased postural control and emerging motor plans such as holding on and using rhythmic, coordinated trunk and leg flexion movements to move the swing. These basic adaptive responses may contribute to the functional behavior of staying seated in an upright position during circle time in the school classroom or participating with peers on a playground swing, thus contributing to engagement in important childhood occupations. In a case study of a child with autism who participated in the Schaaf et al. clinical trial,[216] such improvements in basic adaptive responses are called proximal outcomes of OT-SI.[217] These proximal outcomes are thought to lead to distal outcomes related to participation in daily routines.

Development of Increasingly More Complex Adaptive Responses

Adaptive responses can vary in complexity, quality, and effectiveness.[19] As noted, a simple adaptive response might be simply holding on while sitting on a moving swing. An example of a more complex adaptive response would be releasing grasp while swinging on a trapeze, and then at just the right moment, jumping off to land on a pillow. This type of action requires timing and sequencing, as well as integration of various sensory functions such as proprioceptive awareness of changes in body position, tactile perception in the hands, vestibular sense of motion through space, and visual perception of the intended target. Over time, effective OT-SI intervention is expected to enable the child to make increasingly more complex adaptive responses. This outcome is based on the assumption that sensory integrative procedures promote more efficient organization of multisensory input at elementary levels of functioning, which in turn is expected to enhance functions that are more complex. The result is an improvement in the child's ability to make judgments about the environment, what can be done with objects, and which specific actions need to be taken to accomplish a goal. Increase in complexity of adaptive responses is another example of proximal outcomes, which lead to long-term distal outcomes of OT-SI.[217]

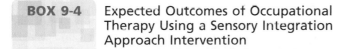

BOX 9-4 Expected Outcomes of Occupational Therapy Using a Sensory Integration Approach Intervention

1. Increase in the frequency or duration of adaptive responses
2. Development of increasingly more complex adaptive responses
3. Improvement in gross and fine motor skills
4. Improvement in cognitive, language, and academic performance
5. Increase in self-confidence and self-esteem
6. Enhanced occupational engagement and social participation
7. Enhanced family life

Improvement in Gross and Fine Motor Skills

The child who makes consistent and more complex adaptive responses shows evidence of improved sensory integration. Moreover, this child meets new challenges with greater self-confidence. A net result of these gains frequently is greater mastery in the motor domain. An example is the child with a vestibular processing problem who exhibits greater competency and interest in playground activities and sports after individual OT-SI intervention, even though these activities were not practiced during therapy. Motor skills may be among the earliest complex skills to show measurable change in response to an OT-SI approach, probably because extensive motor activity is inherent in this intervention approach.[182]

Improvement in Cognitive, Language, or Academic Performance

Although cognitive, language, and academic skills are not usually the specific objectives of OT-SI, improvement in these domains has been detected in some effectiveness studies involving the provision of ASI intervention.[13,19,24,151,194,244] Application of OT-SI therapeutic procedures is thought to generate broad-based changes in these areas secondary to enhancement of sensory modulation, perception, postural control, or praxis.[20,57] For example, a child with autism may be helped through a sensory integrative approach to respond in a more adaptive way to sights, sounds, touch, and movement experiences. This improvement in sensory modulation may lead to a better ability to attend to language and academic tasks; thus, improvements in these areas may follow. A child who has a vestibular processing disorder may improve in postural control and equilibrium, freeing the child to concentrate more efficiently on academic learning, without the distraction of frequent loss of sitting balance or loss of place while copying from the blackboard. This child's vestibular-related improvements are also likely to have a positive effect on playground and sports activities because effects of classic sensory integration intervention are expected to generalize to a wide range of outcome areas.

Increase in Self-Confidence and Self-Esteem

Ayres asserted that enhanced ability to make adaptive responses promotes self-actualization by allowing the child to experience the joy of accomplishing a task that previously could not be done.[20] The outcome of therapy that encourages successful, self-directed experiences is a child who perceives the self as a competent actor in the world. Individual and group programs and direct and indirect services can help the child master the activities that are personally meaningful and essential to success in the world of everyday occupations. Mastery of such activities is expected to result in feelings of personal control that, in turn, lead to increased willingness to take risks and try new things.[20] For example, a child with gravitational insecurity may experience not only fear responses to climbing and movement activities, but also feelings of failure and frustration when limited in participating in the play of peers. In such a case, an increase in self-confidence and comfort in one's physical body is often accompanied by a general boost in feelings of self-efficacy and worth. Cohn, Miller, and Tickle-Degnen noted that parents' perceptions of the benefits of occupational therapy using a sensory integrative approach included enhancing feelings of self-worth, in addition to improving abilities and activities.[70] Parents in this study perceived that this intervention enabled their children to take more risks and try new activities, which opened the door to greater possibilities.

Enhanced Occupational Engagement and Social Participation

Occupational therapy programs that address sensory integrative problems encourage the child to organize his or her own activity, particularly in the OT-SI intervention approach. As the child develops general sensory integrative capabilities and improved strategies for planning action, gains are seen in relation to the ability to master self-care tasks, cope with daily routines, and organize behavior more generally.[20] As a result, the child often is able to participate more fully in the occupations that are typical for peers. Anticipated gains in social participation are often specified as individualized goals. For example, intervention may help the child who is overly sensitive to touch or movement to respond to sensations in a more adaptive manner. As a result, the child approaches and engages in the challenges of everyday occupations, such as getting ready for school in the morning, sharing a table with others in the school cafeteria, behaving appropriately in the classroom, and playing with friends on the playground with greater security and confidence. As noted previously, Cohn et al.[70] reported that parents viewed their children as more willing to try new experiences following intervention, thus enhancing their opportunities for social participation. Not only is participation in daily occupations performed with greater competency and satisfaction, but relationships with others are likely to become more comfortable and less threatening. It is noteworthy that randomized clinical trials of OT-SI using the OT-SI fidelity measure have consistently found significant gains in individualized goals related to social participation and occupational engagement.[170,193,216]

Enhanced Family Life

When children with sensory integrative problems experience positive changes during intervention, their lives and the lives of other family members may be enhanced. One possible by-product of intervention based on OT-SI principles is that parents gain a better understanding of their children's behavior and begin to generate their own strategies for organizing family routines in a way that supports the entire family system. This kind of change can be particularly powerful for parents of children with autism, whose perceptions of child behaviors may be reframed as they become familiar with the sensory integrative perspective. For example, behavior that is interpreted as bizarre, such as insisting on wearing tight rubber bands on the arms, may be reframed as a meaningful strategy that the child uses to obtain deep pressure input for self-calming.[5] Instead of viewing the behavior as a frustrating sign of pathology that should be eliminated, reframing may lead the parents to explore other ways that they could provide the child with the deep pressure experiences that he or she seeks. An important outcome of sensory integrative intervention, then, may include changes in parents' understanding of the child, leading to new coping strategies and alleviation of parental stress.[69] In her studies of parental perspectives, Cohn has found that an important outcome of the sensory integrative approach is that parents tend to "reframe" their view and expectations of their children in a positive manner.[67,68]

Measuring Outcomes of Ayres Sensory Integration Intervention

Because every child with a sensory integrative problem is unique, the expected outcomes of an OT-SI approach are individualized and diverse. As noted in the preceding section on expected outcomes, goals are often stated as objectives that target particular observed behaviors of the child. These objectives should contain a specific description of the desired behavior, including the context of the behavior and an objective way to measure it, for example, by timing how long the child can sustain an activity or with what percentage of success she can perform it after a number of attempts. Some good examples of measurable outcomes that target child-specific behaviors are provided by single subject studies.[59,147]

Additionally, outcomes are sometimes measured using standardized tests. In fact, some of the SIPT tests (e.g., Design Copying, Standing and Walking Balance, and most of the praxis tests) are good measures of change because of their strong test–retest reliability, in addition to being relevant to concerns that are commonly voiced by parents and teachers. However, standardized tests often do not address key occupational issues. When used, care must be taken to select a test that is likely to be sensitive to the kinds of changes expected for the particular child. Sometimes changes in raw scores are more informative than changes in standardized scores, because raw score change is a direct measure of the child's improvement in skill relative to performance at initial assessment. Comparing the child's performance to normative data may not detect actual changes in performance.

Goal attainment scaling (GAS) is an alternative to standardized tests that addresses the uniquely individualized nature of expected outcomes of OT-SI. Goal attainment scaling provides a means to prioritize goals that are specifically relevant to individuals and their families and to quantify the results using a standard metric that allows comparison of achievement across different types of goals (see Chapter 24). Emerging evidence indicates that this approach is useful for capturing outcomes of OT-SI intervention programs.[154] In three randomized, controlled clinical trials, GAS detected significant improvements among children who received OT-SI intervention, compared with those receiving alternative conditions.[170,193,217] This procedure for systematic monitoring of meaningful goals aligns well with current recommendations of the American Academy of Pediatrics[3] regarding sensory integration therapies for children with developmental and behavioral disorders.

Sensory Stimulation Protocols

This section discusses specific sensory protocols that are provided by the therapist or by the teacher or parent under the guidance of the therapist. In this discussion, we use the term *sensory stimulation protocol* to refer to interventions that involve application of specific types of sensory stimuli that are controlled by the therapist and delivered in a predetermined manner, usually according to a prescribed schedule or sequence. Examples include brushing the skin using a specific technique and sequence to provide tactile input, spinning in a prescribed sequence to provide controlled vestibular input, or having the child wear headphones while listening to selected music or other sound stimuli as part of a packaged sequential program. The sensory stimulation is applied in a non-contingent manner, that is, specific procedures used are not dependent on the child's behavior.

As described earlier, sensory stimulation techniques are used on a limited basis within OT-SI intervention sessions, where they are embedded within ongoing activities and are constantly modified based on the child's response. Whenever possible, control of the sensory input is given to the child. Within OT-SI sessions, the common purpose of these strategies is to support the child's sensory and arousal modulation. For example, swinging might be introduced by the therapist to increase or decrease arousal level by constantly adjusting the sensory qualities of the swinging activity (e.g., velocity, direction, intensity, predictability) according to the child's ongoing responses. Another example is the introduction of deep touch-pressure stimulation, such as having the child wear a weighted vest during activities, or playing a game of making a pretend "sandwich" by having the child lie inside two large pillows or mats. This kind of sensory strategy generally has a short-term calming effect, which may serve to help decrease sensory defensiveness, anxiety, or heightened arousal in the immediate situation.[89] Such sensory strategies are usually initiated at moments when the therapist judges that they may help move the child into a more organized state for making adaptive responses. Within the context of an OT-SI session, the therapist constantly monitors the child's response and accordingly adjusts the stimulus, shares control of the stimulus with the child, or discontinues the stimulus.

In contrast, sensory stimulation protocols are often used as stand-alone interventions that are performed in a prescribed manner and sequence, according to a particular schedule or sequenced program. Probably the most regimented examples are the Wilbarger Protocol and the Astronaut Program. The Wilbarger Protocol involves application of touch pressure in a particular sequence via brushing arms and legs with a surgical scrub brush using stroking motions, followed by manual compression of specific joints, every 2 hours.[245] The Astronaut Program is a protocol involving application of rotary vestibular combined with sound stimulation.[129] Expected outcomes for the Wilbarger and Astronaut protocols include improved sensory modulation and self-regulation, and general improvements in attention, learning, and behavior. Evidence on effectiveness of the Wilbarger protocol is inconsistent and limited to a few case studies,[44,77] and evidence regarding the Astronaut protocol currently is not available.

The strongest research support at this time for sensory stimulation protocols is for use of massage protocols. Two randomized controlled trials (RCTs) using a massage protocol developed by Tiffany Field indicated some improvements in tactile modulation and reductions in problem behaviors among children with autism, perhaps related to improved sleep after massage.[91,94] More recently, RCTs of a type of Qigong massage, based in traditional Chinese medicine, have also found positive effects. This intervention was designed to improve sensory processing, physiologic self-regulation, and sleep of children with autism. Significant improvements in behavior of children with autism were indicated after individualized delivery of a Qigong massage regimen over a 5-month period by trained occupational therapists or parents who were trained and coached by occupational therapists.[226,227]

Sound-based interventions (also called sound therapy or auditory programs) involve complex applications of auditory stimulation, specifically music delivered through headphones or other listening systems. These interventions usually involve multiple sessions in which a specific sequence of filtered music is presented over time. Generally, the child is not guided or prompted to make any responses to the stimulation beyond simply listening. Originally developed by physicians as an individual therapy, occupational therapists have used and developed versions that can be used either alone, during OT-SI intervention sessions, or during other sensory-based interventions. Sound-based interventions target a variety of outcomes, including sensory modulation, self-regulation, attention, improved language, and adaptive functioning. These interventions have been tested in single-system studies, small group comparison designs, and RCTs with mixed findings for children with diverse conditions.[45,106,178,202,228]

Sensory-Based Strategies

We use the term *sensory-based strategies* to refer to specific sensory interventions that are less regimented than sensory stimulation protocols, with more flexible guidelines for use in daily life. Examples include wearing a weighted vest for touch pressure and enhanced proprioceptive input, sitting on a therapy ball for augmented vestibular-proprioceptive input, or use of body compression devices such as the Grandin hug machine. In practice, these sensory strategies are usually integrated into daily routines and are delivered by parents or teachers or are self-administered by the child, following instruction by a professional. Expected outcomes vary depending on diagnosis and the specific intervention used, but generally they include better self-regulation, improved attention, and decreased behavior problems such as self-stimulatory or aggressive behaviors.

The sensory strategy that has been researched most often is the use of weighted vests to improve attention to task and in-seat behaviors in the classroom, but most of these single-subject studies did not find expected improvements in behavior.[73,93,119,120,128,145,196] However, positive short-term effects of sitting on a therapy ball chair (also called stability ball) in the classroom have been documented in a few single-system studies of children with autism spectrum or attention deficit disorders, with immediate benefits related to in-seat behavior, attention to task, and productivity in academic tasks for many but not all children.[29,92,218,219] Data from a study conducted by Bagatell and her colleagues suggest that therapy balls may be most effective when used selectively with consideration for the sensory processing characteristics of the individual child.[29] In their study of children with autism, the best responder to a ball chair was a child who demonstrated strong vestibular-proprioceptive sensory seeking. Perhaps this strategy was effective because therapy balls generate more sensory input via vestibular and proprioceptive systems compared with conventional classroom chairs. Conversely, use of a therapy ball was not helpful for a child in this study who had poor postural stability. It may be that, for this child, sitting on a ball chair created stress and distraction owing to the extra challenge on postural control that this strategy imposes. These findings underscore the importance of conducting an assessment of sensory integration before selecting sensory strategies for a particular child. Research on use of therapy cushions (inflatable disks placed in the child's chair to sit upon) has not produced benefits that are as positive as therapy balls, but they may be a more practical alternative to therapy balls in some classrooms.[218,236]

Less well known are sensory interventions that involve self-administration of deep touch pressure across the body using special compression devices. A small RCT evaluated use of the Grandin hug machine for 6 weeks found some reduction in self-perceived anxiety and decreased arousal/reactivity, as measured by electrodermal responses, in children with ASD.[89] An experimental study of a similar device that provided self-administered deep pressure around the circumference of the body showed that it had a calming effect with decreased subjective anxiety and increase in perceived relaxation.[137]

Many sensory strategies used by occupational therapists have not yet been studied systematically. Diana Henry has developed a series of guidebooks for different age groups that describe many of the sensory strategies that therapists have found to be useful and practical.[110,113-115] She also has developed an electronic tool called *Quick Tips* for linking Sensory Processing Measure assessment results to a menu of sensory strategies to consider for the child being assessed.[111,112]

Individual Training in Specific Skills

Although OT-SI intervention is focused on improving foundational neural functions that allow a wide range of capabilities and skills to emerge, therapists will provide interventions that immediately help a child develop specific skills and the family develop short-term coping strategies. For example, a child with poor proprioceptive feedback may need to keep up with handwriting exercises assigned in class. Application of individual OT-SI intervention would aim to help the child develop better body awareness that eventually will help not only with writing but also with catching, throwing, cutting, buttoning, and many other proprioception-dependent skills. However, because of everyday classroom stress from the demands of handwriting, the occupational therapist may provide specific handwriting interventions to help the child develop better handwriting skills. When working on specific skill development, the occupational therapist may find that success is easier to obtain when mindful of the basic assumptions underlying OT-SI intervention (see Box 9-2). For example, the occupational therapist could build on the child's inner drive by encouraging self-direction and active participation, for example, through having the child write words, sentences, or paragraphs related to individual interests and experiences.

Occupational therapists providing OT-SI intervention often reserve a segment of individual therapy sessions to devote to specific skill training, if indicated by the child's presenting problems and by the child and family's goals. Skills often targeted include fine motor skills, dressing skills, sensorimotor oral and eating skills, and games and activities that are popular with peers (e.g., jacks, bike riding). Expected outcomes are specific to the targeted skill. Other chapters in this textbook that address skill therapy programs provide detailed information about specific outcomes and how they are measured.

Group Interventions

Group activity programs may be provided in conjunction with individual OT-SI or after a period of time receiving individual OT-SI. These may include groups that focus on social skills, communication, visual-motor or fine motor skills, gross motor skills or activities, or self-regulation. Group programs are ideal arenas in which the increases in self-confidence made in individual therapy can be tried out in the more challenging context of a social setting.

In some situations, external variables such as funding limitations, availability of staff, or organizational policies create the need for children to receive therapy in a group setting. If a group intervention is the only option, it is important that occupational therapists make recommendations for specific interventions based primarily on the needs of the children being served, rather than allowing the external factors to dictate the type of intervention that is provided in the group setting.

The occupational therapist working with a group of children cannot provide the same level of vigilance to individual responses that takes place during individual therapy. Therefore, some of the highly individualized applications of OT-SI intervention cannot be used within a group, nor can the therapist give the close guidance that is finely tuned to the individual child's needs at every moment of the treatment session. However, the principles of OT-SI outlined in Box 9-3 are important concepts to incorporate into the group format as much as possible.

To apply sensory integration principles to a group program, an occupational therapist should be familiar enough with sensory integration theory to understand precautions and general effects of various sensory and motor activities. Experience and training in working with groups, including how to maintain the attention of children in a group, how to address varying skill and interest levels, and how to deal with behavioral issues, are also recommended for occupational therapists applying sensory integration principles in group programs.

Group programs, compared with individual therapy, tend to place greater demands on children for several reasons, including limited opportunity for individualization of activities, the presence of other children with their unpredictable behaviors, and reduced opportunity for direct assistance from the therapist. Thus, a limitation posed by group programs is that challenges imposed on the group may at times be too great for an individual child, leading to frustration and failure. The therapist who provides a group program needs to be alert to the potential for this undesirable effect and strive to avoid it as much as possible.

On the other hand, working with children in a group provides valuable opportunities to observe some of the ways in which sensory integrative problems disrupt participation in a social context (Figure 9-13). Some problems emerge only in group situations and may not be evident during individual therapy. For example, tactile defensiveness may not be apparent in the safe constraints of individual therapy but may become obvious as a child tries to participate within a group of people who are brushing by in an unpredictable manner. Observing how the group dynamic affects the child can help the therapist know which aspects of the classroom, playground, park, or after-school activities are likely to pose a threat or challenge (Case Study 9-2).

An especially innovative application of sensory integration concepts to groups is reflected in the work of Williams and Shellenberger.[246] Through a group format, their Alert Program helps children learn to recognize how they feel when their levels of alertness and arousal change throughout the day. Using this awareness, participants then learn to monitor their arousal levels in a variety of settings and to identify the sensory experiences that they can use to change their level of alertness to function more optimally. This approach particularly seems to be useful in school settings and as an adjunct to individual OT-SI. In a survey of types of services provided by occupational therapists to children with emotional disturbances in public schools, Barnes and her colleagues found that the most commonly reported intervention was sensory integration, with nearly 47% using the Alert Program individually or in groups.[35] In another study, positive outcomes for children with emotional disturbance were documented following an 8-week long Alert Program delivered within the classroom setting.[36] An RCT showed that children with fetal alcohol spectrum disorders who received a caregiver-child adaptation of the Alert Program made significant gains in executive and emotional functioning compared with the control group.[243]

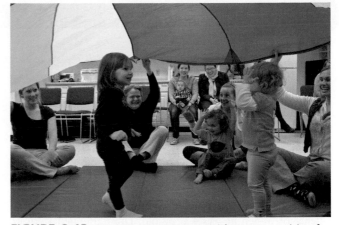

FIGURE 9-13 Group programs provide opportunities for children with sensory integrative disorders to develop coping skills that help them function in social context with peers.

It is important to differentiate between what can be accomplished within a group versus an individual therapy session. Because group programs do not permit the same degree of intensive, individualized work, they generally are not expected to lead to the same outcomes. Goals for group interventions usually address the particular purpose of the group intervention, such as development of particular social or motor skills. Gains in social participation are among the most important and helpful of group intervention outcomes.

Consultation on Modification of Activities, Routines, and Environments

Sensory integrative problems are complex and are often misinterpreted as solely behavioral, psychological, or emotional. Helping family members, teachers, and other professionals to understand the sensory integrative nature of the problem can be a powerful means toward helping the child. When the child's behavior is reframed is sensory terms using everyday language, a new understanding of the child often ensues. Cermak aptly referred to this process as *demystification*.[62] Parents commonly express relief at finally understanding puzzling and frustrating behaviors, and they may experience release from feeling that they have caused these problems through a maladaptive parenting style. This insight opens the door to discovering simple strategies that can be used throughout the day that help the

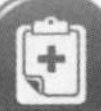

CASE STUDY 9-2 Drew

History

Drew was diagnosed with autism when he was 7 years of age. His cognitive functioning was within age expectations. His mother was a native Korean speaker, and his father was a native English speaker. Both Korean and English were spoken in the home. All of Drew's early developmental milestones were attained within normal limits, except for language acquisition. He did not speak any words until 2 years of age, and by age 3 his family was concerned about his delayed language skills. Drew attended an English-language preschool at 3 years of age and then a Korean-language preschool. He was asked to leave the second preschool because of aggressive behavior. When he was 4 years old, Drew attended a private special-education school where he received speech therapy and participated in a language-intensive playgroup. When Drew reached kindergarten age, he was enrolled in public special education programs.

Reason for Referral

Drew initially was referred by a counselor to an occupational therapy private practice for evaluation when he was nearly 8 years old. His counselor thought that Drew had signs of a sensory integrative disorder, and he believed that Drew might benefit from occupational therapy. Drew's mother reported that her main concerns for Drew were related to his poor socialization skills, his limited ability to play with games and toys, and his tendency to become easily frustrated.

Evaluation Procedures

Although the Sensory Integration and Praxis Tests (SIPT) were attempted during the initial occupational therapy assessment, Drew did not follow the directions or attend to the tests sufficiently to obtain reliable scores. Consequently, his occupational therapy evaluation was guided by the therapist's knowledge of sensory integration theory and comprehensive procedures for assessment of sensory integration. Evaluation procedures consisted of a parent interview, parent completion of a developmental history and sensory questionnaire, and structured as well as unstructured observations of Drew in a clinical therapy setting. At the time of assessment it was not possible to interview Drew's teacher. However, Drew's mother, who often observed him in the classroom, provided information about his performance at school.

Evaluation Results

Drew demonstrated inefficiencies in several areas related to sensory integration. During the assessment, signs of inconsistent responses to tactile input were evident. For example, Drew demonstrated a complete lack of response to some tactile stimuli such as a puff of air on the back of his neck or the light touch of a cotton ball applied to his feet when he was not visually attending. However, he withdrew in an agitated fashion when the therapist attempted to position him. His mother reported that he showed extreme avoidance of certain textures of food and clothing and that he disliked being touched. She also stated that he seemed to become irritated by being near other children at school and sometimes pinched or pushed peers who came close to him. Drew also appeared easily overstimulated by extraneous visual and auditory stimuli. His mother stated that he often covered his ears at home when loud noises were present and that at school he sometimes seemed confused as to the direction of sounds. He was observed to pick up objects and look at them very closely, and he appeared to rely on his vision to complete tasks. In response to movement, he enjoyed swinging slowly but became fearful with an increase in velocity. His mother stated that he often seemed afraid when he was climbing on equipment at the park.

Drew's balance was observed to be poor, and his equilibrium reactions were inconsistent. He also had trouble positioning himself on various pieces of equipment, indicating poor body awareness. During the assessment he appeared to seek touch-pressure stimuli, including total body compression. He was reported to jump a great deal at home and at school. These types of proprioception-generating actions appeared to have a calming effect on Drew.

In the area of praxis, Drew imitated positions and followed verbal directions to complete motor actions, but he had difficulty initiating activities on his own or attempting something that was unfamiliar to him. He also had difficulty timing and sequencing his actions. His mother reported that he tended not to participate in sports or in park activities and that he had trouble throwing, catching, and kicking balls. Drew completed puzzles, strung beads, and wrote his name; however, bilateral activities such as cutting and pasting were difficult for him.

Socially, Drew demonstrated poor eye contact and tended to use repetitive phrases that he had heard in the past. His mother stated that he wanted to play with peers but found it hard to make friends. Drew was independent in all self-care skills, except for tying shoes and managing some fasteners.

Based on the interview and questionnaire with Drew's mother, as well as observation of Drew in the specialized therapy setting, the therapist's evaluation report concluded that his behaviors indicated irregularities in sensory responsiveness, including hyper-responsiveness to some aspects of tactile, vestibular, visual, and auditory stimuli. Perception of tactile and proprioceptive information was also thought to be affected because of signs of poor tactile awareness and inefficient use of position sense. He also demonstrated difficulty with balance, bilateral coordination, and the ideation, timing, and sequencing aspects of praxis. These difficulties were thought to interfere with Drew's ability to play purposefully with toys and to participate in age-appropriate games and sports. These sensory integrative problems, in combination with his language delays, very likely were interfering significantly with his social skills and his ability to make friends, and increasing his tendency to become frustrated, which were the major concerns of his parents.

Recommendation

Individual occupational therapy was recommended to improve Drew's sensory integrative functioning as well as fine and gross motor skills. Because socialization issues were such a major concern for Drew's family and were interfering with his performance at school, the evaluating therapist also

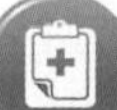

CASE STUDY 9-2 Drew—cont'd

recommended that Drew participate in an after-school group occupational therapy program to facilitate the acquisition of social skills.

Occupational Therapy Program

Drew received individual and group occupational therapy for 1 year in a therapeutic setting designed for the provision of OT-SI. The individual therapy involved OT-SI intervention as well as intervention strategies focused on specific skill development. Over the course of therapy, Drew demonstrated significant gains in sensory integrative functions. Specifically, he no longer exhibited signs of tactile defensiveness and fear of movement activities, and his performance in fine and gross motor activities suggested improved tactile perception and body position awareness. Motor planning of novel actions improved but continued to be of some concern for Drew. However, he made measurable gains in familiar motor tasks such as catching and throwing a ball, writing, and using scissors. Through the group occupational therapy program, Drew developed new social skills that enabled him to initiate and maintain interaction with peers, share objects, and play cooperatively with some assistance and structure from adults.

After this year of individual and group occupational therapy, a combination of consultation and individual therapy at school was recommended and provided. Teacher consultation addressed modification of classroom activities and routines to support Drew's success. The focus of this phase of Drew's occupational therapy program was to help him apply his improved sensory, motor, and social skills within the natural context of school. Because the initial year of therapy using an OT-SI approach had helped Drew tolerate and respond appropriately to sensory information, and because he had developed many of the specific skills that he needed in the classroom during individual therapy, his focus on and mastery of the demands expected of him at school had greatly improved. By the end of the school year, Drew's occupational therapist recommended that occupational therapy be discontinued because she believed that his teacher would continue supports in the areas that had been addressed through the consultation program.

However, when the individualized educational program (IEP) team met to discuss Drew's transition to a new school, they had significant concerns that Drew might regress in a new setting with many new routines and expectations. The IEP team requested that occupational therapy continue to ensure a smooth transition for Drew and to put in place a plan that would continue to help him develop socially.

When school resumed in the fall, the occupational therapist had arranged a "big buddy" program with a local high school. Two high school seniors worked with Drew as part of a social service assignment during recess for the fall semester. The occupational therapist trained the high school students to carry out a socialization program aimed at helping Drew feel comfortable with a new set of peers. Drew seemed to look up to the high school students and responded well to the "big buddy" program.

By the end of the fall semester in the new school, Drew played cooperatively with peers, interacting independently and communicating appropriately. His occupational therapy program was formally discontinued at this time, although the occupational therapist continued to communicate informally with Drew's teacher on occasion. The option for further consultation or direct intervention was available should the need arise, but no further intervention was needed.

child to feel more comfortable and participate more fully in everyday occupations. Teachers also may appreciate having an alternative way to view child behaviors, especially when this new perspective is coupled with classroom strategies that promote responses from the child that are more productive. Children also stand to benefit greatly from understanding their own sensory characteristics. Because individual differences in sensory integration may be lifelong tendencies, it is critical that the child with sensory processing differences learn to construct daily routines and organize the sensory aspects of work and play activities and environments in order to live as comfortably and successfully as possible.[82]

Through consultation and collaboration with those who are in ongoing contact with the child, the therapist can provide critical information and recommend implementation of specific strategies to influence the child's life positively across a variety of settings. Indirect intervention in the form of consultation is often critical for success and should be included in a comprehensive occupational therapy program for the child with sensory integration challenges. Whenever individual OT-SI intervention is provided, consultation with parents and/or teachers should also be provided.

Consultation using the concept of "sensory diet"[244] involves collaboration with parents or teachers to embed individualized sensory experiences at strategic time points throughout the day to support the child's alertness or calming at appropriate times. For example, a sensory diet for a child might include physical activity before school to boost arousal level, chewing gum while in class to support sustained attention, and a deep pressure massage to promote calming on returning home.

In many situations, the first step in the consultation process should be to help caregivers and teachers better understand sensory integration in general, as well as how sensory integration concepts apply to specific children. This can be achieved through individual meetings with parents or teachers, parent/teacher conferences, group experiential sessions, lecture and discussion groups, professional in-services, and ongoing education programs (Figure 9-14). Helping the adults in a child's life to understand their own sensory integrative processes is often an effective way to make new sensory integration concepts meaningful. Williams and Shellenberger use this tactic in their Alert Program.[246] Before implementing the program with children, the adults who will administer the program participate in a training program designed to develop self-awareness and insight into their own sensory characteristics and preferences.

Perhaps the most important component of any consultation program is providing guidance for identifying, preventing, and coping with the specific challenges in everyday life that stem

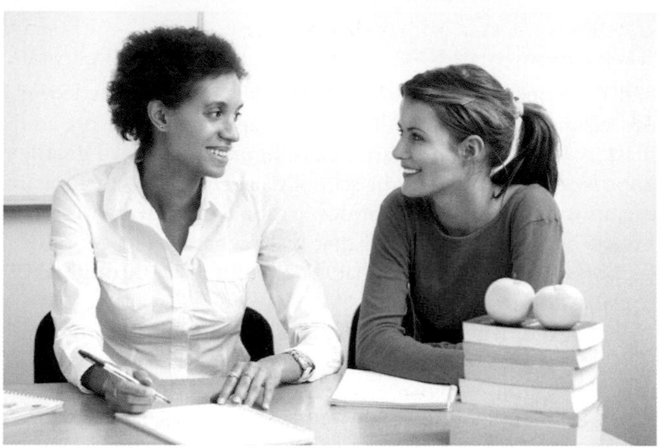

FIGURE 9-14 Consultation in school involves joint problem solving between the occupational therapist and the teacher. (Photo © istock.com.)

from a child's sensory integrative problems. Sometimes specific activities can be suggested that help a child to prepare for a challenging task. For example, a child who has tactile defensiveness may more readily engage in activities such as finger painting or sand play if firm touch-pressure is applied to the skin before the activity. Modifying the activity might involve providing tools to use with the paint or sand to give the child a ready "break" from the unpleasant sensation. A home program that includes gradual introduction of tactile sensation in a safe place, such as the bathtub, can also help to reduce negative reactions. The therapist can also promote success in activities by suggesting individualized ways to help a child through difficult tasks. For example, some children with dyspraxia are likely to be more successful in completing a novel task when they receive verbal directions, whereas others respond optimally to visual demonstrations, and still others need physical assistance with the motions. Determining which method or combination of methods is most likely to help the individual child can assist adults in facilitating success.

Another important way that consultation can support a child's functioning is through recommendations for environmental modifications that aim to manage sound, lighting, contact with other people, environmental odors, and visual distractions in the classroom, playground, cafeteria, and assembly rooms. This is particularly important for children who are generally over-responsive, as they tend to be highly affected by sensory characteristics of their environments that others may not notice. Environmental modifications can make an important difference in a child's attention, behavior, and, ultimately, ability to participate in academic and social activities.

The same therapist qualifications needed to provide individual OT-SI intervention are desirable in providing consultation. The occupational therapist should be well versed in sensory integration concepts in order to explain them in simple yet accurate and meaningful terms. Furthermore, the therapist needs to fully understand the child's sensory integrative difficulties and use this understanding to predict what the child's likely responses will be to various activities and situations. Therefore, the occupational therapist needs to conduct a comprehensive assessment of the child before making any suggestions, in order to identify the sensory strategies that are likely to be most helpful, and to consider any precautions that might apply. Procedures or techniques that require advanced training of an occupational therapist should not be recommended for parents and other professionals. For example, an appropriate consultation program never attempts to train a parent or teacher to provide individual therapeutic activities that require advanced training for monitoring the child's response, such as applying intense sensory stimulation. Also, it is imperative that the occupational therapist have excellent communication skills and respect for the various people and environments that are involved. Bundy provides a helpful description of the communication process involved in a good consultation program.[52]

Expected outcomes of consultation programs depend on the individual child's presenting problems, the family or school team's goals, and the focus of the consultation. For instance, helping a teacher understand how best to seat a child in class (e.g., on a therapy ball chair versus a firm wooden chair, or in the front corner of the room near the teacher's desk versus the back of the room) may make it easier for the child to attend to instruction in the classroom. Desired outcomes might be measured as increased time on task, increased time in seat, decreased number of disruptive behaviors in class, or improved performance in academic tasks.

Limited research has been conducted on outcomes resulting from consultation involving changes to daily environments or routines, but the evidence that exists is consistently positive. In a study of the effectiveness of home-based consultation, Dunn et al.[87] evaluated a contextual intervention in which therapists made regular home visits to provide coaching to parents on issues related to activity settings, family routines, and sensory processing characteristics of their children with autism, all of whom demonstrated atypical sensory processing. Outcomes data from GAS and other instruments indicated that the parents felt more competent and the children demonstrated increased participation in everyday life following 10 intervention sessions. Hall and Case-Smith[106] conducted a pre- post-test study in which 10 young children with moderate to severe sensory modulation and visual-motor problems received a combined sensory diet and sound-based intervention that was individually tailored for each child and administered at home by parents with ongoing occupational therapy consultation. Results indicated improved sensory modulation and visual-motor skills. Kinnealey et al.[131] conducted a single subject study of four adolescent males with sensory over-responsiveness, three of whom had autism, to examine whether modifications to classroom sound and lighting would improve their attention and perceptions of classroom experiences. The intervention consisted of replacing fluorescent with halogen lighting and installing sound-absorbing walls, which decreased the decibel levels within the room. Results indicated that all students demonstrated increased attention to academic tasks. In daily journals students expressed comfort and pleasure with the altered environment. An RCT that compared an 8-week course of school-based movement therapy to standard school routine showed behavioral improvements for the treatment group,[108] and a pre- post-test study of a 4-month manualized morning yoga program produced significant reductions in maladaptive behaviors of children compared with the standard morning routine at school.[133] In all of these studies raters were not blinded to condition, which raises concern that outcome ratings may have been biased, but results are very encouraging and suggest that further evaluation of these interventions is warranted.

Often during consultation for individual children, occupational therapists become aware of sensory features within home, school, or community environments that can be modified in ways that benefit all of the children who live, work, and play there. In such situations, occupational therapists should consider using their knowledge of sensory integration to advocate for environmental changes that will benefit all children. For example, playgrounds or backyards may be modified to stimulate development of praxis and playfulness for all the children by providing equipment and materials that can present sensorimotor challenges at varying levels of complexity and can be played with in many different ways.[54] Adjustments to school environments may be especially important because children spend large amounts of time in this environment. These may include alterations in lighting, sound, or types and amount of sensory stimulation present in different areas. Additionally, daily routines with key sensory components may benefit all children in a classroom. For example, research indicates that children generally better attend to demanding academic tasks when they engage in physical activity breaks throughout the day, which boosts ability to sustain attention to cognitively challenging tasks.[37,124] Initial morning routines involving sensorimotor activity may assist in preparing children for the cognitive work ahead in the school day, and regularly scheduled recess periods allow for physical activity to prepare children to return to the classroom refreshed and ready to work.[122]

Sensory integration is a fascinating, dynamic, and complex area of pediatric occupational therapy practice. In addition to the interventions discussed in this chapter, new applications of sensory integration theory are emerging, for example, collaborations among occupational therapists, psychologists, and other professionals such as art therapists to merge sensory integration knowledge and techniques into psychotherapeutic interventions for children who have experienced trauma.[135] Other emerging applications of sensory integration knowledge aim to promote the well-being of communities as well as individual children, for example, through playground design and school-wide routines that support the emotional, physical, intellectual, and social development of all children. For these as well as established interventions for children with sensory integration difficulties, research will continue to be important in discerning the extent to which an intervention is helpful, how it is helpful, and for whom it is helpful.

Summary

Since the inception of this field 50 years ago, research has played an important role in shaping theory, assessment, and intervention practices that address sensory integration. The existence of different patterns of sensory integration challenges encountered by children has a strong evidence base with a long history. Although more research is needed to discern who are the best candidates for OT-SI, the existing research for this intervention is encouraging and suggests that it produces outcomes related to children's everyday lives. Alternative interventions that build on sensory integration theory also influence today's landscape of occupational therapy practice for children.

Summary Points

- Sensory integration refers to a complex set of neural processes in the brain involving the integration of sensory information for active use in purposeful behavior.
- The term *sensory integration* is also used to refer to a specific practice approach in occupational therapy, that is, OT-SI.
- Sensory integration theory posits that the tactile, proprioceptive, and vestibular sensory systems are influential in early child development and that the child's active engagement to meet challenges by integrating and using sensory information leads to both neuroplastic and behavioral changes that influence further development and engagement in occupations.
- A long history of quantitative research provides evidence for the existence of several patterns of sensory integration problems that arise in childhood (i.e., sensory modulation, discrimination and perception, vestibular-bilateral, and praxis difficulties) that are associated with different effects on the occupational life of a child.
- Clinical assessment of sensory integration should be comprehensive and include history, interviews and questionnaires, naturalistic and structured observations, and standardized testing. Data from these different sources must be integrated to discern whether a recognizable pattern of sensory integration difficulty is present, and if so, what the appropriate course of action should be to help the child and family.
- Occupational therapy using a sensory integration approach (OT-SI) is provided in individual therapy sessions in which the occupational therapist encourages the child's active engagement, collaborates with the child on activity choices, and presents the child with sensory and motor challenges while ensuring success and safety, all within the context of play in a specially designed clinical environment.
- The Fidelity Measure for Ayres Sensory Integration Intervention can be used to ensure that when OT-SI intervention is provided, the process of intervention as well as occupational therapist qualifications and the therapeutic environment are appropriate.
- OT-SI may be appropriate when assessment results indicate a known pattern of sensory integration difficulty for children with learning and behavioral challenges, with autism, with other diagnoses, or with no medical diagnoses.
- Outcomes of OT-SI intervention include achievement of more sustained or complex adaptive responses, improved fine or gross motor skills, improved language or social skills, enhanced self-confidence and self-esteem, better participation in occupations at home and in school, and enhanced family life. These outcomes are evaluated using assessment of specific behaviors as well as standardized tests and methods such as goal attainment scaling.
- Evidence of effectiveness of OT-SI is mixed, but the best evidence uses rigorous research design, including fidelity

checks, and provides encouraging evidence of effectiveness, particularly when goal attainment scaling is used.

- Alternative interventions that are used in conjunction with or instead of OT-SI intervention include sensory stimulation protocols, sensory-based strategies incorporated into daily routines, specific skill training, group interventions such as the Alert Program, and consultation models; outcomes vary for these diverse interventions, and studies of effectiveness are generally more limited.

REFERENCES

1. Ahn, R. R., Miller, L. J., Milberger, S., et al. (2004). Prevalence of parents' perceptions of sensory processing disorders among kindergarten children. *American Journal of Occupational Therapy, 58*, 287–293.
2. American Academy of Cerebral Palsy and Developmental Medicine. (2008). AACPDM methodology to develop systematic reviews of treatment interventions (Revision 1.2). Retrieved February 24, 2014, from: <https://www.aacpdm.org/resources/outcomes/systematicReviewsMethodology.pdf>.
3. American Academy of Pediatrics. (2012). Policy statement: Sensory integration therapies for children with developmental and behavioral disorders. *Pediatrics, 129*(6), 1186–1189.
4. American Occupational Therapy Association. (2008). Occupational therapy practice framework: Domain and process. *American Journal of Occupational Therapy, 62*, 625–668.
5. Anderson, E. L. (1993). Parental perceptions of the influence of occupational therapy utilizing sensory integrative techniques on the daily living skills of children with autism. Los Angeles: University of Southern California. Unpublished master's thesis.
6. Ayres, A. J. (1963). The Eleanor Clark Slagle Lecture. The development of perceptual-motor abilities: A theoretical basis for treatment of dysfunction. *American Journal of Occupational Therapy, 17*, 221–225.
7. Ayres, A. J. (1964). Tactile functions: Their relation to hyperactive and perceptual motor behavior. *American Journal of Occupational Therapy, 18*, 6–11.
8. Ayres, A. J. (1965). Patterns of perceptual-motor dysfunction in children: A factor analytic study. *Perceptual and Motor Skills, 20*, 335–368.
9. Ayres, A. J. (1966). Interrelations among perceptual-motor abilities in a group of normal children. *American Journal of Occupational Therapy, 20*, 288–292.
10. Ayres, A. J. (1966). Interrelationships among perceptual-motor functions in children. *American Journal of Occupational Therapy, 20*, 68–71.
11. Ayres, A. J. (1969). Deficits in sensory integration in educationally handicapped children. *Journal of Learning Disabilities, 2*(3), 44–52.
12. Ayres, A. J. (1971). Characteristics of types of sensory integrative dysfunction. *American Journal of Occupational Therapy, 25*, 329–334.
13. Ayres, A. J. (1972). Improving academic scores through sensory integration. *Journal of Learning Disabilities, 5*, 338–343.
14. Ayres, A. J. (1973). *Sensory integration and learning disorders.* Los Angeles: Western Psychological Services.
15. Ayres, A. J. (1972). *Southern California Sensory Integration Tests.* Los Angeles: Western Psychological Services.
16. Ayres, A. J. (1972). Types of sensory integrative dysfunction among disabled learners. *American Journal of Occupational Therapy, 26*(1), 13–18.
17. Ayres, A. J. (1975). *Southern California Postrotary Nystagmus Test.* Los Angeles: Western Psychological Services.
18. Ayres, A. J. (1977). Cluster analyses of measures of sensory integration. *American Journal of Occupational Therapy, 31*(6), 362–366.
19. Ayres, A. J. (1978). Learning disabilities and the vestibular system. *Journal of Learning Disabilities, 11*(1), 30–41.
20. Ayres, A. J. (1979). *Sensory integration and the child.* Los Angeles: Western Psychological Services.
21. Ayres, A. J. (1985). *Developmental dyspraxia and adult-onset apraxia.* Torrance, CA: Sensory Integration International.
22. Ayres, A. J. (1989). *Sensory Integration and Praxis Tests manual.* Los Angeles: Western Psychological Services.
23. Ayres, A. J. (2004). *Sensory integration and the child* (2nd ed.). Los Angeles: Western Psychological Services.
24. Ayres, A. J., & Mailloux, Z. (1981). Influence of sensory integration procedures on language development. *American Journal of Occupational Therapy, 35*(6), 383–390.
25. Ayres, A. J., Mailloux, Z., & Wendler, C. L. W. (1987). Developmental apraxia: Is it a unitary function? *Occupational Therapy Journal of Research, 7*, 93–110.
26. Ayres, A. J., & Marr, D. (1991). Sensory integration and praxis tests. In A. G. Fisher, E. A. Murray, & A. C. Bundy (Eds.), *Sensory integration: Theory and practice* (pp. 203–250). Philadelphia: F. A. Davis.
27. Ayres, A. J., & Tickle, L. (1980). Hyperresponsivity to touch and vestibular stimuli as a predictor of positive response to sensory integration procedures in autistic children. *American Journal of Occupational Therapy, 34*, 375–381.
28. Bach-Y-Rita, P. (1981). Brain plasticity. In J. Goodgold (Ed.), *Brain plasticity.* St. Louis: Mosby.
29. Bagatell, N., Mirigliani, G., Patterson, C., et al. (2010). Effectiveness of therapy ball chairs on classroom participation in children with autism spectrum disorders. *American Journal of Occupational Therapy, 64*, 895–903.
30. Bagby, M., Dickie, V., & Baranek, G. T. (2012). How sensory experiences in children with and without autism affect family occupations. *American Journal of Occupational Therapy, 66*, 78–86.
31. Baranek, G. T. (1999). Autism during infancy: A retrospective video analysis of sensory motor and social behaviors at 9-12 months of age. *Journal of Autism and Developmental Disorders, 29*(3), 213–224.
32. Baranek, G. T., Foster, L. G., & Berkson, G. (1997). Sensory defensiveness in persons with developmental disabilities. *Occupational Therapy Journal of Research, 17*, 173–185.
33. Baranek, G. T., David, F. J., Poe, M. D., et al. (2006). Sensory Experiences Questionnaire: Discriminating sensory features in young children with autism, developmental delays, and typical development. *Journal of Child Psychology and Psychiatry, 47*(6), 591–601.
34. Baranek, G. T., Little, L. M., Parham, L. D., et al. (2014). Sensory features in autism spectrum disorders. In F. Volkmar, R. Paul, K. Pelphrey, & S. Rogers (Eds.), *Handbook of autism* (4th ed., pp. 378–408). Hoboken, NJ: Wiley.
35. Barnes, K. J., Beck, A. J., Vogel, K. A., et al. (2003). Perceptions regarding school-based occupational therapy for children with emotional disturbances.

American Journal of Occupational Therapy, 57, 337–341.

36. Barnes, K. J., Vogel, K. A., Beck, A. J., et al. (2008). Self-regulation strategies of children with emotional disturbance. *Physical and Occupational Therapy in Pediatrics, 28*(4), 369–387.
37. Barros, R. M., Silver, E. J., & Stein, R. F. K. (2009). School recess and group classroom behavior. *Pediatrics, 123*, 431–436.
38. Beckett, C., Maughan, B., Rutter, M., et al. (2006). Do the effects of early severe deprivation on cognition persist into early adolescence? Findings from the English and Romanian Adoptees Study. *Child Development, 77*, 696–711.
39. Beery, K. E., & Beery, N. A. (2006). *The developmental test of visual-motor integration* (5th ed.). San Antonio, TX: Psychological Corporation.
40. Behen, M. E., Helder, E., Rothermel, R., et al. (2008). Incidence of specific absolute neurocognitive impairment in globally intact children with histories of early severe deprivation. *Child Neuropsychology, 14*, 453–469.
41. Ben-Sasson, A., Cermak, S. A., Orsmond, G. I., et al. (2007). Extreme sensory modulation behaviors in toddlers with autism spectrum isorders. *American Journal of Occupational Therapy, 61*(5), 584–592.
42. Ben-Sasson, A., Hen, L., Fluss, R., et al. (2009). A meta-analysis of sensory modulation symptoms in individuals with autism spectrum disorders. *Journal of Autism and Developmental Disorders, 39*, 1–11.
43. Bennett, E. L., Diamond, M. C., Krech, D., et al. (1964). Chemical and anatomical plasticity of brain. *Science, 146*, 610–619.
44. Benson, J. D., Beeman, E., Smitsky, D., et al. (2011). The deep pressure and proprioceptive technique (DPPT) versus nonspecific child-guided brushing: A case study. *Journal of Occupational Therapy, Schools, & Early Intervention, 4*(3–4), 204–214.
45. Bettison, S. (1996). The long-term effects of auditory training on children with autism. *Journal of Autism and Developmental Disorders, 26*, 361–374.
46. Blanche, E. I. (2002). *Observations based on sensory integration theory.* Torrance, CA: Pediatric Therapy Network.
47. Blanche, E., & Schaaf, R. (2001). Proprioception: A cornerstone of sensory integrative intervention. In S. S. Roley, E. I. Blanche, & R. C. Schaaf (Eds.), *Understanding the nature of sensory integration with diverse populations* (pp. 385–408). San Antonio, TX: Therapy Skill Builders.
48. Blanche, E. I., Bodison, S., Chang, M. C., et al. (2012). Development of the Comprehensive Observations of Proprioception (COP): Validity, reliability, and factor analysis. *American Journal of Occupational Therapy, 66*, 691–698.
49. Bretherton, E., Bates, S., McNew, C., et al. (1981). Comprehension and production of symbols in infancy: An experimental study. *Developmental Psychology, 17*, 728–736.
50. Brown, C., & Dunn, W. (2002). *Adolescent/Adult Sensory Profile.* San Antonio, TX: The Psychological Corporation.
51. Bruininks, R. H., & Bruininks, B. (2006). *Bruininks-Oseretsky Test of Motor Proficiency: Examiner's manual.* Circle Pines, MN: American Guidance Service.
52. Bundy, A. C. (2002). Using sensory integration theory in schools: Sensory integration and consultation. In A. C. Bundy, S. J. Lane, & E. A. Murray (Eds.), *Sensory integration: Theory and practice* (2nd ed., pp. 309–332). Philadelphia: F. A. Davis.
53. Bundy, A. C., & Murray, E. A. (2002). Sensory integration: A. Jean Ayres' theory revisited. In A. C. Bundy, S. J. Lane, & E. A. Murray (Eds.), *Sensory integration: Theory and practice* (2nd ed., pp. 141–165). Philadelphia: F. A. Davis.
54. Bundy, A. C., Luckett, T., Naughton, G. A., et al. (2008). Playful interaction: Occupational therapy for all children on the school playground. *American Journal of Occupational Therapy, 62*, 522–527.
55. Burke, J. P., Schaaf, R. C., & Hall, T. B. L. (2008). Family narratives and play assessment. In L. D. Parham & L. S. Fazio (Eds.), *Play in occupational therapy for children* (2nd ed., pp. 195–215). St. Louis: Mosby.
56. Burleigh, J. M., McIntosh, K., & Thompson, W. M. W. (2002). Central auditory processing disorders. In A. C. Bundy, S. J. Lane, & E. A. Murray (Eds.), *Sensory integration: Theory and practice* (2nd ed., pp. 141–165). Philadelphia: F. A. Davis.
57. Cabay, M., & King, L. J. (1989). Sensory integration and perception: The foundation for concept formation. *Occupational Therapy in Practice, 1*, 18–27.
58. Case-Smith, J. (1991). The effects of tactile defensiveness and tactile discrimination on in-hand manipulation. *American Journal of Occupational Therapy, 45*, 811–818.
59. Case-Smith, J., & Bryan, T. (1999). The effects of occupational therapy with sensory integration emphasis on preschool-age children with autism. *American Journal of Occupational Therapy, 53*, 489–497.
60. Cermak, S. A. (1988). The relationship between attention deficits and sensory integration disorders (Part I). *Sensory Integration Special Interest Section Newsletter, 11*(2), 1–4.
61. Cermak, S. A. (1991). Somatodyspraxia. In A. C. Bundy, S. J. Lane, & E. A. Murray (Eds.), *Sensory integration: Theory and practice* (2nd ed., pp. 137–170). Philadelphia: F. A. Davis.
62. Cermak, S. A. (2001). The effects of deprivation on processing, play and praxis. In S. S. Roley, E. I. Blanche, & R. C. Schaaf (Eds.), *Understanding the nature of sensory integration with diverse populations* (pp. 385–408). San Antonio, TX: Therapy Skill Builders.
63. Chamak, B., Bonniau, B., Jaunay, E., et al. (2008). What can we learn about autism from autistic persons? *Psychotherapy and Psychosomatics, 77*, 271–279.
64. Chang, M. C.-C., Parham, L. D., Blanche, E. I., et al. (2012). Autonomic and behavioral responses of children with autism to auditory stimuli. *American Journal of Occupational Therapy, 66*, 567–576.
65. Chugani, H. T., & Phelps, M. E. (1986). Maturational changes in cerebral function in infants determined by 18FDG positron emission tomography. *Science, 231*, 840–843.
66. Clark, F. A., Mailloux, Z., & Parham, D. (1989). Sensory integration and children with learning disorders. In P. N. Pratt & A. S. Allen (Eds.), *Occupational therapy for children* (2nd ed., pp. 457–509). St. Louis: Mosby.
67. Cohn, E. S. (2001). From waiting to relating: Parents' experiences in the waiting room of an occupational therapy clinic. *American Journal of Occupational Therapy, 55*, 168–175.
68. Cohn, E. S. (2001). Parent perspectives of occupational therapy using a sensory integration approach. *American Journal of Occupational Therapy, 55*, 285–294.
69. Cohn, E. S., & Cermak, S. A. (1998). Including the family perspective in sensory integration outcomes research. *American Journal of Occupational Therapy, 52*, 540–546.
70. Cohn, E. S., Miller, L. J., & Tickle-Degnen, L. (2000). Parental hopes for therapy outcomes: Children with sensory modulation disorders. *American Journal of Occupational Therapy, 54*, 36–43.
71. Cosbey, J., Johnston, S. S., & Dunn, M. L. (2010). Sensory

processing disorders and social participation. *American Journal of Occupational Therapy, 64*, 462–473.
72. Coster, W., Deeney, T., Haltiwanger, J., et al. (1998). *School function assessment.* San Antonio, TX: Therapy Skill Builders.
73. Cox, A. L., Gast, D. L., Luscre, D., et al. (2009). The effects of weighted vest on appropriate in-seat behaviors of elementary-age students with autism and severe to profound intellectual disabilities. *Focus on Autism and Other Developmental Disabilities, 24*, 17–26.
74. Cui, M., Yang, Y., Zhang, J., et al. (2007). Enriched environment experience overcomes the memory deficits and depressive-like behavior induced by early life stress. *Neuroscience Letters, 404*, 208–212.
75. Daunhauer, L., & Cermak, S. (2008). Play occupations and the experience of deprivation. In D. Parham & L. Fazio (Eds.), *Play in occupational therapy for children* (2nd ed.). St. Louis: Mosby.
76. Davies, P. L., & Gavin, W. J. (2007). Validating the diagnosis of sensory processing disorders using EEG technology. *American Journal of Occupational Therapy, 61*, 176–189.
77. Davis, T. N., Durand, S., & Chan, J. M. (2011). The effects of a brushing procedure on stereotypical behavior. *Research in Autism Spectrum Disorders, 5*, 1053–1058.
78. Dowell, L. R., Mahone, E. M., & Mostofsky, S. H. (2009). Associations of postural knowledge and basic motor skill with dyspraxia in autism: Implications for abnormalities in distributed connectivity and motor learning. *Neuropsychology, 23*(5), 563–570.
79. Dru, D., Walker, J. P., & Walker, J. B. (1975). Self-produced locomotion restores visual capacity after striate lesion. *Science, 187*, 265–266.
80. Dunn, W. W. (1997). The impact of sensory processing abilities on the daily lives of young children and families: A conceptual model. *Infants and Young Children, 9*(4), 23–25.
81. Dunn, W. W. (1999). *Sensory Profile: User's manual.* San Antonio, TX: Psychological Corporation.
82. Dunn, W. W. (2001). The sensations of everyday life: Empirical, theoretical, and pragmatic considerations. *American Journal of Occupational Therapy, 55*, 608–620.
83. Dunn, W. W. (2002). *The Infant/Toddler Sensory Profile manual.* San Antonio, TX: Psychological Corporation.
84. Dunn, W. W. (2006). *Sensory Profile school companion manual.* San Antonio, TX: Psychological Corporation.
85. Dunn, W., & Bennett, D. (2002). Patterns of sensory processing in children with attention deficit hyperactivity disorder. *Occupational Therapy Journal of Research, 22*, 4–15.
86. Dunn, W., Myles, B. S., & Orr, S. (2002). Sensory processing issues associated with Asperger syndrome: A preliminary investigation. *American Journal of Occupational Therapy, 56*, 97–102.
87. Dunn, W., Cox, J., Foster, L., et al. (2012). Impact of a contextual intervention on child participation and parent competence among children with autism spectrum disorders: A pretest-posttest repeated-measures design. *American Journal of Occupational Therapy, 66*, 520–528.
88. Dziuk, M. A., Gidley Larson, J. C., Apostu, A., et al. (2007). Dyspraxia in autism: Association with motor, social, and communicative deficits. *Developmental Medicine and Child Neurology, 49*, 734–739.
89. Edelson, S. M., Edelson, M. G., Kerr, D. C. R., et al. (1999). Behavioral and physiological effects of deep pressure on children with autism: A pilot study evaluating the efficacy of Grandin's Hug Machine. *American Journal of Occupational Therapy, 53*, 145–152.
90. Eluvanthingal, T. K., Chugani, H. T., Behen, M. E., et al. (2006). Abnormal brain connectivity in children after early severe socioemotional deprivation: A diffusion tensor imaging study. *Pediatrics, 117*, 2093–2100.
91. Escalona, A., Field, T., Singer-Strunck, R., et al. (2001). Brief report: Improvements in the behavior of children with autism following massage therapy. *Journal of Autism and Developmental Disorders, 31*, 5.
92. Fedewa, A. L., & Erwin, H. E. (2011). Stability balls and students with attention and hyperactivity concerns: Implications for on-task and in-seat behavior. *American Journal of Occupational Therapy, 65*, 393–399.
93. Fertel-Daly, D., Bedell, G., & Hinojosa, J. (2001). Effects of a weighted vest on attention to task and self-stimulatory behaviors in preschoolers with pervasive developmental disorders. *American Journal of Occupational Therapy, 55*, 620–640.
94. Field, T., Lasko, D., Mundy, P., et al. (1997). Autistic children's attentiveness and responsivity improve after touch therapy. *Journal of Autism and Developmental Disorders, 27*, 333–338.
95. Fisher, A. G. (1991). Vestibular-proprioceptive processing and bilateral integration and sequencing deficits. In A. G. Fisher, E. A. Murray, & A. C. Bundy (Eds.), *Sensory integration: Theory and practice* (pp. 69–107). Philadelphia: F. A. Davis.
96. Flanagan, J. E., Landa, R., Bhat, A., et al. (2012). Head lag in infants at risk for autism: A preliminary study. *American Journal of Occupational Therapy, 66*, 577–585.
97. Fredrickson, J. M., Schwartz, D. W., & Kornhuber, H. H. (1966). Convergence and interaction of vestibular and deep somatic afferents upon neurons in the vestibular nuclei of the cat. *Acta Otolaryngologica, 61*, 168–188.
98. Freuler, A., Baranek, G., Watson, L., et al. (2012). Brief report: Precursors and trajectories of sensory features: Qualitative analysis of infant home videos. *American Journal of Occupational Therapy, 66*, e81–e84.
99. Fuentes, C. T., Mostofsky, S. H., & Bastian, A. J. (2011). No proprioceptive deficits in autism despite movement-related sensory and execution impairments. *Journal of Autism and Developmental Disorders, 41*, 1352–1361.
100. Goldsmith, H. H., Van Hulle, C. A., Arneson, C. L., et al. (2006). A population-based twin study of parentally reported tactile and auditory defensiveness in young children. *Journal of Abnormal Child Psychology, 34*(3), 393–407.
101. Grandin, T., & Scariano, M. M. (1986). *Emergence labeled autistic.* Novato, CA: Arena Press.
102. Green, S. A., & Ben-Sasson, A. (2010). Anxiety disorders and sensory over-responsivity in children with autism spectrum disorders: Is there a causal relationship? *Journal of Autism and Developmental Disorders, 40*, 1495–1504.
103. Gregg, C. L., Hafner, M. E., & Korner, A. (1976). The relative efficacy of vestibular-proprioceptive stimulation and the upright position in enhancing visual pursuit in neonates. *Child Development, 47*, 309–314.
104. Gregory-Flock, J. L., & Yerxa, E. J. (1984). Standardization of the prone extension postural test on children ages 4 through 8. *American Journal of Occupational Therapy, 38*, 187–194.
105. Gunnar, M. R., & Barr, R. G. (1998). Stress, early brain development, and behavior. *Infants and Young Children, 11*(1), 1–14.
106. Hall, L., & Case-Smith, J. (2007). The effect of sound-based intervention on children with sensory processing disorders and visual-motor delays. *American Journal of Occupational Therapy, 61*, 209–215.

107. Ham, H. S., Bartolo, A., Corley, M., et al. (2011). Exploring the relationship between gestural recognition and imitation: Evidence of dyspraxia in autism spectrum disorders. *Journal of Autism and Developmental Disorders, 41*, 1–12.
108. Hartshorn, K., Olds, L., Field, T., et al. (2001). Creative movement therapy benefits children with autism. *Early Child Development and Care, 166*, 1–5.
109. Henderson, C., Pehoski, E., & Murray, E. A. (2002). Visual-spatial abilities. In A. C. Bundy, S. J. Lane, & E. A. Murray (Eds.), *Sensory integration: Theory and practice* (pp. 123–140). Philadelphia: F. A. Davis.
110. Henry, D. A. (2000). *Tool chest: For teachers, parents and students.* Flagstaff, AZ: Henry Occupational Therapy Services.
111. Henry, D. A. (2014a). *SPM quick tips.* Torrance, CA: Western Psychological Services.
112. Henry, D. A. (2014b). *SPM-P quick tips.* Torrance, CA: Western Psychological Services.
113. Henry, D. A., & Wheeler, T. (2001). *Tools for parents: A handbook to bring sensory integration into the home.* Flagstaff, AZ: Henry Occupational Therapy Services.
114. Henry, D. A., Wheeler, T., & Sava, D. I. (2004). *Sensory integration tools for teens: Strategies to promote sensory processing.* Flagstaff, AZ: Henry Occupational Therapy Services.
115. Henry, D. A., Wineland, M. K., & Swindeman, S. (2007). *Tools for tots: Sensory strategies for toddlers and preschoolers.* Flagstaff, AZ: Henry Occupational Therapy Services.
116. Hensch, T. K. (2005). Critical period plasticity in local cortical circuits. *Nature Reviews. Neuroscience, 6*, 877–888.
117. Hickman, L. (2001). Sensory integration and fragile X syndrome. In S. S. Roley, E. I. Blanche, & R. C. Schaaf (Eds.), *Understanding the nature of sensory integration with diverse populations* (pp. 385–408). San Antonio, TX: Therapy Skill Builders.
118. Hilton, C., Graver, K., & LaVesser, P. (2007). Relationship between social competence and sensory processing in children with high-functioning autism spectrum disorders. *Research in Autism Spectrum Disorders, 1*(2), 164–173.
119. Hodgetts, S., Magill-Evans, J., & Misiaszek, J. E. (2011a). Weighted vests, stereotyped behaviors and arousal in children with autism. *Journal of Autism and Developmental Disorders, 41*, 805–814.
120. Hodgetts, S., Magill-Evans, J., & Misiaszek, J. E. (2011b). Effects of weighted vests on classroom behavior for children with autism and cognitive impairments. *Research in Autism Spectrum Disorders, 5*, 495–505.
121. Holloway, E. (1998). Early emotional development and sensory processing. In J. Case-Smith (Ed.), *Pediatric occupational therapy and early intervention Andover Medical: Boston* (pp. 163–197).
122. Hopkins, G. (2010). The 4th R: Making the case for recess. Retrieved from: <http://ofprincipalconcern-educationworld.blogspot.com/2010/03/fourth-r-making-case-for-recess.html>.
123. Iwanaga, R., Honda, S., Nakane, H., et al. (2013). Pilot study: Efficacy of sensory integration therapy for Japanese children with high-functioning autism spectrum disorder. *Occupational Therapy International, 21*(1), 4–11.
124. Jarrett, O. S. (2003). Recess in elementary school: What does the research say? *ERIC Digest.* Retrieved from <www.ericdigests.org/2003-2/recess.html>.
125. Salihagic-Kadic, A., Kurjak, M., Medic, W., et al. (2005). New data about embryonic and fetal neurodevelopment and behavior obtained by 3D and 4D sonography. *Journal of Perinatal Medicine, 33*, 478–490.
126. Jacobs, S. E., & Schenider, M. L. (2001). Neuroplasticity and the environment. In S. S. Roley, E. I. Blanche, & R. C. Schaaf (Eds.), *Understanding the nature of sensory integration with diverse populations* (pp. 29–42). San Antonio, TX: Therapy Skill Builders.
127. Jirikowic, T., Olson, H. C., & Astley, S. (2012). Parenting stress and sensory processing: Children with fetal alcohol spectrum disorders. *OTJR: Occupation, Participation, and Health, 32*, 160–168.
128. Kane, A., Luiselli, J. K., Dearborn, S., et al. (2004). Wearing a weighted vest as intervention for children with autism/pervasive developmental disorder: Behavioral assessment of stereotype and attention to task. *The Scientific Review of Mental Health Practice: Objective Investigations of Controversial and Unorthodox Claims in Clinical Psychology, Psychiatry and Social Work, 3*, 19–24.
129. Kawar, M., Frick, S., & Frick, R. (2005) *Astronaut training: A sound-activated vestibular visual protocol for moving, looking, and listening.* Madison, WI: Handbooks for Innovative Practice.
130. Kimball, J. G. (1999). Sensory integrative frame of reference. In P. Kramer & J. Hinojosa (Eds.), *Frames of for pediatric occupational therapy* (pp. 169–204). Baltimore: Williams & Wilkins.
131. Kinnealey, M., Pfeiffer, B., Miller, J., et al. (2012). Effect of classroom modification on attention and engagement of students with autism or dyspraxia. *American Journal of Occupational Therapy, 66*, 511–519.
132. Knickerbocker, B. M. (1980). *A holistic approach to learning disabilities.* Thorofare, NJ: C. B. Slack.
133. Koenig, K. P., Buckley-Reen, A., & Garg, S. (2012). Efficacy of the Get Ready to Learn Yoga Program among children with autism spectrum disorders: A pretest-posttest control group design. *American Journal of Occupational Therapy, 66*, 538–546.
134. Koenig, K. P., & Rudney, S. G. (2010). Performance challenges for children and adolescents with difficulty processing and integrating sensory information: A systematic review. *American Journal of Occupational Therapy, 64*, 430–442.
135. Koomar, J. (2009). Trauma- and attachment-informed sensory integration assessment and intervention. *Special Interest Section Quarterly: Sensory Integration, 32*(4), 1–4.
136. Koomar, J. A., & Bundy, A. C. (2002). Creating direct intervention from theory. In A. C. Bundy, S. J. Lane, & E. A. Murray (Eds.), *Sensory integration: Theory and practice* (2nd ed., pp. 261–308). Philadelphia: F. A. Davis.
137. Krauss, K. E. (1987). The effects of deep pressure touch on anxiety. *American Journal of Occupational Therapy, 41*, 366–373.
138. Lai, J. S., Parham, L. D., & Johnson-Ecker, C. (1999). Sensory dormancy and sensory defensiveness: Two sides of the same coin? *Sensory Integration Special Interest Section Quarterly, 22*, 1–4.
139. Lane, E. A., Dennis, S. J., & Geraghty, M. E. (2011). Brief report: Further evidence of sensory subtypes in autism. *Journal of Autism and Developmental Disorders, 41*, 826–831.
140. Lane, A. E., Young, R. L., Baker, A. Z., et al. (2010). Sensory processing subtypes in autism: Association with adaptive behavior. *Journal of Autism and Developmental Disorders, 40*, 112–122.
141. Lane, S. J., Reynolds, S., & Dumenci, L. (2012). Sensory overresponsivity and anxiety in typically developing children and children with autism and attention deficit hyperactivity disorder: Cause or coexistence? *American Journal of Occupational Therapy, 66*, 595–603.
142. Lee, J. R. V. (1999). Parent ratings of children with autism on the Evaluation of Sensory Processing (ESP). Los

Angeles: University of Southern California. Unpublished master's thesis.

143. Lee, H. W., Shin, J. S., Webber, W. R. S., et al. (2009). Reorganisation of cortical motor and language distribution in human brain. *Journal of Neurology, Neurosurgery, and Psychiatry, 80*, 285–290.
144. Leekam, S., Nieto, C., Libby, S., et al. (2007). Describing the sensory abnormalities of children and adults with autism. *Journal of Autism and Developmental Disorders, 37*, 894–910.
145. Leew, S. V., Stein, N. G., & Gibbard, W. B. (2010). Weighted vests' effect on social attention for toddlers with autism spectrum disorders. *Canadian Journal of Occupational Therapy, 77*, 113–124.
146. Lewis, V., & Boucher, J. (1995). Generativity in the play of young people with autism. *Journal of Autism and Developmental Disorders, 25*, 105–121.
147. Linderman, T. M., & Stewart, K. B. (1999). Sensory integrative-based occupational therapy and functional outcomes in young children with pervasive developmental disorders: A single-subject study. *American Journal of Occupational Therapy, 53*, 207–213.
148. Liss, M., Saulnier, C., Fein, D., et al. (2006). Sensory and attention abnormalities in autistic spectrum disorders. *Autism: The International Journal of Research and Practice, 10*, 155–171.
149. Lundy-Ekman, L. (2013). *Neuroscience: Fundamentals for rehabilitation* (4th ed.). St Louis: Saunders Elsevier.
150. Magalhaes, L. C., Koomar, J., & Cermak, S. A. (1989). Bilateral motor coordination in 5- to 9-year-old children. *American Journal of Occupational Therapy, 43*, 437–443.
151. Magrun, W. M., Ottenbacher, K., McCue, S., et al. (1981). Effects of vestibular stimulation on spontaneous use of verbal language in developmentally delayed children. *American Journal of Occupational Therapy, 35*, 101–104.
152. Mailloux, Z. (2001). Sensory integrative principles in intervention with children with autistic disorder. In S. S. Roley, E. I. Blanche, & R. C. Schaaf (Eds.), *Understanding the nature of sensory integration with diverse populations* (pp. 385–408). San Antonio, TX: Therapy Skill Builders.
153. Mailloux, Z. (2006). Goal writing. In S. Smith Roley & R. Schaaf (Eds.), *SI: Applying clinical reasoning to practice with diverse populations* (pp. 63–70). San Antonio, TX: PsychCorp.
154. Mailloux, Z., May-Benson, T., Summers, C. A., et al. (2007). The issue is—goal attainment scaling as a measure of meaningful outcomes for children with sensory integration disorders. *American Journal of Occupational Therapy, 61*(2), 254–259.
155. Mailloux, Z., Mulligan, S., Roley, S. S., et al. (2011). Verification and clarification of patterns of sensory integrative dysfunction. *American Journal of Occupational Therapy, 65*, 143–151.
156. Mailloux, Z., Leao, M., Becera, T., et al. (in press). Modification of the Postrotary Nystagmus Test for evaluating young children. *American Journal of Occupational Therapy.*
157. Mailloux, Z., & Roley, S. S. (2002). Sensory integration. In H. Miller-Kuhaneck (Ed.), *Autism: A comprehensive occupational therapy approach* (pp. 215–244). Rockville, MD: AOTA Press.
158. Maurer, D., & Maurer, C. (1988). *The world of the newborn.* New York: Basic Books.
159. May-Benson, T. (2001). A theoretical model of ideation in praxis. In E. Blanche, S. Roley, & R. Schaaf (Eds.), *Sensory integration and developmental disabilities* (pp. 163–181). San Antonio, TX: Therapy Skill Builders.
160. May-Benson, T. A., & Cermak, S. A. (2007). Development of an assessment for ideational praxis. *American Journal of Occupational Therapy, 61*, 148–153.
161. May-Benson, T. A., & Koomar, J. A. (2007). Identifying gravitational insecurity in children: A pilot study. *American Journal of Occupational Therapy, 61*, 142–147.
162. May-Benson, T. A., & Koomar, J. A. (2010). Systematic review of the research evidence examining the effectiveness of interventions using a sensory integrative approach for children. *American Journal of Occupational Therapy, 64*, 403–414.
163. May-Benson, T. A., Roley, S. S., Mailloux, Z., et al. (in press). Structural elements of the Ayres Sensory Integration Fidelity Measure. *American Journal of Occupational Therapy.*
164. McCarter, J. A. (2010). Growing up with sensory processing challenges. *Special Interest Section Quarterly: Sensory Integration, 33*(3), 1–2.
165. McCune-Nicolich, L. (1981). Toward symbolic functioning: Structure of early pretend games and potential parallels with language. *Child Development, 52*, 785–797.
166. Melzack, R., & Wall, P. D. (1965). Pain mechanisms: A new theory. *Science, 150*(3699), 971–979.
167. Miller, L. J. (2003). Empirical evidence related to therapies for sensory processing impairments. *National Association of School Psychologist Communique, 31*(5), 34–37.
168. Miller, L. J. (2006). *Miller function and participation scales.* San Antonio, TX: Pearson Education.
169. Miller, L. J., Anzalone, M. E., Lane, S. J., et al. (2007). Concept evolution in sensory integration: A proposed nosology for diagnosis. *American Journal of Occupational Therapy, 61*, 135–140.
170. Miller, L. J., Coll, J. R., & Schoen, S. A. (2007). A randomized controlled pilot study of the effectiveness of occupational therapy for children with sensory modulation disorder. *American Journal of Occupational Therapy, 61*, 228–238.
171. Miller, L. J., Oakland, T., & Herzberg, D. (2013). *The Goal-Oriented Assessment of Lifeskills.* Los Angeles: Western Psychological Services.
172. Miller, L., Reisman, J. J., McIntosh, D. N., et al. (2001). An ecological model of sensory modulation: Performance of children with fragile X syndrome. In S. S. Roley, E. I. Blanche, & R. C. Schaaf (Eds.), *Understanding the nature of sensory integration in diverse populations* (pp. 57–82). San Antonio, TX: Therapy Skill Builders.
173. Miller, L., & Summers, J. C. (2001). Clinical applications in sensory modulation dysfunction: Assessment and intervention considerations. In S. S. Roley, E. I. Blanche, & R. C. Schaaf (Eds.), *Understanding the nature of sensory integration in diverse populations* (pp. 247–274). San Antonio, TX: Therapy Skill Builders.
174. Miller Kuhaneck, H., Ecker, C., Parham, L. D., et al. (2010). *Sensory Processing Measure—Preschool (SPM-P): Manual.* Los Angeles: Western Psychological Services.
175. Miller Kuhaneck, H., Henry, D., & Glennon, T. (2007). *Sensory Processing Measure— Main Classroom Form.* Los Angeles: Western Psychological Services.
176. Minshew, N. J., Sung, K., Jones, B. L., et al. (2004). Underdevelopment of the postural control system in autism. *Neurology, 63*(11), 2056–2061.
177. Mottron, L., & Burack, J. (2001). Enhanced perceptual functioning in the development of autism. In J. Burack, T. Charman, N. Yirmiya, & P. R. Zelazo (Eds.), *The development of autism: Perspectives from theory and research* (pp. 131–148). Mahwah, NJ: Erlbaum.
178. Mudford, O. C., Cross, B. A., Breen, S., et al. (2000). Auditory integration training for children with autism: No behavioral benefits detected. *American Journal on Mental Retardation, 105*(2), 118–129.

179. Mulligan, S. (1998). Patterns of sensory integration dysfunction: A confirmatory factor analysis. *American Journal of Occupational Therapy, 52*, 819–828.
180. Mulligan, S. (2003). Examination of the evidence for occupational therapy using a sensory integration framework with children: Part two. *Sensory Integration Special Interest Section Quarterly, 26*(2), 1–5.
181. O'Neill, M. (2010). Parenting a child with sensory integration challenges. *Special Interest Section Quarterly: Sensory Integration, 33*(3), 2–3.
182. Ottenbacher, K. (1982). Sensory integration therapy: Affect or effect? *American Journal of Occupational Therapy, 35*, 571–578.
183. Parham, L. D. (1987). Evaluation of praxis in preschoolers. *Occupational Therapy in Health Care, 4*(2), 23–36.
184. Parham, L. D. (2002). Sensory integration and occupation. In A. C. Bundy, S. J. Lane, & E. A. Murray (Eds.), *Sensory integration: Theory and practice* (2nd ed., pp. 413–434). Philadelphia: F. A. Davis.
185. Parham, L. D., Cohn, E. S., Spitzer, S., et al. (2007). Fidelity in sensory integration intervention research. *American Journal of Occupational Therapy, 61*, 216–227.
186. Parham, L. D., & Ecker, C. J. (2007). *Sensory Processing Measure—Home Form.* Los Angeles: Western Psychological Services.
187. Parham, L. D., Ecker, C., Miller-Kuhaneck, H., et al. (2007). *Sensory Processing Measure manual.* Los Angeles: Western Psychological Services.
188. Parham, L. D., Roley, S. S., May-Benson, T., et al. (2011). Development of a fidelity measure for Research on Ayres Sensory Integration. *American Journal of Occupational Therapy, 65*, 133–142.
189. Parush, S., Sohmer, H., Steinberg, A., et al. (1997). Somatosensory functioning in children with attention deficit hyperactivity disorder. *Developmental Medicine and Child Neurology, 39*, 464–468.
190. Pediatric Therapy Network [producer] (2003). Applying sensory integration principles where children live, learn and play [motion picture]. Available from Pediatric Therapy Network, 1815 West 213th Street, Suite 100, Torrance, CA 90501.
191. Pfeiffer, B. (2002). The impact of dysfunction in sensory integration on occupations in childhood through adulthood: A case study. *Sensory Integration Special Interest Section Quarterly, 25*(1), 1–2.
192. Pfeiffer, B. A. (2012). Sensory hypersensitivity and anxiety: The chicken or the egg? *Special Interest Section Quarterly: Sensory Integration, 35*(2), 1–4.
193. Pfeiffer, B. A., Koenig, K., Kinnealey, M., et al. (2011). Effectiveness of sensory integration interventions in children with autism spectrum disorders: A pilot study. *American Journal of Occupational Therapy, 65*(1), 76–85.
194. Ray, T., King, L. J., & Grandin, T. (1988). The effectiveness of self-initiated vestibular stimulation in producing speech sounds in an autistic child. *Occupational Therapy Journal of Research, 8*, 186–190.
195. Reeves, G. D. (2001). From neurons to behavior: Regulation, arousal, and attention as important substrates for the process of sensory integration. In S. S. Roley, E. I. Blanche, & R. C. Schaaf (Eds.), *Understanding the nature of sensory integration in diverse populations* (pp. 89–108). San Antonio, TX: Therapy Skill Builders.
196. Reichow, B., Barton, E. E., Sewell, J. N., et al. (2010). Effects of weighted vests on the engagement of children with developmental delays and autism. *Focus on Autism and Other Developmental Disabilities, 25*, 3–11.
197. Reynolds, S., & Lane, S. J. (2008). Diagnostic validity of sensory over-responsivity: A review of the literature and case reports. *Journal of Autism and Developmental Disorders, 38*(3), 516–529.
198. Reynolds, S., & Lane, S. J. (2009). Sensory over-responsivity and anxiety in children with ADHD. *American Journal of Occupational Therapy, 63*, 443–450.
199. Reynolds, S., Lane, S. J., & Richards, L. (2010). Using animal models of enriched environments to inform research on sensory integration intervention for the rehabilitation of neurodevelopmental disorders. *Journal of Neurodevelopmental Disorders, 2*(3), 120–132.
200. Reynolds, S., Shepherd, J., & Lane, S. J. (2008). Sensory modulation disorders in a minority Head Start population: Preliminary prevalence and characterization. *Journal of Occupational Therapy in Schools and Early Intervention, 1*(2), 1–13.
201. Rieke, E. F., & Anderson, D. (2009). Adolescent/Adult Sensory Profile and obsessive-compulsive disorder. *American Journal of Occupational Therapy, 63*, 138–145.
202. Rimland, B., & Edelson, S. E. (1995). Brief report: a pilot study of auditory integration training in autism. *Journal of Autism and Developmental Disorders, 25*(1), 6170.
203. Rogers, S. J., Bennetto, I., McEvoy, R., et al. (1996). Imitation and pantomime in high-functioning adolescents with autism spectrum disorders. *Child Development, 67*, 2060–2073.
204. Rogers, S. J., Hepburn, S., & Wehner, E. (2003). Parent reports of sensory symptoms in toddlers with autism and those with other developmental disorders. *Journal of Autism and Developmental Disorders, 33*, 631–642.
205. Roley, S. S., & Schneck, C. (2001). Sensory integration and visual deficits, including blindness. In S. S. Roley, E. I. Blanche, & R. C. Schaaf (Eds.), *Understanding the nature of sensory integration with diverse populations* (pp. 313–344). San Antonio: TX: Therapy Skill Builders.
206. Roley, S. S. (2002). Application of sensory integration using the Occupational Therapy Practice Framework. *Sensory Integration Special Interest Section Quarterly, 25*(4), 1–4.
207. Roley, S. S. (2006). Evaluating sensory integration function and dysfunction. In R. Schaaf & S. S. Roley (Eds.), *SI: Applying clinical reasoning to practice with diverse populations* (pp. 15–36). San Antonio, TX: PsychCorp.
208. Roley, S. S., Mailloux, Z., & Erwin, B. (2008). Ayres Sensory Integration. Retrieved November 16, 2008, from Sensory Integration Global Network website: <http://www.siglobalnetwork.org/asi.htm>.
209. Roley, S. S., Mailloux, Z., Miller-Kuhaneck, H., et al. (2007). Understanding Ayres Sensory Integration. *Occupational Therapy Practice, 12*(17), CE1–CE8.
210. Román-Oyala, R. (2011). Risk factors associated with sensory modulation disorder: Applications of a vulnerability model. *Sensory Integration Special Interest Section Quarterly, 34*(2), 1–4.
211. Royeen, C. B. (1989). Commentary on "Tactile functions in learning-disabled and normal children: Reliability and validity considerations." *Occupational Therapy Journal of Research, 9*, 16–23.
212. Sanes, J. R., & Jessell, T. M. (2013). Experience and the refinement of synaptic connections. In E. R. Kandel, J. H. Schwartz, T. M. Jessell, S. A. Siegelbaum, & A. J. Hudspeth (Eds.), *Principles of neural science* (5th ed.). New York: McGraw-Hill.
213. Schaaf, R., & Anzalone, M. (2001). Sensory integration with high risk infants and young children. In S. S. Roley, E. I. Blanche, & R. C. Schaaf (Eds.), *Understanding the nature of sensory integration with diverse*

populations (pp. 385–408). San Antonio: TX: Therapy Skill Builders.

214. Schaaf, R. C., Miller, L. J., Seawell, D., et al. (2003). Children with disturbances in sensory processing: A pilot study examining the role of the parasympathetic nervous system. *American Journal of Occupational Therapy, 57*, 442–449.
215. Schaaf, R. C., Benevides, T., Blanche, E., et al. (2010). Parasympathetic functions in children with sensory processing disorder. *Frontiers in Integrative Neuroscience, 4*, 1–11.
216. Schaaf, R. C., Benevides, T., Mailloux, Z., et al. (2014). An intervention for sensory difficulties in children with autism: A randomized trial. *Journal of Autism and Developmental Disabilities. 44*(7), 1493–1506.
217. Schaaf, R. C., Hunt, J., & Benevides, T. (2012). Occupational therapy using sensory integration to improve participation of a child with autism: A case report. *American Journal of Occupational Therapy, 66*, 547–555.
218. Schilling, D. L., & Schwartz, I. S. (2004). Alternative seating for young children with autism spectrum disorder: Effects on classroom behavior. *Journal of Autism and Developmental Disorders, 34*, 423–432.
219. Schilling, D., Washington, K., Billingsley, F., et al. (2003). Classroom seating for children with attention deficit hyperactivity disorder: Therapy balls versus chairs. *American Journal of Occupational Therapy, 57*, 534–541.
220. Schneider, M. L. (1992). The effect of mild stress during pregnancy on birth weight and neuromotor maturation in rhesus monkey infants *(Macaca mulatta). Infant Behavior and Development, 15*, 389–403.
221. Schneider, M. L., Clarke, A. S., Kraemer, G. W., et al. (1998). Prenatal stress alters brain biogenic amine levels in primates. *Development and Psychopathology, 10*, 427–440.
222. Schoen, S., Miller, L. J., Brett-Green, B., et al. (2008). Psychophysiology of children with autism spectrum disorder. *Research in Autism Spectrum Disorders, 2*, 417–429.
223. Shumway-Cook, A., Horak, F., & Black, F. O. (1987). A critical examination of vestibular function in motor-impaired learning-disabled children. *International Journal of Pediatric Otolaryngology, 14*, 21–30.
224. Siaperas, P., Ring, H. A., McAllister, C. J., et al. (2011). Atypical movement performance and sensory integration in Asperger's syndrome. *Journal of Autism and Developmental Disabilities, 5*, 1301–1302.
225. Siengsukon, C. (2013). Neuroplasticity. In L. Lundy-Ekman (Ed.), *Neuroscience: Fundamentals of rehabilitation* (pp. 66–80). St. Louis: Elsevier Saunders.
226. Silva, L. M. T., Schalock, M., Ayres, R., et al. (2009). Qigong massage treatment for sensory and self regulation problems in young children with autism: A randomized controlled trial. *American Journal of Occupational Therapy, 63*, 423–432.
227. Silva, L. M. T., Schalock, M., & Gabrielsen, K. (2011). Early intervention for autism with a parent-delivered qigong massage program: A randomized controlled trial. *American Journal of Occupational Therapy, 65*, 550–559.
228. Sinha, Y., Silove, N., Hayen, A., et al. (2011). Auditory integration training and other sound therapies for autism spectrum disorders (ASD). *Cochrane Database of Systematic Reviews, 12*, doi:10.1002/14651858.CD003681.pub3.
229. Slavik, B. A., & Chew, T. (1990). The design of a sensory integration treatment facility: The Ayres Clinic as a model. In S. C. Merrill (Ed.), *Environment: Implications for occupational therapy practice* (pp. 85–101). Rockville, MD: American Occupational Therapy Association.
230. Slavik, B. A., Kitsuwa-Lowe, J., Danner, P. T., et al. (1984). Vestibular stimulation and eye contact in autistic children. *Neuropediatrics, 15*, 333–336.
231. Solomon, P., Kubzansky, P. E., Leiderman, P. H., et al. (1961). *Sensory deprivation*. Cambridge, MA: Harvard University Press.
232. Spitzer, S., & Roley, S. S. (2001). Sensory integration revisited: A philosophy of practice. In S. S. Roley, E. I. Blanche, & R. C. Schaaf (Eds.), *Understanding the nature of sensory integration with diverse populations* (pp. 3–27). San Antonio, TX: Therapy Skill Builders.
233. Stern, D. N. (1985). *The interpersonal world of the infant*. New York: Basic Books.
234. Su, C.-T., Wu, M.-Y., Yang, A.-L., et al. (2010). Impairment of stance control in children with sensory modulation disorder. *American Journal of Occupational Therapy, 64*, 443–452.
235. Tomchek, S. D., & Dunn, W. (2007). Sensory processing in children with and without autism: A comparative study using the Short Sensory Profile. *American Journal of Occupational Therapy, 61*, 190–200.
236. Umeda, C., & Deitz, J. (2011). Effects of therapy cushions on classroom behaviors of children with autism spectrum disorder. *American Journal of Occupational Therapy, 65*, 152–159.
237. Vanvuchelen, M., Roeyers, H., & De Weerdt, W. (2011). Objectivity and stability of the Preschool Imitation and Praxis Scale. *American Journal of Occupational Therapy, 65*, 569–577.
238. Vargas, S., & Camilli, G. (1999). A meta-analysis of research on sensory integration treatment. *American Journal of Occupational Therapy, 53*, 189–198.
239. Walker, K. F. (1991). Sensory integrative therapy in a limited space: An adaptation of the Ayres Clinic design. *Sensory Integration Special Interest Section Newsletter, 14*(3), 1, 2, 4.
240. Watling, R., Koenig, K. P., Davies, P. L., et al. (2011). *Occupational therapy practice guidelines for children and adolescents with challenges in sensory processing and sensory integration.* Bethesda, MD: AOTA Press.
241. Watson, L., Patten, E., Baranek, G. T., et al. (2011). Differential associations between sensory response patterns and language, social, and communication measures in children with autism or other developmental disabilities. *Journal of Speech, Language, and Hearing Research, 54*, 1562–1576.
242. Weisel, T. N. (1982). Postnatal development of the visual cortex and the influence of environment. *Nature, 299*, 583–591.
243. Wells, A. M., Chasnoff, I. J., Schmidt, C. A., et al. (2012). Neurocognitive habilitation therapy for children with fetal alcohol spectrum disorders: An adaptation of the Alert Program. *American Journal of Occupational Therapy, 66*, 24–34.
244. White, M. (1979). A first-grade intervention program for children at risk for reading failure. *Journal of Learning Disabilities, 12*, 26–32.
245. Wilbarger, P., & Wilbarger, J. L. (1991). *Sensory defensiveness in children aged 2-12*. Denver: Avanti Educational Programs.
246. Williams, M. S., & Shellenberger, S. (1994). *"How does your engine run?" A leader's guide to the Alert Program for Self-regulation*. Albuquerque: TherapyWorks.
247. Wilson, B. N., & Kaplan, B. J. (1994). Follow-up assessment of children receiving sensory integration treatment. *Occupational Therapy Journal of Research, 14*, 244–266.
248. Wilson, B. N., Kaplan, B. J., Fellowes, S., et al. (1992). The efficacy of sensory integration treatment compared to tutoring. *Physical and Occupational Therapy in Pediatrics, 12*, 1–36.

249. Wilson, B. N., Pollock, N., Kaplan, B. J., et al. (2000). *Clinical Observations of Motor and Postural Skills (COMPS)* (2nd ed.). Framingham, MA: Therapro.
250. Windsor, M. M., Roley, S. S., & Szklut, S. (2001). Evaluating sensory integration and praxis within the context of occupational therapy. In S. S. Roley, E. I. Blanche, & R. C. Schaaf (Eds.), *Understanding the nature of sensory integration with diverse populations* (pp. 216–234). San Antonio, TX: Therapy Skill Builders.
251. Wiss, T. (1989). Vestibular dysfunction in learning disabilities: Differences in definitions lead to different conclusions. *Journal of Learning Disabilities, 22*, 100–101.
252. Woodward, A. L. (2009). Infants grasp of others. *Current Directions in Psychological Science, 18*(1), 53–57.
253. Yochman, A., Parush, S., & Ornoy, A. (2004). Responses of preschool children with and without ADHD to sensory events of everyday life. *American Journal of Occupational Therapy, 58*, 294–302.

CHAPTER 10

Cognitive Interventions for Children

Angela Mandich • Jessie Wilson • Kaity Gain

KEY TERMS

Performance Based Approaches
Cognitive Behavior Therapy
Cognitive Orientation to Occupational Performance (CO-OP)
Declarative and Procedural Knowledge
Metacognition
Strategy
Cognitive Strategy: Global and Domain Specific

GUIDING QUESTIONS

1. What theories provide the foundation for cognitive approaches?
2. What do the terms *cognition* and *metacognition* mean?
3. What concepts, principles, and key features define a cognitive intervention?
4. How are cognitive strategies applied in occupational therapy practice?
5. How is Cognitive Orientation to Occupational Performance (CO-OP) applied?

Cognitive interventions have their historical beginnings in the disciplines of education and psychology. Pediatric occupational therapists have begun to realize the effectiveness of cognitive approaches with children who experience various developmental disabilities. These intervention approaches are often referred to as ***performance based approaches*** and also have been called ***top down*** approaches in the occupational therapy literature. The focus of performance-based approaches is to assist the client in identifying, developing, and utilizing cognitive strategies to perform activities of daily living.[41,44] Currently, in the pediatric occupational therapy practice, two main cognitive approaches are being used: cognitive approaches that attempt to change faulty or delayed cognitive processes, such as Cognitive Behavior Therapy, and cognitive approaches that enable occupational performance, such as the Cognitive Orientation to Occupational Performance (CO-OP) approach.

In this chapter we explain the role of cognition and cognitive strategies in supporting occupational performance. The following sections provide an understanding of the common terms used in cognitive interventions, a summary of the history of cognitive approaches, an overview of the theoretical perspectives that guide the use of cognitive interventions. A rationale for using cognitive approaches will then be discussed highlighting the key features of cognitive interventions and the research evidenced supporting the use of these approaches.

Cognitive interventions focus on the development of strategies to accomplish the chosen task. The following table describes general terminology that is used in the cognitive literature and provides an overview of key concepts (Table 10-1).[50]

Theoretical Foundations of Cognitive Approaches

The theoretical foundations of cognitive interventions are rooted in the fields of developmental and educational psychology. L. S. Vygotsky (1896-1932) was a Russian psychologist who made many important contributions to the fields of cognitive and educational psychology. Vygotsky believed that cognitive development occurred through the gradual internalization of concepts and relationships.[63] He noted that younger children used overt speech (talking out loud) when they were problem solving through a difficult task. In contrast, older children seemed to think about a solution internally before acting.[39] When comparing the problem solving dialogs (internal and overt) of the older and younger children he concluded they were similar, and deduced that as development occurs children gradually internalize their thought processes.[63] Vygotsky viewed learning as being embedded in social and cultural contexts. He underscored the necessity of cooperative dialogs between adults and children in the learning process, and saw these communicative opportunities as a way of developing children's internal dialogs.[4] Children must be actively engaged in the learning and developmental process. Vygotsky viewed the learning process as a "circular reaction" in which action and motivation influence one another and contribute to the child's learning and development.[62]

The zone of proximal development is the range of skills that a child can achieve through social interaction with a more competent individual. A child's developmental skills fall into a "zone, or range, of skills which differ contingent upon the social interactions accompanying the activity, rather than a specific skill level"[25] (p. 105). Therefore each stage of a child's development is characterized by different modes of social interaction. In therapeutic practice this concept is most commonly known as scaffolding.

Alexander Luria (1902-1977) was a developmental psychologist who worked closely with Vygotsky to create

TABLE 10-1 Common Definitions In Cognitive Interventions

	Definition	Application to Occupational Therapy
Cognition	Cognition is described as a child's ability to acquire and use information in order to adapt to environmental demands.[27]	Cognitive approaches that teach cognitive skills are focused on working collaboratively with children to enable them to identify and recognize cognitive processes and strategies utilized when completing meaningful daily activities.[50]
Declarative knowledge	Declarative knowledge is knowledge about things; it is the knowledge that is often explicitly known and can be consciously brought to the attention of the learner.[54]	Declarative knowledge includes rules and facts about a skill, and is often used during the initial stages of learning.[54] It is kept within the individual's working memory and can be converted to procedural knowledge through rehearsal and verbalization.
Procedural knowledge	Procedural knowledge is the implicit knowledge about how to complete a task.[54]	Procedural knowledge is often acquired through the repetition of an activity and observed through enhanced task performance.[54]
Metacognition	Metacognition refers to an individual's knowledge concerning their own cognitive processes and products or anything related to them. Through metacognition, children generalize and transfer cognitive skills to meet changing contextual demands.[50] Metacognition is made up of two components: metacognitive knowledge and self-regulation.[12]	Metacognitive strategies are employed when a task becomes too difficult relative to the child's skill level and they are required to select appropriate cognitive strategies, monitor, and evaluate their application.[39] During the implementation of cognitive approaches in occupational therapy, metacognition is the skill that is directly impacted and enhanced through the intervention process.
Metacognitive knowledge	Metacognitive knowledge consists of one's awareness of the cognitive processes that are employed to learn and perform a new task.[12,50]	This is the individual's ability to stop and reflect on how he or she is learning. Is it through the use of mnemonics, rehearsal, or imagery (or other various cognitive strategies that will be discussed later in the chapter) that they are able to retain new information?[60]
Self-regulation	Self-regulation is the individual's influence over their own thought processes, emotional states, motivation and patterns of behavior.[2] It is the process of selecting, monitoring, and evaluating the effectiveness of cognitive strategies.[44]	To demonstrate self-regulation, an individual who encounters a problem pauses, selects a different strategy, applies it and evaluates the performance outcome.[50] The ability to self-regulate allows for skill transfer and generalization to occur.
Cognitive strategies	Strategies are cognitive processes that are more advanced than the outcomes that are a natural consequence of carrying out a task. Strategies are both consciously employed and are controllable by the learner.[48] Goal-directed strategies are used to help the individual achieve a task or fulfill a purpose. Cognitive strategies can be defined as a "mental plan of action that helps a person to learn, problem solve, and perform. The use of cognitive strategies can improve an individual's learning, problem solving, and task performance in terms of efficiency, speed, accuracy, and consistency"[60] (p. 227).	Cognitive strategies support skill acquisition or reacquisition. They help individuals regulate and manage challenges in learning and performance, playing a key role in achieving a higher level of task performance.[60] Strategies include the "how to" knowledge the individual uses when acquiring new skills and problem solving through a difficult situation or navigating contextual challenges.[60] Coping with daily stresses, learning how to take the bus to a new location in the community, and deciding to cook a different meal for dinner all incorporate the use of strategies, and therefore strategies are a typical part of everyday learning and performance.[50]

cultural-historical psychology.[28] Luria believed that a child's development could not be simply explained through a natural inborn process, but that development is a complex and dynamic relationship between many factors including the child's social and cultural environment(s). Luria delineated how individuals explore problems and learn new concepts, identifying five stages in an individual's problem solving process. These included:

1. Discovery of the problem
2. Investigation of the problem
3. Selection of an alternative strategy
4. Attempt to solve the problem
5. Comparison of results of the solution[28,29]

Children use overt verbalization of process steps when learning a new skill, which eventually fades into covert speech as the child rehearses the process steps of the new activity. Luria hypothesized that the speech system is formed in the process of the child's social intercourse with an adult and is a powerful means of systemic organization of human mental processes.[28,29]

Meichenbaum[34,36] further emphasized the importance of speech and adult guidance in driving the development of cognitive strategies. Hypothesizing that internal speech can regulate one's behavior; he proposed that a child could follow self-instructional steps to assist in behavior regulation.[34] This problem-solving pathway included the child identifying a goal, developing a plan, enacting the plan, and then evaluating its success.[34] These steps are modeled by a more competent adult and then verbalized out loud by the child. Through adult guidance and functional practice and rehearsal, the steps of Goal, Plan, Do, Check are internalized and recalled covertly by the child when performing a task.[34] Meichenbaum also utilized scaffolding to help with the generalization of the newly formed cognitive strategies.

Scaffolding

Scaffolding emphasizes communication between adults and children in an effort to develop children's internal dialogs, which help to guide their own actions in the acquisition of new skills.[4] In cognitive approaches the progression of moving skill acquisition from an overt to covert process demonstrates the increasing independence of the child in his or her understanding of task demands, in using problem-solving strategies, and in coping with failures.[35] Through scaffolding the occupational therapist modifies a cognitive intervention to create the just-right-fit between the child's ability level and the task demands. A clinical example of strategies moving from an overt to a covert process is when a child is learning how to hit a baseball. Initially the child may articulate aloud the steps required to successfully make contact with a baseball during practice. "Keep my eye on the ball," "swing through the ball," and "take my time" are examples of self-coaching, a domain-specific strategy that over time fades to an internalized (covert) strategy.[44,45]

Discovery Learning

Discovery learning proposes that children construct their own knowledge by drawing on their past experiences and interacting directly with the task and the environment(s).[8] Discovery learning, in a pure sense, is task exploration; however, through the addition of instructional scaffolding it can more accurately be defined as guided discovery.[49] In guided discovery learning, the therapist assumes the role as a facilitator. Rather than providing direct instruction, the occupational therapist allows the client to generate his or her own answers through tailoring the task and the environment to the individual.[49] Occupational therapists can pose questions to clients as they complete a task, offering them the opportunity to approach an activity differently. In doing so, they are also able to illuminate important components and concepts of the task. As a child engages in guided discovery learning, he/she takes control over his/her performance and the occupational therapist is able to reduce the amount of support/guidance provided.[44,49] Through this increase in competence and the experience of success, guided discovery learning shifts the individual's reinforcement for learning from external to a more internal locus.[8] "The child is now in a position to experience success and failures not as a reward or punishment, but as information"[8] (p. 28). Guided discovery learning offers opportunities for the child to ask questions and generate ideas that can be further tested or researched.[8] Through the shifting of the child's motivation for learning from an external to internal locus of control, guided discovery aids in enhancing the learner's level of self-efficacy.

Metacognition

Bandura[2] believed that a child's experiences performing an activity contribute to his or her self-perceptions. Through the development of metacognitive abilities, children learn to evaluate their performance of a task and reflect on their areas of strength and weakness.[2,39] When setting new goals based on their identified areas of difficulty, children begin to feel empowered. Similar to the foundational elements of guided discovery learning, empowerment fosters increased goal commitment, enhanced performance, and the intrinsic motivation to set new meaningful goals.[2,39]

Like Vygotsky and Bruner, Bandura believed that the individual child was the main motivator for cognitive development and that these intrinsic capabilities emerge through interactions with others.[2,14,61] Therefore engagement of the child in the learning process and to change interaction with social partners are key elements to successful learning.[14] Learning occurs through the result of experience, and information is interpreted through the lens of the individual's values and beliefs. Contributions from the fields of cognitive and educational psychology have brought to light the foundational elements of discovery learning, and the understanding that children display optimal learning when they are allowed to reflect on their participation in their chosen occupations.[61]

Instrumental Enrichment

Feuerstein[3] developed an Instrumental Enrichment program based on the notion that an individual's cognitive performance can be modified through intentional mediated interventions.[24] When an adult selects and organizes environmental stimuli so that it is congruent with the child's level of learning, the child's learning is optimized.[3,39] Children learn when adults are mediators, assisting the child to derive generalized meaning from life experiences.[11] Feurestein and Haywood[17] developed mediation techniques for the adult to use to help children to make sense of their life experiences. These techniques include process questioning, bridging, comparison/describing, modeling, challenging, and elaborated feedback.[11,39] These mediation techniques provide a method through which the child learns to bridge newly acquired cognitive strategies to daily living situations. Occupational therapists can use mediated learning to promote a child's ability to generalize new learning to his or her daily routine.

Rationale for Using Cognitive Approaches

Evidence is beginning to accumulate regarding the functional benefits of using a cognitive approach as an occupational therapy intervention.[44,60] This section provides a rationale for using cognitive approaches.

Motivation

An individual engages in an occupation based on personal choice and motivation.[39,44] The occupations that an individual chooses to engage in define who he or she is, add to the individual's experiences and create new meaning.[9] Participation in occupations directly influences identity and the development of one's self.[9] Motivation also influences learning, persistence, and the willingness to participate in rehabilitation.[10] Intervention goals need to reflect occupations that the child identifies are important and that he desires to improve.[37] These elements resonate with the values and beliefs in client-centered practice, and reflect the views of Meichenbaum who highlighted the importance of the child being an active collaborator in the therapeutic process.[37]

Children who experience illness and/or a disability are often restricted in the occupations in which they can participate. Environmental, physical, and institutional barriers inhibit full engagement in many of the occupations.[18,42] Participating in daily occupations brings meaning to lives, offers a sense of accomplishment, and is a determinant of health.[47] When an individual is unable to participate in a chosen occupation, lower self-esteem or self-efficacy, a decreased sense of independence, and an overall loss of motivation may result.[1,13] Cognitive interventions and adult-guided discovery learning focus on child-generated ideas, maintain the child's internal locus of control, and can promote the child's self-efficacy.[39,44,46] They offer individuals choice and control, which allow the child to derive a sense of self-determination and empowerment.[47]

Generalization and Transfer

Generalization is defined as the ability of an individual to apply what they have learned in therapeutic rehabilitation to different environments and activities.[56,58] Both internal and external factors affect the generalization of skills. External (to the learner) factors include the environmental context, the nature of the task, and the learning criteria of the activity. The internal factors that directly affect generalization are the learner's metacognition, his or her processing strategies, and the learner's characteristics.[7,22,58] A multi-contextual approach can promote skill generalization.[58] Scaffolding through adult feedback can help a child generalize and transfer newly developed skills to different environments and tasks.[39] Cognitive approaches to therapeutic intervention focus on the generalization and transfer of skills through the following means:

- *Maintaining client motivation:* ensures that the child applies the strategies to different tasks. Children are collaborators in the therapeutic process, promoting motivation and aiding in the transfer of skills to the child's natural environments and daily activities.[35,46]
- *Contextually relevant practice:* exposes children to a number of different transfer experiences that allows the child to understand the commonalities among situations/tasks.[58] Finding these commonalities among tasks, environments, and oneself can help the child their cognitive strategies in various environments and tasks.[44,46]
- *Direct exposure to the task:* allows the child to engage directly in the task or occupation he desires to improve.[5,42]

The occupational therapist uses dynamic performance analysis (DPA) to solve performance problems and identify possible solutions. Through DPA the child gains a deeper understanding of the task and environmental demands and explores solutions to performance problems.[44,46] The process of analyzing performance eventually becomes internalized by the child through scaffolding, which allows the child to "check" his or her occupational performance on an on-going basis. The child can then take the newly developed skills and transfer them to other tasks and environments while problem solving performance ongoing.[44]

Lifelong Development

The occupations that individuals participate in over time can be defined as their occupational trajectories.[20] Individual's occupational trajectories are fluid in nature and can change owing to different life transitions.[20] Some examples of life transitions include moving to a different grade in school, leaving home for postsecondary education, or getting a job. As children grow, develop, and mature, they experience different tasks and activities that might become barriers to their occupational success.[20] Using a cognitive approach to guide therapeutic intervention recognizes the importance of children independently applying cognitive strategies to different environments and activities.[44,59]

As children encounter transition points in their lives and as their occupations change, so do the cognitive strategies that they employ. Fluidity and flexibility in the attributes and uses of cognitive strategies enable them to be used over the life course.[59]

Cognitive Interventions

A number of different cognitive approaches have been described in the broader literature. Bouffard and Wall (1990) proposed a five-step problem-solving framework to guide motor skill acquisition.[6] The steps are Problem Identification, Problem Representation, Plan Construction, Plan Execution, and Evaluation of Progress. Henderson and Sugden[18] also proposed an approach to motor skill acquisition, Cognitive Motor Approach, that centered on a three-step information-processing framework.[6] The first step is Movement Planning and requires the child to understand the task and its demands and decide if the task is achievable. In order to do this, the child gains this information through sensory and perceptual processes, including vision and kinesthesia, and then translates this information into a plan.[18,37] The next step is Movement Execution. During the final step, Movement Evaluation, the child monitors her or his progress. The Cognitive Motor Approach is effective in improving the functional skills of children with developmental coordination disorder (DCD).[65] Expanding on these principles, Cognitive Orientation to Daily Occupational Performance (CO-OP) uses a learning-based perspective on skill acquisition and occupational performance.[37,44]

Cognitive Orientation to Daily Occupational Performance

"CO-OP is a client-centered, performance-based, problem solving approach that enables skill acquisition through a process of strategy use and guided discovery."[44] (p. 2).

CO-OP places emphasis on the interaction between individual and environmental factors to promote children's successful participation in daily activities.[39,44] Developed within

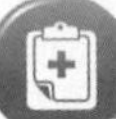

CASE STUDY 10-1 Productivity

Matty is a 9-year-old boy who was referred for an Occupational Therapy assessment within the school setting to address difficulties with his printing skills. Matty displays challenges with baseline placement and spacing between words, which significantly affects the overall legibility of his written work and his overall academic performance. He was seen for eight occupational therapy sessions by his school-based occupational therapist. During this time the occupational therapist worked with him on his printing skills, using the CO-OP approach, and the Goal, Plan, Do, Check framework. Within this framework, Matty was able to identify his own concerns with his printing skills and generate his own solutions to resolve the problematic aspects of his handwriting. With verbal guidance from the occupational therapist, he was able to identify that sometimes all of his letters do not sit on the line and at times all of his words run together. The occupational therapist was then able to guide Matty in identifying domain-specific strategies that can be used to assist with this including: using paper with a highlighted baseline to act as a visual cue for letter placement, using a finger space between words, and securing a "printing checklist" onto his desk to remind him of letter placement and spacing. Using these strategies, Matty improved these specific areas of his printing within the classroom environment.

Application of the CO-OP Approach: Goal and Points of Breakdown

Goal	Breakdown Points
Improve the quality of his handwriting	Poor letter formation Words are too close together Difficulty making sure his letters sit on the line correctly (baseline orientation)

Application of the CO-OP Approach: Strategy Use

Domain Specific Strategy	Specific Strategy/PLAN	Bridging for the Strategy
Task specification/modification	Finish the letter Make the letter larger	Having a writing checklist secured to his desk to prompt him of the important strategies that he had developed
Supplementing task knowledge	"There should always be a finger space between your words."	Teach younger sister how to print: role-playing teacher Making scrapbook of summer vacation
Attention to doing	"Where do you need your letters to sit?"	Teaching student, teacher, and parent to highlight baseline of paper to help with attention to doing

an evidence-based framework, CO-OP draws on behavioral and cognitive psychology, health, human movement science, and occupational therapy to achieve its objectives.[39,44] See Case Study 10-1.

Primary Objectives of CO-OP

There are four objectives of CO-OP: (1) skill acquisition, (2) cognitive strategy use, (3) generalization, and (4) transfer of learning.[44,46] CO-OP uses cognition as a performance support and does not attend to cognitive dysfunction. The primary objective of CO-OP is to enable occupational performance in children.[37,44] In a typical CO-OP program, the child selects three occupations or activities to learn over 10 intervention sessions.[44,46] The occupations are chosen by the child, in collaboration with his or her parents, and may include activities such as handwriting, rollerblading, tying shoe laces, or cutting paper. Through the intervention, cognitive strategies are used to solve the performance problems and enable skill development within the occupations.[43,44,46] The second objective of CO-OP is to teach the child how to use these strategies to achieve his or her goals.[44,46] Over the course of the intervention, children learn a global problem-solving strategy that enables them to discover and identify domain specific strategies that will support their performance.[44,46] The third objective of CO-OP is to facilitate generalization of the occupation to other settings including home and school.[44,46] Once the child has obtained the skills required to perform the identified occupation, the focus of therapy shifts to facilitating generalization of the learning beyond the therapy situation.[44,46] Thus the final objective of CO-OP is the transfer of the learning to other occupations. Because only three occupations are addressed in the course of a CO-OP intervention, it is important that the children learn to adapt their skills and strategies to other new occupations that they confront in daily life.[44,46]

Who Benefits from CO-OP?

Traditionally, the CO-OP approach was developed for use with children with DCD[37,44,46] and CO-OP has been shown to be effective with this population.[5,64] More recently, CO-OP has been used with children with high-functioning autism spectrum disorders (ASD), traumatic brain injuries), attention deficit hyperactivity disorder and motor skill delays.[16,40,51,66] See Research Notes 10-1 and 10-2.

Cognitive interventions have been used to address a variety of client goals including: fine motor skill development such as printing or cutting; gross motor skills such as shooting a basketball or riding a bike; organizational activities; and a variety of ADLs such as getting dressed and meal preparation.[40,65] In order for the CO-OP approach to be successful, research highlights the importance of parent support and inclusion within the therapeutic process as well as the ability for the child to understand the cognitive framework and application of

RESEARCH NOTE 10-1

The Use of Cognitive Interventions for Children with Autism Spectrum Disorders (ASD)

Phelan, S., Steinke, L., & Mandich, A. (2009). Exploring a cognitive intervention for children with pervasive developmental disorder. Canadian Journal of Occupational Therapy, *76(1), 23–28.*

Abstract

Purpose. This study investigated use of CO-OP with children who have PDD (more current term: ASD). CO-OP emphasizes problem-solving strategies and guided discovery of child- and task-specific strategies.

Method. Three goals were established in collaboration with the parents and the child. Pre and post-measures of parents' perceptions of child performance were identified using the Canadian Occupational Performance Measure (COPM). Repeated measures were taken using clinical observations, video analysis, and the Performance Quality Rating Scale (PQRS).

Findings. Improved COPM ratings of performance and satisfaction were observed, and these results were paralleled by improved PQRS scores.

Self-report and PQRS results provide preliminary evidence of the effectiveness of the CO-OP approach with children who have ASD, supporting the use of CO-OP and suggesting further investigation.

Implications for Practice

- When working with children with ASD, it is essential to incorporate their special interests into therapy sessions whenever possible in order to increase motivation and enhance learning opportunities.
- Parent's observations and interaction with their children during the intervention sessions influenced engagement and performance levels.
- The use of additional strategies, which increased structure to the intervention sessions, seemed to benefit the children in the present study. These included verbally and visually outlining the session schedule.

RESEARCH NOTE 10-2

The Use of Cognitive Intervention for Children with Acquired Brain Injury

Missiuna, C., DeMatteo, C., Hanna, S., Mandich, A., Law, M., Mahoney, W. & Scott, L. (2010). Exploring the use of cognitive intervention for children with acquired brain injury. Physical & Occupational Therapy in Pediatrics, 30*(3), 205–219.*

Abstract

Introduction. Children with acquired brain injury (ABI) often experience cognitive, motor, and psychosocial deficits that affect participation in everyday activities.

Objective. This study explored the use of CO-OP with children with ABI.

Method. Children with ABI, experiencing school and self-care difficulties, were identified from a previous study. Six children, aged 6 to 15 years, completed 10 weekly intervention sessions with an occupational therapist. Children and parents rated the child's performance of challenging everyday tasks and their satisfaction with this performance. Task performance was also evaluated objectively through videotape analysis.

Results. Participants showed significant improvement in their ability to perform child-chosen tasks and maintained this performance 4 months later. However, they had difficulty applying extensive problem-solving strategy and discovering cognitive strategies on their own.

Implications for Practice

- Children with ABI were able to identify and sustain motivation to work on child-chosen goals using the CO-OP approach.
- Cognitive strategy use and retention appeared to differ with children with ABI. Children with ABI did use more task-specific cognitive strategies and had more challenges transferring the "Goal, Plan, Do, Check" strategy to other tasks.
- Overall, CO-OP was effective with children who have had an ABI to facilitate skills development of child-chosen goals. Some adaption of the CO-OP approach may be required when working with his population, including increased parent/caregiver involvement.

cognitive strategies.[37,44] Although a certain level of cognitive functioning is required for the CO-OP approach to be successful, cognitive interventions can often be modified based on the client and the specific population.

Key Features of the CO-OP Approach

Essential to the effectiveness of CO-OP is that the child and occupational therapists are fully engaged in the approach as it has been specified in the intervention protocol.[44,46] CO-OP is comprised of seven key elements, referred to as key features (Figure 10-1).

The first key feature is goal identification.[44,46] The client goals are established in collaboration with child and family, and focus on occupations the child wants, needs, or is expected to perform. The child is actively engaged in the goal-setting process to ensure motivation.[1,44] In the CO-OP approach, the child's perspective is integral to the therapy process. As such, the child is actively engaged in choosing the goals.[44,46]

The second key feature of CO-OP is Dynamic Performance Analysis (DPA),[45] which acknowledges that performance is the result of the interaction between the person, environment, and occupation. The occupational therapist analyzes the child performing the task and documents the performance problems or performance breakdowns. In doing so, the occupational therapist focuses on the fit between client abilities, skills, and actions and the task and environmental demands and supports.[44,45] The focus of CO-OP is on performance and correcting performance problems or breakdown, not on underlying component skills.[44] Once the occupational therapist has identified

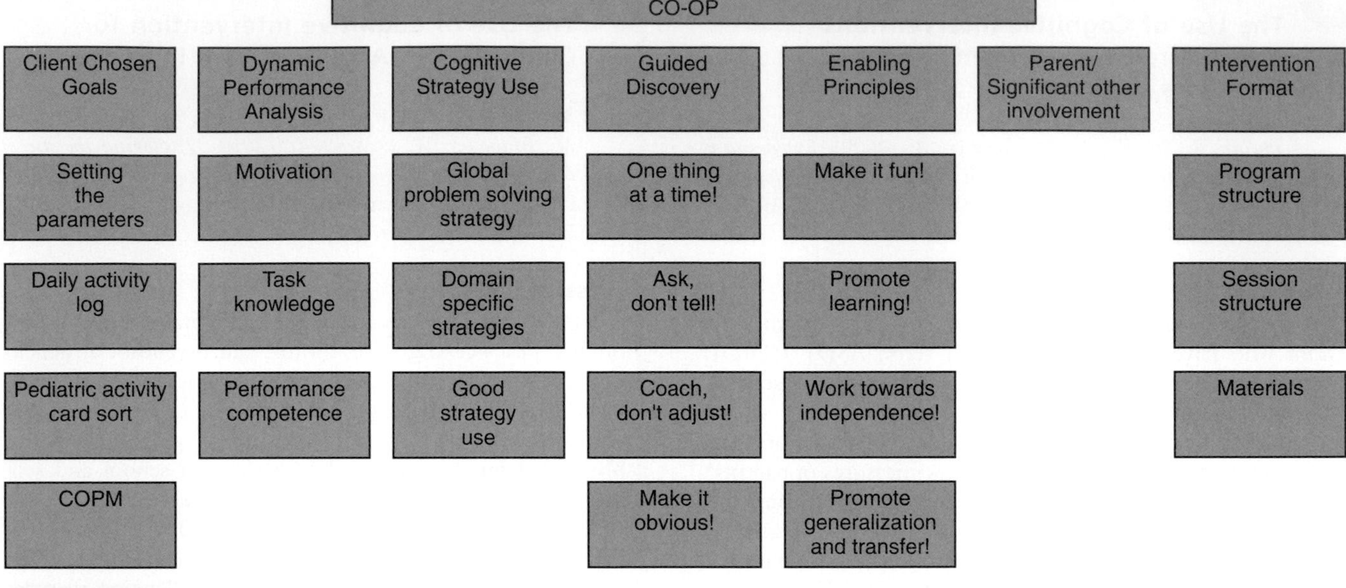

FIGURE 10-1 Key features of the CO-OP approach.[44]

the initial performance breakdown points, the therapist uses cognitive strategies to bridge the gap between ability and skill proficiency.[44,45]

The third key feature is cognitive strategies that are used to support skill acquisition, generalization and transfer.[44,46] As discussed in the previous section, cognitive strategies are cognitive operations beyond those that are inherent to the task itself. In the CO-OP approach, the child uses cognitive strategies to problem solve a performance issue and monitor the outcome.[44-46] In other words, the strategies promote metacognition and thinking about one's thinking.[12,23] Two types of strategies are used in the CO-OP approach: global and domain specific. Global strategies are intended to be used over long periods of time, in a variety of different contexts.[44] The global or executive strategy Goal-Plan-Do-Check used in CO-OP was developed by Camp, Blom, Herbert, and VanDoorwick (1976) and used by Meichenbaum.[35,36]

Goal: What do I want to do?
Plan: How am I going to do it?
Do: Do it!
Check: How well did my plan work? Do I need to revise my plan?

In CO-OP, the child is taught to use the mnemonic Goal-Plan-Do-Check, to support the solving of occupational performance problems.[44] During the first therapy session, the child is introduced to the Goal-Plan-Do-Check strategy and is directly taught how to use it. To ensure that the child understands the global strategy, the child is asked to teach the occupational therapist an activity using this new framework.[44,46] The global strategy frames each intervention session. Initially the occupational therapist takes the lead in using the Goal-Plan-Do-Check strategy. As the child learns the strategy, the child gradually begins to initiate strategy use.[44,46] Through the process of overtly talking oneself through an occupation, the steps become internalized and eventually covert, therefore speech guides behavior (Figure 10-2).[37,44]

The second type of strategies used in CO-OP is domain specific. Domain-specific strategies (DSS) are specific to a particular task or part of a task.[30,37,43,44] See Table 10-2 for a comprehensive list of domain-specific cognitive strategies that can be used within the CO-OP approach. All DSSs are nested in verbal guidance. The goal is to lead the child from early reliance on the occupational therapist's verbal guidance to the independent use of cognitive problem solving strategies through self-talk.[44,46] Therefore, as the intervention progresses, the occupational therapist encourages the child to talk himself through a sequence. Verbalization ensures that the cognitive mechanisms that distinguish it from other approaches are used; that the strategies are brought to the attention of the child; that the child understands the role of the strategies; and that the child can use the strategies independently, in the absence of the occupational therapist.[44] Once the child and occupational therapist have identified the strategies, the therapist reinforces their use during the intervention sessions (Figures 10-3 and 10-4).

The next key feature of CO-OP is guided discovery.[44] In the guided discovery process the learner is helped to identify a problem to solve; she is not given the solution but is provided with hints, coaching, feedback, or modeling to identify a solution.[44,46] In CO-OP the process of guided discovery is closely linked with the process of strategy use. It is used in conjunction with the DPA process primarily to identify when the child becomes "stuck" and elucidate the plan within the Goal-Plan-Do-Check problem-solving process.[44,45] Guiding the child to discover the plans and the DSSs increases the likelihood that he/she will attribute the success of the plans to himself/herself, supporting self-efficacy.[1,45]

Guided discovery supports both skill acquisition and strategy use. Guided discovery has four main elements: (1) One

GOAL
Getting dressed on my own!
CHECK
DO
PLAN
AJ
AJ
Add Text
Add Text

FIGURE 10-2 Concept Map: Goal, Plan, Do, Check.

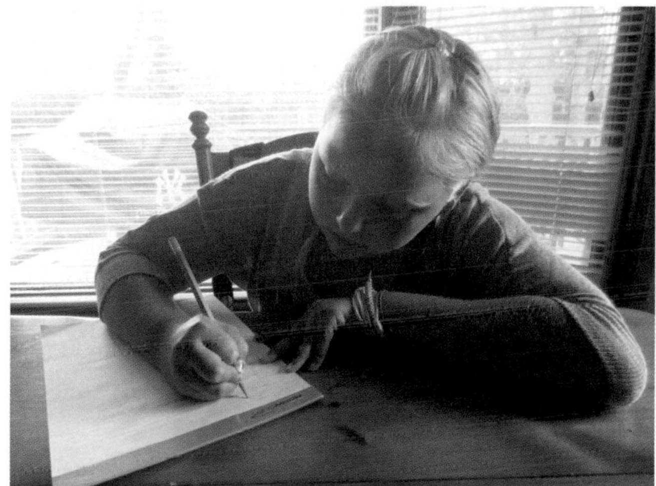

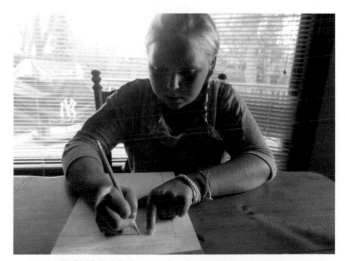

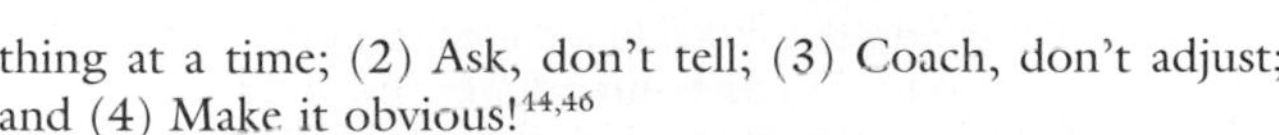

FIGURE 10-3 Productivity: Highlight margins.

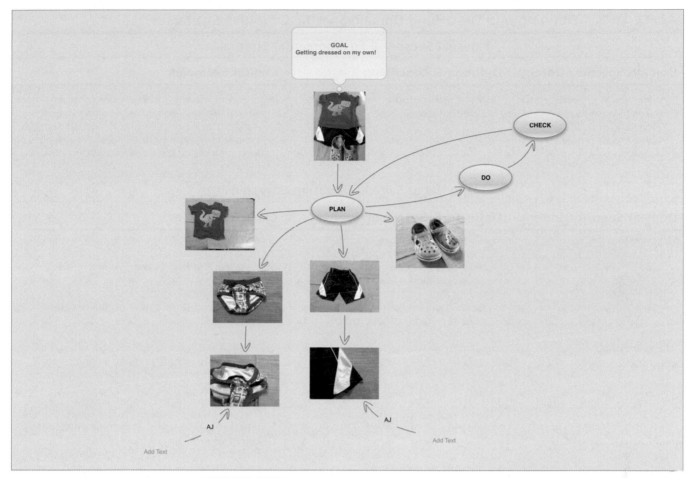

FIGURE 10-4 Productivity: Finger space.

thing at a time; (2) Ask, don't tell; (3) Coach, don't adjust; and (4) Make it obvious![44,46]

- *One thing at a time.* When a child is having difficulty performing an occupation, often several performance problems exist. Because CO-OP is embedded in a learning paradigm and skills are considered to be learned, not developed, it is important to keep the intervention and the client focused on only "one thing at a time."[44,46]
- *Ask, don't tell.* When a child discovers the solution to a performance problem, the child is likely to remember that solution and use more often that when he or she is told the solution. Through Socratic questioning, the child is taught to critically think, analyze, and evaluate solutions. Asking questions helps the child focus on the relevant aspects of the performance and strategy identification is facilitated.[44]

TABLE 10-2 Defining and Describing Domain Specific Cognitive Strategies

External Sensory & Environmental Strategies		
Domain Specific Strategy	**Defining & Describing**	**Clinical Examples**
Sensory cues or prompts from the environment that the individual provides to him/herself to help guide skill acquisition	Tactile, visual, auditory, and/or kinesthetic cues.	Pictures, vibrations (from buzzer or other external device), alarms—any other modality that attracts the learner's attention and guides them through the steps of a task, or prompts their memory or previously learned motor patterns.[60]
Mental or Self-Verbalization Strategies		
Domain Specific Strategy	**Defining & Describing**	**Clinical Examples**
Self-coaching	Encouragement, positive self-talk, strength-based thinking to help increase persistence and/or to control and regulate the learner's emotions	"I can do this!" "Stay calm and focused. ..." "Only a few more times and I will have it!"
Self-guidance	Providing instruction to himself/herself to assist in completing a new/difficult task, cueing oneself and reminders to prepare for or complete an activity	Talking oneself through the steps of an activity, talking aloud through the problem-solving process, self-talk
Self-questioning	Identifying and asking himself/herself or visualizing key questions relating to the activity or task performance	Picturing in the "mind's eye" key transition points of an activity, identifying and asking himself/herself specific areas of difficulty experienced in each task
Imagery	Mental images that are created to represent physical objects, actions, experiences, or events	Creation of images, symbols, or representations that have direct meaning to the client. Can also include imaging textures, sounds, smells, and kinesthetic feelings of movement.
Association	Relating previous knowledge to relevant information about task	Associations can arise from previous experiences, recognition of physical similarities, and knowledge of categories.
Rote-script	A rote pattern of words or phrases that are meaningful to the client and can help to guide a sequence of actions or improve the recall of information	Some motor pattern rote scripts might include: "dribble, dribble, shoot" (basketball), or "slide down, climb up, slide down" (making an "x" in printing)
Elaboration	Increase and add new information and relate it back to previous knowledge.	Can include the expansion and addition of images, symbols, actions, words, or sentences. It also includes verbal and mental processes.
Mnemonic techniques	Associating pictures, words, phrases, or images to cue an action or enhance memory recall	"Bunny ears"—when tying shoes "Helper hand"—when printing and completing bilateral cutting activities
Rehearsal	Repeating information visually or mentally to aid in retention of important information related to the given task/occupation	Repeating key words/actions out loud, creating internalized visual images of the task procedure and visually carrying out the task in a repeated manner
Reconstruction	Involves mental and verbal processes and involves the learner thinking back to a previous task, experience, or context to guide their performance in a new situation	The learner reconstructs experiences, activities, or contexts through imaging, replaying, and/or verbalizing.
Anticipation	Preparing for a new activity through imagining or verbalizing possible outcomes, areas of difficulty, or scenarios the learner might encounter	Before a client goes to school she anticipates loud noises, crowds, visual distractions, and possible "safe spots" to collect her thoughts when feeling overwhelmed.
Knowledge	Identifying, acknowledging, and reflecting on what the individual knows about a given task	Observing the individual completing the task, conducting assessment/interview in an attempt to discover how much the learner knows and understands regarding task sequence and demands

TABLE 10-2 Defining and Describing Domain Specific Cognitive Strategies—cont'd

Mental or Self-Verbalization Strategies—cont'd		
Domain Specific Strategy	**Defining & Describing**	**Clinical Examples**
Translation	Converting written instructions and directions into different mediums in order to meet the individual's unique learning needs	Creating visual images/schedules explaining written information, chunking directions together into smaller steps
Task Modification and Specification Strategies		
Domain Specific Strategy	**Defining & Describing**	**Clinical Examples**
Finger pointing	Similar to attention to doing; however, limited to pointing with one's finger directly at relevant task stimuli to enhancing timing within a task or refocus the learner's attention	As the individual is reading (book, task directions, etc.) have the learner point at each word to slow down the pace at which he or she is acquiring new information and to ensure not to skip ahead.
Task simplification	Simplifying or breaking apart the parts of a task into more manageable pieces	When printing, the learner writes his name, date, and title at the top of the page and then the teacher scribes the rest of the assignment.
Lists	Creating and/or using a list of steps to help guide task performance and/or cue actions	The list can be comprised of audio, visual, or written steps. For example a written list/script that is left by the phone that walks the learner through the socially appropriate steps to carry out when answering the phone
Task specification	Discussion regarding the specifics of a task, its components, or relevant features prior to engaging in the activity	These specifications should highlight those areas that require special attention, planning, or consideration. For example, placing an "x" where the child hangs his book bag or places his lunch bag.
Attention to doing	Identifying the specific and relevant cues or features that need to be attended to when completing the task	An example might be: "Where do you need to start your letters?" (printing)
Pacing strategies	Activities that assist with the timing of tasks	Some examples might include: humming a song, taking breaks, counting out-loud or to oneself, or tapping one's foot.
Stimuli reduction	Removing or decreasing the amount and number of stimuli present at a given time	Covering or removing a part of task stimuli: for example, when reading a page of information, placing a blank sheet over-top of the rest of the lines of text (hiding it) so that the reader can focus on one line at a time
Organization	Restructuring and reorganizing task materials or steps so that they are grouped together in a more logical or meaningful way	Commonly referred to as categorization or association. Reorganizing a list of chores so that all of the ones that need to be completed in the morning are together, and all the ones that need to be completed in the evening are together.

Adapted and Referenced from.[44,59,60]

- *Coach, Don't Adjust.* One of the most important components of the CO-OP approach involves adjusting the task or the environment to support occupational performance and skill acquisition.[44,46] Many occupational therapists intuitively adjust a variety of factors including body positions, chair position, or equipment to ensure success. Often this leads to success within therapy sessions and in the presence of the occupational therapist, but the child may not be aware of these enabling strategies and may find it difficult to achieve success in the absence of the therapist.[44,58] Within the CO-OP intervention, the occupational therapist is required to bring these adjustments to the child's attention by guiding the child to discover the personal, task, or environmental adjustments that will improve occupational performance.[44-46]
- *Make it Obvious.* Often children do not readily learn from observation and may have difficulty identifying the important components of a task.[44] Therefore when working with a child using the CO-OP approach, the part of the occupation the child needs to attend to is "made obvious" by the occupational therapist. As well, the relationship between strategy use and outcome are also "made obvious."[44,46]

The fifth key feature of CO-OP is the four enabling principles that are used throughout the intervention.[44] These four enabling principles include: (1) Make it fun; (2) promote learning; (3) work toward independence; and (4) promote generalization and transfer. These enabling principles are important in engaging the child in therapy.

Parent or caregiver involvement is essential throughout the CO-OP therapeutic process.[15,44,46] The primary role of parents or caregivers is to support the child in learning the occupations and the strategies and to facilitate the generalization and transfer of these to the home, school, and other environments.[21,44,57]

The CO-OP program involves ten intervention sessions.[44,46] In the first phase of the CO-OP process the child identifies three goals to address during intervention and then the occupational therapist assesses the child's baseline performance in each one of the chosen skills.[44,46] Subsequently, the occupational therapist teaches the child the Goal-Plan-Do-Check strategy and then it is applied it to the child's three goals. The Goal-Plan-Do-Check strategy is then used to identify the DSSs.[44,46] Once therapy is complete the occupational therapist re-evaluates the child's performance. See Case Study 10-2.

Evaluations Used in CO-OP

Within the CO-OP intervention, a variety of evaluation tools can be used by the occupational therapist to ensure meaningful goal selection, monitor skill acquisition, and demonstrate improvements in occupational performance (Figure 10-5). These include but are not limited to the following.

- *The Daily Activity Log* is a tool used to record the activities a child identifies as important over the course of a day. In CO-OP, the client is asked to complete the Daily Activity Log, with the assistance of parents/significant others if necessary, thinking about a typical day. The completed Daily Activity Log is used to provide the occupational therapist with information on the client's typical day and is used to initiate the process of goal setting.[44,46]
- *Pediatric Activity Card Sort (PACS)*[31] are picture-based assessments used to determine level of occupational engagement. Organized in four categories, hobbies, chores, sports, and personal care, clients are asked to sort the pictures into those he or she does and those he or she does not do. The PACS may be used to complement the Daily Activity Log in the process of goal setting.
- The *Canadian Occupational Performance Measure (COPM)*[26] is a client-centered, self-report measure designed to identify treatment goals in the areas of self-care, productivity and leisure. Within the CO-OP approach, the COPM is used to identify the three client-chosen goals that are the focal point of the intervention. The occupational therapist uses the information obtained from the Daily Activity Log to initiate the COPM interview and to help guide the questions asked so as to ensure that the best goals are identified. The COPM is administered again at the end of intervention to measure outcome.
- The *Performance Quality Rating Scale (PQRS)*[19,33,37] is an observation-based rating scale used to measure performance and change in performance.

See Case Study 10-3.

Evidence for Using Cognitive Approaches

This chapter describes interventions focused on the role of cognition and cognitive strategies in supporting occupational performance. Research Note 10-3 describes the use of CO-OP with children under 7 years old.

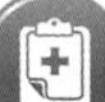

CASE STUDY 10-2 Self-Care

Sarah is a 10-year-old girl who was referred for an occupational therapy assessment of her fine motor skills. Sarah demonstrates difficulties completing a variety of self-care activities such as tying her shoes, buttoning buttons, and zipping zippers. An assessment of Sarah's fine motor skills was conducted, revealing some challenges with in-hand manipulation skills and bilateral motor coordination skills. Sarah's challenges in these areas were impacting her ability to be independent in a variety of areas. Sarah was seen by a private occupational therapist for 12 sessions, in which the CO-OP approach was used to support skill acquisition. Throughout the first sessions, the occupational therapist introduced the Goal, Plan, Do, Check framework and applied it to activities that Sarah was already successful in completing. In doing so, Sarah then understood how the Goal, Plan, Do, Check strategy could be applied. Working with Sarah's parents, the occupational therapist explained this strategy and discussed how to incorporate it into Sarah's daily activities. The occupational therapist then used dynamic performance analysis (DPA) to better understand client motivation, task knowledge, and current occupational performance. The occupational therapist, Sarah, and her parents identified a variety of domain-specific strategies to assist in skill acquisition. Through identifying proper body/hand positioning, feeling the movements, and using verbal instruction and self-guidance, Sarah mastered the three selected skills within the 12 therapy sessions.

Application of the CO-OP Approach: Goal and Point of Breakdown

Goal	Breakdown Points
Tying her shoes	She does not know how to form the loops. She struggles with manipulating the laces in her hands (holding the one still and looping the other around, or holding two loops at the same time). She does not know how to tie the final knot.
Buttoning buttons	Grasping the button while holding the fabric steady with her other hand Aligning the button with the correct hole Pulling the button through the hole

CASE STUDY 10-2 Self-Care—cont'd

Goal	Breakdown Points
Doing up and undoing her zippers	Holding the zipper stable with one hand and manipulating the other side of the zipper with her other hand Pushing the end of the zipper all the way into the pull tab (having it grab so that the zipper does not split)

Application of the CO-OP Approach: Goal and Strategy Use

Domain Specific Strategy	Specific Strategy/PLAN	Bridging for the Strategy
Attention to doing	Making an X Glue my loop to the shoe	Tying soccer cleats and figure skates
Motor mnemonic	Make a bunny ear	Tying her doll's shoes and indoor gym shoes at school
Feeling the movement	"Feel the edge of the button and grip that as you pull it through the hole." "Feel the end of the zipper fit snugly into the pull tab before pulling up."	Buttoning her doll clothing and helping her younger brother with dressing in the morning Putting her sleeping bag back together when camping
Verbal rote script	"Hole one—button one, hole two—button two, hole three—button three"	Buttoning doll clothing and helping her younger brother with dressing in the morning
Body position	"Pinch the pull tab between your index and thumb."	Buttoning (pinching the button to manipulate more effectively)

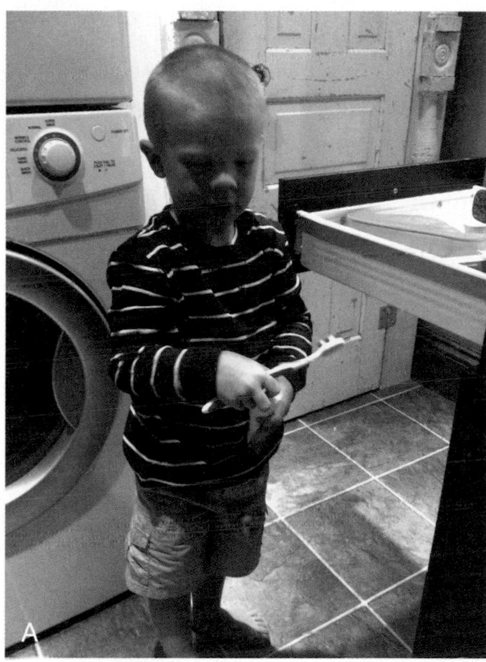

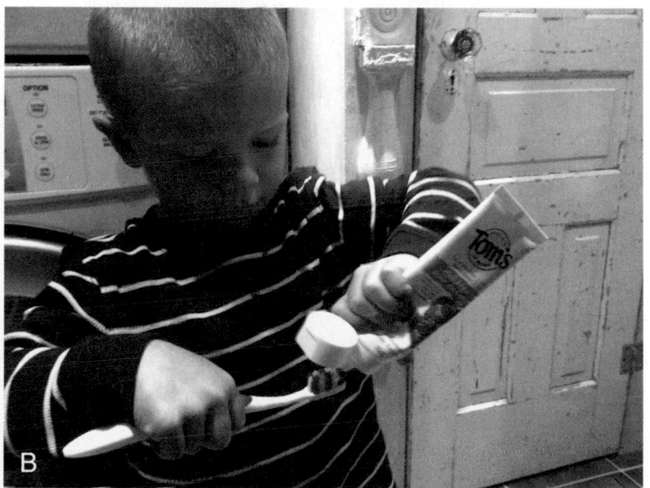

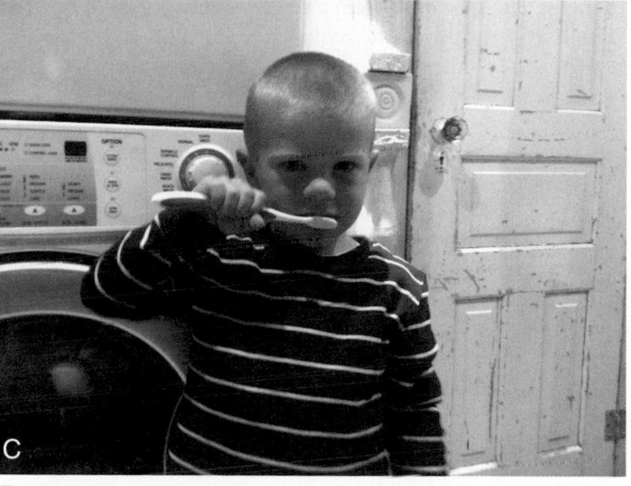

FIGURE 10-5 **A-G,** Brushing teeth.

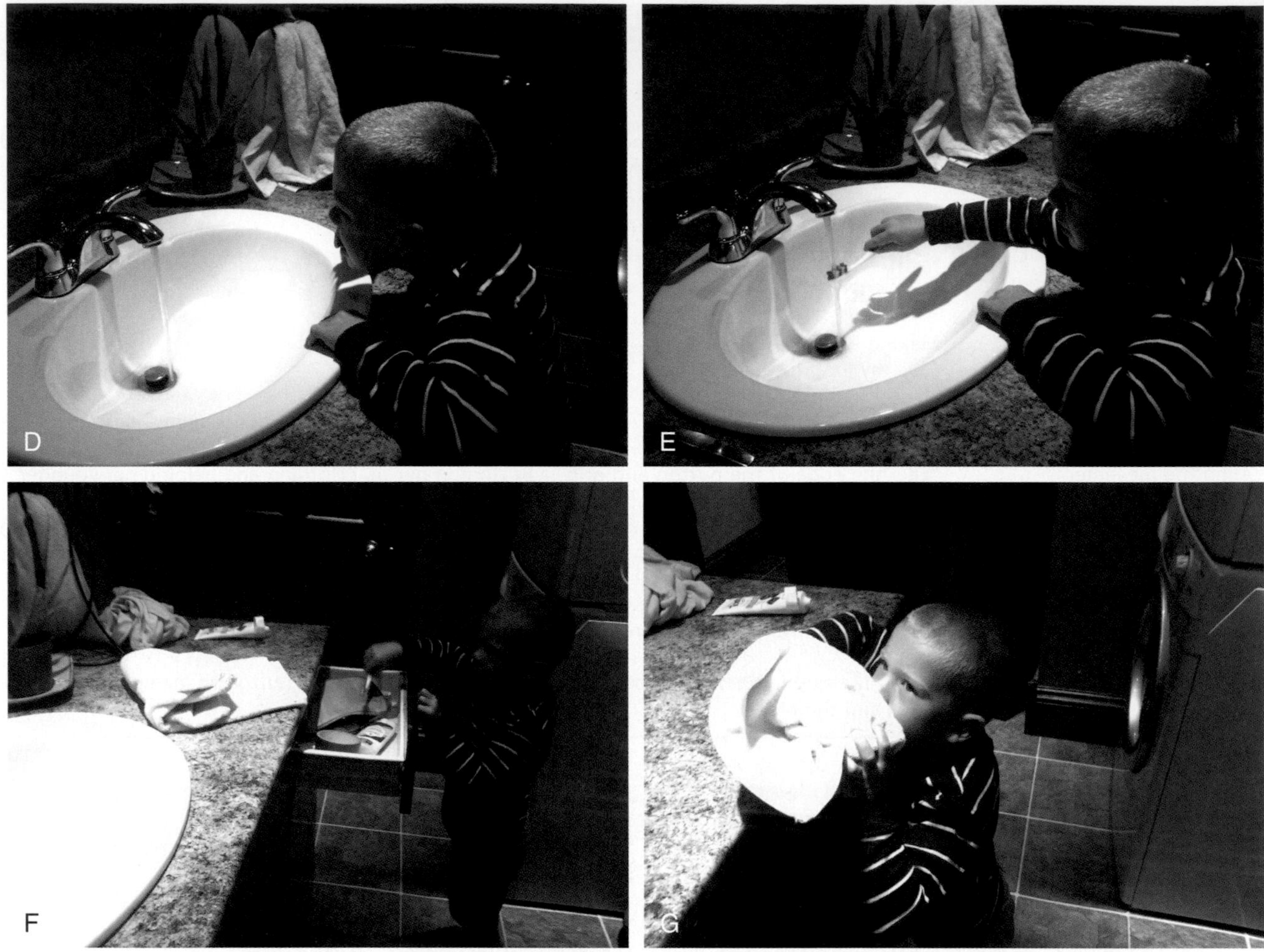

FIGURE 10-5, cont'd

CASE STUDY 10-3 Leisure and Play

Sam is a 7 year old boy who has a diagnosis of Developmental Coordination Disorder. He was referred for private occupational therapy services with one goal in mind: learning to ride his new bike. Through completion of the COPM, the occupational therapist working with Sam and his family realized that Sam was highly motivated to acquire the skills to complete the activity successfully. The occupational therapist used the CO-OP approach as the framework for Sam's 12 therapy sessions. They focused on task components of bike riding as the "just right challenge for him." The occupational therapist modeled the activity of bike riding while using verbal guidance to ensure that Sam had all the information (verbal, visual, and physical) necessary to attempt to complete the task accurately. The occupational therapist used domain-specific cognitive strategies like body position and feeling the movement to help Sam navigate through the motor learning process. Ensuring Sam was an active collaborator in the therapeutic process guaranteed his motivation and improved his skill acquisition and retention. Sam was provided "homework" to practice the skill of bike riding at home, using the cognitive strategies that he learned during his treatment sessions. The home program encouraged the involvement of Sam's family in the learning process, and helped with skill retention, generalization, and transfer. After succeeding at each "step" of bike riding (determined through task analysis), Sam was able to perform the task of bike riding in a controlled environment. The next step for Sam's success was to practice his newly developed skills in an open environment (on his street at home) to learn how to manage environmental obstacles (e.g., street signs, curbs, traffic) using his cognitive strategies.

Application of the CO-OP Approach: Goal and Points of Breakdown

Goal	Breakdown Points
Riding his bike	Taking off from a stopped position (balancing bike and starting to pedal) Turing the bike while pedaling at the same time Remember to pedal backward to stop his bike

CASE STUDY 10-3 Leisure and Play—cont'd

Application of the CO-OP Approach: Strategy Use

Domain-Specific Strategy	Specific Strategy/Plan	Bridging for the Strategy
Body position	Keep my feet moving.	Running, playing volleyball or badminton
Feeling the movement	"Feel your body lean to the side as you turn the corner." "Feel the forward power (motion) as you start pedaling"	Enhancing body awareness and positioning to improve task performance in all sport skills (Figure 10-6)
Attention to doing	"Look ahead to where you are going to turn ... where you are going."	Roller blading and skateboarding
Verbal motor mnemonic	"Step back."	Stopping the bike, stopping when using roller blades
Task-specification modification	Use training wheels until confident with balance and control of the bike.	Understanding that when learning new skills, support from equipment or a person is useful for gaining confidence in task performance.

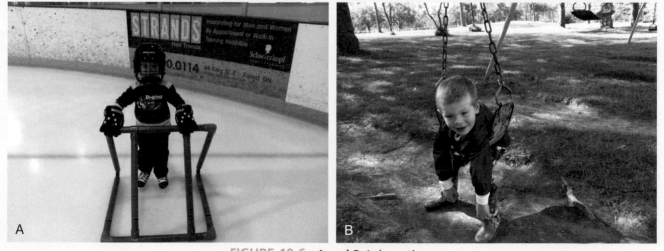

FIGURE 10-6 **A and B,** Leisure time.

RESEARCH NOTE 10-3

Using Cognitive Interventions for Children Under 7

Taylor, S., Fayed, N. & Mandich, A. (2007). CO-OP Intervention for Young Children with Developmental Coordination Disorder. OTJR: Occupation, Participation and Health, *27(4), 124–130.*

Abstract

Children with developmental coordination disorder experience difficulties with fine and gross motor tasks that affect their occupational performance. Research has found Cognitive Orientation to daily Occupational Performance (CO-OP) to be an effective approach for improving skills in daily occupational with children between 7 and 12 years old who have developmental coordination disorder. The purpose of this single-case design was to determine the effectiveness of using the CO-OP approach with children ages 5 to 7 years. Four children chose three different goals to work on during therapy. Child and parent Canadian Occupational Performance Measure (COPM) ratings at follow-up demonstrated the effectiveness of the CO-OP approach, supporting the use of CO-OP with younger children and suggesting further research on the CO-OP with younger children is warranted.

Implications for Practice

- CO-OP was shown to be an effective treatment method to be used with children as young as 5 years.
- Slight modifications to the administration of the CO-OP were necessary with younger children. The younger the child, the more varied each session was required to be to maintain their attention span, and repetition between sessions was important. Reducing the session length with young children and increasing the number of sessions may be beneficial for children in this age group.
- All children reported improvements in their perceived performance of their chosen tasks, with improved ratings of performance by occupational therapists and parents.
- Children ages 5 to 7 with DCD appear to demonstrate the ability to draw on metacognitive strategies to improve on tasks that are meaningful to them. Furthermore, young children may be able to modify their own cognitive processes through training in skills such as planning, checking, and monitoring.

Summary

Cognitive interventions are frequently used by occupational therapists.[55] Research evidence is accumulating that suggests they are effective in enabling occupational performance in children.[43,49,50,55] As well, cognitive strategies can be used to guide the acquisition of new skills and to promote generalize and transfer of these skills.[43,53]

- Cognitive and educational psychology theories have directly informed the development of cognitive approaches in occupational therapy. The key theorists include Vygotsky, Luria, Meichenbaum, Bruner, Bandura, and Feuerstein.[1,4,10,13,29,34-36,38,43,57,58] Each theorist contributes to the foundational concepts, principals, and key features of cognitive interventions in occupational therapy.
- Cognitive strategies are the implicit mental processes that guide learning.[43,55] When the task becomes difficult, relative to the child's skill level, then metacognitive strategies are required to select appropriate cognitive strategies, monitor and evaluate their application.[23,44,60] Once a strategy use becomes automatic and can be efficiently used, then thinking about and monitoring the strategies consciously becomes unnecessary.[39,44]
- Cognitive interventions focus on working on the goals identified by the child and the family, therefore enhancing motivation, skill retention, generalization, and transfer.[21,44,53]
- Scaffolding is intentional and graded adult feedback to promote the skill development of the child. It is a global problem-solving structure that enables learning through everyday activities and helps children to bridge their newly developed skills to different environments and activities.[39,44,62,63]
- Guided discovery is task exploration with purposeful scaffolding. The occupational therapist assumes the role of a facilitator and allows the child to generate her or his own answers (strategies) through tailoring the task and the environment to the individual.[44,46]
- Using DPA, the occupational therapist analyzes the child's performance of the task on an ongoing basis, documenting performance problems and/or areas of skill breakdown. Focus is placed on the fit between client abilities, skills, and actions, paired with the task and environmental demands and supports.[44,46]
- CO-OP's four enabling principles include: (1) Make it fun; (2) promote learning; (3) work toward independence; and (4) promote generalization and transfer. These enabling principles are important in engaging the child in therapy, and prompting cognitive strategy development.[44,46]
- CO-OP is applied through a family- and client-centered framework that focuses on a performance-based problem-solving approach that enables skill acquisition through a process of strategy use and guided discovery.[39,44]
- The CO-OP approach uses the global cognitive strategy Goal-Plan-Do-Check coupled with individually relevant domain-specific cognitive strategies. Emphasis is placed on the child using cognitive strategies developed through guided discovery and the implementation of the enabling principals, to problem solve a performance issue and monitor the outcome.[44]
- Research has shown that children who participate in cognitive interventions demonstrate a higher level of self-efficacy, skill retention, generalization, and transfer.[37,43,44]

REFERENCES

1. Bandura, A. (1982). Self efficacy mechanism in human agency. *American Psychologist, 37*, 122–147.
2. Bandura, A. (1993). Perceived self-efficacy in cognitive development and functioning. *Educational Psychologist, 28*, 117–148.
3. Ben-Hur, M., & Feuerstein, R. (2011). Feuerstein's new program for the facilitation of cognitive development in young children. *Journal of Cognitive Education and Psychology, 10*(3), 224–237.
4. Berk, L. L., & Schanker, S. G. (2006). *Child Development* (2nd ed.). Toronto: Pearson Education Inc.
5. Bernie, C., & Rodger, S. (2004). Cognitive strategy use in school-aged children with developmental coordination disorder. *Physical & Occupational Therapy in Pediatrics, 24*(4), 23–45.
6. Bouffard, M., & Wall, A. E. (1990). A problem solving approach to movement skill acquisition: Implications for special populations. In G. Reid (Ed.), *Problems in movement control.* Amsterdam: Elsevier Science (North-Holland).
7. Bransford, J. D. (1979). *Human cognition: Learning, understanding and remembering.* Belmont, CA: Wadsworth.
8. Bruner, J. S. (1961). The act of discovery. *Harvard Educational Review, 31*, 21–32.
9. Christiansen, C. (2004). Occupation and identity: Becoming who we are through what we do. In C. H. Christiansen & E. A. Townsend (Eds.), *Introduction to occupation the art and science of living* (pp. 121–139). Upper Saddle River, NJ: Prentice Hall.
10. Dweck, C. S. (1986). Motivational processes affecting learning. *American Psychologist, 41*(10), 1040.
11. Feuerstein, R., Hoffman, M., & Miller, R. (1980). *Instrumental enrichment: An intervention program for cognitive modifiability.* Baltimore: University Park Press.
12. Flavell, J. (1979). Metacognition and cognitive monitoring: A new area of cognitive developmental inquiry. *American Psychologist, 34*, 906–911.
13. Gage, M., & Politajko, H. (1996). Enhancing occupational performance through an understanding of perceived self-efficacy. In R. P. Fleming-Cottrell (Ed.), *Perspectives on purposeful activity: Foundation and future of occupational therapy* (pp. 367–371). Bethesda, MD: American Occupational Therapy Association.
14. Goodley, D., & Runswick-Cole, K. (2010). Emancipating play: Disabled children, development and deconstruction. *Disability & Society, 25*(4), 499–512.
15. Graham, F., Rodger, S., & Ziviani, J. (2009). Coaching parents to enable children's participation: An approach for working with parents and their children. *Australian Occupational Therapy Journal, 56*(1), 16–23.
16. Hahn-Markowitz, J., Manor, I., & Maeir, A. (2011). Effectiveness of cognitive–functional (Cog–Fun) intervention with children with attention

deficit hyperactivity disorder: A pilot study. *American Journal of Occupational Therapy, 65,* 384–392.

17. Haywood, H. C. (1987). A meditational teaching style. *The Thinking Teacher, 4*(1), 1–6.
18. Henderson, S. E., & Sugden, D. (1992). *The movement assessment battery for children.* Kent, UK: The Psychological Corporation Ltd.
19. Henry, L., & Polatajko, H. J., (2003). Exploring the inter-rater reliability of the performance quality rating scale. Paper presented at the Canadian Associate of Occupational Therapists Conference, Winnipeg, Manitoba.
20. Humphry, R., & Womack, J. (2013). Transformations of occupations: A life course perspective. In B. A. Boyt Schell, G. Gillen, M. E. Scaffa, & E. S. Cohn (Eds.), *Willard & Spackman's occupational therapy* (12th ed., pp. 60–72). Baltimore: Lippincott Williams & Wilkins.
21. Jaffe, L., Humphry, R., & Case-Smith, J. (2010). Working with families. In J. Case-Smith & J. Clifford O'Brien (Eds.), *Occupational therapy for children* (6th ed., pp. 108–146). Maryland Heights, MO: Mosby Elsevier.
22. Jenkins, R. L. (1979). The influence of children in family decision-making: parents' perceptions. *Advances in Consumer Research, 6*(1), 413–418.
23. Katz, N., & Hartman-Maeir, A. (1997). Occupational performance and metacognition. *Canadian Journal of Occupational Therapy, 64*(2), 53–62.
24. Kozulin, A., Lebeer, J., Madella-Noja, A., et al. (2010). Cognitive modifiability of children with developmental disabilities: A multicenter study using Feuerstein's Instrumental Enrichment-Basic program. *Research in Developmental Disabilities, 31,* 551–559.
25. Larson, E. A. (1995). The occupation of play: Parent-child interaction in the service of social competence. *Occupational Therapy in Health Care, 9*(2/3), 103–120.
26. Law, M. (1998). Does client centered practice make a difference? In M. Law (Ed.), *Client centered occupational therapy* (pp. 19–28). Thorofare, NJ: Slack.
27. Lidz, C. (1987). *Dynamic assessment: An interactional approach to evaluating learning potential.* New York: Guildford Press.
28. Luria, A. (1961). *The role of speech in the regulations of normal and abnormal behaviors.* New York: Liveright.
29. Luria, A. (1959). The directive function of speech in development. *Word, 18,* 341–352.
30. Mandich, A. D., Polatajko, H. J., Macnab, J. J., et al. (2001). Treatment of children with developmental coordination disorder: What is the evidence? *Physical & Occupational Therapy in Pediatrics, 20*(2–3), 51–68.
31. Mandich, A., Polatajko, H., Miller, L., et al. (2004). *The Paediatric Activity Card.* Ottawa, ON: CAOT Publications ACE.
32. Martini, R., Mandich, A., & Green, D. (2014). Implementing a modified cognitive orientation to daily occupational performance approach for use in a group format. *The British Journal of Occupational Therapy, 77*(4), 214–219.
33. Martini, R., & Polatajko, H. J. (1998). Verbal self-guidance as a treatment approach for children with developmental coordination disorder. *Physical and Occupational Therapy in Pediatrics, 20*(2/3), 125–144.
34. Meichenbaum, D., & Goodman, J. (1971). Training impulsive children to talk to themselves: A means of developing self-control. *Journal of Abnormal Psychology, 77,* 115–126.
35. Meichenbaum, D. (1977). *Cognitive-behavioral modification: An integrative approach.* New York: Plenum Press.
36. Meichenbaum, D. (1991). Cognitive behaviour modification: Workshop presented at the Child and Parent Research Institute symposium.
37. Miller, L. T., Politajko, H. J., Missiuna, C., et al. (2001). A pilot trial of a cognitive treatment for children with developmental coordination disorder. *Human Movement Science, 20,* 183–210.
38. Missinna, C., Malloy-Miller, T., & Mandich, A. (1998). Mediational techniques: origins and application to occupational therapy in pediatrics. *Canadian Journal of Occupational Therapy, 65*(4), 202–209.
39. Missiuna, C., Mandich, A. D., Politajko, H. J., et al. (2001). Cognitive orientation to daily occupational performance (CO-OP): Part I—Theoretical foundations. *Physical & Occupational Therapy in Pediatrics, 20*(2/3), 69–81.
40. Missiuna, C., DeMatteo, C., Hanna, S., et al. (2010). Exploring the use of cognitive intervention for children with acquired brain injury. *Physical & Occupational Therapy in Pediatrics, 30*(3), 205–219.
41. Missiuna, C., Malloy-Miller, T., & Mandich, A. (1997). Cognitive, or "top-down," approaches to intervention. *Keeping Current,* 97-1.
42. Perry, S. B. (1998). Clinical implications of a dynamic systems theory. *Neurology Report, 24,* 4–10.
43. Polatajko, H. J., Mandich, A. D., Miller, L. T., et al. (2001). Cognitive Orientation to Daily Occupational Performance (CO-OP) Part II The Evidence. *Physical & Occupational Therapy in Pediatrics, 20*(2–3), 83–106.
44. Polatajko, H. J., & Mandich, A. D. (2004). *Enabling occupation in children: the cognitive orientation to daily occupational performance (CO-OP) approach.* OHawa, Canada: CAOT Publications ACE.
45. Polatajko, H. J., Mandich, A. D., & Martini, R. (2000). Dynamic Performance analysis: A framework for understanding occupational performance. *American Journal of Occupational Therapy, 54,* 65–72.
46. Politajko, H. J., Mandch, A. D., Missiuna, C., et al. (2001). Cognitive approach to daily occupational performance (CO-OP): Part III-Protocol in brief. *Physical & Occupational Therapy in Pediatrics, 20*(2/3), 107–123.
47. Polgar, J. M., & Landry, J. E. (2004). Occupations as a means for individual and group participation in life. In C. H. Christiansen & E. A. Townsend (Eds.), *Introduction to occupation the art and science of living* (pp. 197–220). Upper Saddle River, NJ: Prentice Hall.
48. Pressiey, M. (1994). Embracing the complexity of individual differences in cognition: Studying good information processing and how it might develop. *Learning and Individual Differences, 6*(3), 259–284.
49. Pressley, M., Roehrig, A. D., Raphael, L., et al. (2003). Teaching processes in elementary and secondary education. In W. M. Reynolds & G. E. Miller (Eds.), *Handbook of psychology, Vol. 7: Educational psychology.* Hoboken, NJ: John Wiley & Sons Inc.
50. Pressley, M., & Harris, K. R. (2006). Cognitive strategies introduction: From basic research to classroom instruction. In E. Anderman, P. H. Winne, P. A. Alexander, & L. Corno (Eds.), *Handbook of educational psychology* (2nd ed., pp. 265–286). Mahwah, NJ: Lawrence Erlbaum.
51. Rodger, S., Ireland, S., & Vun, M. (2008). Can cognitive orientation to daily occupational performance (CO-OP) help children with Asperger's syndrome to master social and organisational goals? *British Journal of Occupational Therapy, 71*(1), 23–32.
52. Rodger, S., Springfield, E., & Polatajko, H. (2007). Cognitive orientation for daily occupational performance approach for children with Asperger's syndrome: A case report. *Physical & Occupational Therapy in Pediatrics, 27*(4), 7–22.
53. Sangster, C. A., Beninger, C., Polatajko, H. J., et al. (2005). Cognitive strategy generation in children with

developmental coordination disorder. *Canadian Journal of Occupational Therapy, 72*(2), 67–77.
54. Seger, C. A. (1994). Implicit learning. *Psychological Bulletin, 155*, 163–196.
55. Smits-Engelsman, B. C. M., Blank, R., Van Der Kaay, A. C., et al. (2013). Efficacy of interventions to improve motor performance in children with developmental coordination disorder: A combined systematic review and meta-analysis. *Developmental Medicine & Child Neurology, 55*(3), 229–237.
56. Sufrin, E. M. (1984). The physical rehabilitation of the brain injured elderly. In B. A. Edelstein & E. T. Couture (Eds.), *Behavioral assessment and rehabilitation of the traumatically brain-damaged* (pp. 191–221). New York: Plenum.
57. Sugden, D. (2007). Current approaches to intervention in children with developmental coordination disorder. *Developmental Medicine & Child Neurology, 49*(6), 467–471.
58. Toglia, J. P. (1991). Generalization of treatment: A multicontext approach to cognitive perceptual impairment in adults with brain injury. *The American Journal of Occupational Therapy, 45*(6), 505–516.
59. Toglia, J. P. (2011). The dynamic interactional model of cognition in cognitive rehabilitation. In N. Katz (Ed.), *Cognition, occupation and participation across the life span: Neuroscience, neurorehabilitation and models of intervention in occupational therapy* (3rd ed., pp. 161–201). Bethedsa, MD: AOTA Press.
60. Toglia, J. P., Rodger, S. A., & Politajko, H. J. (2012). Anatomy of cognitive strategies: A therapist's primer for enabling occupational performance. *Canadian Journal of Occupational Therapy, 79*, 225–236.
61. Tudge, J. R. H., & Winterhoff, P. A. (1993). Vygotsky, Piaget, and Bandura: Perspectives on the relations between the social world and cognitive development. *Human Development, 36*, 61–81.
62. Vygotsky, L. S. (1978). Mind in society: The development of higher psychological processes, 14e. Cambridge, MA: Harvard University Press.
63. Vygotsky, L. (1987). Thinking and speech. In R. W. Reiber & A. S. Carton (Eds.), *The collected works of L. S. Vygotsky* (pp. 39–28).
64. Ward, A., & Rodger, S. (2004). The application of cognitive orientation to daily occupational performance (CO-OP) with children 5-7 years with developmental coordination disorder. *British Journal of Occupational Therapy, 67*(6), 256–264.
65. Wright, H. C., & Sugden, D. A. (1998). A school based intervention programme for children with developmental coordination disorder. *European Journal of Physical Education, 3*, 35–50.
66. Zwicker, J. G., & Hadwin, A. F. (2009). Cognitive versus multisensory approaches to handwriting intervention: A randomized controlled trial. *Occupational Therapy Journal of Research: Occupation, Participation and Health, 29*, 40–48.

CHAPTER 11

Interventions to Promote Social Participation for Children with Mental Health and Behavioral Disorders

Claudia List Hilton

KEY TERMS

Anxiety disorders
Mood disorders
Autism spectrum disorders
Fetal alcohol spectrum disorders
Attention-deficit/hyperactivity disorder
Social cognitive
Executive function
Theory of mind
Weak central coherence
Joint attention
Social cognitive
Behavior modification
Self-determination
Peer-mediated intervention
Sensory integration
Applied behavior analysis
Relationship development intervention
Social stories
Mind reading
Video detective
Emotions charades
Power cards
Stress thermometer
Incredible five-point scale
SOCCSS
Video modeling
Social autopsies
Comic strip conversations
Privacy circles

GUIDING QUESTIONS

1. What are the diagnostic categories and potential problems of children who may have social participation deficits?
2. What are the major theories that explain social skill deficits in children?
3. What are the roles of occupational therapists and other team members who provide services to children and youth with social skill impairments?
4. What specific types of skills can be addressed with social skills interventions?
5. How do theories and approaches inform social skills intervention?
6. What are the principles and strategies that occupational therapists use to improve social skills in children?
7. What evidence supports interventions that can be used with children who have social skill impairments?

This chapter discusses the role of occupational therapy in supporting children's social participation. It examines diagnostic categories of children for whom social participation can be problematic and describes various theories explaining the basis for these impairments. It describes types of social goals, approaches, and strategies to help practitioners design intervention.

International Classification of Functioning, Disability, and Health, Occupational Therapy Practice Framework, and Social Participation

The International Classification of Functioning, Disability, and Health: Children and Youth Version (ICF-CY) identifies interpersonal interactions and relationships as one of the domains of activities and participation necessary for children's health.[170] The Occupational Therapy Practice Framework (OTPF) identifies social participation as one of the occupations whereby occupational therapy promotes children's health.[4] Social participation is defined as "organized patterns of behavior that are characteristic and expected of an individual or a given position within a social system."[106] Social participation includes engagement with community, family, and peers or friends in interpersonal interactions and relationships. Promoting social participation for children in natural contexts supports social well-being and is a focus of occupational therapy intervention.

Establishing and maintaining satisfying interpersonal relationships are essential elements of social well-being.[166] Close, confiding, and supportive relationships enhance health by preserving the immune system and encouraging good health habits.[6] Socially sanctioned, approved, and valued occupations are most supportive of a person's health. The qualities of a person's social relationships have been consistently associated with physical health, life satisfaction, and mortality.[7,13,24,75] Therefore, occupational therapy interventions to promote a child's social participation and social well-being can contribute to multiple aspects of health, functional performance, and quality of life.

Importance of Social Skills and Social Participation

Children achieve developmental milestones and occupational goals through social interactions.[38,53] Social skills can be defined as "socially acceptable learned behaviors that enable a person to interact with others in ways that elicit positive responses and assist the person in avoiding negative responses."[54] Social skills

BOX 11-1 Examples of Social Goals

Demonstrate Specific Social Behaviors
- Appropriately greet others.
- Introduce self (to peer and adult).
- Ask someone to play.
- Start a conversation.
- Appropriately give compliments.
- Ask for help.
- Appropriately respond to irritating behaviors of others.
- Participate in conversations.
- Talk about areas outside of special interests.
- Demonstrate cooperative interaction during activities with peers.
- Look at others while engaged in conversation.
- Increase social initiations.
- Participate in conversations.
- Take turns in conversations.
- Start conversations

Awareness of Social Rules
- Demonstrate awareness of unwritten social rules.
- Maintain appropriate physical distance from others.
- Use respectful words when disagreeing with others.
- Stand up for self in an appropriate manner.
- Improve appropriate social responding.
- Use good manners.
- Participate and cooperate in a group project.
- Deal appropriately with irritating behavior by peers.
- Exhibit good manners and good friend behaviors.

Awareness of Others
- Assist others when needed.
- Demonstrate how and when to interrupt.
- Demonstrate how to share a friend with others without becoming jealous or angry.
- When talking, pause appropriately to allow others to talk.
- Differentiate between types and topics of conversation appropriate for different people and situations (e.g., peers, teachers, girls, boys).
- Verbalize understanding of intentions of others.
- Demonstrate increased social motivation.
- Correctly read nonverbal cues.

Executive Function Skills

Self-Management
- Recognize and verbalize uncomfortable sensory feelings.
- Demonstrate strategies to deal with uncomfortable sensory feelings.
- Apply strategies that help to calm self.
- Keep hands and feet to self.
- Participate in activities when rules are made by others.
- Reduce interfering behaviors.
- Use appropriate voice volume.
- Take turns.
- Follow directions given by adults after first time.
- Stay with group while participating in an activity.
- Think before acting.

Problem Solving
- Ask for help when needed.
- Negotiate with friends.
- Deal with bullies appropriately.
- Compromise when you disagree.

are necessary for effective social participation. Participation in educational and social activities is the context in which children and youth make friends, learn social skills and competencies, and develop their sense of purpose.[63,85,108] As a child gains social skills, he or she can participate in the meaningful occupations of childhood with greater competence and satisfaction. Development of these skills facilitates the formation of relationships with others that are comfortable and non-threatening. Children develop moral and social values consistent with those of their cultures through social networks. Social skills have a great impact on improving a child's self-esteem. The importance of social interactions in boosting coping skills and resiliency has been established in studies of children with disabilities.[62,133]

In addition to the direct benefits of social participation for the child and his or her development, parents and children place great importance on socialization.[45,114] Cohn et al.[46] found that one of the parents' main hopes for intervention outcomes was the development of behaviors and skills needed for their child to fit in and be included at school and in the community. Parents identified the need for their children to learn appropriate behaviors so that they can conform to the norms of their environments and can interact fully and form meaningful relationships with siblings, same-aged peers, and other children in general. Therefore, developing a child's social competence benefits the child, satisfies parental goals, and enhances the quality of family life. For occupational therapy to be most effective in providing family- and client-centered services, addressing social participation is an essential part of intervention.

Occupational Therapy Goals for Social Participation and Social Skills

Social participation goals addressed by occupational therapy fall into several categories: those in which the child needs to learn specific behaviors, those that involve becoming aware of social rules, those that involve being more aware of the perspectives of others (theory of mind), and those that involve improvements in executive function, such as self-management and problem solving. Box 11-1 provides examples of social goals.

Social Participation Impairments in Specific Childhood Conditions

Children with mental health or behavioral disorders often exhibit limited social participation. The following sections describe evidence about the types of social impairment seen in children and youth with these conditions.

Autism Spectrum Disorders

Social and communication deficits comprise one of the two core components of autism spectrum disorder (ASD).[5] Problem areas include social awareness, social motivation, social communication, theory of mind (see later section, "Theoretical Basis of Social Deficits"), and executive function. Children with ASD experience profound difficulties in interpersonal communication and social relationships, with relatively poor insight into their own difficulties.[68] Social difficulties contribute to a lack of close, reciprocal relationships with other children. Church et al.[44] reported social problems of being too quiet and unassuming, lacking the social skill of assertion, or being too exuberant and active to the point that the child would violate social boundaries. These behaviors frequently alienate classmates and create patterns of negative interactions that are hard to overcome.

Studies investigating the social skills of individuals with ASD cite lack of friends as a problem.[18,68,86] Children with ASD are usually aware of and interested in others, but often approach them in inappropriate ways.[156] They may express an interest in having friends, but usually become frustrated because of frequent failures. Very few adolescents and adults with autism in one study had friendships with same-aged peers, which included participation in a variety of activities, were reciprocal in nature, and occurred outside prearranged settings.[115] Typically, the greater the demands on spontaneous use of social skills, the greater the level of social disability experienced in individuals with ASD.

Social dysfunction, one of the primary features of ASD, may be its most defining characteristic.[127] Improving social functioning is one of the most important and daunting challenges to professionals working with children who have ASD.[127,159] Social skills and social skill interventions are probably more frequently studied in children with ASD than any other diagnostic group.

Fetal Alcohol Spectrum Disorder

When gestationally exposed to alcohol with a diagnosis of fetal alcohol spectrum disorder (FASD), individuals experience a multitude of sociobehavioral impairments that tend to persist across the life span and may even worsen with age.[90] These include impairments in social competence,[28,34,98] social relationships,[26,151] social problem solving,[144] inappropriate friendliness,[111] and difficulty with peer relationships and socially appropriate interactions.[26] Children with FASD may also experience social withdrawal, teasing or bullying, poor social judgment, difficulties with perceiving or responding to social cues, difficulty exhibiting consideration for others, and difficulty forming reciprocal friendships.[34,147] Children with FASD may benefit from interventions to improve executive function, theory of mind, and social problem solving.

Attention-Deficit/Hyperactivity Disorder

The core symptoms in ADHD are problems with attention, impulsiveness, and hyperactivity.[14,65] Other problem areas include difficulties in the domains of attentional and cognitive functions, such as problem solving, planning, orienting, flexibility, sustained attention, response inhibition, and working memory.[119,134] Additional problems are often seen in affective components, such as emotional regulation,[39,113,136] that are fundamental to children's problems with social skills.[92,160] Children with emotional regulation problems become easily irritated when things do not go their way or they cannot get what they want immediately, which often results in unpleasant social interactions. Intervention goals for these children include improving behaviors that reflect executive function.

Anxiety Disorders

Problems in social skills and social interactions are often seen in children diagnosed with anxiety disorders. In their study of 154 children ages 6 to 11 years, Ginsburg et al.[64] found that highly socially anxious children reported lower levels of social acceptance and global self-esteem and more negative peer interactions. The girls with high levels of social anxiety were also rated by parents as having poor social skills, particularly in the areas of assertive and responsible social behavior. Anxiety disorders can develop into social anxiety disorder (SAD) in the teen years and, without treatment, tend to follow a chronic, unremitting course.[42,84] SAD is characterized by a marked fear or anxiety about one or more social situations in which the individual is exposed to possible scrutiny by others.[5] Cognitive-behavioral therapy (CBT) has been shown to be effective in reducing symptoms and functional impairment and in improving social skills in individuals with SAD.[73,157] CBT is a psychotherapeutic approach that uses a combination of behavioral and cognitive principles to address dysfunctional emotions, maladaptive behaviors, cognitive processes, and contents through a number of goal-oriented, explicit, systematic procedures.[44] Learning specific social behaviors, awareness of others, self-management, and problem solving are areas of intervention to address social problems seen in children with anxiety disorders.

Learning Disabilities

Social impairment is often a barrier to participation in social occupations for children with a learning disability (LD). Many children with an LD have difficulty with interpersonal understanding and social interaction,[3,88] which is often exhibited by misconduct in the classroom,[49] inability to cooperate and establish positive relationships with peers,[116] and marked difficulties in working through rough spots in peer relationships in comparison to typically developing peers.[162] Agaliotis and Goudiras[3] have found that children with LD experience more difficulty than typically developing children in appreciating the components that make up the context of interpersonal conflict, devising alternative solutions to resolve a conflict, and appreciating the consequences of the solutions that they propose. Furthermore, typically developing children select assertive strategies such as compromise, whereas children with LD select unilateral, less acceptable, nonassertive, and powerless strategies, such as avoidance of negotiation, to resolve an interpersonal conflict situation.[35]

Mood Disorders

Problems in self-regulation (see Chapter 13 for more information about self-regulation), coping,[47] and interpersonal difficulties[66,79] are among the factors associated with increased risk for depression. These vulnerabilities increase individuals' chances of encountering stress, another risk factor for depression, and decrease their ability to deal with the stress once it occurs. Therefore, many depression prevention strategies include

TABLE 11-1 Developmental Disorders and Common Social Problems

Diagnosis	Common Social Problems
Autism spectrum disorders	Interpersonal communication, social relationships, relatively poor insight into their own difficulties, being teased or bullied, executive function, theory of mind, social awareness, social motivation, social problem solving
Fetal alcohol spectrum disorder	Social competence, social relationships, social problem solving, inappropriate friendliness, difficulty with peer relationships and socially appropriate interactions, social withdrawal, being teased or bullied, poor social judgment, difficulties with perceiving or responding to social cues, exhibiting consideration for others, forming reciprocal friendships, executive function, theory of mind, social problem solving
Attention-deficit/hyperactivity disorder	Attentional and cognitive functions, such as problem solving, planning, orienting, flexibility, sustained attention, response inhibition, working memory, emotional regulation, executive function
Anxiety disorders	Social skills, social interactions, awareness of others, self-management, problem solving, executive function
Learning disabilities	Social awareness, social interaction, inability to cooperate and establish positive relationships with peers, social problem solving, executive function
Mood disorders	Self-regulation, coping, communication skills, social skills

training in coping, social problem solving, and social and communication skills.[61]

Table 11-1 provides an overview of developmental disorders and associated social problems.

Theoretical Basis of Social Deficits

Several theoretical models have emerged to describe the alterations in thought processes that explain social skills deficits and participation limitations in children. Most of these theories originate from research examining children with ASD. The dominant models include the constructs of *theory of mind*, *weak central coherence*, *joint attention*, and *reduced competence* in a cluster of neuropsychological skills called *executive functions*.[109,155]

The theory of mind hypothesis defines the social dysfunction in ASD as the result of disruptions in processes leading to the acquisition of the capacity to conceive of other people's and one's own mind.[16] In other words, the person is blind to the existence of thoughts, beliefs, knowledge, desires, and intentions that contribute to why people do what they do. This may lead to problems such as misunderstandings about the intentions of others, misreading their facial expressions and body language, getting too close while interacting with them, being perceived as insensitive or inconsiderate, and having difficulty understanding how to take turns in conversation and how to talk about the interests of others.

For example, Sasha is a 10-year-old with FASD. She has impaired theory of mind. When her classmate, Mary, who is frequently very clumsy, accidentally knocks a few books off Sasha's desk, Sasha becomes very upset and yells at Mary to stop being mean to her. In another incident, Ben, a classmate, was very upset one time because his grandmother had just died. Instead of offering words of comfort, Sasha said, "She was old. Old people die," which made Ben feel even worse.

A second explanation is the weak central coherence hypothesis.[73] It describes the problem as a tendency to process all stimuli in a fragmented fashion, focusing on details rather than integrated and meaningful wholes, which results in a piecemeal and disjointed internal social world. This might account for a preoccupation with parts of things rather than the whole, such as spinning the wheels of a toy car instead of play that demonstrates a functional understanding of how a car is used, or with preoccupations with letters or numbers instead of using them for reading words or understanding quantities.

A third explanation for social deficits in children is limitation in joint attention.[29] Joint attention is the process of sharing one's experience of observing an object or event by following gaze or pointing gestures. It is critical for social development, language acquisition, and cognitive development. A child with limited joint attention may not share a toy with his or her sibling, point to pictures of a book, or verbalize to his or her parent who is reading the book. Children with joint attention problems do not usually assimilate others' facial expressions when engaged in a joint activity; therefore, they lack awareness of others' nonverbal communications.

The fourth explanation for deficits in social skills is the executive dysfunction hypothesis, which focuses on the lack of self-organizing elements required in general learning. Executive functions guide attention, inhibit irrelevant responses, abstract rules, and generate goals used for task execution.[122] A child with executive dysfunction has problems with general learning because of perseveration and poor self-regulation, difficulties with change, reduced forward planning, and ineffective problem-solving skills. He or she can usually do well with familiar tasks in familiar contexts with familiar people, but struggles with understanding and dealing with new tasks in unfamiliar contexts with unfamiliar people. Issues with adherence to strict routines and avoidance of new situations can be explained by this hypothesis.

Occupational Therapy Evaluation of Social Participation

Occupational therapists are well qualified to play a primary role in working with children who have mental health and behavioral disorders that limit social participation. With a solid knowledge of social, cognitive, behavioral, and sensory development, occupational therapists use client-centered practice and therapeutic use of self to motivate and empower clients to achieve higher levels of social competence and social participation. Other professionals and paraprofessionals are often involved in social interventions, including clinical psychologists, speech-language pathologists, social workers, and teachers. Each has specific knowledge and skills that contribute to the potential effectiveness of the intervention.

Assessment of Social Participation in Children

Assessment of social skills is included in several comprehensive child development assessments and can also be ascertained by using assessment tools that are specific to social skills and social development. Social skills assessment includes information such as eye contact with others during interaction, understanding of nonverbal communication, social awkwardness, sense of humor, turn-taking or sharing, appropriate voice volume when talking with others, interest in others, and understanding of rules and appropriate proximity when interacting with others.

Occupational therapists can choose from general assessments that include social information and specific assessments of social behaviors (Table 11-2). Examples of comprehensive assessments that include social performance are the Hawaii Early Learning Profile and Pediatric Evaluation of Disabilities Inventory—Computer-Adapted Test for young children and the School Function Assessment for school-age children. Chapter 6 identifies other examples.

Goal Attainment Scaling

Assessment tools for measuring social skills and social participation can be used to measure progress. However, these assessments may not be specific and sensitive enough to capture the stages of improvement in intervention goals. Another option that can be more individualized is Goal Attainment Scaling (GAS).[86] GAS can be a useful tool for measuring social skills progress because of its ability to identify and measure progress toward very individualized goals, which may not be included in standard assessments. It can establish expected levels of improvement to measure progress. See Chapters 12 and 23 for more details.

GAS was introduced in the mental health field to evaluate program effectiveness. It has since been applied in various settings, including rehabilitation and education, and has become a common method of measuring progress in some areas of occupational therapy. GAS can provide an outcome measure that is broad enough to detect meaningful improvements while sensitive enough to the specific goals of the individual child and family.[107] Goals are typically set for each client and are then weighted by clients and their caregivers, depending on importance. The goals are scaled from −2 to +2, in which zero is the expected outcome and +2 greatly exceeds the expected level of performance following intervention.[146] The score of −2 has been defined as an outcome that is "much less than expected" and −1 as "less than expected."[96] The five possible outcomes allow therapists to give credit for partially achieving a goal or exceeding it. The score can be standardized, despite the individual nature of the goals, because each possible outcome is theoretically equally as difficult to achieve.[58] In one study, GAS was found to be more sensitive to intervention-related client change (the change brought about by participation in a specific intervention program) than norm-referenced standardized measures.[132]

Use of the GAS promotes cohesion among the intervention team members, family, and child because they can all be involved in developing and prioritizing the goals.[99] GAS provides focus on intervention outcomes and does not compare the child's performance with that of a typically developing child[86] (Figure 11-1).

Theoretical Models and Approaches for Social Skills Interventions

Elliot and Gresham[54] have identified five factors that contribute to social skills deficits: (1) lack of knowledge, (2) lack of practice or feedback, (3) lack of cues or opportunities, (4) lack of reinforcement, and (5) the presence of interfering problem behaviors. These factors help identify potential strategies for interventions and explain the potential value of social interventions. Five theoretical approaches and models are frequently used by occupational therapists to develop occupational therapy social skills group.[156] The five approaches to facilitate social participation include social cognitive, sensory modulation, behavioral modification, self-determination, and peer-mediated intervention. Each theoretic approach or model guides interventions and aligns with principles widely used in occupational therapy practice (Table 11-3).

Peer-Mediated Intervention

This educational intervention model includes typically developing children who are partnered with children with disabilities to effect some type of behavioral changes in the children with disabilities.[117,128] The use of peer-mediated intervention is based on the belief that peers can be as good as or even more effective than adults at intervention. For many skill domains, the contexts created by peers are closer to the typical environments in which children must be able to function. The abundance of peers in most settings creates natural opportunities for clients to learn from multiple examples, and the natural variability of peers' methods creates many opportunities for clients to learn under variable training conditions. Peer-mediated interventions are believed to facilitate generalized outcomes.[149] Children with autism become more responsive to social interactions and engage in increased peer interactions when increased peer support is present.[17,84]

To capitalize on the benefits of peer mediation, the social skills program includes at least one typically developing child who is the same age or slightly older than the other participants. Occasionally, a younger sibling of one of the participants can also be effective, especially if the two have mostly positive interactions and if the younger sibling is relatively mature in his interactions. Peers can be taught to remind the child with social skills impairments what he or she needs to do in a certain situation. A trial period may sometimes be necessary to determine the appropriateness of using siblings as peers.

TABLE 11-2 Specific Assessments for Social Impairment

Name of Measure	Brief Description of Content
Caregiver-Teacher Report Form (CTRF)[1]	For children ages 1½ to 5 years old, this questionnaire is designed to obtain caregivers' or teachers' reports of children's academic performance, adaptive functioning, and behavioral-emotional problems. Teachers rate the child's academic performance in each subject on a five-point scale ranging from 1 (far below grade level) to 5 (far above grade level). For adaptive functioning, teachers use a seven-point scale to compare the child to typical pupils for how hard he or she is working, how appropriately he or she is behaving, how much he or she is learning, and how happy he or she is.
Teacher Report Form (TRF)[1]	Questionnaire for children ages 6 to 18 years old. See Caregiver-Teacher Report Form for description.
Child Behavior Checklist (CBCL)[1]	Designed to assess the behavioral problems and social competencies of children per parent report for ages 1½ to 5 years and ages 6 to 18 years. Subscales include Social Withdrawal, Somatic, Anxious/Depressed, Social Problems, Uncommunicative, Hyperactive, Delinquent, and Aggressive. The CBCL also includes 20 social competence items covering the child's activities, social relations, and school performance. Questions are easy to understand; items address behaviors found across a wide range of functioning; and probes regarding social behaviors are useful with investigations of children with ASD.
Friendship Qualities Scale[31]	Theoretically grounded, multidimensional measurement instrument to assess the quality of children's and early adolescents' relationships with their best friends according to five conceptually meaningful aspects of the friendship relationship: companionship, conflict, help-aid, security, and closeness.
PKBS–2: Preschool and Kindergarten Behavior Scales[103]	Separate score conversion tables are available for home-based and school-based raters. Completion of the rating form takes about 12 minutes. The Social Skills scale includes 34 items on three subscales: Social Cooperation, Social Interaction, and Social Independence. The Problem Behavior scale includes 42 items on two subscales, Externalizing Problems and Internalizing Problems. In addition, five supplementary problem behavior subscales are available for optional use. The PKBS-2 was standardized with a nationwide sample of ratings of 3317 children ages 3 through 6 years. Ethnicity, socioeconomic status, and special education classification of the standardization sample are very similar to those characteristics of the U.S. population, based on the 2000 census.
School Social Behavior Scales, 2nd edition (SSBS-2)[102]	64-item questionnaire designed to assist school personnel in identifying student deficits in school-related social competence and antisocial behaviors. It can be completed in 5 to 10 minutes by teachers to help identify social skills goals for children 5 to 18 years of age. It provides an inventory of a student's ability to apply the skills necessary to meet with success in school settings and for eventual success in employment settings. It was standardized with a national sample of 2280 students, in grades K-12. Raw scores are converted to T-scores, percentile ranks, and descriptive Social Function Levels.
Social Communication Questionnaire (SCQ)[134]	Brief questionnaire used to evaluate communication skills and social functioning in children older than 4 years who may have autism or autism spectrum disorder (ASD). It is completed by a parent or other primary caregiver in less than 10 minutes. Current and lifetime versions are available.
Social Responsiveness Scale, 2nd edition (SRS-2)[48]	65-item questionnaire that inquires about a child's ability to engage in emotionally appropriate reciprocal social interactions through interpersonal skills and communication. It can be used as a screener or as an aid to diagnose ASD. It uses a quantitative scale to determine where a child falls within the range of social behaviors that are addressed and occur in the population as a whole. The SRS divides these behaviors into five subscales to be used for treatment planning and evaluation of program effectiveness; these include social awareness, social cognition, social communication, social motivation, and autistic mannerisms. A singular T-score is then generated and determines the severity of social deficits.
Social Skills Improvement System (SSIS)[69]	The SSIS provides a broad, multirater standardized assessment of social skills and problem behaviors of students from preschool through high school. Students are rated in areas of how often behaviors occur and how important each behavior is to the respondent. Forms consist of three-point, Likert-type scales reported by the teacher, student, and/or parent. Separate forms are used for preschool, elementary, and secondary levels of school.
Triad Social Skills Assessment, 2nd edition[148]	Designed for children ages 6 to 12 years who have basic reading skills at the first-grade level. It is criterion-based and assesses knowledge and skills in three areas: cognitive, behavioral, and affective. Sources of information are (1) parent report, (2) teacher report, (3) observation, and (4) direct child interaction.

Goal: Take turns in conversation. **Baseline:** Rachel will answer questions that are asked to her with very short answers but no explanations, and will not ask a question or make a statement to continue a conversation with peers.				
Much less than expected outcome	**Less than expected outcome**	**Expected outcome**	**More than expected outcome**	**Much more than expected outcome**
−2	−1	0	+1	+2
Rachel will answer one question asked during an exchange with a peer with an explanation that is more than a few words long.	Rachel will answer two or more questions asked during an exchange with a peer with an explanation that is more than a few words long.	Rachel will ask one question to continue a conversation after being asked a question by a peer.	Rachel will ask two or more questions to continue a conversation after being asked a question by a peer.	Rachel will ask a question to start a conversation with a peer.
Goal: Stress modulation/calm self. **Baseline:** Seth frequently (more than once per day) becomes overwhelmed with situations that occur in school that cause him to have a behavioral meltdown, which is very disruptive and interferes with his social interactions with peers.				
−2	−1	0	+1	+2
Seth will identify his stress level appropriately and apply a modulating tool that has been suggested to him on one occasion during therapy when he is already calm.	Seth will identify his stress level appropriately and apply a modulating tool that has been suggested to him during therapy which calms him on one occasion when he is beginning to feel stressed.	Seth will identify his stress level appropriately and apply one modulating tool during therapy which calms him without being told on one occasion when he is beginning to feel stressed.	Seth will identify his stress level appropriately and apply one modulating tool outside therapy which calms him without being told on one occasion when he is beginning to feel stressed.	Seth will identify his stress level appropriately and apply one modulating tool outside therapy which calms him without being told on two occasions in one day when he is beginning to feel stressed.

FIGURE 11-1 Goal attainment scale examples.

TABLE 11-3 Theoretical Approaches and Models Supporting Social Skills Groups

Intervention Approach or Model	Principles	Strategies
Peer-mediated	Typically developing children are partnered with children who have disabilities to affect behavioral changes in the children with disabilities.	During therapy sessions or social skills groups, a same-age or slightly older peer is included in the session to provide role modeling and help facilitate socially appropriate behaviors in the child who has social impairment.
Sensory integration	Children may need to learn more effective habits for modulating their sensory processing needs in a safe, acceptable manner in social situations through sensory integration.	Activities might include hanging on a trapeze bar upside down and swinging back and forth, jumping into a ball pit, or pulling themselves up a ramp on a scooter board.
Self-determination	This involves satisfaction of the needs for autonomy, competence and relatedness promote well-being.	Children make choices, indicate preferences, problem solve, plan, and initiate activities included in therapy and social skills group sessions.
Social-cognitive	Children learn by observing the behavior of others. Groups based on this theory include two phases, acquisition and performance.	Participant goals are addressed and worked on by the entire group during the didactic social skills segments of the groups. The leaders or other participants describe and demonstrate the social skills, followed by others performing the skill.
Behavioral interventions	Behavior is a response to an environmental stimulus and behavior is reinforced by environmental consequences that follow.	A reward system is used, such as a goal chart, to recognize and reward attempts to work on goals. Rewards are provided at the end of the session if the number of attempts to work on goals meets previously identified quotas.

Sensory Integration Intervention

The use of sensory integration in a social skills group adds an important aspect that is usually only included when groups are developed by occupational therapists (see Chapter 9). Ayres, an occupational therapist, has defined sensory integration as "the neurological process that organizes sensation from one's own body and from the environment and makes it possible to use the body effectively within the environment" (p. 11).[8] Children who have difficulty integrating the continuous stream of sensory input and responding appropriately may also have difficulty with self-esteem, self-actualization, socialization, and play.[32] Many children with ASD have atypical sensory processing that appears to contribute to their social impairment[76] and that can be misinterpreted as a social or behavioral problem.[105] These children may need to learn more effective habits for modulating their sensory processing needs in a safe, acceptable manner in social situations. They may also need to learn to integrate the needs of others with their own needs. For these reasons, principles of sensory modulation can be included in each session to enhance participants' ability to filter sensations, attend to those sensations that are relevant to the activity, and maintain and personally recognize optimal level of arousal throughout sessions.

In a small randomized controlled trial (RCT), children with sensory processing disorders who received sensory integration intervention made significant gains in goal attainment, attention, and cognitive-social skills.[104] In a more recent RCT of sensory integration intervention, Pfeiffer et al.[123] found improvements in autistic mannerisms and self-regulatory behaviors in children with ASD who received the intervention. This reduction was believed to be an indication of improved ability to process sensory stimuli in the environment without needing to resort to self-stimulatory behaviors. Fazlioglu and Baron[56] found a significant reduction in atypical sensory responses in a group of children with ASD after participating in a sensory integration intervention program in which many of the test items referenced social behaviors (e.g., can answer when his or her name is uttered, cannot give answers to simple questions asked, cannot use "yes" or "no" for a specific purpose). Schaaf et al.[137] examined changes in a child with ASD following sensory integration intervention. They found improved regulation and organization in responses to sensory input and improved communication. The parent report described a happier child with less rigid behaviors and increased tolerance of unexpected changes in routine, a decrease in his activity level, distractibility, and impulsivity, with better safety during play, improved play skills, and so much improvement in his attention in the classroom that he did not need an aide for his school work.

Therapists can implement the core elements of sensory integration intervention[120,121] to promote self-regulation at the start of each social skills session by providing participant-initiated sensory modulation activities (see Chapter 9).[123] Examples include hanging on a trapeze bar upside down and swinging back and forth, jumping into a ball pit, or pulling themselves up a ramp on a scooter board. Under the therapist's guidance, the children can build their own obstacle course that incorporates proprioceptive, tactile, and vestibular input. Following the activities to promote self-regulation, the children identify their levels of arousal before and after their chosen activities to help them better recognize their levels of arousal, better understand how to measure the impact of modulation, and determine the best modulating activities for them.[15] Additional discussion regarding identifying and meeting individual needs in a socially appropriate way, without external supports, can be discussed in subsequent groups (Figure 11-2). See Chapter 9 for more information on sensory integration.

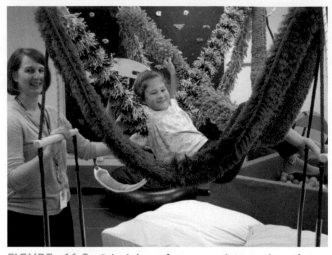

FIGURE 11-2 Principles of sensory integration theory can be included in each session to enhance participants' ability to filter sensations, attend to those sensations that are relevant to the activity, and maintain and personally recognize their optimal levels of arousal throughout sessions. (Photo by Washington University Program in Occupational Therapy.)

Self-Determination

The self-determination theory, from the field of psychology, states that satisfaction of the needs for autonomy, competence, and relatedness promotes well-being.[135] Autonomy refers to having a sense of choice, initiative, and endorsement of one's activities. Competency represents a sense of mastery over one's capacity to act in the environment. Relatedness denotes feelings of closeness and connectedness to significant others. "As young children make choices, indicate preferences, problem solve, plan and initiate, they are making sense of the world around them in a way that can ultimately produce feelings of competence, confidence, and empowerment."[55]

By encouraging children to make their own choices in social skills sessions, therapists support self-determination. As children progress along the continuum, activities become increasingly meaningful, intrinsically motivating, and more satisfying. Participants are involved in the initial selection of social skills goals and identification of focus goal(s) for each session. They take part in brainstorming a name for the group, identifying rules of behavior for the group, making choices about the content of group activities, choosing snacks, and choosing rewards for goal attainment. This model also supports competency in social situations by providing "just-right" challenges. Children apply newly developed social skills in small, less intimidating, peer context, with gradually decreasing external support from therapists. Individual growth and acquisition of skills during sessions is possible because of the connections and

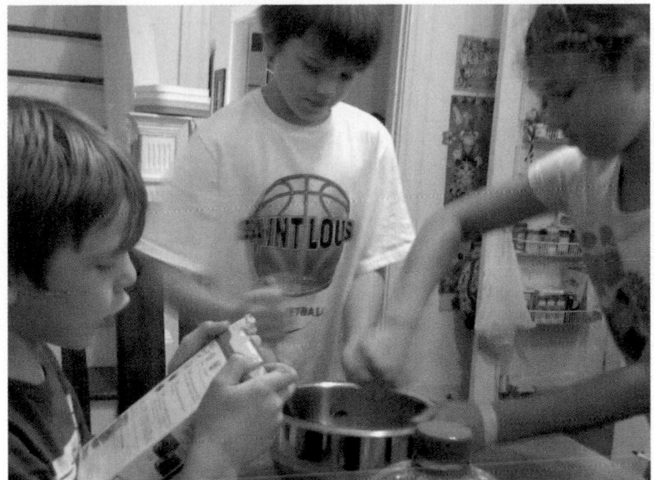
FIGURE 11-3 By encouraging the children to make their own choices in social skills sessions, activities become increasingly meaningful, intrinsically motivating, and more satisfying. (Photo by Claudia Hilton.)

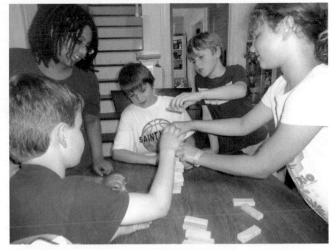
FIGURE 11-4 Children can learn by observing the behavior of others. (Photo by Cheryl Klohr.)

friendships made while relating to other group members (Figure 11-3).

Social Cognitive

This psychological theory, proposed by Bandura,[9-11] is a typical model for social skills groups. This theory supports the idea that children learn by observing the behavior of others. Groups based on this theory include two phases, acquisition and performance. During acquisition, a child observes the behavior of others and its consequences. The child remembers this observation for later use. During the performance phase, the child performs the behavior based on his or her perception of the situation and its consequences.

Participants' goals are addressed and worked on by the entire group during the didactic social skills segments of the groups. The leaders describe and demonstrate the proper social skills, followed by the group members performing the skills. Social interactions can provide opportunities for a child to serve as a role model for others while simultaneously acquiring new behaviors or attitudes through the imitation of others (Figure 11-4).[43,72]

Behavioral Interventions

Founded by psychologist B. F. Skinner,[143,144] behaviorism builds on the theory that all behavior is a response to an environmental stimulus and that behavior is reinforced by environmental consequences that follow. Behavioral interventions use techniques of altering an individual's reaction to stimuli through positive reinforcement and the extinction of maladaptive behavior. A measurable system of reinforcement is established to focus specifically on behavior. The system encourages using positive reinforcement only, thus lessening the emphasis on negative behavior, and is another model commonly used to promote the development of many skills of children with disabilities.

Once social skills goals are established for participants in the group, a chart may be used as a visual reminder. This chart also serves as a record to reward daily efforts toward goal attainment (Figure 11-5). One goal is identified as the most important goal for that session and is indicated on the chart with an arrow. The most important goal changes as one is achieved or if another becomes more important. Each time the child works on any goal, he or she receives a star in the box for that goal. Participants can be encouraged to note or comment on each other's positive behaviors to further facilitate socialization. At the end of each session, each child who earns a specified number of stars for his or her most important goal and at least one star for each of the other goals can then be allowed to choose a small prize (usually a small toy or treat) from the prize bowl, which has already been identified as a good prize by the child so that the reward is readily sought by the child.

Interventions for Social Skills

The ultimate goal for social skills interventions is to participate in group and social situations appropriately. Some children with ASD do not have adequate interest or behavior to interact with others successfully. In this case, social skills can be introduced individually with the therapist. The following activities are appropriate for children who are at least 4 years old, are higher functioning, and who demonstrate some interest in social interaction. According to the child's progress, the child can be introduced to dyads (groups of two children) and then later to social skills groups (Figure 11-6).

Social Interventions

Although the purpose of social interventions is to improve social skills, these interventions can be part of individual or group interventions. The following activities can be introduced to children on an individual basis to prepare or participate in social skills groups.

Promoting Specific Social Behaviors and Adherence to Social Rules

Practitioners can provide social skills training in groups or individually. Most strategies to promote social skills can be used

Name	Goals	Session #1	Session #2	Session #3	Session #4	Session #5
Joshua	1. Identify stress thermometer level and choose tool to adjust	☆☆	☆☆	☆☆	☆☆☆	☆☆
	2. Use appropriate voice volume	☆	☆☆☆	☆☆	☆☆☆	☆☆
	3. Stay with group	☆☆☆	☆☆☆☆	☆☆☆☆	☆☆☆☆☆	☆☆☆☆☆
	4. Follow directions after the 1st request from an adult	☆☆☆☆	☆☆☆	☆☆☆	☆☆☆	☆☆☆☆☆
	5. Attend politely to activity	☆☆☆	☆☆☆☆☆	☆☆☆	☆☆☆	☆☆☆
Sarah	1. Identify stress thermometer level and choose tool to adjust	☆☆☆	☆☆☆☆	☆☆☆	☆☆	☆☆☆
	2.Think before you move, be safe	☆☆☆	☆☆☆	☆☆☆☆	☆☆☆☆☆	☆☆☆☆☆
	3. Use good friend behaviors	☆☆☆	☆☆☆☆	☆☆☆☆☆	☆☆☆☆☆	☆☆☆☆☆
	4. Be cool with things that are irritating	☆☆	☆☆☆	☆	☆☆☆	☆☆☆
	5. Ask for help when needed	☆☆☆☆	☆☆☆☆☆	☆☆☆	☆☆☆☆	☆☆☆
Eli	1. Identify stress thermometer level and choose tool to adjust	☆☆☆	☆☆	☆☆	☆☆☆	☆☆☆☆
	2. Think before you move, be safe	☆☆☆☆☆	☆☆☆☆☆	☆☆☆	☆☆☆	☆☆☆☆
	3. Take turns in conversations	☆☆☆	☆☆☆	☆☆☆☆☆	☆☆☆☆☆	☆☆☆☆☆
	4. Start a conversation to join the group	☆☆	☆☆	☆	☆☆☆☆	☆☆☆☆☆
	5. Deal well with bullying.	☆☆☆	☆☆☆	☆☆☆	☆☆	☆

FIGURE 11-5 Goal chart.

one-on-one or in groups. The strategies in this section, however, were designed for individual use. These interventions were developed for children with ASD; however, they can be effectively used to promote social participation in children with a range of mental health and behavioral disorders.

Video Modeling

The original concept of teaching children to model the behavior of their peers was termed *observational learning* or *modeling*.[9] Video modeling and video self-modeling evolved as technology became more available. Video modeling involves an individual watching a video demonstration of a certain behavior and then imitating the behavior of the model.[21] Video self-modeling is used to allow children to observe and model from their own behavior.[77] The use of these interventions for children with ASD has been extensively examined and found to be effective for improving social communication skills, functional skills, and behavioral functioning.[20] Video modeling promotes skill acquisition; skills are maintained over time and transferred across persons and settings.

The therapist and child identify social or behavioral areas that are difficult for the child to perform (e.g., greetings, introductions, offering help, asking for help, transitions, play skills) and then prepare a script in which the child successfully performs that particular social interaction. The child is videotaped while acting out the script with another individual. The child and therapist view the video and identify how the child acted and the effect of the behavior on the other person. The videotape can be sent home with the child for repeat viewing, if possible. The amount of script preparation completed by the child can be graded, depending on how much the child can

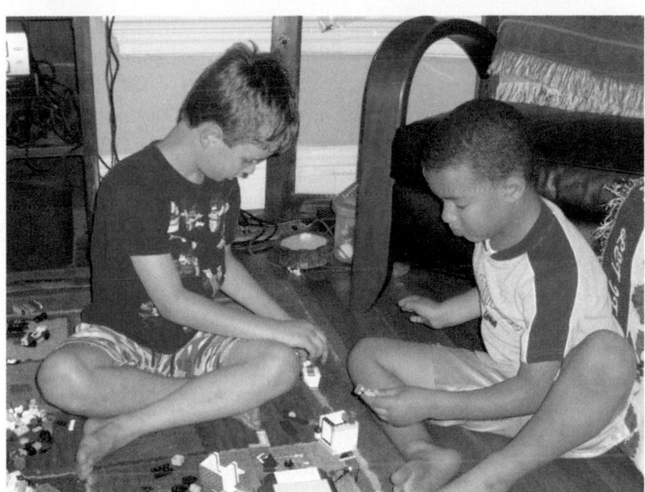

FIGURE 11-6 Some children who may not be ready for social skills groups can benefit from the less threatening structure of a dyad. (Photo by Cheryl Klohr.)

do. This strategy can be used for other social and behavioral areas in which the child has difficulty.

Video self-modeling has been used effectively for treating many conditions, including depression,[81] stuttering,[27] elective mutism,[124] attention disorders,[53,169] behavior disorders,[94] and aggressive behaviors.[101] It is effective for children diagnosed with ASD for improving communication skills,[40,41,141] behavior during transition,[139] and play skills.[30,52,115,154]

Social Scripts

Many human social events have expected sequences of interactions that involve specific verbal routines, termed *social scripts*.[57] Persons with ASD often struggle with these scripts because of their lack of social awareness.[158] Social scripts or scripting can be used in an intervention so that children can practice what to do in those social situations that they find awkward.[60] The therapist helps the child think of an awkward or challenging social situation, such as introducing self, giving help, asking for help, and giving or receiving a compliment. The therapist works with the child to identify a script appropriate for that type of situation. The script is written so that the child can practice it. The child can be paired up with another child to practice the script, simulating a situation in which the script can be used. Then the child practices the script in a real situation. As the child remembers and uses the script consistently, the therapist fades out use of the visual prompt. The child can keep a notebook to record useful scripts to refer to as needed. During intervention, various situations can be presented to the child, who is encouraged to develop a new and appropriate script for each situation. Social scripts can be used for video self-modeling.

Studies examining the effectiveness of social scripts have shown decreased perseverative speech in children with ASD,[61] improved initiation of conversations in children with ASD and Down syndrome,[89,97] and increased length of time spent in conversation in children with ASD.[83] A major limitation of this intervention approach is that the child may become dependent on the script and be unable to engage in spontaneous, unscripted interactions. Script fading has been developed to address this problem.[89]

Power Cards

Power cards recognize a child's special interests or heroes and are used to help facilitate appropriate behaviors in social situations and routines.[59] To implement this strategy, the therapist identifies a social situation or behavior that the child needs to handle better. He or she finds a picture of a favorite hero of the child and adheres to a card. The therapist writes a scenario of the hero advocating the correct behavior (e.g., SpongeBob talking about the appropriate way to act during circle time in the classroom). The desired behavior is divided into steps and written on the card with the picture of the hero (e.g., walk quietly to your carpet square, sit down without touching your classmates, listen to the teacher, sit quietly while the teacher is talking, sing the good morning song with the class). The therapist and child practice acting out the scene, using the information on the card as prompts for appropriate behavior. The therapist can laminate the card so that the child can keep it with him or her to help as a reminder on how to handle the situation. The card can be posted at the location where the behavior is most appropriate, such as posting a hand washing card near the sink.

Because many children with ASD have special interests or heroes and are strong rule followers[159] and because they process visual information better than auditory information,[126] this strategy is effective for many children with ASD. It can also be used for a larger group (e.g., classroom, entire school) to support preferred behaviors, such as walking quietly in the hall, washing hands after using the bathroom, antibullying behaviors, and increasing attendance by using popular characters from movies or television shows. Power cards have been used successfully to increase good sportsmanship behavior in a child with autism[85] and improve disruptive and noncompliant behaviors of children with autism in the classroom setting.[111]

Social Stories

Social stories were developed to teach social skills to children with ASD.[68] One social skill or issue is addressed in each story. This method helps children who take things literally to understand concepts, overcome fears or preoccupations, establish healthy routines, and develop new social skills. The stories consist of four types of sentences[109] that prepare the children for what they can expect to feel and what they should do in certain situations that are difficult for them. The types of sentences are as follows:

1. *Descriptive sentences* explain what occurs and why, who is involved, and provide background for the story. Example: "Kids often need to go to the bathroom at school or public places and so do I."
2. *Directive sentences* provide direction to the child and instruct on how to do something or how to respond. They frequently use the words "I can" or "I will" and never use negative words, such as "I will not." Example: "I can go to the bathroom without flushing all the toilets."
3. *Perspective sentences* describe the reactions of other people and their feelings. Example: "It bothers other people when someone flushes all the toilets in the bathroom."
4. *Control or affirmative sentences* are sometimes written by the student to help him or her recall information. Example: "I will only flush my toilet one time when I go to the bathroom in the school or in a public place."

The story should be kept brief and written in the first person, and visual aids, such as photos and diagrams, can be helpful. Stories can be bound in a small binder so that the child can carry them.

Social stories have been shown to be effective for decreasing inappropriate behaviors and increasing appropriate behaviors in children with various diagnoses. Examples of social stories outcomes for children and youth with ASD include improving mealtime skill,[25] decreasing disruptive behaviors,[118] increasing prosocial behavior,[51] teaching sex education,[153] and increasing game play skills.[127] Other positive effects for social stories include increasing physical activity of developmentally disabled students when used in combination with visual schedules[172] and improving appropriate interpersonal conflict resolution strategies in children with learning disabilities.[82] Box 11-2 on the Evolve website lists websites for social stories.

Applied Behavior Analysis

Applied behavior analysis (ABA) is a didactic approach to help children perform socially significant behaviors through a reinforcement training technique.[155] ABA supervisors are usually licensed clinical psychologists, with training and certification in applied behavior analysis. They often supervise others, including paraprofessionals, who require specialized training. Occupational therapy students are often among those who are ABA providers. Occupational therapists may work in collaboration with the ABA providers.

ABA intervention for children with ASD is often intensive—that is, up to 40 hours per week. ABA is considered a successful behavioral intervention, yielding substantial gains in intelligence quotient, language, academic performance, and adaptive behavior, with significantly better social behavior.[155] ABA currently has many different forms.

Discrete trial training (DTT), from Lovaas' Young Autism Project,[96] is now the most widely recognized form of ABA. DTT works on developing learning readiness by teaching fundamental skills such as attention, compliance, imitation, and discrimination learning as small, individually acquired tasks.[110] It consists of one-on-one instruction to teach skills in a planned, controlled, and systematic manner in small repeated steps. Each trial or teaching session is discrete, having a definite beginning and end. Within DTT, the use of antecedents (prompts) and consequences is carefully planned and implemented. Praise and/or rewards are used to reinforce desired skills or behaviors. Data are collected about beginning skill level, progress and challenges, skill acquisition and maintenance, and generalization of learned skills or behaviors used to support decision making.

ABA, in its various forms, is conducted entirely in a structured teaching environment and has been questioned for its applicability in natural situations. To address these concerns, traditional ABA techniques have been modified in recent years for use in more natural situations.[138] Traditional ABA has long been recognized as the educational treatment of choice for young children with autism, but it is less clear whether this treatment paradigm is the optimal approach for less severely affected, higher functioning individuals.[155]

Privacy Circles

Privacy circles are used to help children identify which topics or activities are appropriate to discuss or to do with different people and in various settings.[130] Privacy circles address the lack of social awareness,[158] mindblindness,[16] and poor knowledge regarding privacy issues.[147] The therapist gives the child a template with eight to ten concentric circles (like a target). The child or therapist puts the child's name in the middle. The child lists people that he or she might interact with regularly, such as mom, dad, brothers, sisters, teacher, friends, neighbors, and people at the grocery store. The therapist helps the child categorize the people in intimacy levels from most intimate to least intimate. These people are then placed in the circles, with the most intimate toward the middle and the least intimate toward the outside. The therapist then gives the child examples of conversation topics or activities that range in levels of intimacy (a concern about a private part of his or her body, new shoes that light up when she or he walks). The therapist then has the child identify in which circle the conversation or activity fits. Redirection may be necessary, and discussion is part of the process. As situations come up, new topics and activities can be added to the privacy circles to help the child understand the contexts of their appropriateness (Case Study 11-1).

Enhancing Social Awareness and Relationships with Others

Mind Reading

Theory of mind explains the social dysfunction in children with ASD, in which the person is blind to the existence of thoughts, beliefs, knowledge, desires, and intentions that contribute to why people do what they do.[16] Mind reading helps children with ASD improve in and increase their theory of mind.

The first level of this strategy uses drawings and photos of faces to determine what a person might be feeling.[78] Drawings and photographs of facial expressions can be used to help

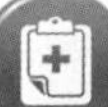

CASE STUDY 11-1 Cedric

Cedric is a 7-year-old with FASD. He has noticed recently that offering details about his father's anatomy brings much attention from other children in his class, which he is constantly seeking. His teacher knows that his parents would be mortified to learn that he was sharing such intimate information about his father and would like to help Cedric be better able to judge what is appropriate to share with whom. The occupational therapist suggested that they might try using privacy circles to help Cedric understand what is appropriate and what is not appropriate. They also discussed the issue with his mother, who was very supportive of the plan. Cedric worked on his privacy circles, kept a copy at his desk, and took a copy home with him. The teacher told him that if he could follow his privacy circle rules each day, he could help her pass out homework papers to the class at the end of each day. He liked the attention that he got from the class and how important he felt for passing out the homework papers. After a few reminders, he was able to follow his privacy circles without needing more reminders.

children identify the emotions expressed in them. Children can make charts of emotions by cutting out photographs of people expressing different emotions and placing them on the chart for each emotion. To make the activity easier, participants can choose from a small list of emotions. Beyond recognizing facial expression of emotions, mind reading can include understanding expectations of emotional responses based on intent (e.g., statement about what Jimmy wanted, statement about what his mother gave him, and question of how he feels about it) and understanding why someone might have a different perspective from the child (e.g., removing the candy from a candy box, replacing it with crayons, and asking a child who did not witness the switch what is in the box).

Measurement tools have been identified for mind-reading competence,[157] and encouraging results were seen in a study of three boys with ASD.[19] Various adaptations of this strategy have also been developed. Interactive computer software has been developed for mind reading to teach individuals to recognize emotions through the use of video clips, photographs, voice recordings, lessons, and games involving individuals displaying a range of emotions.[65,93,142] One study found marked improvement in recognizing emotions in pictures and voices presented similarly in the computer program but showed little improvement when subjects were presented with photographs of the individual's eyes or with film clips.[93] Other studies found improvement beyond the specific areas addressed by the program, including the use of emotion recognition cartoons, understanding strange stories,[142] and face and voice emotion recognition.[93]

Emotions Charades

Emotions charades adds a real-life and present aspect to mind reading. It uses role-playing situations that involve expressions of emotions. Other people guess which emotion is being expressed.[100] The activity can be structured in several ways, depending on the ability levels of the children. The therapist may act out a short situation in which he or she uses facial expressions and body language to express an emotion and then have the children guess the emotion. Students can pair up and select a short scenario in which one person must express one emotion and the other expresses another emotion. The pair then acts out the scene, and others guess which emotions they are expressing. This activity can be graded by changing the complexity, adding or subtracting the number of emotions included, and posting a list of emotions to which the participants can refer as they try to decipher the charade. See Figure 11-7 for a list of emotions that can be acted out through this strategy.

Afraid	Bored
Anxious/Worried	Disgusted
Cautious	Embarrassed
Frightened	Guilty
Terrified	Hopeful
Uncertain	Indifferent
Angry	Innocent
Enraged	Jealous/Envious
Exasperated	Self-conscious
Frustrated	Shocked
Irritated	Shy
Confident	Arrogant
Courageous	Depressed
Optimistic	Disappointed
Confused	Grieving
Curious	Hurt
Interested	Lonely
Amused	Sorry
Ecstatic	Sad
Enthusiastic	Satisfied
Excited	Relieved
Happy	Silly
Proud	

FIGURE 11-7 Suggested emotions for emotions charades.

Video Detective

This strategy adds another dimension to mind reading. It consists of watching video clips to help children increase their skills of interpreting nonverbal communication.[100,112] The therapist first explains concepts of body language and verbal and nonverbal communication. Then a video segment is played, with the volume muted. Children are asked which emotions certain actors appeared to be expressing through their nonverbal behaviors in the video. Each child has a turn to respond and provide explanations for his or her answers. The scene is played again with the volume on, and the children examine their previous answers to see if they still agree. The group discusses the nonverbal behaviors that were helpful, those that they found confusing, and which actors seemed to do the best at nonverbal communication. To make this activity easier, the therapist can give the children choices of which emotions are being expressed, choose clips that have very expressive nonverbalactions (such as silent movies), or choose clips with only a few actors.

Social Autopsies

Social autopsies were originally developed for children with an LD.[95] They can also be effective for children with ASD and FASD because they can address incidents related to theory of mind[16] and provide a nonthreatening way to examine retroactively how the child handled a difficult situation. They also use problem-solving strategies that are useful for children with ADHD, LD, anxiety, and mood disorders. After the situation occurs, the child is asked to describe the event and the possible motivations of others who were involved. The therapist engages the child in a discussion of alternative responses that could have been used. The therapist and child discuss good and poor responses to situations. Using videotapes that demonstrate the behavior and resulting consequences can increase understanding and motivation for the child.

Enhancing Executive Function

Self-Management

Self-management strategies have demonstrated considerable effectiveness for changing behavior in children with behavior disorders,[36] developing academic skills in children with learning disabilities,[74] increasing social interactions in children with ASD,[87,140,150] and decreasing off-task behaviors in children with ASD.[50] Learners are taught to discriminate between appropriate and inappropriate behaviors, monitor and record their own behaviors accurately, and reward themselves for behaving appropriately.[114] Teaching a child to monitor and manage his or her own behavior gradually increases independence and supports generalization of the skills. Self-management can be directed at skills prerequisite to social skills, such as self-regulation. Several types of interventions could be included under the umbrella of self-management. Examples include use of video modeling, checklists, goal charts, stress thermometers, five-point scales, wrist counting devices, and role playing. They might be used by occupational therapists for intervention with children with ASD, FASD, ADHD, anxiety, LD, and mood disorders.

Comic Strip Conversations

Comic strip conversations are similar to social autopsies, but use comic strip drawings to illustrate a social interaction.[67] They are designed to promote theory of mind and improve social interactions in children by facilitating joint attention and understanding intention. The situation is drawn as a comic strip at a calm time, after a difficult situation occurs (Case Study 11-2). The drawing includes the thought bubbles of the various participants' perspectives and intentions. This gives the child practice in attempting to understand the perspectives and intentions of others. For situations that did not go well, the comic strip can be redrawn to show a more ideal interaction and outcome, which instructs and models better social behavior choices for the child.

A limited number of small studies have examined the effectiveness of comic strip conversations. This strategy was found to be effective in increasing social satisfaction and decreasing loneliness in three children with ASD and, when used in combination with social stories, was effective in reducing inappropriate social behaviors of two individuals with ASD.[80]

Stress Thermometer

Scales and thermometers can help children recognize, quantify, and describe different levels of their emotions and behaviors. The scales or thermometers can be introduced to a group of children or an individual child. They can address group behaviors, such as voice volume or stress level, or individual behaviors, such as obsessions or compulsions.

For the anger or stress thermometer, the therapist gives the child a template for a thermometer with graded levels of anger or stress[23] (Figure 11-9). It may include four to ten levels, depending on the understanding of the child. The therapist can list the emotions for the child (e.g., calm, irritated, furious, enraged), and the child can look for pictures of faces in a magazine to match those emotions. The child may code the thermometer with colors, according to the emotion. The child may also use special interests as themes for the thermometer, such as weather (with *hurricanes* at the top level and *calm and breezy* at the bottom) or dinosaurs (with *Tyrannosaurus rex* at the top and *pterodactyl* at the bottom). Children who are not yet proficient at writing can use pictures for the levels. The therapist and child can then determine where the child's level of anger fits on the anger thermometer during a specific situation.

Initial teaching of this technique should be done at a quiet time after an angry event. The therapist asks the child to recall a time when he or she felt like a *tornado* or felt *calm and breezy* and the levels in between (see Figure 11-9 for an example). The therapist and child can also role play and re-enact original words, tone of voice, and actual level of anger to understand the system better. The thermometer can be used to help the child become better aware of his or her responses, regulate responses, and keep track of responses to various situations or interventions (see Figure 11-9).

Incredible Five-Point Scale

The Incredible Five-Point Scale[33] organizes behaviors, such as voice volume, friendly behaviors, and feeling angry or afraid, along a five-point continuum (Figure 11-10). The scales can be used to help children better understand the social impact of their behaviors, regulate their responses, and calm themselves when they overrespond. Like the thermometers, the scales should be introduced at a quiet and calm time after an event in which the child had difficulty with regulation. The scale can be used to quantify the behavior and give the child a way to communicate about the behavior in a quantifiable way. For example, if a child has difficulty with being too loud, a voice volume scale can be used to help the child understand the need to modulate the volume of his or her voice. The therapist can have the child demonstrate the different levels on the scale. Then the scale is shared with others who interact with the child, including parent and teacher. They can then give feedback about the volume level when it is not appropriate for the situation. See Case Study 11-3.

Relationship Development Intervention

Relationship Development Intervention (RDI) is a parent-based, cognitive-developmental approach in which primary caregivers of children, adolescents, and young adults with ASDs and similar developmental disorders are trained to function as facilitators for their children's mental development to provide daily opportunities for successful functioning in increasingly challenging dynamic systems.[70] RDI is designed to teach parents to play an important role in improving critical emotional, social, and metacognitive abilities through carefully graduated, guided interaction. The therapist works with the child and teaches and guides the parent to provide effective social cues to facilitate the child's attention and responsiveness.

One study that examined the progress of 16 children with ASD who participated in RDI over a 5-year period found important changes in the Autism Diagnostic Observation Schedule (ADOS) and Autism Diagnostic Interview-Revised (ADI-R) scores, along with measures of flexibility and school placement.[71] At baseline, all of the children met ADOS and ADI-R criteria for autism prior to treatment, but no child met these criteria at follow-up. Similar positive results were found in relation to flexibility and educational placement. Studies examining the effectiveness of this intensive parent-based intervention are limited but indicate its potential value in addressing social skill deficits in children. Occupational therapists may find that using this approach in collaboration with parents may enhance their ability to support development of social skills in their young clients.

Alert Program: How Does Your Engine Run?

Children often experience stress in response to events that occur in their lives. For certain children, stress may be related to sensory responsiveness. Sensory over-responsiveness and under-responsiveness are common problems for many children with ASD, which can interfere in social participation when not well managed.[2,12,22,76,160]

The Alert Program[167] is a systematic intervention designed to help children who have difficulty staying on task or who become upset because of certain types of sensory input. The aims of the program are to help children with the following:

CASE STUDY 11-2 Stephanie

Stephanie, an 11-year-old girl with ASD, has difficulty understanding slang and expressions that are not meant to be taken literally, a common problem in children with ASD. Wendell, a boy in her class, greeted her with "Hey, Baby!" and she became upset because she thought that he thought she was a baby. She told her occupational therapist about the incident and they made a comic strip conversation of the event. After discussion with the therapist, she realized that the slang term "Baby" was actually meant to be a friendly and endearing expression. They rewrote the comic strip to show how she could handle the situation next time. See Figure 11-8 for this example of using comic strip conversations to improve social interactions.

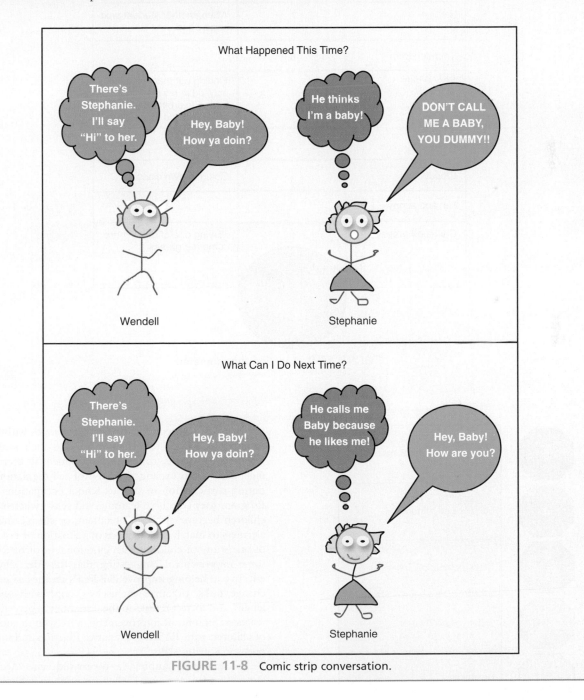

FIGURE 11-8 Comic strip conversation.

Level of Stress Condition	Level Number	When I Feel That Way
Hurricane	10	Missing recess because I argued with the teacher
Tornado	9	
Lightning	8	
Hail	7	When another student said I was weird
Thunderstorm	6	
Very Windy	5	Finding out that I was the only kid in my class not invited to a birthday party of another kid in the class
Rainy	4	
Cloudy	3	Going to gym class
Hot and sunny	2	
Calm and breezy	1	Playing one of my favorite computer games

FIGURE 11-9 Labeling thermometer.

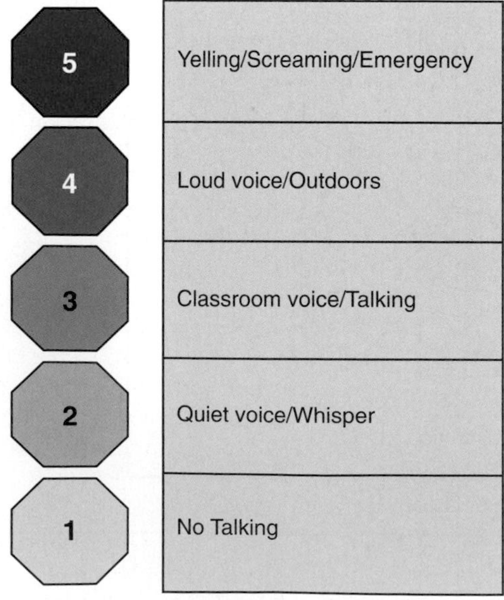

FIGURE 11-10 Voice volume scale.

(1) To learn to recognize their arousal states within the environment as related to behavior, such as their sensitivity and reactions to sounds, touch, and movement in their surroundings; and (2) to expand their use of self-regulation strategies during participation in various school occupations. The Alert Program uses cognitive learning and sensory activities to help children become aware of, maintain, or change their levels of alertness to match the demands of a situation or task.[167] Results of one study of children with emotional disturbance[15] showed some improvement, suggesting that the Alert Program was effective in helping improve children's abilities to self-regulate, change tasks, organize themselves, cope with sensory challenges, and focus on tasks in the classroom as perceived by their teachers. Significant improvements were seen in another group of children with FASD in executive function and interpersonal problem-solving skills.[163]

For example, Aubrey, a 6-year-old with ASD, became stressed and overaroused when he went to school assemblies that were held in the gymnasium at his school. The high noise level and the proximity of all the children often caused him to feel overstimulated, resulting in disruptive behaviors. His occupational therapist worked with him using the Alert Program[167] to identify his arousal level and find activities that would help

CASE STUDY 11-3 Darrius

Darrius is an 8-year-old boy with FASD. He has been having difficulty with touching and being affectionate to others in inappropriate ways, such as kissing and hugging his classmates, and people he does not know very well, such as store clerks or friends of his parents whom he has just met. His teacher was very concerned about this, so she collaborated with the occupational therapist and his mother to come up with a five-point scale addressing this behavior (Figure 11-11). They explained to Darrius that each number on the scale referred to touching others, and each number had a special type of person whom it was okay to touch in that way. They also added a reward system to help encourage him to follow the scale, in which he would have 15 minutes of computer time at the end of the day if he could follow the scale or if he would quickly respond when reminded that he was not following the scale. After 2 weeks using the scale, Darrius was able to follow it without reminders and, after a month, no longer needed to use the scale.

5	Kiss	Family
4	Hug	Family and close friends when you say hello or goodbye after a long time
3	Patting back, Touching arm	Classmates, family, and close friends
2	Shake hands	Anyone when you first meet them or say hello or goodbye after a long time
1	No touching	Anyone

FIGURE 11-11 Who can I touch scale.

to reduce it. He began doing the calming activities before the large school assemblies. He also learned how to detect when his arousal level was getting high and he needed a calming strategy. Aubrey learned how to calm himself enough to be able to tolerate attending the assemblies for longer and longer periods. He was also able to give his teacher a sign that he was becoming overstimulated so that she could remove him from the assembly to a quiet area to calm himself.

Problem Solving

Coaching

Coaching is defined as an interactive process that promotes the care provider's ability to support a child's participation in everyday experiences and interactions across settings by developing new skills, refining existing abilities, and gaining a deeper understanding of their actions.[131] It can also be used directly with children to empower them to organize and execute their responsibilities in an academic setting and in everyday life. Coaching uses questions that elicit reflective thinking and prompt students' ability to plan and carry out their goals. Coaches view the students as creative and resourceful; their role is to help students learn how to take action to accomplish goals that are important to them.[165] Coaching has been used successfully with college-age individuals with ADHD to create structure and execute change by identifying strategies that circumvent their deficits in executive functioning.[152] In another study of coaching college students with ADHD, improvements were seen in motivation, time management, anxiety, test preparation, and self-efficacy.[173]

For example, Jasmine, a 14-year-old with LD, was having difficulty keeping friendships. Jasmine discussed with her occupational therapist the problem of her most recent best friend, Amanda, becoming less responsive to her invitations to participate in social activities. The therapist asked her questions about what happened just before she saw the change in Amanda, and Jasmine reported that she had become very upset and started screaming at Amanda and calling her names because Amanda was going with another friend to the mall when Jasmine invited her to go swimming at the public swimming pool. The therapist asked Jasmine how she might have felt if Amanda had responded the same way to her, and Jasmine stated that it would have made her angry. The therapist asked how she could better handle the situation that would not upset Amanda. Jasmine identified a plan to apologize to Amanda and, for the next time that Amanda has other plans, she will suggest another, later option rather than screaming at Amanda and calling her names.

SOCCSS

Another strategy addresses children's theory of mind limitations and social problem solving by assisting them in identifying problem situations, possible solutions, and possible consequences for each solution. It is known as SOCCSS (*s*ituation, *o*ptions, *c*onsequences, *c*hoices, *s*trategies, *s*imulation).[129] This strategy sequentially organizes social and behavioral concerns for students with social interaction challenges.[112,113] The procedure involves six steps; it is used after a difficult situation has occurred as a way of examining the options for the next time a similar situation comes up or, if possible, to interrupt and examine a current situation before the choice step is made.

1. *Situation*: The therapist and student identify a problem that has arisen. The problem is defined, and a goal is stated through discussion, writing, and drawing (e.g., "Tommy cuts in line in front of me at the drinking fountain. I don't want him to cut in front of me").
2. *Options*: The therapist and student brainstorm to identify possible solutions. The therapist does not evaluate the student's responses. Multiple solutions are encouraged.
3. *Consequences*: The therapist and student evaluate each of the student's responses by answering: "Will the solution get me what I want? Will I be able to do it?"

4. *Choices*: The student prioritizes the options and consequences and selects a solution. The solution selected is the one with the most advantageous consequences.
5. *Strategies*: The student originates a plan of action with guidance from the therapist.
6. *Simulation*: The strategy is practiced through role playing, writing it out, imagery, or talking with a peer.

This strategy can be simplified by offering a range of options for the child to choose from during each step of the process. Studies of the SOCCSS approach have revealed varying degrees of success when used to decrease tantrums, rage, and meltdowns related to misunderstanding social situations by two elementary age boys with Asperger syndrome.[113] See Case Study 11-4.

Description and Evidence for Specific Interventions in Social Skills Groups

Social skills groups have been used to improve social skills and participation in children. Studies have shown that social skills groups can be effective for improving peer relations,[168] improving theory of mind,[119] improving social skills,[91,125] improving greeting and play skills,[171] improving knowledge of social skills,[161] increasing empathy,[75] increasing social interaction,[37] and improving facial recognition.[145]

Most of the studies examining the effectiveness of social skills groups have been small and methodologically weak[164]; criticisms of these studies include inadequate measurement of

CASE STUDY 11-4 Sam

Sam is a 7-year-old with LD. He is not quite as tall as most of the other boys in his class. Sometimes Jeremy, a taller boy in his class, does things that are inconsiderate toward Sam, such as pushing in line in front of him. Sam's social skills group was talking about SOCCSS, and Sam told them of the incident with Jeremy butting in line in front of him at the drinking fountain. He said that he usually tried to hit Jeremy and then either got hurt or got in trouble. The group helped him to think of options, consequences, and his choice (Figure 11-12). They role played the situation with him so that he could practice his response. The next time that Jeremy pushed in front of him, he tried out his choice, and it worked. Jeremy listened to him and let him have his turn first.

SOCCSS **Situations, Options, Consequences, Choices, Strategies, Simulation**		
Situation Who: Jeremy and Sam What: Jeremy butted in line for the drinking fountain in front of Sam When: After recess Why: Sam was watching another classmate when it was his turn		
Options	**Consequences**	**Choice**
Shove or punch Jeremy	I could get in trouble	
	Jeremy could hit back harder	
Tell Jeremy that it is my turn and if he doesn't listen, tell the teacher	Jeremy might listen or the teacher could tell him not to butt in line	X (Sam's choice)
Don't do anything	Jeremy will probably butt again	
Call Jeremy a bad name	Jeremy could hit me or call me a name	
	I could get in trouble	
Strategy The next time Jeremy butts in line, Sam will tell him that it is his turn, not Jeremy's. If Jeremy does not listen, Sam will tell the teacher.		
Simulation Sam will role play this situation with a friend or classmate until he has the confidence to carry it out with Jeremy.		

FIGURE 11-12 Example of SOCCSS—Jeremy and Sam.

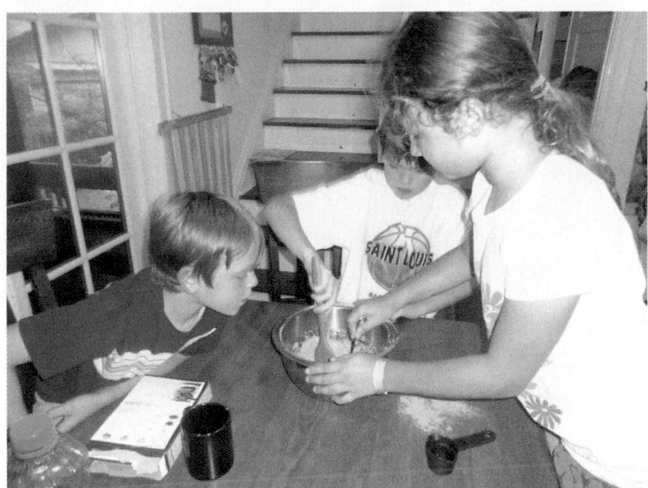

FIGURE 11-13 Social skills group activities allow children opportunities to practice their new skills in a structured environment, with immediate feedback. (Photo by Cheryl Klohr.)

social skills and deficits, small and poorly characterized samples, minimal examination of the degree to which learned skills generalize, inadequate dosage, lack of intervention fidelity, and lack of client-centeredness in matching a strategy to the individual needs of a child.[21] Occupational therapists often conduct social skills groups in collaboration with psychologists, social workers, speech language pathologists, and other professionals (Figure 11-13).

Process of Developing the Social Skills Group

Social skills groups can be developed to be included in a school-based program, outpatient clinic, or after-school program. School-based programs are usually more convenient for families and encourage friendships and continued support for the practice of social skills. The number of children who could potentially participate, availability of space and equipment, and willingness by the school administration to dedicate personnel and time to social skills programming are important considerations. It may be useful to conduct a focus group or discussion group with interested parents to determine the location, frequency, and schedule for potential participants.

When selecting children who could benefit from participating in the groups, the occupational therapist chooses participants who do not have aggressive behaviors that might be dangerous to others, have adequate language to interact with others, and have adequate motivation to interact with others. Children who do not fit these criteria can begin in individual sessions or dyads (with only one other child) until they meet the criteria for participation in a group. It is helpful to publicize the groups through parent communication networks, such as parent support groups, other autism service providers, and Internet parent discussion groups. Fees can be covered directly by families, insurance carriers, special autism funds in certain states, and grants. Funding may be available through the school district or Medicaid.

Social skills groups can be administered in school, after school, or during the summer. For optimal impact, the groups should be scheduled at least twice a week for 60 to 90 minutes over a 14-week session or daily for at least a 2-week session over the summer. Age groups can include children across a 3-year span, but longer age spans may be less effective because social issues change more significantly across a wider age span.

BOX 11-2 Key Elements of Social Skills Groups

- Parents, participants, and therapists should be involved in establishing goals.
- Consistent and predictable format—a visual schedule should be posted at each session.
- Rules for behavior for the group should be determined by the group and then posted.
- Parents should receive intensive training and home programming.
- Clients and parents should be provided with immediate feedback and "homework."

Key Characteristics

Certain important qualities are necessary for a successful social skills group. These include parent involvement, use of schedules, and use of activity themes (Box 11-2).

Parent Involvement

For maximum effectiveness, it is important that parents be very involved in the social skills group.[23] Parents should initially be oriented to the theoretical models, format of the sessions, and what they will be expected to do to support their child. Pretests can be completed using assessments that will be used to measure the effectiveness of the groups. Parents select the goals that they think are important to address by the social skills group. Each participant should also identify goals that he or she thinks are important. These goals are used to guide the therapist in finalizing a list of goals that are developmentally appropriate for the child. The parents are apprised of the activities and goals for each session. When the child returns to the next session, he or she can receive credit on the goal chart for attempts to address the goal at home or at school. Parents may document attempts. Some activity themes can culminate in a presentation that parents can observe, which is another way to include them in the groups.

Schedule

Because of the need for sameness and predictability in children with ASD[122] and because they process visual information better than auditory information,[126] each session should provide similar structural components, which are posted on a daily visual schedule. The schedule may include a sensory modulation segment to promote optimal arousal levels, didactic social skills segment, social skills application activity, and snack (Figure 11-14). Topics to promote development of social skills include the areas of social deficit, which include such items as friendship skills, self-control, conversation skills, understanding the feelings of others, taking turns, and dealing with bullies. Activities are graded to meet each child's needs and ensure success. The therapist tailors discussion topics to address individualized goals.

Social Group Themes and Activities

Activity themes add a playful aspect to the groups and can be helpful to guide the selection of activities. Themes can be identified ahead of time by the leaders or at the beginning of each month by the participants (for the longer groups). Depending on the age and gender mix of children in the group, themes might include grossology, let's build it, aviation, creepy bugs, the wild world, show time, chef school, transporters, make it grow, rock star, and shopping. See Table 11-4 for more details about what could be included for these themes.

The activity theme gives the participants good and enjoyable opportunities in which to practice their developing social skills. Attending a group that uses a child's special interest as a theme can be a strong motivator for participation (Figure 11-15).

Schedule of Activities	
15-20 minutes	Sensory modulation
20-30 minutes	Didactic social theme
20-30 minutes	Activity theme
15-20 minutes	Snack
15-20 minutes	Game
10-15 minutes	Review goals

FIGURE 11-14 Schedule of activities.

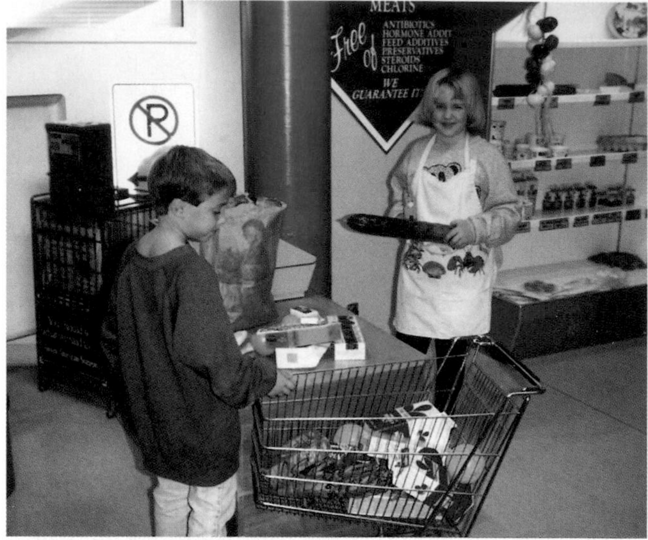

FIGURE 11-15 A shopping theme can give children an opportunity to role play social situations in the community. (Photo by Claudia Hilton.)

TABLE 11-4 Social Skills Group Themes

Theme	Topics That Might Be Covered
Grossology	Making goop, flubber, slime, silly putty, instant worms, or other sticky, gooey, gross materials (recipes can be found on the Internet). Making earthworms, pudding "cake" with chocolate cream-filled cookies (recipe can be found on the Internet) Identifying "body parts" by touch without being able to see them (spaghetti noodles = worms, dried apricot or pear = ear, candy corn = tooth, peeled grape = eyeball, cooked cauliflower = brains, extra dense jello = liver)
Let's build it	Select items that can be built; can start with individual projects and later construct a large group project
Aviation	This could include any aviation project, such as paper helicopters (patterns can be found on the Internet), parachutes made from plastic bags cut into squares and connected to small army men by strings from the corners, paper airplanes. The group can find a balcony or parking lot from which to drop them toward a target placed on the ground.
Creepy bugs	Activities that involve insects, such as making a collage of favorite insects cut from magazines, drawing insects, construction of insects, making no-bake cookies that look like insects, collecting insects
The wild world	This can include activities that involve animals, similar to the insect theme (above).
Showtime	This usually culminates in some type of show that can be presented to parents at the end of the theme segment and may involve acting out a short book or a singing or musical instrument presentation.
Chef school	This can involve any type of food preparation. Caution should be given to safety when using a stove or oven and to prepare items that will be ready by the end of the session. In addition, diet restrictions of the participants need to be considered, so using gluten-free flour or preparing items that do not include milk products, peanuts, or soy may be incorporated into the planning. Some creative and easy recipes are available on the Internet, such as candy sushi, Missouri mud, snack mix, fruit smoothies, pretzels, and tortilla snowflakes.
Transporters	Transportation theme that includes trucks, trains, or other favorite vehicles. It can involve drawing or constructing individual vehicles or making a group train or wall mural.
Make it grow	Any activity involving learning about or growing plants, such as growing sprouts, starting bean plants in pots, and planting plants in an outdoor space.
Rock star	Activities can include making easy percussion instruments, such as rain sticks, tambourines, drums, or chimes (patterns available on the Internet); identifying and making a collage of favorite musicians, performing a musical performance for parents at the end of the segment
Shopping	Activities revolve around various shopping experiences. Participants can make items to sell to each other, parents, and staff; set up a store to sell the items; or set up a simulated store to work on money exchange.

Summary

This chapter examines aspects of social skill impairment in children across several diagnostic categories. It examines theoretical bases of social impairment and theoretical models for intervention. It provides occupational therapists with several specific strategies and methods to use in intervention to address this important area of occupation in children. Evidence for various social participation interventions is included. It suggests that a combination of social, cognitive, behavioral, and sensory strategies can effectively increase social participation in children with mental health or behavioral disorders.

- Social participation problems are often seen in children who have ASD, FASD, ADHD, anxiety disorders, LDs, and mood disorders.
- Theories that explain social skill deficits in children include limited theory of mind, weak central coherence, delayed acquisition of joint attention, and limitations in executive function.
- Occupational therapists play primary roles in working with children who have social impairment and limited social participation. Social skills interventions can be conducted in collaboration with psychologists, social workers, speech language pathologists, and other professionals.
- Social skills interventions can improve specific social behaviors, understanding of social rules, awareness of others, and executive function.
- Theories and approaches used to inform social skills interventions in this chapter include peer-mediated intervention, sensory integration, self-determination, social cognitive, and behaviorism.
- Many principles and strategies that occupational therapists can use to improve social skills in children are addressed in this chapter.
- Evidence for the interventions ranges from no specific evidence to strong evidence.

REFERENCES

1. Achenbach, T. M., & Rescorla, L. A. (2001). *Manual for ASEBA School-Age Forms and Profiles.* Burlington, VT: University of Vermont, Research Center for Children, Youth, and Families.
2. Adamson, A., O'Hare, A., & Graham, C. (2006). Impairments in sensory modulation in children with autistic spectrum disorder. *British Journal of Occupational Therapy, 69*(8), 357–364.
3. Agaliotis, I., & Goudiras, D. (2004). A profile of interpersonal conflict resolution of children with learning disabilities. *Learning Disabilities: A Contemporary Journal, 2,* 15–29.
4. American Occupational Therapy Association. (2008). Occupational therapy practice framework: Domain and process. *American Journal of Occupational Therapy, 62,* 625–683.
5. American Psychiatric Association. (2013). *Diagnostic and statistical manual of mental disorders* (5th ed.). Washington, DC: American Psychiatric Association.
6. Argyle, M., & Crossland, J. (1987). The dimensions of positive emotions. *British Journal of Social Psychology, 26*(Pt. 2), 127–137.
7. Ashida, S. (2008). Differential associations of social support and social connectedness with structural features of social networks and the health status of older adults. *Journal of Aging and Health, 20,* 872–893.
8. Ayres, A. J. (1972). *Sensory integration and learning disorders.* Los Angeles: Western Psychological Services.
9. Bandura, A. (1977). *Social learning theory.* Englewood Cliffs, NJ: Prentice Hall.
10. Bandura, A. (1989). Human agency in social cognitive theory. *American Psychologist, 44,* 1175–1184.
11. Bandura, A. (1982). Self-efficacy mechanism in human agency. *American Psychologist, 37,* 122–147.
12. Baranek, G., Foster, L., & Berkson, G. (1997). Tactile defensiveness and stereotyped behaviors. *American Journal of Occupational Therapy, 51,* 91–95.
13. Barger, S. D., Donoho, C. J., & Wayment, H. A. (2009). The relative contributions of race/ethnicity, socioeconomic status, health, and social relationships to life satisfaction in the United States. *Quality of Life Research, 18,* 179–189.
14. Barkley, R. A. (1998). *Attention-deficit/hyperactivity disorder: A handbook for diagnosis and treatment* (2nd ed.). New York: Guilford.
15. Barnes, K. J., Vogel, K. A., Beck, A. J., et al. (2008). Self-regulation strategies of children with emotional disturbance. *Physical & Occupational Therapy in Pediatrics, 28*(4), 369–387.
16. Baron-Cohen, S. (1995). *Mindblindness: An essay on autism and theory.* Cambridge: MIT Press.
17. Barry, T., Klinger, L., Lee, J., et al. (2003). Examining the effectiveness of an outpatient clinic-based social skills group for high-functioning children with autism. *Journal of Autism and Developmental Disorders, 33*(6), 685–701.
18. Bauminger, N., & Kasari, C. (2000). Loneliness and friendship in high-functioning children with autism. *Child Development, 71*(2), 447–456.
19. Bell, K. S., & Kirby, J. R. (2002). Teaching emotion and belief as mindreading instruction for children with autism. *Developmental Disabilities Bulletin, 30*(1), 16–58.
20. Bellini, S., & Akullian, J. (2007). A meta-analysis of video modeling and video self-modeling interventions for children and adolescents with autism spectrum disorders. *Exceptional Children, 73*(3), 264–287.
21. Bellini, S., & Peters, J. K. (2008). Social skills training for youth with autism spectrum disorders. *Child and Adolescent Psychiatric Clinics of North America, 17,* 857–873.
22. Ben-Sasson, A., Cermak, S., Orsmond, G., et al. (2007). Extreme sensory modulation behaviors in toddlers with autism spectrum disorders. *American Journal of Occupational Therapy, 61,* 584–592.
23. Benson, P., Karlof, K. L., & Siperstein, G. N. (2008). Maternal involvement in the education of young children with autism spectrum disorders. *Autism: The International Journal of Research and Practice, 12*(1), 47–63.
24. Berkman, L. F., & Syme, L. S. (1979). Social networks, host resistance, and mortality: A nine-year follow-up study of Alameda County residents. *American Journal of Epidemiology, 109,* 186–204.
25. Bledsoe, R., Myles, B. S., & Simpson, R. L. (2003). Use of a social story intervention to improve mealtime skills of an adolescent with Asperger syndrome. *Autism: The International Journal of Research and Practice, 7*(3), 289–295.

26. Bishop, S., Gahagan, S., & Lord, C. (2007). Re-examining the core features of autism: A comparison of autism spectrum disorder and fetal alcohol spectrum disorder. *Journal of Child Psychology and Psychiatry, 48*, 1111–1121.
27. Bray, M. A., & Kehle, T. J. (1996). Self-modeling as an intervention for stuttering. *School Psychology Review, 25*, 358–369.
28. Brown, R., Coles, C., Smith, I., et al. (1991). Effects of PAE at school age. II. Attention and behavior. *Neurotoxicology and Teratology, 13*, 369–376.
29. Bruinsma, Y., Koegel, R. L., & Koegel, L. K. (2004). Joint attention and children with autism: A review of the literature. *Mental Retardation and Developmental Disabilities Research Reviews, 10*(3), 169–175.
30. Buggey, T., Toombs, K., Gardener, P., et al. (1999). Training responding behaviors in students with autism: Using videotaped self-modeling. *Journal of Positive Behavior Interventions, 1*, 205–214.
31. Bukowski, W. M., Hoza, B., & Boivin, M. (1994). Measuring friendship quality during pre- and early adolescence: The development and psychometric properties of the friendship qualities scale. *Journal of Social and Personal Relationships, 11*, 471–484.
32. Bundy, A., Lane, S., & Murray, E. (2002). *Sensory Integration: Theory and practice*. Philadelphia: F. A. Davis.
33. Buron, K. D., & Curtis, M. (2003). The incredible 5-point scale. Shawnee Mission, KS: Autism Asperger Publishing Co. from: <http://www.5pointscale.com/stuff_kari_mitzi.htm> Retrieved August 5, 2012.
34. Carmichael Olson, H., Streissguth, A., Sampson, P., et al. (1997). Association of PAE with behavioral and learning problems in early adolescence. *Journal of the American Academy of Child and Adolescent Psychiatry, 36*, 1187–1194.
35. Carlson, C. (1987). Social interaction goals and strategies of children with learning disabilities. *Journal of Learning Disabilities, 20*, 306–311.
36. Carter, J. F. (1993). Self management: Education's ultimate goal. *Teaching Exceptional Children, 25*(3), 28–33.
37. Carter, C., Meckes, L., Pritchard, L., et al. (2004). The friendship club: An after-school program for children with Asperger syndrome. *Family and Community Health, 27*, 143–150.
38. Case-Smith, J. (2005). *Occupational therapy for children*. St. Louis: Elsevier Mosby.
39. Castellanos, F. X., Sonuga-Barke, E. J., Milham, M. P., et al. (2006). Characterizing cognition in ADHD: Beyond executive dysfunction. *Trends in Cognitive Sciences, 10*(3), 117–123.
40. Charlop, M. H., & Milstein, J. P. (1989). Teaching autistic children conversational speech using video modeling. *Journal of Applied Behavior Analysis, 22*, 275–285.
41. Charlop-Cristy, M. H., Le, L., & Freeman, K. A. (2000). A comparison of video modeling with in vivo modeling for teaching children with autism. *Journal of Autism and Developmental Disorders, 30*, 537–552.
42. Chavira, D. A., Stein, M. B., Bailey, K., et al. (2004). Child anxiety in primary care: Prevalent but untreated. *Depression and Anxiety, 20*, 155–164.
43. Christopher, J. S., Nangle, D. W., & Hansen, D. J. (1993). Social-skills interventions with adolescents: Current issues and procedures. *Behavior Modification, 17*, 314–338.
44. Church, C., Alisanski, S., & Amanullah, S. (1999). The social, behavioral, and academic experiences of children with Asperger syndrome. *Focus on Autism and Other Developmental Disabilities, 15*(1), 12–20.
45. Clark, D. M. (1986). A cognitive approach to panic. *Behaviour Research and Therapy, 24*, 461–470.
46. Cohn, E., Miller, L. J., & Tickle-Degnen, L. (2000). Parental hopes for therapy outcomes: Children with sensory modulation disorders. *The American Journal of Occupational Therapy, 54*(1), 36–42.
47. American Occupational Therapy Association. (2010). Scope of practice. *American Journal of Occupational Therapy, 64*(Suppl.), S70–S77. doi:10.5014/ajot.2010.64S 7 0-64S77.
48. Constantino, J., & Gruber, C. (2012). *Social Responsiveness Scale* (2nd ed.). Los Angeles: Western Psychological Services. (SRS-2).
49. Constantino, J. N., & Todd, R. D. (2005). Intergenerational transmission of subthreshold autistic traits in the general population. *Biological Psychiatry, 57*(6), 655–660.
50. Coyle, C., & Cole, P. (2004). A videotaped self-modeling and self-monitoring treatment program to decrease off-task behaviour in children with autism. *Journal of Intellectual and Developmental Disabilities, 29*(1), 3–15.
51. Crozier, S., & Tincani, M. (2007). Effects of social stories on prosocial behavior of preschool children with autism spectrum disorders. *Journal of Autism and Developmental Disorders, 37*(9), 1803–1814.
52. D'Ateno, P., Mangiapanello, K., & Taylor, B. A. (2003). Using video modeling to teach complex play sequences to a preschooler with autism. *Journal of Positive Behavior Interventions, 5*, 5–11.
53. Dowrick, P. W., & Raeburn, J. M. (1995). Self-modeling. In P. W. Dorwrick & J. Higgs (Eds.), *Using video: Psychological and social applications* (pp. 105–124). New York: Wiley.
54. Elliot, S. N., & Gresham, F. M. (1993). Social skills interventions for children. *Behavior Modification, 17*, 287–313.
55. Erwin, E., & Brown, F. (2003). From theory to practice: A contextual framework for understanding self-determination in early-childhood environments. *Infants & Young Children, 16*(1), 77–87.
56. Fazlioglu, V., & Barau, G. (2008). A sensory integration therapy program on sensory problems for children with autism. *Perceptual and Motor Skills, 106*(2), 415–422.
57. Fivush, R., & Slackman, E. A. (1986). The acquisition and development of scripts. In K. Nelson (Ed.), *Event knowledge: Structure and function in development* (pp. 71–96). Hillsdale, NJ: Erlbaum.
58. Forbes, D. A. (1998). Goal attainment scaling: A responsive measure of client outcomes. *Journal of Gerontological Nursing, 24*(12), 34–40.
59. Gagnon, E. (2001). *Power cards: Using special interests to motivate children and youth with Asperger syndrome and autism*. Shawnee Mission, KS: AAPC.
60. Ganz, J. B., Cook, K. T., & Earles-Vollrath, T. L. (2006). *How to write and implement social scripts*. Austin, TX: Pro-ed.
61. Ganz, J., Kaylor, M., Bourgeois, B., et al. (2008). The impact of social scripts and visual cues on verbal communication in three children with autism spectrum disorders. *Focus on Autism and Other Developmental Disabilities, 23*(2), 79–94.
62. Garber, J. (2006). Depression in children and adolescents: Linking risk research and prevention. *American Journal of Preventive Medicine, 31*(6S1), S104–S125.
63. Garmezy, N. (1985). Stress-resistant children: The search for protective factors. In J. E. Stevenson (Ed.), *Recent research in developmental psychopathology: Journal of Child Psychology and Psychiatry, book 4* (pp. 213–233). Oxford, England: Pergamon Press.
64. Ginsburg, G. S., La Greca, A. M., & Silverman, W. K. (1998). Social anxiety in children with anxiety disorders: Relation with social and emotional functioning. *Journal of Abnormal Child Psychology, 26*(3), 175–185, UI: 9650624.

65. Golan, O., & Baron-Cohen, S. (2006). Systemizing empathy: Teaching adults with Asperger syndrome or high-functioning autism to recognize complex emotions using interactive multimedia. *Developmental Psychopathology, 18*, 591–617.
66. Goldman, L. S., Genel, M., Bezman, R. J., et al. (1998). Diagnosis and treatment of attention-deficit disorder in children and adolescents. *JAMA: The Journal of the American Medical Association, 279*(14), 1100–1107.
67. Gray, C. A. (1998). Social stories and comic strip conversations with students with Asperger syndrome and high-functioning autism. In E. Schopler (Ed.), *Asperger syndrome or high-functioning autism?* (pp. 167–194). New York: Plenum Press.
68. Gray, C., & White, A. L. (2002). *My social stories book.* New York: Kingsley.
69. Gresham, F. M., & Elliott, S. N. (2008). *Social skills improvement system: Rating scales manual.* Minneapolis, MN: Pearson.
70. Gutstein, S. E. (2009). Empowering families through relationship development intervention: An important part of the biopsychosocial management of autism spectrum disorders. *Annals of Clinical Psychiatry, 21*(3), 174–182.
71. Gutstein, S. E., Burgess, A. F., & Montfort, K. (2007). Evaluation of the relationship development intervention program. *Autism: The International Journal of Research and Practice, 11*(5), 397–411.
72. Hansen, D. J., Nangle, D. W., & Meyer, K. A. (1998). Enhancing the effectiveness of social skills interventions with adolescents. *Education and Treatment of Children, 21*, 489–513.
73. Happe, F. G., & Frith, U. (1996). The neuropsychology of autism. *Brain, 119*, 1377–1400.
74. Harris, K. R. (1986). Self-monitoring of attentional behavior versus self-monitoring of productivity: Effects on on-task behavior and academic response rate among learning disabled children. *Journal of Applied Behavior Analysis, 19*, 417–423.
75. Hillier, A., Fish, T., Cloppert, P., et al. (2007). Outcomes of a social and vocational skills support group for adolescents and young adults on the autism spectrum. *Focus on Autism and Other Developmental Disabilities, 22*, 107–115.
76. Hilton, C. L., Graver, K., & LaVesser, P. (2007). Relationship between social competence and sensory processing in children with high functioning autism spectrum disorders. *Research in Autism Spectrum Disorders, 1*(2), 164–173.
77. Hosford, R. E. (1981). Self-as-models: A cognitive social-learning technique. *The Counseling Psychologist, 9*, 45–62.
78. Howlin, P., Baron-Cohen, S., & Hadwin, J. (1999). *Teaching children with autism to mind-read: A practical guide.* Chichester, UK: John Wiley & Sons.
79. Humphries, A. (2003). Effectiveness of PRT as a behavioral intervention for young children with ASD. *Bridges practice-based research syntheses, 2*(4), 123–141.
80. Hutchins, T. L., & Prelock, P. A. (2006). Using social stories and comic strip conversations to promote socially valid outcomes for children with autism. *Seminars in Speech and Language, 27*(1), 47–59.
81. Kahn, J. S., Kehle, T. J., et al. (1990). Comparison of cognitive-behavioral, relaxation, and self-modeling interventions for depression among middle-school students. *School Psychology Review, 19*, 196–211.
82. Kalyva, E., & Agaliotis, I. (2009). Can social stories enhance the interpersonal conflict resolution skills of children with LD? *Research in Developmental Disabilities, 30*(1), 192–202.
83. Kamps, D. M., Potucek, J., Lopez, A., et al. (1997). The use of peer networks across multiple settings to improve social interaction for students with autism. *Journal of Behavioral Education, 7*(3), 335–357.
84. Kamps, D. M., Kravits, T., Lopez, A. G., et al. (1998). What do the peers think? Social validity of peer-mediated programs. *Education and Treatment of Children, 21*, 107–134.
85. Keeling, K., Myles, B. S., Gagnon, E., et al. (2003). Using the power card strategy to teach sportsmanship skills to a child with autism. *Focus on Autism and Other Developmental Disabilities, 18*(2), 105–222.
86. Kiresuk, T. J., Smith, A., & Cardillo, J. E. (1994). *Goal attainment scaling: Application, theory and measurement.* Hillsdale, NJ: Erlbaum.
87. Koegel, L. K., Koegel, R. L., Hurley, C., et al. (1992). Improving social skills and disruptive behavior in children with autism through self-management. *Journal of Applied Behavior Analysis, 25*(2), 341–353.
88. Koning, C., & Magill-Evans, J. (2001). Social and language skills in adolescent boys with Asperger syndrome. *Autism: The International Journal of Research and Practice, 5*(1), 23–36.
89. Krantz, P., & McClannahan, L. (1993). Teaching children with autism to initiate to peers: Effects of a script-fading procedure. *Journal of Applied Behavior Analysis, 26*, 121–132.
90. Kravetz, S., Faust, M., Lipshitz, S., et al. (1999). LD, interpersonal understanding, and social behavior in the classroom. *Journal of Learning Disabilities, 32*, 248–256.
91. Kroeger, K. A., Schultz, J. R., & Newsom, C. (2007). A comparison of two group-delivered social skills programs for young children with autism. *Journal of Autism and Developmental Disorders, 37*, 808–817.
92. Kully-Martens, K., Denys, K., Treit, S., et al. (2012). A review of social skills deficits in individuals with fetal alcohol spectrum disorders and prenatal alcohol exposure: Profiles, mechanisms, and interventions. *Alcoholism, Clinical and Experimental Research, 36*(4), 568–576.
93. Golan, O., & Baron-Cohen, S. (2006). Systemizing empathy: teaching adults with Asperger syndrome or high-functioning autism to recognize complex emotions using interactive multimedia. *Developmental Psychopathology, 18*, 591–617.
94. Lasater, M. W., & Brady, M. P. (1995). Effects of video self-modeling and feedback on task fluency: A home-based intervention. *Education and Treatment of Children, 8*, 389–407.
95. Lavoie, R. D. (1994). *Learning disabilities and social skills with Richard Lavoie: Last one picked … first one picked on.* Alexandria, VA: PBS Video.
96. Lovaas, O. I. (Ed.), (2003). *Teaching individuals with developmental delays: basic intervention techniques.* Austin, TX: Pro-Ed.
97. Loveland, K. A., & Tunali, B. (1991). Social scripts for conversational interactions in autism and Down syndrome. *Journal of Autism and Developmental Disorders, 21*, 177–186.
98. Mailloux, Z., May-Benson, T. A., Summers, C. A., et al. (2007). Goal attainment scaling as a measure of meaningful outcomes for children with sensory integration disorders. *American Journal of Occupational Therapy, 61*, 254–259.
99. Maloney, F. P., Mirrett, P., Brooks, C., et al. (1978). Use of the goal attainment scale in the treatment and ongoing evaluation of neurologically handicapped children. *American Journal of Occupational Therapy, 32*(8), 505–510.
100. McAfee, J. (2002). *Navigating the social world.* Arlington, TX: Future Horizons.
101. McCurdy, B. L., & Shapiro, E. S. (1988). Self-observation and the reduction of inappropriate classroom behavior. *Journal of School Psychology, 26*, 371–378.

102. Merrell, K. W. (2002). *School Social Behavior Scales* (2nd ed.). Wood Dale, IL: Stoelting.
103. Merrell, K. W. (2003). *Preschool and Kindergarten Behavior Scales* (2nd ed.). Austin, TX: Pro-ed.
104. Miller, L. J., Coll, J. R., & Schoen, S. A. (2007). A randomized controlled pilot study of the effectiveness of occupational therapy for children with sensory modulation disorder. *American Journal of Occupational Therapy, 61*(2), 228–238.
105. Miller, L. J., Robinson, J., & Moulton, D. (2004). Sensory modulation dysfunction: Identification in early childhood. In R. DelCarmen-Wiggins & A. Carter (Eds.), *Handbook of infant, toddler and preschool mental health assessment* (pp. 247–270). New York: Oxford University Press.
106. Missiuna, C., Pollock, N., & Law, M. (2004). *Perceived efficacy and goal setting for children with disability.* San Antonio, TX: PsychCorp.
107. Mitchell, T., & Cusick, A. (1998). Evaluation of a client-centered paediatric rehabilitation programme using goal attainment scaling. *Australian Occupational Therapy Journal, 45,* 7–17.
108. Mosey, A. C. (1996). *Applied scientific inquiry in the health professions: An epistemological orientation* (2nd ed.). Bethesda, MD: American Occupational Therapy Association.
109. Moyes, R. A., & Moreno, S. J. (2001). Incorporating social goals in the classroom: A guide for teachers and parents of children with high-functioning autism and
110. Myers, S. M., & Johnson, C. P. (2007). Management of children with autism spectrum disorders. *Pediatrics, 120,* 1162–1175.
111. Myles, B. S., Keeling, K., & Van Horn, C. (2001). Results of classroom studies using the power card strategy. In E. Gagnon (Ed.), *Power cards: Using special interests to motivate children and youth with Asperger syndrome and autism.* Shawnee Mission, KS: AAPC.
112. Myles, B. S., & Southwick, J. (1999). *Asperger syndrome and difficult moments: Practical solutions for tantrums, rage, and meltdowns.* Shawnee Mission, KS: AAPC.
113. Myles, B. S., Trautman, M. L., & Schelvan, R. L. (2004). *The hidden curriculum: Practical solutions for understanding unstated rules in social situations.* Shawnee Mission: Kansas: AAPC.
114. Neitzel, J., & Busick, M. (2009). *Overview of self-management.* Chapel Hill, NC: National Professional Development Center on Autism Spectrum Disorders, Frank Porter Graham Child Development Institute, The University of North Carolina.
115. Nikopoulos, C. K., & Keenan, M. (2003). Promoting social initiation in children with autism using video modeling. *Behavioral Interventions, 18,* 87–108.
116. O'Brien, J., Bergeron, A., Duprey, H., et al. (2009). Children with disabilities and their parents' views of occupational participation needs. *Occupational Therapy in Health Care, 25,* 1–17.
117. Odom, S. L., & Strain, P. S. (1984). Peer-mediated approaches to promoting children's social interaction: A review. *American Journal of Orthopsychiatry, 54,* 544–557.
118. Ozdemir, S. (2008). The effectiveness of social stories on decreasing disruptive behaviors of children with autism: Three case studies. *Journal of Autism & Developmental Disorders., 38,* 1689–1696.
119. Ozonoff, S., & Miller, J. N. (1995). Teaching theory of mind: A new approach to social skills training for individuals with autism. *Journal of Autism and Developmental Disorders, 25,* 415–433.
120. Parham, L. D., Cohn, E. S., Spitzer, S., et al. (2007). Fidelity in sensory integration intervention research. *American Journal of Occupational Therapy, 61,* 216–227.
121. Parham, L. D., Roley, S. S., May-Benson, T. A., et al. (2011). Development of a fidelity measure for research on the effectiveness of the Ayres sensory integration intervention. *American Journal of Occupational Therapy, 65,* 133–142.
122. Pennington, B. F., & Ozonoff, S. (1996). Executive functions and developmental psychopathology. *Journal of Child Psychology and Psychiatry, 37,* 51–87.
123. Pfeiffer, B. A., Koenig, K., Kinnealey, M., et al. (2011). Effectiveness of sensory integration interventions in children with autism spectrum disorders: A pilot study. *American Journal of Occupational Therapy, 65,* 76–85.
124. Pigott, H. E., & Gonzales, F. P. (1987). Efficacy of self-modeling in treating an electively mute child. *Journal of Clinical Child Psychology, 16,* 106–110.
125. Provencal, S. L. (2003). The efficacy of a social skills training program for adolescents with autism spectrum disorders. Unpublished doctoral dissertation, University of Utah.
126. Quill, K. (1995). *Teaching children with autism: Strategies to enhance communication and socialization.* New York: Delmar.
127. Quirmback, L. M., Lincoln, A. J., Feinberg-Gizzo, M. J., et al. (2009). Social stories: Mechanisms of effectiveness in increasing game play skills in children diagnosed with autism spectrum disorder using a pretest-posttest repeated measures randomized control group design. *Journal of Autism and Developmental Disorders, 39,* 299–321.
128. Roeyers, H. (1996). The influence of nonhandicapped peers on the social interactions of children with a pervasive developmental disorder. *Journal of Autism and Developmental Disorders, 26,* 303–320.
129. Roosa, J. (1995). SOCCSS (Situations, Options, Consequences, Choices, Strategies, Simulation), a technique for teaching social interaction. Retrieved from: <http://brainspire.org/index.html?/credentials.htm>.
130. Rose-Colley, M., Symons, C. W., & Cummings, C. D. (1989). Privacy circles: An affective teaching technique for controversial topics. *Journal of School Health, 59*(4), 165–166.
131. Rush, D. D., & Shelden, M. L. (2005). Evidence-based definition of coaching practices. *CASEinPoint: Insights into Early Childhood and Family Support Practices, 1*(6), 1–6.
132. Rushton, P. W., & Miller, W. C. (2002). Goal attainment scaling in the rehabilitation of patients with lower-extremity amputations: A pilot study. *Archives of Physical Medicine and Rehabilitation, 83,* 771–775.
133. Rutter, M. (1990). Psychosocial resilience and protective mechanisms. In J. Rolf, A. S. Masten, D. Cicchetti, et al. (Eds.), *Risk and protective factors in the development of psychopathology* (pp. 181–214). Cambridge, UK: Cambridge University Press.
134. Rutter, M., Bailey, A., & Lord, C. (2003). *SCQ: The Social Communication Questionnaire manual.* Los Angeles: Western Psychological Services.
135. Ryan, R., & Deci, E. (2000). Self-determination theory and the facilitation of intrinsic motivation, social development, and well-being. *American Psychologist, 55*(1), 68–78.
136. Rydell, A., Hagekull, B., & Bohlin, G. (1997). Measurement of two social competence aspects in middle childhood. *Developmental Psychology, 33,* 824–833.
137. Schaaf, R. C., Hunt, J., & Benevides, T. (2012). Occupational therapy using sensory integration to improve participation of a child with autism: A case report. *American Journal of Occupational Therapy, 66,* 547–555.

138. Schreibman, L., & Ingersoll, B. (2005). Behavioral interventions to promote learning in individuals with autism. In F. R. Volkmar, R. Paul, A. Klin, & D. Cohen (Eds.), *Handbook of autism and pervasive developmental disorders* (3rd ed., Vol. II, pp. 882–896). Hoboken, NJ: John Wiley & Sons.
139. Schreibman, Whalen & Stahmer (2000).
140. Shearer, D. D., Kohler, F. W., Buchan, K. A., et al. (1996). Promoting independent interactions between preschoolers with autism and their nondisabled peers: An analysis of self-monitoring. *Early Education and Development, 7,* 205–220.
141. Sherer, M., Pierce, K. L., Paredes, S., et al. (2001). Enhancing conversational skills in children with autism via video technology. Which is better, "self" or "other" as a model? *Behavior Modification, 25,* 140–158.
142. Silver, M., & Oakes, P. (2001). Evaluation of a new computer intervention to teach people with autism or Asperger syndrome to recognize and predict emotion in others. *Autism: The International Journal of Research and Practice, 5*(3), 299–316.
143. Skinner, B. F. (1953). Science and human behavior. New York: Free Press.
144. Skinner, B. F. (1976). *Walden two.* New York: Macmillan.
145. Solomon, M., Goodlin-Jones, B. L., & Anders, T. F. (2004). A social adjustment enhancement intervention for high-functioning autism, Asperger's syndrome, and pervasive developmental disorder NOS. *Journal of Autism and Developmental Disorders, 34,* 649–668.
146. Stephens, T., & Haley, S. (1991). Comparison of two methods for determining change in motorically handicapped children. *Physical and Occupational Therapy in Pediatrics, 11*(1), 1–17.
147. Stokes, M. A., & Kaur, A. (2005). High-functioning autism and sexuality: A parental perspective. *Autism: The International Journal of Research and Practice, 9,* 266–289.
148. Stone, W., Ruble, L., Coonrod, E., et al. (2010). *Triad Social Skills Assessment* (2nd ed.). Nashville: Vanderbilt Kennedy Center.
149. Strain, P. S., Kohler, F. W., & Goldstein, H. (1996). Learning experiences: An alternative program: Peer-mediated interventions for young children with autism. In E. D. Hibbs & P. S. Jensen (Eds.), *Psychosocial treatments for child and adolescent disorders: Empirically based strategies for clinical practice* (pp. 573–587). Washington, DC: American Psychological Association.
150. Strain, P. S., Kohler, F. W., Storey, K., et al. (1994). Teaching preschoolers with autism to self-monitor their social interactions. *Journal of Emotional and Behavioral Disorders, 2,* 78–88.
151. Streissguth, A. P., Aase, J. M., Clarren, S. K., et al. (1991). Fetal alcohol syndrome in adolescents and adults. *JAMA: The Journal of the American Medical Association, 265,* 1961–1967.
152. Swartz, S. L., Prevatt, F., & Proctor, B. E. (2005). A coaching intervention for college students with attention deficit/hyperactivity disorder. *Psychology in Schools, 42*(6), 647–656.
153. Tarnai, B., & Wolfe, P. S. (2008). Social stories for sexuality education for persons with autism/pervasive developmental disorder. *Sexuality and Disability, 26*(1), 29–36.
154. Taylor, B. A., Levin, L., & Jasper, S. (1999). Increasing play-related statements in children with autism toward their siblings: Effects of video modeling. *Journal of Developmental and Physical Disabilities, 11,* 253–264.
155. Tchaconas, A., & Adesman, A. (2013). Autism spectrum disorders: A pediatric overview and update. *Current Opinion in Pediatrics, 25*(1), 130–143.
156. Tomchek, S., & Case-Smith, J. (2009). Occupational therapy practice guidelines for children and adolescents with autism. Bethesda: AOTA Press.
157. Tonks, J., Williams, W. H., Frampton, I., et al. (2007). Assessing emotion recognition in 9-15-year olds: Preliminary analysis of abilities in reading emotion from faces, voices and eyes. *Brain Injury, 21*(6), 623–629.
158. Volkmar, F. R., Lord, C., Bailey, A., et al. (2004). Autism and pervasive developmental disorders. *Journal of Child Psychology and Psychiatry, 45*(1), 135–170.
159. Volkmar, F., Klin, A., Siegel, B., et al. (1994). DSM-IV autism/pervasive developmental disorder field trial. *American Journal of Psychiatry, 151,* 1361–1367.
160. Watling, R., Deitz, J., & White, O. (2001). Comparison of sensory profile scores of young children with and without autism spectrum disorders. *American Journal of Occupational Therapy., 55,* 416–423.
161. Webb, B. J., Miller, S. P., Pierce, T. B., et al. (2004). Effects of social skill instruction for high-functioning adolescents with autism spectrum disorders. *Focus on Autism and Other Developmental Disabilities, 19,* 53–62.
162. Weiss, M. J., & Harris, S. L. (2001). Teaching social skills to people with autism. *Behavior Modification, 25,* 785–802.
163. Wells, A. M., Chasnoff, I. J., Schmidt, C. A., et al. (2012). Neurocognitive habilitation therapy for children with fetal alcohol spectrum disorders: An adaptation of the Alert program. *American Journal of Occupational Therapy, 66,* 24–34.
164. Whalen, C. K., & Henker, B. (1985). The social world of the hyperactive (ADHD) children. *Clinical Psychology Review, 5,* 447–478.
165. Whitworth, L., Kimsey-House, K., Kimsey-House, H., 2007). *Co-active coaching: New skills for coaching people toward success in work and life* (2nd ed.). Mountain View, CA: Davies-Black.
166. Wilcox, A. (2006). *An occupational perspective of health* (2nd ed.). Thorofare, NJ: Slack.
167. Williams, M. S., & Shellenberger, S. (1996). *The Alert program: "How does your engine run?".* Albuquerque: TherapyWorks.
168. Williams, T. L. (1989). A social skills group for autistic children. *Journal of Autism and Developmental Disorders, 19,* 143–155.
169. Woltersdorf, M. A. (1992). Videotape self-modeling in the treatment of attention-deficit hyperactivity disorder. *Child & Family Therapy, 14,* 53–73.
170. World Health Organization. (2007). *International classification of functioning, disability and health: Children and youth version.* Geneva: World Health Organization.
171. Yang, N. K., Schaller, J. L., Huang, T., et al. (2003). Enhancing appropriate social behaviors for children with autism in general education classrooms: An analysis of six cases. *Education and Training in Developmental Disabilities, 38,* 405–416.
172. Zimbelman, M., Paschal, A., Hawley, S. R., et al. (2007). Addressing physical inactivity among developmentally disabled students through visual schedules and social stories. *Research in Developmental Disabilities, 28*(4), 386–396.
173. Zwart, L. M., & Kallemeyn, L. M. (2001). Peer-based coaching for college students with ADHD and learning disabilities. *Journal of Postsecondary Education and Disability, 15*(1), 1–15.

CHAPTER

12

Social Participation for Youth Ages 12 to 21

Jessica Kramer • Kendra Liljenquist • Matthew E. Brock • Zachary Rosetti • Brooke Howard • Melissa Demir • Erik W. Carter

KEY TERMS

Social participation	Environment
Transition to adulthood	ICF

GUIDING QUESTIONS

1. How is social participation of adolescents and young adults conceptualized?
2. How is social participation influenced by the environment?
3. How does social participation in adolescence affect future development and the capacity to perform adult responsibilities and roles?
4. How do occupational therapists evaluate social participation in youth and young adults?
5. Which intervention approaches and strategies improve social participation in youth and young adults?

What is Social Participation?

Social participation has broad and varied meanings; examples include connecting with friends electronically via text or virtual chat, volunteering in the community, interacting with co-workers, and completing a school assignment with friends. Occupational therapists may use the term *social participation* to describe all these interactions. Leaders in the fields of rehabilitation, sociology, psychology, and education have proposed different ways of understanding engagement in social contexts. Integrating these varying approaches can provide occupational therapists with a robust understanding of the various ways in which youth involvement in social life situations can enhance development and successful transition to adulthood.

Identity Development and Social Participation

Adolescence is an important time for the development of identity—that is, defining who one is, what to value, and which directions to pursue in life.[42] Identity development was originally conceptualized as a series of linear stages. However, research has suggested that identity development is a dynamic process that occurs throughout adolescence.[89] The development of an identity is important to youth as they transition to adulthood because youth may select career trajectories, social networks, and leisure choices that reflect their developing identity.

Social participation can facilitate the development of identity of all young people, including youth with disabilities. Qualitative work done by Hansen et al.[56] highlighted two important themes about the development of identity that relate to engagement in occupations: *trying new things* and *learning your limits.* Trying new things allows adolescents to discover how these new activities fit or do not fit into their developing identity. New activities may also require youth to use or develop a different set of skills. Thus, participation in activities offers young people a chance to explore their unique abilities and furthers the development of their identity. Occupational therapists can play an important role in the identity development of youth with disabilities by facilitating social participation through skill development and environmental and task modifications.

Social relationships also play an important role in identity development, especially in the development of a positive disability identity. The literature on youth transition to adulthood continually cites peer mentorship, support, and modeling as best practices for youth with disabilities.[13,16,28,43] Youth with disabilities appreciate the opportunity to talk with others who face similar barriers in their daily lives and acquire new skills and insights when exposed to other youth who have resolved similar problems.[60,65,102,124] Connecting with other people with disabilities can also help youth identify and appreciate valuable aspects of their disability, a key step to integrating a disability identity into a positive sense of self.[46] For example, a study of youth attending a disability-only summer camp found that camp participation facilitated personal and group identity formation.[49] Camp provided youth with the opportunity to spend time with other youth with disabilities, manage their time and schedules without assistance from their parents, and explore a range of new activities in a safe and accepting environment. After these experiences, they expressed a positive change in feelings about their disability, identity, and what might be possible in the future. Although inclusion with peers without disabilities and equal access is an important right that must be ensured for young people with disabilities, additional experiences within the disability community may play an essential role in the development of a positive disability identity.

Participation and International Classification of Functioning, Disability, and Health

The World Health Organization's International Classification of Functioning, Disability, and Health (ICF) has defined participation as "involvement in a life situation."[139] This broad definition provides an opportunity and a challenge for the field of rehabilitation. The general conceptualization of participation provides the profession with the opportunity to address areas of involvement that are determined most relevant and important to individuals in rehabilitation. However, the lack of a clear delineation between participation and other related concepts, such as the ICF concept of activity, has made it difficult for researchers and clinicians to measure and intervene at the level of participation.

Rehabilitation scholars have attempted to define participation better as it relates to social interactions with others. The American Occupational Therapy Association (AOTA) Practice Framework has defined social participation as "organized patterns of behavior that are characteristic and expected of an individual or a given position within a social system" that occur in the community, family, and with peers.[4] Khetani and Coster have noted that the ICF terms *participation* and *social participation* have been used interchangeably in rehabilitation, and that "any life situation can be social."[61] Whiteneck and Dijikers[138] suggested that participation requires role performance at the societal level, rather than activities that an individual may perform on his or her own. This chapter will structure the discussion of social participation around the following ICF concepts (Figure 12-1):

- *Interpersonal interactions and relationships.* This concept provides an understanding of social relationships and how they may be enacted across the major life areas and contexts discussed below.
- *Major life areas of education, work, and economic life.* For adolescents, these areas of occupation are often a primary focus of education and other interventions during their transition to adulthood. For our discussion of social participation, we will examine education and postsecondary training, as well as work and prevocational experiences.
- *Community, social, and civic life.* These are participation contexts outside the family in which social interactions are a key component of meaningful participation for adolescents transitioning to adulthood and developing more autonomy. This includes community life, religion, and citizenship, as well as recreation and leisure. For our discussion of social participation, recreation and leisure (a primary concern of occupational therapists) will be discussed separately from community life, religion, and citizenship.

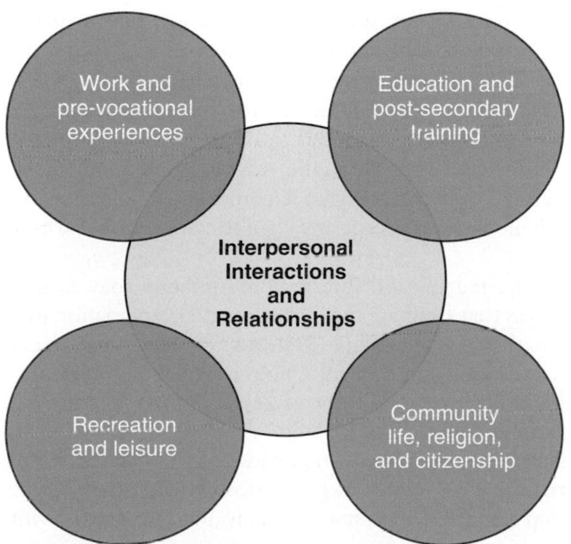

FIGURE 12-1 Conceptualizing social participation based on the International Classification of Functioning, Disability, and Health (ICF).

Role of the Environment and Culture on Social Participation

Social participation, by its very definition, involves an interaction between a person and an individual or group of individuals. These interactions are further influenced by other structural and cultural expectations. Therefore, social engagement is not only an action that occurs between individuals, but also a result of specific environmental opportunities and constraints.[62] For youth with disabilities, limited social participation is as related to environmental barriers as it is to impairments or limited social skills. Research with younger children with disabilities has suggested that after controlling for the effect of impairment on participation, differences in the levels of participation of children with disabilities are explained by the community in which they live.[44,53] Although similar work has not yet been conducted with transition-age youth, these findings point to the potential impact of the environment on the participation of all youth with disabilities.

The field of positive youth development considers the various environmental and personal factors and experiences that can influence the successful development of youth into adulthood. In this field of study, the ongoing interactions, or transactions, between two or more people or groups are conceptualized as *social processes.*[123] These social processes occur in specific settings, such as classrooms, after-school programs, or community centers. Resources in these settings and the organization of those resources dictate how social processes occur in a specific setting and may determine a positive or negative social participation outcome.

One example of the impact of transactions on social participation can be found in the case study about Project TEAM (see later, Case Study 12-4). In this case study, when Emily sought information about a volunteer opportunity, the positive attitude and responsiveness of the staff person at the daycare center facilitated a positive social interaction. This social interaction helped Emily obtain the information she needed to become a volunteer. Emily built on this positive interaction and identified staff at the day-care center as a potential source of support to help her meet future job responsibilities. The outcomes may have been different for Emily if the day-care center had different resources available or chose to organize and use those resources in a different way—for example, if the staff person did not have enough time to answer questions because of his or her job responsibilities or held a negative attitude about disability, or the organization made information available only on their website.

Another way to conceptualize the impact of the environment on participation comes from the field of disability studies.[2,54,96] The social model of disability posits that disability is not the result of impairment but a consequence of inaccessible environments. Instead of viewing disability as a natural consequence of bodily differences (or impairments), the social model of disability of suggests that disability is a result of cultural and social beliefs and expectations about individuals who are different.[95] Cultural and social assumptions about impairment that can lead to the segregation and isolation of youth with disabilities include the following:

- Individuals with different minds, such as those who experience positive psychiatric symptoms (e.g., hallucinations), are labeled as intellectually disabled or unsafe or dangerous without supervision and intervention.[48,104]
- Bodily differences and the resulting functional differences, such as not being able to walk, are tragic or unbearable and lead to a poor quality of life.[81]
- Bodily or mental differences are a manifestation of spiritual differences or have occurred in retribution for spiritual transgressions.[93]

The social model of disability challenges the origin of these types of assumptions. Examples of subcultures in which these assumptions do not exist demonstrate how individuals with disabilities can be fully included in society and are not seen as different or labeled as "disabled." For example, at the beginning of the twentieth century, a small and isolated island off the coast of New England, Martha's Vineyard, had a high proportion of deaf citizens.[51] This was a result of a genetic trait found in many of the families who had settled there. Because so many individuals in this close-knit community were deaf, most individuals on the island were fluent in sign language, leading to a culture in which hearing and deaf individuals attended school, conducted business, and socialized together. This was a stark contrast to life off the island, where individuals who were deaf were treated with suspicion or isolated in special settings, such as institutions or training schools for the deaf. This story illustrates how social inclusion and participation can be facilitated or restricted by cultural structures and beliefs.

Environment and the International Classification of Functioning, Disability, and Health

Occupational therapists can use the ICF framework to identify key resources in the environment systematically.[139] Box 12-1 provides examples of how different environmental factors, as defined by the ICF, can influence social participation. Numerous studies illustrate the impact of these environmental factors on the social participation of youth and young adults with disabilities.[5,72]

The impact of the physical environment on participation of youth with disabilities has been widely documented. Frequently mentioned barriers to participation include the physical layout of spaces, such as the presence of stairs and other structural features that limit mobility, thus affecting youth's ability to participate in the full range of activities.[17,98] In addition, lack of adequate space to provide individualized attention and assistance to youth with disabilities can be a barrier to social participation and lead to misperceptions among peers. One young person explained, "A few teachers took me aside and went through things with me. But we had to work in the canteen, there was nowhere else. Classmates were astonished at me—spending time with a teacher! If they knew what [we] were talking about, they'd know I needed the extra help" (p. 164).[111]

Further logistical issues, such as lack of transportation, often in school-related endeavors outside the typical school day, such as field trips, have also been shown to influence participation.[38,84] Inadequate transportation is a major barrier to social and community participation[127]; 34% of persons with disabilities report a lack of appropriate transportation options compared with 16% of those without disabilities.[57]

Social aspects of the environment also affect how youth with disabilities experience participation in a range of settings. Issues such as close proximity of adults and negative attitudes of others can reduce engagement with peers.[37,25,127] Attitudes, especially misunderstandings regarding the abilities and needs of young people with disabilities, can also be detrimental to successful social participation.[72] For example, when adults overestimate the needs of an individual youth with a disability, they may restrict choices and opportunities for participation. For example, a youth shared how a substitute teacher singled her out as "the only person who could not participate in an activity that she had previously played" (p. 65).[15] However, underestimating the needs of youth with disabilities can be equally dangerous. In another study, a young woman explained how a gym teacher believed that she was not working hard enough. She explained, "He had me walking, jogging, running and I said 'Sir, I can't do this, I'm going to be sick.' I was in such a state, I was blue.... But they still made me do it" (p. 274).[79]

Policies have also been shown, positively and negatively, to affect the participation of youth with disabilities in school, extracurricular activities, and community activities. The lack of needed services and services that are not tailored to the youth's needs and interests are reported as barriers to participation.[72] Service and support systems that provide opportunities for young people to make choices and that involve youth in organizational decision making may support higher levels of social participation.[127] For example, in one study, a youth explained how not integrating his input in decision making led to poor outcomes at school: "He [the teacher] promised to ask and take into consideration what I could and could not do, but actually he did not accept any changes and nothing was done" (p. 159).[6]

Finally, federal and international policies may help create structures that facilitate the inclusion and participation of youth with disabilities. The United Nations Convention on the Rights of the Child stated that all children, including children with disabilities, are entitled to be involved in matters and decisions concerning them.[9,28,45,75,115,121]

These policies can influence federal and state governments, international nonprofit organizations, and other groups to develop practices that systematically include youth with disabilities in society. Legislation such as the Individuals with Disabilities Education Act (IDEA; see Chapter 23) guarantees youth with disabilities the right to be educated next to their general education peers in the least restrictive environment.

BOX 12-1 International Classification of Functioning, Disability, and Health: Environmental Factors and Social Participation

Products and Technology

These are natural or synthetic products or systems of products, equipment, and technology in an individual's immediate environment that are gathered, created, produced, or manufactured.

- Augmentative communication devices can be used to share ideas with other students in a class activity.
- Smartphone apps can be used to help individuals remember the steps of a game or organize their social time.

Natural and Human-Made Changes to the Environment

These are animate and inanimate elements of the natural or physical environment and components of that environment that have been modified by people.

- Weather, such as extreme temperatures, may affect the ability of individuals with chronic medical conditions to move about their community.
- Universal design, such as curb cuts and well-lit signage, can provide access for a broad range of individuals in a community—for example, parents who push strollers, persons who use a wheelchair, or an older adult who may have an unsteady gait.

Support and Relationships

These are the amount of physical or emotional support, nurturing, protection, assistance, and relationships provided by people or animals to other persons in their homes, places of work, schools, at play, or in other aspects of their daily activities.

- A service dog may help a teenager with autism spectrum disorder (ASD) feel more comfortable in a new social setting, such as a community dance.
- An encouraging teacher assists a student with a disability with his college application, providing additional postsecondary opportunities for the student.

Attitudes

These are observable consequences of customs, practices, ideologies, values, norms, factual beliefs, and religious beliefs.

- A coach may think that it is not safe for a youth with a disability to play sports. The coach requires a teenager to obtain extensive medical documentation before allowing him or her to join the team.
- An occupational therapist works under the assumption that skills are best developed during engagement in meaningful occupations, rather than in contrived situations. Instead of pretending to plan a route using the bus, the occupational therapist rides the bus with a young adult to practice going to a new job site.

Services, Systems, and Policies

These include the following: services that provide benefits; structured programs and operations in various sectors of society designed to meet the needs of individuals; systems that exert administrative control and organizational mechanisms and are established by governments at the local, regional, national, and international levels or by other recognized authorities; and policies constituted by rules, regulations, conventions, and standards established by governments at the local, regional, national, and international levels or by other recognized authorities.

- A local center for independent living provides access to personal care attendants. Having assistance to get ready in the morning allows a young adult to move out of his or her parents' house into an apartment with a roommate.
- The Americans with Disabilities Act ensures that persons with disabilities can access businesses in their community such as movie theaters, recreational centers and pools, and restaurants.

Although this policy does not guarantee social participation, it can encourage practices that may lead to increased social participation. This includes regulations such as inclusion in the standard curriculum next to students without disabilities. Similarly, in 2013, the U.S. Department of Education called for educational systems to provide equal opportunities for youth with disabilities to participate in sports. Participating in school sports opens opportunities for youth with disabilities to interact with other students and adults and may also facilitate skills associated with positive development into adulthood (see later, Research Note 12-2).

Another environmental and contextual factor that may have a significant influence on the social participation of youth with disabilities is socioeconomic status. Shattuck and colleagues[110] found that youth with autism spectrum disorders (ASDs), ages 13 to 17 years, with family incomes higher than $75,000, were more likely to be involved in extracurricular activities, have friends, and be invited to activities compared with youth with ASDs with family incomes lower than $50,000. Youths with ASD ages 18 to 21 years were four times more likely to be employed or enrolled in postsecondary education if their families were above the poverty level during early adolescence (ages 13-16 years).[80] For early adolescents with cerebral palsy, lower levels of parent education (which may be associated with lower income) were associated with lower scores of social function.[129]

Social Participation in Adolescence and Young Adulthood

Interpersonal Relationships

The ICF defines interpersonal interactions as carrying out the actions and tasks required for basic and complex interactions with people (from strangers to family members) in a contextually and socially appropriate manner. Thus, these interpersonal interactions are the foundation of social participation. The ICF includes a range of *relationships* in which a youth may engage on a daily basis, including friendships, relating to persons in authority such as teachers and employers, family relationships such as siblings and parents, and brief interactions with strangers within the community. Thus, while completing an individual task such as shopping, the opportunity for social participation may emerge if a young person is shopping with a friend, bumps into a former sports coach, or seeks assistance from a store clerk.

Adolescent relationships are marked by increasing autonomy.[141] Youth social networks expand beyond the family and friendships arranged by parents. Adolescents begin to initiate friendships of their own choosing and begin to form intimate relationships. They also begin to form relationships with adults outside the family and increasingly see teachers, coaches, or other community members as mentors. Thus, transition is a time when adolescents begin to build a larger social network beyond the family.

Friendships and Youth with Disabilities

Many students with disabilities, especially those with intellectual and developmental disabilities, experience far fewer social interactions and social invitations than their peers without disabilities.[114,126,130] A study of youth ages 5 to 17 years found that those without disabilities participated in significantly more social activities with peers compared with those with ASD and intellectual disabilities. Social activities included playing games, sleepovers, and going out to places in the community.[117] Youth with different disabilities also experience a varying amount of social contact and social participation experiences. Of adolescents ages 13 to 17 years with ASD, 43% reported never seeing friends, compared with 15.7% of youth with intellectual disabilities. A common method of communication among teenagers is the phone,[50] yet 47.7% of youth with intellectual disabilities report getting calls from friends once a week, but only 9.6% of youth with ASD report getting calls from friends more than once a week.[110]

High school students with disabilities receiving special education services in public schools often remain socially isolated because of the possibility of disability-related stigma[47] and other barriers to friendship opportunities, such as the presence of adult paraprofessionals and limited inclusion in nonacademic school activities.[72] Central to the concept of friendship for students with disabilities is the distinction that when students without disabilities receive some form of incentive (e.g., money, class credit, volunteer experience) to spend time with a classmate labeled with a developmental disability, it is not friendship.[82,85,109] However, often programs that foster relationships through matching or mentoring are the only opportunities for youth with and without disabilities to interact. Such programs may be an avenue for those without disabilities to begin to understand better that youth with disabilities have interests, feelings, and experiences similar to those of all teenagers.[20,22] Sometimes these programs can lead to meaningful and long-lasting friendships, as in the story of Joshua and Stephanie (Case Study 12-1).

The element of choice is the essential component of friendship between all youth, with and without disabilities.[107,120] Meaningful friendships between high school students with

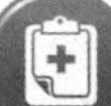

CASE STUDY 12-1 The Friendship of Stephanie and Joshua: Defining Friendship on Their Own Terms

Stephanie and Joshua were sophomores at East High School, a suburban public high school in the northeastern United States with an approximate population of 1100 students. Stephanie is an outgoing young woman with an easygoing nature who does not have a disability. Joshua is an outgoing young man with a playful nature who has Menkes syndrome. He is very expressive with his facial features and watches everything going on around him, constantly looking to interact with people who are close by. He uses a wheelchair, does not speak words, and needs support with most daily tasks because his one consistent movement is to reach out with his left hand. The two have been friends since they met as reading partners in an inclusive fifth grade classroom. From then, Stephanie followed the general education curriculum in classes with her peers while Joshua received special education services in a separate, self-contained class.

One day, Stephanie knelt to the right of Joshua's wheelchair and he reached across his body with his left hand toward her head. He flashed a wry grin, looking as if he knew exactly what he was doing when he tugged at her hair. She said, "Hey! Josh!" She pulled her hair out of his hand and stood back up. He laughed and she shook her head with a friendly and feigned look of exasperation. She smiled at him, and he straightened up with excitement in his wheelchair. They held hands for a moment before leaving.

Joshua displayed intentionality using one of the few movements that he can control to interact playfully with Stephanie. He demonstrated a type of slapstick humor that represents a complex form of nonspoken communication and helped form their connection. Whenever either one of them entered a room, they immediately scanned it to find the other and share a smile. They consistently expressed enjoyment to be together.

However, Stephanie struggled to describe her friendship with Joshua in any way other than with the immediate connection she felt with him:

We just kind of clicked and I felt comfortable with him from the start. Being with him is a lot of fun. He's always smiling and we just really get along. I can't imagine not seeing him.... We just click and it doesn't matter what either of us can do. We just have a close relationship. It shouldn't be compared to others. It's just our relationship.

Later, in an attempt to define friendship generally, she returned to the metaphor of clicking:

Oh, wow. Just having a bond. You can't explain it. You can't explain why you click, but you just do. You just mesh together with someone.

Joshua does not have a way to communicate by speaking words or selecting or typing words and letters. Stephanie stated that she knows what Joshua likes from spending so much time together and reading his facial expressions and reactions:

I know Joshua and I are such good friends because of all the time we spend together. Both of us know a lot about the other. Joshua is really good at sensing what kind of mood I'm in. I know he enjoys seeing me from his expression when I get there, happy, and when I leave, sad. I'd say for any friendship to become a great one you need to spend a lot of time with the friend. I'd say that any good friendship evolves from spending as much time together as possible.

and without developmental disabilities are chosen individually, occur outside friendship programs, and are based on shared interests.[3,11,14,30,35,82,100,107,116,113,118,120]

These relationships are defined by the value of human reciprocity.[64] In a self-report study, almost all adolescents ages 12 to 18 years with ASD (96%) reported having at least one friend, whereas 86% of their parents reported that the same youth had at least one friend.[74] When comparing the names of friends listed by adolescents themselves and their parents, adolescents and parents agreed 60% on the adolescent's best friend; however, 21% of the adolescents and parents listed completely different names of friends.[74] These findings may indicate that youth may define or understand friendship in a way different from adults. For example, one study of friendships between high school students with and without disabilities found that young people did not want friendships to be defined by outside expectations (see Case Study 12-1).

Education and Postsecondary Training

The societal role of student is commonly associated with the time period of adolescence. Our modern conceptualization of education includes a formalized setting in which adults with expertise provide youth with the knowledge and skills needed to be successful in society.[86] Secondary school, vocational training, and higher education are formal education contexts named in the ICF. These educational contexts require youth to engage with others to achieve learning outcomes.

Research on children's participation in school-related settings often varies, making it difficult to draw decisive conclusions in regard to the participation patterns of children with disabilities in school. A national survey of teachers (N = 1180)[112] found that 50% to 60% of students with disabilities were rated as "fully participating" in learning-related activities such as science labs, library use, or art classes, and 69% fully participated in field trips. How do we know if this reported rate of academic participation is problematic or lower than in students without disabilities?

Using the Participation and Environment Measure—Children and Youth, Coster et al.[34] reported on the differences in participation patterns for youth with and without disabilities living in the United States and Canada (Research Note 12-1). Youth with disabilities were less likely to get together with peers outside class and less likely to participate in school-sponsored team activities, clubs, or organizations (Figure 12-5). In addition, in the school context, youth with and without disabilities reported differences in the environmental barriers encountered and environmental supports available to them. Overall, students with disabilities are more likely to encounter features in the environment that make it difficult to engage in school activities (Figure 12-6). These barriers do not appear to be ameliorated by other resources; up to 20% of parents have reported that the school resources are inadequate (Figure 12-7).

Overall, this study paints a picture of school participation disparities for youth with disabilities who are ages 12 to 17 years and highlights the need for supports and services that support optimal social participation and inclusion at school. Such participation disparities could explain why some research finds that youth with disabilities in the United States have a higher dropout or incompletion rate (17%) than students without disabilities (11%).[57]

RESEARCH NOTE 12-1

Community Participation of Children and Youth with and without Disabilities

Using the Participation and Environment Measure—Children and Youth, Bedell and colleagues explored the community participation patterns of children and youth with disabilities compared with their typically developing peers.[12] The study included over 500 children and youth ages 5 to 17 years from the United States and Canada. Half of the sample included youth with disabilities; disability categories ranged from mobility limitations to intellectual and development disabilities. Parents used the PEM-CY to report frequency of participation in a range of activities in the community. The scale ranged from never (0) to daily (7). Parents also reported on the absence or presence of environmental barriers, as well as the adequacy of resources.

The study found that young people identified as having a disability participated in community activities at significantly decreased rates when compared with youth without disabilities (Figure 12-2). In addition, environmental supports and barriers were shown to vary drastically between youth with and without disabilities. Youth with disabilities experience a higher rate of barriers in the community environment (Figure 12-3). Furthermore, parents of youth with disabilities reported inadequate resources to address these barriers. At least 50% or more parents reported that public transportation, programs and services, equipment and supplies, and money were not adequate to support consistent community participation (Figure 12-4).

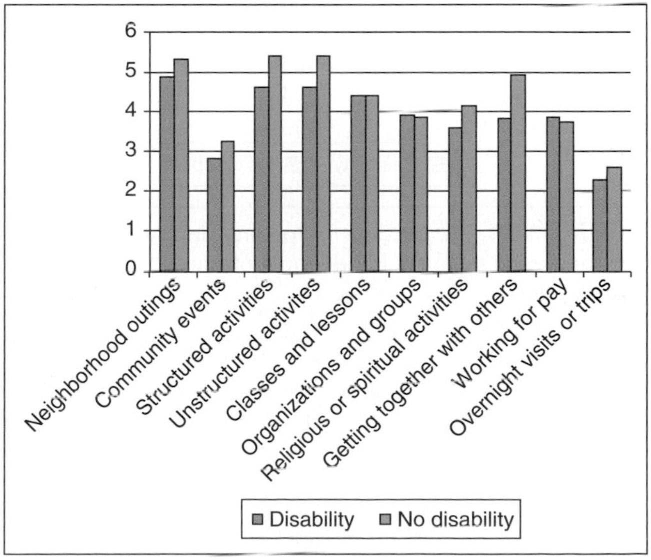

FIGURE 12-2 Mean frequency of participation in Community Participation Involvement of Youth.

Work and Prevocational Experiences

Acquiring and keeping a part-time, full-time, or volunteer job is an important societal role. Many first employment experiences occur during adolescence in informal positions such as

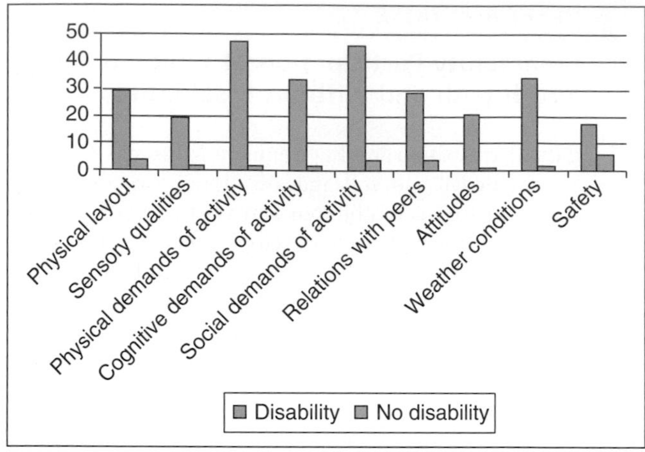

FIGURE 12-3 Percentage of parents indicating that a feature of the environment makes it harder for their child with a disaility to be involved in community activities.

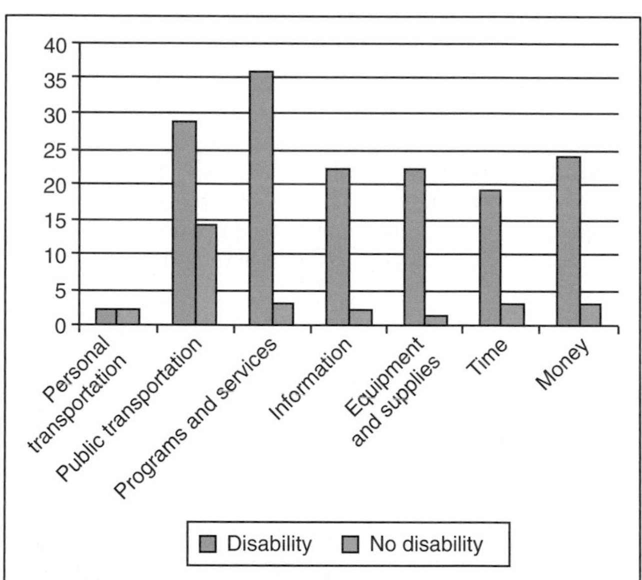

FIGURE 12-4 Percentage of parents indicating that an environmental resource is inadequate to support community participation.

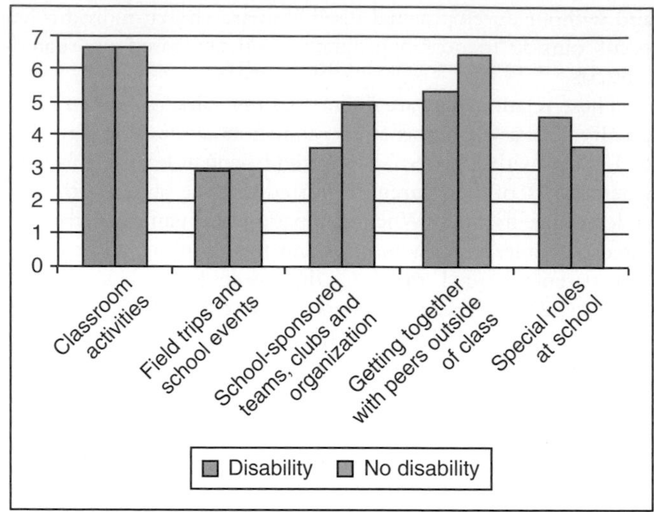

FIGURE 12-5 Mean frequency of participation involvement of school participation of youth with and without disabilities, ages 12-17 years.

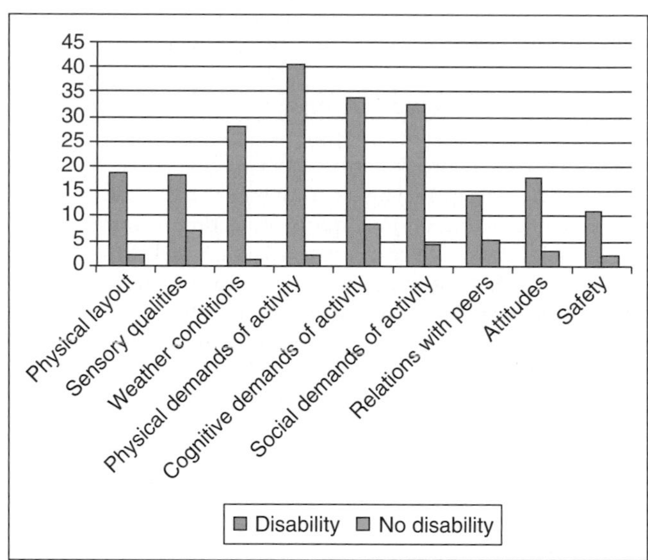

FIGURE 12-6 Percentage of parents of youth ages 12-17 years indicating that a feature of the school environment makes it harder to participate in an activity.

babysitting or landscaping or part-time work in community stores. These experiences provide youth with the opportunity to develop the skills they need to be successful employees after transition to adulthood. Employment also provides youth with an identity and is a mechanism to increase their autonomy from their parents and families.[141] Paid employment also provides them with the opportunity to engage as an economic participant in society, which includes purchasing goods, owning a checking account, and increasing economic self-sufficiency by saving and acquiring resources such as a car.

For adolescents and young adults with disabilities, employment experiences during their transition years may not lead to long-term employment. Recent national surveys have shown that only 21% of working-age adults with disabilities in the United States (ages 18-64 years) are employed, compared with 59% of working-age adults without disabilities.[57] A myriad of factors affect the employment of persons with disabilities, including lack of adequate vocational training, discrimination from others, and provision of essential medical benefits that are dependent on income level.[57] A recent study found that for youth with significant disabilities, such as ASD and intellectual disabilities, one predictor of employment in early adulthood after controlling for disability severity was summer vocational experiences during high school and parent expectations of future employment during high school.[41] Occupational therapists can play an important role in helping adolescents and young adults with disabilities identify, secure, and participate in employment. The Project TEAM case study gives an example of one manualized intervention that supported the career goals of Emily, a young lady with an intellectual disability.

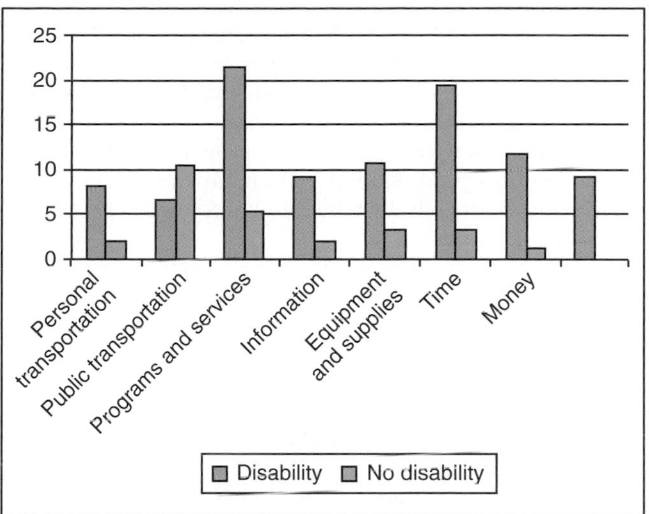

FIGURE 12-7 Percentage of parents of youth ages 12-17 years indicating that an environmental resource was inadequate to support school participation.

Community Life, Religion, and Citizenship

Community organizations such as charities, clubs, and professional organizations provide youth with opportunities to engage in contexts outside their families and schools. Involvement in cultural organizations may also contribute to an adolescent's identity development. Although youth may belong to the same religious community as their family, adolescence may be a time in which young people engage in more independent exploration of their spiritual beliefs, with a deepening or withdrawal from the family's selected spiritual community. They may also become more involved in local civic life as they become increasingly aware of problems in their communities and as they approach voting age. They may become involved in advocating for local or national legislation and policies that reflect their expanding belief systems. A national survey of adults in the United States found that persons with and without disabilities are equally likely to vote in national elections.[57] For an example of the positive impact of group political advocacy on the social participation of young adults with disabilities, see Box 12-2.

BOX 12-2 Group Political Disability Advocacy in Young Adulthood

Desiree Forte, MS.Ed., and Ryan Levia, Disability Advocate

Act Today, Influence Tomorrow (ATIT)* is a youth advocacy group formed to give youth with disabilities an outlet to help promote change and bring attention to issues surrounding disability rights. The group comes together one Saturday a month to focus on issues chosen by the youth, such as state graduation requirements, community issues, disability history, and disability awareness. For many of the young people, this is their first time being fully exposed to the disability community and a way to be out independently. This group also gives them a chance to gain the tools they need to help improve their quality of life by spending one Saturday a month not feeling different or isolated. Disabled youth† who do not have access to a group like this can become uncomfortable and lack the proper etiquette of being around other people with disabilities. This can lead to having poor self-esteem and being uncomfortable about their own situations. By being part of a group such as this, youth have been able to learn how to work with others and deal with some of the issues they face surrounding disability. We are two young adults, Ryan and Desi, who benefited tremendously from being a part of this group in our late teens and early 20s, and we collaborated to write this article.

ATIT was originally created in collaboration between multiple disability agencies (Boston Center for Independent Living and Easter Seals Massachusetts).* This collaboration allowed us to network and connect with other youth programs, giving us the avenues to expand personally and as a group. For example, Ryan later gained employment from a program he learned about by being part of ATIT. The mentor and supporters with and without disabilities who also attended the meetings provided additional networking opportunities. For example, a supporter from the group provided Desi with work experience, helping greatly improve her skills and resume. Both of us gained a wealth of knowledge about how advocacy and working with others can help increase disability awareness and promote positive change.

In 2009, the group decided that a major issue in Massachusetts was lack of a month recognizing disability. The group was also concerned about the lack of disability history and awareness being taught in public schools. The group felt strongly that by teaching students about disability, it would lower the negative stigma and decrease bullying. With the help of the group's mentors, a bill was drafted to establish the month of October as Disability History and Awareness Month in Massachusetts. As a group, everyone worked to promote the bill through word of mouth and social media to build support for the cause. When it came time for the group's voice to be heard at the State House, members of the group testified before the Senate Oversight Committee. The group also held a rally at the State House to make one final push. In less than 1 year of filing, the bill was passed. This means that every year, the governor issues a proclamation declaring October Disability History and Awareness Month in Massachusetts. For everyone, individually and as a group, this proclamation was a huge accomplishment.

Creating and passing a bill was an eye-opening and educational experience for all involved. By working as a group, members of ATIT learned the importance of advocating for what they believe in, along with the effort it takes to have our voices heard. Everyone also learned more about the process of government and that government officials were not as hard to face as initially thought. Although this process became overwhelming at times, the group learned that by working together, the process was more enjoyable and that as a group our voice becomes much louder. The group continues to work today to help spread awareness about Disability History Month and is trying to find a way to mandate that disability history and awareness be taught in public schools and universities. As time goes on, the group dynamics are constantly changing as members become older and new ones join. Still, the positive effects of being part of a group such as this will never change, and youth will continue to learn and grow by working with great peers and mentors.

*ATIT is now the Massachusetts Easter Seals Youth Leadership Network.

†Person first language, such as youth with disabilities, is a respectful way to write about people with disabilities. However, some members of the disability community choose to use the term *disabled* to describe a person to highlight the centrality of disability to their identity. This reflects a positive and empowered disability identity.

The benefits to participating in community service are clear; for example, youth who participate in volunteer service are more likely to have higher grades and graduate from college.[36,108] Providing service learning opportunities in middle school and high school also appears to be associated with reduced disciplinary referrals.[101] Providing youth with disabilities with the opportunities to engage in community service may be one way to increase their social networks and support successful transition to adulthood. However, they may not be as involved in community, civic, and religious organizations as those without disabilities. Only one in six adults with disabilities has participated in a group or organized activity that advocates for the rights of people with disabilities, and those with at least some college education are more likely to participate in advocacy.[57] Youth with disabilities also report low levels of civic engagement; only 35% of youth with autism and 33% of youth with intellectual disabilities ages 13 to 17 years completed volunteer or community service.[110] Innovative programs such as EPIC Service Warriors (Case Study 12-2) can provide unique opportunities for youth with disabilities to build social networks and serve their community.

Persons with and without disabilities also differ in religious participation; 50% of adults with disabilities attend religious services regularly compared with 57% of adults without

CASE STUDY 12-2 EPIC Service Warriors: "Discover Greatness Through Service"

EPIC Service Warriors is a community service and education program for youth with disabilities between the ages of 16 and 23 (Figure 12-8). By creating the change they want to see in the world, the Service Warriors learn more about local communities and develop practical skills that will help them develop as leaders and pursue future goals. This program also flips the switch on assumptions of many community members by changing the position of power; instead of being served, youth with disabilities serve others.

The EPIC Service Warriors Program runs from April to March. During the year, a team of Service Warriors participates in an Opening Day and Orientation in April, completes a minimum of 11 community service and skill-building projects in the greater Boston Area, and attends a graduation celebration at the end of its service year. Graduates of the program have the opportunity to become Service Leaders for future teams of Service Warriors. The Service Warriors are also supported by a staff of persons with and without disabilities.

Each month, the Service Warriors engage in a day of service such as a clean-up of a local park or school, making food at homeless shelters and food kitchens, and wrapping toys for a toy drive. Often, the Service Warriors partner with other service and community organizations for the day of service. Partnering not only increases manpower for the service day, but also increases the other organizations' awareness of the capacity of youth with disabilities and demonstrates how service organizations can become more inclusive (Figure 12-9).

Each service day begins with a team-building activity, such as sharing something "epic" that each warrior has accomplished since the previous service day. The team then begins completing the service task. Although the EPIC Executive Director, Jeff Lafata, ensures that each site is physically accessible so all members can "get in the door," he does not provide any preliminary training or task modification. Instead, the philosophy "if you need us, tell us" guides the day. Together, the Service Warriors figure out how to accomplish their service task. At the end of the service day, the group engages in a critical discussion about the assumptions that others may have toward specific areas of the community or members of the community. Questions such as "What did you expect?" and "What did you see?" help young people reflect. For example, after a park clean-up service day in a neighborhood with a reputation for violence and poverty, the group reflected that many members of the community were spending time at the park, and the neighborhood was vibrant and active.

The stories of two recent graduates of the EPIC Service Warriors program, Lloyd and Pat, illustrate how engagement in community service builds skills, increases self-determination, and enhances social participation.

epic
young leaders with ability

FIGURE 12-8

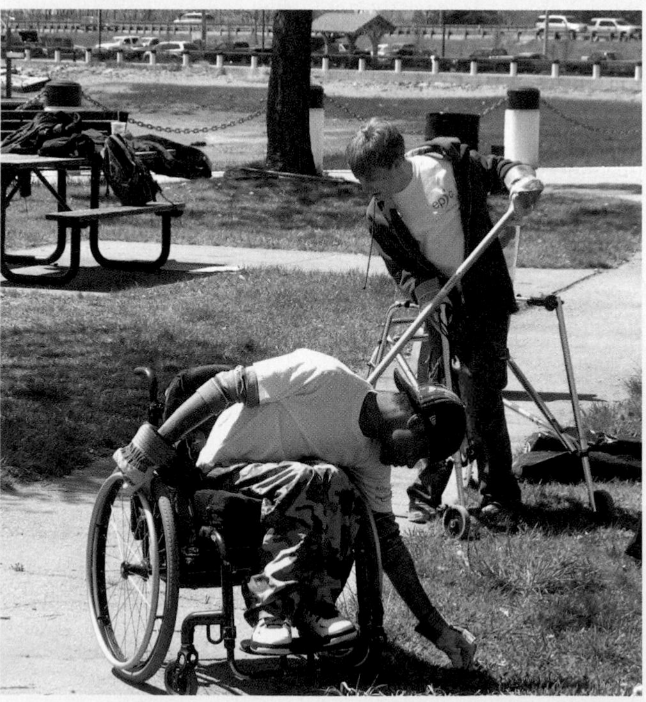

FIGURE 12-9 EPIC Service Warriors clean up their community.

CASE STUDY 12-2 EPIC Service Warriors: "Discover Greatness Through Service"—cont'd

When Lloyd began Service Warriors, he was 20 and experiencing "huge struggle(s)." He had been homeless and received "personal" help through the state Department of Developmental Services (DDS). After securing an emergency placement at a short-term residential facility, Lloyd still had to deal with drama and difficulty with schoolwork and paperwork related to his learning disability. Through a teacher, and after completing a disability awareness training, Lloyd found out about EPIC Service Warriors and signed up because he wanted to "find something to do."

Lloyd's favorite service project was helping at a community farm that grew food for local meal programs and food pantries. During this project, Lloyd pulled weeds and dead plants, removed vegetables that had been destroyed by animals, and prepared an area for future planting. Lloyd explains, "They don't have time to do certain things" because the farm is nonprofit and relies on community volunteers. The EPIC Service Warriors also learned about the cost of food and the resources needed to ship food to people. This is important because "people need food—we have families and group settings" who all need food. Lloyd also tasted his first fresh carrot that day, right out the ground. Working at the community farm helped Lloyd "reflect on what I do" and remember how much he enjoyed working outside. He had a summer job working for the city's housing authority in landscaping and indoor remodeling. He found employment as a bus monitor, supervising a young boy during the long trip from his town to a specialized program several cities away. However, his experiences on the farm led Lloyd to seek assistance from EPIC staff and DDS caseworkers to seek a new job. Lloyd was offered a position in the Department of Public Works in the city where he now lived. Lloyd even met the mayor, who visited the city workers on the first day of training to thank them for their service to the community. Lloyd directly connected his experience with Service Warriors with this new job: "[It made me] realize that values of the community are very important. Being around with people and interacting—making sure our community is clean and safe and making it a better place so everyone can live and be happy. I want to see people be happy about their community, how it's clean. My new job has that same value—it's bunched up into one."

Before coming to Service Warriors, Pat had been in other groups and activities. He was in 11th grade and working on passing standardized tests in English, math, and science required for a high school diploma. Pat shared: "I am one of those types of people that doesn't pick something myself and look around. My mom picks it out and then I try it to see if I like it." He had tried track, basketball, and music group. He also worked in the school store and had janitorial experience working with his uncle. He also was attending an after-school club, "a hangout, chill out club. But it wasn't much, mostly set for kids with disabilities. I felt I didn't have a place."

Service Warriors was different. Pat explained, "We get a different task every time—it's full of variety. And plus it's never boring.... Plus a lot of the Service Warriors are supportive and sociable and they have a lot going for them, like I have. It's one laugh after another." Pat enjoyed giving back to the community on issues that were important to him, like people who are homeless or can't afford food. He enjoyed the day of service at a local agency providing services, supports, and housing to homeless individuals . They made salads and also packed up sandwiches in bags for the visitors. He also enjoyed painting a mural of a school motto during another school clean-up day. Pat described how this service activity was aligned with one of his talents: "I am an art freak. I find painting fascinating and I like to try my hand at it. So when I am given the privilege, it's the most exciting thing that could happen art-wise. I am fond of painting inside the lines."

Pat described how he accomplished all the different service activities throughout the year. "Sometimes when I am new to a position, I kind of do it with other group members to see how they do it, and see if we can help each other. Then when I get the hang of it, I do it by myself. I got help by asking, they demonstrated, and then I handled it pretty decently and independently." However, Pat noted that some of the activities were difficult and didn't always go well, such as when he tried to make a fleece blanket. The blanket took all day to make and required help from the Service Warriors, but by working as a team they were able to finish the blanket.

Programs like Service Warriors can expand the social networks of teenagers and young adults with disabilities. Lloyd explained how the group increased their bonds over time: "Around the middle of the year we started to interact with each other. By the time we hit toward the end of the year I was emotional. We made huge connections.... I am still in touch with some of them, and now that I am a Service Leader, I am with the new team." Pat described how working with others toward common goals can help individuals achieve their personal goals. Pat shared that "being in EPIC extends back to one of my goals since I was younger—to be great to myself, to be great in this world. I was born to be great and I wanted to do something worthwhile for my family to make them proud. In EPIC, every one of us is supportive. I expected [EPIC staff] to support us, but it never ceases to amaze me.... we were all supporting each other." See Figure 12-10.

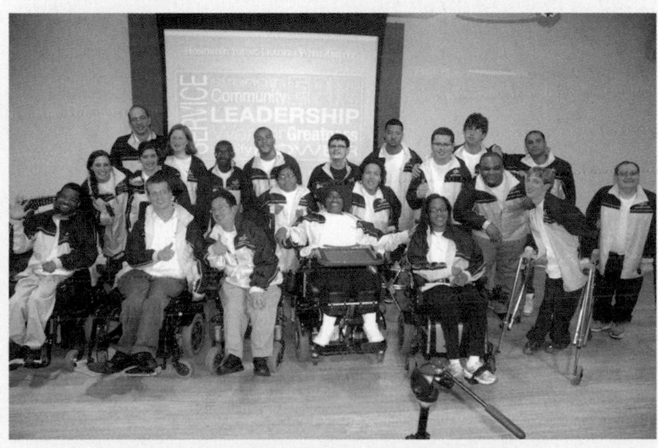

FIGURE 12-10 EPIC Service Warriors.

Continued

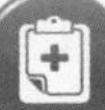

CASE STUDY 12-2 EPIC Service Warriors: "Discover Greatness Through Service"—cont'd

Programs that take a positive approach to disability and provide youth with the opportunity to challenge themselves in a supportive environment can *change how youth with disabilities think about themselves* and their abilities. Lloyd shared the following:

Being in Service Warriors helped me build up confidence and self-advocating for yourself, having strength in you. I need to overcome the situation.... We are living in a situation where it's very tough and there always need to be some resources.... Without us, other groups may not be able to provide help to other people.... You are setting a good example for a community. You are showing young people that you can do it, that you can tell them, "Hey listen, I did this. I want you to take this opportunity and show me." I want to guide them along and show them the steps. You have to accept that you have a disability and it's a natural thing ... back then when I was younger I didn't realize ... I always wanted to be better.... Basically, at the end, you have to share what your talents are.

Lloyd's statement also demonstrates how changes in his self-perception led him to reach out to other youth, further expanding his own social networks as well as the social networks of others.

Pat shared a similar feeling about realizing his capacity through the support of the group:

You kind of use your talents that you never knew before, but then you can unleash. For example, when we were doing a school clean-up around a ball field, there was so much to pick up. I picked up a whole lot more than I could have forced myself to if I was doing it on a regular basis and not with EPIC. But with EPIC you can make it happen in a massive way.

Like Lloyd, Pat's personal experiences with EPIC led to a desire to reach out to others. He is a Service Leader for the next team of Service Warriors and tried to introduce the idea of doing community service to his after-school club: "At one point I was motivated [and] I asked other members if they considered doing so and they said no. But it's different in EPIC.... One purpose is not just making a difference, but to have each of our lives be great, each of our lives epic."

disabilities.[57] Only about 27% of youth with autism or intellectual disability reported that they belonged to a religious youth group,[110] but belonging to a community of faith and incorporating those values into everyday life is important for persons with disabilities.[19] One study about faith participation was conducted with over 400 families that included U.S. youth and young adults with disabilities ages 0 to 30 years. Families reported the following affected the inclusion and participation of families with disabilities in congregations: (1) knowledge of disability and how best to support people with disabilities, (2) practices and supports available in the congregation, (3) attitudes and religious beliefs about disability, and (4) characteristics of the congregation, such as accessibility and size.[62] Engagement in religious communities is not only important for the spiritual well-being and developing identity of young people with disabilities, but can also expand their social networks. For example, families reported that over 60% of youth with disabilities engage in congregational activities with same-age peers. Occupational therapists can provide population-based services by identifying physical and social religious environments that are more likely to facilitate the inclusion and social participation of youth with disabilities and their families.

Recreation and Leisure

As young people better identify their interests and hobbies, they devote more time to self-selected recreational and leisure activities that support their growing skills and identity.[32] The ICF defines recreation and leisure as any form of play, recreation, or leisure activity that is informal or organized. "Hanging out" with friends at a local coffee shop, joining a community sports league, or playing in a band are all ways in which a young person engages in social participation. Often, these recreational activities are supported by youth's increasing economic independence and the money earned in part-time or informal employment.

Research suggests that there may be disparities in the social participation of youth with and without disabilities in recreation and leisure activities. In one study that included youth with autism and intellectual disabilities, 16% to 23% belonged to a sports team and 7% to 10% belonged to a performing group.[110] Research Note 12-1 summarizes the findings of a study comparing the participation of youth with and without disabilities in community activities, which included recreational and leisure activities and unstructured social interactions. Limited involvement in leisure and recreational activities can have a detrimental impact on the future development of young people with disabilities. Research with high school youth has shown that involvement in recreational and leisure activities provides young people with the opportunity to develop social skills, such as negotiation and compromise and emotional regulation (Research Note 12-2). Youth with disabilities may not experience these benefits if they do not participate in recreational and leisure activities.

Changes in Social Participation Over Time

Patterns of changes of social participation over time are less understood for young people with disabilities transitioning to adulthood. Some studies may provide insight about how social participation can change as youth transition to adulthood. For those with significant physical disabilities, such as cerebral palsy, spina bifida, and acquired brain injury, youth in early adolescence ages 12 to 14 years were found to participate significantly less in recreational activities than younger children with similar disabilities.[78] A recent cross-sectional study found that elementary and middle school children with disabilities have significantly greater odds of participating in organized activities in comparison to preschool or high school youth with disabilities.[91] These studies could imply a pattern in which older youth with disabilities have fewer opportunities, supports, or less time or desire to participate in organized activities.

RESEARCH NOTE 12-2

Differing Profiles of Developmental Experiences across Types of Organized Youth Activities

Larson and colleagues[76] asked youth to reflect on the various skills or developmental opportunities that resulted from participation in different organized activities. The youth self-reported using the Youth Experiences Survey (YES) 2.0, which includes items that ask about specific skills and opportunities associated with positive development into adulthood, such as developing positive relationships, initiative, and exploring one's identity. Eleventh-grade students ($N = 2280$) from 19 high schools in Illinois participated in the study.

The authors calculated the mean response for each item on the YES for all 2280 responses. The authors then grouped the responses based on the type of activity youth referenced during their self-reports (e.g., sports, fine arts), and calculated the mean for each item. The means were then compared to determine whether different types of activities were more likely to support different opportunities and skills for youth transitioning to adulthood.

Sports. Youth reported significantly more opportunities to develop initiative and emotional regulation and engage in teamwork while participating in sports compared with other organized activities represented. They reported fewer opportunities to engage in identity work, develop positive relationships, and network with adults during organized sport activities.

Performance and Fine Arts: Youth who participated in fine arts programs reported significantly higher rates of initiative. Compared with other activities, performing arts supported fewer opportunities for teamwork, positive relationships, and adult networking experiences.

Academic Clubs and Organizations: Youth reported significantly fewer opportunities for all skills and developmental experiences during engagement in academic clubs and organizations compared with other activities.

Community-Oriented Activities: Compared with other activities, youth who participated in community-oriented activities reported significantly more opportunities to network with adults but significantly fewer opportunities to engage in teamwork and develop emotional regulation.

Service Activities: Youth in service activities reported significantly more opportunities for teamwork, building positive relationships, and networking with adult compared with other activities. They also reported significantly lower rates of developing emotional regulation through service activities.

Faith-Based Youth Groups: Youth who participated in faith-based youth groups reported significantly more opportunities for all skills and developmental experiences on the YES when compared with other activities.

Negative Developmental Experiences: Stress was reported to be higher than the average in sports and lower in academic, service, and faith-based activities. Regardless of gender, Socio-economic status and ethnicity, youth reported similar rates of both positive and negative experiences in various organized activities.

However, it is difficult to draw these conclusions from cross-sectional research that does not explore change in the same cohort of youth over time. One nationally representative, longitudinal database, the National Longitudinal Transition Study 2 (NLTS2; http://www.nlts2.org) followed students with disabilities over a period of 9 years. Findings from these NLTS2 data indicate significant social participation limitations in youth with disabilities. For example, many young adults with ASD age 17 to 21 years reported that in the previous year they had not gotten together with a friend (55%) or talked with a friend on the phone (64%).[80] Four years later, the same young adults reported more frequent contact with friends; only 38.6% had never seen friends and 47.2% had never received a call from friends.[97] Although social participation seemed to improve in this cohort as they became young adults, other factors, such as loss to follow-up, can affect the findings. Future research is needed in this area to understand how social participation may change during the transition to adulthood and identify how occupational therapists can best support the social participation of young adults with disabilities during this transition.

Evaluating Social Participation

Youth Self-Reports of Social Participation

Often, occupational therapists working with young people rely primarily on other professionals' or parents' perspectives.[31,119,133] However, studies have shown that youth's needs and concerns are not always recognized or shared by parents or other adults.[40,83,88,92,94] Also, parents have expressed difficulty providing proxy reports because they are not always aware of their child's feelings or familiar with what their son or daughter does at school or in the community.[59,68] Use of a parent report may be more problematic for transition-age youth who may not share their feelings with parents or who may engage in many activities without the direct supervision of parents. Thus, it is imperative to use youth self-report to understand and evaluate social participation.[106,125]

Child Occupational Self-Assessment

The Child Occupational Self-Assessment (COSA)[70] is a self-report of competence and value for daily activities based on the Model of Human Occupation.[65] COSA includes 25 items that represent daily activities that most youth encounter at home, school, and in their communities. Several items explicitly rate social participation, such as "doing things with classmates" and "doing things with friends." COSA also includes items that assess self-care, time management, and self-regulation. The primary purpose of COSA is to gather youth's perspectives about their participation and provide a mechanism for them to identify and create goals for occupational therapy.

Each COSA item is rated using two four-point scales: competence—I have a big problem doing this, I have a little problem doing this, I do this okay, I am really good at doing this—and importance—not really important to me, important to me, very important to me, most important of all to me. COSA can be completed in several ways. One form includes rating scale symbols to assist with comprehension; the importance scale uses an increasing number of stars, and the competence scale uses happy or sad faces. COSA also includes a card sort completion option and a summary matrix that may be used for reporting purposes by young people who do not need the symbols to understand the rating scales.

COSA is interpreted by identifying gaps between youth's perceived competence for an activity and the reported level of competence. The Model of Human Occupation posits that youth are at risk for poor occupational adaptation when one's perceived competence for a valued activity is low. Thus, COSA is used to identify potential areas in which social participation may put a youth at risk for poor occupational adaptation at home, in school, and in the community.

Studies have found that COSA items address concerns that are meaningful to youth with disabilities.[66,94] Therapists can use a variety of modifications during administration to ensure youth can access and understand the assessment.[69] COSA can be administered in several sessions, using different forms and simplified rating scales.[68] These types of accommodations are essential to ensuring that young people have a voice in the intervention planning process.

Youth Experience Survey

The Youth Experience Survey (YES) 2.0[55,56] is a self-report instrument designed to capture high school students' developmental experiences in an organized youth activity, such as an extracurricular activity or community-based program. The survey is designed to ask about experiences that have been shown to promote positive development into adulthood.

Items in YES focus mainly on positive developmental experiences. Three domains are related to personal development: identity work, initiative, and basic skills. Three domains measure interpersonal development: teamwork and social skills, positive relationships, and adult networks and social capital. Items from each of these positive domains can be further grouped into subscales for a total of 17 scales. YES also has a negative experiences domain that measures negative experiences that young people may encounter. The domain has a total of five scales that address stress, inappropriate adult behavior, negative influence, social exclusion, and negative group dynamics.

Questions in each domain are worded in the first person and are statements about feelings or things that may have happened during participation in extracurricular activities. Some example questions that can be relevant to social participation are as follows:

- "Learned that my emotions affect how I perform" (emotional regulation scale)
- "Learned that working together requires compromise" (teamwork and social skills scale)
- "Got to know people in the community" (adult networks and social capital scale)

Youth rate each question on a four-point scale to indicate if they experienced the question during participation, from 1, not at all, to 4, yes, definitely. Each scale score is then computed as an average in which scores can range from 1 to 4. These scaled scores can then be aggregated to the domain level.

Other Youth Self-Report Measures

Other youth self-reports, discussed elsewhere in this text, may also be appropriate to assess social participation. One example is the Canadian Occupational Performance Measure (COPM), which is used in the case of Kara. Another example is the recently developed self-report participation measure, the Questionnaire of Young People's Participation (QYPP). This is aligned with the ICF and includes items that capture information about interpersonal relationships; education; employment; and community, social, and civic life. QYPP has been validated with adolescent and young adults with cerebral palsy in England.[122]

Other evidence-based measures that are not explicitly about social participation may provide therapists with information about young people's feelings or perceptions that could affect social participation choices, including the following:

- Measures of self-determination, such as the AIR Self-Determination Scale[140] and Arc Self-Determination Scale,[134] assess youth's perceived abilities to set and achieve goals of personal importance. Higher levels of self-determination in high school have been linked with more successful postsecondary transition outcomes relevant to social participation, including employment and independent living.[135,136]
- The Self-Perception Profile for Adolescents[58] includes subscales of social competence and friendships.
- Assessments of leisure engagement or role participation, such as the Children's Assessment of Participation and Enjoyment (CAPE), Preferences for Activities of Children (PAC), and the Role Checklist, can be used to document areas of interest and identify new activities that may facilitate social participation.
- Goal attainment scaling[63] may be an effective approach to track progress toward individual social participation goals (see Chapter 24). Goal attainment levels can be developed by therapists in collaboration with youth and their families. For example, Project TEAM used goal attainment scaling to evaluate Emily's outcomes after completing the training.

Parent Assessments of Social Participation

Participation and Environment Measure—Children and Youth

The Participation and Environment Measure—Children and Youth (PEM-CY) is a parent report instrument that examines participation and environment across three settings: home, school, and community. Participation items for each setting represent types of activities typically performed in that environment about which the parent would likely have knowledge. There are ten items in the home section, five in the school section, and ten in the community section. Many of the items relate to social participation, for example, "socializing using technology" (home section), "getting together with peers outside of class" (school section), and "community events" (community section). For each activity type, the parent is asked to identify how frequently the youth participates (from daily [7] to never [0]) over the past 4 months; how involved the youth is while participating (five-point response scale ranging from very involved to minimally involved); and whether the parent would like to see the youth's participation in this type of activity change (no or yes; if yes, the parent can select whether he or she would like to see a change in frequency, level of involvement, or variety).

After answering the participation questions for each setting, the parent is then asked whether certain features of the environment help or make it harder for the youth to participate in activities in that setting; response options include not an issue, usually helps, sometimes helps, sometimes makes harder, and usually makes harder. Additional questions are about perceived adequacy of resources such as information, money, or supplies; response options include not needed, usually yes, sometimes yes and sometimes no, and usually no.

Summary scores for the PEM-CY were constructed to provide the most useful information for the intended purpose of the instrument.[33] Most of the summary scores are computed as percentages of a particular response or the maximum percentage possible. The maximum percentage possible is particularly suited for calculation of summary scores in situations in which data are missing because not all items are applicable.

Pediatric Evaluation of Disability Inventory—Computer Adaptive Test: Responsibility Domain

The Pediatric Evaluation of Disability Inventory (PEDI), originally published in 1992, is currently available as the Pediatric Evaluation of Disability Inventory Computer Adaptive Test (PEDI-CAT).[52] This is a clinical assessment for children and youth that can be used across all diagnoses, conditions, and settings.

PEDI-CAT is comprised of a comprehensive item bank of 276 functional activities acquired throughout infancy, childhood, and young adulthood. It can be completed by parent or caregiver report or professional judgment of clinicians or educators who are familiar with the child. PEDI-CAT is recommended for use with children approaching 1 year and up to 21 years of age. PEDI-CAT provides normative T-scores, age percentiles, and a criterion score.

PEDI-CAT includes four domains: daily activities, mobility, social/cognitive, and responsibility. The social/cognitive domain assesses the ability to interact with others in a community and participate in one's family and culture. The items address four content areas: communication, interaction, everyday cognition, and self-management. Some items on the social/cognitive domain assess skills that can facilitate social participation (e.g., "shows positive reactions to friends' success such as congratulating a peer for scoring a goal or doing well on a test"). The items in this domain are rated using four-point difficulty scale, from unable (1) to easy (4).

The responsibility domain is a unique measure of participation and management of higher level tasks essential for independent living and successful transition to adulthood. The responsibility rating scale measures the shift of responsibility from parents to the young person. The responsibility domain addresses overall independence in managing essential life tasks rather than requiring independent performance. Responsible management of essential life tasks may include seeking assistance or resources as needed or directing others to accomplish the task. Thus, the responsibility domain is aligned with the ICF's concept of participation.

The responsibility domain items address four content areas: staying safe, taking care of daily needs, organization and planning, and health management. Some items on the responsibility domain pertain specifically to social participation (e.g., "choosing and arranging all social interactions") and items that assess skills that can support social participation (e.g., "planning and following a weekly schedule" and "traveling safely within in the community"). All items on the responsibility domain are rated using a five-point rating scale that measures the shift of responsibility from parents (1) to shared responsibility (3) to the young person taking all responsibility (5).

Child and Adolescent Scale of Participation

The Child and Adolescent Scale of Participation (CASP) measures the extent to which children participate in home, school, and community activities compared with children of the same age, as reported by family caregivers. It was originally designed to monitor outcomes and needs of children with traumatic and other acquired brain injuries (ABIs). The CASP subsequently has been used to assess children with other diagnoses.[10,105,128,137] CASP has been recommended as an assessment that is aligned with the ICF to measure participation.[1]

The CASP consists of 20 ordinal-scaled items and four subsections, some of which are aligned with social participation: (1) home participation (six items), (2) community participation (four items), (3) school participation (five items), and (4) home and community living activities (five items). The 20 items are rated on a four-point scale: "age expected (full participation)," "somewhat restricted," "very restricted," and "unable." A "not applicable" response is selected when the item reflects an activity in which the child would not be expected to participate because of age (e.g., work). Item, subsection, and total summary scores can be examined for use in research and practice. Higher scores reflect greater age-expected participation. CASP also includes open-ended questions that ask about effective strategies and supports and barriers that affect participation. Parent report and self-report versions are available. See Tables 12-1, 12-2, and 12-3 for descriptions of assessments.

Interventions to Facilitate Social Participation

Following an assessment of social participation, occupational therapists can develop interventions to address social participation difficulties by the following:

- Helping youth with disabilities acquire communication and interaction skills
- Identifying ways to modify the environment to support social participation
- Using peers to encourage social interactions and social participation.

As illustrated by the cases in this chapter, interventions that use these approaches can facilitate the social participation of youth transitioning to adulthood. The interventions featured in these cases are informed by a variety of conceptual models and use a range of strategies. These cases demonstrate that a range of theories and strategies can be integrated into interventions to improve social participation. Occupational therapists should use clinical reasoning to select the principles and strategies most likely to support social participation based on the circumstances, needs, and specific goals of each young person.

Skill-Focused Interventions

A range of interventions is used to improve communication skills of transition-age youth with autism and intellectual disabilities, including cognitive-behavioral approaches to teach self-monitoring, using prompting picture books and social

TABLE 12-1 Youth Self-Report Assessments Related to Social Participation

Instrument	Construct Assessed	Targeted Age	Respondent	Subscales and Domains Relevant to Social Participation	Example Item	Example Rating Scale
Child Occupational Self-Assessment (COSA)	Perceived competence and value for 25 everyday activities; responses can inform intervention planning.	7-18 yr	Youth self-report	Competence for everyday activities Value for everyday activities	Do things with friends. Do things with classmates. Have enough time to do things I like.	Competence: "I have a big problem doing this, I have a little problem doing this, I do this okay, I am really good at doing this" (scale includes happy and sad faces). Value: Not really important to me, important to me, really important to me, most important of all to me
Youth Experience Survey (YES)	Assessing developmental experiences resulting from a range of activities or programs that promote positive development into adulthood	High school	Youth self-report	Positive relationships (diverse peer relationships, prosocial norms) Teamwork and social skills (group process skills) Adult network and social capital (integration with family, linkages to community, linkages to work and college)	"Learned I had a lot in common with people from different backgrounds." "Learned how my emotions and attitude affect others in the group." "Got to know people in my community."	Yes, definitely; quite a bit; a little; not at all
ARC Self-Determination Scale	Identifying strengths and limitations in the area of self-determination	Adolescents to adults	Youth self-report	Autonomy Psychological empowerment	"I make friends with other kids my age." "My friends and I choose activities we want to do." "I will have a hard time making new friends" *or* "I will be able to make friends in new situations."	Autonomy: I do not even if I have the chance; I do sometimes when I have the chance; I do most of the time when I have the chance; I do every time I have the chance. Psychological empowerment: Choose between two statements.
AIR Self-Determination Scale	Assessing the capacity and opportunity to act self-determined in the contexts of home and school	Adolescents to young adults	Youth self-report (parallel parent or professional self-report available)	Items can be grouped into knowledge, ability, and perception for each context. Items are aligned with think-do-adjust process across contexts.	"People at school listen to me when I talk about what I want, what I need, or what I'm good at." "I have someone at home who can tell me if I am meeting my goals."	Never, almost never, sometimes, almost always, always
Self-Perception Profile for Adolescents	Perceived competence and self-worth	Adolescents	Youth self-report	Global self-worth, scholastics, social acceptance, job competence, friendships, behavior	"Some teenagers feel like they could do better at work they do for pay but other teenagers feel that they are doing really well at work they do for pay."	Contrast two statements: Sort of true for me, really true for me

TABLE 12-2 Parent Report Assessments Related to Social Participation

Instrument	Construct Assessed	Targeted Ages (yr)	Respondent	Subscales and Domains Relevant to Social Participation	Example Item	Example Rating Scale (points)
PEDI-CAT	Performance of daily activities Management of daily life tasks	0-21	Parent self-report	Social-cognitive Responsibility	"Shows positive reactions to friend's success such as congratulating a peer for scoring a goal or doing well on a test" "Choosing and arranging all social interactions"	Social-cognitive: Unable, hard, a little hard, easy Responsibility five-point scale: Adult or caregiver has full responsibility; the child does not take any responsibility (1) Child takes full responsibility without any direction, supervision, or guidance from an adult or caregiver (5)
PEM-CY	Participation in daily activities (frequency, involvement, and desire for change) Impact of the environment on participation (barriers and supports, resources)	Children and youth ages 5-17 yr	Parent report	Home participation, home environment School participation, school environment Community participation, community environment	"School-sponsored teams, clubs, and events" "Neighborhood outings (e.g., shopping at the store or mall, going to a movie, eating out at a restaurant, visiting the local library or bookstore)." "The social demands of typical activities (e.g., communication, interacting with others)"	Frequency (eight-point scale): Daily to never Involvement (five-point scale): Very involved to minimally involved Environmental barriers or supports: Not an issue; usually helps; sometimes helps, sometimes makes harder; usually makes harder Environmental resources: Usually yes; sometimes yes, sometimes no; usually no
CASP	Level of participation compared with same-aged peers	Children and youth ages 5-17 yr	Parent report (parallel youth self-report available)	Home participation Community participation School participation	"Social, play or leisure activities with family members at home (e.g., games, hobbies, 'hanging out')" "Communicating with other children and adults in the neighborhood and community"	Age-expected (full participation), somewhat restricted, very restricted, unable

TABLE 12-3 Research Evidence and Psychometric Properties of Featured Assessments

Assessment Name	Assessment Validity	Assessment Reliability	Other Evidence
Child and Adolescent Scale of Participation (CASP)	Both parent and youth report have strong internal consistency (a = 0.95 and 0.87 respectively)[87]	ICC analysis indicated moderate agreement between youth and parent reports (ICC = 0.63; 95% CI = 0.41 to 0.75), although youth reported their activity or participation to be significantly higher than their parents.[87]	
Child Occupational Self-Assessment (COSA)	Assessment items on each scale (competence, importance) form a unidimensional construct, and good item fit indicates the items work well together to measure each construct.[71,73]	Youth who are younger or who have intellectual disabilities are more likely to use the four-point rating scale incorrectly.[73] Parents and children disagreed 63.5% on competency and 61% on value responses. Substantial discrepancies (more than two rating categories) occurred on 20.5% of competency and 19% of value. Parents thought that their children saw themselves as less competent in occupations than the child reported to be.[94]	During administration, therapists reported providing accommodations: scheduling, presentation, and response format. Therapists also reported therapeutic use of self during the administration of COSA by developing rapport and empowering the child.[69]
Participation and Environment Measure—Children and Youth (PEM-CY)	The PEM-CY items work well together to measure participation across contexts. Internal consistency coefficients were 0.59 (home), 0.61 (school), and 0.70 (community) for participation frequency and 0.83 (home), 0.72 (school), and 0.75 (community) for involvement. Cronbach's alpha was ≥0.80 for all scales except home-supportiveness (0.67) and school resources (0.73). The PEM-CY can discriminate among youth with varying levels of participation. Two-way analyses of variance found a significant effect of disability across all settings. Additional analyses showed that these differences were consistent within each age interval. For children without disabilities, there was a significant increase in the range of activities in which children participated as they got older, but this pattern was not seen consistently in the children with disabilities.	Test-retest reliability estimates (intraclass correlation estimates) of the total scores for participation frequency (maximum percentage possible) were moderate for the school setting (0.58) and good for home and community (0.84 and 0.79, respectively). Reliability of the percentage who ever participates score was highest for the home (0.92) and school (0.82) settings, and lower for the community (0.66). Test-retest reliability for mean participation involvement scores was moderate to good: 0.71 for home, 0.76 for school, and 0.69 for the community. Test-retest reliability for the desire for change total score was consistently good (>0.75). Test-retest reliability estimates for the environment section summary scores were all good; intraclass correlation coefficients for supportiveness totals were 0.76 for the home, 0.87 for school, and 0.96 for the community. All reliability estimates for the environmental resources scores were >0.80, indicating good agreement across occasions in each setting.	The design of the instrument was based on results from focus groups and in-depth interviews with parents of children and youth with and without a variety of disabilities who helped define the relevant dimensions for measurement, activity types that were most applicable and important in each setting, and relevant features of the environment that affected their child's participation.[11]
Pediatric Evaluation of Disability Inventory—Computer Adaptive Test (PEDI-CAT)	Confirmatory factor analysis and item fit to a two-parameter item response theory model confirm that 60 items on the social-cognitive domain and 51 items making up the responsibility domain are unidimensional.[52]	Scores obtained on the social-cognitive and responsibility domain using the full item bank of 51 items and CAT of 15 items were highly correlated (both 0.99), indicating that CAT can produce an accurate measure in fewer items.[52] Test-retest reliability of the CAT was very high (ICC = 0.98 social cognitive; 0.96 responsibility).[39]	Parents reported satisfaction with the PEDI-CAT format.[39]
Youth Empowerment Survey (YES)	Items on each scale work well together to provide an acceptable measure of youth empowerment. Cronbach's alpha was ≥0.80 for all scales except negative group dynamics (0.75). The positive scales of the YES 2.0 (personal and interpersonal experiences) were moderately intercorrelated (15 of the 18 scales ranged from 0.50 to 0.60). The negative scales were also intercorrelated, ranging from 0.46 to 0.77.[55,56]	Significant and moderate correspondence was found between the students' and the leaders' responses on most of the YES scales. Emotional regulation and two subscales on the adult network domains were not significant.[55,56]	N/A

stories to facilitate interactions with others, and practicing specific communication skills in the context of games.[22,26] These interventions target youth's ability to initiate social interactions, take turns during conversation, engage in an increased variety of conversation topics, and enhance interaction quality.[22,26,103] Although these studies have found positive effects, the researchers examined specific social skills or measured communication skills on a second-by-second basis and did not consider social participation in the context of sustained social interactions.[26]

Occupational therapy interventions extend beyond working on social skills and target other factors to support successful social participation. Such interventions may include the following:

- Transportation and mobility training to increase youth's ability to access social activities
- Gathering information through print, the Internet, and over the phone about available social activities and programs
- Developing time and money management skills that facilitate continued participation in social activities
- Identifying self-regulation strategies that can make social participation more enjoyable for young people with anxiety, poor attention, or repetitive behaviors

Kara's case (Case Study 12-3) illustrates how an adolescent uses goal setting and metacognitive strategies in combination with skills training (e.g., managing a bank account, community mobility) to achieve higher level social participation. Kara was empowered to set her own goals that were meaningful and motivating to her. The therapist used a metacognitive approach, which allowed Kara to set her own goals and become the change agent as she took on more responsibilities and gained more independence. With support and guidance, Kara replicated the approach and achieved subsequent goals. With time, she began to internalize the process so that she could replicate it without assistance. This shift allowed her to continue to set and achieve her own social participation goals as she made her way into the adult world.

Environment-Focused Interventions

Understanding social participation as a *social process* may help occupational therapists implement interventions that go beyond communication and social skill building. Models such as the ICF (see earlier) stress that the environment is a primary contributor to participation and disability. Modification of the environment is a central component of occupational therapy practice.[4] During most occupational therapy interventions, parents or professionals adapt the environment on behalf of youth with disabilities, rather than teach youth with disabilities the skills needed to identify and advocate for environmental modifications. Thus, the young people remain dependent on the assistance of professionals. Environment-focused interventions need to involve youth themselves in actively generating and working to achieve solutions to challenges. As a result, modifications are more likely to be acceptable, and through the process of self-generating solutions, youth gain the knowledge and skills to be effective self-advocates.

Project TEAM (***T****eens making* ***E****nvironment and* ***A****ctivity* ***M****odifications*) is an occupational therapy intervention that is research-based, theoretically grounded, and developed in collaboration with youth with disabilities.[67] Project TEAM empowers youth with developmental disabilities to systematically identify environmental barriers and supports, generate modification strategies, and request reasonable accommodations. Skills that enable youth with disabilities to act as their own advocates include self-evaluation, problem solving, goal setting, and self-reinforcement skills. Project TEAM fosters the development of these skills using a self-monitoring process informed by a cognitive-behavioral approach called the Game Plan.[90] The Game Plan is a problem-solving and self-monitoring process that follows the steps of Goal-Plan-Do-Check. These new problem-solving skills facilitate youth's participation in postsecondary education and training, employment, and community living as they transition to adulthood.

Project TEAM is a manualized, group-based intervention designed to be cofacilitated by an experienced leader with a disability (disability advocate) and a licensed service provider (e.g., occupational therapist, social worker, educator). Project TEAM includes eight group sessions and two experiential learning field trips for each participant. Each trainee who begins Project TEAM identifies an activity or role (e.g., applying for a job or volunteer position, identifying a new role in an existing job, attending a leisure or social event (e.g., attending a rock concert, going out to dinner), or joining a community organization (e.g., sports team, theater group) that he or she strives to complete by the end of the 12-week self-advocacy intervention. The activity goal emphasizes participation, not independent performance, and is achieved by removing environmental barriers to participation. Case Study 12-4 provides an example of how Project TEAM facilitated social participation in the area of employment.

Emily's case illustrates how a self-advocacy and problem-solving training such as Project TEAM can support the social participation of transition-age youth with disabilities. By attending to the aspects of the environment that posed a challenge, Emily realized she could advocate about her abilities and needs. For example, regarding the barrier of opening tight objects, Emily identified that co-workers could help her with this task. Despite having previously considered this to be a personal impairment, Emily now understood how the environment affects achievement of her goal. By identifying and addressing the environmental barriers, she realized that she could participate in infant childcare if the right supports and modification strategies were in place. Her use of the Game Plan helped her identify and resolve barriers to beginning a volunteer role and enabled her to work toward beginning this new role in her community (Box 12-3).

Peer Support Interventions

Although peer relationships are important aspects of comprehensive secondary schooling, the approaches used to support students with disabilities to participate in classrooms, clubs, and other school activities sometimes limit these important social connections. When youth with disabilities receive most or all of their support from adults (e.g., related service providers, paraprofessionals, special educators), they may have few opportunities to get to know their peers without disabilities. Peer support interventions offer an evidence-based alternative to reliance on adult-delivered support in school and community settings. This approach involves equipping one or more peers

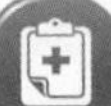

CASE STUDY 12-3 Skill-Focused Interventions for Social Participation: Kara

Kara is a 21-year-old woman diagnosed with high-functioning autism and anxiety disorder. Until she was 19, she received a traditional education through a combination of integrated and substantially separate classrooms supported by an individualized education program (IEP) that included pull-out sessions for occupational therapy and speech language pathology services. Kara passed the required standardized exams in her state to obtain her diploma at age 18. However, her parents advocated to keep her in a specialized school through her 22nd birthday to focus on life skills, vocational skills, and social participation, all of which were severely affected by her autism and anxiety symptoms. When Kara turned 19, her anxiety increased and she became unable to attend school because of severe agoraphobia. Within a few months, her symptoms became so severe that she withdrew from school completely and received tutoring at home. Kara subsequently experienced significant feelings of depression, and her family grew increasingly hopeless as they faced her future.

Despite her often paralyzing anxiety, Kara was motivated to reach her long-term goals—make new friends, find a job she liked, and attend a college course. She also made a personal goal to travel to New York to see a show on Broadway, something she had done in years past but not since her anxiety had worsened. To do that, she needed to make some money, improve her ability to manage her anxiety, and gain some life skills to plan, organize, and execute her trip. Kara was evaluated using the Canadian Occupational Performance Measure (COPM)[77] and the Adult/Adolescent Sensory Profile[18] (for more information, see Chapter 9). Kara identified the following goals after completing the COPM:

- Manage money (specifically to save and budget money for a trip to New York).
- Use a cell phone (especially to send and receive text messages).
- Diversify leisure (decrease time on Internet, increase social time).
- Take public transportation.
- Get a job.
- Take a college-level class.
- Prepare own meals.
- Do more chores around the house.

Kara gave the most disparate ratings for managing money: 3 for performance, 1 for satisfaction, and 9 for importance. Thus, Kara and the therapist decided that managing money would be the first goal they addressed. Kara's sensory sensitivity (more than most people) and sensory avoiding (more than most people) scores also indicated that she might have difficulty in social situations. She reported having trouble concentrating in a noisy environments, preferred to be alone, and avoided situations where unexpected things might happen. She specifically mentioned that despite her interest in plays, she has difficulty in many theaters because of the slope, stating that she feels "claustrophobic." She stated that she has a few coping strategies for dealing with her anxiety and sensory discomfort, namely, listening to familiar music, repeating familiar phrases to herself, and rocking in her chair. She expressed an interest to broaden her coping strategies to enable her to tolerate a wider variety of environments.

Kara was seen by an occupational therapist twice weekly for 45-minute sessions. Her IEP goals incorporated her COPM goals, with an initial focus on money management and identifying sensory-based strategies to support her social participation in multiple contexts. The therapist worked with her in her classroom once a week during their banking and budgeting block and once per week outside the classroom.

Kara's therapy was primarily guided by the metacognitive strategy, *Goal-Plan-Do-Check*.[99] This particular metacognitive strategy requires the participant to set a goal, make a plan to achieve that goal, follow through with the plan, given support as needed, and then review her performance. Kara applied this framework to increasingly more complex tasks, beginning with the goal of opening a bank account and progressing over the year to her ultimate goal of using a budget to save enough money to fund her trip to see a Broadway performance. During the process, the occupational therapist provided Kara with guidance and support as she completed each step. For example, based on her COPM ratings, Kara's first goal was to open her own bank account, which would support her ultimate goal to go with family or a friend on a trip. Her plan was to do the following:

1. Identify a bank that had a branch close to her home and to her school. She planned to do this by searching online.
2. Contact the bank and find out the steps for opening an account. Included in this was identifying materials she might need to have prior to opening the account.
3. Gather the materials and information required
4. Travel to the bank and meet with a representative to open the account.

For the *do* portion of this intervention, Kara carried out each step during an occupational therapy session, and the therapist collaborated with Kara's family, her social worker, and her classroom teacher to ensure that she was following through with agreed-on tasks and was receiving the support she needed to be successful. After each step, Kara and the therapist reviewed her performance and the outcomes to make explicit the process, the strategies she was using, and the types of supports she felt were beneficial. This same approach, *Goal-Plan-Do-Check,* was applied to most of Kara's goals and was very effective at facilitating her success.

Kara's therapy sessions also gave her opportunities to explore different sensory strategies, such as a weighted blanket and deep pressure. The occupational therapist presented Kara with the strategies, and together they made a plan about when and where to use them and how to assess their effectiveness. With the involvement of Kara's family, she tested the strategies in different environments to determine when and where they were beneficial.

In a year, Kara earned enough to take her trip to New York with a cousin. In addition to attending a Broadway show, she visited the zoo, using the sensory strategies she identified. Using the *Goal-Plan-Do-Check* and sensory strategies, she achieved other social participation goals, including conversing with two friends via text message and Facebook, enrolling in a class at a local community college, and securing a job at a local museum orienting visitors when they arrived. During her annual assessment, Kara rated her performance of money management at a 7, her satisfaction at an 8, and importance as a 7.

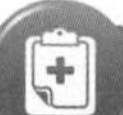

CASE STUDY 12-4 Project TEAM Case: Emily

Emily, an 18-year-old Project TEAM trainee, has a mild intellectual disability and hypotonia. She is currently in her junior year of high school. This case will follow the steps of the Game Plan to illustrate how Emily identified and resolved physical and social environmental barriers to employment.

First Base Goal: What Activity Would I Like to Do?

When Emily spoke with the facilitator during their initial assessment, she was excited about creating her own activity goal. Taking on the formal position of a childcare volunteer became Emily's activity goal. Through this role, Emily would have greater interactions with members of her community. She would also gain experiences that would support her future vocational goals and help her become more familiar with the organizational structure and procedures of day-care centers, such as background checks and staff training requirements. Emily and the facilitator decided her goal would be to identify a center and shadow other staff members while helping to provide childcare to infants. She would also strive to babysit for longer than 1 hour, allowing her to become more involved and engaged with the children. This information was used to create a series of goal attainment levels that would be used at the completion of Project TEAM to evaluate Emily's success (See Figure 12-12).

Second Base Plan Step 1: What Parts of the Environment Help Me or Make It Hard for Me?

As Emily began learning about environmental supports and barriers, she began to identify a range of factors that would help or make it harder for her to reach her goal to volunteer in infant childcare. She identified two parts of the environment as barriers using the Game Plan worksheet, services and organizations, and signs and information (Figure 12-11). These barriers made it challenging to find local community organizations that offered babysitting, accepted childcare volunteers, and readily described the application processes. Because of her hypotonia, Emily also noted that she was concerned about opening tightly closed objects, such as lids or bottles, which would likely be a responsibility of a childcare volunteer. Thus, she also identified *things* as a potential barrier while engaged in childcare.

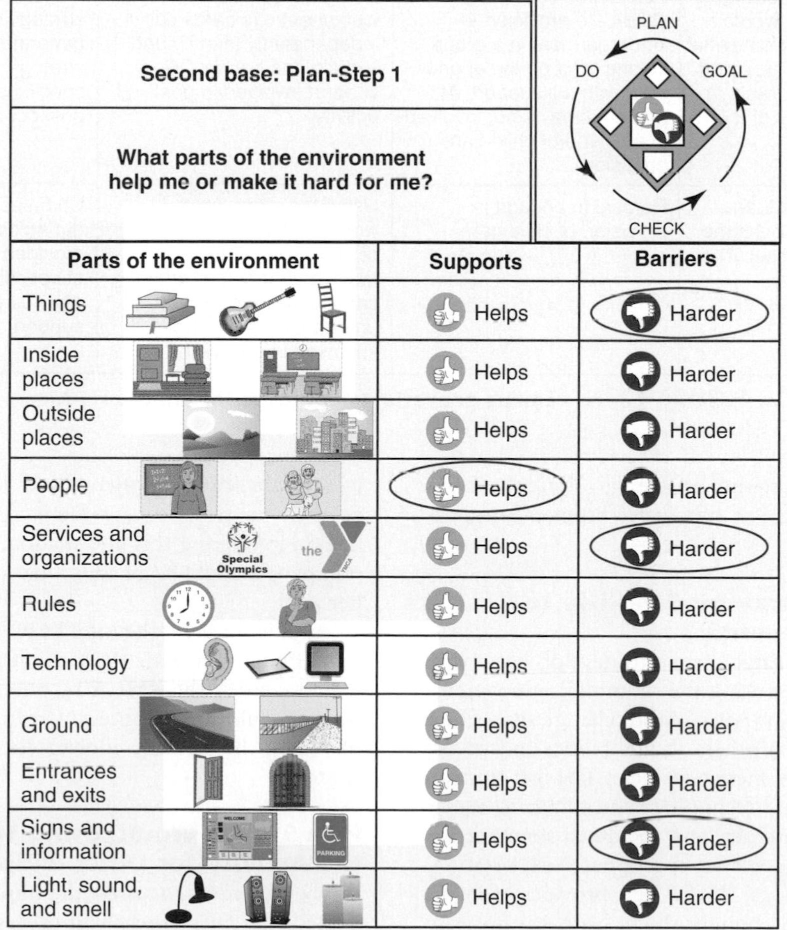

FIGURE 12-11 Emily's completed Plan Step 1 of the Game Plan worksheet.

Continued

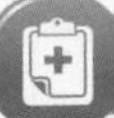

CASE STUDY 12-4 Project TEAM Case: Emily—cont'd

Rating	Level	Personal activity goal	Environment Factors goal	Strategy goal
+2	Much more than expected outcome, likely to occur 7% of the time	Providing assistance to younger children in a group setting for one hour with support on more than one occasion.	Can spontaneously and independently identify and explain barriers and supports involved in goal activity.	Using game plan worksheet, considers consequences of strategy use with support IN ADDITION TO activities in level +1.
+1	Somewhat more than expected outcome, likely to occur 21% of the time	Providing assistance to younger children in a group setting for one hour with support on one occasion.	Using the game plan worksheet/ cue cards can independently identify and explain barriers and supports for goal activity.	Spontaneously and independently names at least one appropriate strategy category and/or generates a specific strategy idea; AND uses the strategy during goal activity with support.
0	Expected outcome, likely to occur 43% of the time	Observing younger children in a group setting for at least one hour.	Using the game plan worksheet/cue cards [as needed] with orienting or guiding questions from facilitators, can identify and explain barriers and supports involved in goal activity.	Using the game plan worksheet independently names at least one appropriate strategy category and/or generates a specific strategy idea; AND uses the strategy during goal activity with support.
−1	Baseline/current, unless no worse is possible. Somewhat less than expected outcome, likely to occur 21% of the time.	Possesses knowledge of child-care provision to kindergartners in a group setting for a period of one hour with full support. At present time, is not involved in any type of child-care provision.	Using the game plan worksheet/cue cards can independently identify and explain one barrier OR support involved in goal activity.	When provided with a strategy category generates an appropriate strategy; AND uses a specific strategy during goal activity with support.
−2	Much less than expected outcome, likely to occur 7% of the time	Refusal to engage in provision of child-care.	Using the game plan worksheet/cue cards with orienting or guiding questions from facilitators can identify and explain one barrier OR support involved in goal activity.	Chooses one strategy during goal activity when provided with examples of specific strategy ideas, AND uses the strategy with support during goal activity.

FIGURE 12-12 Emily's goal attainment levels for Project TEAM.

Emily also noticed that several people, including the facilitator and her mother, acted as supportive listeners and provided suggestions.

Plan Step 2: What Strategy Can I Use to Change the Environment?

Through Project TEAM, Emily began to develop her ability to change the environment using the six modification strategies taught in the curriculum: plan ahead, change spaces, use technology or things, teach others about abilities and needs, change the rules, and ask someone for help. The first strategy she implemented was to use technology and things to search for information on the Internet, and she asked someone for help (her mother) to pinpoint an appropriate organization. She finally identified the local YMCA as a provider of infant childcare. However, Emily thought the website was not easy to navigate, and she made a phone call to contact the center. This approach provided her with specific information about when babysitting is offered and how the overall childcare program works. Because the staff at the day-care site was helpful in offering this information, Emily also identified that staff people could be an additional support to help her achieve her goal.

After identifying the local YMCA as her targeted organization, Emily met with the facilitator to brainstorm how she would contact the YMCA by phone to share her interest in being a childcare volunteer. Creating a script in preparation of calling the director allowed Emily to use the plan-ahead strategy.

Plan Step 3: Would Using This Strategy Change the Activity for Other People?

Emily wanted to focus on the implications of using the two related strategies of teaching others about abilities and needs (to share information with her co-workers about her disability and why it is difficult for her to open bottles and lids) and

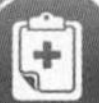

CASE STUDY 12-4 Project TEAM Case: Emily—cont'd

ask for help (by asking co-workers for help opening bottles and lids). Emily acknowledged that using these strategies would add to her co-workers' responsibilities because they would have to assist Emily in providing care to the other children. Additionally, Emily imagined that these strategies might make babysitting more difficult if she is working with only one staff member. However, with support from the facilitator, Emily identified that co-workers generally share responsibilities when they care for children. For example, if a co-worker is tying the shoelaces of a child who is upset, Emily may be able to help by making silly faces to help the child cheer up. Emily also considered the impact that using her strategies may have on the children. She wondered if children may become confused or have less fun if she could not provide all primary responsibilities. With support from the facilitator, Emily concluded that the children would have more fun if she volunteered with them because she knows how to be playful with children and encourage fun interactions.

Do: Who Do I Talk to About This Change?

With assistance, Emily logged onto the Internet on a computer and identified an e-mail and phone number for the Director of Child Care at her local YMCA. Emily noted that the director was the correct person to speak to obtain an application because the director has authority. Therefore, Emily decided that the script she wrote with the facilitator would now be intended for the director and that she would follow the script when she called this person.

Check: Am I Able to Do This Activity Now?

During an end of the year meeting with her IEP team, Emily shared her interest in volunteering with the YMCA during the summertime. As a result, the team provided her with the opportunity to shadow childcare with a class at school and actively participate in providing care to children. This placed her final level of goal attainment at +2. In addition, her ability to identify environmental barriers and supports and generate strategies to resolve environmental barriers gave her a goal attainment level of +2 for learning goals related to environmental factors and modification strategies. Emily intends to continue to work toward her goal to volunteer with the YMCA with support from her parents and IEP team (Figure 12-12).

BOX 12-3 Supporting Social Participation for Teens and Young Adults with Significant Multiple Disabilities

- Modify positioning equipment so the young person can sit at the dinner table with family.
- Use picture schedules to structure a trip to the mall with friends that provides options for the beginning, middle, and end of the outing.
- Modify a line dance routine done at the prom so that all attendees can participate.
- Suggest that youth transport water and snacks for a team on his or her wheelchair tray or by pulling a cart.
- Partner with a local small business undergoing remodeling to include an accessible main entrance and/or accessible layout and signage.
- Provide education and training to the local Better Business Bureau about serving customers with disabilities.
- Create an adaptive digital camera that a young person can use to document events such as sports, school service projects, or arts programming.
- Implement a low-key lunch day in the office building's break room by lowering lights and limiting noise.
- Design a buddy system in a local arts production to pair actors with supporters who can help with lines, blocking, and staging.
- Program a student's speech-generating device to deliver the daily weather for the morning news program at a high school.
- Help a young person and their family complete applications for city paratransit services.

without disabilities to provide ongoing social and/or academic support to their classmate with a disability while accessing needed assistance from school staff.[21] These interventions are undertaken through the following steps:

- A plan is developed for how peers will offer support in various school settings.
- Peers are invited to participate.
- An orientation meeting is held to equip peers for their new roles.
- School staff provide needed assistance and feedback as students work together.
- Adults gradually reduce their involvement and proxmity as the student and peer gain confidence and experience together.

Research suggests peer support interventions can be effective and feasible to implement within secondary schools.[23,27] For students with disabilities, these interventions have been associated with higher rates of social interaction, increased access to social support, improved social skills, expanded friendship networks, and greater participation in the life of the school. However, it is the reciprocal benefits of these interventions that are particularly compelling. Peers without disabilities who have been involved in providing support report gaining a deeper appreciation of diversity, stronger commitment to the importance of inclusion and social justice, increased understanding of disability, enhanced self-esteem, stronger advocacy skills, and improved attitudes.[24] School staff also reported that these peer-mediated approaches are effective, easy to implement, and regularly used in their schools.[25] The flexibility of peer support interventions makes it possible to individualize them to for use within a wide variety of classrooms and with a diverse range of students. Case Study 12-5 describes how a peer support

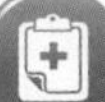

CASE STUDY 12-5 Peer Support Intervention: Dylan

Like many other seniors at his high school, Dylan is a fan of stock car racing and enjoys listening to country music. Dylan also has autism. He communicates using sign language or a program on his iPad through which he can select or spell out words. Although he spends most of his school day in a special education classroom, he attends a general education environmental science class every morning.

At first, Dylan had fairly limited participation in his environmental science class. He sat toward the back of the room next to Ms. Collins, an individually assigned paraprofessional. Ms. Collins worked to create activities for Dylan that were related to class content and could be completed successfully (e.g., word searches, matching worksheets). With help from Ms. Collins, Dylan completed these worksheets as his classmates participated in lectures, engaged in class discussions, and completed other individual and group assignments. Dylan's classmates were never unkind to him, but they hardly ever talked to him. Dylan did not complain about the class, but as soon as he finished a worksheet, he looked at Ms. Collins and pointed to his wrist—his way of asking her if he could return to the special education classroom.

Ms. Collins heard about an opportunity in her district to learn about peer support arrangements, an intervention strategy for fading adult support and empowering peers to provide academic and social support in inclusive classrooms. She was especially excited about learning strategies for engaging Dylan more fully in the class and building new social connections with his peers. Ms. Collins took steps to establish a peer support arrangement in Dylan's class. First, she identified peers who might be willing to participate. On a day when Dylan was absent, she spoke with the class about the purpose of peer supports and how this might be a fun opportunity to work with Dylan and get to know him better. She was pleasantly surprised by the number of students who expressed interest and she decided to initially involve three students—Chris, Alisha, and Sarah—as Dylan's peer supports.

Next, Ms. Collins held a brief orientation session with the peers to tell them more about Dylan and discuss how they might help support and interact with him during class. When she shared how Dylan liked stock car racing and listening to particular popular country music artists, Chris was surprised. He had no idea he and Dylan had so many shared interests. Ms. Collins explained that Dylan used his iPad and some sign language to communicate. She showed the peers the various signs Dylan uses most often and demonstrated how to program new words or phrases into Dylan's iPad. Ms. Collins then showed the peers a support plan she created for Dylan. She explained that the plan offered a starting point for the peers to interact with Dylan and support him during various class activities, but she also encouraged the students to come up with their own ideas for how Dylan could become more actively involved in the class. Excited, Sarah asked if they could all begin working together with Dylan the next day.

The following day, Ms. Collins talked with the classroom teacher about rearranging the seating chart so Dylan could work next to Chris, Alisha, and Sarah in the midst of the rest of the class. Ms. Collins told Dylan he would be sitting in a new seat with some new friends who were excited to get to know him. At first Dylan seemed hesitant because he was not used to sitting with anyone other than Ms. Collins. But when Chris greeted him and started talking about a recent NASCAR race, Dylan excitedly followed Chris to his new seat.

Over the next few months, Chris, Alisha, and Sarah found creative ways to interact with Dylan. They introduced Dylan to other students, and soon many others were greeting Dylan in the hallways and in class. Alisha noticed Dylan's iPad did not include the vocabulary used in class discussions during environmental science class, so she asked Ms. Collins if it would be okay to help Dylan program in new words. Ms. Collins worked with the teacher to get a list of key words each week so Alisha could help Dylan program in these words on a regular basis. Knowing Dylan has access to content-related words on his device, Dylan's teacher began to call on him to answer questions for the very first time. Sarah helped Dylan find a correct response on his iPad and Chris started prompting Dylan to raise his hand in class to share answers. Before long, Dylan volunteered to answer questions on his own, and was noticeably excited when he knew the right answer.

Dylan was not the only person to benefit from being part of the peer support arrangement. At the end of the semester, the peers shared what a positive experience it had been to get to know Dylan, help him meet others, and participate more fully in the class. Alisha said, "I now understand Dylan's disability in a different way than before, and I have developed a friendship with him." Sarah noted the experience had changed "how I view people with disabilities. I learned that they do understand what is going on a lot of the time and can be great friends." Chris was very glad he had an opportunity to "get to know Dylan as a person" and emphasized that Dylan "opened up a ton after we began getting to know one another." Ms. Collins was especially excited about how well things had gone. She reflected on her experience by saying, "Coming to class is more enjoyable. Dylan comes on his own now and looks for his peers." She says that implementing peer support has "benefited everyone—even me."

intervention helped one young man, Dylan, develop social relationships with other high school students.

In the case of Dylan, a paraprofessional identified and created peer support opportunities. However, an occupational therapist could play a vital role in working at the school level to structure a peer support system, identify and train paraprofessionals to facilitate peer support, and create opportunities for peer interactions through special activities. This intervention approach is a type of tier I intervention that can enhance the social participation of all students (see Chapter 23).

Summary

This chapter reviews conceptualizations of participation from a variety of fields, including rehabilitation, education, and sociology, to illustrate the complexity of social participation during adolescence and transition to adulthood.

- A framework based on the ICF grounded our discussion of social participation in interpersonal interactions and relationships and identified four participation contexts that are particularly relevant for adolescents in which social interactions can occur: work; education; community life, religion, and citizenship; and recreation and leisure.
- This chapter also described how the physical, social, cultural, and political environment can affect social participation by shaping the opportunities available to young people with disabilities.
- The research review demonstrated the developmental benefits of participation in these contexts for future success as adults. However, we also highlighted the social participation disparities experienced by adolescents with disabilities and potentially negative developmental implications.
- Occupational therapy can play an important role in facilitating the social participation of transition-age youth with disabilities and their successful transition to adulthood.
- Occupational therapists have at their disposal a range of youth self-report and parent report assessments that can be used to identify needs related to social participation.
- Interventions that target youth skills, the physical and social environment, or that use peers may be used to increase social networks and enhance the social participation experiences of young people with disabilities transitioning to adulthood.

REFERENCES

1. Adolfsson, M., Malmqvist, J., Pless, M., et al. (2011). Identifying child function from an ICF-CY perspective: Everyday life situations explored in measures of participation. *Disability and Rehabilitation, 33,* 1230–1244.
2. Albrecht, G. L., Seelman, K. D., & Bury, M. (Eds.), (2001). *Handbook of disability studies.* Thousand Oaks, CA: Sage.
3. Amado, A. N. (1993). *Friendships and community connections between people with and without developmental disabilities.* Baltimore: Paul H. Brookes.
4. American Occupational Therapy Association. (2008). Occupational Therapy Practice Framework: Domain and process. *American Journal of Occupational Therapy, 62*(6), 625–683.
5. Anaby, D., Hand, C., Bradley, L., et al. (2013). The effect of the environment on participation of children and youth with disabilities: a scoping review. *Disability and Rehabilitation, 35*(19), 1589–1598.
6. Asbjornslett, M., & Hemmingsson, H. (2008). Participation at school as experienced by teenagers with physical disabilities. *Scandinavian Journal of Educational Research, 15,* 153–161.
7. Ault, M. J., Collins, B. C., & Carter, E. W. (2013a). Factors associated with participation in faith communities for individuals with developmental disabilities and their families. *Journal of Religion, Disability, & Health, 17,* 184–211.
8. Ault, M. J., Collins, B. C., & Carter, E. W. (2013b). Congregational participation and supports for children and adults with disabilities: Parent perceptions. *Intellectual and Developmental Disabilities, 51*(1), 48–61.
9. Bearman, M., Bowes, G., & Jolly, B. (2005). Looking for the child's perspective. *Medical Education, 39,* 757–759.
10. Bedell, G. (2009). Further validation of the Child and Adolescent Scale of Participation (CASP). *Developmental Neurorehabilitation, 12,* 342–351.
11. Bedell, G. M., Khetani, M. A., Cousins, M., et al. (2011). Parent perspectives to inform development of measures of children's participation and environment. *Archives of Physical Medicine and Rehabilitation, 92,* 765–773.
12. Bedell, G., Law, M., Coster, W., et al. (2013). Community participation, supports and barriers of school age children with and without disabilities. *Archives of Physical Medicine and Rehabilitation, 92*(2), 315–323.
13. Beresford, B. (2004). On the road to nowhere? Young disabled people and transition. *Child: Care, Health and Development, 30*(6), 581–587.
14. Berndt, T. J. (1982). The features and effects of friendship in early adolescence. *Child Development, 53,* 1447–1460.
15. Blinde, E. M., & McCallister, S. G. (1998). Listening to the voices of students with physical disabilities. *Journal of Physical Education, Recreation, and Dance, 69,* 64–68.
16. Britner, P. A., Balcazar, F. E., Blechman, E. A., et al. (2006). Mentoring special youth populations. *Journal of Community Psychology, 34*(6), 747–763.
17. Borell, L., & Hemmingson, H. (2002). Environmental barriers in mainstream schools. *Child: Care, Health and Development, 28,* 57–63.
18. Brown, C., & Dunn, W. (2002). *Adult/Adolescent Sensory Profile: User's Manual.* San Antonio, TX: Psychological Corporation.
19. Carter, E. W. (2013). Supporting inclusion and flourishing in the religious and spiritual lives of people with intellectual and developmental disabilities. *Inclusion, 1*(1), 64–75.
20. Carter, E. W., Cushing, L. S., Clark, N. M., et al. (2005). Effects of peer support interventions on students' access to the general curriculum and social interactions. *Research and Practice for Persons with Severe Disabilities, 30,* 15–25.
21. Carter, E. W., Cushing, L. S., & Kennedy, C. H. (2009). *Peer support strategies for improving all students' social lives and learning.* Baltmore, MD: Paul H. Brookes.
22. Carter, E. W., & Hughes, C. (2005). Increasing social interaction among adolescents with intellectual disabilities and their general education peers: Effective interventions. *Research and Practice for Persons with Severe Disabilities, 30*(4), 179–193.
23. Carter, E. W., & Kennedy, C. H. (2006). Promoting access to the general curriculum using peer support strategies. *Research and Practice for Persons with Severe Disabilities, 31,* 284–292.
24. Carter, E. W., Moss, C. K., Hoffman, A., et al. (2011). Efficacy and social validity of peer support arrangements for adolescents with disabilities. *Exceptional Children, 78,* 107–125.
25. Carter, E. W., & Pesko, M. J. (2008). Social validity of peer interaction intervention strategies in high school classrooms: Effectiveness, feasibility, and actual use. *Exceptionality, 16,* 156–173. doi:10.1080/09362830802198427.
26. Carter, E. W., Sisco, L., Brown, L., et al. (2008). Peer interactions and academic engagement of youth with developmental disabilities in inclusive middle and high school classrooms. *American Journal of Mental Retardation, 113*(6), 479–494.

27. Carter, E. W., Sisco, L. G., Chung, Y.-C., et al. (2010). Peer interactions of students with intellectual disabilities and/or autism: A map of the intervention literature. *Research and Practice for Persons with Severe Disabilities, 35*(3–4), 63–79.
28. Cavet, J., & Sloper, P. (2004). Participation of disabled children in individual decisions about their lives and in public decisions about service development. *Children and Society, 18*, 278–290.
29. Cella, D., Yount, S., Rothrock, N., et al. (2007). The Patient-Reported Outcomes Measurement Information System (PROMIS): Progress of an NIH roadmap cooperative group during its first two years. *Medical Care, 45*(Suppl. 1), S3–S11.
30. Chappell, A. L. (1994). A question of friendship: Community care and the relationships of people with learning difficulties. *Disability and Society, 9*, 419–434.
31. Chen, C. C., Heinemann, A. W., Bode, R. K., et al. (2011). Impact of pediatric rehabilitation services on children's functional outcomes. *American Journal of Occupational Therapy, 58*(1), 44–53.
32. Coatsworth, J. D., Sharp, E. H., Palen, L.-A., et al. (2005). Exploring adolescent self-defining leisure activities and identity experiences across three countries. *International Journal of Behavioral Development, 29*(5), 361–370.
33. Coster, W., Bedell, G., Law, M., et al. (2011). Psychometric evaluation of the participation and environment measure for children and youth (PEM-CY). *Developmental Medicine and Child Neurology, 53*, 1030–1037.
34. Coster, W., Law, M., Bedell, G., et al. (2013). School participation, supports and barriers of students with and without disabilities. *Child: Care, Health and Development, 39*(4), 535–543.
35. Day, M., & Harry, B. (1999). "Best friends": The construction of a teenage friendship. *Mental Retardation, 37*, 221–231.
36. Davila, A., & Mora, M. (2007). *Civic engagement and high school academic progress: An analysis using NELS data.* College Park, MD: University of Maryland School of Public Policy, Center for Information and Research on Civic Learning and Engagement (CIRCLE).
37. Diez, A. M. (2010). School memories of young people with disabilities: An analysis of barriers and aids to inclusion. *Disability and Society, 25*(2), 163–175.
38. Dudgeon, B. J., Massagli, T. L., & Ross, B. W. (1997). Educational participation of children with spinal cord injury. *American Journal of Occupational Therapy, 51*, 553–561.
39. Dumas, H., Fragala-Pinkham, M. A., Haley, S., et al. (2012). Computer adaptive test performance in children with and without disabilities: Prospective field study of the PEDI-CAT. *Disability and Rehabilitation, 34*(5), 393–401.
40. Dunford, C., Missiuna, C., Street, E., et al. (2005). Children's perceptions of the impact of developmental coordination disorder on activities of daily living. *British Journal of Occupational Therapy, 68*(5), 207–214.
41. Erik, W., Austin, D., & Trainor, A. A. (2012). Predictors of postschool employment outcomes for young adults with severe disabilities. *Journal of Disability Policy Studies, 23*(1), 50–63.
42. Erikson, E. H. (1968). *Identity, youth, and crisis.* New York: Norton.
43. Field, S., & Hoffman, A. (2002). Preparing youth to exercise self-determination: Quality indicators of school environments that promote the acquisition of knowledge, skills, and beliefs related to self-determination. *Journal of Disability Policy Studies, 13*(2), 114–119.
44. Forsyth, R., Colver, A., Alvanides, S., et al. (2007). Participation of young severely disabled children is influenced by their intrinsic impairments and environment. *Developmental Medicine and Child Neurology, 49*, 345–349.
45. Garth, B., & Aroni, R. (2003). "I value what you have to say": Seeking the perspective of cihldren with a disability, not just their parents. *Disability and Society, 18*(5), 561–576.
46. Gill, C. J. (1997). Four types of integration in disability identity development. *Journal of Vocational Rehabilitation, 9*, 39–46.
47. Goffman, E. (1963). *Stigma: Notes on the management of spoiled identity.* New York: Simon & Schuster.
48. Goodley, D. (2001). "Learning Difficulties," the social model of disability and impairment: Challenging epistemologies. *Disability and Society, 16*(2), 207–231.
49. Goodwin, D. L., & Staples, K. (2005). The meaning of summer camp experiences to youths with disabilities. *Adapted Physical Activity Quarterly, 22*, 159–178.
50. Gray, L., Thomas, N., & Lewis, L. (2010). *Teachers' use of educational technology in U.S. public schools: 2009*, (NCES publication no. 2010-040). Washington, DC: National Center for Education Statistics, Institute of Education Sciences, U.S. Department of Education.
51. Groce, N. E. (1985). *Everyone here spoke sign language: Hereditary deafness on Martha's Vineyard.* Cambridge, MA: Harvard University Press.
52. Haley, S. M., Coster, W. J., Dumas, H. M., et al. (2012). *The PEDI-CAT*, version 1.3.6. Boston: CRECare.
53. Hammal, D., Jarvis, S. N., & Colver, A. F. (2004). Participation of children with cerebral palsy is influenced by where they live. *Developmental Medicine & Child Neurology, 46*, 292–298.
54. Hammel, J., Charlton, J., Jones, R. A., et al. (2014). Disability rights and advocacy: Partnering with disability communities to support full participation in society. In B. A. Boyt Schell, G. Gillen, & M. E. Scaffa (Eds.), *Willard and Spackman's occupational therapy* (pp. 1031–1050). Philadephia: Wolters Kluwer/Lippincott Williams & Wilkins.
55. Hansen, D. M., & Larson, R. (2005). *The Youth Experiences Survey 2.0: Instrument revisions and validity testing.* University of Illinois, Champaign-Urbana.
56. Hansen, D. M., Larson, R., & Dworkin, J. (2003). What adolescents learn in organized youth activities: A survey of self-reported developmental experiences. *Journal of Research on Adolescence, 13*, 25–56.
57. Kessler Foundation/National Organization on Disability. The 2010 Survey of Americans With Disabilities. <http://www.2010DisabilitySurveys.org>. Accessed June 18, 2014.
58. Harter, S. (1982). The perceived competence scale for children. *Child Development, 53*, 87–97.
59. Irwin, D. E., Gross, H. E., Stucky, B. D., et al. (2012). Development of six PROMIS pediatrics proxy-report item banks. *Health and Quality of Life Outcomes, 10*(1), 22.
60. Joseph Rowntree Foundation. (2003). *An evaluation of a young disabled people's peer mentoring/ support project.* York, UK: Joseph Rowntree Foundation.
61. Khetani, M., & Coster, W. (2014). Social participation. In B. A. Boyt Schell, G. Gillen, M. E. Scaffa, & E. Cohn (Eds.), *Willard and Spackman's occupational therapy* (pp. 731–744). Philadelphia: Wolters Kluwer/Lippincott Williams & Wilkins.
62. Kielhofner, G. (2007). *A model of human occupation: Theory and application* (4th ed.). Baltimore: Lippincott, Williams, & Wilkins.
63. Kiresuk, T. J., Smith, A., & Cardillo, J. E. (Eds.), (1994). *Goal attainment scaling: Applications, theory, and measurement.*

Hillsdale, NJ: Lawrence Erlbaum Associates.

64. Kliewer, C. (1998). *Schooling children with Down syndrome: Toward an understanding of possibility.* New York: Teachers College Press.
65. Kotzer, E., & Margalit, M. (2007). Perception of competence: Risk and protective predictors following an e-self-advocacy intervention for adolescents with learning disabilities. *European Journal of Special Needs Education, 22*(4), 443–457.
66. Kramer, J. (2011). Using mixed methods to establish the social validity of a self-report assessment: An illustration using the Child Occupational Self-Assessment (COSA). *Journal of Mixed Methods Research, 5*, 52–76.
67. Kramer, J. M., Barth, Y., Curtis, K., et al. (2013). Involving youth with disabilities in the development and evaluation of a new advocacy training: Project TEAM. *Disability and Rehabilitation, 35*(7), 614–622.
68. Kramer, J., Coster, W., Kao, Y. C., et al. (2012). A new approach to the measurement of adaptive behavior: Development of the PEDI-CAT for children and youth with autism spectrum disorders. *Physical & Occupational Therapy in Pediatrics, 32*(1), 34–47.
69. Kramer, J., Heckmann, S., & Bell-Walker, M. (2012). Accommodations and therapeutic techniques used during the administration of the Child Occupational Self-Assessment. *British Journal of Occupational Therapy, 75*(11), 495–502.
70. Kramer, J. M., Kafkes, A., Basu, S., et al. (2005). *The Child Occupational Self Assessment (COSA), version 2.1.* Chicago: University of Illinois at Chicago.
71. Kramer, J., Kielhofner, G., & Smith, E. V., Jr. (2010). Validity evidence for the Child Occupational Self-Assessment (COSA). *American Journal of Occupational Therapy, 64*(4), 621–632.
72. Kramer, J. M., Olsen, S., Mermelstein, M., et al. (2012). Youth with disabilities' perspectives of the environment and participation: A qualitative meta-synthesis. *Child: Care, Health and Development, 38*(6), 763–777.
73. Kramer, J., Smith, E. V., Jr., & Kielhofner, G. (2009). Rating scale use by children with disabilities on a self-report of everyday activities. *Archives of Physical Medicine and Rehabilitation, 90*(12), 2047–2053.
74. Kuo, M. H., Orsmond, G. I., Cohn, E., et al. (2013). Friendship characteristics and activity patterns of adolescents with an autism spectrum disorder. *Autism: The International Journal of Research and Practice, 17*(4), 481–500.
75. Lansdown, G., & Karkara, R. (2006). Children's right to express views and have them taken seriously. *Lancet, 367*, 690–692.
76. Larson, R. W., Hansen, D. M., & Moneta, G. (2006). Differing profiles of developmental experiences across types of organized youth activities. *Developmental Psychology, 42*, 849–863.
77. Law, M., Baptiste, S., Carswell, A., et al. (2005). *The Canadian Occupational Performance Measure.* Toronto, Canada: Canadian Association of Occupational Therapists.
78. Law, M., King, G., King, S., et al. (2006). Patterns of participation in recreational and leisure activities among children with complex physical disabilities. *Developmental Medicine and Child Neurology, 48*, 337–342.
79. Lightfoot, J., Wright, S., & Sloper, P. (1999). Supporting pupils in mainstream school with an illness or disability: Young people's views. *Child: Care, Health and Development, 25*(4), 267–283.
80. Liptak, G. S., Kennedy, J. A., & Dosa, N. P. (2011). Social participation in a nationally representative sample of older youth and young adults with autism. *Journal of Developmental and Behavioral Pediatrics, 32*, 277–283.
81. Longmore, P. K. (2003). *Why I burned my book: And other essays on disability.* Philadelphia: Temple University Press.
82. Lutfiyya, Z. M. (1991). "A feeling of being connected": Friendships between people with and without learning difficulties. *Disability, Handicap and Society, 6*, 233–245.
83. Majnemer, A., & Limperopoulos, C. (2002). Importance of outcome determination in pediatric rehabilitation. *Developmental Medicine and Child Neurology, 44*, 773–777.
84. Mancini, M., & Coster, W. (2004). Functional predictors of school participation by children with disabilities. *Occupational Therapy International, 11*(1), 12–25.
85. Martin, J., Jorgensen, C., & Klein, J. (1998). The promise of friendship for students with disabilities. In C. Jorgensen (Ed.), *Restructuring high schools for all students: Taking inclusion to the next level* (pp. 145–181). Baltimore: Paul H. Brookes.
86. Mayall, B. (2004). Sociologies of childhood. In M. Holborn (Ed.), *Developments in Sociology: An Annual Review* (Vol. 20, pp. 37–57). Ormskirk, Lancashire, UK: Causeway Press.
87. McDougall, J., Bedell, G., & Wright, V. (2013). The youth report version of the Child and Adolescent Scale of Participation (CASP): Assessment of psychometric properties and comparison with parent report. *Child: Care, Health and Development, 39*, 512–522.
88. McGavin, H. (1998). Planning rehabilitation: A comparison of issues for parents and adolescents. *Physical and Occupational Therapy in Pediatrics, 18*, 69–82.
89. Meeus, W., Iedema, J., Helsen, M., et al. (1999). Patterns of adolescent identity development: Review of literature and longitudinal analysis. *Developmental Review, 19*, 419–461.
90. Meichenbaum, D. (1977). *Cognitive-behavioral modification: An integrative approach.* New York: Plenum Press.
91. Mirza, M. (2013). Assessing person-environment-occupation interactions through epidemiological research: Individual, household, and community-level correlates of social participation for low-income children with and without disabilities. Chicago: Presented at the Second Summit of Occupational Therapy Scholars, University of Illinois at Chicago.
92. Missiuna, C., Pollock, N., Law, M., et al. (2006). Examination of the Perceived Efficacy and Goal Setting System (PEGS) with children with disabilities, their parents, and teachers. *American Journal of Occupational Therapy, 60*(2), 204–214.
93. Mitchell, D. T., & Snyder, S. L. (2000). *Narrative prosthesis: Disability and the dependencies of discourse.* Ann Arbor: University of Michigan Press.
94. O'Brien, J. C., Bergeron, A., Duprey, H., et al. (2009). Children with disabilities and their parents' views of occupational participation needs. *Occupational Therapy in Mental Health, 25*, 164–180.
95. Oliver, M. (1996a). *Understanding disability from theory to practice.* New York: St. Martin's Press.
96. Oliver, M. (1996b). *Understanding disability from theory to practice.* New York: St. Martin's Press.
97. Orsmond, G. I., Shattuck, P. T., Cooper, B. P., et al. (2013). Social participation among young adults with an autism spectrum disorder. *Journal of Autism and Developmental Disorders, 43*(11), 2710–2719.
98. Pivik, J., McComas, J., & LaFlamme, M. (2002). Barriers and facilitators to inclusive education. *Exceptional Children, 69*(1), 97–107.
99. Polatajko, H. J., & Mandich, A. (2004). *Enabling occupation in children: The Cognitive Orientation to daily Occupational Performance (CO-OP)*

approach. Ottawa, ON: CAOT Publications.

100. Pogrebin, L. C. (1987). *Among friends: Who we like, why we like them, and what we do with them*. New York: McGraw-Hill Book.
101. Potts, S., Kirkham, M., Monsour, F., et al. (2001). *Sustaining service learning in Wisconsin: What principals, teachers and students say about service-learning*. Madison: Wisconsin Department of Public Instruction.
102. Powers, L. E., Garner, T., Valnes, B., et al. (2007). Building a successful adult life: Findings from youth-directed research. *Exceptionality, 15*(1), 45–56.
103. Rao, P. A., Beidel, D. C., & Murray, M. J. (2008). Social skills interventions for children with Asperger's syndrome or high-functioning autism: A review and recommendations. *Journal of Autism and Developmental Disorders, 38*, 353–361.
104. Rapley, M. (2004). *The social construction of intellectual disability*. Cambridge, UK: Cambridge University Press.
105. Robertson, C. M. T., Suave, R. S., Joffe, A. R., et al. (2011). The registry and follow-up of Complex Pediatric Therapies Program: A mechanism for service, audit, and research after life-saving therapies for young children. *Cardiology Research and Practice, 2011*, 1–11.
106. Rosenbaum, P., & Stewart, D. (2007). Perspectives on transitions: Rethinking services for children and youth with developmental disabilities. *Archives of Physical Medicine and Rehabilitation Research, 88*, 1080–1082.
107. Rubin, L. (1985). *Just friends: The role of friendship in our lives*. New York: Harper & Row.
108. Scales, P. C., Blyth, D. A., Berkas, T. H., et al. (2000). The effects of service learning on middle school students' social responsibility and academic success. *Journal of Early Adolescence, 20*(3), 332–358.
109. Schaffner, C. B., & Buswell, B. (1992). *Connecting students: A guide to thoughtful friendship facilitation for educators & families*. Colorado Springs, CO: PEAK Parent Center.
110. Shattuck, P. T., Orsmond, G., Wagner, M., et al. (2011). Participation in social activities among adolescents with an autism spectrum disorder. *PLoS ONE, 6*(11), e27176.
111. Shevlin, M., Kenny, M., & McNeela, E. (2002). Curriculum access for pupils with disabilities: An Irish experience. *Disability and Society, 17*(2), 159–169.
112. Simeonsson, R. J., Carlson, D., Huntington, G. S., et al. (2001). Students with disabilities: A national survey of participation in school activities. *Disability and Rehabilitation, 23*(2), 49–63.
113. Siperstein, G., Leffert, J., & Wenz-Gross, M. (1997). The quality of friendships between children with and without learning problems. *American Journal on Mental Retardation, 102*, 111–125.
114. Siperstein, G. N., & Parker, R. C. (2008). Toward an understanding of social integration: A special issue. *Exceptionality, 16*(*3*), 119–124.
115. Sloper, P., & Lightfoot, J. (2003). Involving disabled and chronically ill children and young people in health service development. *Child: Care, Health, & Development, 29*(1), 15–20.
116. Snell, M. E., & Janney, R. (2000). *Social relationships and peer support*. Baltimore: Paul H. Brookes.
117. Solish, A., Perry, A., & Minnes, P. (2010). Participation of children with and without disabilities in social, recreational and leisure activities. *Journal of Applied Research in Intellectual Disabilities, 23*(3), 226–236.
118. Staub, D. (1998). *Delicate threads: Friendships between children with and without special needs in inclusive settings*. Bethesda, MD: Woodbine House.
119. Taylor, H. G. (2004). Research on outcomes of pediatric traumatic brain injury: Current advances and future directions. *Developmental Neurology, 25*(1), 199–225.
120. Taylor, S. J., & Bogdan, R. (1989). On accepting relationships between people with mental retardation and non-disabled people: Towards an understanding of acceptance. *Disability, Handicap and Society, 4*(1), 21–35.
121. Tisdall, E. K. M., & Davis, J. (2004). Making a difference? Bringing children's and young people's views into policy-making. *Children and Society, 18*, 131–142.
122. Tuffrey, C., Bateman, B. J., & Colver, A. C. (2013). The Questionnaire of Young People's Participation (QYPP): A new measure of participation frequency for disabled young people. *Child: Care, Health and Development, 39*, 500–511.
123. Tseng, V., & Seidman, E. (2007). A systems framework for understanding social settings. *American Journal of Community Psychology, 39*, 217–228.
124. Valnes, B., Hare, R., Block, J., et al. (2003). *Future directions agenda for youth with disabilities, 2003*. Portland, OR: National Youth Leadership Network.
125. Varni, J. W., Burwinkle, T. M., Sherman, S. A., et al. (2005). Health-related quality of life of children and adolescents with cerebral palsy: Hearing the voices of the children. *Developmental Medicine and Child Neurology, 47*, 592–597.
126. Vaughn, S., Elbaum, B., & Boardman, A. G. (2001). The social functioning of students with learning disabilities: Implications for inclusion. *Exceptionality, 9*(1–2), 47–65.
127. Verdonschot, M. M. L., De Witte, L. P., Reichrath, E., et al. (2009). Impact of environmental factors on community participation of persons with an intellectual disability: A systematic review. *Journal of Intellectual Disability Research, 53*(1), 54–64.
128. Voll, R. (2009). Social participation and vocational integration as an objective of child and adolescent psychiatric rehabilitation. *Zeitschrift für Kinder- und Jugenpsychiatrie und Psychotherapie, 37*(5), 421–429.
129. Voorman, J., Dallmeijer, A., Van Eck, M., et al. (2010). Social functioning and communication in children with cerebral palsy: Association with disease characteristics and personal and environmental factors. *Developmental Medicine and Child Neurology, 52*, 441–447.
130. Wagner, M., Cadwallader, T. W., Garza, N., et al. (2004). *Social activities of youth with disabilities. A report from the National Longitudinal Transition Study-2 (NLTS2)*. Menlo Park, CA: SRI International.
131. Wagner, M., Newman, L., Cameto, R., et al. (2007). Perceptions and expectations of youth with disabilities. A special topic report on findings from the National Longitudinal Transition Study-2 (NLTS2). Executive Summary. *Journal for Vocational Special Needs Education, 30*(1), 13–17.
132. Wainer, H., Dorans, N. J., Eignor, D., et al. (2000). *Computerized adaptive testing: A primer* (2nd ed.). Mahwah, NJ: Lawrence Earlbaum Associates.
133. Wallen, M., O'Flaherty, S. J., & Waugh, M.-C. A. (2007). Functional outcomes of intramuscular botulinum toxin type A and occupational therapy in the upper limbs of children with cerebral palsy: A randomized controlled trial. *Archives of Physical Medicine and Rehabilitation, 88*, 1–10.
134. Wehmeyer, M. L., & Kelchner, K. (1995). *The Arc's Self-Determination Scale*. Arlington, TX: Arc National Headquarters.
135. Wehmeyer, M. L., & Palmer, S. B. (2003). Adult outcomes for students with cognitive disabilities three-years after high school: The impact of self-determination. *Education and Training in Developmental Disabilities, 38*, 131–144.

136. Wehmeyer, M. L., & Schwartz, M. (1997). Self-determination and positive adult outcomes: A follow-up study of youth with mental retardation or learning disabilities. *Exceptional Children*, *63*(2), 245–255.
137. Weintraub, N., Rot, I., Shoshani, N., et al. (2011). Participation in daily activities and quality of life in survivors of retinoblastoma. *Pediatric Blood Cancer*, *56*, 590–594.
138. Whiteneck, G., & Dijkers, M. P. (2009). Difficult to measure constructs: Conceptual and methodological issues concerning participation and environmental factors. *Archives of Physical Medicine and Rehabilitation*, *90*(11 Suppl. 1), S22–S35.
139. World Health Organization. (2008). *International Classification of Functioning, Disability, and Health—Children and Youth version (ICF-CY)*. Geneva: WHO.
140. Wolman, J. M., Campeau, P. L., DuBois, P. A., et al. (Eds.), (1994). *AIR Self-Determination Scale and user guide*. Washington, DC: American Institutes for Research.
141. Zimmer-Gembeck, M. J., & Collins, W. A. (2006). Autonomy development during adolescence. In G. Adams & M. Berzonsky (Eds.), *Handbook of Adolescence* (pp. 175–204). Malden, MA: Blackwell.

CHAPTER

13

Interventions and Strategies for Challenging Behaviors

Renee Watling

KEY TERMS

Challenging behaviors
Contingency methods
Functional behavioral analysis
Positive behavioral support
Prevention

GUIDING QUESTIONS

1. What are the four functions of challenging behaviors?
2. How can a therapist *prevent* challenging behaviors from occurring?
3. What are strategies for *supporting* positive behaviors in children?
4. What are principles and strategies to reduce challenging behaviors?
5. How are positive behavior support and functional behavioral analysis used to support student behaviors in school contexts?

Strategies for Managing Difficult Behavior

All children display inappropriate or challenging behaviors as they grow through the various ages and stages of childhood. Special attention must be given when such behaviors interfere with the child's ability to engage and participate in daily life activities, when they are disruptive to the engagement and participation of others, or when the behaviors place the child or others at risk for injury (Case Study 13-1). It is important for occupational therapists to be familiar with and skilled at using therapeutic strategies designed to prevent and reduce challenging behaviors to diminish the negative impact of such behaviors on the child's occupational performance. This chapter introduces behavior management concepts and presents evidence-based strategies for preventing and reducing challenging or unacceptable behavior in children.

Much of what is known about challenging behavior and the strategies to facilitate behavior change has emerged from the fields of education and psychology. In recent years, behavioral intervention methods have gained increasing popularity as their effectiveness has been demonstrated in programs for children with autism spectrum disorders and other conditions. Robust research investigating these methods provides a wealth of knowledge that occupational therapists can apply to help understand why challenging behavior occurs, how to prevent challenging behavior, and how to intervene when a child exhibits challenging behavior.

Behavior Happens

Behavior is an expressive act by an individual that can have many different forms and meanings (Figure 13-1). Whether a certain behavior is appropriate and acceptable is dependent on the context and contextual norms for the given situation. For example, in a public school building, it would be inappropriate and unacceptable for a student to leave the classroom and go to the playground when the teacher passes out a work assignment; however, the same behavior would be appropriate and desirable in response to the recess bell or a clanging fire alarm. Similarly, it is considered inappropriate and unacceptable for a child to scream and withdraw when his or her dinner plate loaded with green beans is placed on the table, but screaming and withdrawal are acceptable and possibly even anticipated when a child receives an immunization shot. Humans are dynamic organisms with constantly active neurologic, physiologic, and physical systems who interact with environments, materials, and other dynamic organisms. With so many variables at play, the possibility of a mismatch between two or more variables is likely. When such a mismatch occurs between person and contextual variables, the likelihood of undesired or inappropriate behavior increases.[35]

Inappropriate behavior can take many forms. Passive behaviors such as noncompliance, withdrawal, avoidance, inattention, and lack of response are not overtly disruptive but still interfere with occupational performance and participation. Active behaviors such as direct refusal to engage, opposition, aggression toward people or property, or self-injurious behavior not only interfere with occupational performance and participation, but can also be disruptive or harmful to self or others. Passive and active forms of inappropriate behavior can be difficult to manage and require attention and intention by caregivers and service providers.

Behavior Always has a Purpose

In many, if not most, daily situations, inappropriate or challenging behavior is seen as an inconvenience and an irritant to others in the surrounding environment. Have you ever been seated in a restaurant at a table next to a screaming toddler? Or in the movie theater behind a person using a cell phone?

CASE STUDY 13-1 Sam and Eli

Sam is a 2½-year-old boy who lives with his mother, father, and 6-year-old brother. Sam enjoys staying at home to play with his toys or watch movies. He plays by himself for unlimited periods of time. He spends many hours a day driving his cars and trucks back and forth while lying prone and watching the wheels turn. If his brother plays with the cars, Sam screams uncontrollably until the car is returned to him. Another of Sam's favorite activities is playing with balls. He pulls the basket of balls to the top of the stairs, where he bounces them off the wall and down the stairs into the family room over and over. If someone else retrieves one of the balls or tries to engage Sam in a ball game, an ear-piercing scream is heard before Sam deteriorates into a kicking, screaming tantrum.

Sam's brother, Eli, is 6 years old. He attends kindergarten 5 days each week, where he follows the classroom routine, engages with teacher-directed activities, and plays side by side with his peers. At home, Eli plays by himself for up to 30 minutes at a time. He prefers activities such as coloring and playing with dinosaur figurines. His favorite color is blue and his coloring pictures show all shades of the hue. His favorite dinosaur is a *Tyrannosaurus rex*, and Eli can recite a number of known facts about this creature. When a visitor comes to the family home, Eli inundates the person with incessant talk about the *T. rex*. His eye contact is spontaneous but fleeting. He is easily distracted, looking away from a task to investigate all noise or movement around him. When approached by others, Eli gives a quick "Hi" and then directs his gaze to the person's shoulder and begins reciting facts about the *T. rex*.

Sam eats approximately 10 different foods. His diet is restricted by his own preferences for certain tastes and textures and also by intolerance for gluten. His mother is careful to prepare foods that are gluten-free and that she knows Sam will eat. He is able to use a spoon and fork moderately well but prefers to use his fingers for self-feeding. He refuses all fruits, vegetables, and dairy products. His mother has expressed concern about Sam's nutrition. His behavioral rigidity considerably affects the family's daily life. He does well on weekdays during the school year while his brother is at school. On school days, Sam accompanies his mother on errands to one familiar place at a time if his mother brings favorite toys and a snack. If his mother tries to combine two errands into one trip, Sam has tantrum and refuses to exit the car. Sam's behavior is much more erratic on weekends and holidays when the schedule is inconsistent and more people are at home.

Both Sam and Eli are diagnosed with developmental disabilities.

FIGURE 13-1 All behavior serves a purpose. A child ready to strike out could be acting aggressively, seeking attention, or protecting himself from a source of harm. Determining the purpose the behavior serves for the child is the first step in managing challenging behavior.

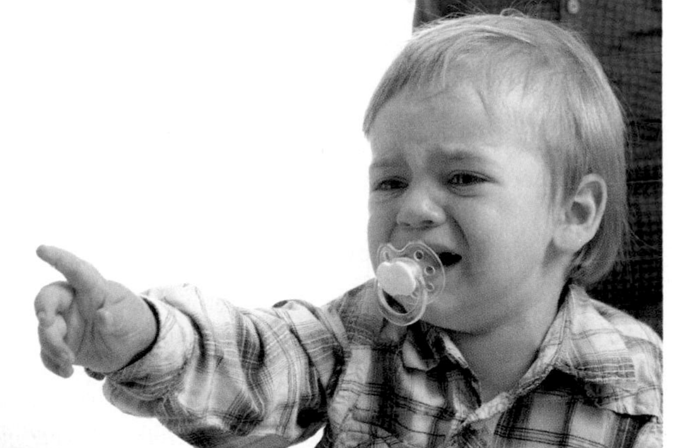

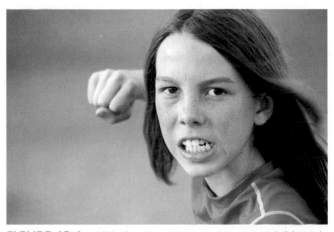

FIGURE 13-2 The child in this figure is demonstrating two behaviors: crying and pointing. Crying often allows a person to avoid an undesired event, while pointing is a method of obtaining a desired item or event. (Photo © istock.com)

How about needing to get a child dressed to leave the house for a doctor's appointment, but when you try to help, the child repeatedly hits his or her ears?

To manage difficult behavior effectively, it is critical to remember that all behavior serves a purpose. The purpose of a given episode of challenging behavior can be most accurately identified only by the person executing the behavior. However, while engaged in challenging behavior, a child is unlikely to be in a state in which he or she can verbalize the purpose of the behavior. Decades of research has identified four primary purposes of challenging behavior: (1) obtaining a desired object or event; (2) avoiding a situation; (3) escaping from an undesired object, event, or demand[14]; and (4) sensory functions[30] (Figure 13-2).

These four functions may be influenced by a range of factors. Some of these are internal and emerge from a lack of skill or ability to perform in a desired manner. Others are external factors that are outside a child's control. Box 13-1 identifies

BOX 13-1 Factors That Influence Behavior

Internal Factors
Desire for control
Fatigue
Illness
Ineffective communication
Pain
Poor emotional regulation
Poor self-regulation
Poor sensory processing

External Factors
Task demands greater than skill level
Change in schedule
Unfamiliar person
Unfamiliar place

some of the internal and external factors that can influence behavior.

Functional behavioral analysis (FBA) is a formal process for evaluating the factors influencing behavior to understand why a challenging behavior is occurring. It is widely used in school systems; the process is usually directed by professionals with specialized training in behavioral analysis methods. The FBA process aims systematically to identify a behavior's antecedents (events occurring before and triggering the behavior) and consequences (events after the behavior that reinforce the behavior). An FBA can be resource-intensive and often is reserved for situations in which extreme or dangerous behaviors are occurring. The formal FBA process is described later in the chapter. For less severe situations, a modified FBA can be conducted informally by determining mismatches between the person's skills and abilities and the contextual factors that are in effect when the challenging behavior occurs.

Being Prepared for Problem Behavior

To be best prepared to manage the range of behaviors likely to be experienced in a pediatric setting, the occupational therapist should give special attention to developing knowledge and skills specific to behavior management. This includes becoming familiar with a variety of general strategies that can be implemented to help create a context in which challenging behaviors are less likely to occur and more readily managed if they do occur. The following methods are suggested as general approaches to being prepared for problem behavior. These strategies are recommended as first steps in reducing the likelihood that problem behavior will occur. As a child grows and develops greater knowledge and skills, it is appropriate to adjust the type, structure, frequency, and intensity of supports provided.

Ruling Out Pain or Illness

Children experiencing pain or illness can act out in a variety of ways.[3] Pain-based behaviors can be especially difficult to identify in children who are nonverbal. Behaviors associated with pain or illness may have a sudden onset, be associated with a certain body position, be cyclic, or occur frequently for no apparent external reason. If behaviors appear to be associated with pain, the occupational therapist should work with the child's family and other service providers to determine whether the behavior is driven by pain and, if appropriate, should follow through with recommendations to remediate the source of pain.

Establishing Predictability and Consistency

Maintaining a consistent context in relation to schedule, environment, people, and demeanor helps allay a child's anxiety about what is going to happen next.[13] When anxiety is diminished, the child has more resources available to direct toward self-management and productivity. Children are more successful when expectations, environments, people, and situations are familiar. As much as possible, the occupational therapist should work to increase the known and decrease the unknown. Strategies include scheduling activities in a similar order and location from day to day, keeping the physical arrangement and furnishings in the environment consistent, offering the same type of activities, establishing consistent social expectations, and arranging to have the same people interact with the child during the same activities.

Creating a Calm Atmosphere

Keeping the physical environment clean and organized creates a sense of order and predictability. Children know where to find desired items and which areas to avoid if certain items are off limits. In addition, maintaining a calm demeanor when mishaps occur can help minimize chaos and preserve a sense of order. Children often react to the stress and anxiety displayed by others with a disorganization of their own behavior. When adults remain calm, a sense of order is maintained, and the child is at ease.

Praise for Appropriate Behaviors

It is recommended that for every negative comment, a child should hear at least eight positive comments.[16] Adults should consistently reward and reinforce appropriate behaviors by attending to them, complimenting the child on his or her behavior, and identifying specifically what the child did that was appreciated. Specific feedback can increase the child's awareness of the desired behaviors. Although general feedback can help a child build confidence in his or her ability to produce desired behaviors, specific feedback helps the child know exactly what to do the next time and increases the likelihood that the desired behaviors will occur again.

Using "Do" Statements

Similar to providing specific feedback, using "do" statements tells a child exactly what is desired. Rather than telling a child "Don't pull Susie's hair," the occupational therapist rephrases the statement to direct the child to do a behavior that is desired, for example, "Use your hands for nice touching." In contrast with the "don't" statement, the "do" statement appeals to the child's desire to please and helps keep a positive atmosphere. Modeling the instructed behavior while saying the instruction helps reinforce what is being communicated.

Keeping Perspective

Challenging behavior happens despite preventive measures. As children learn and grow through new stages of development and independence, they continually seek to discover where

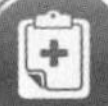

CASE STUDY 13-2 Dominic

Dominic has an extensive collection of train engines that he keeps arranged in a row on his bedroom floor. A new train engine is a treasure to Dominic. He carries it with him for days after receiving it and carefully determines its placement in his collection at bedtime. His satisfaction with determining each train's placement is celebrated with laughter, clapping, and jumping. If the trains are disrupted, as when the floor is vacuumed, Dominic becomes upset, making guttural vocalizations of increasing intensity while rocking back and forth. When he recovers from being upset, Dominic meticulously works to ensure that each train engine is in the correct order and placement.

The challenging behaviors that Dominic displays when his trains are disrupted can be avoided by giving careful attention to the situation. First, Dominic should be prepared in advance for the need to move the trains. For example, his mother should inform him that she needs to vacuum the floor and allow Dominic time to move his trains carefully on his own. Second, support and assistance should be offered when the trains are disrupted. For example, Dominic should be informed when the trains become disrupted, and the person responsible should offer to assist Dominic in replacing the trains. The assistance should be provided in a manner meaningful and acceptable to Dominic, whether it is handing the trains to him one at a time, pointing to the place in line where each train should be placed, or simply being near Dominic as he works on replacing each train.

limits exist, where their capabilities lie, and what they are allowed to do. It is important for the occupational therapist to be prepared to respond whenever the challenging behavior occurs so that expectations for appropriate behavior are quickly and effectively reestablished.

Behavior Management Approaches

Management of challenging behavior can take various forms, and the specific approach chosen will depend on the context, knowledge, skill, and available resources. Behavior management may occur at the individual level in the home, community, or clinic environment. School programs typically use a system-wide positive behavior support (PBS) approach to addressing challenging behaviors in children and youth. PBS combines a range of prevention and intervention methods to reduce challenging behaviors and increase appropriate behaviors.[27] The overarching goal of PBS is to improve quality of life for children. Many of the methods used in PBS are described below. Research support for PBS has demonstrated its effectiveness at reducing behaviors for children and youth who demonstrate disruptive or negative behaviors, those at risk of being identified as having a behavior disorder, and those with a variety of disabilities.[4,5,9,21,26,34]

The PBS approach is described in more detail in the section on intervening when challenging behaviors already exist.

Three primary approaches to managing challenging behavior are presented in this chapter: (1) preventing challenging behavior from occurring, (2) supporting desired behaviors, and (3) intervening when challenging behaviors already exist. Strategies associated with each of these approaches are discussed in this section.

Preventing Challenging Behavior

Strategies for preventing challenging behavior are similar to the general strategies for supporting appropriate behavior described earlier. However, these strategies become extremely useful when a child is known to have a repertoire of challenging behaviors, and the goal is to prevent those behaviors from emerging.

Minimizing Aversive Events

Children often demonstrate inappropriate behaviors in response to events that they find aversive (Case Study 13-2).[14] To minimize aversive events, situations and scenarios must be perceived through the child's eyes. In other words, the occupational therapist should think about what it is that the child finds aversive. Often, these are things that adults or other children do not consider problematic. Careful consideration of a particular child's temperament, personality, likes, dislikes, skills, abilities, and sensory processing tendencies can be helpful in identifying which conditions and events the child finds aversive. When an aversive condition is identified, minimizing the frequency, intensity, or duration of the condition can help reduce the child's reactive behaviors. For example, if a child is known to act out when he or she enters a classroom full of children, an adjustment can be made so that the child arrives earlier and enters a relatively empty classroom. Other examples include decreasing the amount of time that the child accompanies the parent on errands and reducing the volume at which the radio is played if these situations are known to result in displays of challenging behavior. If the correct events or conditions are not identified and addressed, no change in the behavior should be expected.

Sharing Control

Children often have very little control over their environments and the situations that surround them throughout the day. By allowing the child to choose activities, determine the order of events, or contribute ideas about what should happen, the occupational therapist can instill a sense of value and build self-esteem. The experiences of making acceptable choices, contributing to a collaborative effort, and giving valued input not only help the child feel important but can foster a sense of commitment to the therapeutic relationship. In turn, this can create the desire to preserve the relationship through effective and appropriate behaviors. See Research Note 13-1.

Providing an Environment That Promotes Successful Engagement

Challenging behaviors often occur when a child is bored or unoccupied. Providing an environment that promotes

RESEARCH NOTE 13-1

Benefits of Providing Activity Choices

Rispoli, M., Lang, R., Neely, L., Camargo, S., Hutchins, N., Davenport, K., & Goodwyn, F. (2013). A comparison of within- and across-activity choices for reducing challenging behavior in children with autism spectrum disorders. Journal of Behavior Education, 22, *66–83.*

Four children with autism whose challenging behaviors served the purpose of escaping from the task demands placed on them. Participants ranged in age from 5 to 11 years old. Two children were in self-contained classrooms, one in an inclusive classroom and one in a resource room setting. Data collection included in vivo recording for two students and video recording for the other two. Between one and five challenging behaviors were targeted per student. These included screaming, aggression, elopement, verbal protesting, delayed echolalia, and property destruction. During the baseline phases of the study, each child received adult-selected schoolwork to complete at a table. The work was removed for a brief period if the child demonstrated one of the target behaviors. During the intervention phases, the children experienced two different choice conditions. Each child was given the opportunity to choose (1) the type of schoolwork he or she would do while seated at the table or (2) the manner in which he or she would complete schoolwork selected by the adult. Available choices were location, materials, and vocal quality of spoken responses. The interventionist used prompting to encourage task engagement (baseline) or choice making (intervention) and positive reinforcement to acknowledge engagement or choice making. Data analysis revealed that all children displayed lower levels of challenging behavior when given choices for activities and methods of engagement.

Clinical Application

- Challenging behaviors often can be reduced by offering activity choices. Types of choices include the following:
  - Selecting between preferred and nonpreferred activities
  - Selecting the method of engagement, such as using crayons, markers, or chalk for writing or drawing
  - Selecting where to engage in the task—for example, completing puzzles on a swing or doing oral-motor activities while seated on a therapy ball
- Choices can be offered at the beginning of a session, allowing the child to help establish the sequence of activities to occur, or offered throughout a session, providing the child with multiple choice-making opportunities.

engagement can reduce boredom and thereby reduce occurrences of challenging behavior.[15] Environments that promote engagement offer structured and unstructured activities that are appropriate to the child's level of development, are enjoyed by the child, and allow the child to experience success. Supplies and materials should be readily available to the child in locations that allow independent access (Figure 13-3). Strict rules about how and where materials are used should be relaxed to allow creativity and ingenuity. A child who is dynamically engaged in productive activity is less likely to engage in inappropriate or challenging behaviors.

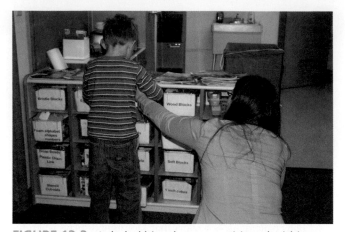

FIGURE 13-3 Labeled bins that are positioned within easy reach for the child allow him to access materials without hindrance. This supports positive behaviors by increasing his independence.

Increasing Communication Effectiveness

Children who do not have an effective means of communication often use behavior to deliver a message. Messages about pleasant experiences or enjoyable activities may be communicated through a smile, hug, or clapping. However, messages about pain, an undesired activity or location, frustration, or an unpleasant situation may be communicated through a variety of inappropriate methods such as screaming, hitting, throwing, or destroying property. Being attentive to a child's efforts to communicate is a first step in preventing situations that lead to frustration with communication barriers. Providing a means for the child to express positive and negative messages effectively and efficiently can reduce inappropriate behaviors associated with lack of functional communication.[11] Working with a speech-language pathologist to identify and implement the most effective and appropriate communication system is highly recommended. Strategies that can be helpful include using physical gestures or sign language and exchanging written symbols or icons. Strategies should be appropriate for the child's ability level and should be portable for easy accessibility in all environments and situations.

In addition to providing an effective means for the child to communicate, it is equally important that the child receive and comprehend messages directed to him or her. This responsibility often falls to the speaker because many children are not able to express that they do not understand a message. Awareness by the receiver that a message has been communicated but not understood can be very frustrating. When the message is not acted on, the sender becomes frustrated at the lack of response. The receiver is not only at a loss to decipher the message, but may also receive verbal and/or nonverbal communication about the sender's growing frustration. This scenario can result in increased anxiety, which may lead to behavioral outbursts. Using simple language to convey messages, allowing additional time for processing of information, and supplementing verbal information with gestures or visual information can increase the

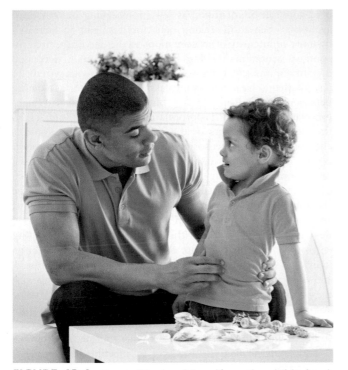

FIGURE 13-4 By positioning himself on the child's level, the adult is better able to speak directly to the child. Simple language, allowing additional time for processing, and inclusion of gestural or physical cues can also promote effective communication and help to decrease challenging behaviors.

possibility that messages are received and understood by the child, reducing the likelihood of frustration and resulting behavioral reactions[19] (Figure 13-4).

Clarifying Expectations

When activities or schedules are similar from day to day, assumptions may be made that expectations are known. Children, while sensing the comfort of a familiar environment, schedule, and social structure, do not necessarily attach performance expectations to environments or situations. Uncertainty about what is expected may lead the child unknowingly to act in inappropriate ways or to act out to test the limits. Many children respond best when rules are clearly established and limits are defined. Explicitly communicating expectations about what the child is supposed to do and how he or she is expected to act can alleviate any misconceptions or misunderstandings and help ensure that the child and therapist have the same expectations.[35]

Supporting Self-Regulation

Many children who demonstrate challenging behaviors also have difficulty managing responses to environmental stimuli (see Chapter 9 on sensory integration). Ambient noise, flickering lighting, constant movement of others, inadvertently being bumped, and other unpredictable or intense environmental stimuli can be anxiety-producing for persons who are sensitive to these stimuli. The result can be physiologic overarousal such that the individual's sympathetic fight-or-flight response occurs. This response can manifest as behaviors such as aggression toward others, hyperactivity, violence, self-injurious behaviors,

BOX 13-2 Environmental Modifications to Support Child's Self-Regulation

- Minimize ambient noise by adding carpeting, closing the classroom door, turning off appliances, and/or removing fluorescent lighting.
- Reduce visual stimulation by removing decorations from walls, closing curtains on windows, closing the classroom door, and providing a study carrel.
- Reduce situations that may result in accidental bumping or brushing against the child. Pay attention to stationary activities as well as activities requiring movement.
- Create zones for specific types of activities (e.g., quiet work, messy work, moving bodies).
- Install dimmer switches for lighting.
- Provide a hideout so the child can withdraw from overstimulating conditions.
- Arrange seating to minimize the possibility of the child being bumped or jostled.
- Rearrange the schedule to allow moving through the school building or visiting a community location at a time when it is not crowded.

and immediate and intense withdrawal from the situation. For these children, disorganized behavior may be a precursor to problem behavior.

The occupational therapist should watch for disorganized behavior and help the child identify when behavior is becoming dysregulated. This may include informing the child of the disorganized behavior by specifically describing the behavior that was observed, identifying the context in which the behavior occurred, and describing what behavior would have been more appropriate to the context. In addition, the therapist should help the child develop a repertoire of more appropriate responses. Careful attention to and management of stimuli present in the environment can prevent the "fight, flight, or fright" response from occurring, allowing the individual to participate in the environment successfully. Box 13-2 identifies some suggested environmental modifications.

Matching Demands to Abilities

When performance demands exceed an individual's abilities, that person can become frustrated, angry, avoidant, or aggressive. Conversely, when performance demands are too low and do not match or challenge an individual's abilities, the person can become bored or uninterested in a task or activity. Either of these situations can result in challenging behavior as the individual expresses frustration with the mismatch between demands and abilities.[1] Creating individualized expectations and adjusting activities so that the child experiences an appropriate level of challenge can help alleviate frustration and create a just-right match between each child's performance demands and performance abilities (Figure 13-5).

Supporting Positive Behavior

Strategies for supporting positive behaviors can be powerful tools in preventing situations that elicit problem behaviors. Some of the strategies are global and can be particularly useful for group situations in which more than one child requires assistance in managing appropriate behavior.[29] Other strategies are individualized to a particular child. All the strategies should be implemented consistently and predictably to create a context that supports the child's ability to be successful.

General Strategies

Meeting Sensory Needs

Sensory input is an inherent part of life. Every experience and situation is saturated with sensation. Sensory information is received, interpreted, and managed by the central nervous system through a variety of chemical and electrical mechanisms. The central nervous system produces behavioral and emotional responses to this input. When an individual's processing of sensory information is ineffective or inaccurate, erratic behaviors that are inappropriate to the context or situation can be displayed.[2] These behaviors can take many forms. Often, the behaviors can be identified as sensation-seeking or sensation-avoiding.[10] Sensation-seeking behaviors result in an increased quantity or intensity of sensory input to the nervous system. In contrast, sensation-avoiding behaviors result in a decreased quantity or intensity of sensory input to the nervous system. In and of themselves, sensation-seeking and sensation-avoiding behaviors are not inappropriate, but they may occur with inappropriate intensity, at inappropriate times, and without regard for the safety of others or the environment. For example, a child who is seeking sensory input may frequently touch other objects or people, press so firmly with a pencil that it breaks, or hug others so tightly that they feel discomfort. In contrast, a child who avoids sensory input may attempt to leave the classroom if the overall sensory stimulation level of noise, lights, and activity becomes too high and may strike out at others if he or she is not allowed to withdraw from an overly stimulating environment. By being aware of and taking efforts to meet an individual's sensory needs, such situations can be avoided, allowing individuals to have greater success in interacting with the people, objects, and situations around them. This can be accomplished through a variety of strategies ranging from intense, one-on-one intervention to a range of sensory-based strategies that are embedded in the daily routine. An example of addressing challenging behavior by meeting sensory needs is presented in Case Study 13-3. In addition, see Chapter 9 for a discussion of sensory integration disorders and strategies to meet sensory needs.

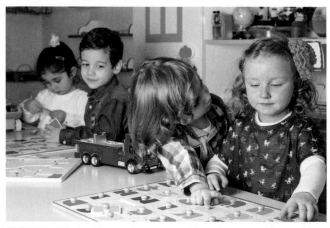

FIGURE 13-5 Therapists can easily adapt puzzles so that all children experience success by altering the complexity of the puzzle. This allows all children to participate.

Building New Skills

Children who have deficits in performance areas can become frustrated with the frequent experience of poor performance or lack of success. As noted, frustration can lead to a demonstration of undesired behaviors as a way of expressing or dealing with the frustration.[17] Thus, it is important that occupational therapists incorporate efforts to build new skills into their intervention plans. When developing the intervention plan, those skills that appear to pose the greatest barriers to independence

CASE STUDY 13-3 Stephen

Stephen is a 10-year-old boy enrolled in the third grade. His teacher states that Stephen often has difficulty with attention to tasks, following directions, and completing his work. He constantly fidgets with his clothing and does not sit still in his chair. He is frequently sent to the principal's office for disrespecting a teacher's authority and having an uncooperative attitude. He often has a scowl on his face and does not greet others or participate in social interactions. His comments are negative and demeaning toward others. He does not receive compliments or praise but deflects these comments by highlighting a rule that was broken or promise not kept. A recent psychological evaluation resulted in a diagnosis of oppositional defiant disorder.

The classroom teacher requested an occupational therapy evaluation to address Stephen's difficulty in performing the handwriting required to complete his schoolwork. In addition to poor development of intrinsic hand musculature, the occupational therapy evaluation identified difficulties in processing visual, auditory, and tactile sensation such that behavior and fine motor performance were affected. The occupational therapist recommended modifications to Stephen's classroom to address his sensitivity to bright lights, ambient noise, and unexpected touch. The placement of his desk was moved from the center of the classroom to the side, near the teacher's desk, a study carrel was brought into the classroom, and Stephen was allowed to wear sunglasses in class during work time. The occupational therapist collaborated with the classroom teacher to develop an activity plan incorporating regular opportunities for movement and physical effort to help meet Stephen's need for increased proprioceptive input. In addition, she conducted an in-service for the school staff, instructing them on the relationship between poor sensory processing and ineffective behavioral regulation, the importance of addressing sensory needs as a first step in helping children regulate behavioral responses to others more effectively, and the need to teach and reinforce those behavioral skills intentionally that the child needs to develop.

BOX 13-3 Skills That Promote Social Participation

Communicating wants, desires, dislikes
Compliance with requests
Cooperation with adults and peers
Flexibility
Giving an object on request
Independent play
- Ability to initiate
- Ability to sustain
- Ability to conclude

Making choices
Parallel play
Social play
Variety in play
Sharing
Turn-taking
Waiting

in self-care, physical mobility, play, or education are often prioritized. However, it also is important to include the development of skills that enable the child to experience success in the regular daily occupations of social interaction and participation. Box 13-3 identifies skills that are easily overlooked but are important to social participation. These should be incorporated into the occupational therapy intervention plan in an effort to build new skills and reduce frustration and the resulting problem behaviors.[35]

Specific Strategies

Increasing Compliance Through Contingency Methods

Many children resist engaging in tasks that they do not enjoy. Resistance can take many forms, including, but not limited to, withdrawal, refusal, avoidance, and aggression. Contingency methods such as offering rewards or using a token economy can help elicit participation in nonpreferred activities. Contingency methods are based on the principle of allowing access to a desired event contingent on performance of or compliance with a directive, instruction, or rule. For example, during intervention, a child who enjoys blowing bubbles would be allowed to play with bubbles only after he or she has completed a therapist-directed task, such as pencil and paper work. Contingency approaches are commonly used in everyday life for children; for example, access to outdoor play is not granted until the child puts on a coat, or dessert is not served unless the child finishes dinner (Figure 13-6). By withholding the desired item or activity until after the child completes the mandatory task, motivation is increased and compliance is gained.

Use of contingencies can be complicated when a child unfamiliar with contingencies tries to negotiate the demands or displays undesired behaviors in an effort to avoid the contingency. It is important that the therapist avoid engaging the child in power struggles during these times. Instead, the adult should, in a matter-of-fact manner, adhere to the contingency in place and ensure that the child does not gain access to the desired event or activity unless the required task is completed.

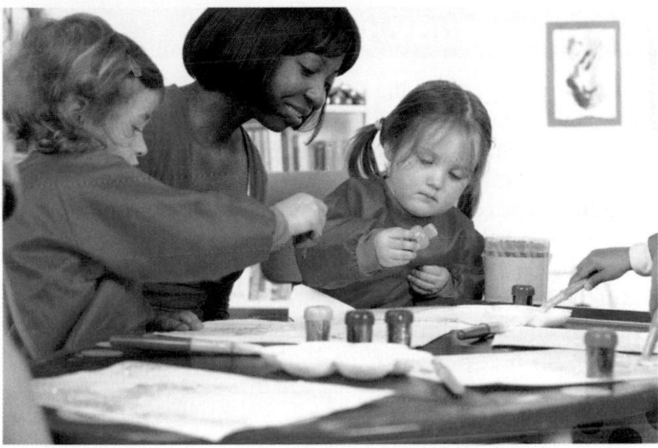

FIGURE 13-6 The child in this figure is resistant to using tools, including paintbrushes. Her typical approach is to fingerpaint. The adult is positioned close enough to the child to facilitate the required behavior of paintbrush use, after which the child is allowed to fingerpaint.

Token Economies

Token economies are similar to withholding strategies but are more complex. A system in which the child earns tokens for desired behaviors is established and taught. Examples of behaviors that are reinforced are compliance with a rule, completion of a certain task or part of a task, and keeping hands out of the mouth. The tokens can be exchanged for privileges such as 2 minutes of play with a preferred toy, a piece of candy, or the opportunity to play a game on the computer. In essence, certain privileges are withheld from the child until he or she has sufficient tokens to buy them. The tokens are earned through performance of desired tasks, engagement in prescribed activities, or demonstration of an appropriate behavior. In establishing the token economy, the specific behavior for which tokens can be earned should be specified, as should the number of tokens each behavior is worth. For example, a child might earn one token for engaging in seat work for 3 minutes without needing redirection, or earn two tokens for spontaneously sharing art supplies with another child (Figure 13-7). In addition, the privileges or items that the child can purchase with the tokens and the cost of each should be established at the outset of establishing the token economy.

The complexity of token economies can be adjusted depending on the child's developmental and cognitive age. A very simple system may involve merely the earning of tokens and purchasing of rewards, whereas a complex system may incorporate having the child relinquish tokens for episodes of undesired behaviors (Case Study 13-4). In one type of system, the child earns one color of token (often green or white) for desired behaviors and another color (often red) for undesired behaviors. The tokens for desired behavior have purchasing value, and those for undesired behavior decrease purchasing value. For example, a child might earn one green token for each 2 minutes that he or she remains seated during independent work time and one red token each time he or she moves out of the chair. At the end of a 10-minute work period, the child has four green tokens and two red tokens. Each red token cancels out one green token, leaving the child with two tokens for that period of time.

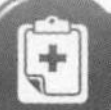

CASE STUDY 13-4 Stephen

In addition to addressing Stephen's sensory needs, the occupational therapist worked with Stephen and his teacher to develop a behavior contract outlining expectations for appropriate interactions with the teacher, school staff, and other children. The contract includes a token economy and specifies the positive behaviors that Stephen is expected to display. He earns a green token for each desired behavior, a red token for undesired behavior, and specific graduated consequences for not abiding with the contract. Green tokens are earned for specific occurrences of appropriate interactions with others and for maintaining an appropriate on-task classroom behavior for a specified duration of time. Red tokens are given to Stephen for occurrences of inappropriate social interactions, off-task behavior, swearing, and noncompliance with the teacher's instructions. Tokens are counted and exchanged at the end of each school day for a choice from the school prize box, 5 minutes of free choice from a specified set of activities, or opportunities for special activities, such as ice cream with the principal.

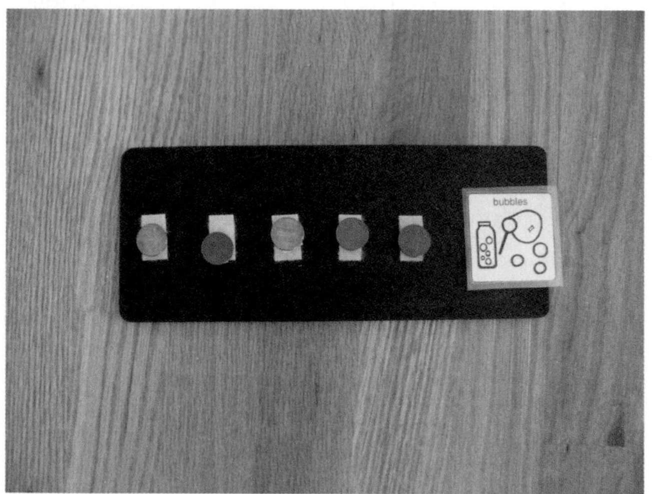

FIGURE 13-7 A token board is a variation on the token system. The child earns one token for a specified amount of work such as putting one piece in a puzzle. Once the token board is full, the child earns the opportunity to engage with the activity represented in the picture.

Positive Reinforcement

Positive reinforcement is a specific strategy that has been established as a powerful behavior change technique. Positive reinforcement is the contingent presentation of a type of consequence that when presented immediately after a behavior, increases the probability of that behavior occurring again.[24] In other words, a consequence that strengthens a behavior functions as a positive reinforcer for that behavior. Consider the mother who gives in and hands her child a cookie to stop the crying that began when the mother first denied the child's request for the cookie. Although the mother's purpose in giving the cookie was to stop the crying, the crying resulted in the child obtaining a desired object. In other words, from the child's perspective, the crying worked. The likelihood that the child will behave in the same manner in the future (crying) has been increased by the positive reinforcer (obtaining the cookie). The power of positive reinforcement to effect behavior change has more than 40 years of empirical support[22,23,37-39]; however, occupational therapists typically are not trained in these techniques.[36] Strategic and effective use of positive reinforcement can increase desired behaviors and reduce challenging behaviors, thereby supporting client engagement in therapeutic activities.

Alternate Preferred and Nonpreferred Activities

At times, all children need to participate in or complete tasks or activities that they do not enjoy. Attempts to gain the child's compliance in a nonpreferred task can lead to opposition, withdrawal, or outright refusal. If the adult keeps pressing the child to comply, challenging behaviors can escalate. One strategy for gaining compliance is to alternate the nonpreferred activity with one or more preferred activities. This strategy is similar to the contingency approaches in which a desired activity or event is withheld until the child performs a therapist-directed task. To implement this strategy successfully, the nonpreferred activity should seamlessly follow the preferred activity and should be presented in a matter-of-fact manner that does not highlight the child's lack of preference for the activity. By strategically and seamlessly sequencing the nonpreferred activity to come immediately after a preferred activity, the child is more likely to comply because the activity seems to flow from the one that was just completed (Case Study 13-5).

Addressing Transitions

Transition between activities or environments can be a particularly problematic time during which challenging behaviors emerge. In school situations, the classroom schedule often dictates when children transition between activities. Adults have strategies such as watching the clock and having an awareness of how much time has passed, which helps them anticipate a pending transition. Children do not have the same strategies, and transitions can appear to be arbitrarily imposed. Some practical strategies can support children to anticipate and make transitions; these help minimize noncompliance, refusals, or behavioral outbursts.

A *transition routine* can help set the stage for a positive transition. Transition routines consist of using the same set of events each time a transition needs to occur. Singing a particular song and using a hand-clapping pattern are simple, distinct events that can be used to signal transitions. Using the same strategies for each transition provides familiarity, establishes context, and communicates expectations, all of which can help children transition successfully (Figure 13-8).

Visual schedules are a commonly used and effective method for supporting successful transitions.[8,33] These are particularly useful in situations in which the schedule remains relatively similar from day to day or week to week or to represent changes

CASE STUDY 13-5 Anastasia

Anastasia is a 5-year-old girl with a diagnosis of developmental delay. She demonstrates many signs of sensory processing disorder, including sensory-seeking behaviors, distractibility, and high frequency of movement. These behaviors result in poor engagement in tabletop activities. Anastasia's mother has brought her to occupational therapy with concerns about readiness for school, specifically her unwillingness to engage in pencil and paper activities. During the evaluation, Anastasia refused to complete the writing activities on standardized testing of fine motor and visual-motor skills. During observations, Anastasia used a static tripod grasp while drawing on a chalkboard. She approximated continuous circles, but no other shapes. Her attention was fleeting and she did not return to the chalkboard spontaneously or on request.

Evaluation results identified significant deficits in fine motor and visual motor skills as well as poor processing of vestibular, tactile, and proprioceptive input. The occupational therapist began intervention using a sensory integration approach. As part of therapy sessions, Anastasia participated in obstacle courses in which she was challenged to push, pull, climb, swing, jump, ride a scooter board around obstacles, and crawl. As Anastasia's distractibility decreased and her willingness to engage in therapist-directed activities increased, the occupational therapist began to incorporate pencil and paper tasks into the obstacle courses. After using a hand-over-hand motion to pull herself up a ramp while riding prone on a scooter board, and then jumping off the ramp platform into a mountain of pillows and crawling through a tunnel, Anastasia sat on a therapy ball and drew straight lines on paper mounted on a slant board. Anastasia was not allowed to continue the obstacle course until she completed the pencil and paper task. Over time, the occupational therapist gradually increased the complexity of drawing, duration of the drawing task, and quality of work expected. As she alternated between the sensory-based activities she needed to become prepared and organized for table work with the table work activities, Anastasia's willingness to engage and her duration of engagement increased, allowing her to develop new skills.

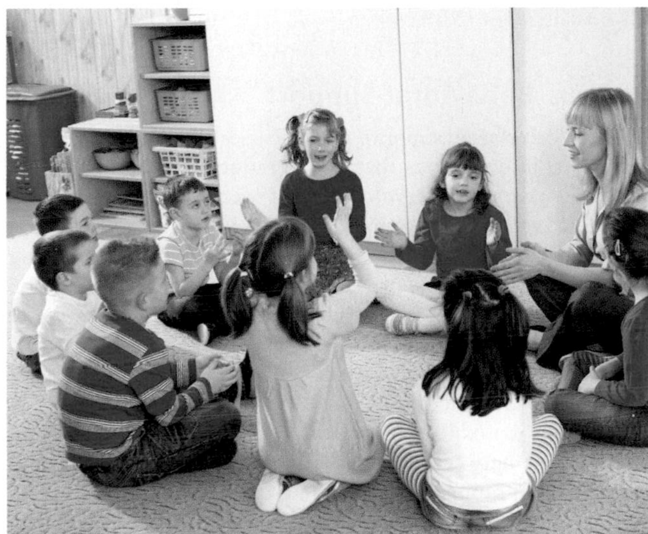

FIGURE 13-8 This class of students is engaged in a song accompanied by clapping, which indicates that it is time to transition from circle time to the next activity.

in the schedule for a child who has difficulty tolerating change. Picture icons or word cards can be arranged on a schedule board to represent the sequence of activities or events that is going to occur. Children can follow the visual representation of the sequence. Depending on a given child's abilities, he or she can learn to use the visual schedule independently, consulting it when one activity is completed or when a transition is indicated. Some visual schedules merely represent activity sequences, with no time allotted. Other schedules are time-based and indicate the day of the week, time of day, and activity that will be occurring. Many visual schedules use removable cards so that the schedule can be modified easily if the schedule changes. Some schedules are written on poster board mounted to the wall; others are secured in a binder or notebook that is easily transported from one setting to another. The form of the schedule and amount of support given to the child in using the schedule are individualized to the child's capabilities.

Timers provide an objective signal that something is about to occur.[12] Once it is set, a timer operates independently of an adult, so the implication that changes are arbitrarily imposed by the adult is reduced. To implement the use of a timer, the occupational therapist shows it to the child and informs him or her about what will happen (e.g., "The timer will make a beeping sound. When you hear the beeping sound, it will be time to clean up the blocks and come to the table for snack"). The occupational therapist trains the child on how to turn the timer off. When the timer signals, the occupational therapist cues the child that the timer is beeping, helps the child turn off the timer, and reminds the child what the sound meant (Case Study 13-6).

Once an occupational therapist establishes use of the timer, it can be applied in a variety of contexts and situations. Children can learn to operate the timer themselves as a way to self-monitor use of time and compliance with time limits. Alarm clocks can be used in a similar manner as timers to indicate events that occur at a specific time of day, such as time to go to the bus stop, time to get ready for bed, and time to leave for an appointment.

Another strategy for supporting transitions is the use of *representational objects.* In this method, concrete objects that clearly represent the various activities or events that make up the child's day are assembled. When the child needs to transition to a new activity, he or she is shown or given the relevant representational object and a simple verbal instruction. For example, the occupational therapist may hand the child a crayon and say, "It is time for art." The child may take the object and carry it to the location where the next activity will occur. The use of representational objects is flexible and can be paired with the other strategies of transition routines, visual

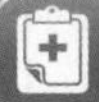

CASE STUDY 13-6 Meg

Meg is a 4-year-old girl with autism. She enjoys playing with alphabet blocks and her toy piano. Meg has extreme difficulty concluding her play to transition to a different activity. When a transition is imposed on her, Meg demonstrates one of two predictable responses: a complete lack of response, as if she did not hear the instruction, or extreme refusal to transition, expressed by screaming and stamping her feet. At times, the behavior can escalate into a full-blown tantrum including hitting, kicking, dropping to the floor, and throwing toys.

Meg is enrolled in a preschool classroom for children with developmental disabilities. Transition between activities occurs multiple times each day as the children engage in different play centers, circle time, snack time, and outdoor play. Meg's difficulties with transitions often disrupt the class. The occupational therapist works with Meg on a weekly basis and introduces a timer to help her learn how to conclude an activity. Within 3 days, Meg consistently responds when the timer signals. She alerts to the sound, discontinues her activity, and turns the timer off. Sometimes she returns to her activity and reengages, but when cued by the teacher or occupational therapist, she is able to transition to the next activity. By the end of nine school days, Meg reliably alerts to the sound of the timer, discontinues her activity, and consults a visual schedule to determine what she is to do next. She then activates the timer for a preset duration of time and transitions to the activity indicated on her schedule.

schedules, and timers in the manner that best supports the child's success.[33]

General Support Strategies

Many challenging or inappropriate behaviors can be ameliorated through the use of general positive strategies. These strategies are examples of the therapeutic use of self.

- Providing extra time for a child to process a verbal instruction or organize an appropriate response to a stimulus can alleviate anxiety and stress and the resulting behavioral reaction.
- Providing encouragement that communicates belief in the child's ability to succeed can improve self-esteem and a sense of self-worth.[25]
- Giving explicit instructions on how to approach or complete a task can alleviate fears of failure that may cause a child to withdraw or disengage from an activity.
- Providing specific feedback about the child's efforts and what could be done differently next time can also build confidence and motivate a child to try again, rather than walk away from a task with a feeling of despair.

The occupational therapist uses the therapist-client interactions strategically to support the child in whatever challenge he or she is experiencing and to communicate belief in the child's ability to achieve his or her desires. Effective therapeutic use of self leads to a partnership between the occupational therapist and client that is empowering and encouraging.[32] The power of these experiences can help prevent misbehaviors that are associated with feelings of despair and low self-esteem.

Intervening When Children are Known to Have Challenging Behaviors

When challenging behaviors are known to exist, the occupational therapist should collaborate with the child's caregivers and other service providers to understand the frequency, intensity, and purpose of the behaviors before intervening. It is important that the team of service providers have a unified approach across environments and providers to address the behavior most effectively and efficiently. Because all behavior serves a purpose, it is critical that the intervention be preceded by a systematic evaluation of the behavior. This systematic process identifies the function of the behavior and contextual factors that support and maintain the behavior, both of which are crucial for selecting relevant interventions. Systematic evaluation of the behavior is best accomplished through an FBA. An FBA is one component of a comprehensive approach to behavior management (PBS).

Positive Behavioral Support

Positive behavioral support encompasses a range of positive behavioral interventions that aim to reduce challenging behaviors while promoting development of socially important behaviors. The overarching goal of PBS is to improve the quality of life for children by increasing desired behaviors and reducing challenging behaviors.[6,31] The primary strategies of PBS emerged through decades of educational research and involve environmental adjustments of those factors that may trigger, reinforce or maintain the challenging behaviors.[28] Sugai and colleagues[31] identified four foundations of PBS that govern its use. PBS is based on *behavioral science* and emphasizes the relationships between behavior and environmental factors and the belief that human behavior can be changed through manipulation of those factors. The PBS approach uses *practical interventions*, such as redesign of environment or curriculum, to address the goodness of fit between contextual factors, problem behaviors, and the interventions implemented.[1] For PBS to be considered effective, the *outcomes* must be socially significant, and behavior must change to a degree that enhances the quality of life of the individual. In addition, PBS adheres to a *systems perspective* that addresses the multiple contexts and social partners of the individual, as well as the policies that govern each context. See Research Note 13-2.

PBS can have a highly significant and positive effect on reducing the behavioral challenges of students with disabilities in schools.[5] The Individuals with Disabilities Education Act (IDEA) amendments of 1997, which were reaffirmed in 2004,[20] specifically identify PBS as an effective preventive program for children whose behaviors impede their own learning or the learning of others (20 U.S.C. § 1414(d)(3)(B)(i)). The use of behavioral interventions within a PBS model is always based on an FBA, a systematic process that analyzes problem behavior to define the behavior operationally, identifies the events that

RESEARCH NOTE 13-2

Effects of Positive Behavioral Support

Chitiyo, M., Makweche-Chitiyo, P., Park, M., Ametepee, L. K. & Chitiyo, J. (2010). Examining the effect of positive behavior support on academic achievement of students with disabilities. Journal of Research on Special Educational Needs, 11, *171–177.*

In a meta-analysis of studies published from 1996 to 2006, Chitiyo et al.[7] found support for a relationship among problem behavior, positive behavior support, and academic performance. Five published studies met the inclusion criteria and were included in the analysis. The resulting population was 25 participants between 5 and 14 years of age with diagnoses of attention-deficit/hyperactivity disorder (ADHD), autism, developmental disorder, emotional and behavior disorders, and students at risk of delay. Inclusion criteria required that the studies addressed problem behavior in school settings, used positive behavior support at an individual or classroom-wide level, and measured behavior and academic performance. Results identified a positive correlation (r = .40) between behavioral outcomes and academic achievement, suggesting that as problem behaviors improved, so did academic performance. Outcomes were more favorable for participants with emotional or behavior disorders and those with ADHD.

Application to Practice

- Positive behavior supports can support positive outcomes in academic performance. In addition to measuring change in students' challenging behaviors, occupational therapists should include cognitive outcomes when measuring the effectiveness of these strategies within classroom and school wide intervention programs.
- Positive behavior supports produced stronger effects in behavior change and academic performance for students with emotional and behavioral disorders and those with ADHD. Careful consideration of client characteristics is warranted when considering PBS as an intervention and developing goal statements for measuring progress.
- Students with autism demonstrated milder changes in response to positive behavior support strategies, so it may be important to include PBS as only one component of a comprehensive program of intervention to support students with autism.
- Individual outcomes should be closely monitored and the intervention program modified if desired outcomes are not achieved.

reliably predict the occurrence and nonoccurrence of those behaviors, and those factors that maintain the behaviors across time.[31] FBA is mandated by IDEA in the following situations:

- A child who does not have a behavior intervention plan is removed from their current placement for more than 10 school days (e.g., suspension) for behavior that turns out to be a manifestation of the child's disability (20 U.S.C. § 1415(k)(1)(F)(i)).
- (It is) appropriate to address any behavior that results in a long-term removal (20 U.S.C. § 1415(k)(1)(D)).

As a systems-wide approach, PBS includes three levels of strategies.[28] The first level aims to *prevent* challenging behaviors from occurring. Strategies may include creating an organized environment to support learning, arranging the physical environment to promote engagement and positive behavior, and providing instruction in communication and social skills to support social interaction and participation. If challenging behaviors emerge or continue after the first wave of supportive strategies are in place, more targeted methods are used. This second level of intervention may include group instruction in school success strategies or skill development, establishment of a support network throughout the school, or implementation of corrective teaching. A third level of intervention is implemented on a student by-student basis for challenging behaviors that are resistant to the first two levels of intervention. This level of intervention provides intensive individualized strategies, including the following: (1) an FBA resulting in a comprehensive behavior plan, (2) implementation of targeted methods during daily routines and activities to decrease challenging or interfering behaviors, and (3) further development of communication and social skills to support participation. The Evolve site lists resources for positive behavior support.

Functional Behavioral Analysis

FBA is a five-step process consisting of the following: (1) team building and goal setting, (2) functional assessment of the behavior, (3) hypothesis development, (4) development of the comprehensive support plan, and (5) implementation and outcome monitoring of the plan, including refining the plan as needed.[4] Occupational therapists may be part of the FBA process because they often have personal knowledge of the client and direct experience with the targeted behavior. Each of the five steps of the FBA process is described briefly here.

The first step of the FBA process is to gather a team of individuals who collaborate to work together for the child's best interest. Ideally, the team includes the child's parents or caregivers as recognized experts on the child and as partners in the intervention process. Together with the caregivers, the team works first to identify desired outcomes for the child.[4] Team planning considers the child as a "whole" person, including the child's capacities and areas needing further development. This process creates a foundation on which the intervention and support plans are built.

The second step involves the comprehensive functional assessment of the specific behavior. Efforts focus on clearly describing the challenging behavior, the context(s) in which it occurs, antecedents and consequences that maintain the behavior, and functions of the behavior. The goal of this step is to understand the purpose of the behavior and determine when the behavior is most or least likely to occur. Data collection is the best method for understanding the purpose of the behavior and the events that maintain the behavior. Data can be gathered by interviewing people who have direct knowledge of the child and experience with the behavior, observing the child where and when the behavior is most likely to occur, reviewing records in which the behavior has been documented, and gathering information about contextual variables such as health or changes in other environments or activity schedules.

The third step in the FBA process is to develop hypotheses about the behavior, including the antecedents (factors that trigger the behavior), consequences (responses to the behavior), and function of the behavior (e.g., requesting something, avoiding or escaping from something, meeting a sensory need). Hypotheses statements are generated based on the information gathered in the second step.

In the fourth step, a comprehensive behavior support plan is developed. The plan itself has four elements: (1) functional assessment of behavior, including hypothesized functions of the behavior; (2) specific individualized intervention strategies to be used; (3) strategies to be applied throughout the day; and (4) evidence that the plan is consistent with the values and resources of the child receiving support and of those providing support.[18]

The collaborative effort of the team to gather data about the behavior and develop hypotheses about the function and reinforcing events surrounding the behavior is used to understand the behavior and functional purpose that it serves for the child. This understanding is used to develop the intervention component of the plan, which includes positive behavioral strategies aimed at preventing the challenging behavior from occurring and strategies aimed at helping the child develop new skills that effectively and efficiently achieve the same function as the challenging behavior. The new skills are taught to the child as replacement strategies for the challenging and undesired behavior. The PBS plan may incorporate the strategies identified earlier in this chapter if they are appropriate for the factors that are influencing the target behavior(s). The plan also includes contingencies for the challenging and replacement behaviors. The contingencies for demonstration of the replacement behavior are designed to reinforce and strengthen use of the new behavior, whereas the contingencies for the challenging behavior are designed to discourage its use.

The final step of the PBS process is implementation of the plan and measurement of outcomes. Once the plan is developed, it is tested for goodness of fit with the personal, physical, and social contexts of the child, family, and other service providers to ensure that all persons involved in implementing the plan are equally comfortable using the plan in their respective situations. Ensuring goodness of fit is a critical step in increasing the likelihood that the plan is used.

As the plan is implemented, the team evaluates the effectiveness of the plan in producing the desired results: reduction of the challenging behavior and demonstration of the replacement behaviors. The team meets periodically to review the plan's effectiveness and the child's progress. Modifications and adjustments are made as needed, followed by implementation and monitoring of the revised plan (Case Study 13-7).

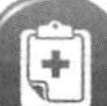

CASE STUDY 13-7 Jessie

Seven-year-old Jessie was suspended from his second-grade classroom because of uncontrollable aggressive outbursts that included yelling at the teacher, refusing to complete schoolwork, overturning desks, and throwing school supplies. The behaviors had been building throughout the fall and culminated with punching the teacher in early December. An FBA was initiated in November and revealed that Jessie's behaviors escalated when work demands involved extended writing and during collaborative group work activities. The occupational therapist had observed Jessie's handwriting abilities in October at the request of the classroom teacher. Jessie used a mature tripod grasp, formed letters correctly, and exhibited good upper extremity positioning and postural support for handwriting tasks. Jessie performed handwriting activities without difficulty when copying from a sample or when writing personal information, such as his name. The occupational therapist observed signs of anxiety when Jessie was asked to write creatively, documenting that he "seemed unable to generate ideas or topics to write about and he became flushed, fidgeted with his pencil, and stated that the assignment was 'stupid.'"

During the FBA, it was discovered that signs of anxiety often preceded Jessie's behavioral outbursts and that the outbursts were worse later in the day, during the creative writing lessons. Jessie also showed signs of anxiety during collaborative work activities. When group work was assigned, Jessie fidgeted with materials in his desk and did not join his group until specifically instructed by the teacher. He did not join in the group discussions or participate in work activities. Rather, he remained at the fringe of the group. If his participation was requested by a peer or instructed by the teacher, Jessie shifted his weight and looked around anxiously, often giving excuses for not working. If pushed to participate, he verbally refused with increased vocal intensity and volume, and sometimes shoved a desk or chair. The FBA team hypothesized that the behaviors were a result of poor ability to cope with anxiety and that writing and social situations were anxiety-producing for Jessie.

The FBA team worked together to develop a plan to match writing and social demands to Jessie's abilities better, provide support during writing assignments, and provide intervention to develop social skills that would support his ability to participate in group learning activities.

In addition to modifications the teacher made to assignments, the occupational therapist provided recommendations for modifying the classroom environment to decrease anxiety-producing situations and add coping supports. She also designed a program aimed to help Jessie develop improved self-regulation of behavior, body scheme, fine motor coordination, and social skills. Some classroom-wide strategies included seated isometric exercises for the entire class at key times during the school day, regularly scheduled dimmed lighting and whispered voice times, and a "cozy corner" for independent use by students. The occupational therapist also worked with Jessie, his teacher, and the school counselor to identify two peers with whom Jessie could work to build his social skills. She provided training sessions with the students, teacher, and counselor, including instruction on teamwork, complimenting, turn-taking, and collaboration. Data collection forms were used to track Jessie's behavior. A change in the frequency and intensity of Jessie's behavior was seen almost immediately, and within 3 weeks of implementing the program, Jessie's inappropriate behavior had diminished to occasional verbal outbursts, with no physical aggression.

Summary

- Challenging and inappropriate behaviors are demonstrated by children with a wide range of developmental disabilities and can interfere with engagement in occupation, prevent participation in context, and create situations that are potentially harmful.
- Intervention includes prevention of challenging behaviors, support of positive behaviors, and system-wide and individualized interventions for existing problem behaviors.
- Challenging behaviors always have a function, and understanding that function is the first step of planning intervention. When problem behaviors exist, reducing the problem behavior should be a primary focus of occupational therapy intervention.
- Using familiar activities in a predictable sequence can be an effective strategy for reducing the anxiety that often precedes inappropriate withdrawal, refusal, or aggressive behaviors.
- Effective management of challenging behavior includes not only improving an individual's behavioral competence, but also creating contexts that support positive behaviors and intentionally managing consequences.
- A child with poor sensory processing and integration may have considerable difficulty regulating behavior in highly stimulating environments. Addressing a child's sensory needs can be a key part of a program to prevent challenging behaviors.
- Contingency methods in which a child gains access to a preferred activity, object, person, or event only after engaging in or completing a specified activity can be useful in helping the child build or develop new skills. Use of contingency methods must be individualized and customized to the child and to the behavior being addressed.
- The therapeutic use of self, which is an inherent part of occupational therapy service delivery, is an essential aspect of building therapeutic relationships that support positive behaviors. Occupational therapists working with children with challenging behaviors should be intentional about building the therapeutic relationship and using it as an intervention strategy.
- Because all behavior is purposeful, it is important to analyze and identify the function of each challenging or undesired behavior systematically using a functional behavior analysis. Occupational therapists can participate in this process by contributing their observations of behavior and its relationship to occupational performance and contextual factors for the individual child.
- Occupational therapists have knowledge and skills in task analysis, human behavior, and occupational engagement and participation, enabling them to collaborate with caregivers and other service providers effectively to analyze problem behavior, develop behavioral intervention plans, and implement behavior management strategies. These attributes make occupational therapists key contributors to designing and implementing positive behavioral support programs in home, school, and community environments.

REFERENCES

1. Albin, R. W., Lucyshyn, L. M., Horner, R. H., et al. (1996). Contextual fit for behavior support plans: A model for a goodness-of-fit. In L. K. Koegel, R. L. Koegel, & G. Dunlap (Eds.), *Positive behavior support: Including people with difficult behavior in the community* (pp. 81–89). Baltimore: Brookes.
2. Baker, A. E., Lane, A., Angley, M. T., et al. (2008). The relationship between sensory processing and behavioural responsiveness in autistic disorder: A pilot study. *Journal of Autism and Developmental Disorders, 38,* 867–875.
3. Bauman, M. (2008). Autism: Emotion and behavior—is it all in the brain? Paper presented at R2K: Research 2008 Sensory Integration, Emotions, and Autism, Long Beach, CA.
4. Buschbacher, P. W., & Fox, L. (2003). Understanding and intervening with the challenging behavior of young children with autism spectrum disorder. *Language, Speech, and Hearing Services in Schools, 34,* 217–227.
5. Carr, E. G., Horner, R. H., Turnbull, A. P., et al. (1999). *Positive behavior support for people with developmental disabilities: A research synthesis.* Washington, DC: American Association on Mental Retardation.
6. Carr, E. G., Dunlap, G., Horner, R. H., et al. (2002). Positive behavior support: Evolution of an applied science. *Journal of Positive Behavior Interventions, 4,* 4–16.
7. Chitiyo, M., Makweche-Chitiyo, P., Park, M., et al. (2010). Examining the effect of positive behavior support on academic achievement of students with disabilities. *Journal of Research on Special Educational needs, 11,* 171–177.
8. Dettmer, S., Simpson, R. L., Myles, B. S., et al. (2000). The use of visual supports to facilitate transitions of students with autism. *Focus on Autism and Other Developmental Disabilities, 15,* 163–169.
9. Dunlap, G., & Fox, L. (1999). A demonstration of behavioral support for young children with autism. *Journal of Positive Behavior Interventions, 1*(2), 77–87.
10. Dunn, W. (1997). The impact of sensory processing abilities on the daily lives of young children and their families: A conceptual model. *Infants and Young Children, 9*(4), 23–35.
11. Durand, V. M., & Carr, E. G. (1992). An analysis of maintenance following functional communication training. *Journal of Applied Behavior Analysis, 25,* 777–794.
12. Ferguson, A., Ashbaugh, R., O'Reilly, S., et al. (2004). Using prompt training and reinforcement to reduce transition times in a transitional kindergarten program for students with severe behavior disorders. *Child and Family Behavior Therapy, 26,* 17–24.
13. Flannery, K. B., & Horner, R. H. (1994). The relationship between predictability and problem behavior for students with severe disabilities. *Journal of behavioral Education, 4,* 157–176.
14. Foxx, R. M. (1996). Twenty years of applied behavior analysis in treating the most severe problem behavior: Lessons learned. *Behavior Analyst, 19*(2), 225–235.
15. Foxx, R. M., & Meindl, J. (2007). The long-term successful treatment of the aggressive/destructive behaviors of a preadolescent with autism. *Behavioral interventions, 22,* 83–97.
16. Grazier, P. B. (1995). Starving for recognition: Understanding recognition and the seven recognition do's and don'ts. Retrieved from: <http://

www.teambuildinginc.com/article_recognition.htm>.

17. Horner, R. H. (2000). Positive behavior supports. *Focus on Autism and Other Developmental Disabilities, 15*, 97–105.
18. Horner, R. H., & Carr, E. G. (1997). Behavioral support for students with severe disabilities: Functional assessment and comprehensive intervention. *The Journal of Special Education, 31*, 84–104.
19. Horner, R., Carr, E., Strain, P., et al. (2002). Problem behavior interventions for young children. *Journal of Autism and Developmental Disorders, 32*, 423–446.
20. Individuals with Disabilities Education Act of 2004, P.L. 108-446.
21. Iovanne, R., Dunlap, G., Huber, H., et al. (2003). Effective educational practices for students with autism spectrum disorders. *Focus on Autism and Other Developmental Disabilities, 18*, 150–165.
22. Koegel, R. L., Koegel, L. K., Frea, W. D., et al. (1995). Emerging interventions of children with autism: Longitudinal and lifestyle implications. In R. L. Koegel & L. K. Koegel (Eds.), *Teaching children with autism: Strategies for initiating positive interactions and improving learning opportunities* (pp. 1–16). Baltimore: Brookes.
23. Koegel, R. L., O'Dell, M., & Dunlap, G. (1988). Producing speech in nonverbal autistic children by reinforcing attempts. *Journal of Autism and Developmental Disorders, 18*, 525–538.
24. Malott, R. W., Malott, M. E., & Trojan, E. A. (2000). *Elementary principles of behavior* (4th ed.). Upper Saddle River, NJ: Pearson Education.
25. McMinn, L. G. (2000). *Growing strong daughters.* Grand Rapids, MI: Baker.
26. National Research Council. (2001). *Educating children with autism.* Washington, DC: National Academy Press.
27. Neitzel, J. (2010). Positive behavior supports for children and youth with autism spectrum disorders. 1. Preventing school failure. Retrieved from <http://eric.ed.gov/?id=EJ884650>.
28. Odom, S. L., Collet-Klingenberg, L., Rogers, S. J., et al. (2010). Evidence-based practices in interventions for children and youth with autism spectrum disorders. Retrieved from: <http://eric.ed.gov/?id=EJ903737>.
29. OSEP Technical Assistance Center on Positive Behavior Supports and Intervention. (2008). School-wide PBS. Retrieved from: <http://www.pbis.org/school/default.aspx>.
30. Reese, R. M., Richman, D. M., Belmont, J. M., et al. (2005). Functional characteristics of disruptive behavior in developmentally disabled children with and without autism. *Journal of Autism and Developmental Disorders, 35*, 419–428.
31. Sugai, G. S., Horner, R. H., Dunlap, G., et al. (2000). Applying positive behavior support and functional behavioral assessment in schools. *Journal of Positive Behavior Interventions, 2*, 131–143.
32. Taylor, R. R. (2008). *The intentional relationship: Occupational therapy and use of self.* Philadelphia: F. A. Davis.
33. Thelen, P., & Klifman, T. (2011). Using daily transition strategies to support all children. *Young Children, 66*, 92–98.
34. Turnbull, A., Edmonson, H., Griggs, P., et al. (2002). A blueprint for schoolwide positive behavior support: Implementation of three components. *Exceptional Children, 68*, 377–402.
35. Watling, R. (2005). Interventions for common behavior problems in children with disabilities. *OT Practice, 10*, 12–15.
36. Watling, R., & Schwartz, I. S. (2004). Understanding and implementing positive reinforcement as an intervention strategy for children with disabilities. *American Journal of Occupational Therapy, 58*, 113–116.
37. Williams, J. A., Koegel, R. L., & Egel, A. L. (1981). Response-reinforcer relationships and improved learning in autistic children. *Journal of Applied Behavior Analysis, 14*, 53–60.
38. Wolf, M., Risley, T., & Mees, H. (1964). Application of operant conditioning procedures to the behaviour problems of an autistic child. *Behavior Research and Therapy, 1*, 305–312.
39. Zanolli, K., & Daggett, J. (1998). The effects of reinforcement rate on the spontaneous social initiations of socially withdrawn preschoolers. *Journal of Applied Behavior Analysis, 31*, 117–125.

CHAPTER

14

Feeding Intervention

Kimberly Korth • Lauren Rendell

KEY TERMS

Aspiration
Cleft lip and palate
Differential attention for behavioral intervention
Dysphagia
Esophageal motility
Esophageal pH probe
Food or liquid bolus
Fiberoptic endoscopic evaluation of swallowing (FEES)
Gastric emptying or gastric motility
Gastroesophageal reflux
Gastrointestinal endoscopy
Gastrostomy tube
Laryngeal penetration
Modified barium swallow study
Nasogastric tube
Phases of swallowing (oral preparatory, oral, pharyngeal, esophageal)
Rooting reflex
Tracheoesophageal fistula
Upper GI series

GUIDING QUESTIONS

1. Which medical conditions are commonly associated with feeding and swallowing disorders?
2. Which cranial nerves influence oral motor control and swallowing?
3. What are the typical developmental sequences for oral feeding and self-feeding skills?
4. How do occupational therapists evaluate feeding, eating, and swallowing?
5. What are the supplemental diagnostic tests used to evaluate underlying causes for feeding disorders?
6. What are the major components of a comprehensive intervention plan for pediatric feeding, eating, and swallowing problems?
7. How does positioning influence self-feeding and swallowing skills?
8. Why do occupational therapists modify foods and liquids in the feeding intervention plan?
9. What are the theoretical principles and strategies associated with behavioral interventions for selective eating or food refusal?
10. What are the safety considerations for occupational therapists working with children with feeding and swallowing disorders?

The process of feeding, eating, and swallowing is critical for health and wellness and plays an integral part in a child's social, emotional, and cultural maturation. At the most basic level, the process of taking in adequate nutrition is essential for normal growth and development. Feeding, eating, swallowing, and participation in mealtimes are all important occupations for infants and children.

Feeding, eating, and swallowing are complex processes, with multiple underlying medical, sensory, motor, behavioral, positioning, and environmental influences. A holistic approach is required during evaluation and intervention planning, often accompanied by collaboration with other professionals. This chapter will assist the occupational therapist in recognizing and understanding these complex processes and underlying influences to help develop safe and effective intervention plans.

Feeding: Definition and Overview

Throughout childhood, from infancy through adolescence, dietary requirements are constantly changing. At the same time, a child's feeding development gradually moves from complete dependence toward independent self-feeding. This dynamic process is integrally dependent on the acquisition of a multitude of skills, including overall muscle tone and stability, gross motor and upper extremity development, fine motor skills, and complex oral motor and swallowing skills. Mealtimes allow a child to explore new tastes and textures while concurrently encouraging the development of motor skills through finger feeding and the use of utensils.

Of equal importance, the feeding process is marked by social contact with other children, parents, and family members, and it is essential for the development of social interaction skills in the child. Children learn to communicate needs and desires through verbal and nonverbal cues. Feeding is one of the earliest instances in a child's life in which he or she learns to signal needs and desires, such as hunger, satiety, and thirst. Finally, because this complex process is shaped by cultural and social norms, it often lays the foundation for the acquisition of certain customs and rules of sociocultural behavior.

Feeding—sometimes called *self-feeding*—is defined as the process of setting up, arranging, and bringing food from the table, plate, or cup to the mouth. *Eating* is the ability to keep and manipulate food or fluid in the mouth and swallow it. *Swallowing* is a complex act in which food, fluid, medication, or saliva is moved from the mouth through the pharynx and the esophagus and into the stomach.[4]

Incidence of Feeding Disorders

Feeding and swallowing disorders are relatively common among children. Feeding and swallowing problems are reported in 10% to 25% of all children, 40% to 70% in premature infants, and

70% to 80% in children with developmental delays or cerebral palsy.[43,44,48,52] Feeding and swallowing disorders can have significant health implications, including adverse effects on nutrition, overall development, and general well-being.

Common Medical Diagnoses Associated with Feeding Disorders

Children develop difficulties with feeding, eating, and/or swallowing as a result of medical, oral, sensorimotor, and behavioral factors, either alone or in combination.[44] A variety of medical conditions can influence a child's ability and willingness to participate in oral feeding. Some of the most common medical diagnoses associated with feeding dysfunction include prematurity, neuromuscular abnormalities, structural malformations (such as cleft lip and/or palate), gastrointestinal conditions, visual impairments, and tracheostomies. The diagnosis of autism spectrum disorder (ASD) has a high prevalence of feeding difficulties due to sensory, motor, or behavioral challenges influencing the child's food preferences and willingness to eat.

Children with developmental disabilities may fail to meet basic nutritional needs because of delayed or deficient oral motor and self-feeding skills. Oral motor dysfunction causing poor nutrition is strongly associated with poor growth and adverse health outcomes.[24,51] These children may exhibit food refusal or selectivity behaviors, vomiting, swallowing difficulty, prolonged mealtimes, poor weight gain, and failure to thrive.

Behavioral problems are very common in children with feeding disorders. Food refusal and/or food selectivity can relate to multiple factors, including anxiety, hypersensitivities, behavioral rigidity or need for routine, or behavior dysregulation. Selective eating may also relate to underlying medical causes, such as gastroesophageal reflux disease (GERD) and food allergies.

A child who has frequent or chronic vomiting after feeding may be diagnosed with GERD. It is important to note that reflux is not uncommon, and most babies spit up on an occasional basis as their gastrointestinal system matures. This occasional spitting up or vomiting is not harmful to the baby, and, generally, no adverse effects on feeding or growth should be identified. The infant likely will outgrow these symptoms as he or she gains postural control and stability and maturation of the gastrointestinal system. GERD becomes problematic, however, when chronic spitting up and vomiting leads to problems with the infant's or child's health, ability to eat successfully, and poor growth or inadequate weight gain.[38]

Food allergies are also a common medical condition that can influence a child's success with feeding. Food allergies may create significant discomfort, resulting in a negative experience associated with eating. Some of the most common food allergies include milk, eggs, soy, wheat, and peanuts. The presence of food allergies may cause esophagitis, vomiting, skin rash, itchiness, pain, breathing difficulties, and/or discomfort during eating, contributing to the child's unwillingness to eat and subsequent negative behavior.

Depending on the severity of a child's feeding dysfunction, children with medical, oral, sensorimotor, and/or behavioral factors may ultimately require supplemental enteral feeding support to meet his or her nutritional needs for adequate growth and development. This enteral feeding support can be delivered via nasogastric, gastrostomy, or orogastric tubes. For children needing sustained enteral nutrition support (longer than a few weeks), health care providers often recommend a gastrostomy tube, which is considered optimal for long-term use. The decision to provide enteral nutritional support for a child is often not easy and should be determined in coordination with the child's primary caregivers and medical team.

Feeding Development and Sequence of Mealtime Participation

Anatomy and Development of Oral Structures

Intact oral structures and cranial nerves are prerequisites for eating and drinking. Various aspects of oral motor development emerge as the child begins to control movements of the tongue, cheeks, and lips. The anatomic structures of the mouth and throat change significantly during the first 12 months of life. The growth and development of the oral structures allow for increasingly mature feeding patterns.

The oral cavity houses the structures that enable successful management of foods and liquids during oral feeding. These structures consist of the mandible, maxilla, upper and lower lips, cheeks, tongue, teeth, floor of the mouth, hard palate, soft palate, uvula, and anterior and posterior faucial arches and aid in sucking, biting, chewing, and food bolus formation in preparation for swallowing. Table 14-1 outlines the functions of oral structures in feeding.

TABLE 14-1 Functions of Oral Structures in Feeding

Structure	Parts	Function During Feeding
Oral cavity	Hard and soft palates, tongue, fat pads of cheeks, upper and lower jaws, and teeth	Contains the food during drinking and chewing and provides for initial mastication before swallowing
Pharynx	Base of tongue, buccinator, oropharynx, tendons, and hyoid bone	Funnels food into the esophagus and allows food and air to share space; the pharynx is a space common to both functions.
Larynx	Epiglottis and false and true vocal folds	Valve to the trachea that closes during swallowing
Trachea	Tube below the larynx supported by cartilaginous rings	Allows air to flow into bronchi and lungs
Esophagus	Thin and muscular esophagus	Carries food from the pharynx, through the diaphragm, and into the stomach; collapses at rest and distends as food passes through it

Adapteded from Wolf, L. S., & Glass, R. P. (1992). *Feeding and swallowing disorders in infancy: Assessment and management.* Tucson, AZ: Therapy Skill Builders.

The newborn has a small oral cavity filled with fat pads inside the cheeks and tongue. The small and tight oral cavity allows the child to grasp and easily compress the nipple during breast-feeding and achieve automatic suction. The negative pressure caused by the sucking movements of the jaw extracts liquid from the nipple.[38] Thus, a full-term, healthy newborn can suck easily and successfully from a breast or bottle nipple. Between 4 and 6 months of age, the infant's oral structures begin to change, influenced by growth and maturation of postural control and overall motor systems. The oral cavity becomes larger and more open, the tongue becomes thinner and more muscular, and the cheeks lose much of their fatty padding. With the increase in oral cavity space, the tongue, lips, and cheeks provide greater control of liquid and food within the mouth. New sucking patterns develop, enabling the infant to handle liquid without the structural advantages of early infancy. These include up and down movements of the tongue to extract liquid from the nipple.

During this time, sucking patterns become more voluntary, and oral motor control begins to support lumpy foods and spoon feeding. This maturation continues as the child grows and acquires teeth to allow effective mastication and improved management of food textures.

Multiple cranial nerves support sensory and motor functions during oral feeding. Cranial nerves (CNs) V, VII, and XII innervate the sensory-motor pathways required to suck and extract liquid from a nipple. The trigeminal nerve (CN V) influences the oral motor function of mastication, as well as the lower jaw and palatal elevators. It also enables sensory function of the face, teeth, tongue, palate, nose, and nasal sinuses. The facial nerve (CN VII) provides motor function to specific muscles of the face and sensory innervations to the tongue. Lastly, the hypoglossal nerve (CN XII) enables motor function of the tongue.[38,58] Table 14 2 lists the cranial nerves associated with eating and swallowing.

Pharyngeal Structures and Function

The pharynx consists of distinct structures important to management of air flow for respiration and control of food or liquid during swallowing. The pharynx, comprised of the nasopharynx, oropharynx, and laryngopharynx, plays an integral role in the proper timing of breathing and swallowing during oral feeding.

The structures in the infant's throat are also in close proximity to one another. The epiglottis and soft palate are in direct approximation. As a result, the liquid from the nipple safely passes from the base of the tongue to the esophagus. During swallowing, the larynx elevates and the epiglottis falls over the opening to the upper airway. Therefore, aspiration is less likely before 4 months of age, and the infant can safely feed in a reclined position.

As the infant grows, the hyoid, epiglottis, and larynx descend, creating space between these structures and base of the tongue. The hyoid and larynx become more mobile during swallowing, elevating with each swallow. The greater complexity of the suck-swallow-breathe sequence leads to greater coordination among these structures. The elongated pharynx increases the risk of aspiration during feeding in a reclined position, as the pull of gravity accelerates the flow of liquid into the entrance of the esophagus. During this time, most children are fed in a more upright position as they generally transition away from bottle feeding to cup drinking, and more advanced food textures are introduced. Figure 14-1 depicts the anatomic structures of the mouth and throat.

Phases of Swallowing

There are four defined phases of swallowing. The oral preparatory phase is often reflexive in young infants and under voluntary control in older children. During this phase, oral manipulation of food occurs, using the jaw, lips, tongue, teeth, cheeks, and palate. This results in the formation of a food bolus. The amount of time spent in this phase varies, depending on the texture of the food or liquid.

The second phase is the oral phase, which is also generally reflexive in young infants and under voluntary control in older children. This phase begins when the tongue elevates against the alveolar ridge of the hard palate, moving the bolus posteriorly, and ends with the onset of the pharyngeal swallow.

The third phase, the pharyngeal phase, is primarily reflexive. During this phase, the swallow is triggered at the anterior

TABLE 14-2 Cranial Nerves Associated with Eating and Swallowing

Cranial Nerve	Type	Function
I (olfactory)	Sensory	Sensory fibers for smell
V (trigeminal)	Mixed	Sensory fibers from cheek, nose, upper lip, and teeth Sensory fibers from skin over mandible, lower lip, and teeth Motor fibers to the muscles of mastication
VII (facial)	Mixed	Sensory fibers from taste receptors to the anterior two thirds of the tongue Motor fibers to the muscles of facial expression and salivary glands
IX (glossopharyngeal)	Mixed	Sensory fibers from taste receptors on the posterior third of the tongue Motor fibers to the muscles used in swallowing and to the salivary glands
X (vagus)	Mixed	Sensory fibers from the pharynx, larynx, esophagus, and stomach Motor fibers to the muscles of the pharynx and larynx Autonomic fibers to the smooth muscles and glands to alter gastric motility, heart rate, respiration, and blood pressure
XII (hypoglossal)	Motor	Motor fibers to the muscles of the tongue

Adapteded from Morris, S. E., & Klein, M. D. (2000). *Pre-feeding skills* (2nd ed., p. 49, Table 4.2). Tucson, AZ: Therapy Skill Builders.

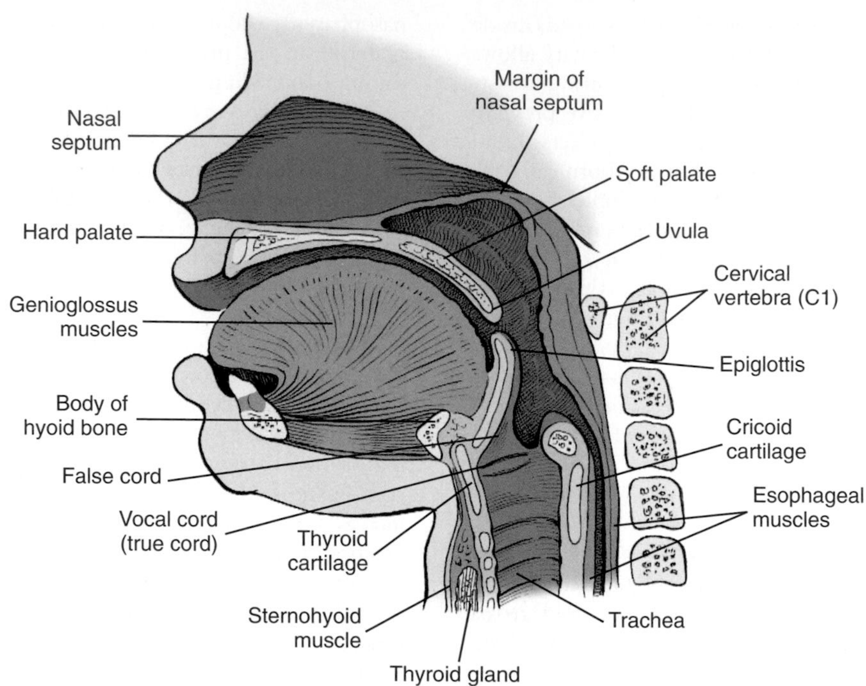

FIGURE 14-1 Anatomic structures of the mouth and throat.

faucial arches. The hyoid and larynx move upward and anteriorly, and the epiglottis retroflexes to protect the opening of the airway. It ends with the opening of the upper esophageal sphincter.

The final phase is the esophageal phase, which, along with the pharyngeal phase, is not under voluntary control. It starts with relaxation of the cricopharyngeus muscle to open the upper esophageal sphincter and ends with relaxation of the lower esophageal sphincter at the distal end of the esophagus, allowing foods to enter the stomach.

The glossopharyngeal nerve (CN IX) and vagus nerve (CN X) are the primary cranial nerves providing innervation for reflexive swallow functions. The glossopharyngeal nerve provides motor and sensory function to the pharynx. The vagus nerve enables motor function of the pharynx, larynx, and esophagus and innervates sensory function of the pharynx, larynx, trachea, and lungs.[38,58]

Stages and Ages of Feeding Development

Before a child is even born, the fetus develops necessary feeding skills that will support functional and successful oral feeding after birth. Initial early feeding reflexes such as the swallowing reflex have been known to develop between 10 and 14 weeks of gestational age. This reflex helps regulate amniotic fluid and aids in the maturation of the fetus' gastrointestinal tract. Around 16 to 20 weeks gestational age, the fetus mouths his or her thumb in early, non-nutritive oral stimulation. As early as 15 to 18 weeks, sucking is observed; however, not until after birth does the infant learn to coordinate suck, swallow, and breathing patterns for successful oral feeding.

Infants born preterm may lack the oral motor development required for effective oral feeding. Because technologic advances have been made in the medical field in the past several decades, infants are able to survive outside the womb at a very young gestational age, often as early as 22.5 or 23 weeks postconception. Depending on the infant's age, many factors must be taken into consideration when determining if a premature infant is ready to begin the process of oral feeding. As a result, it is imperative to understand the development of feeding skills in utero, as well as feeding readiness cues, when assessing an infant's ability to engage in oral feeding experiences. Cues such as skin color, state, breathing, and motor changes, as well as coordination of swallowing and breathing, are all factors to take into consideration when determining the premature infant's readiness to feed. Working with the fragile neonatal population requires advanced learning activities and mentored clinical experiences.

An infant born healthy and full term is typically ready to take on oral feeding, whether by breast or bottle. Infants are born with significant physiologic flexion, which enables them to continue to coordinate a successful sucking pattern outside the womb. Early reflexes such as the rooting reflex, sucking reflex, and synchronized suck-swallow-breathe patterns typically aid in the infant's success with initial oral feeding. During the first 3 months of life, infants feed using symmetric oral motor sucking movements. When fed, they are typically held by their caregiver and cradled in a flexed position, which allows them to bring the hands to midline and eventually to the mouth. During this period, infants experience a variety of sensory stimulation that prepares them for further sensory experiences. They feel input from the caregiver's hands, clothing, and other surfaces. They hear their parents' voices, experience eye contact, feel rhythmic heartbeats against the caregiver's chest, and experience a variety of smells during early feeding experiences. These early sensory and social activities during feeding may become a foundation for parent-infant bonding and later social development.

Between 3 and 6 months of age, the infant has developed improved head and neck control and is now able to lift and turn the head to maintain head position in supported sitting. As a result of this improved motor control, infants at this age are often positioned more upright for feeding. During this period, infants are becoming more interested in their surroundings and reach and grasp for toys and items of interest. The 3- to 6-month-old infant is still breast- or bottle-fed, but now brings hands to midline to help hold the bottle or embrace the caregiver. During this stage, oral reflexes (see earlier) are fading, and the infant develops voluntary control over sucking and swallowing patterns. The infant continues to use symmetric oral motor movements to suck and extract liquids; however, increased mobility of the tongue is often seen as the infant begins to explore toys and other items orally. This oral exploration plays a critical role in preparing the infant's oral sensory and oral motor development for further food texture introductions. During this stage, some infants demonstrate readiness for puréed food; however, this is not consistent across all infants.

The healthy 6- to 12-month-old infant should now be ready for the introduction of more advanced food textures. At this stage, motor skill development has significantly progressed. Typically developing infants should be sitting up independently and ready to sit in a high chair for feedings. Further refinement of fine motor skills has also occurred and the infant is beginning to use radial digital and then pincer grasps to pick up small items, such as a piece of solid food. The 6- to 12-month-old infant is continually engaging in a greater variety of sensory experiences. During this time, with the aid of tooth eruption, an explosion in oral sensory mouthing behavior is often observed, further aiding in readiness and developmental skills for more advanced feeding and eating activities.

The 6-month-old infant continues to be fed by breast or bottle. However, at this stage, the infant is now ready for the introduction of spoon feeding with purées and should be ready for meltable finger foods at around 8 months of age. Throughout this age range, the infant opens his or her mouth in response to presentation of the spoon and, with practice and experience, learns to close the mouth around the spoon to clear the purée into the mouth. A continued suckle transit pattern is used to swallow.

Chewing patterns also develop at this stage, first with munching, using symmetric up and down movements characterized by the jaw and tongue moving together in unison. Later, between 8 and 12 months, the infant begins to develop vertical chewing movements, characterized by disassociation between the jaw and tongue. Tongue lateralization is emerging at this stage, contributing to greater control of food within the oral cavity. Cup drinking is often introduced during this stage as well. Significant anterior fluid loss can be expected as the infant first begins to explore a cup, straw, or sippy cup.

By 12 to 24 months of age, the young toddler is now able to feed himself or herself independently because of further development and refinement of gross, fine, and oral motor skills. The toddler uses a mature pincer grasp and release pattern to pick up small finger foods and successfully place them in the mouth. Although a 12-month-old can bring a loaded spoon to the mouth, mastery of spoon feeding develops between 18 and 24 months as the child learns to scoop with the spoon successfully and orient the spoon correctly to feed with minimal spilling. Throughout this year, cup drinking has also progressed because bottle feeding and breastfeeding are typically fading. Further development of postural stability enables the toddler to transition from the high chair to a less supportive booster seat. By 12 months of age, the toddler is able to bite through a soft food with the front teeth and has developed more rotary chewing skills, characterized by diagonal jaw movements and the presence of lateral tongue movements. These more advanced oral motor skills enable the toddler to manage more challenging food textures, such as soft and coarsely chopped table foods, with more difficult chewable foods being managed by 24 months.

Some foods present a high choking risk in toddlers, such as some raw fruits and vegetables, seeds, nuts, and small round foods. These foods should be avoided or cut into small pieces during this stage of development. At this age, the toddler is engaging in sensory exploration with a variety of foods and textures, enabling him or her to learn about foods (through taste, smell, temperature, and texture).

At 24 months through 5 years of age, children develop significantly improved core stability and postural control. Because of this skill development, they are able to sit at the table without further adaptations or assistance. They are independently self-feeding with fingers, utensils, and cups. As a result of further refined rotary jaw movements, the 2- to 3-year-old child is now successfully eating a wide variety of table foods. At this age, highly chokeable foods should still be avoided but can be introduced with caution at 3 years. By 5 years, fully functional adult patterns have developed, and intake is generally based on personal preference, exposure, and experience. Tables 14-3 and 14-4 summarize the developmental sequences for oral feeding and self-feeding skills in infants and young children.

Mealtime: An Overview

Often, mealtime is a family time that provides physical, cognitive, and emotional nourishment to all members. Meals arrange the day temporally, organize it into periods, and signal that certain activities end and new ones begin. Mealtimes provide routine and structure and offer a time for relaxation, communication, and socialization. At mealtimes, parents and children communicate symbolically and emotionally while at the same time satisfying very basic nourishment needs.[19] Many believe that "to nourish a child is to nurture a child." Thus, mealtimes are cultural rituals and, as such, an integral part of a family's life and a time for bonding and sharing.

Caregivers and children engage in shared and individual roles during mealtime. Usually, the child is expected to remain seated, attend to the caregiver, feed himself or herself (when age appropriate), communicate with others at the table, and follow family rules for table manners and routines. The caregiver is expected to provide food in quantities sufficient to satisfy hunger, assist in feeding younger children, communicate and interact with other family members, and establish mealtime norms and routines.

A child's mealtime participation changes as he or she goes through the different stages of growth and development, from infancy to adulthood. During infancy, parents are responsible for feeding or assisting the child. During preschool and school-age years, the parents' role shifts toward oversight, communication, and discipline. Almost all parents try to create a pleasant and relaxing family atmosphere during meals. Families frequently have ever-changing dynamics that create busy

TABLE 14-3 Developmental Sequence of Eating Skills

Age (mo)*	Type of Food	Sucking and Drinking Skills	Swallowing	Biting and Chewing
1-4	Liquids only	Uses a suckling or sucking pattern	Tongue moves in anterior-posterior movement to swallow	Does not bite or chew
5	Liquids and beginning puréed foods; formula or breast milk remains primary source of nutrition	Uses a sucking or suckling pattern; tongue moves up and down	Choking on breast or bottle is rare; sequences 20 or more sucks from bottle or breast	Uses a primitive phasic bite and release pattern; biting not yet controlled or sustained; jaw moves up and down in munching and biting
6	Liquids and puréed foods	No longer loses liquids during sucking; introduction of sippy cup or small sips from open cup or straw; tongue moves in anterior-posterior pattern with cup drinking; may have anterior liquid loss when drinking from cup or straw	Swallows thin puréed foods; uses long sequences of coordinated sucking, swallowing, and breathing with breast or bottle; may cough or choke when using a cup	Up and down jaw movements more variable and less automatic; some tongue lateralization when food is placed to the side
8-9	Soft foods, mashed table foods, meltable solids.	Strong sucking pattern, no liquid loss with bottle; continuing introduction of sippy cup or straw	Uses long sequences of sucking during cup drinking; takes one to three sucks before stopping to swallow or breathe; swallows thin or thick purées	Uses lateral movements to transfer food from the center to the sides of the mouth; munches with diagonal movement; voluntary biting on food and objects; lips active with jaw during chewing
12	Easily chewed foods including soft meats, coarsely chopped table foods	Most of liquid now from a cup; uses a sucking pattern (up and down tongue movement); may lose liquid when using an open cup	Swallows liquids and semisolid foods with tongue tip elevation; at times exhibits tongue protrusion while swallowing; lips often closed during swallowing	Controlled sustained bite with soft cookie; easily transfers food from the center to both sides; begins rotary chewing movements; lips active during chewing
18	Coarsely chopped table foods, some raw fruits, most cooked meats	Mature sucking patterns; jaw is stable when drinking from cup	Uses tongue tip elevation with swallowing; swallows solid foods with easy lip closure; no loss of food	Uses controlled sustained bite on hard cookie; chews with lips closed; demonstrates rotary chewing
24	Most table food; use caution with raw vegetables, foods with skins, tough meats, or small round foods that increase risk of choking	Adult-like drinking pattern	No liquid loss; swallows solid foods with easy lip closure; tongue tip elevation used for swallowing	During chewing, can transfer food from both sides of the mouth; uses circular rotary movements when transferring food; lips closed during chewing

*Ages are approximate and may vary among infants.
Adapted from Glass, R., & Wolf, L. (1998). Feeding and oral motor skills. In J. Case-Smith (Ed.), *Pediatric occupational therapy and early intervention.* Boston: Butterworth Heinemann; and Morris, S. E., & Klein, M. (2000). *Pre-feeding skills* (2nd ed.). San Antonio, TX: Therapy Skill Builders.

environments, often not allowing time to create these important mealtimes, with consistent structure and routine. Creating a pleasant family atmosphere during mealtime can be challenging if a child has a disability that affects eating performance. The child's temperament, health, and disposition and the parents' health and moods are all important factors contributing to mealtime social interactions.

Contextual Influences on Mealtime: Cultural, Social, Environmental, and Personal

Contextual (environmental) factors must be taken into consideration when working with children who have feeding disorders and with their families. In some cases, feeding problems are based primarily on contextual issues, including physical, social,

TABLE 14-4 Developmental Continuum in Self-Feeding

Age (mo)	Eating and Feeding Performance	Concurrent Changes in Performance Components: Sensorimotor	Cognition	Psychosocial
5-7	Takes cereal or puréed baby food from spoon	Has good head stability and emerging sitting abilities; reaches and grasps toys; explores and tolerates various textures (e.g., fingers, rattles); puts objects in mouth	Attends to effect produced by actions, such as hitting or shaking	Plays with caregiver during meals and engages in interactive routines
6-8	Attempts to hold bottle but may not retrieve it if it falls; needs to be monitored for safety reasons		Object permanence is emerging and infant anticipates spoon or bottle	Is easily distracted by stimuli (especially siblings) in the environment
6-9	Holds and tries to eat cracker but sucks on it more than bites it; consumes soft foods that dissolve in the mouth; grabs at spoon but bangs it or sucks on either end of it	Good sitting stability emerges; able to use hands to manipulate smaller parts of rattle; guided reach and palmar grasp applied to hand-to-mouth actions with objects	Uses familiar actions initially with haphazard variations; seeks novelty and is anxious to explore objects (may grab at food on adult's plate)	Recognizes people once regarded as strangers; emerging sense of self
9-13	Finger feeds self a portion of meals consisting of soft table foods (e.g., macaroni, peas, dry cereal) and objects if fed by an adult	Uses various grasps on objects of different sizes; able to isolate radial fingers on smaller objects	Has increased organization and sequencing of schemas to do desired activity; may have difficulty attending to events outside visual space (e.g., position of spoon close to mouth)	Prefers to act on objects than to be passive observer
12-14	Dips spoon in food, brings spoonful of food to mouth, but spills food by inverting spoon before it goes into mouth	Begins to place and release objects; likely to use pronated grasp on objects like crayon or spoon	Recognizes that objects have function and uses tools appropriately; relates objects together, shifting attention among them	Has interest in watching family routines
15-18	Scoops food with spoon and brings it to mouth	Shoulder and wrist stability demonstrate precise movements	Experiments to learn rules of how objects work; actively solves problems by creating new action solutions	Internalizes standards imposed by others for how to play with objects
24-30	Demonstrates interest in using fork; may stab at food such as pieces of canned fruit; proficient at spoon use and eats cereal with milk or rice with gravy with utensil	Tolerates various food textures in mouth; adjusts movements to be efficient (e.g., forearm supinated to scoop and lift spoon)	Expresses wants verbally; demonstrates imitation of short sequence of occupation (e.g., putting food on plate and eating it)	Has increasing desire to copy peers; looks to adults to see if they appreciate success in an occupation; interested in household routines

temporal, and cultural factors. Understanding the contextual factors that influence mealtimes and feeding performance helps determine the basis for problems and possible solutions.

A family's culture can be described as a set of beliefs, values, and traditions that guides their actions, often including what types of foods a family eats and specific mealtime routines and roles. In some cultures, children are fed by a caregiver throughout the preschool years, whereas in others, infants are encouraged to self-feed, despite the ensuing mess. Cultural beliefs also determine the amount and type of food that parents believe that their children should eat and where and when mealtime occurs. As occupational therapists, it is imperative to respect a family's cultural beliefs and social norms to provide the best support of their mealtime routines and the values they hold around eating.

A family's socioeconomic status also has an impact on mealtime and feeding patterns. Families in poverty may be unable to provide sufficient food or may eat less nutritious foods, which often tend to be high in carbohydrates and fat. A parent's educational level, which can be related to socioeconomic status, can affect a child's diet because an undereducated parent may lack knowledge of basic nutrition. In these situations, it is important to help families not only with knowledge of feeding and development, but also to involve other resources and providers who may assist with these challenging situations. Occupational therapists can refer families to resources such as social workers and the Women, Infants, and Children (WIC) program (also called the Special Supplemental Nutrition Program).

A caregiver's personality traits and other individual factors can also shape mealtime and affect a child's ability to feed. When the caregiver does not enjoy feeding a child or approaches it as a chore, the task can lose much of its meaning, changing the mealtime experience for the adult and child. For example, some caregivers are anxious about feeding and tend to be controlling when the child is a poor eater. The caregiver may have preconceived ideas about how much the child should eat and may engage in force feeding or maladaptive feeding routines to compensate for the child's disinterest in eating. A controlling parent may find that the child desires control of what he or she eats, and a battle of wills may result. Controlling parents may also have difficulty with allowing the child freedom to explore and interact with foods as they learn to participate in self-feeding. They may have difficulty allowing their children to become messy, limiting their overall sensory experiences with foods.

Comprehensive Evaluation of Feeding and Swallowing Skills

The process of analyzing and identifying feeding and swallowing challenges in children is complex. Comprehensive evaluation requires clinicians to question, observe, and analyze multiple factors within the child's abilities and family's routines that influence the mealtime structure and limit or enhance success with oral feeding.

Initial Interview and Chart Review

When initiating a feeding and swallowing evaluation, it is important to begin this complex process by gathering as much background information as possible. The team reviews the child's medical chart and may request that the caregiver complete a feeding, developmental, and/or nutritional intake questionnaire prior to the appointment. The child's developmental status and health history are also important in identifying feeding problems and guiding decisions about subsequent evaluation and intervention needs. The written reports from physicians, occupational and physical therapists, speech-language pathologists, early childhood specialists, and teachers provide fundamental information about the child. For example, a child with a past history of prolonged hospitalization may not have had typical feeding, motor, or sensory opportunities. A child with a history of motor delays may have had restricted upper extremity movements, resulting in limited oral exploration and influencing sensory systems and delayed self-feeding skills. Understanding the child's developmental course and rate of change in other occupational performance areas such as object play and social interactions is important for the occupational therapist to set realistic goals, prioritize objectives, and choose appropriate intervention strategies.

The occupational therapist then gathers general information about the family's concerns with oral feeding and mealtimes. The occupational therapist obtains information about current feeding practices, cultural norms, social rules, and mealtime routines by asking the parents to describe the child's feeding over the course of a typical day. This open-ended inquiry, as opposed to multiple-choice questions, allows the occupational therapist to identify potential areas of concerns that were not reported during the initial description of the child's feeding problems.

A discussion of the feeding problem from the parents' perspective is critical because it helps identify the primary concerns. For example, are the parents most concerned about weight gain, or is it the length of time required for feeding that poses a problem? Does the child seem to lose most of the food consumed during feeding (e.g., through vomiting or reflux)? Is the child's behavior during feeding causing distress for the entire family during mealtimes? Although the parents' expressed concerns become the focus of the subsequent intervention, the occupational therapist should always consider other concerns expressed by health care professionals (e.g., physicians or other health care providers) when developing a feeding plan, especially when these concerns differ from those expressed by the parents.

The parents also provide information about the child's development and feeding history, including feeding milestones. Obtaining this information may help the occupational therapist identify the root of the feeding problem (e.g., long-standing sensory or behavioral issues may have affected feeding). Inquiring about remediation strategies used with the child in the past may be helpful in identifying appropriate next intervention strategies. Parents whose child has been seen by other medical or therapy providers may have important information to share regarding interventions that worked and those that did not.

Although these issues are discussed separately, feeding problems are seldom attributable to a single cause and usually are the result of delays, impairments, medical concerns, or behavioral challenges in multiple areas. For example, children with severe sensory problems may have subsequent oral motor skill delays, and children with neuromotor impairments may also experience swallowing disorders. Often, because of past feeding challenges, families will modify routines, mealtime structure, and behavioral expectations, thus creating maladaptive contextual challenges, which must be addressed. Box 14-1 provides an example of guiding questions that may be used to evaluate the contexts of feeding.

After the therapist has completed a comprehensive interview, initial impressions are often formed about the child's feeding difficulties, the family's routines and structure around eating and mealtimes, and any additional areas that may help determine the cause of the feeding problem. The next step is to complete a hands-on evaluation of generalized muscle tone, neuromuscular status, sensory processing development, and general developmental level. Observations of movement initiation, play, and transition patterns allow the occupational

BOX 14-1 Guiding Questions to Evaluate the Contexts for Feeding

Physical
- Is seating and positioning adequate? Supportive? Does it provide stability?
- Are head, neck, shoulders, and pelvis well aligned?
- Is space adequate for eating activities?
- Are noise and activity levels conducive to eating?

Social
- Who feeds the child?
- Who is present during the meal?
- What is the nature of the social interaction among family members during the meal?
- What communication or interaction occurs between the caregiver and child during feeding?

Temporal
- Is sufficient time allotted and available for a relaxing meal?
- How often is the child fed?
- How long does it take?

Cultural
- How do cultural beliefs and values influence mealtime?
- What foods does the family eat?

therapist to observe muscle tone, sensory processing, and postural control. Low postural muscle tone can interfere with the ability to maintain upright posture and head and neck alignment. Hypotonicity or hypertonicity can lead to difficulty grading or sustaining oral motor patterns, uncoordinated breathing, drooling, decreased oral exploration, and limited self-feeding. Sensory processing difficulties may influence the child's ability to sit successfully for meals, progress with food textures, or tolerate other typical mealtime experiences.

Structured Observation

Once an evaluation of the child's motor systems, sensory development, and muscle tone has been completed, the next step in the evaluation process is to complete structured observations of the child's oral structures and oral motor patterns. Initial observations should include assessments of symmetry, size, tone, and range of motion of the outer oral structures, including the jaw, and then proceeding intraorally to the lips, gums, dentition, hard and soft palates, and tongue.

Once observations of oral structures are complete, the evaluator should then progress with observations of the child eating a snack or a meal with the parent or caregiver. This observation enables the occupational therapist to get a sense of mealtime routines, feeding practices, and social or behavioral interactions typically occurring at home. Observing the parent-child interaction provides insight into the everyday context of feeding. For example, does the parent talk to the child? Does the child send clear cues regarding readiness to eat, satiation, or food preferences? Does the parent respond to the child's verbal and nonverbal cues?

Objective observations of the parent-directed mealtime enable further assessment of the child's motor, sensory, cognitive, and communication skills. It is often recommended that parents bring foods that the child typically accepts at home, as well as foods that are more challenging for the child. This allows the occupational therapist to observe the child in an optimal and less optimal performance. The occupational therapist also encourages the caregiver, when possible, to use the seating system, plates, and utensils that are typically used at home.

After all interviews, observations, and assessments have been completed, the occupational therapist interprets all assessment findings, prioritizes concerns, and develops initial recommendations to assist the family. It is important to mention that evaluation of a child's feeding and eating, for most children, relies on structured interview and observations. To date, few standardized assessments and reliable outcome measures to evaluate the complex process of oral feeding are available.

Additional Diagnostic Evaluations

When a child exhibits feeding difficulties, a variety of medical procedures may be recommended to evaluate feeding and swallowing skills further. The upright modified barium swallow study (MBSS), also called a videofluoroscopic swallow study, is the radiographic procedure of choice for assessing the oral, pharyngeal, and upper esophageal anatomy and function during feeding and swallowing. It is most useful in identifying aspiration or the risk of aspiration and in tailoring treatment for infants and children with feeding disorders. This evaluation can also be helpful for detecting problems related to head and neck positioning, bolus characteristics, rate and sequence of feeding, and safe food or liquid consistencies. The results of the test can be helpful in identifying compensatory techniques to minimize the risk of aspiration and maximize eating efficiency.[8] The occupational therapist selects the types of food and liquid textures based on the child's current diet and level of feeding performance and mixes them with liquid, powder, or barium paste.[47] It is important to remember that the MBSS only captures a brief sample of swallowing, and positioning, food or liquid amount, and order of presentation are up to the therapy team conducting the study.[7] Typically, during this evaluation, radiation exposure is limited to 5 minutes or less, thus requiring occupational therapists to determine clinically the most important food and liquid textures to examine during this brief period.

The MBSS is used to analyze the swallow mechanism and is particularly important for children who aspirate or are at a high risk for aspiration because of severe motor, neurologic, developmental, or structural abnormalities. Clinical observations that may suggest swallowing problems include gagging, coughing, choking, nasopharyngeal reflux, increased congestion, wet vocal quality, and frequent occurrence of respiratory infections and/or pneumonias. Aspiration may be silent, so a thorough history and feeding observation are critical.

During the MBSS, the occupational therapist should distinguish aspiration from laryngeal penetration. Aspiration refers to food or liquid entering the airway before, during, or after a swallow. The presence of aspiration is an abnormal finding and may lead to chronic lung disease, pneumonia, and other medical problems. Laryngeal penetration describes the flow of food or liquid underneath the epiglottis into the laryngeal vestibule, but not into the airway. It does not pass through the vocal folds. The frequency and severity of laryngeal penetration may vary and may not always correlate to an increased risk of aspiration. Infants and children may have intermittent episodes of mild laryngeal penetration (also called epiglottic undercoating) during swallowing, which do not increase the risk for aspiration.[23] The presence of deep laryngeal penetration, characterized by food or liquid entering the laryngeal vestibule to the level of the vocal cords, is correlated to an increased risk factor for aspiration episodes.[23]

Because the MBSS recording shows food traveling through the mouth and pharynx, the occupational therapist receives real-time, detailed information about the child's oral motor and pharyngeal function. The results of the MBSS indicate the safety and appropriateness of oral feeding and guide the occupational therapist's recommendations.[59] These may include modified feeding positions and/or food and liquid textures for the parents to use during feeding that appear to result in optimal swallowing patterns, without aspiration. Although the MBSS gives the occupational therapist important information and insight about the swallowing problem, it may not always be representative of the child's typical feeding in a more natural environment.

Similar to the MBSS, a fiberoptic endoscopic evaluation of swallowing (FEES) also evaluates a child's swallow function. In contrast to the MBSS, the FEES uses a flexible endoscope with a light and camera that is inserted into a nostril and down the throat. With this evaluation, the camera then records the pharyngeal swallow function from the inside as the child eats or drinks. This allows for direct visualization of the larynx and pharynx to observe for penetration, aspiration, and residual material. It is important to note that the child must be awake and willing to cooperate with eating while the endoscope is in place.

An upper gastrointestinal (GI) series is a common evaluation used to screen for anatomic differences, such as GI malrotation, stricture, vascular ring, and/or fistulas or pouches, which may cause vomiting and other feeding problems. An upper GI series is helpful in evaluating for the presence of gastroesophageal reflux (GER). It is important to note that the upper GI series evaluates one moment in time and, according to expert clinical guidelines, is not usually helpful in diagnosing the presence or severity of GER.[56] The upper GI series typically does not assess swallow function or the presence of aspiration.

Medical providers often recommend an esophageal or pH probe to discover the presence and severity of GER. With this evaluation, a probe is inserted into the esophagus though the nose to monitor abnormal acid levels, typically over a 24-hour period. However, a pH probe test may be difficult to complete because it often requires an overnight stay in the hospital, and the probe may be poorly tolerated by young infants and children.

An endoscopy may be used to evaluate the esophagus, stomach, and duodenum, referred to as an esophagogastroduodenoscopy (EGD). This test involves passing a flexible endoscope through the nose and visualizing the structures for the presence of esophagitis or other abnormalities. Tissue biopsies may be taken from the esophagus, stomach, or duodenum to evaluate for the presence of eosinophils. Eosinophils are present in abnormally large numbers when a child is experiencing food allergies. They contribute to esophagitis and discomfort during eating. It is important to note that a child needs to be sedated to participate in an EGD.

Table 14-5 provides a comparison of the most commonly used diagnostic procedures for children with feeding disorders.

Intervention: General Considerations

Problems with feeding, eating, and swallowing are often caused by multiple underlying factors. If feeding problems persist as the child grows older, new problems or skill impairments may appear that further complicate the intervention needs. For example, children with dysphagia who require nonoral feeding for an extended period may experience subsequent developmental delays in self-feeding skills because of limited experience. Occupational therapists can provide direct intervention for children with feeding, eating, and swallowing disorders to improve functional participation in mealtimes. Throughout the intervention process, occupational therapists must consider medical and nutritional problems that often coexist with the child's feeding disorder, prioritize areas of focus, and collaborate with physicians, nutritionists, and other health care professionals to create an optimal intervention plan.

Feeding activities occur multiple times throughout the day in a variety of natural environments, and occupational therapists must work closely with families and other caregivers to ensure carryover within the daily routine. Children with oral feeding difficulties often require one-on-one attention or increased caregiver time and effort throughout each day. Mealtimes may be quite stressful for parents or caregivers, especially when the child's oral feeding difficulties create ongoing problems with nutrition and growth. Whenever possible, typical family mealtime routines should be preserved within the intervention program. Occupational therapists should consider the caregivers' time investment and provide realistic recommendations that do not significantly increase the burden of care within the family system. Parents of children with feeding, eating, and swallowing disorders may benefit from peer support groups, which have been shown to strengthen caregivers' abilities to cope with stressful problems on a daily basis.[15]

Occupational therapists use a holistic approach when developing an intervention plan for children with feeding, eating, and swallowing disorders. Consideration is given to many different overlapping areas, including child factors, performance skills, activity demands, environmental contexts, and family patterns.[5] A comprehensive occupational therapy intervention plan may include environmental adaptations, positioning recommendations, adaptive equipment, food texture or liquid modifications, sensory development activities, behavioral strategies, neuromuscular handling techniques, and/or suggestions to improve independence in self-feeding. When implementing new recommendations or interventions, occupational therapists may encourage parents to try a technique a number of times before determining that it is successful or unsuccessful. Occupational therapists may also recommend that parents implement only one or two key changes at a time to determine which interventions are more successful than others.

A variety of intervention models are used to treat children with feeding problems, including specialized inpatient

TABLE 14-5 Comparison of Most Commonly Used Diagnostic Procedures for Children with Feeding Disorders

Test	Indications	Advantages	Limitations
Upright modified barium swallow study (MBSS); videofluoroscopic swallow study	• Analyze the swallow mechanism • Rule out aspiration • Determine point of aspiration • Identify safe food and liquid consistencies	• Fluoroscopy, not a single-picture x-ray • Videotaped • Upright position simulates feeding • Primary feeder often presents food • Familiar feeding utensils (bottle, cup, spoon) • Use of liquid, purée, and/or solid • Lateral and anterior/posterior view • Can determine when aspiration occurs • Investigation of treatment options	• May be difficult to simulate normal feeding in radiology examination room • Child must be able to swallow appropriate amount of barium • Results reflect that particular date and time • Study environment may increase child stress, resulting in aspiration • Radiation exposure from fluoroscopy
Upper GI series	• Diagnose structural abnormalities of the esophagus, stomach, or intestines, such as malrotation or stricture	• Clear contrast image of upper GI anatomy • Documents gastroesophageal reflux (GER) events if they occur during study • Observes esophageal motility and mechanism for stomach emptying	• X-ray radiation exposure • Supine positioning • Barium flow rate may not simulate bottle feeding • Primary feeder often not present • Limited accuracy in capturing or diagnosing GER
Esophageal pH probe	• Quantifies frequency, acidity, and duration of GER	• Prolonged evaluation of GER over 24 hours • Documents effect of movement, sleep, and meals on GER • Documents frequency and severity of GER events • Can be combined with other assessments, such as pulse oximetry, or documentation of choking episodes • Established guidelines for normal and abnormal results	• Invasive procedure, often requiring overnight stay in a hospital • May not correlate with clinical symptoms (e.g., coughing, vomiting, wheezing)
GI endoscopy, esophagogastroduodenoscopy (EGD)	• Provides a direct view of GI tract to diagnose inflammation or structural abnormalities	• Direct observation of esophageal and stomach tissues for changes that may have occurred with chronic GER • Tissue biopsies often studied for presence of eosinophils, which may indicate food allergies	• Invasive procedure, requiring anesthesia • Presence of inflammation or abnormalities may not correlate with clinical symptoms (e.g., vomiting, other feeding problems) • Cannot determine frequency of GER
Fiberoptic endoscopic evaluation of swallowing (FEES)	• Analyze the swallow mechanism • Rule out aspiration • Identify safe food and liquid consistencies • Visualize anatomic structures during swallowing	• Allows variability in positioning the child during eating or drinking • No x-ray radiation exposure • Can be combined with traditional laryngoscopy	• Requires child to be awake and cooperative while having small tube inserted in the nose and pharynx while swallowing • Often requires coordination between swallowing therapist and otorhinolaryngologist or ear, nose, and throat physician • Visualization while swallow is occurring can be difficult because structures close and contract.

Adapted from from Morris, S. E., & Klein, M. (2000). *Pre-feeding skills* (2nd ed.). San Antonio, TX: Therapy Skill Builders.

programs, intensive outpatient programs, direct weekly therapy, and periodic consultative services. Many pediatric hospitals and outpatient centers have multidisciplinary feeding clinics for additional support, allowing access to a number of health care professionals from different medical backgrounds. In general, children with mild feeding difficulties often do well with weekly therapy or consultative therapy. Children with more severe feeding problems may require more intensive models of therapy.

Safety and Health

Basic safety guidelines should be followed when providing occupational therapy intervention. Children who demonstrate clinical signs of aspiration may require additional assessment with an upright MBSS to determine appropriate feeding goals. Occupational therapists must also consider the child's nutritional status and prioritize treatment goals to maximize a child's ability to meet basic nutritional needs. Some interventions may require implementation outside regular meal sessions so as not to disrupt the child's ability to meet oral intake requirements.

Universal precautions are followed during therapy activities when the occupational therapist will potentially contact food, mucous, or structures within the child's mouth. These precautions include the use of gloves to prevent the spread of infection.[39] Another critical factor when working with different food textures is the understanding that certain foods carry a high choking risk and require modifications or close supervision with young children. Occupational therapists must also understand and follow any dietary restrictions for children with food allergies, metabolic disorders, diabetes, or religious or cultural beliefs.

Intervention Strategies

Environmental Adaptations

Occupational therapists often recommend changes to the mealtime structure or environment to promote success with oral feeding. Environmental adaptations may be recommended to modify the child's daily mealtime routines. Specifically, occupational therapists may provide intervention recommendations for scheduling and location of meals, length of meal periods, sensory stimulation within the environment, and/or changes to the order of mealtime activities (e.g., solid foods before liquids, nonpreferred foods before preferred foods).

Children often benefit from regularly scheduled meals at consistent times or locations from day to day. Consistently scheduled meals and snacks allow the child to experience periods of time without eating, which may promote hunger cues and more interest in eating.[38] When parents allow children to snack or consume liquids throughout the day, children may have little opportunity to become hungry at mealtimes, when more nutritious foods are presented. Children should also have a consistent location for meals, such as sitting in a high chair or at a specific table. Wandering around while eating or having meals in different locations every day may be distracting for young children and does not help establish positive mealtime behaviors.[33]

Some children may require modifications to the length of their meal periods. Children with neuromuscular impairments may eat slowly and have a long meal period because of oral motor or self-feeding difficulties. Parents of children with poor growth may prolong mealtimes to try to encourage more food intake. When mealtimes are longer than 30 to 40 minutes on a regular basis, the demands on the child and caregiver become extremely high. Children who become fatigued during prolonged meals may expend increased energy to sustain the feeding, outweighing any benefits from additional oral intake.[26] Children with delayed gastric emptying or GER may benefit from smaller, shorter, more frequent meals throughout the day.[38] Larger meals may create more discomfort or episodes of vomiting in children with GI disorders. In typical children without feeding problems, meal periods of 15 to 30 minutes are usually ideal, depending on the age of the child and complexity of the food being offered.

The amount of sensory stimulation and number of distractions within the environment may also affect a child's oral feeding skills. Many children show improved oral feeding when environmental distractions are limited. Limiting the sensory stimuli in the environment may be beneficial for children who are concentrating on independent self-feeding, children who are hypersensitive to environmental stimuli, and infants with disorganized suck-swallow-breathe coordination. A calming sensory environment can be created with dim lights, reduced noise, soft or rhythmic music, and limited interruptions. Alternatively, some children may eat better when environmental distractions are present during mealtimes. Active toddlers may consume more food or have improved ability to remain seated at a meal when they are allowed access to a favorite toy or television show. When distractions are present, toddlers may not focus on the actual eating activity and may need more assistance from caregivers. The use of distraction may also help some children with sensory defensive behaviors to reduce the child's focus on the discomfort of the oral feeding activity.[40]

Occupational therapists may also consider the order of presenting foods and liquids during meal sessions. Some children have more success when challenging oral feeding activities are presented at the beginning of the meal, when the child is feeling hungry. Alternatively, when the challenging feeding task creates disruption or distress and impacts the child's oral intake for the remainder of the meal, occupational therapists can recommend a new intervention outside meals or during a smaller snack session.

When considering a variety of environmental modifications, occupational therapists can often use information obtained during the initial feeding assessment to assist with clinical reasoning for these interventions. Often, a period of trial and error may occur to determine ultimately the best environmental modifications for each individual child.

Positioning Adaptations

Oral motor and feeding activities require skilled movement and coordination of many small muscle groups, which are supported by overall gross motor control and stability. Children with postural instability and neuromuscular impairments have difficulty with oral motor control if they do not have adequate positioning support. Positioning changes may have an immediate impact on some difficult oral motor problems, such as tonic bite and tongue thrust movement patterns. When an occupational therapist is making positioning adaptations, proximal support (support at the trunk and neck) influences distal movement and control. Thus, occupational therapists consider positioning throughout the child's whole body. Positioning of the feet, legs, and pelvis influences the child's trunk stability. Stability, muscle tone, and postural control in the trunk muscles will affect the child's head and neck position. The position and graded muscle control of the child's head and neck influence jaw movements. Finally, good jaw stability and freedom of movement influence the child's tongue and lip control.[38] Providing external support, stability, and alignment through the use of positioning adaptions will often improve comfort and optimize oral motor skills and oral intake during mealtimes.

Infants may be supported in a variety of positions during oral feeding. Side-lying in the caregiver's arms is a common position during breastfeeding. This position may also be recommended for children who have difficulty coordinating sucking, swallowing, and breathing, because the impact of gravity does not immediately draw the liquid into the pharyngeal space. It may be difficult for the caregiver to hold a child comfortably in a side-lying position for prolonged periods, especially with older children or infants with hypotonia. Infants may also be supported in an elevated supine or sitting position in the caregiver's arms or on a caregiver's thighs, facing the caregiver. This elevated supine position (Figure 14-2) provides excellent alignment and midline orientation for infants who take formula from a bottle. An infant seat, car seat, or Tumble Forms Feeder Chair (Figure 14-3) may be adapted with small rolls to provide head and trunk support or slight shoulder protraction to help an infant hold his or her own bottle. Both these positioning options allow the feeder to have two hands free, creating opportunities to provide oral motor support or implement handling techniques. Occupational therapists should monitor whether these positions contribute to a slouched or compressed posture in the trunk and make adjustments if excessive slouching is present.

Allowing infants or young toddlers to drink a bottle while lying in a flat supine position (e.g., in a crib, on the floor) is generally not recommended. Positioning that includes propping the bottle on the young infant's chest should also be discouraged.

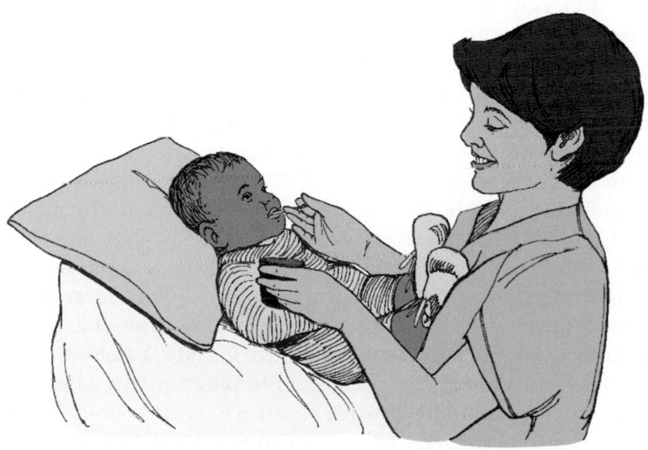

FIGURE 14-2 Face-to-face positioning for feeding.

For older infants and toddlers who are engaging in spoon-feeding activities, additional positioning options are available (Figure 14-4). A regular high chair may provide adequate trunk support for some children and can be easily adapted with small towel rolls for additional foot support or lateral support. The height of a standard high chair also allows caregivers to sit comfortably at the table, promoting social interaction between the child and family.

Older children with neuromuscular impairments may require a wheelchair or an adaptive stroller, such as a Kid Kart or Rifton chair, to provide optimal support during oral feeding. A variety of options and accessories are available for customization of these positioning devices. Within a seated position, the child should have supported feet and neutral pelvic alignment. Lateral trunk or arm supports, pelvic strap or seat belt, head

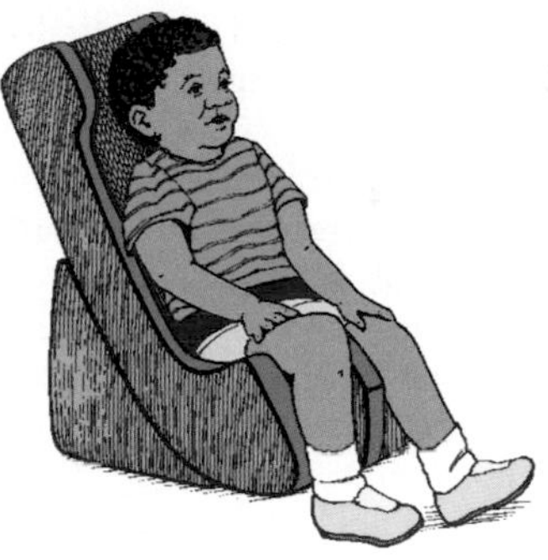

FIGURE 14-3 Tumble Forms Feeder Chair offers support and an adjustable feeding angle.

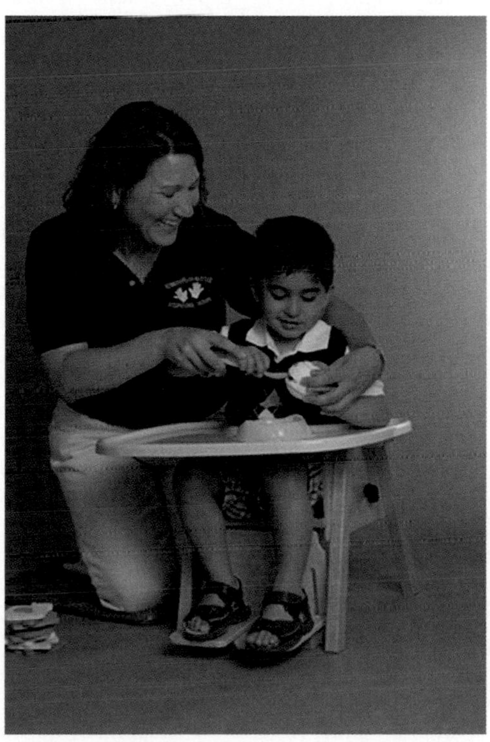

FIGURE 14-4 Adaptive positioning provides a firm base of support to the trunk and feet during self-feeding.

rests, specialized chest straps, or a tray may help provide more stability for the pelvis, trunk, and head. Children with neuromuscular impairments demonstrate improved head control, reaching, grasping, sitting posture, and visual tracking when using positioning devices during activities of daily living.[31] Optimal positioning includes vertical head and trunk position, hip flexion greater than 90 degrees, knee flexion at 90 degrees, and feet supported on a flat surface.[31]

Occupational therapists may need to work with families to determine whether positioning equipment will fit comfortably in the home and evaluate caregiver perceptions about adaptive equipment. Reilly and Skuse studied positioning during mealtimes in the home for children with cerebral palsy.[42] They found that positioning problems were common among children with cerebral palsy; however, only 50% of parents who received adaptive positioning devices routinely used the equipment.

In general, positioning adaptations aim to provide stability in the trunk and support the child in a midline orientation, with the head and neck aligned in neutral or slight flexion during oral feeding. The child's age, size, neuromuscular status, and self-feeding skills must be considered, as well as the caregiver's position and comfort. Finally, positioning adaptations should promote social interaction and communication during mealtimes. Occupational therapists must evaluate each child and caregiver individually to determine the best options for positioning during oral feeding, provide education about the benefits of proper positioning, and suggest alternatives to positioning equipment when necessary.

Adaptive Equipment

A variety of adaptive equipment is available for feeding activities, including adaptive spoons, forks, cups, and straws. Adaptive equipment may promote improvement in oral motor control, increase independence in self-feeding, and/or compensate for a motor or sensory impairment.

Occupational therapists should consider the properties of the spoon or fork used in feeding activities. A spoon with a shallow bowl may help a child with decreased lip closure. A spoon with bumps or ridges on the bottom of the bowl or a chilled metal spoon may provide additional sensory input for a child with decreased sensory registration. A rubber-coated or dense plastic spoon may be used as an alternative to a metal spoon for a child who bites down on the utensil. Utensils with shorter handles, curved handles, or larger grip diameters may help a child self-feed more independently.[33]

A child first learning to drink from a straw may do well with a shorter or smaller straw, such as one that typically comes with a juice box. These straws require less oral suction and may deliver a smaller liquid bolus that is easier to control in the mouth. Children who require thickened liquids or those with decreased lip closure may benefit from the use of a relatively short straw with a standard diameter. Therapists may also consider using a straw with a specialized one-way valve. When liquid is pulled into a straw with a valve, it does not fall back into the cup if the child loses suction, thus allowing the child with weakness to put forth less effort and achieve more success. A cup with a handle may help a child with poor fine motor skills to drink more independently. U-shaped cut-out cups help maintain a neutral head position when drinking liquid. Clear cut-out cups also allow the therapist or caregiver to see liquid entering the child's mouth easily when physical assistance is provided for drinking activities.

Typically, most young children use sippy cups as a transition between the bottle and an open cup or straw. Sippy cups are perceived as being easy to use and comforting to children. A variety of sippy cups are commercially available for children. They may have hard plastic spouts or soft spouts and permanent or removable nonspill valves. They may be fast-flowing, with little suction required, or slower flowing, requiring more oral suction. Occupational therapists working with children with feeding and swallowing disorders must carefully consider how different sippy cup properties affect the child's oral motor control and swallowing function.

Interventions to Improve Self-Feeding

Children experience delays in self-feeding skills because of physical weakness, abnormal muscle tone, cognitive delays, visual impairments, sensory processing difficulties, behavioral refusal, or poor motivation to eat. Each of these underlying causes creates different challenges for the intervention plan. Children will have the most success when they have begun to demonstrate an interest in self-feeding and an interest in exploring food more independently. Within each intervention plan, the occupational therapist's goal is to facilitate the child's success and gradually decrease the amount of caregiver assistance required during mealtime.

For children with physical or neuromuscular deficits, it is particularly important to create a balance between the effort of self-feeding and the impact on oral motor skills, swallowing safety, overall length of the meal, and child's nutritional needs. Therapists may implement self-feeding activities for only a portion of the meal, or during a smaller snack session, to allow practice and skill development opportunities without creating lengthy meal periods or causing reduced food intake for the child.

Adaptive positioning can be used to facilitate grasp patterns or hand to mouth movements. Adaptive positioning to support self-feeding activities may include a chair that provides good postural support and allows access to a stable tray or table for increased arm stability. A raised tray or table surface may provide more trunk and shoulder stability while decreasing the distance the child needs to move the spoon or fork from the bowl to the mouth. Stabilizing the elbow on the table or tray can also help reduce the physical demands of self-feeding, extending the child's endurance.

A Dycem mat or a nonskid placemat may help prevent movement of the dish or bowl to compensate for uncoordinated arm movements. Children may have improved independence when self-feeding with foods that stick to the spoon or with a scoop dish that has raised edges. Some dishes also have a suction cup on the bottom to help secure them to the table.

Children with upper extremity weakness or poor grasping skills may benefit from simple adaptations, such as a utensil with a lightweight, built-up handle or universal cuff (a palm strap that secures the utensil to the hand in a stable position). More complex options for severe weakness include a deltoid aid, mobile arm support, and electronic feeding systems activated by a simple push button switch.

A variety of adaptations can be made to help children drink liquids more independently. Cups with a wide base or cups with lids may help reduce spillage when the child is placing the cup on a table. Some children may benefit from a long straw placed into a cup that is secured in a cup holder, reducing the need to lift or move the cup with the hands.

Children with cognitive or behavioral problems may benefit from backward chaining of self-feeding, with gradually decreasing levels of assistance provided. During the first step of this backward chain, a child may be required only to move the spoon with the hand for the last few inches before it reaches the mouth. The child then advances to lifting a spoon from the plate to the mouth after the occupational therapist has provided assistance to scoop the food. The last step encourages total independence with both scooping and bringing the food to the mouth. The occupational therapist praises and encourages the child for each step of his or her progress toward independent self-feeding.

When encouraging self-feeding in children with a visual impairment, occupational therapists may recommend consistent orientation of food and drink on the placemat. For example, placing the cup in the 2 o'clock position next to the plate or placing different foods in consistent locations in the dish may improve the child's awareness of the mealtime environment for improved independence. Occupational therapists may also use contrasting colors with plates, cups, and placemats to improve visual discrimination.

Children with tactile hypersensitivity may be less willing to explore food with their hands to finger-feed independently or they may become upset with food that spills during initial attempts at spoon feeding. Therapy activities to reduce generalized hypersensitivity outside mealtimes are indicated to prepare the child for self-feeding. During mealtimes, occupational therapists may try a variety of spoons, such as those with a small diameter or smooth handle, to improve a child's success and tolerance. Some hypersensitive children may be more willing to try self-feeding when they are simply provided with a napkin or moist cloth to reduce their discomfort if the feeding activity becomes messy.

Modifications to Food Consistencies

Different textures and sensory properties of foods may be considered in an intervention plan. Foods with a smooth, even, cohesive consistency, such as yogurt and strained fruits or vegetables, are easier to manage when a child has oral sensory and oral motor impairments. Thick, lumpy, or pasty foods such as oatmeal require more oral motor strength and sensory tolerance when compared with smoother and thinner puréed foods. Foods that are dense, crunchy, sticky, or uneven in consistency are more difficult to manage and require more advanced chewing skills. Table 14-6 provides examples of food progressions based on texture and consistency.

The National Dysphagia Diet, published in 2003, was an effort to provide standardized terminology when describing food texture modifications in dysphagia management.[3] Although pediatric therapists often use additional descriptors for food textures, such as "stage 3," "junior," or "ground," some institutions have begun using the terminology from the National Dysphagia Diet (Box 14-2).

When presenting foods and liquids, therapists may alter the size of the bite or sip of liquid. When first beginning to advance with a new skill for the child, occupational therapists may present a food or liquid in a small, consistent bolus size. For example, offering one teaspoon of liquid (5 mL) from a small cut-out cup may help the occupational therapist to evaluate the child's oral motor and swallowing skills clearly when compared with unmeasured, free access sips. Similarly, offering a smaller food bolus when trying a new taste or texture may result in greater success for the child.

Consideration should be given to other sensory properties of foods, such as taste and temperature. Cold foods or foods with strong flavors, including tangy, salty, or sour foods, may be beneficial for children with decreased oral sensory awareness. Bland, room temperature, or slightly warm foods may be more tolerable for children with oral hypersensitivity.

BOX 14-2 Levels of Food Texture for Dysphagia Management

Level 1: Puréed—puréed foods that are homogeneous, cohesive, or pudding-like.
Level 2: Mechanically altered—cohesive, moist, semi-solid foods that may require some chewing; ground or minced meats and fork-mashed soft fruits and vegetables included in this diet level; most bread products, crackers, dry foods excluded
Level 3: Advanced—soft-solid foods that require more chewing ability, such as crackers, breads, cooked vegetables, soft fruits, and meats; excludes some fruits with skins, hard or crunchy vegetables, tough meats such as beef or pork steak, and foods that are very sticky or dry
Level 4: Regular—no food restrictions

Modifications to Liquids

Different consistencies of liquid require different oral motor and oral sensory demands. Thin liquids presented from an open cup are the most difficult to control in the mouth and pharynx during swallowing. Occupational therapists may recommend modifications to the thickness of liquid to compensate for a variety of swallowing, oral motor, and oral sensory deficits.

Thickened liquid is easier to control with the lips and tongue, moves more slowly in the mouth, and allows the child more time to organize a bolus for effective swallowing, without early spillage into the pharyngeal cavity. Children with dysphagia may not be able to coordinate swallowing with thin liquids, and aspiration and penetration events are more common with thin liquids when evaluated with MBSS.[13,23,37] Thickened liquids may also be used to compensate for oral motor skill deficits when a child is first learning to drink from an open cup, even when the child has pharyngeal competence with thin liquids from a bottle or sippy cup. See Box 14-3 for descriptions of the three most commonly used liquid consistencies.

A variety of foods and supplements can be used to thicken liquids. SimplyThick is one type of commercial gel thickener, made with xanthan gum, that may be recommended for older children. Other commercial powder thickeners typically contain modified food starch and/or cornstarch. Note that important new precautions and warnings have been issued by the U.S. Food and Drug Administration (FDA) for the use of xanthan

TABLE 14-6 Food Progression Based on Texture and Consistency

	Puréed	Junior, Coarse Puréed	Wet-Ground, Mashed	Soft, Dissolved	Chopped, Soft Solid	Full Diet
Meat and meat substitutes	Strained meats or proteins; foods are blenderized to a smooth, even consistency	Commercial junior foods; soft meats finely ground in a food grinder with added liquids; scrambled eggs are mashed; hummus	Ground meats with gravy; scrambled soft eggs; mashed tofu	Ground meats; regular scrambled eggs; tofu	Small pieces of soft meats; hard-cooked eggs, deli-sliced turkey or ham	Cut-up meats; stew; almonds or nuts
Dairy products	Thinned pudding; plain yogurt; strained cottage cheese	Fork-mashed cottage cheese; tapioca pudding; thickened cream soups	Cottage cheese	Yogurt with soft fruits; American cheese slices	Cheddar or Swiss cheese	All dairy products
Bread and cereals	Infant cereals thinned with milk	Thicker infant cereals; Cream of Wheat	Cooked cereals such as oatmeal	Breads, muffins, crackers, cereal (without milk), pancakes; well-cooked pasta or rice	Dry cereals with milk; sandwiches with smooth filling cut into small pieces; firmer pasta or rice	Sandwiches with various fillings
Fruits and vegetables	Strained fruits and vegetables	Junior fruits; junior vegetables; regular unstrained applesauce; mashed potatoes or yams	Fork-mashed, soft canned fruits without skins; soft ripe mashed fresh fruits; fork-mashed, well-cooked vegetables	Canned fruits (peaches, pears) or soft ripe fruits cut into small pieces (peeled); well-cooked vegetables	Canned fruits or increased texture (fruit cocktail); regular bite-sized pieces of cooked vegetables cut into small pieces	Raw fruits; dried fruits; raw vegetables with fibers or skins (corn, celery, peppers); vegetable soups, mixed salads

BOX 14-3 Liquid Consistencies (from Thinnest to Thickest)

- Thin—consistency of water or juice
  Many formulas and milk products have a slightly higher viscosity than that of clear liquids; however, they are still considered thin liquids. Soup broth and foods that melt are also considered thin liquids.
- Nectar—consistency of tomato juice, including many natural fruit nectars (e.g., apricot nectar, pear nectar) and some store-bought yogurt smoothies
- Honey—consistency of honey, which slowly drips off a spoon

gum thickeners with young infants, premature infants, and older children who have a history of necrotizing enterocolitis.[10,54,55] Necrotizing enterocolitis (NEC) is a serious medical condition related to necrosis of tissue in the intestines or bowel. Current xanthan gum precautions have a significant impact on treatment options for young infants with swallowing disorders. Occupational therapists are urged to become knowledgeable about these FDA warnings and provide education to other medical providers.

Regular fruits and vegetables, baby foods, yogurt, and pudding may be blenderized to make thickened smoothies or shakes for older children. Dried infant cereals or mashed potato flakes may be added to thicken pediatric formula or nonhuman milk. Infant cereals are not effective to thicken expressed human breast milk because the starches contained in the cereal are broken down by the amylase in breast milk, quickly returning the milk to a thin liquid. Each thickener has different sensory, nutrition, and thickening properties, all of which should be considered in an occupational therapist's recommendations.

Interventions for Dysphagia

When aspiration or pharyngeal dysphagia affects a child's ability to eat safely, the availability of well-researched intervention

RESEARCH NOTE 14-1

Bulow, M., Olsson, O., & Ekberg, O. (2003). Videoradiographic analysis of how carbonated thin liquids and thickened liquids affect the physiology of swallowing in subjects with aspiration on thin liquids. Acta Radiologica, 44, *366–372.*

Abstract

The purpose of this study was to evaluate how carbonated thin liquids affected swallowing physiology during videofluoroscopic assessments. Participants were evaluated with a variety of liquid consistencies during a videofluoroscopic swallow study. Forty adults who demonstrated aspiration with thin liquids were then included in this study and received additional assessment with carbonated thin liquids. Of the 40 participants, 36 had a diagnosed neurologic impairment. Data were analyzed to compare carbonated liquids with thin and thickened liquids regarding the frequency of aspiration or penetration, pharyngeal transit time, and pharyngeal retention during swallowing. The results indicated that carbonated liquids significantly reduced aspiration and penetration events and demonstrated faster pharyngeal transit time when compared with thin and thickened liquids. Carbonated liquids also demonstrated significantly decreased pharyngeal retention when compared with thickened liquids. When thickened liquids were compared with thin liquids, significantly fewer penetration and aspiration events were noted with the thickened liquids.

Implications for Practice

The use of thickened liquids and carbonated thin liquids by those who demonstrate aspiration or penetration with thin liquids is supported by this descriptive study. Although this study has not yet been duplicated with a pediatric population, the results suggest that carbonated liquids may reduce aspiration in children known to aspirate thin liquids. Carbonated liquids may be an alternative to thickened liquids.

options is limited. Historically, occupational therapists recommended food or liquid consistency adaptations, such as thickened liquids for children who aspirate with thin liquids. Although this continues to be a popular recommendation, it may not be suitable for young infants.

When thickened liquids are recommended for children of any age, the child's liquid intake and hydration status must be closely monitored to ensure that the child is meeting daily fluid requirements. Some children who are prescribed thickened liquids have poor acceptance of the new liquid and reduce their oral intake. Studies have suggested alternatives to thickeners, such as carbonated liquids, to reduce aspiration or penetration (Research Note 14-1). Comprehensive caregiver training is needed to ensure understanding of aspiration, methods for modifying food or liquids, and safety precautions during oral feeding.

As noted earlier, supportive positioning can have a major impact on the child's oral motor and swallowing skills. A chin tuck position may be recommended when the child has delayed swallow initiation. During an MBSS, a delay is typically seen as pooling of food or liquid in the pharyngeal space located close to the opening of the larynx. When the child is positioned with a slight chin tuck, the laryngeal opening may become smaller, reducing the risk of aspiration or penetration. Occasionally, a chin tuck position may be contraindicated for young infants who have laryngomalacia or tracheomalacia (softening of the cartilage in the larynx or trachea) because their soft tissues may be more prone to collapse.[46] Garon also reported problems associated with the chin tuck position in dysphagic adults with abnormal epiglottic movement patterns after a neurologic insult.[25] Occupational therapists need to make individualized positioning recommendations based on a comprehensive assessment and, when available, information obtained from an MBSS.

Adaptations to the mealtime structure may be made to compensate for dysphagia. Occupational therapists may recommend reducing the meal length to compensate for weakness or muscle fatigue. Some children with poor oral control require multiple swallows to clear one bite of food. If a child is unable to complete a subsequent swallow in response to a verbal prompt, an empty spoon offered in the same way as a bite of food may stimulate oral movements to prompt a second swallow. Therapists may also provide recommendations for the pace of oral feeding to allow the child sufficient time to swallow all the food between each bite. More difficult foods, liquids, or self-feeding activities may need to be limited or presented within the first few minutes of a meal session, when the child is less fatigued. Children may also benefit from smaller bites of food or sips of liquid. This can be achieved through the use of a controlled-flow cup, smaller diameter straw, single discrete sips, slow-flow bottle system, or smaller spoon.

Research studies have been completed with adult and pediatric clients evaluating the use of neuromuscular electrical stimulation (NMES) in the treatment of dysphagia. Although the overall evidence is still considered inconclusive, especially in pediatric populations, some studies have shown that NMES produces significant improvements in swallow function when other traditional interventions have failed.[17,22] NMES is provided to strengthen or reeducate muscles on the face and anterior neck. The use of NMES has precautions and contraindications, and this type of therapy should be administered only by occupational therapists who have obtained additional specialty training and/or certification.

In many cases, aspiration is silent and cannot be detected during clinical observations. Because of the potential medical complications resulting from chronic aspiration and the limited number of effective treatment options, alternative, nonoral feeding methods may be required for some children. Occupational therapists are urged to work collaboratively with physicians, nutritionists, and other professionals to individualize each intervention plan for children with dysphagia.

Interventions for Sensory Processing Disorders

In most young children, oral exploration and gradual adaptation to new sensations are natural processes. Abnormal sensory processing, such as hypersensitivity to food tastes, textures, or smells, can create significant problems with oral feeding. Children with oral hypersensitivity often react negatively to touch near or within the mouth. They may turn away from feeding or toothbrushing activities, restrict food variety, gag frequently, or have difficulty transitioning to age-appropriate food textures. Children diagnosed with generalized tactile defensiveness have a significantly higher incidence of oral hypersensitivity and oral feeding difficulties compared with their typical peers.[50] Oral hypersensitivity is also common in children who have received extensive medical interventions. Medical interventions such as endotracheal intubation, orogastric or nasogastric tube feeding, tracheostomy, or frequent oral suctioning may have caused ongoing distress, gagging, or pain, affecting the development of the sensory systems. Early feeding problems experienced in infancy, such as GER or swallowing difficulties, can create negative associations between food consumption and sensory discomfort.[49] The child's sensory system becomes overprotective, and hypersensitivities may continue long after the noxious stimuli has been eliminated. Children with developmental and neurologic conditions, including autism, pervasive developmental disorders, cerebral palsy, traumatic brain injury, genetic conditions, and sensory processing disorders, commonly exhibit oral hypersensitivity.

During intervention, occupational therapists create opportunities for gradual oral sensory exploration through play and positive experiences to reduce oral hypersensitivity. Children may tolerate greater sensory input if the activity is under the child's control and provided in the context of a motivating, developmentally appropriate play activity.[14] Occupational therapists provide access to textured objects, teethers, or vibrating toys and playfully encourage the child to explore them with his or her hands, face, and mouth. Occupational therapists may also engage the child in songs or games to encourage self-directed touch to the face or play dress-up with hats, scarves, or sunglasses. Children with oral hypersensitivity may benefit from generalized deep pressure or calming strategies such as slow linear rocking before oral stimulation. Infants may be encouraged to soothe themselves with hand-to-mouth activities or a pacifier. Occupational therapists often aim to create a balance of stimulating and calming sensory input to elicit an adaptive, more normalized response from the child.

Children may gradually improve acceptance of occupational therapist–directed touch with firm pressure that is first applied distally on the body, such as on the arms or shoulders, before moving to touch near the face. A variety of tools can be used to provide stimulation within the mouth, including a gloved finger, vibrating toy, warm washcloth, Nuk brush, infant or child toothbrush, or teething ring. Applying firm pressure to the child's gums or palate may help reduce oral hypersensitivity. Older children with more mature oral motor skills may enjoy whistles, oral sound-making games, bubbles, and blow toys to improve oral sensory processing.

During feeding activities, the occupational therapist introduces new flavors and textures gradually. A lollipop or teething ring can be dipped into a new flavor of food. Children may advance their oral feeding skills when slight changes are made to their current preferred foods. The occupational therapist can gradually thicken a food, combine strained baby foods with puréed table foods for stronger flavors, or change food temperatures to expand the child's sensory experiences. The occupational therapist or parent should provide consistent praise and encouragement for the child's oral exploration and feeding attempts.

Some children with sensory processing disorders have low sensory registration and may demonstrate poor oral sensory awareness. These children may frequently seek oral sensory stimulation by mouthing their hands, toys, or clothing. They may have decreased awareness of drooling or try to overstuff their mouths when eating. Occupational therapists may establish a treatment program to provide enhanced oral sensory input intermittently throughout the day. Oral activities with a rubber massage brush, cold washcloth, or vibrating device can be used to provide oral sensory stimulation.[33] During mealtimes, foods with strong flavors and cold temperatures may help the child take appropriately sized bites of food. Children who consistently overstuff their mouths when eating may require foods that are cut into pieces and close supervision for safety.

Behavioral Interventions

Food refusal often begins with the presence of underlying medical or skill problems. Children with GER, constipation, or food allergies may feel uncomfortable when eating and develop food refusal behaviors as a result.[49] Children who gag with textured foods or refuse cup drinking may not have adequate sensory or motor skills to manage these feeding activities. However, a child's refusal behaviors and oral aversion may persist long after the initial medical, sensory, or skill problems have been adequately managed. Children with ASD may exhibit selective eating or refuse to try new foods, given their propensity for rigid and repetitive behaviors and olfactory, gustatory, or tactile sensitivities (see later). When children exhibit food refusal or selective eating, behavioral power struggles may develop during mealtimes. Behavioral inconsistencies may be seen in which the child accepts cup drinking in the preschool setting but refuses to drink from a cup at home. In many cases, occupational therapists may need to include behavioral intervention strategies to promote successful advancement of oral feeding.

A child's refusal to eat may contribute to caregiver stress, and mealtimes may become a battleground, with increasing levels of negative or stressful interactions.[28] Occupational therapists try to create new positive interactions and child associations around feeding activities and mealtimes. Occupational therapists and caregivers should have a relaxed, confident, and caring demeanor when implementing behavioral interventions during oral feeding and therapy activities. Offering choices and turn taking during an activity may help a child feel a sense of control and increase his or her willingness to participate during mealtimes. For example, a caregiver may offer a choice of two different foods, or the occupational therapist may allow the child to choose which activity is performed first.

Behavior management interventions include the use of positive reinforcement to increase desired behaviors and ignoring or redirecting negative behaviors. Multiple research studies have supported the use of differential attention during mealtimes, during which positive reinforcement is combined with ignoring or redirection of inappropriate behaviors to improve oral intake.[9,32,41] Positive reinforcement and regular exposure to nonpreferred foods can significantly improve oral consumption and self-feeding skills.[57] The use of punishment or negative reinforcement is not recommended. When possible, occupational therapists are encouraged to consult with psychologists and other professionals with knowledge and experience treating behavioral problems in children.

When implementing behavior management strategies, the occupational therapist carefully determines an appropriate form of praise or reinforcement for each individual child. Examples of positive reinforcement include social attention, verbal praise, music, favorite toy, stickers, access to a small prize box, video games, or television. If the child is not motivated to earn the reinforcement item or activity, the intervention will have limited success. Furthermore, toys or activities that are used to praise a child for positive eating behaviors should not be readily available outside feeding sessions. If the child is allowed free access to the reinforcement outside feeding activities, the child will not be motivated to earn the item during the mealtime.

During behavioral interventions, the occupational therapist should break the activity down into small achievable steps and provide clear expectations. When the expectations are small and achievable, the child has the opportunity to experience praise and positive reinforcement for participation and success. Consistent success with an activity should be attained before the expectation is increased.[21] If the performance expectation increases too rapidly, or the activity is continued indefinitely, until the child's refusal behaviors intensify, the child may quickly learn to refuse more strongly to escape the activity the next time it is presented. When behavioral strategies are implemented with gradual progression of new skills, positive reinforcement, and clear expectations, the child learns to trust the occupational therapist or caregiver, and the negative behaviors may quickly decrease in frequency and intensity.

It is not unusual for children with feeding disorders to experience negative behaviors when trying new oral feeding activities. Negative behaviors may include crying, pushing the spoon or cup away, and spitting out food. Occupational therapists can intentionally ignore these behaviors, calmly persist with the meal, and redirect the child without focusing too much attention on the disruptive behavior. When parents or occupational therapists react strongly to negative or disruptive behaviors and immediately end the activity, the child's behaviors tend to increase in response to the attention and removal of the nonpreferred feeding activity. Occupational therapists may suggest the use of a visual schedule or timer set in advance to help the child clearly understand when the activity is finished, rather than having the parent end the meal when the child's behavior has escalated. This clear end to the activity may also help the child transition from the difficult or new task back to the usual routine of feeding or postmealtime activity.

Interventions for Food Refusal or Selectivity

Many typical children refuse new foods when they are first introduced as toddlers. Evidence has been reported that it takes multiple presentations of a food before a child feels comfortable with it and before a true food preference can be determined.[34] Some caregivers will encourage their child to try a new food once or twice and then give up. Occupational therapists should educate parents to continue offering small amounts of a new food across multiple meal sessions to allow the child sufficient time to adapt to the new taste or texture. As noted, some children referred to occupational therapists are highly selective, or picky, eaters. Parents of children with ASD frequently report selective eating behaviors, rigidity surrounding mealtime routines, delayed transitions to textured foods, and concerns for nutrition and gastrointestinal problems. Children with ASD may struggle with changes in mealtime routines, refuse foods that are a specific color, texture, or temperature, and be less responsive to positive eating behaviors modeled by others. Over time, children with ASD or severe food selectivity may become progressively more restrictive in their food preferences, raising concern for nutritional deficiencies.[2,20]

Initial recommendations may include consultation with physicians to consider GERD, food allergies, digestive problems, or structural abnormalities. Occupational therapists may also need to address underlying skill deficits or swallowing safety concerns, which may contribute to food refusal behaviors. When management of medical or skill problems has been optimized, children may continue to demonstrate ongoing food refusal or selective eating behaviors.

In addition to using behavioral strategies described earlier, children with food refusal or selectivity often benefit from environmental adaptations, including mealtime structure for consistent feeding times, reducing grazing or excessive liquid consumption outside meals, consistent eating locations, and consistent length of meals. These environmental strategies will promote hunger cues, limit access to less nutritious foods, and create structure within the meal to establish positive eating patterns.

Occupational therapists should also consider interventions to reduce tactile, gustatory, or olfactory hypersensitivity by introducing new smells and tastes carefully and gradually and by allowing children to explore foods using a playful approach. Foods that are similar to the child's preferred foods can be introduced before completely novel foods. Nonpreferred foods can be paired with preferred foods at mealtime, or interventions to reduce olfactory, gustatory, and oral tactile hypersensitivity can be applied outside meal sessions. The occupational therapist helps the family to balance meeting the child's nutritional needs while introducing a variety of foods to his or her diet.

A variety of alternative nutritional interventions has been proposed to help treat ASD, such as high-dose vitamin supplements and/or dietary restrictions. Scientific evidence for the effectiveness of these alternative interventions is inconclusive or not available.[2,20] A thorough review of these interventions is beyond the scope of this chapter, but occupational therapists are encouraged to consider the impact of these interventions for children with severe food selectivity and food refusal behaviors. For example, children with ASD may not be willing to eat the foods or supplements recommended in the alternative diet.[59] The diet may further restrict the limited variety of food that the child is willing to eat, and consultation with a registered dietitian or physician may be necessary to monitor for negative side effects from high-dose supplements.

Delayed Transition to Textured Foods

Children who are unable to transition to age-appropriate food textures frequently have a combination of oral sensory and oral motor problems, and some may also demonstrate behavioral refusal. Occupational therapists may implement non-nutritive oral motor activities to reduce hypersensitivity and improve oral motor coordination. Jaw strengthening and repetitive chewing activities without the demand for swallowing may help the child build oral motor skills. Figure 14-5 illustrates a child engaging

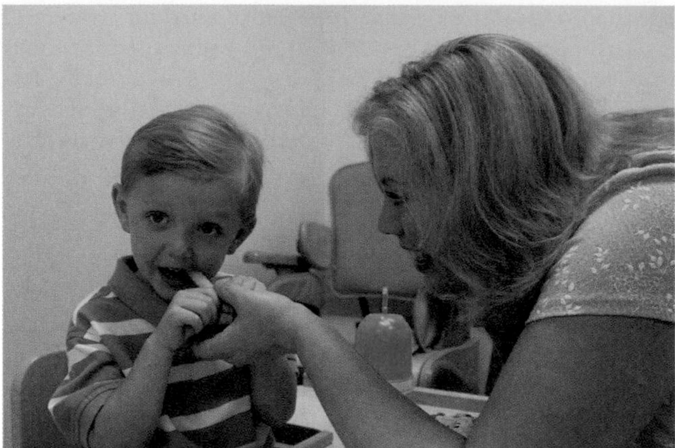

FIGURE 14-5 Using a resistive device to improve oral motor skills for advanced food textures.

in a jaw-strengthening activity. Increased tolerance for food textures can be addressed by placing crumbs on a piece of chewy tubing or slowly adding rice flakes to a puréed food. Children who consume baby foods should begin to transition to puréed table foods, allowing adjustment to stronger flavors and encouraging acceptance of a wider variety of oral sensations. Children may practice chewing foods encased in a mesh feeding bag to experience repetitive chewing with less risk for gagging or choking. Occupational therapists may provide praise or behavioral reinforcement for the child's participation in challenging new activities. When a child takes a few small bites of textured food safely outside primary meal sessions, occupational therapists may begin to integrate these new skills slowly during meals, such as during the first five to ten bites. Rapidly increasing demands during the meal session, before the child has adequate motor or sensory skills, may affect oral intake or nutritional status and create stressful child-caregiver interactions. Box 14-4 is helpful in recognizing the foods that may be indicated and contraindicated in children with immature oral motor skills.

Delayed Transition from Bottle to Cup

A child may also have difficulty transitioning from breastfeeding or bottle feeding to drinking from a cup. Efficient cup drinking requires more mature oral motor skills than bottle feeding. Difficulty transitioning from the bottle to the cup can be caused by poor jaw stability or delayed lip and tongue control, affecting the child's ability to manage a liquid bolus. Children with a history of failure to thrive may have prolonged dependence on bottle feeding or breastfeeding as the most reliable method to meet their nutritional or hydration needs. When a child is orally hypersensitive, he or she may dislike the intermittent touch of the cup on the outside of the lips or the spillage that often occurs during early cup drinking activities.[33] Hypersensitive children may also seek the calming, organizing sensory input that comes from sucking during bottle or breast feeding.

To help children prepare for cup drinking activities, occupational therapists may initially work on jaw stability, lip closure, tongue movements, and oral sensitivity through positioning, handling, and oral motor activities. Cups with nonspill valves in the lid require stronger lip closure and oral suction abilities and may be more difficult to use by children with neuromuscular impairments. A spouted cup may initially make it easier for a child to suck the liquid or form a bolus in the mouth. Spouted cups may also provide similar sensory input to bottle feeding for children with sensory defensiveness. When drinking from a cup with a spout, the child may need to tilt the head back, which may create additional difficulties if the child has extensor posturing, poor head control, or pharyngeal swallowing problems. Use of a cut-out cup may help reduce head and neck extension and allows the occupational therapist to observe the flow of liquid and the child's mouth movements easily during drinking activities.

With free-flowing liquid from an open cup or nonvalved spouted cup, children should be positioned in a more upright position to encourage bolus formation in the mouth, without the impact of gravity creating an uncontrolled flow into the pharyngeal space. Children may also benefit from thickened liquids when first learning to drink from a cup to compensate for decreased oral control or pharyngeal swallowing skills.

External jaw support can be provided by the occupational therapist whose index finger placed underneath the lower mandibular bone and the thumb is placed on the anterior chin. Providing jaw support while sitting beside the child with the arm around the back of the child's neck may allow the occupational therapist to provide additional stability for the child to maintain adequate head alignment (Figure 14-6). Children often bite on the rim or spout of the cup to gain additional jaw stability. They also may push the cup into the corners of their lips or rest their tongue on the rim of the cup for additional sensory input.[33] These patterns should decrease over time

BOX 14-4 Properties of Foods for Children with Immature Oral-Motor Skills

Indicated Foods

Even consistency
Increased density and volume
Thick (liquids)
Uniform texture
Stays together (will not break up in the mouth)
Easy to remove and suck

Contraindicated Foods

Multiple textures and consistencies (e.g., tacos, vegetable soup, stews, salads)
Sticky (e.g., peanut butter)
Greasy (e.g., fried foods)
Tough (e.g., red meat, processed meats, diced fruit)
Fibrous and stringy (e.g., celery, citrus fruits, raw vegetables)
Skins (raw fruits, peanuts)
Spicy (pepper and horseradish)
Seeds and nuts (plain or in breads and cakes)
Thin liquids (e.g., water, broth, coffee, tea, apple juice)
Quickly liquefying (e.g., Jell-O, ice cream, and watermelon)
Foods that break up in the mouth (e.g., some cookies and flaky pastries)
Hard, crunchy (e.g., carrots)

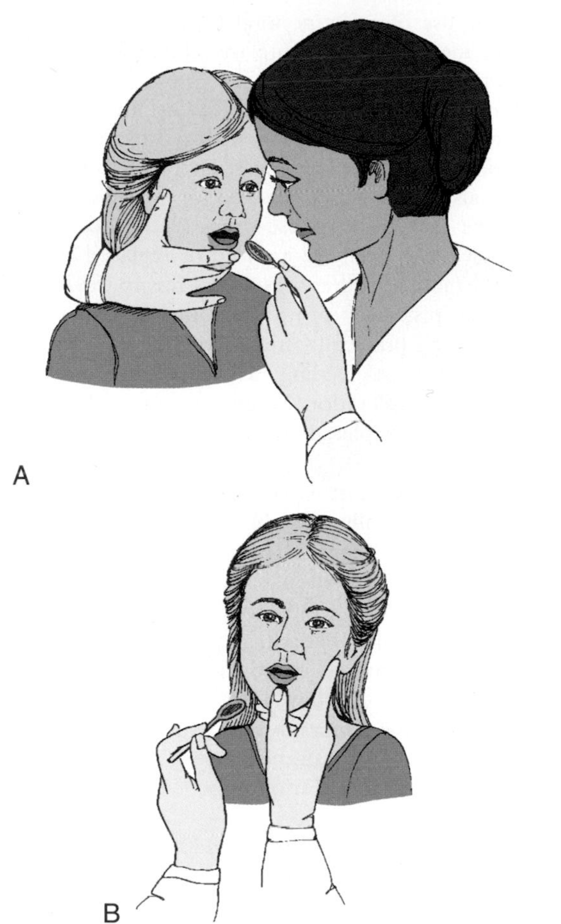

FIGURE 14-6 Jaw control and oral support. **A,** From the side. **B,** From the front.

as the child becomes more skilled in managing liquids from a cup.

Neuromuscular Interventions for Oral Motor Impairments

A wide range of children demonstrate oral motor impairments that affect the development of feeding skills. Oral motor problems are seen frequently in children with global neuromuscular impairments caused by cerebral palsy, traumatic brain injury, prematurity, or genetic conditions such as Down syndrome. Children without neuromuscular impairments may also demonstrate oral motor problems when they are delayed in transitioning from a bottle to a cup or from puréed foods to textured foods. Inexperience with normal feeding activities may contribute to oral motor weakness and coordination difficulties. Oral hypersensitivity may cause a child to retract the tongue into the mouth to avoid stimulation, contributing to maladaptive oral movement patterns. Occupational therapists include oral motor activities within a comprehensive intervention plan to promote strength and coordination for the development of more advanced oral feeding skills.

Whenever possible, oral motor activities should include foods or flavors to incorporate taste receptors and facilitate the integration of sensory and motor skills for a functional response. Hypersensitive children may tolerate non-nutritive activities initially, before they are able to accept the additional sensory input that food flavors provide.

Jaw weakness is often seen in children with oral feeding difficulties. This may contribute to an open-mouthed posture at rest, drooling, food loss during feeding, difficulty with chewing a variety of age-appropriate foods, or poor stabilization when drinking from a cup. Jaw weakness and instability may also affect lip closure for spoon feeding and control during swallowing. Occupational therapists may facilitate jaw strength with a variety of non-nutritive or nutritive activities. Non-nutritive strengthening activities may include sustained biting or repetitive chewing on a resistive device or flexible tubing before the introduction of food textures. Nutritive jaw strengthening activities may include biting or chewing on fruits or vegetables encased in a mesh pouch or progressive resistive activities with a variety of solid or chewy foods placed over the molar surfaces.[45]

Children with neuromuscular impairments may have strong patterns of abnormal oral movement. The child may exhibit a tonic bite by biting down forcefully in response to a stimulus and demonstrate subsequent difficulty opening or relaxing the jaw. A strong tongue thrust movement pattern may also be present, in which the tongue forcefully protrudes beyond the border of the lips during oral feeding activities. A well-supported and slightly flexed head position reduces these abnormal movement patterns. Children with tongue thrust may also benefit from oral motor activities to facilitate tongue lateralization and placement of the spoon or food bolus to the sides of the mouth, rather than at midline.[11]

Children may demonstrate immature forward-backward tongue movements during feeding, poor dissociation of the tongue from the jaw, and poor tongue lateralization to control textured food over the molar surfaces. Occupational therapists may engage the child in activities to facilitate tongue movements, such as encouraging the child to make silly faces in a mirror or lick lollipops, frosting, or whipped cream from the corners of the mouth or within the cheeks. Stimulating the sides of the tongue and inside the cheeks with a Nuk brush or oral motor tool may also encourage tongue lateralization.

Problems affecting the lips and cheeks include abnormal tightness or weakness. A child may demonstrate lip or cheek retraction, making it difficult for the child to assume or sustain lip closure. Good lip closure and lip seal are needed to assist the child with oral food control and prevent anterior spillage during feeding. It is also very difficult to swallow with retracted lips and cheeks because the lips seal the oral cavity to create pressure to propel the food bolus into the pharyngeal cavity. Slow perioral and intraoral cheek stretches can help promote lip closure before initiating functional activities with spoon feeding or whistles.

Researchers and clinicians suggest that oral motor therapy is an important component of a global treatment approach for children with feeding problems.[6,16,35] A recent systematic review by Howe and Wang[30] has indicated that research evidence supports the use of oral motor and physiologic interventions for preterm infants, children with neuromuscular impairments, and children with oral structure abnormalities such as cleft palate (see later). Research Note 14-2 also describes a study evaluating oral motor intervention in children with cerebral palsy.

RESEARCH NOTE 14-2

Gisel, E.G. (1994). Oral-motor skills following sensorimotor intervention in the moderately eating-impaired child with cerebral palsy. Dysphagia, 9, *180–192.*

Abstract

This study looked at the efficacy of oral sensorimotor treatment in children with cerebral palsy. Outcomes were reported for nutrition anthropometrics, such as weight and skin fold parameters. Additional outcomes were reported for functional oral feeding activities, including spoon feeding, biting, chewing, cup drinking, straw drinking, swallowing, and drooling. Twenty-seven American toddlers and school-age children with cerebral palsy completed the 20-week study. Comparisons were made among treatment groups; protocols comprised 20 weeks of oral sensorimotor treatment, 20 weeks of chewing-only treatment, and 10 weeks of no treatment followed by 10 weeks of treatment. During the treatment phase, oral motor therapy or chewing was completed daily for 5 to 7 minutes prior to snack or lunch. Oral motor treatment interventions were described in detail and included activities to stimulate tongue lateralization, lip closure, and chewing skills. The results showed a positive treatment effect at the end of the 20-week period for all three treatment groups, with improvements noted in the areas of spoon feeding, chewing, and biting skills. Each group showed improvements in different functional oral feeding skills; however, improvements were noted in the third group only after treatment was initiated in the second 10-week period. Improvements in nutrition anthropometrics, cup drinking skills, and videofluoroscopic swallowing results were not significant for any of the three treatment groups.

Implications for Practice

Oral motor and chewing interventions may be effective to improve some oral feeding activities; however, the research evidence continues to be limited. Occupational therapists should carefully, objectively, and regularly evaluate whether progress is being demonstrated in their patients. They may also supplement oral motor therapy with a variety of interventions, including food texture modifications, sensory-based activities, postural and respiratory activities, positioning adaptations, and behavioral techniques as part of a comprehensive treatment plan to improve feeding skills in this population.

Transition from Nonoral Feeding to Oral Feeding

Nonoral feeding with a gastrostomy, nasogastric tube, or other method is indicated when a child is unable to meet his or her nutrition or hydration needs by mouth. Nonoral feeding methods may be used when the child has dysphagia; complex heart, respiratory, or other medical conditions; or GI problems. Other children require nonoral feeding simply because they are unable to consume enough food or liquid by mouth for adequate growth and hydration. Inadequate nutrition or hydration can severely limit a child's motor development, cognitive development, and health.[26] The placement of a gastrostomy tube or the use of other nonoral feeding methods can be a temporary measure to promote the child's nutritional status and growth.[53]

When children receive nonoral feeding, they are at risk for developing oral motor and oral sensory impairments because of limited oral feeding experiences. Nasogastric and orogastric tubes may also create sensory distress for the child during placement of the tube. When these tubes are needed over a long period, they are typically re-inserted or replaced at least once per month, causing further sensory distress to the child. Occupational therapists may provide an intervention program to provide ongoing oral exploration activities and social engagement during nonoral feeding. The goal is to create positive social and oral exploration experiences on a daily basis and ultimately link these pleasurable experiences with the satiation of hunger.

If the child has a history of aspiration dysphagia or if oral feeding is not medically safe, the child may suck on a pacifier or engage in mouth play with teethers, spoons, and toys during nonoral feeding. Occupational therapists and caregivers can engage in games that include touch and exploration around the face and mouth. Children may also benefit from games that encourage them to make different sounds with their mouth, give kisses, or blow whistles or bubbles. Whenever possible, occupational therapists should encourage families to include their child in mealtime routines, such as sitting with the family at the table during tube feedings and oral play activities.

When the child is medically cleared to have nutritive stimulation, occupational therapists and caregivers can provide flavors or tastes of foods by dipping a finger, pacifier, spoon, or toy into juice, formula, or puréed foods. Children who receive nonoral feeding may have limited opportunities to experience typical feelings of hunger. This is especially true when children require nonoral feedings on a continuous schedule, across many hours during the day. Children who are able to tolerate more compressed bolus feedings may have more opportunities to experience hunger, which may increase the child's motivation to consume some foods by mouth. As the child begins to advance oral intake skills, occupational therapists need to collaborate with physicians or nutritionists who can determine appropriate schedule changes and reductions in nonoral nutrition.

Children who have a tracheostomy often require nonoral feeding methods. The risk and complications of aspiration are significantly increased in a child with a tracheostomy because of the fragility of the respiratory system.[1] Increased risk of aspiration may occur in children with a tracheostomy, related to the changes in pressure created by the new opening in the laryngeal cavity or poor laryngeal mobility. Children with a tracheostomy may be ready for nutritive stimulation when they are able to manage their own saliva without frequent suctioning and can tolerate a speaking valve or cap, which may help create more normalized pharyngeal swallowing coordination.[29] Occupational therapists must collaborate with physicians and complete comprehensive assessments of swallowing before initiating nutritive oral feeding activities in children with a tracheostomy. Before receiving medical clearance for oral feeding, children with a tracheostomy will benefit from oral exploration and desensitization activities when oral feeding is not possible.

When children are medically cleared and have sufficient oral motor and swallowing skills to consume larger amounts of food by mouth, they may continue to demonstrate strong oral aversions, hypersensitivity, or refusal to engage in oral feeding activities. Transitioning from nonoral to oral feeding is a gradual process and may require a variety of oral sensory, skill development, and behavioral intervention activities over a period of time. This process is often complex and requires collaboration with physicians, nutritionists, and other professionals.

Cleft Lip and Palate

Approximately 1 in 700 infants is born with a cleft lip and/or cleft palate.[12] A cleft lip or palate is a separation or hole in the oral structures usually joined together at midline during the early weeks of fetal development. A cleft lip is separation of the upper lip, which may be seen as a small indentation, or a larger opening that extends up to the nostril. A cleft palate is a separation of the anterior hard or posterior soft palate and may occur with or without a cleft lip. Clefts in the lip and palate range in severity, may be unilateral or bilateral, and may be part of a larger constellation of medical problems associated with a specific syndrome, such as Pierre-Robin sequence, CHARGE association, Smith-Lemli-Opitz syndrome, Wolf-Hirschhorn syndrome, fetal alcohol syndrome, and orofaciodigital syndrome.[36] Children born with clefts typically require one or more surgical procedures to repair the lip or palate. These surgeries may be scheduled at various times in the young child's life, depending on other medical problems, growth and nutrition status of the child, and growth of the lip and/or palatal tissues.

Children born with cleft lip and/or palate often have oral feeding difficulties, including problems latching onto the bottle or breast, inefficient milk transfer, prolonged feeding times, milk leaking from the nose, and poor weight gain. Because of the lack of closure between the oral and nasal cavities, young infants with cleft lip or palate have difficulty creating suction to express liquid during breastfeeding or bottle feeding.[27] Infants born with clefts in the lip and palate, bilateral clefts, and syndromes that include other medical problems typically have more severe feeding problems. Infants born with only a minor cleft lip are often successful with breastfeeding or bottle feeding, with only a few simple adaptations.[36]

Occupational therapists recommend compensatory positioning, adaptive feeding techniques, and specialized bottles for young infants with cleft lip or palate. Feeding the child in a more upright position (>60 degrees) may help improve milk transfer to the posterior oral cavity. Cheek and/or lip support may be recommended to help with gentle closure of a cleft lip to improve latching or suction during feeding. A variety of specialized bottles and nipples are available that use up and down compression movements (rather than suction) or allow the caregiver to squeeze the bottle to help deposit milk into the infant's mouth. The Special Needs Feeder (previously called the Haberman Feeder) and the Mini Special Needs Feeder both have soft nipples and one-way valves that can deliver milk with little to no oral suction.[36] Longer nipples may help deposit liquid toward the back of the infant's mouth, beyond the cleft. Soft squeezable bottles, such as the Mead-Johnson Cleft Lip and Palate Nurser, allow the parent to deposit small amounts of milk into the mouth in synchrony with the infant's sucking efforts. Infants with severe cleft lip and palate may require additional medical interventions, such as a nasal trumpet or palatal obturator, to be successful with oral feeding. These devices are costly, require custom fitting, often need replacing as the infant grows larger, and may be challenging to use.[36] Therefore, it is often suggested to try positioning adaptations and specialized bottle systems as a first approach.

After surgical repair of a cleft, occupational therapists may perform scar massage, initiate therapy activities to reduce oral hypersensitivity, and reassess the oral feeding method. Some children may have ongoing problems with food or liquid entering the nasal cavity during oral feeding. Interventions for this problem include evaluating which food or liquid textures are more challenging for the child, alternating bites of food with sips of liquid, suggesting positioning changes during feeding, and recommending smaller sized bites of food or sips of liquid.

Other Structural Anomalies

Other structural anomalies affecting the feeding process include micrognathia and macroglossia. *Micrognathia* is defined as a small recessed jaw. *Macroglossia* is a term used when the tongue is disproportionately large in comparison with the size of the mouth or jaw. Occupational therapists need to consider the impact of the size and position of oral structures on respiration and oral movement patterns during feeding. They may use different nipples, utensils, or positioning adaptations to help compensate for these structural differences. For example, infants with micrognathia may benefit from a prone or side-lying position to help draw the tongue into a more forward position, allowing improved respiration and nipple compression during bottle feeding. Infants with macroglossia may require adaptations to reduce tongue-thrusting movements and anterior food loss during feeding.

Structural anomalies of the larynx and esophagus include laryngeal clefts, esophageal strictures, tracheoesophageal fistula, and esophageal atresia. Laryngeal clefts vary in severity and are the result of a malformation of the tracheoesophageal septum in utero.[18] Tracheoesophageal fistula and esophageal atresia are both repaired surgically, often within the first few days of life. Children with a history of surgical repair to the esophagus are at increased risk of later developing esophageal stricture, a narrowing of the esophagus. Although these diagnoses are rare, children with structural anomalies of the esophagus are at increased risk for aspiration during swallowing, food refusal behaviors, delayed transition to textured foods, and poor esophageal motility.

Esophageal motility describes how quickly foods and liquids move through the esophagus and empty into the stomach. Liquids and smooth, runny foods empty into the stomach more quickly than thick, fibrous, or more solid foods. Children who have a history of esophageal structural anomalies may have problems advancing to higher food textures as a result of decreased esophageal motility. Occupational therapists may recommend adapting food textures to maximize oral intake, alternating bites of food with sips of liquid to help clear the esophagus, slowing the pace of feeding, or encouraging a subsequent dry swallow after each bite of food to help compensate for delayed esophageal motility.

Summary

The causes of pediatric feeding, eating, and swallowing disorders are diverse and complex. Occupational therapists consider the whole child during the assessment and intervention process, including multiple overlapping child factors and performance skills, activity demands and contexts, and family patterns (Case Study 14-1).

- A competent occupational therapy practitioner who provides services for feeding, eating, and swallowing has knowledge and skills in the following:
  - Anatomy and physiology of oral motor and swallowing functions
  - Growth and developmental milestones for oral feeding and self-feeding skills
  - Nutrition and medical conditions that influence the assessment and intervention process
  - Diagnostic tests used with children with feeding and swallowing disorders
  - Social, emotional, and behavioral factors that affect feeding and mealtimes
  - Sensory processing skills that support feeding transitions
  - Safety considerations for feeding and swallowing
  - Environmental influences and adaptations
  - Positioning modifications
  - Adaptive equipment and oral motor techniques used in feeding intervention plans
- The assessment and treatment of pediatric feeding disorders often require interprofessional collaboration between the occupational therapist and other members of the child's treatment team.
- Inclusion of parents and other primary caregivers in all stages of the assessment and treatment program is mandatory to ensure the child's ultimate success in eating across environments.

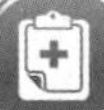

CASE STUDY 14-1 Marco

Marco was a 4½-year-old boy referred for an evaluation of feeding, eating, and swallowing. His problems with oral feeding began early in infancy. He had difficulty latching on during breastfeeding attempts and did not have adequate weight gain, so he was transitioned to bottle feeding at 1 month of age. He coughed and sputtered during bottle feeding in infancy, often at the end of the feeding. Marco was very particular about what type of nipple was used with his bottle and did not take his bottle whenever a different nipple was attempted. Baby foods were first introduced at 6 months of age. With baby foods, Marco gagged, refused to open his mouth, and turned away after the first few bites. His parents stopped trying baby foods for a few weeks, and then they would try again. Marco demonstrated similar refusal behaviors with every attempt. Marco's parents later insisted that Marco sit at the dinner table at the start of family meals, where he was encouraged to try some new foods. When Marco refused to eat, his parents would allow him to leave the table after a few minutes.

As a toddler, Marco continued to be dependent on formula from a bottle, and he continued to have difficulty growing and gaining weight. At the advice of the primary care physician, Marco's mother stopped bottle feeding and only offered a cup and a variety of foods when Marco was 4 years old. Marco then refused to eat or drink anything for 3 days. He was admitted to the hospital for dehydration, and he started nasogastric tube feedings. After the tube feeding started, he never returned to accepting the bottle. After 3 weeks of nasogastric feeding, a gastrostomy tube was placed.

Marco lived in a rural community and had limited access to medical specialists and therapy services. Marco had never had a modified barium swallow study. He had no history of pneumonia, but he had occasional unexplained low-grade fevers, which the parents attributed to teething. Marco received a private speech-language evaluation approximately 2 months prior to the occupational therapy feeding evaluation, and concerns were reported with receptive language, expressive language, and articulation. Marco was scheduled to enroll in a preschool class in the fall.

Evaluation Findings

At the time of the evaluation, Marco received 100% of his nutrition from PediaSure via his gastrostomy tube on a continuous schedule over 16 hours. He was unable to tolerate an increase in his tube feeding rate, with leakage around the gastrostomy tube site and behavioral discomfort noted.

Marco licked a potato chip during the parent-directed feeding observation. He refused to bite, chew, or swallow any foods or liquids that were encouraged by his mother. Marco grimaced during the occupational therapy oral-motor assessment, but he was able to participate with encouragement, clear expectations, and praise. He gagged when stimulation was provided on his tongue or palate and demonstrated retraction in his cheeks and tongue. Marco used a weak, nonrhythmic, immature munching pattern, with simulated chewing. He had a positive tongue lateralization response and a closed-mouth posture at rest, with no evidence of drooling. Oral-facial muscle tone appeared to be within normal limits.

Marco was ambulatory, alert, sociable, and able to communicate basic needs. During observations of play, he did not want to explore "squishy balls" with his hands during the evaluation, and he pulled away during a scissors activity when the paper began to touch the back of his hand.

Intervention Considerations

Prior to the start of treatment, Marco was referred for an evaluation by a gastroenterologist. An endoscopy was completed, which showed significant esophagitis and gastroesophageal reflux disease, but no evidence of allergies. Marco began antireflux medication. Marco was not referred for a videofluoroscopic swallow study because of the severity of his refusal to consume food or liquid by mouth. Marco was

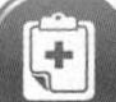

CASE STUDY 14-1 Marco—cont'd

monitored throughout his treatment program for clinical signs of dysphagia.

Because Marco's family lived in a rural area, with limited availability of treatment services, he was referred for an intensive day treatment program to improve his oral feeding skills. He received intervention from an occupational therapist, behavioral psychologist, and speech-language pathologist. He also received consultations with a nutritionist, gastroenterologist, and social worker. Occupational therapy services were provided three or four times per week for 30- to 60-minute sessions for a total of 5 weeks. Occupational therapy sessions integrated sensory, motor, and behavioral treatment techniques to improve Marco's ability to consume a variety of foods, manage liquids from a cup, and improve self-feeding skills. Specific occupational therapy activities included the following:

Sensory

Marco demonstrated oral hypersensitivity, with symptoms of generalized tactile defensiveness. During treatment, Marco engaged in play-based sensory activities with finger paint, craft activities, squishy balls, Play-Doh, clay, rice, and water play. Oral sensory preparatory activities included slow, deep pressure touch beginning on the arms and shoulders before progressing to the outer cheeks and lips.

Behavior

Marco often refused to try new feeding and oral motor activities. The occupational therapist implemented behavioral strategies to offer choices when possible and set clear, consistent expectations. Enthusiastic praise and other reinforcements (e.g., favorite toy or game) were provided after participation in oral feeding and difficult activities. A timer was used to signal the end of the meal or therapy session. Activities were graded to provide a gradual increase in demands that were consistent with the child's oral-motor and oral-sensory skill levels. Toward the end of the treatment program, external toy reinforcements were gradually decreased to encourage self-motivated participation.

Oral Motor

Marco had oral motor impairments limiting his ability to manage a variety of foods. He demonstrated jaw weakness and tightness or retraction in his cheeks, lips, and tongue. Initially during meal sessions, Marco was offered puréed foods to maximize his oral intake and compensate for his oral motor and oral sensory difficulties. During occupational therapy sessions (e.g., outside mealtimes), Marco quickly improved his tolerance for oral motor activities when they were combined with behavior management and sensory processing techniques. The occupational therapist was able to complete cheek and lip stretches to improve management of food in the buccal cavity during chewing. After these stretches, Marco was encouraged to activate these muscles by exploring a variety of whistles. Intraoral activities were provided with a Nuk brush, vibration, toothette sponge, flavor sprays, lollipops, and a regular toothbrush. Marco also participated in jaw-strengthening activities. Expectations were increased gradually when Marco's oral motor skills were adequate to manage more textured foods. Initially, Marco mashed small amounts of cracker crumbs placed in his mouth for mashing. He then began biting and munching small pieces of dissolvable solid foods and progressed to a wider variety of soft solids, such as cooked vegetables and canned fruits. Marco's cup drinking skills were also advanced gradually, with small single sips at first, leading up to consecutive sips and swallows from an open cup.

Discharge Status

At the time of discharge from the feeding program, Marco consumed 100% of his nutrition needs by mouth, ate a wide variety of foods, and self-fed almost all his food. He continued to be anxious when a new food was introduced and needed some physical prompts and behavioral strategies to "try it out" before he would attempt to eat the food independently. He demonstrated significantly improved jaw strength, oral motor coordination, and oral sensory responses. He consumed ½-inch pieces of soft solid foods during snack sessions. He continued to be somewhat slow with his chewing, so he ate fork-mashed texture in meal sessions. Marco was referred for weekly speech and occupational therapy services after discharge for continued work on higher food textures and language skills. Marco's mother was also provided with a comprehensive program to continue his oral feeding development at home.

REFERENCES

1. Abraham, S. S., & Wolf, E. L. (2000). Swallowing physiology of toddlers with long-term tracheostomies: A preliminary study. *Dysphagia, 15*, 206–212.
2. Ahearn, W. (2001). Why does my son only eat macaroni and cheese?: Dealing with feeding problems in children with autism. In C. Maurice, R. Foxx, & G. Green (Eds.), *Making a difference: Behavioral intervention for autism.* Austin, TX: Pro-ed.
3. American Dietetic Association: National Dysphagia Diet Task Force (2002). *National dysphagia diet: Standardization for optimal care.* Chicago: American Dietetic Association.
4. American Occupational Therapy Association (2006). *Specialized knowledge and skills in feeding, eating, and swallowing for occupational therapy practice.* Bethesda, MD: American Occupational Therapy Association.
5. American Occupational Therapy Association. (2008). Occupational therapy practice framework: Domain and process. *American Journal of Occupational Therapy, 62*(6), 609–639.
6. Arvedson, J. C. (1998). Management of pediatric dysphagia. *Otolaryngologic Clinics of North America, 31*, 453–476.
7. Ardveson, J. C., & Brodsky, L. (2002). Instrumental evaluation of swallowing. In J. C. Arvedson & L. Brodsky (Eds.),

Pediatric swallowing and feeding: Assessment and management (2nd ed.). Albany, NY: Singular/Thomson Learning.

8. Arvedson, J. C., & Lefton-Greif, M. A. (1998). *Pediatric videofluoroscopic swallow studies: A professional manual with caregiver guidelines.* San Antonio, TX: Communication Skill Builders.
9. Babbitt, R. L., Hoch, T. A., Coe, D. A., et al. (1994). Behavioral assessment and treatment of pediatric feeding disorders. *Journal of Developmental and Behavioral Pediatrics, 15*, 278–291.
10. Beal, J., Silverman, B., Bellant, J., et al. (2012). Late-onset necrotizing enterocolitis in infants following use of a xanthan gum-containing thickening agent. *Journal of Pediatrics, 161*(2), 354–356.
11. Beckman, D. (2000). *Oral motor assessment and intervention.* Presented at the Oral Motor Assessment and Intervention I conference, Charlotte, NC.
12. Bessell, A., Hooper, L., Shaw, W. C., et al. (2011). Feeding interventions for growth and development in infants with cleft lip, cleft palate, or cleft lip and palate. *Cochrane Database of Systematic Reviews, 2*, 1–23.
13. Bulow, M., Olsson, R., & Ekberg, O. (2003). Videoradiographic analysis of how carbonated thin liquids and thickened liquids affect the physiology of swallowing in subjects with aspiration on thin liquids. *Acta Radiologica, 44*, 366–372.
14. Bundy, A. C., & Koomar, J. A. (2002). Orchestrating intervention: The art of practice. In A. C. Bundy, S. J. Lane, & E. A. Murray (Eds.), *Sensory integration: Theory and practice* (2nd ed.). Philadelphia: F. A. Davis.
15. Chamberlin, J., Henry, M. M., Roberts, J. D., et al. (1991). An infant and toddler feeding group program. *American Journal of Occupational Therapy, 45*, 907–911.
16. Christensen, J. R. (1989). Developmental approach to pediatric neurogenic dysphagia. *Dysphagia, 3*, 131–134.
17. Christiaanse, M., Glynn, J., & Bradshaw, J. (2003). *Experience with transcutaneous electrical stimulation: A new treatment option for the management of pediatric dysphagia.* Winston-Salem, NC: Wake Forest School of Medicine, University Health Sciences.
18. Cohen, M. S., Zhuang, L., Simons, J. P., et al. (2011). Injection laryngoplasty for type 1 laryngeal cleft in children. *Otolaryngology—Head and Neck Surgery, 144*(5), 789–793.
19. DeVault, M. L. (1991). *Feeding the family: The social organization of caring as gendered work.* Chicago: University of Chicago Press.
20. Feucht, S., Ogata, B., & Lucas, B. (2010). Nutrition concerns of children with autism spectrum disorders. *Nutrition Focus, 25*(4), 1–13.
21. Fischer, E., & Silverman, A. (2007). Behavioral conceptualization, assessment, and treatment of pediatric feeding disorders. *Seminars in Speech and Language, 26*, 223–231.
22. Freed, M. L., Freed, L., Chatburn, R. L., et al. (2001). Electrical stimulation for swallowing disorders caused by stroke. *Respiratory Care, 46*, 466–474.
23. Friedman, B., & Frazier, J. B. (2000). Deep laryngeal penetration as a predictor of aspiration. *Dysphagia, 15*, 153–158.
24. Fung, E. B., Samson-Fang, L., Stallings, V. A., et al. (2002). Feeding dysfunction is associated with poor growth and health status in children with cerebral palsy. *Journal of the American Dietetic Association, 102*, 361–368.
25. Garon, B. (2003). Swallow dysfunction: New research evidence. Paper presented at Keep Pace Seminars conference, Baltimore.
26. Gisel, E. G., Applegate-Ferrante, T., Benson, J. E., et al. (1995). Effect of oral sensorimotor treatment on measures of growth, eating efficiency and aspiration in the dysphagic child with cerebral palsy. *Developmental Medicine and Child Neurology, 37*, 528–543.
27. Glass, R. P., & Wolf, L. S. (1999). Feeding management of infants with cleft lip and palate and micrognathia. *Infants and Young Children, 12*, 70–81.
28. Greer, A. J., Gulotta, C. S., Masler, E. A., et al. (2008). Caregiver stress and outcomes of children with pediatric feeding disorders treated in an intensive interdisciplinary program. *Journal of Pediatric Psychology, 33*, 612–620.
29. Gross, R. D., Mahlmann, J., & Grayhack, J. P. (2003). Physiologic effects of open and closed tracheostomy tubes on the pharyngeal swallow. *Annals of Otology, Rhinology, and Laryngology, 112*, 143–152.
30. Howe, T. H., & Wang, T. N. (2013). Systematic review of interventions used in or relevant to occupational therapy for children with feeding difficulties ages birth-5 years. *American Journal of Occupational Therapy, 67*(4), 405–412.
31. Hulme, J. B., Gallacher, K., Walsh, J., et al. (1987). Behavioral and postural changes observed with the use of adaptive seating by clients with multiple handicaps. *Physical Therapy, 67*, 1060–1067.
32. Kerwin, M. E. (1999). Empirically supported treatments in pediatric psychology: Severe feeding problems. *Journal of Pediatric Psychology, 24*, 193–214.
33. Klein, M. D., & Delaney, T. A. (1994). *Feeding and nutrition for the child with special needs.* Tucson, AZ: Therapy Skill Builders.
34. Koivisto Hursti, U. K. (1999). Factors influencing children's food choice. *Annals of Medicine, 31*(Suppl. 1), 26–32.
35. Logemann, J. A. (1998). *Evaluation and treatment of swallowing disorders* (2nd ed.). Austin, TX: Pro-Ed.
36. Miller, C. K. (2011). Feeding issues and interventions in infants and children with clefts and craniofacial syndromes. *Seminars in Speech and Language, 32*(2), 115–126.
37. Miller, C. K., & Willging, J. P. (2003). Advances in the evaluation and management of pediatric dysphagia. *Current Opinion in Otolaryngology & Head and Neck Surgery, 11*, 442–446.
38. Morris, S. E., & Klein, M. D. (2000). *Pre-feeding skills* (2nd ed.). Tucson, AZ: Therapy Skill Builders.
39. Occupational Safety and Health Administration. (1991). *Federal Register, 56*(235).
40. Palmer, M. M., & Heyman, M. B. (1993). Assessment and treatment of sensory- versus motor-based feeding problems in very young children. *Infants and Young Children, 6*, 67–73.
41. Piazza, C. C., Patel, M. R., Gulotta, C. S., et al. (2003). On the relative contributions of positive reinforcement and escape extinction in the treatment of food refusal. *Journal of Applied Behavior Analysis, 36*, 309–324.
42. Reilly, S., & Skuse, D. (1992). Characteristics and management of feeding problems of young children with cerebral palsy. *Developmental Medicine and Child Neurology, 34*, 379–388.
43. Reilly, S., Skuse, D., & Poblete, X. (1996). The prevalence of feeding problems and oral motor dysfunction in children with cerebral palsy: A community survey. *Journal of Pediatrics, 129*(6), 877–882.
44. Rommel, N., DeMeyer, A. M., Feenstra, L., et al. (2003). The complexity of feeding problems in 700 infants and young children presenting to a tertiary care institution. *Journal of Pediatric Gastroenterology and Nutrition, 37*, 75–84.
45. Rosenfeld-Johnson, S. (2005). *Assessment and treatment of the jaw.* Tucson, AZ: Talk Tools Innovative Therapists International.
46. Ruark McMurtrey, J. (2007). Best practices for behavioral management of pediatric dysphagia. *Pediatric Feeding and Dysphagia Newsletter, 7*, 1–5.
47. Schuberth, L. M. (1994). The role of occupational therapy in diagnoses and management. In D. N. Tuchman &

R. Walter (Eds.), *Disorders of feeding and swallowing in infants and children* (pp. 115–130). San Diego, CA: Singular.

48. Schwarz, S. M. (2003). Feeding disorders in children with developmental disabilities. *Infants and Young Children, 15*, 29–41.
49. Skuse, D. (1993). Identification and management of problem eaters. *Archives of Disease in Childhood, 69*, 604–608.
50. Smith, A. M., Roux, S., Naidoo, N. T., et al. (2005). Food choice of tactile defensive children. *Nutrition, 21*, 14–19.
51. Sullivan, P. B., Juszezak, E., Lambert, B. R., et al. (2002). Impact of feeding problems on nutritional intake and growth: Oxford feeding study II. *Developmental Medicine and Child Neurology, 44*, 461–467.
52. Sullivan, P. B., Lambert, B., Rose, M., et al. (2000). Prevalence and severity of feeding and nutritional problems in children with neurological impairment: Oxford feeding study. *Developmental Medicine & Child Neurology, 42*(10), 674–680.
53. Tarbell, M. C., & Allaire, J. H. (2002). Children with feeding tube dependency: Treating the whole child. *Infants and Young Children, 15*, 29–41.
54. U.S. Food and Drug Administration (2011). FDA press release: Do not feed Simply Thick to premature infants. Retrieved from: <http://www.fda.gov/NewsEvents/Newsroom/PressAnnouncements/ucm256253.htm>.
55. US Food and Drug Administration (2012). FDA expands caution about Simply Thick. Retrieved from: <http://www.fda.gov/ForConsumers/ConsumerUpdates/ucm256250.htm>.
56. Vandenplas, Y., Rudolph, C. D., Di Lorenzo, C., et al. (2009). Pediatric gastroesophageal reflux clinical practice guidelines: Joint recommendations of the North American Society for Pediatric Gastroenterology, Hepatology, and Nutrition (NASPGHAN) and the European Society for Pediatric Gastroenterology, Hepatology, and Nutrition (ESPGHAN). *Journal of Pediatric Gastroenterology & Nutrition, 49*(4), 498–547.
57. Werle, M. A., Murphy, T. B., & Budd, K. S. (1993). Treating chronic food refusal in young children: Home-based parent training. *Journal of Applied Behavior Analysis, 26*, 421–433.
58. Wolf, L. S., & Glass, R. P. (1992). *Feeding and swallowing disorders in infancy: Assessment and management.* Tucson, AZ: Therapy Skill Builders.
59. Wood, B. K., Wolery, M., & Kaiser, A. P. (2009). Treatment of food selectivity in a young child with autism. *Focus on Autism and Other Developmental Disabilities, 24*(3), 169–177.

CHAPTER 15

Activities of Daily Living and Sleep and Rest

Jayne Shepherd

KEY TERMS

- Activities of daily living (ADLs)
- Performance context
- Grading techniques
- Backward chaining
- Forward chaining
- Cues
- Prompts
- Video self-modeling (VSM)
- Assistive devices
- Environmental adaptations
- Adaptive positioning
- Partial participation
- Sleep

GUIDING QUESTIONS

1. What factors affect performance of the activities of daily living (ADLs) and sleep habits of children?
   - How do the environment and context of where the activity is occurring help or hinder performance?
   - How do body structures and functions, performance skills, performance patterns, and activity demands contribute to a child's ADL performance and sleep and rest?
2. How and when do you evaluate ADL skills?
   - When do children typically perform ADL and sleep tasks independently?
   - What formal or informal evaluations are available?
3. Which general intervention strategies and approaches are used to promote ADL skills and healthy sleep and rest?
4. What evidence is available to support the use of specific intervention techniques with specific groups of children with disabilities?
5. How can I modify the environment, equipment, or techniques to support ADL development and sleep in children with disabilities?
6. What are the effects of context on a child's performance and parental expectations for ADL, sleep, and rest?

Activities of daily living (ADLs) encompass some of the most important occupations children learn as they mature. Self-care, or ADLs, include learning how to take care of one's body, such as toilet hygiene, bowel and bladder management, bathing and showering, personal hygiene and grooming, eating and feeding, dressing, and functional mobility.[3] Other ADL tasks include caring for a personal device and learning to express sexual needs.[3] As the child matures, he or she learns to perform ADLs in socially appropriate ways so that he or she can engage in the other occupations within the family unit and community, such as education, play, leisure, rest and sleep, social participation, instrumental activities of daily living (IADLs), and work. Often, when a child is young, he or she performs ADLs as co-occupations of caregivers and children, especially when the child has a disability. Parents often establish the routines for bathing, dressing, feeding, and delegate more complex ADLs to others.[3] In addition, rest and sleep occupations often affect ADL performance.

This chapter discusses the dynamic interaction of child factors, contexts, activity demands, and performance skills and patterns that allows a child to engage in ADL occupations in a variety of environments. Evaluation methods, intervention approaches, and evidence-based strategies for improving outcomes in ADL activities are reviewed. Typical development, limitations, and modifications for toileting, dressing, bathing, grooming, and performing other related ADL tasks are described (feeding is discussed in Chapter 14). Examples of adaptations to physical and social environments are provided, with consideration given to cultural, temporal, virtual, and personal influences.

Importance of Developing ADL Occupations

The foundations for mastering ADLs begin in infancy and are refined throughout the various stages of development. As unique individuals living in certain contexts, children learn these activities at varying rates and have occasional regression and unpredictable behaviors. Cultural values, parental expectations, social routines, and the physical environment influence when children begin to bathe, dress, groom, and toilet themselves. Overall, society and families assume that children develop increasing levels of competence and self-reliance to meet their own ADL needs. Growth and maturity allow the child to participate in various roles and environments, with decreasing levels of adult supervision for ADLs.[65,119]

When a child is born with or acquires a disability, parental and child expectations for ADLs and daily living independence are modified. Occupational therapists are instrumental in collaborating with parents and children to learn how to modify activity demands and routines so that children perform ADL tasks in their everyday environments. Active participation in ADLs has several benefits for the child, including maintaining and improving bodily functions and health (e.g., strength, endurance, range of motion [ROM], coordination, memory, sequencing, concept formation, body image, cleanliness, hygiene) and problem solving while mastering tasks that are meaningful and purposeful to the child. This task mastery leads to increased self-esteem, self-reliance, and self-determination and gives the child a sense of autonomy.[33,97] When children dress themselves, they may choose their own clothing, participate in dress-up during playtime, put on a coat when going outside, change clothes for gym class, and/or dress in a uniform to participate in band or work at a restaurant. As the child learns new ADL tasks, he or she develops a sense of accomplishment and pride in his or her abilities. This increasing independence also gives parents, teachers, and other caregivers more time and energy for other tasks[47] while the child contributes to the family unit.

As a child learns new ADL tasks, routines or patterns of observable behaviors develop. These repetitive routines (e.g., morning routine for getting ready for school, bedtime routine) are embedded within the family culture and environment.[38,144] Occupational therapists ask parents about daily routines and customs at home or school that may influence a child's ADL performance. Some examples of questions to consider asking are as follows:

- When are children expected to be toilet-trained or independent in brushing their teeth?
- How is your child expected to get from room to room in your house or in school?
- Can you please describe your morning routine?

Routines help satisfy or promote the completion of ADL tasks to meet role expectations in home, school, community, and work environments. They are culturally based and often are a combination of what is expected but also what is practical.[43] Each family, teacher, employer, or community organization may follow a unique routine for self-care tasks. For example, the family may require a toilet break whenever they are going somewhere, and teachers may allow students to use the toilet at fixed times during the day. Sometimes routines become damaging and hinder the performance of ADLs.[1,38,144] For example, a child with autism or obsessive-compulsive disorder may be quite rigid about how he or she performs grooming tasks and is inflexible when Aunt Lou visits and the placement of items in the bathroom changes.[170] He or she also may routinely wash the hands after touching any object. These patterns of behavior now interfere, instead of support, ADL performance. Families may or may not have routines that affect ADL performance (e.g., when they eat, when bathing occurs, how often laundry is done, how children are expected to manage personal items such as glasses or retainers). As a child matures, he or she becomes more responsible for developing and maintaining routines that become habits to prevent further illness and maintain health and well-being. Checking skin conditions, maintaining cleanliness during toileting or bathing, preventing cavities through tooth brushing, maintaining personal care devices such as orthotics or catheters, and developing consistent bedtime and sleep habits are some of the healthy living routines that help the child meet role expectations for community living.

Factors Affecting Performance

Child factors, performance environment, contextual aspects, and specific demands of the self-care activity, as well as the child's performance skills, affect the child's ability to participate successfully in ADL occupations. ADLs are performed in a context of interwoven internal and external conditions, some from within the child (e.g., bodily functions and body structures related to the disability, personal and cultural contexts) and others around the child (e.g., social and physical environments; virtual, cultural, and temporal contexts).[1] As occupational therapists consider these factors, they determine the knowledge and performance skills (goal-directed actions) and patterns that the child needs to learn self-care.

Child Factors and Performance Skills

Occupational therapy intervention to increase ADL function considers what the child and family value and the context in which tasks occur. The levels of independence, safety, and adequacy of occupational performance of the child and expectations of the family determine the child's ADL occupations in various contexts.

Specific child factors (body structures and functions), performance skills, and performance patterns will affect ADL performance. For example, children with tactile hypersensitivity may cry during dressing and refuse to dress, despite having the motor and cognitive skills to do so. Children with visual impairments may need to use their sense of touch when brushing the hair. A child with cerebral palsy may not have the postural control to sit up during dressing but may have the sensory perceptual skills (e.g., right-left discrimination, figure/ground) to dress in a side-lying position. A child with attention-deficit/hyperactivity disorder (ADHD) may have all the motor and sensory perceptual skills to complete a self-care task, but his or her cognitive organization, sequencing, and memory may interfere with adequate and safe performance.[143]

Interest level, self-confidence, and motivation are strong forces that help children attain levels of performance that are above or below expectations. Children with intellectual disabilities, traumatic brain injury, or multiple disabilities may have impairments in coordination, initiative, attention span, sequencing, memory, safety, and ability to learn and generalize activities across environments. However, with instruction and opportunity, ADLs sometimes become the tasks that these children perform most competently.[111]

The child's disability or health status may affect the ability to perform ADL tasks and may also affect caregiver-child interaction during ADL tasks. The child's capacity for learning and ability to complete difficult tasks safely are considered. Pain, fatigue, amount of time the child needs to complete the task, and the child's satisfaction with his or her performance influence the choice of ADL occupations.[67] Children who have had pain caused by medical procedures may avoid ADL tasks because they think that they will hurt.[11,176] Rehabilitation studies of children with cerebral palsy (CP)[119,169] have found that the severity of CP was the greatest predictor of a person's self-care (e.g., eating, grooming, bathing, dressing, toileting), mobility function (e.g., transfers, locomotion), and social function, as measured by the Pediatric Evaluation of Disability

CASE STUDY 15-1 Karina: Partial Participation

Four-year-old Karina is hospitalized every 2 months because of respiratory complications related to a muscular disorder. Like most 4-year-old girls, Karina has an opinion about and preference for how her hair is styled, and she likes to wear barrettes, ribbons, jewelry, and pretend makeup. Karina has a tracheotomy, poor endurance, limited strength, and limited postural control to sit independently. Although sitting independently in bed to groom is limited by these client factors, with partial participation, Karina is still part of the activity. She can sit up and bend forward with physical support from the occupational therapists, reach and choose her barrettes, and, with assistance, comb her hair.

Inventory (PEDI). When gross and fine motor skills were less affected, the child's functional skills increased and the amount of caregiver assistance decreased.[119]

Providing intervention for foundational gross and fine motor skill development, including developing core strength and balance, may improve ADL outcomes for children.[9] Recent rehabilitation research also suggests that constraint-induced movement therapy (CIMT) may improve and maintain functional upper extremity performance that may affect ADL participation.[19,136]

Children who are acutely ill or who have multiple disabilities that require numerous procedures throughout the day (e.g., tube feeding, tracheotomy care, bowel and bladder care) may not have the time or energy to perform ADL tasks independently. For example, Jenna, a 10-year-old child with a C6 spinal cord injury and quadriplegia, can dress herself independently in a 45-minute period, but she and her family prefer that someone else dress her so that she has more energy for school tasks. Children with multiple disabilities may be physically unable to do all or any part of ADL tasks, but they can partially participate or direct others on how to care for them (Case Study 15-1). When children are hospitalized for long periods, they often need to have some control over their participation in self-care routines. Figure 15-1 shows how doing a small part of self-care routines is possible and meaningful for children in the hospital with acute illnesses.

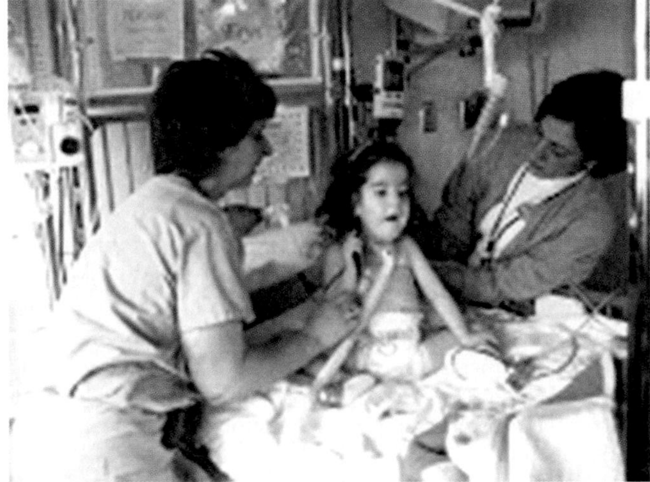

FIGURE 15-1 **Partial participation.** This child partially participates in hair combing and chooses her barrettes while therapists support her in her hospital bed.

Performance Environments and Contexts

The initiation and completion of ADL tasks are influenced by the context of the tasks, including interwoven conditions internal and external to the child (e.g., personal, cultural, temporal, and virtual contexts) and around the child (physical and social environments). Children in early and middle childhood often perform ADLs in different settings. The four primary settings that children experience are home, school, community, and work. Once the occupational therapist understands the contexts in which occupation occurs, intervention strategies congruent with the demands of the activity are chosen or aspects of the environment that are barriers to the child's performance of ADL tasks are modified. Although this section has divided the contexts into various areas, all the areas are interrelated.

Personal and Temporal Contexts: Family Life Cycle and Developmental Stage

Age, gender, education, and socioeconomic status define the personal context for ADL occupations.[1] In assessing dressing, awareness of the personal context is critical in choosing age- and gender-appropriate clothing within the family's budget. The time of day or year, life stage of the child or other family members, family routines and occupations, and duration, sequence, or past history of the activity are included in the temporal context.[1] Consider Cory, who is learning to tie his shoes. A routine method is established so that he does the task the same way every time he tries it at home and school—first pull both laces tight, then make an X. Cory practices it every time he tries to tie his shoes but becomes frustrated easily. If mom and dad work, practicing shoe tying before going to school works if they all get up 15 minutes earlier in the morning, and Cory doesn't become frustrated with the time constraints. When the seasons change, Cory must not only tie his shoes, but also don boots and extra clothes (e.g., mittens, snow pants). With these additional time constraints, his parents may decide to practice shoe tying at a different time of the day or on the weekend.

Children typically master ADLs in a sequence, achieving specific tasks as overall competency increases. The sequence of ADL development helps occupational therapists and families form realistic expectations for children at different ages and helps determine the appropriate timing for teaching these occupations. By considering the child's age, occupational therapists determine when it is time to stop working on specific preparatory or therapeutic activities. For example, 6-year-old Tilly has received occupational therapy for 5 years to enhance eating by trying to increase her lip closure and develop a more efficient suck-swallow pattern. If she has not learned this over the past 5 years, what are her chances of learning it this year? It may be time for the occupational therapist to work on self-feeding strategies or on an IADL activity, such as operating an appliance with a switch for meal preparation.

Families vary in their ability and availability to assist and encourage their child to perform ADLs. This ability often depends on where the family and child are in the family life cycle, personal factors or characteristics of the child, and family's ability to spend time and be flexible in everyday routines.[10,14,148,170] When the child is an infant, parents often seek instruction on feeding, dressing, and bathing. By 3 years of age, the child's self-feeding, dressing, and toileting skills may become issues for parents. For example, if Mary is the youngest of seven children, increased ADL independence in feeding or dressing may be less important because her older siblings love to feed and dress Mary. As Mary transitions into a day-care setting or another sibling is born, learning basic ADL skills may become a priority.

Mothers of very-low-birth-weight children or children at risk tend to adjust to their child's motor and cognitive needs by giving more directive and positive emotional and social assistance during ADLs than parents of children who were born full term.[76] Sometimes, parental overinvolvement in a child's self-care provokes increased anxiety in the child.[176] Occupational therapists need to consider how caregivers actively support or hinder ADL participation by modifying the social and physical environment or by changing the demands of the ADLs.[76] First-hand knowledge of parents and caregivers about strategies that "work" with their child and within their family routines is essential to consider in planning ADL intervention.[14,43,144]

When the child enters elementary school, typically by 6 years of age, functional mobility in the school environment, dressing (especially outerwear), toileting, socialization with peers, grooming (e.g., washing the hands and face), and functional communication (e.g., writing, drawing, expressing needs) become increasingly important. As older siblings become more aware of and sensitive to the child's disability, they may ignore their brother or sister in community settings or be more motivated by the occupational therapist to help the child learn ADL tasks.

During adolescence (13-21 years), parents and child can begin to have different concerns and goals for therapy. Both may be concerned about the adolescent's independence in ADL; however, adolescents may have more concerns about fitting in with a social group.[103] When children who require maximum physical assistance in ADLs approach adulthood, they may become a great concern to parents. For the first time, parents may not have the physical strength to handle the daily care needs of their child or may voice concerns about the child's safety if someone else provides the caretaking.

Increasing independence in ADL tasks during adolescence often determines whether a child will fit in with peers, obtain a job, or go to college outside the school and family environment. The child takes on increased responsibility for managing ADL routines, caring for personal devices, and perfecting grooming skills (e.g., shaving, hair styling, skin care, braces). During this stage, families further investigate current community resources as they think about future living arrangements, vocational opportunities, and the availability of other recreational activities for their child.[166] Additional IADL tasks are introduced to promote independence during this stage, including caring for clothing, preparing meals, shopping, managing money, and maintaining a household.[62] Parent issues may focus on the child's ability to express sexual needs, be safe in many environments, and respond appropriately to emergencies.

Social Environment

The social environment, family, other caregivers, and peers provide encouragement and support ADL independence. They also shape expectations regarding the child's ADL occupations. In large families, different members may be assigned to perform or help with specific ADL tasks for a child with a disability; in other families, the parent may be the sole person responsible for the daily living needs of the child. Family expectations, roles, and routines for managing daily living needs also influence the child's development of ADL and performance patterns.[166] For example, parents living on a farm may expect their child to get up at dawn, put on overalls and boots, do chores such as feeding the animals, receive home schooling, and help sell eggs to augment the family income.

When planning treatment, the occupational therapist considers personal characteristics of family members, such as temperament, coping abilities, flexibility, and health status (see Chapter 5).[166] For example, the mother may place her older child in the "mothering" role if she is depressed and unable to get out of bed and begin the morning routine. Parents with intellectual disabilities or mental health problems may need to see an occupational therapist modeling a behavior to learn how to cue and structure a task for their children.[37,166] Parents with physical problems may need instructions and practice in using specific techniques and assistive devices safely.

An analysis of social routines helps determine when and how ADLs are taught. Routines may differ significantly across home, school, community, and recreational environments. The variation in routine may confuse or be disorganizing to children with intellectual disabilities, autism, or ADHD disorders but may be motivating to children without attention, sensory, or cognitive problems. When tasks are taught or practiced at times and places where they occur naturally, they more quickly become part of the child's behavior repertoire. For example, school-based occupational therapists may meet children at the bus to work on functional mobility and may be present as the child removes his or her coat to work on dressing. When tasks are embedded throughout all environments, children have multiple opportunities to practice activities and learn how to use the natural cues in the environment to modify their behavior. Social interactions and networks of peer buddies are extremely powerful in motivating children[70] and helping them succeed in self-care. Judie Schoonover, an occupational therapist and assistive technology specialist in Virginia, describes creative routines to practice ADL tasks within the school routine[59]:

Rehearsing routines such as dressing and undressing for toileting with students with limited cognition is not meaningful when practiced separate from their daily routines. They do not understand why they are undressing, then pulling their pants right up without using the toilet! Instead, I have asked their mothers to send snacks to school in something that snaps, unbuttons, or zips. Guess what? Undoing fasteners to get a snack out is far more engaging, and doesn't require weekly OT sessions in the therapy room. Another strategy I've used for a child working on an IEP goal of shoe tying or buttoning (but who doesn't wear buttons or tie shoes!) is to talk with her teacher about incorporating tying a bow as part of her behavior plan. Whenever the child accomplishes a task in class, she buttons a button on an incentive chart or ties a bow on a special dowel rather than put[ting] a sticker on a chart (p. 10).

Cultural Context

As occupational therapists work with children and families in an array of service provision models, they must be aware of their own and others' cultural beliefs, customs, activity patterns, and expectations for performance in ADLs.[94] An occupational therapist may become involved with a family because someone else believes that services are needed, and the family may not welcome the occupational therapist's personal questions about the child's and family's self-maintenance occupations and routines. Cultural expectations of the family, caregivers, and social group as a whole may determine behavior standards. Family beliefs, values, and attitudes about child rearing, autonomy, and self-reliance influence how parents perceive ADLs. In Anglo-European cultures, parents usually are concerned about children meeting developmental milestones,[61] whereas other cultures (e.g., Hispanic) may be more relaxed about milestone attainment.[179] Children may not be taught to button their coats, tie shoes, or cut food until a later age because parents may value this role as part of their caregiving and affection for the child.

Social role expectations and routines are influenced by culture. In a study by Horn, Brenner, Rao, and Cheng, African American parents expected toilet training routines to begin at an earlier age (18 months) than white parents at a higher income level (25 months).[69] Many Anglo-European parents encourage children to become independent and self-reliant.[61] In contrast, many Hispanic families[179] and Asian families may encourage dependency or interdependency in the family. Routines for dressing, feeding, bathing, going to bed, and carrying out household tasks vary among cultural groups. For example, bathing may occur less than once a day in some cultures, and hairstyles and head garments may be worn for different occasions, depending on the child's cultural group.

Culture also influences the type and availability of tools, equipment, and materials that a child uses to perform ADLs. Customs and beliefs may determine how parents dress their children, what they feed them, which utensils are used for self-feeding, how they prepare food, which type of adaptations are acceptable to them, and how they meet health care needs. For example, by custom, Muslim or non-Muslim families from the Middle East may only use their left hand for toileting.[93] Economic conditions, geographic location, and opportunities for education and employment can help determine the types of resources and supports available to families. Economics influence ADL tasks in many ways—shoes may be old and the wrong size, indoor plumbing may be nonexistent, or a nanny may be expected to dress, groom, and/or feed a young child with disabilities.

Physical Environment

Barriers in the physical environment, including terrain, furniture, and other objects, may hinder the child's ability to improve ADL performance. Inaccessible buildings and rooms crowded with furniture limit how children in wheelchairs move throughout the environment. On the other hand, a large open space may be too much room to allow a preschooler to contain his or her excitement and complete ADL tasks. Differences in surfaces also affect mobility; for example, rugs can make using a walker or wheelchair more difficult. Other physical characteristics that the therapist assesses relate to the type of furniture, objects, or assistive devices in the environment and whether they are usable and accessible. What is usable in one environment (e.g., a particular type of toilet at home) may not be usable in other environments, such as a hospital or job site. Sensory aspects of the physical environment often influence performance (e.g., type of lighting, noise level, temperature, visual stimulation, tactile or vestibular input of tasks). In particular, children with autism or ADHD are often overly sensitive to and distracted by the sensory aspects of an environment.[10,12]

The objects used to perform ADL tasks may help or hinder ADL performance. Clothing items (e.g., clothes with snaps, hook and loop shoes), grooming items (e.g., toothbrush, size and design of toothpaste dispenser), or bathing items (e.g., type of soap, bathing mitt, feel of towel) may motivate or distract the child. ADL objects or assistive devices need to be accepted, fit the child and family's preferences, and meet the demands of the social, cultural, and physical environment.

Activity Demands

The activity demands in certain contexts facilitate or impede the quality of ADL performance. A task analysis helps the occupational therapist understand the complexity and various aspects of the activity. This evaluation involves analyzing the objects used, space and social demands, sequencing and timing, and required actions and skills.[1] Activity demands vary in the clinic, home, school, and community. For example, when an adolescent with a traumatic brain injury is learning to style her hair, her performance skills may vary significantly in the occupational therapy clinic from those observed in her hospital or home bathroom. The child's unfamiliarity with the set up of the sink or bathroom may disrupt the flow of motor skills, and the spatial arrangements, lighting, and surface availability may cause process skill problems. For the activity, specific steps are followed and sequenced according to time requirements.

Verbal instruction in sequencing will support performance of ADL tasks. For example, "First you comb the knots out of your hair, then you part the hair and comb it. After a minute of brushing the hair, use the curling iron."

If the adolescent is doing this with friends, the demand on performance skills increases as the number of tasks or steps and social demand to share supplies and to converse increase. In summary, grading ADL performance involves considering adaptations to the environment, type of activity or interactions required, and sequence of the activity. Occupations are viewed according to the environments in which they occur, demands of the activity, and the child's abilities.

Evaluation of Activities of Daily Living

Families and their children play key roles in determining which evaluation procedures are used. By working collaboratively with families, occupational therapists learn about the child,

TABLE 15-1 Rating of Self-Care Skill Independence During Task Analysis

Level of Independence	Definition	Bathing Example
Independent	Child does 100% of the task, including setup.	Child gets out needed supplies and equipment and bathes, rinses, and dries himself or herself without assistance.
Independent with set up	After another person sets up the task; child does 100% of the task.	Caregiver places bathtub seat in tub and organizes bath supplies; child bathes, rinses, and dries himself or herself without assistance.
Supervision	Child performs task by himself or herself but cannot be safely left alone; he or she may need verbal cueing or physical prompts for 1%-24% of task.	Child bathes, rinses, and dries himself or herself without assistance but needs monitoring when getting into and out of tub and when washing lower extremities because of poor balance and judgment.
Minimal assistance or skillful	Child does 51%-75% of task independently but needs physical assistance or other cueing for at least 25% of task.	Child bathes and rinses body parts independently but needs physical assistance getting into and out of tub; he or she is cued to monitor water temperature and to dry body parts.
Moderate assistance (26%-50% partial participation)	Child does 26%-50% of task independently but needs physical assistance or other cueing for at least 50% of task.	Child adjusts water temperature and washes and rinses face, torso, and upper extremities independently; he or she needs physical assistance getting into and out of tub and for washing and rinsing lower extremities and back.
Maximal assistance (1%-25% partial participation)	Child does 1%-25% of task independently but needs physical assistance or other cueing for 75% of task.	Child independently washes, rinses, and dries face but needs verbal cues to wash torso; he or she needs physical assistance getting into and out of tub and for washing other body parts.
Dependent	Child is unable to do any part of the task.	Caregiver physically picks up child, places him or her in tub, and washes, rinses, and dries child's body parts; child does not lift body parts to be washed or dried.

Adapted from Trombly, C. A., & Quintana, L. A. (1989). Activities of daily living. In C. A. Trombly (Ed.), *Occupational therapy for physical dysfunction* (3rd ed., p. 387). Baltimore Williams & Wilkins.

various environments in which ADLs occur, demands of the activities, and expectations and concerns of the family. When children get older and are able to communicate, the occupational therapist includes them in determining which areas of ADLs are important to them. The parents and child often become more vested in the results if the occupational therapist gives them a chance to select or refuse evaluations and choose where and when the evaluation is completed.[48] This approach also gives occupational therapists a better understanding of the contexts in which the child performs occupations and of current performance patterns that may be valued by the family.

Evaluation Methods

Evaluation of ADLs begins with an analysis of occupational performance, which may involve collecting data from numerous sources. Interviews, inventories, and structured and naturalistic observations are evaluation methods typically used to measure ADL performance in occupational therapy. The occupational therapist uses these methods alone or in combination to analyze occupational performance (abilities and limitations), develop collaborative goals with children and their families, plan intervention strategies, and measure outcomes of treatment. The choice of instrument depends on the reason for the evaluation. Some instruments interview the caregiver or can be completed as an inventory, whereas others are scored while observing the child.

For ADL independence, the child must not only complete the task but also obtain and use the supplies the task requires. The occupational therapist generally rates performance according to the child's ability to set up and complete a task and may assess performance by grading the child's level of independence. Table 15-1 presents one example of how the occupational therapist might rate a child's independence in bathing.

Ecologic or environmentally referenced assessments are appropriate for all children and are particularly useful for children with moderate to severe disabilities who have difficulty generalizing tasks from one environment to another.[114] A *top-down approach* considers the contexts in which the child per forms valued occupations in addition to what the child can or cannot perform.[23] With this approach, the therapist can do the following:

- Ask the parent and child what they want or need to do.
- Identify the environments or context in which the task occurs, the steps of the task, and the child's capabilities.
- Compare the demands of the task with the child's actual performance skills while completing the task.
- Identify and prioritize the discrepancies to develop an intervention plan.

With naturalistic or ecologic observation, the occupational therapist gathers information in the typical or natural setting in which the activity occurs. Usually, the occupational therapist completes a task analysis to identify the steps of the activity, sequence of these steps, and how the child adapts to the demands of the environment. For example, when observing a child's ability to use the toilet at school, the occupational therapist notes accessibility barriers and sensory characteristics of the environment. How the child adapts to these factors, the typical classroom routines and expectations for toileting, and any cultural aspects of the toileting process (e.g., type of clothing the child is wearing, which hand is acceptable for wiping) are also noted. After identifying these contexts and the steps and sequence needed to complete the task, the occupational therapist chooses appropriate intervention strategies according to the demands of the activity in the school context.

Environmental observation is time-consuming but provides an abundance of information when used in a team effort.[118,126] In addition to evaluating the performance skills and patterns used, the therapist identifies the level of assistance and the number of modifications needed to improve the child's independence. Anderson et al.[6] have written *Self-Help Skills for People with Autism: A Systematic Teaching Approach,* which gives specific methods for collecting data set-up tasks and collect data, which is useful for all children.

Team Evaluations

Curriculum-referenced or curriculum-guided assessments are often used by interdisciplinary teams in settings such as early intervention or school system practice. Self-care is often an area of assessment. The Carolina Curriculum for Infants and Toddlers with Special Needs (CCITSN),[73] Carolina Curriculum for Preschoolers with Special Needs (CCPSN),[74] and Hawaii Early Learning Profile[42] are typical curriculum-referenced assessments used in early intervention. Specific information about these assessments is found in Chapter 6.

Giangreco et al. have developed a useful transdisciplinary, curriculum-based assessment and guide, Choosing Options and Accommodations for Children (COACH).[48] Therapists use COACH to identify areas of concern (not specific skills) for school-age children with moderate to severe disabilities and help plan inclusive educational goals with a family prioritization interview and environmental observations. The team identifies priorities, outcomes, and needed supports for specific environments and across environments in the areas of communication, socialization, personal management, leisure and recreation, and applied academics. Team members plan goals together, write interdisciplinary goals, and then decide which services the child needs. The team may decide that an occupational therapist is needed only as a consultant if the special education teacher is able to address the ADL task adequately.

Measurement of Outcomes

Health care and educational systems are demanding evidence-based practice and cost-effectiveness for therapy intervention. Within the past decade, professionals in the fields of rehabilitation and occupational therapy have developed universal assessments to measure the outcomes of therapy designed to enhance ADL skills. Outcomes may include improved occupational performance, adaptation, role competence, health and wellness, satisfaction, prevention, or self-determination and self-advocacy.[1] In addition to providing a means to evaluate children individually, the collection of aggregated ADL assessment results or outcome measures can help justify program expansion or changes in intervention strategies.

In rehabilitation, four primary assessments, which are valid and reliable, are used to measure occupational performance and adaptation to ADL tasks in children and adolescents. Occupational therapists can use the Functional Independence Measure (FIM; ≥8 years) and Functional Independence Measure-II for Children (WeeFIM-II; ≤7 years).[58] The Pediatric Evaluation of Disability Inventory Computer Adaptive Test (PEDI-CAT)[57] is used for children from birth to 21 years of age.[25] Kothari, Haley, Gill-Body, and Dumas found the PEDI to be a valid measure of outcomes in children with brain injury.[84]

The Assessment of Motor and Process Skills (AMPS) assesses ADL and IADL performance skills in various environments, familiar (home or school) and unfamiliar (occupational therapy clinic).[36,40] It has been used in outcome studies with children older than 3 years and adolescents from different cultural backgrounds and with an array of disabilities.[39,54] While the child performs a chosen task according to the instructions given, the occupational therapist rates the 16 ADL motor and 20 ADL process skills. The AMPS tasks use a top-down approach that gives a comprehensive view of how efficiently, safely, and independently the child is functioning in performance contexts.[39,40] The AMPS is sensitive in identifying deficits in motor and process skills for children with ADHD (e.g., coordination, calibration, sequencing, memory).[122]

School therapists may not find the PEDI-CAT, WeeFIM-II,61, or FIM to be a useful outcome assessment of school performance. As discussed in Chapter 23, the School Function Assessment (SFA) evaluates the child's participation in six different environments: transportation, transitions, classroom, cafeteria, bathroom, and playground.[24] This assessment gives the therapist a profile of valuable information about self-care performance and role performance in the school environment, which is used to develop individualized education program (IEP) outcomes. The Child Occupation Self-Assessment (COSA) is a self-rating tool that a child uses to describe his or her competence ("How well I do the task?") and the importance or value of doing a task ("How important is this to me?") in school, home, and community settings.[81] Observations of ADL and IADL tasks, as well as managing emotions and cognitive tasks, are part of this assessment. Two versions are available, a checklist with visual symbols and a card sort version. For example, one item is "Keep my body clean." The child then rates how well he or she does the task and how important it is to him or her.

The Canadian Occupational Performance Measure (COPM) assesses a client's perception of his or her ADL skills, productivity, and leisure occupations over time and is useful for assessment and reassessment.[87] The self-assessment part of the COPM makes it more appropriate for children older than 8 years.[87] Another method to measure outcomes in ADL performance is using goal attainment scaling (GAS).[4,15,95,105] This method allows the child, family, and occupational therapist to set goals and criteria for success and may be used in combination with the Canadian Occupational Performance Measure.[28,52,94,104,135] It is an appropriate outcome measurement tool if standardized testing is not available or if outcomes are variable.[102]

Before intervention, outcome measures are defined after talking with the child and family to find out what type of change would be meaningful. Data are collected over time and then goals are modified for incremental differences. Research Note 15-1 describes a review of the literature on GAS in pediatric rehabilitation[158] and gives suggestions for using GAS.

RESEARCH NOTE 15-1

Steenbeek, D., Ketelaar, M., Galama, K., & Gorter, J. W. (2007). Goal attainment scaling in paediatric rehabilitation: A critical review of the literature. Developmental Medicine and Child Neurology, 49 *(7), 550–556.*

Abstract

In this article, a literature review of goal attainment scaling (GAS) was completed. Three studies in pediatric rehabilitation were reviewed to assess the psychometric properties of GAS. The authors concluded that additional research is needed because only one study investigated inter-rater reliability (found to be good), and only one study investigated content validity (found to be acceptable). Low concurrent validity was found in one study, and no construct validity or content reliability was reported. In six additional studies reviewed by the authors, the use of GAS demonstrated "good sensitivity to change." The authors concluded that GAS is a promising, responsive method to use in pediatric rehabilitation to evaluate individual goals and progress. However, the authors suggested that additional research is needed related to the reliability of this method when used with children of different ages and types of disabilities and by therapists of different disciplines.

Implications for Practice

- GAS is a sensitive, practical, and easy way to measure small individual changes in ADL occupations using occupational therapy intervention.
- Goals are formulated by parents and children first and then clearly defined on a scale. Goals chosen should represent desired functional changes for performing future ADL tasks.
- Training in GAS is necessary to ensure that goals are objective, discrete, measurable, relevant, and realistic and use equal intervals for performance on the scale.
- If multiple raters are going to use GAS for measuring progress, interrater reliability should be checked by having the raters watch a video of children doing the task and then having them rate performance.

Intervention Strategies and Approaches

When planning intervention procedures, the occupational therapist considers the child's characteristics, performance skills, and patterns in relation to the context and demands of the activity. Occupational therapists need to be sensitive to parents' and other caregivers' needs and concerns. It is helpful to listen to and reassure these individuals while engaging them in observations and problem solving. When planning treatment for children with performance problems in ADLs, the occupational therapist must ask himself or herself the following questions[153]:

- Which ADLs are *useful* and *meaningful* in current and future contexts?
- What are the *preferences* of the child and/or the family?
- Are the activities *age-appropriate* (used by peers without disabilities)?
- Is it *realistic* to expect the child to perform or master this task?
- Which *alternative methods* can the child use to perform tasks (e.g., including the use of activity modifications or assistive technology)?
- Does learning this task *improve the child's health, safety, and social participation?*
- Do *cultural issues* influence how tasks are taught?
- Can the task be assessed, taught, and *practiced in a variety of environments?*

Therapists use various approaches to improve ADL skills in children, including the following: (1) promoting or creating; (2) establishing, restoring, and maintaining performance; (3) modifying or adapting the task, method, and/or environment; and (4) preventing problems and educating others.[1] Occupational therapists often use a combination of these approaches and various theoretical orientations to help children participate in ADL occupations. Table 15-2 gives examples of these approaches and possible theoretical orientations for the occupational therapist to use when teaching a child to button his or her shirt. These approaches are discussed throughout each area of ADL tasks later in this chapter.

Promoting or Creating Supports

Occupational therapists often create supports within the environment that offer all children the opportunity to engage in ADL occupations that are age-appropriate and not related to a disability status.[1] This approach offers team or system supports for schools without focusing on the child with a disability.[59,126] When using this approach, occupational therapists design a program in which school or community groups participate. Possible activities include the following: creating a module or center activity requiring zipping, snapping, and/or buttoning; developing a box of fine motor and self-care activities to distribute to all kindergarten classrooms in the district; giving an in-service presentation to the church or school about self-care development or healthy sleep habits; or participating as a building committee member to make recommendations about a universal design for the new bathrooms or gyms being built. When working with families, occupational therapists may promote opportunities in which everyone can participate using a morning checklist for self-care routines. A visual picture board may help all the children in the family to understand which tasks are needed for a morning routine.

Establishing, Restoring, and Maintaining Performance

The occupational therapist may attempt to establish ADL performance and patterns using a developmental approach or, if this is not possible, may try to restore or remediate the child's abilities that interfere with performance. To establish ADL patterns, the occupational therapist establishes the child's developmental and chronologic age and plans treatment according to a typical developmental sequence. In this approach, the occupational therapist examines underlying body structures and functions (e.g., strength, tactile discrimination), selects age-appropriate tasks and habits to target in intervention, and gives parents some expectations for skill development. During interventions to establish or restore performance, occupational

TABLE 15-2 Approaches to Improving the Performance of Activities of Daily Living

Approach	Appropriate Frame of Reference	Problem: Buttoning Buttons Without Use of the Right Hand
Create or promote	Person-environment-occupation (PEO) Developmental	Suggest opportunities to help all students learn skills needed for buttoning. Use activities such as dress-up clothes, smocks, lunch bags with buttons or snaps. Provide calendars or number lines with a button or snap activity. Provide a variety of fine motor activities for center time.
Establish, restore, and maintain	Developmental Motor control Biomechanical Neurodevelopmental treatment Sensory integration PEO	Use specific activities to establish hand use and prehension patterns for buttoning. Use coins in a piggy bank, board games with small, thin game pieces, and craft activities (e.g., friendship bracelets, mosaics) to work on hand strength and coordination before beginning with buttons. Provide tasks to develop, improve, or restore body functions (e.g., ROM of hand; weight bearing to decrease tone; increase sensory input by playing with foam or PlayDoh); use dexterity activities to improve motor skills (coordinate, manipulate, flow, calibrate, grip). Maintain performance patterns by using a dressing routine or other tasks that provide practice opportunities for buttoning on a regular basis (e.g., have a calendar on which the day of the week has to be buttoned to the calendar); maintain dexterity and strength through a daily exercise routine.
Modify, adapt	PEO Human occupation Rehabilitation Biomechanical Sensory integration Neurodevelopmental treatment	Revise current activity demands or the context to compensate for body function and body structure limitations that affect performance skills and performance patterns. Adapt the task method: Child uses one-handed buttoning technique, uses a pullover shirt so that buttoning is not an issue, or uses an extra-large shirt with buttons already buttoned; he or she wears the button shirt over a pullover shirt like an open jacket. Cueing performance may include verbal, gestural, physical, or visual prompts. Adapt the object or use assistive technology: Buttons are replaced with other buttons that have long shanks or that match the child's tactile preference; child uses a button hook, elastic sewn-on buttons, or pressure-sensitive tape; child and devices are positioned for stability during activity (e.g., child sits in a chair with arms to button a shirt). Adapt the task environment: Child practices buttoning in the bedroom, away from distracting toys or siblings; parent, sibling, or peer is asked to button the shirt; shirt with buttons is used because it is culturally important to a teenager not to wear a pullover shirt.
Prevention, education	Human occupation Developmental Rehabilitation Biomechanical Sensory integration Coping	Educate and prevent failure at buttoning. Occupational therapist models and teaches the child and parent how to use the above approaches and lets them practice the approach while he or she watches. Occupational therapist provides home ideas for developing opportunities to practice games or tasks and gives written, pictorial, verbal, or video instructions. Occupational therapist consults with day-care provider or teacher to ensure carryover of the method used. Occupational therapist helps child anticipate possible problems when purchasing clothing with different fasteners and how to ask for help if needed.

Adapted from American Occupational Therapy Association (AOTA). (2008). Occupational therapy practice framework: Domain and process. *American Journal of Occupational Therapy, 62*, 625–683; and Dunn, W., Brown, C., & McGuigan, A. (1994). Ecology of human performance: A framework for considering the effect of context. *American Journal of Occupational Therapy, 48*(7), 595–607.

therapists identify gaps in skills and intervene to teach or remediate the underlying problem that is interfering with a child's ADL performance. This approach focuses on the child's deficits in body function and structure to perform ADL activities.

Occupational therapists often use biomechanical, motor control, cognitive orientation, neurodevelopmental therapy (NDT), sensory integration, and/or behavioral approaches to restore performance skills. For preschoolers with moderate fine motor delays, some ways to increase self-care skills are to provide play and targeted fine motor and praxis interventions, which require in-hand manipulation, grasp strength, and eye-hand coordination. Using an NDT approach, the occupational therapist encourages the mother to relax the child and lower spastic muscle tone before dressing. In this case, the occupational therapist models by holding the child's pelvis when supine, slowly rolling the child's hips from one side to the other to reduce the tone and encourage trunk rotation. After this preparation improves the child's task performance, the occupational therapist encourages the parent to hold the child at the pelvis while helping him or her pull up his or her pants. When using this approach, occupational therapists provide parents and children with suggestions on how to practice these rotational movement patterns in various tasks.

In a motor learning approach, a child may learn how to put on shoes through practicing the whole task in a variety of activities (e.g., dress-up, relay races, morning dressing routine) or environments (e.g., home, school, therapy session, gym class). During practice, the child receives specific feedback (e.g., "Pull the back of the shoe up when pushing the heel down in the shoe"). Jarus and Ratzon found that mental practice increased the acquisition of new bimanual motor skills for children faster than just physical practice.[71] This technique may also help children acquire ADL skills (e.g., mental rehearsal of putting the shoe on the foot).

Mobility Opportunities Via Education (MOVE) is a structured interdisciplinary program that helps establish and restore sitting, standing, and walking skills for children with severe motor limitations.[16] The MOVE team plans and provides motor intervention using a motor control or task-oriented approach. Primary goals are eating, toileting, and motor skills; progress is monitored; and goals are updated through systematic data collection.[16,165,173] Child-centered goal setting helps the team target functional outcomes (e.g., to stand to pull up pants at the toilet). Activities are used to develop ADL skills for the context in which they are used. Teams are trained together, and it is often difficult to distinguish between occupational therapists and teachers. This approach is used with those in any age group with moderate to severe motor limitations and is appropriate for children with and without intellectual impairments. Some research studies have supported the effectiveness of this program for children and adults with severe motor disabilities.[16,172,173]

Occupational therapists also use behavioral approaches to establish and restore ADL skills. They may use backward or forward chaining to teach the tasks. In *backward chaining*, the occupational therapist performs most of the task, and the child performs the last step of a sequence to receive positive reinforcement for completing the task. Practice continues, with the occupational therapist performing fewer steps and the child completing additional steps. This method is particularly helpful for children with a low frustration tolerance or poor self-esteem because it gives immediate success. In forward chaining, the child begins with the first step of the task sequence, then the second step, and continues learning steps of the task in a sequential order until he or she performs all steps in the task. *Forward chaining* is helpful for children who have difficulty with sequencing and generalizing activities. The occupational therapist gives varying numbers of cues, or prompts, before or during an activity. Therapist or person cues and environment or task cues may occur naturally or artificially in an environment. Occupational therapists can use verbal, gestural, or physical cues or a combination of all three.[154,168]

Environmental or task cues may include picture sequences or checklists, color coding, positioning, and modifying the sensory properties of the environment or materials used in a task. Figure 15-2 illustrates a visual picture sequence for hand washing. Reese and Snell[125] have described a hierarchic approach to presenting artificial cues from least intrusive (verbal cues) to more intrusive (verbal and gestural cues) to most intrusive (verbal and physical cues). For example, they described this hierarchy of physical cues: (1) shadowing the child's movements, (2) using two fingers to guide the child, and (3) using a hand-over-hand approach to guide movement. The occupational therapist or parent uses the fewest cues necessary and fades out cues to promote independence. Figure 15-3 shows examples of these different types of cues, which can be used as a child performs various self-care occupations. Research Note 15-2 presents a review of studies that used different cues

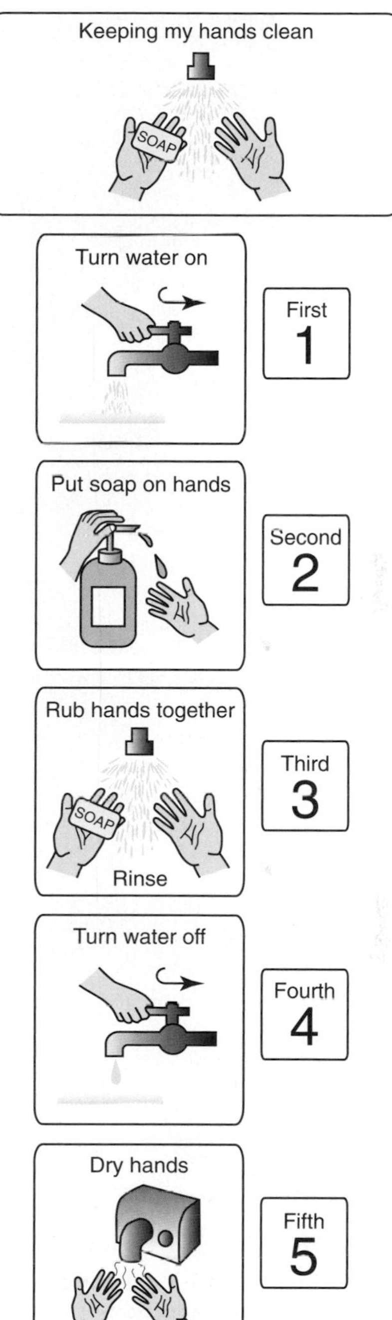

FIGURE 15-2 This simple picture sequence gives Adam the needed cues to wash his hands independently. (Courtesy Judith Schoonover, Loudoun County Public Schools, Loudoun County, Virginia; Picture Communication Symbols from Mayer-Johnson, Solana Beach, CA.)

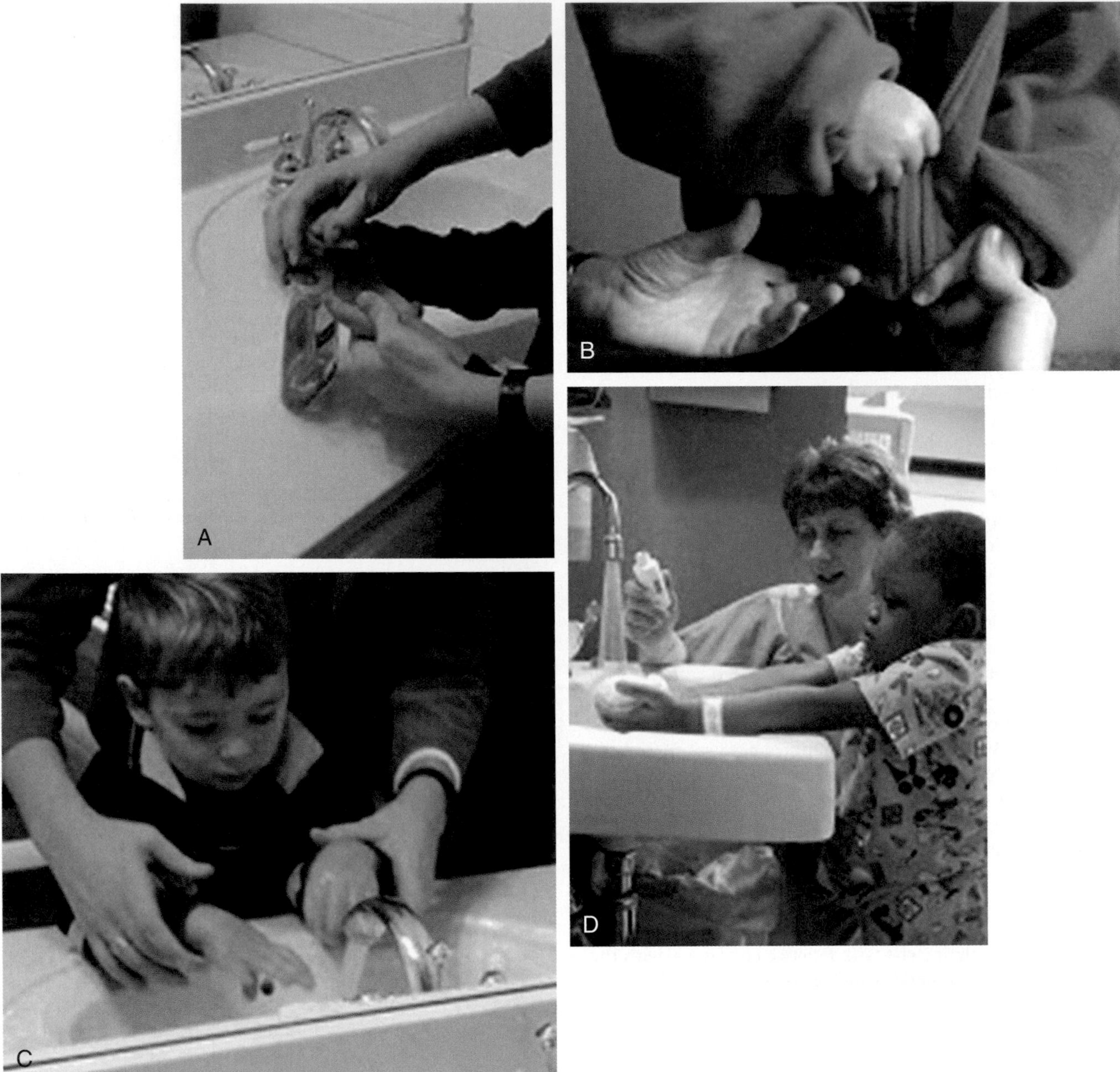

FIGURE 15-3 **Hierarchy of cues, from most intrusive to least intrusive. A,** A hand-over-hand approach is used for squirting soap onto the child's hands. **B,** Two fingers are used to guide zipping of the child's coat. **C,** The occupational therapist shadows her hand over the top of the child's hands to cue hand movements for hand washing. **D,** The occupational therapist verbally cues the child on how to wash the hands.

for persons with severe and profound disabilities and gives practical suggestions to consider.

Once self-care routines and patterns have been developed, it is important to maintain them and any of the environmental supports that promote continued ADL success. Repetition and the development of habits and routines are essential organizers, particularly for children who take a long time to learn new skills, have a poor memory, or thrive on routine or practice. Schedules for toileting or dressing, visual prompts displayed on the wall, a set place for items when grooming, and a checklist for how to clean a splint or contacts are all examples of contextual supports. Health maintenance activities (e.g., self-catheterization, wheelchair push-ups, ROM exercises, taking medication regularly, eating nutritious meals) support task performance in all occupations, including ADLs such as maintaining a bowel and bladder routine, transferring to the toilet, and dressing.

Adapting the Task or Environment

When adapting or modifying an activity (using a compensatory approach), the occupational therapist uses alternative physical

RESEARCH NOTE 15-2

Lancioni, G. E. & O'Reilly, M. F. (2001). Self-management of instruction cues for occupation: Review of studies with people with severe and profound developmental disabilities. Research in Developmental Disabilities, 22, *41–65.*

Abstract

Learning and maintaining occupations is often difficult for children with severe and profound developmental disabilities. The authors of this paper reviewed studies about this population for the last 15 to 20 years and identified five main strategies of instructional cues: (1) cards with picture cues, (2) computer-aided and stored picture cues, (3) cards with object cues attached, (4) audio recording equipment that stores verbal cues, and (5) self-verbalization of what is being done. The effectiveness of these strategies and the practicality of using the different types of instructional cues were discussed.

Implications for Practice

- When choosing cues to facilitate ADL performance, occupational therapists need to consider the effectiveness and practicality of the cues.
- It is important not to infer that all children with moderate to severe disabilities respond the same way to different prompts or that only one type of prompt is appropriate.
- Ask the child and caregivers their preferences for the type of cue to be given for completing the task. Attitudes can sabotage the effectiveness of cue use.
- After learning one cue for one step, try to use one cue to do two steps of the self-care task. This helps decrease dependency on the cues for a multistep ADL task.
- Collect data to see which cueing system works best. For example, does the child remember the steps for dressing with picture card cues or cues stored in a recording device or PDA, or a combination of cues?
- For complex tasks, consider using other types of cues such as videos, video monitoring, video self-monitoring, or verbal cues. Take baseline data and data during the intervention to see if performance is improving.

techniques, substitute movement patterns, or other adaptive performance patterns to enable the child to complete a task. Adaptation strategies may include modification of the task or task method, use of assistive technology, and/or modification of the environment. Occupational therapists often use a combination of these strategies to improve a child's performance, considering the performance context. Table 15-3 provides examples of typical adaptation approaches used with different functional problems in ADLs.

Occupational therapists practice adaptation or compensatory strategies in various contexts and modify them until they become functional. For example, a child with a bilateral upper extremity amputation may use several compensatory strategies for ADL tasks. As an adapted method, the child may use the feet or mouth to write or dress or may learn new movement patterns to operate a prosthetic arm (assistive device) for manipulating objects. Adapting the social environment by using a personal assistant or peer in the home or school environment is another adaptation strategy. Modification of the bedroom set up for easier accessibility and placement of clothes in lower drawers that are reachable from a wheelchair can increase dressing independence.

Adapting or Modifying Task Methods

The occupational therapist often modifies tasks by using grading techniques. Grading is the adaptation of a task or portions of a task to fit the child's capabilities. By using a task analysis, the occupational therapist rates subtasks of the activity and varies them according to their degree of ease or difficulty for the child. The occupational therapist may modify the activity demands to compensate for limited capabilities and performance skills. He or she may grade the tasks according to specific qualities (e.g., simple to complex). Grading a task may include gradually increasing the number of steps for which the child is responsible, fading the amount of personal assistance or cueing the child receives, and reducing the strength needed or length of time the child takes to complete an activity.[154]

Each ADL involves a series of task steps that are performed together in a specific sequence. When a child cannot complete a task independently or when completion of the task requires too much of the child's energy, occupational therapists may suggest *personal assistance,* which the child directs.[152] *Partial participation* occurs when a child performs some steps of the task and a caregiver completes the remaining steps; this allows the child to practice and often improves performance of the ADL task.

Adapting the Task Object or Using Assistive Technology

Assistive devices are commercially available or are custom-made by the occupational therapist, skilled orthotist, or rehabilitation engineer. By using local and national databases, publications, and Internet searches on product comparison, occupational therapists can keep informed about the availability of new assistive devices to find equipment for unique or specific problems.

The choice of an assistive device is a cooperative decision made by the child, parents, therapists, and other team members who work with the child.[22] Together, these individuals systematically evaluate what the child needs to do, his or her performance contexts, the child's abilities and limitations, the capabilities of the device itself, and the child's perception of using the device.[63,124] Teams choose the device that has the best environmental fit. The occupational therapist and team offer comprehensive support, education, and coaching to the family, caregivers, child, and others about how to use the device.[124] Adolescents who are striving to identify with their peers tend to reject devices that call attention to their disabilities. To be worthwhile, an assistive device should meet the following requirements:

- *Assist in the task* the child is trying to complete without being cumbersome.
- Be *acceptable* to the child and family and in the contextual environments in which it will be used (e.g., in terms of appearance, functions, upkeep, storage, amount of time to set up or learn how to use the device).
- Be *practical and flexible* for the environments in which it will be used (e.g., have acceptable dimensions, portability, and positioning, be usable with other assistive devices).
- Be *durable* and easy to clean.

TABLE 15-3 Typical Adaptation Principles Used with Children and Adolescents with Disabilities

Behavior or Disability	Adaptation Principles
Low vision or hearing (or both)	Use intact or residual senses. Amplify sensory characteristics of objects (e.g., color, size, tactile and auditory features). Give cues consistently to determine whether activity is beginning or ending. Use tactile, verbal, visual, or object cues (e.g., put hand on washcloth or say, "It's time to wash your face"). Use gestures (e.g., point to arm that is put in sleeve first). Decrease auditory and visual distractions.
Dislike of being touched (tactile defensive)	Prepare child for touch by giving deep pressure and applying organized, rhythmic touch. Give choices for tactile preferences (e.g., clothes, washcloths, brushes). Let child perform touching on himself or herself (e.g., use toothbrush or wash face or body). Allow child to wear snug clothing (e.g., turtleneck) or loose clothing in accordance with his or her preference.
Inability to find clothes or understand top, front, or bottom	Amplify characteristics. Reduce distracters (e.g., place only one utensil on countertop for cooking activity). Use visual or gestural cues (e.g., mark medial border of shoes with "happy faces" to keep shoes on correct feet). Use systematic scanning when searching for objects (e.g., clothes in closet).
Inability to sit up or maintain balance	Provide support externally (e.g., use positioning device). Change position of child (e.g., have child sit to put on shoes or dress in side-lying position). Change position of activity (e.g., keep grooming items together in a bucket on top of the sink).
Limited reach	Reduce amount of reach needed. Change position of activity. Lengthen handles (e.g., use long-handled bath sponge or reacher).
Difficulty grasping objects	Build up handles of objects (e.g., brushes, spoons). Substitute assistive devices so that grasping is not necessary (e.g., use universal cuffs or straps). Stabilize objects with other body parts (e.g., in teeth or between legs).
Weakness, with little endurance	Eliminate gravity (e.g., prop elbow or dress in side-lying position). Use lightweight objects. Use power equipment.
Difficulty controlling movement	Provide stable base of support (e.g., sit on floor with wide base). Eliminate need for fine control (e.g., use an enlarged zipper pull). Use weighted devices to give proprioceptive feedback (e.g., weighted toothbrushes and cups).
Poor memory; inability to remember sequences or directions	Establish and practice set routines and sequences. Use partial participation, grading techniques, and backward and forward chaining. Use visual cues (e.g., pictures, labels, checklists, color coding). Substitute assistive technology (e.g., alarm on watch or timers). Use verbal cues (e.g., "First, then second"; jingles, rhymes, songs). Use real-life materials in the setting in which the occupation occurs.
Tendency to become easily frustrated; outbursts	Identify purpose of "problem behavior" (e.g., escape, avoid, attention, obtain, transition, or stimulate) by analyzing antecedents and consequences. Limit exposure to context associated with misbehavior. Use preferred tasks and give choices. Reinforce, coach, and expand appropriate alternate behaviors. Avoid personal assistance and coaching (use partial participation). Use grading, prompting, fading prompts, and generalization.

Adapted from Geyer, L. A., Kurtz, L. A., & Byram, L. E. (1998). Prompting function in daily living skills. In J. P. Dormans & L. Pellegrino (Eds.), *Caring for children with cerebral palsy: A team approach* (pp. 323–346). Baltimore: Paul H. Brookes; and Koegel, L. K., Koegel, R. L., Kellegrew, D., & Mullen, K. (1996). Parent education for prevention and reduction of severe problem behaviors. In L. K. Koegel, R. L. Koegel, & G. Dunlap (Eds.), *Positive behavioral support: Including people with difficult behavior in the community* (pp. 3–30). Baltimore: Paul H. Brookes.

- Be *expandable*—that is, able to meet the child's needs now and when the child has grown and has more sophisticated abilities.
- Be *safe* for the child to use (e.g., physical, behavioral, or cognitive child factors such as drooling, throwing, or difficulty with sequencing do not interfere with use of the device).
- Have a *system of maintenance or replacement* with continued use.
- *Meet the cost constraints* of the family or purchasing agency.

Overall, the child should complete tasks at a higher level of efficiency using the device than he or she could without it. Trial use of a device is highly recommended; this helps determine the feasibility of its use and demonstrates its value to the child and primary caregivers. Caregiver roles are lightened by using assistive devices and modifications.

Computers and cognitive prosthetic devices have come into use to give children the visual and/or auditory prompts needed

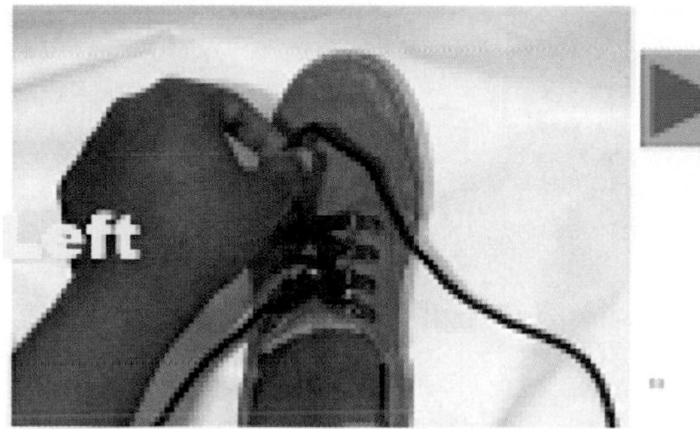
Use your left hand to pick up the right lace close to the knot and slide your fingers up the lace.
Left

FIGURE 15-4 **Sample talking book.** This frame from *Talking Shoes* was created with Microsoft PowerPoint. (Courtesy Laura Pal and Kelly Showalter, Virginia Commonwealth University, Richmond, VA.)

to initiate, sequence, sustain, and terminate ADL and work activities.[29] For example, a talking book from Microsoft's PowerPoint helps a child learn how to tie a shoe, dress himself or herself, and set a table if the technology is nearby. As shown in Figure 15-4, for tying shoelaces, the child or adolescent uses the talking book as a visual and auditory prompt on his or her computer, tablet, personal digital assistant (PDA), or smartphone. Other cognitive prosthetic devices that assist in ADL tasks include portable memory aids (e.g., checklists, voice-activated tape recorders), medication alarm pill boxes, watches with specialized features (alarms, schedules, talking), alarm organizers, pagers, sound-activated key rings, and simple switches that program up to three steps.

Assistive technology for ADLs includes videos, computers, tablets, televisions, PDAs, smartphones, and digital memo devices. Talking books, visual schedules, stories using digital pictures, computer-generated checklists, or CDs may be used as cues to improve dressing, toileting, hand washing, and other ADL skills.[80,148,156,158] These electronic devices give the prompts needed to help children and adolescents begin the ADL task and sequence the routine so the task is completed.[45,46,77,78] Recent research has demonstrated the effectiveness of using video modeling of others (VMO) or videos of the child performing a task (video self-modeling [VSM]).[15,99] These may be played on an MP3 player, PDA, computer, tablet, or smartphone and uploaded to a website for use at other times. Video modeling has been used successfully with hand washing[132] and toileting.[80]

Adapting the Physical Environment

In all the approaches discussed, the occupational therapist uses the interactions among the child, environment, and contexts to improve performance. Adaptation of the physical environment may include simple modifications to lighting, floor surface, amount and type of furniture or objects, and overall traffic pattern of the room or building. For some children, occupational therapists minimize sensory stimuli and eliminate visual and auditory distractions. Other children may require increased environmental stimulation (e.g., color or music) to cue their performance. Table 15-4 presents adaptation examples of the physical environment to promote ADL performance.

Work Surface

The work surface supports the child, materials, tools, and assistive devices in an activity. The boundaries of the work space help children keep within usable or safe environments. For example, a cut-out surface on a table or a lip on a wheelchair tray or sink countertop can serve as a boundary. The occupational therapist adds various textures, colors, and pictures to the work surface area to give sensory cues about boundaries or to structure the task. Even with these modifications, some children (e.g., those with weakness in one side of the body) need assistance in stabilizing objects. Table 15-5 presents suggestions for stabilizing objects when they are placed on the work surface or held by the child.

Characteristics of the work surface amenable to adaptation include height, angle of incline, size, distance from the body, distance from other work areas, and general accessibility. Changes in these features enhance the child's function in various ways, including improving arm support, increasing the visual orientation of a task, adapting seat height for easier transfers, and optimizing table height for wheelchair access. See Chapter 20 for more specifics of positioning

Positioning

Occupational therapists consider the position of the child and of the materials or activity when planning intervention. When possible, the occupational therapist uses the most typical position for a given activity, with the fewest restrictions or adaptations to stabilize the body for function. Children who have problems with posture and movement often lack sufficient control to assume or maintain stable postures during activity performance and thus benefit from adaptive positioning. Adaptive positioning may include using different positions (e.g., sitting instead of standing), low-technology devices (e.g., lap boards, pillows, towel rolls), or high-technology devices (e.g., customized cushions, wheelchairs, orthotics). If an adaptive device or orthotic is used, the occupational therapist needs to consider systematically whether the device assists or hinders ADL performance. Chafetz et al. have found that some children wearing a thoracolumbosacral orthosis had better posture but actually performed less efficiently with dressing when wearing the orthosis.[20]

Alternative body positions are extremely helpful to children with disabilities. These changes help compensate for physical limitations in body functions such as strength, joint movement, control, and endurance and provide relief to skin areas and bony prominences. The occupational therapist considers positions that maximize independent task performance. Key points for stability that enable the child to use available voluntary movement are the pelvis and trunk, head, and extremities. The following questions guide decision making about positioning:

- Is the child aligned properly? Are the hips, shoulders, and head in aligned with each other?
- Which positions or devices increase trunk stability (e.g., using a hard seat insert or lateral or orthotic supports, using a surface to support the feet, widening the sitting base by abducting the legs)?
- Is support adequate to maintain an upright posture, with the head in the midline?
- Can the child use his or her hands and visually focus on the task?

TABLE 15-4 Environmental Adaptations for the Home When Accessibility Is Limited

Architectural Barrier	Structural Changes	Possible Assistive Devices	Task Modifications
Entrances and exits	Hand rails Hand stairs Ramp Built-up terrain to door height Stair lift In-home elevator Increased door width (33-36 inches minimum) Step-back hinges Door rehinged to open in or out Pocket or folding door Electric door openers	Straps or loop door handle Lever handles Portable doorknob Built-up key holders Combination locks Environmental control unit	Use different entrance. Remove inside doors. Use curtains for privacy. Use hip or wheelchair to open doors.
Bathroom	Increased door width (33-36 inches minimum); French doors or accordion door Enlarged room Sink mounted low Open space under cabinet Showers with built-in seat Placement of tub faucets changed Ramped shower stall Toilet bidet installed Linen closet shelves with no door	Safety rails Seat reducer Raised commode seat Step placed in front of commode Wheelchair commode Insulated pipes Single-lever faucets Tub seats Wheelchair shower chair Hydraulic lifts Toilet paper tongs Toilet paper mounting Angled mirror Wall-mounted hair dryer with switch Suction-cupped bucket to hold supplies	Freestanding commode in secluded area Urinal bed bath Sponge bath Liquid soap Soap on a string Shampoo pump Dry shampoo
Bedroom	Downstairs bedroom Enlarged space Enlarged closet doors Low closet pole Closet storage system with shelves Built-in bookshelves at low and medium heights Holes cut in work surfaces for holding objects and electrical cords Built-in dressers or dressers bolted to the wall Special glides for wall drawers	Leg extenders Bed rails Firm mattress Straps or rope ladders Mounted shoe rack Environmental control units or switches for television, radio, and light access Enlarged drawer handles or loops added Positioning devices Adaptive chairs	Place bed on floor. Keep most-used clothes in accessible drawers. Use shelves instead of dresser drawers for clothes. Store toys in shoe bag.
Kitchen	Enlarged space Lowered countertops Lowered cabinets No cabinets under sink Built-in range top Sliding drawers and organizers in cabinets Wall-mounted, side-by-side oven Dishwasher mounted higher or has front opening Front-opening washing machine		Keep most-used items in low cupboards or on accessible surfaces. Hang bowls and pans on wall instead of storing in cabinets. Eat on wheelchair lap tray instead of table. Keep water in insulated pump bottle on table. Use a stool for washing dishes.

Sitting and sometimes standing are the most appropriate positions for the child to perform ADL tasks. In addition to postural alignment, the therapist recommends positions that provide the child with the following: (1) good orientation of his or her body to the work surface and the materials being used; (2) good body and visual orientation to the therapist (if instruction is being given); and (3) the ability to get to the place where the ADL occurs independently, maintain the necessary position, and leave. The occupational therapist modifies chair heights so that the child's feet are touching the floor to support postural stability and facilitate transfers. If the occupational therapist raises the seat height, a foot rest is also provided. The occupational therapist shortens or lengthens chair legs with blocks or leg extenders.

Kangas advocates a task-ready position for children with moderate to severe motor disabilities.[79] Instead of positioning the child's hips, knees, and ankles at 90-degree angles, Kangas positions them so that they are ready to move. In the task-ready

TABLE 15-5 Stabilization Materials and Application Procedures

Material	Application Procedures
Tape	Applies quickly but often is a temporary solution; includes masking, electrical, and duct tapes (duct tape is sturdy and has holding power).
Nonslip, pressure-sensitive matting	Fits under objects or around them and can be glued to objects; friction between materials minimizes slipping and sliding of objects; available in rolls or pads.
Suction cup holders	Hold lightweight materials, maintaining suction between object and work surface; single-faced suction cups can be applied permanently to objects (e.g., with nails, screws, or glue); double-faced suction cups can be moved from object to object.
C-clamps	Secure flat objects to lap trays, table edges, and other surfaces.
Tacking putty	Sticks posters onto walls; holds lightweight objects on surfaces such as tables, lap trays, angle boards, and walls.
Pressure-sensitive hook and loop tape (Velcro)	Sewn to cloth or glued to the base of objects and work surfaces; soft loop tape is used on areas that will contact the child's skin or clothing.
Wing nuts and bolts	Secure objects to a table surface or lapboard when holes are drilled through the object and holding surface; sturdy and more permanent.
Magnets	Affix to an object; stabilize objects on metallic surfaces such as refrigerator doors, metal tables, and magnetic message boards.
L-brackets	Hold objects in an upright plane; holes are drilled in the work surface and object to correspond with the L-bracket holes; objects are secured with nuts and bolts.
Soldering clamps	Hold small items for intricate work (e.g., mending a shirt, sewing on a button, putting on a bracelet); mounted to free-standing base; bases are weighted, suction cupped, or held to the surface with a C clamp.
Elastic or webbing	Attach to or around objects or positioning devices to hold them down; they also secure flat objects straps onto a work surface; straps are secured by tying, pressure-sensitive hook and loop tape, D rings and buckles, grommets, or screws.

position, the pelvis is secure, the trunk and head are slightly forward so that the shoulders are in front of the pelvis, the arms and hands are in front of the body, and the feet are flat on the floor or behind the knees. The occupational therapist removes or loosens as many restraints or chair adaptations as safely possible so that the child has maximal potential for movement. Such movement, even when subtle, provides visual, vestibular, proprioceptive, and kinesthetic feedback. A carved or molded seat and seat belt across the thighs give additional sensory feedback and are used for positioning the pelvis and for safety.

Prevention and Education

Problem Solving: Cognitive Approach

Anticipatory Problem Solving

Children learn and perform ADL tasks in a variety of environments, not just in the clinic or where the task typically occurs. Anticipatory problem solving is a preventive approach that prepares children and their families for unexpected events that may occur during self-care occupations.[123] Typically, parents do this with young children during toilet training. They anticipate that the child will have accidents in the beginning and bring two changes of clothes in case this does occur. In a study by Bedell, Cohn, and Dumas, parents used anticipatory problem solving to help prevent meltdowns for their children with brain injuries.[14] By thinking ahead (e.g., remembering not to have the child dressed in overalls on gym day, having children wear splints on the weekend and not during the week), parents ensure that their children can actively participate in school activities.

Children and youth also need to be part of anticipatory problem solving. By anticipating problems and generating solutions ahead of time, children can often reduce the anxiety they experience when trying a new task or entering a new environment.[140] Using contextual cues, such as noticing the floor is wet in the bathroom, and practicing different scenarios may be helpful. Schultz-Krohn suggested asking the following questions[140]:

1. What is the task to be completed and where will it occur?
2. What are the objects needed to complete the task?
   a. Are these objects available and ready to be used?
   b. If the objects are not available (e.g., misplaced, broken, being used by someone else), what else could be used, and who and how will the child ask for help?
3. What safety risks or hazards are within the environment or related to the objects being used by this student or other students? How can these risks be avoided?

Planning a natural teaching incident to occur during an activity ("sabotage")[159] gives the child, caregivers, teachers, and occupational therapists a good idea of how well the child can adapt and possibly use the anticipatory problem-solving solutions generated (Case Study 15-2). Giving the child an opportunity to choose a different way to complete or adapt a task promotes self-determination.

Cognitive Orientation Approach

In a similar model, occupational therapy researchers have developed a model of intervention called the Cognitive Orientation to daily Occupational Performance (CO-OP).[120] Researchers have studied the application of the CO-OP model in occupational therapy intervention on children with brain injuries, developmental coordination disorders (DCDs), and autism. These studies have demonstrated improvement in skills using the CO-OP approach.[120,129,130] In this model, children learn verbal problem-solving approaches and cognitive strategies to apply when they incur performance challenges. Talking about the task first, practicing it, and then practicing and talking about the task (dual tasking) are the three main steps used in

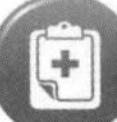

CASE STUDY 15-2 Nadia

Nadia was injured in a car accident and is now using a wheelchair for functional mobility in middle school while her femur and tibia fractures mend. Before Nadia's injury, she was identified as having a learning disability, with problems with spatial relations. Using the anticipatory problem-solving questions from Schultz-Krohn,[124] the outlined questions were answered during therapy. Mom is transporting Nadia to and from school, and her tasks to complete are to move safely around the school environment in the halls, classroom, band room, school nurse's office, restroom, and cafeteria. She needs a wheelchair, lap tray, and/or book bag, map of the school, and a way to keep her schoolwork organized.

If these objects do not work or are unavailable, the occupational therapist and Nadia generated some solutions. If a wheelchair does not fit within a small classroom space, she could use her crutches for short distances or a rolling computer chair and ask someone else to push her closer to the table. The occupational therapist, teacher, and mother discuss how to transfer from the wheelchair to a rolling chair or separate bench, and Nadia practices these transfers in case she needs to make these transfers. In addition, the occupational therapist and Nadia discuss her seating arrangements in each class and decide that a change in desk placement is needed. If a lap tray is not available, she asks others to carry her cafeteria tray or classroom materials. A divided book bag, which should help with organization, is placed on the back of her wheelchair. A side pocket on the armrest is used for pencils, money, and personal grooming items. Because of Nadia's poor spatial relations, time is taken to review and practice how to use the wheelchair without running into walls or other people. A safe distance from people is established, and she asks her teachers to be excused 5 minutes before classes end so she is not in the crowded hallways. Wheelchair maintenance and safety also are discussed, as well as deciding who may assist with the wheelchair. To enhance Nadia's anticipatory problem solving, the occupational therapist may place a barrier to her mobility performance and provide a natural teaching incident by moving classroom chairs to impede her pathway.

the CO-OP model. Research Note 15-3 describes a small study that used the CO-OP approach with boys with DCD.

Coaching and Education

Child and caregiver collaborative education is essential in all therapy for children. By developing collaborative partnerships through coaching, role modeling, and problem solving with others, the occupational therapist helps prevent injuries and possible failure in occupational performance and provides emotional support to caregivers.[124,150,174] This collaboration helps children perform ADLs in their environments and helps teachers, caregivers, and children learn safety information, specific techniques, and coping strategies. When providing information, occupational therapists consider the learning capacity, preferences, and environmental contexts of children and their families and caregivers, as well as the demands of the activity.[67]

Hanft, Rush, and Shelden have suggested using a coaching approach with children, parents, caregivers, and teachers based on an understanding of their knowledge, skills, and desired outcomes.[60] This requires asking the right questions and having all parties reflect on their progress. Questions that are reflective, comparative, and interpretive are used throughout the coaching process. Questions to reflect (e.g., what, who, when, where), compare (how), and interpret (e.g., Why did this work? What other issues may arise?) give the occupational therapist needed information to help coach the child and family. Hanft et al. suggest observing, listening, responding, and planning collaboratively with all parties involved in the task.[60] Observing the child where the task naturally occurs is essential. Observing the child and caregiver and then the child and occupational therapist, and using self-observation via videotape of all or any of the parties, helps everyone reflect and understand how the child completes the ADL task. Occupational therapists need to listen respectfully and objectively to all parties to understand preferences, concerns, and areas of need when working together. Responding to concerns, giving feedback, and collaboratively deciding how to proceed with a task helps all parties. Finally, coaching requires careful planning:

- Which strategies will they try this week?
- How will the occupational therapist modify the routine if this does not work?
- How will the teacher and the therapist give each other feedback?

Graham, Rodger, and Ziviani used occupational performance coaching (OPC) to give a structured approach for goal setting and specific instruction while providing emotional support.[52,53] This approach helps parents identify ways to promote more successful occupational performance by considering how the child, environment, and task interact with each other. Preliminary results found that OPC for ADL performance for children ages 5 to 12 years and their parents improved occupational performance and was sustained for 6 weeks postintervention. The mother's self-competence and occupational performance in coaching also appeared to generalize to goals other than ADL.

Occupational therapists present child or caregiver education in various ways by using coaching and other educational methods. They often demonstrate, or model, how to do the task (e.g., tub transfers) when instructing. In addition, the occupational therapist may use visual aids, written instructions, audiotapes, videotapes, and checklists. Drahota, Wood, and Sze Van Dyke used cognitive restructuring to help parents see the necessity of children doing their own self-care skills at developmentally appropriate times and to see small gains as success.[32]

An educational approach provides parents and children with the chance to make informed choices about the services, methods, assistive technology, and environmental adaptations they will use.[4] Grading, forward and backward chaining, partial participation, and modeling help train caregivers.[167] In this chapter, anticipatory problem solving or CO-OP, as well as coaching and educating caregivers and children, is assumed to

RESEARCH NOTE 15-3

Rodger, S., & Liu, S. (2008). Cognitive Orientation to (daily) Occupational Performance: Changes in strategy and session time use over the course of intervention. OTJR: Occupation, Participation and Health, 28 *(4), 168–179.*

Abstract

In this study, the authors used the Cognitive Orientation to daily Occupational Performance (CO-OP) intervention to help improve the motor performance of four 6- to 9-year-old-boys with developmental coordination disorder (DCD) in daily occupations. Ten treatment sessions were videotaped for each subject, and a computer analysis examined the cognitive strategies and changes in strategies used during the sessions. "Session time use referred to the duration of Talking About Task (describing the task or plans that will be executed), Practicing Task (actually doing the task or activity), and Dual Tasking (both talking and doing) coded during video segments observations" (p. 168). The authors examined the use of cognitive strategies within the subjects and across all four subjects during the 10 individual sessions. Each subject had varied results, and no patterns of cognitive strategy use were evident. The authors concluded that each child has a unique way of interacting with a task and the environment, and this emphasized the need for client-centered intervention that is individualized, which is the purpose of the CO-OP model.

Implications for Practice

- ADL instruction must be individualized for children and is dependent on the interaction of the child factors, interests, and performance skills with the demands of the task and characteristics of the environment.
- When planning ADL intervention, such as washing the face of a child with DCD, consider using some of these CO-OP strategies:
  1. Talking about the task: Determine which face cleanser and cloth to use; where, when, and how it will be used; and which safety precautions are needed for face washing (e.g., water too hot, soap in the eyes).
  2. Practicing the task: Grade the set up of the activity by the occupational therapist doing it first; practice first with a washcloth with no soap, then practice with soap; try it in an isolated environment without distractions, try it within therapy sessions, then try it at home.
  3. Dual tasking: While face washing, discuss how he or she is or is not following safety precautions, and what is working, such as the pressure he or she is using or the pattern he or she is using to wash the entire face.

be integral to intervention approaches for helping children develop ADL skills.

Specific Intervention Techniques for Selected ADL Tasks

Specific intervention strategies for toilet hygiene and bowel and bladder management, dressing, bathing and showering, personal hygiene and grooming, and sexual activity are described in this section. Interrelationships among child factors, contexts, and activity demands are considered. Combinations of approaches and strategies that help children become as independent as possible in ADL occupations are presented. As with all occupational therapy, the therapeutic use of purposeful and meaningful activities, consultation, and education are methods used to help others learn ADL occupations.

Toilet Hygiene and Bowel and Bladder Management

Typical Developmental Sequence

Independent toileting is an important self-maintenance milestone, and its achievement varies widely among children. It carries considerable sociologic and cultural significance. Self-sufficiency is often a prerequisite for participation in day-care centers, school programs, recreational and community opportunities, and secondary school vocational programs. Like other ADL tasks, toileting is a complex task requiring a thorough analysis of the demands of the activity and how the context and child's capabilities influence performance skills and patterns. To begin to learn this task, a child must be physically and psychologically ready. In addition, parents or caregivers need to be ready to devote the time and effort to toilet training the child. A communication system between caregivers and the child is essential:

- What cue, word, or gesture is used to say it is time to urinate or defecate?
- What is expected before, during, and after the toileting task?
- Is there consistency in how caregivers in different environments help the child manage the task?

At birth, a newborn voids reflexively and involuntarily. As the child matures, the spinal tract is myelinated to a level that allows for bowel and bladder control at the lumbar and sacral areas, and the child learns to control sphincter reflexes for volitional holding of urine and feces. Children are often physiologically ready for toileting if they have a pattern of urine and feces elimination.

Bowel control precedes bladder control, and studies indicate that girls are trained an average of 2.5 months earlier than boys.[141] Independence in toileting requires that the child be able to get on and off the toilet, manage fasteners and clothing, clean after toileting, and wash and dry hands efficiently, without supervision. Children progress in a developmental sequence, according to each child's unique maturational pattern. The typical developmental sequence for toileting is presented in Table 15-6.

Typical Factors That Interfere with Toileting Independence

Children with spinal cord injury, spina bifida, or other conditions that produce full or partial paralysis require special management for bowel and bladder activities. Loss of control over these bodily functions and the odor that results can cause embarrassment and reduce self-esteem. School-age children are characteristically modest about their bodies, and adolescents are struggling with identity issues and the need to be like their peers.

The type of bladder problem depends on the level and type of neurologic impairment. When the lesion is in the lumbar

TABLE 15-6 Typical Developmental Sequence for Toileting

Approximate Age (yr)	Toileting Skill
1	Indicates discomfort when wet or soiled Has regular bowel movements Sits on toilet when placed there and supervised (<5 min)
1½	Urinates regularly Shows interest in potty training
2	Stays dry for 2 hours or more Flushes toilet by self Achieves regulated toileting with occasional daytime accidents (32.5-35 mo) Rarely has bowel accidents
2½	Tells someone that he or she needs go the bathroom (31.9-34.7 mo) May need reminders to go to the bathroom May need help with getting on the toilet Wakes up dry at night Washes hands independently (29-31 mo) Wipes urine independently (32 mo)
3	Goes to the bathroom independently; seats himself or herself on toilet (33-39 mo) May need help with wiping May need help with fasteners or difficult clothing
4-5	Independent in toileting (e.g., tearing toilet paper, flushing, wiping effectively, washing hands, managing clothing)

Adapted from Coley, I. (1978). *Pediatric assessment of self care assessment* (pp. 145, 149). St. Louis: Mosby; and Orelove, F., & Sobsey, D. (1996). Self-care skills. In F. Orelove & D. Sobsey (Eds.), *Educating children with multiple disabilities* (2nd ed., pp. 342-). Baltimore: Paul H. Brookes; and Schum, T. R., Kolb, T. M., McAuliffe, T. L., et al. (2002). Sequential acquisition of toilet-training skills: A descriptive study of gender and age differences in normal children. *Pediatrics, 109*(3), E48.

region or below, the reflex arc is no longer intact, and the bladder is flaccid (lower motor neuron bladder). When the lesion is above the level of bladder innervation, the result is an automatic bladder (upper motor neuron bladder). The child undertakes training programs to develop an automatic response for the upper motor neuron bladder. In children with a flaccid bladder, training will be ineffective because the bladder has insufficient tone and requires assistance in emptying.

The occupational therapist works with physicians and nurses to determine bladder training and management programs after medical testing and collaborative discussions with children and their parents. Four main methods are used to manage urine: (1) condom catheterization (for males), (2) indwelling catheters, (3) intermittent catheterization (every 4 to 6 hours), and (4) ileal conduits. Parents are asked to restrict the child's fluid intake before program sessions to prevent bladder distention. When girls have partial control of bladder function, they wear disposable diapers or incontinence pads.

A basic principle for success in bowel re-education is to have a regular and consistent evacuation of the bowel. Bowel program timing is a matter of choice, but a consistent schedule is needed. In some cases, the child receives suppositories and a warm drink before evacuation. This stimulates contraction and relaxation of muscle fibers in the walls of the intestine, moving the contents onward. Other techniques include digital stimulation, massage around the anal sphincter, and manual pressure using the Credé method on the abdomen. Occasionally, removal of the stool by hand or by a colostomy is recommended. As with an ileostomy, colostomy collection bags are emptied and cleansed on a regular basis. and the child learns to do this independently as soon as possible.

Children with congenital or acquired neurologic disorders often undergo catheterization or bowel programs. Compared with the toileting practices of their peers, these additional bowel and bladder tasks require more time, higher cognitive functions to plan, organize, and remember to perform the procedure, and established routines.[162] In addition, children may have difficulty in any of the following areas: maintaining a stable yet practical position; hand dexterity (praxis and speed); perceptual awareness; strength, ROM, and stability; and accuracy in emptying collection devices. Memory, safety, and sensory awareness are needed for many of these procedures. Although nurses are often the professionals who teach bowel and bladder control methods, the occupational therapist may help establish the hand skills necessary, adapt the context by providing assistive devices or adapted methods, and/or establish a routine that becomes habitual and easy for the child and helps prevent future infections or embarrassment. Levan, an occupational therapist, has described a "penis paddle" made to assist a young man with self-catheterization.[90] By collaborating with the school nurse, the device was incorporated into the self-catheterization routine.

Closely associated with bowel and bladder care is perianal skin care. The skin is cleansed thoroughly to protect the tissue against the effects of contact with waste matter and eliminate odor. All children with decreased sensation are susceptible to *decubitus ulcers,* pressure sores that develop rapidly when blood vessels are compressed (e.g., around a bony prominence, such as the ischial tuberosity). Daily inspection of the buttocks with a long-handled mirror is needed.

Children with Limited Motor Skills and Bodily Functions

Diapering becomes a difficult task when infants or children have strong extensor and adduction (muscle and movement function) patterns in their legs. Occupational therapists teach the mother restorative or remedial methods to decrease extensor patterns before diapering and to incorporate these methods into the diapering routine. For example, the mother may first place a pillow under the child's hips, flex the hips, and slowly rock the hips back and forth before she helps the child abduct the legs for diapering.

Toileting independence may be delayed in children of all ages with limitations in strength, endurance, range of motion, postural stability, and manipulation or dexterity. With an unstable sitting posture, the child has difficulty relaxing and maintaining a position for pressing down and emptying the bowels.

With weakness and limited ROM, the child may be unable to manage fastenings because of hand weakness or may have problems sitting down or getting up from the toilet seat because of hip-knee contractions or quadriceps weakness.

Cleansing after a bowel movement is difficult if the child cannot supinate the hand, flex the wrist, or internally rotate and extend the arm. An anterior approach may work. The occupational therapist must caution girls against contamination from feces, which causes vaginitis. If possible, girls should wipe the anus from the rear. Solutions to cleansing problems are difficult and often discouraging. These children may require remediation strategies to improve body capacities (e.g., active ROM) or adaptation strategies (e.g., wiping tongs, use of a bidet) to perform the toileting task.

Children with Intellectual Limitations

Children with intellectual disabilities take longer to learn toileting, but they often become independent.[114] Problems with awareness, initiation, sequencing, memory, and dexterity in managing their clothes are typical. As with all children, physiologic readiness for toileting is a prerequisite for training programs. The occupational therapist uses task analysis to determine which steps of the process are problems, and he or she then determines which cues and prompts are needed to achieve the child's best performance. The occupational therapist also evaluates which methods work as successful reinforcement.[168]

According to a large longitudinal study by Joinson et al., school-age children with developmental delay, difficult temperament, and/or who have mothers with depression or anxiety are at risk for problems with bowel and bladder control during the day.[75] Occupational therapists need to consider if any of these factors are interfering with toilet training and if additional time, procedures, suggestions, or referrals are needed. Some parents of children with developmental delay or autism may use a behavioral approach to incontinence.[89] The Azrin and Foxx[8] training method for toileting is behaviorally based and requires the child to be at least 20 months of age and able to complete prerequisites (e.g., sit independently, imitate, stay dry a couple of hours.). Caregivers spend 4 to 6 hours training in the bathroom with their child while giving positive reinforcement and overcorrection for errors. A few studies have reported success with the Azrin and Foxx method, but studies that compare the effectiveness of different toilet training methods for children with disabilities are limited.[87] The Evolve website gives additional resources on toileting.

Adaptation Strategies for Improving Toileting Independence

Adaptation strategies include remodeling or restructuring the environment, selecting assistive devices or different types of clothing, or devising alternative methods to enhance independence. The occupational therapist also addresses caregiver needs as the child becomes heavier and more difficult to assist with toileting.

Characteristics of physical and social environments at home or school influence how a child manages toileting hygiene. Privacy is particularly important for the older child and adolescent; helping children determine where to perform the procedure and how to manage it in school and recreational environments is often a challenge. Social routines and expectations are also important variables for the occupational therapist to consider when making recommendations for managing toileting. These expectations depend on the child's age and abilities and how the family perceives the child's ability to manage this aspect of his or her ADLs.

Social Environment and Temporal Context

Of all ADL tasks, toileting requires the most sensitive approach on the part of those who work with the child on a self-maintenance program. Children may purposely restrict their fluid intake at school to avoid the need for elimination. Unfortunately, limited fluid intake promotes infections, which increases the difficulty of regulating the bowel and bladder. Families, teachers, nurses, and paraprofessionals work with occupational therapists to evaluate the social environment and find the best place, time, and routine for the child. When self-catheterization is done in the school or community environment, the child can ensure privacy by using the health room or a private bathroom stall or perform this ADL when children are usually not taking bathroom breaks. Carrying catheterization supplies in a fanny pack or a small nylon (nontransparent) bag also protects the child's privacy.

Occupational therapists help children who lack bowel and bladder control to develop routines and health habits that eliminate possible odors. By focusing on performance patterns, the occupational therapist reinforces and incorporates regular cleansing and changing of appliances (collection bags for ileal conduits and colostomies) and urine collection bags into daily schedules. A good fluid intake also is recommended to prevent odors and bacterial growth.

Children with autism often have a difficult time with toileting practices. Wheeler has offered a practical guide to toilet training for children with autism and related disorders.[171] The discussion of support strategies, such as modeling and social stories, and numerous examples of common problems and solutions associated with training individuals with autism are excellent. Wheeler used social context and many visual prompts to structure the steps for toileting. In a small study of preschoolers with autism, video modeling with operant conditioning was more successful in establishing toileting than operant conditioning by itself.[80] Table 15-7 defines methods to adapt toileting and improve toileting independence.

Physical Environment

The bathroom often is the most inaccessible room in the house, yet it is essential that every family member have access to it. The floor space may be insufficient to allow the child to turn a wheelchair for a toilet transfer. The location and height of the sink, faucets, towels, soap, and toilet paper may make them inaccessible to young children. Children with olfactory hypersensitivity may have difficulty tolerating bathroom odors (e.g., air freshener, perfumed toilet paper or soap). Therefore, the bathroom's space, equipment, and objects may need to be adapted or modified.

Toileting Adaptations

Numerous adaptations are available to assist the child in positioning and maintaining cleanliness after toileting. Urinals, catheters, leg bag clamps, long-handled mirrors, positioning devices to provide postural stability or hold the legs open, and universal cuffs with a catheter or digital stimulator attached are some examples of assistive devices that occupational therapists may provide. For children with good postural control but limited ROM or grasp, simple inexpensive aids include various types of toilet paper tongs and toilet paper–holding devices.

TABLE 15-7 Analysis and Interventions for Toileting

Area	Analysis	Intervention Ideas
Required (task analysis)	Recognizes signal to go to the bathroom (visual or sensation) Goes to bathroom and closes door Pulls clothes down (only as much as needed) Sits or stands at toilet Urinates or defecates (or words child uses) Gets toilet paper Wipes, then throws toilet paper in toilet Flushes once Pulls clothes up Washes and dries hands Throws away trash Leaves bathroom	Have visual routine on wall (objects, pictures, or action words). Make tasks smaller or larger, depending on child's abilities (e.g., separate washing and drying of the hands). Add task if child is omitting it or is having trouble (e.g., if child is smearing feces, use "wipe" as one of the steps). Child uses too much toilet paper: (1) Remove toilet paper roll and use Kleenex, or pull off correct amount to be used and hand it to child; or (2) place a tape mark on the wall of how much paper to roll out. Child does not sit: Use timer and instruct child to stay "seated" until timer rings; use potty that is close to the floor.
Client factors (body functions and structures)	Sensations (bladder fullness, voluntary control, emptying bladder, wet or dry, toilet paper texture, noise of flushing) Physiologic readiness Strength, coordination, and endurance to manage clothing and fasteners Balance to stand at or sit on toilet Emotional readiness—fears of flushing or disease, need for privacy, attitude toward toileting	Use habit training if no pattern is evident: Go at the same times every day. Have child dress in easy-to-manipulate clothing. Use preparatory activities at other times to build strength and coordination for fasteners. Support child's body (e.g., grab bars, foot support, ring reducer, potty chair on floor). Change toilet papers or use different material, such as wet wipes or cloth.
Environment, contexts (cultural, social, physical, personal, temporal, cognitive)	*Cultural*: Family and societal expectations of toileting; words used; whether child uses a public bathroom and sits on the toilet seat; institutional practices (e.g., co-toileting in preschool, language used) *Social*: Acceptance of use of a diaper; how child indicates need to toilet (e.g., pee-pee, gestures), others in bathroom, flushing, gender-specific public bathroom rules *Physical*: Size, temperature, sounds; set up; way to flush, height of toilet, adaptations (toilet seat or potty chair; grab bars or safety frame around toilet); faucets and other fixtures *Personal*: Chronologic age, grade in school, gender *Temporal*: Previous experiences, fears of flushing or disease, need for privacy, attitude toward toileting	Spell out expectations in the beginning. Dedicate a bathroom to toilet training, if possible. Play soft music or toilet song on a tape player. Public bathrooms: Boys need cueing for bathroom behavior and may need a social story: leave a space between yourself and someone else at a urinal; keep your pants up over your buttocks while urinating at a urinal; don't talk or look others in the eye while at the urinal; be quick and leave when you are finished; only you will touch your body while in the bathroom (unless catheterization training). If child dawdles in bathroom, have him or her go with a peer buddy or go at a less busy time. If child is fearful, have him or her open door for escape, then flush.
Performance skills (sensory—perceptual, motor—praxis, cognitive, emotional regulation, communication, social)	Posture, mobility, coordination, strength, and effort needed *Cognitive*: Initiate, sequence, and terminate How child communicates need to go to bathroom (e.g., physically or by speaking)	Provide way to indicate a need to go: • Picture cues of entire sequence • Object cues or transitional object • Social story • Timer • Spoken cues • Positioning body on toilet • Sensitivity to smells and sounds • Physical, gestural cues • Ear plugs, timing, not after another person used the toilet

TABLE 15-7 Analysis and Interventions for Toileting—cont'd

Area	Analysis	Intervention Ideas
Performance patterns (habits, routines, roles)	Recognizes typical routines in the family for eating and drinking Recognizes typical times and patterns when child urinates or defecates Uses habit training to go at a certain time of the day, every day Cleans up accidents by himself or herself without harsh reprimanding Behavior challenge may be provoked by changes in routines	Limit or increase liquids. Use wet-dry chart to determine typical times for toileting. Use visual schedule for toileting steps (including wiping) and times, as well as times for drinking fluids. Use same routine and rituals for toileting (e.g., particular times or when waking, before trips, after meals). Urge family, school, and day-care center all to follow the same routine and collect data.
Activity demands (objects, spatial, social, sequencing, timing)	Placement of potty chair or toilet seat; height of toilet, flushing mechanism, toilet paper dispenser Space in bathroom, arrangement of items Door shut or closed; whether child announces it's time to go Steps to toileting, flushing after going potty; when to close door, get toilet paper or paper towel Public bathroom social expectations	Change layout of objects or accessibility of environment. Include "shut the door" as part of toileting sequence. Discuss public bathroom expectations; have social story available to talk about them. Public bathroom (boys): Use private stall first, then move to urinal.

Adapted from Wheeler, M. (1998). *Toilet training for individuals with autism and related disorders.* Arlington, TX: Future Horizons.

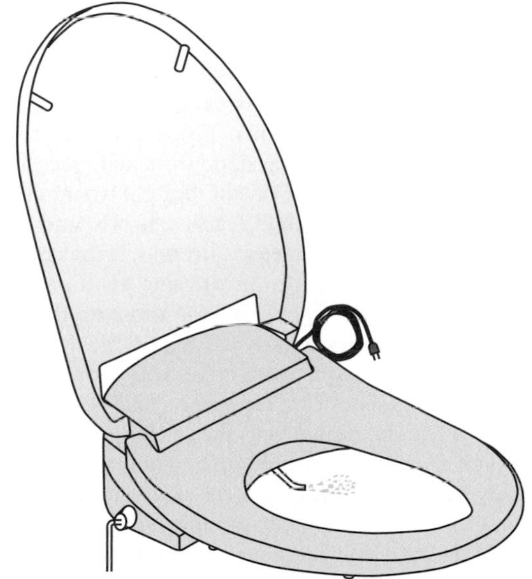

FIGURE 15-5 Electrically powered bidet makes it possible to clean the perianal area independently, without using hands or paper.

A combined bidet and toilet offers a means of total independence. Several models are available that attach to a standard toilet bowl. A self-contained mechanism spray washes the perianal area with thermostatically controlled warm water and dries it with a flow of warm air. The child operates the controls with the hand or foot (Figure 15-5). Various special cushions designed to prevent tissue trauma are available commercially.

The type of clothing worn during toileting often hinders the child's independence or caregiver's ability to promote independence. Tight stretch garments are often recommended to help with postural control, but these may result in problems with toileting independence or incontinence.[112] For children who wear diapers, a full-length crotch opening with a zipper or hook and loop (e.g., Velcro) closure makes changes easier. When children are first learning toilet training, the use of elastic-waisted diapers that pull up gives them the opportunity to practice this part of the toileting sequence while protecting clothing from accidents. As children mature, they may be responsible for changing their own diapers or caring for their appliances and equipment. Girls may wear wraparound or full skirts because these are easy to put on and adjust for diaper changes or toileting. The child reaches and drains leg bags with greater ease when the pants have zippers or hook and loop closures along the seams. Flies with long zippers or hook and loop closures make it easier for boys to urinate or catheterize themselves when in wheelchairs.

Adaptations for Unstable Posture

When children sit on the toilet, they need postural security. When toilet seats are low enough that the feet rest firmly on the floor, the abdominal muscles that aid in defecation effectively fulfill their function. Reducer rings are used for small children to decrease the size of the toilet seat opening and thus improve sitting support. A step in front of the toilet helps small children get onto it. Safety rails that attach to the toilet or wall can assist with balance and allow free use of the child's hands. For the child who has outgrown small training potties, freestanding commodes may be useful when wheelchair access to the bathroom is impossible. A toilet chair that rolls into place over the toilet is another option. Commodes that feature such modifications as adjustable legs, safety bars, angled legs for stability, and padded, upholstered, and adjustable back rests and head rests are often helpful to caregivers. Commodes are also available with seat reducer rings, seat belts, and adjustable footrests.

Menstrual Hygiene

In adolescence, girls need to learn how to care for their menstrual needs. As puberty begins, hormones increase and moodiness, emotional turmoil, irregular bleeding, menstrual cramps, and poor hygiene may emerge.[123] For girls with intellectual disabilities, understanding the changes in their body and learning new hygiene skills may be difficult. Depending on the child's disability, puberty may occur between 9 and 16 years of age, and avoiding abuse and reproductive concerns require consideration. These topics are discussed in this chapter's section on sexual activity.

Puberty is often a difficult time for parents, and they may approach their child's physician for menstrual suppression medication and contraception.[123] Options for gynecologic care are important to discuss with parents and the youth. A pelvic or breast examination is part of maintaining health and is necessary to detect possible health problems. The California Department of Developmental Services has developed a manual for physicians about how to conduct a gynecologic examination for women with disabilities and is a helpful resource for parents.[149] Menstrual management is part of toileting hygiene, and many skills, routines and habits, and adaptations may be recommended for the young adolescent girl with a disability and her caregivers. Similar to girls with normal development, young girls with disabilities need to be prepared before menarche for the changes that will occur to their body. They need reassurance that bleeding and sometimes cramps are part of growing up and are normal. Parents and occupational therapists may work with the young adolescent to understand changes in the body and moods, as well as the methods and hygiene habits necessary for managing menstruation (e.g., wearing pads or tampons).

Teaching Methods for Girls with Limitations in Cognition

For girls with autism, Wrobel suggests using stories and visual cues to help girls learn about menstruation and advising them to inform their teacher or parent when bleeding occurs.[177] Techniques suggested are using photosequencing cards, red food coloring placed on a sanitary pad, repetitive practice of how to place the pad in the panties, wearing the pad for a few days at a time before the onset of menarche, and instructions in proper wrapping and disposal of the pad. Specific stories, pictures, and examples are given related to the hygiene of menstruation, changing pads at school, getting cramps, and keeping menstruation private. These same techniques and ideas are applicable for girls with intellectual disabilities, and practicing the actual hygiene task during menses is most effective.[34] Alarms on watches, PDA timers, or cues can be used to help the adolescent change her pad every 3 to 4 hours or remind her that her period may begin this week. Using anticipatory problem solving, parents and caregivers can ensure that the adolescent has extra supplies or clothing to manage any mishaps.

Teaching Methods for Physical Limitations

For girls with significant physical and/or cognitive disabilities, therapists can train caregivers to help with menstrual care ADLs.[56] Adaptive devices for menstrual care are similar to aids used for toilet hygiene. Long-handled mirrors, positioning devices to provide postural stability (e.g., grab bars, toilet safety frames) or hold the legs open, toilet paper tongs, and universal cuffs with a tampon inserter attached are some examples of assistive devices that occupational therapists may provide. If a bidet is available, it may help with cleanliness during menstruation. In Australia, occupational therapists are involved with the Health and Well-Being Network and provide intervention strategies to address menstrual needs of adolescents and women with disabilities. Together with other team members, they created a booklet and kit to help families and professionals explore attitudes, practical strategies, and other options for managing menstrual care.[30]

Dressing

Typical Development

For a typical child, achieving independence in dressing usually takes 4 years of practice. Characteristically, learning to undress comes before learning to dress. Caregivers introduce self-dressing in a natural way, at bedtime, by allowing the child to complete the final step in pulling off a garment. Similarly, when the child becomes more goal-directed and motivated to be independent, he or she is ready to try the more difficult tasks of learning to put on clothing. Often, the caregiver uses backward chaining by putting the garment on the child and allowing the child to complete the action. Gradually the child performs more of the task, and the caregiver performs less. A parent-friendly book that assists caregivers in using backward chaining and collecting data has been written by Turner, Lammi, Friesen, and Phelan.[167] Table 15-8 presents the typical development of dressing.

Dressing requires children to use a variety of performance skills and patterns to meet the unique demands of the activity. They need to know where their bodies are in space and how body parts relate while they use visual and kinesthetic systems to guide arm and leg movements. Visual and somatosensory systems enable the child to understand form and space and how clothing conforms to and fits on the body. Dynamic postural stability is important as the child reaches, bends, and shifts his or her center of gravity while getting dressed. If the child avoids crossing the midline and performs dressing tasks on the right side of the body with the right hand and those on the left with the left hand, he or she most likely will have difficulty with tasks that require both hands to work together, such as fastening clothing and tying shoelaces. How the child coordinates the two sides of the body, manipulates the clothing, grips fasteners, and calibrates the amount of strength and effort determine how the activity is completed. Cognitive skills such as choosing appropriate clothing, temporally organizing and remembering the steps of the task, and adapting to contextual changes (e.g., new materials, noise in the environment, placement of clothing) also affect dressing outcomes.

Typical Problems and Intervention Strategies

Limitations in Cognitive and Sensory Perceptual Skills

Children who have underlying cognitive and perceptual deficits may also have problems in processing performance skills. They may demonstrate problems with choosing, using, and handling clothing. These may include difficulty distinguishing the right and left sides of the body, putting a shoe on the correct foot, turning the heel of a sock, differentiating the front of clothing from the back, or identifying the correct leg or sleeve. Temporal organization, especially initiating, continuing, sequencing, terminating, and organizing the dressing task, is often problematic

TABLE 15-8 Typical Developmental Sequence for Dressing

Age (yr)	Self-Dressing Skills
1	Cooperates with dressing (holds out arms and legs)
	Pulls off shoes, removes socks
	Pushes arms through sleeves and legs through pants
2	Removes unfastened coat
	Removes shoes if laces are untied
	Helps pull down pants
	Finds armholes in pullover shirt
2½	Removes pull-down pants with elastic waist
	Assists in pulling on socks
	Puts on front-buttoning coat or shirt
	Unbuttons large buttons
3	Puts on pullover shirt with minimal assistance
	Puts on shoes without fasteners (may be on wrong foot)
	Puts on socks (may be with heel on top)
	Independently pulls down pants
	Zips and unzips jacket once on track
	Needs assistance to remove pullover shirt
	Buttons large front buttons
3½	Finds front of clothing
	Snaps or hooks front fastener
	Unzips zipper on jacket, separating zipper
	Puts on mittens
	Buttons series of three or four buttons
	Unbuckles shoe or belt
	Dresses with supervision (needs help with front and back)
4	Removes pullover garment independently
	Buckles shoes or belt
	Zips jacket zipper
	Puts on socks correctly
	Puts on shoes, needs assistance in tying laces
	Laces shoes
	Consistently identifies the front and back of garments
4½	Puts belt in loops
5	Ties and unties knots
	Dresses unsupervised
6	Closes back zipper
	Ties bows
	Buttons back buttons
	Snaps back snaps

Adapted from Klein, M.D. (1983). *Pre-dressing skills.* Tucson, AZ: Communication Skill Builders.

for children with intellectual disabilities or autism. When children have difficult organizing the task, the occupational therapist often recommends modifying the demands of dressing in various environments. Artificial cues such as color coding or labeling dressers or bins with pictures or words help children locate objects for dressing in the bedroom environment. Picture charts and checklists help the child remember the sequence of steps in a task and provide a routine for completing it.

Behaviorally, the child may become frustrated with the complexity of certain dressing tasks. Language deficits may restrict the child's ability to express personal preferences or frustrations. Frustration may increase when the child is faced with tasks that require fine manipulations if coordination is limited or the child has sensory modulation problems. Often, a behavioral approach helps the child acquire independence. After making a baseline assessment, the occupational therapist carefully analyzes the demands of each dressing task. Once he or she determines the limitations and strengths in performance skills and patterns, partial participation and backward and forward chaining methods are used. Environmental and task adaptations include visual charts or pictures, social stories, checklists, video modeling, and clothing that is easy to manipulate (e.g., slightly larger clothing, stretchy materials, pullover shirts, loafers). Simultaneous prompting in the dressing activity itself helps children learn the task.[145] Figure 15-6 presents an example of a visual story used for a child who has sensory deficits and who dislikes changes in routines or dressing for outside play. It is purported that the repetition of positive statements makes the child more ready to follow the routine in the story and initiate the task. When using social stories, it is important to use the criteria set by Gray to construct the story.[55] Read the story to the child before he or she begins the task and suggest that it be read daily. Similar to any prompting, the occupational therapist needs to fade the story as the child's abilities or behavior improves or increase use of the story if progress is limited. Evidence for the use and effectiveness of using social stories is limited, although they are frequently used with children who have behavior issues, intellectual disabilities, or autism spectrum disorder (ASD).[127,137] Teachers rate improvement in a child's ability after using a social story, but this is confounded by the inconsistency in following the guidelines set by Gray[55] and reporting how outcomes are measured.

VMO and VSM are well-researched techniques used by a variety of professionals to teach children with autism and intellectual disabilities and may be helpful in promoting ADLs.[15,98,101] By giving children the visual role model, they are motivated to try the task themselves. For children with intellectual limitations, video modeling is helpful because reading is not necessary.[98] In the VMO technique, a child learns a specific skill (e.g., dressing skill) by watching a video of a peer or an adult do the task (putting on a coat). In the VSM technique, by contrast, videos are edited so a child watches himself or herself putting on the coat correctly. The VSM method is labor-intensive; it takes skill to produce and edit a 2- to 3-minute video of the child doing the task. A meta-analysis of video modeling case studies suggested that using an adult as a model (VMO) for children with autism is more effective than VSM, particularly when reinforcement is paired with VMO.[100] Research Note 15-4 describes a review of these techniques and provides suggestions for using VMO and VSM collaboratively with teams.

Physical or Motor Limitations

Children with various conditions find dressing difficult because of the coordination, ROM, and strength required for pulling clothes on and off and connecting fasteners. Children with DCD can have difficulty completing dressing (and managing toileting and utensil use) because of slowness, disorganization, frustration, and a history of depending on others to do the task.[109] Dunford, Missiuna, Street, and Sibert found that children with DCD (5-10 years of age) reported concerns about their self-care skills, even though occupational therapists and parents did not identify these concerns.[33] Children with the use of only one hand find it difficult to zip trousers, tie shoelaces, and button shirts or blouses. Establishing or restoring the child's

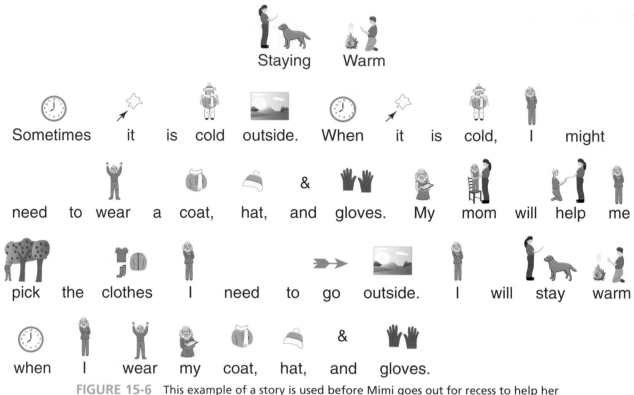

Staying Warm
Sometimes it is cold outside. When it is cold, I might
need to wear a coat, hat, and gloves. My mom will help me
pick the clothes I need to go outside. I will stay warm
when I wear my coat, hat, and gloves.

FIGURE 15-6 This example of a story is used before Mimi goes out for recess to help her rehearse what she is going to do and help her understand why. (Courtesy Rebecca E. Argabrite Grove, Loudoun County Public Schools, Loudoun County VA.)

strength or coordination may help, but in most cases the child learns adaptive techniques, often through his or her own experimentation or the use of assistive technology. Children with cerebral palsy often have difficulty balancing and controlling arm and leg movement when donning and removing clothing. Limited dexterity may also interfere with dressing. Occupational therapists can suggest methods to modify the demands of the activity, such as supportive positioning or the use of adaptive aids such as button hooks, rings on zippers, one-handed shoe fasteners, or hook and loop closures. Because clothing manufacturers recognize the value of universal design, many of these adaptations are now available commercially.[142] Table 15-2 gives other examples of how to adapt or improve fastening skills.

Adaptive Methods for Dressing Children with Motor Limitations

Although it is common to dress an infant while he or she is lying in the supine position, this position frequently increases extensor tone in infants with neurologic impairment. For this reason, some occupational therapists advocate placing the infant prone across the knees, with the infant's hips flexed and abducted, thereby inhibiting leg extensor and adduction tone. When the infant gains head and trunk control, the caregiver dresses him or her in a sitting position, with the child's back resting against and supported by the caregiver's trunk. In this position, the infant has an opportunity to observe his or her own body during dressing.

When dressing an infant with increased extensor tone, the caregiver carefully bends the infant's hips and knees before putting on shoes and socks (Figure 15-7) and brings the infant's shoulders forward before putting the arm through a sleeve. Flexing the child's hip and knee decreases postural tone and makes dressing easier. When a child achieves sitting balance,

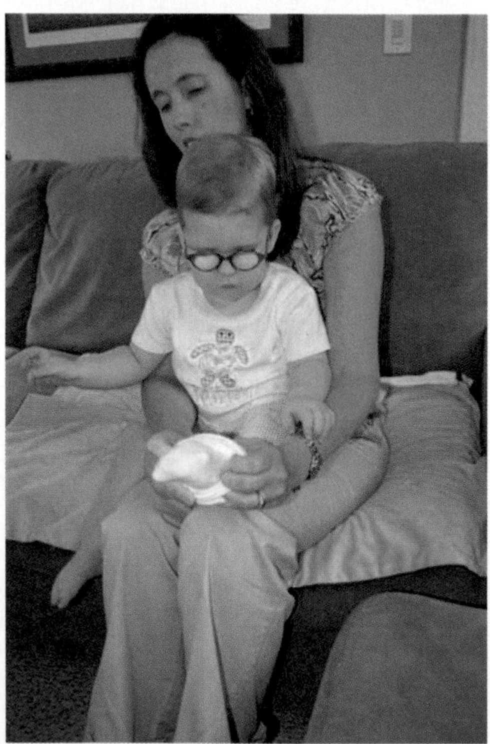

FIGURE 15-7 When dressing a child who is hypertonic, the caregiver should carefully flex the child's hips and knees before putting on socks and shoes.

RESEARCH NOTE 15-4

Mason, R. A., Ganz, J., B., Parker, R.I., Burke, M.D. & Camargo, S. (2012). Moderating factors of video-modeling with other as model: A meta-analysis of single-case studies, Research in Developmental Disabilities, 33, *1076–1086.*

Abstract

A meta-analysis of 42 studies (single-subject design) of children and young adults with autism spectrum disorder (ASD) and developmental disabilities was completed by the authors. Video modeling of others (VMO) effectiveness was reviewed because this is a less complicated technique to use than video self-modeling (VSM). The participant age, diagnosis, and targeted outcomes were analyzed. The results of the meta-analysis suggest that video modeling of others meets evidence-based practice criteria as a strategy to address behavioral functioning, social communication skills, and functional skills across settings.

Implications for Practice

- Video modeling of others (VMO) or video self-modeling (VSM) is a successful technique for increasing the success of the intervention for play and social communication across all ages for students with ASD and is most effective for children ages 6 to 10 years.
- For children with ASD, a short video (2-3 minutes) of another peer or adult doing the task (e.g., putting on a shirt) prior to working on the task itself may help make learning the task sequence go more quickly and improves when paired with positive reinforcement.
- For children, adolescents, and young adults with developmental disabilities, VMO is moderately effective and appears to be more effective when paired with other programming such as prompting, error recognition, and positive reinforcement.
- Videos of ADL skills placed on home or school tablets, PDAs, phones, computers, or television incorporates this intervention strategy into home or school routines to increase the rate of improvement.

a good way to proceed with dressing is to place the child on the floor and later on a low stool, continuing to provide support where needed from the back. Orientation to the child's body parts should remain a focus in the social interaction. The caregiver helps the child understand how the body relates to the clothes and to the various positions (e.g., "The arm goes through the sleeve" and "The head goes through the hole at the top of the shirt").

When the child is older and heavier, there may be no alternative but to dress the child while he or she is in the side-lying or supine position, placing a hard pillow under the child's head. If it is possible to maintain the child in a side-lying position, this posture may make it easier for the caregiver to manage the child's arms and legs and for the child to assist in the dressing task (Figure 15-8).

Adaptive Methods for Self-Dressing

The child who has hand coordination but poor balance may be able to take advantage of the function that he or she possesses when in a side-lying position, with the effect of gravity lessened. For the child who sits but is unstable, a corner of two adjoining walls or a corner seat on the floor may provide enough postural support for independent dressing. Sitting balance is more precarious as the child reaches when donning overhead garments or pants and shoes; therefore, the child needs additional external support. Sitting in chairs with arms or sitting on the floor against a wall may improve performance.

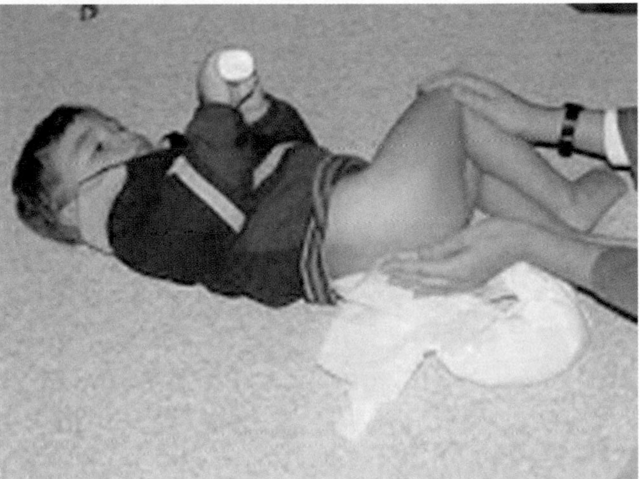

FIGURE 15-8 The side-lying position may reduce stiffness and make dressing easier.

The occupational therapist helps improve the child's dressing by offering the parent and child various problem-solving strategies from which the child and parents may choose. Once the method is chosen, anticipatory problem solving is used to help prepare the child for unexpected events in the environment. Table 15-9 offers choices in problem solving that are used for putting on and taking off different garments. Clothing selection, assistive technology, and adaptations to the task are methods for improving a child's performance in self-dressing.

Attention to the needs of individuals with disabilities has increased over the past decade, with some adaptive clothing becoming available through catalogue supply companies. These companies generally offer attractive fashionable clothing that meets functional requirements but conforms in appearance to the child's peer group standards and fashion trends. When possible, clothing should conceal physical disabilities, or at least should not attract attention to them, and hence contribute to the wearer's sense of well-being. Functionally, the clothing design should enable the wearer to take care of personal needs, help maintain proper body temperature, and provide freedom of movement.

Most clothing is made for individuals in a standing position. For those who spend long hours in a wheelchair, the sitting position causes pulling and straining on some areas of the garment and a surplus of fabric in others. The caregiver makes alterations to provide more comfort in sitting (e.g., pants that are cut higher in the back and lower in the front and cut larger to give additional room in the hips and thighs).[142] A longer inseam also allows the proper hem height for pants when sitting (rests on top of shoe). Pockets in the back may cause shearing or skin breakdown with prolonged sitting. Instead, pockets are placed on the top of the thigh or on the side of the calf for easy access. Front and side seams are sewn with hook and loop fasteners or zippers and wrist loops to assist in donning. Pullover tops with raglan and gusset sleeves allow more room when

TABLE 15-9 Adaptation Strategies for Dressing with Different Types of Garments

Garment	Design Features of Clothing or Assistive Technology Adaptations for Easier Dressing	Adaptations to Task Method
Pull-up garments	Large size Stretchy material Loops sewn into waistband Elastic waistbands, but not too tight Pressure-sensitive tape Zipper pulls Dressing sticks	Sit on chair. Lie on floor. Lie on side and roll side to side to pull up pants. Use chair or grab bar to stabilize oneself while pulling up pants. Put weak or affected extremity in first.
Pullover garments	Large, easy opening for head Flexible knit fabric Large armholes and sleeve openings; raglan sleeves Elastic cuffs and waistbands	Lay garment on lap, floor, or table, front side down; put arms in and flip over head. Use a template to position garment as above. Pull garment over head, then put arms in first. Put weak or affected extremity in second.
Front-opening garments	Loose style Fullness in back of garment On shirt or jacket, collar of different color from main garment Short-sleeve garments first, proceeding to long-sleeve garments Raglan sleeves Garment with no closures or one or two buttons (e.g., sweater, jacket)	Lay garment on lap, floor, or table, with neck of garment toward child; put in arms, duck head, extend arms, and flip garment over the head; shrug shoulders and use arms to help garment fall into place. Put weak or affected arm in first, pull up to shoulder; follow collar, then put in other arm. Use a template for placement of garment.
Buttons	Flat, large buttons Buttons contrast in color with garment Buttons with shanks (easier to grasp) Buttons sewn on loosely Buttons sewn on one side; hook and loop tape on both sides to close shirt or pants Front buttons first, proceeding to side and back buttons	Use pullover styles instead of those with buttons. Button all but the first two or three buttons and put shirt on like a pullover. Begin buttoning with bottom button (easier to see and align). Use a button hook. Use elastic thread to sew on sleeve buttons; put on sleeve without buttoning. Use backward chaining.
Zippers	Nylon zippers (easier than metal) Zipper tabs or rings Zipper pulls Hook and loop tape instead of zipper while pulling up zipper tab with other hand Longer zippers (more space for donning and doffing clothes) Front zippers first, proceeding to side and back zippers	Sit to gain stability. Stand to keep jacket zipper flat. Hold zipper taut with one hand at bottom of zipper. For side zipper, lean against wall to hold bottom of zipper.
Socks	Soft, stretchy socks Large size Tube sock (no set place for heel) Ankle socks first, proceeding to calf or over the calf Loops sewn into socks Sock aide or donner	Sit on stable surface (e.g., chair, floor). Lie on back and prop foot on opposite knee. Fold or roll sock before putting it over the toes and pulling up. Use backward chaining.
Shoes	Long-opening shoes (many eyes) with loose laces Broad shoe (not tight) Slip-on shoes Hook and loop tab closures Elastic laces already tied Elastic curly laces that do not need tying Tabs at heels for pulling shoes on Long-handled shoehorns	Sit on stable surface (e.g., chair, floor). Prop up foot on stool or chair. Lie on back and prop foot on opposite knee. Flex legs and point toes downward. Use gravity to help push heel into shoe (e.g., push down on a hard surface).

maneuvering a wheelchair. If the shirt is cut longer in the back and shorter in the front, it is easier to keep a neat appearance. Rain or winter capes are comfortable in a wheelchair. They are cut longer in the front to cover the child's legs and feet and shorter in the back so that they do not rub against the wheel of the wheelchair.[142]

For children who wear orthoses for spinal support, front openings that extend from the neck to the lower abdomen make self-dressing easier, whereas back openings are easier when others dress the child.[88,142] Caregivers should use larger clothing that fits over orthoses but should avoid loose sleeves for children who push wheelchairs. The child who wears an ankle-foot orthosis may need to have clothing reinforced to protect against rubbing. This is done by sewing fabric patches inside the garment where friction and stress occur and by adapting pants with side seams and hook and loop closures so that the pants fit easily over the orthosis.

When children require gastrostomy feedings, tracheotomy care, catheterization, or diapering, they need clothing that allows easy access. Caregivers can sew moisture-resistant fabric into the seat of pants, on collars, on attaching bibs, and on sleeve cuffs (if the child bites clothing).[161] Jumpsuits or shirts with hook and loop closures at the gastrostomy site, neckline, shoulder, crotch, or pant leg allow caregivers to perform medical procedures without removing the child's clothing.[88,142,161] Refer to the Evolve website for Internet resources on dressing methods, clothing, and other suggestions.

Bathing or Showering

Typical Development

A child's interest in bathing begins before 2 years of age, when he or she begins to wash while in the tub. By 4 years of age, children wash and dry themselves with supervision. It is not until 8 years of age that children independently prepare the bath and shower water (e.g., the appropriate depth and temperature) and wash and dry themselves independently.

Good grooming habits are important for all children but take on added significance for children with disabilities. At an early age, the caregiver needs to encourage and help the child with a disability to achieve cleanliness to maintain his or her health. Bathing should be a pleasurable activity. For the parent of a child who lacks postural stability, bathing becomes a tedious task that requires constant attention and alertness. The work involved multiplies as the child grows and becomes larger and heavier.

Cultural expectations and social routines for bathing vary, and the occupational therapist should consider them when assessing a child's independence. He or she must respect family preferences as to how often a person bathes and with whom (e.g., parent and child bathing together).

Establishing or Restoring Performance

Occupational therapists often use bathing therapeutically to improve body capabilities that interfere with independence. A warm bath may calm a child who is distressed and may decrease tonicity and increase ROM and independent movement. When a child is hypersensitive, water play, rubbing with a washcloth, and deep pressure or rubbing while drying the child may help reduce the child's sensitivity to touch. For children who have difficulty interacting with others or the environment, bath play may motivate the child to explore objects, engage in pretend play, and interact with a sibling or parent.

For children with motor limitations, the occupational therapist may prepare the child to participate more fully in self-bathing. The occupational therapist may use activities to improve ROM, bilateral coordination, grasp, postural control, and motor planning before teaching bathing. Activities or games (e.g., "Simon Says") that require a child to reach above or behind or down to the toes may give him or her the body awareness and necessary movement for self-bathing. While the child is in the tub, many bath toys (e.g., pour, squeeze or wind-up toys, soap crayons, floating boats) are useful to increase ROM, coordination, play skills, and interactions with others. Body paints are useful in cueing and motivating the child to "wash the part with the paint or X on it."

Adapting the Task or Environment

The caregiver's positioning and handling are prime considerations in adapting bathing of children. Children with cerebral palsy may lose their balance when startled. Keeping the child's head and arms forward when lifting and lowering him or her into the tub prevents a reaction of full extension. The caregiver should use slow gentle movements with the child and provide simple verbal cues about the steps of bathing. Draining the tub and wrapping the child in a towel before lifting him or her from the tub makes the child feel more secure.

Parents often need suggestions for bathing a child who is hypersensitive to touch or temperature. This child may avoid bathing at all costs and is at risk of getting hurt while in the tub. Understanding the child's sensory needs and using adaptive techniques may help bathing become a positive experience for parent and child. Preparatory activities that give the child deep pressure before bathing are sometimes helpful, especially deep pressure to the head before shampooing. The child may prefer washing the back and extremities first, and then the stomach and face, using rhythmic, organized, deep strokes. Some parents and children find a hand-held shower with an eye guard hat useful for removing soapsuds (especially during hair washing) and avoiding getting soap in the eyes. Adjusting the water flow or temperature of the hand-held shower and allowing the child to operate it gives the child more control over the direction of the water pressure on his or her body. Sometimes, with children who have tactile sensitivity, using a cup with water is a more relaxing way to rinse off than a shower spray. Wrapping the child in a tight towel after bathing and holding the child with deep pressure also helps.

Adaptive positioning or special equipment may provide support that helps the child feel safe and secure. Bath hammocks hold the body fully and enable the parent to wash the child thoroughly (Figure 15-9, *A*). A light inconspicuous bath support offers design features well adapted to the needs of children with motor deficits (see Figure 15-9, *B*). The front half of the support ring swings open for easy entry and then locks securely, holding the child at the chest to give trunk stability. Various types of bath seats and shower benches (see Figure 15-9C) are available to the older child for help in bathtub seating and transfers. For the child with severe motor limitations who is lying supine in the tub in shallow water, a horseshoe-shaped inflatable bath collar supports the neck and keeps the child's head above water. A bath stretcher is constructed like a cot and fits inside the bathtub at rim or midtub

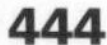

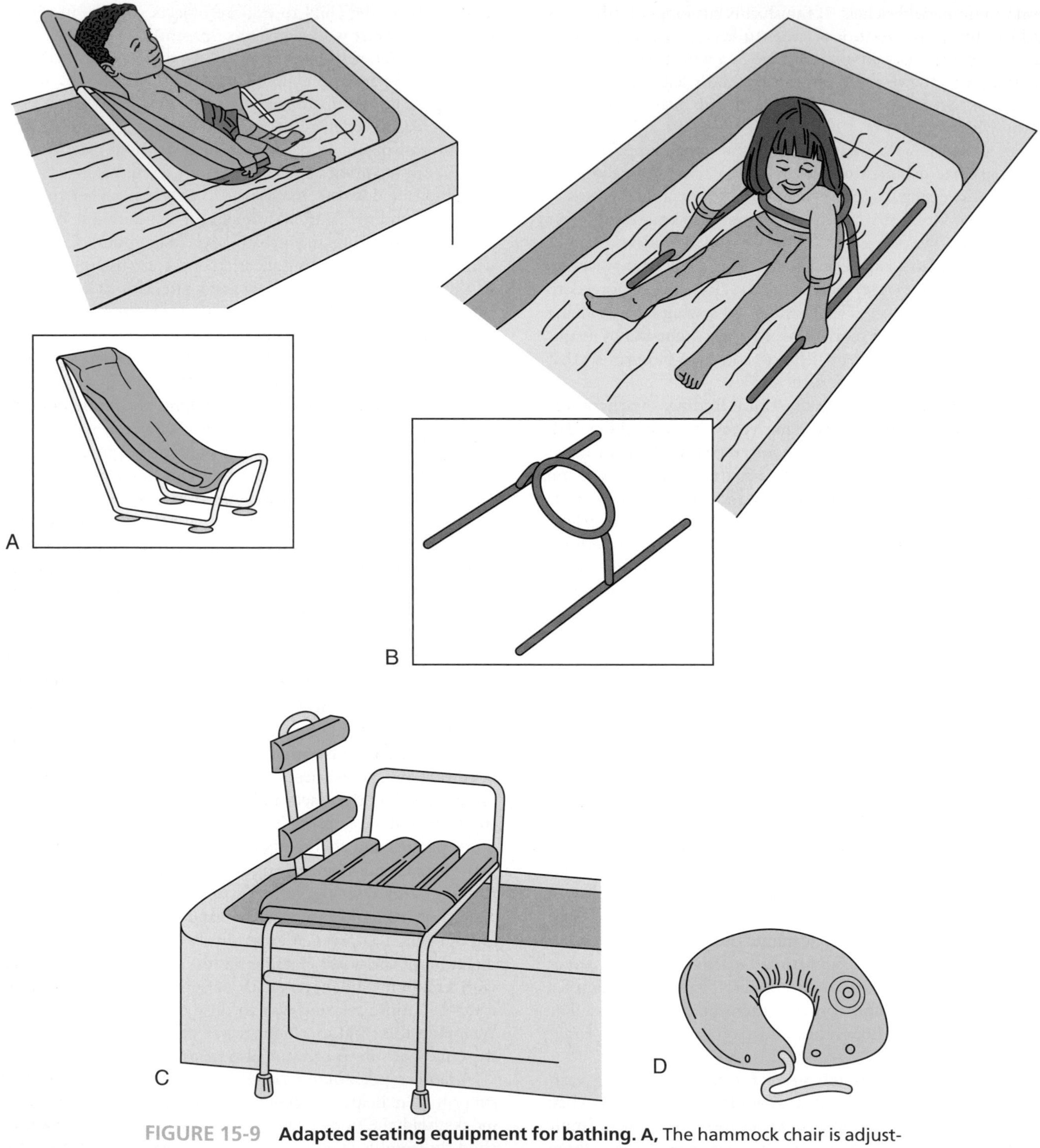

FIGURE 15-9 **Adapted seating equipment for bathing. A,** The hammock chair is adjustable and equipped with oversized suction feet. It fully supports the child who has no sitting balance and poor head control. **B,** A trunk support ring is lightweight and compact and fits all bathtubs. **C,** A shower bench aids seating and transfers. **D,** An inflatable bath collar can be used when the child is in either the supine or the prone position.

level to minimize the caregiver's bending while transferring and bathing the child. As noted, sometimes home modifications such as rolling shower stalls or built-in bath benches are better solutions to increase independence and/or protect the caregiver's back.

Prevention and Education for Bathing Safety

Parent and child education about bathing safety helps prevent injury. Constant monitoring until the child demonstrates safety in the tub is necessary. Sometimes, parents do not teach independence in bathing because they worry that the child may injure himself or herself if left alone. Following a safe routine for bathing, teaching the child what he or she is and is not allowed to do in the tub or shower, and grading the amount of assistance and monitoring help develop independence. Nonslip bath mats beside and in the tub are essential for safety. Grab bars and their placement require careful thought and planning in each individual case. A rubber cover for the bathtub faucet prevents injury if the child touches it or slips and hits the head. Faucets need to be marked for temperature, and children can be directed to begin running their own bath water by first putting on the cold water and then slowly adding hot water.

Through coaching and/or educational materials, parents are taught to use good body mechanics during bathing to prevent back injury. To lessen strain, it is best for the adult to sit on a stool beside the tub or kneel on a cushion. Lifting is done with the knees bent and the back straight, with the legs used for power. As children get older and heavier, a Hoyer lift or an easily accessed shower stall arrangement may be necessary. Parents may need assistance in planning renovations that will assist the child in being independent and/or assist them for the future growth of the child.

Personal Hygiene and Grooming

Skill Development

By 2 years of age, children imitate their parents when brushing their teeth. Supervision of tooth brushing continues until about 6 years of age. Tooth brushing is especially difficult for the child with oral sensitivity. The child should use his or her preferred brushing methods until tolerance improves and he or she accomplishes more thorough cleaning. A small soft brush is easier to move around in the mouth, especially if the child has a tongue thrust or gag reflex. When the child's gums are tender, the caregiver may substitute a soft, sponge-tipped Toothette for a brush. For the child who brushes independently, an electric toothbrush allows more thorough cleaning. This is a good solution for children with limited dexterity, although for children with weakness, an electric toothbrush may be too heavy to manage.

If a child has problems with a weak grasp, the caregiver can enlarge the toothbrush handle with sponge rubber or add a hook and loop strap. One-handed flossing tools are available in large and small sizes and can be adapted by increasing the width or length of the handle. A hand-over-hand technique helps a child learn how to direct the toothbrush in the mouth and reach all teeth (Figure 15-10). As the child starts doing the movement, gestures or only verbal prompts may be needed. As always, a routine sequence for tooth brushing, gradual fading out of cues, and visual pictures about the process assist the child with underlying memory or performance skill problems.

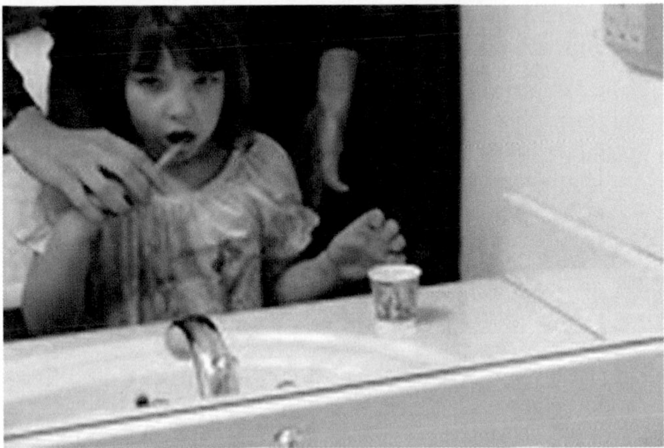

FIGURE 15-10 A hand-over-hand approach works well for Lydia, who is sensitive to tooth brushing. She is participating in the activity and directing which part of the teeth she wants to brush first.

Face washing, hand washing, and hair care are typical grooming activities taught to preschoolers and young children. The family's culture and values and individual interests strongly influence the timing of the development of grooming independence. Adolescence begins at the onset of puberty and is a period of remarkable growth toward physical, sexual, emotional, and social maturity. The physiologic changes that occur at puberty are attributable in part to the increased output of hormones by the pituitary gland. For example, body hair grows, and the sebaceous glands become more active, producing oily secretions. With these physical changes and different social expectations (depending on the culture), new self-maintenance tasks emerge, including skin care, hair styling, hair removal, and application of cosmetics.

In their book, *Caring for Myself*,[44] Gast and Krug give verbal and visual sequences for brushing teeth, getting a haircut, hand washing, bathing, and going to the doctor. The book offers practical prompts, optional considerations for working with sensory issues, and ways to generalize skills and embed self-care activities within a routine. Templates for social stories, which are modifiable for different children, can be used for children who need a script or visual cuing to initiate, sequence, and complete grooming tasks.

Intervention

Grooming is an aspect of ADLs that is highly influenced by cultural values. The occupational therapist must respect the child and family's preferences in regard to hairstyle, cosmetics, and routines. The family and child or adolescent need to take the lead in identifying their concerns and priorities. Problem solving follows the principles and approaches identified in the first sections of this chapter. Case Study 15-3 is an example of an adolescent who desires independence in grooming.

Sexual Activity

While the therapist is working with children on ADL tasks such as bathing or personal hygiene, sexuality questions may arise. Sexuality includes the physical and psychological nature of feeling attractive and/or engaging in intimacy through touch,

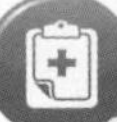

CASE STUDY 15-3 Josie

Josie demonstrates incoordination, poor memory, and limited judgment, but she wants to be independent in her grooming. Josie has worked on improving her coordination so that she can brush her own hair or manipulate the grooming materials, but adaptation strategies are essential to increase her independence in grooming. The occupational therapist recommends that Josie use a brush with a built-up handle, rest her elbow on the table while brushing her hair to stabilize her ataxic movements, use a checklist and visual model, and ask a peer to help style her hair. Josie and her parents are educated about ways to incorporate grooming tasks into everyday routines by placing visual and natural cues in the environment, such as keeping the deodorant on the dresser. Leaving facial cleansing equipment out on the sink gives Josie a visual cue to use it before applying makeup.

kissing, hugging, or intercourse.[11] Although society often still views persons with disabilities as asexual beings,[106] children and adolescents of all disabilities are sexual beings, and adolescence is a critical time when sexual identity is developed.[110] Adolescents with chronic health care conditions may have delayed puberty and growth, as well as observable physical disabilities that make them feel unattractive.[91]

Sexual activities need to be discussed to prevent social exploitation, abuse, sexually transmitted diseases, and pregnancy.[157] Children with developmental disabilities are more prone to the risk of exploitation, often because of the following: (1) they must depend on others for basic needs; (2) they frequently have multiple caregivers; (3) their connection with authority figures is one of learned helplessness or nondiscriminatory compliance; and (4) they have difficulty with social, reasoning, judgment, and problem-solving skills.[31,160] Children with limited communication are at high risk for exploitation, and specific phrases or comments may need to be programmed into their augmentative communication device to protect them from exploitation.[21]

For occupational therapists working with children on very personal daily living activities, it is important to help children differentiate between necessary touch (e.g., diaper changing, catheter instruction, menstrual care, hygiene) and intimate touch. Hinsburger has suggested that occupational therapists and parents always do the following[64]:

- Ask permission before touching.
- Describe what they are doing and why.
- Facilitate participation when performing necessary touch activities.
- Communicate with the child about what was done and why and about any feelings after intimate touch.

Parents may be receptive to discussing their child's sexuality, or they may feel unprepared to address these issues. If parents and professionals begin talking about sexuality education in early childhood (e.g., body, gender, touching, privacy, expressing affection, boundaries), the need to approach complex subjects such as refusal behavior, dating, birth control, and sexuality rights will not be as difficult a transition.[110] Melberg-Schwier and Hingsburger have written an excellent book to guide parents as they embark on this topic.[104] If the child is younger than 18 years, occupational therapists must obtain parental permission to discuss sexuality issues. Occupational therapists need to consider the contextual aspects of the child's family and social groups and determine whether it is appropriate to discuss sexuality and who should discuss it (receiver and informant). Occupational therapists who decide to enter a discourse on sexuality must consider their own knowledge, beliefs, and attitudes so that they give children and their families the correct information nonjudgmentally. They may refer the child to someone who is more knowledgeable about sexuality and more comfortable discussing it. Responsible occupational therapists are careful to separate their personal values with regard to sexuality from those of the client and family. The Evolve website gives a number of online resources for talking about sexuality with children with disabilities.

Children and adolescents with cognitive problems related to intellectual disabilities or a traumatic brain injury often need guidelines for expressing their sexuality appropriately in various contexts.[26,27] Appropriate touch from others, dress and hygiene, masturbation, touching of others, and appropriate interactions with the opposite gender are areas in which education is required to prevent abuse and prosecution for sexual misconduct. Adolescent girls and boys need preparation for the changes that will occur in their bodies at puberty. As children are transitioning into adolescence, questions about how a specific disability (e.g., spina bifida, spinal cord injury) affects sexual abilities and activities often emerge.[138] Older adolescents with chronic health conditions need specific answers and ideas for expressing sexuality in a healthy way.[91] An adolescent may question the physical and psychosocial aspects of sexuality and his or her ability to conceive. Information about contraceptive use and techniques for avoiding intercourse are essential for the adolescent to avoid unwanted pregnancies. As adolescents with disabilities consider conceiving and bearing children in the future, it may be helpful to talk to other parents with disabilities or become aware of online support groups and resources. Table 15-10 presents the information that children need about sexual activity across the age span.

Annon has developed the PLISSIT model to teach people with disabilities about sexuality.[7] This model is based on four phases of information giving: (1) Permission to ask about sexuality, (2) Limited Information given, (3) Specific Suggestions, and (4) Intensive Therapy (usually provided by a trained counselor or psychologist who understands sexuality in individuals with disabilities). This model teaches staff about sexuality issues and informs clients about who is willing to discuss sexuality with them. Taylor and Davis have proposed using an extended PLISSIT model, in which giving permission to talk about each phase is required before proceeding.[163] In some settings, staff members wear a button saying "I'm askable" to designate comfort in talking about sexuality. While practicing bed mobility, dressing, personal hygiene, positioning, and communication and interaction skills, the adolescent often asks sexuality

TABLE 15-10 Typical Sexuality Concepts Discussed with Children and Adolescents with Disabilities

Age (yr)	Typical Behaviors or Concepts to Learn
Birth-2	Touches genitals for sensory pleasure Experiences affection and touch
3-5	Shows interest in genitals of the opposite sex Learns proper names of genitals (social demands) Plays "show me" games with other children Understands that others should not touch his or her genitals Learns that some behaviors are acceptable in public, others to be done in private (e.g., masturbation, undressing) Begins to learn privacy rights (e.g., close doors, knock and wait to enter, close blinds) Begins to learn rules for touch and affection boundaries and authority figures
6-8	Knows differences between boys and girls Names body parts correctly Learns basic elements and language of reproduction and pregnancy Learns about relationships (e.g., friends, mutual respect) and decision making Thinks about social responsibility Understands appropriate and inappropriate social and sexual behaviors Understands necessary (e.g., personal hygiene) and intimate touch Avoids and reports sexual exploitation (understands necessary touch and intimate touch)
9-11	Shows interest in social relationships Discusses body image Discusses sexuality within family Understands personal boundaries Knows how to use refusal skills Understands body changes that will occur during puberty (and any impact on his or her disease or disability) Knows about reproduction and pregnancy Learns about sexually transmitted diseases and the need to abstain from sexual intercourse Avoids or reports sexual abuse (understands necessary touch and intimate touch)
12-18	Is sensitive and private about body Compares body with others and may be critical Asks questions about changes occurring (physical and emotional) Shows more interest in caring for body (e.g., hair, face, exercise) Discusses sexuality and sexual identity with friends Uses preventive health care routinely (e.g., breast, gynecologic, testicular examinations) Begins dating and learning about communication and love Uses values to guide actions in intimacy Expresses sexuality through dress, body movement, or intercourse Understands reproduction, pregnancy, and birth control Knows how to use contraceptives and prevent diseases (safe sex) Asks for or is given genetic counseling Identifies and uses community sexual health services

Adapted from Couwenhoven, T. (2001). Sexuality education: Building a foundation of healthy attitudes. *Disability Solutions, 4*(6), 1–8; Lawrence, K. E., & Niemeyer, S. (1994). Behavior management and psychosocial issues: Sexuality issues. In K. E. Lawrence & S. Niemeyer (Eds.), *Caregiver education guide for children with developmental disabilities* (pp. 236-245). Frederick, MD: Aspen; and National Information Center for Children and Youth with Disabilities (NICHCY). (1992). Sexuality education for children and youth with disabilities. *NICHCY News Digest, 1*(3), 1–6.

questions. Depending on the situation and therapy setting, occupational therapists address these questions in the context in which the questions are asked.[91] For example, while practicing bed mobility, 17-year-old Belinda, who recently suffered a spinal cord injury, asks, "How can I ever have sex with a guy? Can I have a baby?" With prior parental permission, this may be an opportune time to discuss contraceptives, positioning, use of intact senses, control of distracting environmental stimuli, and the medical need to empty her bladder or bowels before sexual activity. Referral to her physician or a gynecologist is appropriate, as is referral to her psychologist or counselor.

If the parents approve, occupational therapists give additional information in a written, oral, or video format and provide the adolescent with the opportunity to talk to older adolescents or adults who have similar disabilities. Sexuality education needs a team approach, and occupational therapists may work with physicians, nurses, or pharmacists to discuss the use of certain medicines and how they affect sexual function. Memory aids for medicine schedules or contraceptive use may also be helpful.

Care of Personal Devices

With maturity, children learn to take care of their personal devices, such as hearing aids, glasses, contact lenses, orthotics, prosthetics, catheters, and/or a variety of pieces of assistive technology used for toileting, grooming, feeding, and dressing. As the child learns how to use these devices, it is essential that he or she know how to clean and maintain them. How many glasses are lost or broken because they are not put back in a case, and how many splints melted by being left in a car? By encouraging children to take responsibility for these devices, perhaps many of these mishaps could be avoided.

Performance Patterns

Developing routines and habits for maintaining items helps children care for their assistive devices. In collaboration with the child, parent, or teacher, occupational therapists can help establish a routine for daily or weekly maintenance of items. Embedding this routine at a naturally occurring time helps the child remember to do the task. For example, the child cleans her or his catheter when getting home from school; before bed, he or she places it back in the fanny pack for the next day. This is often an opportune time to discuss health maintenance activities and routines. Table 15-11 gives an example of health care maintenance for typically developing children and children with spina bifida. Case Study 15-4 shows how developing a routine can help a child care for an assistive device.

Directing Others

Not all children have the motor and praxis skills to clean their glasses, wash their adaptive utensils, or fill a wheelchair cushion with air. Asking someone else to do the task or put equipment away and directing others on how to care for an adaptive aid are possibilities. The child may say, "My wheelchair is riding rough. Would you mind checking the tire pressure?" or "My splint strap is broken." Educating children about their adaptive devices gives them a feeling of responsibility for the device and may help prevent breakdown or nonuse of the device. This also incorporates the skills needed for self-determination and self-efficacy.

Sleep and Rest

Sleep and rest are essential for a child's growth and well-being because it allows children and their parents to restore energy for everyday occupations, including ADLs. Lack of sleep may compromise a child's occupational performance and their physical growth, health, and ability to behave.[139,178] When

TABLE 15-11 Health Care Maintenance for Typically Developing Children and Children with Spina Bifida

Age (yr)	Health Care Maintenance with Typical Development*	Additional Health Maintenance Issues for Child with Spina Bifida
5-9	Follows safety rules at home and school Informs others of emergencies Uses basic first-aid techniques for minor injuries Tells other when he or she is sick Cares for health care items with reminders (e.g., glasses, toothbrush) Routinely washes hands; takes a bath and washes hair with reminders Assists in getting medicine ready	Does pressure reliefs and checks for skin breakdown (e.g., legs, buttocks, and feet) with reminders Tells others when he or she is injured or feels sick (e.g., headache, pain, swelling, change in bowel and bladder patterns) Cares for personal adaptive devices (e.g., crutches, wheelchair, catheters) with reminders Performs self-catheterization at home and school Carries a list of current medicines and doctors' names
10-14	Recognizes when he or she is getting sick or needs to see a doctor Knows emergency procedures (e.g., phone numbers, who to call, what to do) Cares for health care items (e.g., glasses, braces, retainers, facial scrubs) Uses first-aid procedures Eats nutritious meals with supervision Exercises with supervision Takes medicine with supervision Avoids cigarettes, drugs, and sexual abuse	Recognizes when he or she is injured or feels sick (e.g., headache, pain, swelling, change in bowel and bladder pattern) Knows dosage of medications Knows names of doctors (e.g., primary care, urologist, neurologist, orthopedist) Cares for personal adaptive devices (e.g., wheelchair, walker, braces) or instructs others in how to maintain devices Performs self-catheterization in community environments Prevents further health care problems (e.g., drinks to avoid bladder infection, exercises [push-ups]; avoids latex; maintains good hygiene, eating, and exercise practices)
15-18	Recognizes when a change in medicine or health intervention is needed Makes appointment to see doctors Eats nutritious meals Exercises regularly Cares for personal hygiene and follows good health habits Uses first-aid procedures for major and minor injuries Takes medicine when needed Uses birth control as needed	Takes medications independently and knows side effects Knows how to access therapy, doctors, and other health care services Knows how to obtain and pay for medical supplies Prevents secondary disabilities (e.g., manages weight, follows routine medical care, skin care, equipment maintenance)

*Adherence to protocols for medicines, personal devices, health routines, and so on.
Adapted from Ford, A., Schnorr, R., Meyer, L., et al. (1989). *The Syracuse community-reference curriculum guide* (pp. 324–327). Baltimore: Paul H. Brookes; and Peterson, P. M., Rauen, K. K., Brown, J., & Cole, J. (1994). Spina bifida: The transition into adulthood begins in infancy. *Rehabilitation Nursing, 19*(4), 229–238.

CASE STUDY 15-4 Feddah

Feddah is 9 years old and has worn hearing aids for 2 years, after having viral meningitis. Until last month, her parents cared for the hearing aids until Feddah "wanted to do it herself." Because her parents are encouraging Feddah to be self-determined, they thought this was a good idea. Unfortunately, last week, Feddah had a very severe ear infection that the doctor attributed to improper cleaning of her hearing aids. Mom happened to mention this problem to the occupational therapist, who was seeing Feddah to increase her written production and dexterity in manipulating objects. The therapist collaborated with Mom, the audiologist, and Feddah to develop a routine and visual schedule to clean her hearing aids. Feddah's hearing aid case is left on the dresser as a naturally occurring cue to remind her to remove, clean, and put away the hearing aids each night. By using anticipatory problem solving,[124] the therapist and Feddah discussed the task and where the wipes and hearing aid case should be kept. They also discussed how to clean the hearing aids when wipes were not available and how she would handle the care of her hearing aids when on a sleepover. Feddah anticipated that her friend's little sister might try to play with her hearing aids and that she had better ask her friend's mother to help her find a safe place for her hearing aid box. If she forgot her hearing aid box, she would ask for a baggie to store the aids. Figure 15-11 gives an example of a task analysis and data collection sheet for tracking Feddah's routine and success in caring for her own hearing aids. By means of this tracking sheet, the occupational therapist could see if Feddah's performance was improving.

Name: Feddah Week of: May 21st

Activity: Cleaning hearing aid Environment: Home, in bedroom

Verbal cue: "Time to go to bed and take out your hearing aids"

Physical set up: Feddah is at her dresser that is waist high.

Visual cues: Tissues, wipes, hearing aid box is out on dresser top as a visual reminder to do this every night.

Steps	Task analysis	Dates					Comments
		5/21	5/22	5/23	5/24	5/25	
1	Turn off hearing aid	✓-	✓-	✓	✓	✓	
2	Remove hearing aid from ear before bathing or bed	✓	✓	✓	✓	✓	Consistent!
3	Wipe ear mold surfaces with a tissue	A (V)	A (V)	✓	✓	✓	
4	Disinfect the ear mold surface with a disinfectant towelette (non-alcohol based)	A (P)	A (P)	A (V)	✓-	✓-	Rubs hearing aid too vigorously.
5	Check batteries of hearing aid	0	0	A (V)	✓-	✓-	Added a visual picture to remember this.
6	Place hearing aid back in hearing aid box for storage	A (V)	✓-	✓-	✓-	✓-	
7	Keep in a safe and cool place	✓	✓	✓	✓	✓	
Total steps completed this day	Target ✓ = Did it	2	2	4	4	5	Making progress this week!! She is really learning the task.
	Target ✓- = Did most of it	1	2	1	2	2	
	A = Did with verbal (V) or physical prompt (P)	1P 2V	1P 1V	2V	1V	0	
	0 = Didn't do it	1	1	0	0	0	

FIGURE 15-11 Sample task analysis for hearing aid maintenance.

inadequate sleep occurs, cycles of REM (rapid eye movement) and NREM (non–rapid eye movement) sleep are shortened, and memory, muscle repair, and hormone release are stunted. As a result, an illness or its symptoms may be exacerbated.[50,92,117] Babies who are more easily awakened have more episodes of apnea when they are sleep-deprived.[41] Recent studies have shown that sleep deprivation affects cognitive, attention, and social skill development.[117,133,164] Chronic deprivation of sleep may result in a propensity for depression or suicidal ideation.[116,133] In addition, when parents and other household members become sleep-deprived because a child has difficulty sleeping, their ability to meet role expectations (at school, home, work, or in the community) may be affected.[85,121,178]

Sleep disturbances are often tolerated for a few days. They may occur with children occasionally because of illness or special events and emotions (e.g., special party or upcoming concert, moving to a new classroom, staying up later than usual). When sleep is chronically disrupted for weeks at a time, negative effects are inevitable, and possible causes for the sleep disturbance need to be determined.[36,115]

Evaluation of Sleep and Sleep Needs at Different Ages

The International Classification of Sleep Disorders has identified more than 80 different types of sleep disorders.[2] The National Sleep Foundation[111] recommends regular sleep routines and patterns, with similar amounts of sleep each night.[86] Sleep disorders in children are identified as five main problems: bedtime resistance or falling asleep, awakening during the night, irregularity of amount of time in sleep, snoring, and sleepiness during the day.[115] Occupational therapists have a vital role in helping parents develop the bedtime and self-care routines needed to promote healthy habits and patterns for sleep.[4] Table 15-12 describes the typical amount of sleep needed for children and youth at different ages and lists possible factors impeding sleep.

Sometimes, parents are so concerned with the medical needs of their child that sleep is low on their priority list to discuss with physicians or occupational therapists. Physicians and health care professionals need to ask all parents and/or children about their sleep habits.[108] If a caregiver or child reports sleep difficulties consistently to a physician, a sleep screening questionnaire may be given, as well as a nocturnal polysomnography or actigraphy.[83] Screening questionnaires help identify what may be interfering with a child's sleep. A variety of screening questionnaires for sleep disturbances in infants, children, and adolescents have been developed.[146] The Evolve website lists sleep questionnaires most commonly used in research.

Polysomnography measures brain wave, muscle, cardiovascular, and breathing activity during sleep by placing 16 electrodes on the body. Figure 15-12 demonstrates what this might look like for a child. For some children with sensory sensitivities, these procedures are invasive and difficult to tolerate. Actigraphy uses an actimeter that is worn on the wrist or sewn into clothing to measure circadian rhythms and muscle movements during sleep and wake periods.[134] Research suggests that actigraphy and polysomnography results are similar in identifying the quality of sleep.[66]

Assessment of a child's activity level, bedtime routines, sleep habits, and sleep environments often indicates what may be hindering sleep. As always, it is important first to determine the routines and whether cultural considerations influence the sleep habits of the family or child.[147] For example, some parents may sleep in the same room or bed with the infant or child, or the infant sleeps in the family living area instead of a bedroom. Some parents place the sleeping baby in a hammock or in a tightly swaddled prone position. Asking caregivers questions about sleep is essential to begin to understand their values and understanding of sleep hygiene:

- Does your child have regular sleep patterns (bedtime, naptimes, amount of uninterrupted sleep)?
- Where does the child sleep?
- With whom or what (e.g., stuffed animal) does the child sleep?
- When is the child put to bed or to sleep?
- What are typical bedtime routines?
- How long does it take your child to fall asleep?

Table 15-13 gives definitions of quality of sleep, assessment ideas, and questions to ask parents or caregivers to determine if a child has a sleep problem.

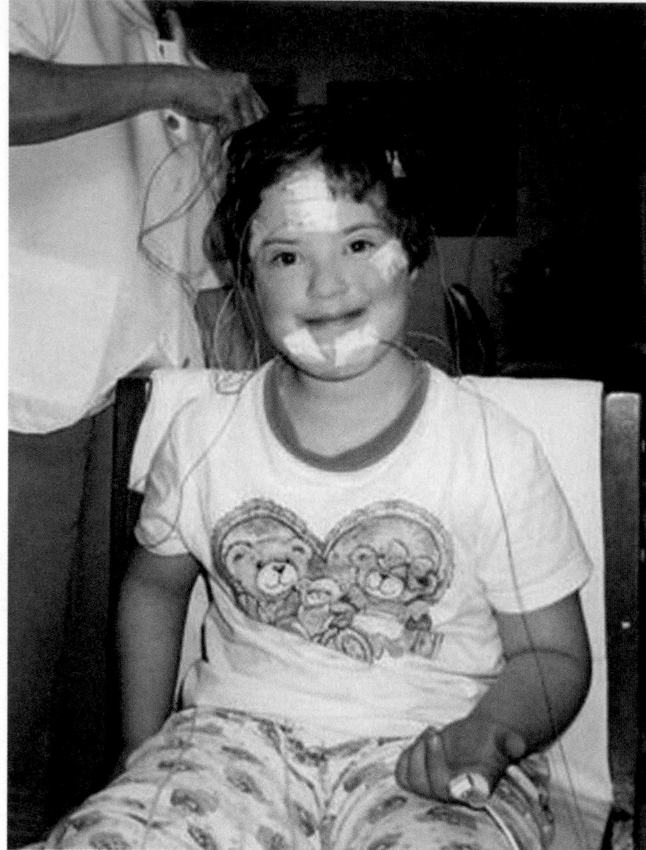

FIGURE 15-12 Bella is having electrodes attached to have a nocturnal polysomnography test.

Sleep Issues for Children with Disabilities

Children with disorders such as asthma, ADHD, allergies, diabetes, cerebral palsy, epilepsy, sickle cell disease, obesity, or brain injury often have sleep disturbance issues.[50,92,117] Children

TABLE 15-12 Typical Amount of Sleep Needed at Different Ages and Possible Factors Impeding Sleep

Age	Amount of Sleep Needed	Naps	Factors to Consider When Child Has Sleep Problems
Newborn, 1-2 mo	12-18 hr 50-60 min REM-NREM cycle	Throughout day	No established sleep/wake cycle Interrupted sleep related to feeding, comfort needs (diaper changes), medical procedures, sleep apnea alarms (if used), or too much sleep during the day When asleep and put to bed, baby wakes up with change in position
3-11 mo	12-18 hr	Three or four times daily, 30 min-2 hr	Usually cannot sleep through the night without feedings until 6 mo of age 70%-80% sleep through the night by 9 months Separation anxiety interferes with sleep Has not learned to self-soothe and is dependent on parents (needs to be drowsy or already asleep to be placed in crib) May be insecure with attachment or always wants to engage with others
Toddler, 1-3 yr	12-14 hr	Once or twice daily (18 mo, once a day), 1-3 hr	Fewer naps needed Needs independence Anxiety about going to sleep (may relate to separation anxiety, inability to self-soothe, imagination, fear of being alone, nightmares) Difficulty with transitions Gets out of bed independently
Preschoolers 3.1-4.11 yr	11-13 hr	Once daily	Bed wetting Nighttime fears or nightmares because of imagination developing (e.g., fear of being alone, the dark, tigers under the bed) Peak age for sleepwalking and sleep terrors Television watching too close to bedtime Outgrown the need for naps and not sleepy when put to bed
School age, 5-10 yr	10-11 hr	0	Bed wetting (typical until age 7) Medical issues—tonsils enlarged, facial profile is convex, has cross bite, reflux or medical procedure (e.g., positioning, suction) Unaware of social cues for calming down to go to sleep Increased demands for schoolwork or other extracurricular activities More interest in computers and internet Caffeine consumption or eating close to bedtime Electronic use in the bedroom or too close to bedtime (e.g., computers, televisions, tablets, video games) Erratic sleep schedule Lack of understanding of the importance of healthy routines for sleep
Teens, 10.1-17 yr	8.5-9.25 hr		Increased demands of school, work, social life, or other activities Anxiety or emotional event during the day Caffeine consumption or eating close to bedtime Electronic use in the bedroom or too close to bedtime (e.g., computers, televisions, tablets, video games, smartphones) Erratic sleep schedule especially weekend versus weekday nights Internal clock of teens—like late nights and waking up later in the morning Lack of understanding of importance for healthy routines for sleep

Data from Mindell, J. A., Meltzer, L. J., Carskadon, M. A., & Chervin, R. (2009). Developmental aspects of sleep hygiene: Findings from the 2004 National Sleep Foundation Sleep in America Poll. *Sleep Medicine, 10,* 771–779; National Sleep Foundation (2013). *Children and sleep.* Retrieved from http://www.sleep foundation.org/article/sleep-topics/children-and-sleep; and National Sleep Foundation (2013). *Understanding children's sleep habits.* Retrieved from http://www.sleepforkids.org/html/habits.html.

who are typically developing have a prevalence of sleep disorders ranging from 10% to 50%, whereas 50% to 80% of children with ASD have sleep disorders.[1,68,128] Parents report that anxiety or resistance to going to sleep often disrupts their child's sleep.[49,51,72,96,117,155]

Children who are recently adopted or who are abused may have sleep latency and awakening problems because they may feel anxious and insecure when going to sleep or waking up.[18] Parents of children with physical disabilities identified concerns about child comfort and safety, and more than 50% thought that positioning aids or orthotics during bedtime hindered sleep.[178]

Occupational Therapy Interventions for Sleep Disorders

Occupational therapists work with physicians, other health care professionals, parents, teachers, and the child to help determine

TABLE 15-13 Sleep Quality Definitions and Assessments for Children with Sleep Issues

BEARS Algorithm (Measurement of Sleep Quality)	Definition	Assessment	Questions to Ask Parents, Caregivers, or Child	Possible Reasons for Sleep Issue
*B*edtime or sleep latency	Time between trying to sleep and actually going to sleep	Sleep log Routines used when going to bed Consistent bedtime? Nocturnal polysomnography or actigraphy Sleep questionnaires	How long does it take your child to fall asleep? Is your child resistant to go to bed or has difficulty going to bed? Does he or she get out of bed frequently prior to sleeping? Does he or she seem anxious when going to bed?	Lack of routines Too early or too late to bed Family discord Social, emotional issues
*E*xcessive tiredness during the day	Ability to stay awake during the day	Parent, child, or teacher questionnaire Youth self-report Actigraphy Sleep questionnaires	Is your child hard to wake up in the morning? Does your child fall asleep during the day outside of scheduled naps? Does he or she complain of being tired or is he or she drowsy, moody, irritable, and/or looks tired to you?	Not enough sleep Irregular sleep Sleep apnea Illness Stress or anxiety
*A*wakenings at night	After going to sleep, number of times the child awakens at night	Sleep log by parents Sleep log by youth, if able Nocturnal polysomnography or actigraphy Sleep questionnaires	Does your child wake up at night? What interrupts his or her sleep? How many times does he or she wake up? Does he or she go back to sleep? Does he or she sleep walk or talk?	Sleep terrors or nightmares Environment is noisy or overstimulating Lack of exercise during the day Eating too close to bedtime Restless leg syndrome Illness
*R*egularity and duration of sleep	Time child goes to sleep and amount of time sleeping (when sleep began and ended)	Sleep log by parents or youth, if able Environmental assessment Nocturnal polysomnography or actigraphy Sleep questionnaires	How many hours does your child sleep? Does he or she have a regular bedtime on weekdays and weekends? What is the bedtime? How many hours does your child sleep?	
*S*noring	Amount and loudness of gasping, choking, or snoring while sleeping	Observation of parents while child sleeps Reports of youth or sibling who sleeps in same room Testing for sleep apnea Sleep questionnaires	Does your child snore at night? Does he or she gasp for air or choke while sleeping? How often? Is the snoring loud or has it changed?	Sleep apnea
Movement or sleep efficiency	Amount of movement during sleep (may have restless leg syndrome)	Observation of parents or siblings who sleep in same room Report of youth, if able Nocturnal polysomnography or actigraphy Sleep questionnaires	When your child sleeps, are the legs restless or move a lot? Are the covers in disarray? Does your child change positions frequently when sleeping? Does your child end up at the other end of the bed after being asleep?	Restless leg syndrome

Adapted from National Sleep Foundation (2013). *Children and sleep.* Retrieved from http://www.sleep foundation.org/article/sleep-topics/children-and-sleep; and Owens, J., & Mindell, J. (2005). *Take charge of your child's sleep: The all-in-one resource for solving sleep problems in kids and teens.* New York: Marlowe.

what interventions may help a child sleep better. Physicians may prescribe medication to sleep, and the parent may have tried a variety of strategies that have already worked. Nurses, respiratory therapists, and psychologists may have similar or additional ideas to promote healthy sleep habits. Children and youth often describe what distracts them when they are trying to go to sleep. Contextual modifications may make a difference in a child's sleep, such as establishing bedtime and wake-up routines and habits.[4,5] Occupational therapists are often aware of the sensory aspects of the routine or environment and may suggest modifications.

Bedtime Routines and Habits

Bedtime routines related to ADLs can support or hinder sleep, based on the individual preferences of the child or caregiver. For example, if Johnny hates taking a bath, giving him a bath may have an alerting effect prior to bedtime, and he will be resistant to going to sleep. Meanwhile, Taniqua enjoys bathing, becomes calm after bathing, and gets very drowsy while reading a book after her bath. As noted, children with sensory processing disorders may find tooth brushing; face washing; texture, weight, or tightness of clothing or blankets; or donning and doffing splints as being aversive, which may affect the child's readiness to go to sleep, bed, or the mat for naptime. If healthy self-care routines are aversive to a child, these activities can be completed after dinner (or after a snack at school), and then a more relaxed child can experience a quiet and enjoyable time prior to naptime or bedtime.[131] In addition, medications, eating, or exercising immediately before bedtime may disrupt the onset of sleep.

Occupational therapists can help caregivers, teachers, children, and youth develop a routine for naptime, rest time, or bedtime that works for them. They can emphasize the need for a consistent routine and similar times and amounts of sleep during naps (if age-appropriate) and during the night (for weekends and weekdays). The following suggestions related to the social and temporal environment may be helpful to caregivers, children, and youth to develop a routine[4,35,111,113,107,147,175]:

- Establish a quiet time prior to bedtime for reading, rocking together in a chair, singing quiet rhythmic songs, or giving the child a back rub (no electronics, television, roughhousing, eating, or exercising right before bed)
- Use checklists, visual schedules, social stories, pictures, video modeling, or object cues (e.g., favorite stuffed animal or blanket used as a transitional object for going to bed).
- Keep the routine and environment the same each time the child goes to sleep (e.g., lights, music or noise machine, door open or closed, transitional object, small drink of water, singing), and keep the wake-up routine the same.
- Use a routine for going back to sleep if the child wakes up during the night.
- Avoid activities prior to bed that are upsetting or alerting to children.
- Put children to bed alone when drowsy but not asleep so they learn to self-regulate.
- Keep the same schedule for bedtime and wake-up time during the week and weekend.
- As children get older and more responsible, have them keep a log of their sleep and a checklist of healthy habits (e.g., television watching, caffeine use, what they are doing prior to bed, exercise during the day). (See Evolve website for different resources for this.)
- Adjust bedtimes according to the day's activity level (e.g., days when the child slept all day in the car or was outside for field day).

Physical Aspects of the Environment

The location and sensory aspects of the sleep environment and type of bedding and clothing may facilitate or hinder the quality of sleep. In addition, as children grow, they may need different firmness in a mattress or type of bed (e.g., from a crib to a youth bed [once a child is 35 inches tall], or a longer bed for the teen who is now 6 foot 4 inches tall!). The sleeping area needs to be quiet and away from noise and activity. Bedrooms should be used for sleeping and not for other activities or punishment. The following suggestions relate to modifying the physical sleep environment, if needed[4,111,147,175]:

- Limit the amount of auditory stimulation during sleep that arouses the child or teen (e.g., music box or CD, white noise, or are they listening to fast beat or loud music on an electronic device while trying to sleep?). Use a story on tape or calm music if not distracting.
- Keep the temperature consistent and determine if vents, windows, or fans that are near the bed are problematic or if the child may be too cold or hot (may need a sleeper pajama versus a nightgown).
- Consider if smells are alerting or calming in the room (e.g., kitchen smells, deodorant in a diaper pail, smell of sheets or clothing).
- Reduce visual stimulation. Use dim or frosted night lights if needed. Keep lights off and remove pictures or mirrors in the bed or on the wall that are reflecting light, toys in bed, lights in hallway, and visually stimulating sheets or blankets.
- Consider the weight, texture, and visual attractiveness of clothing and bedding and the personal preference of the child.
- Use pillows or stuffed animals in the bed to help children feel more secure (not for babies).
- Raise the head of the bed slightly if the child has reflux or difficulty breathing.
- Secure outside doors or windows if sleep walking or escape from the house are issues. Sometimes alarms are installed so that parents are alerted if children are leaving the sleep environment (Case Study 15-5).

Sleep and rest are essential for children with disabilities, and educational programs about healthy bedtimes and sleep hygiene are beneficial to all children at school, home, and rehabilitation centers, and to their teachers and caregivers. AOTA[4,5] materials on sleep may be used as part of handouts for parents, as part of an article for a Parent Teacher Organization or Early Intervention newsletter or part of health fairs given by local hospitals or centers. In addition, obesity prevention materials or programs about healthy eating and daily exercise or activity suggestions may be helpful to educate caregivers and children and youth.[4,13,17,151] See the Evolve website for more information.

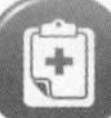

CASE STUDY 15-5 Carson, the Ever-Ready Bunny, Day and Night

Carson is an extremely active 5-year-old who is seen in an outpatient clinic for evaluation. Mom complained about his high activity level and aversive reactions to bathing and tooth brushing and identified problems with Carson's irregular sleep patterns and his inability to stay in bed or asleep for more than 2 or 3 hours. On evaluation, Carson's Vineland II scores were above average for communication and motor skills, but below average in socialization and daily living skills.

Carson had difficulty with sleep latency (getting to sleep) and night awakenings (remaining asleep). Sensory modulation issues appeared to be one issue, but there was also was no regular bedtime in the household. Because Carson continually got out of bed and refused to go to sleep, Mom brought Carson to bed with her so that she could keep "an eye on him." Mom also revealed that she was involved in continuous conflict with Carson's father regarding custody and support, which could be adding stress to bedtime, because they often talked in the evening, after she put Carson to bed.

A variety of approaches were used to address Carson's activity level, his sensory modulation difficulties, and lack of consistent, calming routines at bedtime. Sleep patterns were addressed by educating Mom about the need for consistent meal times and sleep routines to help Carson know what to expect and function better the next day. Some suggestions included having Mom and Carson take Buffy, their dog, for a short walk to get a little exercise. Ideas about reducing food and drink consumption at nighttime and a checklist were developed for the routine after dinner. Tooth brushing was done immediately after dinner becausee Carson became irritated during this activity, and then Mom and Carson would play a quiet board game. A regular bedtime routine was developed to allow Carson time to wind down and prepare to sleep. The television was turned off; "sandwich activities" hugs for deep pressure and a calming bathing routine was developed. Deep pressure was given during the washing and drying-off process and when applying lotion after the bath. Special soaps (with smells that Carson liked), washcloths, rhythmic songs (e.g., "This is the way we wash our face…"), and checklists for bathing were used to give Carson some control and cues for bathing. One parent read a nightly bedtime story while Carson rested under heavy blankets (Figure 15-13). Blankets were left in place to provide deep pressure and proprioceptive input throughout the night. A small nightlight in the hallway and a white noise machine seemed to comfort Carson but not distract him from sleep. His bed was moved away from the vent that blew air directly on him. Mom worked hard to keep Carson in his own bed for sleeping and gave him stickers for staying in his own bed each night. When Carson earned enough stickers, he was able to buy the favorite Disney movie that he was wanting.

Carson was also referred for a psychological assessment because his activity level continued to be high and his attention span was limited during the day at school. This assessment was also important because of the stress of the family going through a custody hearing. In addition, because Carson seemed to appear bored and unchallenged during the day and was not getting enough exercise or activity, his parents enrolled him in different camps during the summer months.

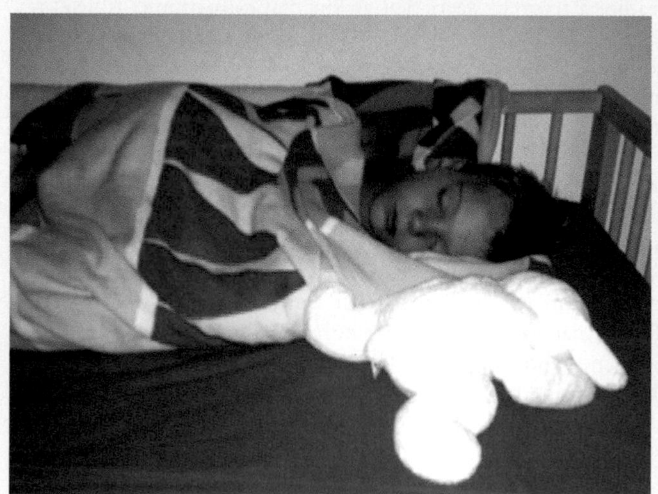

FIGURE 15-13 Carson sleeps with his bunny and heavy blanket for sensory input.

Contributed by Audrey Kane, PhD, OTR/L.

Summary

This chapter presents a wide range of options for enhancing ADL skills and sleep in children and adolescents with disabilities. Occupational therapists collaborate with children, parents or caregivers, and teachers to problem solve which method works best for each individual child. Summary points when promoting ADL function and healthy sleep habits include the following:

- Typical developmental sequences are useful in determining what children need to learn.
- Assessing ADL and sleep habits requires a variety of informal and formal methods related to the caregiver and child's preferences, environment and context in which the task occur, child's capabilities, and demands of the task.
    - Observing children and youth in the natural environment and during the typical routine of the family, school, or worksite is useful.
- Re-evaluation of ADL skills is needed as children develop, and new expectations occur (e.g., puberty or declining health, change in schools).
- Body functions and structures, performance skills, parent or teacher expectations, and performance patterns and routines at home, school, or work influence ADLs and sleep.
    - Establishing or restoring strength, balance, or gross or fine motor skills may influence a child's ability to perform ADL skills.

- Developing healthy habits and routines for ADL and sleep may improve the child's overall health and quality of life.
- As children get older and continue to have difficulty with ADLs, goals for partial participation or instructing others may become more important.
- Intervention strategies for ADL and sleep include positioning, task adaptation, visual supports, assistive technology, and environmental modifications.
- Research supports using visual supports, video modeling, prompting, and cognitive and collaborative approaches to teach ADL tasks.
- Occupational therapists offer adaptations to routines, activities, and sleep environment to promote healthy sleep habits.

Whatever the pediatric setting, occupational therapists have the essential skills needed to evaluate ADLs and sleep and collaborate with others to suggest meaningful and useful interventions.

REFERENCES

1. Allik, H., Larsson, J., & Smedje, H. (2008). Sleep patterns in school-age children with asperger Syndrome or high-functioning autism: A follow-up study. *Journal of Autism and Developmental Disorders, 38*(9), 1625–1633.
2. American Academy of Sleep Medicine. (2005). *International Classification of Sleep Disorders* (ICSD-2). Darien, IL: American Academy of Sleep Medicine.
3. American Occupational Therapy Association. (2008). Occupational therapy practice framework: Domain and practice (2nd ed.). *American Journal of Occupational Therapy, 62*, 625–683.
4. American Occupational Therapy Association (2013a). *Tips for living life to its fullest: Establishing bedtime routines for children.* Retrieved June 1, 2013 at: <http://www.aota.org/-/media/Corporate/Files/AboutOT/consumers/Youth/BedroomRoutineTipSheet.pdf>.
5. American Occupational Therapy Association (2013b). *Tips for living life to its fullest: Establishing morning routines for children.* Retrieved November 1, 2013 at: <http://www.aota.org/-/media/Corporate/Files/AboutOT/consumers/Youth/MorningRoutineTipSheet.pdf>.
6. Anderson, S. R., Jablonski, A. L., Thomeer, M. L., et al. (2007). *Self-help skills for people with autism: A systematic teaching approach.* Bethesda, MD: Woodbine House.
7. Annon, J. (1976). The PLISSIT model: A proposed conceptual scheme for the behavioral treatment of sexual problems. *Journal of Sex Education and Therapy*, 1–15.
8. Azrin, N. H., & Foxx, R. M. (1974). *Toilet training in less than a day.* New York: Simon & Schuster.
9. Bartlett, D. J., Chiarello, L. A., McCoy, S. W., et al. (2010). The Move & PLAY study: An example of comprehensive rehabilitation outcomes research. *Physical Therapy, 90*, 1660–1672.
10. Bagby, M. S., Dickie, V. A., & Baranek, G. (2012). How sensory experiences of children with and without autism affect family occupations. *American Journal of Occupational Therapy, 66*(1), 78–86.
11. Baker, C. P., Russell, W. J., Meyer, W., 3rd, et al. (2007). Physical and psychologic rehabilitation outcomes for young adults burned as children. *Archives of Physical Medicine and Rehabilitation, 88*(Suppl. 2), S57–S64.
12. Baranek, G., David, F., Poe, M., et al. (2006). Sensory Experiences Questionnaire: discriminating sensory features in young children with autism, developmental delays, and typical development. *Journal of Child Psychology & Psychiatry, 47*(6), 591–601.
13. Bazyk, S. (2011). Enduring challenges and situational stressors during the school years: Risk reduction and competence enhancement. In S. Bazyk (Ed.), *Mental health promotion, prevention, and intervention with children a youth: A guiding framework for occupational therapy* (pp. 119–139). Bethesda, MD: American Occupational Therapy Association.
14. Bedell, G. M., Cohn, E. S., & Dumas, H. M. (2005). Exploring parents' use of strategies to promote social participation of school-age children with acquired brain injuries. *American Journal of Occupational Therapy, 59*, 273–284.
15. Bellini, S., & Akullian, J. (2007). A meta-analysis of video modeling and video self-modeling interventions for children and adolescents with autism. *Exceptional Children, 73*, 264–287.
16. Bidabe, D. L., Barnes, S. B., & Whinnery, K. W. (2001). M.O.V.E.: Raising expectations for individuals with severe disabilities. *Physical Disabilities: Education and Related Services, 19*(2), 31–48.
17. Cahill, S. M., & Suarez-Balcazar, Y. (2009). Promoting children's nutrition and fitness in an urban context. *American Journal of Occupational Therapy, 63*, 113–116.
18. Carno, M. A., Hoffman, L. A., Carcillo, J. A., et al. (2003). Developmental stages of sleep from birth to adolescence, common childhood sleep disorders: Overview and nursing implications. *Journal of Pediatric Nursing, 18*(4), 274–283.
19. Case-Smith, J., DeLuca, S. C., Stevenson, R., et al. (2012). Multicenter randomized controlled trial of pediatric constraint-induced movement therapy: 6 month follow-up. *American Journal of Occupational Therapy, 66*, 15–23.
20. Chafetz, R. S., Mulcahey, M. J., Betz, R. R., et al. (2007). Impact of prophylactic thoracolumbosacral orthosis bracing on functional activities and activities of daily living in the pediatric spinal cord injury population. *Journal of Spinal Cord Medicine, 30*(Suppl. 1), S178–S183.
21. Collier, B., McGhie-Richmond, D., Odette, F., et al. (2006). Reducing the risk of sexual abuse for people who use augmentative and alternative communication. *Augmentative and Alternative Communication, 22*, 62–75.
22. Copley, J., & Ziviani, J. (2004). Barriers to use assistive technology for children with multiple disabilities. *Occupational Therapy International, 11*, 229–243.
23. Coster, W. J. (1998). Occupation-centered assessment of children. *American Journal of Occupational Therapy, 52*, 337–344.
24. Coster, W., Deeney, T. A., Haltiwanger, J. T., et al. (1998). *School Function Assessment: User's manual.* San Antonio, TX: Therapy Skill Builders.
25. Coster, W. J., Haley, S. M., Ni, P., et al. (2008). Assessing self-care and social function using a computer adaptive testing version of the Pediatric Evaluation of Disability Inventory. *Archives of Physical Medicine and Rehabilitation, 89*, 622–629.

26. Couwenhoven, T. (2001). Sexuality education: Building a foundation of healthy attitudes. *Disability Solutions, 4*(6), 1–8.
27. Couwenhoven, T. (2007). *Teaching children with Down syndrome about their bodies, boundaries, and sexuality.* Bethesda, MD: Woodbine Books.
28. Cusick, A., McIntyre, S., Novak, I., et al. (2006). A comparison of goal attainment scaling and the Canadian Occupational Performance Measure for paediatric rehabilitation research. *Pediatric Rehabilitation, 9*, 149–157.
29. Davies, D. K., Stock, S. E., & Wehmeyer, M. L. (2002). Enhancing independent task performance for individuals with mental retardation through use of a handheld self-directed visual and audio prompting system. *Education and Training in Mental Retardation & Developmental Disabilities, 37*, 209–218.
30. Disability Office of South Australia. (2008). Managing menstrual care: A resource guide about managing menstruation for women with intellectual disabilities. Retrieved from: <http://www.dfc.sa.gov.au/pub/tabid//185/itemid/634/School-age-and-youth-820-years-with-a-disabilit.aspx>.
31. Donovan, J., (Interviewer), & Gerhardt, P., (Interviewee) (2012). *Learning to love and be loved, with autism [Interview transcript].* Retrieved November 13, 2013 from: <http://www.npr.org/2012/01/18/145405658/learning-to-love-and-be-loved-with-autism>.
32. Drahota, A., Wood, J. J., Sze, K. M., et al. (2011). Effects of cognitive behavioral therapy on daily living skills in children with high functioning autism and concurrent anxiety disorders. *Journal of Autism and Developmental Disorders, 41*, 257–265.
33. Dunford, C., Missiuna, C., Street, E., et al. (2005). Children's perceptions of the impact of developmental coordination disorder on activities of daily living. *British Journal of Occupational Therapy, 68*, 207–214.
34. Epps, S., Stern, R. J., & Horner, R. H. (1990). Comparison of simulation training on self and using a doll for teaching generalized menstrual care to women with severe mental retardation. *Research in Developmental Disabilities, 11*, 37–66.
35. Evans, J., & Rodger, S. (2008). Mealtimes and bedtimes: Windows to family routines and rituals. *Journal of Occupational Science, 15*, 98–104.
36. Fehlings, D., Weiss, S., & Stephens, D. (2001). Frequent night awakenings in preschool children referred to a sleep disorders clinic: The role of non-adaptive sleep associates. *Children's Health Care, 3*(1), 43–55.
37. Feldman, M. A. (1999). Teaching child-care and safety skills to parents with intellectual disabilities through self-learning. *Journal of Intellectual and Developmental Disability, 24*(1), 27–44.
38. Fiese, B. H., Tomcho, T. J., Douglas, M., et al. (2002). A review of 50 years of research on naturally occurring family routines and rituals: Cause for celebration? *Journal of Family Psychology, 16*, 381–390.
39. Fisher, A. G. (2006). *Assessment of Motor and Process Skills: Vol. 1. Development, standardization, and administration manual* (6th ed.). Fort Collins, CO: Three Star Press.
40. Fisher, A. G. (2006). *Assessment of Motor and Process Skills: Vol. 2. User manual* (6th ed.). Fort Collins, CO: Three Star Press.
41. Franco, P., Scaillet, S., Groswasser, J., et al. (2004). Increased cardiac autonomic responses to auditory challenges in swaddled infants. *Sleep, 27*(8), 1527–1532.
42. Furuno, S., O'Reilly, K., Hosaka, C. M., et al. (2004). *Hawaii Early Learning Profile* (2nd ed.). Palo Alto, CA: Vort.
43. Gallimore, R., & Lopez, E. M. (2002). Everyday routines, human agency, and ecocultural context: Construction and maintenance of individual habits. *Occupational Therapy Journal of Research, 22*, 70–77S.
44. Gast, C., & Krug, J. (2008). *Caring for myself.* Philadelphia: Jessica Kingsley.
45. Gentry, T., & Wallace, J. (2008). A community-based trial of PDAs as cognitive aids for individuals with acquired brain injury: Outcome findings. *Brain Injury, 33*, 21–27.
46. Gentry, T., Wallace, J., Kvarfordt, C., et al. (2010). Personal digital assistants as cognitive aids for high school students with autism: Results of a community-based trial. *Journal of Vocational Rehabilitation, 32*(2), 101–107.
47. Gevir, D., Goldstand, S., Weintraub, N., et al. (2006). A comparison of time use between mothers of children with and without disabilities. *Occupation, Participation and Health, 26*, 117–127.
48. Giangreco, M., Cloninger, C., & Iverson, V. (1997). *Choosing options and accommodations for children (COACH)* (2nd ed.). Baltimore: Paul H. Brookes.
49. Giannotti, F., Cortesi, F., Cerquiglini, A., et al. (2006). An open-label study of controlled-release melatonin in treatment of sleep disorders in children with autism. *Journal of Autism Developmental Disorders, 36*, 741–752.
50. Goldman, S. E., Surdyka, K., Cuevas, R., et al. (2009). Defining the sleep phenotype in children with autism. *Developmental Neuropsychology, 34*(5), 560–573.
51. Goldman, S., Richdale, A., Clemons, T., et al. (2012). Parental sleep concerns in autism spectrum disorders: Variations from childhood to adolescence. *Journal of Autism & Developmental Disorders, 42*(4), 531–538.
52. Graham, F., Rodger, S., & Zivani, J. (2009). Coaching parents to enable children's participation: An approach for working with parents and their children. *Australian Occupational Therapy Journal, 56*(1), 16–23.
53. Graham, F., Rodger, S., & Ziviani, J. (2013). Effectiveness of occupational performance coaching in improving children's and mothers' performance and mothers' self-competence. *American Journal of Occupational Therapy, 67*, 10–18.
54. Granberg, M., Rydberg, A., & Fisher, A. G. (2008). Activities in daily living and schoolwork task performance in children with complex congenital heart disease. *Acta Pædiatrica, 97*, 1270–1274.
55. Gray, C. (2000). *The new social story book: Illustrated edition.* Arlington, TX: Future Horizons.
56. Griffin, J., Carlson, G., Taylor, M., et al. (1996). An introduction to menstrual management for women who have an intellectual disability and high support needs. *International Journal of Disability, Development and Education, 41*, 103–116.
57. Haley, S. M., Coster, W. J., Dumas, H. M., et al. (2011). Accuracy and precision of the Pediatric Evaluation of Disability Inventory Computer-Adaptive Tests (PEDI-CAT). *Developmental Medicine & Child Neurology, 53*, 1100–1106.
58. Hamilton, B. B., & Granger, C. U., 2000 *Functional Independence Measure for Children (WeeFIM-II).* Buffalo, NY: Research Foundation of the State University of New York.
59. Hanft, B., & Shepherd, J. (2008). 2…4…6…8…How do you collaborate? In *Collaborating for student success: A guide for school-based occupational therapy* (pp. 1–34). Bethesda, MD: American Occupational Therapy Association.
60. Hanft, B. E., Rush, D. D., & Shelden, M. L. (2004). *Coaching families and colleagues in early childhood.* Baltimore: Paul H. Brookes.
61. Hanson, M. (2004). Families with Anglo-European roots. In E. W. Lynch & M. J. Hanson (Eds.), *Developing cross-cultural competence* (3rd ed.,

pp. 93–126). Baltimore: Paul H. Brookes.

62. Healy, H., & Rigby, P. (1999). Promoting independence for teens and young adults with physical disabilities. *Canadian Journal of Occupational Therapy, 66*, 240–248.
63. Hemmingsson, H., Lidstrom, H., & Nygard, L. (2009). Use of assistive technology devices in mainstream schools: Students' perspective. *American Journal of Occupational Therapy, 63*, 463–472.
64. Hingsburger, D. (1993). *I openers: Parents ask questions about sexuality and children with developmental disabilities.* Vancouver, Canada: Family Support Institute Press.
65. Sandberg, J. F., Hofferth, S. L. (2001). Changes in parental time with children. *Demography, 38*(3), 423–436.
66. Holloway, J. A., & Aman, M. G. (2011). Sleep correlates of pervasive developmental disorders: A review of the literature. *Research in Developmental Disabilities, 32*(5), 1399–1421.
67. Holm, M. B., Rogers, J. C., & James, A. B. (2003). Interventions for daily living. In E. B. Crepeau, E. Cohn, & B. Schell (Eds.), *Willard and Spackman's occupational therapy* (10th ed., pp. 491–554). Philadelphia: J. B. Lippincott.
68. Honomichl, R., Goodlin Jones, B., Burnham, M., et al. (2002). Sleep patterns of children with pervasive developmental disorders. *Journal of Autism and Developmental Disorders, 32*(6), 553–561.
69. Horn, I. B., Brenner, R., Rao, M., et al. (2006). Beliefs about the appropriate age for initiating toilet training: Are there racial and socioeconomic differences? *Journal of Pediatrics, 149*, 151–152.
70. Hughes, C., & Carter, E. W. (2000). *The transition handbook: Strategies high school teachers use that work!* Baltimore: Paul H. Brookes.
71. Jarus, T., & Ratzon, N. Z. (2000). Can you imagine? The effect of mental practice on the acquisition and retention of a motor skill as a function of age. *Occupational Therapy Journal of Research, 20*, 163–178.
72. Johnson, C. R., Turner, K. S., Foldes, E. L., et al. (2012). Comparison of sleep questionnaires in the assessment of sleep disturbances in children with autism spectrum disorders. *Sleep Medicine, 13*(7), 795–801.
73. Johnson-Martin, N., Attermeier, S. M., & Hacker, B. (2004). *The Carolina curriculum for infants and toddlers with special needs* (3rd ed.). Baltimore: Paul H. Brookes.
74. Johnson-Martin, N., Hacker, B., & Attermeier, S. M. (2004). *The Carolina curriculum for preschoolers with special needs* (2nd ed.). Baltimore: Paul H. Brookes.
75. Joinson, C., Herson, J., von Gontard, A., et al. (2008). Early childhood risk factors associated with daytime wetting and soiling in school-age children. *Journal of Pediatric Psychology, 33*, 739–750.
76. Kadlec, M. B., Coster, W., Tickle-Degnen, L., et al. (2005). Qualities of caregiver-child interaction during daily activities of children born very low birth weight with and without white matter disorder. *American Journal of Occupational Therapy, 59*, 57–66.
77. Kagohara, D. M., Sigafoos, J., Achmadi, D., et al. (2011). Teaching students with developmental disabilities to operate an iPod Touch to listen to music. *Research for Developmental Disabilities, 32*(6), 2987–2992.
78. Kagohara, D. M., van der Meer, L., Ramdoss, S., et al. (2013). Using iPods and iPads in teaching programs for individuals with developmental disabilities: A systematic review. *Research in Developmental Disabilities, 34*(1), 147–156.
79. Kangas, K. (1998). Using your head: Access and integration of independent mobility and communication "head first." Presented at TechKnowledgy '98 Conference, Children's Hospital. Richmond, VA, October 28, 1998.
80. Keen, D., Brannigan, K. L., & Cuskelly, M. (2007). Toilet training for children with autism: The effects of video modeling. *Journal of Development and Physical Disabilities, 19*, 291–303.
81. Keller, J., Kafkes, A., Baso, S., et al. (2005). *Child Occupational Self-Assessment (COSA; Version 2.1.).* Chicago: MOHO Clearinghouse.
82. Klassen, T. P., Kiddoo, D., Lang, M. E., et al. (2006). *The effectiveness of different methods of toilet training for bladder and bowel control.* Rockville, MD: Agency for Healthcare Research and Quality. Publication No. 07-E003.
83. Kotagal, S., & Broomall, E. (2012). Sleep in children with autism spectrum disorder. *Pediatric Neurology, 47*(4), 242–251.
84. Kothari, D. H., Haley, S. M., Gill-Body, K. M., et al. (2003). Measuring functional change in children with acquired brain injury (ABI): Comparison of generic and ABI-specific scale using the Pediatric Evaluation of Disability Inventory (PEDI). *Physical Therapy, 83*, 776–785.
85. Krakowiak, P., Goodlin-Jones, B., Hertz-Picciotto, I., et al. (2008). Sleep problems in children with autism spectrum disorders, developmental delays, and typical development: A population-based study. *Journal of Sleep Research, 17*(2), 197–206.
86. Kryger, M. H., Roth, T., & Dement, W. C. (2006). *Principles and practice of pediatric sleep medicine* (4th ed.). Baltimore: Elsevier.
87. Law, M., Baptiste, S., Carswell, A., et al. (2005). *Canadian Occupational Performance Measure* (3rd ed.). Toronto: Canadian Association of Occupational Therapists.
88. Lawrence, K. E., & Niemeyer, S. (1994). *Home care issues/activities of daily living: Caregiver education guide for children with developmental disabilities* (Vol. 4, pp. 31–46). Gaithersburg, MD: Aspen.
89. LeBlanc, L. A., Carr, J. E., Crossett, S. E., et al. (2005). Intensive outpatient behavioral treatment of primary urinary incontinence of children with autism. *Focus on Autism and Other Developmental Disabilities, 20*, 98–105.
90. Levan, P. (2008). A male toileting aide: The penis paddle. *Journal of Occupational Therapy, Schools & Early Intervention, 1*, 68–69.
91. Linkie, C., & Hattjar, B. (2012). Adolescents with disabilities and sexuality. In B. Hattjar (Ed.), *Sexuality and occupational therapy: Strategies with persons with disabilities* (pp. 229–284). Bethesda, MD: American Occupational Therapy Association.
92. Liu, X., Hubbard, J., Fabes, R., et al. (2006). Sleep disturbances and correlates of children with autism spectrum disorders. *Child Psychiatry and Human Development, 37*(2), 179–191.
93. Lynch, E. (2004). Developing cross cultural competence. In E. Lynch & M. Hanson (Eds.), *Developing cross-cultural competence* (3rd ed., pp. 41–78). Baltimore: Paul H. Brookes.
94. Lynch, E., & Hanson, M. (Eds.), (2004). *Developing cross-cultural competence* (3rd ed.). Baltimore: Paul H. Brookes.
95. Mailloux, Z., May-Benson, T. A., Summers, C. A., et al. (2007). Goal attainment scaling as a measure of meaningful outcomes for children with sensory integration disorders. *American Journal of Occupational Therapy, 61*, 254–259.
96. Malow, B., Adkins, K. W., McGrew, S. G., et al. (2012). Melatonin for sleep in children with autism: A controlled trial examining dose, tolerability, and outcomes.

Journal of Autism and Developmental Disorders, 42(8), 1729–1737.

97. Mandich, A. D., Polatajko, H. J., & Roger, S. (2003). Rites of passage: Understanding participation of children with developmental coordination disorder. *Human Movement Science, 22*, 583–595.
98. Marcus, A., & Wilder, D. A. (2009). A comparison of peer versus self video modeling to teach textual responses in children with autism. *Journal of Applied Behavior Analysis, 42*, 335–341.
99. Mason, R. A., Ganz, J., Parker, B., et al. (2012). Moderating factors of video-modeling with other as model: A meta-analysis of single-case studies. *Research in Developmental Disabilities, 33*, 1076–1086.
100. Mason, R. A., Ganz, J. B., Parker, R. I., et al. (2013). Video-based modeling: Differential effects due to treatment protocol. *Research in Autism Spectrum Disorders, 7*, 120–131.
101. McCoy, K., & Hermansen, E. (2007). Video modeling for individuals with autism: A review of model types and effects. *Education and Treatment of Children, 30*, 183–213.
102. McDougall, J., & King, G. (2007). *Goal attainment scaling manual: Description, utility and applications in pediatric therapy* (2nd ed.). Retrieved from: <http://www.tvcc.on.ca/images/stories/All_PDFs/OurServices/Research/gasmanual2007.pdf>.
103. McGavin, H. (1998). Planning rehabilitation: A comparison of issues for parents and adolescents. *Physical and Occupational Therapy, 18*, 69–82.
104. Melberg-Schwier, K., & Hingsburger, D. (2000). *Sexuality: Your sons and daughters with intellectual disabilities.* Baltimore: Paul H. Brookes.
105. Miller, L. J., Schoen, S., James, K., et al. (2007). Lessons learned: A pilot study of occupational therapy effectiveness for children with sensory modulation disorder. *American Journal of Occupational Therapy, 61*, 161–169.
106. Milligan, M. S., & Neufeldt, A. H. (2001). The myth of asexuality: A survey of social and empirical evidence. *Sexuality & Disability, 19*, 91–109.
107. Mindell, J. A., Owens, J. A., Alves, R., et al. (2011). Give children and adolescents the gift of a good night's sleep: A call to action. *Sleep Medicine, 12*, 203–204.
108. Mindell, J. A., Meltzer, L. J., Carskadon, M. A., et al. (2009). Developmental aspects of sleep hygiene: Findings from the 2004 National Sleep Foundation Sleep in America Poll. *Sleep Medicine, 10*, 771–779.
109. Missiuna, C., Moll, S., Law, M., et al. (2006). Mysteries and mazes: Parents' experiences of children with developmental coordination disorder. *Canadian Journal of Occupational Therapy, 73*, 7–17.
110. Murphy, N. A., & Ellias, E. R. (2006). Sexuality of children and adolescents with developmental disorders. *Pediatrics, 118*(1), 398–403.
111. National Sleep Foundation. (2013). Children and sleep. Retrieved from: <http://sleepfoundation.org/sleep-topics/children-and-sleep>.
112. Nicholson, J. H., Morton, R. E., Attfield, S., et al. (2001). Assessment of upper-limb function and movement in children with cerebral palsy wearing Lycra garments. *Developmental Medicine and Child Neurology, 43*, 384–391.
113. O'Connell, A., & Vannan, K. (2008). Sleepwise: Addressing sleep disturbance in young children with developmental delay. *Australian Occupational Therapy Journal, 55*, 212–214.
114. Orelove, F., & Sobsey, D. (1996). ADL skills. In F. Orelove & D. Sobsey (Eds.), *Educating children with multiple disabilities* (3rd ed., pp. 333–375). Baltimore: Paul H. Brookes.
115. Owens, J., & Mindell, J. (2005). *Take charge of your child's sleep: The all-in-one resource for solving sleep problems in kids and teens.* New York: Marlowe.
116. Park, J. H., Yoo, J. H., & Kim, S. H. (2013). Associations between non-restorative sleep, short sleep duration and suicidality: Findings from a representative sample of Korean adolescents. *Psychiatry Clinical Neuroscience, 67*(1), 28–34.
117. Park, S., Cho, S.-C., Cho, I. H., et al. (2012). Sleep problems and their correlates and comorbid psychopathology of children with autism spectrum disorders. *Research in Autism Spectrum Disorders, 6*, 1068–1072.
118. Payne, S., & Howell, C. (2005). An evaluation of the clinical use of the assessment of motor and process skills with children. *British Journal of Occupational Therapy, 68*, 277–280.
119. Phipps, S., & Roberts, P. (2012). Predicting the effects of cerebral palsy severity on self-care, mobility, and social function. *American Journal of Occupational Therapy, 66*, 422–429.
120. Polatajko, H. J., Mandich, A. D., Miller, L. T., et al. (2001). Cognitive Orientation to daily Occupational Performance (CO-OP): Part II—the evidence. *Physical and Occupational Therapy in Pediatrics, 20*, 83–106.
121. Polimeni, M. A. R. (2005). A survey of sleep problems in autism, Asperger's disorder and typically developing children. *Journal of Intellectual Disability Research, 49*(4), 260–268.
122. Prudhomme-White, B., & Mulligan, S. E. (2005). Behavioral and physiologic response measures of occupational task performance: A preliminary comparison between typical children and children with attention disorder. *American Journal of Occupational Therapy, 59*, 426–436.
123. Quint, E. H. (2003). The conservative management of abnormal bleeding in teenagers with developmental disabilities. *Journal of Pediatric and Adolescent Gynecology, 16*, 54–56.
124. Reed, P., & Bowser, G. (2012). Consultation, collaboration, and coaching: Essential techniques for integrating assistive technology use in schools and early intervention programs. *Journal of Occupational Therapy, Schools and Early Intervention, 5*(1), 15–30.
125. Reese, G. M., & Snell, M. E. (1991). Putting on and removing coats and jackets: The acquisition and maintenance of skills by children with severe multiple disabilities. *Education and Training in Mental Retardation, 26*, 398–410.
126. Rempfer, M., Hildenbrand, W., Parker, K., et al. (2003). An interdisciplinary approach to environmental intervention: Ecology of human performance. In L. Letts, P. Rigby, & D. Stewart (Eds.), *Using environments to enable occupational performance* (pp. 119–136). Thorofare, NJ: Slack.
127. Reynhout, G., & Carter, E. (2011). Evaluation of the efficacy of Social Stories using three single subject metrics. *Research in Autism Spectrum Disorders, 5*(2), 885–900.
128. Reynolds, A. M., & Malow, B. A. (2011). Sleep and autism spectrum disorders. *Pediatric Clinics of North America, 58*(3), 685–698.
129. Rodger, S., & Liu, S. (2008). Cognitive orientation to (daily) occupational performance: Changes in strategy and session time use over the course of intervention. *OTJR: Occupation, Participation and Health, 28*, 168–179.
130. Rodger, S., Springfield, E., & Polatajko, H. J. (2007). Cognitive orientation for daily occupational performance approach for children with Asperger's syndrome: A case report. *Physical and Occupational Therapy in Pediatrics, 27*, 7–22.
131. Rodger, S., & Zivani, J. (2012). Autism spectrum disorders: Isn't a spectrum a rainbow? In S. J. Lane & A. Bundy (Eds.), *Kids can be kids: A childhood occupations approach* (pp. 483–506). Baltimore: F. A. Davis.

132. Rosenberg, N. E., Schwartz, I. S., & Davis, C. A. (2010). Evaluating the utility of commercial videotapes for teaching hand washing to children with autism. *Education & Treatment of Children, 33*(3), 443–455.
133. Rzepecka, H., McKenzie, K., McClure, I., et al. (2011). Sleep, anxiety and challenging behaviour in children with intellectual disability and/or autism spectrum disorder. *Research in Developmental Disabilities, 32*(6), 2758–2766.
134. Sadeh, A., & Acebo, C. (2002). The role of actigraphy in sleep medicine. *Sleep Medicine Reviews, 6*(2), 113–124.
135. Sakzewski, L., Boyd, R. N., & Ziviani, J. (2007). Clinimetric properties of participation measures for 5-13 years old children with cerebral palsy: A systematic review. *Developmental Medicine and Child Neurology, 49*, 232–240.
136. Sakzewski, L., Ziviani, J., Abbott, D. F., et al. (2011). Randomized trial of constraint-induced movement therapy and bimanual training on activity outcomes for children with congenital hemiplegia. *Developmental Medicine in Child Neurology, 53*(4), 313–320.
137. Sansosti, F. J., Powell-Smith, K. A., & Kincaid, D. (2004). A research synthesis of Social Story interventions for children with autism spectrum disorders. *Focus on Autism and Other Developmental Disabilities, 19*(4), 194–204.
138. Sawin, K., Buran, C. F., Brei, T. J., et al. (2002). Sexuality issues in adolescents with a chronic neurological condition. *Journal of Perinatal Education, 11*, 22–34.
139. Schreck, K., Mulick, J., & Smith, A. (2004). Sleep problems as possible predictors of intensified symptoms of autism. *Research in Developmental Disabilities, 25*(1), 57–66.
140. Schultz-Krohn, W. (2004). Session 10: Addressing ADLs and IADLs within the school-based practice. In Y. Swinth (Ed.), *Occupational therapy in school-based practice: Contemporary issues and trends*. Bethesda, MD: American Occupational Therapy Association Online Course.
141. Schum, T. R., Kolb, T. M., McAuliffe, T. L., et al. (2002). Sequential acquisition of toilet-training skills: A descriptive study of gender and age differences in normal children. *Pediatrics, 109*(3), E48.
142. Schwarz, S. P. (2000). *Attainment's dressing tips and clothing resources for making life easier*. Verona, WI: Attainment.
143. Segal, R. (2000). Adaptive strategies of mothers with children with attention deficit hyperactivity disorder: Enfolding and unfolding occupations. *American Journal of Occupational Therapy, 54*, 300–306.
144. Segal, R. (2004). Family routines and rituals: A context for occupational therapy interventions. *American Journal of Occupational Therapy, 58*, 499–508.
145. Sewell, T. J., Collins, B. C., Hemmeter, M. L., et al. (1998). Using simultaneous prompting within an activity-based format to teach dressing skills to preschoolers with developmental delays. *Journal of Early Intervention, 21*, 132–142.
146. Shahid, A., Shapiro, C. M., Wilkinson, K., et al. (2013). *STOP, THAT, and one hundred other sleep scales*. New York: Springer.
147. Shepherd, J. (2012). Self-care: A primary occupation. I can do it myself! In S. J. Lane & A. Bundy (Eds.), *Kids can be kids: A childhood occupations approach* (pp. 125–158). Baltimore: F. A. Davis.
148. Shipley-Benamou, R., Lutzker, J. R., & Taubman, M. (2002). Teaching daily living skills to children with autism through instructional video modeling. *Journal of Positive Behavior Interventions, 4*, 165–175.
149. Simpson, E., & Lankasky, K. (2001). Table manners and beyond: The gynecological exam for women with developmental disabilities and other functional limitations. Retrieved from: <http://www.bhawd.org/sitefiles/TblMrs/cover.html>.
150. Skiffington, S., Washburn, S., & Elliott, K. (2011). Instructional coaching: Helping preschool teachers reach their full potential. *Young Children, 66*(3), 12–20.
151. Smallfield, S., & Anderson, A. J. (2009). Using after-school programming to support health and wellness: A physical activity engagement program description. *Early Intervention Special Interest Section Quarterly, 16*(3), 1–4.
152. Smith, R., Benge, M., & Hall, M. (2000). Using assistive technologies to enable self-care and daily living. In C. Christiansen (Ed.), *Ways of living: ADL strategies for special needs* (2nd ed., pp. 57–81). Bethesda, MD: American Occupational Therapy Association.
153. Snell, M. E., & Brown, F. (2000). Development and implementation of educational programs. In M. E. Snell & F. Brown (Eds.), *Instruction of students with severe disabilities* (5th ed., pp. 115–165). Upper Saddle River, NJ: Prentice-Hall.
154. Snell, M. E., & Vogtle, L. K. (2000). Methods for teaching self-care skills. In C. Christiansen (Ed.), *Ways of living: ADL strategies for special needs* (2nd ed., pp. 57–81). Bethesda, MD: American Occupational Therapy Association.
155. Souders, M. C., Mason, T. B., Valadares, O., et al. (2009). Sleep behaviors and sleep quality in children with autism spectrum. *Sleep, 32*(12), 1566–1578. PMCID: PMC2786040.
156. Spriggs, A. D., Gast, D. L., & Ayres, K. M. (2007). Using picture activity schedule books to increase on-schedule and on-task behaviors. *Education and Training in Developmental Disabilities, 42*(2), 209–223.
157. Stalker, K., & McArthur, K. (2012). Child abuse, child protection and disabled children: A review of recent research. *Child Abuse Review, 21*(1), 24–40.
158. Steenbeek, D., Ketelaar, M., Galama, K., et al. (2007). Goal attainment scaling in paediatric rehabilitation: A critical review of the literature. *Developmental Medicine and Child Neurology, 49*, 550–556.
159. Stowitchek, J. J., Laitinen, R., & Prather, T. (1999). Embedding early self-determination opportunities in curriculum for youth with developmental disabilities using natural teaching incidents. *Journal of Vocational Special Needs Education, 21*, 15–26.
160. Sullivan, P. M., & Knutson, J. F. (2000). Maltreatment and disabilities: A population-based epidemiological study. *Child Abuse and Neglect, 4*, 1257–1273.
161. Sweeney, J. (1989). *Clothing for children with severe disabilities: A guide to adaptive garments for use in the institutional setting*. Alexandria, VA: Special Clothes.
162. Tarazi, R. A., Mahone, E. M., & Zabel, T. A. (2007). Self-care independence in children with neurological disorders: An interactional model of adaptive demands and executive dysfunction. *Rehabilitation Psychology, 52*, 196–205.
163. Taylor, B., & Davis, S. (2007). The extended PLISSIT model for addressing the sexual well-being of individuals with an acquired disability or chronic illness. *Sexuality & Disability, 25*(3), 135–139.
164. Taylor, M. A., Schreck, K. A., & Mulick, J. A. (2012). Sleep disruption as a correlate to cognitive and adaptive behavior problems in autism spectrum disorders. *Research in Developmental Disabilities, 33*, 1408–1417.
165. Thomson, G. (2005). *Children with severe disabilities and the MOVE curriculum: Foundations of a task oriented therapy approach*. Chester, NY: East River Press.
166. Turnbull, A. P., Turnbull, H. R., Erwin, E. J., et al. (2004). *Families, professionals, and exceptionality: Positive outcomes through partnerships and trust*

(5th ed.). Columbus, OH: Merrill/ Prentice Hall.

167. Turner, L., Lammi, B., Friesen, K., et al. (2001). *Dressing workbook: The backward chaining strategy.* Ontario, CA: CanChild Centre for Childhood Disability Research. Retrieved on November 7, 2013 from: <http://www.canchild.ca/en/canchildresources/resources/chaining.pdf>.
168. Vogtle, L. K., & Snell, M. E. (2011). Methods for teaching basic and instrumental activities of daily living. In C. Christiansen (Ed.), *Ways of living: ADL strategies for special needs* (4th ed., pp. 105–129). Bethesda, MD: American Occupational Therapy Association.
169. Voorman, J. M., Dallmeijer, A. J., Schuengel, C., et al. (2006). Activities and participation of 9- to 13-year-old children with cerebral palsy. *Clinical Rehabilitation, 20*(11), 937–948.
170. Werner DeGrace, B. (2004). Families, children with autism and everyday occupations. *American Journal of Occupational Therapy, 58,* 543–550.
171. Wheeler, M. (1998). *Toilet training for individuals with autism and related disorders.* Arlington, TX: Future Horizons.
172. Whinnery, S. B., & Whinnery, K. (2011). Effects of functional mobility skills training for adults with severe multiple disabilities. *Education and Training in Autism and Developmental Disabilities, 46*(3), 436–453.
173. Whinnery, K. W., & Whinnery, S. B. (2007). MOVE systematic programming for early motor intervention. *Infants and Young Children, 20,* 102–108.
174. Wilson, K. P., Dykstra, J. R., Watson, L. R., et al. (2012). Coaching in early education classrooms serving children with autism: A pilot study. *Journal of Early Childhood Education, 40,* 97–105.
175. Williamson, G., & Anzalone, M. (2001). *Sensory integration and self-regulation in infants and toddlers: Helping very young children interact with their environment* (p. 82). Washington, DC: Zero to Three.
176. Wood, J. J. (2006). Parental intrusiveness and children's separation anxiety in a clinical sample. *Child Psychiatry and Human Development, 37,* 73–87.
177. Wroble, M. J. (2003). *Taking care of myself: A hygiene, puberty and personal curriculum for young people with autism.* Arlington, TX: Future Horizons.
178. Wright, M., Tancredi, A., Yundt, B., et al. (2006). Sleep issues in children with physical disabilities and their families. *Physical & Occupational Therapy in Pediatrics, 26*(3), 55–72.
179. Zuniga, M. E. (2004). Families with Latino roots. In E. W. Lynch & M. J. Hanson (Eds.), *Developing cross-cultural competence* (3rd ed., pp. 209–250). Baltimore: Paul H. Brookes.

SUGGESTED READINGS

Anderson, S. R., Jablonski, A. I., Knapp, V. M., et al. (2007). *Self-help skills for people with autism: A systematic teaching approach.* Bethesda, MD: Woodbine House.

Baker, B., & Brightman, A. (2003). *Steps to independence: Teaching everyday skills to children with special needs* (5th ed.). Baltimore: Paul H. Brookes.

Coucouvanis, J. A. (2007). *The potty journey: Guide to toilet training children with special needs, including autism and related disorders.* Shawnee Mission, KS: Autism Asperger Publishing.

Ducharme, S. H., & Gill, K. M. (1997). *Sexuality after spinal cord injury: Answers to your questions.* York, PA: Brookes, Maple Press Distribution Center.

Durand, V. M. (1998). *Sleep better: A guide to improving sleep for children with special needs.* Baltimore: Paul H. Brookes.

Lehman, J., Klaw, R., & Peebles, G. (2003). *From goals to data and back again: Adding backbone to developmental intervention for children with autism.* Philadelphia: Jessica Kingsley.

Mayer, T. K. (2007). *One-handed in a two-handed world* (3rd ed.). Boston: Prince Gallison Press.

Owens, J., & Mindell, J. (2005). *Take charge of your child's sleep: The all-in-one resource for solving sleep problems in kids and teens.* New York: Marlowe.

Schwier, K. M., & Hingsburger, D. (2000). *Sexuality: Your sons and daughters with intellectual disabilities.* Baltimore: Paul H. Brookes.

Walker-Hirsch, L. (Ed.), (2007). *The facts of life ... and more: Sexuality and intimacy for people with intellectual disabilities.* Baltimore: Paul H. Brookes.

CHAPTER

16

Instrumental Activities of Daily Living, Driving, and Community Participation

M. Louise Dunn • Kathryn M. Loukas

KEY TERMS

Instrumental activities of daily living
Community participation
Self-determination
Family chores
Adult role acquisition
Social cognition
Disability awareness
Objectives

GUIDING QUESTIONS

1. What are the instrumental activities of daily living during childhood?
2. How does participation in instrumental activities of daily living (IADL) and community activities contribute to occupational development for children and youth of all abilities?
3. What are the developmental opportunities and expectations for participation in IADL and community participation for children and youth?
4. What are the theoretical foundations of occupation-based interventions for improving participation and performance of IADL and community activities? What evidence supports these interventions?
5. What assessments specifically evaluate IADL and community participation for children and youth? How do practitioners select a measurement tool?
6. What approaches/strategies does an occupational therapy practitioner use to increase participation and performance of IADL and community activities for children and youth with special needs?
7. How would an occupational therapy practitioner apply information about development of IADL and community participation to case descriptions of children and youth?
8. How are emotional well-being, health, peer relationships, and life satisfaction associated with IADL and community participation?

Peter is a 14-year-old boy who has autism. His parents are worried about how he will take care of himself in the future. They are unsure about his role in the home and how much to ask of him. At school, the occupational therapy practitioner uses a sensorimotor approach to Peter's intervention, yet she now sees the need for more skills in independent living for Peter. The education team wonders how much to include Peter in life skills and vocational programming.

Kayla is a 12-year-old girl with spastic quadriplegic cerebral palsy. Her occupational therapy practitioner applies a motor control/neurodevelopmental treatment (NDT) and adaptation/compensation approach to her physical needs during her K-6 schooling. Since her transition to middle school, psychosocial concerns have become a priority for her family and teachers. Kayla has expressed concerns regarding her future: Will she ever be able to leave her parents' home? Will she ever be able to have a boyfriend or marry? Can she work or go to college after high school? Will she live independently or interdependently and meet her daily living needs as well as financial, food shopping and preparation, laundry, and other responsibilities of adult life?

Instrumental activities of daily living (IADL) are the more complex aspects of daily living that children and youth develop as they reach adolescence and begin to participate in the community with more autonomy. These activities include care of others, care of pets, child rearing, use of a communication device, community mobility, financial management, health management and maintenance, home management, meal preparation and clean-up, shopping, safety procedures, and emergency responses.[4] Occupational therapists are experts in IADL, task analysis, and independent/interdependent living (Figure 16-1).

Children typically acquire more skill with IADL when they reach adolescence and begin to participate in the community with more autonomy. They continue to develop competence in these activities through adolescence into young adulthood. Instrumental activities of daily living and community participation include activities that promote self-determination, self-sufficiency, health, and social participation for children/youth of all abilities. Instrumental activities of daily living competence can be categorized as part of the "magnificent mundane"[16] and is noted more by its absence than its presence. The magnificent mundane refers to the everyday presence of these tasks and reflects the tacit manner in which children/youth learn and understand their roles in these occupations. As preparation for independent living in the community, IADL include home management (e.g., clothing care, cleaning, and household maintenance), shopping and money management, meal preparation and clean up, community mobility, health maintenance (e.g., taking medications, exercise and nutrition), care of pets and care of others, and safety procedures and emergency responses.[4]

An integral relationship exists between IADL and community participation. For example, shopping is an IADL task that requires interaction with others in the community. Methods for learning to participate in the community may be tacit, such

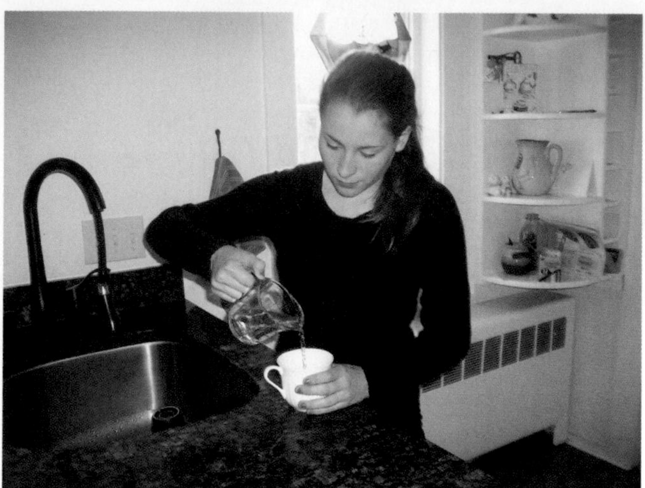

FIGURE 16-1 Precise pouring is necessary in the IADL of meal preparation and clean up.

as learning through observation and assisting with shopping, or more explicit, such as finding and enrolling in community activities. Community participation includes social, play, and leisure activities with peers, and structured activities within the neighborhood and community.[8,52]

Recent studies contribute to our understanding of the diverse and complex challenges involved in preparing youth for optimal community participation. A recent analysis of secondary transition indicates that nonacademic behaviors associated with transition to adult roles include disability awareness and activities that lead toward employment and independence. Youth and adults with physical disabilities reported that they lacked opportunities to direct their health care services such as making their own appointments and asking questions of medical and health personnel.[33,40] Adults with physical disabilities reported dependence in shopping, home cleaning, laundry, and use of public transportation.[6] Youth in foster care often lacked knowledge and experience with independent living, especially safety and home and health maintenance.[61,62] Children and youth with cognitive/behavioral disorders such as traumatic brain injury (TBI), intellectual disability, and autism spectrum disorder (ASD) often lacked opportunities to engage in household tasks and community activities such as shopping and recreational activities.[9,10,55]

Parents and caregivers reported that engagement in domestic tasks, recreation and leisure activities, and community activities was critical and important to health for children and youth of all abilities.[1,11] These parental/caregiver perspectives support the importance of examining participation in home and community activities for children with and without disabilities. However, Bedell and colleagues found that parents and caregivers of children with disabilities (e.g., both physical and cognitive/behavioral) had more barriers to participation in community activities. These barriers included the physical environment, the social environment, and resources for families and programs. These findings support a need to monitor and promote children's participation in these activities from preschool age and through young adulthood.

This chapter provides an overview of the development of IADL skills and community participation, and a description of theoretical tenets, models, and approaches that guide practices to promote competence in IADL and full participation in community living. It further explains how emotional well-being, health, peer relations, social cognition, and life satisfaction are associated with competence and independence in IADL and community living skills. Evaluation and intervention are discussed and illustrated using case examples.

Occupational Development of Instrumental Activities of Daily Living and Community Participation

Successful independent/community living is measured by outcomes related to employment, residing in the community, and community participation. A large longitudinal study demonstrated that 2 years after leaving school, youth with special needs were more likely to be unemployed, live with their parents, and lack engagement in community activities with peers than youth without disabilities.[90] In a second longitudinal study, youth with special needs showed increased employment and engagement in community activities; however, their involvement lagged behind that of their peers without disabilities.[90] Youth with special needs continued to lag behind nondisabled peers in living independently in the community.

Self-determination has been identified as a factor that promotes independent community living. Defined as "a combination of skills, knowledge, attitudes, and behaviors that enable a person to engage in goal-directed, self-regulated, autonomous behavior,"[28] self-determination encompasses many of the behaviors and attitudes often referred to as *life skills* that are both innate and learned.[53] These skills include managing personal care and health needs, taking care of one's belongings and space, managing home repairs, arranging transportation, and living interdependently with others. Opportunities to develop problem-solving skills, understand one's own strengths and limitations, and make choices are critical to developing these skills. The importance of self-determination to independent community living has strong research evidence. In fact, youth with mild intellectual and/or learning disabilities who have higher self-determination had greater employment rates, earned higher wages, and had more community involvement at 1 and 3 years out of school than similar youth with low self-determination.[92,93]

To illustrate IADL expectations for children and adolescents, we present a description of typical IADL function in four age groups starting with late adolescence. We present this information in reverse developmental order because late adolescence is the time when most attention is drawn to IADL function. The use of this reverse developmental order illustrates a progression of skill development from the most complex tasks that require more cognitive and motor skills to less complex tasks. As we progress backward, you will note the many opportunities exist even for younger children to develop IADL skills used for both home and community participation.

Late Adolescence (16 to 18 Years)

By late adolescence, youth are more autonomous and show greater breadth in their IADL and community participation than do early adolescents (Figure 16-2). Many spend most of their time outside the home, driving or taking public transportation, arranging transportation for community events, working a part-time job or volunteering, shopping, managing money, and maintaining a healthful regimen (e.g., taking responsibility for medications, exhibiting awareness of healthful behavior with partners).[22,57,79,84] At this age, many youth prepare hot and cold meals, help with clean up, and manage their laundry. Box 16-1 provides IADL and community participation expectations for older adolescents.

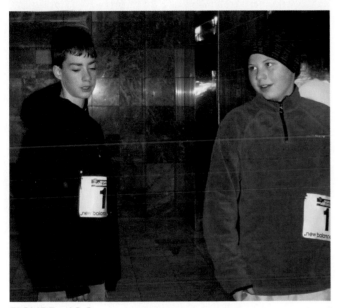
FIGURE 16-2 Two adolescents participate in a local running event as community participation.

Client factors may limit opportunities to engage in IADL tasks and community participation for many youth with physical and/or cognitive disabilities; but with adaptations and accommodations, many become competent in occupational performance. Behavioral concerns such as lack of confidence, dependency, or weak social skills may also influence task performance of youth with physical disabilities, especially in community activities.[56] Coaching, technology, and visual supports for youth with TBI promote adaptation and compensation for their difficulties with memory, problem solving, and self-management to initiate and complete tasks, sustain focus on tasks, and interact with others when completing work.[27] For example, youth with TBI are likely to need specialized coaching and assistance to manage the social demands of using public transportation on their own, to maintain and shift focus within this noisy and stimulating background, and to multitask (e.g., find a seat, count money, greet and respond to others).

Youth with autism spectrum disorder (ASD) may do well with household tasks such as making a snack, yet require supports to accomplish tasks that require more interaction, such as shopping. Cognitive/behavioral interventions assist these youth to manage tasks that involve relating to others, as would be needed to manage health care needs. Supports and opportunities for engaging in structured and unstructured leisure activities such as recreation, team sports, shopping, or

BOX 16-1 Instrumental Activities of Daily Living and Community Participation: Older Adolescents (16-21 Years)

Meal Preparation and Clean Up
- Plans and prepares simple hot and cold meals
- Puts dishes in dishwasher/puts dishes away
- Safely operates stove, oven, toaster, blender, microwave, and dishwasher

Community Mobility
- Can obtain driver's license
- Uses public transportation on own

Health Management and Maintenance
- Transfer to adult health care provider
- Responsible for managing medications
- Attends part of medical appointments alone
- Keeps record of medical history

Household Maintenance and Management
- Looks into housing choices
- Attendant services and supported living options
- Does home repairs (e.g., replaces light bulb, replaces fuses)

Clothing Management
- Launders own clothes
- Mends clothes as needed

Use of Communication Devices
- Keeps in touch with friends by phone, texting, and computer (webcam, e-mail)

Shopping and Money Management
- Practices budgeting and banking skills
- Purchases

Safety and Emergency Response
- Knows how to use fire extinguisher
- Knows what to do in case of fire or emergency

Community Participation
- Makes plans with peers for informal leisure and recreation activities
- Engages in community programs for youth/adults that match leisure or athletic interests
- Works part time and/or volunteers in community

Performance Skills
- Motor and sensory skills well developed or adaptations and accommodations identified
- Emphasis more on psychological, social, and cognitive skills
- Takes more responsibility for own routines

Data from Dunn, L., Coster, W. J., Orsmond, G. I., & Cohn, E. S. (2009). Household task participation of children with and without attentional problems. *Physical and Occupational Therapy in Pediatrics, 29*(3), 234–251; Bloorview Life Skills Institute. (2007). Growing up ready timetable & checklists. Retrieved June 3, 2009, from http://www.bloorview.ca/resourcecentre/familyresources/growingupready.php; Nollan, K. A., Wolf, M., Ansell, D., Burns, J. Barr, L., Copeland, L., et al. (2000). Ready or not: Assessing youth's preparedness for independent living. *Child Welfare, 79*(2), 159–618; Rodger, S. (2006). I can do it: Developing, promoting, and managing children's self-care needs. In S. Rodger, & J. Ziviani (Eds.), *Occupational therapy with children* (pp. 200–221). Oxford, UK: Blackwell.

volunteer activities facilitate participation for youth with ASD.[30] Coaching, peer mentors, and reverse inclusion are client-centered interventions to increase participation of youth with disabilities to seek out and to engage in IADL tasks and community activities. Many late adolescents with disabilities can arrange transportation to get together with friends, access community activities, and perhaps learn to drive through use of technology, assistance, and supports.

Early Adolescence (12 to 15 Years)

For young adolescents, teachers and parents emphasize not only learning from academics and vocational exploration, but also home and health management, shopping and meal preparation, and community participation[33,66,79] (Figure 16-3). School programs attempt to establish adolescents' independence and interdependence working with others. Young adolescents have increased responsibility for caring for others, managing their laundry, and preparing simple, hot meals and snacks.[57,79,84] Technology, such as the microwave, cell phones, e-mail, and instant messaging/texting, increases young adolescents' opportunities for communication and community participation. Box 16-2 provides IADL and community participation expectations for young adolescents.

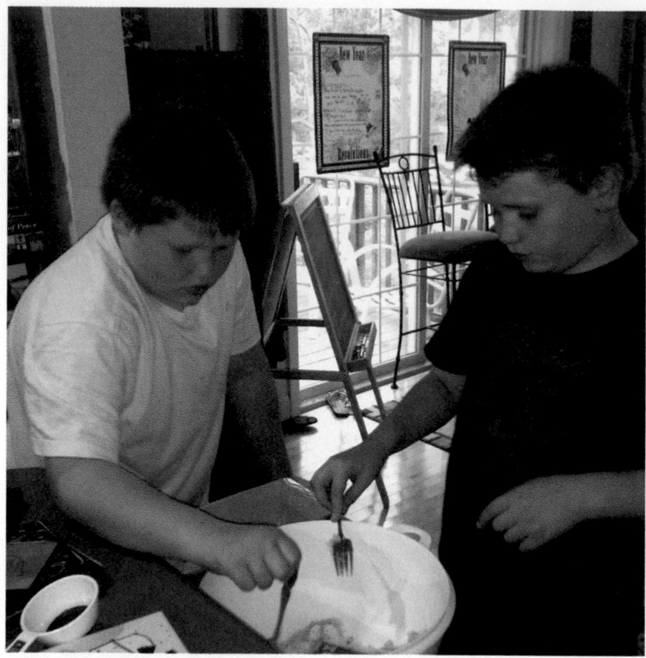

FIGURE 16-3 Children participate in the IADL of meal preparation in their home.

BOX 16-2 Instrumental Activities of Daily Living and Community Participation: Younger Adolescents (12-15 Years)

Meal Preparation and Clean Up
- Plans and prepares simple hot and cold meals
- Puts dishes in dishwasher/puts dishes away

Community Mobility
- Starts to find way around local community
- Arranges rides to friends' houses
- Arranges rides to structured leisure and recreational activities
- Uses public transportation without assistance

Health Management and Maintenance
- Begins to look for adult health care providers
- Attends some medical appointments alone
- Assists with making medical and dental appointments
- Takes more responsibility for managing medications

Household Maintenance and Management
- Participates in discussions with parents about where he or she might live as an adult
- Cleans own space and shared (family) space
- May look after or babysit others or younger siblings
- Vacuums, dusts family space
- Puts away own laundry

Use of Communication Devices
- Uses phone, pens, and computers to send and receive information

Shopping and Money Management
- May use bank card to deposit or withdraw money
- Purchases items with bank card or money
- May receive allowance, earn money from part-time work
- May purchase own goods at store

Safety and Emergency Response
- May take course in basic first aid
- Educates self about what to do in case of fire or emergency
- Responsible for personal safety when crossing street, obeying traffic and road signs

Community Participation
- Engages in informal and structured leisure and recreation with peers
- Keeps in touch with friends by phone, e-mail
- May volunteer in community

Performance Skills and Patterns
- Motor and sensory skills developed or adaptations and accommodations identified
- Emphasis more on psychological, social, and cognitive skills
- Has developed routines for daily activities, yet may need prompting

Data from Dunn, L., Coster, W. J., Orsmond, G. I., & Cohn, E. S. (2008). Household task participation of children with and without attentional problems. *Physical and Occupational Therapy in Pediatrics, 29*(3), 234–251; Growing up ready timetable and checklists. Retrieved June 3, 2009, from http://www.bloorview.ca/resourcecentre/familyresources/growingupready.php; Nollan, K. A., Wolf, M., Ansell, D., Burns, J. Barr, L., Copeland, L., et al. (2000). Ready or not: Assessing youth's preparedness for independent living. *Child Welfare, 79*(2), 159–618; Rodger, S. (2006). I can do it: Developing, promoting, and managing children's self-care needs. In S. Rodger, & J. Ziviani (Eds.), *Occupational therapy with children* (pp. 200–221). Oxford, UK: Blackwell.

Youth with disabilities often need additional practice and opportunities to promote autonomy with IADL and community participation.[9,26] Coaching and role playing help prepare young adolescents with physical disabilities to direct others or seek assistance as needed with IADL and community tasks. Some may be reluctant to express their lack of knowledge about how to prepare a meal and simply wait until someone does it for them. Participating in the planning needed to perform tasks such as moving around the home and community helps young adolescents develop more autonomy despite their cognitive/behavioral and social skill deficits.[56] Addressing assertiveness in interventions helps these young adolescents increase their engagement in leisure and recreational activities.

Similar client factors and various levels of functioning may also impede participation and performance of youth with TBI, ASD, and learning and/or intellectual disabilities. Client factors that include communication challenges and rigid occupational patterns may make it difficult for young adolescents with TBI and ASD to participate in volunteer work or arrange transportation to structured recreational activities. Lack of safety awareness and difficulty understanding the needs of others may make taking care of younger siblings or others difficult for young adolescents with disabilities. For example, clients with autism who insist on rigid routines and tend to be inflexible around changes, make negotiating with others difficult, a skill needed in many recreational activities such as group outings.

Youth at the early adolescent levels are often interested in driving and gaining independence in the community. For youth with disabilities, learning to drive often occurs later if at all. Driving involves factors such as vision, attention, motor control, and executive functioning. Limitations in safety awareness and motor coordination can make learning to drive and, therefore, accessing the community, more difficult for young adolescents with disabilities.

Middle Childhood (6 to 11 Years)

In middle childhood (6 to 11 years), children participate in household chores and neighborhood activities. However, other than school systems that offer a formal Life Skills program, few formal learning opportunities related to IADL and community participation are available. Children in the middle years prepare for future independent/community living through their engagement in everyday family, afters-chool, community, and school activities.[51,67] These occupations give children opportunities to make choices, solve problems, and identify interests and skills that help them develop self-determination, social skills, and competency with IADL and community activities.[72,85,91]

In middle childhood, many children engage in family and household routines; however, diversity in what they do and with whom is common. Parents report that they expect their children to take care of their space and materials, help with clean up after meals, prepare simple cold meals, help with putting away groceries, and care for siblings with supervision[22] (Figure 16-4). As they engage in these tasks, children develop communication, cognitive, and social interaction skills (e.g., problem solving on encountering difficulty). Community activities include formal structured activities such as sports or music lessons, as well as informal unstructured activities such as riding bikes. Box 16-3 provides IADL and community participation expectations for children of middle childhood age.

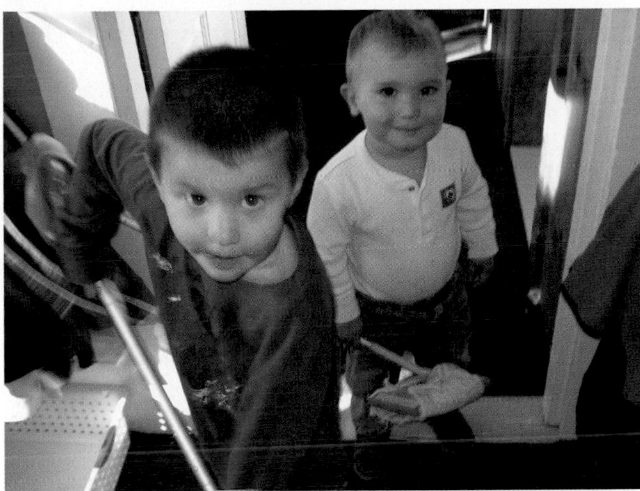

FIGURE 16-4 Children engage in household chores, an important part of occupational development.

Physical, cognitive, and social functioning deficits may make it difficult for children with disabilities to develop the skills necessary to participate in these activities. Children with physical disabilities may participate in recreational activities by observing rather than doing.[78] Some may not assist with IADL such as setting or clearing the table because of the time it takes them to do these tasks or because their physical impairments limit their participation.[18] For children with physical and/or cognitive/behavioral disabilities, generalization of learning to different settings may require specific cognitive and behavioral strategies.[74,76] Children with cognitive/behavioral disabilities such as attention-deficit/hyperactivity disorder (ADHD) may clean up after preparing food in a community setting yet not carry over this learning to their home life.[38] Supports to help children with ADHD transfer skills to the home environment include educating parents on increasing expectations and modifying the environment to cue the child to complete the steps of the task (e.g., using a visual schedule).

Client- and family-centered interventions may increase participation of children with TBI in family routines such as preparing simple cold meals and picking up shared areas. Coaching, visual cues, and opportunities for practice and repetitions may increase their participation in routines so that they can organize their belongings for school and non–school-related activities. Accommodations such as use of social stories for preparation and shopping at less busy times and in smaller stores may help to create an environment of success and reduce emotional outbursts at the supermarket or mall for children/youth who exhibit over-responsiveness to sounds, sights, and smells.

Preschool (3 to 5 Years)

In preschool, participation in home, day care, and community activities frequently occurs with supervision from caregivers or parents. Therefore family involvement is essential to development of IADL and community participation.[42,80,83]

Availability of free play allows children the opportunity to identify interests, make choices, and learn how to share and

BOX 16-3 Instrumental Activities of Daily Living and Community Participation: Middle Childhood (6-11 Years)

Meal Preparation and Clean Up
- With supervision, puts dishes in dishwasher/puts dishes away
- Gets own snacks
- Sets and clears table

Community Mobility
- Rides bicycle, uses rollerblades, scooter around neighborhood
- Makes arrangements with parent for rides to friends' houses, video store, etc.
- Uses public transportation with supervision

Health Management and Maintenance
- Participates in medication routines (as needed)
- Assists with naming medical concerns (e.g., allergies, asthma, seizures)

Household Maintenance and Management
- Puts away own materials, vacuums and dusts own room
- Puts away groceries, helps with recycling
- Organizes materials for school and after-school events

Use of Communication Devices
- Keeps in touch with friends by phone, e-mail
- Answers phone, takes messages

Shopping and Money Management
- May have a savings account
- Shops with parent or caregiver
- Finds items on shelves at supermarket

Safety and Emergency Response
- Can name places to find help or be safe
- Aware of safety with food, fire, and strangers

Community Participation
- With assistance, gets together with peers for leisure activities, hobbies, movies
- May participate in after-school programs, community center activities
- Visits with friends or relatives in neighborhood

Performance Skills and Patterns
- Motor planning and sensorimotor skills continue to develop and are further refined, may be problem areas
- Starting to follow routines for daily activities but requires prompting

Data from Dunn, L., Coster, W. J., Orsmond, G. I., & Cohn, E. S. (2008). Household task participation of children with and without attentional problems. *Physical and Occupational Therapy in Pediatrics, 29*(3), 234–251; Growing up ready timetable and checklists. Retrieved June 3, 2009, from http://www.bloorview.ca/resourcecentre/familyresources/growingupready.php; Nollan, K. A., Wolf, M., Ansell, D., Burns, J. Barr, L., Copeland, L., et al. (2000). Ready or not: Assessing youth's preparedness for independent living. *Child Welfare, 79*(2), 159–618; Rodger, S. (2006). I can do it: Developing, promoting, and managing children's self-care needs. In S. Rodger, & J. Ziviani (Eds.), *Occupational therapy with children* (pp. 200–221). Oxford, UK: Blackwell.

take turns. In Head Start programs, much emphasis is placed on promoting self-determination by assisting children to identify when they need help and guiding them to solve problems on their own.[32,83] Furthermore, children with and without disabilities are involved in many naturally occurring learning opportunities through community activities such as shopping, going to neighborhood playgrounds, attending library story hours, taking walks in the neighborhood, or participating in events at community centers.[25] In the home, preschool children assist with many household tasks such as putting away their own toys, making their beds, putting away their clothes, helping to set the table, and preparing cold snacks.[79] Most families emphasize the child's learning to accomplish basic self-care routines and to take care of his or her belongings.

Instrumental activities of daily living participation for preschool children with disabilities has not been researched. For children with physical disabilities, opportunities to perform tasks such as picking up one's toys, making choices about snacks, or pointing to items at the supermarket may provide ways to develop routines and be part of the family. With coaching and positive supports, children with TBI, ADHD, or ASD can learn to pick up their toys and to make choices about snacks or community activities.

In summary, age and functional abilities contribute to the extent of children's and youth's participation and performance of IADL and community activities. Instrumental activities of daily living and community participation are both the means and ends for development of motor and process performance skills.

Personal and Contextual Influences on Instrumental Activities of Daily Living and Community Participation

Multiple inter-related internal and external factors influence children's and youth's engagement in IADL and community activities. The occupational therapist addresses personal and contextual factors that may support or limit the child's or youth's participation in IADL and community activities.

Personal Influences

Personal influences for children and youth include their *interests*, *preferences*, and *motivation* to engage in activities. Engagement in IADL and community activities requires interest and motivation. Initially, motivation may be promoted with external support; however, to continue to engage in tasks and use skills, children and youth must internalize reasons to engage in IADL.[75] A client-centered approach that targets client interests and choices may increase internal motivation for performing IADL tasks. This, in turn, can lead to increased responsibility and opportunities to engage in occupations of choice or to earn money in the home and/or community.[13,40] For example, a client who initially only wishes to engage in swimming in the community, may be inclined to work folding towels for the pool to pay for his admission. This interest in swimming could also be used to motivate the client to access public transportation or contact others for transportation support.

Contextual Influences

Contextual influences, external to the child, include (1) the natural and built environment (physical context); (2) supports and relationships (social context); (3) attitudes, values, and beliefs (cultural context); (4) computers and assistive technology (virtual); (5) stages of life, time of year, and duration (temporal); and (6) service systems and policies.[2,95] Service systems and policies—eligibility and insurance coverage—also influence opportunities available to children and youth. These contextual influences can either support or limit children's and youth's participation IADL and community activities.

The natural and built environment (physical context) includes the sensory and physical qualities of the setting (e.g., noise, lighting, temperature, terrain, crowding), building design, and accessibility to materials.[56] Within the home, access to different areas and materials supports participation of children and youth in family activities. In the community, buildings that have accessible entrances and activities on a flat terrain support inclusion of children and youth with physical limitations. Examples of barriers are homes without access to all areas and community centers with activities on multiple levels that lack ramps or elevators. Crowding (e.g., group size) and sensory aspects of the environment are potential barriers for children and youth with physical, sensory, cognitive, and intellectual disabilities.[43,65] For children and youth with TBI, ADHD, ASD, and intellectual disability, the noise from people talking and the movement of people in a crowd may contribute to behavioral outbursts, anxiety, and aggression, thus decreasing their participation. Noise, visual stimulation, and crowding limit participation because these factors interfere with balance, mobility, and communication for children and youth with physical disabilities.[65]

Supports and relationships (social context) are particularly salient factors that influence participation of children and youth in IADL and community activities. At home, support is crucial for participation with family members in everyday activities. Families provide children with opportunities and encouragement to learn household tasks such as mealtime preparation and care of common spaces. Modeling of task performance and discussion of tacit planning processes make learning and understanding these tasks more tangible to children and youth. For example, at home children can observe not only their parents but also their siblings. In addition, children may be mentors to their siblings and guides for their parents. As children mature, they may take on the role of caring for their siblings when parents are out of the home. In the community, children may begin by attending structured after-school activities such as sports or recreation groups (see Figure 16-2), or they may meet with peers to socialize at the mall. As they approach older adolescence, they may also take on roles as mentors at recreational centers or scouting events.

The social environment for IADL participation varies by setting (e.g., school, home, community, or work). Children observe parents and siblings doing household tasks and often attempt to model their actions. For example, social outcomes from participating in mealtime preparation and household tasks include promoting a sense of family, interacting with family members, and demonstrating positive social behaviors.[22,66] A long-term social outcome includes preparation for adult roles with preparing meals and engaging with family members. Lack of support and diminished opportunities for participation in these mundane everyday tasks can impede development of community living skills (e.g., such as the example of youth in foster homes).[57]

Cultural values and beliefs significantly influence opportunities for IADL and community participation. Family beliefs about routines and perspectives on how children spend their time influence participation of children and youth in the home and community.[28,34,88] For example, parents of Asian background tend to value academics and place much less emphasis on IADL activities and autonomy for their children.[97] In contrast, Latino and Navajo families tend to focus on interdependency and promote engagement in household and IADL tasks.[81]

The value of interdependency versus autonomy may influence a family's willingness to support the independence of a child or youth with a disability. Families from African American and Hispanic backgrounds are more likely to plan to have their children with developmental disabilities live with them when the children become adults.[13] These values may also influence the opportunities to engage in IADL tasks and community activities for children and youth with disabilities. Parents of children with disabilities, particularly those from lower socioeconomic levels, were less likely to involve their children in household tasks and in interacting with others in the community.[97] Values for engaging in interdependent activities also influence participation in household tasks. For example, parents of children with ADHD tend to emphasize household tasks that involve managing one's own belongings with less focus on shared tasks such as helping at mealtimes.[25]

Community programs that include children and youth of all abilities are supports for community participation.[65] Inclusive community participation opportunities may include recreation, summer camps, sports programs and teams, inclusive arts, and other community programs. Occupational supports may include access to physical space and equipment, modifications in rules to support skill levels, social supports such as a buddy system, and behavioral coaching to design activities and programs that include children of all abilities. The occupational therapy practitioner should take into consideration and prepare youth and families for the possibility of social stigma, bullying, and marginalization.[56,65]

Technology, computers, online resources, and assistive and augmentative communication devices are supports used commonly with children and youth who have disabilities to promote their participation in IADL and community activities. Technology and online resources afford opportunities for children and youth of all abilities to connect with others. Information about community activities, employment, shopping, banking, meal planning, public transportation, and health are available online. A growing number of support groups for children and youth with many differing disabilities have set up websites that provide peer mentoring for learning how to live in the community and care for their own needs.

Examples of *service systems* that promote inclusion of children and youth with disabilities are inclusive aftercare and recreational programs, programs with adaptive equipment, and transportation. *Policies*, rules, and standards that govern these services ensure that they are accessible and enable optimal participation of persons with disabilities.[56,95] For children and youth with disabilities, lack of transportation or length of time required to transition to programs can be a barrier to participation in community activities.[43] Another barrier is the lack of policies and funding to cover costs of additional supports that may be needed for inclusion of children and youth with disabilities in out-of-school activities.[43]

Evaluation of Instrumental Activities of Daily Living and Community Participation

Children, youth, and their families or caregivers play strategic roles in the evaluation process. Parents and caregivers provide relevant information about the settings and contexts in which the children or youth engage in IADL and community activities. Providing youth with opportunities to engage in the evaluation process increases their autonomy and prepares them for decision making and management of their health, IADL, and community participation. In addition, families may increase IADL and community participation expectations of the child/youth as a result of the evaluation process and discussions.

Occupational therapists evaluate IADL and community participation using a combination of the following methods: chart review/history, observation, occupational profile/interview, inventory/questionnaire, performance measures, and interest checklists. The evaluation may be part of a school-based triennial evaluation required under IDEA, a transition plan at the request of a pediatrician or health care practitioner, a request from the parent as part of a hospital-based assessment, or a community program such as foster care. Occupational therapists administer evaluations individually with the child/youth and caregiver, as a team evaluation, or as part of a program evaluation. At school, this process may occur when the educational team, which includes the youth and family, develops the individual transition plan (ITP). This evaluation process also may occur when children and youth return to school after hospitalization secondary to medical concerns such as traumatic brain or spinal cord injury. Interdisciplinary team evaluations often occur in psychiatric facilities, foster care programs, juvenile justice programs, and as part of community system services. Team members often include, but are not limited to, children and youth, caregivers, occupational and physical therapists, speech language pathologists, nurses, psychologists, social workers, and physiatrists. Interprofessional information is helpful for a holistic and realistic appraisal of the child or youth's performance and potential in a variety of settings. Table 16-1 provides a listing of measures used by occupational therapists to assess IADL.

Measurement of Outcomes

Occupational scientists and therapists along with professionals in rehabilitation and health have developed assessments to measure outcomes of IADL and community participation (see

TABLE 16-1 Instruments for Assessing Instrumental Activities of Daily Living and Community Participation for Children and Youth

Instrument	Areas, Method, Age range	Description
AMPS *Assessment of Motor and Process Skills* (5th ed.) Fisher (2003a,b) AMPS Project International P. Box 42 Hampton Falls, NH 03844 www.ampsintl.com	**Areas addressed** Person Task **Method** Observation **Age range** 3 years to adult	• AMPS is a criterion-referenced test for activities of daily living (ADL) and instrumental activities of daily living (IADL) tasks that assess underlying motor and process performance skills used to perform the task. • Examiner training—formal training procedure through course attendance, observation, and calibration of scoring through AMPS International required. • Established reliability and validity with normative data for typical individuals
Ansell-Casey Life Skills Inventory Nollan et al. (2000) Online assessment available at www.casselifeskills.org	**Areas assessed** Person Task **Method** Interview Observation **Age range** 8-18 years	• Assessment of life skills, developed on children and youth in foster care, that is completed online and then automatically scored. • Life skills categories include home and money management, health, safety and emergency, transportation • Criterion-referenced • Good reliability and validity
ASK *Activity Scale for Kids* Young et al. (2000) Nancy Young, PhD nancyyoung@sickkids.on.ca ASK manual (1996) The Hospital for Sick Children Toronto, Ontario	**Areas assessed** Person Task **Methods** Interview Questionnaire Observation **Age range** 5-15 years	• Measures performance (what child does) and capacity (what child is capable of doing) for personal care, dressing, eating, locomotion, stairs, play, transfers, and standing skills • Excellent reliability and validity • Child and/or parent report • Takes ≈30 minutes first time, 10 minutes for repeat tests • Summed scores allow comparison of individuals across time

TABLE 16-1 Instruments for Assessing Instrumental Activities of Daily Living and Community Participation for Children and Youth—cont'd

CHORES *Children Helping Out: Responsibilities, Expectations and Supports* Dunn (2004) Contact Louise Dunn, ScD OTR/L ldunn@brenau.edu	**Areas assessed** Person Environment Task **Methods** Interview Questionnaire **Age range** Grades 1-8 ≈6-14 years	• Parent report measure that examines children's participation in household tasks • Has excellent internal consistency and test-retest reliability for school-aged children (Dunn, 2004) and youth (Dunn, in preparation) • Takes ≈15-20 minutes to complete • Scoring: summary scores allow comparison of individuals across time. • Additional open-ended questions about parents' perspectives on importance and satisfaction with their children's household task participation
COACH *Choosing Options and Accommodations for Children* (2nd ed.) Giangreco, Cloninger, & Iverson (1997) Paul Brookes Publishing PO Box 10624 Baltimore, MD 21285 www.brookespublishing.com	**Areas assessed** Person Task **Methods** Interview/questionnaire Observation **Age range** 3-21 years	• COACH is a curriculum-referenced transdisciplinary team assessment and curriculum with four domains: personal management, community, home, and vocational • Used as a team planning tool; does not assess specific skills • Intended for children with moderate, severe, or profound disabilities but has been used with children with mild disabilities
LIFE-H *Life Habits Questionnaire* Noreau et al. (2007) Contact Luc Noreau, PhD Luc.Noreau@rea.ulaval.ca	**Areas assessed** Person Environment Task **Methods** Interview Questionnaire **Age range** 5-18 years	• Parent and youth report measure based on ICF participation. Excellent reliability and validity. • Examines 6 categories of participation: interpersonal relationships, communication, personal care, mobility education, and recreation. Examines daily activities (e.g., personal care, mobility, nutrition) and social roles (e.g., recreation, responsibility) • Takes ≈15-20 minutes to complete. Youth may complete as part of interview. • Summary scores permit individual comparison over time
Participation and Environment Measure for Children and Youth (PEM-CY) Coster et al. (2011) Available at: http://participation-environment.canchild.ca/en/participation_environment_measure_children_youth	**Areas assessed** Person Environment Task **Methods** Questionnaire—electronic, paper **Age range** 5-17 years	• Parent/caregiver report measure based on ICF classification of participation at home, school, and in community. Excellent reliability and validity. • Takes ≈25-30 minutes to complete. Youth may complete as part of interview. • Population-based measure. Summary scores permit individual comparison over time.
Pediatric Evaluation of Disability Inventory-Computer Adaptive Test (PEDI-CAT) Haley, Coster, Dumas, Fragala-Pinkham, Moed, et al. (1992; 2012) Available at: http://www.Pedicat.com Cost ~ $99	**Areas assessed** Person Environment Task **Method** Questionnaire Electronic **Age range** Birth to 20 years	• Revised with increased attention to ICF classification of participation at home, school, and in community. Excellent reliability and validity. • Takes ≈30 minutes to complete • Summary scores permit individual comparison over time

Table 16-1). Using the International Classification of Functioning, Disability, and Health for Children and Youth, health-related outcomes include participation patterns, activity performance, quality of life, client satisfaction, and contextual supports and barriers.[95]

Assessments for IADL and community participation are relatively few; most are inventories that are completed by a caregiver. The Assessment of Motor and Process Skills (AMPS) is standardized and appears to be sensitive to the progress that children make.[30,31] Studies demonstrated that the AMPS can identify differences in IADL for children with and without ADHD[38] and for children with hemiplegic cerebral palsy.[89]

Several new participation assessments have recently become available (see Table 16-1). The Participation and Environment Measure for Children and Youth (PEM-CY)[19] and the Life Habits Questionnaire (LIFE-H)[68] measure participation at home, school, and in the community. These measures produce change scores that can be used to examine outcomes from individual intervention or programmatic outcomes. Measures may be completed by the caregiver or teacher and by the child or youth for comparison of perspectives.

The PEM-CY has been used to obtain information about participation for children of all abilities from 5 to 17 years.[19] Some examples of PEM-CY home items include socializing

Household tasks (SC = Self-care) (FC = Family-care)	Not expected (1)	Child cannot (2)	Lot of assistance (3)	Some assistance (4)	With supervision (5)	When asked (6)	On own initiative (7)
Puts away own clothes (SC) ☐ Yes ☐ No							
Makes self a cold meal (SC) ☐ Yes ☐ No							
Puts own laundry in hamper (SC) ☐ Yes ☐ No							
Sweeps or vacuums own room (SC) ☐ Yes ☐ No							
Feeds pet (FC) ☐ Yes ☐ No							
Sets or clears the table (FC) ☐ Yes ☐ No							
Takes out garbage/recycling (FC) ☐ Yes ☐ No							
Cares for younger sibling (FC) ☐ Yes ☐ No							

FIGURE 16-5 Examples of items and ratings for the Children Helping Out: Responsibilities, Expectations, and Supports (CHORES) Program.

with technology, household chores, homework, indoor play and games, and computer and video games.[55]

The LIFE-H obtains information about social participation for 5- to 13-year-old children and youth with physical disabilities, TBI, or developmental disabilities.[68] *Life habits* refer to participation in valued everyday activities, such as nutrition, fitness, communication, and personal care, and valued social roles such as responsibility and community life.

Educational personnel, health professionals, and caregivers often address preparation for independent and interdependent living during adolescence; however, research supports monitoring and assessing these performance areas before adolescence. Because children and youth with disabilities often require additional support to learn and perform these tasks, assessment and planning before adolescence are needed. The Children Helping Out: Responsibilities, Expectations, and Supports (CHORES) program was developed for these purposes and provides information about participation in household tasks and some aspects of IADL.[21] In CHORES, household tasks include domestic tasks as well as caring for others. Household tasks are organized into two groups: self-care tasks and family-care tasks.[94] Self-care refers to household tasks for which the outcomes primarily affect the individual, such as picking up one's clothing or making a cold meal for oneself. Family care refers to household tasks for which the outcomes primarily affect others, such as caring for pets and preparing meals (see Figure 16-3).

Scoring on CHORES provides a way to measure change for individuals across time. Changes are measured by comparing the number of tasks performed and the assistance required to perform household tasks. Two open-ended items provide information about the importance of household task participation to parents and parents' satisfaction with their children's household task participation. Refer to Figure 16-5 for examples of items and rating scales for CHORES.

The information gathered from CHORES contributes to development of intervention goals for household task performance and family participation. This information can promote discussions about expectations and opportunities and preparation for independent living for children and youth of all abilities.

Transition Planning

Inclusion of the families or caregivers of children with disabilities promotes and reinforces positive self-esteem and self-determination skills.[35,60,86,93,96] Occupational therapists facilitate psychosocial skills and community participation–based interventions in elementary grades and well before formal transition planning. Occupational therapists often provide services in the school setting to children who experience difficulties with occupational performance of self-care or functional mobility, rendering a prime opportunity for therapists to implement needed skills for independent living. In addition, the school-based occupational therapist understands both the assets and functional challenges of the youth and family, making them the ideal professional to facilitate the transition to adult roles.[46] The American Occupational Therapy Association (AOTA) promotes the role of occupational therapy in transitions. Specific roles for occupational therapists for clients in transition to adulthood include preparation of student and families for changes in roles and routines; representing and advocating for the needs of the student; evaluating and implementing supports for employment and/or continuing education; building skills for employment and volunteer roles; facilitation of self-determination and social integration into the community; evaluation and intervention for occupation-based mobility, including the possibility of driving or using public transportation; and promoting and fostering self-advocacy skills.[3]

As children begin their transition to adult roles, occupational therapy practitioners focus on independent or interdependent community living.[18] This is best accomplished by engagement in meaningful IADL occupations in the natural environment. Ideas include use of cottage industries, student-led planning and implementation of community events, providing support groups for young adults and families, use of public transportation as an intervention activity, and simulated activities such as money exchange and social interactions. As Orentlicher and Michaels note, the adolescent's goal is to achieve full status as an adult:

> *Disability is a natural part of human experiences and it does not diminish the right of the individual to live independently, enjoy self-determination, make choices, contribute to society, pursue meaningful careers, and enjoy full inclusion and integration in the economic, political, cultural and educational mainstream of American society (p. 2).*[69]

Transition planning is concerned with the continuing process of moving from a supported home environment to a role of living in the adult community. Adolescents with disabilities or those who are at risk may require more planning, intervention, and support than a typical student.[44,45,64,69,70]

Occupational therapists understand and appreciate the important link between occupations and identity.[17,49] Desired outcomes for adolescents with lifelong disabilities include safe, independent or interdependent engagement in occupation in the natural occurring contexts of IADL in the home or community[2] and the formation of a strong, positive disability identity (Case Study 16-1).[48]

Theoretical Models and Intervention Approaches

Occupational therapy practitioners use a number of overarching *philosophical tenets* in intervention for individuals, groups, and populations. Overarching tenets pertinent to IADL and community participation include client- and family-centered practice, engagement in occupation to promote health and identity formation, and occupation as means and ends. In different contexts and according to the client pattern of strengths and limitations, *intervention approaches* such as remediation, skill acquisition, adaptation/compensation, environmental modification, education, and/or prevention approaches are applied.[36] In addition, occupational therapists use *Models of Practice* and *Frames of Reference* to guide their clinical reasoning or decision making when planning and implementing intervention.[14] For more information on practice models in occupational therapy with children, see Chapter 2.

Family- and Client-Centered Models of Practice

Family- and client-centered involvement and decision making are an essential part of intervention planning and implementation in IADL and community participation as adolescent and young adult clients move forward in their occupational development. Client-centered practice implies a strong collaborative approach with the client/family, mutual respect and open communication, and facilitation of family/client choice in intervention planning.[36] Examples of client-centered interventions include helping families connect to support groups, offering choices and opportunities to participate, and involving clients in goal writing and documentation of progress. This empowerment is essential in building IADL and community participation occupational performance skills.

Self-Determination and Advocacy

Occupational therapy practitioners and the interdisciplinary team often use a client-centered model or approach to enhance the child's or youth's sense of control and his or her independence. Empowering an adolescent toward self-determination can facilitate independence.[33,84,92,96] One way the occupational therapy practitioner promotes self-determination is by including the child/youth in intervention planning, making choices, and problem solving. Collaborative decision making with the youth and family can foster an intentional relationship that leads to increased occupational performance.[87] This strategy can be replicated in any area of the child or adolescent's program. Health care and education professionals provide supported opportunities to prepare youth for taking care of their daily needs (e.g., taking medications), making appointments, and assessing accessibility in the community.[86] Decision making and increasing independence are crucial to the adolescent feeling competent and in control. These feelings can create "strands of coherence" (p. 236)[73] as the adolescent becomes an adult.

Self-determination can be facilitated through interventions that emphasize self-advocacy, goal setting and attainment, self-awareness, and problem solving.[73] For example, the occupational therapy practitioner can facilitate positive changes to the client's physical appearance, IADL skills, and self-empowerment by encouraging or adapting use of make-up, jewelry, or fashionable clothing. Encouraging involvement in school-based, recreational, and/or Special Olympics sports or athletics can improve performance and social participation.[58] When using group sessions, the occupational therapist can enhance and facilitate positive peer relationships and social roles. Davidson and Fitzgerald advocate for a client-centered approach that includes exploring realistic potential careers and facilitating all areas of adult independence.[20]

Discounting and empowering are complementary strategies that help to empower adolescents and young adults with disabilities. Discounting, or reframing, is a technique that redefines a disability in terms of what a person can do versus what

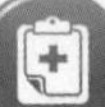

CASE STUDY 16-1 Kayla

Kayla is a 12-year-old girl who is spirited and full of life. She is a child with athetoid cerebral palsy that affects her movement in all areas of motor performance, yet her process skills are intact. She is small and thin for her age and has some significant postural control difficulties and fine motor challenges. Occupational therapy services primarily used an ecological model and sensorimotor interventions during her primary school years. The occupational therapist made modifications for her to participate in a therapy swim group and used modifications and adapted strategies for eating and feeding, clothing management, writing, physical education, music, and art-based activities. She was fully included in school classes with modifications and the assistance of an intervention aide.

As Kayla entered middle school, she was less tolerant of occupational therapy in the inclusive setting. She no longer wanted to use her adaptations for eating and feeding in the cafeteria and often did not wear her ankle foot orthotics. Once happy and fun-loving, she became sullen, was rude to her intervention aide, was abrupt with other children, and would often sit and cry. The occupational therapist implemented an intervention plan based on a client-centered model with emphasis on self-determination in a revised intervention plan.

Self-Perception and Increasing Disability Awareness

Kayla was discouraged after being the only child with significant physical disabilities in her school for 6 years. She felt different from others. She was frustrated and angry about not being able to perform activities independently. She was self-conscious about her physical differences and did not want to stand out in any way.

Kayla had developed habits of being somewhat dependent on others. As she entered adolescence, she developmentally wanted to be more independent and break away, but physically could not. Having an aide kept her feeling dependent and not in control of her life and social activities. She also began having more difficulty keeping up with her peers academically.

Kayla was beginning to understand the "lived body" experience and to develop a "disability identity,"[35] but she had no one to talk to about this emerging identity. She understood the need for adaptations but did not want them to stand out. She was torn between wanting to perform well at school and not wanting to have things done "differently."

In the assessment interview, the occupational therapist helped Kayla vent her frustrations and talk about her current and future roles. It became apparent that she was concerned about her future and doubted her own capacities. In an educational team meeting, more comprehensive occupational therapy services were put in place to improve Kayla's independence, IADL skills, and psychosocial functioning. Goals were written to improve life skills and community participation.

1. Given support group, psychosocial facilitation, and increased responsibility in the home and school, Kayla will improve self-perception, disability awareness, and self-advocacy as measured by self-report.
2. Given graded increased expectations for home chores, clothing management, small meal preparation, pet care, money management, cell phone use, and shopping, Kayla will gain independence in IADL skills as measured by a checklist.
3. Given alternative mobility options including a power scooter, Kayla will successfully access three community events as measured by self and family report.
4. To transition to adult roles, Kayla will develop a realistic plan for future continuing education, interdependent living, and employment.
5. Using adaptations in the school environment, Kayla will effectively identify, manage, and advocate for her own needs/modifications in a polite and responsible manner as reported by aide and occupational therapist observation.

Intervention Strategies

Support Group and Responsibility

Kayla was asked if she would like to train her new teacher and aide about her use of equipment and her writing, dressing, eating, and reading adaptations. She practiced with her occupational therapist during a summer session, and then she presented her needs to her new teachers the day before school began. This increased her sense of control and improved her compliance with her adaptations. In addition, her family was committed to improving her independence and began involving Kayla in family chores. Chores selected by Kayla and her family included setting the table, dusting, vacuuming, and pet care. Kayla also worked with the occupational therapist to gain the skills to make her own lunch and to use the stove, oven, and dishwasher. This improved meaning and responsibility in her family role identity. In addition, the occupational therapist consulted with the family in assisting Kayla with the fine motor use of her cell phone. These skills increased to the point that Kayla began using her cell phone for programming numbers and emergency contacts. She also learned how to monitor her minutes and keep the phone costs within the billing plan. The use of the cell phone created new access to socialization outside of school and she became more involved in after-school events.

Discounting and Empowering

One issue that had emerged was that Kayla did not want to wear her ankle-foot orthotics (AFOs) and would come to school in mid–high-heeled shoes. This caused her to lose her balance and slip, to the point of its being dangerous. Through community events, the occupational therapist helped Kayla realize it was much safer to be comfortable and stable. The occupational therapist persuaded Kayla to try some sports activities for people with disabilities. Kayla tried Special Olympics, and she excelled in horseback riding and swimming. School sports were discounted, and adapted sports were highlighted. This improved her community participation as well as her ADL and IADL skills as she traveled. The outcome was positive and reinforcing once she started winning medals. The

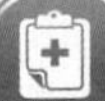

CASE STUDY 16-1 Kayla—cont'd

school supported her by congratulating her over the intercom and displaying her ribbons and medals in a school trophy case.

Developing a Disability Identity[48]

Kayla's occupational therapist was able to arrange for her to visit Jim, an occupational therapist colleague who had cerebral palsy. Kayla, her mother, and the occupational therapist visited Jim at his outpatient clinic. Kayla watched him work doing hand therapy and conversed easily with him and his client. Jim talked about his wife and two children and how he really learned about independence by going to an Easter Seals camp when he was about her age. He talked about choosing hand therapy because he felt that he could not perform mobility-based occupational therapy. He talked about being a better therapist because clients respected his own disability experience. Kayla and Jim continued to e-mail each other after that visit. Kayla confided to the occupational therapist that she asked him about things she would not discuss with others.

Sexuality and Body Image

Kayla's physical development during adolescence provided opportunities for the occupational therapist and Kayla to problem solve the logistical problems and wonderful opportunities of becoming a woman. Her mother helped her find fashionable clothing that was functional for her to put on independently. She decided to cut her hair stylishly short, because it was difficult to take care of her long hair. The occupational therapist consulted with Kayla's mother about discussing sexuality with Kayla. These natural, dynamic, and developmental techniques supported her IADL skills of self-care and independent living.

Exclusive and Inclusive Programming

As mentioned, Kayla attended the Special Olympics two to three times a year and went to Easter Seals Camp in the summer for 2 weeks. Attending camp away from her family was an important step in the development of independence and disability identity. The occupational therapist also encouraged her to participate in school-based activities such as the school play. Academic support was added that included more small-group learning. In the small groups, Kayla was granted the time with assignments to effectively use her adapted computer and keep work output at a reasonable pace. With more support and a more reasonable pace, Kayla's frustration decreased and her school success increased. She improved in her written communication and numerical abilities when engaged in community activities where these skills were necessary.

Developing a Future Vision

The local college added a group home–based dormitory that helped college students with disabilities. Kayla, her occupational therapist, and her family discussed an article about the dorm, and Kayla was very interested; in fact, her aunt was attending that college. Kayla understood that she might always need assistance but could live an interdependent life. She became more tolerant of her intervention aide's assistance and they developed good communication about how and when to assist. She began to take more initiative in her ADL and IADL in the home environment. In collaboration with the occupational therapist, she organized her bedroom and clothing, began a filing system that was large and open to accommodate her fine motor needs, and began online banking with her adapted computer.

Community Mobility

Occupational therapy practitioners arranged for Kayla, her family, and team members to attend a wheelchair clinic, and she obtained a scooter for community mobility. She also had a technology consultation to ensure that her academic technologic support was optimal for future education needs. Kayla used her power scooter in the community for longer travel such as field trips, shopping, and sporting events. These were important steps in establishing her capacity to participate in the community. Kayla again began to thrive.

Outcomes

Individual education program goal areas of community participation, improved independence, and disability identity increased 100% as measured by the educational team. After occupational therapy consultation, the aide in the classroom, although still needed for adaptive assignments and programming, took a less central role and covered the needs of children other than Kayla. Through interviewing and self-assessment, Kayla listed the most significant strategies to her success as her time at summer camp, Special Olympics, and establishment of the mentorship with the occupational therapist with cerebral palsy. She indicated that she felt more in control of her life and more positive about the future. Kayla's family also reported positive outcomes from the comprehensive intervention plan to increase IADL and community participation, noting that their perception of Kayla's future had shifted toward more independence. Kayla's IADL skills in home management, telephone/cell phone use, money management, food preparation, shopping, social interaction, and community mobility had improved along with her confidence, self-determination, self-advocacy, and positive disability identity.

he or she cannot do.[35,50,62] For example, Evans, McDougall, and Baldwin found that participation of youth with disabilities in many community-based activities at their level of ability, fostered development of relationships and social behaviors.[26] The fact that the young people with disabilities are not doing the same work as typical peers is "discounted" and "reframed" as productive work. The researchers found that involvement of youth with disabilities in community participation correlated with increased employment and self-determination in young adulthood. Reframing can be applied to other areas that may be difficult for a child or adolescent to succeed in (e.g., sports and other physical activities). Placing less importance on one skill may close the gap between values and perceived competence, a strategic element to self-esteem and self-identity.[46]

The research literature supports the importance of self-determination to youth's development of self-image, independent living skills, problem solving, and active involvement.[87] Inclusive services that are strength based and widely accessible give adolescents opportunities to succeed in social relations and life tasks. Examples of this type of programming are the Community Capacity-Building project, which provided a forum that brought together youth, families, and community stakeholders to increase a youth's communication and opportunities.[96] A second example is an occupational therapy program that created a "Life Skills Institute" as a comprehensive framework to support youth with disabilities and their families in the transition to adult services.[33]

Incorporation of Sexuality and Body Image

Adolescents are developing physically and psychologically, and occupational therapists support these positive moves toward adulthood. Noticing and appreciating the growth, changes, new interests, moves toward independence, and physical attractiveness can help build self-esteem in children and adolescents. Comments about growth and positive changes can be incorporated into personal care, because both male and female clients may have new personal hygiene needs as well as evolving desires to dress and groom themselves differently. It is important to understand that adolescents with disabilities experience the same hormonal changes as in typical adolescents and perhaps have more questions about what these changes may bring. Families often struggle as their child with a disability becomes a sexual being. The occupational therapist has a key role in supporting this area of occupational performance and adolescent development.[76] One strategy to accomplish this is to establish clear boundaries in youths' relationships and personal space with caregiving adults versus strangers or acquaintances. This is an essential safety strategy for young people with disabilities, who are recognized to be vulnerable to sexual abuse as they move toward further levels of independent living.[76]

The Circles Program facilitates the establishment of physical boundaries for adolescents with developmental disabilities.[86] (See Chapter 12 for further information on social participation.) By teaching safe relationships, appropriate personal space, and sexuality to adolescents with developmental challenges, the practitioner can demonstrate to clients with intellectual disability how close to let people into their personal space. The concepts of personal space are taught with actual circles around the client: The closest circle indicates the space of closeness with family, the middle circle at forearm length indicates friends, and a wider circle of a full arm's length is taught for keeping personal space between the youth and acquaintances and strangers.[86]

Occupation as Identity

Many youth with disabilities do not know what their future might hold. Occupational therapy practitioners work with clients and their families to recommend possible avenues for prevocational and vocational programming, as well as independent living. Through this process, adolescents may see a hopeful and positive future leading to behaviors that support transitions.[63] Although inclusive programs have expanded the opportunities for children and youth with disabilities, inclusion also separates youth from role models with similar disabling conditions. To develop a disability awareness of their own, youth with disabilities need exposure to role models of adults with disability working and thriving in the community. Visiting work sites and group homes can help youth with disabilities and their families form a positive future vision.[33,96]

The use of mentors or positive role models for IADL and community participation skill development is an intervention strategy that can be effectively used to help the youth with disability gain perspective and increase positive self-regard.[5] The adolescent client may also serve as a mentor for others by assisting in a younger classroom, tutoring students in simple reading or math subjects, or bringing cookies to elders in the community. An adolescent can be encouraged to mentor a younger child with a similar disability. A mentoring program that pairs a successful adult from the community with an adolescent with a similar disability can also help to increase the adolescent's confidence.[5,63] Peer and cross-age tutoring in reading or other academic tasks can assist with positive role identity and improve behavior in youth with disabilities.[5,81]

Emphasizing adolescents' assets and abilities is essential. Changing the context from one in which the adolescent client struggles to one in which he or she can succeed is essential to this strategy.[42] For instance, cooking may be an area in which clients with cerebral palsy or other physical impairment have difficulty. Beginning an IADL session with a safe and physically simple task such as wiping the kitchen surfaces may lead to greater success. The adolescent can be encouraged to compare him- or herself with other adolescents with similar disabilities, instead of with typically developing peers. Special Olympics camps for children with special needs or support groups are places in which adolescents can experience more success and less competition. Inclusion within the community is positive, but it is also important to establish esteem and disability identity with like peers.[48] Individualized and person-centered programming such as Special Olympics, specialized summer camp experiences, handicapped ski programs, adaptive sports, support groups, and other avenues should be explored to help the adolescent client develop a disability identity.[48,86] Bedell and colleagues emphasize the importance of creating opportunities for learning daily tasks and social skills for school-aged children with brain injuries.[11] These authors advocate for involving parents in creating opportunities in the community to teach youth cognitive functions and behavioral regulation within the context of daily life occupations.[11]

Support Groups

A number of studies showed positive outcomes from a family/client-centered, peer-run support group for parents of children transitioning to adulthood.[53,77] A peer support group may help parents gain new knowledge and became future oriented in preparing for their child's transition into adulthood. Loukas and co-workers (in process) found that use of a parent support group as part of transition planning programs enhanced IADL participation in the home and led to greater involvement in the community for young adults with high functioning autism.

Creating community connections for support is an important transition component to adulthood for youth with disabilities.[96] Creation of networks that include parents, teachers, occupational therapists, and community agencies can facilitate and support the process of transition to adulthood and entry to the workforce for clients with disabilities.[54,96] When communities have support networks, virtual support groups and websites can be helpful, although an adult should monitor the adolescent's online activity. In addition a growing number of technological tools are available to enhance independence and function, including software apps. (See Chapter 19 for more information on assistive technology.)

Ecological Models

Ecological models that emphasize adaptation/compensation and environmental modifications are frequently used to facilitate participation of individuals with disabilities in IADL and community life. In ecological models, the child's physical and social environments are adapted to improve occupational performance. See Table 16-2 for specific ideas for adaptive success for common physical, cognitive, and psychosocial challenges.

Our introductory client, Peter, is a 14-year-old youth with autism. Occupational therapy services in the middle school used an ecological model to promote Peter's acquisition of skills that are needed in the adult roles of employment and independent living.[15] The practitioner established a lunch group and obtained the adaptive equipment and assistive technology that Peter needed to make lunch with his peers. Environmental adaptations included use of ear protectors in the noisy kitchen, picture symbols in his schedule, and a scripting mechanism for communication. Peter worked with money, interacted with customers, and used adaptive strategies for a new skill in sandwich making. These skills can directly transfer to future employment in a lunch preparation cottage industry.

In addition, Peter became more involved in adapted leisure activities. He competed in Special Olympics in skiing,

TABLE 16-2 Adapted Instrumental Activities of Daily Living

Common Client-Based Challenges	Adaptive Strategies	Application Physical Challenges
Physical Challenges		
Decreased range of motion	Position for limited motion Change the task Provide assistance or interdependence	Write a check Provide stable seating and position hand on inclined tabletop Use online banking Have joint checking account
Decreased strength, endurance, and/or functional mobility	Use work simplification/energy conservation techniques Consider time management to work in small chunks of time Use modern energy-saving devices Plan out tasks to maximize energy	Shop Use a scooter or cart Determine best time of day and shop in small increments of time Use a reacher or other device Pay using debit card Plan with list and determine most efficient route in store
Decreased hand function	Build up utensils or use adapted equipment Use universal cuff or other grip substitute Buy precut or prepared items or energy-saving devices	Prepare a meal Use proper equipment Slide items if necessary Use scissors or devices for opening prepared foods Buy items that are pre-prepared
Cognitive Challenges		
Safety awareness	Develop strict rules and reinforce them Use of equipment such as wire gloves when cutting in the kitchen Use of a "buddy system" Have a safety plan	Use the bus system Follow directions Travel with a friend Learn bus etiquette, including making sure the bus is stopped before entering Alert the driver to safety needs Have an emergency phone
Difficulty with judgment and decision making	Provide an outline or structure to planning Role play outcomes of decisions Decrease impulsivity through use of strategies such as counting before acting Budget money	Go on an outing Plan the outing Budget money needs Role play possible social scenarios, including a sexual advance from a stranger (use the Circles Program, described in text discussion of sexuality and body image) Identify possible scenarios for decision making
Decreased overall cognitive ability	Simplify tasks Simplify instructions or use pictures Repeat needed information Present information in small steps and have the client practice	Cook Choose prepared foods Simplify directions by using pictures Keep kitchen organized with pictures on cabinets Work in small groups with small steps to the task Reinforce needed concepts

Continued

TABLE 16-2 Adapted Instrumental Activities of Daily Living—cont'd

Common Client-Based Challenges	Adaptive Strategies	Application Physical Challenges
Psychosocial Challenges		
Difficulty engaging in social communication	Use scripted-language role play	Go to a movie Script and practice asking for a ticket and stating the name of the show Practice asking for popcorn and managing the conversation and money
Behavioral outbursts	Structured routine Positive behavioral supports Reinforcement system for positive behavior Relaxation techniques	Practice money management Review finances at a prescribed weekly time Set up a reinforcement system to review finances without outburst Use breathing techniques for relaxation
Anxiety	Preparation ahead of time Role play Relaxation techniques Sensory diet (if applicable)	Personal grooming Shave (face, legs), put on deodorant/make-up Set up a routine Provide tactile brushing before shaving Use guided imagery during grooming
Overly friendly or flirtatious behavior	Use Circles Program to learn proper boundaries Reinforcement for positive behavior Role play appropriate behavior Monitor clothing	Go to a dance Review Circles Program Plan clothing Social stories to reinforce safe and appropriate behavior Sexual education at client's level

Adapted from Kieckhefer, G. M. (2002). Foundations for successful transition: Shared management as one critical component. Keynote presentation at the Hospital for Sick Children, Toronto, Canada.

swimming, and track and field. These outings required community participation to practice in various venues. The traveling with families to compete also afforded Peter and his family new modeling and opportunities to use IADL and community participation skills in natural environments. Using a contextual approach, occupational therapists see the "development of everyday activities as embedded in and inseparable from societal effort to offer occupational opportunities and social processes that are part of participation in everyday activities" (p. 261).[42] Therefore occupational therapy practitioners facilitate IADL and community participation by creating accessible contexts for performance. Humphry and Wakeford advocate for the creation of niches or small communities that foster development of roles, patterns, and skills.[42] The use of therapy techniques in the context of real experiences and natural environments enables the generalization and transfer of these skills. By adapting and modifying natural physical and social contexts to enhance children's development, occupational therapy practitioners give children natural opportunities to observe, imitate, and practice new skills (Case Study 16-2; Research Note 16-1).

Reverse Inclusion

Although inclusion is an important aspect to school-based practice, sometimes the special needs and accomplishments of young people with disabilities are best met in an alternative context. Reverse inclusion involves bringing typical children into a program designed for children with special needs, instead of including one child with a disability into a program designed for the skill level of typical children. This opportunity for peer modeling can improve age-appropriate behaviors and social skills targeted in the goals and objectives for the children with

RESEARCH NOTE 16-1

Dunn, W., Cox, J., Foster, L., Mische-Lawson, L., & Tanquary, J. (2012). Impact of a contextual intervention on child participation and parent competence among children with autism spectrum disorders: A pretest-posttest repeated-measures design. American Journal of Occupational Therapy, *66(5), 520–528.*

Dunn et al. (2012) examined the feasibility of a contextual intervention to increase participation of children with ASD in everyday life situations and to increase parental competence. The researchers collaborated with caregivers on identifying goals and on exploring strategies to address each caregiver's selected goals for his or her children (aged 3 through 10) with ASD. Results from this 10-session intervention yielded significant clinical gains in the children's participation in home and community activities and a significant increase in caregiver's parenting competence.

- Although children with ASD received services through school, caregivers reported a significant need for support for their children in home and community settings. Often these services were not provided through school programs.
- Findings support use of coaching to build on caregivers' strengths and problem-solving abilities to increase participation of their children in everyday activities at home
- Findings support use of interventions within natural contexts
- Promoting problem solving and planning around intervention strategies with caregivers by practitioners trained in coaching methods offers promise for occupational therapy interventions.

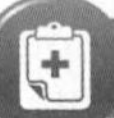

CASE STUDY 16-2 Brenda

Brenda is an experienced school-based occupational therapist. Her practice has evolved to include a group of children with disabilities in the middle and high schools. Brenda has a large caseload and has provided services to these middle school students for many years. She knows the children very well and has a positive relationship with the families. After many transition plans for her middle school students, Brenda decided to increase her use of ecologic approaches and to work more actively with families and clients to write goals that target their future aspirations, including IADL skills, independent or interdependent living, and community participation, including prevocational skills.

In collaboration with the speech therapist, Brenda designed a program for a life skills group. This group began with kitchen tasks, in which students planned, implemented, and worked together. She implemented safety rules and supervision and targeted the unique needs of each of the four students involved. Brenda designed the kitchen program to meet each student's client factor needs. Randy, a boy with muscular dystrophy, needed adaptations for his physical disabilities; Amanda, a girl with autism, required scripting to communicate with others; Troy, a youth with intellectual disability and associated behavioral problems, was assisted by use of a behavioral report card; and Susan, a girl with intellectual disability, followed recipes through a picture-based cookbook. The cooking group required planning and supervision to meet the individual needs of each student as the various IADL skills (e.g., planning a meal; shopping; safe use of cutting utensils; following a recipe; use of the stove, oven, and dishwasher; and safe handling and storage of food) were developed by each youth. In addition, working as a team, communication, social skills, hygiene, table manners, and polite eating were enhanced in the kitchen group participants.

The kitchen group that planned, shopped, prepared, and sold lunches to the school community worked so well that Brenda and the team of students decided to expand the group's activities to working and caring for plants. She convinced the school administration to add a greenhouse to the middle school. The students and Brenda traveled to a greenhouse and performed prevocational activities with a local farmer. They chose the plant varieties and followed directions to help the plants grow in their own greenhouse. This evolved into a school and community sale in which the students gained the IADL skills of pricing items, budgeting, and managing money. The greenhouse program also assisted with communication skills. The students took great pride in their accomplishments. With input from the students, school team, and parent volunteers, Brenda now plans to add a cottage industry of making greeting cards with photographs and stamping. The students find great meaning in these activities, and their IADL skills have improved significantly. In addition, the school community has embraced these endeavors, and the students have improved their self-esteem and future visions of success.

Occupational therapy becomes identity building when therapists provide environments that help persons explore possible selves and achieve success in tasks that are instrumental to identities they strive to achieve, and when it enables them to validate the identities that they have worked hard to achieve in the past (p. 55).[17] This case example was used to demonstrate how occupation as means and ends can meet individual needs in an occupation-based group context.

disabilities.[82] In reverse inclusion, typical peers become participants in occupational therapy groups, special recreation, adapted physical education, or other groups. Benefits have been documented both for typical peers serving as role models and for youth with disabilities.[82]

Supported Inclusion

Young people with disabilities can be supported in natural environments through the use of assistants, peer partners, and educated classmates. To promote participation, supported inclusion usually requires adapted coursework and activities that are consistent with the physical and cognitive abilities of the client.[46] An example of supported inclusion in IADL is partnering a youth with intellectual disability with a peer partner for a community outing. The occupational therapist facilitates the partners to support the student with a disability to make his or her own decisions while role modeling appropriate decisions and behavior in the community.

Chores and Household Tasks

Occupational therapy practitioners can consult with families regarding ways to include young people with disabilities in household activities. Participation in household activities, including chores, facilitates skills and helps the youth to develop a family role through productive participation in home management and caring for others.[21] Parents and caregivers teach children to use the telephone and cell phone, manage their health, and handle and manage money. They also teach children safe interaction with strangers and use of public transportation systems. Parents may need information and assistance from occupational therapists on how to adapt these skills or modify the environment so that their children can gain competence and confidence in IADL. Occupational therapists can also help families understand the link between the child's independence in IADL and eventual employment.[77]

Community Participation

Occupational therapy practitioners advocate for increased community participation for children and youth through shopping, attending school or community events, recreational activities, and/or other avenues of involvement. Practitioners can consult with the family and teachers on strategies to facilitate the child's telephone use, money management, and public transportation access. The practitioner can challenge the youth's physical, cognitive, and social skills through incremental, planned activities in the school and community.

Many IADL and community participation skills are dynamic, complex, and multistep activities, such as cooking, doing laundry, shopping, childcare, driving, and accessing transportation. These tasks are further developed when they are applied in a context that holds meaning for the client. Therefore finding a task that is meaningful and social and serves a purpose of importance to society will enhance performance. The occupational therapy practitioner can create occupational opportunities as part of educational curriculum or programs through establishing cottage industries whereby the adolescents create and sell merchandise, establish a work-based role, or plan and implement an outing, party, or celebration.

Driving and Community Mobility

Occupational engagement and participation in everyday occupations require young people to safely and effectively access the community. Social participation is greatly enhanced when young people can access communities and social gathering places (Figure 16-6). Safe and effective participation in occupational performance is the goal of such intervention. Driving evaluation and intervention for teens is an emerging niche for occupational therapy practice.[4] Occupational therapists evaluate the client to facilitate decisions about driving potential and to develop an intervention plan, which can include assessment of complex vision, visual perception, cognition, motor, and emotional skills.

Other aspects of community mobility to consider during the teen years are use of power mobility to access the community for longer distances and amounts of time. Often young people with mobility impairments should consider a scooter or other power means of mobility in order to access sporting events, shopping malls, field trips, college campuses, and travel destinations. This adaptive approach should be complemented by continued ambulation for those clients who are capable, to assure that the power mobility device does not inhibit ambulatory status, but rather facilitates access to the community.

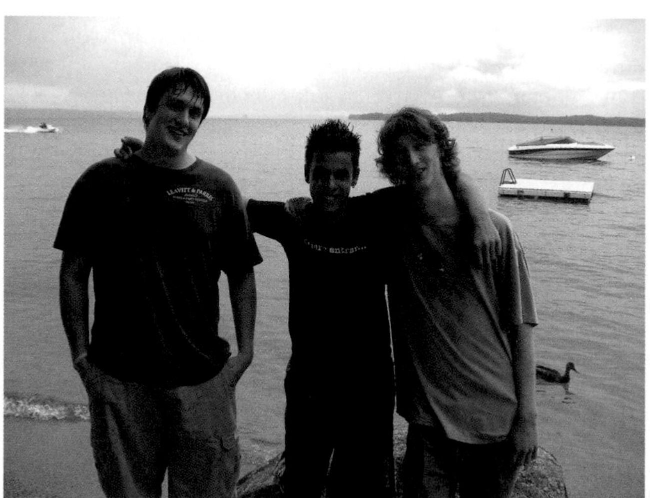

FIGURE 16-6 Adolescents enjoy occupations outdoors as part of community mobility and participation.

Summary

Occupational therapists provide services to enhance the complex processes of IADL and community participation in the lives of children, youth, and their family/support systems. Through the occupational therapy process of evaluation, intervention, and outcomes analysis, the occupational therapy practitioner uses critical thinking to facilitate IADL skills and community participation into practice. Occupational development is unique to each individual and leads to the acquisition of roles, interests, independence/interdependence in community living, and meaningful and productive vocation. As children and youth develop maturity and skills, the roles of parents, professionals, and the youth themselves also evolve. See Table 16-3 for the developmental role continuum.

Professional reasoning that includes the philosophical tenets, broad theoretical models, and intervention approaches guide the practitioner to facilitate occupational performance in IADL and community participation for youth with disabilities. Family and client-centered models provide a collaborative springboard and facilitate adult roles. Ecological models help the practitioner focus on creating contexts to support

TABLE 16-3 The Developmental Role Continuum

Stages	Occupational Therapy Practitioner or Other Professional	Parent/Family	Young Person
Late adolescence	Resource for future planning and implementation of adult roles, routines, and community participation	Consultant to youth; supports and guides decisions. Ensures a safety net.	The youth leads and supervises the program through self-determination.
Early adolescence	Consultant for school success, community participation, vocational programming, empowering client, advocacy, transition, and family planning	Supervises and monitors program, advocates for the child/youth. Implements IADL and community programming.	Active involvement in direction, plan, and method of programming. Input is given and received. Independence and advocacy are facilitated.
Middle childhood	School- or community-based intervention for education and life skills	Manages and monitors education program. Begins chores and roles in the home.	Participates in program and intervention planning.
Early childhood	Direct intervention and support to child and family	Provides care and makes decisions.	Receives care and follows directions.

occupational performance through establish/restore, adapt/modify, alter, prevent, and create techniques.[15] Finally it is the core tenet of engagement in meaningful and age-appropriate occupations as an agent of change that drives occupational therapy practice.[36] Use of active engagement of the client in occupation as means and ends in the IADL and community participation across life contexts is best practice.

Summary Points

- Instrumental activities of daily living that develop during childhood include meal preparation, community mobility, health management and maintenance, household maintenance, clothing management, use of communication devices, shopping, money management, safety and emergency response, driving and community mobility, and community participation.
- Participation in instrumental activities of daily living (IADL) and community activities prepares children and youth for work, vocational roles, and independent and interdependent community living.
- Occupational profile, self/caregiver report, and observational assessments specifically evaluate IADL and community participation.
- Theoretical models that include family/client-centered, ecological, and occupation-based models are used in the professional reasoning of occupational therapy practitioners to improve participation and performance of IADL and community activities for children and youth with special needs.
- Specific, evidence-based, intervention approaches/strategies have emerged from the theoretical foundations for improving participation and performance of IADL and community activities for children and youth.
- Use of strength-based approaches, self-determination, self-advocacy, social participation skills, and social relationships supports youth's independent or interdependent IADL performance and community participation.

REFERENCES

1. Adolfsson, M., Malmqvist, J., Pless, M., et al. (2011). Identifying child functioning from an ICF-CY perspective: Everyday life situations explored in measures of participation. *Disability & Rehabilitation, 33*(13/14), 1230–1244.
2. American Occupational Therapy Association. (2008). Occupational therapy practice framework: Domain and process (2nd ed.). *The American Journal of Occupational Therapy, 62*, 609–639.
3. AOTA. (2008). *Transitions for children and youth: How OT can help*. Bethesda, MD: AOTA Press.
4. AOTA. (2013). *Driving for teens.* Retrieved August 29 from: <http://www.aota.org/Practcie/Children-Youth/Emerging-Niche/Driving-for-teens.aspx>.
5. Anderson, L. B. (2007). A special kind of tutor. Professional development and classroom activities for teachers. *Teaching prek-8, 37*(5). Retrieved June 13, 2008, from: <http://www.teachingk-8.com>.
6. Andrén, E., & Grimby, G. (2004). Activity limitations in personal, domestic and vocational tasks: A study of adults with inborn and early acquired mobility disorders. *Disability and Rehabilitation, 26*, 262–271.
7. Aviles, A., & Helfrich, C. (2004). Life skill service needs: Perspectives of homeless youth. *Journal of Youth and Adolescence, 33*, 331–338.
8. Bedell, G. M. (2004). Developing a follow-up survey focused on participation of children and youth with acquired brain injuries after discharge from inpatient rehabilitation. *Neurorehabilitation, 19*, 191–205.
9. Bedell, G. M., Cohn, E. S., & Dumas, H. M. (2005). Exploring parents' use of strategies to promote social participation of school-aged children with acquired brain injury. *American Journal of Occupational Therapy, 59*, 273–284.
10. Bedell, G., Coster, W., Law, M., et al. (2013). Community participation, supports, and barriers of school-age children with and without disabilities. *Archives of Physical Medicine & Rehabilitation, 94*(2), 315–323.
11. Bedell, G. M., & Dumas, H. M. (2004). Social participation of children and youth with acquired brain injuries discharged from inpatient rehabilitation: a follow-up study. *Brain Injury, 18*, 65–82.
12. Blackorby, J., & Wagner, M. (1996). Longitudinal postschool outcomes of youth with disabilities: Findings from the National Longitudinal Study of Youth. *Exceptional Children, 62*, 399–413.
13. Bowes, J. M., Flanagan, C., & Taylor, A. J. (2001). Adolescents' ideas about individual and social responsibility in relation to children's household work: Some international comparisons. *International Journal of Behavioral Development, 25*, 60–68.
14. Boyt Schell, B. A. B., & Gillen, G. (2014). Overview of theory guided intervention. In B. A. B. Boyt Schell, G. Gillen, & M. E. Scaffa (Eds.), *Willard and Spackman's occupational therapy* (12th ed., pp. 746–749). Philadelphia: Lippincott Williams & Wilkins.
15. Brown, C. E. (2014). Ecological models in occupational therapy. In B. A. B. Boyt Schell, G. Gillen, & M. E. Scaffa (Eds.), *Willard and Spackman's occupational therapy* (12th ed., pp. 494–504). Philadelphia: Lippincott Williams & Wilkins.
16. Chandler, B. E., Schoonover, J., Clark, G. F., et al. (2008). The magnificent mundane. *School System Special Interest Section Quarterly, 15*(1), 1–4.
17. Christiansen, C. H. (1999). Defining lives: occupation as identity: An essay on competence, coherence and creation of meaning. *The American Journal of Occupational Therapy, 53*, 547–558.
18. Conaboy, K. S., Davis, N. M., Myers, C., et al. (2008). *FAQ: Occupational therapy's role in transition services and planning*. Bethesda, MD: American Occupational Therapy Association.
19. Coster, W., Bedell, G., Law, M., et al. (2011). Psychometric evaluation of the Participation and Environment Measure for Children and Youth. *Developmental Medicine & Child Neurology, 53*(11), 1030–1037.
20. Davidson, D. A., & Fitzgerald, L. (2001). *Transition planning for students: OT practice.* Bethesda, MD: American Occupational Therapy Association.
21. Dunn, L. (2004). Validation of the CHORES: A measure of children's participation in household tasks. *Scandinavian Journal of Occupational Therapy, 11*, 179–190.
22. Dunn, L., Coster, W. J., Orsmond, G. I., et al. (2009). Household task participation of children with and without attentional problems in household tasks. *Physical and Occupational Therapy in Pediatrics, 29*, 258–273.

23. Dunn, W., Cox, J., Foster, L., et al. (2012). Impact of a contextual intervention on child participation and parent competence among children with autism spectrum disorders: A pretest-posttest repeated-measures design. *American Journal of Occupational Therapy, 66*(5), 520–528.
24. Dunn, L., & Gardner, J. (2013). Household task participation for children with and without a physical disability. *American Journal of Occupational Therapy, 67,* e100–e105.
25. Dunst, C. J., Bruder, M. B., Trivette, C. M., et al. (2005). Young children's natural learning environments contrasting approaches to early childhood intervention indicate differential learning opportunities. *Psychological Reports, 96,* 231–234.
26. Evans, J., McDougall, J., & Baldwin, P. (2006). An evaluation of the "Youth En Route" program. *Physical & Occupational Therapy in Pediatrics, 26*(4), 63–87.
27. Feeney, T., & Ylvisaker, M. (2006). Context-sensitive cognitive-behavioural supports for young children with TBI: A replication study. *Brain Injury, 20,* 629–645.
28. Field, S., Martin, J., Miller, R., et al. (1998). *A practical guide for teaching self-determination.* Reston, VA: Council for Exceptional Children.
29. Fiese, B. H., Tomcho, T. J., Douglas, M., et al. (2002). A review of 50 years of naturally occurring family routines and rituals: Cause for celebration? *Journal of Family Psychology, 16,* 381–390.
30. Fisher, A. J. (2003). *Assessment of motor and process skills:* Vol. 1. *Development, standardization, and administration manual* (5th ed.). Fort Collins, CO: Three Star Press.
31. Fisher, A. J. (2003). *Assessment of motor and process skills:* Vol. 2. *User manual* (5th ed.). Fort Collins, CO: Three Star Press.
32. Forness, S. R., Serna, L. A., Nielsen, E., et al. (2000). A model for early detection and primary prevention of emotional or behavioral disorders. *Education & Treatment of Children, 23*(3), 325–345.
33. Gall, C., Kingsnorth, S., & Healy, H. (2006). Growing up ready: A shared management approach. *Physical & Occupational Therapy in Pediatrics, 26*(4), 47–62.
34. Gallimore, R., Goldenberg, C. N., & Weisner, T. (1993). The social construction and subjective reality of activity settings: Implications for community psychology. *American Journal of Community Psychology, 21,* 537–559.
35. Gill, C. J., Kewman, D. G., & Brannon, R. W. (2003). Transforming psychological practice and society: Policies that reflect the new paradigm. *American Psychologist, 58,* 305–332.
36. Gillen, G. (2014). Occupational therapy interventions for individuals. In B. A. B. Boyt Schell, G. Gillen, & M. E. Scaffa (Eds.), *Willard and Spackman's occupational therapy* (12th ed., pp. 322–341). Philadelphia: Lippincott Williams & Wilkins.
37. Glidden, L. M., & Jobe, B. M. (2007). Measuring parental daily rewards and worries in the transition to adulthood. *American Journal on Mental Retardation, 112,* 275–278.
38. Gol, D., & Jarus, T. (2005). Effect of a social skills training group on everyday activities for children with attention-deficit-hyperactivity disorder. *Developmental Medicine & Child Neurology, 47,* 539–545.
39. Goodnow, J. J., & Delaney, S. (1989). Children's household work. Task differences, styles of assignment, and links to family relationships. *Journal of Applied Development Psychology, 10,* 209–226.
40. Healy, H., & Rigby, P. (1999). Promoting independence for teens and young adults with physical disabilities. *Canadian Journal of Occupational Therapy, 66,* 240–249.
41. Hillier, A., Fish, T., Cloppert, P., et al. (2007). Outcomes of a social and vocational skills support group for adolescents and young adults on the autism spectrum. *Focus on Autism and Other Developmental Disabilities, 22,* 107–115.
42. Humphry, R., & Wakeford, L. (2006). An occupation-centered discussion of development and implications for practice. *American Journal of Occupational Therapy, 60,* 258–267.
43. Jinnah, H. A., & Stoneman, Z. (2008). Parents' experiences in seeking child care for school age children with disabilities: Where does the system break down? *Children and Youth Services Review, 30,* 967–977.
44. Johnson, D. R. (2007). Challenges of secondary education and transition services for youth with disabilities. Impact: The Institute of Community Integration. Retrieved September 9, 2007, from: <http://iciumnedu/products/impact/163/overs.html>.
45. Johnson, D. R., Stodden, R. A., Emanuel, E. J., et al. (2002). Current challenges facing secondary education and transition services: What research tells us. *Exceptional Children, 68,* 519–531.
46. Journey, B. J., & Loukas, K. M. (2009). Adolescents with disability in school-based practice: Psychosocial intervention recommendations for a successful journey to adulthood. *Journal of Occupational Therapy, Schools, & Early Intervention, 2*(2), 119–132.
47. Keller, J., Kafkes, A., Basu, S., et al. (2005). *Child Occupational Self Assessment (COSA) (version 2.1).* Chicago: MOHO Clearinghouse.
48. Kielhofner, G. (2005). Rethinking disability and what to do about it: Disability studies and its implications for occupational therapy. *The American Journal of Occupational Therapy, 59,* 487–496.
49. Kielhofner, G. (2008). *Model of human occupation: Theory and application* (4th ed.). Philadelphia: Lippincott Williams & Wilkins.
50. Kinavey, C. (2006). Explanatory models of self-understanding in adolescents born with spina bifida. *Qualitative Health Research, 16,* 1091–1107.
51. King, G., Law, M., Hanna, S., et al. (2006). Predictors of the leisure and recreation participation of children with physical disabilities: A structural equation modeling analysis. *Children's Health Care, 35*(3), 209–234.
52. King, G., Law, M., King, S., et al. (2003). A conceptual model of the factors affecting the recreation and leisure participation of children with disabilities. *Physical and Occupational Therapy in Pediatrics, 23*(1), 63–90.
53. Kingsnorth, S., Healy, H., & Macarthur, C. (2007). Preparing for adulthood: A systematic review of life skill programs for youth with physical disabilities. *Journal of Adolescent Health, 41,* 323–332.
54. Krieger, B., Kinebanian, A., Prodinger, B., et al. (2012). Becoming a member of the work force: Perceptions of adults with Asperger syndrome. *Work: A journal of Prevention, Assessment. Rehabilitation, 43*(2), 141–157.
55. Law, M., Anaby, D., Teplicky, R., et al. (2013). Participation in the home environment among children and youth with and without disabilities. *British Journal of Occupational Therapy, 76*(2), 58–66.
56. Law, M., Petrenchik, T., et al. (2007). Perceived environmental barriers to recreational, community, and school participation for children and youth with physical disabilities. *Archives of Physical Medicine & Rehabilitation, 88,* 1636–1642.
57. Lemon, K., Hines, A. M., & Merdinger, J. (2005). From foster care to young adulthood: The role of independent transition programs in supporting successful transitions. *Children and Youth Services Review, 27,* 251–270.
58. Loukas, K. M., & Cote, T. (2005). *Sports as occupation: OT practice.*

Bethesda, MD: American Occupational Therapy Association.

59. Loukas, K. M., Raymond, L., Perron, A., et al. (in press). Occupational transformation: Parental influence and social cognition of young adults with autism. *Work: A Journal of Prevention, Assessment & Rehabilitation.*
60. Magill, J., & Hurlbut, N. L. (1986). The self esteem of adolescents with cerebral palsy. *The American Journal of Occupational Therapy, 40*, 402–407.
61. Massinga, R., & Pecora, P. J. (2004). Providing better opportunities for older children in the welfare system. [electronic version]. *Future of Children, 14*(1), 150–173.
62. Mayberry, W. (1990). Self-esteem in children: Considerations for measurement and intervention. *The American Journal of Occupational Therapy, 44*, 729–734.
63. McConnell, A. E., Martin, J. E., Juan, C. Y., et al. (2012). Career development and transition for exceptional individuals. Hammill Institute on Disabilities. Retrieved from: <http://cde.sagepub.com/content/early/2012/12/13/2165143412468147>.
64. Michaels, C. A., & Orentlicher, M. L. (2004). The role of occupational therapy in providing person centered transition services: Implications for school based practice. *Occupational Therapy International, 11*(4), 209–228.
65. Mihaylov, S. I., Jarvis, S. N., Colver, A. F., et al. (2004). Identification and description of factors that influence participation of children with cerebral palsy. *Developmental Medicine and Child Neurology, 46*, 299–304.
66. Moore, K. A., Chalk, R., Scarpa, J., et al. (2002). Family strengths: Often overlooked, but real. *Child Trends Research Brief*, 1–8.
67. Nollan, K. A., Wolf, M., Ansell, D., et al. (2000). Ready or not: Assessing youth's preparedness for independent living. *Child Welfare, 79*(2), 159–176.
68. Noreau, L., Lepage, C., Boissiere, L., et al. (2007). Measuring participation in children with disabilities using the Assessment of Life Habits. *Developmental Medicine & Child Neurology, 49*, 666–671.
69. Orentlicher, M. L., & Michaels, C. A. (2000). Some thoughts of the role of occupational therapy in the transition from school to adult life: Part I. *Developmental Disabilities Special Interest Section Quarterly, 7*(2), 1–4.
70. Orentlicher, M. L., & Michaels, C. A. (2000). Some thoughts of the role of occupational therapy in the transition from school to adult life: Part II. *Developmental Disabilities Special Interest Section Quarterly, 7*(3), 1–4.
71. Orsmond, G. I., Krauss, M. M., & Seltzer, K. K. (2004). Peer relationships and social and recreational activities among adolescents and adults with autism. *Journal of Autism and Developmental Disorders, 34*, 245–256.
72. Palmer, S., & Wehmeyer, M. (2003). Promoting self-determination in early elementary school. *Remedial and Special Education, 24*, 115–126.
73. Peloquin, S. M. (2006). Occupations: Strands of coherence in a life. *The American Journal of Occupational Therapy, 60*, 236–239.
74. Polatajko, H. J., & Mandich, A. (2005). Cognitive Orientation to daily Occupational Performance with children with developmental coordination disorder. In N. Katz (Ed.), *Cognition and occupation across the life span* (2nd ed., pp. 237–260). Bethesda, MD: American Occupational Therapy Association Press.
75. Poulsen, A. A., Rodger, S., & Ziviani, J. M. (2006). Understanding children's motivation from a self-determination perspective: Implications for practice. *Australian Occupational Therapy Journal, 53*(2), 78–86.
76. Preston, L., & Lewin, J. E. (2006). Understanding issues of sexuality and privacy for individuals with developmental disabilities. *OT Practice, 11*, Bethesda, MD: American Occupational Therapy Association.
77. Raymond, L., & Loukas, K. M. (2012). Creating collaborative lifelong solutions: person, family, professionals, and community. *The NADD Bulletin: The Official Publication of the Association for Persons with Developmental Disabilities and Mental Health Needs, 15*(1), 3–7.
78. Richardson, P. (2003). From roots to wings: Social participation for children with physical disabilities. *Developmental Disabilities Special Interest Section Quarterly, 26*(1), 1–4.
79. Rodger, S. (2006). I can do it: Developing, promoting, and managing children's self-care needs. In S. Rodger & J. Ziviani (Eds.), *Occupational therapy with children* (pp. 200–221). Oxford, UK: Blackwell.
80. Rogoff, B. (2003). *The cultural nature of human development.* Oxford, UK: Oxford University Press.
81. Savage, S. L., & Gauvain, M. (1998). Parental beliefs and children's everyday planning in European-American and Latino families. *Journal of Applied Developmental Psychology, 19*, 319–340.
82. Schoger, K. D. (2006). Reverse inclusion: Providing peer social interactions opportunities to students placed in self-contained special education classrooms. *TEACHING Exceptional Children, Plus, 2*(6). Retrieved September 8, 2008, from: <http://escholarship.bc.edu/education/tecplus/vol2/iss6/art3>.
83. Shogren, K. A., & Turnbull, A. P. (2006). Promoting self-determination in young children with disabilities: The critical role of families. *Infants & Young Children, 19*, 338–352.
84. Simons, D. (2005). Adolescent development. In A. Cronin & M. B. Mandich (Eds.), *Human development and performance* (pp. 216–246). Clifton Park, NY: Thomson Delmar Learning.
85. Spence, S. H. (2003). Social skills training with children and young people: Theory, evidence and practice. *Child & Adolescent Mental Health, 8*, 84–96.
86. Stewart, D., Stavness, C., King, G., et al. (2006). A critical appraisal of literature reviews about the transition to adulthood for youth with disabilities. *Physical & Occupational Therapy in Pediatrics, 26*(4), 5–24.
87. Taylor, R. R. (2008). *The intentional relationship: Occupational therapy and use of self.* Philadelphia: F. A. Davis.
88. Turnbull, H. R., & Turnbull, A. P. (2001). Self-determination for individuals with significant cognitive disabilities and their families. *Journal of the Association for Persons with Severe Handicaps, 26*, 56–62.
89. Van Zelst, B., Miller, M., Russo, R., et al. (2006). Activities of daily living in children with hemiplegic cerebral palsy: A cross-sectional evaluation using the Assessment of Motor and Process Skills. *Developmental Medicine & Child Neurology, 48*, 723–727.
90. Wagner, M., Cameto, R., & Newman, L. (2003). *Youth with disabilities: A changing population. A report of findings from the National Longitudinal Transition Study (NLTS) and the National Longitudinal Transitions Study-2 (NLTS2).* Menlo Park, CA: SRI International.
91. Wehmeyer, M. L., Sands, D. J., & Doll, B. (1997). The development of self-determination and implications for educational interventions with students with disabilities. *International Journal of Disability, Development, and Education, 44*, 305–328.
92. Wehmeyer, M. L., & Palmer, S. B. (2003). Adult outcomes for students with cognitive disabilities three years after high school: The impact of self-determination. *Education and Training in Developmental Disabilities, 38*, 131–144.
93. Wehmeyer, M. L., & Schwartz, M. (1997). Self-determination and positive adult outcomes: A follow-up study of youth with mental retardation or learning

disabilities. *Exceptional Children, 63*, 245–255.
94. White, L. K., & Brinkerhoff, D. B. (1981). Children's work in the family: Its significance and meaning. *Journal of Marriage and the Family, 43*, 789–798.
95. World Health Organization (2007). *International Classification of Functioning: Child and Youth version (ICF-CY)*. Geneva.
96. Wynn, K., Stewart, D., Law, M., et al. (2006). Creating connections: A community capacity-building project with parent and youth with disabilities in transition to adulthood. *Physical & Occupational Therapy in Pediatrics, 26*(4), 89–103.
97. Zhang, D. (2005). Parent practices in facilitating self-determination skills: The influences of culture, socioeconomic status, and children's special education status. *Research & Practice for Persons with Severe Disabilities, 30*(3), 154–162.

CHAPTER

17 Play

Kari J. Tanta • Susan H. Knox

KEY TERMS

Form
Function
Meanings
Playfulness
Play assessments
Play as an intervention modality
Play as an intervention goal

GUIDING QUESTIONS

1. What is the relationship of play to occupational therapy?
2. Which play theories have shaped occupational therapy's lens on play?
3. Which assessment tools do occupational therapists use for evaluation and intervention planning purposes?
4. What are hallmarks of play at different ages?
5. How do individual and environmental factors facilitate and/or inhibit play?
6. How is play used in occupational therapy intervention?
7. How do occupational therapists advocate for play in today's society?

That's the real trouble with the world, too many people grow up. They forget. They don't remember what it's like to be twelve years old.

—Walt Disney

In today's fast-paced world, the ponderings of Walt Disney become all the more relevant for adults and children. In some ways it seems that society is losing sight of the importance of play, for it is through play that we keep mind and body healthy, cultivate social relationships, and learn about ourselves and the world around us. Occupational therapists have a critical role in helping children and families embrace the value of play throughout their lives.

Play ... is the way the child learns what no one can teach him. It is the way he explores and orients himself to the actual world of space and time, of things, animals, structures, and people. Through play he learns to live in a symbolic world of meanings and values, of progressive striving for deferred goals, at the same time exploring and experimenting and learning in his own individualized way. Through play the child practices and rehearses endlessly the complicated and subtle patterns of human living and communication, which he must master if he is to become a participating adult in our social life (pp. v-vi).[37]

Watching children play is like looking through a window into their very being. Play has been identified as one of the primary occupations in which people engage.[3] Parham and Fazio define play as "any spontaneous or organized activity that provides enjoyment, entertainment, amusement or diversion" (p. 448) and "an attitude or mode of experience that involves intrinsic motivation, emphasis on process rather than product and internal rather than external control; an 'as-if' or pretend element; takes place in a safe, unthreatening environment with social sanctions" (p. 448).[76]

There are two sides of play: the science of play, in which play is a critical aspect of human development that deserves serious study, and the art of play, in which the therapist and the child are players, where there is joy, pleasure, and freedom. Occupational therapists need knowledge and skill in both aspects, and in order to facilitate playfulness in a child an occupational therapist must be playful him- or herself.[69] This chapter describes play as the child's occupation from a historical perspective, defines hallmarks of play at different ages, explains the use of play in occupational therapy assessment and intervention, and proposes that occupational therapy practitioners advocate for children's play opportunities in today's society.

Play Theories

As a field, the profession of occupational therapy has built on the work of other disciplines, such as psychology and anthropology, in a quest to address the occupational nature of play. As with other occupations, the occupation of play can be explained through the substrates of form, function, meaning, and context[25]:

- As an activity having certain characteristics (i.e., its form, including motor skill requirements and products)
- As a developmental phenomenon contributing to a child's development and enculturation (i.e., its function, including purposes, processes, and experiences)
- As an experience or a state of mind (i.e., its meaning, including what motivates or satisfies the individual)

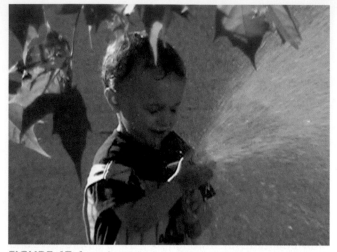

FIGURE 17-1 Infants and toddlers enjoy sensory play such as water play. Exploratory play allows them to learn about their environment.

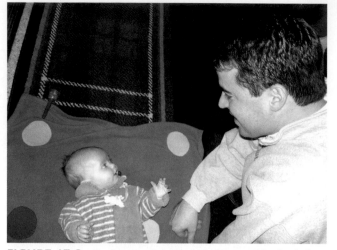

FIGURE 17-2 Social play begins in infancy with the infant looking at parent's face.

Play, like any other activity, takes place within context, which denotes the individual's environments and the personal, physical, and social elements of each environment.

Form

Many play theorists describe play as categories of activities in which children engage.[12,23,26,33] These may include such activities as games, building and construction, social play, pretend, sensorimotor play, symbolic or dramatic play, team sports, and digital play. Children's play activities change over time and reflect their development,[12,73] as well as in response to changes in their own interests and abilities, and societal norms.

Sensorimotor and exploratory play predominate in infancy as infants develop mastery over their own bodies and learn the effect of their actions on objects and people in the environment.[79,88] Sensorimotor play peaks in the second year of life and then declines. Children continue to use sensorimotor play when they learn new motor skills. Exploratory play begins in infancy, and by the end of the first year, infants actively explore their surroundings, demonstrate a beginning understanding of cause and effect, and are interested in how things work (Figure 17-1). In the second year, play centers on combining objects and learning their meaning. Children begin to classify objects and develop purpose in their actions. Exploratory play gradually declines through the preschool years, but it reappears when the child is learning new skills.[12]

Constructive play has identifiable outcomes and predominates during the preschool years, as seen in activities such as sandbox, puzzle, and block table play. Constructive play remains high during middle childhood and adolescence but becomes more abstract. It may develop into arts and crafts. Symbolic play and pretense develop at the end of the first year and through the second, peaking at around 5 years of age and evolving into dramatic and socio-dramatic play. These make-believe games form the foundation for self-regulation, civility, and empathy and enhance a child's capacity for creativity and cognitive flexibility.[91] During middle childhood, symbolic play and fantasy play are seen in mental games, secret clubs, and daydreaming, and in language play such as riddles or secret codes.[12] Television, computer and video games, and movies are also ways of engaging in fantasy play.

Social play begins very early with interaction between the infant and parent (Figure 17-2), and by age 3 children are able to engage in complex social games. Children use role play to learn about social systems and cultural norms. Garvey described four types of roles seen in group play:

1. Functional roles, such as pretending to be a doctor or barista
2. Relational roles, such as pretending to be mother and baby
3. Character roles, such as those from television, movies, and video games
4. Roles with no specific identity[38]

Social play combined with motor play develops into rough-and-tumble play such as play-fighting, pillow fights, or wrestling.[12]

Games with rules teach children to take turns and to initiate, maintain, and end social interactions.[49] This type of play predominates during the school-age years.[12] Social play and games with rules are particularly influenced by the culture. The physical environments available for play, peer groups, and the types of play encouraged by parents have changed as our society has become more urbanized.[73] Currently, time, places, and types of play are more planned and structured, such as with organized sports and "play dates" (Figure 17-3).[56] Additionally, "screen time" as play time has also increased and has been identified as the primary free time activity.[92] It is estimated that in North America, children over the age of 2 average 13 hours per week of video game play.[46]

Adolescents are concerned with autonomy and being socialized into adult roles. (See Chapter 4 for more on adolescents.) This is a period of transition as obligations, time available for play, changes and refinements of interests, family, and peer pressures all affect teen activity.[73] In a study by Csikszentmihalyi and Larson, the most frequent single activity of adolescents was socializing.[30] Second was television and third was sports, games, hobbies, reading, and music. More recently, "screen time" (television, computers, smart phones, video games,

CASE STUDY 17-1 Play as a Modality: Trevor

Trevor is a 14-year-old boy who is an eighth grader at a suburban middle school. He is highly capable but displays difficulties with social interaction, inability to stay focused in the classroom, and a lack of consistently appropriate social skills. He goes about his days at school generally alone and does not participate in school or extracurricular sports or other activities. His parents both work outside the home and his older siblings are generally too busy with their own lives as high school students to engage in positive interaction with him on a regular basis. Trevor spends most of his out-of-school free time engaged in virtual social interaction on X-Box Live with other teens. For hours each day he dons his headset to enthusiastically joke with other kids, talk about his day, and collaborate on gaming strategies with other teens. These conversations have evolved into friendships, regular online play dates, and insider jokes. They have helped Trevor develop important social competencies and self-esteem.

This case example illustrates the use of play through technology to improve social participation.

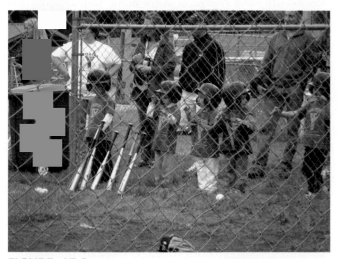

FIGURE 17-3 Play today is often highly structured; for example, young children participate in tee-ball.

tablets), has taken center stage for adolescent leisure time and social interaction as teens interact with each other virtually on their phones and through online gaming portals.

The prevalence of digital technology is altering the way children are learning and playing, blending physical, social, and digital play for children of all ages[62] (Case Study 17-1). The Lego Learning Institute identified six areas of play that are distinctly different from past generations of children, including:

- *Sharism*: Children are more likely to engage in co-creation of ideas at a fast pace versus individual construction. Such play can be seen in video games such as Minecraft played on X-Box Live with friends.
- *Shifting identities*: Boundaries between "mine" and "yours" are blurring. Platforms for movie making and video editing are examples of boundary blurring in the digital realm.
- *Border crossing*: Children are moving between virtual and physical worlds constantly, resulting in a more global view of the world. Games such as Skylanders allow children to integrate online gaming with physical characters that they can connect to others anywhere in the world.
- *Literacies beyond print*: Children are engaging in more active reading and writing with processes such as "earmarking" and "tagging" and are using mix-and-match media rather than creating. E-readers and a multitude of apps make it appealing for youth to read and create on digital devices they can take anywhere.
- *Gaming culture*: Children expect for their worlds to be forgiving and responsive, that they can always press an "undo" button. The child whose Lego Star Wars character has been blown apart can make the character come back to life.
- *Bricoleur culture*: Children are eager to hack and modify, program, and recycle. The explosion of robotics and programming opportunities for children allows them to become engineers.[62]

As society continues to embrace digital technology, occupational therapists can embed meaningful play using digital media, tablet and computer games, and virtual social networks into intervention sessions.

It may be said that play is easy to see, but hard to define, and scholars have found this to be true through the years as many have attempted to categorize play by lists of attributes and by specific types of play. To date, scholars of play have not identified a single characteristic common to all kinds of play but have suggested many qualities or characteristics that differentiate play from non-play. These characteristics include intrinsic motivation (the child engages in play by her own desire), suspension of reality (the child escapes into her imagination fully—she really IS a princess!), internal locus of control (play is child directed), and being spontaneous, fun, flexible, totally absorbing, an end in and of itself, nonliteral, and challenging.[26,33,45,63,74,85]

Most recently, Burghardt (2011)[26] proposed a set of five essential criteria that behavior must meet in order to be confidently identified as play within any species or culture, that embrace the qualities and characteristics identified by earlier scholars but that can provide a more succinct method of identifying play within occupational therapy. These include:

- Behavior is incompletely functional within the context it is performed (play is an end in and of itself)
- Behavior is spontaneous, voluntary, rewarding, or pleasurable (fun and intrinsically motivated)
- Behavior differs from other behaviors in form or timing (e.g., the behavior may only occur in infancy or may be extremely exaggerated)
- Behavior is repeated, though not rigidly (flexible)
- Behavior is initiated when one is relaxed and in the absence of stress (totally absorbing)

Function

Another way of looking at play is in relation to function, or how play influences adaptation. Play functions include processes, experiences, and purposes. Historically, play has been described as the way a child develops the skills necessary for life,[88] as a way of expending surplus energy,[89] or for recreation and relaxation.[88] Modern or contemporary theories emphasize the value of play in contributing to the child's development or to acculturation. They include using play to achieve optimal arousal[13,33] and develop ego function[34] and cognitive skills.[18,79,100] Sociocultural explanations include the development of social abilities,[77,94] role development,[85] and play's contribution to culture.[45,90] As presented in the prior section of this chapter, Burghardt (2011)[26] challenges us to look at play in a broader context using criteria that transcend a more limited view of play behavior. By using criteria to identify play as a whole construct, rather than an isolated behavior, such as play with a toy or engagement in a single leisure pursuit, occupational therapists using such criteria can better address the occupation of play within context.

Occupational therapists are interested in the first-hand experiences of players as a means of identifying what constitutes play through the eyes of the player. Miller and Kuhaneck conducted interviews on the perceptions of play experiences and play preferences in 10 children between the ages of 7 and 11.[69] The children described "fun" as the core category, with four categories of characteristics that explained their play choices: relational, activity, child, and contextual. The authors developed the Dynamic Model for Play Choice to describe four characteristics—child, activity, relational, and contextual—that affect the child's perception of fun and can be used to create play in occupational therapy intervention. Using dynamic systems theory, this model conceptualizes how choice, emotion, meaning, preference, mastery, challenge, and the characteristics of the child, environment, and activity are inter-related and influence child's perception of play. Miller and Kuhaneck further stressed the need for therapists to be playful, choose play as a meaningful goal, remember the importance of fun in therapy, and weave a child's preferences into the session.

Meaning

Play meaning refers to the quality of the experience, a person's state of mind, and the value that the play experience has for the individual. The attitude a person assumes during play is termed *playfulness* and is closely related to the development of cognitive abilities.[7-10] Each person has an internal disposition to play and playfulness that could be described along five dimensions: physical spontaneity, cognitive spontaneity, social spontaneity, manifest joy, and sense of humor.[64] Children give and receive social cues to denote they are playing, lying along a continuum of three elements of playfulness: intrinsic motivation, internal control, and the ability to suspend reality.[19,20] Bundy theorizes that "it is the sum contribution of these three elements that tips the balance toward play or nonplay, playfulness or nonplayfulness" (p. 219).[19,20]

Knox, in a qualitative study of preschool children's play, identified actions and behaviors that characterized playful children.[54] The playful children showed flexibility and spontaneity in their play and in social interactions, curiosity, imagination, creativity, joy, the ability to take charge of situations, the ability to build on and change the flow of play, and total absorption. Nonplayful children were less flexible and had difficulty with transitions or changes, expressed negative or immature affect or speech, often withdrew either physically or emotionally from play sequences, did not have control over situations, and tended to prefer adults or younger children for play.

Children have been found to readily identify environmental and motivational factors that add meaning to their play and facilitate engagement in play activity. Children in one study mentioned that active outdoor play was facilitated through use of a mobile phone to keep in touch with parents, and they were motivated to engage in active play to prevent boredom, be free from adult control and rules, "be themselves," and socialize with friends.[17] For maximum effectiveness, occupational therapy practitioners must engage in active dialog with children and their parents to determine their meaning of play when designing intervention programs and play spaces.[22]

Context

Play also obtains meaning through context. Children's activities can never be isolated from the environment within which they are playing nor from familial, social, and cultural influences.[3] The presence or absence of other persons or animals, the physical setting, and the availability of toys and other objects with which to interact all have a profound effect on children's play (Figure 17-4). Play context includes cultural and societal expectations of play. The environment, quality of care, and types of interactions between caregivers and children can affect play behavior. For example, higher socioeconomic status links to greater levels of imaginary play; permissive home environments encourage creativity; and in childcare centers, high program quality improves children's social interaction and level of play.[10,12,44,48] Access to a variety of materials and opportunities with which to explore and interact and children's ability to control their activities are associated with improved quality of play. In addition, caregivers and peers who are emotionally and verbally responsive help to improve the child's quality of play. Cultural and ecologic factors, such as child-rearing and parental

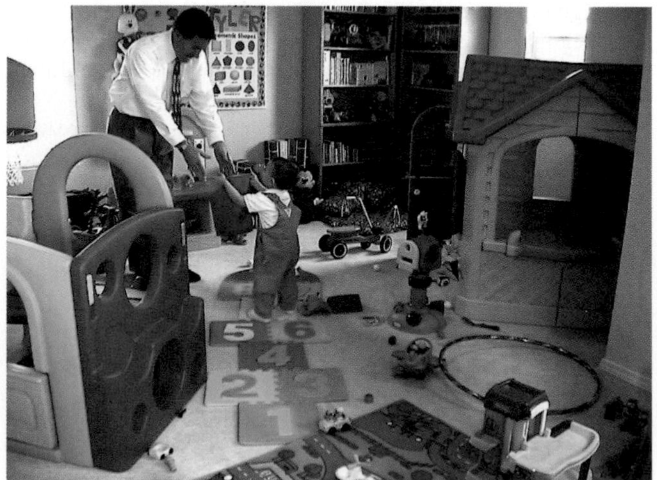

FIGURE 17-4 Playful environments with age-appropriate toys allow children to play.

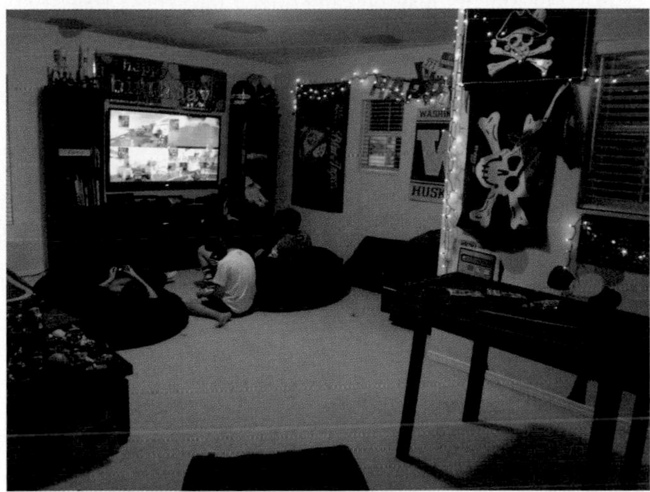

FIGURE 17-5 Teens enjoy technology as a form of play.

influences, peer experiences, the physical environment, the schools, and the media (Figure 17-5),[11,92] also influence the way children play.[49,88]

Indoor play venues for children warrant special attention. In addition to children playing in their own homes and in the homes of their peers, businesses and nonprofit organizations have also identified this shift in play context and have responded. Franchise operations such as Little Gym, Gymboree Play and Music, Jump Planet, and a host of others offering everything from laser tag to indoor skydiving offer spaces for children of all ages to engage in play at a price. Children's museums across the United States have also been increasing in popularity, creating inspiring venues for imaginative play. Environments such as these can be especially beneficial for families seeking out safe and novel play contexts with enhanced opportunities for social interaction.[42]

All environments offer affordances for and constraints to an individual's behavior. Factors that promote play include the availability of objects and persons, freedom from stress, provision of novelty, and opportunities to make choices.[53,68] Factors that may inhibit play include external constraints, too much novelty or challenge, limited choices, and overcompetition. Contextual components that appear to promote play and playfulness include:

1. Familiar peers, toys, and other materials
2. Freedom of choice
3. Adults who are nonintrusive or directive
4. Safe and comfortable atmosphere
5. Scheduling that avoids times of fatigue, hunger, or stress[88,92]

With recent technological advances in the "digital world," it has been suggested that with the ready availability of electronic media and toys, such digital play is replacing the less structured outdoor play of the past and indoor spaces are becoming more prevalent as play venues.[17,62] It is also important to note that the context of play in today's society is rapidly changing and it is no longer as simple as indoor or outdoor play. In the "digital realm," the environment in which a child learns, plays, socializes, and creates is a hybrid of physical and virtual activity and an environment, it could be argued, that is fully immersive.[46,62] Such immersion may be seen when children wear headphones to engage in online gaming.

Play in Occupational Therapy

Play has always been a part of the pediatric occupational therapist's repertoire, although its importance has altered over the years.[92] It is important to know how the profession has evolved related to the occupation of play in order to successfully plan for the future. Adolph Meyer wrote of work, play, rest, and sleep as being the four rhythms that shape human organization.[67] In one of the earliest articles on play in the occupational therapy literature, Alessandrini referred to play as a "serious undertaking, not to be confused with diversion or idle use of time. Play is not folly. It is purposeful activity, the result of mental and emotional experiences" (p. 9).[1] Richmond spoke of play as the vehicle for communication and growth of the child.[86] Play in the early years of occupational therapy was used for a variety of purposes, such as diversion, development of skills, or remediation.

Mary Reilly was instrumental in bringing play into the forefront of occupational therapy in the late 1960s. She described play along a continuum that she called occupational behavior.[85] Through play, children learn skills and develop interests that later affect choices and success in work and leisure. Play is the arena for the development of sensory integration, physical abilities, cognitive and language skills, and interpersonal relationships. In their play, children practice adult and cultural roles and learn to become productive members of society.[12,63,85] Reilly felt that play is a multidimensional system to adapt to the environment and that the exploratory drive of curiosity underlies play behavior. This drive has three hierarchic stages: exploration, competency, and achievement. Exploratory behavior is seen most in early childhood and is fueled by intrinsic motivation. Competency is fueled by *effectance motivation*, a term defined by White as an inborn urge toward competence.[101] This stage is characterized by experimentation and practice to achieve mastery. Achievement is linked to goal expectancies and is fueled by a desire to achieve excellence. Using this frame of reference, other scholars studying under Reilly expanded the concepts of play. Florey offered a developmental framework of play and explored the concept of intrinsic motivation as being central to play.[36] Takata developed a taxonomy of play and described play epochs based on Piagetian stages,[97,98] and Knox examined play in relation to development for the purposes of evaluation.[53] Robinson described how play is used for the child to learn rules and roles.[87]

Occupational science developed in the late 1980s as an academic discipline to study the nature of occupation and how it influences health. Because play is the primary occupation of children, a number of researchers have studied various aspects of play. In studies of parent-child routines and how play is orchestrated into daily routines, Primeau proposed that parents use two types of play strategies: segregation and inclusion.[82] In the segregated strategy, play times were separate from other daily routines, whereas in the inclusion strategy, play was incorporated into daily routines. Parents use play routines to support their children's learning. Pierce studied object play in infants.[80,81] She described three types of object rules learned by children: (1) object property rules (the child's internal representation of the properties of objects), (2) object action rules (the repertoire of actions on the objects), and (3) object affect rules (those factors affecting object choice and keeping play enjoyable).

Play Assessment

Although play is considered the child's major occupation, and most occupational therapists would agree that it is important to the child, few therapists routinely evaluate it.[27,29,60] In a 1998 study, Couch et al. found that 62% of pediatric occupational therapists who responded to her questionnaire stated that they evaluated play, but less than 20% used criterion-referenced play assessments.[28] Play was usually evaluated through clinical observations or as a part of developmental tests.[27] A decade later, Kuhaneck et al. replicated the survey, finding that 38% or 24% fewer of respondents assessed play. Furthermore, few occupational therapists used play assessment tools, with 4% using the Knox Preschool Play Scale and 3% using the Test of Playfulness[59] (Research Note 17-1).

RESEARCH NOTE 17-1

Kuhaneck, H., Tanta, K. C., Coombs, A., & Pannone, H. (2013). A survey of pediatric occupational therapists' use of play. Journal of Occupational Therapy, Schools, and Early Intervention, *6(3), 213–227.*

Abstract

In a 1998 study, Couch, Dietz, and Kanny surveyed pediatric occupational therapists with regard to the use of play in their practice. Results indicated that play was primarily used as a modality to address skills in other developmental areas, not play itself. In the years following this study a significant body of literature promoting the use of play in occupational therapy was published. Kuhaneck et al. (2013) adapted the original Couch et al. mail survey to study whether or not practice patterns had changed. The researchers randomly surveyed 500 pediatric occupational therapists, who were AOTA members of the school system and sensory integration special interest sections, working with children age 3 to 7 years. Results of the survey, with a 40% response rate, yielded similar findings to the original survey by Couch et al. Few therapists focused on play as a therapeutic outcome or assessed play specifically, and most used play as a modality when working on other skill areas. The researchers concluded that minimal changes have occurred since the original Couch et al. study related to the role of play in pediatric occupational therapy, despite the promotion of play within the occupational therapy profession.

Application to Practice

- Occupational therapy practitioners need to advocate for the role of play in the lives of children.
- Play is a child's primary occupation and evidence supports the importance of play to child development.
- Occupational therapists need to seek out continuing education opportunities, including review of the research and literature, to expand their knowledge of play.
- Occupational therapists need to include play in their assessments and intervention plans to positively impact a child's overall development, health, and well-being.
- Along with using play and playfulness as a modality to reach intervention goals, practitioners should target play and playfulness as intervention goals.

Play assessments may be categorized into those that assess developmental competencies and those that assess the way a child plays, including playfulness and play style.

Developmental Competencies

Using a developmental frame of reference, the Revised Knox Preschool Play Scale is an observational assessment designed to describe play competency in children through 6 years of age.[16,52,53,55,57] Revised recently by Knox,[52] the scale describes play in terms of 6-month increments through age 3 and yearly increments through age 6. Four dimensions are examined: space management, material management, pretense/symbolic, and participation. Space management is the manner in which the child learns to manage his or her body and the space around it. Material management assesses how the child manages his or her material surroundings. The pretense/symbolic dimension rates how the child learns about the world through imitation and the development of the ability to understand and separate reality from make-believe. Participation is the amount and developmental level of social interaction. Children are observed indoors and outdoors and rated on all four dimensions.[76]

Other assessments rate the developmental skills of the child through play, such as the Transdisciplinary Play-Based Assessment, which assesses the child in cognitive, social-emotional, language, physical, and motor development through naturalistic play.[65] This assessment and its complementary curriculum are used by inter-professional teams in early childhood programs.

Play, Playfulness, and Play Style

The third way therapists assess play is to analyze the child's experience or state of mind when playing (i.e., playfulness and play style). Bundy developed the Test of Playfulness (ToP) to assess the individual's degree of playfulness.[20,21] The scale contains 34 items representing four elements of playfulness: intrinsic motivation, internal control, ability to suspend reality, and framing. The child is rated on scales of extent, intensity, and skill. The ToP can be scored from direct observations or videotapes of children engaged in free play.[93]

Bundy and her associates also developed an assessment of the environment's capacity to support playfulness, the Test of Environmental Supportiveness (TOES).[93] The primary purpose of the TOES is for consultation with caregivers to determine a player's motivation for play, and it is meant to be administered along with the ToP.[93] Extensive information on utility in practice and case studies is found in Parham and Fazio's *Play in Occupational Therapy for Children*, 2nd ed.[76]

The previous assessments are based on behavioral observation and parent interviews. Because play is unique to the individual, it is important to obtain the child's own perspective of his or her play, and this is usually done through self-report. The Pediatric Interest Profiles consist of three age-appropriate profiles of play and leisure interests and participation for children from 6 to 9 years of age, from 9 to 12 years, and from 12 to 21 years.[41] The profiles assess what activities the child is doing, the child's feelings about the activity, how skilled they perceive themselves, and with whom they play. They can be used in evaluation to (1) identify children and adolescents who may be at risk for play-related problems, (2) establish play-related goals, and (3) identify play or leisure activities to use in intervention. Although this assessment holds promise for use by occupational therapists, particularly with regard to obtaining information on meaning of play activity for children, recent surveys do not show that it is being used in practice.[59]

The recently revised Child Occupational Self-Assessment (COSA, version 2.2) helps practitioners find out from the child what he or she finds interesting and meaningful.[58] The COSA also provides a structure to determine how a child perceives his or her competency. Children identify their interest in a variety of occupations (including play, self-care, chores) and rate how well they feel they perform this activity. This flexible format allows the practitioner to hear from the child directly, helps in establishing a rapport, and aids in intervention planning. This tool can be effective in helping practitioners design play sessions.[75]

Interpreting Play Assessments

Assessment of play should be a part of every occupational therapy evaluation to develop a complete picture of an individual's competence in his or her occupational performance and to plan intervention that focuses on helping that individual participate in meaningful and self-satisfying occupations. Play assessments provide the therapist with a picture of how the individual engages in play in his or her daily life. An analysis of children's play is also helpful in assessing physical and cognitive abilities, social participation, imagination, independence, coping mechanisms, and environment.[12,38]

Play may be informally evaluated in routine, self-chosen, familiar activities in naturalistic settings, providing the therapist with a picture of everyday competencies. Identifying what the child can do in play enables the therapist to focus on the child's abilities rather than disabilities. Because play is an interaction between the child and the environment, the human and physical factors in the environment can substantially influence the child's play.[56] The Revised Knox Preschool Play Scale is a good example of a play assessment that can be used in a naturalistic environment. Play assessments that are designed to take place in standardized settings, such as those that are embedded within developmental assessments with standardized toys, significantly alter and may inhibit the child's play. In addition, although play specifies its own purpose, observed behaviors may have different meanings and serve different purposes for different people. It is difficult for an observer to assess the meaning of play to the participant; therefore practitioners may benefit by interviewing children. The COSA is an assessment tool that helps practitioners understand the meaning the child ascribes to occupations, such as play and school.[58]

Therapists must determine whether the sample of behavior is sufficient, typical, and representative of true play. When observed over a prolonged time, a child's play can vastly differ at different times.[56] To capture a variety of play behaviors, a therapist may need to observe a child multiple times and in a variety of settings. An analysis of play is especially helpful in assessing a child who does not respond well to standardized developmental testing. Knowledge of the individual's play skills, interests, and play style assists in intervention planning. The questions listed in Box 17-1 may help practitioners observe play to develop intervention goals.

BOX 17-1 Questions to Examine Play and Playfulness

- In which activities does the child become totally absorbed?
- What does the child get from these activities?
- Does the child engage routinely in activities in which he or she feels free to vary the process and outcome in whatever way he or she sees fit?
- Does the child have the capacity, permission, and support to do what he or she chooses to do?
- Is the child capable of giving and interpreting messages that convey "This is play; this is how you should interact with me now"?[20]
- Where does the child play? Indoors? Outdoors?
- With whom does the child play? What are the ages and abilities of their peers?
- Does the child have a place of his or her own to escape?
- How does the caregiver support the child's play?
- Is the child rigid or rough with toy use? Does the child use the toys in a traditional or nontraditional manner?

Constraints to Play

The effects of the environment on play can be seen in children who have experienced neglect or long hospitalizations. Extreme examples of constraints to play have been seen in some of the reports of children in Romanian orphanages.[30] These children showed severe sensory problems, extreme delay in developmental skills, and difficulties in interacting with others. Children who experience severely deprived environments also exhibit self-stimulation, limited repertoire of activities, decreased social play, and either increased or decreased fantasy play.[31]

When children are hospitalized, they often experience stress of separation, fear of illness, painful procedures, enforced confinement, and disruption of routines.[50] Some of the effects on play behavior include regression to earlier stages of development; decreased endurance and movement; decreased attention span, initiative, and curiosity; decreased resourcefulness and creativity; qualitative decrease in playfulness; decreased affect; and increased anxiety.[51,61] Occupational therapy and Child Life services may overlap with children in hospital settings, and such teamwork can be beneficial to helping children cope with medical procedures.

Effects of Disability on Play Behavior

The play of children with varying disabilities has been described often in the literature.[50,71] However, problems arise in attempts to generalize across or within disabilities. Children are individuals and respond uniquely in different situations, whether or not they have a disability.

Descriptions of the play of children with disabilities must be interpreted cautiously.[50] Although it is helpful to examine some of the problems that certain conditions may impose on the child, in actual practice, each child must be considered individually. Bundy stated that although a child's play may not be typical, it was more important for "children to be good at what they want to do" (p. 218).[20]

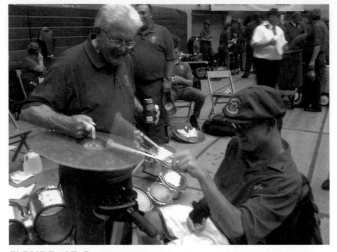

FIGURE 17-6 Matthew, who has cerebral palsy, shows playfulness as he participates in the pregame rally by playing the drum. (Courtesy Jill McQuaid.)

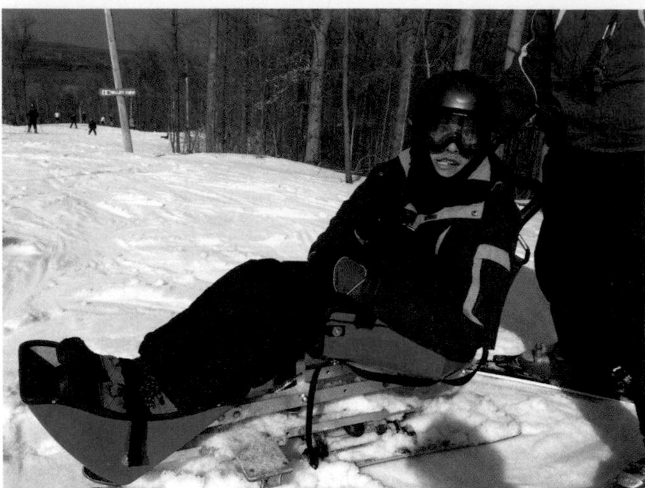

FIGURE 17-7 Matthew takes to the snow using an adapted sled. (Courtesy Jill McQuaid.)

Children may have conditions that limit physical interaction with the environment, toys, and people. The child with a physical impairment may display limited movement, strength, and pain when performing daily activities. Social contacts with family and peers may be disrupted by hospitalizations.[49] The play characteristics of children with physical limitations may include fear of movement, decreased active play, and preferences for sedentary activities. The child may also have problems with manipulating toys and show decreased exploration. Interestingly, children with physical disabilities may actually demonstrate higher levels of playfulness—the positive and pleasurable attitude of play—than children without physical disabilities[1,35] (Figure 17-6).

Children with cognitive impairment often show delayed or uneven skills, difficulty in structuring their own behavior, or lack of sustained attention. These characteristics may be manifested in play preferences for structured play materials, limited or inflexible play repertoires, decreased curiosity, destructive or inappropriate use of objects, decreased imagination, decreased symbolic play, decreased social interaction, decreased language, and increased observer play.[50,71] These children may need more structure and external cues to develop their play skills.

Children with visual impairment have delays in developing an integrated perception of the world caused by lack of vision and delayed motor exploration of surroundings and objects. Children often have difficulty in constructive play, delays in developing complex play routines with others, and decreased imitative and role play.[50,71]

The child with a hearing impairment is believed to have problems with decreased inner language, decreased social interactions, and decreased understanding of abstract concepts. Imagination becomes more restrictive with age and increased time is spent in noninteractive construction play. Children with hearing impairments demonstrate decreased symbolic play and increased solitary play.[50,71]

Children who have difficulty interpreting and integrating sensory input often have a limited or distorted perception of themselves and their world, decreased ability to plan and execute motor and cognitive tasks, and poor organization of behavior. Play characteristics of these children include either excessive movement or avoidance of movement, decreased exploration, decreased gross motor or manipulative play, increased observation or solitary play, increased sedentary play, a restricted repertoire of play, resistance to change, distractibility, or destructiveness.[4,5,19,75]

Children with an autism spectrum disorder (ASD) generally follow a different course of play development than other children and can be at risk for a lack of reciprocal relationships throughout their life span.[99] Their play is characterized by a lack of inner and expressive language, stereotyped movements or types of play, decreased imitation and imagination, lack of variety in play repertoires, motor planning problems, decreased play organization, decreased manipulation of toys, decreased construction and combining of objects, and decreased social play.[6,95] Children with ASD appear to have a fundamental deficit in play greater than what would be expected in examining specific skills. Incidental teaching, integrated playgroups, peer-mediated intervention, and community integration have been well documented as strategies to improve the play skills of children with an ASD.[99]

Children with cerebral palsy may show difficulties across skill areas. They may show limited and abnormal movement, sometimes have decreased cognitive abilities, exhibit multisensory impairments, and often lack opportunities for social play.[35] In play, cognitive abilities are the most decisive factor in limiting play, and children with good cognitive abilities can make adaptations to their physical limitations. Other problems include decreased physical interaction with environment and less interactive play time.[14,15] Therefore occupational therapists must evaluate each child carefully and individualize intervention to the child's strengths and limitations.

Most of the studies of the play of children with disabilities stress the obstacles that the disabling conditions place on the children. The occupational therapy practitioner explores supports for play and begins intervention with the child's play strengths. With adaptations, a child can overcome great obstacles to engage in a favorite activity (Figure 17-7).

CASE STUDY 17-2 Play as a Modality: Sarah and Her Magic Beads

Sarah is a 2½-year-old girl with mild spastic diplegia. She is playful, talkative, and extremely imaginative. A former premature infant, her primary motor impairment is independent ambulation, and despite the ability to walk, she is generally fearful of taking more than a few steps. Her favorite activity in occupational therapy is to play dress-up and direct everyone in the play theme of the day. Costumes are always involved for both Sarah and her therapist, as are long strings of colorful beads. Most of the time she crawls around in costume with her beads dragging along the therapy mats, or she walks holding her occupational therapist's hand. As a means of improving Sarah's confidence with walking, and to decrease her reliance on others, her occupational therapist begins using a string of Sarah's beads to gradually wean her from holding hands. First, the occupational therapist simply holds the beads in her palm as she holds Sarah's hand. Next, the occupational therapist has Sarah help her hold the beads between their clasped hands. Then, the occupational therapist begins to lengthen the beads from a ball in the palms to a single strand of bead, one end held by Sarah and one by the therapist. As Sarah's confidence grows, the occupational therapist gradually lengthens the bead fully out between them—a distance of about 18 inches—and then she eventually lets go of the bead chain completely! Sarah keeps walking with a big smile on her face, waving her "magic beads"!

This case example illustrates the use of play as a treatment modality (e.g., to meet performance goals).

Play in Intervention

What differentiates free play from therapeutic play? Free play is intrinsically motivated, fun, and performed for its own sake rather than having a purpose. The child directs the play. However, in therapy, goals and objectives are established by the therapist (with input from parents and child), who directs the play. However, when external constraints are placed on play, it may be perceived as work and no longer contains playful elements. How then can play be used successfully in intervention?

Rast stated:

> *Play offers a practical vehicle to enlist a child's attention, to practice specific motor and functional skills, and to promote sensory processing, perceptual abilities, and cognitive development. It also serves to support social, emotional, and language development. In the therapeutic setting, play often becomes a tool used to work towards a goal, despite the fact that the goal-oriented, externally controlled aspects of the therapy situation conflict with the essence of play itself. (p. 30)*[84]

Play and leisure activities are used in occupational therapy in two primary ways:

1. As intervention modalities (e.g., using a play activity to improve specific skills in an area other than play) (Case Study 17-2)
2. As an intervention goal (to improve the occupation of play itself)

For play to be used successfully in intervention, the child should feel that he or she is choosing or directing the play episode. This is particularly important when the goal is to increase competence in play development. Play and leisure activities are important methods for promoting a child's performance and skills because they have meaning to the individual. See Box 17-2 for sample goals.

In their 1998 study, Couch et al. found that 91% of pediatric occupational therapists rated play as important to their interventions.[28] For 95% of the respondents, play was used primarily to elicit motor, sensory, or psychosocial outcomes; only 2% used play as an outcome by itself. The therapists also primarily used adult-directed play versus child-directed play. In a replication of this study a decade later, Kuhaneck et al. found similar results, with 88% of respondents reporting a predominant use of play as a means of improving skills in an area other than play (such as fine motor). Only 4% reported the predominant use of play as an intervention outcome.[59]

The way play is used in intervention is influenced by a number of factors: the therapist's frame of reference, the institution's emphasis on improving performance components and skills, and the family's values and concerns for the physical aspects of the child's disability. Goals and objectives are established in accordance with how the child's disability affects his or her daily occupations and on analysis of occupational performance.[3] A major barrier for children with disabilities is the ability to participate in play and leisure activities on par with their peers. Occupational therapists have a key role in facilitating play and leisure participation for children and youth (Case Study 17-3).

BOX 17-2 Sample Play and Playfulness Goals

Overall Area	Sample Measurable Goal
Work cooperatively with peers.	Child will enter a play session without disrupting the play of his or her peers at least twice during a 30-minute play session.
Take turns when playing a game.	Child will share toy with a peer at least three times during a 30-minute play session.
Use play scripts of social stories.	Child will complete two out of four steps of the social story during the 30-minute play session.
Follow the rules to a game.	Child will follow three out of three rules to a simple board game during a 10-minute session.
Engage in rough-house play without hurting others.	Child will exhibit increased body awareness by gently tagging peers (so they do not fall or experience pain) while engaged in outside playground game of tag for 30 minutes.

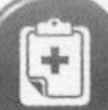

CASE STUDY 17-3 Play as the Goal: Rachel

Rachel is a 9-year-old child in the third grade. Rachel has been diagnosed with generalized anxiety disorder, bipolar disorder, and attention deficit disorder. Her home environment is unstable and Child Protective Services is involved with the family, who struggles financially. Rachel lives with her mother (who has depression, substance abuse, and bipolar disorder) and brother (who was recently incarcerated because of substance abuse). Rachel enjoys arts and crafts and likes to be involved in afterschool activities. She can be pleasant and talkative to adults, but seems to stand on the sidelines with peers and has episodes in which she gets very angry with peers when waiting her turn. Rachel exhibits good gross and fine motor skills. However, she sometimes completes schoolwork quickly and shows poor attention to details. She is struggling in the classroom.

The occupational therapist completed the Child Occupational Self-Assessment (COSA) with Rachel and found that she was not good at socializing with peers. However, Rachel said this was not important to her. After further conversation, Rachel admitted she would like to have some friends at school. The occupational therapist designed intervention to help Rachel learn to play with peers and express her frustration in appropriate fashion. The occupational therapist modeled play behaviors, engaged Rachel in some individual sessions with arts and crafts, and later invited peers to join. Rachel began to share objects with peers once she realized these items would also be available to her. She began to interact with peers and complete arts and crafts projects together. The occupational therapist focused sessions on increasing Rachel's belief in her own abilities (self-competency) to increase her ability to play with peers.

This case illustrates the use of play as the goal of the intervention session.

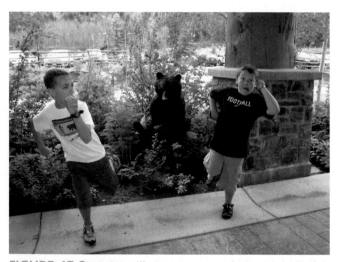

FIGURE 17-8 Being silly is an aspect of play and playfulness. These boys show playfulness as they tease that they are being chased by the bear!

Playfulness in Occupational Therapy

Play is used therapeutically to facilitate playfulness, development of play skills, and acquisition of new behaviors. Often what individuals play with and how they play may not be as important as the affective quality of their play. Some children with significant or multiple disabilities manage to get great joy and benefit out of play. On the other hand, therapists often see children who are not playful and do not derive pleasure out of even the simplest play interaction (Figure 17-8). Facilitating playfulness in the child can be an important goal of therapy.

Morrison and Metzger stated:

The more playful child may generalize this flexible approach into environmental interaction beyond play and into other aspects of his or her life. For the child with a condition that impedes his or her ability to interact with the social or physical environment, a flexible (playful) approach may enable the child to succeed more frequently in these difficult situations. (p. 540)[72]

The therapist should express a playful attitude through speech, body language, and facial expressions. Novelty and imaginary play can be used to facilitate playful participation on the part of the child. Bundy stated that the therapist must know how to play to be able to model play for the child.[19] To develop playfulness, the child must develop intrinsic motivation, internal control, ability to suspend reality, and ability to give and read verbal and nonverbal cues when interacting with peers and caregivers.

Facilitating playful interactions is important for a child of any age. For example, therapists working in a neonatal intensive care unit or with infants in the community can help parents learn to read their infant's cues and adapt to the infant's behavioral tempo to develop mutually positive experiences that form the basis for playful processes as the infant matures.[43] For those who work in schools or who provide consultation for mixed-age programs, therapists can teach educators, parents, and childcare providers the value of having children engage in mixed-age play and interaction, which yields increased leadership skills in older children and creativity and imagination in their younger playmates.[40]

Play Spaces and Adaptations

Critical to creating a play atmosphere for children is considering the environment and the objects, equipment, and opportunities within it. To foster play, environmental spaces, toys, and equipment should have some flexibility in usage (Figure 17-9).

Bundy et al. examined changes in playfulness in a group of typically developing children, ages 5 to 7 years, after new materials (e.g., cardboard boxes, bicycle tires, hay bales, plastic barrels, wood, foam) were introduced to the playground.[22] They found that scores on the Test of Playfulness rose significantly after the intervention, and the teachers felt that the

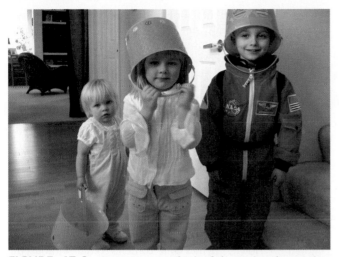

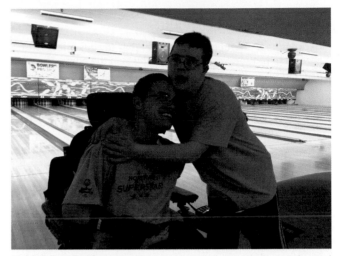

FIGURE 17-9 One aspect of playfulness involves using objects in unconventional ways. These toddlers have used buckets for space helmets.

FIGURE 17-10 Matthew and his friend enjoy adapted bowling and participating in games with friends. (Courtesy Jill McQuaid.)

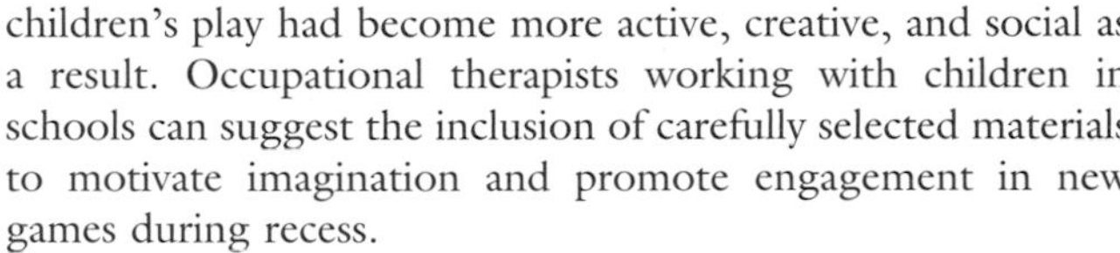

children's play had become more active, creative, and social as a result. Occupational therapists working with children in schools can suggest the inclusion of carefully selected materials to motivate imagination and promote engagement in new games during recess.

In addition, toys and play equipment may need to be adapted for the child to access them optimally. Adaptation of toys and the environment is an important role of the occupational therapist, particularly for the severely involved child. Play spaces should offer a variety of experiences and allow for creativity, illusion, change, and chance. Children need to be able to control the space, that is, have objects, toys, and people to move and change and the freedom to move them.[24] The therapist must know the properties of toys as well as how to adapt them appropriately. Switches, adaptive keyboards, or provisions for sensory impairment may be necessary for the child to benefit from and be more independent in play. Play can be enhanced through a variety of augmentative devices ranging from very simple adaptations to complex electronic devices.[32]

Indoor and outdoor playgrounds and group play spaces need to be designed to promote universal access for children with physical limitations and to encourage socialization (Figure 17-10). Therapists working in school-based practice need to advocate for school playgrounds that are accessible and that offer opportunities for physical exercise, sensory exploration, motor and cognitive skill development, and social skill practice.[96]

In designing playful spaces for children, occupational therapists should consider the following key points:

- Use of color and texture
- Novelty of equipment and supplies
- Attention to the senses (sight and sound options)
- Consideration of age and developmental levels
- Convertibility of play spaces to allow for varied levels of ability and interest
- Comfort, size, and safety (smaller spaces are typically best)
- Ability to suggest themes or allow for varied thematic play
- Therapeutic use of self and others (playfulness is best facilitated by others who are playful!)

Parent Education and Training

Working with parents in relation to play is important for carryover of the skills and abilities learned in therapy into the child's everyday life. Children with physical disabilities may be involved in therapeutic regimens throughout the day and consequently may be deprived of play opportunities. Four barriers to free play in children with physical disabilities are:

1. Limitations imposed by caregivers
2. Physical and personal limitations of the child
3. Environmental barriers
4. Social barriers[70]

Interventions that support the child's free play and include recommendations about play things and play spaces help support the importance of play in overall development. For example, occupational therapists can help parents perform "toy inventories" (Box 17-3) and suggest that parents create play spaces throughout the home (e.g., a special cupboard in the kitchen or a toy workbench in the garage or craft area).

Helping parents understand the importance of play for their child and helping them to interact with their child playfully are key goals of therapy. Parents may need guidance in creating a balance between doing things for their child and allowing the child to form and carry out his or her own intentions. The therapist may need to model play behavior for the parent, encourage the parent to enter into and contribute to play sequences without directing or controlling them, and help the parent organize or adapt the play environment to meet the needs of the child. By actively involving the parents or caregivers, the therapist helps them appreciate their child's strengths, learn the fun of playing with their child, and develop play skills that match their child's interests.

Societal Concerns

As society continues to rely more heavily on technology, and virtual play opportunities increase, parents and caregivers need to have the necessary tools to be able to embrace and integrate potential new opportunities for play and social engagement,

BOX 17-3 Toy Inventory

Occupational therapists can share this toy inventory with parents to promote play and playfulness in the home. Parents often ask for ideas of gifts for their children before a child's birthday or holiday. This inventory may help educate others on the play needs of the child.

Step 1
Explain that "good toys" have the following qualities:
- Are appropriate for the child's age and developmental level
- Keep the child's interest
- Have longevity (in other words they are toys that will stand the test of time and can be used by the child in a variety of ways for years, such as Legos)
- Are safe and durable
- Stimulate learning

Step 2
Encourage parents to create a list of toys in their home by the following categories:
- Active toys (ride-on toys, outdoor or sports equipment)
- Manipulative toys (construction toys, puzzles, dressing toys, beads, blocks, bath toys, and sand or water toys)
- Make-believe (dolls, stuffed toys, puppets, role play, transportation toys)
- Creative toys (musical toys, arts and crafts materials, digital music or tablet devices with creativity apps)
- Learning toys (games, specific-skill toys such as science models, computer or tablet devices with learning applications, books)

Step 3
Review toy inventory with the parent. Make suggestions for home play spaces and play things that relate to the child's intervention goals.

while balancing the technology with real-world, physical play and interaction.

In the last few years, play for all children has diminished. The amount of unscheduled time in the day of an average school-aged child continues to decline as families' work and extracurricular demands rise.[66,92] Because of changing family lifestyles, challenges in education, technology, and safety concerns, children today have little time and space for free play. Singer et al. examined the role of play and experiential learning in 16 nations, divided into developed countries, newly industrial countries, and developing countries.[92] They gathered information from mothers of 2400 children. They found similarities in all nations, with mothers describing the lack of free play and experiential learning opportunities. A major portion of children's free time was spent watching television.

Other studies have shown many barriers to play. One is overstructuring and overscheduling of the child's day.[39,56,66,78] Children's afterschool hours are filled with classes, planned activities, and homework. Another barrier is an overemphasis on early academic achievement. Schools are increasingly moving to eliminate the "playful" parts of school, including recess, gym, sports, and art programs.[39,78] Some states have eliminated recess altogether because it is not considered academic. Academics are being stressed earlier in our educational systems, and parents often feel that, for play to be worthwhile, the adults need to "teach" things during play. A third barrier to play results from parents' concerns for the safety of their children in a culture they perceive as increasingly violent. Outdoor play has decreased markedly and parents schedule "play dates," or planned play experiences. Places for play have decreased also. Many metropolitan areas are severely lacking in park space,[66] and many school playgrounds are often simply asphalt pads with no playground equipment.

The decreases in unstructured, physical play have had a dramatic effect on children. The rise in childhood obesity, as well as in the health problems that accompany obesity, is a major problem facing parents. The over-reliance on television and computers has changed the type of play that children choose and leads to more passivity and reliance on others for entertainment. The increased media exposure has also exposed children to violent themes and content, often without the benefit of parental supervision. Active video games are becoming increasingly popular and offer increased energy expenditure over passive gaming, but the level of physical activity afforded does not match the equivalent of real-world physical activity.[46]

Many organizations, including the American Academy of Pediatrics,[40] the Association for Childhood Education International, and the American Association for the Child's Right to Play,[1,41,47] have issued declarations promoting the importance of and need for active play for children.

Occupational therapy practitioners are in a unique position to act as advocates for play, not only for their clients but also for children in general. In 2008, AOTA published a societal statement on play including the following recommendations:

> *Occupational therapy practitioners support, enhance, and defend children's right to play as individuals and as members of their families, peer groups, and communities by promoting recognition of play's crucial role in children's development, health, and well-being; establishing and restoring children's skills needed to engage in play; adapting play materials, objects, and environments to facilitate optimal play experiences; and advocating for safe, inclusive play environments that are accessible to all. (p. 707)*[82]

Occupational therapists can advocate for play in many ways to respond to the AOTA statement, including:
- Presenting in-services for school personnel and playground monitors
- Offering community classes for parents
- Volunteering to serve on community and school playground building committees
- Working with children's museums to develop play venues
- Distributing the AOTA Tip Sheets "Learning Through Play," which can be found at http://www.aota.org/Play-Skills, and "Recess Promotion," which can be found at http://www.aota.org/Practitioners-Section/Children-and-Youth/New/Recess.aspx.FT-.pdf
- Working with organizations such as the Starlight Children's Foundation to provide playful family experiences for children with chronic and critical health conditions.
- Working with state and national occupational therapy associations and other organizations that promote early learning

and childhood development to advocate for play and play spaces in the community.
- Collaborating with community organizations that provide play opportunities, such as YMCAs, scouts, playrooms, swimming programs, and gymnastic programs, to enhance their accessibility and provide accommodations for all children.

Summary Points

- Play is the primary occupation of childhood and its place within occupational therapy practice ranges from a focus on the development of play skills themselves to a modality to address skills in a variety of developmental domains.
- Occupational therapists' view of play stems from the theoretical underpinnings of many fields, with a focus on the form, function, meaning, and context of play as childhood occupation.
- Occupational therapists use a variety of assessment tools for evaluative and treatment planning purposes. These include the Revised Knox Preschool Play Scale and the Test of Playfulness, both developed by occupational therapists.
- Play is a developmental phenomenon that relates to skills across sensory, motor, cognitive, communication, and social domains. Occupational therapists need to have knowledge of typical play development to effectively evaluate play skills and plan intervention. Play development is influenced by context, including personal, social, cultural, virtual, and societal factors.
- Occupational therapists are in a unique position to advocate for the preservation of play in today's society, including opportunities for the creation of safe and accessible playgrounds, the preservation of recess in schools, and education related to the need for unstructured, physical play to reduce incidence of childhood obesity.

REFERENCES

1. American Association for the Child's Right to Play (2007). IPA declaration of a child's right to play. Retrieved on July 31, 2014 from http://ipaworld.org/about-us/declaration/ipa-declaration-of-the-childs-right-to-play/.
2. American Occupational Therapy Association. (2008). Occupational therapy practice framework: Domain and process. *American Journal of Occupational Therapy, 62*, 625–683.
3. Anderson, J., Hinojosa, J., & Strauch, C. (1987). Integrating play in neurodevelopmental treatment. *American Journal of Occupational Therapy, 41*, 421–426.
4. Ayres, A. J. (1972). *Sensory integration and learning disorders.* Los Angeles: Western Psychological Services.
5. Ayres, A. J. (1979). *Sensory integration and learning disorders.* Los Angeles: Western Psychological Services.
6. Baranek, G., Reinhartsen, D., & Wannamaker, S. (2001). Play: Engaging young children with autism. In R. Huebner (Ed.), *Autism: A sensorimotor approach to management* (pp. 313–351). Gaithersburg, MD. Aspen.
7. Barnett, L. (1990). Playfulness: Definition, design, and measurement. *Play and Culture, 4*, 319–336.
8. Barnett, L. (1991). The playful child: Measurement of a disposition to play. *Play and Culture, 4*, 51–74.
9. Barnett, L., & Kleiber, D. (1982). Concomitants of playfulness in early childhood: Cognitive abilities and gender. *The Journal of Genetic Psychology, 141*, 115–127.
10. Barnett, L., & Kleiber, D. (1984). Playfulness and the early play environment. *The Journal of Genetic Psychology, 144*, 153–164.
11. Bazyk, S., Stalnaker, D., Llerena, M., et al. (2003). Play in Mayan children. *American Journal of Occupational Therapy, 57*, 273–283.
12. Bergen, D. (1988). *Play as a medium for learning and development.* Portsmouth, NH: Heinemann.
13. Berlyne, D. (1966). Curiosity and exploration. *Science, 15*, 25–32.
14. Blanche, E. (2008). Play in children with cerebral palsy: Doing with—not doing to. In L. D. Parham & L. Fazio (Eds.), *Play in occupational therapy for children* (2nd ed., pp. 375–394). St. Louis: Elsevier.
15. Blanche, E., & Knox, S. (2008). Learning to play: Promoting skills and quality of life in individuals with cerebral palsy. In A. Eliasson & P. Burtner (Eds.), *Improving hand function in children with cerebral palsy: Theory, evidence, and intervention* (pp. 357–370). London: Mac Keith Press.
16. Bledsoe, N., & Shepherd, J. (1982). A study of reliability and validity of a preschool play scale. *American Journal of Occupational Therapy, 36*, 783–788.
17. Brockman, R., Jago, R., & Fox, K. R. (2011). Children's active play: Self-reported motivators, barriers, and facilitators. *BioMed Central Public Health, 11*, 461. doi:10.1186/1471-2458-11-461.
18. Bruner, J. (1972). Nature and uses of immaturity. *American Psychologist, 27*, 687–708.
19. Bundy, A. (1991). Play theory and sensory integration. In A. G. Fisher, E. A. Murray, & A. C. Bundy (Eds.), *Sensory integration: Therapy and practice* (pp. 46–68). Philadelphia: F. A. Davis.
20. Bundy, A. (1993). Assessment of play and leisure: Delineation of the problem. *American Journal of Occupational Therapy, 47*, 217–222.
21. Bundy, A. (1997). Play and playfulness: What to look for. In L. D. Parham & L. Fazio (Eds.), *Play in occupational therapy for children* (pp. 52–66). St. Louis: Mosby.
22. Bundy, A., Luckett, T., Naughton, G., et al. (2008). Playful interaction: Occupational therapy for all children on the school playground. *American Journal of Occupational Therapy, 62*, 522–527.
23. Caillois, R. (1958). *Man, play, and games.* Glencoe, NY: Free Press.
24. Chandler, A. (1997). Where do you want to play? Play environments; an occupational therapy perspective. In B. Chandler (Ed.), *The essence of play* (pp. 159–174). Bethesda, MD: American Occupational Therapy Association.
25. Clark, F., Parham, D., Carlson, M., et al. (1991). Occupational science: Academic innovation in the service of occupational therapy's future. *American Journal of Occupational Therapy, 45*, 300–310.
26. Cohen, A. (1987). *The development of play.* New York: New York University Pres.
27. Couch, K. (1996). *The role of play in pediatric occupational therapy.* Seattle:

University of Washington, unpublished master's thesis.

28. Couch, K., Deitz, J. C., & Kanny, E. M. (1998). The role of play in pediatric occupational therapy. *American Journal of Occupational Therapy, 52*, 111–117.
29. Crowe, T. (1989). Pediatric assessments: A survey of their use by occupational therapists in northwestern school systems. *Occupational Therapy Journal of Research, 9*, 273–286.
30. Csikszentmihalyi, M., & Larson, R. (1984). *Being adolescent.* New York: Basic Books.
31. Daunhauer, L., & Cermak, S. (2008). Play occupations and the experience of deprivation. In L. D. Parham & L. Fazio (Eds.), *Play in occupational therapy for children* (2nd ed., pp. 251–262). St. Louis: Elsevier.
32. Deitz, J., & Swinth, Y. (2008). Accessing play through assistive technology. In L. D. Parham & L. Fazio (Eds.), *Play in occupational therapy for children* (2nd ed., pp. 395–412). St. Louis: Elsevier.
33. Ellis, M. J. (1973). *Why people play.* Englewood Cliffs, NJ: Prentice Hall.
34. Erikson, A. (1963). *Childhood and society.* New York: Norton.
35. Finnie, N. (1975). *Handling the young cerebral palsied child at home* (2nd ed.). New York: E. P. Dutton & Company.
36. Florey, L. (1971). An approach to play and play development. *American Journal of Occupational Therapy, 25*, 275–280.
37. Franz, L. (1963). Introduction. In R. Hartley & R. Goldenson (Eds.), *The complete book of children's play.* New York: Cornwall Press.
38. Garvey, A. (1977). *Play.* London: Fontana/Open Books.
39. Ginsburg, K. (2007). The importance of play in promoting healthy child development and maintaining strong parent-child bonds. *Pediatrics, 119*, 182–191.
40. Gray, P. (2011). The special value of children's age-mixed play. *American Journal of Play, 3*(4), 502–522.
41. Henry, A. (2008). Assessment of play in children an adolescents. In L. D. Parham & L. Fazio (Eds.), *Play in occupational therapy for children* (2nd ed., pp. 71–94). St. Louis: Elsevier.
42. Hoffman, J., & Boettrich, S. (2009). Setting the stage for free play: Museum environments that inspire creativity. *Hand to Hand: Association of Children's Museums, 22*(4), 3–5.
43. Holloway, A. (2008). Fostering parent-infant playfulness in the neonatal intensive care unit. In L. D. Parham & L. Fazio (Eds.), *Play in occupational therapy for children* (2nd ed., pp. 335–350). St. Louis: Elsevier.
44. Howes, A., & Stewart, P. (1987). Child's play with adults, toys, and peers: An examination of family and child care influences. *Developmental Psychology, 23*, 423–430.
45. Huizinga, J. (1950). *Homo ludens.* Boston: Beacon Press.
46. Irwin, J., & Biddiss, E. (2010). Active video games to promote physical activity in children and youth: A systematic review. *Archives of Pediatric and Adolescent Medicine, 164*(7), 664–672.
47. Isendberg, I., & Quisenberry, N. (2002). Play: Essential for all children. A position paper of the Association for Childhood Education International. Retrieved on April, 2009 from <http://www.acei.org/playpaper.htm>.
48. Jacobs, B., & White, D. (1994). The relationship of child-care quality and play to social behavior in the kindergarten. In H. Goelman & E. Jacobs (Eds.), *Children's play in child care settings* (pp. 85–101). New York: State University of New York Press.
49. Johnson, J., Christie, J., & Yawkey, T. (1999). *Play and early childhood development.* New York: Longman.
50. Kaplan-Sanoff, M., Brewster, A., Stillwell, J., et al. (1988). The relationship of play to physical/motor development and to children with special needs. In D. Bergen (Ed.), *Play as a medium for learning and development* (pp. 137–162). Portsmouth, NH: Heinemann.
51. Kielhofner, B., Barris, R., Bauer, D., et al. (1983). A comparison of play behavior in nonhospitalized and hospitalized children. *American Journal of Occupational Therapy, 37*, 305–312.
52. Knox, S. (1968). Observation and assessment of the everyday play behavior of the mentally retarded child. Los Angeles: University of Southern California, unpublished master's thesis.
53. Knox, S. (1974). A play scale. In M. Reilly (Ed.), *Play as exploratory learning* (pp. 247–266). Beverly Hills: Sage.
54. Knox, S. (1996). Play and playfulness in preschool children. In R. Zemke & F. Clark (Eds.), *Occupational science: The evolving discipline* (pp. 81–88). Philadelphia: F. A. Davis.
55. Knox, S. (1997). Development and current use of the Knox Preschool Play Scale. In L. D. Parham & L. Fazio (Eds.), *Play in occupational therapy for children* (pp. 35–51). St. Louis: Mosby.
56. Knox, S. (1999). Play and playfulness of preschool children. Los Angeles: University of Southern California, unpublished doctoral dissertation.
57. Knox, S. (2008). Development and current use of the Revised Knox Preschool Play Scale. In L. D. Parham & L. Fazio (Eds.), *Play in occupational therapy for children* (pp. 55–70). St. Louis: Mosby.
58. Kramer, J., Velden, M., Kafkes, A., et al. (2005). *The Child Occupational Self Assessment (COSA)* (version 2.2). Chicago: MOHO Clearinghouse, Department of Occupational Therapy, College of Applied Health Sciences, University of Illinois at Chicago.
59. Kuhaneck, H., Tanta, K. J., Coombs, A. K., et al. (2013). A survey of pediatric occupational therapists' use of play. *Journal of Occupational Therapy, Schools, and Early Intervention, 6*(3); 23–27.
60. Lawlor, M., & Henderson, A. (1989). A descriptive study of the clinical practice patterns of occupational therapists working with infants and young children. *American Journal of Occupational Therapy, 43*, 755–764.
61. LeBlanc, M., & Ritchie, M. (2001). A meta-analysis of play therapy outcomes. *Counseling Psychology Quarterly, 14*, 149–163.
62. LEGO Learning Institute (2009). The changing face of children's play culture: Children's play, learning, and communication in a technology driven world. Retrieved from <http://www.legolearning.net/download/Play_Culture.pdf>.
63. Levy, J. (1978). *Play behavior.* Malabar, FL: Robert E. Kruger.
64. Liebermann, J. (1977). *Playfulness: Its relationship to imagination and creativity.* New York: Academic Press.
65. Linder, T. (1993). *Transdisciplinary play-based assessment.* Baltimore: Paul H. Brookes.
66. Louv, R. (2005). *Last child in the woods.* Chapel Hill, NC: Algonquin Books.
67. Meyer, A. (1922). The philosophy of occupational therapy. *Archives of Occupational Therapy, 1*, 1–10.
68. Michelman, S. (1974). Play and the deficit child. In M. Reilly (Ed.), *Play as exploratory learning* (pp. 157–208). Beverly Hills: Sage.
69. Miller, B., & Kuhaneck, H. (2008). Children's perceptions of play experiences and play preferences: A qualitative study. *American Journal of Occupational Therapy, 62*, 407–415.
70. Missiuna, A., & Pollock, N. (1991). Play deprivation in children with physical disabilities: The role of the occupational therapist in preventing secondary disability. *American Journal of Occupational Therapy, 45*, 882–888.
71. Mogford, K. (1977). The play of handicapped children. In B. Tizard & D. Harvey (Eds.), *Biology of play* (pp. 170–184). Philadelphia: J. B. Lippincott.

72. Morrison, A., & Metzger, P. (2001). Play. In J. Case-Smith (Ed.), *Occupational therapy for children* (4th ed., pp. 528–544). St. Louis: Mosby.
73. Neulinger, J. (1981). *The psychology of leisure* (2nd ed.). Springfield, IL: Charles C Thomas.
74. Neumann, A. (1971). *The elements of play.* New York: MSS Information.
75. O'Brien, J., Asselin, L., Fortier, K., et al. (2010). Using therapeutic reasoning to apply the Model of Human Occupation in pediatric occupational therapy practice. *Journal of Occupational Therapy, Schools, & Early Intervention, 3,* 348–365.
76. Parham, L. D., & Fazio, L. S. (2008). *Play in occupational therapy with children* (2nd ed.). St. Louis: Elsevier.
77. Parten, M. (1933). Social play among pre-school children. *Journal of Abnormal and Social Psychology, 28,* 136–147.
78. Pellegrini, A. (2008). The recess debate. *American Journal of Play, 1,* 181–191.
79. Piaget, J. (1952). *Play, dreams and imitation in childhood.* London: William Heinemann.
80. Pierce, A. (1991). Early object rule acquisition. *American Journal of Occupational Therapy, 45,* 438–449.
81. Pierce, D. (1997, 2008). The power of object play. In L. D. Parham & L. S. Fazio (Eds.), *Play in occupational therapy with children* (2nd ed., pp. 86–111). St. Louis: Elsevier.
82. Primeau, L. (1995). Orchestration of work and play within families. Los Angeles: University of Southern California, unpublished dissertation.
83. Primeau, L. (2008). AOTA's societal statement on play. *American Journal of Occupational Therapy, 62,* 707–708.
84. Rast, M. (1986). *Play and therapy, play or therapy. Play: A skill for life.* Rockville, MD: American Occupational Therapy Association.
85. Reilly, M. (1974). *Play as exploratory learning.* Beverly Hills: Sage.
86. Richmond, J. B. (1960). Behavior, occupation, and treatment of children. *American Journal of Occupational Therapy, 14,* 183–186.
87. Robinson, A. (1977). Play: The arena for acquisition of rules for competent behavior. *The American Journal of Occupational Therapy, 31,* 248–253.
88. Rubin, K., Fein, G., & Vandenberg, B. (1983). Play. In P. Mussin (Ed.), *Handbook of child psychology* (Vol. IV, pp. 694–774). New York: John Wiley & Sons.
89. Schiller, C. (1957). *Innate motor activity as a basis of learning, instinctive behavior.* New York International Universities Press.
90. Schwartzman, B. (1978). *Socializing play: Functional analysis, transformations: The anthropology of children's play.* New York: Plenum Press.
91. Singer, D. G., & Singer, J. L. (2005). *Imagination and play in the electronic age.* Cambridge, MA: Harvard University Press.
92. Singer, D., Singer, J., D'Agostino, H., et al. (2009). Children's pastimes and play in sixteen nations: Is free play declining? *American Journal of Play, 1,* 283–312.
93. Skard, A., & Bundy, A. C. (2008). In L. D. Parham & L. S. Fazio (Eds.), *Play in occupational therapy with children* (2nd ed., pp. 71–94). St. Louis: Elsevier.
94. Smilanski, S. (1968). *The effects of sociodramatic play on disadvantaged preschool children.* New York: John Wiley & Sons.
95. Spitzer, S. (2008). Play in children with autism: Structure and experience. In L. D. Parham & L. S. Fazio (Eds.), *Play in occupational therapy with children* (2nd ed., pp. 351–374). St. Louis: Elsevier.
96. Swinth, Y., & Tanta, K. (2008). Play, leisure, and social participation in educational settings. In L. D. Parham & L. S. Fazio (Eds.), *Play in occupational therapy with children* (2nd ed., pp. 301–317). St. Louis: Elsevier.
97. Takata, N. (1969). The play history. *American Journal of Occupational Therapy, 23,* 314–318.
98. Takata, N. (1974). Play as a prescription. In M. Reilly (Ed.), *Play as exploratory learning* (pp. 209–246). Beverly Hills: Sage.
99. Tanta, K. (2010). Encouraging play and promoting peer interactions in young children with an autism spectrum disorder. In H. M. Kuhaneck & R. Watling (Eds.), *Autism: A comprehensive occupational therapy approach* (3rd ed.). Bethesda, MD: AOTA Press.
100. Vygotsky, L. (1966). Play and its role in the mental development of the child. *Soviet Psychology, 12,* 62–76.
101. White, R. (1959). Motivation reconsidered: The concept of competence. *Psychological Review, 66,* 297–333.

CHAPTER

18 Prewriting and Handwriting Skills

Colleen M. Schneck • Jane Case-Smith

KEY TERMS

Literacy
Handwriting readiness
Functional written communication
Legibility
Domains of handwriting
Models of practice
Handwriting intervention outcomes

GUIDING QUESTIONS

1. What is the role of the occupational therapist in evaluation of and intervention for children with handwriting difficulties?
2. Which factors contribute to handwriting readiness for young children?
3. How would an occupational therapist evaluate handwriting and functional written communication?
4. How do performance skills, client factors, performance patterns, and context influence the student's participation in the writing process?
5. How does handwriting fit into the educational writing process?
6. How do remedial and compensatory strategies improve a student's written communication?
7. How do occupational therapy practitioners use pediatric occupational therapy models of practice and handwriting intervention programs to improve children's handwriting?
8. Which handwriting interventions and programs are supported with research evidence?

Occupational therapy practitioners view the occupations of children to be activities of daily living, education, work, play, and social participation. In the area of education, school-aged children's occupations encompass academic skills such as literacy (including reading and writing), calculation, and problem solving, as well as nonacademic or functional tasks. Functional tasks may include navigating around classroom furniture and classmates, sharing school supplies with a peer, placing a notebook into a locker, constructing a papier-mâché planet, cutting with scissors, and writing words on paper—all of which support a student's academic performance in the classroom. These academic skills and functional tasks are expected to evolve and strengthen throughout a student's school years.[21]

Writing is a tool for communication; it provides a means to project thoughts, feelings, and ideas. Writing is required when children and adolescents compose stories, complete written examinations, copy numbers for calculations, and write messages to friends and family members. Although computers allow students to type letters and reports, they continue to need legible handwriting to complete forms, write personal notes and messages, and maintain records. Handwriting is more than a motor skill; it requires connecting the letter name with a letter form and recalling a clear visual picture of the letter form from memory, as well as being able to execute the motor pattern for each form.[38] Writing is a complex process requiring the synthesis and integration of memory retrieval, organization, problem solving, language and reading ability, ideation, and graphomotor function. The functional skill of handwriting supports the academic task of writing and allows students to convey written information legibly and efficiently while accomplishing school assignments in a timely manner.[16,48]

Handwriting consumes much of a student's school day and is an essential skill for students to master.[20] In a study of elementary grade classrooms, McHale and Cermak[77] found that 31% to 60% of a child's school day consisted of fine motor activities. Most of these fine motor activities (85%) were paper-and-pencil tasks, indicating that students may possibly spend up to one fourth to one half of their classroom time engaged in paper-and-pencil tasks.

When children are having difficulty with handwriting, problems with written assignments follow. Students with neurologic impairments, learning problems, attention deficits, and developmental disabilities often expend extensive time and effort learning to write legibly.[4] Consequences of handwriting difficulties at school may include the following: (1) teachers may assign lower marks for the writing quality of papers and tests with poorer legibility but not poorer content[28,52]; (2) students' slow handwriting speed may limit compositional fluency and quality[49,64,121]; (3) students may take longer to finish assignments than their peers[46]; (4) students may have problems with taking notes in class and reading them later[46]; (5) students may fail to learn other higher-order writing processes such as planning and grammar; (6) writing avoidance may develop, contributing later to arrested writing development; (7) students may omit details of what they know[79]; or (8) students submit shortened or incomplete written responses because of the intense concentration and motor effort required to correctly form letters.[23] The ability to write legibly remains an important skill beyond elementary years; for example, the College Board SAT test requires students to handwrite the essay portion of the test.

Berninger et al.[17] explain that it is critical for children to learn to write automatically to accomplish the extensive written composition required of them in later elementary grades. Handwriting instruction is important to ensure that children learn the "building blocks of written discourse automatically so that they can focus on other important aspects of writing, such as choosing and spelling words, constructing sentences, and organizing the discourse of composing written texts" (p. 4).[17] Studies support the importance of a direct and structured approach to handwriting instruction.[60,100] Because of curriculum demands for increased literacy and math instruction, handwriting instruction has decreased in recent years, resulting in more students struggling with handwriting skills.[35,36]

Teachers often request that occupational therapists evaluate a student's handwriting when it interferes with performance of written assignments. In fact, poor handwriting is one of the most common reasons for referring school-aged children to occupational therapy.[7,73]

The role of the occupational therapist is to view the student's performance, in this case handwriting, by focusing on the interaction of the student, the school environment, and the demands of school occupations.[2] During the evaluation and intervention processes, the practitioner stays focused on (1) the occupation of handwriting, determining which domains of handwriting (e.g., near-point copying or dictation) and which components (e.g., spacing or letter formation) are problematic for the student; (2) the school context (e.g., the curriculum or physical classroom arrangement related to the child's performance); (3) the student's personal context (e.g., cultural, temporal, spiritual, and physical aspects); and (4) student experiences that are interfering with handwriting production. Occupational therapy offers a variety of services to improve handwriting. Therapists provide intervention directly to the child or through consultation with the teacher. In addition, the approach may focus on remediating potential causes of handwriting (i.e., impaired hand strength) or concentrate on the activity of handwriting itself.

The Writing Process

The No Child Left Behind (NCLB) Act of 2001[85] increased the emphasis on literacy and the contributions of school professionals to developing literacy skills in children. Literacy begins with the basic ability to read and write (functional literacy), which is required in everyday life, and proceeds to advanced literacy, which includes reflecting on knowledge of significant ideas, events, and values of a society.[58] Based on an occupation-focused approach,[3] occupational therapists strive to improve children's access to and engagement in early literacy activities.[12] When practitioners consider writing as an important early literacy communication skill, in addition to it being a complex motor task, their approaches to supporting writing expand and easily integrate into the curriculum.[25,42] Occupational therapy intervention focused on supporting writing within the context of meaningful literacy experiences improves not only writing but also a broad set of literacy skills.[9]

Preliteracy Writing Development of Young Children

Handwriting is a complex skill that develops over years of practice. Many children begin to draw and scribble on paper shortly after they are able to grasp a writing tool (Figure 18-1). As young children mature, they write intentionally meaningful messages, first with pictures and then with scribbles, letter-like forms, and strings of letters.[77] The development of a child's writing process in the early elementary grades includes not only mastering the mechanical and perceptual processes of graphics, but also the acquisition of language and the learning of spelling and phonology. Furthermore, early writing competence is highly correlated with later success in reading.[84] Typically, children's writing and reading skills develop in parallel processes with one another.[77] Consequently, if a young child is unable to recognize letterforms and understand that these letterforms represent written language, occupational therapists and educators cannot expect the child to write. Although children vary in the rate they progress through these stages, all children, including those with special needs, progress through these stages.[19]

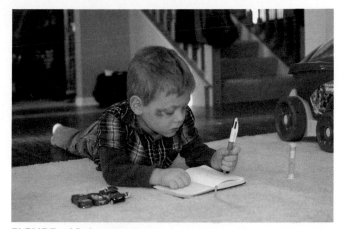

FIGURE 18-1 Three year old imitating writing after observing the therapist.

As children develop, their scribbling and pictures evolve into the handwriting (i.e., language symbols) specific to their culture. Children progress through the following stages of prewriting and handwriting: (1) controlled scribbles; (2) discrete lines, dots, or symbols; (3) straight-line or circular uppercase letters; (4) uppercase letters; and (5) lowercase letters, numerals, and words.[108] Table 18-1 details the development of prewriting and handwriting with approximate age levels for children in the United States.

Writing Development of School-Aged Children

Most children learn to write letters in kindergarten but do not develop fluency until the third or fourth grade, and they do not demonstrate adult speed in writing until the ninth grade.[49] Handwriting requires the integration of both lower-level perceptual-motor processes and higher-level cognitive processes.[53] Correlational studies have found that handwriting skill is linked to eye-hand coordination[23] and is moderately associated with dexterity.[29] A number of correlational studies found that visual-motor integration is the strongest predictor of handwriting legibility.[114,120] The perceptual-motor processes of handwriting include visual perception (e.g., when copying from a model), auditory processing (e.g., when words are dictated),

TABLE 18-1 Development of Prewriting and Handwriting in Young Children

Age Level	Performance Task
10-12 mo	Scribbles on paper
2 yr	Imitates horizontal, vertical, and circular marks on paper
3 yr	Copies a vertical line, horizontal line, and circle
4-5 yr	Copies a cross, right oblique cross, some letters and numerals, and may be able to write own name
5-6 yr	Copies a triangle, prints own name, copies most lowercase and uppercase letters

Bayley, N. (2005). *Bayley scales on infant development* (rev. ed.). San Antonio: Psychological Corporation; Beery, K. E., & Beery, N. (2005). *The Development Test of Visual-Motor Integration.* Cleveland: Modern Curriculum Press; Weil, M., & Amundson, S. J. (1994). Relationship between visual motor and handwriting skills of children in kindergarten. *American Journal of Occupational Therapy, 48,* 982–988.

and visual motor integration (e.g., when combining the components to write). The cognitive processes involved include executive planning and use of working memory. Handwriting also requires specific language processes,[114] including the ability to hear a word and identify which letters form that word (i.e., turning spoken language into written language).

When young children first learn to write their letters, they use their vision to guide their hand movements. Although adults rely more on kinesthetic input when writing,[14] children learn the skills by visually analyzing form and space, then linking the image of a letterform to a motor plan. With practice in visually guiding their hand movement, children develop a kinesthetic memory of letterforms. At this point in their learning, writing becomes automatic.[14] In primary grades, when students are learning handwriting by copying letters, visual-motor coordination and motor dexterity are critical skills.[116] In older students, who are required to produce substantial amounts of writing, cognitive processes become more important (e.g., planning and linguistic skills). The association between lower level (perceptual-motor) handwriting skills and higher-level (memory and cognition) skills was documented by Graham,[45] who found that difficulties with handwriting can interfere with the execution of the composing processes. Because handwriting requires perceptual-motor processes and cognitive processes, students with illegible handwriting may have deficits in either area.

Graham et al.[48] found that handwriting fluency is a predictor of compositional fluency and quality. Once a student has achieved automatic writing, he or she can focus on other aspects of writing (e.g., spelling, grammar, planning, organizing information for writing tasks) and therefore improve composition quality.

Handwriting Readiness

Some controversy exists as to when children are ready for formal handwriting instruction. Differing rates of maturity, environmental experiences, and interest levels are all factors that can influence children's early attempts and success in copying letters. Some children may exhibit handwriting readiness at 4 years of age, whereas others may not be ready until they are 6 years old.[116] Researchers recommend that children master handwriting readiness skills before handwriting instruction is initiated, suggesting that when children are taught handwriting before they are ready they may become discouraged and develop poor writing habits.[114,115]

Letter formation requires the integration of the visual, motor, sensory, and perceptual systems. Performance components associated with handwriting include kinesthesia, motor planning, eye-hand coordination, visual-motor integration, and in-hand manipulation. As described in the previous section, kinesthesia provides the ongoing feedback about movement errors, creates memory of motor patterns, and allows automaticity to develop. In addition, it provides information about directionality during letter formation. Kinesthetic perception also influences the amount of pressure applied to the writing implement. Sufficient fine motor coordination is also needed to form letters accurately.

Benbow[14] described six developmental classifications that underlie skilled use of the hands that contribute to greater adeptness in operating a pencil: (1) upper extremity support, (2) wrist and hand development, (3) visual control, (4) bilateral integration, (5) spatial analysis, and (6) kinesthesia. Other authors define readiness for handwriting on the basis of a child's ability to copy geometric forms. Researchers suggest that handwriting instruction be postponed until after the child masters the first nine figures in the Developmental Test of Visual-Motor Integration (VMI), that is, a vertical line, a horizontal line, a circle, a cross, a right oblique line, a square, a left oblique line, an oblique cross, and a triangle.[10,30,118] Most typically developing kindergarten children should be ready for handwriting instruction in the latter half of the kindergarten school year.

Problems in Handwriting and Visual Motor Integration

Handwriting requires the ability to integrate the visual image of letters or shapes with the appropriate motor response. Visual-cognitive abilities may affect writing in a variety of situations. Children with problems in attention may have difficulty with correct letter formation, spelling, and the mechanics of grammar, punctuation, and capitalization. They also have difficulty formulating a sequential flow of ideas necessary for written communication.[78] For a child to write spontaneously, he or she must be able to re-visualize letters and words without visual cues. A child with visual memory problems may have difficulty recalling the shape and form of letters and numbers. Other problems seen in the child with poor visual memory include mixing small and capital letters in a sentence, writing the same letter many different ways on the same page, and being unable to print the alphabet from memory. In addition, legibility may be poor, and the child may need a model to write.

Visual discrimination problems may also affect the child's handwriting.[102] The child with poor form constancy does not recognize errors in his or her own handwriting. The child may be unable to recognize letters or words in different prints and therefore may have difficulty copying from a different type of print to handwriting. The child may also show poor recognition of letters or numbers in different environments, positions, or sizes. If the child is unable to discriminate a letter, he or she may have difficulty forming it. A child with figure-ground problems may have difficulty copying because he or she is unable to determine what is to be written; the child therefore may omit important segments or may be slower than peers in producing written products.

Visual-spatial problems can also affect a child's handwriting. The child may reverse letters such as *m*, *w*, *b*, *d*, *s*, *c*, and *z* and numbers such as *2*, *3*, *5*, *6*, *7*, and *9*. If the child is unable to discriminate left from right, he or she may have difficulty with left-to-right progression in writing words and sentences. The child may over space or under space between words and letters and may have trouble keeping within the margins. The most common spatial errors in handwriting involve incorrect and inconsistent spacing between writing units and variability in orientation of major letter features when the letter is written repeatedly.[117] A child with visual-spatial difficulties may be unable to relate one part of a letter to another part and may demonstrate poor shaping or closure of individual letters or a lack of uniformity in orientation and letter size.[123] The child may have difficulty placing letters on a line and adapting letter sizes to the space provided on the paper or worksheet. Researchers have not demonstrated strong relationships between handwriting skills and visual perceptual functions, and further research is necessary to better understand the role of visual perception in handwriting.[114]

Failure on visual-motor tests may be caused by underlying visual-cognitive deficits, including visual discrimination, poor fine motor ability, or inability to integrate visual-cognitive and motor processes, or by a combination of these disabilities. Evaluating visual motor skills may help pinpoint children who need close monitoring or specific interventions to prevent the development of handwriting problems.[75] Therefore careful analysis is necessary to determine the underlying problem.

Pencil Grip Progression

The development of pencil grip in young children follows a predictable course for typically developing children but may vary among cultures.[112] Children commonly begin by holding the pencil with a primitive grip—characterized by holding the writing tool with the whole hand or extended fingers, pronating the forearm, and using the shoulder to move the pencil. Between 18 and 30 months, children use a transitional pencil grip, with the pencil being held with flexed fingers, and the forearm is pronated (thumb side downward) or supinated (Figure 18-2*A,B*). In the mature pencil grip, the pencil is stabilized by the distal phalanges of the thumb and index, middle, and possibly ring fingers; the wrist is slightly extended yet dynamic; and the supinated forearm rests on the table.[103,112]

Mature pencil grips include the dynamic tripod grasp, the lateral tripod, the dynamic quadripod, and the lateral quadripod.[32,68] Schneck and Henderson[103] reported in their study of 320 typically developing children that by the age of 6.5 to 7 years, 95% had adopted a mature pencil grasp, either the dynamic tripod (72.5%) or the lateral tripod (22.5%). Outside the United States, Tseng[112] noted that Taiwanese children use the lateral tripod grip (42.9%) almost as frequently as the dynamic tripod (44.1%). In 120 typically developing and

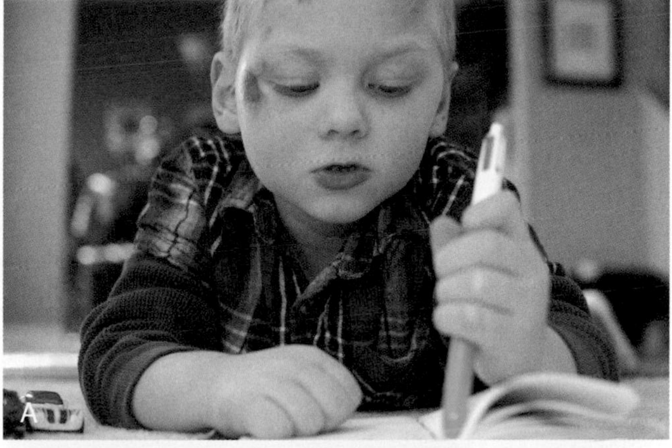

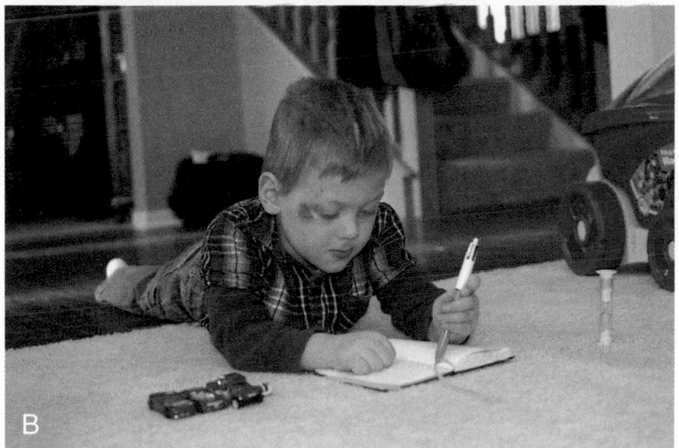

FIGURE 18-2 Primitive and transitional grasps of the marker.

nonproficient fourth grade students, Schwellnus et al.[104] found no difference in perceived effort during a sustained handwriting task for different pen grips from dynamic tripod to lateral tripod (Figure 18-3).

Handwriting Evaluation

When a child with poor handwriting has been referred to occupational therapy, the methods to gather evaluation information must be carefully selected and sequenced. A comprehensive evaluation of a child's handwriting includes (1) the occupational profile and (2) the analysis of occupational performance.

Initially the student's performance in the context of classroom standards should be the focus (before moving toward standardized testing). Assembling data and information from various sources gives the occupational therapist an integrated picture of the child's written communication.

Occupational Profile

The occupational profile describes the student's occupational therapy history, experiences, patterns of daily living, interests, values, and needs. It is designed to gain an understanding of the client's perspective and background.[82] The information for the occupational profile can be gathered by interviewing the child, parent(s), teacher, and other team members.

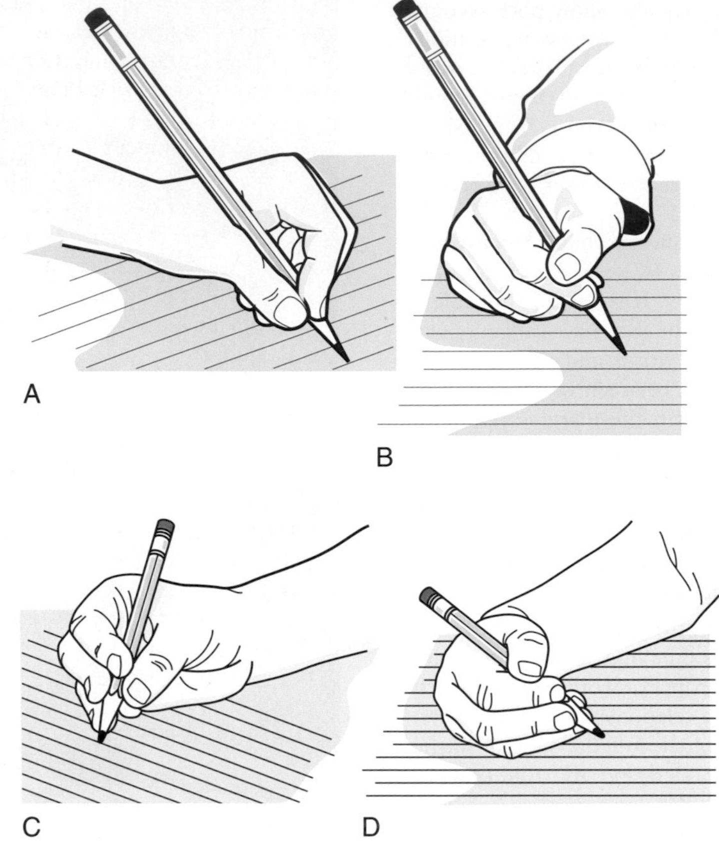

FIGURE 18-3 Mature pencil grips in elementary school children. ***A,*** Dynamic tripod; ***B,*** lateral tripod; ***C,*** dynamic quadripod; and ***D,*** lateral quadripod.

Interviews

Interviewing the child helps the therapist to understand what is important and meaningful to the child. This information helps the therapist gain an understanding of the child's perspective and background. Because teachers observe their students' daily performance in class, they can share information about the student's abilities and achievements and how the student responds to instruction. A sampling of questions to facilitate discussion between the teacher and the occupational therapist is listed in Box 18-1. The educator provides a background picture of the student's capabilities, behavior, and struggles at school. Teachers report that they evaluate students' handwriting by comparing it with that of classroom peers (37%) or comparing it with student handwriting in a book (35%).[54]

Parents provide a different perspective on the child and the child's handwriting abilities. Not only can parents describe the child's developmental, medical, and familial background to the educational team, but they can share invaluable information about the child's interests, social competence, and attitudes toward learning and school.

As members of the educational team, parents also provide important perspectives regarding the child's home activities, resources, and supports, and the child's participation in contexts outside school. To facilitate discussion about the child and his or her writing, therapists may ask parents: (1) Do you expect the child to complete school assignments or written work at home? (2) What is the child's response to written homework? (3) How does the child perform his or her written assignments at home and at school? (4) Which other writing tasks are expected of the child at home (e.g., corresponding with relatives, recording telephone messages)?

BOX 18-1 Questions to Facilitate Discussion among Educational Team Members

1. What are the student's educational strengths and concerns?
2. What is his or her handwriting performance compared with that of peers?
3. Which handwriting method (D'Nealian, Zaner-Blöser, Palmer, Italics) is being used and what is the student's history with this method?
4. What are the learning standards or curriculum of his or her grade?
5. What seems to be causing the poor handwriting?
6. When does he or she do his or her best written work?
7. When does the performance break down?
8. Which strategies for improvement have been tried? Have they worked?
9. Is a student portfolio available on the student's writing development and progress?
10. Are there other daily tasks (e.g., using scissors, getting along with peers, keeping organized) that raise concern for the teacher?

Analysis of Occupational Performance

In addition to interviewing teachers, parents, and the child, a comprehensive evaluation of a child's handwriting includes (1) examining written work samples, (2) reviewing the child's educational and clinical records, (3) directly observing the child when he or she is writing in the natural setting (i.e., school, home), (4) evaluating the child's handwriting legibility and speed, and (5) assessing performance skills suspected to be interfering with handwriting.

Work Samples

As part of the evaluation process, the occupational therapist accesses the child's handwritten class work or homework. Written work samples may include spelling lessons, mathematical problems, or stories. Ideally these samples should represent a typical handwriting performance of the child. When reviewing the child's written product, a comparison of the writing samples of the child's peers can clarify the classroom standards and teacher expectations. Informal evaluation of the work samples for alignment, size, letter formation, legibility, and slant may indicate the need for further evaluation. The use of non-letters may indicate a lack of motor skills or letter knowledge, because both skills are needed for creating accurate letter formations.[43]

File Review

Relevant information regarding past academic performance, special testing, or receipt of special services can be found in the referred child's educational cumulative file. Medical or clinical reports related to the child's education may also be located in the child's regular or special education files. The child's parents may share academic records and reports with clinic- and hospital-based occupational therapists. This documentation may trigger further conversations among the child's parents and team members.

Direct Observation

Observing the student during a writing activity in the classroom is an essential step in the evaluation process (Figure 18-4). The therapist focuses on task performance, attention to task, problem solving, and behavior of the child. Practitioners also note the student's organizational abilities, interactions with the teacher and peers, transitions between activities, and overall performance of other school tasks. School contextual features (e.g., the classroom arrangement, lighting, noise level, instructional media), as well as the teacher's instruction, should be considered in relationship to the student's performance. In addition to a structured protocol for direct observation, the occupational therapist may ask the teacher:

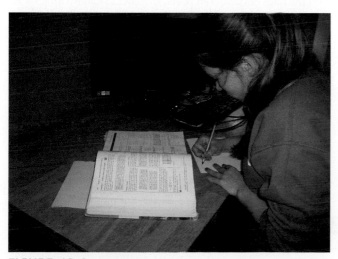

FIGURE 18-4 A student completes a written assignment at her desk.

1. Which writing tasks (e.g., copying sentences from the chalkboard, composing a story) are most problematic for the child?
2. Which writing tasks does the child enjoy?
3. Which behaviors are manifested when the child is required to write? For example, does the child chew on the eraser of the pencil or blow the pencil across the desktop to avoid writing?
4. Can the child engage independently in the task of writing or does he or she need physical and verbal cues from the teacher or educational assistant?
5. How does the child interact with and access writing materials?
6. Is the child easily distracted by visual and auditory stimuli during writing, such as a delivery truck driving by the school window?
7. Where does the child sit in the classroom?
8. What is the writing curriculum (that may or may not include handwriting)?
9. Where is the teacher located when he or she gives assignment directions?
10. How does the observed difficulty interfere with the child's learning?

Measuring Handwriting Performance

In evaluating the actual task of children's handwriting, the following areas need to be examined: (1) domains of handwriting, (2) legibility components, (3) writing speed, and (4) ergonomic factors. Whether the student writes in manuscript (print), cursive (joined script), or both, these four aspects will help the educational team and parents uncover problematic areas of handwriting and establish a baseline of handwriting function. With accurate and relevant handwriting assessment data, the occupational therapist, the child's parents, and the educational or clinical team identify specific goals and objectives for the development of written communication.

Domains of Handwriting

Evaluating the various domains of handwriting allows the occupational therapist to determine which tasks the child may be having difficulty with and address those tasks in the intervention plan. Handwriting tasks demanded of students, and helpful for intervention planning, include the following:

- Writing the alphabet in both uppercase and lowercase letters along with numbers requires the child to remember the motor engram, form each individual letter and numeral, sequence letters and numbers, and use consistent letter cases.

- Copying is the capacity to reproduce numerals, letters, and words from a similar script model, either manuscript to manuscript or cursive to cursive.
- *Near-point copying* is producing letters or words from a nearby model, commonly on the same page or on the same horizontal writing surface, as when a student copies the meaning of a word from a nearby dictionary.
- Copying from a distant vertical display model to the writing surface is termed *far-point copying*, demonstrated by students writing the words "Happy Valentine's Day" on construction paper cards from these words on the class chalkboard.
- More advanced than copying, manuscript-to-cursive transition requires a mastery of letterforms in both manuscript and cursive as the child must transcribe manuscript letters and words to cursive letters and words.
- Writing dictated words, names, addresses, and telephone numbers is a skill children use at school and at home. A higher-level handwriting task combining integration of auditory directions and a motoric response is dictation.
- Composition is the generation of a sentence or paragraph by the child demonstrated by writing a poem, a story, or a note to a friend. The composing process uses the cognitive functions of planning, sentence generation, and revision and requires complex integration of linguistic, cognitive, organizational, and sensorimotor skills.

Legibility

Legibility is often assessed in terms of its components—letter formation, alignment, spacing, size, and slant.[5] However, the bottom line of legibility is readability. Of primary importance is whether what was written by the child can be read by the child, parent, or teacher. Letter formation may be the most critical element to determine legibility.[53] Five features affecting legibility include: (1) improper letterforms, (2) poor leading in and leading out of letters, (3) inadequate rounding of letters, (4) incomplete closures of letters, and (5) incorrect letter ascenders and descenders.[1] *Alignment*, or baseline orientation, refers to the placement of text on and within the writing guidelines. *Spacing* includes the dispersion of letters within words and words within sentences[69] and text organization on the entire sheet of paper. Another component of legibility, *size*, refers to the letter relative to the writing guidelines and to the other letters. Finally, the uniformity or consistency of the *slant* or the angle of the text should be observed. Figure 18-5 illustrates errors of letter formation and size in a child's cursive writing. Typically, legibility is determined by counting the number of readable written letters or words and dividing it by the total number of written letters or words in a writing sample. Therefore if a child produces 20 legible letters when writing the lowercase alphabet, his percentage legibility is 77% (20/26). Experts suggest "cut-off" legibility percentages for poor and good handwriting. Occupational therapy practitioners often use the range of 75% to 78% to discriminate between satisfactory and unsatisfactory handwriting legibility. Students who score above 75% on the Evaluation Tool of Children's Handwriting tend to achieve satisfactory handwriting grades and those below 75% tend to receive unsatisfactory grades.[67] In a large study of 900 students, legibility scores were found to be consistent across grades one through four, improve between fourth and sixth grade, and to maintain in middle school.[49]

Determining appropriate educational and therapeutic services for children requires assessment beyond legibility scores and involves an entire team, including the child's parents. Thus, the occupational therapist must carefully and comprehensively assess the nature of the child's handwriting problems and give recommendations based on this process.

Writing Speed

In addition to legibility, a child's rate of writing, or the number of letters written per minute, is a cornerstone of functional handwriting. Students may take longer to complete written assignments, have difficulty taking notes in class,[46] lose their train of ideas for writing,[74] and become frustrated when their handwriting speed is slower than that of their peers. Writing speed typically decreases when the amount of written work or complexity of the writing task increases.[119] Upper elementary and older students need not only an adequate writing speed, but also the ability to adjust their speed from a hurried, rough draft to a neat, well-paced final one.[119]

Studies of handwriting speed in elementary age students show that handwriting speed increases gradually, becoming faster in each succeeding grade.[49,55,90,124] However, the studies' findings also suggest that the increase in speed may not be linear but marked by various spurts and plateaus. Handwriting speed per grade level has been found to be highly variable when different study designs and writing conditions are used.

Because of the wide range of handwriting speeds, children's writing rates need to be considered individually within the context of their classroom. Teacher expectations and classroom standards may influence children's writing speeds. Thus, it is appropriate to compare a student's writing speed performance with the rates of classroom peers. In general, handwriting speed is problematic when a student is unable to complete written school assignments in a timely manner.

Ergonomic Factors

Ergonomic and environmental factors influence handwriting performance, and therefore the biomechanics of writing posture, upper extremity stability and mobility, and pencil grip are analyzed as the child writes. The therapist observes the student's typical sitting posture when writing. Does the child rest his or her head on the forearm or desktop when writing? Is the child falling out of or slumping in his or her chair? Does

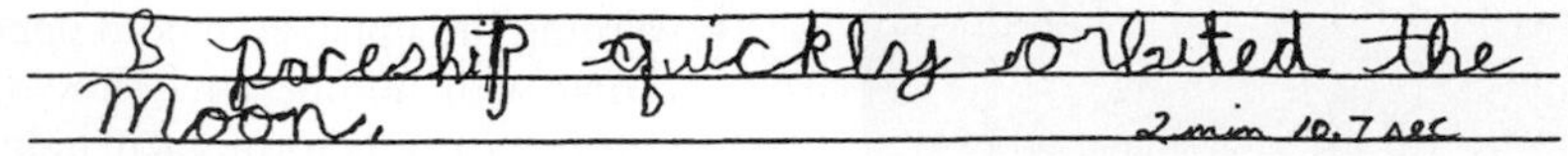

FIGURE 18-5 Cursive handwriting sample exemplifies improper letterforms and disproportionate letter size.

the child stand beside the desk or kneel in the chair? Are the desktop and the chair at suitable heights?

Stability and mobility of the upper extremities (i.e., the ability to keep the shoulder girdle, elbow, and wrist stable) allow the dexterous hand to manipulate the writing instrument. Does the child write with whole-arm movements? What are the positions of the trunk and writing arm? Does the nonpreferred hand stabilize the paper? Does the child apply excessive pressure to the writing tool?

Which grasping pattern is used? Does the student use a variety of atypical grasps or mature, dynamic grasps, as defined? When biomechanical and ergonomic factors are optimal the efficiency in handwriting performance significantly improves.[98]

Handwriting Assessments

Formal or standardized tests are important for assessing the performance of children, as they provide objective measures and quantitative scores, aid in monitoring a child's progress, help professionals communicate more clearly, and advance the field through research. Assessment tools commonly used by occupational therapists in the United States are listed in Box 18-2.

Each of these assessment tools possesses various features regarding domains of handwriting tested (e.g., far-point copying, dictation), age or grade of child (e.g., first and second grades), script examined (e.g., cursive), scoring procedures of the writing performance (e.g., legibility of manuscript), and scores obtained (e.g., percentiles). Typically, tests measure handwriting legibility and speed of handwriting. Scoring procedures for legibility use rating techniques ranging from global and subjective to detailed and specific.[113] For tool selection, the occupational therapist should keep in mind the characteristics of each assessment as well as the strengths and limitations of the tests regarding normative data, reliability, validity, and other psychometric properties (see Chapter 7). Because scoring legibility always has a subjective element, most legibility assessments have low inter-rater reliability.[34] The assessment chosen should provide information about child's handwriting concerns, analyze handwriting performance, and allow for effective intervention planning among the occupational therapist, the child's parents, and other team members.

Interplay of Factors Restricting Handwriting Performance

To understand more fully which element may be interfering with a child's ability to produce text, the occupational therapist considers a child's *performance skills*, *client factors*, *performance patterns*, and *contextual elements*.[3] The example in Case Study 18-1 illustrates how various factors may restrict a child's handwriting performance. This example illustrates the complex interactions that determine which factors influence a child's ability to engage in an occupation such as handwriting.

Like Natasha, children with poor handwriting typically have a web of factors that restrict their handwriting performance. For example, Natasha's client factors (i.e., short attention span,

BOX 18-2 Handwriting Assessments

Evaluation Tool of Children's Handwriting (ETCH)
Description: Criterion-referenced test measuring a child's legibility and speed of children's handwriting in grades 1 through 6. Domains (manuscript or cursive) include alphabet writing of lowercase and uppercase letters, numeral writing, near-point copying, far-point copying, manuscript-to-cursive transition, dictation, and sentence composition.
Author: Susan J. Amundson, MS, OT (1995)[5]
Publication: O.T. KIDS, Inc.

Here's How I Write: A Child's Self-Assessment of Handwriting and Goal-Setting Tool (HWII)
Description: Criterion-referenced tool for students in the second through fifth grade, which uses the students' own assessments of handwriting to set goals for improvement. Interviews are conducted using picture cards to assess handwriting performance, feelings about handwriting, and physical factors related to handwriting.
Authors: Sarina Goldstand, Debbie Gavir, Sharon A. Cermack, and Julie Bissell (2013)[44]
Publication: Therapro Inc., www.therapro.com

Minnesota Handwriting Assessment (MHA)
Description: Norm-referenced test that looks at quality and speed of manuscript handwriting of a near-point copying task. Models are in Zaner-Blöser or D'Nealian script for children in grades 1 and 2.
Author: Judith Reisman, PhD, OT (1999)[95]
Publication: Therapy Skill Builders/ Psychological Corporation

Shore Handwriting Screening for Early Handwriting Development
Description: Screening tool that examines handwriting skills for students from ages 3 to 7 by assessing postural control, head control, letter and number formation, and environmental factors.
Author: Leann Shore (2003)[105]
Publication: Pearson Shorehandwriting.com

Test of Handwriting Skills
Description: Norm-referenced test that examines both manuscript and cursive handwriting through dictation, near-point copying, and alphabet writing from memory. Normative data are provided for children 5-11 years old.
Author: Morrison F. Gardner (1998)[41]
Publication: Psychological and Educational Publications, Inc.

The Print Tool
Description: The Print Tool is a complete printing assessment for students age 6 and older. The Print Tool assesses capitals, numbers, and lowercase letter skills. The skills evaluated include memory, orientation, placement, size, start, sequence, control, and spacing.
Authors: Jan Z. Olsen, OTR and Emily F. Knapton, OTR/L (2006)[87]
Publication: Handwriting Without Tears, www.hwtears.com

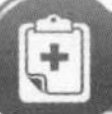

CASE STUDY 18-1 Natasha

Natasha, a 9-year-old girl with a traumatic brain injury, has an illegible script marked by overlapping letters, poor use of writing lines, and many dark erasures. When evaluating Natasha's writing performance in her classroom, the occupational therapist observes that her performance skills, particularly her fine motor coordination, are limited. In-hand manipulation skills are poor as Natasha struggles to turn her pencil from the writing position to the erasing position, manage her worksheet, and use her eraser for correcting errors. When she engages in classroom activities, the occupational therapist observes that Natasha demonstrates a short attention span and impulsiveness. Natasha has difficulty sustaining her attention to desktop work and the teacher's verbal instructions. Furthermore when the occupational therapist examines a story that Natasha wrote earlier during the day, it is apparent that she has not incorporated the habit of writing her text on the lines of the paper. Because she does not adopt this performance pattern, Natasha's text bumps above and below the writing baseline on her paper, resulting in an unreadable story. Finally, the occupational therapist is told by a classroom paraprofessional that Natasha uses English as a second language because of her recent emigration to the United States. Consequently the occupational therapy practitioner recognizes that her cultural context may be affecting her overall performance in the classroom.

impulsiveness) and cultural context (i.e., English as a second language) interact with one another to restrict her handwriting performance. Natasha's short attention span diminishes not only her ability to learn handwriting, but also her ability to learn new concepts, including her second language, English. Because she has limited understanding of language symbols, words, and syntax of the English language, she has difficulty reading English. Furthermore, because reading and writing are parallel learning processes, it is probable that Natasha's handwriting is limited. Natasha's handwriting is more likely to improve once effective compensatory and remedial techniques are in place to improve her attention span and her knowledge and use of the English language.

Educator's Perspective

State standards for written language and literacy, as well as the district curriculum, should be used to guide evaluation and intervention. When educators speak of the writing or composing process, they view it as a goal-directed activity using the cognitive functions of planning, sentence generation, and revision. The actual text production occurs in sentence generation; thus, the child who needs to pay considerable attention to the mechanical requirements of writing may interrupt higher-order writing processes, such as planning or content generation. Hence, most educators view the mechanical requirements of handwriting as an integral subset of the writing process.

Handwriting Instruction Methods and Curricula

During the past decade, an educational debate has focused on teaching handwriting systematically through commercially prepared or teacher-developed programs, or learning it through a "whole-language" approach. The whole-language philosophy purports that both the substance (meaning) of writing and the form (mechanics) of writing are critical for learning to write.[46] Thus, when using the whole-language method as children are learning and mastering handwriting, the teacher gives advice and assigns practice on an individual, as-needed basis. For example, if an educator sees a first-grader struggling to form the letter *m* while writing a story about monsters, he or she may instruct the child regarding the correct letter formation of *m* and encourage extra practice of the letter during the story composition period. Conversely, in a traditional handwriting instruction approach, students are introduced to letter formations and practice them outside the context of writing. For children with learning disabilities and mild neurologic impairments, regular practice in forming letters is essential in the early stages of handwriting development, yet handwriting should have a meaningful context. Thus, a combination of systematic handwriting instruction and whole-language methods may be most beneficial to this group of children.[46]

In the United States, traditional handwriting instruction programs vary among school districts, schools, and grades. It is not uncommon for occupational therapy practitioners to receive a referral for a child with poor handwriting who has never had handwriting instruction! See Table 18-1e on the Evolve website for evidence on classroom instruction.

The most common instruction methods include Palmer, Zaner-Blöser, Italics, and D'Nealian. Unlike the United States, a few countries, such as the United Kingdom, New Zealand, and Australia,[1,63,124] have adopted national curricula for handwriting to improve the standards of handwriting assessment and instruction within their school systems (see Table 18-2e on the Evolve website for handwriting curricula). Early childhood handwriting curricula should include at least six skill areas: (1) small muscle development, (2) eye-hand coordination, (3) holding a writing tool, (4) basic strokes, (5) letter perception, and (6) orientation to printed language. See Table 18-3 for research on handwriting programs. What appears to be important is the implementation of a formal curriculum that allows for ongoing handwriting instruction and practice. Hoy et al.,[61] in an extensive literature review, supported that effective handwriting interventions require 20 or more instructional sessions.

Several handwriting programs have been developed by occupational therapists, which include the Write Start program, Handwriting Without Tears, and Loops and Other Groups.[13] Write Start is a classroom-embedded, co-taught handwriting program for first grade children that can be implemented with high fidelity by a trained occupational therapists and teachers (see Case Study 18-2). This program links handwriting and writing, emphasizes frequent feedback to students, and encourages self-evaluation and self-regulation. Using a small group format for practicing handwriting and writing, the teacher and

TABLE 18-2 Activities to Promote Handwriting Readiness

Areas of Handwriting Readiness	Selected Readiness Activities
Improving fine motor control and isolated finger movements	Roll one-fourth– to one-eighth–inch balls of clay or Silly Putty between the tips of thumb and the index and middle fingers. Pick up small objects (e.g., Cheerios or raisins) with a tweezers. Pinch and seal a Ziploc bag using the thumb opposing each finger. Twist open a small tube of toothpaste with the thumb and index and middle fingers. Move a key from the palm to the fingertips of one hand.
Promoting graphic skills	Draw lines and copy shapes using shaving cream, sand trays, or finger paints. Draw lines and shapes to complete a picture story on blackboards. Form and color pictures of people, houses, trees, cars, or animals. Complete simple dot-to-dot pictures and mazes.
Enhancing right-left discrimination	Connect dots at the chalkboard with left-to-right strokes.
Improving orientation to printed language	Label children's drawings based on the child's description. Encourage book-making with child's favorite topics (e.g., special places, favorite foods). Label common objects in the classroom.

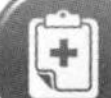

CASE STUDY 18-2 Write Start Handwriting/Writing Program for First Grade Students

Write Start is a classroom-embedded handwriting and writing program that is co-taught by the first grade teacher, an assistant, and an occupational therapist. This team plans and implements 24 sessions (12 weeks) in the first half of the first grade year. All students, with and without individualized educational programs (IEPs), are included. The program incorporates evidence-based instruction, small group activities to promote practice and learning of handwriting, and individualized interventions for students with handwriting difficulties. The sessions follow the following format:

Session One

- The therapist teaches two to three lowercase letters, modeling and using consistent verbal cues (e.g., basement letters, tallies and smallics)
- The students practice the letters on small white-boards.
- The students work in small groups (six to eight students) on handwriting-related activities that reinforce skills (e.g., motor planning, visual motor integration)

Session Two

- The therapist leads a review of the letters learned in session one.
- The students complete a writing sample to evaluate their progress.
- The teacher leads a writing workshop (based on the first grade writing curriculum) with all students participating.
- Students write stories to practice their best handwriting and "publish" their stories.

The interventions emphasized in this co-taught program are:

1. Students practice handwriting and writing with intense repetition.
2. Using the small group format, the teachers and therapist provide immediate and specific feedback to students.
3. The teachers and therapist encourage students' self-evaluation.
4. The teachers and therapist encourage and facilitate peer evaluation, peer modeling, and peer supports during the handwriting activities.
5. Each session is based on evaluation of individual and group progress in handwriting and writing (from the weekly writing sample and writing workshop products).

The goals of the Write Start program are to prevent handwriting problems, promote students' interest in writing, help students understand that legible handwriting enables others to read their stories, and provide inclusive services to students who need additional supports to achieve legible handwriting.

See Case-Smith, J., White, S., & Holland, T. (2014). Effectiveness of a co-taught handwriting program for first grade students. *Physical and Occupational Therapy in Pediatrics, 34*, 30–43.

occupational therapist encourage peer support and peer evaluation of handwriting.[26] Students who participated in the 12-week program made highly significant gains in handwriting legibility and speed and writing fluency.[25,27] Handwriting Without Tears (HWT), developed by an occupational therapist for multiple grade levels, is a full curriculum for developing prewriting and writing skills. This program emphasizes multisensory activities presented in developmentally appropriate sequences.[88] The HWT pre-K program for preschool children promotes prewriting skills by incorporating playing and singing. The activities are designed to enhance sensorimotor skills, social and emotional development, body awareness skills, cognitive and language skills, and visual-perceptual skills that are foundations for handwriting.[88] Lust and Donica[71] found that supplementing the Head Start Curriculum with HWT Pre-K significantly improves handwriting readiness. See Table 18-2 for activities to promote handwriting readiness.

Text continued on p. 513

TABLE 18-3 Handwriting Programs Research

Author(s)	Age/Grade and No. of Children	Program(s)/Frameworks Used	Time	Measures	Effectiveness
Benson, Salls, & Perry (2010)[15]	6 first grade teachers	Handwriting Without Tears (HWT) (used by 3 teachers) Peterson Directed Method (previously used by all 6 teachers; currently used by only 3)	2007-2008 school year	Quarterly journals regarding teachers' experiences and thoughts about curriculum, students' engagement, and garner perceptions were completed by each participant.	Teachers reported that both programs were effective and easy to use but felt each method failed to fully meet their needs and expectations. Less satisfaction was reported with the Peterson method than HWT. Teachers using the Peterson method felt that they had to make more adaptations to the program than those using HWT.
Berninger, Vaughan, Abbott, Rogan, Brooks, Reed, & Graham (1997)[16]	144 first graders	Handwriting styles used: D'Nealian or standard ball and stick Treatment Groups: 1. Motor imitation 2. Visual cue 3. Memory retrieval 4. Visual cue + memory retrieval 5. Copy 6. Control group Rosner's Auditory Analysis Program	Twice a week in 20-min sessions for 24 lessons	Timed measures of handwriting; 6 finger function tasks; 3 timed handwriting tasks; 3 other tasks; Writing Fluency subtest of the Woodcock-Johnson Psycho-educational Battery-Revised; Vocabulary subtest of the Wechsler Intelligence Scale for Children-3rd ed.; Word Attack subtest of the revised Woodcock Reading Mastery Test	Combining numbered arrows and memory retrieval was the most effective treatment for improving handwriting and compositional fluency.
Case-Smith, Holland, & Bishop (2011)[24]	19 first grade students	Pilot program	12 weeks	Write Start program—a co-teaching model with OT and teachers	Students made large gains in handwriting legibility (25%) that were maintained through the end of the school year.
Case-Smith, Holland, Lane, & White (2012)[25]	36 first grade students	Write Start Intervention implemented as a co-teaching model with occupational therapist and teachers.	12 weeks	Evaluation Tool of Children's Handwriting-Manuscript (ETCH-M); Woodcock-Johnson Fluency and Writing Samples subtest of Woodcock Johnson III Test of Achievement (WJIII)	Students showed highly significant improvement in legibility of lowercase letters. There was also significant improvement in speed of lowercase letters and legibility of uppercase letters. Students also made significant gains in writing fluency and written expression. Students performing lower on subtests showed greater improvement.
Case-Smith, Holland, & White (2014)[27]	67 first-grade students, 37 in Write Start classrooms, and 30 in standard classroom instruction	Write Start and standard handwriting instruction	24 45-min sessions that were implemented 2x/week for 12 weeks	Evaluation Tool of Children's Handwriting manuscript, Woodcock Johnson Fluency, and writing samples	Students in Write Start improved significantly in legibility and fluency over regular instruction. Gains in speed and written expression did not differ significantly between groups.

Donica, Coins, & Wagner (2013)[37]	58 Head Start students	Fine Motor and Early handwriting Pre-K curriculum (FMEW) HWT-Get Set for School Program	16 weeks	Shore Handwriting Screening for Early Handwriting Development	Handwriting readiness programs are a positive addition to Head Start Center Time
Delegato, McLaughlin, Derby, & Schuster (2013)[31]	5 preschool students	HWT Program with and without a teacher-made handwriting racetrack	6 weeks	Worksheets scored 0-10	Performance was higher when HWT and racetrack were used than HWT alone.
Graham & Harris (2006)[50]	30 first-grade students (15 were chosen for program)	CASL First Grade Handwriting/ Spelling Program described in article	48 20-min lessons divided into 8 units, with 6 lessons in each unit	Not specified	Students who participated in program made greater gains in spelling, handwriting legibility and fluency, sentence writing, and vocabulary diversity in their compositions immediately after instruction
Howe, Roston, Sheu, & Hinojosa (2013)[60]	72 public school elementary students in first and second grade	Examine effectiveness of two approaches: intensive HW practice and visual-perceptual-motor activities	12 weeks	Handwriting club on HW speed, legibility, and visual-motor skills	Students in the intensive handwriting practice group demonstrated significant improvements in handwriting legibility compared with the visual-perceptual motor group
Lust & Donica (2011)[71]	Preschool students ages 4-5 in one of two rural Head Start classes	HWT-Get Set for School (HWT-GSS) (intervention group) Standard Head Start curriculum (control group)	Three times a week, for 20 min, from October to March (total of 47 sessions)	Pre Writing Domain of the Learning Accomplishment Profile, 3rd ed. (LAP-3); Check Readiness; Bruininks-Oseretsky Test of Motor Proficiency, 2nd ed. (BOT-2)	Improvements in scores for both groups on all measures. Significantly higher levels of improvement in these skills among students in the intervention group.
Keller (2001)[65]	Third- and fourth-grade boys	HWT; use of many sensory integration activities including the program How Does Your Engine Run?	Twice a week for 30-min sessions (reported as not being long enough)	Not specified	Students improved cursive writing skills and social skills. They learned which sensory activities helped them to focus and self-regulate. Students felt more confident in handwriting abilities.
Mackay, McCluskey, & Mayes (2010)[72]	32 children in Australia; ages 6-8 (first and second grade); received a score of 30 or less on the Minnesota Handwriting Assessment (MHA)	Long Handwriting Program (LHP), which utilizes task-specific training	8 weekly sessions, lasting 45 min, conducted in groups of two or three	Minnesota Handwriting Assessment	Evidence that the approach is clinically worthwhile based on statistically significant improvements in legibility, form, alignment, size, and space. No improvements in speed.

Continued

TABLE 18-3 Handwriting Programs Research—cont'd

Author(s)	Age/Grade and No. of Children	Program(s)/Frameworks Used	Time	Measures	Effectiveness
Marr & Dimeo (2006)[74]	26 students ages 6.2-11.9 Grades 1-6	HWT	1 hour per day for 2 weeks	Evaluation Tool of Children's Handwriting (ETCH); Likert ratings provided by parents pretest, posttest, and 3 months posttest	Significant changes in legibility of writing the uppercase and lowercase alphabets. Improvements in two subtests of ETCH and in parent ratings.
McGarrigle & Nelson (2006)[76]	16 first-grade students (13 completed end-program testing)	Interventions developed by third-year occupational therapy students. Frameworks used: sensorimotor, biomechanical, teaching-learning principles, and principles of practice when working with indigenous children.	80-min sessions once a week for 6 weeks	Beery-Buktenica Developmental Test of Visual-Motor Integration (VMI); Conners' Abbreviated Symptom Questionnaire (ASQ); non-standardized handwriting measures; non-standardized scissor skills measure	Significant improvements in sitting posture, pencil grasp, pencil pressure, and paper stabilization/positioning. Students improved their tracing and copying accuracy and letter inclusion, legibility, and formation when writing their names and letters of the alphabet. Improved in aspects of handwriting, scissor skills, and behavior.
Peterson & Nelson (2003)[89]	59 first graders (30 selected for intervention group) Students' mean age: 7.1 yr	D'Nealian handwriting; frameworks: biomechanical, sensorimotor, and teaching-learning principles	30-min sessions, twice a week, for 10 week	Minnesota Handwriting Test	Intervention group demonstrated a significant increase in scores on the posttest of the Minnesota Handwriting Test when compared with scores of the control group.
Ratzon, Efraim, & Bart (2007)[94]	52 first-grade students (24 participants in intervention group)	Graphomotor intervention program developed by Efraim (2002) Activities and tools based on Benbow's recommendations. Frameworks: motor learning, multisensory, and research that found associations between dexterity skills and normal development of visual-motor proficiency	12 sessions, once a week, for 45 min	Beery-Buktenica Developmental Test of Visual-Motor Integration (VMI); Developmental Test of Visual Perception (DTVP-2); Motor Development Scale of the Bruiniks-Oseretsky Test of Motor Proficiency	Students in intervention group made significant gains in the total score on the graphomotor test (DTVP-2) and on the fine motor test (Bruininks-Oseretsky Motor Development Scale)
Roberts, Siever, & Mair (2010)[96]	72 fourth to sixth grade students identified by teachers as having handwriting difficulties	Remediation group based on the Loops and Other Groups Program provided by occupational therapist in small groups after school	60-min sessions, once a week, for 7 weeks	Copying a Phrase; Handwriting subtest of the Test of Written Language; Alphabet Samples; Test of Writing Language (TOWL) Handwriting subtest, Handwriting Evaluation Scale (HES), Speed of copying task, Development of the Attitude Scale to measure satisfaction, Parent/Teacher Report	Improvements in scores on the TOWL that were not found to be related to grade, gender, or amount of homework. Improvements in HES for connected alphabet and all areas except size in unconnected alphabet. Increases in speed and personal satisfaction scores. Improvements more substantial for copying than composition.

Salls, Benson, Hansen, Cole, & Pielielek (2013)[100]	31 typically developing first grade children	Compared the effects of HWT and Peterson Directed Handwriting Curriculum	9-month school year	Print Tool, VMI, Minnesota Handwriting Assessment	Implementation of a structured curriculum may be key to developing good handwriting skills
Shimel, Candler, & Neville-Smith (2009)[105]	50 third grade students without identified handwriting problems	Compared the effects of cursive handwriting programs in improving letter legibility and form	10-15 min per day for 6 weeks	A shift in instruction using either HWT, Loops and Other Groups, or a control (continued use of Zaner-Blöser)	All improved with no significant differences between groups—a shift in handwriting instruction method did not interfere with learning
Taras, Brennan, Gilbert, & Reed (2011)[109]	211 students in 14 kindergarten classes from 12 schools in San Diego (participating in program) 171 students from similar classes (not participating in program)	Write Direction handwriting skill development program used for treatment group	30-min lessons, once a week for 14 weeks	Routine district-level functional measurement tool which included: • Legibility • Formation • Line approximation • Line orientation • Proportion • Directionality and reversals • Spacing	Statistically significant improvement in letter tasks (approximation, line orientation, proportion, and directionality) and sentence tasks (line orientation and proportion) for those participating in the Write Direction program
Weintraub, Yinon, Hirsch, & Parush (2009)[121]	55 second to fourth grade students in Israel, with handwriting difficulties (scored 1 SD below the mean on the Brief Assessment Tool for Handwriting [BATH])	Sensorimotor intervention: • Focused on lower and higher level functions • Preparatory activities focused on motor based skills • Letters taught using multisensory techniques Task-oriented intervention: • Focused on higher level functions • Direct practice and feedback • Focused on writing words and sentences Nontreatment control group	Programs offered in altering order, four times a year for 2 years. Each program consisted of 8 weekly 1-hour sessions.	BATH; Motor Accuracy Test (MAC) subset of SIPT; Developmental Test of Visual Perception-2 (VTVP-2); Balance and Upper-Limb subtests of Bruninks-Oseretsky; Test of Motor Proficiency; Pediatric Examination of Educational Readiness at Middle Childhood; HHE as outcome measure	Control group did not show significant improvements. Both groups found to significantly improve legibility and formation. Long-term measures (4 months after intervention) found significantly higher scores for task-oriented group than sensorimotor group only with spatial organization.

Continued

TABLE 18-3 Handwriting Programs Research—cont'd

Author(s)	Age/Grade and No. of Children	Program(s)/Frameworks Used	Time	Measures	Effectiveness
Zwicker & Hadwin (2009)[124]	72 first and second grade students referred to occupational therapist for handwriting	Random assignment to one of the following groups: Cognitive Intervention Group: • Naming letters • Modeling letters • Tracing letters • Discussion to compare letters • Practice • Evaluation Multisensory Intervention Group: • Naming letters with demonstration • Copying letters from board • Skywriting sand-tray • Traced over textured letters • Traced/copied on worksheet • Traced on regular Paper Control group: No intervention	30-min groups, once a week for 10 weeks	Beery-Buktenica Developmental Test of Visual-Motor Integration (VMI) used for inclusion/exclusion criteria Evaluation Tool of Children's Handwriting (ETCH) used for pre/post-test measures	More positive results to cognitive intervention noted through secondary analysis. Handwriting improvements found in all three groups for first grade students. No uniform improvement. Second graders showed greater improvement with cognitive intervention than sensory intervention.

Benson, J. D., Salls, J., & Perry, C. (2010). A pilot study of teachers' perceptions of two handwriting curricula: Handwriting Without Tears and The Peterson Directed Handwriting Method. *Journal of Occupational Therapy, Schools, & Early Intervention*, *3*, 319–330; Berninger, V., Vaughan, K. B., Abbott, R. D., Abbott, S. P., Rogan, L. W., Brooks, A., et al. (1997). Treatment of handwriting problems in beginning writers: transfer from handwriting to composition. *Journal of Education Psychology*, *89*, 652–666; Case-Smith, J., Holland, T., & Bishop, B. (2011). Effectiveness of an integrated handwriting program for first-grade students. *American Journal of Occupational Therapy*, *65*, 670–678; Case-Smith, J., Holland, T., Lane, A., & White, S. (2012). Effect of a coteaching handwriting program for first graders: one-group pretest-posttest design. *The American Journal of Occupational Therapy*, *66*, 396–405; Case-Smith, J., Holland, T., & White, S. (2014). Effectiveness of a Co-Taught Handwriting Program For First Grade Students. *34*(1), 30–43; Delegato, C., McLaughlin, K., Derby, M., & Schuster, L. (2013). The effects of using handwriting without tears and a handwriting racetrack to teach five preschool students with disabilities pre-handwriting and handwriting. *Journal of Occupational Therapy, Schools, & Early Intervention*, *6*, 255–268; Donica, D.K., Goins, A., & Wagner, L. (2013). Effectiveness of handwriting readiness programs on postural control, hand control, and letter and number formation in head start classrooms. Journal of Occupational Therapy Schools & Early Intervention, *6*(2), 81–93. doi:10.1080/19411243.2013-810938; Graham, S., & Harris, K. R. (2006). Preventing writing difficulties: providing additional handwriting and spelling instruction to at-risk children in first grade. *TEACHING Exceptional Children*, *38*, 64–66; Howe, T.-H., Roston, K. L., Sheu, C.-F., & Hinojosa, J. (2013). Assessing handwriting intervention effectiveness in elementary school students: a two-group controlled study. *American Journal of Occupational Therapy*, *67*, 19–27; Lust, C. A., & Donica. D. K. (2011). Effectiveness of handwriting readiness program in Head Start: a two-group controlled trial, *American Journal of Occupational Therapy*, *65*, 560–568; Keller, M. (2001). Handwriting club: using sensory integration strategies to improve handwriting. *Intervention in School and Clinic*, *37*, 9–12; Mackay, N., McCluskey, A., & Mayes, R. (2010). The Log Handwriting Program improved children's writing legibility: a pretest–posttest study. *American Journal of Occupational Therapy*, *64*, 30–36; Marr, D., & Dimeo, S. B. (2006). Outcomes associated with a summer handwriting course for elementary students. *American Journal of Occupational Therapy*, *60*, 10–15; McGarrigle, J., & Nelson, A. (2006). Evaluating a school skills programme for Australian Indigenous children: a pilot study. *Occupational Therapy International*, *13*, 1–20; Peterson, C. Q., & Nelson, D. L. (2003). Effect of an occupational intervention on children with economic disadvantages. *American Journal of Occupational Therapy*, *57*, 152–160; Raton, N. Z., Efraim, D., & Bart, O. (2007). A short-term graphomotor program for improving writing readiness skills of first-grade students. *American Journal of Occupational Therapy*, *61*, 399–405; Roberts, G. I., Siever, J. E., & Mair, J. A. (2010). Effects of a kinesthetic cursive handwriting intervention for grade 4–6 students. *American Journal of Occupational Therapy*, *64*, 745–755; Salls, J., Benson, J., Hansen, M., Cole, K., Pielielek, A. (2013). A comparison of the handwriting without tears program and Peterson directed handwriting program on handwriting performance in typically developing first grade students. *Journal of Occupational Therapy, Schools, & Early Intervention*, *6*, 131–142; Shimel, K., Candler, C., & Neville-Smith, M. (2009). Comparison of cursive handwriting instruction programs among students without identified problems. *Physical and Occupational Therapy in Pediatrics*, *29*, 170–181; Taras, H., Brennan, J., Gilbert, A., & Reed, H. E. (2011). Effectiveness of occupational therapy strategies for teaching handwriting skills to kindergarten children. *Occupational Therapy, Schools, & Early Intervention*, *4*, 236–246; Weintraub, N., Yinon, M., Hirsh, I. B.-E., & Parush, S. (2009). Effectiveness of sensorimotor and task-oriented handwriting intervention in elementary school-aged students with handwriting difficulties. *OTJR: Occupation, Participation, & Health*, *29*, 125–134; Zwicker, J. G., & Hadwin, A. F. (2009). Cognitive versus multisensory approach to handwriting intervention: a randomized control trial. *OTJR: Occupation, Participation, & Health*, *29*, 40–48.

Manuscript and Cursive Styles

In most elementary schools, manuscript writing is taught in grades one and two, and cursive writing is taught at the end of grade two or the beginning of grade three.[8] The need for manuscript writing may continue throughout life, when students label maps and posters, adolescents complete job or college applications, and adults complete federal income tax forms. By middle school, many students blend manuscript and cursive to form their own style of handwriting. To date, no research has decisively indicated the superiority of one script style over the other.

Both manuscript and cursive possess complementary features, and these should be considered when the occupational therapist, child, child's parent, and educational team are collaboratively deciding which style might best serve the child.

Manuscript is endorsed for the following reasons:

1. Manuscript letterforms are simpler, easier to visually discriminate, and hence easier to learn.
2. It closely resembles the print of textbooks and school manuals.
3. It is needed throughout adult life for documents and applications.
4. It is more readable than cursive.
5. The traditional vertical alphabet is more developmentally appropriate, easier to read, and easier to write for young children, as well as easier for educators to teach, than the slanted alphabet.

Advocates of cursive writing point out the following:

1. Cursive movement patterns allow for faster and more automatic writing.
2. Reversal of individual letters and transpositions of words are more difficult than in manuscript.
3. One continuous, connected line enables child to form words as units.

Handwriting Intervention

In school settings, if the referred student's educational team decides that functional written communication is a priority for the student's individualized educational program (IEP), the occupational therapist may be instrumental in directing and guiding this aspect of the program. Typically, the team uses either a remedial or a compensatory intervention approach, or both, to improve the child's written communication. Compensatory strategies improve a student's participation in school with accommodations, adaptations, and modifications for certain tasks, routines, and settings,[6,66,107] whereas remedial approaches improve or establish a student's functional skills in a specific area.

When the team focuses on the occupation of written communication, generally both remedial and compensatory techniques are concurrently used. For example, Hunter, a second-grader, has manuscript handwriting that is unreadable; about 60% of his written letters are not legible; and his writing speed is at the bottom of his class. Although he participates in an intensive handwriting remediation program, he needs accommodations and strategies that help him achieve functional written communication in the classroom. Consequently his teacher decided to adjust the time required to complete assignments, allow him to use oral reporting for certain class assignments, or require a lower volume of work to be accomplished than that of his peers. The teacher and the occupational therapist select specific techniques to assist him with legibility, such as spacing between words, sizing letters, and placing text on lines. Readiness activities that are easy to incorporate into the classroom can be embedded in his daily routine. Providing varied and interesting writing materials in the classroom and home allow the opportunity to embed meaningful writing experiences into activities.[85]

When a child's handwriting is both illegible and slow, team members may occasionally decide to incorporate assistive technology, such as a computer, tablet, or portable word processor. E-mail and texting are increasingly important methods for personal communication.[42] The student and the team, particularly the occupational therapy practitioner, must work to find a technologic system that allows the student proficiency in text generation.[106] As in handwriting, computer use requires adequate attention, motor control, sensory processing, visual functioning, and self-regulation from the student. Small studies show that word processing with word prediction can improve the legibility and spelling of written assignments.[56] However, the computer is not a magical tool but one that allows the child to acquire keyboarding and word processing skills through planning, routine instruction, and practice. In this age of technology, it is important for all students to develop keyboarding skills for computer use in the classroom, workplace, and home. However, handwriting skills continue to be needed throughout student and adult life. Table 18-4 lists the assistive technology features and the potential benefits of word processing for the student who struggles with handwriting. Table 18-3e on the Evolve website lists forums that occupational therapists can access to learn about specific applications and programs.

Models of Practice to Guide Collaborative Service Delivery

Models of practice and strategies used by occupational therapists may be unfamiliar to children, educators, parents, and other school personnel. Therefore the occupational therapist must be able (1) to clearly articulate intervention techniques, activity modifications, and classroom accommodations being used; (2) to collaborate with the teacher and others to provide service in the least restrictive environment; (3) to implement therapeutic strategies for improving written communication; (4) to train others to work with children with handwriting problems; and (5) to closely monitor the progress of the child and change aspects of the program to continue improvement.

The overall focus of the educational program is the improvement of student performance in a particular area (e.g., written communication). Occupational therapy models of practice that guide services to improve handwriting include (1) acquisitional/motor learning, (2) sensorimotor, (3) biomechanical, (4) cognitive, and (5) psychosocial. Surveys of occupational therapists in the United States[121] and Canada[40] indicate that the most frequently applied theoretical approaches to children's handwriting intervention are multisensory (92%, United States) and sensorimotor (90%, Canada). However, occupational therapists most often combine various theoretical approaches for handwriting intervention,[40] and this use of multiple approaches is advocated in the pediatric occupational

TABLE 18-4 Assistive Technology to Support Handwriting Skills

Assistive Technology	Description
Text to speech	Speaks as the student types letters, words, and sentences. Speaks if text is selected and text-to-speech is then activated. May highlight word and/or sentence as it speaks. Voice (e.g., male/female) can be selected as well as speed of speech.
Electronic spell check	Provides immediate feedback about what has been typed and allows opportunities for self-correction. Spell check after production of writing. In-line spell check with visual supports. In-line spell check with visual and auditory cues. Phonetic spell check. Talking spelling suggestions for misspelled words.
Picture-supported text or picture library	Pictures appear as the students type words for building a sentence or story with pictures only. Pictures can be sized and location can often be selected (above or below text). Some programs will allow a choice of picture libraries used with the text including GIFs (animated pictures). Picture-supported text often has text-to-speech feature.
Abbreviated expansion	Freestanding or embedded software that allows users to create their own shortened abbreviations for commonly used words or phrases. The abbreviation is often expanded by using a modifier key after the abbreviation is typed into the document. The purpose of abbreviation expansion is to reduce the number of keystrokes needed to create a typed document.
Word prediction	Software-embedded word prediction. Independent word prediction. Frequency-weighting word prediction. Grammatically based word prediction (use of syntactic rules). Phonetic word prediction. Content-specific word prediction (e.g., custom dictionaries, extraction of text from digital reading materials). Adjustable number of word prediction choices displayed. Auditory preview of words predicted before selection. In-line versus stationary word prediction. Picture-supported word prediction.
Electronic word and sentence banks	When selected, pictures, words, or sentences contained in a cell/button can be placed in a word processing document. Cells/buttons can be combined together to create a grid/toolbar. Cells/buttons/toolbars/grids can be linked so they can be dynamically displayed onscreen at different times. Cells/buttons/toolbars/grids can be scanned so that switch users can have alternate access for writing activities. Some programs will allow "drag and drop" features of words within the word processor so that cells/buttons/grids/toolbars are not needed.
Voice recognition software	The user speaks into a microphone and the words are converted by the computer into text. Users must "train" and "correct" the system for their unique speaking style. Training and correction can be time consuming, but has improved in the last 5 years. Users need to be able to remember specific commands to direct the computer. Environmental noise can be an issue for reliable detection of text. It is a hands-free text entry system.

therapy literature.[23,89] Current research suggests that motor learning approaches using task-oriented interventions appear to have efficacy.[27,121]

The occupational therapist must be skillful in the use of one or several models of practice concurrently and in teaching others to implement strategies originating from these models of practice. By remaining focused on the child's occupational outcome related to writing and applying various models of practice in the child's educational program, the occupational therapy practitioner can provide appropriate opportunities for the child to learn and master the skill of written communication. A systematic review of handwriting interventions that are considered within the domain of occupational therapy practice concluded that handwriting intervention is effective only if it includes handwriting instruction and practice.[61] Further research to identify effective components of handwriting instruction and efficient means of delivering sufficiently intensive intervention is warranted. Table 18-3 describes the evidence for handwriting intervention effectiveness.

Acquisitional and Motor Learning Approaches

Handwriting may be viewed as a complex motor skill that "can be improved through practice, repetition, feedback, and reinforcement" (p. 70).[59] Researchers have demonstrated that children develop functional handwriting skills when direct handwriting instruction is (1) individualized to the child, (2) planned and changed based on evaluation and performance data, and (3) overlearned and used in a meaningful manner by the child. When therapists and educators employ these conditions in a positive, interesting, and dynamic learning environment, children are more likely to become efficient, legible writers.[8] Therapeutic practice was more effective at improving handwriting performance than sensorimotor-based intervention.[33]

For occupational therapy practitioners, motor learning theories apply to handwriting instruction. Learning a new motor skill has been described as progressing through three phases: cognitive, associative, and autonomous. First, in the *cognitive phase*, the child is attempting to understand the demands of the handwriting task and develop a cognitive strategy for performing the necessary motor movements. Visual control of fine motor movements is thought to be important at this phase. A child learning handwriting in this phase may have developed strategies for writing some of the easier manuscript letters, such as *o*, *l*, or *t*, but may have more difficulty writing complicated letters, such as *b*, *q*, or *g*.

In the *associative phase*, the child has learned the fundamentals of performing handwriting and continues to adjust and refine the skill. Proprioceptive and kinesthetic feedback becomes increasingly important during this phase, whereas reliance on visual cues declines. For example, in the associative phase a child may have mastered the formation of letters but is engaged in improving the handwriting product by learning to space words correctly, to write letters within guidelines, or to maintain consistent letter slant. Children continue to need practice, instructional guidance, and self-monitoring strategies of handwriting performance.

In the *autonomous phase*, the child can perform handwriting automatically with minimal conscious attention. Variability of performance is slight from day to day and the child is able to detect and adjust for any small errors that may occur.[100] Once the child has reached this level of handwriting, his or her attention can be expended on other higher-order elements of writing[46] or it can be saved to alleviate fatigue.[100] Repetition and practice are important elements enhancing children's handwriting skills. Students in an intensive practice group improved significantly more than students in the visual-perceptual-motor activity group.[60]

Implications and strategies for handwriting instruction and remediation evolve from reviews of handwriting studies[62] as well as motor learning theory.[72] Many handwriting intervention programs are commercially available. (See Table 19-4e on the Evolve website for brief descriptions of and ordering information for these programs and a list of Internet resources.) Each should contain a scope and sequence of letter and numeral formations along with successive instructional techniques. To date, no empiric evidence reveals one commercial handwriting program to be more effective than another.

The scope and sequence of the handwriting intervention program should focus on a structured progression of introducing and teaching letter and numeral forms. Frequently, letters with common formational features are introduced as a family, such as the lowercase letters *e*, *i*, *t*, and *l*. After the child has mastered these letters, he or she can use them immediately to write the words *eel*, *tile*, and *little*. Whether the chosen handwriting intervention method is a commercially available or a teacher- or therapist-prepared method, each child's program should be individualized with focus on the child's specific delays. Thus, the focus of the child's program is to sequentially introduce new letters and use them with mastered letters. The therapist also guides, reinforces, and monitors the child in relearning letters formed incorrectly.[24] Combining newly acquired letters with already mastered letters allows the child to write in a meaningful context (i.e., the formation of words and sentences). This immediate reinforcement of writing words is more powerful and purposeful for the child than writing strings of letters repeatedly.[25]

Instructional approaches of handwriting intervention programs vary but tend to comprise a combination of sequential techniques including modeling, copying, stimulus fading, composing, and self-monitoring.[48,52] When acquiring new letterforms, initially the child often needs many visual and auditory cues. However, the service provider fades out the cues as soon as the child can successfully form the letter without them. Next, the child proceeds to copying letters and words from a model and then to writing letters and words from memory as they are dictated. Finally, the child advances to generating words and sentences for practice. In each phase, the child is encouraged to correct his or her own work, also known as self-monitoring. Students can identify their best letters or words, can read what they have written to identify words difficult to read, and can share their self-reflection with peers or the therapist.[27,57]

Acquiring handwriting skills and applying them in school means the educational team focuses not only on letter formation but also on the legibility and speed of the student's handwriting. In addition to correct letterforms, other components of legibility include spacing, size, slant, and alignment. Spacing between letters and words, text placement on lines, and sizing letters often need direct modeling and instruction.

Sensorimotor Interventions

The parameters for this model of practice, when applied by the occupational therapist with children with handwriting problems, include providing multisensory input through selected activities to reinforce learning. When given various meaningful sensory opportunities at a level that permits assimilation, the child's nervous system can integrate information more efficiently to produce a satisfactory motor output (e.g., legible letters in a timely manner). All sensory systems, including the proprioceptive, tactile, visual, and auditory, can be accessed and reinforced within a handwriting intervention program. For example, providing novel and interesting materials for children to practice letterforms may keep students motivated, excited, and challenged, thereby enhancing student success and learning. Children with handwriting difficulties who have experienced frustration with commonly used paper-and-pencil drills may respond more favorably to handwriting instruction using a multisensory format. Although, fundamentally, multisensory approaches provide students with more information for learning and can increase motivation, a study that compared sensorimotor interventions with therapeutic practice of handwriting found that children received handwriting practice improved more in handwriting performance.[33]

Writing tools, writing surfaces, and positions for writing are all integral parts of a sensorimotor approach. Examples of writing tools to be used are felt-tip pens (regular, overwriter, changeable-color), crayons (scented, glittered, glow-in-the-dark), paintbrushes, grease pencils or china markers, weighted pens, mechanical pencils, wooden dowels, vibratory pens, and chalk. Children's interest in and feelings about writing might

TABLE 18-5 Strategies for Handwriting Problems

Handwriting Problems	Potential Solutions
Spacing between letters	Use finger spacing with index finger. Use fingerprint spacing by pressing on an inkpad before finger spacing. Teach the "no touching rule" of letters.
Spacing between words	Use adhesive strips (e.g., Post-It Notes) as spacers between words. Make spaces with a rubber stamp. Use a dot or a dash (Morse code) between words.
Spacing on paper	Use grid paper. Write on every other line of the paper. Draw colored lines to mark (e.g., green is left, red is right).
Placing text on lines	Use pictorial schemes on writing guidelines. Provide raised writing lines as tactile cues for letter placement. Remind students that unevenly placed letters are "popcorn letters."
Sizing letters and words	Use individualized boxes for each letter. Name letters with ascending stems, no stems, and descending stems, "birds," "skunks," and "snakes," respectively.
Near-point copying	Highlight the text on the worksheet to be copied. Teach the students to copy two or three letters at a time.
Far-point copying	Enlarge print for better viewing. Start with copying from nearby vertical models. Position the student to face the chalkboard.
Dictation	Attach an alphabet strip to the desktop for the student who cannot remember letterforms. Dictated spelling words can contain several but not all letters.
Composition	Be certain that students can form letters from memory. Provide magnetic words to write short poems or stories.
Speed	Allow students to begin projects early to finish with peers. Photocopy math problems from textbook to reduce copying. Preselect volume of work to be done that may be different from that of peers.

Modified from Amundson, S. J. (1998). *TRICS for written communication: Techniques for rebuilding and improving children's school skills.* Homer, AK: O.T. KIDS.

improve when allowed to use a variety of writing tools. Writing with chalk, grease pencils, or a resistive tool also provides additional proprioceptive input to children, because more pressure for writing is required than with the traditional tools of paper and pencil. Unconventional writing tools and writing on textured surfaces can be easily incorporated into classroom assignments.

Colored lines on the paper or paper with raised lines can be helpful for the child who has difficulty knowing where to place the letters on the page. In addition, green lines drawn to symbolize *go* on the left side of the paper and red lines to symbolize *stop* on the right side may help a child know which direction to write his or her letters and words. Upright orientation of the writing surface may also lessen directional confusion of letter formation (*up* means up and *down* means down) versus orientation at a desk on a horizontal surface, where *up* means away from oneself and *down* means toward oneself.[101]

Biomechanical Approaches

Ergonomic factors such as sitting posture, paper position, pencil grasp, writing instruments, and type of paper influence handwriting quality and speed. Therapists implement compensatory strategies, including adaptive devices, procedural adaptations, and environmental modifications, to improve the interaction and fit between a child's capabilities and the demands of the handwriting task. This model emphasizes modifications to the student's context to improve handwriting and written production. Various strategies for addressing handwriting problems that combine sensorimotor, biomechanical, and compensatory approaches are listed in Table 18-5.

Sitting Posture

Although standing and lying prone may be encouraged as alternative writing positions, students continue to spend much of the school day seated at a desk. Therefore the occupational therapist should immediately address the student's seated position in the classroom. An optimal writing posture includes the student sitting with the feet planted firmly on the floor, providing support for postural shifts and adjustments.[14] The table surface should be 2 inches above the flexed elbows when the child is seated in the chair. In this position, the student can experience both symmetry and stability while performing written work. To facilitate appropriate seating for students, the occupational therapy practitioner may recommend adjusting heights of desks and chairs, providing footrests for children, adding seat cushions and inserts, or repositioning a child's desk to face the chalkboard in the classroom. Compared with standard school furniture, the use of specialty school furniture did not lead to immediate gains in printing legibility for children with cerebral palsy.[99]

Paper Position/Writing Surface

Paper should be slanted on the desktop so that it is parallel to the forearm of the writing hand when the child's forearms are resting on the desk with hands clasped.[70] This angle of the paper enables the student to see his or her written work and to avoid smearing his or her writing. Right-handed students may slant the top of their paper approximately 25 to 30 degrees to the left with the paper just right of the body's midline. Conversely, a slant of 30 to 35 degrees to the right and paper placement to the left of midline are needed for students using a left-handed tripod grasp. For the student with a left-handed "hooked" pencil grasp lacking lateral wrist movements, slanting the paper to the left is appropriate. The writing instrument should be held below the baseline, and the nonpreferred hand should hold the writing paper.

Writing on slanted surface (20- to 30-degree slant) can improve the child's pencil grasp. The slant automatically positions the hand in wrist extension and tends to angle the hand into some supination. A wrist-extended position facilitates finger flexion and grasp. In addition, the hand on a slanted surface is positioned closer to the eyes, which can facilitate the eyes' tracking of the hand's movement. Use of a vertical or semi-vertical surface can also promote more upright posture. Figure 18-6 shows an example of a slant board used in a first grade classroom.

Pencil Grip

Benbow[14] defined the ideal grasp as a dynamic tripod with an open web space. With the web space open (forming a circle), the thumb and index and middle fingers make the longest flexion, extension, and rotary excursions with a pencil during handwriting. Current researchers agree common grasp patterns include the lateral quadripod, dynamic quadripod, and lateral tripod.[32,103] Educational team members may consider encouraging a student to modify the pencil grasp when he or she (1) experiences muscular tension and fatigue, also known as writer's cramp; (2) demonstrates poor letter formation or writing speed; (3) demonstrates a tightly closed web space that limits controlled precision finger and thumb movements; or (4) holds the pencil with too much pressure or exerts too much pencil point pressure on the paper.

A variety of prosthetic devices and therapeutic strategies are available to assist the child in positioning the digits for better manipulation of the writing instrument.[6] The occupational therapist should be knowledgeable about hand functions to determine which adaptive devices and techniques are most appropriate for each individual child. Stetro grips, triangular pencils, moldable grips, and the pencil grip may facilitate tripod grasps. Writing muscle tension and fatigue may be reduced for some children by using a wide-barreled pencil. To gain more mobility of the radial digits, children may hold a small eraser against the palm with the ulnar digits, allowing for more dynamic movement of the pencil. Older children with hand hypotonicity may achieve a viable pencil grasp by holding the pencil shaft between the web space of the index and middle fingers with thumb opposition.[14] Other techniques to encourage the delicate stability-mobility balance of a functional pencil grasp include the use of external supports such as microfoam surgical tape, ring splints, and neoprene splints and should be used with a working knowledge of hand anatomy and kinesiology. A rubber band sling that encourages the student to use a slanted and relaxed pencil position for writing is shown in Figure 18-7.

In attempting to modify a grip pattern, the educational team needs to carefully consider a child's age, cooperation, and motivation along with the child's acceptance of a new grip pattern or prosthetic device before attempting to reposition the child's fingers. Modifying a grasp pattern may be more successful with younger children, and once grip positions have been established, they are very difficult to change.[14]

Writing Tools

The type of writing instruments children use in the classroom also warrants consideration. Bralecki and Rice[18] found that the diameter of a pencil does not have an effect on legibility of a child's handwriting when compared with the size of his or her hand. In general, children should be allowed to choose among a variety of writing tools; parents and teachers may help the individual child determine which writing utensil

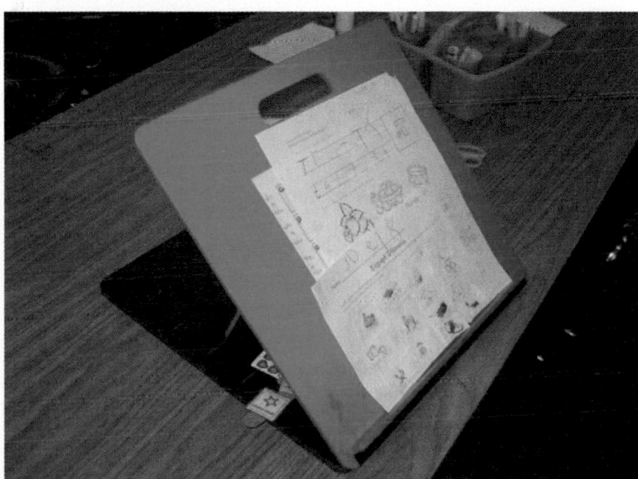

FIGURE 18-6 A slant board can be helpful when a student is first learning handwriting because it promotes wrist extension and an efficient pencil grasp. Eye-hand coordination may be easier with the hand closer to the child's eyes.

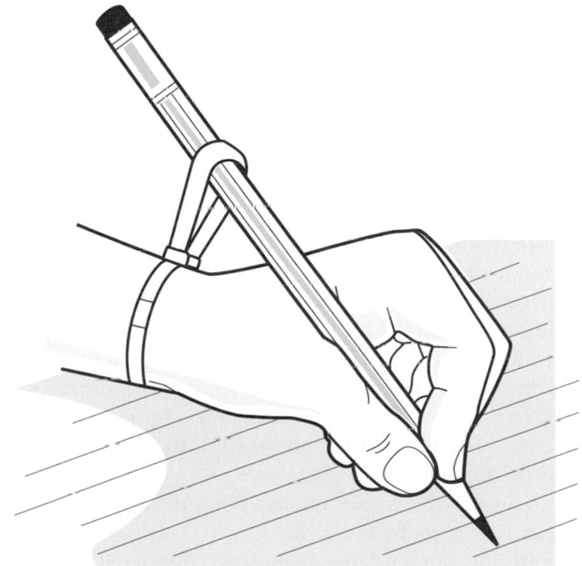

FIGURE 18-7 A rubber band sling allows for a slanted, relaxed pencil position.

is most efficient and comfortable. Traditionally, kindergarten and primary grade classroom teachers have promoted the use of a wide primary pencil for beginning writers. Carlson and Cunningham[22] examined tool usage among preschool children performing drawing, tracing, and writing tasks. They found that the readability of their written work was not enhanced by the use of a wider diameter pencil. This study suggests that the pervasive use of the primary pencil is probably not warranted for all kindergarten children because some children perform better with a no. 2 pencil, whereas others do well with a primary pencil.

Cognitive Interventions

Cognitive interventions for handwriting are based on learning theories that involve self-instruction and verbal mediation,[80] as well as strategies of imitation, practice, self-evaluation, and feedback.[53,90] One top-down cognitive approach is the Cognitive Orientation to (daily) Occupational Performance (CO-OP).[81,91] The therapist uses verbally based, highly individualized problem-solving techniques to facilitate motor skill acquisition (see Chapter 11). In this approach the child, facilitated by the therapist, generates his or her own solutions to resolve problematic aspects of task performance using a combination of strategies.[91] The global strategy Goal-Plan-Do-Check provides a problem-solving framework that can be generalized to any task. Within this framework, the child applies domain-specific cognitive strategies to master occupational performance goals.[92]

For students with cognitive limitations that affect attention, activities to compensate include (1) placing a black mat that is larger than the worksheet underneath it to increase high contrast, thereby assisting visual attention to the worksheet; (2) drawing lines to group materials; and (3) reorganizing worksheets.[110] Visual stimuli on a worksheet or in a book can be reduced by covering the entire page except the activity on which the student is working or by using a mask that uncovers one line at a time (Figure 18-8). Reducing competing sensory input in both the auditory and visual modalities can be helpful for some students with poor visual attention. For example, headphones can be worn when working on a visual task. Good lighting and use of pastel-colored paper helps reduce glare. Practice of visual searching techniques, such as using *Where's Waldo?* and similar books, can encourage development of search strategies and visual attention.

Other suggestions include cueing the child to important visual information by using a finger to point, a marker to underline, or therapist verbalization to help the child maintain visual attention. For example, children tend to look at a picture when it is named. Visual work should be presented when the student's energy is highest and not when he or she is fatigued.[97] In addition the teacher can devise and teach the student time-pressure management strategies.

Strategy training can be used to control distractibility, impulsivity, or a tendency to lose track or to overfocus.[111] Intervention strategies that are taught to the student may include the following[39]:

- Attending to the whole situation before attending to parts
- Taking timeouts from a task
- Monitoring the tendency to become distracted
- Searching the whole scene before responding

A handwriting program should support the student's learning style. The student whose preferred learning style is based on an auditory system can benefit from verbal cues or self-talk when writing. A student who is a visual learner can benefit from a writing strip on the desk, "word walls," modeling, and visual cues on the paper for start points. In addition, the therapist can develop cue cards for the student to place on his or her desk with common reversals. Directional cues can be paired with verbal cues for the child who commonly reverses letters and numbers. These cognitive cues rely on visual images for distinguishing letters and include the following:

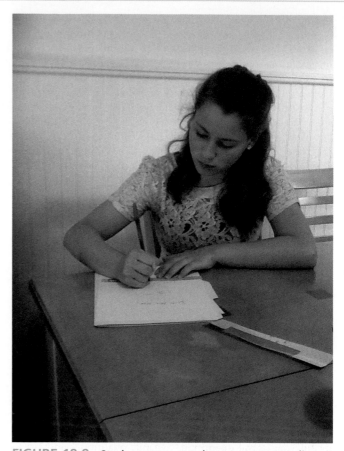

FIGURE 18-8 Student uses a mask to uncover one line at a time.

1. With palms facing the chest and thumbs up, the student makes two fists. The left hand will form a *b* and the right hand will form a *d*.
2. Lower case *b* is like *B*, only without the top loop.
3. To make a lower case *d*, remember that *c* comes first, and then add a line to make a *d*.

Children with visual-cognitive problems often overspace or underspace words. The correct space should be slightly more than the width of a single lowercase letter. When a child has handwriting spacing problems, the occupational therapist may recommend using a decorated tongue depressor or a pencil to space words, or simply have the child use his or her finger as a guide. The child can also imagine a letter in the space to aid in judging the distance.

An effective writing surface for assisting students with text placement and size is a color-coded, laminated sheet. When accompanied by verbal cues from the service provider, this sheet provides immediate visual cues to the child learning letterforms. Beneath the solid, red writing baseline, the color brown represents the "soil" or "ground"; the space above the

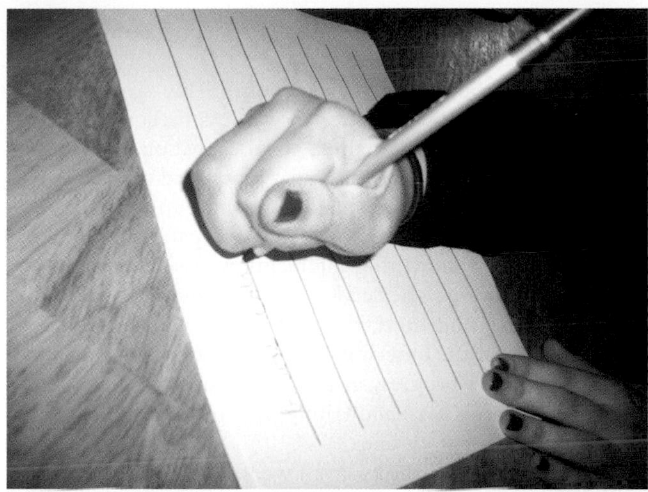

FIGURE 18-9 Lined paper with diagrams helps with letter size and the placement of text.

solid baseline and dashed black middle guideline are green for the "grass"; and the space above the dashed guideline to the top solid writing line is blue for the "sky." For example, the letter *h* would start at the top of the sky, head downward, and end in the grass. This same pictorial scheme can be applied to lined paper for classroom assignments, allowing students strong cues for learning letter placement and size (Figure 18-9).[6]

When students need additional help to stop at lines, templates with windows can be used in teaching handwriting. These templates can be made out of cardboard with three windows; one for one-line letters (*a*, *c*, *e*, *i*, *m*, and *n*), one for two-line letters (*b*, *d*, *k*, *l*, and *t*), and the third for three-line letters (*f*, *g*, *j*, *p*, *q*, *z*, and *y*). It is important to consider that visual memory is used to recognize the letters or words to be written, and motor memory starts the engram for producing the written product. Therefore it may be that motor memory, not visual memory, is the basis for the problem.

Various types of writing paper are available in the educational setting. Unlined paper and lined paper with a dashed middle guideline between the lower baseline and upper line are both commonly used in the early elementary grades. Studies of handwriting suggest kindergartners who use paper with lines and those who use paper without lines do not differ in legibility.[30,118] Children typically first practice writing letters using wide-spaced (1-inch) lines. As handwriting proficiency improves, usually in third or fourth grade, children use paper with narrow-spaced (⅜-inch) lines.[8] The occupational therapist and educator can allow the student the opportunity to experiment with paper with different lines and line spacing to determine which supports optimal handwriting.

Psychosocial Approaches

Psychosocial approaches used for children's handwriting intervention typically focus on improving the student's self-control and coping skills. Psychosocial approaches also create social contexts for practicing and learning handwriting, recognizing the importance of peer supports, peer modeling, and social interaction to student learning. Occupational therapists reinforce the importance of handwriting for communicating with others, sharing written stories, and sharing personal messages. The therapist uses social communication as a context for practicing handwriting (e.g., writing a note to parents and addressing an envelope to his or her residence). Sharing with children the importance of readable handwriting and the rationale for intervention, as well as providing positive, meaningful, everyday experiences using handwriting, helps children value the act of handwriting and increases motivation to produce good handwriting. When a child presents a neatly drawn and written (relative to the child's ability) Thanksgiving Day card at home, the parents can provide social reinforcement. In addition, teachers might reward the child with typically poor handwriting with a special certificate for improved handwriting on receipt of a readable spelling paper or written class assignment. By offering children choices, success, responsibility, and encouragement within the natural setting, therapists teach children to view handwriting as a functional and socially valid skill.

Occupational therapy practitioners also use small groups as a context for handwriting interventions. In Case-Smith et al.,[25] students practiced handwriting in small groups, then shared their papers with each other to "circle the best letter." Peer evaluation appeared to motivate the students and reinforce their best handwriting. By using integrated groups of students with high and low level handwriting, the therapist encouraged peer modeling and natural peer supports (e.g., peer-to-peer encouragement). Occupational therapists have also created handwriting clubs to motivate students and to support handwriting practice by encouraging fun and positive social interactions.[60]

Service Delivery

According to the research, children with disabilities have less instructional time with literacy. The quantity and quality of literacy experiences are dramatically different from those of their peers.[83] Providing occupational therapy services to children with handwriting difficulties should be based primarily on the needs of the individual child as determined by the educational or clinical team. Currently many educational teams use a continuum of service delivery that allows for more flexibility, fluidity, and responsiveness to an individual child's needs (see Chapter 24). Case Study 18-3 illustrates a continuum of services to promote written expression.

Some children are good candidates for improving their manuscript or cursive handwriting through remediation. However, other children are not. The occupational therapist and the child's clinical and educational teams need to consider compensatory strategies that allow the child with poor handwriting the greatest opportunity for functional written communication. Alternatives to handwriting include keyboarding and word prediction, adapting and reducing the amount of written assignments, dictating assignments, and having study buddies to assist with written expression. In school settings, the educational team, along with the parent(s), determines which type of written communication is or will be most functional for the child and develop a short-term plan (e.g., learning essential manuscript words) and a long-term plan (e.g., learning word processing).

Consultation and training others to implement intervention strategies are often the most appropriate service delivery models to improve children's handwriting. Alternative service providers (e.g., educators, educational assistants, volunteers, high school students, and parents) can implement techniques and programs when the occupational therapist assumes responsibility for

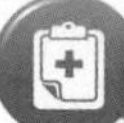

CASE STUDY 18-3 Continuum of Occupational Therapy Services for Tara

At the beginning of second grade, Tara, a girl with a learning disability, was assessed by the occupational therapist for poor handling of classroom materials and tools (e.g., glue stick, scissors, computer mouse) and illegible handwriting. After a comprehensive occupational therapy evaluation, Tara's parents and the educational team decided to focus on assisting her to become a more proficient writer, with the occupational therapist and the regular education teacher spearheading the intervention program.

The therapist and the teacher met to develop classroom strategies to be implemented. These strategies included positioning Tara's desk directly in front of the chalkboard, reducing the length of her written assignments, and providing her with an alphabet strip attached to her desktop and placed at the recommended angle of her writing paper.

The educator also requested the help of the occupational therapist in implementing motivating exercises to prepare the entire class for their daily creative writing period. The occupational therapist scheduled a time with the teacher and spent 10 to 15 minutes per week (for 4 weeks) teaching the entire class hand-dexterity games before a classroom writing activity. She also provided the teacher with a written handout of games, so the teacher could ask questions and have a later reference.

Because of the extremely poor legibility of Tara's writing, the team chose to have her join an ongoing handwriting intervention group in the classroom. This group held 25-minute sessions twice a week for three consecutive weeks. During this direct service time, the occupational therapist further assessed individual children. She trained the teacher's assistant to coordinate the handwriting group and address some of the individual problems. The occupational therapist returned to the handwriting intervention session once every 2 weeks to supervise the service provider, monitor the children's progress, and modify the programs when needed. A regular consultation time was established with the educator to evaluate Tara's progress in class, strategize regarding new situations affecting her handwriting performance, and write a progress note to her parents.

In Tara's case, during the first 4 weeks after the initial team meeting, the occupational therapist implemented direct service, training of a teaching assistant, and consulting with the teacher. However, the provision of services was not locked into a set schedule (e.g., two 25-minute sessions per week of direct therapy). By using a continuum of service provision, the occupational therapist initially worked with the teacher, orchestrated an ongoing intervention program that another service provider could implement after training, and continued to make regular contact with Tara and the educational team members, including Tara's parents.

organizing, modeling, and teaching the methods. When intervention methods are implemented by others, the occupational therapist regularly monitors, provides feedback, and adjusts techniques as needed. Practicing through homework should be used on an individual basis, after consideration of how this fits with the child's interests, ability, and occupational engagement.[61] Consultation appears most successful when the occupational therapist models the strategies for the services provider, clearly articulates the rationale for the methods and approaches used in the program, and designs a well-organized program that can be applied easily.

A user-friendly program that the teacher or aide can easily implement within the classroom is more likely to be followed. For example, by supplying (1) specific written and oral directions of the program; (2) a container, such as a basket, full of materials for the handwriting intervention program (e.g., Thera-Band, in-hand manipulation games, sequenced writing lessons, clay trays, different writing tools); (3) data management sheets; and (4) a system to provide reinforcement and rewards, the program can be administered easily. Handwriting interventions for one student can also benefit other children in the classroom who may be struggling with handwriting. For students to benefit, therapists must give teachers guidance and instruction in how to appropriately use these tools and should monitor how they are used.

In addition, meaningful writing activities that enhance handwriting can be embedded throughout the school day. For example, teachers can emphasize good handwriting when students use interesting paper and writing tools in writing centers, write shopping lists in the kitchen center, create class books, survey peers about their favorite ice cream and graph the results, or write letters to peers and family. "Capitalizing on the meaning that is the heart of all writing" is essential to promote writers who want to share their thoughts through writing.[42]

Summary

Handwriting is an important academic occupation for children. Children with neuromuscular impairments, learning disabilities, and developmental delays are often referred to occupational therapy for handwriting problems.

- The role of the occupational therapist includes evaluating the child's functional performance of prewriting and handwriting skills, along with the related client factors, task demands, and environmental features.
- The occupational therapist assists the educational or clinical team in planning an integrated approach to promote a functional written communication means for the child.
- Handwriting intervention programs should be comprehensive, incorporating activities and therapeutic techniques from the acquisitional/motor learning, sensorimotor, biomechanical, cognitive, and psychosocial models of practice.
- Handwriting programs and interventions should be provided in the child's natural setting and should be explicitly linked to the writing curriculum.
- For many children with handwriting difficulties, compensatory strategies and computer keyboarding can augment handwriting and enable success in functional written communication.

REFERENCES

1. Alston, J. (1991). Handwriting in the new curriculum. *British Journal of Special Education, 18*, 13–15.
2. Alston, J. (1995). Assessing writing speeds and output: Some current norms and issues. *Handwriting Review*, 102–106.
3. American Occupational Therapy Association. (2008). Occupational therapy practice framework: Domain and process second edition. *American Journal of Occupational Therapy, 62*, 609–639.
4. Amundson, S. J. (1992). Handwriting: Evaluation and intervention in school settings. In J. Case-Smith & C. Pehoski (Eds.), *Development of hand skills in the child*. Rockville, MD: American Occupational Therapy Association.
5. Amundson, S. J. (1995). *Evaluation tool of children's handwriting*. Homer, AK: OT KIDS.
6. Amundson, S. J. (1998). *TRICS for written communication: Techniques for rebuilding and improving children's school skills*. Homer, AK: O.T. KIDS.
7. Asher, A. V. (2006). Handwriting instruction in elementary schools. *American Journal of Occupational Therapy, 60*, 461–471.
8. Barchers, S. I. (1994). *Teaching language arts: An integrated approach*. Minneapolis: West Publishing.
9. Bazyk, S., Michaud, P., Goodman, G., et al. (2009). Integrating occupational therapy services in a kindergarten curriculum: A look at the outcomes. *The American Journal of Occupational Therapy, 63*(2), 160–171. doi:10.5014/ajot.63.2.160.
10. Beery, K. E. (1997). *The developmental test of visual-motor integration* (5th ed.). Austin, TX: Pro-Ed.
11. Beery, K. E., & Beery, N. (2005). *The Development Test of Visual-Motor Integration*. Cleveland: Modern Curriculum Press.
12. Bell, B., & Swinth, Y. L. (2005). Defining the role of occupational therapy to support literacy development. *School Systems Special Interest Quarterly, 12*(3), 1–9.
13. Benbow, M. (1990). *Loops and other groups*. Tucson, AZ: Therapy Skill Builders.
14. Benbow, M. (2006). Principles and practice of teaching handwriting. In A. Henderson & C. Pehoski (Eds.), *Hand function in the child: Foundations for remediation* (2nd ed.). St. Louis: Mosby.
15. Benson, J. D., Salls, J., & Perry, C. (2010). A pilot study of teachers' perceptions of two handwriting curricula: Handwriting Without Tears and The Peterson Directed Handwriting Method. *Journal of Occupational Therapy, Schools, & Early Intervention, 3*, 319–330.
16. Berninger, V., Vaughan, K. B., Abbott, R. D., et al. (1997). Treatment of handwriting problems in beginning writers: Transfer from handwriting to composition. *Journal of Education Psychology, 89*, 652–666.
17. Berninger, V., Yates, C., Cartwright, A., et al. (1992). Lower-level developmental skills in beginning writing. *Reading and Writing: An Interdisciplinary Journal, 4*, 256–280.
18. Bralecki, S., & Rice, M. (2012). Quality of handwriting and scaling of hand size to pencil size in typically developing children. Poster presented at American Occupational Therapy Association Annual Conference.
19. Cabell, S. Q., Justice, L. M., Zucker, T. A., et al. (2009). Emergent name-writing abilities of preschool-age children with language impairment. *Language, Speech, and Hearing Services in Schools, 40*(1), 53–66.
20. Cahill, S. (2009). Where does handwriting fit in strategies to support academic achievement. *Intervention in School and Clinic, 44*, 223–228.
21. Cahill, S. (2009). Where does handwriting fit in? *Intervention in School and Clinic, 44*, 223–228.
22. Carlson, K., & Cunningham, J. (1990). Effect of pencil diameter on the graphomotor skill of preschoolers. *Early Childhood Research Quarterly, 5*, 279–293.
23. Case-Smith, J. (2002). Effectiveness of school-based occupational therapy intervention on handwriting. *American Journal of Occupational Therapy, 56*, 17–25.
24. Case-Smith, J., Holland, T., & Bishop, B. (2011). Effectiveness of an integrated handwriting program for first-grade students: A pilot study. *American Journal of Occupational Therapy, 65*, 670–678.
25. Case-Smith, J., Holland, T., Lane, A., et al. (2012). Effects of a coteaching handwriting program for first graders: One-group pretest-posttest design. *American Journal of Occupational Therapy, 66*, 396–402.
26. Case-Smith, J., Weaver, L., & Holland, T. (2014). Effects of a classroom-embedded occupational therapist-teacher handwriting program for first-grade students. *American Journal of Occupational Therapy, 68*, 1–9.
27. Case-Smith, J., White, S., & Holland, T. (2014). Effectiveness of a co-taught handwriting program for first grade students. *Physical and Occupational Therapy in Pediatrics, 34*, 30–43.
28. Connelly, V., Campbell, S., MacLean, M., et al. (2006). Contribution of lower order skills to the written composition of college students with and without dyslexia. *Developmental Neuropsychology, 29*, 175–196.
29. Cornhill, H., & Case-Smith, J. (1996). Factors that relate to good and poor handwriting. *American Journal of Occupational Therapy, 50*, 732–739.
30. Daly, C. J., Kelley, G. T., & Krauss, A. (2003). Relationship between visual-motor integration and handwriting skills of children in kindergarten: A modified replication study. *American Journal of Occupational Therapy, 57*, 459–462.
31. Delegato, C., McLaughlin, K., Derby, M., et al. (2013). The effects of using handwriting without tears and a handwriting racetrack to teach five preschool students with disabilities pre-handwriting and handwriting. *Journal of Occupational Therapy, Schools, & Early Intervention, 6*, 255–268.
32. Dennis, J. L., & Swinth, Y. (2001). Pencil grasp and children's handwriting legibility during different-length writing tasks. *American Journal of Occupational Therapy, 55*, 175–183.
33. Denton, P., Cope, S., & Moser, C. (2006). Effects of sensorimotor-based intervention versus therapeutic practice on improving handwriting performance in 6- to-11-year-old children. *American Journal of Occupational Therapy, 60*, 6–27.
34. Diekema, S. M., Deitz, J., & Amundson, S. J. (1998). Test-retest reliability of the evaluation of children's handwriting—manuscript. *American Journal of Occupational Therapy, 52*, 248–254.
35. Donica, D. (2010a). A historical journey through the development of handwriting instruction (Part1): The historical foundation. *Journal of Occupational Therapy, Schools, and Early Intervention, 3*(1), 11–31.
36. Donica, D. (2010b). A historical journey through the development of handwriting instruction (Part 2): The occupational therapists' role. *Journal of Occupational Therapy, Schools, and Early Intervention, 3*(1), 32–53.
37. Donica, D. K., Goins, A., & Wagner, L. (2013). Effectiveness of handwriting readiness programs on postural control, hand control, and letter and number

formation in head start classrooms. *Journal of Occupational Therapy Schools & Early Interventions*, *6*(2), 81–93.

38. Edwards, L. (2003). Writing instruction in kindergarten. *Journal of Learning Disabilities*, *36*, 136–148.
39. Fasotti, L., Kovacs, F., Eling, P., et al. (2000). Time pressure management as a compensatory strategy training after closed head injury. *Neuropsychological Rehabilitation*, *10*, 47–65.
40. Feder, K., Majnemer, A., & Synnes, A. (2000). Handwriting: Current trends in occupational therapy practice. *Canadian Journal of Occupational Therapy*, *67*, 197–204.
41. Gardner, M. F. (2006). *Test of handwriting skills-revised*. Austin: Pro-Ed.
42. Gerde, H. K., Foster, T. D., & Skibbe, L. E. (2014). Beyond the pencil: Expanding the occupational therapists role in helping young children to develop writing skills. *The Open Journal of Occupational Therapy*, *2*(1), 5.
43. Gerde, H. K., Skibbe, L. E., Bowles, R. P., et al. (2012). Child and home predictors of children's name writing. *Child Development Research*, *2012*, 1–12.
44. Goldstand, S., Gavir, D., Cermak, S., et al. (2013). *Here's how I write: A child's self-assessment of Handwriting and Goal Setting Tool*. Framingham, MA: Therapro.
45. Graham, S. (1990). The role of production factors in learning disabled students' compositions. *Journal of Educational Psychology*, *82*, 781–791.
46. Graham, S. (1992). Issues in handwriting instruction. *Focus on Exceptional Children*, *25*, 1–14.
47. Graham, S. (2009). Want to improve children's writing? Don't neglect their handwriting. *American Educator*, (Winter 2009/2010), 20–40.
48. Graham, S., Berninger, V., Abbott, R., et al. (1997). The role of mechanics in composing of elementary school students: A new methodological approach. *Journal of Educational Psychology*, *89*, 170–182.
49. Graham, S., Berninger, V., Weintraub, N., et al. (1998). The development of handwriting fluency and legibility in grades 1 through 9. *Journal of Educational Research*, *92*, 42–52.
50. Graham, S., Harris, K. R., & Macarthur, C. (2006). Explicitly Teaching Struggling Writers: Strategies for Mastering the Writing Process. *Intervention in School and Clinic*, *41*, 290.
51. Graham, S., & Harris K. R. (2009). Almost 30 years of writing research: making sense of it all with The Wrath of Khan. *Learning Disabilities Research & Practice*, *24*(2), 58–68.
52. Graham, S., Harris, K. R., & Fink, B. (2000). Is handwriting causally related to learning to write? Treatment of handwriting problems in beginning writers. *Journal of Educational Psychology*, *92*, 620–633.
53. Hammerschmidt, S. L., & Sudaswad, P. (2004). Teacher's survey on problems with handwriting: Referral, evaluation, and outcomes. *American Journal of Occupational Therapy*, *58*, 185–191.
54. Hamstra-Bletz, L., & Blöte, A. (1990). Development of handwriting in primary school: A longitudinal study. *Perceptual and Motor Skills*, *70*, 759–770.
55. Handley-More, D., Deitz, J., Billingsley, F. F., et al. (2003). Facilitating written work using computer word processing and word prediction. *American Journal of Occupational Therapy*, *57*, 139–151.
56. Harris, K. R., Graham, S., & Mason, L. H. (2006). Improving the writing, knowledge and motivation of struggling young writers: Effects of self-regulated strategy development with and without peer support. *American Educational Research Journal*, *43*, 295–340.
57. Henry, D. (2005). *Tools for tots: Sensory strategies for toddlers & preschoolers*. Glendale, IL: Henry OT Services.
58. Holm, M. B. (2000). Our mandate for the new millennium: Evidence-based practice, 2000 Eleanor Clarke Slagle lecture. *American Journal of Occupational Therapy*, *54*, 575–585.
59. Howe, T., Roston, K. L., Sheu, C., et al. (2013). Assessing handwriting intervention effectiveness in elementary school students: A two-group controlled study. *American Journal of Occupational Therapy*, *67*, 19–25.
60. Hoy, M. M. P., Egan, M. Y., & Feder, K. P. (2011). A systematic review of interventions to improve handwriting. *Canadian Journal of Occupational Therapy*, *78*, 13–25.
61. Hoy, M., Egan, M., & Feder, K. (2011). A systematic review of interventions to improve handwriting. *Canadian Journal of Occupational Therapy*, *78*(1), 13–25.
62. Jarman, C. (1990). A national curriculum for handwriting? *British Journal of Special Education*, *17*, 151–153.
63. Karlsdottir, R., & Stefansson, T. (2002). Problems in developing functional handwriting. *Perceptual and Motor Skills*, *94*, 623–662.
64. Keller, M. (2001). Handwriting club: Using sensory integration strategies to improve handwriting. *Intervention in School and Clinic*, *37*, 9–12.
65. Kemmis, B., & Dunn, W. (1996). Collaborative consultation: The efficacy of remedial and compensatory interventions in school contexts. *American Journal of Occupational Therapy*, *50*, 709–717.
66. Koziatek, S. M., & Powell, N. J. (2002). A validity study of the Evaluation Tool of Children's Handwriting—Cursive. *American Journal of Occupational Therapy*, *56*, 446–453.
67. Koziatek, S. M., & Powell, N. J. (2003). Pencil grips, legibility, and speed of fourth-graders' writing cursive. *American Journal of Occupational Therapy*, *57*, 284–288.
68. Larsen, S. C., & Hammill, D. D. (1989). *Test of legible handwriting*. Austin, TX: Pro-Ed.
69. Levine, K. J. (1991). *Fine motor dysfunction: Therapeutic strategies in the classroom*. Tucson, AZ: Therapy Skill Builders.
70. Lust, C., & Donica, D. (2011). Effectiveness of a handwriting readiness program in head start: A two-group controlled trial. *American Journal of Occupational Therapy*, *65*, 560–568.
71. Mackay, N., McCluskey, A., & Mayes, R. (2010). The Log Handwriting Program improved children's writing legibility: A pretest–posttest study. *American Journal of Occupational Therapy*, *64*, 30–36.
72. Magill, R. A. (1985). *Motor learning concepts and applications*. Dubuque, IA: William C. Brown.
73. Marr, D., & Dimeo, S. B. (2006). Outcomes associated with a summer handwriting course for elementary students. *American Journal of Occupational Therapy*, *60*, 10–15.
74. McAvoy, C. (1996). Making writers. *Closing the gap newsletter*, *15*(1), 9.
75. McGarrigle, J., & Nelson, A. (2006). Evaluating a school skills programme for Australian Indigenous children: A pilot study. *Occupational Therapy International*, *13*, 1–20.
76. McGee, L. M., & Richgels, D. J. (2000). *Literacy's beginnings: Supporting young readers and writers* (3rd ed.). Boston: Allyn & Bacon.
77. McHale, K., & Cermak, S. (1992). Fine motor activities in elementary school: Preliminary findings and provisional implications for children with fine motor problems. *American Journal of Occupational Therapy*, *46*, 898–903.
78. Medwell, J., & Wray, D. (2008). Handwriting—A forgotten language skill? *Language and Education*, *22*, 34–37.

79. Meichenbaum, D. (1977). *Cognitive-behavior modification: An integrative approach.* New York: Plenum Press.
80. Missiuna, C., Mandich, A. D., Polatajko, H. J., et al. (2001). Cognitive Orientation to daily Occupational Performance (CO-OP): Part I. Theoretical foundations. *Physical and Occupational Therapy in Pediatrics, 20,* 69–81.
81. Mulligan, S. (2003). *Occupational therapy evaluation for children: A pocket guide.* Philadelphia: Lippincott Williams & Wilkins.
82. Musselwhite, C., & King-DeBaun, P. (1997). *Emergent literacy success: Merging technology and whole language for students with disabilities.* Park City, UT: Creative Communicating.
83. National Early Literacy Panel (NELP) (2008). *Developing early literacy: Report of the National Early Literacy Panel.* Washington, DC: National Institute for Literacy.
84. Neuman, S. B., Roskos, K., Wright, T. S., et al. (2007). *Nurturing knowledge: Building a foundation for school success by linking early literacy to math, science, art, and social studies.* New York: Scholastic.
85. No Child Left Behind Act of 2001 (Elementary and Secondary Education Act Amendments) Pub. L. 107-110, 115 Stat. 1425 (2002).
86. Olsen, J., & Knapton, E. (2006). *The print tool evaluation and remediation package.* Cabin John, MD: Handwriting Without Tears.
87. Olsen, J., & Knapton, E. (2008). *Handwriting without tears Pre-K teachers guide.* Cabin John, MD: Handwriting Without Tears.
88. Peterson, C. Q., & Nelson, D. L. (2003). Effect of an occupational intervention on children with economic disadvantages. *American Journal of Occupational Therapy, 57,* 152–160.
89. Phelps, J., & Stemple, L. (1987). The children's handwriting evaluation scale for manuscript writing. In T. C., Dallas (Ed.), *Texas Scottish Rite Hospital for Crippled Children.*
90. Polatajko, H. J., & Mandich, A. D. (2004). *Enabling occupation in children: The Cognitive Orientation to daily Occupational Performance (CO-OP) approach.* Ottawa: CAOT.
91. Polatajko, H. J., Mandich, A. D., Miller, L. T., et al. (2001a). Cognitive Orientation to daily Occupational Performance (CO-OP): Part II. The evidence. In C. Missiuna (Ed.), *Children with developmental coordination disorder: Strategies for success.* New York: Haworth Press.
92. Polatajko, H. J., Mandich, A. D., Missiuna, C., et al. (2001b). Cognitive Orientation to daily Occupational Performance (CO-OP): Part III. The protocol in brief. In C. Missiuna (Ed.), *Children with developmental coordination disorder: Strategies for success.* New York: Haworth Press.
93. Ratzon, N. Z., Efraim, D., & Bart, O. (2007). A short-term graphomotor program for improving writing readiness skills of first-grade students. *American Journal of Occupational Therapy, 61,* 399–405.
94. Reisman, J. (1999). *Minnesota handwriting test.* San Antonio, TX: Psychological Corporation.
95. Roberts, G. I., Siever, J. E., & Mair, J. A. (2010). Effects of a kinesthetic cursive handwriting intervention for grade 4–6 students. *American Journal of Occupational Therapy, 64,* 745–755.
96. Rogow, S. M. (1992). Visual perceptual problems of visually impaired children with developmental disabilities. *Re:View, 24,* 57–64.
97. Rosenblum, S., Goldstand, S., & Parush, S. (2006). Relationships among biomechanical ergonomic factors, handwriting product quality, handwriting efficiency, and computerized handwriting process measures in children with and without handwriting difficulties. *American Journal of Occupational Therapy, 60,* 28–39.
98. Ryan, S., Rigby, P., & Campbell, K. (2010). Randomised controlled trial comparing two school furniture configurations in the printing performance of young children with cerebral palsy. *Australian Occupational Therapy Journal, 57,* 239–245.
99. Salls, J., Benson, J. D., Hansen, M. A., et al. (2013). A comparison of the handwriting without tears program and Peterson directed handwriting program on handwriting performance in typically developing first grade students. *Journal of Occupational Therapy, Schools, & Early Intervention, 6,* 131–142.
100. Schmidt, R. A. (1982). *Motor control and learning.* Champaign, IL: Human Kinetics.
101. Schneck, C. M. (2014). Best practices in visual perception and academic skills to enhance participation. In G. Frolek Clark & B. Chandler (Eds.), *Best practices for occupational therapy in schools.* Bethesda, MD: AOTA Press.
102. Schneck, C. M., & Henderson, A. (1990). Descriptive analysis of the developmental progression of grip position for pencil and crayon control in nondysfunctional children. *American Journal of Occupational Therapy, 44,* 893–900.
103. Schwellnus, H., Carnahan, H., Kushki, A., et al. (2012). Effect of pencil grasp on the speed and legibility of handwriting after a 10-minute copy task in grade 4 children. *Australian Occupational Therapy Journal, 59,* 180–187.
104. Shimel, K., Candler, C., & Neville-Smith, M. (2009). Comparison of cursive handwriting instruction programs among students without identified problems. *Physical & Occupational Therapy in Pediatrics, 29,* 170–181.
105. Shore, L. (2003). *Shore handwriting screening for early handwriting development: Examiner's manual.* Chaska, MN: Psych Corporation.
106. Swinth, Y., & Anson, D. (1998). Alternatives to handwriting: Keyboarding and text-generation techniques for schools. In J. Case-Smith (Ed.), *AOTA self-study series: Making a difference in school system practice.* Bethesda, MD: AOTA.
107. Tan-Lin, A. S. (1981). An investigation into the developmental course of preschool/kindergarten aged children's handwriting behavior. *Dissertation Abstracts International, 42,* 4287–A.
108. Taras, H., Brennan, J., Gilbert, A., et al. (2011). Effectiveness of occupational therapy strategies for teaching handwriting skills to kindergarten children. *Occupational Therapy, Schools, & Early Intervention, 4,* 236–246.
109. Temple, C., Nathan, R., Temple, F., et al. (1993). *The beginnings of writing.* Boston: Allyn & Bacon.
110. Toglia, J. P. (2003). Cognitive-perceptual retraining and rehabilitation. In E. B. Crepeau, E. S. Cohen, & B. A. B. Schell (Eds.), *Willard and Spackman's occupational therapy* (10th ed.). Philadelphia: Lippincott Williams & Wilkins.
111. Tseng, M. H. (1998). Development of pencil grip position in preschool children. *Occupational Therapy Journal of Research, 18,* 207–224.
112. Tseng, M. H., & Cermak, S. A. (1991). The evaluation of handwriting in children. *Sensory Integration Quarterly, 19,* 1–6.
113. Tseng, M. H., & Cermak, S. A. (1993). The influence of ergonomic factors and perceptual-motor abilities on handwriting performance. *American Journal of Occupational Therapy, 47,* 919–926.
114. Tseng, M. H., & Chow, S. M. (2000). Perceptual-motor function of school age children with slow handwriting speed. *American Journal of Occupational Therapy, 54,* 83–88.
115. Vreeland, E. (1998). *Handwriting: Not just in the hands.* Springfield, NH: Maxanna Learning Systems.

116. Volman, M. J. M., Van Schendell, B. M., & Jongmans, M. J. (2006). Handwriting difficulties in primary school children: A search for underlying mechanisms. *American Journal of Occupational Therapy, 60*, 451–460.
117. Weil, M., & Amundson, S. J. (1994). Relationship between visual motor and handwriting skills of children in kindergarten. *American Journal of Occupational Therapy, 48*, 982–988.
118. Weintraub, N., & Graham, S. (1998). Writing legibly and quickly: A study of children's ability to adjust their handwriting to meet classroom demands. *Learning Disabilities Research and Practice, 13*, 146–152.
119. Weintraub, N., & Graham, S. (2000). The contribution of gender, orthographic, finger function, and visual-motor processes to the prediction of handwriting status. *Occupational Therapy Journal of Research, 20*, 121–140.
120. Weintraub, N., Yinon, M., Hirsh, I. B.-E., et al. (2009). Effectiveness of sensorimotor and task-oriented handwriting intervention in elementary school-aged students with handwriting difficulties. *OTJR: Occupation, Participation, & Health, 29*, 125–134.
121. Woodward, S., & Swinth, Y. (2002). Multisensory approach to handwriting remediation: Perceptions of school-based occupational therapists. *American Journal of Occupational Therapy, 56*, 305–312.
122. Ziviani, J. (2006). The development of graphomotor skills. In A. Henderson & C. Pehoski (Eds.), *Hand function in the child: foundations for remediation.* St. Louis: Mosby.
123. Ziviani, J., & Watson-Will, A. (1998). Writing speed and legibility of 7- to 14-year-old school students using modern cursive script. *Australian Occupational Therapy Journal, 45*, 59–64.
124. Zwicker, J. G., & Hadwin, A. F. (2009). Cognitive versus multisensory approaches to handwriting intervention: a randomized controlled trial. *OTJR: Occupation; Participation & Health, 29*, 40–48.

CHAPTER

19

Influencing Participation Through Assistive Technology and Universal Access

Judith W. Schoonover • Rebecca E. Argabrite Grove

KEY TERMS

Assistive technology service
Universal design
Universal Design for Learning (UDL)
Input
Output
Alternative and augmentative communication
Electronic aids for daily living
Learned helplessness
Self-determination
Electronic books
Computer-based communication system
Electronic communication aids
Non-electronic communication aids
Self-advocacy
Positioning and ergonomics
Digitized speech
Synthesized speech

GUIDING QUESTIONS

1. What are the purposes of assistive devices and services and their relevance to the practice of occupational therapy?
2. How do legal mandates influence assistive technology service delivery?
3. Which guiding frameworks/models influence decisions about assistive technology?
4. How do teams collaborate to provide assistive technology services?
5. How can assistive technology enhance childhood occupations?
6. Which assessments are used to evaluate the need for, selection of, and effects of assistive technology?
7. How do sociocultural differences influence the acceptance of assistive technology?
8. What is the continuum of and interrelationship between no-tech and high-tech solutions?
9. How are evidence-based practices used throughout the service delivery process?
10. What are resources for continued competence in the evaluation, selection, and implementation of assistive technology?

"Not every child has an equal talent or an equal ability or equal motivation; but children have the equal right to develop their talent, their ability, and their motivation."
—John F. Kennedy

Introduction

Assistive technology (AT) has been an important tool since the origins of the occupational therapy profession, as well as throughout its history, to improve function and participation. Traditionally, occupational therapists have used different types of adaptive equipment, such as reachers, buttonhooks, and pencil grips, to promote functional independence in their clients. However, the explosion of technology into everyday life has changed the way (and offers possibilities for where) children receive, interact with, and apply information. Technology provides new and exciting options for people in general, but for children with disabilities it is often a necessity. Judiciously selected AT affords users creative solutions, which allows them greater independence and opportunities for participation at home, at school, in the workforce, in the community, and in society. Occupational therapy practitioners (OTPs) use a wide range of electronic devices, from simple switches to tablets to complex robotics, to support meaningful occupational engagement. Stoller described AT as "special devices or structural changes that promote a sense of self-competence, the further acquisition of developmental skills into occupational behaviors, and/or an improved balance of time spent between the occupational roles in an individual's life as determined by the individual's goals and interests and the external demands of the environment" (p. 6).[105]

"Occupational therapy practitioners' understanding of their clients' daily occupational needs, abilities, and contexts make them ideal collaborators in the design, development, and clinical application of new or customized technological devices" (p. 678).[3] Assistive technologies may unlock human potential and optimize human performance throughout the life span and across contexts, and allow individuals to assume or regain valued life roles. The selection of the "right tool for the job" bridges the gap between what people *want* to do and what they *can* do to participate in activities that are meaningful and life sustaining. Assistive technologies can serve a variety of needs and can be part of the educational, habilitative, and/or rehabilitative process depending on the environments in which services are provided.

Congress enacted legislation designed to support the procurement and use of AT for individuals with disabilities. This expansion in the use of AT opens new doors, creates opportunities, and enables individuals with disabilities to realize functional goals that were previously unattainable. Although the materials, structure, and form of devices used continue to evolve over time, above all other considerations the primary emphasis of AT across the life span continues to be on functional outcomes for AT users.[32]

Ideas about disability are shifting. The practice of occupational therapy acknowledges the impact of the environment in intervention, recognizing its effect on performance and participation. Assistive devices and services are only as effective as the environment in which they are implemented. The World Health Organization[116] states that disability is a condition that is based on the interaction between persons with health conditions and their environment. Emphasis is placed on the removal of environmental barriers preventing inclusion and participation rather than trying to change the individual. If children with disabilities are to enjoy their right to participate at school, work, play, and in the community and to have the opportunity to realize their full potential, creating and maintaining an accessible environment are essential. Occupational therapy practitioners "make recommendations to structure, modify, or adapt the environment and context to enhance and support performance" (p. 357).[4] With the influx of technology into the daily lives of all individuals comes the increased responsibility for OTPs to keep abreast of current trends so that the tools they recommend and implement can produce the best outcomes for the clients they serve.

Influencing Children's Growth and Development with Assistive Technology

Children have an "inborn drive to discover and learn" (p. 1)[21] that motivates them to understand the world around them, strive for independence, establish a sense of self, and connect socially with others. When a disabling condition is present, children may have difficulty with accessing play, learning, or self-care activities. Burkhart offered four "secrets" to support children's successful engagement: (1) create motivating activities, (2) develop opportunities for active participation, (3) present information and materials using multiple modalities, and (4) use authentic learning scenarios in natural contexts.[21] Research indicates that AT can be instrumental in helping young children with disabilities learn valuable life skills such as social skills, including sharing and taking turns, communication skills, attending, fine and gross motor skills, self-confidence, and independence.[9,63,85,109,111] As children grow they may use technology to develop independence in many activities of daily living and instrumental activities of daily living, complete school assignments, develop prevocational and vocational skills, increase opportunities for social participation, and play games or participate in leisure activities. The use of AT can create novel opportunities for children to explore, interact, and function in their environments.

For children with disabilities, introducing the appropriate types of technology systems as early as possible may enable the child to participate in important learning situations that otherwise, because of his or her disabilities, may not be possible. For more than 20 years, researchers and clinicians have documented and discussed the unique opportunities that all types of AT offer for teaching and for advancing the life choices of children with disabilities.[11,12,39,51,63,70,93,106,109]

Because technology is constantly changing, this chapter presents problem-solving approaches, principles, and frameworks for decision making versus in-depth descriptions of specific devices or systems. The frameworks and guidelines for decision making that are presented should not be viewed as limiting strategies. Rather, they are meant to be a starting point. Each practitioner needs to adjust the concepts, given the individual needs of the client and family, other team members involved, availability of resources, and factors unique to each situation.

Definition and Legal Aspects of Assistive Technology

Assistive technology comprises a broad range of devices, services, strategies, and practices used to address functional problems encountered by individuals who have disabilities.[27] *Assistive technology* is legally defined by Public Law (PL) 108-364, The Assistive Technology Act of 2004, as "any item, piece of equipment or product system whether acquired commercially off the shelf, modified, or customized that is used to increase, maintain or improve functional capabilities of individuals with disabilities."

Public Law PL 108-364 further defined an AT service as any service that directly assists an individual with a disability in the selection, acquisition, or use of an AT device. The law includes several clarifications to enhance the definition of AT service: (1) evaluating needs and skills for AT; (2) acquiring assistive technologies; (3) selecting, designing, repairing, and fabricating AT; (4) coordinating services with other therapies; and (5) training both individuals with disabilities and those working with them to use the technologies effectively.

In a similar manner, the Individuals with Disabilities Education Improvement Act (IDEA) (PL 108-446) defines both AT devices and services as a means of providing a free and appropriate public education. IDEA 2004 requires that individualized education program (IEP) and individualized family service plan (IFSP) teams consider a child's need for AT devices and services at least annually during the development of the IEP/IFSP. Additional information regarding other legislation related to AT can be found in Table 19-1e on the Evolve website.

In practice and research, *assistive technology* is used as a broad term that encompasses devices ranging from low technology to high technology. Low-tech devices (e.g., pencil-and-paper communication boards and built-up foam handles) are inexpensive, simple to make, and easy to obtain. High-tech devices (e.g., wheelchairs, augmentative communication devices, and specialized computer software and peripherals) are generally expensive, more difficult to make, and may take longer to obtain. Mid-tech devices fall somewhere in between and may consist of hand-made or commercially available items. Other descriptors of AT include "soft" and "hard" technologies, representing the human components (decision making, strategizing, training) involved in the provision of AT and the actual, tangible devices.[32]

This chapter discusses general information regarding the use of AT with children, followed by specific examples of application. Many of the principles and decision-making strategies discussed in this chapter can be generalized to all areas of AT.

Models for Assistive Technology Assessment and Decision Making

"When matching person and technology, you become an investigator, a detective. You find out what the different alternatives are within the constraints."

—*From* **Living in the State of Stuck: How Technology Impacts the Lives of People with Disabilities**

The OTP uses a variety of theories and principles to guide the occupational therapy process (evaluation, intervention, and outcome monitoring). Models specifically related to AT help OTPs make decisions regarding its use and facilitate the integration of AT within the practice of occupational therapy.

Assessment tools and models to guide AT evaluation and service delivery have been developed by a number of professionals.[9,32,98,113,117] Each of these models provides a framework for evaluating needs, making decisions, and implementing intervention. Using a model for service delivery helps to ensure that the evaluation process is systematic and complete. Three models are described in this chapter. The Human Activity Assistive Technology (HAAT) model,[32] the Student Environment Task Tool (SETT) framework,[117] and the Matching Person and Technology assessment process[97] follow the person-environment-occupation model[75] and emphasize an occupation-based approach to AT practice. These models provide frameworks for decision making regarding the selection, implementation, and evaluation of AT.[32]

Human Activity Assistive Technology

The HAAT model (Figure 19-1) is a dynamic and interactive model in which three factors—the human, activity, and AT—form a collective whole that is then placed within the context of participation.[32] The human component includes physical, cognitive, and emotional elements. Activities are synonymous with occupations (e.g., self-care, productivity, leisure), and AT refers to a device and/or service. The context is strongly emphasized as a determining factor for outcomes.[32]

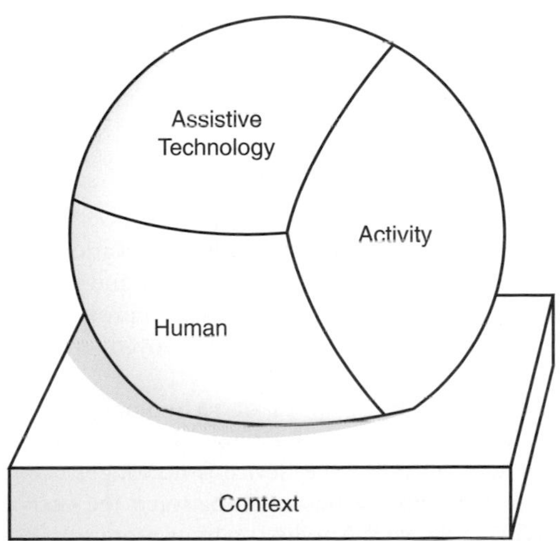

FIGURE 19-1 The Human Assistive Technology (HAAT) model. (From Cook, A., & Polgar, J. [2008]. *Cook & Hussey's assistive technologies: Principles and practice* [3rd ed.]. St. Louis: Elsevier.)

Student Environment Task Tool

A framework developed specifically for school settings is referred to as the SETT framework: student, environment, task, and tools. It is designed to be used by educational teams to develop good decision making that promotes collaboration, communication, sharing of knowledge and perspectives, flexibility, and ongoing processes among educational team members,[117] resulting in student-centered, environmentally specific, and task-focused tool systems to support a student's participation in curricular and extracurricular activities throughout the school day. SETT includes a series of questions that are designed to guide discussion, evaluation, and intervention. Teams may choose to use a few or all of the questions, depending on the needs of the student. Table 19-1 outlines the SETT

TABLE 19-1 SETT Framework Questions

Context	Questions
Student	What does the student need to do? What are the student's special needs and current abilities?
Environments	What are the instructional and physical arrangements? Are there special concerns? What materials and equipment are currently available in the environments? What supports are available to the student and the people working with the student on a daily basis? How are the attitudes and expectations of the people in the environment likely to affect the student's performance?
Tasks	What activities occur in the student's natural environments that enable progress toward mastery of identified goals? What is everyone else doing? What are the critical elements of the activities? How might the activities be modified to accommodate the student's special needs?
Tools	What no-tech, low-tech, and high-tech options should be considered for inclusion in an AT system for a student with these needs and abilities doing these tasks in these environments? What strategies might be used to invite increased student performance? How might the student try out the proposed system of tools in the customary environments in which they will be used?

questions. Many of these questions are consistent with the type of information that an OTP gathers as part of the occupational profile and occupational performance analysis, and they are applicable to a variety of settings. The Wisconsin Assistive Technology Initiative publication, *Assessing Students' Needs for Assistive Technology (ASNAT)*, 5th Edition,[55] is a comprehensive, process-based, systematic approach to providing a functional evaluation of the student's need for assistive technology in his or her environment using the SETT format.

Matching Person and Technology

The Matching Person and Technology model and assessment process are designed to help individualize the process of matching each person with the most appropriate AT. This model and process consider three factors: milieu (i.e., characteristics of the environment and psychosocial setting in which the person uses the technology), personality (i.e., personality, temperament, and preferences), and technology (i.e., functions and features).[97]

Occupational therapy practitioners consider the dynamic and constant interaction of the person with the environment through engagement in occupation during all aspects of AT service delivery.[67] Environmental interventions and modifications should be considered first or in tandem with any devices or services required to ensure engagement and participation. Additionally, social, spiritual, and cultural factors should be examined as potential contributors to outcomes of AT intervention.

Child- and Family-Centered Approach

The social context of AT use can be considered the most influential and important, because it is often the social environment, including the attitude of others, that creates a disability more than the physical barriers in the environment.[32] Any person (e.g., parent, sibling, teacher) who interacts with an individual using AT, either directly or indirectly, is considered part of the social context. The simple presence of a disability can be socially stigmatizing, and the introduction of AT can add an additional burden, particularly when individuals within the social environment do not support use of the technology. When consistent individuals support the child in using AT across environments (e.g., home, school, work), the use of the technology is likely to be more effective and more linked to enhanced participation. Each person's unique culture influences the manner in which he or she interacts with others and the importance of participation and engagement in various activities and life roles.[32] Some cultures do not value the independence that AT provides individuals with disabilities, or an AT device may be abandoned if it replaces an important life function of another family member. For example, the grandmother who views communicating for a child with cerebral palsy as one of her roles may resist the child's use of an augmentative communication system. Cultural factors must be considered in providing AT devices and services. Box 19-1 summarizes some sociocultural factors that the occupational therapist may need to consider when evaluating, designing, and selecting AT systems for children.

In addition to recognizing the impact of the social and cultural environment from the standpoint of AT acceptance, it is important to communicate the purpose of the AT and to provide training and support to those in the environment who will facilitate implementation. A study of caregiver perspectives of AT use with young children on the autism spectrum revealed that caregivers had misconceptions about what AT is and received little support from early intervention providers in understanding the function of AT.[18] Assistive technology service includes teaching caregivers how to use AT devices in naturally occurring activities. Effective training begins by determining factors that need to be considered during the planning stage of the training, moves to strategies and techniques to use during the training, and concludes with strategies for follow-up after the training has ended (Research Note 19-1).[45]

Competent AT service provision involves communicating the intent of the device, how it will assist the child, and why it is important to use it via demonstration, modeling, and practice. Even when AT devices are intuitive and easy to understand, additional training assists teachers, related service providers, paraprofessionals, administrators, parents, and/or other caregivers in determining appropriate times and places to use the technology and strategies to increase both use and *usefulness*.

BOX 19-1 Cultural Factors That Affect Assistive Technology Delivery

Use of time
Balance of work and play
Sense of personal space
Values regarding finance
Roles assumed in the family
Knowledge of disabilities and sources of information
Beliefs about causality
View of the inner workings of the body
Sources of social support
Acceptable amount of assistance from others
Degree of importance attributed to physical appearance
Degree of importance attributed to independence
Sense of control over things that happen
Typical or preferred coping strategies
Style of expressing emotions

From Cook, A., & Polgar, J. (2008). *Cook and Hussey's assistive technologies: Principles and practice* (3rd ed.). St. Louis: Elsevier.

Technology Abandonment

"We are fascinated with technology. We expect it to make a difference in our lives, and particularly in education. We see its effects as beneficial. We look for it to change and improve what has come before. We await technological improvements in our lives, from better toaster ovens to improved, more efficient schools..." (p. 3).[66]

Despite the many promises of technology, one third or more of individuals discontinue use of their AT devices.[97] Abandonment can mean the device is no longer needed, but more often it signifies a mismatch between the user and the device. When a device fails to live up to its promise of potential, freedom, and independence, disillusionment with the idea of AT may result. Failure to take into consideration the user's preferences, ideas, and desires for an AT device is a primary reason for abandonment.[86,97] Users of AT, their families, and/

RESEARCH NOTE 19-1

Dunst, C. J., Trivette, C. M., Meter, D., & Hamby, D. W. (2012). Influences of contrasting types of training on practitioners' and parents' use of assistive technology and adaptations with infants, toddlers and preschoolers with disabilities. Research Brief, *6(1). Tots-n-Tech Institute: http://www.tnt.asu.edu.*

Abstract

This systematic review included 35 studies examining adult learning methods and practices relative to the provision of assistive technology (AT) training for children between the ages of 0 and 8.75 years. Six operationally defined adult learning characteristics were used to code and analyze results for practitioner, parent, and child outcomes. Results indicate that greater positive benefits were gained by adult learners and children when AT devices were described, explained, and demonstrated by trainers; learners had input and direct practice with the devices; trainer feedback and strategies for real life application were provided; and learners engaged in a standards-based self-assessment for mastery.

Implications for Practice

- Acceptance and sustained use of AT is likely to be most effective when recipients of AT training are involved in all phases of the learning process, including planning, application, reflection, and self-assessment.
- Effective methods for AT training should include trainer and learner joint engagement in activities with real-life application, learner input, guided practice and feedback, and standards-based self-assessment for mastery of use.
- AT training should be focused and concentrated with a small number of learners (<15) and child AT users (<10) during initial learning phases.

or educational staff may have high expectations for an AT device and can be devastated when expectations are not fully met. Assistive technology is abandoned for many reasons. According to Copley and Ziviani,[34] barriers to AT implementation and integration in the educational setting include lack of appropriate staff training and support, negative staff attitudes, inadequate assessment and planning processes, insufficient funding, difficulties with procuring and managing equipment, and time constraints. Lauer, Longnecker Rust, & Smith[73] propose replacing the term "abandonment" with the term "discontinuance," suggesting that it provides a more accurate reflection of the AT utilization process. When service providers have more insight into AT discontinuance, they do a better job of updating, revising, and improving AT services for users and their family members, which in some cases results in the device no longer being necessary as the individual's health, function, and well-being improve.

Learned Helplessness and Self-Determination

When children perceive that they have little control over outcomes within their environments, the phenomenon of learned helplessness can result. Learned helplessness is a secondary disability and is the belief that one cannot exert personal control over outcomes experienced when interacting with the environment.[2,79] Children with learned helplessness exhibit low self-esteem, directly affecting how they interact and perform functional skills. They may demonstrate a lack of initiation and an inability to cope with the events around them. In addition, when opportunities for integrating basic cognitive and perceptual skills are missed in early childhood, these children do not develop a foundation for learning higher-level concepts. Therefore it is essential to create an environment that provides guided practice, strategies, and adaptations to allow children to become independent as early as possible.

The opposite of learned helplessness is self-determination. Self-determination is defined as "acting as the primary causal agent in one's life and making choices and decisions regarding one's quality of life free from undue external influence or interference" (p. 24).[114] Self-determination encompasses self-efficacy (outcome and efficacy expectations) and self-advocacy. Efficacy expectations are personal beliefs regarding one's capability to realize a desired behavior in a specific context (judgment of what one can do with the skills one has). Outcome expectations are personal beliefs about whether a particular behavior will lead to a particular consequence (being able to determine if one's goals are realistic). Self-advocacy refers to an individual's ability to speak for him- or herself, make decisions for him- or herself, and voice his or her rights, particularly when those rights have been violated or diminished. The individual is able to take ownership of his or her needs, rather than expecting someone else to take responsibility for them.[108,114] Appreciating and being able to function with a sense of interdependence are crucial parts of self-determination.

Self-determination is a set of skills that can be taught and learned. Key characteristics and components include autonomy, self-awareness, choice making, decision making, problem solving, goal setting and attainment, internal locus of control, positive attributions of efficacy and outcome expectations, and self-knowledge.[114] OTPs promote the development of self-determination, providing services that develop skills of interdependence and independence, enhancing the participation and productivity of children, and recognizing that self-determination can mean different things to different people and strongly influences quality of life. AT devices can help with the development, practice, and effective use of self-determining behaviors for children with disabilities.

Self-determination has been identified as a critical component of successful transition from cradle to college and/or career, as well as for supporting the continued use of assistive technology after transition out of high school.[25] Several online resources support the users of assistive technology in determining and articulating their needs. (See Box 19-1e on the Evolve website for transition portfolios and materials.)

Setting the Stage for Assistive Technology Service Provision

Practice Settings

"The institutional context refers to larger organizations within a society that are responsible for policies, decision-making processes, and procedures" (p. 43).[32] The International Classification of Functioning, Disability and Health categorizes

TABLE 19-2 Practice Settings in Which Assistive Technology Services Are Provided

Setting	Services Provided
Hospital or medical center	Primary role is evaluation that is typically provided on an outpatient basis for a series of assessments (1-2 visits); may require an inpatient stay of 2-3 weeks Referrals and recommendations made directly to agencies or third party payers Limited access to child for follow-up and training; limited opportunities to consult with parents and teachers May provide direct treatment, particularly for children under the age of 3 years or those who have an acquired disability (e.g., spinal cord injury)
Regional center	Developed in response to legislation, funded by the Department of Education or other agencies for individuals with disabilities Often has AT lending library for borrowing equipment on a short-term basis Team has broad-based experience with various diagnoses, resources for obtaining equipment, types of AT, and adapted methods of use Also involved in advocacy, consumer awareness, focus groups Limited follow-up care and minimal input into training the child, family, and educational team
Public school	Most children receive AT services at a school Daily problem solving related to AT use can occur and child receives support in the natural environment in which AT is to be used School-based team has easy access to child and understands educational curriculum but may lack expertise or experience with more complex AT systems
Home and community setting	May provide direct treatment, especially for children under the age of 3 years Direct training available to child and family Problem solving related to AT use can occur and child receives support in the natural environment in which AT is to be used Can provide carryover to other practice settings such as school or work May have limited opportunities to consult with others

Adapted from Beukelman, D. R., & Mirenda, P. (1992). *Augmentative and alternative communication: Management of severe communication disorders in children and adults*. Baltimore: Brookes.[13]

economic, legal, and political components as services, systems, and policies.[116] This institutional overlay has major implications for both the acquisition and use of AT with regard to funding, legislation related to environmental and community access, as well as standards that govern product design, function, and safety.[32]

Differences in practice settings in which OTPs who provide AT may be employed are outlined in Table 19-2. The role of the OTP in each of these settings is governed by a combination of professional scope of practice, the expertise of other members of the team, and the agency or funding source.

Occupational Therapy Process and Assistive Technology in the Schools

According to the most recent statistics published by the U.S. Department of Education, Office of Special Education Programs,[112] as required under the IDEA, an estimated 6.5 million children from birth to 21 years of age receive special education services. Most children who need AT receive those services in school. AT devices and services are provided if necessary for a child to receive free and appropriate public education in the least restrictive environment. The need for AT must be considered, at least annually, for all children who receive services under IDEA. When AT is a necessary part of the student's program, the school district is responsible to make sure that it is available to the child. It is not uncommon for the expertise of an OTP to be requested when the team is considering AT for a student. Guides and models for considering AT for students in special education are available online (see Appendix 19-A on the Evolve website for Internet resources).

Baush, Ault, and Hasselbring indicated that appropriate AT devices and services can help a student improve, increase, or maintain performance of functional skills (e.g., self-help, mobility, or communication), access curriculum (e.g., multimedia presentations or books on tape), become a more efficient learner (e.g., pencil grips and raised lined paper to improve writing legibility), or compensate for lack of skills (e.g., word prediction software to assist with spelling or reduce keystrokes).[10] The roles and responsibilities of IEP team members, including the OTP, providing AT services within a school setting are listed in Box 19-2.

The Interprofessional Team

The provision of AT services occurs across disciplines, and the training and experience of the service providers has not been widely studied (see Research Note 19-1).[115] Several universities offer certificate programs and advanced degrees in AT. In addition, the Rehabilitation Engineering and Assistive Technological Society of North America (RESNA) has established a mechanism for verifying a minimum level of competence for individuals serving as AT providers through an examination process that provides credentialing for persons working as assistive technology professionals. The assistive technology professional usually has a background in a rehabilitation discipline such as occupational therapy, physical therapy, speech-language pathology, or engineering.

BOX 19-2 Roles and Responsibilities of School Assistive Technology Teams

1. Consider AT devices and services as an integral and necessary part of the IEP process as outlined by IDEA 2004.
2. Become familiar with different types of AT and a variety of tools that support student needs.
3. Assess each student's need for devices and services to support educational performance and access to curricular and extracurricular activities.
4. Seek additional resources and assistance from other educational professionals such as the members of an IEP.
5. Gather and analyze data about a student and his or her customary educational environments, goals, and tasks when considering AT needs. Student performance in core academic areas, social skills and behavior, communication, independent living, and organizational skills, along with demands of the task and environmental features, exist in a dynamic relationship and may all be considered in combination during the AT assessment process.
6. Consider a range of AT options from no-tech to high-tech and use of existing resources, the procurement of new devices, or both.
7. Organize the physical space where AT is used, establish routines that support use of AT, and support consistent use of AT in all appropriate environments.
8. Communicate and document the AT process in the IEP, with rationale for the decisions made and scientific evidence to support devices and services. Supporting evidence may include AT assessments, device trials, student achievement with and without AT, student-based preferences, and teacher observations.

From Baush, M. E., Ault, M. J., & Hasselbring, T. S. (2006). QIAT Consortium (2007). Quality indicators for assistive technology services. Retrieved August 2008 from http://natri.uky.edu/assoc_projects/qiat.

RESEARCH NOTE 19-2

Watson, A. H., Ito, M., Smith, R. O., & Andersen, L. T. (2010). Effect of assistive technology in a public school setting. American Journal of Occupational Therapy, 64, *18–29.*

Abstract

Given the lack of outcomes research in assistive technology (AT), as provided in the public school setting and required by the Individuals with Disabilities Education Act (IDEA), this quasi-experimental repeated-measures study examined the effectiveness of AT as a result of a specific service delivery model utilizing a multidisciplinary team approach. Thirteen students with varied educational disabilities were provided with AT to target academic and communication goals over the course of a school year within a special education setting. Results indicate that a multidisciplinary approach may have a significant effect on individualized education program (IEP) goals. These findings support the use of AT by occupational therapists to achieve students' individualized educational goals.

Implications for Practice

- AT provided by a multidisciplinary team may be helpful in promoting attainment of IEP goals and objectives in a public school setting.
- The Student Performance Profile has potential as an effective tool for collecting AT outcomes.
- Data collection and analysis of student outcome measures may improve service delivery and provide justification for AT services.

As with many other specialty areas in pediatrics, the successful implementation of AT requires a cohesive and effective team that emphasizes shared vision and ownership. The team's input is critical to making decisions regarding AT because devices are used across the child's environments and address multiple performance goals that cross professional boundaries. See Research Note 19-2.

Collaboration among children, parents, teachers, and occupational therapists enables the team to determine the best match of AT to strengths and needs and provides a supportive environment for measuring, learning, and reviewing the use of the AT. Decisions that the interprofessional team and the family make together are most likely to meet the multifaceted needs of the child.

The specific members of the team may vary depending on the type of device being introduced to the child, the expertise of the individuals involved, and the specific setting. For example, in a clinical setting the team may include the child and family, occupational therapist, physical therapist, speech-language pathologist, doctor, nurse, rehabilitation engineer, and social worker. In school-based practice the team may include the child and family, occupational therapist, physical therapist, speech-language pathologist, educator, administrator, and psychologist.

In some settings, occupational therapy assistants and aides provide some of the AT services. Assistants are particularly helpful in training a child to use a system once the occupational therapist has planned and established the program. Assistants and aides may also be involved in practicing use of the device with the child and helping others use the systems. Occupational therapists working in AT service delivery must determine which activities are appropriate to delegate and which activities are specialized and require the training and skills of a therapist.[5]

Assistive Technology Evaluation and Intervention: A Dynamic Process

The OTP has a key role on the AT evaluation team. The unique perspective on occupation and engagement in meaningful activities offered to the team is helpful in determining needs, problem-solving potential solutions, and evaluating outcomes. The assessment of client satisfaction is a key factor in determining the effective implementation and usefulness of AT in the lives of individuals with disabilities.[36,37,97,99,108]

In addition to evaluation and intervention services, AT services may also include device procurement, training, skill acquisition, monitoring, and other services that support and enable the child's participation in home, school, and community activities. Because of the complexity of many AT systems, specifically those that are high-tech, the OTP needs a systematic procedure for follow-up and adjustments to help ensure the viability of the system over time. These steps of the process are dynamic rather than linear and sequential. For example, intervention may begin by addressing prerequisite skills for AT use before completing the AT evaluation and procuring a specific device. Once a system has been chosen and purchased, evaluation, monitoring, and decision-making processes continue throughout intervention.

Evaluation

According to IDEA (1997; 2004), school divisions are required to provide assistive technology evaluations and services; however, the Federal Register (July 10, 1993) distinguishes between assessment and evaluation as follows: Evaluation: A group of activities conducted to determine a child's *eligibility* for special education. Assessment: A group of activities conducted to determine a child's *specific needs.* The implication of this language is that an evaluation might be a one-time event, whereas an assessment is an ongoing event.

When considering AT needs, the OTP closely examines the child's abilities and difficulties, demands of the environment and task, and the child's goals. The first step of the assessment is to identify key activities that the child or family needs or wants him or her to do. The Canadian Occupational Performance Measure is a useful tool to assist with the identification of client-centered goals and the importance of the goals.[74] The importance that an individual assigns to an activity helps predict whether he or she will accept technology that enables participation in that activity.[103]

A number of inventories, checklists, and processes have been developed to assist with assessment. When an assessment is requested, observation should occur in the student's natural environment, which might include home, school (e.g., classroom, playground, lunchroom, bathroom, extracurricular areas), and community settings (e.g., work settings or other relevant locations). When conducting the evaluation, practitioners consider all factors influencing a child's participation in given activities, including how often and for how long the child engages in them (Box 19-3). During the assessment, existing technology used by the child and its effectiveness in the customary environment are documented. A complete occupational therapy evaluation may or may not be a component of the AT process, depending on the practice setting in which it occurs. Formal and informal evaluation tools that may be used during the assessment process are described in Table 19-3.

The AT assessment may be completed by the team who will also provide the intervention (e.g., fitting and training of the device) or a team that has been formed specifically for the purpose of completing AT assessments. Many hospitals, clinics, and some community agencies and schools have a designated AT team because of the complexity of many AT systems. The OTP who does not work with AT on a regular basis may have difficulty maintaining expertise on all the systems and devices available because of the number of devices and the rapid development of new systems. When separate teams are responsible for evaluation and intervention, ideally these teams collaborate to make decisions and recommendations.

In addition to a comprehensive assessment, a trial period with different types of AT is needed to achieve a good match between the AT device or system and the child and family. The trial period may be one of the most important aspects of the AT evaluation. These trials can help prevent the costly procurement of an incorrect device. The cost of AT includes not only the purchase of the device but also the ongoing expenses for maintenance, upgrades to the system, and repairs. Throughout assessment and intervention, consideration should be given to the family's financial resources, access to repair services, whether the AT device significantly increases the child's level of participation, whether the AT device will "grow" with the child, and whether a less complex device will meet the same needs.[109]

The team discusses these issues and others unique to each family in deciding whether the system is a reasonable and appropriate investment for the family that will result in increasing the child's functional independence. The team presents the

BOX 19-3 Guiding Questions in Evaluating a Child for Assistive Technology

Motor
- Which body parts are capable of reliable, accurate, and controlled movement?
- Can the child be positioned adequately in and maintain an upright sitting posture?
- Does the child have sufficient range of motion, finger dexterity, strength, and endurance?
- What is the child's overall endurance and strength?
- What is the child's level of independence in daily living skills?

Sensory and Perceptual
- Can the child attend to visual feedback on the monitor?
- Can the child respond to auditory feedback?
- What are the child's strengths and limitations in visual perception and visual motor skills?
- Is the child easily distracted by visual stimuli?

Cognitive and Communication
- What is the child's cognitive level?
- What is the child's attention span?
- What are the child's receptive and expressive language skills and potential?
- What are the child's face-to-face and written communication needs?
- Can the child sequence multiple-step directions?

Psychosocial
- Does the child seem motivated to use AT?
- Which activities does the child enjoy?
- Does the child see AT use as meaningful and rewarding?
- Will the child and family tolerate the influence of this AT device?

Context
- Where will the child use the AT device?
- How can the AT device or interface be positioned for optimal use?
- Do classroom or home environments allow for safe and easy access to educational materials and use of the AT devices?
- Does the child have any previous experience with AT?
- Are the individuals who work with the child (family and professionals) willing to use AT?
- What are the short- and long-term goals with the AT device?

TABLE 19-3 Assistive Technology Assessments

Assessment	Description
Assessing Students' Needs for Assistive Technology: A resource manual for school district teams from the Wisconsin Assistive Technology Initiative (WATI), updated June 2009; http://www.wati.org/?pageLoad=content/supports/free/index.php	Not designed as a test protocol but provides a comprehensive process-based systematic approach to assessment. Package includes WATI Assessment forms together with the *Consideration Guide, Student Information Guide, Environmental Observation Guide, Decision Making Guide, AT Checklist,* and *Trial Use Guide.*
Georgia Project for Assistive Technology (GPAT), http://www.gpat.org/	GPAT has developed lists of assistive technology devices by attribute (e.g., writing support) and resources pertaining to legal mandates for assistive technology, considering assistive technology for students with disabilities, documenting need for assistive technology, implementation and integration, and evaluation of effectiveness of assistive technology.
MPT Assessment Instruments, http://www.matchingpersonandtechnology.com/mptdesc.html	Each instrument is actually a pair of instruments: one designed for the provider of technologies (counselor, occupational therapist, teacher, employer, trainer, etc.) and the other designed for the technology user. *Survey of Technology Use (SOTU)*—helps identify technologies an individual feels comfortable with or successful in using so new technology can be built around existing comfort or success *Assistive Technology Device Predisposition Assessment (ATD PA)*—helps people select AT *Educational Technology Predisposition Assessment (ET PA)*—helps students use AT to attain educational goals
Functional Evaluation for Assistive Technology, http://www.nprinc.com/assist_tech/feat.htm	Five scales are completed by various members of the AT team to allow for an ecologic assessment of needs: Contextual Matching Inventory; Checklist of Strengths and Limitations; Checklist of Technology Experiences; Technology Characteristics Inventory; and Individual-Technology Evaluation Scale.

BOX 19-4 Criteria for Evaluating Assistive Technology Devices

1. *Effectiveness.* How much the device improves the user's living situation and enhances functional capability and independence
2. *Affordability.* The extent to which a person can purchase, maintain, and repair a device without financial hardship
3. *Reliability.* The degree to which a device is dependable, consistent, and predictable in its performance and levels of accuracy for a reasonable amount of time
4. *Portability.* The influence of the device's size and weight on the user's ability to move, carry, relocate, and operate it in varied locations
5. *Durability.* The extent to which a device delivers continued operation for an extended period of time
6. *Securability.* How well a consumer believes that a device affords physical control and is secure from theft or vandalism
7. *Safety.* How well a device protects the user, care provider, or family member from potential harm, bodily injury, or infection
8. *Learnability.* The ease of assembly, initial learning requirements, and time and effort to master use
9. *Comfort and acceptance.* The extent to which a user feels physically comfortable with the device and does not experience pain or discomfort with use; how aesthetically appealing the user finds the device and the user's psychologic comfort when using it in private or public
10. *Maintenance and repairability.* The degree to which the device is easy to maintain and repair (by the consumer, a local repair shop, or a supplier)
11. *Operability.* The extent to which the device is easy to use, is adaptable and flexible, and affords easy access to controls and displays

From Scherer, M. J., & Lane, J. P. (1997). Assessing consumer profiles of "ideal" assistive technologies in ten categories: An integration of quantitative and qualitative methods. *Disability and Rehabilitation, 19,* 528-535.

child and family with objective and realistic information regarding investment in and use of AT.

Given a complete description of the options and alternatives, the family and the team make the final decision as to which AT is implemented and how it is incorporated into the child's routines. Box 19-4 presents 11 criteria, developed by more than 700 AT consumers, that the team should use to evaluate different AT devices. In summary, AT evaluations should be conducted (1) as part of an ongoing process linked to educational and/or therapeutic planning, (2) by a team within the natural setting where the child needs to engage in his or her occupations, (3) with trials with potential AT devices, and (4) with meaningful follow-through involving all team members.[92]

Decision Making

Occupational therapy practitioners use problem solving and clinical reasoning skills throughout the process of procurement,

TABLE 19-4 Assistive Technology (AT) Outcome Measures

AT-Specific Tools	General Tools
Efficiency of Assistive Technology and Services (EATS) Includes several assessments that target achievement of objectives (effectiveness) and individual perception of their value (utility); http://www.siva.it/research/eats/index.htm	**Canadian Occupational Performance Measure (COPM)** Client-centered measure used to detect self-perceived change in occupational performance over time Is completed by the caregiver for young child or child with limited ability to respond; http://www.caot.ca/copm/index.htm
Matching Person and Technology (MPT) Series of instruments that measure the fit between a person and technology; http://members.aol.com/IMPT97/mptdesc.html	**Occupational Self-Assessment (OSA)** Self-rated measure of occupational performance and environmental adaptation Explores performance, habits, roles, volition, interests, and environment; http://www.moho.uic.edu/assess/osa.html
Psychosocial Impact of Assistive Devices Scale (PIADS) Self-rating scale that measures the impact of rehabilitation products on quality of life in the areas of adaptability, competence, and self-esteem; http://www.piads.ca	**Occupational Therapy Functional Assessment Compilation Tool (OT FACT)** Can compare and summarize longitudinal re-evaluation information following intervention Highlights skills and deficits, resulting disabilities, and profiles of function in daily living, educational, vocational, and recreational activities; http://www.r2d2.uwm.edu/otfact/
Quebec User Evaluation of Satisfaction with Assistive Technology (QUEST) Structured and standardized measure that allows one to rate degree of satisfaction with AT and importance ascribed to it; http://members.aol.com/IMPT97/orderform.html#QUEST	**School Function Assessment, AT Supplement (SFA-AT)** Focuses on how AT impacts a student's ability to complete functional tasks covered in the SFA; http://www.r2d2.uwm.edu/atoms/idata/detail-idata.cfm?idata_id=43

From Argabrite Grove, R., Broeder, K., Gitlow, L., Goodrich, B., Levan, P., Moser, C., et al. (2007, April). *Assistive technology in the schools: From start to finish.* Pre-Conference Institute at AOTA's Annual Conference and Expo, St. Louis, MO.

implementation, and follow-up with AT. Problem solving involves defining the situation or problem, determining the short- and long-term goals, and brainstorming potential processes to reach the determined goals. In addition to the assessment tools described in Table 19-4, see Box 19-2e on the Evolve website for resources that support AT decision making. When working with children, the team, including the occupational therapy practitioner, considers short- and long-term goals in terms of what the child's needs are at present, 1 year later, 3 to 5 years later, and 7 to 10 years later. This can be difficult when working with young children, but the information can facilitate decision making, especially in addressing AT needs. In working with an adolescent, the focus becomes a successful transition plan, independence in the community, and participation in work roles. The procurement and use of the AT can be a critical part of a successful transition into future life roles for an adolescent.[20,72,104] The team revisits and rewrites goals systematically as the child grows and matures, as contexts change, as child and family needs and desires change, and if the child's medical condition changes.

Lahm and Sizemore interviewed AT teams to identify factors that influenced decision making in selecting AT.[71] Important factors included client goals, environmental demands, family/client demands, and client diagnosis. Funding was considered but was lower in importance. Because an awareness of environmental demands was another important factor, evaluations should include strategies for gathering information about the environmental demands (e.g., site visits, checklists, photos, interviews) to facilitate the best decision making.

Device Procurement

It can take up to several months to procure an AT device. When funding issues stall the process, members of the team may be involved in writing letters of justification to insurance companies and other third-party payers. Careful documentation during the trial periods with different devices can help with this process. Documentation can include videos or pictures of the child using the system that demonstrate how the system helps improve his or her function.

Once the system has arrived, the team works to put the system together, test the system, and begin training. Some companies provide representatives who can help with the process, and others have videos that come with the system. However, it is not uncommon for a system to be delivered with minimal instructions. This can be daunting to the family and other support providers. Comprehensive intervention and education help the child and family incorporate the device into their daily lives.

Funding

Occupational therapy practitioners working in the area of AT are often involved in helping procure the appropriate devices. In particular, they often provide the documentation used in applying for funding. Funding can come from various sources, including Medicaid, grants, private insurance, nonprofit agencies such as United Cerebral Palsy, private foundations, schools, and individual payment. In some states, funds are available through the Department of Developmental Disabilities, the

Department of Health, or the Department of Social Services to help purchase AT devices. As students enter high school and begin the transition to work and career sites, the state's vocational rehabilitation agency may also assist with the funding of devices. In addition, the team can consider alternative sources of funding.[23] Community service organizations, equipment loan programs, used and recycled equipment, and technical assistance projects can provide funds for AT. Often these alternative sources can take additional time and effort to research and contact. However, when a family or system has limited resources, pursuing creative funding options can result in the successful procurement of a device. When families cannot afford new devices or secure funding, they may explore AT reuse programs such as the *Pass It On Center* coordinated by the U.S. Department of Education's Office of Special Education and Rehabilitative Services, because these programs often do not have eligibility requirements.[84] OTPs should learn about the different funding options available within their state and region to contribute to the team's effort to obtain funding for AT devices. See Research Note 19-3.

Funding of AT in school districts raises unique issues. The school district is the payer of last resort, but it is ultimately responsible for AT devices that the child needs to learn in the school environment.[23,110] Public or private insurance can be applied to obtain AT devices and services when they are determined to be medically necessary.[102] The use of these funds must be voluntary on the part of the parents and with their written consent. School districts can also work with community service organizations or associations (e.g., the Muscular Dystrophy Association) to purchase AT devices or pay for services. If the AT device is purchased with the parents' funds or insurance, then the device belongs to the child and the child's family. However, if the school district purchases the device, then the school district owns the device.[82,113]

The occupational therapist may write or assist with writing a letter of justification to support the funding of an AT device. Strong supporting documentation is based on the assessment data gathered by the team and takes into consideration the language and priorities of the funding agency that clearly demonstrates the necessity of the device to strengthen the child's engagement in occupation is an important part of the process.[23] If the letter is written to a health insurance agency, then medical necessity must be emphasized; if it is directed to an education-related funding source, then it must address the child's ability to access and participate in educational programming. Requests to vocational agencies must address employment potential and work skills.[23,100,113] Other key elements in the letter may include information about the child, the device, the assessment procedures including results of any trials conducted, and the environment(s) in which it will be used; how the child will benefit from the device; alternatives to or potential outcomes of not being provided with the device; supporting photos or measurements; and information about the cost of the device and other options considered.

RESEARCH NOTE 19-3

Long, T. M., Woolverton, M., Perry, D. F., & Thomas, M.J. (2007). Training needs of pediatric occupational therapists in assistive technology. American Journal of Occupational Therapy, 61, *345–354.*

Abstract

The training of providers working with children who need AT devices or services has not kept pace with the variety and complexity of AT devices available. This article reports on a survey of pediatric occupational therapists who responded to questions about their training needs in the area of AT and delivering AT services. A large number of respondents reported less-than-adequate training in policies governing AT services and the organization and function of the service delivery system. Therapists reported a need for and interest in accessible and affordable training in the areas of funding of technology and services; collaborating with families and other service providers; and accessing reliable, knowledgeable vendors.

Implications for Practice

- Policy and practice context for providing AT services has become more complex, and practitioners are faced with, or unaware of, new and more sophisticated devices that might promote more opportunities for meaningful participation in their clients with disabilities.
- A majority of pediatric occupational therapists in this national sample rated their preparation in the area of AT as being less than adequate and rated their confidence in terms of delivering AT and AT services as low.
- Training in identification of funding sources and use of high-tech devices is among the most pressing training needs.

Implementation of Assistive Technology Services

An AT implementation plan is part of the service aspect of AT delivery and should include person(s) responsible, conditions of use, frequency of use, and duration of use. The team considers all of the tasks and contexts in which the AT will be used. For example, if a student requires a voice output communication system, it should be readily available at all times throughout his or her day (e.g., at lunch or recess to socialize, during instruction to ask or answer questions, during independent work to indicate needs and wants, and at home to interact with his or her family).

The introduction of an AT device, especially a complex device, can change the focus of a child's program. Time must be spent on training and practice within the child's natural environments (i.e., school, home) as the family and professionals make efforts to integrate use of the device into the child's everyday activities. Thus the development of skills needed to use the device often becomes the focus of intervention. Involvement by every member of the team encourages skill generalization to various settings and situations of the child. When staff are encouraged to work as a team and time is provided for them to communicate, the effectiveness of AT is likely to increase. AT devices should be readily accessible; if the device or strategy takes longer than 60 seconds to access and set up, it is less likely to be used. Examples of forms used to document an implementation plan (e.g., the NATRI Assistive Technology

Implementation Plan and the QIAT Plan for Evaluation of Effectiveness of AT Use) can be accessed in Appendix 19-B on the Evolve website.

Bowser and Reed[17] identified key points to assist educational teams in making decisions regarding the use of AT services and identifying resources that can be written into the child's IEP. Implementation and periodic review of the plan will help avoid the potential discontinuance of recommended AT devices and services.

Measuring Progress and Outcomes

Not only does good AT decision making require an eye on the future, but evaluating the outcomes of AT takes a long-term commitment[38] to ensure that it continues to support the child's engagement and participation in purposeful activities. Often it is difficult to operationalize and define global outcomes specific to AT.[52] The goal of outcome measurement is to determine the efficacy and utility of AT devices and implications for discontinued use. It is important that occupational therapists as members of AT teams select appropriate outcome measures to determine whether devices and services have the intended effect.

Data collection is critical to evaluating AT's success. The team should be involved in a collaborative discussion regarding how data will be collected. Data collection should be simple and straightforward enough for all team members including family members to understand and complete with ease. Outcome measures should be individualized to how the child will access and use the equipment. For example, when designing a data sheet for switch use, one considers which part of the body will be used to activate the switch, how much wait time will be allowed before a prompt is given, the type of prompt to be given (e.g., visual, verbal, hand-over-hand), and objectively what constitutes success for the given task (e.g., single switch activation, activation or deactivation of an electronic device, holding a switch for a specified amount of time). The occupational therapist can guide the team in a discussion of how to measure the child's performance.

Data collected over time can support the continued use of AT devices or justify the need for follow-up assessment. Often data are collected on targeted goals and objectives and are dependent on the service settings in which the device is used. Possible factors to measure include changes in the child's performance or level of function, change in level of participation, how often the device is used and under what circumstances, overall consumer satisfaction, goal achievement, quality of life, and cost analysis/savings. Table 19-4 outlines a number of assessments that may be used to evaluate outcome measures for AT.[7]

Once the child and family have a basic understanding of the AT system and begin to use it independently, the child may be discharged from direct services. However, discharge from a regular routine of intervention should include a follow-up plan. Follow-up can occur in several ways, from a telephone call to an extended clinic visit or simple review and analysis of data collected. The type of follow-up and when it should occur depends on the complexity of the system and the skills of the child, family, and other professionals working with the child. A predetermined schedule for follow-up (e.g., at intervals of 6 months or less or sometimes 1 year or more) is a component of effective service delivery. Problems and delays in service can be prevented with planned periodic review.

In addition to outcomes for individual users of AT, instruments are available to assist AT teams in conducting quality assurance studies for the services that they provide. Quality Indicators for Assistive Technology (QIAT)[89] and the School Profile of Assistive Technology Services[90] are both used in school settings to support the development and delivery of AT services. Use of these indicators as guidelines can support outcomes for the child, the family, the classroom, and the system.

Universal Design and Access

Because it encompasses such a broad spectrum of services, the definition of AT is elusive; therefore, some OTPs fail to recognize that the familiar tools in their "toolboxes" are really AT devices (Figure 19-2). Occupational therapy practitioners working with children with special needs, their families, and educators often create, individualize, or adapt devices to enable independent participation for students with physical, communication, or developmental challenges to learning.[105]

Professionals and consumers have a common misconception that AT is complicated and expensive. Often, simple low-tech solutions are overlooked. Mistrett found that given a range of low- to high-tech solutions, families generally choose to use low-tech solutions more often, perhaps because their appearance is similar to typically found toys and materials and calls less attention to the disability.[80] Assistive technology can be viewed as a barrier rather than a bridge, or "just one more thing to do," unless it is intuitive and its value is revealed in everyday successes. Assistive technology can help to level the playing field for children with disabilities, enhancing physical, instructional, and social inclusion opportunities.

Access

Providing physical access to homes and schools may include both devices and services.[65] Modifications to buildings, rooms, and other facilities allow children with physical or sensory

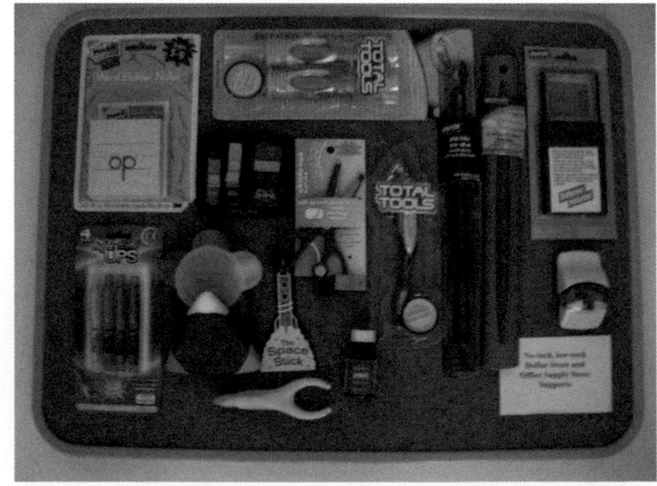

FIGURE 19-2 Examples of readily available, universally designed low-tech tools. (Photo courtesy Judith Schoonover.)

impairments to navigate both inside and outside of buildings using curb cuts, ramps, and door openers; labeling of key areas with pictures, text, and Braille; the provision of accommodations for individuals of varying sizes or those who use wheelchairs to access restrooms, water fountains, or elevators. Occupational therapy practitioners are trained to identify ways to improve performance and safety in the natural context to arrange resources and to modify the environment to decrease or eliminate barriers.

Bus modifications for entry and exit and safe and appropriate seating can help with transportation to and from school or community and school-related activities including field trips, sports, and recreation. Within the building, doors, walkways, handles, light switches, and stairs can be modified to provide equal access to all students. Outside the building, seating and playground modifications can allow or enhance safe mobility and participation in recreational activities.[54]

Schools and clinics have established guidelines for ensuring universal access as they update and expand their computer systems. When all children, including those with disabilities, have equal access to technology, costly modifications for individuals can be avoided. Often the complexity of AT is not considered when general technology is purchased, so that computers do not support some of the software programs or adaptive peripherals needed by children with disabilities. A team of professionals, consumers, technology developers, and standards organizations must plan together to ensure that technology is accessible to all.

Universal Design

"We must create spaces at all times that all can use, no matter their abilities, age or size."

—Ron Mace, architect, founder and program director of the Center for Universal Design[29]

Ron Mace was a visionary who used the term *universal design* (UD) to describe the concept of making all products and the built environment physically pleasing and usable to the greatest extent possible by everyone, regardless of their age, ability, or status in life. His work on accessible design was instrumental in the passage of national legislation prohibiting discrimination against people with disabilities, the Fair Housing Amendments Act of 1988, and the Americans with Disabilities Act of 1990. The principles of universal design are outlined in Box 19-5.

According to the Center for Universal Design, "the intent of UD is to simplify life for everyone by making products, communications, and the built environment more usable by as many people as possible at little or no extra cost."[29] Universal design is a proactive approach that can eliminate many barriers but does not replace the need for individualized AT. Although typical furnishings, toys, and instructional materials found in homes and classrooms may meet the needs of many, items that are "easier to handle, larger, less slippery, color coded, or in some ways more inviting and functional" (p. 5)[91] may be required for others.

BOX 19-5 Principles of Universal Design

Principle One:
Equitable Use
The design is useful and marketable to people with diverse abilities.

Principle Two:
Flexibility in Use
The design accommodates a wide range of individual preferences and abilities.

Principle Three:
Simple and Intuitive Use
Use of the design is easy to understand, regardless of the user's experience, knowledge, language skills, or current concentration level.

Principle Four:
Perceptible Information
The design communicates necessary information effectively to the user, regardless of ambient conditions or the user's sensory abilities.

Principle Five:
Tolerance for Error
The design minimizes hazards and the adverse consequences of accidental or unintended actions.

Principle Six:
Low Physical Effort
The design can be used efficiently and comfortably and with a minimum of fatigue.

Principle Seven:
Size and Space for Approach and Use
Appropriate size and space are provided for approach, reach, manipulation, and use regardless of user's body size, posture, or mobility.

Connell, B. R., Jones, M., Mace, R., Muller, J., Mullick, A., Ostroff, E., Sanford, J., Steinfeld, E., Story, M., & Vanderheiden, G. The Center for Universal Design (1997). The Principles of Universal Design, Version 2.0. Raleigh, NC: North Carolina State University. Retrieved September 2014 from http://www.ncsu.edu/ncsu/design/cud/about_ud/udprinciples.htm.

Positioning and Ergonomics

Positioning and ergonomics include the physical positioning of the child for comfort, function, and work; location of the child within the environment; and location of supports in relationship to the child. Seating, positioning, and mobility devices are often the foundation for successful use of AT, and they may be used to improve body stability, provide proximal trunk and head support, allow for exploration of the environment, and reduce localized skin pressure.[87]

Positioning should never be static in nature. The right seating and positioning equipment allow users to interact with their environment and perform tasks that are meaningful and life sustaining. "A task performance position is one that the person must be able to assume and maintain and in which the person can move" (p. 3).[64]

The environment cannot and should not come to the child; the child should be able to enter into and interact within the environment. One size does not fit all (Figure 19-3). With variances in physical size and stature, standard furniture can make it a challenge to provide adjustability to fit everyone comfortably. Individually designed seating and positioning allows users of AT to work in neutral, relaxed positions that

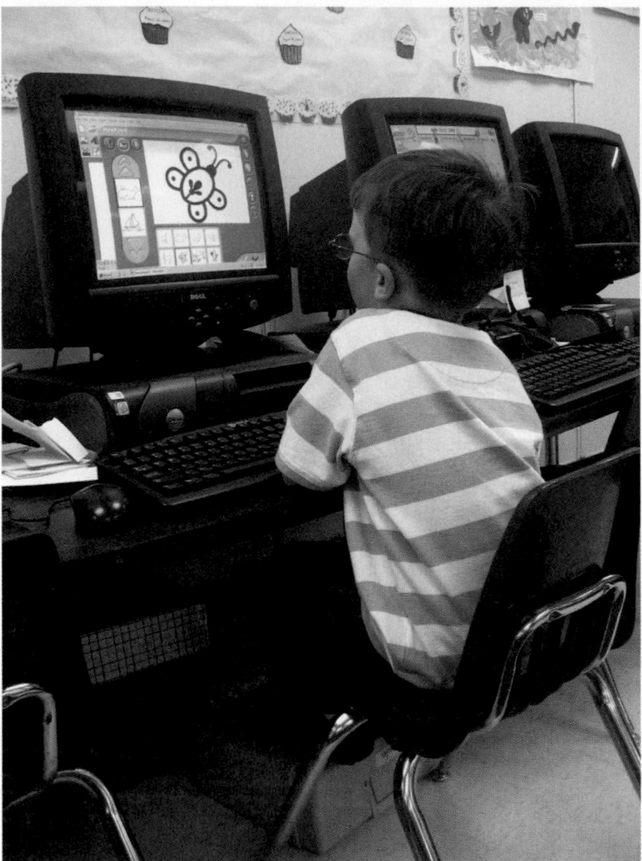

FIGURE 19-3 One size does not fit all. It is important to adjust learning environments to promote health and productivity. (Photo courtesy Judith Schoonover.)

consider energy conservation, which is important to maximize productivity while protecting health and minimizing the risk of injury. As technology becomes a more important part of children's lives, so does the need to pay attention to the health aspects of using computers, tablets, and mobile devices. American children typically spend between 1 and 3 hours a day at a computer, putting them at high risk for wrist, neck, and back problems.[35] If children, or those advocating on their behalf, learn at an early age how to adjust a workstation, they will make similar adjustments later in life. These habits and skills can be established as early as the preschool years. Many schools have chosen not to include ergonomics programs because of the costs often associated with implementation. Box 19-6 outlines some minor changes that have minimal or no costs associated with them.

BOX 19-6 Ergonomics: Budget-Minded Solutions/Tips for Home and School

Evaluate current equipment to determine whether it can be adjusted at all. If adjustable equipment is available, ensure that all users understand the need for it and how to adjust it. Educate and empower students to make their own workstation modifications by providing them with the tools and materials they require.

Recognize that lighting, glare, and proximity of the computer monitor to the user can all have negative impact on vision. The computer monitor should be at or slightly below eye level and approximately 24 inches away. Provide document holders at eye level to minimize eyestrain when copying.

Good ergonomic habits are best learned when modeled.

One size does not fit all. Provide a number of seating options and footrests for the user to choose from.

Never use the "legs" that many keyboards have attached on the bottom surface of the keyboard because they place the keyboard at a positive slope (slant the keyboard toward the operator). This position forces the user to bend wrists to touch the keys rather than maintaining a neutral position. If a slanted plane is desirable for visibility purpose, place keyboard on binder so that user's wrists are supported.

Obtain or make footrests—investigate whether your school or a local high school can make footrests as part of their woodworking program.

Make adjustments to the equipment as needed—providing several heights of work surfaces or sizes of chairs may be warranted.

If a mouse tray is unavailable, make sure that the mouse is close to the side of the user's body. This is necessary to ensure that the upper arm can remain relaxed and posture can remain as neutral as possible. In some cases, a lap tray can be used.

Costs can be minimized by involving school maintenance staff, woodworking classes, parent organizations, or service clubs to make adjustments to equipment.

Stretching programs (i.e., to stretch neck, spine, shoulders) can be downloaded from many reputable websites at no charge. If no changes can be made to the workstation, ensure that all students are educated on taking appropriate breaks and are given stretches.

Modified from Office ergonomics reminder sheet (2003). *Options Quarterly Online Newsletters*. Available at http://www.oiweb.com/pages/newsarchive03.html.

Participation: Supporting Life Skills with Assistive Technology

Occupational therapy practitioners work with children with significant disabilities. Although prerequisite skills may be necessary for successful use of certain devices, many children use a range of AT to address life skills such as communication, mobility, self-help, play and leisure, and work.[118]

Switch Use to Operate Toys and Appliances

Low technology, such as the use of simple switches and cause and effect toys/appliances or software, may be the initial AT system of choice. Occupational therapists may use these devices to help a child learn cause and build foundational skills for future AT systems. For some children with significant disabilities, simple devices that provide sensory input (e.g., fans, vibrators, music, lights) may be more motivating than some of the cause-effect toys or software. These devices can be hooked into an electronic aid to daily living (EADL) and then a switch can be used to turn them on and off. The EADL can run electronically operated toys or appliances and has functions that allow the child to control how the switch is used (e.g., a timer can be used so the child has to hit the switch every 30 seconds).

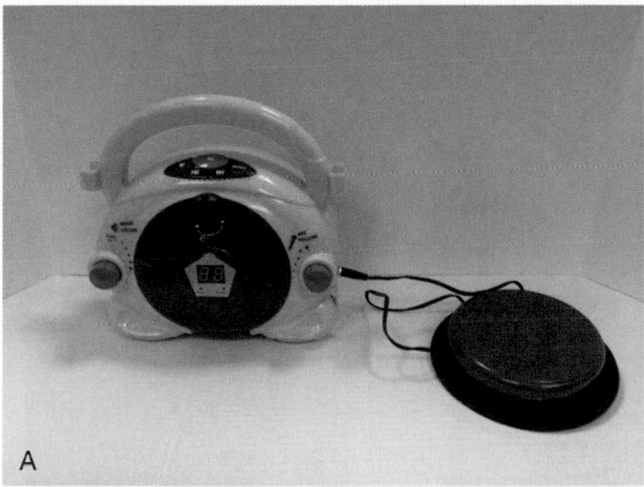

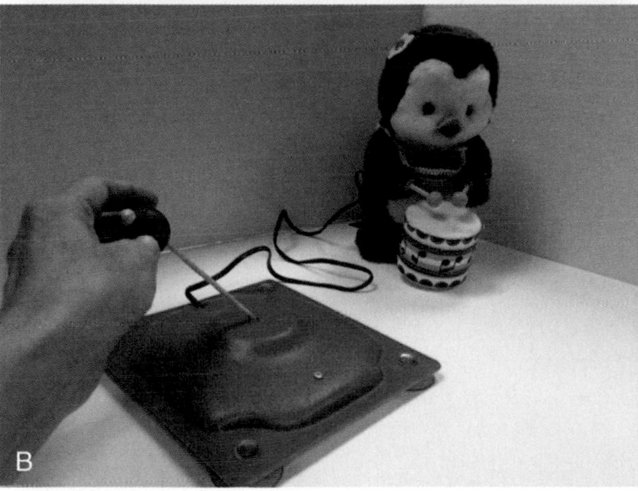

FIGURE 19-4 **A,** An example of a touch switch: the jelly bean switch. **B,** An example of a switch that is activated by pulling on the multicolored ball. (**A,** Photo courtesy Enabling Devices. **B,** Photo courtesy Judith Schoonover.)

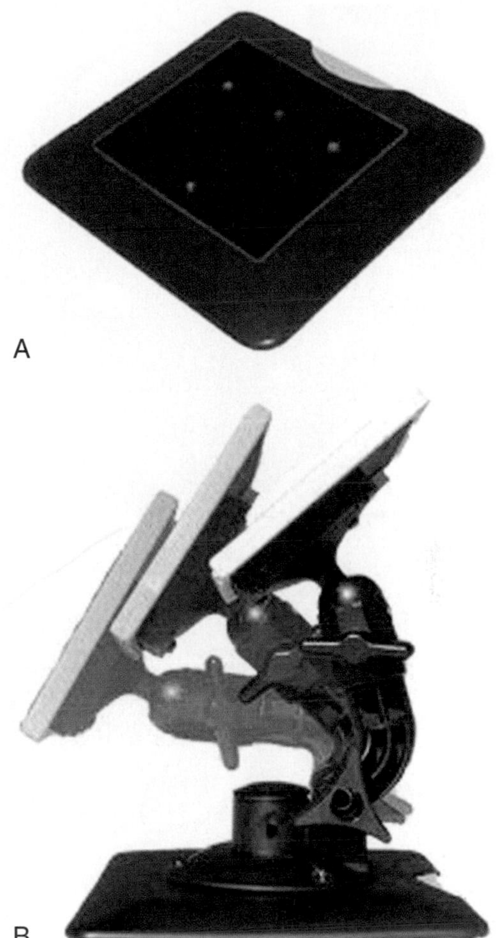

FIGURE 19-5 **A,** The Sensitrac flat pad switch. Switch is activated by a simple touch. **B,** The Sensitrac flat pad switch can be easily positioned for a child to access. (Photos courtesy Ablenet.)

Often, low-tech solutions are controlled through a single switch. Typically, a touch switch that requires a press and release is used (Figure 19-4*A*). However, for some children this type of switch may not be motivating, or the student may not have the physical skills needed to access the switch. Figure 19-4*B* shows an example of a switch that helps a student learn cause-effect relationships. Some children may not have the physical skills to press or pull against resistance and may use a switch that is activated through a light touch (Figure 19-5*A*). Switches can be mounted so that the position can be easily adjusted to improve access for a student (Figure 19-5*B*). Although this switch requires minimal controlled movement, its cognitive demand is greater than that for the switches pictured. The touch-free switch may be too abstract for students with low cognitive skills.[31]

Through the use of low-tech tools, switches, and simple cause-effect activities, all children can participate in a variety of learning activities at home and in the classroom. Figure 19-6*A* shows an option for participation in a water play activity through a switch toy. Figure 19-6*B* shows an option for participation in a gardening activity, and Figure 19-6*C* illustrates an option for game play with peers. Switches may allow partial participation, in which the student uses a switch to complete one step of the task. For example in Figure 19-6*B*, the student pressed the switch to turn on the Waterpik; then another student used the Waterpik to water the flowers.

Switch Use with Computers

Many of the switches that can be used to access low-tech solutions (see Figures 19-4 and 19-5) can also be used to access the computer. More complex switch systems use indirect selection. In deciding on a switch-driven system, consideration should be given to the motoric and cognitive requirements of the system.[31] For example, a child who is able to accurately and reliably hit a switch at 9 months of age does not have the cognitive skills to understand the concept of scanning. In addition, research suggests that the placement of the switch (e.g., a head switch versus a switch that is struck with the hand) may have a cognitive component that affects a child's accuracy.[56] A single (or dual) switch can be used to run systems such as scanning.

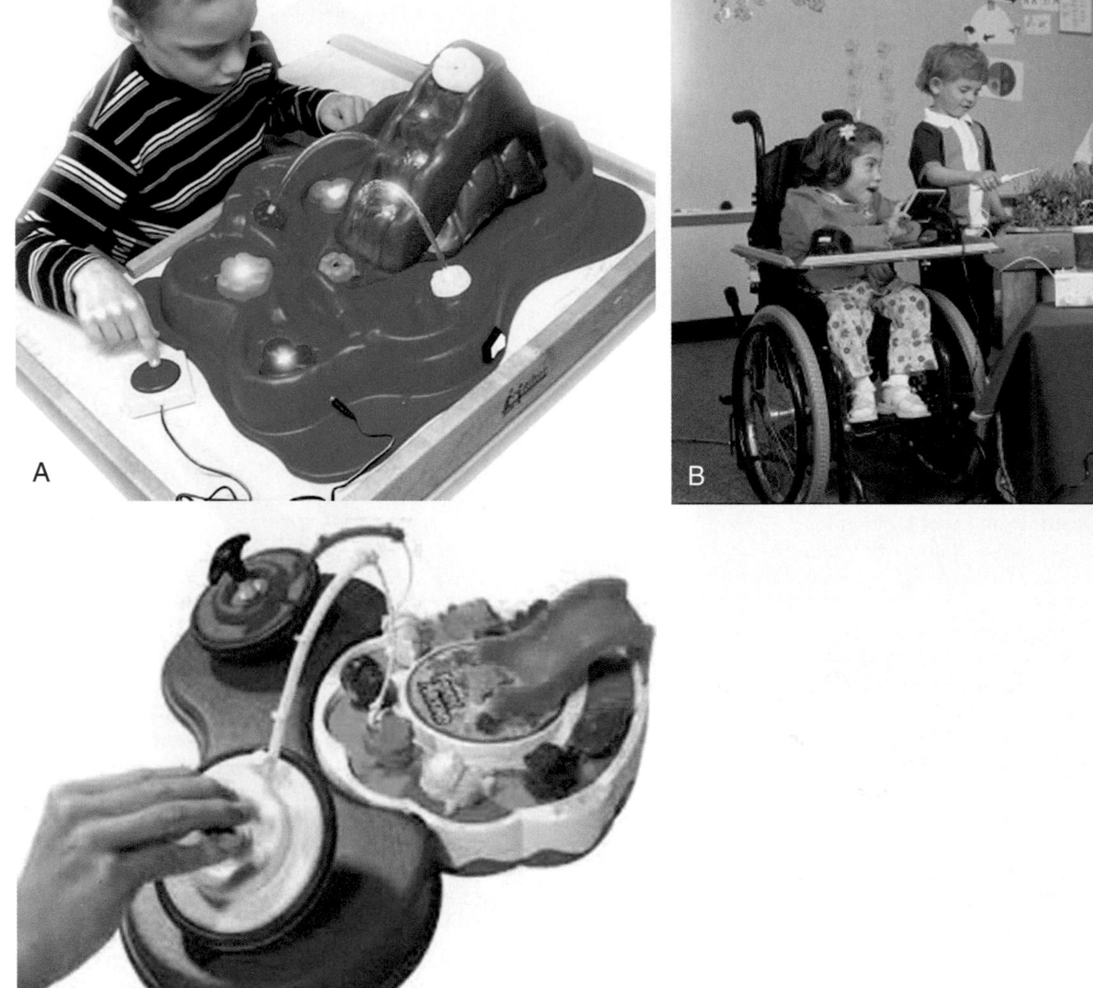

FIGURE 19-6 **A,** The child uses the switch to play with the water toy. **B,** The child uses the switches to participate in a gardening activity with her peers. **C,** The child uses the switch to turn on the Bed Bugs game. (**A** and **C,** Photo courtesy Ablenet; **B,** Photo courtesy Enabling Devices.)

Alternative and Augmentative Communication

"If all my possessions were taken from me with one exception, I would choose to keep the power of communication, for by it I would soon regain all the rest."

—Daniel Webster, 1822

Verbal communication is an inherent function of human beings and lends quality and detail to social interactions with others. Communication is not designed to be a solitary activity, because the purpose of communication is to exchange and share information with another individual. Children with disabilities may present with a range of performance levels related to receptive and expressive language. The National Joint Committee for the Communications of Persons with Severe Disabilities states, "all persons, regardless of the extent or severity of their disabilities, have a basic right to affect, through communication, the conditions of their own existence."[81] In addition to this basic right, the committee has outlined specific communication rights that should be ensured during all daily communication acts with persons with disabilities (Box 19-7).

Alternative and augmentative communication (AAC) is defined as communication that does not require speech and that can be individualized to the unique needs of the child. An AAC system uses a combination of all the methods of communication available to a child. This can include "any residual speech, vocalizations, gestures, and communicative behaviors in addition to specific communication strategies and communication aids" (p. 7).[40] The overall purpose of AAC is to enable the transmission of a message to another individual. Research indicates that individuals with complex communication needs who do not gain successful access to AAC are at high risk for abuse, crime, unemployment, and limited social networks.[19,26]

Alternative and augmentative communication interventions should be dynamic and include not only the individual child, but also his or her primary communication partners. Beyond

BOX 19-7 Basic Communication Rights

1. The right to request desired objects, actions, events, and persons and to express personal preferences or feelings
2. The right to be offered choices and alternatives
3. The right to reject or refuse undesired objects, events, or actions, including the right to decline or reject all proffered choices
4. The right to request and be given attention from and interaction with another person
5. The right to request feedback or information about a state, object, person, or event of interest
6. The right to active treatment and intervention efforts to enable people with severe disabilities to communicate messages in whatever modes and as effectively and efficiently as their specific abilities will allow
7. The right to have communication acts acknowledged and responded to, even when the responder cannot fulfill the intent of these acts
8. The right to have access at all times to any needed augmentative and alternative communication devices and other assistive devices and to have those devices in good working order
9. The right to environmental contexts, interactions, and opportunities that expect and encourage persons with disabilities to participate as full communicative partners with other people, including peers
10. The right to be informed about the people, things, and events in one's immediate environment
11. The right to be communicated with in a manner that recognizes and acknowledges the inherent dignity of the person being addressed, including the right to be a part of communication exchanges about individuals that are conducted in his or her presence
12. The right to be communicated with in ways that are meaningful, understandable, and culturally and linguistically appropriate

From National Joint Committee for the Communication Needs of Persons with Severe Disabilities. (1992). Guidelines for meeting the communication needs of persons with severe disabilities. *ASHA, 34* (Suppl. 7), 1–8.

the obvious function of self-expression, AAC supports the development of language and emerging literacy skills, enhances participation in educational settings, facilitates friendships, and supports interactions with family members and people in the greater community.[32] When one family member relies on AAC, it always has an impact on the entire family unit.[57] For this reason, it is imperative to use a collaborative approach when evaluating and implementing AAC supports. Various members of the team will bring different levels of expertise to share: child and parents will have the best knowledge of daily communication needs and routines; teachers will have knowledge related to literacy and instruction; speech-language pathologists are experts in language development; and occupational and physical therapists provide services related to positioning, accessing, and physically using the AAC system.

Attitude and acceptance of AAC play a role in its impact on the quality and function of interactions. AAC systems are designed with layout and components that match the desires, preferences, abilities, skills, and environmental contexts of the child. Many parents are fearful that AAC will interfere with speech development, when in fact it has been found to enhance it.[16] A family-centered approach should be used when AAC is integrated into the child's daily experiences and interactions, to ensure caregiver support of its use.[78]

BOX 19-8 Strategies to Facilitate Communicative Interaction

1. Structure the environment to foster interaction.
2. Attend to the child. Solicit a shared focus.
3. Provide meaningful opportunities for communication.
4. Have realistic expectations for the child.
5. Provide appropriate language input.
6. Avoid yes/no questions and "test" questions.
7. Pace the interaction. Give the student time to communicate. WAIT.
8. Follow the child's lead. Respond to his or her attempts to communicate.
9. Provide models for the child's expressive modes of communication. Coach the child as needed.
10. Prompt if necessary. Remember to fade out prompts to natural cues. Enjoy communication.

Adapted from Special Education Technology Center, Ellensburg, WA.

Communicative interaction has four purposes[77]: expression of wants and needs, information transfer, social closeness, and social etiquette. There are three types of AAC communicators[38]: emergent communicators who have no reliable method of symbolic expression, context-dependent communicators who do have symbolic communication but are limited to specific contexts because they are intelligible only to familiar partners or may have insufficient vocabulary, and independent communicators who can communicate with anyone on any topic. Children who use AAC are most frequently identified as "responders," whereas typically developing peers consistently act as the "initiators" of communication.[30] These classifications can serve as a foundation for identifying and establishing an AAC system in conjunction with the use of strategies that facilitate communication (Box 19-8).

Types of Alternative and Augmentative Communication Devices

AAC devices can be viewed on at least two continua, including no-tech to high-tech systems and aided or unaided communication methods. Depending on their age, contexts, and skills, children may use a combination of aided and unaided communication and a combination of low- and high-tech devices. Unaided or body-based communication is no-tech and consists of vocalizations, gestures, facial expressions, sign language, pantomime, eye gaze, and/or pointing. All people use some combination of unaided communication. Children with disabilities often use gestures, facial expressions, and body language as allowed by their functional skills.

Aided communication systems are distinguished as either nonelectronic or electronic communication aids and require the child to be able to use a symbol system.[32] Nonelectronic aids are considered low-tech and include communication boards or books, picture-based systems, or paper and pencil. Picture-based systems are used increasingly with children in preschool, children with significant disabilities, and children with autism (Figure 19-7). Some children may find it easier to

FIGURE 19-7 Example of a low-tech communication board. (Photo courtesy Judith Schoonover.)

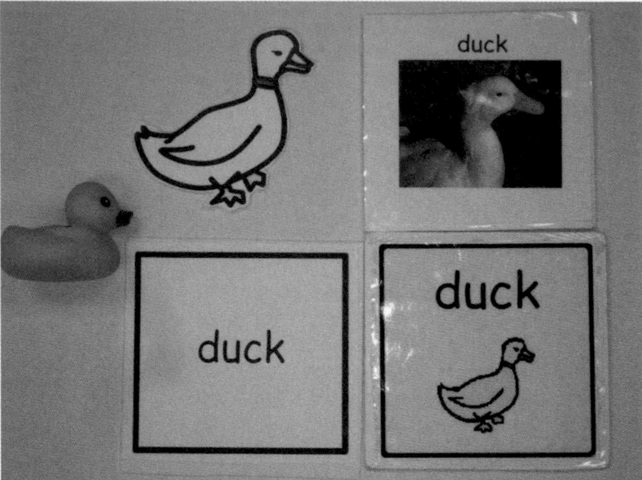

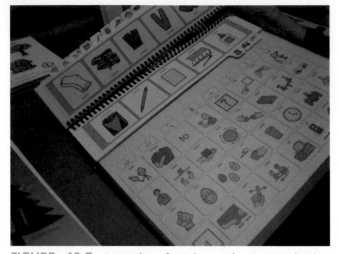

FIGURE 19-8 Multiple means of representation clockwise from left: an object, a TOBI, a photo, a picture symbol, and a word. (Photo courtesy of Judith Schoonover.)

use visual-based systems of communication and to process content delivered using such systems.

Picture Exchange Communication System (PECS) is a form of ACC often used with individuals with a variety of communicative, cognitive, and physical difficulties, including preschoolers, adolescents, and adults who have little or no verbal ability. Visual representation such as objects, photographs, realistic drawings, line drawings, and written words can be used to increase understanding, communication, and social connectedness and can take many forms depending on the environment and the circumstances under which they are used. Visual bridges[62] can be designed to assist students to communicate about themselves using a combination of written words, objects, photos, computer-generated picture symbols, clip art, or other visual cues. Visual bridges can also be used during reading and writing activities. Emergent readers benefit from graphics paired with text to reinforce the meaning of print.

For individuals who have difficulty understanding two-dimensional visual representation systems such as photos, drawings, and graphics, PECS can be useful. For example, a True Object Based Icon (TOBI)—a drawing, picture, or photo cut out in the actual shape or outline of the item that is represented (Figure 19-8)—can be used with these individuals. Another example of providing symbolic representation of language, allowing communicators to relate to objects and experiences, are tangible symbols,[95] two- and three-dimensional manipulatives that can be objects, parts of an object, or an associated object that conveys meaningful information to the user or represents their communicative intent. For example, a small bit of chain might indicate time to swing, or a circle formed from a pipe cleaner may indicate "morning circle" (Figure 19-9).

Electronic communication aids or devices are generally considered more high-tech and may include speech generating devices (SGDs), talking frames, cell or smart phones, tablets, or computers. Speech-generating devices may produce digitized or synthesized speech output.[32] Digitized speech records a person's actual voice and allows flexibility in selecting a child, male, or female voice; however, it requires a lot of memory for storage and is limited to only what is recorded and stored. Synthesized speech is generated electronically but has the

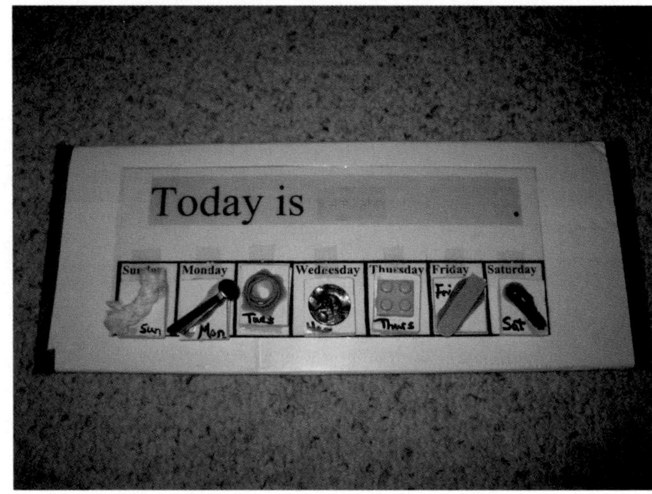

FIGURE 19-9 Example of a tactile symbol communication board. (Photo courtesy Judith Schoonover.)

advantage of text-to-speech capabilities. The intelligibility of synthesized speech can vary depending on the type of system.

Different types of simple AAC devices are available. One example can be seen in Figure 19-10*A*. This device can be used for communication, by containing a recorded message that is activated each time the user presses the switch (Figure 19-10*B*). Another simple AAC device for individuals who are ambulatory is shown in Figure 19-10*C*; it is worn like a watch and can have several prerecorded messages. These messages are easy to change and symbols can be used to help the user remember the messages. Using symbols when shopping can help users remember items (Figure 19-10*D*). Devices like those in Figure 19-10*E* benefit children who may eventually use more high-tech AAC.

High-tech electronic communication aids generally are either computer-based systems or dedicated systems. Computer-based systems are often considered in addition to a communication system. Computer-based systems are made up of computers that can perform as a communication system through the use

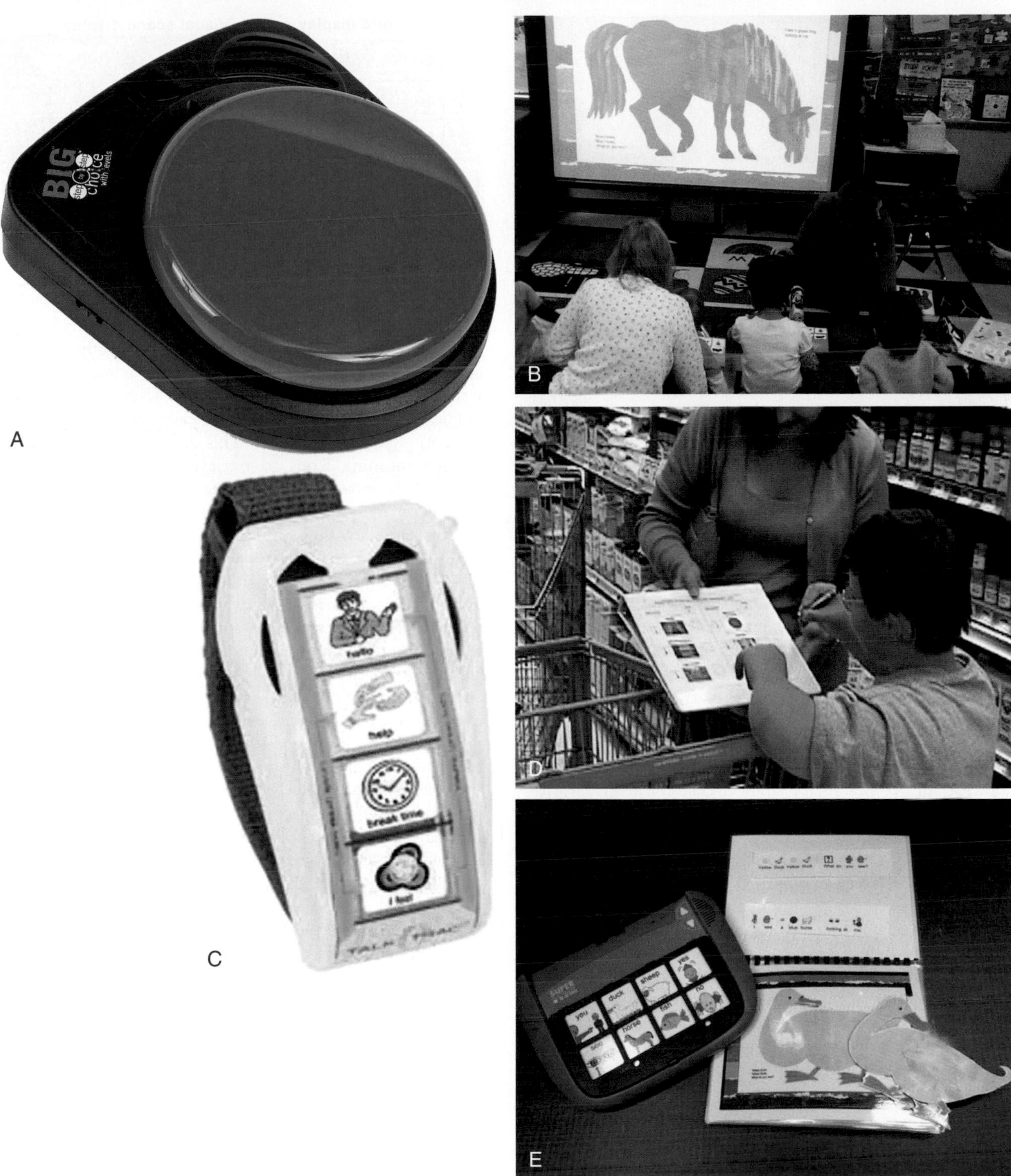

FIGURE 19-10 AAC devices. **A,** BIGMack communication device. **B,** Using a continuum of communication supports to participate in storytime. **C,** Talk Trac communication device. **D,** Using symbols while shopping to help the user remember. **E,** Supertalker to retell story. (Photos courtesy Judith Schoonover.)

of specialized software and other modifications, but can also carry out other functions such as environmental control. Ideally, computer-based systems should be able to be mounted on wheelchairs or easily portable in some other manner. Dedicated systems operate primarily as electronic communication aids (Figure 19-11) with hardware and software features specifically designed for communication purposes. These systems are available in various sizes and weights and provide auditory, visual, or printed output. All electronic communication devices are programmed with individualized overlays. The board's

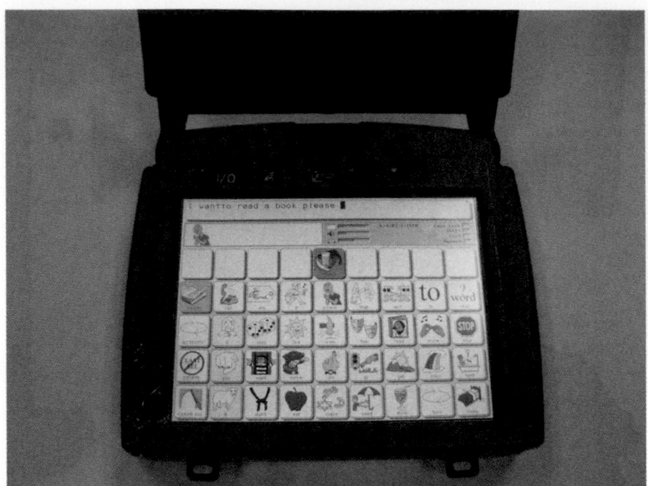

FIGURE 19-11 Example of a dedicated, dynamic display augmentative and alternative communication device. (Photo courtesy of Judith Schoonover.)

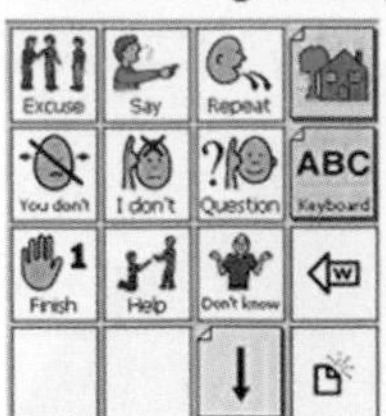

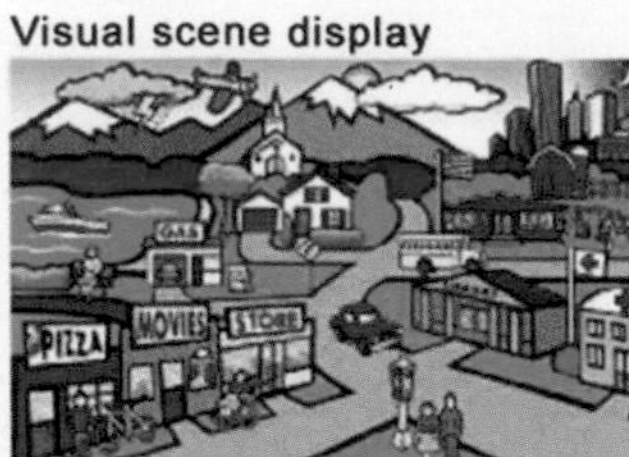

FIGURE 19-12 Visual scene display versus grid. (From Blackstone, S. [2004]. Visual scene displays. *Augmentative Communications News, 16*, 1–5.)

overlays can provide as few as two and as many as 128 choices to the child.

In recent years, relatively inexpensive mobile technology from touch-screen phones to tablet devices has become a popular and sometimes controversial alternative to more traditional and often more expensive speech-generating devices. Mobile apps provide many of the vocabulary building and text-to-speech features of other AAC devices and some have features that allow programming "on the fly." Although mobile technology may be smaller and more portable, work faster, and have a more socially acceptable appearance, customizability, learnability, durability, and supports for training may be compromised.[1] Access considerations include turning on the device, navigation between programs or screens, and icon selection. Because of their mainstream popularity, many people are aware of mobile devices as possible systems to be considered to deliver communication-related systems. Caution must be exercised to avoid making the user fit the device as opposed to determining the right device for the individual. With new technologies come new approaches to providing communication devices, including one developed by a speech-language pathologist and an occupational therapist that tries to integrate and use multisensory convergence (motor, auditory, visual) to promote the development of language.[58]

Selecting an Alternative and Augmentative Communication System

A number of factors are considered in designing a high-tech AAC system, the first of which is to assess understanding of symbolic representation.[14] Receptive understanding of functional objects, visual matching, and spelling and literacy skills related to word recognition are all cognitive skills that help define the symbol system that is necessary. Examples of symbol systems include real objects, photographs, symbols, and traditional orthography (use of letters and words).

The control interface or manner in which the device is accessed may include use of a keyboard; single, dual, or multiple switch arrays; and joystick, mouse, or other alternative pointing devices.[32] Selections can be made directly by pointing or touching or via an indirect method such as auditory or visual scanning, directed scanning, or coded access. To allow communication faster than the rate of keying in text, encoding (or symbol) systems are used. This language uses sequenced multiple-meaning icons to retrieve words, phrases, or sentences. Like word prediction, many communication systems come with message prediction. Some of the more advanced systems can learn the communication "style" of the user and begin to predict with greater accuracy.

In addition to the input method, AAC devices use two visual display types (screens). A dynamic communication display offers thousands of graphics (some that are electronically animated) and text options. The display changes (using the same message-formation process that produces natural speech) based on the choices of the user. They are often accessed via a touch screen; however, alternatives are available. Dynamic displays, such as the one in Figure 19-11, are helpful for children who may have difficulties with memory, but they do require a high level of visual attention, constant decision making, and the need for mastery of object permanence. The second type, visual scene displays, offer "hot spots" that are contextually embedded within graphics that provide more meaningful and individualized interactive displays (Figure 19-12). Drager[44] made a comparison of visual scene displays and more traditional grid layouts used by typically developing 2½-year-old children during communicative tasks during a birthday party. Findings indicated that performance was better using the visual scene display.

Once a device has been obtained, programming of the device and training of the child and all communication partners are essential for success. Collaborative efforts should be taken to identify vocabulary that includes conversational messages (greetings, information sharing, and requests), core vocabulary (for literate or preliterate children to encourage language and cognitive development), and fringe vocabulary (unique to the individual child's activities, preferences, family, environments, favorite expressions, etc.).[32] Vocabulary needs will vary by context, communication mode, and individual characteristics.[15] Specific functions of communication, such as requesting; rejecting/protesting; gaining attention; engaging in greetings, farewells, and other social niceties; commenting; achieving social closeness; asking for information; and confirming/denying,[43] must be taught to optimize communication competence (Box 19-9).[77] As with all other AT, communication systems are constantly being upgraded and changed. Continuing education courses and additional training can help

BOX 19-9 Communication Competence

Linguistic Competence: adequate mastery of the native language (i.e., vocabulary and grammar) plus mastery of the code (e.g., signs or symbols) required to operate the AAC system.

Operational Competence: mastery of technical skills required to operate the system, i.e., the motor and cognitive skills required to signal a message or to operate specific device features (e.g., pointing, signing, visual scanning, operating switches, controlling cursors, editing).

Social Competence: knowledge and skill in the social rules of communication (e.g., making appropriate eye contact, sharing the balance of talking and listening), and using communication for a range of different purposes (e.g., social chatting, requesting items, responding to others, contradicting people).

Strategic Competence: flexibility to adapt communicative style to suit the receiver (e.g., signing more slowly to strangers, turning up the volume on the communication aid).

From Light, J. (1989). Toward a definition of communicative competence for individuals using augmentative and alternative communication systems. *Augmentative and Alternative Communication, 5*, 137–144.

therapists become familiarized with the terminology, communication strategies, and available hardware and software.

Computers

Use of personal computers is becoming more prevalent in school, home, and work settings. The computer is a flexible, motivating, and powerful instructional tool that can facilitate individualized teaching and learning. Computers with or without specialized software provide multiple means of communicating, playing, exploring, self-expression, interacting with the environment, learning cause and effect, and completing school and work-related tasks with greater degrees of independence. Most children with and without disabilities have had some exposure to a computer system by the time they enter school. At home, the computer might be used for recreation, entertainment, communication, work, and study. Social connections with others can be formed through e-mail, instant messaging, and social networking sites. For example, some adolescents with disabilities describe social networks and friendships that they have been able to develop using the computer, Internet access, and appropriate software programs.[108]

A computer can motivate children to learn and develop a large repertoire of skills. It provides simulations of experiences that some cannot otherwise experience. The computer is also infinitely patient with drill and practice and can provide the repetition needed for some children to learn. An almost endless variety of software programs, input devices, and output devices are available to customize computers to meet individual needs.[6] Young children can be introduced to a progression of systems that follows their developmental and functional needs. Success using simple systems precedes the use of more complex systems. Table 19-5 outlines benefits of computer use for children.

At school, children typically use word processing programs, the Internet, e-mail, and virtual classrooms in some aspect of their education. Software programs cover most academic subjects as well as recreational and competitive activities. The multimedia features of the computer can support learning rules, turn taking, and social skills. Math software and Internet sites include features such as virtual manipulatives or drills; creative writing software has recording features, sound, graphics, and animations; and keyboarding software teaches typing, as software and website designers continue to add features that make their products and sites accessible to a growing range of people and abilities.

The judicious use of computers and software can help develop literacy or strengthen skills through the use of games, screen readers, and online books. "Virtual field trips" make it possible to visit and explore environments that might otherwise be inaccessible, and computer simulations can provide preparation for social situations, academic tasks, prevocational training, and driver education. For children who are unable to recognize print in traditional formats, modifications to access the same text as that for their peers can decrease their dependence on the support of others in the environment to read or write for them. When, as a result of motor, emotional, or attention difficulties, children are challenged to produce art products or written work, the computer can assist in generating digital artwork or text that is neat and uniform in appearance. Producing more accurate, legible, or attractive work can increase self-esteem and self-expression and decrease frustration. As with any tool, the user must be aware of its features and trained in its applications and maintenance to receive full benefits. Successful computer access requires a means to provide input into the system, receive output (or information) from the computer, and process that information to use it in a functional, meaningful manner. Various types of computers (e.g., Macintosh or personal computer [PC]) are available in the home, school, clinical, and work settings. Before recommending the purchase of software programs or adapted access devices, the memory and technology of the system must be evaluated to determine its compatibility with the program. Now, many software programs are both PC and Mac compatible. For example, alternative keyboards can be used on either machine without significant reconfiguration. However, because certain hardware and access devices remain specific to either the PC or the Mac, therapists should attend to these specifications. Competencies that school-based occupational therapists should possess include the ability to operate major computing systems used in public schools and troubleshoot system problems, establish networks using telecommunications systems, operate general application programs, apply teacher utility tools, and provide computer-based instruction.[59]

Input

In considering different input systems for accessing computers or tablets, the "least change" principle should be applied. This means that a standard keyboard and standard workstation with some modifications are preferred over an expanded keyboard or other type of input device if the child can use them (Figure 19-13), exemplifying the concept of least restrictive environment (Table 19-6). Interventions to enable computer access are listed in Table 19-7.

Output Systems and Information Processing

Output is the product or outcome that is produced when using a computer. Like input, output can also accommodate the needs of individuals with disabilities. Information (output)

TABLE 19-5 Benefits of Computers for Young Children

Benefit	Examples
Put child in control	Use child-directed software
	Allow child to move at his or her own pace
	Are accessible to children with limited motor control
	Use two-switch step scanning for simple cognitive interface
Engage the child cognitively	Use two-switch software whereby each switch has a distinct function
	Provide trial-and-error learning
	Provide logical consequences to the child's efforts
	Use of patterns and use of surprise
	Provide experiences with familiar objects and tasks
	Allow for active versus passive learning
Provide opportunities for choice making	Sustain attention—increase opportunity for control and cognitive engagement
	Further expand awareness of consequences
	Provide error-free learning environment
Provide language immersion	Provide voice-output feedback describing child's actions
	Use simple but functional language
	Provide opportunities for sound play
	Offer predictable repeated lines with periodic surprise lines to go along with the action
	Relate three-dimensional experiences with objects and toys to two-dimensional screen
Provide opportunities for joint attention and shared interaction	Give opportunity for adult-child interaction
	Encourage pointing, showing, and shared enjoyment
	Provide opportunity for the child to take the lead and the adult to follow along and support
	Provide opportunities for child-child interaction
Facilitate communicative interaction	Allow the child to express ideas
	Provide voice-output and visual information that may be used to communicate to someone else
Provide multisensory feedback with consistency and repetition of language and cognitive concepts	Allow virtual manipulation of objects to develop cognitive skills
	Provide immediate feedback to child
	Allow child to control repetition as desired
	Reinforce emerging literacy skills
	Reinforce emerging mathematical skills or sequence, numbers, and patterns within a play context—not adult directed
Ensure cognitive simplicity	Present concepts in small steps
	Help child maintain attention by providing immediate success
	Help child stay out of a random "guessing mode" or "trying to please mode," which could lead to inaccurate or confusing consequences

From Burkhart, L. J. *Effective use of computers with young children.* Available at http://www.lburkhart.com/handcomp.html.

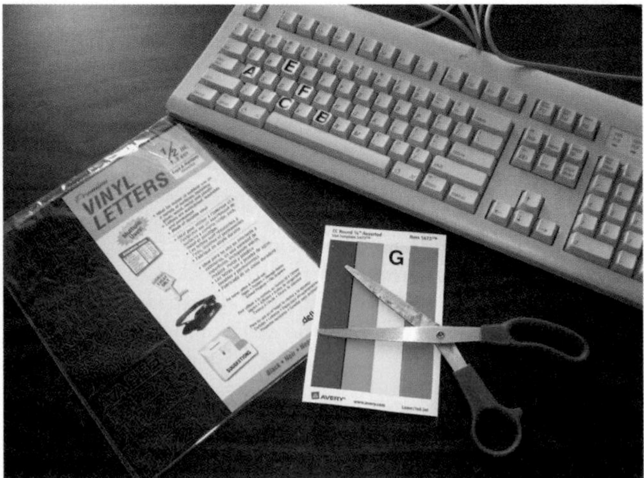

FIGURE 19-13 Example of low-tech keyboard modifications including color-coding and enlarging letters on keys. (Photo courtesy Judith Schoonover.)

from the computer is displayed visually on the monitor or printed from the printer. For a child with visual, perceptual, or cognitive impairment, adaptations to the monitor may need to be considered. Some printers provide braille output, and several software programs provide voice output. Some of these programs read text, whereas others provide output regarding all the functions of the computer. Voice output systems can help support learning and computer use and exploration for students with learning disabilities, cognitive delays, autism, and visual impairments.

The computer's output and the user's successful processing of information are often closely related. If the user cannot successfully process and use the information received from the computer in a meaningful and functional manner, he or she will abandon the system. With the increased screen resolution and the complexity of graphics now available in computers, some users with visual-perceptual difficulties find the visual information they receive distracting or overwhelming. For example, a child who has poor figure-ground skills may have difficulty with graphics that are cluttered and complex.

TABLE 19-6 Problem Solving for Computer Access (Starting with a Standard Computer Workstation)

Problem	Potential Solutions
Difficulty pressing one or more keys	Change height of table or chair Change position of keyboard Change sensitivity of key or active delayed acceptance Use a keyguard Use an expanded keyboard with larger keys Use a stylus, mouthstick, or headstick Change size of letters on keyboard
Tendency to produce multiple characters rather than one	Change height of table or chair Change position of keyboard Change sensitivity of key or active delayed acceptance Deactivate auto-repeat
Difficulty holding down more than one key simultaneously	Use Sticky Keys feature or utility Use a mechanical key latch
Ability to use only one hand	Teach student to use one-handed typing techniques for standard keyboard Use a chord keyboard Reconfigure the keyboard to use one-handed pattern Use onscreen keyboard and mouse for typing
Difficulty with the standard mouse	Use a trackball Use a trackpad Create a mouse track template Use MouseKeys feature of operating system
Slow or inefficient input	Increase keyboarding practice so that motor patterns are more automatic Set up templates for standard formats Use macros and abbreviation expansion for repeated words and phrases Use word prediction software programs
Drooling	Use a keyboard cover (Safe Skin) Use alternative keyboards that are not moisture sensitive
Difficulty seeing the screen or highlights	Ensure that the monitor is not facing a window or that the blinds are drawn Use an antiglare filter Reduce glare by turning down overhead lights Change size of font Change font (serif fonts are better for reading text; sans serif fonts are better for letter recognition) Change attributes of font (bold) Change color of background or text for greater contrast Set screen to monochrome Use a large screen or lower screen resolution Use a screen magnifier (hardware or software)
Difficulty reading text	Ensure that the monitor is not facing a window or that the blinds are drawn Use an antiglare filter Reduce glare by turning down overhead lights Change size of font Change font (serif fonts are better for reading text; sans serif fonts are better for letter recognition) Change attributes of font (bold) Change color of background or text for greater contrast Set screen to monochrome Use a large screen or lower screen resolution Use a screen magnifier (hardware or software) Use a voice output tool (screen reader)
Tendency to be distracted by sound	Turn off sound features of application Turn down volume from system control panel
Difficulty hearing feedback	Use hearing protectors or noise-canceling ear protectors Turn up volume (can use headphones) Use amplified speakers
Difficulty finding correct key on the keyboard	Use stickers or enlarged key letters to highlight correct keys Increase size or contrast of keyboard caps Use color coding for "landmark" keys Use Kids Keys Keyboard (for younger students) Mask nonapplicable keys

TABLE 19-6 Problem Solving for Computer Access (Starting with a Standard Computer Workstation)—cont'd

Problem	Potential Solutions
Difficulty shifting between information on the screen, the keyboard, and the desktop	Use document clip to suspend printed page next to monitor Change position of keyboard Change position of monitor Use a touch screen and on-screen keyboard
Difficulty remembering keyboard functions	Develop a "cheat sheet" of keyboard shortcuts to keep close by Develop keyboard mnemonics to aid memory of keyboard functions
Decreased motivation	Recheck student goals to ensure student involvement in goal-making process Try a different software program to address goal Change the purpose for which the computer is being used Change the access method Decrease the amount of time on the computer Scale the activity to the student's skills (up or down)

From Swinth, Y. L., & Anson, D. (1998). Alternatives to handwriting: Keyboarding and text-generation techniques for schools. In J. Case-Smith (Ed.), *AOTA self-paced clinical course: Occupational therapy: Making a difference in school system practice.* Rockville, MD: AOTA.

TABLE 19-7 Computer Access

Input	Ergonomic keyboard Disabling auto-repeat function Keyboard adaptations (color-coded, alphabetic, keyguards) Direct (expanded) and indirect (letter scanning, switch) selection
Alternate keyboards	Membrane: require less pressure to activate and allow customization of overlays Miniature: smaller and lighter; designed for users with decreased strength and range of motion Chord: designed to minimalize finger travel; require multiple simultaneous keystrokes to produce letters and phrases Onscreen keyboards: provide image of keyboard that can be accessed via mouse, touch, trackball, joystick, eyegaze
Mouse emulators	Devices that simulate mouse movement and selection, including arrow keys, touch pads, trackballs, head pointers, interactive whiteboards, and touch windows and screens
Voice recognition	The computer or tablet recognizes and translates voice sounds into text or commands (refer to Evolve website for more information)
Other input	Other types of input systems used with children include eye-gaze systems, braille, TouchFree Switch, and a Tongue Touch Keypad. Once the user activates the keys, a signal is sent to an interface box connected to the computer

Software

Careful decisions must be made to find programs that match interests and skills. With the burgeoning number of software programs available, from simple to highly complex, many with disabilities can use common software programs that are available to everyone. Often software programs require that the user make specific, discrete responses to visual, auditory, or tactile stimuli. The user must be able to attend briefly and have the interest and motivation to activate a toy or a computer purposefully. Computer activities and programs, including public domain software, can be used to teach basic skills, such as object permanence, sustained attention, and cause-and-effect relationships. Other computer programs teach skills in discrimination, matching, and directionality. The OTP can determine whether and how the software customizes the video and audio display to meet students' individualized needs.

Because computers operate using different input and output methods and a large variety of software programs are available, they are useful tools to promote children's functional independence in life roles. Children can have opportunities to use computers throughout their school years and into their work settings; they can also use computers as environmental control devices and for play and leisure exploration.

Electronic Aids for Daily Living

Originally EADLs were known as environmental control units (ECUs). These are systems that allow the child to interact with and manipulate one or more electronic appliances, such as a television, radio, CD player, lights, telephone, or fan, using voice activation, switch access, a computer interface, or adaptations such as X-10 units (transmitters and receivers) that use a communications "language," allowing compatible products to interact with each other using the existing electrical wiring. The EADL should meet primary needs as well as any long-range goals. The system should also be fairly easy to assemble, learn to use, and maintain. As mentioned previously, EADLs can be integrated into a computer system. They also can be standalone systems. Some of these systems have a discrete control interface (an electronic device is turned either on or off, such

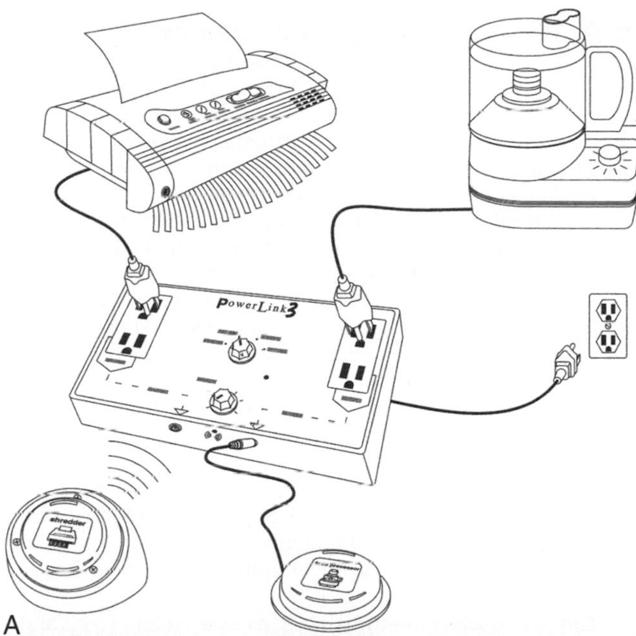

A

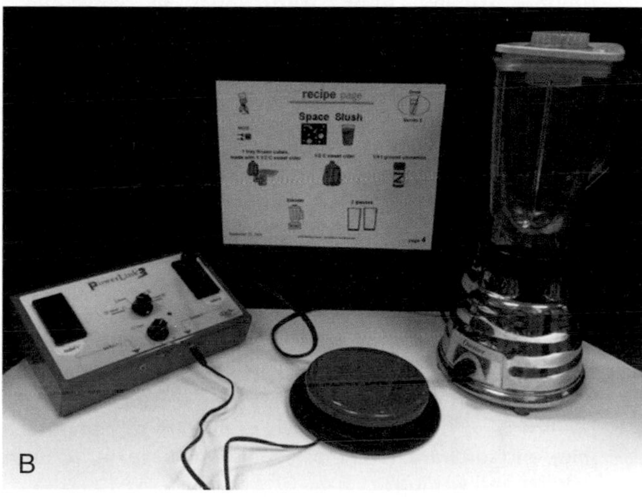

B

FIGURE 19-14 Schematic of an EADL setup with the Powerlink. (Drawing courtesy Ablenet.)

as a light, fan, or television), and others are capable of continuous control interface (devices that operate in successively greater or smaller degrees of control). Lowering and raising the volume on a television and dimming a light are examples of continuous control. A common EADL setup used with children is shown in Figure 19-14. Many EADL options are available for a variety of settings.

Changing the Landscape in Education: Planning for Every Student in the Twenty-First Century

Universal Design for Learning

One aspect of universal access that is gaining increased attention in the schools is universal design for learning (UDL).[94] UDL is defined in the Higher Education Opportunity Act (P.L.110-315) as:

A research-based framework for designing curriculum—including goals, methods, materials, and assessments—that enables all individuals to gain knowledge, skills, and enthusiasm for learning. Universal design for learning provides curricular flexibility (in activities, in the ways information is presented, in the ways students respond or demonstrate knowledge, and in the ways students are engaged) to reduce barriers, provide appropriate supports and challenges, and maintain high achievement standards for all students, including those with disabilities (HEOA, P.L. 110-315, §103[a][24]).

The concept of universal design (UD) was referred to by the Center for Applied Special Technology[28] as a framework for educational reform based on decades of brain research and focused on providing curriculum and materials to support learners with diverse needs in today's schools. Principles of UD in the educational environment assume that students with a variety of skills and needs will be participants in learning and that the goals, curriculum, instructional materials, and assessments need to proactively anticipate and address this diversity through alternatives, options, and adaptations. School administrators have placed increased emphasis on the development and implementation of a universally designed curriculum that allows all children equal opportunity to learn and demonstrate what they have learned. UDL advocates for more than one way to represent content (the "what" of learning), plan and execute learning activities (the "how" of learning), and achieve and maintain learner engagement (the "why" of learning). It involves developing and improving learning environments where all children are included.

Three principles form the framework of UDL[27]:

1. Multiple means of representation to give learners various ways to acquire information and knowledge (e.g., more than one example, critical features highlighted, use of media and formats, use of background context)
2. Multiple means of actions and expression to provide learners with options to demonstrate what they know (e.g., flexible models of skilled performance, opportunities to practice with supports, ongoing, relevant feedback, flexible opportunities for demonstrating skill)
3. Multiple means of engagement to tap into learners' interests, offer appropriate challenges, and increase motivation (e.g., choices of content and tools, adjustable levels of challenge, choices of rewards, choices of learning context).

Assistive technology and accessible software are important elements of a universally designed curriculum.[61] Through their professional assessment and unique understanding of the relationship between the environment, the person, and demands of occupational engagement, OTPs in school settings have practiced UDL principles and provided interventions that include multiple means of representing what they want the student to learn or do, accommodating for differences in perception; engaging the student to maintain that "just-right" challenge of attention motivation and self-regulation; and allowing students to "show what they know," as well as assessing the effectiveness of their intervention.[101] UD, UDL, and AT share the goal of reducing barriers and facilitating participation, yet UD and UDL do not replace the need to provide AT *devices* and particularly AT *services.* Assistive technology is based on an individual need, whereas UDL is approached from an educational environment standpoint in which instructional design meets a diverse population of learning style and needs. Students may require individually selected AT devices in the form of communication devices, visual aids, mobility supports, particular software, and adapted toys and tools in order to meaningfully participate in their roles as learners.

Instructional Technology

The influx of technology into our daily lives has resulted in dynamic and continuously changing tools altering the way we work, play, and socialize. The National Technology Plan for Education 2010 calls for schools to infuse curriculum and teaching methodology with technology skills. One of the many goals (and benefits) of the National Educational Technology Standards is designing student-centered, project-based, and online learning environments to meet the learning styles and needs of a wide range of students.

Schools use many kinds of instructional technology, providing software in most academic areas and for students of all ages. Examples include literacy software to develop letter-to-sound correspondence, math software for drill and practice of math facts, keyboarding software, and content-area software to reinforce concepts of science and social studies. Student assignments may include copying or producing written work using a word processor, research using the Internet, and e-mail. The inherent flexibility of technology offers opportunities for differentiation and scaffolding consistent with educational initiatives such as UDL and Response to Intervention with potential for improving the learning and achievement of all students. For example, use of a technology-based graphic organizer can provide nonreaders and readers with visual representation of a concept with text, images, and/or graphics and sound recordings. Educators can embed recorded directions and specific details to further enhance the graphics and support student learning.

This same technology plays an additional role for persons with disabilities by providing access to the learning environment. Features in software applications including adjustable user settings and alternate keyboard access can help reduce barriers and positively influence participation. Occupational therapy practitioners who are aware of the accessibility needs of their clients can advocate for the purchase of accessible instructional software. The National Center on Accessible Information Technology in Education promotes the use of electronic and information technology for individuals with disabilities in educational institutions at all academic levels and features a searchable database of questions and answers regarding accessible educational and instructional technology on its website (http://www.washington.edu/accessit/). Features to consider in evaluating accessibility of instructional software are outlined in Box 19-10.

Sometimes students with disabilities *require* technology that is helpful or sometimes used by students without disabilities such as calculators and word processors. Students with disabilities might *need* to use calculators or word processors or use them with modifications to participate in math or writing activities. This need redefines common classroom tools as AT that may be a required service in the IEP; therefore it is important to consider how important the tool is to the student's learning and participation.

BOX 19-10 Key Features to Consider In Evaluating Accessibility of Instructional Software

- Does the documentation describe accessibility features such as keyboard access to functions and features, options to change display settings such as size and font, options to turn off animation or blinking, and information about how to turn on captioning for video content of the software program?
- Is documentation available in electronic text so that it can be converted easily to braille or audio formats and can be read easily by people who use a screen reader or screen magnification program?
- Are all commands and functions available from the keyboard? Keyboard commands or shortcuts provide a simplified method for navigating through menus and dialogues and making selections. These features are important for individuals who may not see the cursor on screen or who have difficulty with mouse control.
- If information is conveyed in color, is it also conveyed using text?
- Can users select features such as size, color, font, and contrast to aid those with visual or perceptual difficulties?
- If the software uses animation such as flashing, rotating, or moving displays, is all information available when animation is turned off to support users who might become distracted or visually overwhelmed?
- Is information that is conveyed with sound such as music, narration, or tones also conveyed in another way?
- If a software program uses video to convey important information, is that information available in other formats such as a transcript or audio version? If the software program requires timed responses, can the response times be adjusted or disabled to meet user needs?
- Does the software program allow and support use of AT such as screen reading software, screen magnification software, voice recognition software, word prediction software, alternative keyboards or computer mice, and software that helps people who have difficulties reading and writing?

National Center on Accessible Information Technology in Education (AccessIT). (2004). Accessible Instructional Software in Education (Publication #6). University of Washington. Retrieved September 2014 from http://adasoutheast.org/ed/edpublications/itseries/6_Instructional_Software.pdf.

Occupational therapy practitioners should have knowledge of the accessibility features of computer operating systems and networked software; an awareness of the attributes available in instructional tools such as overhead projectors, interactive whiteboards, digital cameras, and tablet computing; an ability to use the Internet; and programs or software to connect with others electronically.

Assistive Technology for Literacy Skills

Literacy skills include the complicated processes of reading, writing, and spelling as forms of communication; reading is the communication process of constructing meaning from written text, and writing is the communication process of composing meaningful text.

The primary goals of IDEA 2004 and the No Child Left Behind Act of 2001 are improving student achievement and providing students who have disabilities with access to the general education curriculum; however, providing access does not guarantee increased participation, especially for children who have reading and writing difficulties. Public educational institutions must ensure that communications with persons with disabilities "are as effective as communications with others" as mandated by Title II of the ADA by the federal Office of Civil Rights (OCR) (28 C.F.R. § 35.160[a]). In this context "communication" means: "The transfer of information, including (but not limited to) the verbal presentation of a lecture, the printed text of a book, and the resources of the Internet."

Children who struggle with learning to read and write need to be supported by individuals who can accurately assess their strengths and weaknesses and select and apply AT tools and strategies effectively. Assistive technology can help children with disabilities in language acquisition by learning to attend to words and enhancing their interest in listening to stories. Most important, they can increase their opportunities for social engagement. Koenig and Holbrook define functional literacy as "the application of literacy skills and the use of a variety of literacy tools to accomplish daily tasks in the home school, community, and work setting" (p. 265).[69] A multitude of software, word processors, text readers, and electronic books are available on the Internet to support children's literacy. An essential element related to the effectiveness of technology in supporting literacy is its interactive quality, which allows children to get involved with the content as they manipulate the media.[50] Literacy software programs interact with children, similar to a parent's reading to children and involving them in the book by turning the pages, looking at pictures, and asking questions. Technology allows children to control the process by "hooking" their interest. Koenig reiterates the importance of starting early with children "regardless of the severity" of their disability.[68] For additional information, refer to the Literacy Support Software Comparison Chart from Spectronics Inclusive Learning Technologies available on the Evolve website.

Reading Skills

Children most at risk for reading difficulties are those with less verbal skill, phonologic awareness, letter knowledge, and familiarity with the basic purposes of and mechanisms for reading.[22] Research on early reading development emphasizes the pairing of written words and sounds for helping children's decoding skills. For children with physical, visual, communication, or cognitive delays, traditional books may restrict their abilities to interact with and access books. One of the methods that can be used to provide successful literacy experiences is through adapting books.[33] Adapted books provide print access that follows the UDL framework. Adaptations can include making books easier to use (turning pages or holding) and text easier to read (simplified, changed) and remember. The original story or subject is maintained but may contain modified language, clear visual representations, and manageable page layouts to increase the potential for participation. Adapted books can be prop- or paper-based or created electronically with software or apps. Adapted books can be used by themselves or with AT

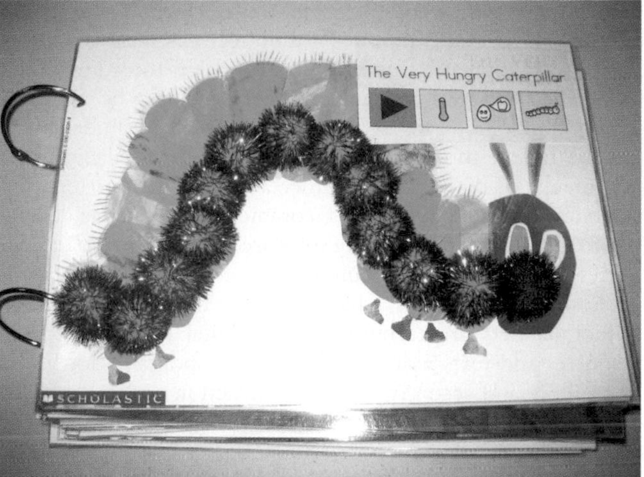

FIGURE 19-15 Example of an adapted book with tactile and rebus symbol support. (Photo courtesy Judith Schoonover.)

ranging from low-tech homemade devices to switches, voice output communication aids, braille or large print materials, sign language, or adapted props. For more information on how to create, publish, and share free e-books, see Box 19-3e on the Evolve website.

Copyright laws allow the creation and use of books in an alternate format solely for the purpose of making the book accessible to persons with disabilities; however, it is important to review copyright laws and how they pertain to each situation in which an adapted book is being contemplated. A copy of the original book is required when using an adapted book. Books can be adapted to provide physical access to text by creating space between pages with page "fluffers" (foam, weather stripping, sponges, giant paper clips, clothespins), using book holders for stabilization (recipe book holders, card holders, acrylic display frames, easels), or reproducing them so that they can be listened to or viewed with technology (Figure 19-15). Accommodations for print difficulties include change in font size and color, magnification, contrast, audio output, tactile display, icon-enhanced text, scaffolded information, and multimedia. Altering the spacing between characters, words, lines of text, and in margins can affect a reader's ability to more easily view and interpret print. Electronic books combine reading, writing, listening, and speaking and provide a multisensory approach with related pictures, sound, and video, and appeal to different learning styles. The ability to read is essential for many daily life activities and participation in varied environments at home, school, work, and in the community. Reading contributes to play and leisure, academics and world knowledge, communication and social awareness, following directions and schedules, shopping and meal preparation, and work-related tasks. Edyburn proposed a process of scaffolding digital text to meet the varied reading and cognitive needs of children by reducing the amount of text, as well as adding additional visual cues in the form of pictures or symbols. He used the term *cognitive rescaling* to describe "a process of altering the cognitive difficulty of information" (p. 10).[47] (See Evolve website for resources on cognitive rescaling.) Print materials can be designed or transformed with supports embedded to ensure that all learners have access to information through the use of common software features such as evaluating readability level, summary tools, voice recordings, and autocorrect in novel ways. Comprehension can be aided by inserting graphic organizers, photos, and video. Students can also be taught to alter the amount, cognitive challenge, and appearance of digital text.[83] Other accommodations for print disabilities include the use of commercially available talking photo albums, specific reading software, e-books, audio recordings, screen readers, and multimedia.

Although trends in education are changing, and more school districts are turning toward digital textbooks, many resources and texts written and published primarily for use in elementary and secondary school instruction and required by the state education agency or local education agency for use by students in the classroom are print-based. Some students may have difficulty accessing these materials, such as those with low vision or blindness or those with physical challenges who are unable to hold a book or turn pages. Provisions within the IDEA require state and local education agencies to provide the same information found in textbooks or handouts in specialized formats called "accessible instructional materials" ("AIM") such as braille, large print, audio, and digital text to students with disabilities who require them in a timely manner (Section 300.172, Final Regulations of IDEA 2004). The website of the National Center on Accessible Instructional Materials (http://aim.cast.org/) serves as a resource to educators, parents, publishers, conversion houses, accessible media producers, and others interested in learning more about implementing AIM and National Instructional Materials Accessibility Standards. Occupational therapy practitioners working as a part of a team can assist in the identification of needed learning opportunities for students with print disabilities, assist students in using the materials provided in alternative formats, and collect data on the effectiveness of the provided supports. Based on their ability to assess motor, cognition, language/processing, and sensory strengths and weaknesses, OTPs can assist with selection of the appropriate technology (interface/input, processing, output, properties), instruction, training, accommodations, and/or modifications associated with AIM.

Assistive Technology for Writing

The act of writing not only requires motor and sensory skills but also includes cognitive processes in the form of recognizable language and vocabulary; generation of ideas; organization of ideas; expression of ideas; and use of correct grammar, punctuation, and spelling. With handwriting as the most common reason for referrals to occupational therapy in school-based practice, practitioners are well aware that writing skills can be enhanced with no-tech or low-tech aids and devices. Simple adaptations, like smooth-writing pens that are comfortable to hold or adapted paper, can make the difference between needing physical assistance and working independently. Service delivery in the natural context, using tools that are intuitive, may mean borrowing or adapting tools that already exist in the classroom.

For individuals who may have motor difficulties that affect the ability to write for function, alternatives to written production should be explored such as the use of a keyboard and mouse (or alternative mouse), portable word processor, or notebook computer. Technology competencies should not be limited to teaching keyboarding as an alternative to handwriting, but rather encompass the accessibility features of computer operating systems and networked software; an awareness of the attributes available in instructional tools such as overhead projectors, interactive whiteboards, digital cameras, and tablet computing; and an ability to use the Internet or connect with others electronically. Beyond the physical components, writing can be conceptualized as a cognitive process that includes the following steps: prewriting/brainstorming ideas, drafting/composing and organizing initial ideas, editing, and, finally, publishing the final product.[32]

Standard word processing and multimedia software, often available in the classroom, features sizable and colored fonts, margin and line spacing options, spell and grammar checking, opportunities for outlining and highlighting, use of tables to organize information, use of macros and abbreviation expansion, general accessibility features, and incorporation of multimedia to represent ideas. More specifically, concept-mapping software allows the user to conceptualize information graphically using a combination of pictures and/or text. It is helpful for planning, organizing, and drafting and frequently offers templates for getting started.

Other software products allow the child to complete a written assignment with visual and/or auditory feedback. Word prediction and word completion can reduce the number of keystrokes necessary and as a result may increase overall speed.[32] After a child types in the first few letters of a word, the program will attempt to predict whole words and presents a list of choices for the child to scan and select (Figure 19-16). Many word prediction programs include customizable dictionaries that suggest alternative word selections, which can facilitate improvement in the quality of a child's written work. These features are beneficial to support spelling for children who have good word recognition skills. Spell-checking programs have proved to be helpful editing tools, specifically when integrated into a word processing program; however, grammar checkers have not.[76] Other options may include use of a traditional or electronic dictionary or thesaurus for children who have word retrieval deficits.

In combination with visual supports, some children benefit from the use of auditory feedback. Text-to-speech software converts printed digital text to synthetic speech and is available in a number of software applications, free Internet downloads, and in Windows and Macintosh operating systems. Synthesized text-to-speech screen readers support drafting and editing, which can help detect errors by reviewing what is written and listening to individual letters, words, or sentences. Most

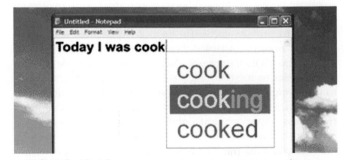

FIGURE 19-16 Example of word prediction software.

text-to-speech applications feature highlighting functions providing audio as well as visual support. They also reduce the visual load for individuals with visual processing deficits and are a valuable alternative for auditory learners. Users with print disabilities can also access contents of web pages, e-mail, e-books, or printed documents when paired with digital speech output, which is available in a number of applications. The age and gender of the "voice," reading rate, dynamic highlighting, and color of font and background can be manipulated to address the individual needs or preferences of the user. In addition, word processing applications often include a voice recording feature to support the writing process. Ideas can be captured through recording, then listened to in order to transcribe, or an educator can relay directions or offer instructional prompts within the text document.

Some children require speech-to-text (or voice recognition) options that allow them to dictate thoughts and commands to a program that produces written text for them. Speech input technology responds to the human voice by producing text or executing verbally dictated commands to navigate through computer applications.[32] Speech recognition presents words through speech, so to produce accurate dictation the user must have appropriate breath support and oral mechanisms.[60] The process results in a multisensory written language experience. Voice quality, pitch, volume, and articulation have a direct impact on the quality of the product generated, as well as set up and positioning of the user. In addition to specific dictation software products and apps, Windows and Macintosh operating systems include speech recognition features. A substantial training component is required to use this type of technology, and the environmental context in which it is used must be examined closely. Speech input can be accomplished by dictating to another individual or to a tape recorder or by using the record feature in various operating systems or applications as a less costly alternative. This allows individuals with intelligible speech to express themselves, even when writing is problematic for attention, motoric, or cognitive reasons.[26]

Assistive Technology for Math

Mathematics is a part of typical school curriculum and is considered a functional life skill. Mathematical concepts include sorting, numbers, differences in attributes (color, shape, size), patterns, counting, sequence, graphing, and numeration. Ideally, a combination of individualized instructional strategies and numerous opportunities to use and manipulate concrete objects to count, sort, compare, and combine is used to reinforce concepts of same/different and greater than/less than/equal to. Additional support (e.g., grippers, nonskid materials), access to a calculator (Figure 19-17), or alternatives to hands-on manipulation such as "virtual manipulation" (http://nlvm.usu.edu/en/NAV/vlibrary.html) allows active participation in math exploration for all.[8]

To determine whether a child needs AT in the area of mathematics, the IEP team should consider whether the child can effectively participate in math instruction and complete math requirements of the curriculum or work setting without the use of aids/devices. If not, then a determination must be made regarding which tools would most effectively reduce barriers to accessing the curriculum. Refer to Table 19-8 for a description of math supports.

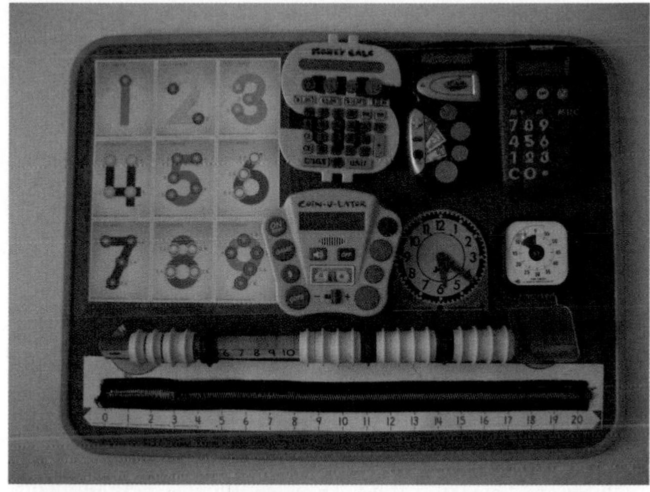

FIGURE 19-17 Examples of no-tech, low-tech math supports including TouchMath, number lines and counters, coin calculators, a calculator with enlarged buttons, a Time Timer, and a standard Judy Clock math manipulative. (Photo courtesy Judith Schoonover.)

TABLE 19-8 Assistive Technology Supports for Math

Number line/ruler	Provides visual support for writing numbers correctly as well as basic computation
TouchMath	Multisensory teaching approach that links manipulation with memorization of math facts
Enlarged or masked math worksheets	Reduces visual clutter and provides additional space for showing work
Graph or grid paper	Supports alignment of problems
Alternative response methods	Number stamps, stamps for drawing graphs, clocks, and number lines
Handheld calculator	Provides visual support for writing numbers correctly or in sequential order as well as computation
Talking calculator	Vocalizes data and resulting computations through speech synthesis
Special features calculator	Options to speak and simultaneously display numbers, functions, entire equations, and results
On-screen calculator	Features such as speech synthesis and adjustment to display including size and color of keys and numbers
Specialized calculator	Realistic money bill and coin buttons to count money or teach value of different coins

Assistive Technology as a "Cognitive Prosthetic"

Assistive technologies for overcoming challenges associated with focus, memory deficits, ability to organize, and task completion is an important emerging field. Portable organizers can be used as cognitive aids and assist in organization and self-regulation by providing self-directed electronic task management support for vocational and nonvocational activities.[53] Tablet-based computing devices and their associated applications enhance the lives of students with cognitive challenges by providing them with academic, communication, leisure, employment, and transition support and access to vital information in a socially acceptable format. Edyburn[49] defines cognitive prosthetics as assistive technology that helps a person use compensatory strategies to perform daily activities.

Typically electronic in nature, cognitive prosthetics include personal digital assistants, pocket personal computers, watches with alarm features, mobile devices including cell phones with reminder features, etc. Personal digital assistants and other mobile devices have touch screens that allow a person to input, save, and retrieve information. These devices offer a portable solution for keeping track of assignments, appointments, reminders, and contact information, as well as deliver prompts or access preferred stimuli, and may include microphones, forward- and backward-facing cameras, and touch-screen capabilities. Pictures and videos can be used to provide social cues, step-by-step directions, and more. Personal calendars and daily planners can be used to manage time and complete tasks. Global positioning system receivers can help with independent navigation within the community. The multiple function capabilities of mobile device platforms may permit a consolidation of tools. Apps, software, and free Internet sites can help organize daily and monthly activities. Online tutorials and apps can deliver training that can be repeated many times. Software that is multisensory, can be personalized, is reinforcing, and can motivate is preferable. It is important to consider the limitations of mobile devices, including the need for technical competencies in order use them independently, and the possibility of disruption owing to damage, malfunction, or theft.

Not all cognitive supports are high tech in nature. Structuring the environment can also enhance performance. For example, shields or color codes on equipment can help with focus and sequencing; using carrels around work areas can reduce visual distractions; and earphones can help block out sound distractions. Other simple solutions include portable timers, alarm clocks, social scripts, and watches with alarms.

Assistive Technology and Transition

Transition planning is essential to pave the way to successful change. Transitions are an inevitable part of life, yet the passages from preschool to elementary school, elementary school to high school, and high school into early adulthood can result in a loss of continuity. For an individual with disabilities, transitions can be especially challenging if the supports that provide access to participation are not available or prove unsuitable in the new environment. Critical information, as well as competencies, can be lost if positioning, teaching methodologies, and information regarding specialized technology are not passed along from one stage and setting to the next. IDEA mandates the provision of both AT services and transition services for students with disabilities. When a student with a disability requires AT to accomplish one or more functional skills, the use of that AT must be included in effective transition planning. Transition plans for AT users address the ways the student's use of devices and services are transferred from one setting to another. AT transition involves people from different classrooms, programs, buildings, or agencies working together to ensure continuity. In addition to ensuring that AT devices and support services accompany students during transitions, service providers should assist clients and their families in becoming responsible users of AT. The goal of self-management and independent use should begin the first time a child uses AT, steering him or her onto a path of optimal independence as an adult. Competencies should be developed in the area for which the AT device was chosen (e.g., communication, writing) as well as in how to use and care for the device, when to use it, and the social implications and responsibilities of using the device.[24] Development of self-determination skills to ensure that AT becomes an integrated part of typical routines will aid in successful transitions from home to school and from school to the community.[24]

BOX 19-11 Components of Effective Transition Plans for Assistive Technology Users

- Address the AT needs of the student, including roles and training needs of team members, subsequent steps in AT use, and follow-up after transition takes place.
- Empower the student using AT to participate in the transition planning at a level appropriate to age and ability.
- Recognize advocacy, as related to AT use, as critical to the plan's success.
- Identify the AT requirements in the receiving environment.
- Proceed according to an individualized timeline.
- Address specific equipment, training, and funding issues such as transfer or acquisition of AT, manuals, and support documents.

The QIAT Community (Revised, 2012). Quality Indicators for Assistive Technology Transition. Retrieved September 2014 from http://indicators.knowbility.org/indicators.html.

For individuals beginning or ending their public school education, transition planning is included in legal mandates; therefore transition plans should contain a statement of needed AT devices and services and indicate agency responsibilities and linkages, if appropriate. Various agencies may be involved, and the decision regarding who is responsible for providing the AT services needed for successful postgraduation activities should be determined in advance by the transition team.

The QIAT Consortium has identified areas of best practice for AT transition[88] (Box 19-11), and although their guidelines focus mainly on the late high school transition to postsecondary and work placement, they serve as a reminder of the goals of the transition process and help identify key elements that need to be addressed in a transition plan. The FCTD Family Information Guide to Assistive Technology and Transition Planning, available online and in printable (pdf) format, was last updated in 2009 and includes sections on transition planning and AT, laws governing accommodations and transition in birth to 12 years, postsecondary settings, resources, and more.

Evidence-Based Practice and Assistive Technology

Research of AT services and outcomes is limited.[46,48,96,107] Because of the ever-changing nature of this field, the

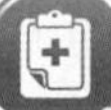

CASE STUDY 19-1 Assistive Technology Problem Solving

Jeremy

Jeremy is a 2-year-old with Down syndrome. His family wants to provide every opportunity for him to develop cognitive skills. They plan for him to attend general education classrooms as he gets older. They were recently at a conference and heard about tablet technologies as tools for supporting learning and educational performance for some children with Down syndrome. They asked the early intervention team to recommend a tablet and apps to use with Jeremy. Would you recommend a tablet for 2-year-old Jeremy? If so, what criterion would you use to determine which apps to recommend?

Linnea

Linnea is a third grade student with spinal muscular atrophy. She is fully included in her neighborhood school with support from related services as needed. Recently she has been complaining to her parents and therapists that her hand gets tired when writing and that her handwriting looks "sloppy." Her teacher also has noticed that she seems irritable and lacks concentration during class. Linnea, her family, and her therapists have discussed using computers for written communication in the past, but Linnea and her family have always been reluctant to explore this at length because she does not want to "look different." Linnea has had experience with computers since kindergarten. Her class goes to the computer lab three times a week, and she began learning basic keyboarding skills in second grade. Her classroom has two computers that students use for drill, practice, and special projects. How would you address written language requirements in the context of Linnea's classroom using a UDL approach?

Margy

Margy is 17 years old and has cognitive impairments and attention-deficit/hyperactivity disorder (ADHD). During her last individualized transition plan, her family expressed the desire for Margy to get a job in the family carpet cleaning business. Margy enjoys greeting people, and others enjoy her bubbly and outgoing personality, so her parents felt it would be good if she could work with the receptionist in the front office of their business. Her father felt that she should have more responsibility than simply greeting customers. Challenges reported by her teacher include being on time to class, remaining focused on tasks, and organizing herself and materials. In addition, Margy has a difficult time communicating when she gets nervous, which can affect her intelligibility. After further discussion, the team agreed that this could be a reasonable expectation for Margy and worked to develop a plan to reach this goal. Which AT and/or environmental modifications might you consider for Margy?

complexity of the devices, and the need for individualized decisions, it is difficult to build a large evidence base in this area of practice that is consistent with the available technology.[48] Some AT companies are adding research information regarding their products and AT outcomes to their websites; however, research published in peer-reviewed journals may be of higher quality and avoids the bias often found in research used to promote products to consumers. Whenever possible, AT research should guide and support decision making and provide further foundational knowledge about AT devices and services. When evidence is not available, OTPs working in this area must engage in data-based decision making with each client to document whether the use of the device results in increased participation and engagement across environments. Occupational therapy practitioners should be good consumers of AT research and should also measure and document AT outcomes as part of best practice services. Ongoing research examining the effectiveness of AT as an intervention is needed.

Summary

Assistive technologies can diminish the impact of disabilities and allow children improved alternatives to participate.[80] Occupational therapy practitioners who work with children and youth are ideally suited to evaluate and determine an appropriate match of AT tools to the child and should become familiar with the continuum of AT options available on the Evolve website (see Table 19-8e). Recent advances in AT allow many devices to grow and expand with the child during the developmental years and into adolescence and adulthood as they undergo transition into higher education and community work experiences. With the current pace of progress and research, future AT will offer greater ease of use, wider application, assistance in additional areas of function, and more availability as a result of lower costs (Case Study 19-1). The responsibility of those who implement AT intervention is to provide a health-promoting balance between occupational roles and activities consistent with the individual's valued goals and interests, as well as the demands of society.[105]

Most people could not escape technology if they tried. Cell phones, tablets, and social media affect all aspects and contexts of everyday life, including work, leisure, self-help, and interpersonal relationships. Most important, *assistive* technology changes and reshapes attitudes about what people *do* and *can do*. With this influx of new tools, it is crucial to determine the "right tool for the job." Occupational therapy practitioners have the opportunity, challenge, and responsibility to educate themselves and others about the possibilities offered by new technologies, while not forgetting that the best solution might be the easiest and least complex.

Collaboration among team members and professional development are necessary practice components of AT that require both time and commitment. Barriers to collaboration include finding time and a place to meet. Technology can be used by practitioners to bridge time and distance gaps such as use of an electronic survey to schedule meetings or to post planning documents online in order for all shareholders to contribute thoughts and ideas. Although meeting in real time may be preferable, use of conference calls, multimedia, video conferencing, e-mail, "cloud storage" of documents, and chat rooms can support productivity on behalf of the children and families served. Care should be taken that the modalities chosen meet the learning style and comfort level of the participants.

The direct connection between occupational therapy and AT allows us to unlock human potential and optimize human performance through the promotion of participation in activities that are personally meaningful, relevant, and life sustaining. The challenge is to increase collaborative practices, insist on opportunities for professional development, advocate for the provision of appropriate AT, and continue to define the role of occupational therapy in the provision of AT.

- Children who use AT at an early age have the advantage of developing with and using it to benefit them throughout their lives.
- Occupational therapy practitioners should become familiar with the continuum of AT options and engage in ongoing professional development to maintain competency.
- The combination of occupational therapy and AT services together can promote success across all areas of occupation.
- It is important to recognize how the physical, academic, social, and virtual environments contribute to functional performance.
- AT is both a device and a service and must be matched appropriately to the child and family's needs.
- Collaboration with other team members is essential.
- UDL allows access for all while simultaneously meeting the needs of children with disabilities, thus creating an inclusive climate for social participation.

REFERENCES

1. AAC-RERC. (2011). Mobile devices and communication apps. Retrieved from <http://aac-rerc.psu.edu/index.php/pages/show/id/46>.
2. Abramson, L. Y., Seligman, M. E. P., & Teasdale, J. D. (1978). Learned helplessness in humans: Critique and reformation. *Journal of Abnormal Psychology*, *87*, 49–74.
3. American Occupational Therapy Association. (2004). Assistive technology within occupational therapy practice. *American Journal of Occupational Therapy*, *58*, 678–680.
4. American Occupational Therapy Association. (2010b). Occupational therapy's perspective on the use of environments and contexts to support health and participation in occupations. *American Journal of Occupational Therapy*, *64*, S57–S69.
5. American Occupational Therapy Association. (2010a). Specialized knowledge and skills in technology and environmental interventions for occupational therapy practice. *American Journal of Occupational Therapy*, *64*, S44–S56.
6. Anson, D. K. (1997). *Alternative computer access: A guide to selection.* Philadelphia: F. A. Davis.
7. Argabrite Grove, R., Broeder, K., Gitlow, L., et al. (2007). *Assistive technology in the schools: From start to finish.* St. Louis, MO: Pre-Conference Institute at AOTA's Annual Conference and Expo.
8. Assistive Technology Training Online (ATTO) Project. (2000–2005). Retrieved on July 30, 2014 from <http://atto.buffalo.edu/registered/ATBasics/Curriculum/Math/printmodule.php>.
9. Bain, B. K., & Leger, D. (1997). *Assistive technology: An interdisciplinary approach.* New York: Churchill Livingstone.
10. Baush, M. E., Ault, M. J., & Hasselbring, T. S. (2006). *Assistive technology planner: From IEP consideration to classroom implementation.* Lexington, KY: National Assistive Technology Research Institute.
11. Behrmann, M. M. (1984). A brighter future for early learning through high tech. *The Pointer*, *28*, 23–26.
12. Behrmann, M. M., Jones, J. K., & Wilds, M. L. (1989). Technology intervention for very young children with disabilities. *Infants and Young Children*, *1*, 66–77.
13. Beukelman, D. R., & Mirenda, P. (1992). *Augmentative and alternative communication: Management of severe communication disorders in children and adults.* Baltimore: Brookes.
14. Beukelman, D. R., & Mirenda, P. (2005). *Augmentative and alternative communication: Management of severe communication disorders in children and adults* (3rd ed.). Baltimore: Brookes.
15. Beukelman, D. R., McGinnis, J., & Morrow, D. (1991). Vocabulary selection in augmentative and alternative communication. *Augmentative and Alternative Communication*, *7*, 171–185.
16. Blackstone, S. (2006). False beliefs, widely held. *Augmentative Communication News*, *3*, 1–6.
17. Bowser, G., & Reed, P. (2012). *Education TECH points: A framework for assistive technology planning* (3rd ed.). Winchester, OR: Coalition for Assistive Technology in Oregon.
18. Cardon, T. A., Wilcox, M. J., & Campbell, P. H. (2011). Caregiver perspectives about assistive technology use with their young children with autism spectrum disorders. *Infants and Young Children*, *24*(2), 153–173.
19. Bryen, D. N., Cohen, K., & Carey, A. (2004). Augmentative communication employment training and supports: Some employment outcomes. *Journal of Rehabilitation*, *70*, 10–18.
20. Burgstahler, S. (2003). The role of technology in preparing youth with disabilities for postsecondary education and employment. *Journal of Special Education Technology*, *18*, 7–20.
21. Burkhart, L. (2002). Getting past learned helplessness for children who face severe challenges: Four secrets for success. Retrieved from <http://www.lburkhart.com>.
22. Burns, M. S., Griffin, P., & Snow, C. E. (1999). *Starting out right: A guide to promoting children's reading success.* Washington, DC: National Academy Press. Retrieved from: <http://www.nap.edu/html/sor/>.
23. Carlson, S. J., Clarke, C. D., Harden, B., et al. (2003). *Assistive technology and IDEA: Effective practices for related services personnel.* Rockville, MD: American Speech-Language-Hearing Association (ASHA).
24. Castellani, J., & Bowser, G. (2006). *Transition planning: Assistive technology supports and services. Technology in action* (Vol. 2). Arlington, VA: Center for Technology in Education, Johns Hopkins University, and Technology and Media Division of the Council for Exceptional Children.
25. Castellani, J. D., & Bowser, G. (2007). *Transition planning: Assistive technology supports and services.* Arlington, VA: Technology and Media Division of the Council for Exceptional Children.
26. Cavanagh, C. A. (2008). Speech recognition trial protocol. *Closing the Gap*, *26*(5), 8–11.

27. Center for Applied Assistive Technology (2011). *Universal design for learning guidelines version 2.0.* Wakefield, MA: Author.
28. Center for Applied Special Technology. (2012). About CAST. Retrieved from <http://www.cast.org/about/index.html>.
29. Center for Universal Design. (1997). About universal design. Retrieved from <http://www.ncsu.edu/ncsu/design/cud/about_ud/udprinciples.htm>.
30. Clarke, M., & Kirton, A. (2003). Patterns of interaction between children with physical disabilities using augmentative and alternative communication systems and their peers. *Child Language Teaching and Therapy, 19,* 135–151.
31. Cole, J., & Swinth, Y. L. (2004). Comparison of the touch-free switch to a physical switch, children's abilities and preferences: A pilot study. *Journal of Special Education Technology, 19*(2), 19–30.
32. Cook, A., & Polgar, J. (2008). *Cook and Hussey's assistive technologies: Principles and practice* (3rd ed.). St. Louis: Elsevier.
33. Cooper-Duffy, K., Szedia, P., & Hyer, G. (2010). Teaching literacy to students with significant cognitive disabilities. *Teaching Exceptional Children, 42*(3), 30–39.
34. Copley, J., & Ziviani, J. (2007). Use of a team-based approach to assistive technology assessment and planning for children with multiple disabilities: A pilot study. *Assistive Technology, 19,* 109–125.
35. Cornell University. (1999). Computers in schools are putting elementary schoolchildren at risk for posture problems, says Cornell study. *Science Daily.* Retrieved August 2008 from <http://www.sciencedaily.com/releases/1999/02/990202071806.htm>.
36. Demers, L., Weiss-Lambrou, R., & Ska, B. (2002). The Quebec User Evaluation of Satisfaction with Assistive Technology (QUEST 2.0): An overview and recent progress. *Technology and Disability, 14,* 101–105.
37. Demers, L., Wessels, R. D., Weiss-Lambrou, R., et al. (1999). An international content validation of the Quebec User Evaluation of Satisfaction with Assistive Technology (QUEST). *Occupational Therapy International, 6,* 159–175.
38. DeRuyter, F. (1995). Evaluating outcomes in assistive technology: Do we understand the commitment? *Assistive Technology, 7,* 3–16.
39. Dickey, R., & Shealey, S. H. (1987). Using technology to control the environment. *American Journal of Occupational Therapy, 41,* 717–721.
40. Doster, S., & Politano, P. (1996). Augmentative and alternative communication. In J. Hammel (Ed.), *AOTA self-paced clinical course: Technology and occupational therapy: A link to function.* (pp. 2–47). Rockville, MD: AOTA.
41. Douglas, J., Reeson, B., & Ryan, M. (1988). Computer microtechnology for a severely disabled preschool child. *Child: Care, Health and Development, 14,* 93–104.
42. Dowden, P., & Cook, A. M. (2002). Choosing effective selection techniques for beginning communicators. In J. Reichle, D. Beukelman, & J. Light (Eds.), *Exemplary practices for beginning communicators* (pp. 101–124). Baltimore: Brookes.
43. Downing, J. (2005). *Teaching communication skills to students with severe disabilities* (2nd ed.). Baltimore: Brooke.
44. Drager, K. (2003). Light technologies with different system layouts and language organizations. *Journal of Speech, Language, and Hearing Research, 46,* 289–312.
45. Dunst, C. J., Trivette, C. M., Meter, D., et al. (2012). *Influences of contrasting types of training on practitioners' and parents' use of assistive technology and adaptations with infants, toddlers and preschoolers with disabilities.* Research Brief, 6*(1). Tots-n-Tech Institute:* <http://www.tnt.asu.edu>.
46. Edyburn, D. L. (2000). 1999 in review: A synthesis of the special education technology literature. *Journal of Special Education, 15,* 7–18.
47. Edyburn, D. L. (2002). Cognitive rescaling strategies. *Closing the Gap, 21,* 1–4.
48. Edyburn, D. L. (2003). Assistive technology and evidence-based practice. *ConnSENSE Bulletin.* Retrieved July 30, 2014 from <http://connection.ebscohost.com/c/articles/11002897/assistive-technology-evidence-based-practice>.
49. Edyburn, D. L. (2006). Cognitive prostheses for students with mild disabilities: Is this what assistive technology looks like? *Journal of Special Education Technology, 21*(4), 62–65.
50. Farmer, L. (1998). Turn on to reading through technology. *Library Talk,* (Sept./Oct.), 16–17.
51. Foulds, R. A. (1982). Applications of microcomputers in the education of the physically disabled child. *Exceptional Children, 49,* 143–162.
52. Gelderblom, G. J., & deWitte, L. P. (2002). The assessment of assistive technology outcomes, effects and costs. *Technology and Disability, 14,* 91–94.
53. Gentry, T., Wallace, J., Kvarfordt, C., et al. (2010). Personal digital assistants as cognitive aids for high school students with autism: Results of a community-based trial. *Journal of Vocational Rehabilitation, 32,* 101–107.
54. George, C. L., Schaff, J. I., & Jeffs, T. L. (2005). Physical access in today's schools: Empowerment through assistive technology. In D. Edyburn, K. Higgins, & R. Boone (Eds.), *The handbook of special education technology* (pp. 355–378). Whitefish Bay, WI: Knowledge by Design.
55. Gierach, J. (Ed.), (2009). *Assessing students' needs for assistive technology: A resource manual for school district teams* (5th ed.). Milton, WI: Wisconsin Assistive Technology Initiative.
56. Glickman, L., Deitz, J., Anson, D., et al. (1996). Effect of switch control site on computer skills of infants and toddlers. *American Journal of Occupational Therapy, 50,* 545–553.
57. Goldbart, J., & Marshall, J. (2004). "Pushes and pulls" on the parents of children who use AAC. *Augmentative and Alternative Communication, 20,* 194–208.
58. Halloran, J., & Halloran, C. (2012). *LAMP: Language acquisition through motor planning.* Wooster, OH: The Center for AAC and Autism.
59. Hammel, J., & Niehues, A. (1998). Integrating general and assistive technology into school-based practice: Process and information resources. In J. Case-Smith (Ed.), *Occupational therapy: Making a difference in school system practice.* (Lesson 11). Rockville, MD: AOTA.
60. Higgins, E. L., & Raskind, M. H. (2000). Speaking to read: The effects of continuous vs. discrete speech recognition systems on the reading and spelling of children with learning disabilities. *Journal of Special Education Technology, 15,* 19–30.
61. Hitchcock, C., & Stahl, S. (2003). Assistive technology, universal design, universal design for learning: Improved learning opportunities. *Journal of Special Education Technology, 18,* 45–52. IDEA Practices. (2004). Retrieved on July 30, 2014 from <https://erlc.wikispaces.com/file/view/Hitchcock%20%26%20Stahl%202003.pdf/332661338/Hitchcock%20%26%20Stahl%202003.pdf>.
62. Hodgdon, L. A. (1995). *Visual strategies for improving communication (vol 1). Practical supports for school and home.* Troy, MI: Quirk Roberts Publishing.

63. Judge, S. L. (2001). Computer applications in programs for young children with disabilities: Current status and future directions. *Journal of Special Education Technology, 16*(1), 29–40.
64. Kangas, K. M. (2000). The task performance position: Providing seating for accurate access to assistive technology. *Physical Disabilities Special Interest Section Quarterly, 23*, 1–3.
65. Kelker, K., & Holt, R. (2000). *Family guide to assistive technology.* Cambridge, MA: Brookline Books.
66. Kerr, S. T. (1996). *Technology and the future of schooling: Ninety-fifth yearbook of the National Society for the Study of Education, part II.* Chicago: University of Chicago Press.
67. Kielhofner, G. (2008). *Model of human occupation: Theory and application* (4th ed.). Baltimore: Lippincoot Williams & Wilkins.
68. Koenig, A. J. (1992). A framework for understanding the literacy of individuals with visual impairments. *Journal of Visual Impairment and Blindness, 86*, 277–284.
69. Koenig, A. J., & Holbrook, M. C. (2000). Literacy skills. In A. J. Koenig & M. C. Holbrook (Eds.), *Foundations of education: Instructional strategies for teaching children and youth with visual impairments* (Vol. 2, pp. 265–329). New York: American Foundation for the Blind.
70. Lahm, E. A. (1989). *Technology with low incidence populations: Promoting access and learning.* Reston, VA: The Council for Exceptional Children.
71. Lahm, E. A., & Sizemore, L. (2002). Factors that influence assistive technology decision-making. *Journal of Special Education Technology, 17*(1), 15–26.
72. Lamb, P. (2003). The role of the vocational rehabilitation counselor in procuring technology to facilitate success in postsecondary education for youth with disabilities. *Journal of Special Education Technology, 18*(4), 53–63.
73. Lauer, A., Longenecker Rust, K., & Smith, R. O. (2006). Factors in assistive technology device abandonment: Replacing “abandonment” with “discontinuance” (ATOMS Project Technical Report). Retrieved from <http://www.r2d2.uwm.edu/atoms/archive/technicalreports/tr-discontinuance.html>.
74. Law, M., Baptiste, S., Carswell, A., et al. (2005). *Canadian Occupational Performance Measure* (4th ed.). Toronto: Canadian Association of Occupational Therapy Inc.
75. Law, M., Cooper, B., Strong, S., et al. (1996). The person-environment-occupation model: A transactive approach to occupational performance. *Canadian Journal of Occupational Therapy, 63*, 9–23.
76. Lewis, R. (2005). Classroom technology for students with learning disabilities. In D. Edyburn, K. Higgins, & R. Boone (Eds.), *Handbook of special education technology research and practice* (pp. 324–334). Whitefish Bay, WI: Knowledge by Design.
77. Light, J. (1989). Toward a definition of communicative competence for individuals using augmentative and alternative communication systems. *Augmentative and Alternative Communication, 5*, 137–144.
78. Light, J. C., & Drager, K. (2002). Improving the design of augmentative and alternative technologies for young children. *Assistive Technology, 14*, 17–32.
79. Maier, S. F., & Seligman, M. E. (1976). Learned helplessness: Theory and evidence. *Journal of Experimental Psychology. General, 105*, 3–46.
80. Mistrett, S. (2004). Assistive technology helps young children with disabilities participate in daily activities. *Technology in Action, 1*(4), 1–8.
81. National Joint Committee for the Communication Needs of Persons with Severe Disabilities. (1992). Guidelines for meeting the communication needs of persons with severe disabilities. *ASHA, 34*, 1–8.
82. Neighborhood Legal Services, Inc. (2003). Funding of assistive technology: The public school’s special education system as a funding source: The cutting edge. Retrieved October 10, 2008 from <http://www.nls.org>.
83. Norton-Darr, S., & Schoonover, J. (2012). Spreading the word about cognitive rescaling as a tool for inclusion. *Closing the Gap Solutions*, 7–13.
84. Office of Special Education and Rehabilitative Services, U.S. Department of Education. Reuse your assistive technology. Retrieved July 2008 from <http://www.ed.gov/print/programs/atsg/at-reuse.html>.
85. Parette, H. P., & VanBiervliet, A. (1990). A prospective inquiry into technology needs and practices of school-aged children with disabilities. *Journal of Special Education Technology, 10*, 198–206.
86. Phillips, B., & Zhao, H. (1993). Predictors of assistive technology abandonment. *Assistive Technology, 5*, 36–45.
87. Post, K. M., Hartmann, K., Gitlow, L., et al. (2008). AOTA’s Centennial Vision for the future: How can technology help? *Technology Special Interest Section Quarterly, 18*, 1–4.
88. QIAT Consortium. (2007). AT in transition. Retrieved June 2008 from <http://natri.uky.edu/assoc_projects/qiat/documents/6%20QIAT%20QIs%20Transition.doc>.
89. QIAT Consortium. (2007). Quality indicators for assistive technology services. Retrieved August 2008 from <http://natri.uky.edu/assoc_projects/qiat/>.
90. Reed, P. (2000). School profile of assistive technology services. Retrieved August 2008 from <http://www.wati.org/AT_Services/schoolprofile.html>.
91. Reed, P. (2003). *Designing environments for successful kids.* Oshkosh, WI: Wisconsin Assistive Technology Initiative.
92. Reed, P. (2004). The WATI assessment package. Retrieved October 2005 from <http://www.wati.org/Materials/pdf/wati%20assessment.pdf>.
93. Robinson, L. M. (1986). Designing computer intervention for very young handicapped children. *Journal of the Division for Early Childhood, 103*, 209–213.
94. Rose, D. H., & Meyer, A. (2002). *Teaching every student in the digital age: Universal design for learning.* Alexandria, VA: Association for Supervision and Curriculum Development.
95. Rowland, C., & Schweigert, P. (2000). *Tangible symbol systems: Making the right to communicate a reality for individuals with severe disabilities* (2nd ed.). Portland, OR: OHSU Design to Learn Projects.
96. Scherer, M. J. (1996). Outcomes of assistive technology use on quality of life. *Disability and Rehabilitation, 18*, 439–448.
97. Scherer, M. J. (2000). *Living in the state of stuck: How technology impacts the lives of people with disabilities.* Cambridge, MA: Brookline Books.
98. Scherer, M. J., & Craddock, G. (2002). Matching person and technology (MPT) assessment process. *Technology and Disability, 14*, 125–131.
99. Scherer, M. J., & Lane, J. P. (1997). Assessing consumer profiles of “ideal” assistive technologies in ten categories: An integration of quantitative and qualitative methods. *Disability and Rehabilitation, 19*, 528–535.
100. Schmeler, M. R. (1997). *Strategies in documenting the need for assistive technology: An analysis of documentation procedures. AOTA technology special interest section quarterly Vol. 7.* Bethesda, MD: American Occupational Therapy Association.
101. Schoonover, J. (2013). Best practices in universal design for learning. In

G. Frolek-Clark & B. Chandler (Eds.), *Best practices in school occupational therapy*. Bethesda, MD: AOTA Press.

102. Sibert, R. I. (1997). Financing assistive technology: An overview of public funding sources. *AOTA Technology Special Interest Section Newsletter, 7,* 1–4.
103. Spencer, J. (1998). Alternative meanings of assistive technology. In D. B. Gray, L. A. Quatrano, & M. L. Lieberman (Eds.), *Designing and using assistive technology: The human perspective*. Baltimore: Brookes.
104. Stodden, R. A., Conway, M. A., & Chang, K. B. T. (2003). Findings from the study of transition, technology and postsecondary supports for youth with disabilities: Implications for secondary school educators. *Journal of Special Education Technology, 18*(4), 29–43.
105. Stoller, L. C. (1998). *Low-tech assistive devices: A handbook for the school setting.* Framingham, MA: Therapro, Inc.
106. Sullivan, M. W., & Lewis, M. (2000). Assistive technology for the very young: Creating responsive environments. *Infants and Young Children, 12*(4), 34–52.
107. Swanson, H. L. (1999). Instructional components that predict treatment outcomes for students with learning disabilities: Support for a combined strategy and direct instruction model. *Learning Disabilities Research and Practice, 14,* 129–140.
108. Swinth, Y. L. (1997). *The meaning of assistive technology in the lives of high school students and their families.* Seattle: University of Washington.
109. Swinth, Y. L. (1998). Assistive technology in early intervention: Theory and practice. In J. Case-Smith (Ed.), *Pediatric occupational therapy and early intervention* (2nd ed., pp. 277–298). Woburn, MA: Butterworth-Heinemann.
110. Swinth, Y. L., & Anson, D. (1998). Alternatives to handwriting: Keyboarding and text-generation techniques for schools. In J. Case Smith (Ed.), *AOTA self-paced clinical course: Occupational therapy: Making a difference in school system practice.* Rockville, MD: American Occupational Therapy Association.
111. Todis, M., & Walker, H. M. (1993). User perspectives on assistive technology in educational settings. *Focus on Exceptional Children, 46*(3), 1–16.
112. U.S. Department of Education, National Center for Educational Statistics (2012). Retrieved from <http://nces.ed.gov/fastfacts/display.asp?id=64>.
113. Assistive Technology Industry Association (ATIA) Funding Guide. Retrieved on July 30, 2014 from <http://www.atia.org/i4a/pages/index.cfm?pageid=4219>.
114. Wehmeyer, M. L. (1996). Self-determination as an educational outcome: Why is it important to children, youth, and adults with disabilities? In D. J. Sands & M. L. Wehmeyer (Eds.), *Self-determination across the life span: Independence and choice for people with disabilities* (pp. 17–36). Baltimore: Brookes.
115. Weintraub, H., Bacon, C., & Wilcox, M. (2004). *AT and young children: Confidence, experience and education of early intervention providers. Research brief Vol. 1.* Tots n Tech Research Institute. Retrieved February 2008 from <http://tnt.asu.edu>.
116. World Health Organization (2002). *International Classification of Functioning, Disability and Health (ICF).* Geneva: Author.
117. Zabala, J. S. (2010). The SETT framework: Straight from the horse's mouth. Retrieved on July 30, 2014 from <http://www.joyzabala.com/uploads/CA_Kananaskis__SETT_Horses_Mouth.pdf>.
118. Zabala, J. (2007). 10 things everyone needs to know about assistive technology in schools in 2006. Presented at the national conference of the Assistive Technology Industry Association (ATIA), Orlando, FL.

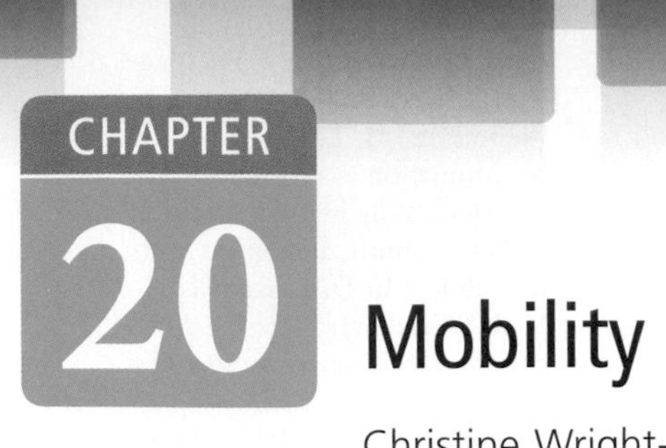

CHAPTER 20

Mobility

Christine Wright-Ott

KEY TERMS

Functional mobility
Community mobility
Developmental theory of mobility
Augmentative mobility
Manual wheelchairs
Power wheelchairs
Powered mobility evaluation
Seating
Positioning

GUIDING QUESTIONS

1. How is mobility important to a young child's development?
2. What factors should be considered during an evaluation for seating and mobility equipment?
3. How is mobility assessed and categorized for different levels of motor function?
4. What are alternative methods of mobility appropriate to meet the child's developmental and functional needs?
5. What are wheelchair features and designs that meet the needs of children with various levels of motor control?
6. What power mobility devices are currently available?
7. How do occupational therapists and family determine the most appropriate device?
8. How is technology used to assess seating and positioning?
9. What devices are available to children with unique seating and position needs?
10. How do positioning and seating affect function and successful use of a mobility device?
11. How are biomechanical principles applied to position and seating?

This chapter presents an overview of the importance of mobility for growth and development and the implications of impaired mobility. Responsibilities of the occupational therapist for evaluating and recommending appropriate mobility devices are emphasized. Guidelines and criteria for selecting mobility equipment are defined, and descriptions of mobility devices are provided. This chapter also describes the importance of positioning and other factors that influence successful use of assistive devices.

Mobility is fundamental to an individual's overall development and functioning in the occupations of self-care, work, and play and is essential to quality of life. The definition of *functional mobility* includes moving from one position or place to another (e.g., bed mobility, wheelchair mobility, and transfers [wheelchair, bed, car, tub or shower, toilet, or chair]), performing functional ambulation, and transporting objects. *Community mobility* is defined as moving oneself in the community and using public or private transportation (e.g., driving or accessing buses, taxicabs, or other public transportation systems). This chapter addresses primarily mobility as a means of locomotion, with an emphasis on evaluation and intervention principles.

Developmental Theory of Mobility

The newborn has little independent control of any part of the body. Motor and sensory symmetry and midline orientation develop gradually, followed by controlled purposeful movements and the beginning of alternating coordinated movements. The first form of mobility that the infant experiences is rolling, first from side to supine, then prone to supine, and finally in either direction. The 6-month-old infant achieves mobility by pivoting in the prone position. The infant continually becomes more active against gravity (Figure 20-1). Most 8-month-old infants creep and move from sitting to quadruped positioning and back. By the ninth to tenth month, the infant has a strong desire to move upward. First, infants pull to stand and cruise along furniture, such as a coffee table; then they hold onto someone or something as they take their first steps. The average age at independent walking is 11.2 months, and most children achieve independent upright ambulation between 9 and 15 months of age.[11,18]

Developmental theorists accept that physical and psychological developments are interrelated and that early experiences influence subsequent behavior. "Through their motor interactions infants and toddlers learn about things and people in their world and also discover they can cause things to happen" (p. 18).[15] During the first months of life, children seek physical control of their environment and continue to do so by building and enhancing their motor skills day by day.

Children gain various learning experiences as they move about.[36] Locomotion and other motor skills, which develop rapidly during the first 3 years of life, become the primary vehicles for learning and socialization and for the growth of a healthy sense of independence and competence. A typical

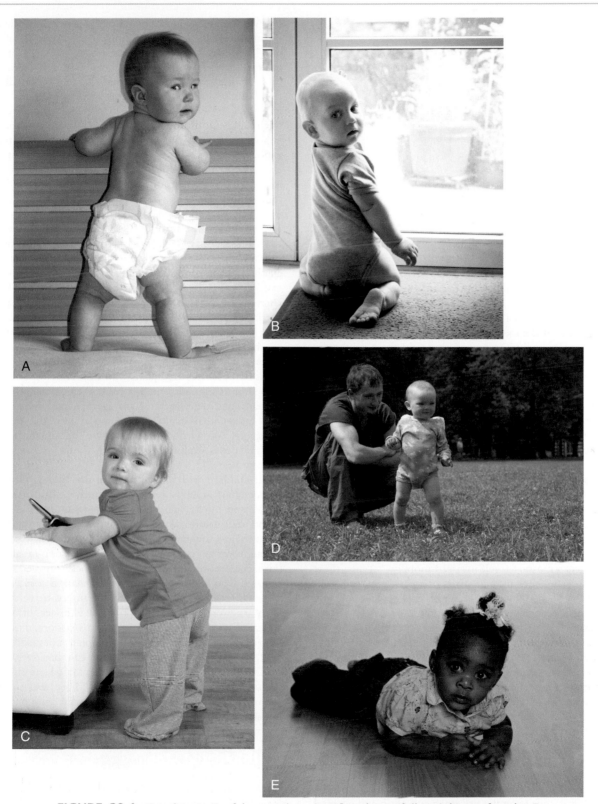

FIGURE 20-1 Development of locomotion. **A,** Infant bears full weight on feet by 7 months. **B,** Infant can maneuver from sitting to kneeling position. **C,** Infant can stand holding onto furniture at 9 months. **D,** While standing, Infant takes deliberate step at 10 months. **E,** Infant crawls with abdomen on floor and pulls self forward, and then (**F**) creeps on hands and knees at 9 months. (From istock.com.) *Continued on next page*

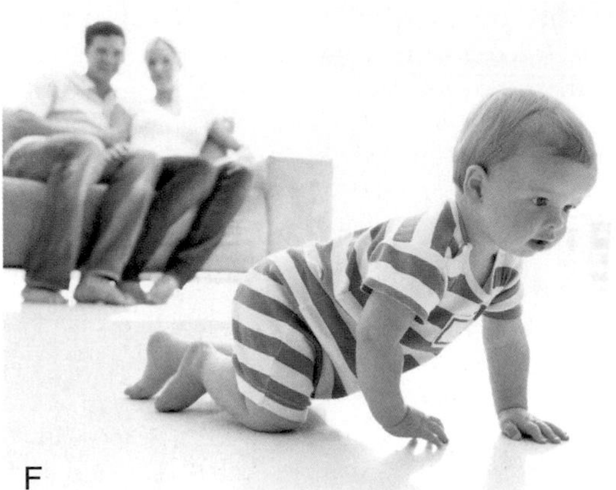

FIGURE 20-1, cont'd

toddler travels more than 39 football fields per day and accumulates an average of 15 falls an hour.[2] Piaget viewed self-produced movement as a crucial building block of knowledge. He theorized that the intercoordination of vision and audition with movements, including locomotion, laid the basis for the child's understanding of space, objects, causality, and self.[65] The ability of children to influence their environment and to affect or alter it through their own actions is intrinsically motivating. Early experiences are believed to foster curiosity, exploration, mastery, and persistence, and are therefore important for later intellectual functioning.

Impaired Mobility

Children with physical disabilities who have difficulty achieving independent motor control are often deprived of opportunities for self-initiated or self-produced mobility. Palisano found that very few children with severe cerebral palsy between ages 4 and 12 years have a means for self-initiated mobility.[62] When these children do experience mobility, it is of a passive nature, as in being held or pushed in a stroller. Children with cerebral palsy spend more time sitting than their peers.[66] Because they lack the necessary movements to explore and act on their environment, important learning opportunities are hindered. Mobility-impaired toddlers who cannot move across a room to reach out and touch an object or interact with a person are at a great disadvantage. They cannot experience the sensorimotor and developmental activities of their peers who have achieved upright mobility, such as pushing and pulling toys, opening and closing drawers, or moving around and under objects. Psychologists who have studied typical development have observed improvements in social-emotional, cognitive, and visual spatial development in infants when they first gain mobility.[1,8,17,19] Self-initiated mobility also affects motor functioning and the ability to develop mature reach and grasp and postural control.[49,50] Researchers who have studied the impact of early exploration on a child's development have also suggested that self-produced locomotion and active choice are important for the development of perception and cognition.[16,31,60,72,81] Young children who at 3 years old were high stimulation–seeking demonstrated increased cognitive, scholastic, and neuropsychological test performance at 11 years.[69]

"When development along any line is restricted, delayed, or distorted, other lines of development are adversely affected as well" (p. 66).[14] Restricted experiences and mobility during early childhood can have a diffuse and lasting influence. Long-term physical restriction during infancy or early childhood can significantly alter and disrupt the entire subsequent course of emotional or psychological development in the involved child.[45] Such deprivation of physical and social contingencies can lead to secondary developmental problems, including limiting motivation to explore the environment. Infants born with significant motor impairments quickly "begin to lose interest in a world which they do not expect to control" (p. 113).[12] This motivational effect is termed *learned helplessness,* a condition in which the child gives up trying to control his or her own world because of motor disability and diminished expectations of caregivers.[29,72] Butler found that children whose mobility is limited during early childhood develop a pattern of apathetic behavior—specifically, a lack of curiosity and initiative.[14] These character traits are believed to have a critical influence on intellectual performance and social interaction. The detrimental effects of limited early exploration were identified in a study comparing shortcut choices in a simulated maze of able-bodied teenagers with those of teenagers who had varying histories of mobility impairment. Despite equivalent levels of mobility, participants whose mobility was more limited early in development were poorer in the task than those whose mobility had deteriorated with age. The results suggest that early independent exploration is important in the development of spatial knowledge and that the detrimental effects of limited early exploratory experience may persist into the teenage years.[74]

In children with severe physical disabilities, newly gained independent mobility can have a positive effect on emotional, social, and intellectual states.[26,35] Paulsson and Christoffersen found that children with disabilities using mobility devices became less dependent on controlling their environment through verbal commands, more interested in all mobility skills, and more active in peer activities.[63] Butler found that children who had some means of ambulation could and would make choices, but those who did not ambulate were much less likely to exercise available options.[13] The lack of ambulation appeared to severely restrict the child's opportunities to practice decision making and express an opinion or desire. Guerette et al. found that powered mobility can positively influence cognitive and psychosocial development of young children who are unable to move independently.[40] They also suggest that self-initiated powered mobility for a young child has a positive impact on the family.[80]

Self-Initiated Mobility

Intervention for young children with physical disabilities often includes the provision of adapted equipment: supported chairs, standers, bath seats, and adapted strollers. This equipment provides a means for properly and safely positioning a child, but it does not provide a means for accessing the environment or experiencing the stages of development that occur with self-initiated mobility. Children who have a means for self-initiated mobility decide where, when, and how to move. It is the responsibility of the occupational and physical therapist to

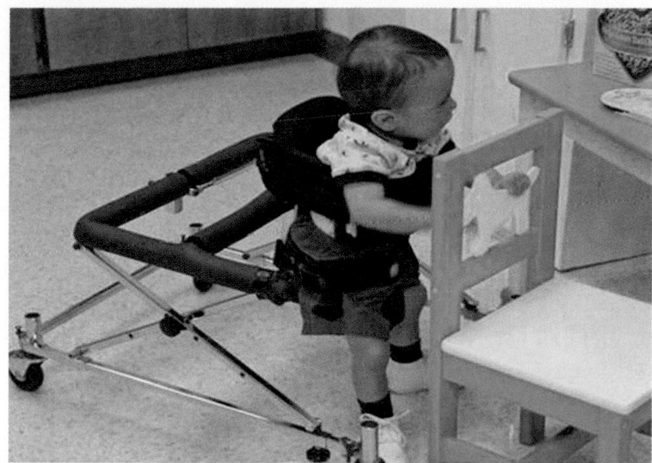

FIGURE 20-2 The FCI Walker Mini allows an 18-month-old child with a developmental delay to explore his environment. (Courtesy Freedom Concepts Inc.)

determine how young children with disabilities can access their environment, explore their surroundings, and experience developmentally appropriate activities. Mobility devices, which provide a physically disabled child with a means to access and explore the environment, not only provide a means for mobility but also facilitate psychosocial, visual spatial, language, and cognitive development. Such devices include prone scooters, handheld walkers, support walkers, manual and power wheelchairs, and alternative powered mobility devices.

The current trend is for mobility devices to be recommended at young ages, when typical children are first ambulating (Figure 20-2). Many professionals believe that if self-initiated mobility does not occur in the first year, the use of devices for mobility should be considered. Mobility is often a priority issue for children with disabilities and others in their environment. When researchers surveyed the occupational performance needs of school-age children with physical disabilities in the school system and community, most teachers, parents, and children identified mobility as their greatest area of concern.[68] However, professionals lack agreement when and if mobility devices for very young children, particularly support walkers and powered mobility devices, are appropriate.

A support walker differs from a handheld walker in that it typically includes a seat with postural supports for the pelvis, trunk, and sometimes the head. In the past, occupational therapists were reluctant to recommend support walkers for children with cerebral palsy because they would often use undesirable postures during ambulation, and they believed it might increase the child's spasticity. However, many support walkers are now designed with features that complement the child's therapeutic goals.[58,60,91] In addition, several studies have demonstrated that resistive exercise does not increase spasticity in individuals with cerebral palsy.[10,27,32,53] Although further study is needed, several studies of persons with cerebral palsy concluded that a progressive strength-training program can improve muscle strength and walking ability without increasing spasticity.[4,10]

Professionals and third-party payers may resist providing a powered mobility device to a young child with physical disabilities, particularly before the age of 5 years. Indeed, most children born with congenital mobility impairments are not given their first wheelchair until the age of at least 3 years, and most of these do not receive a chair they can propel independently until age 5.[33,35] Children with a physical disability under the age of 5 years are often denied the opportunity for using a powered mobility device because they are considered too young to have the cognitive skills to understand how to use it. However, "Clinical experience and research projects have established that powered mobility devices offer children at least as young as 17 months of age a safe and efficient method of independent locomotion" (p. 18).[15,37] Galloway studied the ability of infants as young as 7 months to use a motorized robotic device for self-generated mobility.[37] Research continues to substantiate the fact that children as young as 18 months can achieve independent skills in powered mobility.[33,35]

However, it can be a challenging task for an occupational therapist to suggest consideration of a mobility device, particularly a power wheelchair, to the family of a young mobility-impaired child. Many caregivers consider the suggestion as a symbol of giving up hope for independent ambulation. For this reason, use of a walker, support walker, or alternative powered mobility device may be more accepted by the families of very young children. The occupational therapist must convey to the family the concept that all children need a means of mobility to access the environment for exploration to encourage development in the visual, perceptual, language, social, and cognitive domains. The mobility device is intended to assist the child in achieving independence in exploration until and if another method is acquired.

Caregivers may believe that use of a power wheelchair will reduce the likelihood of their child's achieving independent mobility through ambulation. Research has not demonstrated that use of a powered mobility device prevents or delays the child's acquisition of motor skills. On the contrary, researchers find positive changes in children's development after the introduction of a powered mobility device.[55,63,88] During mobility training, children with severe motor disabilities demonstrated improved head control and trunk stability, increased motivation, and greater self-confidence in movement.[13] Deitz, Swinth, and White concluded that for some young children with severe motor impairments and developmental delay, use of a powered mobility device may potentially increase self-initiated movement occurrences during free play.[25] Nilsson and Nyberg analyzed case studies of preschool children with profound cognitive disabilities participating in power wheelchair training experiences.[55] They concluded that the training experiences increased wakefulness and alertness, stimulated a limited use of arms and hands, and promoted the understanding of very simple cause-and-effect relationships.

In another study, children 15 months to 5 years of age with physical disabilities who participated in a 2-week mobility exploration day camp demonstrated a variety of positive behavioral changes.[88] The children experienced mobility by using the Mini-Bot, a standing powered mobility device, to explore the environment (Figure 20-3). They participated in daily 1½ hour sessions for 2 weeks. Behavioral changes that caregivers and occupational therapists observed in some children included increased eye contact, increased verbalization and communication, improved sleeping patterns, increased active arm use, and a more positive disposition.

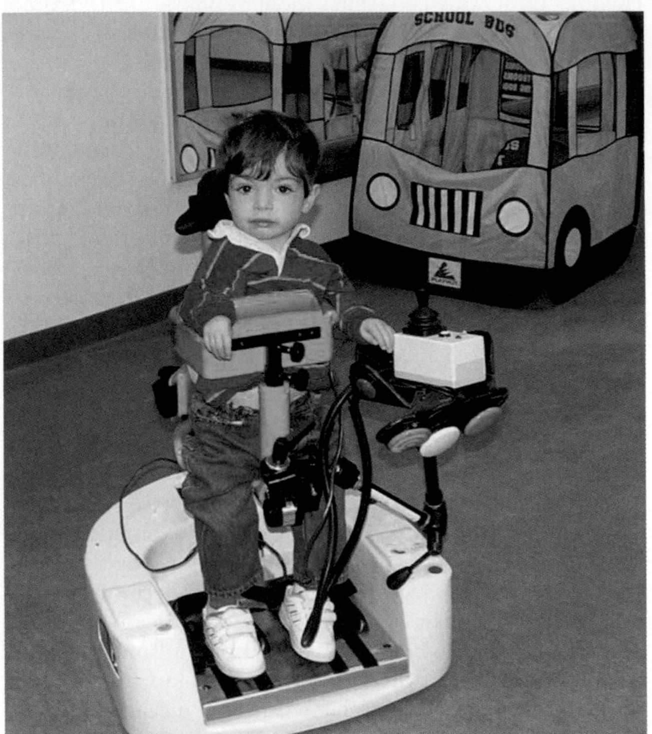

FIGURE 20-3 A 2-year-old child with arthrogryposis experiences self-initiated mobility while standing and moving in the powered Mini-Bot, with the option to drive it with a joystick or switches. (Courtesy Innovative Products, Inc.)

Augmentative Mobility

Butler introduced the term *augmentative mobility* to describe all types of mobility that supplement or augment ambulation. "Given augmentative mobility, disabled children can experience more success in directly controlling their environment, thereby reducing or avoiding secondary social, emotional and intellectual handicaps" (p. 18).[15]

The concept of augmentative mobility for functional mobility can be expanded to include transitional mobility. Transitional mobility allows the child to use a mobility device to have self-initiated movement without the expectation that it must be functional. The child may not consistently move the mobility device in a desired direction but uses it as a means for exploring the effects of movement and learning how to move. The occupational therapist can best provide transitional mobility by allowing the child to move the device in a large room with open space in which the child is free to explore. These experiences can then help the child make the transition to a more functional level of purposeful mobility. Not all children are able to achieve functional mobility; in these instances transitional mobility remains an important means for the child to explore the environment.

Ideally, a mobility-impaired child should have more than one type of mobility device for use in indoor and outdoor environments. Any methods that are chosen for mobility require close cooperation among all professionals working with the child and family.

Assessment and Intervention

Classification of Mobility Skills

Children's mastery of functional mobility skills has been classified and categorized in several ways. Hays examined current existing diagnostic conditions of children without locomotion and divided them into four functional groups[43]:

1. *Children who will never ambulate.* This category includes children with cerebral palsy with severe involvement and spinal muscular atrophy types I and II. Generally, these children have no opportunity for independent mobility.
2. *Children with inefficient mobility who ambulate but are unable to do so at a reasonable rate of speed or with acceptable endurance.* This category includes children with cerebral palsy with less involvement and myelomeningocele with upper-extremity involvement. For these children, assisted mobility may provide an efficient means of mobility above that which they are capable of producing themselves. Warren uses the term *marginal ambulators* for this group.[86]
3. *Children who have lost their independent mobility.* This category includes victims of trauma and children with progressive neuromuscular disorders. The developmental implications may be less critical than in the first two groups, and the issue is acceptance of assisted mobility as an adaptation to the acquired disability.
4. *Children who temporarily require assisted mobility and often progress to independent mobility with age.* This category includes many children with osteogenesis imperfecta and arthrogryposis. Functional considerations in this group are both developmental and practical.

There are significant differences among these groups that may have implications for mobility and its integration into the child's overall concept of disability, as well as for evaluation and intervention. Group I children may achieve independent mobility through the use of a support walker and power wheelchair. Group II children may be able to independently propel a manual wheelchair, ambulate in a support walker indoors, and use a power wheelchair for community mobility. Children in groups III and IV will use a variety of mobility methods during the transition period.

Mobility Assessments

Evaluation of children has traditionally focused on the achievement of developmental milestones. Occupational therapists have discussed the limitation of such evaluations because underlying impairments (e.g., motor control deficits) cannot fully explain the extent and form of functional difficulties seen in children with disabilities.[22] Furthermore, the tasks that are most relevant for daily independence in mobility function have not been well defined in traditional developmental milestone tests. The team considers several factors before selecting the type of mobility device that is appropriate for a child. These factors include:

- Purpose and goals for using the device
- Environments for intended use
- Child's physical and psychosocial abilities and limitations.
- Advantages and disadvantages of the device across environments
- Modifications that may be needed for comfort and control

- Congruence to intervention goals
- Cost-benefit ratio

Using a top-down evaluation process, the occupational therapist focuses on what the child needs or wants to do, the context in which he or she typically engages in occupations, and the limitations that he or she may experience.[22,30] Therapists assess underlying performance abilities only to the extent that is needed to help clarify the possible sources of limitations in occupational performance. In mobility evaluation, occupational therapists focus on the child's overall pattern of locomotion and transfer skills in relation to a particular performance context.

Occupational therapy models of practice, such as the Person, Environment, Occupation, and Performance model of human occupation or the Canadian Occupational Performance Model, may provide the overarching framework to view the child's performance in daily living and mobility. These models provide the framework for semi-structured interviews to identify the child's strengths and weaknesses within their family and environment. After understanding the child, practitioners may decide to examine mobility more specifically.

Three instruments that evaluate children's functional abilities, including mobility, are the Pediatric Evaluation of Disability Inventory Computer Adaptive Test (PEDI-CAT),[41] the Functional Independence Measure for Children (WeeFIM),[84] and the School Function Assessment.[22]

- The PEDI-CAT assesses daily activities, mobility, social/cognitive, and responsibility domains. The functional mobility subscale measures basic transfer skills (e.g., getting in and out of a car) and body transportation activities (e.g., walking up and down stairs).
- WeeFIM is based on the Functional Independence Measure and is for children from 6 months to 7 years of age. This scale measures the child's independence in mobility—transfers, locomotion, and stairs—and provides useful information for progress assessment, program planning, and communication with caregivers.
- The School Function Assessment identifies the adaptations that benefit a student to perform functional tasks in the school environment K-6. It is a criterion-based instrument intended to facilitate collaborative program planning as it relates to elementary school students with disabilities. Part I measures the student's participation levels during six school activities: regular or special education classroom, recess or playground, transportation to and from school, bathroom and toileting activities, transitions to and from the classroom, and mealtime or snack time. Part II measures the types of task supports provided to the student (assistance from adult) or adaptation (e.g., a wheelchair); Part III examines how the student performs during specific school-related tasks in the areas of Physical Activity Performance and Cognitive Behavioral Activity Performance.

The Pediatric Powered Wheelchair Screening Test (PPWST) and the Powered Mobility Program (PMP) were developed as a cognitive assessment battery and a wheelchair mobility training and assessment program to help clinicians determine a young child's readiness to drive a power wheelchair.[77,78] The PPWST and PMP were validated for children ages 20 to 36 months with orthopedic disabilities who used a joystick to control the wheelchair.[38,39] The cognitive domains of spatial relations and problem solving were found to be significant predictors of power wheelchair mobility performance.

Occupational therapists evaluate client factors (e.g., motor, perceptual, and cognitive factors) that influence mobility. Human functions important to mobility include neuromotor status (vision, hearing, and seizure disorders), orthopedic conditions, and psychosocial variables. Occupational therapists also consider both chronologic and developmental age and the child's environments. The therapist must make potential mobility devices and positioning systems available during the evaluation process so that the child and the caregivers have an opportunity to gain experience using potential mobility devices. These trials provide the caregivers and the child with information and experience that will assist them in becoming informed consumers and full participants in deciding which mobility device best meets their needs.

Mobility Evaluation Teams

Selection of the most appropriate positioning and mobility device requires the skills of a therapy team working in close collaboration with the school team, prescribing physician, child, parent or caregiver, and assistive technology professional (ATP). The ATP is "a service provider who analyzes the needs of individuals with disabilities, assists in the selection of the appropriate equipment, and trains the consumer on how to properly use the specific equipment. This equipment may include manual and power wheelchairs, alternate computer access, augmentative and alternative communication devices and other technology to improve the function and quality of life for an individual with a disability" (http://resna.org). The ATP is credentialed through the Rehabilitation Engineering and Assistive Technology Society of North America (RESNA). Occupational and physical therapists who make recommendations for assistive technology equipment often seek an ATP credential. An ATP may also be certified as a Seating Mobility Specialist through RESNA, which recognizes and identifies rehabilitation professionals with advanced knowledge and experience in the field of seating and mobility. RESNA also provides certification for a Rehabilitation Engineering Technologist, who designs, customizes, and modifies assistive technology (AT). The ATP is responsible for maintaining updated knowledge of available equipment and assisting in identifying choices of mobility devices according to the features that the child requires to use it optimally.

The physical or occupational therapist, together with the child, family, and school team, determine the needs of the child and establish goals to identify the features and options in a mobility device or devices that will meet the desired outcomes and assist the family in setting appropriate functional goals and expectations for using the mobility device. The child's school team should be included in the evaluation process to determine the needs of the child for accessing the school environment, the physical space, the curriculum, communication technology, and educational materials. Once the needs are identified, the purpose for using the device is determined, and the environments in which it will be used are considered, the therapist or family requests a local supplier of durable medical equipment or ATP to bring the mobility devices under consideration to the therapy session. The ATP offers input about what features and options are available on the device and how to adjust it properly. The ATP provides a variety of mobility devices during the evaluation with features that meet the mobility needs of the child, family, and school team.

Some medical equipment suppliers may have a limited selection of devices available for demonstration, so only one device may be evaluated at each session. Therefore the occupational therapist may not have the opportunity to compare the child's performance in various types of mobility devices. Without direct comparison of the mobility devices, decisions about which devices are optimal for the child are difficult for the occupational therapist to make. The decision is less risky when side-by-side comparisons of different devices are available during the evaluation. This method enables evaluation of performance with each mobility device under consistent child and environmental conditions. If a supplier is not able to bring the requested devices, the manufacturer's representative may be able to provide the device and expertise for the evaluation.

Once the mobility device and options are recommended in a written report and justified to the funding agency for authorization, actual delivery may take 3 to 9 months. It is imperative that the ATP and occupational therapist work together during the delivery and fitting of the equipment, which typically takes up to an hour, to assure that the mobility device meets the needs of the child and expectations of the team. Most funding agencies do not approve replacement of a mobility device, such as a wheelchair, within 3 to 5 years of the purchase date. If the equipment is not appropriate, the child and family may not have another option for several years. The limitations in reimbursement become critical when a misunderstanding during the evaluation or ordering process results in a device that does not meet the predetermined outcomes. It is imperative that the occupational therapist, ATP, and family immediately decide how to best resolve these issues. The therapist is responsible for periodically (every 4-6 months) reevaluating the fit and function of the device to determine if it meets the stated goals and growth of the child.

Mobility Devices

Selection of a specific type of a mobility device depends on several factors. The therapy team first decides on the purpose for using the mobility device or devices. Does the child need a means for exploring and accessing the environment (self-propelled manual, power wheelchair, or hands-free support walker) or do the caregivers need a convenient way to transport the child (stroller or manual wheelchair)? The next, most critical aspect of evaluating a mobility device is to consider the environments in which it is to be used by the child and caregivers. If the child's home has high pile carpet, propelling a manual wheelchair or using a walker with wheels smaller than 5 inches in diameter will be quite difficult. The force needed to move a wheelchair over various surfaces has been measured. Using concrete as the baseline, the increase in force needed to cross each surface is 3% for linoleum, 20% for low-pile carpet, and 62% for high-pile carpet.[3] The effort required by the individual to use the device will affect functional performance. If the mobility device is too complicated or the child must exert too much effort, it will not be used.

The occupational therapist must consider the features, adaptations, and hardware options needed for optimal use across all environments such as school, home, and community; the system must not reduce performance in functional activities such as eating, personal hygiene, transfers, and augmentative communication. The needs and concerns of the caregivers and school personnel who will be transferring the child into and out of the device, transporting it, and maintaining the equipment must be considered. The cost/benefit ratio is considered in decision making.

The occupational therapist must use his or her skills as an investigator during the mobility assessment process. Thoughtful planning and careful analysis of person-device-environment fit are necessary for the therapist to ensure that the child and family receive the optimal device. When a device is ordered without a comprehensive team mobility evaluation, the child may end up with a wheelchair that will not fit into the family van with the user in it, tips over when the speech-generating device is mounted on it, cannot be self-propelled outside because the family lives in a hilly area, is too large to maneuver efficiently in the classroom environment, or is too tall to fit under the tables and desks. Case Study 20-1 provides an example of a child whose need for a mobility device—a support walker—was not evaluated properly.

Alternative Mobility Devices

Tricycles

Tricycles (Figure 20-4) are a means for mobility, although third-party funding is typically not available because tricycles are not considered a medical necessity. However, they can provide community mobility outdoors and on playgrounds.

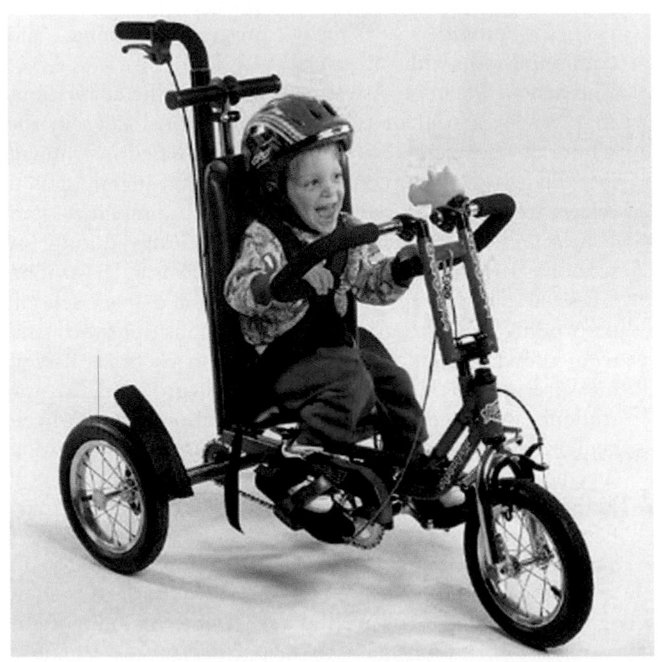

FIGURE 20-4 The Discovery Trike can fit a child as young as 12 months. An adult can assist the child by steering the front wheel with the push handle. (Courtesy Freedom Concepts.)

CASE STUDY 20-1 Brian

Brian is 5 years old and has severe spastic cerebral palsy. He is dependent on others for mobility in his manual wheelchair. He is fully included in a kindergarten classroom. His mother believes Brian will have more peer interaction if he can use a support walker in the classroom, which places him at his peer's height. She also believes he had better digestive function when he previously used a walker at a younger age. Brian was evaluated at his medical therapy session to determine what type of walker would provide him with mobility in the classroom. His parents expressed interest in a particular walker, and the occupational therapist borrowed one from a medical equipment provider for Brian to use during the evaluation at the medical therapy unit. The family was excited when they observed Brian slowly propelling the walker forward. The therapist recommended the walker for purchase with custom modifications, which included a headrest and a custom thigh-length seat to reduce adduction. The family ordered the walker and Brian began to use it in his classroom.

After 5 months of trying to use the support walker in the classroom, he could not take more than three steps in it. The occupational therapist determined that he did not have the ability to maneuver the walker in the classroom because of a high degree of resistance from the carpeted surface. The therapist initially evaluated Brian in a room with linoleum, without consideration of the classroom environment. The therapist reevaluated Brian in another walker that had large 20-inch wheels, which made it easier for him to maneuver over carpet. At this time, additional funding to purchase another walker is not available. He would have benefited from a side-by-side evaluation of several types of walkers with consideration of the characteristics of all the environments in which he would use the walker and consultation with all team members.

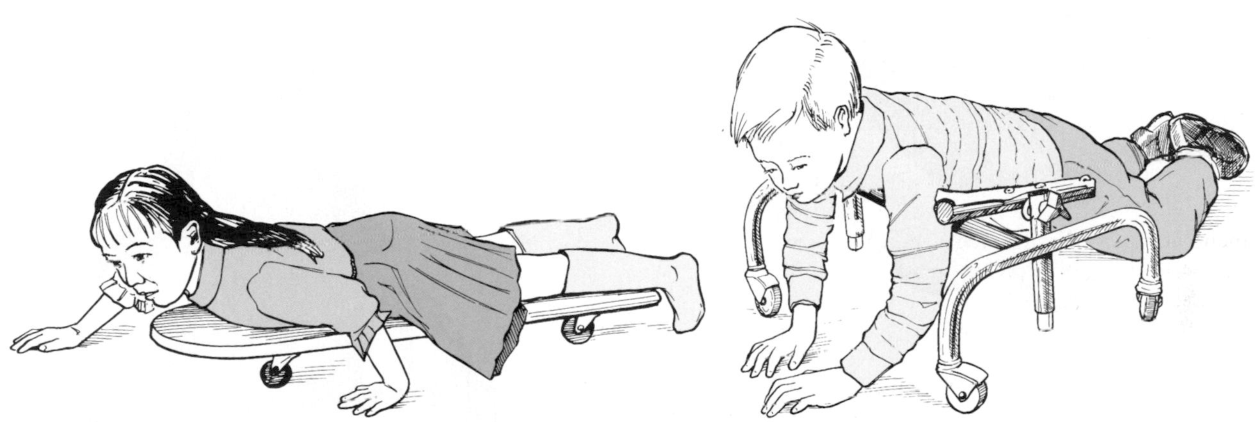

FIGURE 20-5 Prone scooter mobility devices.

Many types of tricycles are available with adaptations, such as trunk supports, and hand-propelled models are available for children who do not have the ability to pedal with their legs (e.g., children with spina bifida). A unique and helpful feature for both the child and the care provider is a handle at the back of the Freedom Concepts tricycle, which enables the adult to steer the front wheel while the child pedals. This assists a child with limited upper extremity function who may not have the ability to hold onto the handle bars to steer the tricycle.

Prone Scooters

Prone scooters (Figure 20-5) require use of the arms and the ability to lift the head while moving. The advantages of using a prone scooter include access for participating in play activities on the floor, the ability to get on and off independently, and the ability to change direction more easily than with other types of manual mobility devices. Disadvantages include fatigue from maintaining neck and back extension, vulnerability of the head to hitting objects, the possibility of the hands getting caught in the casters or rubbed on rough surfaces, and difficulty viewing the environment above the ground level. Children with spina bifida may find the prone scooter functional because they have the upper extremity function and strength to propel it and the scooter can support their legs.

Caster Carts

Caster carts offer another means of mobility to children with upper-extremity function (e.g., those with spina bifida) (Figure 20-6*A*). Children can use caster carts indoors or on flat outdoor surfaces. Some children may be able to transfer on and off independently because of the close proximity to the floor. The device requires a considerable amount of energy expenditure for propelling long distances because of the small diameter of the wheels. Children with lower-extremity muscle contractures or tightness, such as in the hamstring muscles, may find it difficult to sit comfortably and securely because they are often unable to tolerate long-leg sitting. These children may feel more comfortable with a triangular-shaped wedge placed under the knees to support their legs in knee flexion. A battery-powered multidirectional scooter board from Enabling Devices allows a child to move either in a circular motion with one switch input or in all directions using several switches or a joystick (Figure 20-6*B*).

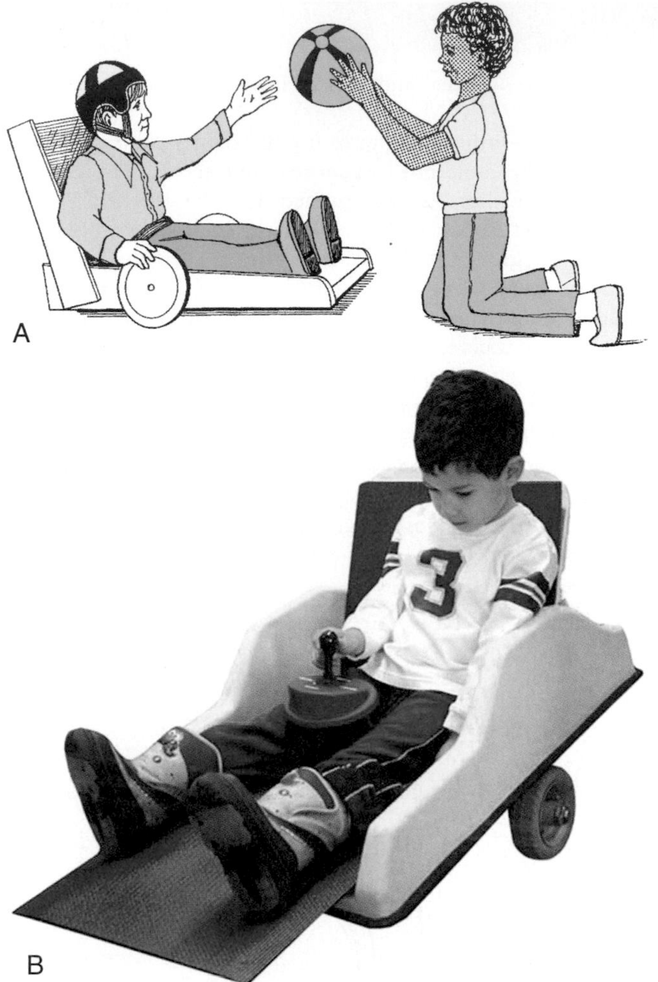

FIGURE 20-6 **A,** Caster cart mobility device. **B,** Joystick- or switch-controlled multi-directional scooter board. (Courtesy Enabling Devices, Hastings-on-Hudson, NY.)

Aeroplane Mobility Device

The aeroplane mobility device was designed by an occupational therapist for children with cerebral palsy who can move their legs but need support of the upper body (Figure 20-7*A*). The device provides developmentally appropriate positioning, particularly for children with spasticity, because the child is positioned with hip abduction and extension with knee flexion, and the upper extremities are in a weight-bearing position. This position often assists in reducing undesirable posturing in children who have spastic cerebral palsy, especially for children who exhibit extensor posturing in standing. Other advantages include ease in viewing the environment, the handmade nature of the device, and acceptance by parents because it looks like a toy rather than an assistive device. The aeroplane mobility device is not available commercially but can be fabricated from wood. Disadvantages include lack of adjustability for growth, difficulty turning and moving backward, and heaviness.

Mobile Stander

If a child has upper extremity function to push and maneuver wheels, a mobile stander may provide another means for mobility. These devices allow the child to experience lower extremity weight bearing in a standing position while achieving mobility by using large hand-held wheels for self-propulsion (Figure 20-7*B*).

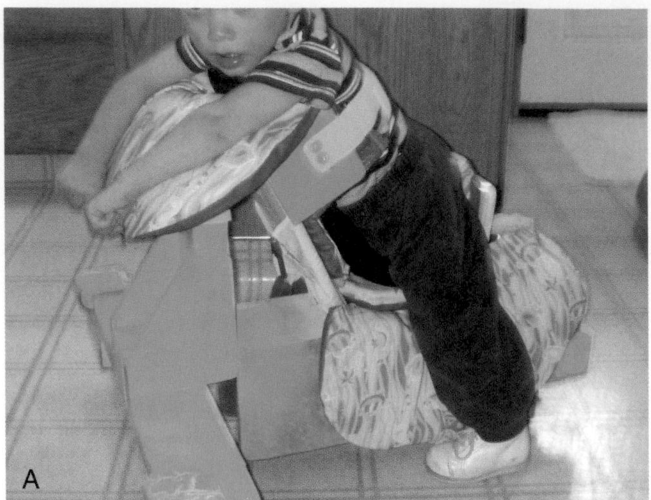

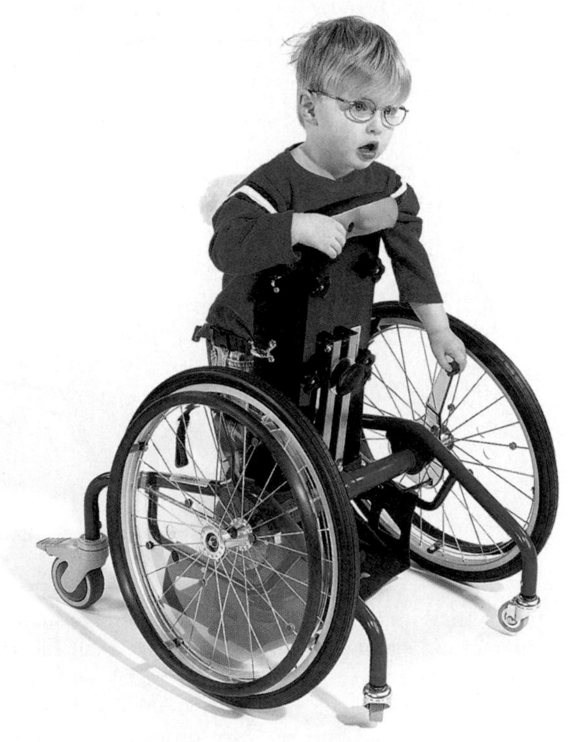

FIGURE 20-7 **A,** The aeroplane mobility device can be handmade and is designed for children younger than 3 years of age. **B,** The Rifton Dynamic Stander provides standing mobility in prone which clients can self-propel with their upper extremities. (Courtesy Rifton Equipment.)

Walkers

Children who have the ability to pull to a standing position, maintain a grip on a handle, and steer with their arms may be

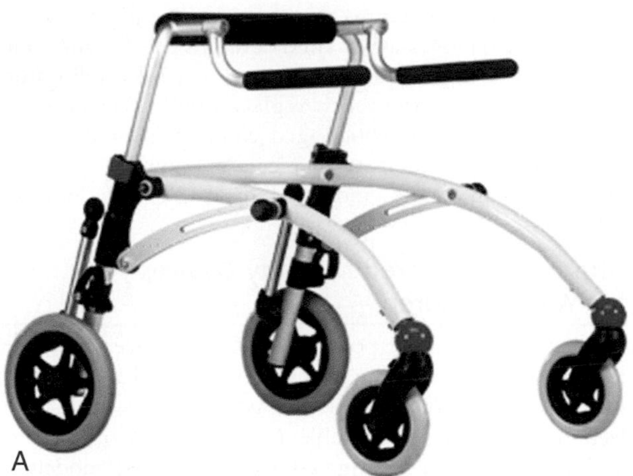

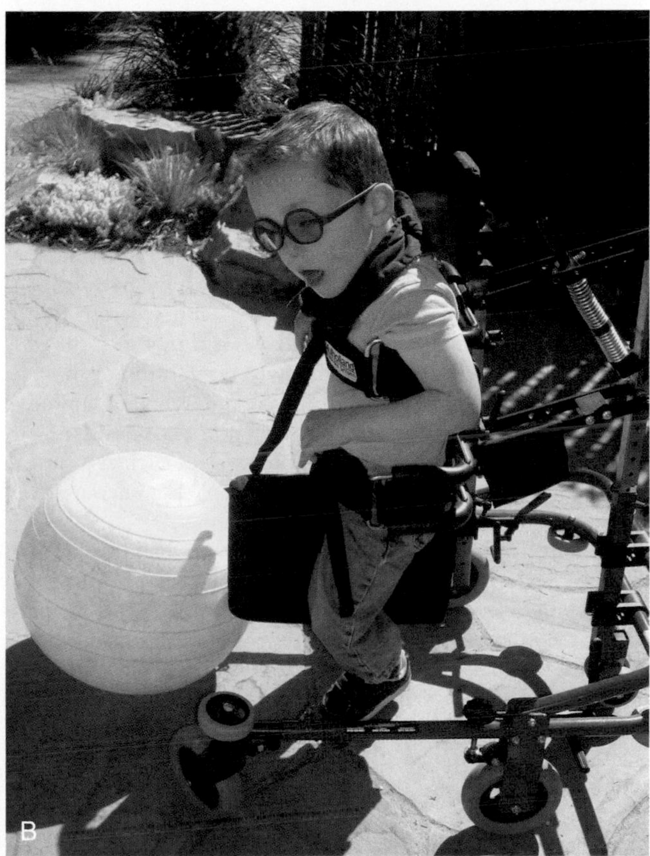

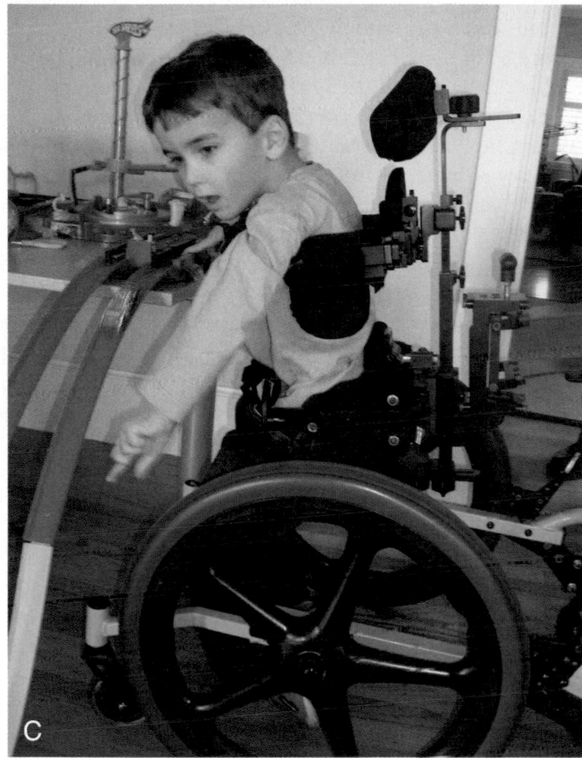

FIGURE 20-8 **A,** The Crocodile walker is a hand-held walker designed for children who can hold onto the frame without pelvic or trunk supports (Snug Seat). **B,** A preschooler plays ball in his WalkAbout. **C,** A young child accesses his favorite race car toy at home by walking up to it in his KidWalk.

able to use a hand-held walker. These walkers are designed for use either in front of (anterior walker) or behind (posterior walker) the child (Figure 20-8*A*). Children with mild to moderate cerebral palsy or lower levels of spina bifida with leg bracing most commonly use hand-held walkers. Walkers can have three or four wheels and are available in various wheel sizes. The smaller the caster, the more difficult it is for use outdoors and over uneven surfaces. Posterior walkers are available with a feature in which the casters lock when the walker is pushed backward. This feature enables the child to stand and lean against the walker or the seat during rest periods. However, this feature makes maneuvering the walker more difficult because the child cannot move the walker in a reverse direction, which is needed when backing away and turning, without lifting it up to overcome the anti-rollback mechanism. Casters can be fixed rather than swiveled, which allows movement only in the forward direction so the user must lift the walker to turn it. Swivel casters allow the child to turn the walker without lifting it, but this feature requires more postural control from the child to direct the walker. The advantages of hand-held walkers are their low cost and convenient transportability. The disadvantages for some users include poor body alignment when pushing a walker and the fact that the hands are not free for performing tasks.

Support walkers are designed for children who have some ability to move their legs reciprocally but need support at the pelvis, chest, and possibly the upper extremities and head. It is critical to identify the purpose for using the support walker and the environments where it will be used, to achieve maximum benefit for the child. If the purpose of the support walker is to provide self-initiated mobility for a child to access the indoor home environment, allowing the child to reach objects and people, then features should include wheels that are a minimum of 5 inches in diameter, which move more efficiently over carpets and thresholds than smaller wheels, and a design that does not include hardware, arm troughs, or a tray in front of the child, which would limit the ability to reach during exploratory activities (Figure 20-8*C*). However, children with limited arm and hand function as a result of hypotonia or spasticity may require modifications to the support walker such as a tray, which limits getting close to objects and people but encourages spatial awareness through movement.

Decisions regarding available options and features on a walker are made based on the child's physical function and the environment. Selection of appropriate features and adjustments that provide optimal positioning will increase functional use of these types of walkers. Children who adduct or scissor their legs as a result of spasticity may propel the walker more efficiently if a wider and longer padded seat is provided to reduce adduction and maintain leg alignment during ambulation. A young child with hypotonia or weakness may be more successful using a lightweight walker with all swivel casters over smooth flat surfaces such as linoleum (see Figure 20-2). Adjustable posterior tilt, a feature that positions the child slightly behind vertical, may also assist a weak child in maintaining an upright trunk and head position. Children with spastic cerebral palsy may need to be tilted in a slightly forward lean position, which along with a properly positioned pelvis (in neutral or anteriorly tilted position) assists in placing the feet behind the pelvis and trunk, thereby making it easier for the child to initiate movement in a forward direction. However, forward tilt can also make it significantly more difficult for the child to keep the head upright.

Support walkers can provide children with the opportunity to explore their environment in an upright, hands-free position while providing capability for active range of motion. Therapists are encouraged to promote more activity in children with cerebral palsy by using mobility-enhancing devices.[23] However, many support walkers have limitations in maneuverability, particularly indoors, because they require a large turning radius. The KidWalk was designed by an occupational therapist to promote use of the upper extremities during exploration.[60] It has minimal hardware in front of the child so the child can use self-initiated mobility to be within arm's reach of people and objects to access and explore the environment and perform developmental activities such as pushing, pulling, opening and closing drawers, reaching, and carrying objects to achieve occupational therapy goals. The KidWalk allows a high degree of maneuverability, particularly over carpeted surfaces and thresholds, because of the placement of a large wheel located at the vector of the child's body, which also encourages rotation of the upper body over the pelvis, a more desirable movement. It incorporates a mechanism for weight shifting during ambulation and a dynamic swivel seat to encourage reciprocal leg movements and does not depend on upper body function to maneuver it. The upper body supports can be removed as the child develops balance and control. Because of its large mid-wheel design, it works well outdoors and over uneven surfaces such as playgrounds. Benefits of using a support walker for school-aged children include the ability to exercise and participate in recess by running and chasing or kicking, throwing, and catching balls while interacting with peers.

Alternative Powered Mobility Devices for Young Children

A variety of alternative powered mobility devices are available for children who cannot achieve self-initiated mobility using reciprocal leg movements or by pushing large wheels. Motorized toy vehicles are available for children to provide early mobility experiences using a joystick; adapted models with special electronics for using up to four switches are also available. From the caregiver's perspective, the greatest advantage for use of these toy vehicles is that they look like a toy that any other child would use, rather than an assistive device. They are also an option for providing a child with the opportunity to learn how to drive a motorized device in preparation for using a power wheelchair. Disadvantages include difficulty using these vehicles indoors because of limited maneuverability; large size, which prevents the child from getting close to objects in the environment for reaching, exploring, and interacting with others; and sometimes noisy operation.

The MiniBot and the GoBot were developed by an occupational therapist (see Figure 20-3).[89,90] Each is a powered mobility device designed to enable physically challenged preschool children from 12 months to about 8 years of age to move in an upright position and explore the environment by getting close enough to objects and peers to reach and touch. It is intended for transitional mobility indoors or for use outdoors on flat surfaces. The child can be positioned in either a standing, semi-standing, or seated position. A joystick or multiple switches can be positioned at any location at which the child can reach the controls for driving the device. The MiniBot is not a power wheelchair; it is a therapeutic and educational tool intended to provide developmental opportunities equivalent to those experienced by able-bodied peers, such as pushing or pulling toys, kicking balls, moving quickly, moving slowly, and problem solving. The MiniBot can increase the child's opportunities for hands-free exploration and provide new sensory experiences (particularly vestibular, visual motor, and spatial relations). It is intended for children who would otherwise spend their early developmental years passively sitting in a stroller or manual wheelchair.

Wheeled Mobility Systems

Wheeled mobility systems include dependent mobility systems or transit wheelchairs, independent manual mobility systems such as self-propelling wheelchairs, and independent powered mobility systems that are battery powered. The first mobility system most children acquire is a stroller, which is considered to be a transit dependent mobility system because the user is depending on others for mobility. Parents often prefer the ease of use of a stroller and feel the appearance is more acceptable than that of a wheelchair when the child is very young.[20]

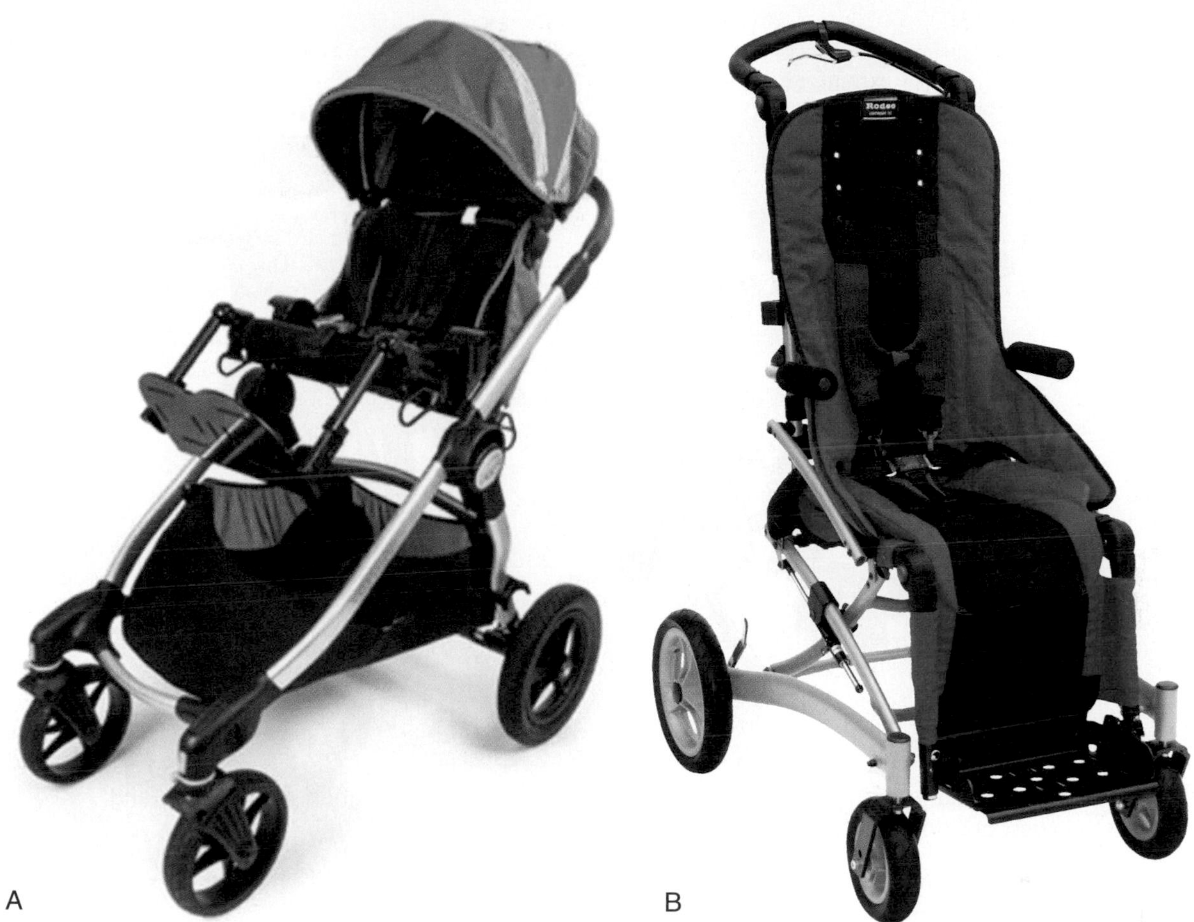

FIGURE 20-9 Strollers. **A,** The Zippie Voyage Stroller™ provides tilt, recline, and seating components in a foldable base. **B,** The Convaid Rodeo chair is a light weight, crash tested transit model with tilt-in-space, size-adjustable frame, and optional thoracic lateral supports. (**A,** Courtesy Snrise Medical; **B,** Courtesy Convaid, Inc.)

However, a stroller may not provide supportive seating for a child with moderate to severe disabilities. Mobile positioning systems, which provide more support than a stroller, while still being lightweight and easily foldable, are available through medical equipment providers. Some of these models include bus or van anchors for transporting the child in a vehicle, such as the Convaid Rodeo (Figure 20-9*B*), and lightweight foldable strollers with a seating system, like the Zippie Voyage by Sunrise Medical (Figure 20-9*A*).

Other dependent seating and positioning systems offer an adjustable height chassis to position the child close to the floor or up to various table heights (Figure 20-10*A*). The seating system is fully adjustable by the occupational therapist to accommodate the needs of a variety of users so a custom seating system is not necessary, but modifications may be required to meet individual needs. These types of adjustable positioning chairs are meant to primarily be used indoors and are not designed for transporting because they are quite heavy. Dependent mobility systems can provide convenience for care providers and teachers, as well as optimal positioning for function. The seating system can also be removed on some models and transferred to another type of base such as an outdoor or stroller base. The greatest disadvantage of a dependent mobility system is that the child must depend solely on others for mobility and has no means for self-initiated mobility and exploration. Peers may also perceive an older child with a disability who uses a dependent mobility system such as a stroller as being less able and less approachable than a child of similar age who sits in a wheelchair. Dependent mobility systems that can be retrofitted into a larger wheel base should be considered if the team believes that the child will be able to self-propel within the next few years. However, if the child appears to have some ability to eventually propel the wheels but does not have repeated opportunities early in development to learn how to reach and push, then the likelihood of doing so may be lessened.

Manual Wheelchairs

Manual mobility systems are either independent manual wheelchairs that allow the user to self propel by pushing two large wheels or dependent manual wheelchairs with small wheeled bases that do not provide opportunities for independent mobility (Figure 20-11*F*). A manual wheelchair is appropriate for a child who has the ability to functionally and efficiently propel it. It is also used as a means of transportation by caregivers or as a backup wheelchair when the child's power wheelchair is

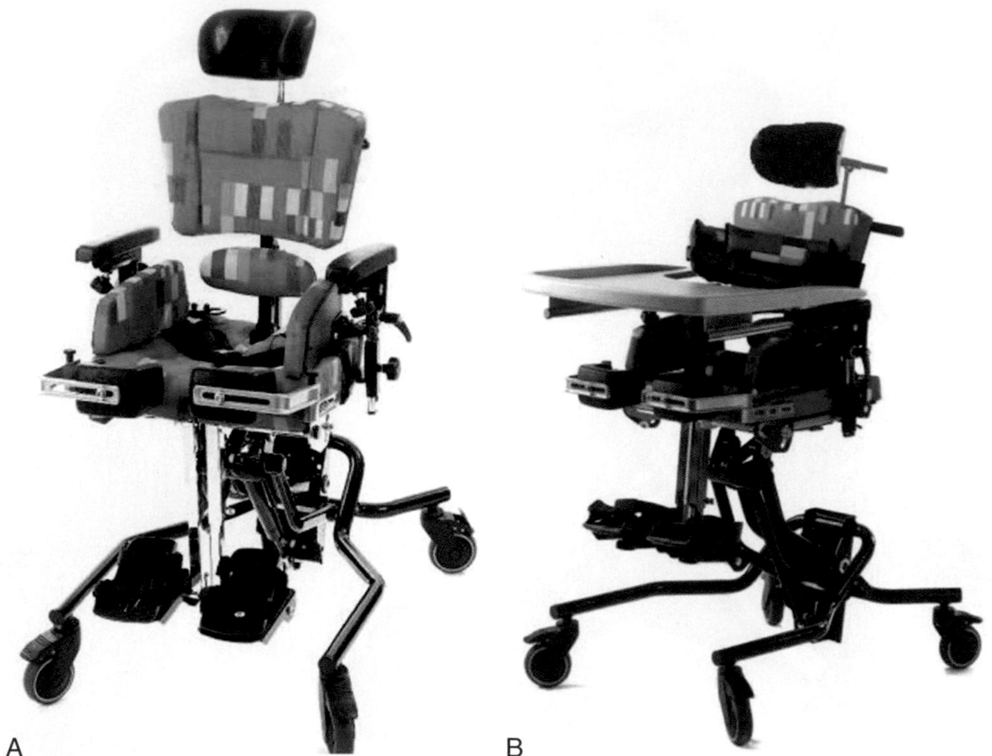

FIGURE 20-10 The Leckey Contoured Advance Seat in the highest position (**A**) and lowest position (**B**). (Distributed by Ottobock USA.)

not working. Great strides in design and material selection have resulted in lighter frames than the standard 35-pound wheelchair such as the TiLite Twist (Figure 20-11*A*). Weights can range as low as 14 pounds for lightweight, ultra-lightweight, and high-performance manual wheelchairs.[51] Manual wheelchairs for playing court sports such as tennis and basketball or racing are designed specifically for the sport.[21] These wheelchairs have a rigid frame and a high degree of camber in the rear wheels and use small rollerblade-type casters in front.

Wheelchairs with large rear tires are most common but models with large front tires and small back casters are available (Figure 20-11*B*). Propelling a wheelchair with large front tires may be more efficient for the child because more surface area of the tire is exposed for gripping the wheel and pushing. However, the large front tires can limit access to the environment, such as when transferring and sitting at tables. The wheelchair with large front tires is also more difficult to push over curbs and uneven surfaces because of interference from the rear casters.

If the user has a single functional arm for wheelchair propulsion, such as a child with hemiplegia, an adapted manual wheelchair with a one-arm drive feature can provide independent mobility. The wheelchair is designed with two rims on the wheel the child uses to propel. One of the rims is connected through an axle to the other wheel. If either rim is pushed separately, it turns the wheelchair. If both rims are pushed simultaneously, the wheelchair moves forward or backward. A manual wheelchair can also be propelled with the feet if the wheelchair has a low seat-to-floor height, known as *hemi-height*.

A power assist unit, designed into the hub of a special wheel attached to a manual wheelchair, provides the convenience of a manual wheelchair without the extra effort involved with propulsion (Figure 20-11*C*). The LEVO Kid wheelchair includes a powered sit-to-stand feature, which can provide peer height interaction and the benefits of convenient standing throughout the day (Figure 20-11*D*).

A new concept in mobility systems is the Kids ROCK2 Reaction™ Dynamic Seating wheelchair, which allows the child to move into trunk flexion or extension in the wheelchair while maintaining proper pelvic positioning. When the child moves using hip and knee extension, the backrest reclines and the footrests move in an upward direction extending in a 35-degree range. When the child relaxes, the compressed springs move the backrest and footrests to the starting position (Figure 20-11*E*).

Power Wheelchairs

Powered mobility wheelchairs have a battery-operated motorized unit that the user drives by means of a joystick or alternative controls such as pneumatic sip-and-puff, ultrasonic head controls, proximity switches that operate by the user moving close to the switch but not touching it, or multiple push switches. If a child cannot propel a wheelchair long distances at the same speed and efficiency as demonstrated by the average person walking, then the occupational therapist should consider recommending a power wheelchair to increase the child's independence and function. The advantages of a power wheelchair over a manual one are increased speed capability, ease

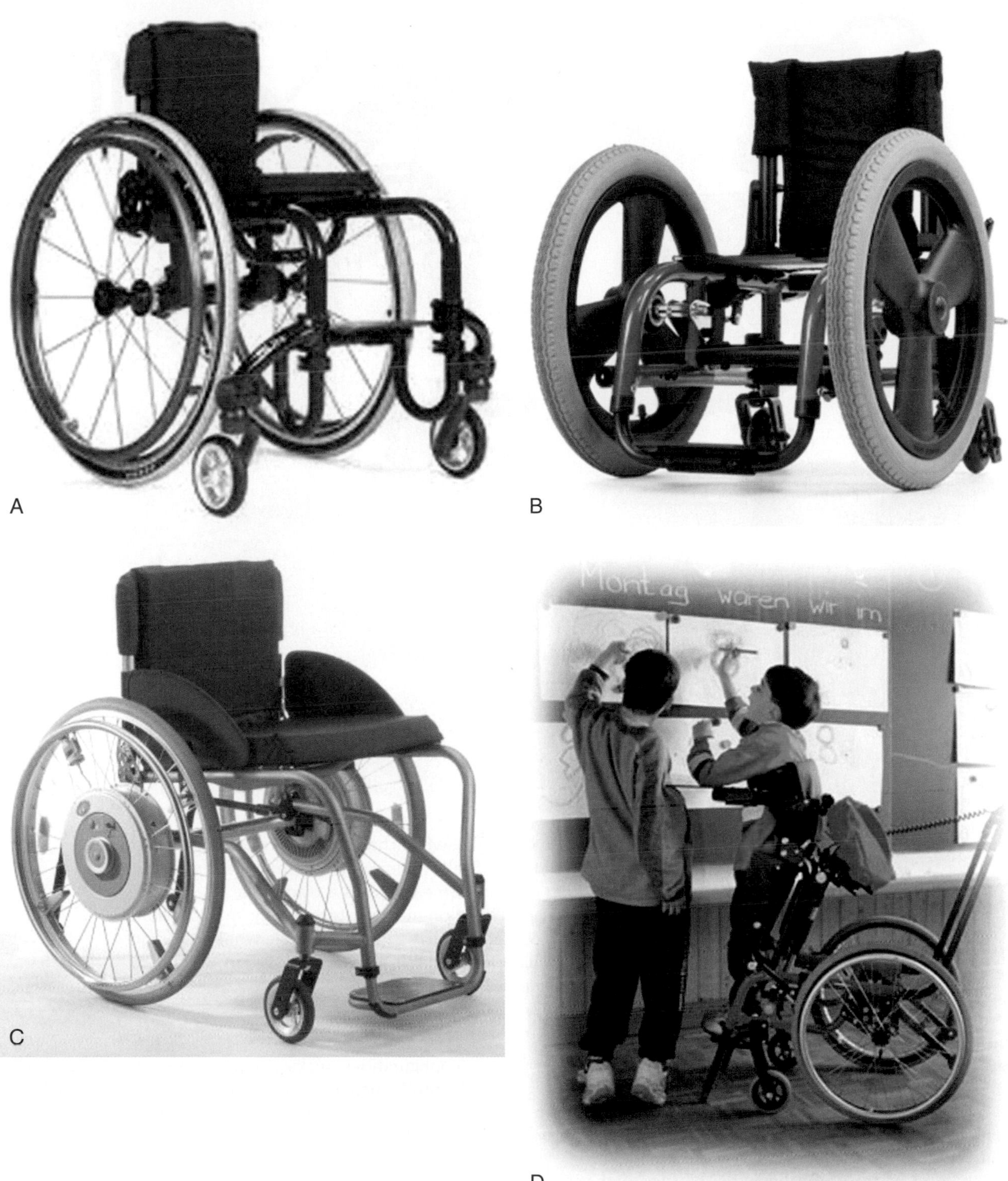

FIGURE 20-11 **A,** The TiLite Twist. **B,** The Zippie Kidz manual wheelchair is available in a reverse wheel configuration for young growing toddlers. **C,** Emotion by Frank Mobility provides a power assist unit in the hub of the wheels for ease in propelling a manual wheelchair. **D,** The LEVO KID wheelchair provides a sit-to-stand feature in a manual wheelchair with the touch of a button.

Continued on next page

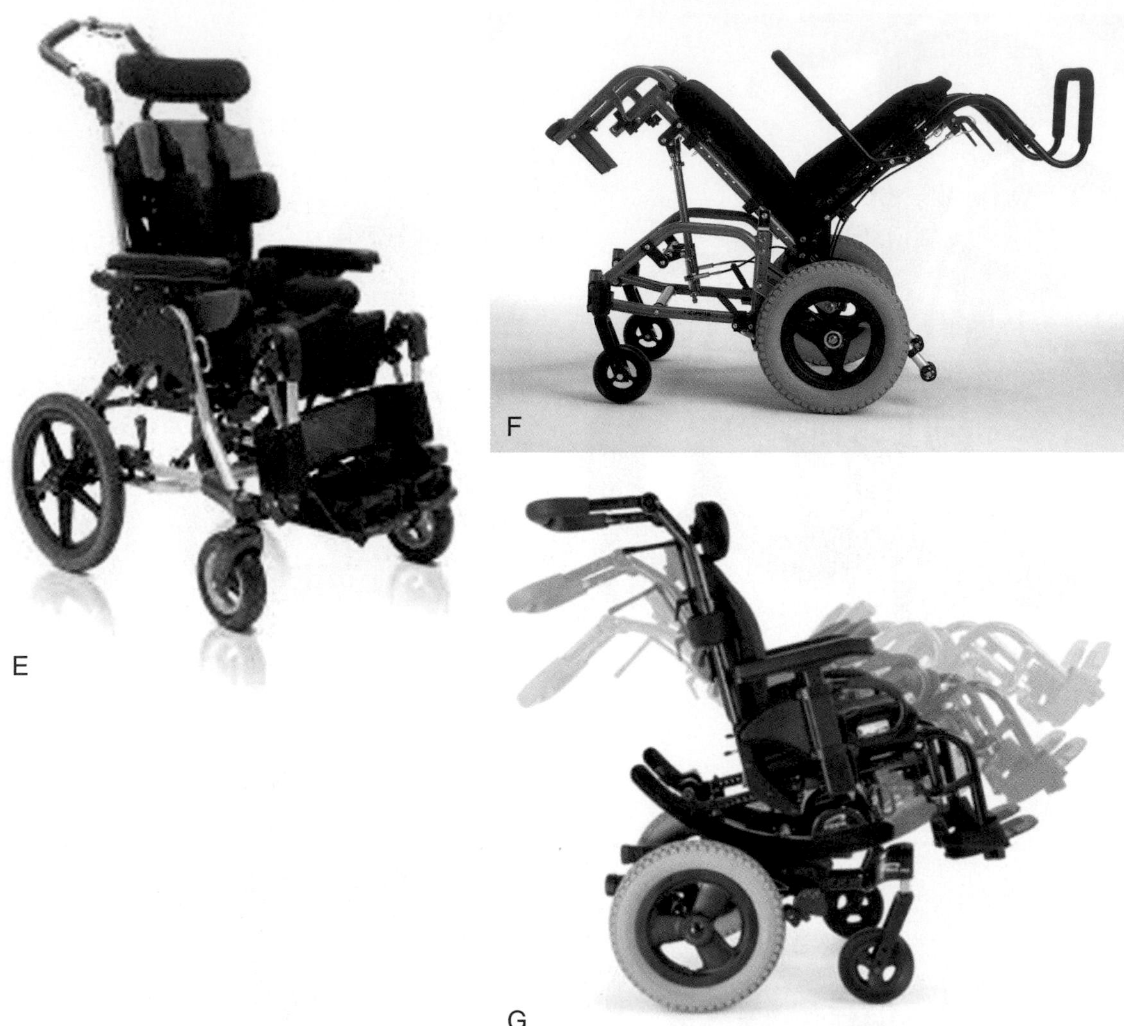

FIGURE 20-11, cont'd **E,** The KidsROCK2 manual wheelchair with Reaction TM Dynamic Seating. **F,** The Zippie TS tilt-in-space chair is specifically designed to accommodate pediatric growth. It is available in either a folding or rigid frame and uses a traditional tilt-in-space feature. **G,** The Zippie IRIS utilizes advanced rotation-in-space technology that provides smooth and controlled tilt rotation up to 55 degrees, the shortest possible wheelbase, and an extremely low weight. (A, courtesy TiLite; D, available through LEVO USA, Inc.; E, by Quantum Rehab for Kids; F and G, from Sunrise Medical.)

of maneuvering, and less energy expenditure required for moving, particularly for long distances. Some children who use a power wheelchair also have a manual wheelchair for use in environments that are not accessible to a power wheelchair or when the power wheelchair is being repaired.

Power wheelchairs are available in several styles with various options and are differentiated by the electronics, control systems, and placement of the drive wheel, which may be rear-wheel drive (Figure 20-12*A*), mid-wheel (Figure 20-12*B*), or front-wheel (Figure 20-13*A*). Attributes that are affected by the drive wheel position include maneuverability, stability, traction, and performance (speed, efficiency, obstacle climbing, and crossing a side slope). Maneuverability depends on the turning radius.

- Rear-wheel drive wheelchairs are designed with the drive wheels located at the rear of the wheelchair and caster wheels in front. It tracks straighter than other wheel configurations, making it easier to steer if using alternative controls such as switches. It works well over rough terrain and has less hardware extending in back of the wheelchair than the mid-wheel drive configuration.
- Mid-wheel drive wheelchairs tend to have greater maneuverability because of the smaller turning radius.[46] Some mid-wheel power wheelchair manufacturers claim to have a 19-inch turning radius, versus a minimum 33-inch radius with a rear-wheel drive. However, mid-wheel drive wheelchairs require a third set of stabilizing caster wheels, which may extend up to 17 inches behind the user. This feature may make it difficult for users to turn around without catching the casters on objects, particularly if spatial awareness is not optimal.
- Front-wheel drive works well over various types of terrain, uphill and downhill, because power in the front wheels pulls

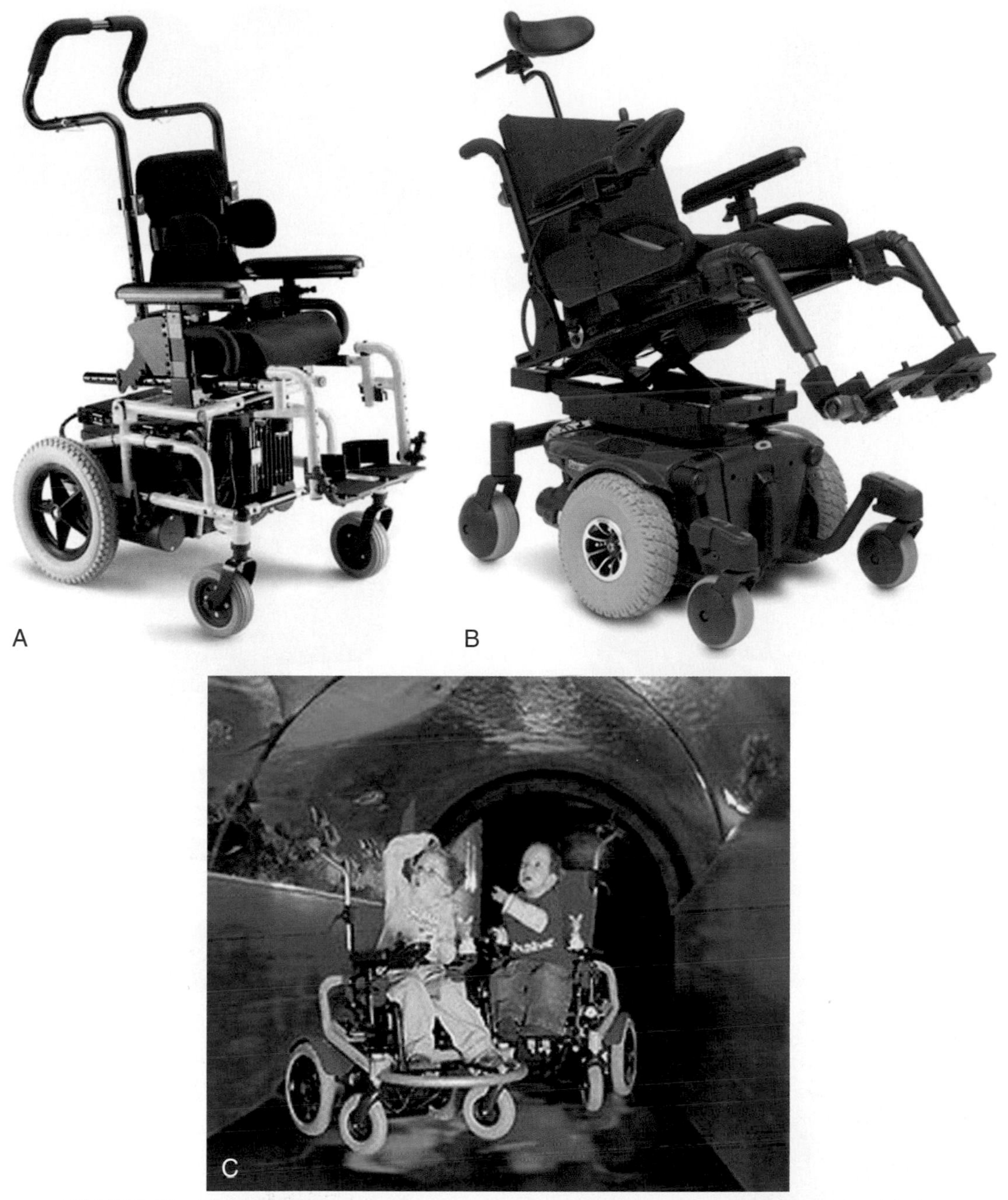

FIGURE 20-12 **A,** The Power Tiger is a rear wheel drive pediatric power wheelchair. **B,** The Q610, a mid-wheel drive power wheelchair with tilt-in-space. **C,** Skippi power wheelchair. (A, manufactured by Invacare; B, by Quantum Rehab; C, manufactured by Otto Bock.)

the user over obstacles. Children who have used a rear-wheel drive wheelchair may find maneuvering a front-wheel drive wheelchair more challenging because the back end of the wheelchair may fishtail at higher speeds.

The recent trend in power wheelchair design is to provide a full suspension system in the front and rear casters or tires. This allows the user to move over a variety of terrains and drive up 3-inch curbs, even at slow speeds. Standard rear-wheel drive wheelchairs are optimal for children who have limited vision and spatial awareness difficulty, because most of the wheelchair hardware is within their field of vision. Most wheelchair manufacturers provide a choice of several models that are intended for joystick operation and models that include sophisticated microcomputer electronics for alternative input methods for driving and for remotely operating environmental devices. Features of power wheelchair electronics can accommodate the needs of various users. Such features include adjustments for torque, tremor dampening for children having difficulty directing the joystick, a short-throw joystick option for users with muscle weakness who do not have the strength to push the

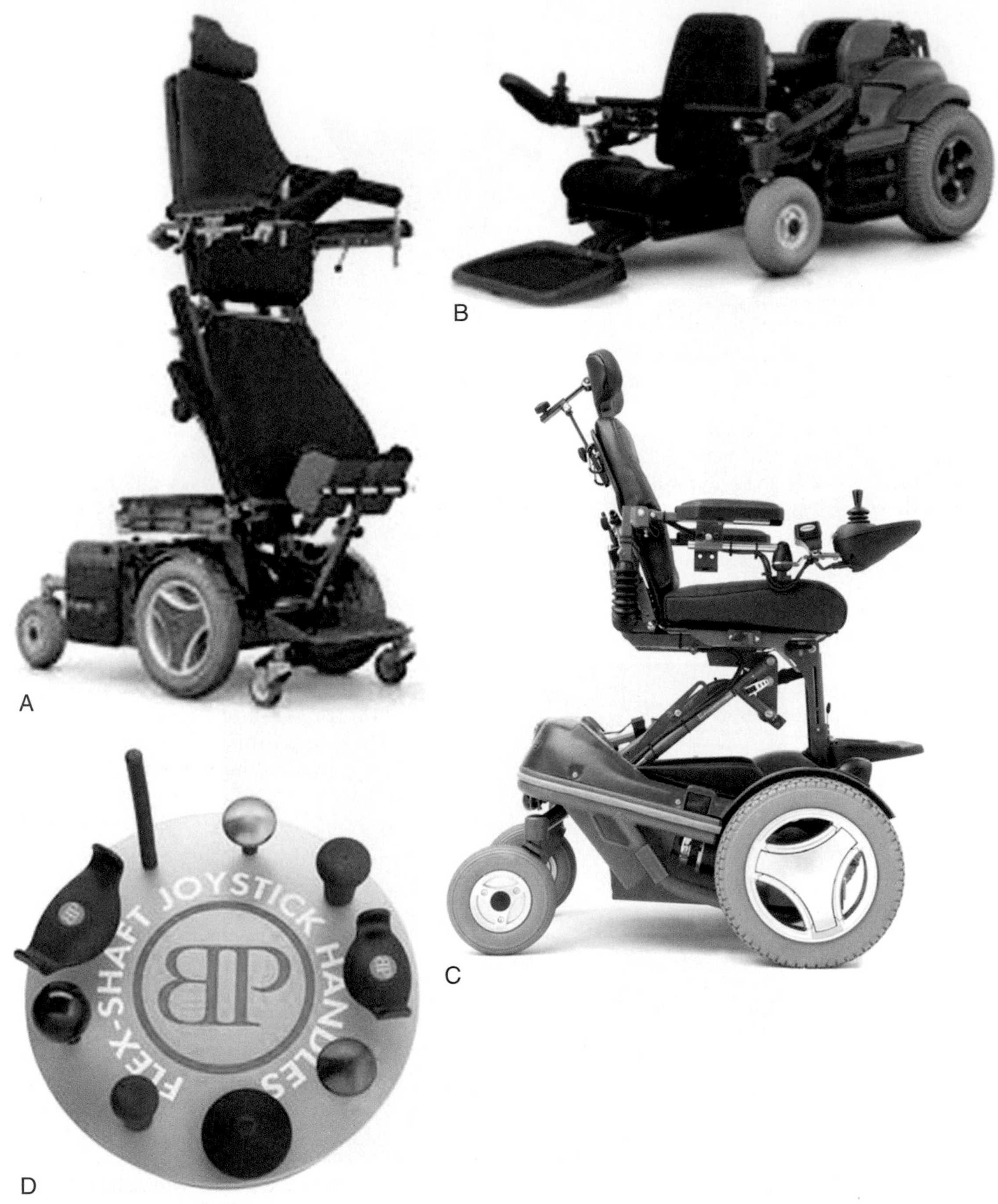

FIGURE 20-13 **A,** The C400 VS Jr. is designed specifically for children. This front wheel drive power wheelchair allows standing to be achieved from a horizontal or seated position. The user can drive while in a standing position. **B,** The K450 MX power seat-to-floor function lets children get down on the ground, perfect for story time, transfers and playing with peers. **C,** The Koala Mini Flex seat elevator reaches up to 8″. **D,** Joystick Knob display by Body Point. (A-C, Courtesy Permobil, Lebanon, TN; D by Body Point.)

joystick to its end range, speed adjustments, and acceleration settings so that the wheelchair can be set to increase speed rapidly or gradually. Some manufacturers now offer electronics, such as the True Track Technology (Invacare Corp.), that enable the wheelchair to track straight on slopes and uneven surfaces. Speeds can be as high as 15 mph, but typically range from 3 to 10 mph. Distance traveled on one battery charge can be as far as 25 miles.

Several features can be made available on power wheelchairs to increase a child's function and level of independence. Technology-dependent children who require oxygen support can become mobile by using portable ventilator carts attached to the wheelchair.[7] Another useful feature for accessing the environment enables the child to independently move from a sitting to a standing position and drive around while standing (see Figure 20-13*A*). A seat that lowers to the floor may assist children to independently transfer into the wheelchair and play with peers (Figure 20-13*B*). A powered elevating seat, which raises the child to various heights for greater accessibility in the environment, is also available (Figure 20-13*C*). Additional features include power tilt-in-space, which tilts the seat backward to about 45 degrees while maintaining the same seat-to-back angle (see Figure 20-12*B*), and power recline, which places the child in the supine position by reclining the back of the chair. These two features are useful for individuals who need frequent relief of pressure under their buttocks, such as those with spinal cord injury and muscle weakness or for those with hip, back, and neck pain.

Power wheelchairs are typically controlled with a joystick. A proportional joystick allows the driver to increase acceleration and speed of the wheelchair in relation to the distance the joystick is moved. The farther the user pushes the proportional joystick, the more rapidly the wheelchair moves. A nonproportional joystick (digital or microswitch) does not affect the wheelchair's speed; any amount of force used to push the joystick results in the same speed. An attendant joystick is another option for a power wheelchair. It is typically a small joystick mounted to the back of the wheelchair and is accessed by the caregivers who need to drive the power wheelchair when accuracy is required, such as moving up a narrow ramp.

Power wheelchairs do not typically fold for transporting in a vehicle. Accessible vans that have been modified with a lift are required for transporting the user and power wheelchair in a vehicle. However, there is a pediatric power wheelchair, the Skippi from Ottobock Kids, that can be disassembled so that it can be transported in a vehicle without the need for a van (Figure 20-12*C*). If the child can be transferred to a car seat, a covered trailer can be hitched to the back of a vehicle for transporting a power wheelchair.

Powered mobility scooters are another option for powered mobility. The individual who uses a scooter typically has good sitting balance, requires minimal positioning adaptation, and can understand and physically operate the tiller handle bar controls.

A manual wheelchair can be converted to a power wheelchair by purchasing an add-on unit such as the E-Fix by Frank Mobility Systems Inc. The unit includes two motors that are placed inside the hub to rotate the tires, an electronic control unit, and a joystick. The manual wheelchair can still remain foldable. The electronic controls for the add-on units are not as sophisticated or adjustable as those found on standard power wheelchairs. This makes it more difficult for some children with impaired motor responses to accurately operate the chair. Add-on units are also not highly recommended for individuals who use their wheelchairs outdoors and over rough terrain because they are not designed to withstand the forces that a power wheelchair must endure.

The power wheelchairs today offer sophisticated electronics that provide opportunities to integrate mobility with speech-generating devices and electronic aids to daily living so the child can use the power from the wheelchair to continuously charge the speech-generating device, turn on lights, operate the television, and wirelessly access a computer through the power wheelchair electronics.

Selection of Wheelchair Features

If the child's goal is to independently propel a manual wheelchair, it is critical that the wheelchair and seating be designed to allow proper biomechanics for efficient propulsion. The occupational therapist achieves this by recommending the proper size of wheelchair frame and an appropriate seating system. Most wheelchair manufacturers include wheelchair growth kits, which accommodate the need to widen or lengthen the frame without entirely replacing the wheelchair. It is critical to select a wheelchair that fits the child's present needs, rather than a wheelchair that is too large with the goal that the child will "grow into" it. A wheelchair that is too wide is more difficult for the child to propel. If the seat is too long, the child's pelvis cannot achieve a neutral position; it will be pulled into a posterior tilt, reducing upper extremity function and causing the child to sit on the sacrum with a rounded back, which contributes to the risk of sliding out of the seat. If the backrest is too tall, it will be difficult to position a headrest at the occipital area behind the neck or use shoulder straps.

The occupational therapist simultaneously considers what type of seating or positioning system is needed and how it will interface with the mobility base for optimal function and performance. For example, in ordering a seat cushion, the child's functional mobility skills, the frame size of the manual wheelchair, and the desirable seat to floor height must be considered. If the cushion is placed on top of the wheelchair frame, the child may be positioned too far from the wheels for reaching and propelling them efficiently. To prevent this situation, the occupational therapist considers the height of the wheelchair seat when ordering the cushion; a workable alternative in this instance is a narrower cushion that can be recessed into the wheelchair frame.

Another common situation that reinforces the need to assess seating and wheelchair mobility simultaneously is recommending a backrest cushion for a child without considering the features of the wheelchair. The cushion may position the child too far forward of the axle's wheel. If the child's center of gravity is forward of the rear wheels instead of directly over the rear wheel axle, propulsion is more difficult and inefficient. Many wheelchairs have a standard axle plate whereby the hub of the wheel is mounted to the frame and the wheels cannot be relocated within the child's reach. However, if the occupational therapist recommends an adjustable axle plate for the wheelchair in combination with the appropriate front caster size, the wheels can be relocated and mounted in the best location for the child to reach the wheels for propulsion.

Wheelchair features are recommended based on needs in the areas of mobility (being able to reach and propel the wheels of a manual wheelchair or reach the floor to propel with the feet), accessibility (moving through doorways, maneuvering in small spaces, and fitting under tables), transfer techniques (dependent or independent), seating and positioning, communication (which may include mounting a speech-generating device to the wheelchair), and transportation (if the child will be transported while sitting in the wheelchair in a motor vehicle, certain options such as transport tie-downs need to be included on the wheelchair). The features available in a manual wheelchair that may affect the child's posture and function include the ability to mount an appropriate seating system; the frame's diameter size for attaching a mounting bracket to position a speech-generating device; and options such as tilt-in-space, recline, and capability for multiple axle positions for adjusting the wheel location.

Wheelchairs are available in standard or custom sizes as measured by the seat width and depth, height of the seat from the floor, and backrest height. The occupational therapist must consider seating systems and wheelchairs that will accommodate the child's growth, physical changes, and functional needs while also considering the needs of the caregivers. The therapist should begin selection of a wheelchair by evaluating and documenting the child's current physical and functional abilities, with consideration of physical changes that may occur and the positioning and mobility goals for the child. Wheelchair selection depends on the type of seating and positioning system the individual requires. For example, if a child needs to sit with a medial thigh pad or abductor to keep the knees apart, then a wider space between the leg rest hangers will be required. Wheelchairs are typically designed with equal distance between the footrest hangers, but some models have a footrest hanger that flares out to accommodate wider foot placement. The occupational therapist must also consider the environments in which the child will use the wheelchair, which method the child will use for propelling the wheelchair, how the caregivers will transport it, and which sources of funding are available. The therapist is often responsible for providing a medical justification for the seating and mobility system.

Once the child's needs have been identified, the occupational therapist matches them to the specific features available in a wheelchair:

- *Style of frame:* Folding manual wheelchair (has lots of flexibility; folds side to side or forward onto the seat), nonfolding or rigid manual wheelchair (lightest weight, has "tightest" responsive ride, back folds down, and wheels are removable), modular folding (frames come apart, separating the seating system from the base, which folds for manual and power wheelchairs), modular nonfolding (can be disassembled into several parts for manual and power wheelchairs).
- *Tilt-in-space:* Tilt is when the seat orientation to the ground can be changed while the seat-to-back angle remains constant.[24] This allows the seat to be tilted backward or forward as an entire unit while maintaining the same seat-to-back angle. It can be manual or powered for independent operation by the user. Tilt ranges are 45 to 65 degrees. Tilt can accommodate users with insufficient head and trunk control, individuals who require pressure relief under the pelvis, or those with back or hip pain. The greater the degree of tilt, the more weight is distributed from the pelvis to the back (see Figure 20-12*B*). The occupational therapist must be aware that the tilt-in-space position may restrict the child's field of vision. When tilted backward, the child's visual field is directed upward toward the ceiling. In this position the child must flex the head forward to view the surroundings. This tilted position may also stimulate the sleep mechanism and limit the development of head control. A tilt-in-space feature can also provide a few degrees of anterior tilt to position the child slightly forward, which may encourage trunk and neck extension for a more work-ready position. Manufacturers offer a traditional tilt-in-space wheelchair, with tilt occurring at a fixed pivot point (see Figure 20-11*F*) or a rotation-in-space wheelchair (Figure 20-11*G*).
- *Recline:* Recline is when the angle between the seat and the back can be changed while the angle between seat and ground remains the same.[24] This feature positions the user in a reclined position in which the seat-to-back angle opens from the seated angle to about 170 degrees. It can be operated manually by a caregiver or operated with power by the user. Some children with gastrointestinal issues may need to recline after a meal. This feature may also assist the care provider by allowing a reclined position for diaper changes.
- *Footrest style:* Footrests support the user's feet and may act as a step for transfer in and out. Features include single plate or double plate, fixed, pull-up, swing-in or swing-out, and manual and powered elevating leg rests. The typical angle of footrests is 70 or 90 degrees to accommodate fixed positions of the legs and feet. Many children sit more upright with 90-degree footrest hangers to accommodate tight hamstring muscles. If footplates are too far in front, placing a stretch on tight hamstrings, the pelvis will be pulled into a sacral sit position, thereby promoting a rounded trunk, which will adversely affect the child's head position. Footrest hangers that are angled less than 90 degrees make the length of the wheelchair frame longer, thereby decreasing maneuverability in tight places. Foot positioning options include shoe cups, ankle straps, or toe straps to secure the feet onto the foot rest, which may be necessary for added stability or when an extended leg position interferes during transport of the child.
- *Armrest style:* Armrest styles can be full length, which makes it difficult to get close to a table or desk, or arm length, which incorporates a notched area in the frame of the armrest for getting under surfaces. Armrests can be height adjustable, fixed, or removable, with pull-out or swing-away options. Some users may benefit from wider, contoured armrest pads for more arm support, particularly when using a joystick for driving a power wheelchair. Tubular style swing-up armrests, which are narrow, are often recommended for individuals who can reach the wheels for propelling.
- *Backrest height:* A high backrest may be needed to support the seating and positioning needs of a client with a severe disability or for tilt and recline. A low backrest may be more functional for a client with good upper body function. A backrest that ends at the top of the shoulders is preferred so an adjustable height-contoured headrest can be positioned under the child's occiput.
- *Backrest adjustability:* An angle-adjustable back provides the ability to set the seat-to-back angle to accommodate the child's position. A child who extends or pushes backward may benefit from a decreased back angle, whereas a child who is hypotonic and has difficulty maintaining a vertical head position may benefit from a greater than 90-degree seat-to-back angle. A biangular backrest is comprised of two back cushions hinged together: a pelvic pad that ends just below the posterior superior iliac spine is attached by a hinge to the upper back cushion. This allows the pelvic pad to be angled forward to encourage an anterior or neutral pelvic position while the upper back cushion is tilted rearward to allow the upper back to be positioned slightly behind the

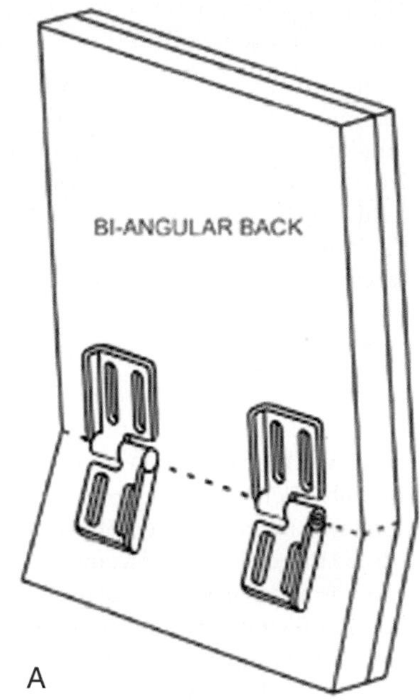

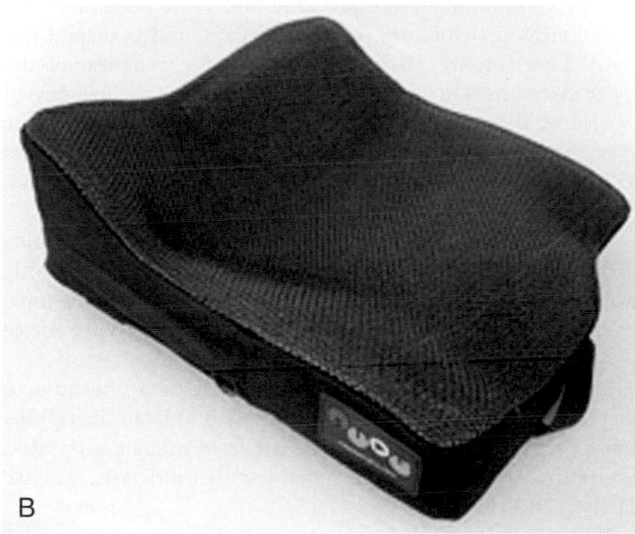

FIGURE 20-14 A, The Freedom Designs Inc. Ergo Adjustable Bi-Angular Back Cushion. B, Ride Designs cushion can be custom molded for an individual.

pelvis to accommodate the natural curves of the spine (Figure 20-14*A*). This is in contrast to a flat back rest cushion, which does not accommodate the natural spinal curves.

- *Height and adjustability features* of push handles for the adult pushing the wheelchair. If a manual wheelchair will be pushed primarily by a tall caregiver, then the push handle height will need to be adjustable or extended.
- *Floor-to-seat height:* Seat height is important for transfers and getting under surfaces such as tables. A lower seat height is typically preferred for younger children, particularly if a seating system will be integrated into the chair, which may raise the user higher. A lower seat height may facilitate self-transfers. A high seat height may place the child closer to peer height.
- Style and location of wheel locks or brakes. If the child has the strength and understanding to lock the brakes independently, then they need to be within reach. Some brakes are under the wheelchair and operated by pushing a lever with the foot. A push button brake can be positioned on the back of the wheelchair frame behind the push handles, a convenience for the caregivers and an option for a child who should not be releasing the brake intentionally.
- *Type, size, and placement of wheels and casters* on a manual wheelchair for maximum efficiency during propulsion and to accommodate weight distribution: An adjustable axle plate can provide individualized wheel placement for the child to reach the tires. This may also assist children who are positioned forward of the push wheel because of a short seat depth, which places too much weight over the forward casters, thereby increasing resistance during propulsion. Tires can be pneumatic (air filled for a cushioned ride), semi-pneumatic (gel insert for flat-free maintenance), or solid (no maintenance but provides the stiffest ride and may add extra weight).
- *Additional features* include sit-to-stand in a manual wheelchair (see Figure 20-11*D*) or a power wheelchair, whereby the child can move independently from a seated position to standing (see Figure 20-13*A*). The advantage of this feature is the ability to reach various heights, bear weight, and stretch throughout the day, and for some boys, the efficiency of standing without needing to transfer for toileting needs, as when using a urinal.

Powered Mobility Evaluation and Intervention

To determine which power mobility device is appropriate for a child, the occupational therapist, teacher, child, and caregivers must first define the goals for using powered mobility (Box 20-1). The team also considers how the child will access or drive the power wheelchair, and which power wheelchairs provide the control interface methods that the child needs now and may need in the near future, if change in motor performance is expected. The occupational therapist begins an evaluation of the child's ability to drive a power wheelchair by assessing the child's position, to determine how to optimize motor function for efficient and accurate access of the controls. It may be necessary to use an evaluation seating system or interim modifications to the child's own seating system during the powered mobility evaluation. The child must feel secure, comfortable, and stable, particularly in the pelvis, trunk, and head, before attempting to operate a power wheelchair.

Selecting the Control Device

A joystick is the standard and often the preferred method for the individual who can maneuver it efficiently and accurately. The user can operate a joystick using a hand, foot, forearm, chin, head pointer, or even the back of the head, by using an adaptation that connects the joystick to a bracket that is attached to a movable headrest. Some children may find it difficult to accurately use a joystick placed in its traditional location at the front end of the armrest. These children may have

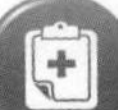

CASE STUDY 20-2 Trevor

Trevor, a 4-year-old child who is unable to communicate, was having difficulty driving the power wheelchair using a joystick placed at the end of his right armrest. The teacher questioned Trevor's ability to drive safely and accurately, believing that his bumping into objects was purposeful. The occupational therapist observed Trevor's arm and hand movements and noted that he seemed to have difficulty pushing the joystick forward and to the right side. He tended to internally rotate his arm and pull it toward his body. The joystick was then mounted on an adjustable bracket that positioned it in midline, close to his chest. The midline position also enabled the joystick box to be rotated about 30 degrees toward his body. After several more attempts at driving, Trevor's accuracy improved immediately. Once the most reliable placement was located, he became a functional driver.

BOX 20-1 Questions to Guide Mobility Device Selection

- Are the goals to provide functional and independent home, school, and community mobility, or are the goals to provide transitional mobility experiences so that the child can have new opportunities to learn how to move, explore, and interact within the environment?
- Which maneuverability features of the powered device are important in considering the various environments in which the device will be used (such as indoors in limited spaces in a classroom or home, outdoors over rough terrain, or on a playground)?
- What are the table heights the wheelchair must fit under at school, the home, and community?
- Is it necessary for the child to reach various heights in the wheelchair? Should a powered lift seat be considered?
- Will the child need the ability to tilt-in-space or recline?
- How will the child transfer into and out of the wheelchair?
- How will the mobility device be transported? Will it need to be disassembled to fit inside the trunk of a vehicle?
- If the wheelchair is to be transported in a van, is head clearance sufficient for the child when entering the vehicle and can the wheelchair be secured to the van for transport?
- Will the environments need to be made accessible with ramps into doorways or powered lifts into vehicles?
- Will the child need an environmental control option included in the power wheelchair electronics for using the joystick or alternative access method to wirelessly access an alternative electronic device such as a speech-generating device or computer?

better motor control if the joystick is placed inside the armrest, in midline, or rotated several degrees toward the body (Case Study 20-2). A micro joystick, or attendant joystick, which is smaller in size than a standard joystick, may be necessary for these types of situations and are available for most power wheelchairs. The small joystick is easier to position in midline or under the chin. Another feature that can assist in improving control or efficiency during joystick use is a support (such as a wide armrest or trough) under the elbow, forearm, or wrist. If the child has difficulty moving the joystick in the desired direction, the occupational therapist can place a template with a cross shape cut out inside the control box to limit deviation of the joystick to the desired directions. The therapist can also position the joystick with proper hardware to another location in which control will be enhanced. During the evaluation for joystick operation, the therapist not only must evaluate the positioning needs of the child and placement of the joystick, but must consider the type of joystick, type of joystick knob, and desired location of the on-off switch for either independent access or to avoid unintentional access by the user.

Joystick knobs are available in various styles, shapes, and sizes to accommodate various hand and wrist positions. The most common shapes are round, T-shaped, and U-shaped like a goal post (Figure 20-13*D*). A child with weakness of the upper extremities may find it more efficient to use a U-shaped joystick so that the hand is supported in the palm and at the sides. Another access method is the use of an interface tablet device that senses finger movement on a tablet device to navigate a power wheelchair.[59]

Selection of the most appropriate style of joystick and its placement directly affects the ability to accurately and efficiently drive a power wheelchair. Case Study 20-3 provides an example of a child whose position is evaluated for more accurate use of a powered mobility device.

Children with severe physical disabilities may be able to operate a power wheelchair but often are not given the opportunity because they are physically unable to operate a joystick. Alternative control interfaces or access methods are available for these individuals.

If a child does not have the physical ability to control a joystick, the occupational therapist should consider alternative control interfaces or access methods such as switch operation, particularly for individuals with cerebral palsy. Multiple switch access is available in which switches are placed around the body part that is able to reach the switches, typically using three or four switches. The wheelchair is driven in one of four directions, depending on which switch is activated. Many types of switches are available, for example, battery-powered electronic and proximity sensors, activated by getting near the switch, and mechanical switches that require different levels of pressure to activate, that vary in size, or that include auditory feedback. Switches can be placed at the head, hand, elbows, knees, or feet, where the child has the ability to make contact with the switches and release them or move close to the switches if they are in proximity. An adjustable mounting bracket, such as that available through AbleNet Inc., is extremely helpful for positioning a switch consistently in multiple locations.

Before selecting the type of switch, the occupational therapist first identifies the most reliable movements the child can voluntarily use to access a switch, utilizing the least amount of

CASE STUDY 20-3 Amanda

Amanda is a 9-year-old girl who has a diagnosis of cerebral palsy quadriplegia with athetosis (see Figure 20-15). Her trunk stability is limited such that she cannot sit independently; she extends her hips and back, causing her to slide forward in her seat; she has minimal control of arm and hand movements but can voluntarily move her arms toward her side; she has fair to good head movements when her pelvis and trunk are stable. Efficient and reliable operation of a power wheelchair is not possible because the positioning seat belt slips, causing her to slide forward on the seat, adversely affecting motor control of her arms and head.

She now sits in a custom seating system comprised of a contoured seat cushion, which is soft under the pelvis and moderately firm under her thighs to reduce extensor thrust posturing; a biangular back cushion with lateral hip and trunk pads; an occipital neck rest; and a sub-ASIS (defined below) padded bar.[52] The seat belt alone did not provide a stable pelvis that she needed to reduce extraneous body and head movements. The sub-ASIS bar is placed across the lap where the seat belt would be placed. It is hinged on one end of the seat cushion and connects to a bracket on the other end, which provides consistent but comfortable hip placement. It is positioned just below (sub) the anterior superior iliac spine (ASIS) of her pelvis, which provides a consistent pelvic position and, therefore, upper body position, rather than depending solely on a positioning belt, which loosens and allows her pelvis to slide forward on the seat, decreasing stability and increasing extraneous movements. The positioning belt remains in place for her to use instead of the sub-ASIS bar when stability of the pelvis is not necessary.

These seating components have increased her stability such that she can move her head accurately to activate three proximity switches from Adaptive Switch Labs (ASL) to drive a power wheelchair. She independently accesses two switches placed on the side of her armrest to change modes of operation for speed and moving in reverse. A third switch placed on the right side of her armrest allows her to turn her wheelchair on and off independently. She accesses her speech generating device, a Vmax by DynaVox mounted to her power wheelchair, by using a head tracking-mouse emulation method that uses a camera to track her head movements. She wears a reflective dot on her forehead, which the camera tracks while she moves her head to position the cursor on the screen over a letter or symbol. Her communication device can also be programmed to work remotely with electronic devices around her house. She can use it as a universal remote for her television and DVD player and to operate light switches in a room. She also has access to a telephone with an additional accessory on her Vmax.

active range and therefore energy expenditure. Children may have experience using a switch to operate a modified battery-operated toy or single-switch computer game, which requires one activation of the switch with a quick release.[87] The child may be able to use the same movements for switch access to drive a power wheelchair, but most children will use an access method that requires them to maintain contact and activation on the switch during the time they are driving the power wheelchair and move off the switch in time for stopping.

If the child can nod "yes" and "no," then he or she may have the ability to use the same movements for activating switches placed in back and to the sides of the head. The head-switch sensing array from Adapted Switch Labs (ASL) consists of proximity switches embedded into a headrest that detect head movements for driving the wheelchair (Figure 20-15). Users may have more optimal control of the head array if they also use a suboccipital neck support to increase stability. These switches are operated not by making contact on the switch, but rather by getting close or proximal to the switch. The head array can also be mounted near the hand or foot for use with movements of the arm or leg. An array of fiber optic switches from ASL can be embedded in a lap tray so the child can wave an arm above each switch to operate the wheelchair or other electronic device.

Switches can be used in a momentary or latched mode through the wheelchair electronics. Momentary switches require the user to maintain contact on the switch to activate it. The child needs to be able to maintain contact on the switch long enough to move the wheelchair in a desired direction. A latching mode allows the user to press the switch one time to activate it, rather than holding it in the "on" position. A second

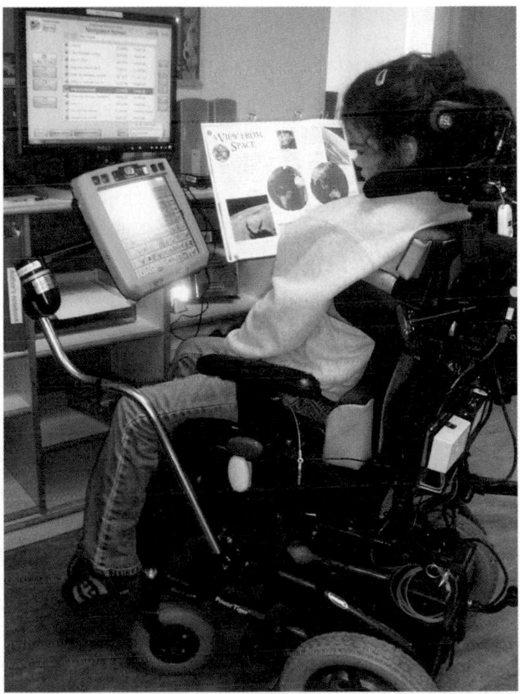

FIGURE 20-15 A 9-year-old girl in Power Tiger from Invacare using an ASL head array for driving and for mouse emulation on her computer.

activation turns the switch "off." If the child needs to use switches to drive a power wheelchair, at least three switch sites are preferred: for driving forward and turning both directions. Reverse can be operated by a fourth switch or the adult. If the child can operate only one or two switches, the occupational therapist may need to consider a scanning method, which the child uses through a scanning menu on a display; however, the scanning method requires a higher degree of concentration requiring visual and cognitive function because of the complexity of the task.

An input method used frequently by individuals with spinal cord injuries is pneumatic sip 'n' puff, which the user activates by gently inhaling or exhaling into a straw-like device held in the mouth. This method requires oral motor control and the ability to build pressure in the mouth.

The Tongue Drive System uses sensors imbedded in a dental retainer and a magnet pierced onto the tongue that makes contact with the sensors to drive the power wheelchair. The Rolltalk Nova is an interface for driving a power wheelchair using eye gaze, which is intended for individuals with very little active movement.

Once the occupational therapist has determined a preferred motor response, the child can assess the switch on a powered mobility device. However, the quality of motor control and accuracy is directly dependent on the child's body position and the extent to which the position influences stability, mobility, muscle tone, and energy expenditure. Therefore, an evaluation of power wheelchair mobility control must simultaneously include a seating evaluation to determine how the child's motor control is influenced by body position.

Assessing Driving Performance

Several factors can interfere with a person's ability to drive a powered mobility device. If a child has difficulty, the occupational therapist should first consider if the wheelchair, electronics, and interface, such as switches, are working properly. The brakes must be released and the wheels must be engaged. If the child continues to have difficulty, the type and placement of the controls should be re-evaluated. Simultaneously, the therapist evaluates the child's position to determine whether changes in the child's posture influence motor control. Other considerations include undetected visual and perceptual difficulties, impairment in hearing, processing and response time, seizures, motivation, and behavior. Children with visual impairment often find it difficult to drive a power wheelchair outdoors in bright sun, preferring to do so indoors in large areas such as a clinic or classroom.

Many children may not initially be successful using a power wheelchair because of the overwhelming amount and degree of sensory input that is required. Imagine being a child with a severe disability who has difficulty with motor planning, coordination, visual perception, and communication, and is experiencing movement in a powered device for the first time. It would be overwhelming to experience the excitement and vestibular sensation of moving while trying to view the surroundings, which are quickly passing by, and simultaneously listen to an adult telling you how and where to move.

The occupational therapist should assess a young child for powered mobility, whenever feasible, by providing a method that promotes exploration, problem solving, and self-learning for the child. Such a method requires an open space with activities and toys strategically placed around the room to facilitate experiences in movement and exploration.

The most common method for evaluating a person's ability to use a powered mobility device is to have the device available for trial use during the evaluation. A facility typically cannot afford to purchase power wheelchairs for evaluation purposes. Fortunately, ATPs often lend power wheelchairs to a clinical therapy unit for short-term evaluation purposes. The positioning and mobility equipment with the specific features that the child will need to operate the device should be available during the evaluation. Equipment used during an evaluation should be in optimal working condition. The occupational therapist should begin the evaluation by test-driving the equipment to learn the forces and movements required to drive it, select the best speed for the client, and set any other adjustments, such as sensitivity of the controls. If a powered mobility device is not actually available, the switches can be mounted on the child's manual wheelchair and when the switch is pressed by the child, the therapist can move the wheelchair accordingly, as if the child is in control of driving.

It may also be beneficial to lend or rent a power wheelchair to children and their families for an extended evaluation. This allows more time for the child to learn how to use the controls and for the family to become familiar with the features of a power wheelchair to assist them in becoming more informed consumers. It provides an opportunity for the family to experience the responsibilities of maintaining and transporting a power wheelchair.

Power Mobility Training

Children may initially prefer spinning in circles seeking the vestibular and sensory input rather than listening to directions or driving to a target. This should be part of the training as it provides sensory input they would otherwise not experience. Learning to drive a power wheelchair, particularly with alternative controls, takes practice, and those children who can be exposed to the experiences on a daily basis in a natural environment will have an advantage over children who can only receive training once a week in a clinical setting.

The occupational therapist should "limit physical and verbal commands as much as possible to avoid sensory overload on the part of the child" (p. 85).[76] If a child is trying to move toward an object, the therapist should state the desired outcome, such as "come closer," rather than specific commands, such as "push the joystick left" or "push the red switch and come over here." Feedback should also be positive, such as "You found the wall," rather than "Oops, you crashed again."[88] If further assistance is needed to help the child understand the operation of the control, the therapist can facilitate the proper response by physically guiding the child's movements for the desired response. The therapist must understand that children respond to visual, auditory, and sensory demands at different rates. A child with spastic cerebral palsy or quadriplegia may require much longer to make a visual motor response than a child with athetoid cerebral palsy, a spinal cord injury, or muscle disease.

Computer programs are available for powered mobility assessment and training.[75] R. J. Cooper and Associates has developed a power wheelchair simulation program as well as software for joystick and mouse training. The program displays a power wheelchair on the screen that the user must navigate through a maze or room. Hasdai, Jessel, and Weiss studied whether a driving simulator would help a child master skills that are comparable with those required to drive a power wheelchair.[42] Their results indicated benefits from using such a program to prepare children for powered mobility.

Seating and Positioning

Positioning is critical to the successful use of any mobility device because posture and task performance are inter-related.[21] How an individual is positioned in a mobility device, whether it be standing or sitting, can have an effect on several physiologic factors, including visual and motor performance, postural control,[54] ranges of movement, muscle tone,[56] endurance, comfort, respiration, and digestion. These factors can affect functional performance activities such as hand function,[57] levels of independence in mobility, self-care, activities of daily living such as transfers, and social interaction with others.[44]

Understanding the Biomechanics of Seating

To identify the positioning needs of a child, the occupational therapist must first have a thorough understanding of the biomechanical forces and neurophysiologic factors that can influence posture and movement. Biomechanical considerations are critical to obtaining proper alignment of the pelvis, spine, and head when postures are flexible or when accommodating individuals who have fixed postures and no longer have active or passive range of motion as a result of contractures. The position and stability of the pelvis provide a foundation for movements that occur above and below the pelvis. Box 20-2 presents exercises that stress the importance of good alignment in sitting. Neurophysiologic factors include the child's reaction to tactile input, body reactions to orientation in space, and movement.

BOX 20-2 Exercises to Understand the Biomechanics of Seating

Sitting in Posterior Pelvic Tilt

While in a sitting position, place your hands on the anterior crest of your pelvis (the two hip bones). Bend forward by rounding your back. You will feel your pelvis rolling backward into a posteriorly tilted position. Hold your pelvis in this position and try to sit upright by extending your back. You may be able to move your head upright, but moving your trunk into a vertical position is dependent on placing your pelvis in a neutral or anteriorly tilted position. To view your environment with your pelvis in the posteriorly tilted position, you would need to either hyperextend your neck (an undesirable position) or slide your pelvis forward in the seat until your head achieves an upright position. Try maintaining a rounded or kyphotic back position and slide your pelvis forward in the seat. Feel the excessive pressure at the cervical and upper thoracic levels and the coccyx. Imagine being positioned like this for hours at a time and experiencing the discomfort, fatigue, and limited range of your upper extremities if you were in a wheelchair without a proper positioning system to improve or accommodate your posture.

Pelvic Position Stability

Place your buttocks at the edge of your seat, lean only onto one side of your pelvis, and lift your feet so they are unsupported. Hold your pencil at its top edge and try to write. It is difficult to perform accurate and efficient movements of your arm and hands because you do not have a stable base for the movements to occur. Imagine trying to accurately and safely operate the joystick of a power wheelchair in this position.

Seating Guidelines

The goals of seating are to provide alignment (in the presence of flexible postures) or accommodation (in the presence of fixed or static postures); stability to improve distal motor function while minimizing undesirable tone and reflexes that interfere with alignment and stability; distribute seated pressures to maintain skin integrity; improve physiologic function such as breathing, swallowing, and digestion; increase independence in electronic activities of daily living and activities of daily living; increase seating tolerance; decrease fatigue; and provide comfort.

There are basically three types of seating system cushion surfaces: planar, contoured, and custom molded. *Planar seating* consists of flat surfaces with no contours. This type of seating may be more appropriate for individuals with mildly affected development who require only minimal body contact with the support surfaces of the seat. *Contoured seating* systems allow the body to have more contact with the support surface because its shape conforms to the curves of the spine, buttocks, and thighs. A contoured seat can be fabricated by layering various densities of foam that respond to the shape and weight of the person, thereby contouring around the bony prominences and other body curves (Figure 20-16*A*). A molded seating system is custom made for an individual who has fixed contractures and asymmetries of the pelvis and spine, such as scoliosis. The seating specialist uses a seat simulator to take an impression of the individual in the preferred seated posture which accommodates the asymmetrical position of the legs, pelvis, and spine. The impression is either electronically scanned or actually sent to the manufacturer for fabrication of the cushions (Figure 20-16*B*).

Cushions can also be custom molded using foam-in-bag technology, in which liquid foam is poured into a plastic bag that is positioned around the person's body and, once formed, provides a molded cushion that is then upholstered. This technique is more difficult to fabricate, because the individual's position must be held in place while the foam is being formed. If the child moves, the quality of the foam mold is negatively affected.

Optimal seating provides a stable place for the child's pelvis and spine, from which a range of movements for achieving functional tasks can occur. Seating is not static. Rather, it is a series of active movements or postures an individual uses to accomplish a series of motor tasks, such as maintaining the pelvis, trunk, and head upright against gravity while using the movements of the eyes, arms, and hands to access the controls of a power wheelchair or push the wheels of a manual wheelchair. For this reason, a series of postures must be made available to the child, not by restraining the child with straps and harnesses, but rather by supporting and guiding the child's

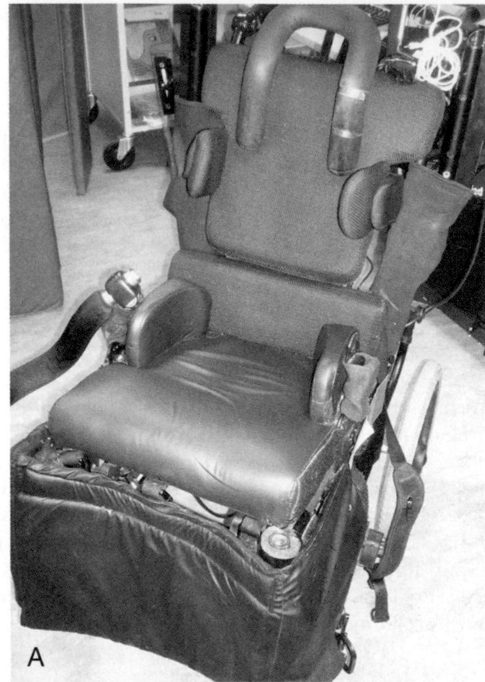

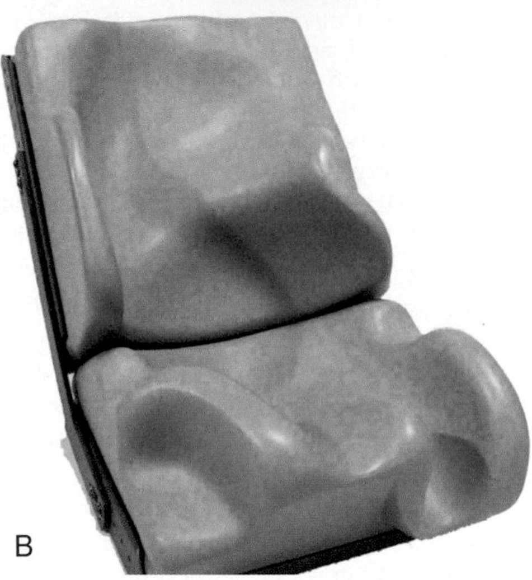

FIGURE 20-16 **A,** A custom seating system includes a biangular back cushion, contoured seat cushion, lateral hip and trunk pads, a Subasis bar, an occipital ring headrest and custom padding around the frame of the tilt-in-space wheelchair for a child with athetoid cerebral palsy. **B,** A custom molded seating system accommodates an individual's asymmetrical fixed position. (By Prairie Seating Corporation.)

movements with an appropriate seating and mobility system. The occupational therapist needs to consider the biomechanical forces of an individual's movements to determine what may be contributing to undesirable postures and, therefore, limited function.

The key points in achieving functional seating are the position and stability of the pelvis. A pelvis in a slight anterior tilt or neutral position is preferred. The angle of hip flexion can also affect postural control in sitting. Some children with extensor posturing may have a reduction of muscle tone with less than 90 degrees of hip flexion combined with hip abduction,

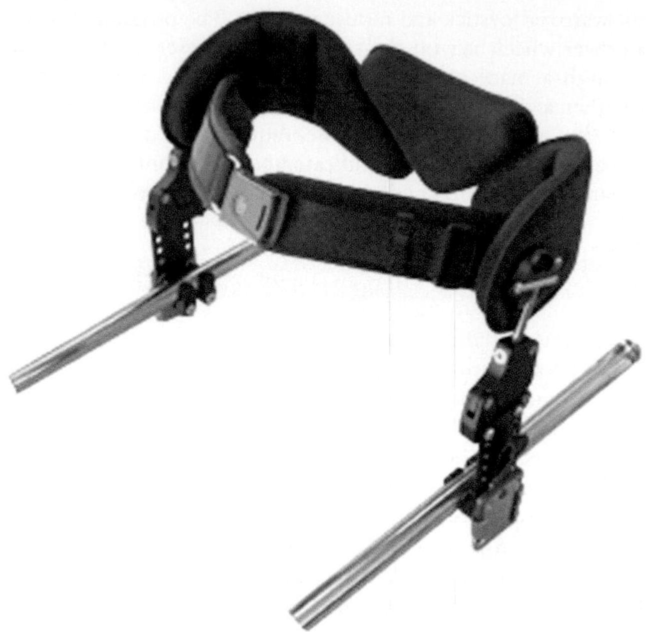

FIGURE 20-17 Hip Grip, a dynamic pelvic stabilization device.

whereas others may prefer an anteriorly tilted seat with the knees lower than the hips and weight over the feet. Stability at the pelvis can be achieved through contact points around the pelvis. These include the surfaces under and at the sides and the forces on top of the pelvis. The occupational therapist must determine how a child responds to various types of seat surfaces and contours under the pelvis such as a flat seat surface or a contoured seat (a seat cushion that provides a recessed pocket for the pelvis and blocks forward movement of the ischial tuberosities).

The occupational therapist can also improve stability of the pelvis and trunk by ensuring that the femur is properly supported along its entire length, from the back of the pelvis to approximately 1 inch from the popliteal area under the knee. One exception to this is to use a much shorter seat depth for a client who can propel a wheelchair using the legs and feet. In this situation, a shorter seat with a slight anterior tilt would be preferred. Contoured lateral hip pads placed on the seat cushion in contact with the pelvis can assist in maintaining a symmetrical position and reduce pelvic shift to either side. Stability can be provided above the pelvis to reduce sliding in an upward and forward direction. This is typically accomplished by placing a positioning belt at a 45-degree angle to the seat or closer to the thighs. Positioning belts come in several styles and include a standard 2-point attachment as well as a 4-point attachment belt, which provides support on top of the thighs as well as a 45-degree angle around the pelvis. A new device for dynamically positioning the pelvis while allowing for functional pelvic movements is the Hip Grip pelvic stabilization device from Body Point (Figure 20-17). Made of a contoured padded harness, the Hip Grip attaches to the lower part of the wheelchair backrest and around the sacral area of the pelvis. A positioning belt with sub-ASIS pads is secured in front of the pelvis. A rotational mechanism at the sides of the Hip Grip maintains postural stability while allowing the user to move the pelvis in the anterior and posterior directions, as when reaching or propelling the wheelchair. For children who consistently slide and push out of the seat and may have skin irritation from the position belt slipping, the Subasis bar is another seating component for providing a consistent pelvic position. It consists of a padded contoured positioning bar that is mounted on the seat cushion in front of the pelvis just below the individual's anterior superior iliac spine (ASIS), in front of the pelvis. It is hinged on one side, allowing it to swing into place over the pelvis where it is snapped into place with hardware mounted to the other side of the seat (Figure 20-16*A*). Lateral contoured hip pads are also used in conjunction with the sub-ASIS bar to assure that the pelvis is positioned in midline, and it is most frequently used in conjunction with a biangular backrest. Fit and function must be checked weekly when using a sub-ASIS bar to assure an optimal fit (placed snugly under the ASIS but can be rotated when in place), which is critical for successful implementation.

Other components, such as footplates, lap trays, arm rests or arm troughs, a contoured backrest, and headrests, can provide additional support to the pelvis and trunk. Proper support of the head is as important as supporting the pelvis. A headrest that completely supports the entire head may limit the child's ability to see and hear. A lower profile head rest that provides support in the suboccipital area of the head may allow for greater range of head movements to accommodate vision, hearing, and use of switches around the head for accessing devices for communication and mobility.

The use of orthotics, or devices for bracing the extremities or body, may also assist in achieving optimal positioning in the seated and standing positions. Ankle-foot orthoses are most commonly recommended to align the foot and ankle and assist in either reducing muscle tone or supporting a weak limb. For a child who uses an ankle-foot orthosis when ambulating in a support walker, a hinged orthosis that allows for ankle movement may provide more function than a static design. A thoracic-lumbar-sacral orthosis, or body jacket, may be another alternative for individuals with scoliosis to use for support in the seated position.

Young children who exhibit an increase in extensor movements and asymmetry when being evaluated for a seating system may benefit from using a "barrier" vest as proposed by Kangas.[48] The vest is made from Plastazote foam, which is not strong enough to totally support the child and allows the child to have some movement. It is worn to decrease the child's sensitivity to individual points of contact from hands touching the body during handling or from pads on a seating system, which can set off the extensor body reaction. The child wears the vest for up to 6 months while developing greater postural stability.

Seating Evaluation

The therapist should begin the initial assessment by observing the child using any existing seating and mobility systems to note posture, movements, comfort, satisfaction with the equipment, and other factors that may affect function. During the seating evaluation, the occupational therapist will need to consider:

1. The angle between the seat and the back surfaces
2. The tilt of the system in space (orientation)
3. The type of surface on which the child will be seated
4. The seating components that will provide stability and affect postures[9]

The occupational therapist should begin the evaluation by positioning the child on a low mat table so that he or she can complete a postural assessment to determine whether any limitations in ranges of movement exist that may interfere with the upright and seated positions. The therapist obtains further information by positioning the child in a sitting position while using the hands to support the child to identify key points of control and positions that provide a desirable change in posture, muscle tone, and movements. These key points become the necessary components of the seating system. The positions, such as the angle of hip flexion and the orientation in space of the child, become the pitches and angles of the components necessary in the seating system and wheelchair hardware.[21]

Once the occupational therapist gathers information from the postural assessment, other methods are also available that use evaluation equipment for assessment of the child's position to determine which components, angles, and sizes are needed in a seating system. Simulators are self-contained, with chairs that the therapist can adjust to fit a child or an adult to determine which type of seating components and angles are appropriate.[82] The simulator allows the therapist to "evaluate the client in the system, alter angles of the seat to the back, try varying positions in space, and determine component sizes and accessories that are required before making recommendations for a particular system" (p. 73).[83]

The occupational therapist and the ATP can use simulators to evaluate planar, contoured, and molded seating (see Figure 20-18). The therapist first completes a postural evaluation of the individual to determine which seating components are necessary and then adjusts the simulator to the individual's size. The therapist selects angles, which include seat-to-back and tilt. Further adjustments can be made to determine how position influences movement and function. The advantages of using a seating simulator include (1) use as a single evaluation tool for various ages, sizes, and diagnoses; (2) source of information about the various types of seating systems, such as planar versus molded; and (3) options to motorize simulators to evaluate powered mobility access and the effect of positioning on motor control. The problem that the assessment team often encounters when using simulators is difficulty in transferring the information from the simulator into an actual seating system and knowing how that system will integrate into a mobility base. Children may also respond negatively to the simulator evaluation because its mechanical appearance and large size may intimidate them.

Another method for evaluating seating and positioning is use of a modular mockup or adjustable evaluation seat system that can be placed in a mobility base. These are typically available in planar or contoured seating devices rather than in custom-molded devices. The main advantage of using this method is that the child can use the actual mobility device while seated in the mockup seat. A trial using an adjustable evaluation seat system is particularly important because positioning can influence body movements and therefore functional outcomes. The disadvantages are that more equipment must be available to fit a range of individuals, and pitches and angles cannot always be accurately assessed.

Children with hypotonia, such as those with muscle disease or cerebral palsy, have specific needs. A useful positioning

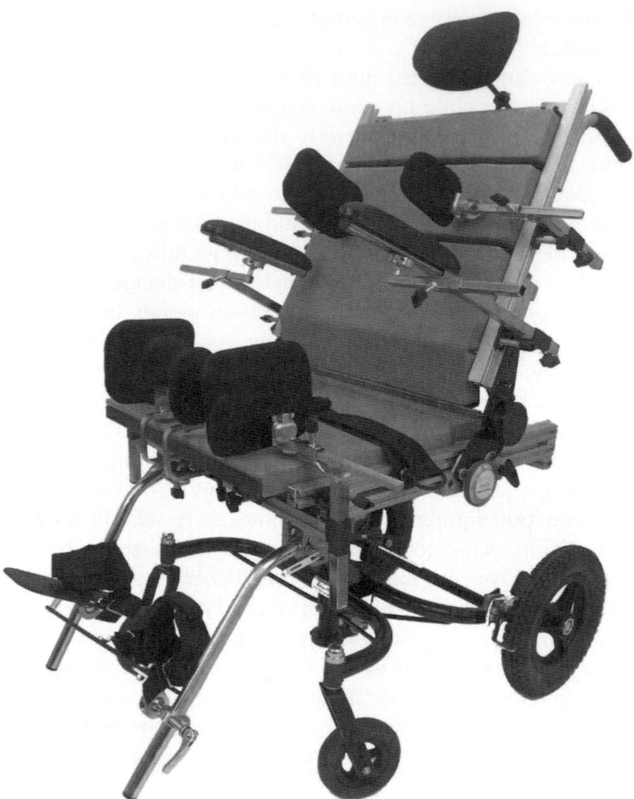

FIGURE 20-18 Prairie Seat Simulator. A clinician can use the fully adjustable Prairie Seat Simulator to evaluate a client for wheelchair seating components, pitches, and angles.

system includes a biangular back design that supports the sacrum in a neutral position but angles the remaining backrest about 15 degrees away from the back at the posterior superior iliac spine. This provides a resting position of the trunk behind the pelvis and accommodates the forces of gravity in the upright position (see Figure 20-16*A*). Consideration of a tilt-in-space feature in the mobility base and an adjustable seat-to-back angle may also provide the hypotonic or weak child with greater tolerance for sitting upright.

Children with increased muscle tone and spasticity who adduct their legs and extend their hips and spine are often more difficult to position. The occupational therapist must identify key points of control for positioning these children. For example, the therapist determines the desired degree of hip and knee flexion or extension, hip abduction, and reduction of asymmetrical positioning that positively influences muscle tone and control of extremity movement. The critical factor for reducing the degree and frequency of extensor posturing is to determine which factors contribute to these movements. Kangas observed that certain children become more asymmetrical as hypertonus increases and that this increase in muscle tone is stimulated when they feel pressure behind their head or neck from a headrest.[48] These children may also have better postural control in the upright position rather than reclined or tilted.[56] In other children who extend forcibly in combination with rotation of one side of the body forward, the resulting pelvic obliquity may place strain on the soft tissue when the child is positioned symmetrically with both legs forward. These

BOX 20-3 Gross Motor Function Classification System

LEVEL I—Walks without Limitations
LEVEL II—Walks with Limitations
LEVEL III—Walks Using a Hand-Held Mobility Device
LEVEL IV—Self-Mobility with Limitations; May Use Powered Mobility
LEVEL V—Transported in a Manual Wheelchair

For additional description of the levels, see: http://www.canchild.ca/en/measures/gmfcs_expanded_revised.asp.

children often prefer to have one leg abducted (almost off the seat cushion) and one leg forward. This often reduces the strength and frequency of hip extension and rotation of the upper body as the child extends.

The occupational therapist must frequently re-evaluate a child's position, particularly in a seated mobility device, to accommodate postural, developmental, and physiologic changes. Once a child receives a seating mobility system, the therapist should re-evaluate its fit and function every 4 to 6 months. Positioning and mobility literature and support materials are available,[20,28,82,83] and more specific information and techniques on positioning are available through additional reading and workshops.

Mobility Devices and Diagnoses

Children with cerebral palsy achieve most of their gross motor abilities before the age of 5 years and peak in their motor performance by adolescence.[71] Children in Level III of the Gross Motor Function Classification System (GMFCS)[61] may walk with aids, but like children in Levels IV and V they will depend on wheelchair mobility for most of their mobility needs. See GMFCS levels defined in Box 20-3. To achieve a high level of independent mobility, both manual and power wheelchairs should be considered at an early age for children with impaired walking ability.[70] Children at GMFCS Levels III-V benefit from using a support walker at an early age to explore their surroundings, exercise, and access physical education and recess activities, such as running, and interactive games like chase and soccer.

Children with spina bifida are provided with mobility devices such as a caster cart at a very early age. Because it is low to the ground, young children's use of caster carts for indoor mobility on smooth surfaces allows peer interaction and self-transfers. Many of these children may achieve ambulation with assistive devices including braces and hand-held walkers, depending on the level of the lesion, ability to stand upright, and their support systems.[64] Because children can propel a manual wheelchair independently, their functional performance and self-determination can increase. Appropriate wheelchairs for preschool children include small sizes that are low to the ground and have large wheels in front for greater access to push. As the child gets older, rigid lightweight or ultra-lightweight manual wheelchairs are appropriate. It is important to include a pressure-relief seat cushion, particularly for older children. Some children may need to depend on powered mobility to keep up with their peers for long distances. A power wheelchair that lowers the young child to the floor and back up to seat height may be appropriate for independent transfers (see Figure 20-13*B*).

Children with neuromuscular disorders such as spinal muscular atrophy (SMA) and muscular dystrophy typically need powered mobility from an early age. Children as young as 20 months old with SMA can learn to drive a power wheelchair independently.[47] Most children can initially operate a joystick, but options for alternative access should be built into the electronics when initially recommending the power wheelchair to accommodate changes in physical ability if the child is no longer able to independently operate the joystick. A tilt-in-space feature on the wheelchair and a pressure-relief cushion are often needed for later stages during the course of the disease.

Children with a mid to high level spinal cord injury require a power wheelchair, some with a ventilator attached to the back of the wheelchair. The occupational therapist considers weight-relieving features of a wheelchair, such as tilt-in-space, reclining back, and pressure-relief cushions. Alternative controls such as sip 'n' puff or switch arrays may be needed if upper extremities are immobile. Electronic aids for daily living and computer access strategies can be integrated into the electronics of the power wheelchair. Children with lower level spinal cord injuries may be able to propel an ultralight wheelchair.

Transportation of Mobility Systems

Manufacturers of wheelchair mobility systems do not recommend using them as a seat in a motor vehicle. However, most families do not recognize this warning and allow the child to travel while seated in the wheelchair in a motor vehicle or school bus. Manufacturers are now providing safer options for transporting a wheelchair with the child in it because of a voluntary ANSI/RESNA standard called WC-19, Wheelchairs Used as Seats in Motor Vehicles.[5] Wheelchairs are considered WC-19 compliant if they have four accessible and identifiable points to secure the chair to the vehicle, as well as seating, a frame, and other components designed to allow better fit of a lap and shoulder belt. The standard requires wheelchairs to be dynamically crash-tested at 30 miles per hour and 20*g* crash conditions, which are the standards used to test child safety seats.

It is important that occupational therapists recommend wheelchairs that are WC-19 compliant and educate clients and families on safe methods for transporting a wheelchair in a motor vehicle. Standards have also been developed to recognize the safety of a specialized seating system that may be used in another manufacturer's wheelchair bases. The ANSI/RESNA WC-20 standards are for seating devices for use in motor vehicles.[6] One standard requires that all students being transported in a wheelchair on a bus must face forward. Wheelchairs that are transported in a side-facing position are more likely to deform and collapse in a crash, and the shoulder belt is ineffective.[73] School-based occupational therapists must work with transportation personnel to educate them on the importance of forward-facing positions for wheelchair riders, as well as the proper use of tie-downs. The lap belt must be snug and low on the pelvis and the shoulder belt positioned over the middle of the clavicle and across the sternum, where it connects to the pelvic belt over the hip. Any device such as an augmentative communication device or computer and lap tray must be removed and tied down separately.

Factors That Influence the Successful Use of Mobility Devices

Successful use of mobility devices depends on the fit of the child to the device, the features of the device, and the physical and social environments. Specific functional performance tasks correlate with the ability to use a power wheelchair. Preliminary findings indicate a relationship between specific cognitive scales and readiness for powered mobility, particularly in the areas of spatial relations and problem solving.[34,79,85]

Another factor that influences a child's ability to use a powered device is the ability of the professional or the caregiver to determine the most accurate and efficient means for the child to access the device. If a child is having significant difficulty in maneuvering a powered mobility device successfully, the occupational therapist must first re-evaluate the position of the child and the access method to determine whether it is the most effective means. The longer it takes a child to successfully demonstrate use of a control, the more likely it is that either the access method is inappropriate or the child's seating needs have not been met. Case Study 20-4 describes this type of situation.

The occupational therapist must consider changes that the child will have in the future, both expected and unexpected, when recommending equipment. For example, the therapist must determine whether the system can be easily changed as the child gains new skills, grows, or changes physically. This is particularly important for the therapist to consider when ordering a power wheelchair. For example, a child with a progressive disability may be able to operate a joystick at the time the chair is ordered. However, electronic options need to be included, such as the ability to readily change the input method, if the child's functional status changes and use of a joystick is no longer feasible. It is more economical in most cases to initially order options on equipment rather than retrofit the equipment at a later date.

The occupational therapist may also need to determine where and how a speech-generating device can be mounted to the child's wheelchair. Selection of the appropriate mounting bracket depends on the tube size of the wheelchair frame and locations on the wheelchair where it can be attached. A problem that therapists often encounter with manual wheelchairs is positioning the child or rear wheels too far forward of the wheelchair's center of gravity, which often causes the wheelchair to tip forward when the communication device is mounted. The most frequent problem encountered with mounting a speech-generating device on power wheelchairs is finding a place to mount the bracket on the frame and making certain it does not interfere with moving through doorways.

The therapy team and ATP have a responsibility to assist the family and child in becoming informed consumers by identifying seating and mobility issues and needs, then presenting several alternatives during the evaluation. The family should make the final decision on the specific type of mobility device after considering the options that the team presents. The most important and significant contribution that the occupational therapist can make is to evaluate access methods and help

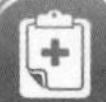

CASE STUDY 20-4 Stephanie

Stephanie is a 15-month-old girl with cerebral palsy who successfully used a switch-operated GoBot to maneuver and explore her surroundings. It took her about 5 hours to become proficient at using a set of four press switches with her hand and to understand the relationship to directionality. However, when she entered another therapy program, the occupational therapist did not consider information on her ability to use switches for driving. Instead, the therapist placed her in a wheelchair training program using the only equipment available, a joystick-operated power wheelchair. After 6 months of training for 3 hours each week, Stephanie demonstrated no improvement in her ability to drive the power wheelchair. Upon re-evaluation of her access method, the therapist provided her with four switches at her hand and evaluated a switch array behind her head. She was able to use both access methods but when questioned, preferred using switches behind her head. The head switch array provided her with immediate success in driving the power wheelchair. Had the therapist provided her with the appropriate control method (switch access instead of a joystick, which she could not operate because of her impaired motor function), she might have demonstrated the ability to use the power wheelchair in significantly less time.

caregivers develop and implement strategies to meet identified goals. The therapist must re-evaluate the outcome as the child progresses. This includes providing periodic evaluations of fit and function of the equipment.

Summary

The literature indicates that independent mobility plays a facilitative role in cognitive, language, and social development.[47] Therefore when mobility is severely delayed or restricted, emotional and psychosocial development are affected. Augmentative mobility devices can provide young children with functional or transitional mobility. They allow children with physical disabilities greater opportunities to become initiators and active participants in daily occupations and experiences. Occupational therapists emphasize methods of adapting the child's environments to maximize his or her functional mobility. The occupational therapist is responsible for ensuring that children with physical receive opportunities for mobility at the earliest age possible to promote participation and development more equal to their able-bodied peers.

Case Studies 20-5, 20-6, and 20-7 include comprehensive information about the children's equipment and adapted environments. These descriptions demonstrate how mobility equipment is integrated with other AT and environmental adaptations to best meet the children's functional needs.

Summary Points

- Self-initiated mobility allows young children with physical disabilities the opportunity to access and explore their surroundings, significantly contributing to visual spatial, sensory motor, social, emotional, and cognitive development.
- Several factors must be considered during an evaluation for seating and mobility equipment, including the purpose or goals for using the device, environments in which the device will be used, features and adaptations that will meet the desired outcomes across all environments, factors that might reduce function in other areas (hardware that interferes with transfers, eating, personal hygiene, or communication), needs and concerns of the care providers and school personnel, options for transporting the device, and cost versus benefits.
- Occupational therapists consider features and options on a mobility device to allow the child's optimal function given his or her abilities and limitations in everyday environments.
- If a child cannot propel a manual wheelchair at the same speed and efficiency as ambulatory peers, then a power wheelchair should be considered to increase independence and function.
- Self-propelling manual wheelchairs are typically recommended over dependent mobility bases, because they offer large wheels for self-propulsion, a frame that can be adapted for growth, more options for mounting speech-generating devices, more adjustments for posture, a range of tilt and seat-to-back angles, and a variety of seating components for postural support.
- Power wheelchairs are designed with a front-wheel, mid-wheel, or rear-wheel configuration and each has advantages and disadvantages.
- The evaluation team should select a wheelchair that fits the child's present body size and needs but also take into account the potential for growth.
- The occupational therapist must consider the features of a seating and positioning system that meet the needs of the client before considering the wheelchair base. Because posture and task performance are inter-related, positioning is critical to the successful use of any mobility device. The therapist must consider positioning components, pitches, angles, and surface contours that affect posture and movement.
- For a child who is prone to pressure-related problems when sitting in a wheelchair, pressure-relief cushions, tilt-in-space, and or recline should be considered. A tilt-in-space feature of a wheelchair functions by maintaining the same seat-to-back angle while tilting the seat backward or forward, and a reclining feature reclines the seat back, increasing the seat-to-back angle and allowing for hip extension.
- Manufacturers of power wheelchairs offer electronic options to adapt joystick functions and to remotely access other devices such as a computer, speech-generating device, telephone, or television through the electronic controls of the wheelchair.
- Occupational therapists need to be aware of wheelchair transportation safety and WC-19 compliant mobility equipment, which indicates that the manufacturer has designed the wheelchair for use as a seat in a moving vehicle.

CASE STUDY 20-5 David and Eric

David

David is an 11-year-old boy diagnosed with Duchenne's muscular dystrophy at 4 years of age. Shortly afterward, his little brother, Eric, was diagnosed with the same condition at 5 months of age. The two brothers and an older sister live with their parents in a small town.

Duchenne's muscular dystrophy is an inherited X-linked disease that affects the voluntary skeletal musculature, with progressive weakness and degeneration of the muscles that control movement. The muscle weakness begins in the proximal and axial musculature and slowly progresses distally. Frequently, children with Duchenne's muscular dystrophy require a wheelchair by 12 years of age. Breathing becomes affected during the later stages of the disease, leading to severe respiratory problems. Respiratory infections commonly cause death during the person's early twenties.

When receiving David's diagnosis, the family was introduced to a team of professionals who specialize in different aspects of musculoskeletal weaknesses. The family received support to help them deal with the initial shock and necessary information about the disease. Twice a year, the family continued to meet with the team for medical and orthopedic evaluations. They also received counseling services to support their social and psychological well-being.

Last year, David had an Achilles tendon lengthening to release a tight heel cord, and shortly thereafter began to use a long-leg orthosis. It is important to lengthen the walking phase in boys with Duchenne's muscular dystrophy to delay hip and knee flexion deformities and equinovarus deformity of the foot and ankle. For 2 years David used a standard lightweight manual wheelchair for traveling long distances or when he was fatigued. Currently the therapy team and David's family are considering a power wheelchair for David, to allow him to conserve energy for social and educational activities. The team plans on spinal stabilization when David's scoliosis exceeds 25 degrees and normal forced vital capacity pulmonary function drops below 50%.

Eric

Eric is now 7 years of age. The progression of his disease is following the same course as David's, although somewhat slower. The early signs of Duchenne's muscular dystrophy are becoming prominent, such as the waddling gait, tendency to fall, and difficulty rising from a sitting or lying position.

At the time of Eric's diagnosis, the family lived in an apartment but soon decided to build a house. The occupational therapist provided recommendations for designing the house for wheelchair accessibility to maximize function and independence.

The family has been living in the house for 2 years, and they are pleased with the features that enable the boys to be independent. The outdoor surfaces (sidewalks and ramps) are firm, stable, and slip resistant. The floor plan is spacious, doorways are wide, and there are no thresholds. A few sliding doors have been installed to allow maximum door width and to eliminate floor swing space requirements. Controls, levers, and switches are placed low to be within reach from a wheelchair. The windows' lower edges are only 20 inches above the floor for the same reason. The bathrooms are spacious, with both a bathtub and a shower. The boys love taking baths because they stay warmer and move more freely in the water. The sink is freestanding so the boys can get close to it. An automatic faucet has been installed, which turns on when the hands are placed under the faucet. A full-length mirror is on the wall.

The family continues to need extensive support and assistance to adjust to new challenges. In addition to direct service to the family, the occupational therapist continues to work closely with the schools to ensure that accessibility is available.

CASE STUDY 20-6 Jason

Jason is a 7-year-old boy with cerebral palsy, which has affected his ability to speak, move his body with control, and eat. Although he demonstrates severe delays in his motor skills, he is alert and attentive and understands what is said to him. From his early days, his family was motivated to ensure that Jason have a childhood as normal as possible. They were creative in designing simple devices and tools to accomplish these goals. His grandfather designed the first mobility device for him. Using a pushcart to hold golf clubs, he mounted a car seat to the frame with foam pieces in the seat to help align Jason's body and prevent him from leaning over. His mother used it to push him around the neighborhood during her daily jogging routine. He also used a standard stroller but required a positioning system to assist him in sitting upright by providing support at the pelvis, trunk, and head. The first seating system was made of Tri-Wall, a three-layer-thick cardboard that can be used to fabricate temporary seat inserts for children. Another seat insert was fabricated from Tri Wall and placed on a dining room chair so that he could eat at the family table instead of in a high chair.

By the time he was 12 months of age, Jason's family built him an aeroplane mobility device (see Figure 20-7*A*) to use at home. When he outgrew this by 2 years of age, his occupational therapist evaluated him for a support walker and found that he could effectively use the KidWalk by Prime Engineering (see Figure 20-8*C*). He continued to use this device for indoor mobility and for playing in Little League for special needs children when he was 5 years of age. He and his teammates used an automatic device to hit the ball, and Jason ran around the field using his walker.

When Jason was 3 years old, his family decided that the walker alone did not adequately meet his community mobility needs. His occupational therapist evaluated him for a power wheelchair and found that he could operate the joystick once

Continued

CASE STUDY 20-6 Jason—cont'd

he was positioned with maximal support at his feet, pelvis, trunk, and head. His therapist and family determined the features he would need to operate a power wheelchair. He needed a molded seating system for support and alignment, and, to increase independence, the system needed to include the capability to elevate the seat from the floor to various heights. The therapist identified a power wheelchair with these features and recommended a custom-molded seating system.

The family made the home environment accessible to Jason in many ways. When he was 2 years of age, they decided that it was important for him to roll out of bed in the morning and try to roll on the floor. They placed a low-height mattress on the floor in the corner of his bedroom and made it his bed. They lined the sides of it with his stuffed toys to protect him from unintentionally hitting his arms against the walls. This arrangement allowed him to get out of bed on his own. They also lowered the light switch in his room so that he could reach it from his walker or wheelchair.

Positioning him in the bathtub when he was a toddler was a challenge, but his mother made a bath seat for him from a milk crate. She placed foam around the edges and the seat for comfort. When he outgrew this, his family acquired a bath seat designed for children with disabilities. His occupational therapist recommended an adapted toilet seat with a high backrest. It provided Jason with the ability to begin toilet training at 2 years of age. His family also installed a flip-down bar in front of the toilet so Jason could stand at the toilet "like his dad."

During these early years, Jason's occupational therapist introduced him to augmentative communication symbols and aids. By the time he was 12 months of age, he could point to symbols in his communication book using his fist and soon progressed to using a speech-generating device with voice output by accessing it with a head tracking system. The speech-generating device was mounted on his power wheelchair. Today Jason is fully included in a second grade class. He uses AT to do his schoolwork and has an attendant with him throughout the day. Both simple and sophisticated AT devices have enabled him to function within a regular education classroom and to participate in most of the activities of his peers.

CASE STUDY 20-7 Jet

Jet is an inquisitive, happy and interactive 6-year-old boy who has cerebral palsy. He began attending preschool seated in his first wheelchair, a Zippie TS, a tilt-in-space dependent base, which he had outgrown. His therapy and preschool team, understanding the benefits of self-initiated mobility, recommended an evaluation to include a lightweight manual wheelchair he might learn to propel himself with optimal seating and positioning. The wheelchair had to easily disassemble to fit into the family car and be light enough to help him learn to propel it in spite of his hypotonia. He also required seating options that would stabilize his pelvis to prevent it from sliding forward into hip extension when he would use his arms and hands. He used a speech-generating device (SGD) with a key guard for communication and accessed it by pointing with either hand. It would need to be mounted to the frame of the new wheelchair. Seating options were evaluated first by having him borrow a wheelchair for several weeks with a seating system temporarily designed for him. The trial system allowed him some experience with new seating components so he could be part of the decision-making process and allowed the team to observe his function to determine how the components contributed to or interfered with functional tasks. After the trials, Jet, his family, school, and therapy team with the ATP decided that the most appropriate seating components for him would include a Jay backrest with lateral trunk pads, a contoured custom seat cushion with contoured lateral hip pads, a Subasis bar to provide hip stability, and a HAWC headrest to provide occipital and lateral support of his neck to assist in separating shoulder movements from body and head movements (Figure 20-19). Without the HAWC headrest, he leaned to either side when he tried to use his hands, which affected his visual field, endurance, and accuracy when selecting targets on his SGD. The headrest also provided midline support during feeding and allowed him to feed himself finger foods and drink from a straw more efficiently. The ATP

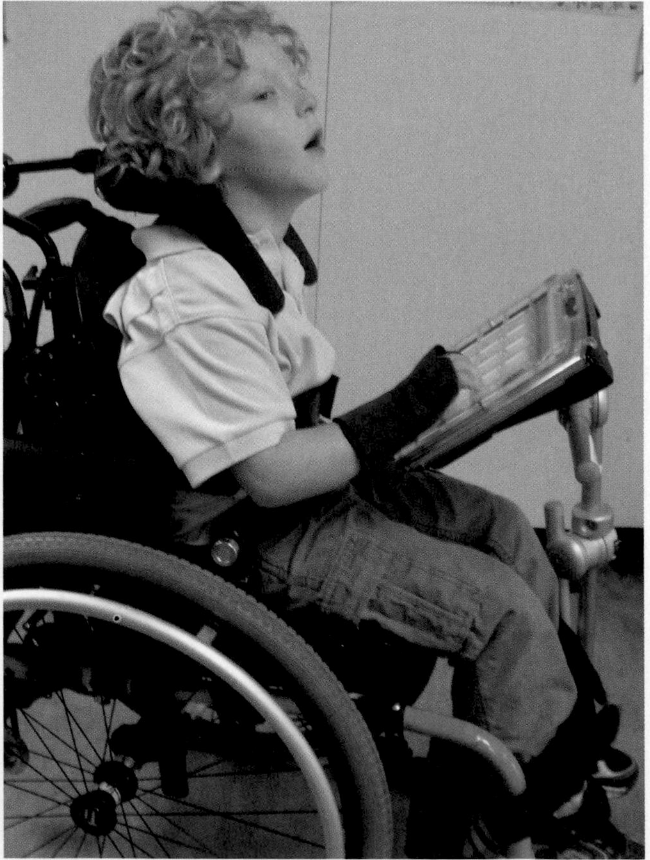

FIGURE 20-19 A 6 year old boy wears wrist splints to access his speech generating device mounted to his wheelchair while seated in his TiLite manual wheelchair and positioned in a Jay back, HAWC headrest, a custom seat cushion and subasis bar at his pelvis.

CASE STUDY 20-7 Jet—cont'd

presented several lightweight manual wheelchairs at the evaluation and the family/team decided that the features of the TiLite Twist best met his needs because of the accessible wheels he could learn to propel, 1-inch tubing (which made it easier to mount his SGD), ability to adjust pitch through the caster, flip-back footrest, and foldable backrest for transport and growth adjustments.

Jet also had to access his environments in preschool, at home, and in the community as well as to have a means for dynamic weight bearing and exercise. After evaluating several dynamic standing mobility devices, he was able to most efficiently maneuver a KidWalk owing to its ability to allow for weight shift, its compact turning radius, and large wheels for independent mobility on the playground turf surface. It was recommended and authorized. The KidWalk provides him with the opportunity to independently choose center time activities in preschool, run at recess with his peers, and begin learning how to jump. His family acquired the KidWalk for home use and Jet learned to walk to his local park, surprising his family by learning how to open the gate, drink from a fountain independently for the first time (Figure 20-20), and help with activities such as washing the family car (Figure 20-21). He is learning to self-propel the wheels of his manual wheelchair across a room and recently self-propelled outdoors over his backyard deck to pick a flower. His most efficient means for mobility is walking in his KidWalk. His next mobility goal is to learn to access a powered mobility wheelchair for distance mobility, which he is learning to do in weekly therapy sessions.

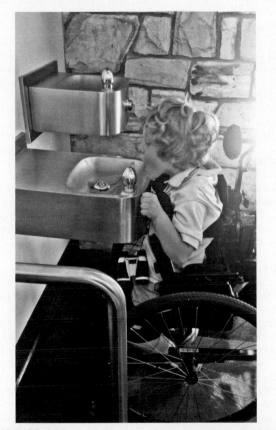

FIGURE 20-20 Jet walks up to a drinking fountain in his KidWalk standing mobility device and learns how to take a drink for the first time.

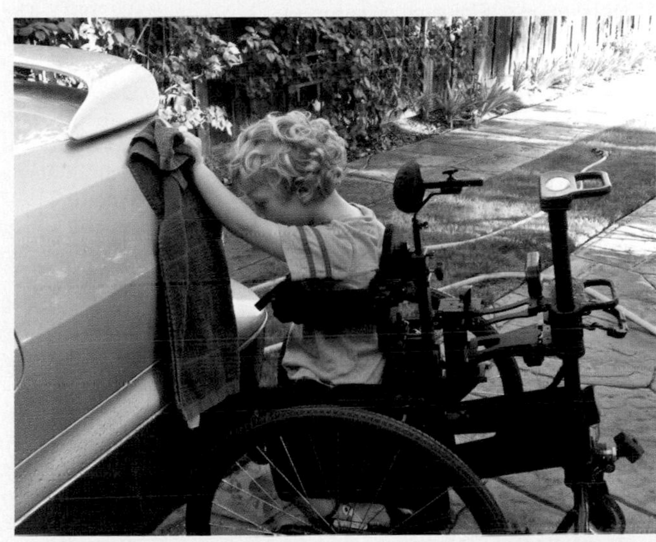

FIGURE 20-21 Jet washes his family's car while standing and moving in the KidWalk.

REFERENCES

1. Acredolo, L., Adams, A., & Goodwyn, S. (1984). The role of self-produced movement and visual tracking in infant spatial orientation. *Journal of Experimental Child Psychology, 38*, 312–327.
2. Adolph, K. E. (2008). Learning to move. *Current Directions in Psychological Science, 17*(3), 213–218.
3. Americans with Disabilities Act and Accessible Information Technology Center. (2003). Bulletin #4. Retrieved July 2009 from <http://www.adaproject.org>.
4. Andersson, C., Grooten, W., Hellsten, M., et al. (2003). Adults with cerebral palsy: Walking ability after progressive strength training. *Developmental Medicine and Child Neurology, 45*, 220–228.
5. ANSI/RESNA Subcommittee on Wheelchairs and Transportation. (2000). *ANSI/RESNA WC, Vol.1/Sect. 19. Wheelchairs used as seats in motor vehicles.* Arlington, VA: RESNA.
6. ANSI/RESNA Subcommittee on Wheelchairs and Transportation. (2008). *ANSI/RESNA WC. Vol. 4/Sect. 20. Seating systems used in motor vehicles.* Arlington, VA: RESNA.
7. Backer, G., & Howell, B. (1997). Physical therapy goals and intervention for the ventilator-assisted child or adolescent. In L. Driver, V. Nelson, &

S. Warschausky (Eds.), *The ventilator assisted child.* San Antonio, TX: Communication Skill Builders.
8. Benson, J., & Uzgiris, I. (1985). Effect of self-initiated locomotion on infant search activity. *Developmental Psychology, 21,* 923–931.
9. Bergen, A., Presperin, J., & Tallman, T. (1990). *Positioning for function: Wheelchairs and other assistive technologies.* New York: Valhalla Rehabilitation Publications.
10. Blundell, S., Shepherd, R., Dean, C., et al. (2003). Functional strength training in cerebral palsy: A pilot study of a group circuit training class for children aged 4–8 years. *Clinical Rehabilitation, 17,* 48–57.
11. Bly, S. L. (1994). *Motor skills acquisition in the first year.* Tucson, AZ: Therapy Skill Builders.
12. Brinker, R. P., & Lewis, M. (1982). Making the world work with microcomputers: A learning prosthesis for handicapped infants. *Exceptional Children, 49,* 163–170.
13. Butler, C. (1986). Effects of powered mobility on self-initiated behaviors of very young children with locomotor disability. *Developmental Medicine and Child Neurology, 28,* 325–332.
14. Butler, C. (1988). High tech tots: Technology for mobility, manipulation, communication, and learning in early childhood. *Infants and Young Children, 2,* 66–73.
15. Butler, C. (1988). Powered tots: Augmentative mobility for locomotor disabled youngsters. *American Physical Therapy Association Pediatric Publication, 14,* 21.
16. Campos, J. J., & Bertenthal, B. I. (1987). Locomotion and psychological development in infancy. In K. M. Jaffe (Ed.), *Childhood powered mobility: Developmental, technical, and clinical perspectives* (pp. 11–42). Proceedings of the RESNA First Northwest Regional Conference. Washington, DC: RESNA Press.
17. Campos, J., Bertenthal, B., & Kermoian, R. (1992). Early experience and emotional development: The emergence of wariness of heights. *Psychological Science, 3,* 61–64.
18. Cech, D., & Martin, A. (1995). *Functional movement development across the life span.* Philadelphia: Saunders.
19. Clearfield, M. (2004). The role of crawling and walking experience in infant spatial memory. *Journal of Experimental Child Psychology, 89*(3), 214–241.
20. Cook, A., & Polgar, J. (2008). Technologies that enable mobility. In A. Cook & J. Polgar (Eds.), *Assistive technologies: Principles and practice* (3rd ed., pp. 408–442). St. Louis: Mosby.
21. Cooper, R. (1998). Biomechanics and ergonomics of wheelchairs. In R. Cooper (Ed.), *Wheelchair selection and configuration.* New York: Demos.
22. Coster, W. (1998). Occupation-centered assessment of children. *American Journal of Occupational Therapy, 52,* 337–344.
23. Damiano, D. L. (2006). Activity, activity, activity: Rethinking our physical therapy approach to cerebral palsy. *Physical Therapy, 86,* 1534–1540.
24. Dicianno, B. E., Arva, J., Lieberman, J. M., et al. (2009). RESNA position on the application of tilt, recline, and elevating legrests for wheelchairs. *Assistive Technology, 21*(1), 13–22.
25. Deitz, J., Swinth, Y., & White, O. (2002). Powered mobility and preschoolers with complex developmental delays. *American Journal of Occupational Therapy, 56,* 86–96.
26. Douglas, J., & Ryan, M. (1987). A preschool severely disabled boy and his powered wheelchair: A case study. *Child: Care, Health and Development, 13,* 303–309.
27. Eagleton, M., Iams, A., McDowell, J., et al. (2004). The effects of strength training on gait in adolescents with cerebral palsy. *Pediatric Physical Therapy, 16,* 22–30.
28. Engstrom, B. (1993). *Ergonomics, wheelchairs and positioning.* Hasselby, Sweden: Posturalis Books.
29. Everand, L. (1997). Early mobility means easier integration. *Canadian Review of Sociology and Anthropology, 34,* 224–234.
30. Fisher, A. G. (1998). Uniting practice and theory in an occupational framework. *American Journal of Occupational Therapy, 52,* 509–519.
31. Foreman, N., Foreman, D., Cummings, A., et al. (1990). *Journal of General Psychology, 117,* 195–233.
32. Fowler, E. G., Ho, T. W., Nwigwe, A. I., et al. (2001). The effect of quadriceps femoris muscle strengthening exercises on spasticity in children with cerebral palsy. *Physical Therapy, 81,* 1195–1223.
33. Furumasu, J., Guerrette, P., & Tefft, D. (1996). The development of a powered wheelchair mobility program for young children. *Technology and Disability, 5,* 41–48.
34. Furumasu, J., Guerrette, P., & Tefft, D. (2004). Relevance of the Pediatric Powered Wheelchair Screening Test (PPWST) for children with cerebral palsy. *Developmental Medicine and Child Neurology, 46,* 468–474.
35. Furumasu, J., Tefft, D., & Guerette, P. (1996). Pediatric powered mobility: Readiness to learn. *Team Rehabilitation,* October, 29–36.
36. Galloway, J. C. (2011). *Babies gone wild: Unleashing the exploratory power of infants.* Sykes Symposium on Pediatric Physical Therapy, Health and Development, conducted at the University of Southern California.
37. Galloway, J. C., Ryu, J., & Agrawal, S. K. (2008). Babies driving robots: Self-generated mobility in very young infants. *Journal of Intelligent Service Robotics, 1,* 123–134.
38. Guerette, P., Tefft, D., & Furumasu, J. (2005). Pediatric powered mobility: Results of a national survey of providers. *Assistive Technology, 17,* 144–158.
39. Guerette, P., Tefft, D., Furumasu, J., et al. (1999). Development of a cognitive assessment battery for young children with physical impairments. *Infant-Toddler Intervention: The Transdisciplinary Journal, 9,* 169–181.
40. Guerette, P., Furumasu, J., & Tefft, D. (2013). The positive effects of early powered mobility on children's psychosocial and play skills. *Assistive Technology, 25*(1), 39–48.
41. Haley, S. M., Coster, W. J., Ludlow, L. H., et al. (1992). *Pediatric evaluation of disability inventory (PEDI).* San Antonio, TX: Psychological Corp.
42. Hasdai, A., Jessel, A. S., & Weiss, P. L. (1998). Use of computer simulator for training children with disabilities in the operation of a powered wheelchair. *American Journal of Occupational Therapy, 52,* 195–220.
43. Hays, R. (1987). Childhood motor impairments: Clinical overview and scope of the problem. In K. M. Jaffe (Ed.), *Childhood powered mobility: Developmental, technical, and clinical perspectives.* Proceedings of the RESNA First Northwest Regional Conference. Washington, DC: RESNA Press.
44. Hulme, J., Poor, R., Schulein, M., et al. (1983). Perceived behavioral changes observed with adaptive seating devices for multi-handicapped developmentally disabled individuals. *Physical Therapy, 62,* 204–208.
45. Hundert, J., & Hopkins, B. (1992). Training supervisors in a collaborative team approach to promote peer interactions of children with disabilities in integrated preschools. *Journal of Applied Behavior Analysis, 25,* 385–400.
46. Hune, K., Guarrera-Bowlby, P., & Deutsch, J. (2007). The clinical decision-making process of prescribing power mobility for a child with cerebral palsy. *Pediatric Physical Therapy, 19,* 254–260.
47. Jones, M. A., McEwen, I. R., & Hansen, L. (2003). Use of power mobility for a young child with spinal muscular atrophy. *Physical Therapy, 83,* 253–262.
48. Kangas, K. (2001). *Chest supports: Why they are not working.* Presented at the

Seventeenth International Seating Symposium (pp. 41–44). February 22-24.

49. Kermoian, R., & Meng, D. (1992). *How cultural practices mediate the onset of crawling.* Miami, FL: Proceedings of the Eighth International Conference on Infant Studies.

50. Kermoian, R. (1998). Locomotor experience facilitates psychological functioning: Implications for assistive mobility for young children. In D. Gray, I. Quatrano, & M. Lieberman (Eds.), *Designing and using assistive technology: The human perspective* (pp. 251–268). Baltimore: Brookes Press.

51. Lange, M. (2008). Manual wheelchairs: Understanding these general categories can help therapists meet individual needs. *ADVANCE, 24*(6), 31–33.

52. Margolis, S. A., Jones, R. H., & Brown, B. E., (1985). *The sub-ASIS bar: An effective approach to pelvic stabilization in seated positioning* (pp. 45–47). The Proceedings of the 8th Annual Conference on Rehabilitation Engineering.

53. McBurney, H., Taylor, N. F., Dodd, K. J., et al. (2003). A qualitative analysis of the benefits of strength training for young people with cerebral palsy. *Developmental Medicine and Child Neurology, 45,* 658–663.

54. Myhr, U., & Wendt, L. (1991). Improvement of functional sitting position for children with cerebral palsy. *Developmental Medicine and Child Neurology, 33,* 246–256.

55. Nilsson, L., & Nyberg, P. (2003). Driving to learn: A new concept for training children with profound cognitive disabilities in a powered wheelchair. *American Journal of Occupational Therapy, 57,* 229–233.

56. Nwaobi, O. (1986). Effects of body orientation in space on tonic muscle activity of patients with cerebral palsy. *Developmental Medicine and Child Neurology, 28,* 41–44.

57. Nwaobi, O. (1987). Effect of unilateral arm restraint on upper extremity function in cerebral palsy. In *Proceedings of the Annual RESNA Conference* (pp. 311–313). Washington, DC: RESNA Press.

58. Paleg, G. (1997). Made for walking: A comparison of gait trainers. *Team Rehab Report,* July, 41–45.

59. Paleg, G. (2007). What's new in mobility accessories. *Rehab Management, 20*(2), 24–27.

60. Paleg, G. (2008). Moving forward. *Rehab Management, 21*(5), 16, 18–19.

61. Palisano, R., Rosenbaum, P., Walter, S., et al. (1997). Development and reliability of a system to classify gross motor function in children with cerebral palsy. *Developmental Medicine and Child Neurology, 39*(4), 214–223.

62. Palisano, R. J., Tieman, B. L., Walter, S. D., et al. (2003). Effect of environment setting on mobility methods of children with cerebral palsy. *Developmental Medicine and Child Neurology, 45,* 113–120.

63. Paulsson, K., & Christoffersen, M. (1984). Psychological aspects of technical aids: How does independent mobility affect the psychological and intellectual development of children with physical disabilities. In *Proceedings of the Second Annual Conference on Rehabilitation Engineering* (pp. 282–286). Washington, DC: RESNA Press.

64. Pauly, M., & Crener, R. (2013). Levels of mobility in children and adolescents with spina bifida-clinical parameters predicting mobility and maintenance of these skills. *European Journal of Pediatric Surgery, 23*(2), 110–114.

65. Piaget, J. (1954). *The construction of reality in the child.* New York: Basic Books.

66. Pirpris, M., & Graham, H. K. (2004). Uptime in children with cerebral palsy. *Journal of Pediatric Orthopedics, 5,* 521–528.

67. Ploughman, M. (2008). Exercise is brain food: The effects of physical activity on cognitive function. *Developmental Neurorehabilitation, 11*(3), 236–240.

68. Pollock, N., & Stewart, D. (1998). Occupational performance needs of school-aged children with physical disability in the community. *Physical and Occupational Therapy in Pediatrics, 18,* 55–68.

69. Raine, A., Reynolds, C., Venables, P. H., et al. (2002). Stimulation seeking and intelligence: A retrospective longitudinal study. *Journal Personality and Social Psychology, 82,* 663–674.

70. Rodby-Bousquet, E., & Hagglund, G. (2010). Use of manual and powered wheelchair in children with cerebral palsy: A cross-sectional study. *BMC Pediatrics, 10,* 59.

71. Rosenbaum, P. L., Walter, S. D., Hanna, S. E., et al. (2002). Prognosis for gross motor function in cerebral palsy: Creation of motor development curves. *Journal of the American Medical Association, 288*(11), 1357–1363.

72. Seligman, M. (1975). *Helplessness: On depression, development, and death.* San Francisco: Freeman.

73. Shutrump, S., Manary, M., & Buning, M. (2008). Safe transportation for students who use wheelchairs on the school bus. *Occupational Therapy Practice,* 8–12.

74. Stanton, D., Wilson, P. N., & Foreman, N. (2002). Effects of early mobility on shortcut performance in a simulated maze. *Behavioral Brain Research, 136,* 61–66.

75. Taplin, C. S. (1989). Powered wheelchair control, assessment, and training. In *RESNA '89: Proceedings of the 12th Annual Conference* (pp. 45–46). Washington, DC: RESNA Press.

76. Taylor, S., & Monahan, L. (1989). C. Brubaker (Ed.), Considerations in assessing for powered mobility. *Wheelchair IV: Report of a conference on the state of the art of powered wheelchair mobility, December 7–9, 1988.* Washington, DC: RESNA Press.

77. Tefft, D., Furumasu, J., & Guerette, P. (1993). Cognitive readiness for powered wheelchair mobility in the young child. In *Proceedings of the RESNA 1993 Annual Conference* (pp. 338–340). Washington, DC: RESNA Press.

78. Tefft, D., Furumasu, J., & Guerette, P. (1995). Development of a cognitive assessment battery for evaluating readiness for powered mobility. In *Proceedings of the RESNA 1995 Annual Conference* (pp. 320–322). Washington, DC: RESNA Press.

79. Tefft, D., Guerette, P., & Furumasu, J. (1999). Cognitive predictors of young children's readiness for powered mobility. *Developmental Medicine and Child Neurology, 41,* 665–670.

80. Tefft, D., Guerett, P., & Furumasu, J. (2011). The impact of early powered mobility on parental stress, negative emotions and family social interactions. *Physical and Occupational Therapy in Pediatrics, 31*(1), 4–15.

81. Telzrow, R., Campos, J., Shepherd, A., et al. (1987). Spatial understanding in infants with motor handicaps. In K. M. Jaffe (Ed.), *Childhood powered mobility: Developmental, technical and clinical perspectives* (pp. 62–69). Proceedings of the RESNA First Northwest Regional Conference. Seattle, WA: RESNA Association for the Advancement of Rehabilitation Technology.

82. Trefler, E. (1999). Then and now: Saving time with simulators. *Team Rehabilitation,* (February), 32–36.

83. Trefler, E., Hobson, D., Taylor, S., et al. (1993). *Seating and mobility.* Tucson, AZ: Therapy Skill Builders.

84. Uniform Data System for Medical Rehabilitation. (1999). *Functional independence measure for children (WeeFIM).* Outpatient version 5.0. Buffalo, NY: State University of New York at Buffalo.

85. Verburg, G., Field, D., & Jarvis, S. (1987). Motor, perceptual, and cognitive factors that affect mobility control. In *Proceedings of the 10th Annual Conference on Rehabilitation Technology.* Washington, DC: RESNA Press.

86. Warren, C. G. (1990). Powered mobility and its implications. *Journal of Rehabilitation Research and Development. Clinical Supplement, 27*, 74–85.
87. Wright, C., & Nomura, M. (1995). *From toys to computers, access for the physically disabled child.* San Jose, CA: Don Johnston.
88. Wright-Ott, C. (1997). The transitional powered mobility aid: A new concept and tool for early mobility. In J. Furumasu (Ed.), *Pediatric powered mobility* (pp. 58–69). Washington, DC: RESNA Press.
89. Wright-Ott, C. (1998). Designing a transitional powered mobility aid for young children with physical disabilities. In D. Gray, L. Quatrano, & M. Lieverman (Eds.), *Designing and using assistive technology: The human perspective* (pp. 285–295). Baltimore: Brookes.
90. Wright-Ott, C. (1999). A transitional powered mobility aid for young children with physical disabilities. Presented at ICORR 99 Sixth International Conference on Rehabilitation Robotics, July 1999, Stanford, CA.
91. Wright-Ott, C., Escobar, R., & Leslie, S. (2002). Encouraging exploration. *Rehabilitation Management. 15*, 30–35.

SUGGESTED READING

Bertenthal, B. I., Campos, J. J., & Barrett, K. C. (1984). Self-produced locomotion: An organizer of emotional, cognitive, and social development in infancy. In R. N. Emde & R. J. Harmon (Eds.), *Continuities and discontinuities in development* (pp. 175–210). New York: Plenum Press. doi:10.1007/978-1-4613-2725-7_8

Cook, A., & Polgar, J. (2008). *Assistive technologies: Principles and practice* (3rd ed.). St. Louis: Mosby.

Fuhrman, S., Buning, M., & Karg, P. (2008). Wheelchair transportation: Ensuring safe community mobility. *Occupational Therapy Practice*, (October), 10–13.

Sunny Hill Health Centre. Seating and mobility. <http://www.seatingandmobility.ca>.

Tefft, D., Furumasu, J., & Guerette, P. (1996). *Ready, set, go: Pediatric powered mobility with young children training video and manual.* Downey, CA: LAREI.

Tefft, D., Furumasu, J., & Guerette, P. (1997). Pediatric powered mobility: Influential cognitive skills. In J. Furumasu (Ed.), *Pediatric powered mobility: Developmental perspectives, technical issues, clinical approaches* (pp. 70–91). Washington, DC: RESNA Press.

University of Pittsburgh Department of Rehabilitation Science and Technology. http://wheelchairnet.org.

Zollars, J. *Special seating: An illustrated guide.* Revised Edition. Available at: <http://www.seatingzollars.com/jeanannezollars.html>.

CHAPTER 21

Neonatal Intensive Care Unit

Jan Hunter • Anjanette Lee • Leslie Altimier

KEY TERMS

- Neonatal intensive care unit
- Nursery classifications (levels of care)
- Neonatal developmental specialist
- Mastery skill levels, novice to expert
- Preterm infants
- Very-low-birth-weight infants
- NICU models of care
- Healing environment (physical and sensory)
- Individualized, family-centered, developmentally supportive care
- Neuroprotection
- Neuroprotective core measures
- Epigenetics
- Sleep and brain development
- Preterm infant neurobehavioral organization
- Synactive theory of development
- States of arousal
- Neuromotor development
- Therapeutic positioning
- Nutritive sucking
- Non-nutritive sucking
- Cue-based, infant-driven feeding
- Kangaroo care and skin-to-skin holding

GUIDING QUESTIONS

1. What is the scope of knowledge and what are the various roles required for competent practice in the neonatal intensive care unit (NICU)?
2. What is meant by "potentially better practices (PBPs) to support neurodevelopment in the NICU," as developed by the collaborative Vermont Oxford Network project?
3. How do the intrauterine and NICU extrauterine environments differ?
4. What are protective interventions to reduce avoidable stimulation from excessive or inappropriate light, sound, and caregiving practices in the NICU?
5. Why is protected sleep so important to an infant in the third trimester, whether in the womb or the NICU?
6. What factors are considered in evaluating an infant in the NICU?
7. What are the six neurobehavioral states, as defined by Brazelton and Als?
8. How and why do posture and movement patterns differ between term and extremely preterm infants?
9. What are common positional deformities of preterm infants, and how do these iatrogenic deformities potentially influence future development?
10. What factors are considered in therapeutic positioning?
11. What key factors facilitate successful breastfeeding in the NICU?
12. Why is non-nutritive sucking beneficial to preterm infants?
13. What are the primary differences between a traditional feeding approach and a cue-based, infant-driven feeding approach with NICU infants?
14. What are challenges in parenting a preterm infant in the NICU?

Kimberly underwent an emergency cesarean delivery at 25 weeks' gestation when intrauterine circulation problems developed in two of her three triplets. Adyson was born prematurely to a 15 year-old student who concealed her pregnancy from her parents. Tonya, with a history of three previous miscarriages, had a cerclage (a surgical procedure to help keep the cervix closed during pregnancy), and was able to carry Darren until 32 weeks' gestation. Brittney was born at 28 weeks to a mother being treated with methadone. Dylan, born at term to a febrile mother, became critically ill with pneumonia and developed respiratory failure during his first day of life. Myesha was delivered by an emergency cesarean section following a motor vehicle accident in which the placenta was partially torn from the uterine wall. Maria's prenatal ultrasound revealed an infant with multiple congenital anomalies.

These real-life examples represent the urgency and wide range of skilled medical care necessary to optimize survival and functional outcome in preterm and high-risk infants. Each of these infants was admitted to a neonatal intensive care unit (NICU) following delivery; all but one baby survived.

Overview of the NICU and Developmental Care

A neonatal intensive care unit is a stimulating and rewarding practice area for therapists with a passion for at-risk infants.

Experienced NICU clinicians are convinced that many long-term functional problems can be minimized or eliminated with appropriate developmental support from birth, a very motivating concept.

Because the NICU is a complex setting, with the most vulnerable patients and little or no room for error, it can also be overwhelming and intimidating for someone new to the NICU. Everything is relevant and interrelated—just where does one start to build knowledge and skills? A NICU primer, a short illustrated introduction to the world of the NICU, is available on the Evolve website.

This chapter includes a basic medical foundation, the changing role of a neonatal developmental specialist, the scope of knowledge and skills required, basic fetal development and the impact of birth requiring neonatal intensive care, environmental considerations, neuroprotective developmentally supportive care applications, neuromotor development, feeding in the NICU, and partnering with families. The final section discusses practical suggestions and approaches to becoming an essential member of the NICU team and attaining proficiency as a neonatal developmental specialist.

Nursery Classification and Regionalization of Care

While the NICU primer (available on the Evolve website) provides a historical overview of the NICU; this section describes the current status. The spiraling expense and complexity of medical care created a growing discrepancy between newborn death rates at major medical centers and those at smaller hospitals. In the early 1970s, regionalization of perinatal care emerged to provide advanced levels of health care to any mother or infant within an identified perinatal care region while avoiding unnecessary duplication of services. Patient care was generally provided at the nearest hospital, with transfer to a higher level facility as needed for more complex problems. Initially three levels of neonatal care were identified: level I (routine newborn care), level II (intermediate care), and level III (neonatal intensive care). Subcategories were added in 2004 but not consistently used. The latest revision in 2012 includes four levels of neonatal care, as described in Box 21-1.[13,129]

BOX 21-1 Nursery Classifications (2012)

- *Level I*: A hospital nursery that is able to provide neonatal resuscitation and postnatal care of healthy newborn infants and stable late-preterm infants born at 35 to 37 weeks' gestation. Sufficient expertise and experience to stabilize ill newborns or infants born at less than 35 weeks' gestation prior to transfer to a higher level facility are also necessary.
- *Level II*: This hospital special care nursery provides care to infants born at or less than 32 weeks' gestation with birth weight ≤ 1500 g who have physiologic immaturity issues that are expected to resolve rapidly with continued maturation (e.g., apnea of prematurity, inability to maintain body temperature, inability to take oral feedings) or who are convalescing from a higher level of care. A level II NICU can provide continuous positive airway pressure and may provide mechanical ventilation for brief periods (e.g., 24 hours).
- *Level III*: This is a hospital NICU able to provide continuous life support and comprehensive care for extremely high-risk newborn infants and those with critical illness, including infants born extremely preterm. Level III units can provide critical medical and surgical care and ongoing assisted ventilation (e.g., high-frequency ventilation, inhaled nitric oxide). Level III units have ready access to a full range of pediatric medical subspecialists; advanced imaging with interpretation on an urgent basis; access to pediatric ophthalmologic services for the monitoring, treatment, and follow-up of retinopathy of prematurity; and pediatric surgical specialists and pediatric anesthesiologists on site or at a closely related institution to perform major surgery. Level III units can facilitate transfer to higher level facilities or children's hospitals, as well as back-transport recovering infants to lower level facilities.
- *Level IV*: These units have the capabilities of a level III NICU and are located in institutions that can provide on-site surgical repair of serious congenital or acquired malformations. Level IV units can facilitate transport systems and often provide outreach education to other area NICUs.

Adapted from American Academy of Pediatrics, Committee on the Fetus and Newborn. (2012). Levels of neonatal intensive care. *Pediatrics, 130*, 587–597; and Stokowski, L. A. (2012). Noteworthy professional news: Four levels of neonatal care. *Advances in Neonatal Care, 12*, 326–328.

Developmental Specialists Emerge as Integral Members of the NICU Team

Infant survival was the original indicator of NICU success. As the survival rate increased for younger, smaller, and sicker infants, an increased awareness of environmental and caregiving influences on the vulnerable newborn has enlarged the scope of NICU care to encompass infant development and family issues, in addition to primary medical concerns.[71] Consequently, a unique neonatal developmental specialist role has emerged, which transcends traditional discipline boundaries. Neonatal developmental specialists in a specific NICU may variably be an occupational therapist, physical therapist, speech pathologist, nurse, and/or child life specialist with advanced training and a passion to help babies and their families function at an optimal level in the NICU and beyond. A neonatal developmental specialist can be expected to provide direct patient care, collaborative consultation with families and the medical team, staff and family support and education, facilitation of system changes in the NICU environment, and/or caregiving practices that are neuroprotective to the infant and supportive of family as partners in care.[10,115]

Traditional neonatal therapy in the 1980s (and still persisting in some NICUs) consists solely of rehabilitation and developmental stimulation for infants identified with developmental risk factors (e.g., extreme prematurity, prenatal drug exposure, genetic syndrome), pathology with inherent neurodevelopmental risks (e.g., central nervous system [CNS] abnormalities), and atypical performance (e.g., abnormal tone, poor feeding, chronic illness with developmental delay). Traditional therapy targets specific problems such as limited range of motion, atypical muscle tone, extreme irritability, poor feeding, and developmental delay. Remediation and rehabilitation continue to be appropriate for NICU infants with pathology affecting development and function.

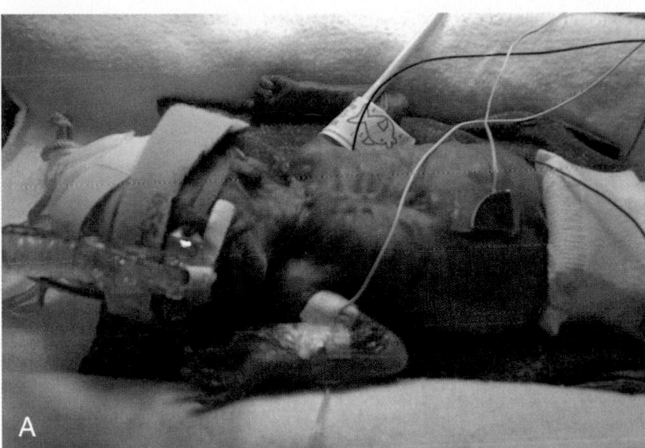

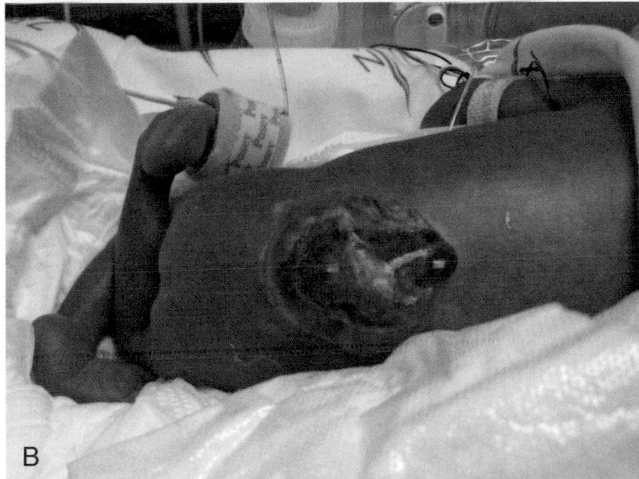

FIGURE 21-1 A critically ill extremely preterm newborn **(A)** and an infant with multiple congenital anomalies **(B;** hydrocephalus, a large myelomeningocele, and lower extremity arthrogryposis) illustrate the range of infants cared for in a neonatal intensive care unit. (Courtesy Infant Special Care Unit, University of Texas Medical Branch, Galveston, TX. Photographs by Jan Hunter.)

Currently, state-of-the-art developmentally supportive care is neuroprotective and begins at birth to help promote physiologic stability and optimal neurodevelopment, rather than waiting for a baby to first become medically stable.[81] This approach acknowledges that any infant who requires neonatal intensive care has inherent developmental risks and vulnerabilities, parenting an infant in the NICU is stressful and difficult, environmental and caregiving factors interact and affect each baby's evolving status, and both the infant and family must receive individualized support throughout the NICU hospitalization for optimal outcomes (Figure 21-1).

The early neuroprotective and preventive component of developmental support is not necessarily inherent in the traditional rehabilitation model. In contrast with the rehabilitation emphasis of direct hands-on contact, the current practice of protecting the fragile newborn from excessive or inappropriate sleep disruption and sensory input is often a more urgent priority than direct interventions or interactions with the infant.

Becoming a Developmental Specialist

The advanced practice area of the NICU requires specialized knowledge and skills that take time and intentional effort to acquire. These include the following: familiarity with relevant neonatal medical conditions, procedures, and equipment; understanding the unique developmental abilities and vulnerabilities of term, preterm, and ill infants; familiarity with evolving neonatal behavioral organization, family systems, NICU ecology; current models of practice; and appreciation of the manner in which these factors interact to influence infant and family behavior and development.[15,132,133,136]

Despite the degree of experience in other practice areas, everyone initially enters the NICU as a novice. Trust, acceptance, and respect are gradually earned from protective NICU staff as each neonatal developmental specialist achieves and consistently demonstrates competency in knowledge, skills, and interpersonal professional relationships. It helps to understand the progression from novice to expert, with the traditional Dreyfuss definitions that were operationalized by Hunt[42,63] (see Table 21-1e on the Evolve website).

Developing a Medical Foundation

Abbreviations and Terminology

Learning the language of the NICU is essential for the neonatal developmental specialist. Although changing documentation requirements specify that practitioners eliminate abbreviations and spell out terms, NICU language continues to contain many abbreviations, as illustrated by the following medical summary:

> Cody is a 39 wk pma wm born at 25 WBD, 24 WBE by SVD to a 19 y/o now G2P1Ab1, A+, VDRL-mom with h/o of IVDA, smoked 1 PPD, PIH, PTL, PPROM 72° PTD. Pt. had TCAN ×1 (reduced PTD), AGA at 545 gms, Apgars 1^1, 3^5, $6.^7$ Significant medical complications have included RDS, CLD, PIE, AOP, PDA (ligated), hyperbilirubinemia, anemia, MRSE and CONS sepsis, medical NEC, BIH (repaired), R gr. 3 and L gr. 4 IVH with frontal and temporal lobe PVL, ROP stage III OD (regressing) and stage III with plus disease OS (s/p Avastin injection OS). Pt. required HFOV with iNO, for 22 days, SIMV for 8 days, BiPAP for 14 days, NCPAP for 9 days, and remains on HFNC with FiO2 0.5 at 0.5L.

Understanding abbreviations and the terms they represent is a prerequisite to beginning a neonatal practice. See Box 21-2 for a list of some common NICU abbreviations.

Classifications for Age

For consistency, the American Academy of Pediatrics' Committee on the Fetus and Newborn (2004) has established the following definitions.[12]

Gestational age (or menstrual age) refers to the total time elapsed between the first day of the last normal menstrual period and the day of birth. Gestational age (GA) is calculated as completed weeks; a 26-week and 5-day fetus is considered 26 weeks GA. The range used for a full-term pregnancy in the United States is generally 38 to 42 weeks. Any infant born before 38 weeks is considered preterm; an infant born between 34 and 37 weeks is called late-preterm, with increasing recognition that such infants are still immature and vulnerable; and an

BOX 21-2 Common Medical Abbreviations in the Neonatal Intensive Care Unit

A
A—apnea
AAP—American Academy of Pediatrics
Ab—abortions (includes spontaneous)
ABG—arterial blood gas
ABR—auditory brainstem response
AD—right ear
AEP—auditory evoked potential
AGA—appropriate for gestational age
A-line—arterial line
AOP—apnea of prematurity
APIB—Assessment of Preterm Infant Behavior (Als)
AROM—assisted rupture of membranes
AS—left ear
As & Bs—apnea and bradycardia
ASD—atrial septal defect
AU—both ears
B
B—bilateral; bradycardia
BAEP—brainstem auditory evoked potential
BAER—brainstem auditory evoked response
BIH—bilateral inguinal hernia
BPD—bronchopulmonary dysplasia
bpm—beats/min (pulse)
BSER—brainstem evoked response (same as ABR, AEP, BAER, or BAEP)
BW—birth weight
C
CAN—cord around neck (nuchal cord)
CBC—complete blood count
CDH—congenitally dislocated hip
CHD—congenital heart disease
CHF—congestive heart failure
CLD—chronic lung disease
CMV—cytomegalovirus
CNGF—continuous nasogastric feeding
CNS—central nervous system
COGF—continuous orogastric feeding
CPAP—continuous positive airway pressure
CPT—chest physical therapy
C/S—cesarean section
CSF—cerebrospinal fluid
CTF—continuous tube feeding
CXR—chest x-ray
D
dB—decibels
DIC—disseminated intravascular coagulation
DTGV—transposition of the great vessels
D_5W—5% glucose solution
$D_{10}W$—10% glucose solution
E
ECMO—extracorporeal membrane oxygenation
ELBW—extremely low birth weight (<1000 g)
F
FC—foot-candle
FEN—fluids, electrolytes, nutrition
FHR—fetal heart rate
FiO_2—fraction of inspired oxygen (percentage of oxygen concentration)
FT—full term
G
G—gravida (pregnancies)
GA—gestational age
GBS—group B streptococcus
GER—gastroesophageal reflux
GERD—gastroesophageal reflux disease
H
HAL—hyperalimentation (same as TPN)
HC—head circumference
HFJV—high-frequency jet ventilation
HFV—high-frequency ventilation
HFOV—high-frequency oscillating ventilation
HIE—hypoxic-ischemic encephalopathy
HMD—hyaline membrane disease
HR—heart rate
HSV—herpes simplex virus
HTN—hypertension
HUSG—head ultrasound
I
ICH—intracranial hemorrhage
ICN—intensive care nursery
IDC—Integrative Developmental Care model
IDM (or IODM)—infant of a diabetic mother
IDV—intermittent demand ventilation
IH—inguinal hernia
IMV—intermittent mandatory ventilation
iNO—inhaled nitric oxide
I/O—intake/output
IPPB—intermittent positive pressure breathing
IRV—inspiratory reserve volume
IUGR—intrauterine growth retardation
IV—intravenous
IVDA—intravenous drug abuse
IVF—in vitro fertilization; intravenous feeding
IVH—intraventricular hemorrhage
K
kcal—kilocalories
KMC—kangaroo mother care
L
L (or LC)—living children
LA—left atrium
LBW—low birth weight (<2500 g)
LGA—large for gestational age
LMP—last menstrual period
L/S ratio—lecithin-to-sphingomyelin ratio
LTGV—physiologically corrected transposition of the great vessels
LV—left ventricle
M
MAP—mean airway pressure
MAS—meconium aspiration syndrome
MCA—multiple congenital anomalies
MDU—maternal drug use
MRSA—methicillin-resistant *Staphylococcus aureus*
MRSE—methicillin-resistant *Staphylococcus epidermidis*
N
NB—newborn
NBAS—Neonatal Behavioral Assessment Scale (Brazelton)
NC—nasal cannula
NCPAP—nasal continuous positive airway pressure
ND—nasoduodenal
NEC—necrotizing enterocolitis
NG—nasogastric
NGT—nasogastric tube
NICU—neonatal intensive care unit
NIDCAP—Neonatal Individualized Developmental Care and Assessment Program (Als)
NNNS—NICU Network Neurobehavioral Scale

BOX 21-2 Common Medical Abbreviations in the Neonatal Intensive Care Unit—cont'd

NNS—non-nutritive sucking
NO—nitric oxide
NP—nasopharyngeal
NPA—National Perinatal Association
NPCPAP—nasopharyngeal continuous positive airway pressure
NPO—nothing by mouth
NREM—non-rapid eye movement
NS—nutritive sucking
NTE—neutral thermal environment

O

O_2 sats—oxygen saturation
OD—oral-duodenal; right eye
OG—oral gastric
OGT—oral gastric tube
OS—left eye
OU—both eyes

P

P—pulse; para (births)
P_1—primipara (first birth)
$Paco_2$—arterial partial pressure of CO_2 (concentration of CO_2 in peripheral arteries)
PAL—peripheral arterial line
Pao_2—arterial partial pressure of O_2 (concentration of O_2 in peripheral arteries)
PBPs—potentially better practices
PCA—postconceptional age (old term; now PMA, postmenstrual age)
PDA—patent ductus arteriosus
PEEP—positive end-expiratory pressure
PFC—persistent fetal circulation (old term; now PPHN, persistent pulmonary hypertension of the newborn)
PICC—percutaneously inserted central catheter
PIE—pulmonary interstitial emphysema
PIH—pregnancy-induced hypertension (preeclampsia, eclampsia)
PIP—pulmonary insufficiency of the preterm; peak inspiratory pressure
PMA—postmenstrual age
PO—by mouth
PPD—packs per day (refers to smoking)
PPHN—persistent pulmonary hypertension of the newborn (previously called persistent fetal circulation, PFC)
PPROM—prolonged premature rupture of membranes
PPS—peripheral pulmonic stenosis
PROM—passive range of motion
PROM—premature rupture of membranes
PS—pulmonic stenosis
PT—preterm
PTL—preterm labor
PVL—periventricular leukomalacia

Q

q—every
qh—every hour
qid—four times a day

R

RA—right atrium
RBC—red blood cell
RDS—respiratory distress syndrome
REM—rapid eye movement
ROM—rupture of membranes
ROP—retinopathy of prematurity (formerly called retrolental fibroplasia, RLF)
RPR—rapid plasma reagin (test for syphilis)
RRR—rate, rhythm, respiration
RV—right ventricle

S

SA—substance abuse
Sao_2—oxygen saturation
sats—oxygen saturation levels
SCN—special care nursery
SGA—small for gestational age
SIMV—synchronized intermittent mandatory ventilation
s/p—status post
SROM—spontaneous rupture of membranes
SSC—skin-to-skin care
SVD—spontaneous vaginal delivery

T

TA—truncus arteriosus
TAPVR—total anomalous pulmonary venous return
TCAN—tight cord around neck
TCM—transcutaneous monitor
$Tcpo_2$—transcutaneous oxygen pressure
TLC—total lung capacity
TOF—tetralogy of Fallot
TORCH—congenital viral infections (***to***xoplasmosis, ***r***ubella, ***c***ytomegalovirus, and ***h***erpes)
TPF—toxoplasmosis fetalis
TPN—total parenteral nutrition
TPR—temperature, pulse, respiration
TRDN—transient respiratory distress of the newborn
TTN—transient tachypnea of the newborn

U

UAC—umbilical artery catheter
UAL—umbilical artery line
UDC—Universe of developmental care model
ULBW—ultralow birth weight (<750 g)
URI—upper respiratory infection
USG—ultrasound
UTI—urinary tract infection
UVC—umbilical venous catheter

V

VDRL—Venereal Disease Research Laboratory
VEP (VER)—vision evoked potential (response)
VLBW—very low birth weight (<1500 g)
VSD—ventricular septal defect

W

WBC—white blood cell
WBD—weeks by dates (for gestational age assessment)
WBE—weeks by examination (gestational age assessment)
WBU—weeks by ultrasound (gestational age assessment)

infant born after 42 weeks is post-term. Once the infant is born, the GA remains the same.

Postmenstrual age (PMA) refers to the infant's increasing age in relation to the first day of the last menstrual period, and thus continually changes over time. PMA is obtained by adding the weeks since birth to the infant's gestational age. When the infant born at 27 weeks reaches his or her expected due date, the PMA is 40 weeks (27 weeks of gestation plus 13 weeks since birth). PMA is commonly used until 40 to 44 weeks, equivalent to term or 1-month corrected age, respectively.

Chronologic age refers to the infant's actual age since birth. Chronologically, the infant born at 27 weeks' gestation is 3 months old on the expected due date and 12 months old on the first birthday. Chronologic age of preterm infants is usually corrected for prematurity to correlate better with developmental expectations and performance (e.g., the infant born at 27 weeks' gestation will not developmentally look the same at 3 months' chronologic age as the infant born at term).

Corrected age refers to how old the infant would be if born at term rather than prematurely. The number of weeks of prematurity is first determined (GA is subtracted from the term equivalent of 40 weeks) and then subtracted from the chronologic age. The infant born at 27 weeks' gestation was born 13 weeks prematurely (40 weeks – 27 weeks GA = 13 weeks early). The corrected age of this infant on the first birthday is 9 months because the actual birth was 3 months earlier than the expected due date. Corrected age is variably used for 1 to 3 years in children born preterm when assessing developmental status.

Classifications by Birth Weight

Infants born weighing more than 2500 g (5.5 pounds) are considered average in size. A birth weight of 1500 to 2500 g is termed *low birth weight* (LBW). A very-low-birth-weight (VLBW) infant is 1000 to 1500 g, extremely low birth weight (ELBW) is less than 1000 g, and ultralow birth weight (ULBW) is less than 750 g.

Birth weight between the 10th and 90th percentiles on a standardized growth chart is appropriate for gestational age (AGA). Birth weight below the 10th percentile is small for gestational age (SGA), and birth weight above the 90th percentile is large for gestational age (LGA). These categories apply equally to preterm, term, and post-term infants. Any infant growing normally in utero will be AGA. An infant of a mother with severe pregnancy-induced hypertension (PIH) who experienced intrauterine growth restriction (IUGR) may be born SGA, whereas the infant of a mother with diabetes is often LGA.

Medical Conditions and Equipment

Medical complications and technology both have profound effects on preterm and high-risk infants, with subsequent implications and precautions for neonatal therapists. Developing a basic medical foundation and learning NICU medical terminology is an ongoing process that progresses from a general familiarity with terms and definitions to gradually understanding the pathophysiology of diseases and biomechanics of equipment. Recognizing that medical technology and interventions are constantly evolving, Table 21-1 lists common medical equipment in the NICU.

Models of Care in the NICU

Developmentally supportive care is a philosophy and approach to caregiving intended to improve neurodevelopmental outcomes in preterm and sick infants who lack the maturity, health, or competence necessary to cope with life in the NICU easily. Incorporating rapidly growing scientific knowledge from multiple disciplines, ***developmental care*** is an inclusive term applied to environmental modifications, changes in caregiving practices, and efforts to increase family involvement.

Developmentally supportive care has historical roots. In the nineteenth century, Florence Nightingale emphasized the importance of nurturing healing environments for patient recovery and improved outcomes.[98] With the survival of increasingly preterm infants and the creation of neonatal intensive care as a medical specialty, conceptual frameworks have emerged to guide understanding and provision of neuroprotective developmentally supportive care with this uniquely vulnerable population.[3,5,89]

Universe of Developmental Care Model

The universe of developmental care (UDC) model reformulated neonatal developmental care theory to portray a patient- and family-centered environment within the health care universe.[46] Because the skin and brain both develop from the embryonic ectoderm, in the UDC model, the skin acts as a shared sensory interface between the infant's brain and the current environment. This approach recognizes the interactive link between all developing systems and the caregiver and family while simultaneously providing a practical basis for formulating individualized patient care plans within the NICU's complex technologic environment.

With its inclusion of assessment and documentation, this approach also can address the increasing emphasis on core measures of quality control required by regulatory organizations (e.g., Centers for Medicare and Medicaid Services and the Joint Commission). The UDC model includes five developmental care core measures focused on care actions essential to promoting healthy growth and development of the preterm infant and family. These developmental care core measures include the following: (1) protected sleep, (2) pain and stress assessment and management, (3) activities of daily living (positioning, feeding, and skin care), (4) family-centered care, and (5) healing environment.[41]

Neonatal Integrative Developmental Care Model

The neonatal integrative developmental care (IDC) model expanded the five core measures described above into seven distinct family-centered developmental core measures for neuroprotective neonatal care. This expansion enables additional focus on developmentally appropriate positioning and handling, optimizing nutrition and feeding, and protecting skin, all areas that are fundamental to neonatal developmental care.[9] The seven neuroprotective core measures for family-centered developmental care described in the IDC model include the following: (1) healing environment, (2) partnering with families, (3) positioning and handling, (4) safeguarding sleep, (5) minimizing stress and pain, (6) protecting skin, and (7) optimizing nutrition. The simplified neonatal IDC model depicts the seven core measures as overlapping petals of a lotus demonstrating the integrative nature of developmental care[6] (Figure 21-2).

The IDC is the most current and comprehensive model for NICU developmental care. Most of the remaining chapter content can be placed within this framework; the reader is

TABLE 21-1 Common Medical Equipment in the NICU

Equipment	Description	Purpose
Thermoregulation Equipment		
Radiant warmer	Open bed with overhead heat source	Typically used during medical workup of new admission or for critically ill infants requiring easy access for frequent or complicated medical care
Incubator (Isolette)	Clear plastic heated box enclosing mattress and infant	Used to provide warmth (and sometimes humidity); allows calories to be used for growth and healing Preferred location for attempting to reduce environmental stimuli, discourage unnecessary handling, and protect sleep. Infant may or may not be dressed and swaddled, depending on specific NICU protocol. Depending on design, access is through portholes or a door on the front, or the entire top of the Isolette raises up.
Open crib	Bassinet-style bed; no external heat source provided; infant dressed in clothes and swaddled in blankets	Used for larger and more stable infants; caregivers (including occupational therapist) must be careful to avoid cold stress during baths, assessments, and procedures.
Oxygen Therapy with Assisted Ventilation		
Bag and mask ventilation	Bag attached to face mask is rhythmically squeezed to deliver positive pressure and oxygen.	Used for resuscitation of an infant at delivery or during acute deterioration or to increase oxygenation if necessary after an apneic spell.
CPAP	Steady stream of pressurized air given through an endotracheal tube, nasopharyngeal tube, nasal prongs, or small nasal mask; supplemental oxygen may or may not be used.	Positive pressure is used to keep the alveoli and airways from collapsing (to keep them open) in an infant who is breathing spontaneously but has a disorder such as RDS, pulmonary edema, or apnea. CPAP is now commonly used from birth (when effective) to reduce potential problems from mechanical ventilation.
Mechanical ventilation (CMV, HFOV, HFJV)	Machine controls or assists breathing by mechanically inflating the lungs, increasing alveolar ventilation, and improving gas exchange. Conventional mechanical ventilation forces can contribute to lung damage; high-frequency ventilation (oscillators and jets) use different mechanics to cause less barotrauma to the lungs.	Used for infants with depressed respiratory drive, pulmonary disease with increased work of breathing and suboptimal oxygenation and ventilation (e.g., MAS, RDS), and frequent apnea despite CPAP; infant is usually orally or nasally intubated but may have a tracheostomy if ventilator dependence will be prolonged.
ECMO	Sophisticated life support system that uses a modified heart-lung bypass to provide nearly total lung rest and minimize barotrauma (lung damage that can occur with prolonged high ventilator settings)	Used as a rescue technology for qualifying infants in critical respiratory failure who are unresponsive to conventional medical management or sometimes for preoperative support during cardiac surgery. Use of ECMO has decreased with the advent of therapies such as high-frequency ventilation and inhaled nitric oxide (pulmonary vasodilator drug).
Oxygen Therapy without Assisted Ventilation		
High-flow nasal cannula (HFNC)	Warmed and humidified oxygen or room air (21% oxygen) delivered at higher flow rates (>1 L/min) by flexible NC with small prongs that fit into the nares; a HFNC can be set up from ventilators or many CPAP machines; Vapotherm (Vapotherm, Exeter, NH) is a separate respiratory therapy device attached to a nasal cannula that allows very high nasal flows of supersaturated (saturated without condensation) air-oxygen blends.	Used to improve gas exchange or reduce work of breathing. High flow rates may reduce the need for intubation and mechanical ventilation or replace less well-tolerated nasal CPAP. Very high humidity allows higher flow rates (compared with those possible with nasal cannula) without drying nasal mucosa.
Nasal cannula	Humidified oxygen delivered by flexible nasal cannula with small prongs that fit into the nares	Used for infants requiring supplemental oxygen without positive pressure support, generally for prolonged periods. Handling and portability are easier with a nasal cannula than with an oxyhood.
Oxygen hood (oxyhood)	Plastic hood with flow of warm humidified oxygen placed over infant's head and possibly upper trunk	Used for infants who are breathing independently but need a higher concentration of oxygen than 21% room air; higher humidification allows oxygen delivery that is less drying to nasal mucosa than oxygen by a nasal cannula (not as commonly used since HFNCs became available).

CPAP, Continuous positive airway pressure; *ECMO,* extracorporeal membrane oxygenation; *HFJV,* high-frequency jet ventilation; *HFOV,* high-frequency oscillating ventilation; *MAS,* meconium aspiration syndrome; *RDS,* respiratory distress syndrome.

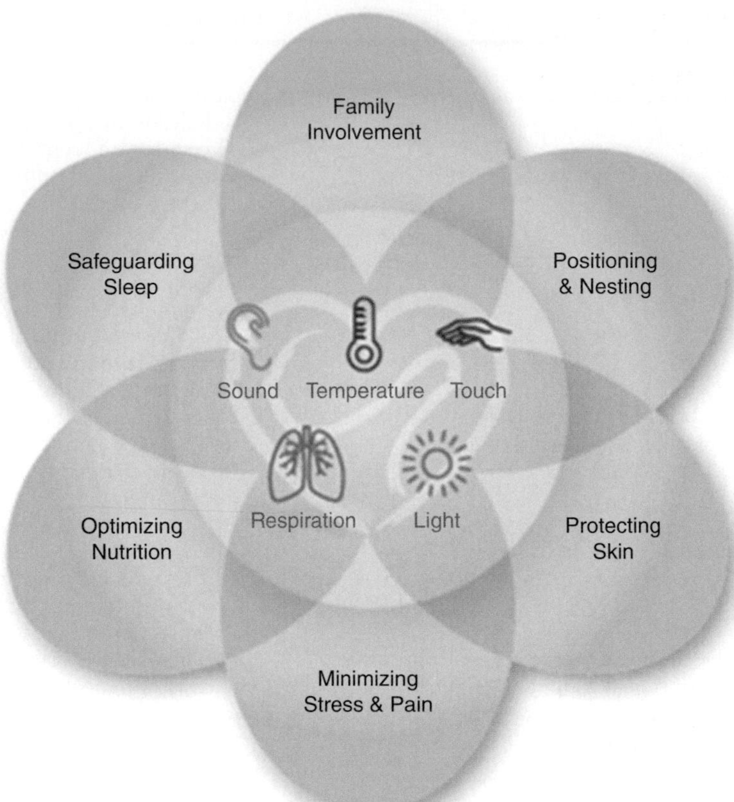

FIGURE 21-2 A simplified schematic diagram of the neonatal integrative developmental care model depicts the seven core measures as overlapping petals of a lotus, demonstrating the integrative nature of developmental care. (Courtesy Leslie Altimier.)

encouraged to refer often to the schematic diagram of the IDC model to help organize information.

NICU Environment and Caregiving

Evidence-Based Practice and Potentially Better Practices to Support Neurodevelopment in the NICU

The scientific method is a cyclic process of inquiry based on observations, synthesis, hypothesis, and predictions that lead to more observations. Evidence-based practice (EBP) traditionally rests on the gold standard of randomized controlled trials (RCTs). However, not all aspects of NICU neuroprotective developmental care can be methodologically or ethically captured in RCTs, and EBP is not intended to rely only on RCTs to the exclusion of other potentially innovative strategies gained from practice.[105] Browne[29] noted that EBP integrates clinical expertise and systematic clinical research; external clinical evidence informs but does not replace individual clinical expertise

A collaborative hospital project by the Vermont Oxford Network (VON) conducted a comprehensive review of relevant neonatal literature.[76,81] The researchers reviewed a vast amount of literature and synthesized the information to identify 16 potentially better practices (PBPs), with an emphasis on potential (rather than definitive) benefit. The group concluded PBP's that are known to be safe but have limited clinical evidence for long-term benefit become more compelling when compared with existing practices with uncertain safety and no evidence of benefit.

The VON group divided the identified PBPs into two bundles, with the first cluster of interventions to be implemented for all infants on admission and the second bundle of interventions to be added by 31 to 32 weeks. Caregiving interventions were bundled because they are all necessary and more effective as a group than if implemented separately, and omission of any one of these practices may lessen the ultimate benefit. The extensive literature review, application to brain development and sensory systems, evidence-based conclusions, and implementation strategies make these two articles valuable developmentally supportive care resources for the NICU developmental specialist or caregiver. These 16 PBPs are summarized in Table 21-2.

"Mismatch" of an Immature Infant in the High-Tech Environment

Sensory components of the typical intrauterine and NICU extrauterine environments are significantly different (Table 21-3). Barring complications, the fetus develops in a warm, snug, darkened environment in which basic needs are met and a normal sequence of development is supported.

The intrauterine environment of the maternal womb protects a developing fetus against harsh outside stimulation while

TABLE 21-2 Potentially Better Practices to Support Neurodevelopment in the NICU

System	Potentially Better Practice	Benefits
Cluster I		
Full implementation recommended for all NICU admissions beginning at 23 weeks' gestation		
T-1	Containment and body flexion	T, S
T-2	Positive oral stimulation, non-nutritive suck	T
T-3a	Gentle touch, hand grasping, facial stimulation	T, S
T-4	Decrease painful and negative stimulation	T, S
C-1	Exposure to mother's scent	C, S
C-2	Minimizing exposure to noxious odors	C, S
A-1	Noise abatement	A, S
V-1	Minimizing ambient light exposure	V, S
V-2	Avoiding direct light exposure	V, S
S-1	Developing strategies that preserve normal infant sleep cycles Supporting family involvement in care practices that promote sleep Nonemergent care provided at appropriate times; minimizes disruption of sleep (with diurnal implementation, as possible, after 30-wk gestation)	S
S-2	Minimizing exposure to narcotics and other medications that may disrupt or disturb sleep cycles	S
Cluster II		
Full implementation recommended for all NICU admissions beginning at 31-32 wk		
T-3b	Infant massage, diurnal implementation	T
T-3c	Skin-to-skin care	T, C, S
A-2	Exposure to audible maternal voice, diurnal implementation	A
V-3	Cycled lighting: minimum of 1-2 hr	A, V, S
V-4	Provide more complex visual stimulation after 37 wk (term gestation)	V

A, Auditory development; *C*, chemosensory development; *S*, preservation of sleep; *T*, somatesthetic-kinesthetic-proprioceptive development; *V*, visual development.
NOTE: A potentially better practice may affect multiple developing sensory systems (T, C, A, V, S).
Data from Laudert, S., Liu, W. F., Blackington, S., Perkins, B., Martin, S., MacMillan-York, E., et al.; NIC/Q 2005 Physical Environment Exploratory Group. (2007). Implementing potentially better practices to support the neurodevelopment of infants in the NICU. *Journal of Perinatology, 27*, S75–S93; and Liu, W. F., Laudert, S., Perkins, B., MacMillan-York, E., Martin, S., & Graven, S.; NIC/Q 2005 Physical Environment Exploratory Group. (2007). The development of potentially better practices to support the neurodevelopment of infants in the NICU. *Journal of Perinatology, 27*, S48–S74.

TABLE 21-3 Comparison of Intrauterine and Extrauterine Sensory Environments

System	Intrauterine	Extrauterine
Tactile	Constant proprioceptive input; smooth, wet, usually safe and comfortable; circumferential boundaries	Often painful and invasive; dry, cool air; predominance of medical touching, with relative paucity of social touching
Vestibular	Maternal movements, diurnal cycles, amniotic fluid create gently oscillating environment, flexed posture with boundaries to movements	Horizontal, flat postures; rapid position changes; influence of gravity, restraints, and equipment
Auditory	Maternal biologic sounds, muffled environmental sounds	Loud, noncontingent, mechanical, frequent (sometimes constant), harsh intermittent impulse noise
Visual	Dark; may occasionally have very dim red spectrum light	Bright lights, eyes unprotected Often no diurnal rhythm
Thermal	Constant warmth, consistent temperature	Environmental temperature variations, high risk of neonatal heat loss

providing a variety of tactile, vestibular, chemical, visual, and auditory sensory stimuli in a controlled and integrated fashion.[79] The intrauterine environment of a developing fetus is characterized by limited light exposure, muted noise through fluid, sleep cycle preservation, and unrestricted access to the mother via somatosensory auditory and chemosensory pathways.[10] The uterine wall provides secure yet flexible boundaries with generalized extremity flexion and containment for the developing fetus. Vestibular and tactile stimuli come from maternal and fetal movements, immersion in warm amniotic fluid, and contact with the fetus's own body parts and the uterine wall. Hormonal cycles of the mother provide rhythmic stimulation and cyclic organization. Nutritional and oxygenation needs of the fetus are met by the placenta. Auditory inputs include the maternal voice, bowel sounds, blood flow through the placenta and umbilical cord, and filtered sounds from the extrauterine environment, transmitted through amniotic fluid and maternal body tissues.[95]

After birth, demands are suddenly made on the preterm newborn to breathe, regulate body temperature, move against the effects of gravity, activate immature gastrointestinal (GI) function, adjust to bright light and unmuffled noise, cope with invasive or painful procedures, and endure frequent sleep disruptions and deprivation. The preterm infant's immature CNS is generally competent for protected intrauterine life but not sufficiently developed to adjust to and organize the overwhelming stimuli and demands of the NICU. Negative and random sensory inputs replace meaningful positive sensory inputs into the developing brain and can permanently alter normal brain development. This creates a so-called mismatch of the neonate with the high-tech world now necessary for survival.

The ***animate*** environment refers to the presence and activities of people in the NICU, both medical (hospital staff and caregiving practices) and social (primarily family and friends). The ***inanimate*** environment usually refers to the physical properties of light and sound in the NICU, although other factors such as gravity and temperature are also significant. Continual overwhelming stimuli in the NICU may stress the highly sensitive preterm infant's already vulnerable CNS, cause repeated hypoxic episodes, contribute to abnormal structural and functional changes of the brain, and create maladaptive behaviors that contribute to later poor developmental outcome.[48,110] Events, stimuli, and environmental factors can support the processes of organized sensory development or create significant interference. Sensory interference may occur when immature sensory systems are stimulated with inappropriate stimuli or out of turn—because sensory systems develop in a predetermined order, sensory stimulation that is excessive or disrupts this order may cause sensory interference (interference with expected normal sensory system development).[79] The healing environment referred to in the IDC model addresses physical and sensory components of the NICU.

Physical Environment

A multidisciplinary NICU committee, under the auspices of the Physical and Developmental Environment of the High-Risk Infant Project, regularly updates and publishes a consensus on recommended standards for NICU design. This comprehensive set of minimum design standards is based on clinical experience and an evolving scientific database. The intent is to optimize NICU design within the constraints of available resources, facilitate excellent neuroprotective developmental health care for the infant in a setting that provides adequate space and facilities to support the central role of the family, and meet the needs of the NICU staff.[128] The latest recommendations are used worldwide and are available online (www.nd.edu/~nicudes).[143]

Sensory Environment

Creating and monitoring a healing sensory environment involves issues related to tactile (touch and thermoregulation), vestibular, olfactory, gustatory, auditory, and visual sensory systems of the neonate. The proficient neonatal developmental specialist understands emerging strengths and vulnerabilities of early sensory system development and the impact of direct and indirect sensory stimulation on the vulnerable NICU infant.

Development of fetal sensory systems occurs in a chronologic but overlapping order. The limbic system (emotions) and systems of touch (somatosensory), movement (kinesthetic, proprioceptive, vestibular), smell (olfactory), and hearing (auditory) are structurally complete but functionally immature at the earliest age of viability. They all respond to external stimuli by 25 to 28 weeks' gestation and exhibit in utero learning; developmentally supportive care will respond to the developmental needs of each of these systems.[49] Visual system structures and function are not complete because their earliest use is ideally at term gestation.

Because the sick preterm infant experiences significant stress (e.g., agitation, autonomic instability, excessive use of calories) when incoming stimuli exceed the ability of the immature CNS to respond and adapt, reducing avoidable stressors (including unnecessary therapy interventions) to help the infant remain calm, organized, and asleep becomes a priority.[81] Examples of developmental interventions that support neonatal physiologic stability and brain development include practices such as preservation of sleep, NICU light and sound modifications, therapeutic positioning, nurturing touch, non-nutritive sucking, alteration of caregiver timing and handling techniques, and increased family involvement.[10,64,76,81]

Temperature (Thermoregulation)

As the newborn moves from a warm, fluid-filled, floating intrauterine environment with flexible constraints to a dry, cool environment influenced by gravity and loss of consistent boundaries, a major goal of neonatal care is to provide a neutral thermal environment in which the infant is neither gaining nor losing heat at the expense of energy expenditure.[7] Preterm infants are predisposed to excessive heat loss and are vulnerable to cold stress from several causes. Extended postures, thin skin, immature thermoregulation, and reduced insulating subcutaneous fat in very premature infants allow heat to transfer from the body to the air. A specialized brown fat used by newborns to metabolize heat is not produced until the last trimester of gestation. Pulmonary dysfunction, CNS immaturity, and frequent caregiving interventions may also contribute to heat loss. The infant may lose heat by convection (heat loss to surrounding air), conduction (body contact with cooler solid surface), radiation (heat loss to cooler solid object not in direct contact with the infant, such as incubator walls), and evaporation (heat lost as liquid from the respiratory tract and permeable skin, which is converted into a vapor).

The optimal environment for any newborn, especially a preterm infant, is kangaroo care, or skin-to-skin holding on the bare chest of mother (or father; Figure 21-3). The term *thermosynchrony* refers to a process during skin-to-skin contact in which the temperature of a mother's chest has been shown to increase by 2° C to warm a cool infant and decrease by 1° C to cool an overheated infant. Skin-to-skin contact with the mother meets the premature infant's needs for touch in the most natural environment possible outside the womb and also supplies needed proprioceptive sensory input to the infant's developing brain. When the parents are unavailable for skin-to-skin holding, or it is not possible, attention should focus on thermoregulation of the infant's individual bed space. To maintain a constant central temperature within narrow limits (36.5°-37.5° C), VLBW or premature infants should be cared for in incubators or radiant warmers.[7]

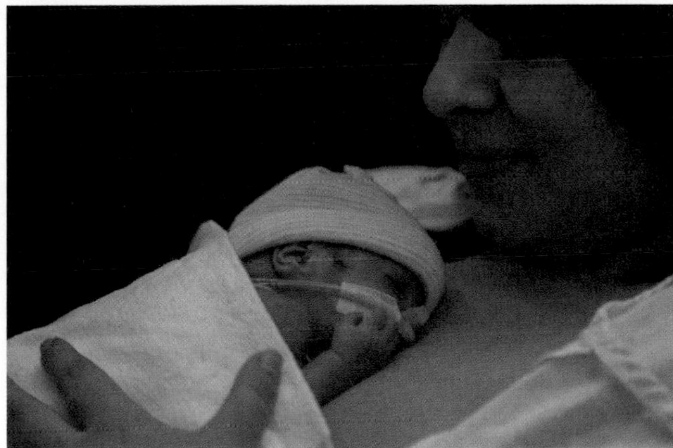

FIGURE 21-3 Skin-to-skin holding (kangaroo care) involves placing the unclothed baby (except for diaper) against the bare chest of the mother or father. Numerous benefits have been documented for infant and parent (specifically the mother), and an international initiative is under way to increase the initiation and frequency of this practice. (Courtesy NICU, Memorial Hermann Hospital Southwest, Houston. Photograph by Beverly Edwards.)

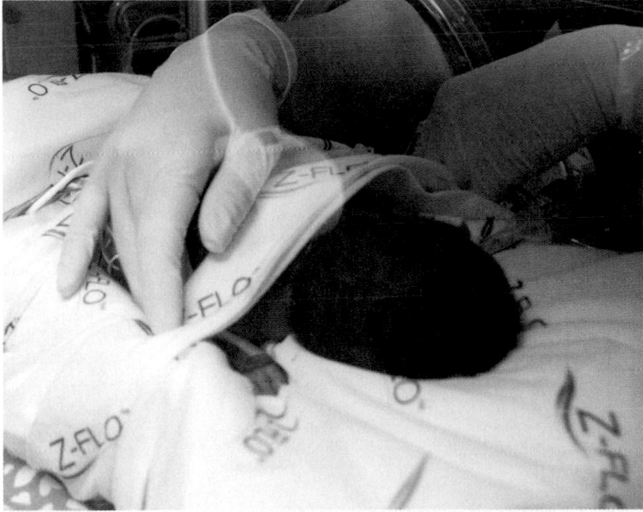

FIGURE 21-4 Three-dimensional nesting in a fluidized positioner that conforms to each infant reduces body exposure and heat loss mechanics in this extremely preterm infant born at 22 weeks' gestation, now 24 weeks' PMA. (Courtesy Infant Special Care Unit, University of Texas Medical Branch, Galveston, TX. Photograph by Jan Hunter).

Positioning an infant in a midline, flexed, and contained position with the assistance of therapeutic positioning aids and swaddling decreases the surface area of the infant exposed to environmental air, thus reducing radiant and convective heat losses. This flexed and contained position offers additional temperature stability for the infant by minimizing extraneous movement and energy expenditure. Fluidized positioners magnify these benefits by allowing the infant to be immersed in a three-dimensional conformational positioner that assumes the same ambient temperature as the incubator or radiant warmer[64] (Figure 21-4).

The developmental specialist must diligently protect NICU infants from heat destabilization during each and every contact. Cold stress and overheating can cause complications in NICU infants.

Touch and Proprioception

The percentage of human touch in the NICU is overwhelmingly medical, and even noninvasive touch can be perceived as painful when it follows another painful procedure. Physical support of the infant during caregiving handling and procedures, kangaroo care (described briefly earlier), holding by a parent, and infant massage attempt to balance medical with nurturing touch.

Massage is an art and a science, best performed by a caregiver specifically trained in infant massage techniques, precautions, and warning signs. Massage is an active engagement between the infant and the caregiver; it is done with (rather than to) the baby. As with any type of stimulation, the developmental specialist should closely monitor the infant's physiologic and neurobehavioral responses, with handling modified accordingly. Specialized training, such as the Neonatal Touch and Massage Certification (http://www.neonatalcertification.com) is recommended to ensure that the developmental specialist adapts well-baby massage techniques to the unique medical and neurobehavioral sensitivities of the NICU infant.

Traditional infant massage can be physiologically stressful and behaviorally disorganizing to preterm infants younger than about 32 weeks' postconception and those who are not yet medically stable. These younger or medically fragile infants may benefit more from the gentle human touch of a static hand swaddle (facilitative tuck). Preterm infants with the prerequisite degree of medical stability for more traditional infant massage are often approaching hospital discharge; developmental specialists can teach parents infant massage techniques for home use (Figure 21-5). Studies have shown that massage is associated with multiple physiologic, neurologic, behavioral, and neuromuscular benefits for infants; parents report decreased stress, increased attachment, improved self-esteem, and a more active role in caregiving.[144]

Massage is increasingly recommended as an intervention to promote growth and development of preterm and low-birth weight infants in the NICU. However, some have raised concerns as to whether infant massage can produce overstimulation and therefore cause adverse effects. Further research through controlled trials is recommended to determine the benefits, risks, and optimal application of this nurturing human touch.[70] As with all interventions, precautions are needed to carefully guard against cold stress.

Sound and Noise in the NICU

Early auditory development involves the structural parts of the ears that develop in the first 20 weeks of gestation and the neurosensory part of the auditory system that is in a critical period of development from 25 weeks' gestation to approximately 5 to 6 months post-term.[50] An infant's ear structures (outer, middle, and inner ear) and cortical auditory center are formed and functioning by 25 weeks' gestation, although they remain functionally immature and continue to develop during the last trimester.

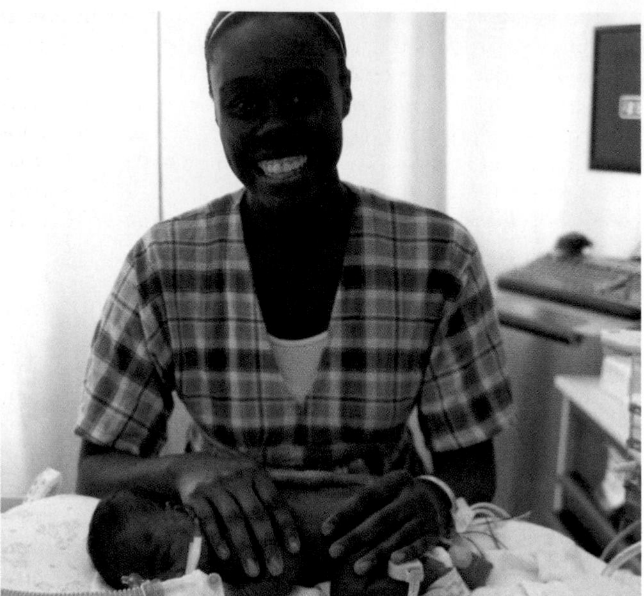

FIGURE 21-5 Mother using a static hand swaddle to provide nurturing touch to her NICU infant prior to adding selected massage strokes as tolerated. (Courtesy Kara Ann Waitzman, Creative Therapy Consultant, Neonatal Touch and Massage Certification.)

Neurosensory auditory development is sensitive to extrauterine differences in the NICU environment.[52] In the womb, sounds are muted through a fluid-filled environment. In contrast, NICU infants have historically been bombarded with noise (undesirable sound) that may be relatively constant throughout the day and night, predominantly mechanical rather than social, and often noncontingent to individual infants. Sound inside the incubator is characterized by continuous white noise and nonspeech sounds; harsh mechanical noises penetrate clearly and reverberate, whereas speech sounds are indistinct. NICU infants are exposed to vibration and noise during transport and when on high-frequency ventilation; noise and vibration combined may have a synergistic effect.

An infant born prematurely is exposed to low- and high-frequency sound without the protective noise attenuation of the mother's body. The hearing threshold of the infant has been reported as 40 decibels (dB) at 28 to 34 weeks' gestation, 30 dB at 35 to 38 weeks' gestation, and less than 20 dB at term; these thresholds are greatly exceeded in the NICU.[73] Loud or prolonged sounds may damage the delicate hair cells in the developing cochlea, with resultant hearing loss in the same frequency range as that of the damaging sound; preterm infants are at risk for hearing loss in low-frequency (speech) and high-frequency ranges.[52]

Sensory interference may occur when immature sensory systems are stimulated out of order or bombarded with inappropriate stimuli. Background noise in the NICU may also interfere with the infant's ability to discriminate speech of parents and other caregivers.[52,92] Long-term difficulties in auditory processing can occur in the presence of normal intelligence and hearing sensitivity; behaviors associated with disturbed auditory processing have been noted in NICU graduates. Auditory processing problems may manifest as poor listening skills, difficulty following multistep directions, poor discrimination of specific auditory signals amid other background or impulse noise, distractibility, short attention span, and/or poor reading and spelling skills.[67]

Infant stress from environmental noise may be observed as a decrease in oxygenation and an increase in vasoconstriction, blood pressure, intracranial pressure, heart rate, respiratory rate, apnea, and bradycardia.[140] Sound is registered by the brain even during sleep, and intense impulse noise is known to increase visible arousals and arousals detected by changes in sleep brain wave patterns. Sleep disruption is a major concern in the NICU,[48] with major negative impacts on the neural circuitry formation essential to early brain and sensory system development. Sleep deprivation also impedes the infant's medical recovery.[48]

Sound Recommendations for the NICU Infant

Early auditory system development occurs when nerve cells in the brain, sensory organs, and peripheral nerves fire independently of outside stimulation; this spontaneous endogenous stimulation can be blocked by exposure to drugs, alcohol, and toxic chemicals. Unlike the visual system, however, the auditory system also requires outside auditory stimulation (voice, music, and meaningful environmental sounds) during the last trimester.[52] Auditory learning and memory requires the following: (1) a low background noise level (see NICU design standards[143]) for the infant to (2) hear and recognize differences in pitch, pattern, intensity, and rhythm within (3) protected sleep cycles, with emphasis on rapid eye movement (REM) sleep, especially after 32 weeks' gestation.[50]

The NICU staff needs to be diligent to provide an appropriate supportive environment for early auditory environment. Single-patient room designs reduce noise overflow. The staff in NICUs with pods or larger rooms can move bed spaces of sensitive infants away from loud or high-traffic areas and hold conversations, including medical rounds, away from the bedside. Auditory alarms can be reduced in volume and silenced quickly to reduce infant exposure to piercing impulse noise; remote control devices to silence alarms and visual alarms are also available. Respiratory tubing and water traps can be positioned to promote drainage; accumulated water should be emptied frequently to prevent bubbling (60-70 dB). Incubator covers can significantly reduce the noise level in an incubator.

In addition to controlling background noise, staff should arrange the timing of caregiving to support and protect sleep cycles and REM sleep. Neonatal developmental specialists can model appropriate voice and interaction for parents. Parents who understand the value and benefits of sleep are less likely to frequently awaken and overstimulate their infant. Emotional memories, comfort, and attachment are linked to auditory learning in even young infants; this is another incentive for educating and including parents in infant care. In contrast, an environment with loud low-frequency noise, unusual vibration and motion, and frequent sleep disruptions can interfere with optimal auditory development.

High noise levels in NICUs affect staff and families as well as infants, elevating the stress level in an already stressful environment. Goals of a quieter NICU include prolonged periods of undisturbed sleep for the infant, providing an environment for discernment of an audible maternal voice at 31 to 32 weeks' gestation and beyond, and providing a more comfortable and safe work environment for staff.[81]

Music therapy is a current NICU 'hot topic', and initial research shows benefit to infants. Music therapy intervention has been shown to "deepen infant sleep-state, support infant self-regulation, assist in the stabilization of breathing and heart rates, enhance parent/infant bonding, sooth irritability, re-enforce feeding/sucking rhythms and weight gain, and promote a sense of safety during painful procedures" (http://nicumusictherapy.com/Nicumusictherapy/Welcome.html).

Evidence continues to be gathered about what source, type, intensity, or duration of music can be beneficial to preterm infants. Any intervention must consider the infant's state and stability, timing in relation to other demands on the infant, potential disruption to (or enhancement of) infant sleep (best tested with sleep electroencephalography), and impact on any nearby infants. Musical toys and tape recordings, which can reverberate inside the incubator and continue playing regardless of infant cues, do not qualify as controlled and sensitive music therapy and are not recommended in the NICU. Headphones are also not recommended because of variable decibel levels and the noncontingent obligatory nature of the stimulation.

Light in the NICU

Lighting requirements in the NICU are very different for NICU infants and their adult caregivers.[114] The NICU staff needs variable light levels and sources for personal biorhythms (e.g., arousal and alertness, mood, temperature, hormone levels, sleep cycles) and for work-related tasks such as charting, infant assessments, and intricate procedures. Lighting needs generally increase with caregiver age.

Conversely, the fragile immature infants generally need protection from NICU light sources. The visual system of the preterm infant is functionally and structurally incomplete before term birth and requires dimness and sleep for continued optimal development.[48,49] The growth of the eye in utero is genetically coded and needs no light prior to 40 weeks; the infant's visual system continues to develop normally without external stimuli during the last trimester of gestation, with significant maturation and differentiation occurring in the retina and visual cortex.[48,49]

In infants born early, the eyelids remain fused until 24 to 26 weeks' gestation, with little spontaneous eye opening until after 29 weeks, emphasizing that the eyes of the preterm infant are not yet ready to process visual input at this stage of development. Preterm infants are unable to protect themselves from room light because they cannot close their eyelids tightly until after 30 weeks; their thin eyelids do not adequately filter light; and the iris does not significantly constrict until 30 to 34 weeks.[44]

Sensory interference can occur when one developing sensory system is stimulated out of turn or bombarded with inappropriate stimuli. For example, auditory system maturation typically occurs without strong competing sensory stimuli during the last trimester. Early birth with premature exposure to light may precipitate earlier visual system function, but preterm infants exposed to light in the NICU during the last trimester have an increased incidence of auditory processing dysfunction at school age. Premature stimulation of the visual system appears to compete and interfere with optimal development of the auditory sensory system during this critical period.[48] Although early light exposure has not been shown to increase the incidence of retinopathy of prematurity,[111] ambient NICU illumination may be implicated in subtle visual pathway sequelae and visual processing problems.[44,49,79]

Increased light intensity has been shown to increase heart rate and respiratory rate and decrease oxygen saturation for preterm infants in the NICU. Light levels and abrupt fluctuations can disrupt sleep of the premature infant, an important consideration because vast sensory system and early brain developments occur during sleep.[50]

Environmental Modifications of Light in the NICU

In contrast with the darkened womb, many NICUs have chaotic and unpredictable lighting patterns. Neither continuous dim or bright light has been demonstrated to be optimal for the development of preterm babies, and often the youngest and sickest infants are exposed to the highest levels of light for monitoring and medical procedures. Guidelines for appropriate NICU lighting are available from the regularly updated recommended standards for newborn ICU design.[143] Light intensity (illuminance) is measured with the metric unit lux (preferred term) or the English unit, foot-candle. One foot-candle equals approximately 10 lux (more precisely, 1 foot-candle = 10.764 lux).

Flexibility in lighting options accommodates the variable needs of caregivers and babies at differing stages of development and at various times throughout the day. Combinations of direct and indirect deflected lighting, adjustable ambient lighting at each bedside, no light source in an infant's direct line of sight, focused adjustable task lighting, and separate, well-lit areas for tasks such as charting or medication preparation are beneficial.[143] At least one source of natural daylight visible from each patient care area provides psychological benefits to NICU families and staff and assists with day-night cycled lighting.[2]

Circadian cycles are individual biorhythms over a period of approximately 24 hours. A third-trimester fetus has a functioning biologic clock (suprachiasmatic nuclei in the hypothalamus) capable of generating circadian rhythms, such as hormone secretion, activity patterns, and feeding cycles, in response to maternal day-night cues. These maternal circadian signals are disrupted in the infant who is born prematurely.[81] Light influences the infant's circadian system by a different neuronal pathway from that used for vision and becomes important for regulating circadian biorhythms after preterm birth. It has been suggested that the circadian system of a preterm infant is responsive to light very early (perhaps by 25-28 weeks' gestation) and that low-intensity light can entrain the developing circadian clock.[113,120] Cycled lighting in neonatal care has been shown to establish circadian cycles with beneficial effects on infant's fussing and crying behavior and growth in the first weeks of life.[56]

Because bright lights can disrupt sleep, current recommendations suggest a baseline (ambient) level for the patient care area of 10 to 20 lux.[87] This continuous dim lighting is probably best for infants younger than 28 weeks' gestation.[48] After 28 weeks' gestation, diurnally cycled lighting (dim lighting at night, with daytime levels increased to 250-500 lux) shows evidence of potential benefits for the infant (e.g., longer sleep, improved growth, more stable breathing, decreased levels of stress hormones), and cycled lighting in the NICU shows no evidence of harm.[81,113] A recent Cochrane review compared the effectiveness of cycled lighting (CL; ≈12 hours of light on and

BOX 21-3 Guidelines for Supporting Visual Development in the NICU

The infant's visual system is designed to develop in utero in darkness until term birth, devoid of external images or light stimulation. NICU care practices need to protect the endogenous processes needed for visual development carefully and prevent interference with the development of the other sensory systems

22-28 Weeks

The eyes of a very preterm infant (22-28 weeks' gestation) should always be protected from bright and direct light. Only low-level indirect ambient lighting should be used for preterm infants who cannot block out light through their thin eyelids, may not be able to turn away from light, and cannot communicate their needs. The developmental specialist should also be aware that some sedative and CNS depressant drugs can interfere with the endogenous neuronal activity necessary for early visual development; nonpharmacologic pain management and secure supportive positioning may decrease the need for high doses or frequency of these drugs.

28-36 Weeks

Care of the 28- to 36-weeks'-gestation preterm infants should focus on protecting sleep cycles, especially REM sleep. During this time, intense stimulation from NICU noises, vibrations, and other disturbing stimuli of other sensory systems can greatly interfere with the processes of visual system development and also disrupt sleep cycles and necessary REM sleep.[79] Because the infant's circadian clock can respond to light by 28 weeks, some daily exposure to shorter wavelength light can help entrain a circadian rhythm.

The ability to attend visually emerges at 32-34 weeks PMA and is enhanced in low ambient light. Although we cannot prevent an infant from using emerging visual skills, this does not mean that we should encourage it at this young age. Sensory interference and unnecessary competition with auditory development remains a concern. In addition, attempts by parents and caregivers to stimulate visual engagement and interaction at this age often create stress and disturb sleep cycles and endogenous brain activity.

36-40 Weeks

At 40 weeks' gestation, the human visual system has intact retinal development and pathways to the visual cortex and now requires regular external and interactive visual stimulation. Visual experiences for healthy visual development requires ambient light (not direct light), focus, attention, novelty, movement, and, after 2 to 3 months, color.

State Organization

State organization prior to term age equivalency does not require vision, but instead develops in response to gentle nurturing input (e.g., warmth, skin-to-skin holding, soft voice or music, pleasant and familiar taste and smell, gentle motion). For infants in this age range, social and emotional context and atmosphere are just as important as the visual experience; parents need to be involved and trained to understand the type and content of interaction necessary for continued development in these early post-term months.

Adapted from Graven, S. N. (2011). Early visual development: Implications for the neonatal intensive care unit and care. *Clinics in Perinatology,* 38, 693–706.

12 hours of light off) with irregularly dimmed light (DL) or near-darkness (ND) and with continuous bright light (CBL) on growth in preterm infants at 3 and 6 months of age. Trends for many outcomes favored CL compared with ND and CBL.[93]

Graven[49] has emphasized three primary areas of care in the NICU that can adversely affect visual development in the preterm infant. These include interference with endogenous brain cell activity, sleep deprivation, and intense light exposure. Box 21-3 summarizes implications for supporting visual development in the NICU.

Supplemental Sensory and Developmental Stimulation

Much of the early research on supplemental stimulation with preterm infants was based on the sensory deprivation theory and the subsequent desire to provide additional stimuli. This research has been criticized because of the use of small samples, exclusive application to healthy preterm infants, wide age span of infants treated as a homogenous group, failure to take into account individual differences of infants, and methodologic discrepancies that preclude comparisons among studies.

Although much remains unknown, sleep protection remains a top priority. Concerns exist about the immediate and long-term impact of sensory stimuli in the NICU on the preterm infant's still-developing sensory systems. When considering sensory stimulation in the NICU, protecting the fragile newborn from excessive or inappropriate sensory input is a more compelling priority than direct intervention or interaction with the infant. Stimulation is not therapeutic if it disrupts sleep or stresses the infant; an infant may respond to stimuli, but at a physiologic cost, with no sum benefit. Developmental specialists must continually modify sensory stimulation in the NICU according to each infant's postconceptional age, medical status, current state of readiness and responsiveness, ongoing cues of stress or stability, and current sleep cycle. In other words, the developmental specialist provides graded sensory input when the infant is ready and seeking, not because it is time for therapy.

Early stimulation for these younger preterm infants may be safest if it replicates normal parenting activities, such as being held, listening to the caregiver's soft voice, and looking at the caregiver's face. Young infants tolerate stimulation best if it is unimodal (one sensory input at a time). Ideally, family members provide this contact (Figure 21-6).

Stable infants approaching or exceeding term age equivalency often become bored or uncomfortable and demand more attention. Fluidized positioners (Sundance Solutions, White Plains, NY) allow increased positioning comfort and variability in bed and with developmental equipment. The developmental specialist may provide mobiles, mirrors, and/or musical toys for auditory and visual stimulation. Baby swings or vibrating, bouncy infant seats can provide gentle vestibular input and a different view of the world. Even the variety of being placed in a standard infant seat may calm some infants. Portable infant carriers may be options for stable infants who can be

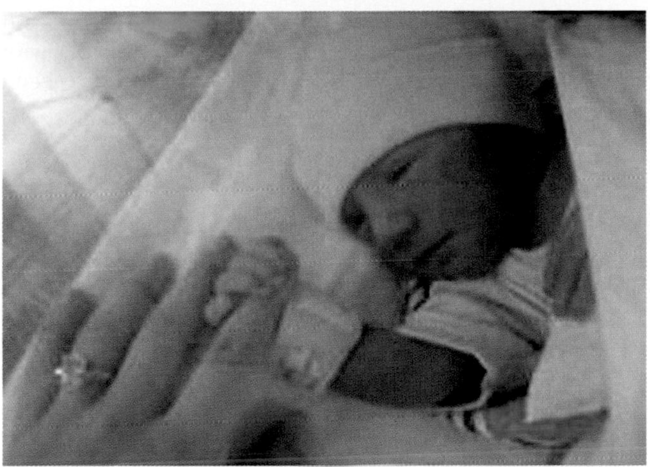

FIGURE 21-6 The support provided by containment, suckling, and grasping helps this preterm infant establish eye contact with her mother for a time of quality interaction.

temporarily separated from (or have portable) medical equipment. Supporting families to be available, involved, and knowledgeable is the best way to meet the infant's developmental and emotional needs both in the NICU and after discharge.

Potential Impact of the NICU Environment on Brain Development in the Preterm Infant

The brain and sensory systems of the neonate are intimately inter-related. Every sensory experience is recorded in the brain, creating a behavioral response and thereby leading to yet another sensory experience. This cyclic interdependent action and reaction is the basis for neurobehavioral and neurosensory development.

The developing brain forms three distinctive structural layers: the brainstem, limbic system, and cerebral cortex.[83] The brainstem (medulla, cerebellum, pons) is nearly complete around the seventh month of gestation.[19,43,112] The brainstem receives sensory messages and relays sensory information to the cerebral cortex. An example is the processing of vestibular sensations necessary for hearing, balance, vision, and focusing attention.[83] The brainstem also regulates autonomic functions of internal organs, such as breathing, heartbeat, and digestion.[19]

The limbic system is located by the thalamus, under the cerebrum. In addition to involvement in smell, the multiple structures comprising the brain's limbic system are directly involved with emotion, behavior, motivation, and formation of long-term memory.

With continued maturation (to adulthood), the highly specialized cerebral cortex (cerebrum, or cognitive brain) performs complex organization of sensory input, contains specific areas to control volitional function, and develops plasticity to adapt throughout the life span.[19,43]

Nervous system basic functions include autonomic, sensory, motor, and state regulation. Autonomic function includes self-regulation of respirations, heart rate, blood pressure, temperature, and nutritional intake. The infant must adapt and respond to many changes simultaneously to survive and thrive in the extrauterine environment after birth.[25,138] Although autonomic regulation is usually sufficiently mature for the full-term infant to adapt successfully after birth, the preterm infant often requires assistance.

Multiple factors interact to influence both structural and functional brain development. The development of early brain architecture and function before the youngest age of viability (cell differentiation and migration, initial cell location, primitive neuronal pathways, response to early stimulation) is primarily guided by a genetic blueprint and influenced by spontaneous internal (endogenous) or maternal hormonal stimulation. After birth, at any viable age, external (exogenous) experiences from the environment now stimulate sensory organs of variable maturity. The resulting interaction when external environmental stimulation influences are sufficient to alter gene expression (not gene sequence) is a process termed *epigenetics*.[35,88] Alterations in gene expression following maternal exposure to stress, environmental toxins, and nutritional modifications have been associated with physiologic and behavioral changes in offspring.[94]

The interaction among low birth weight, prenatal adversity, and postnatal environmental conditions has been associated with low cognitive function, behavioral disorders, and psychiatric disorders.[121] The impact of preterm birth on the developing brain, along with associated painful and unpredictable procedures, environmental stress, and maternal separation, may contribute not only to injury but also to lasting epigenetic consequences.[88] The field of epigenetics may provide critical information about how early experiences, prenatal and postnatal, may affect long-term development.

The fetal neurologic system is in a highly active stage of development during the third trimester of gestation. Young children and adolescents who were VLBW infants have pronounced structural abnormalities demonstrated as smaller volumes of cerebral white matter and neocortical grey matter, smaller surface area of the corpus callosum, larger lateral ventricles, and smaller cerebellar and brainstem volumes.[135] Focal injuries such as periventricular hemorrhagic infarction and cystic periventricular leukomalacia are highly correlated with motor impairment; however, an apparently normal cranial ultrasound does not imply a reduced risk for major neurosensory deficits.[21,22,65,74,139] Subtle alterations in the volume or architecture of brain wiring (neuronal pathways and connections) may not be visible on radiologic imaging but can still lead to neurodevelopmental or learning differences.[72]

The statistics of survival and of long-term neurodevelopmental problems are generally correlated with the degree of prematurity, although exceptions exist on both ends of the spectrum. Last-trimester brain and neurosensory development outside the protective development of the womb increase the risk for motor impairments, cerebral palsy, visual impairment, auditory dysfunction, learning difficulties, and behavioral disorders.[4,57,130,134] Additionally, preterm infants demonstrate increased risk for language delays, visual processing difficulties, and executive dysfunction.[20,66]

Extremely preterm (<26 weeks' gestation) and LBW infants are also at increased risk for a variety of behavioral problems, such as attention deficit, attention-deficit/hyperactivity disorder, autism spectrum disorders, anxiety, and other emotional disorders.[24,68,80,119] Of growing concern is the prevalence of neurodevelopmental impairments in preterm survivors, which include a constellation of cognitive, language, and behavioral outcomes without major neurosensory deficits.[1,2,18] Although the causes of these impairments remain unclear, it is thought that early stressful environmental influences on the brain during critically sensitive developmental periods may contribute to these adverse outcomes,[30] a concept that is well supported by animal research.

With research documenting increased risk for subtle and significant long-term sequelae in children born prematurely, efforts to support the preterm infant's fragile neurologic system become essential to decrease the negative effects of continuing development within the extrauterine environment of the NICU.[76,81] This goal is the basis of neuroprotective developmentally supportive care, with the hope and promise of improved outcomes for future infants.

Box 21-4 summarizes the highlights of fetal brain and sensory system development at advancing gestational ages, with corresponding implications for environmental and caregiving modifications.

Safeguarding Sleep

Medical literature is unequivocal on the divergent and profound effects of sleep deprivation and improved sleep on NICU infants.[50,81] At 23 weeks' gestation, the fetal brain is smooth, with undeveloped synaptic connections, which subsequently develop within the context of the NICU experience for the prematurely born infant. A last-trimester fetus has undisturbed

BOX 21-4 Fetal Sensory System Development: Implications for Environmental and Caregiving Modifications

Basic Brain Development

First trimester: Formation of neural tube and prosencephalon. Disruption of normal development during this period can cause major malformations, such as neural tube defects and agenesis of corpus callosum.

2-4 months' gestation: Proliferation of neuronal and glial cells, which are stored in the germinal matrix.

3-8 months' gestation: Migration of cells from germinal matrix to cerebral cortex.

5 months' gestation through childhood: Organization (alignment, orientation, layering) of cortical neurons, arborization (differentiation and branching of axons and dendrites to increase cell connection possibilities), increased complexity in brain surface convolutions (sulci) as different areas develop for specific functions.

8 months' gestation (peak time): Myelinization.

Most Fetal Sensory Systems (Tactile, Vestibular, Taste, Smell) Are Functioning at the Age of Viability

Tactile: Even the youngest NICU infant has sophisticated perioral sensation and perceives pressure, pain, and temperature. The back and legs are very sensitive to touch, especially prior to 32 weeks, when modulation improves.

Vestibular: System structurally complete but still functionally immature. Movement and position changes can be overstimulating and stressful.

Taste: Withdraws from bitter taste at 26-28 weeks. Calms to sweet taste at 35 weeks. Taste can be affected by sense of smell.

Smell: Responds to odors with approach or avoidance. Noxious odors can prompt physiologic instability and behavioral stress. He or she can recognize mother via smell.

NICU Implications

Coordinate care among disciplines to reduce handling, minimize sleep disturbances, and accommodate feedings. Help support the infant during examinations and procedures:

- Contain extremities (use hands, blanket, positioning aid).
- Encourage sucking on pacifier or on own hand.
- Brace feet against boundaries or palm of caregiver hand.
- Have baby grasp tubing, strap, adult finger.
- Shield infant's eyes from room or procedure light.
- Observe for signs of overstimulation. Can you pause and help infant reorganize before proceeding?
- Contain infant's extremities flexed against his or her body during smooth, slow position changes.
- Use soft fluid boundaries; amount of support needed will vary but is greater for younger, sicker infants.
- Firm steady touch (containment) is better tolerated than light moving touch (stroking).
- Young infants may tolerate holding better skin-to-skin (versus swaddled) and without vestibular stimulation (rocking).
- Protective gloves may have unpleasant taste; wash and rinse first if inserting finger into infant's mouth.
- Oral medication—consider gavage, mixing with feeds.
- Protect infant from noxious smells (e.g., disinfectant).
- Placing a soft cloth infused with the parent's scent near the infant may be calming and facilitate feeding.

Auditory-Visual Sensory System Fetal Development (at Age of Viability) with NICU Implications

Auditory System

24 weeks: Ear (outer, middle, inner) and cortical auditory center essentially formed and functional.

26 weeks: Can elicit brainstem evoked potentials.

NOTE: Preterm infants have increased incidence of sensorineural hearing loss. Auditory processing problems also occur; some animal studies implicate sensory interference (inappropriate timing and intensity of exposure to sensory stimuli related to critical periods of development).

NICU Implications

Preterm infants are sensitive to NICU noise. Auditory overstimulation can cause physiologic stress.

"People" noise is the hardest to reduce and control.

Isolettes can be protective.

NOTE: Mechanical noises penetrate incubators better than speech sounds.

Efforts to reduce noise can occur at many levels:

- Environmental modifications (e.g., sound-absorbing ceiling tiles, carpet, padding bottoms and lids of trash cans, padded Isolette covers, no radios)
- Activity relocation (clerk, main phone, medical rounds all moved away from bedside areas)
- Caregiving practices (silence alarms quickly, speak softly, close Isolette doors quietly)
- Technology (visual alarms, vibrating beepers)
- Neonates demonstrate preference for mother's voice.
- Relaxing music may be effective with older infants.

BOX 21-4 Fetal Sensory System Development: Implications for Environmental and Caregiving Modifications—cont'd

Visual System

Weeks	Development
22	All retinal layers present
25	Can distinguish rods and cones Light elicits blink reflex
25-26	All neurons of visual cortex present
26-28	Eyelids open (no longer fused)
27	May have brief spontaneous wakefulness Unable to visually focus
28-30	Eyes may remain open occasionally Eye movements typically rapid and jerky
30-32	Closes eyes to bright light Brief quiet alert state Visual attention still often stressful Monocular vision
32-35	Demonstrates visual preference Visually tracks horizontally past midline Efforts at visual attention may fatigue infant.
36-40	Retinal vascularization and optic nerve development complete Visually tracks in horizontal, vertical, and circular directions Head and eye movements not well coordinated Preference for curved lines and shapes (versus angular, straight) Can see colors

NICU Implications

The visual system is the least mature of all sensory systems at preterm birth; infant must consistently be protected while visual maturation continues.

- Eyelids are thin and do not block out all room light. Decrease NICU room light, cover bed space, and/or shield eyes of individual infants from direct or bright lighting (including during procedures).
- Avoid abrupt increases in lighting levels.
- Lower light helps reduce staff noise, activity, and stress.
- Studies suggest benefits in altering NICU light levels to provide day-night cycles.
- Supplemental visual stimulation does not seem to accelerate visual system maturation, can fatigue young premies, and can create significant neurobehavioral stress, including apnea and bradycardia.
- Allow infant to indicate readiness for visual stimulation (in quiet alert state, already attending to environment).
- Lower light levels facilitate eye opening for attention.
- Black and white designs are overstimulating for immature infants; the human face is the best model for visual stimulation when the baby is mature and stable.
- Black and white may be therapeutic for infants with significant visual impairments.
- Brainstem visual evoked potentials in preterm infants are difficult to interpret because of visual system immaturity.

sleep in a protected environment; an NICU infant has frequent sleep disruptions in a stressful environment.[23,53]

The primary activity in brain development during the last trimester is synaptogenesis (neurons connecting to others neurons at an amazing rate of 1 to 2 million connections/second), which forms the primitive neuronal pathways that are later refined by experience.[48,50] Synaptogenesis at this stage is endogenous (occurs spontaneously within the brain in the absence of external stimulation) and forms the early brain architecture that is later refined by exogenous (external) stimuli. Endogenous synaptogenesis produces brain complexity and plasticity, only occurs during sleep, and occurs only during REM sleep after 28 weeks' gestation.[48,50]

Prior to 28 weeks, the only sleep state seen on an electroencephalogram (EEG) is an immature sleep stage termed *indeterminate sleep*. Indeterminate state and arousals are associated with less stable oxygenation and hypoxemic episodes, conditions frequently observed in this very immature population. The indeterminate sleep state is gradually replaced by the EEG-identifiable sleep states of active sleep (REM sleep) and quiet sleep (non-REM [NREM] sleep). Normal sleep organization demonstrates maturation. REM sleep may initially comprise up to 75% of total sleep time in the 30- to 36-week infant; REM and NREM sleep are almost equal as the infant approaches term, and by 8 months of age NREM sleep occupies almost 80% of total sleep time.[48,50,88]

Sleep preservation and organization are important determinants of an infant's developmental outcome. REM and NREM sleep cycling are essential for early neurosensory development, learning and memory, and preservation of brain plasticity (neuronal adaptability to new situations and demands) for the life of the individual.[88] Premature infants during childhood are known to have smaller brains than their full-term counterparts, with increased risks for problems with sensory processing, learning disorders, abstract thinking, behavior, coping, adaptability, and attention; brain wiring can be disturbed, even in the absence of structural brain pathology.[24,48] Undisturbed sleep is absolutely essential for normal development of the infant brain and sensory systems during the last trimester, so interventions to protect and prolong sleep should be a top caregiving priority (Figure 21-7).

Minimizing Pain

From the first moments after birth, the premature infant is subjected to noxious sounds, bright lights, and a multitude of

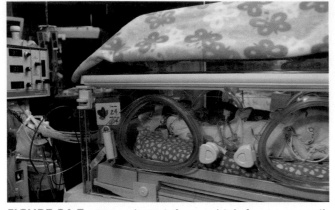

FIGURE 21-7 24-week GA infant on high-frequency oscillating ventilation (HFOV). Efforts to protect sleep include placement of the infant in an incubator to decrease random handling and stimuli, clustered care, covering the Isolette to block overhead light (cover folded back for this picture), and supportive positioning in an individually contoured fluidized positioner. (Courtesy Sundance Enterprises, White Plains, NY; http://www.sundancesolutions.com.)

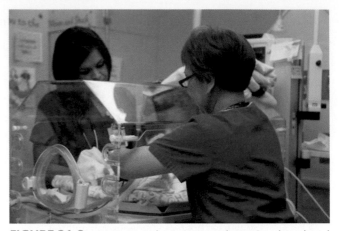

FIGURE 21-8 A nurse and respiratory therapist plan ahead to coordinate their care. The infant benefits from fewer sleep disruptions (vital to sensory system and brain development) and is continuously supported by one caregiver as the other completes necessary tasks. (Courtesy NICU, Memorial Hermann Hospital Southwest, Houston. Photograph by Beverly Edwards.)

painful procedures, along with repetitive, non-nurturing handling and separation from the mother. Seemingly benign handling and caregiving by the NICU staff, such as bathing, weighing, and diaper changes, are perceived as stress by the infant.[37,77] This altered sensory experience is inherently stressful and has negative effects on the infant's brain development.

Consequences of neonatal stress include increased energy expenditure, decreased healing and growth, impaired physiologic stability, and altered brain development. NICU stressors and painful interventions may raise cortisol levels, limiting neuroplastic reorganization and therefore learning and memory of motor skills. Infants who are exposed to repeated painful experiences can have negative short- and long-term consequences for brain organization during sensitive periods of development.[54] Minimizing stress in preterm infants may have many neurologic benefits, such as reducing the likelihood of programming abnormal stress responsiveness, which may help preserve existing neuroplastic capacity.[107] Infants have demonstrated markedly improved outcomes when the stress of environmental overstimulation is reduced. Pharmacologic and nonpharmacologic management of pain is a top priority in NICU caregiving. Non-nutritive sucking is often successful for soothing and self-regulation; a pacifier dipped in a 24% sucrose solution can be used to help manage minor procedural pain.[142]

Preterm infants are extremely vulnerable to pain. Decreased ability to attenuate pain may allow even relatively benign procedures to be perceived as painful, especially when occurring just after handling or another painful experience.[65] Immediate consequences of severe or repetitive painful experiences in the NICU may include physiologic instability, medical complications, sleep disturbances, feeding problems, and poor self-regulation. Painful procedures may result in heightened pain sensitivity to routine handling, as well as delayed recovery from noxious and routine caregiving procedures.[142] Repetitive or prolonged pain has been implicated in enhanced neuronal cell death in the immature brain, with concerns for future neurodevelopmental outcome.[7] Although pain scores have typically been used to evaluate the effects of pain relief interventions, sleep structure has been documented as a more objective measure for prolonged effects of pain and its management.[17] Preserving infants' sleep and relieving their pain are both important for their health; however, clinicians tend to disregard preterm infants' sleep needs because they cannot verbalize their need for sleep. Clinicians should provide preterm infants with neuroprotective interventions, not to only relieve pain but also to preserve sleep organization.[78]

NICU Caregiving

Minimizing Stress

NICU caregiving patterns differ significantly from those in the fetal intrauterine environment and the normal home setting. The sense of touch is highly developed in utero, with gentle human touch normally providing consistent positive tactile input after term birth. Touch in the NICU, however, is usually related to medical care rather than social nurturing. NICU interventions are often intrusive or aversive and are typically constant throughout a 24-hour span.

Caregiving procedures may contribute to an infant's physiologic instability (e.g., increased heart rate, fluctuations in blood pressure, alterations in cerebral blood flow, hypoxemia), motor stress, energy depletion, and agitation. Caregiving based primarily on external criteria, such as fixed schedules for vital signs and feeding, often ignores or delays the caregiver's response to the infant's cues that indicate that he or she needs care.[45] Conversely, coordinating care among disciplines can reduce sleep disruptions and provide an extra set of hands and eyes to support the infant during caregiving (Figure 21-8).

Developmentally supportive caregiving in the NICU strives to minimize avoidable stressors, facilitate infant medical and neurobehavioral stability, provide therapeutic positioning, facilitate and protect sleep, promote self-regulation, foster normal developmental sequences, and encourage family participation.[76,81] The individual infant's cues, sleep state, and ongoing medical status should determine the timing and sequencing of caregiving. Procedures and interventions for each infant should be based on necessity rather than nursery routines (including therapy schedules), avoiding unnecessary or rough handling and movement.

Caregiving based on ongoing infant cues is an integral part of developmentally appropriate care.[51] Although seemingly efficient, the idea of clustering care may need modification because infants do not always tolerate all the care that is being clustered into one caregiving period. Infant-driven cues, rather than routinely clustered care, should be used for optimal caregiving practices. These cues can communicate an infant's needs and status at any given time, potentially indicating timing for interventions or opportunities for sensory input and interaction, as well as infant tolerance to stimulation. Frequent handling and touching can disturb sleep, leading to decreased weight gain, decreased state regulation, and significantly detrimental effects on brain development.

Moving preterm infants suddenly and quickly can be a negative and stressful experience that often results in autonomic deterioration with apnea, bradycardia, and/or increased oxygen requirement. A general rule of thumb for caregiving in the NICU is to use a slow interactive approach, with a single sensory input at a time. Caregivers prepare the baby for touch or movement by speaking softly and containing extremities during movement and lifting (Figure 21-9). Table 21-4 summarizes considerations for caregiving related to the infant's state of arousal. Caregiving is frequently controlled by the nurse, but developmentally appropriate caregiving can be achieved by effective collaboration of all therapists to negotiate timing, intensity, and appropriateness of interventions, tests, and procedures. Continuous observation and response to infant cues require caregivers to alter routines according to developmentally supportive principles.[127] A paradigm shift from task-oriented and scheduled care to infant-responsive care must occur to carry out optimal caregiving practice. Every caregiver must stay in the present and be mindful when interacting with the infant.

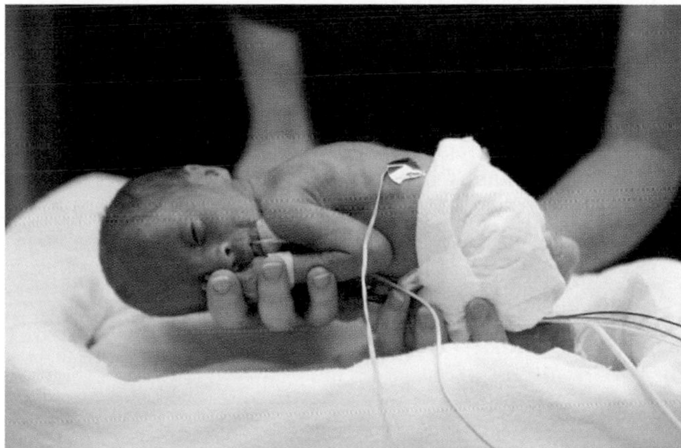

FIGURE 21-9 Lifting an infant in a prone or side-lying position allows gravity to help keep the infant's arms and legs in midline, making it easier for the caregiver to support a fetal tuck position fully. This infant remained calm and restful during lifting. In contrast, infants lifted in a supine position are more difficult to contain, frequently showing extension, with flailing and agitation. (Courtesy NICU, Memorial Hermann Hospital Southwest, Houston. Photograph by Beverly Edwards.)

Skin Protection

The IDC core measure of protecting skin is inherent in NICU caregiving; skin care practices defining bathing practices, emollient use, humidity practices, use of adhesives, and overall caregiving touch for babies in each stage of development should be incorporated into unit practices and policies. The skin of very preterm infants (<30 week' gestation) is fragile, with an increased risk of epidermal stripping and a predisposition to edema; handling and positioning that minimizes forces of pressure, friction, and shear can help protect skin integrity.[61] With skin considered to be the sensory interface of the brain with the external environment,[41] therapeutic positioning, interface surfaces, and comfort assume greater significance.

Bath time is frequently stressful and exhausting to NICU infants. If the infant's body is well supported, with extremities contained, bathing by immersion in warm water is usually more soothing than sponge bathing. Swaddled bathing has proved successful, even with irritable and disorganized infants. The swaddled infant is immersed to the shoulders in a tub of warm water, and the face is washed first with clean water. Next, one body section is unwrapped for bathing and rinsing and then rewrapped in the wet cloth before proceeding to washing another section of the body—right upper body, then left upper body, then legs and buttocks.[108] The warmth and proprioceptive weight of a wet blanket seem calming, and infants are usually quiet and alert throughout this bath, making swaddled bathing a successful and enjoyable caregiving experience for parents (Figure 21-10). Not only does swaddled tub bathing promote more organized infant behavior, infants also show overall higher and less variability in body temperature.[82]

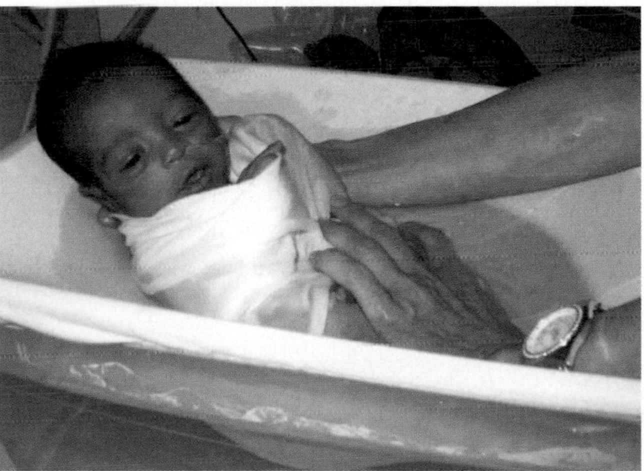

FIGURE 21-10 Swaddled bath. A swaddled preterm infant is immersed in a tub of warm water for a developmentally supportive bath. (Courtesy NICU, Medical Center of Plano, Plano. TX. Photograph by Dana Fern.)

TABLE 21-4 Newborn States and Considerations for Caregiving

Newborn State	Comments
Sleep States	
Deep Sleep (Non–Rapid Eye Movement [NREM] Sleep)	
Slow state changes Regular breathing Eyes closed; no eye movements No spontaneous activity except startles and jerky movements Startles with some delay and suppresses rapidly Lowest oxygen consumption	Infant is very difficult if not impossible to arouse. Infant will not breast-feed or bottle-feed in this state, even after vigorous stimulation. Infant is unable to respond to environment; frustrating for caregivers. Term infants may exhibit a slow heart rate (80-90 beats/min), which may trigger heart rate alarms and result in unnecessary stimulation by neonatal intensive care unit staff. At birth, preterm infants have altered states of consciousness:
Light Sleep (Rapid Eye Movement [REM] Sleep) Low activity level Random movements and startles Respirations irregular and abdominal Intermittent sucking movements Eyes closed; rapid eye movement Higher oxygen consumption	Early dominant states are light sleep, quiet, and active alert. "Protective apathy" enables the preterm infant to remain inactive, unresponsive, and in a sleep state to conserve energy, grow, and maintain physiologic homeostasis. Full-term infants begin and end sleep in active sleep; preterm infants are more responsive than term infants to stimuli in active sleep. Infants may cry or fuss briefly in this state and be awakened to feed before they are truly awake and ready to eat. Lower and more variable oxygenation states
Awake States	
Drowsy or Semidozing	
Eyelids fluttering Eyes open or closed (dazed) Mild startles (intermittent) Delayed response to sensory stimuli Smooth state change after stimulation Fussing may or may not be present Respirations—more rapid and shallow	Infant may awaken further or return to sleep if left alone. Quietly talking and looking at the infant, or offering a pacifier or an inanimate object to see and listen to, may arouse the infant to the quiet alert state. Less mature infants (30 wk) demonstrate a drowsier quiet alert state than older infants (36 wk).
Quiet Alert, with Bright Look Focuses attention on source of stimulation Impinging stimuli may break through; may have some delay in response Minimal motor activity	Immediately after birth, term newborns exhibit a period of quiet alertness, their first opportunity to take in their parents and the extrauterine environment. Dimmed lights, quiet talking, and stroking optimize this time for parents. Best state for learning to occur because infant focuses all attention on visual, auditory, tactile, and sucking stimuli; best state for interaction with parents—baby is maximally able to attend and respond reciprocally to parents.
Active Alert—Eyes Open	
Considerable motor activity—thrusting movements of extremities; spontaneous startles Reacts to external stimuli with increase in movements and startles (discrete reactions difficult to differentiate because of general higher activity level) Respirations irregular May or may not be fussy	Infant has decreased threshold (increased sensitivity) to internal (hunger, fatigue) and external (wet, noise, handling) stimuli. Infant may quiet self, may escalate to crying, or, with consolation by caregiver, may become quiet, alert, or go to sleep. Infant is unable to attend to caregiver or environment maximally because of increased motor activity and increased sensitivity to stimuli.
Crying—intense and difficult to disrupt with external stimuli Respirations rapid, shallow, and irregular	Crying is infant's response to unpleasant internal and/or external stimulation—infant's tolerance limits have been reached (and exceeded). Infant may be able to quiet self with hand to mouth behaviors; talking may quiet a crying infant; holding, rocking, or putting infant upright on caregiver's shoulder may quiet infant.

Infant Neurobehavioral and Neuromotor Development

Evaluation of the Infant

The golden rule for developmental evaluation and intervention with all NICU infants is "Above all, do no harm!" The following guidelines consider that goal.

1. Safety for the infant takes priority over convenience for the occupational therapist in all aspects of care. Review applicable medical conditions and equipment, be very aware of stress cues, and never perform an evaluation item simply to fill in a blank space on a form if the information obtained will not benefit the care plan for the baby.
2. Learn an evaluation tool thoroughly before touching an infant and be constantly aware of changes in an infant's stress level. Many occupational therapists use a structured assessment supplemented with data gathering and clinical observations. Administration of some structured neonatal

assessments requires specialized training and/or certification of reliability (e.g., Neonatal Individualized Developmental Care and Assessment Program [NIDCAP]); others may be used after independent study of the manual and practice (e.g., Hammersmith Neonatal Neurological Examination).

3. Appreciate the nurse's role in protecting the infant and use astute clinical observations of the infant and surrounding environment before any touching. Very fragile infants can be assessed entirely by skilled observation, with no additional touching.
4. Weigh the value of any hands-on evaluation procedures against potential stressful effects on the infant. Co-assessments with other disciplines may reduce unnecessary duplication of items that require handling.
5. Avoid fitting a baby into a convenient opening in your schedule. Instead, make it your priority to observe and respect the infant's sleep cycle, feeding schedule, caregiving routine, and medical status. Respect the infant's signs of stress during handling; switch to an observational assessment if the infant does not readily return to a calm organized state, even with caregiver assistance.
6. Performing an evaluation is easier than accurately analyzing the results; overinterpretation and mistaking immaturity for pathology are frequent errors of inexperienced developmental specialists. Preterm infants, especially those born at an extremely young gestational age, often differ in neuromotor and neurobehavioral progression from infants born at term.

Routine ongoing reassessment in the NICU and in a follow-up clinic as infants mature and recover is essential for developing sound clinical judgment about the meaning of early clinical findings.

Infant Neurobehavioral Development

Neurobehavioral Organization of the Preterm Infant

In-Turning, Coming-Out, and Reciprocity

An early description of preterm infant behavioral organization by physicians in the 1970s helped provide rule-of-thumb guidelines for developmental specialists in their approach to infants and in their supporting successful parenting in the NICU.[47] Infants in the in-turning stage are generally immature or critically ill; they require minimal handling, with maximal environmental and caregiving protection. Infants in the coming-out stage remain fragile and vulnerable but have brief periods of availability to attend to their environment; graded unimodal stimulation may be appropriate for brief periods based on observed infant state and tolerance. The more mature and stable infant in the reciprocity stage attends and interacts when in an appropriate quiet alert state, but the caregiver must respect approach and avoidance signals. Advancing postconceptional age and medical status (acuity and chronicity) affect an individual infant's progression throughout these stages.

Synactive Theory of Development

The research of Dr. T. Berry Brazelton in the 1970s focused primarily on the reactions and interactions of healthy term infants to environmental and social stimuli.[28] Heidilese Als built on Brazelton's earlier work and adapted the model specifically to preterm infants.

Because preterm infants are continually affected by and responsive to environmental influences, Als proposed a model for understanding these emerging capabilities of preterm infants to organize and control their behavior.[3] Als' synactive theory of development identified five separate but interdependent subsystems—autonomic, motor, state, attention-interaction, and self-regulation in the infant. These subsystems are in constant interaction with each other (the neonate's internal functioning), the environment, and caregivers. Through recognizable approach and avoidance behaviors occurring in these subsystems, infants continually communicate their level of stress and stability in relation to what is happening to and around them (Table 21-5). Maturation and improved (or declining) health are reflected in sequential observations of subsystem development, although very preterm infants often do not reflect the same performance capabilities as an infant born at the equivalent older age (Table 21-6).

Synactive theory forms the basis for individualized developmentally supportive and family-centered care. Caregivers are trained to be sensitive to each infant's fragility and stress behaviors versus robustness and stability behaviors (Figure 21-11). The caregiver then uses these observations to modify the environment and caregiving practices to facilitate the infant's organization and well-being. Each infant's attempts to maintain or return to a calm, organized state are also noted and encouraged. The infant and family are seen as an integral unit, with parents supported in assuming an active role with their infant in the NICU.

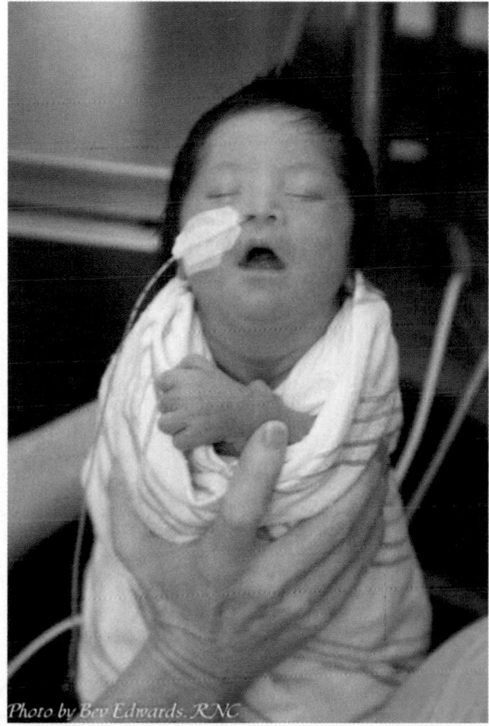

FIGURE 21-11 Reading an infant's neurobehavioral cues: This infant's gape face is indicative of low muscle tone, low arousal, and lack of readiness to interact or feed orally. It is important for caregivers and parents to learn to read and respect infant behaviors to avoid pushing (stressing) the infant and frustrating the adult. (Courtesy NICU, Memorial Hermann Hospital Southwest, Houston, TX. Photograph by Beverly Edwards.)

TABLE 21-5 Synactive Theory of Development: Neurobehavioral Subsystems, Signs of Stress, and Stability*

Subsystem	Signs of Stress	Signs of Stability
Autonomic	**Physiologic instability**	**Physiologic stability**
Respiratory	Pauses, tachypnea, gasping	Smooth, regular respiratory rate
Color	Changes to mottled, flushed, pale, dusky, cyanotic, gray, or ashen	Pink, stable color
Visceral	Hiccups, gagging, spitting up, grunting, straining (as if producing bowel movement)	Stable viscera with no hiccups, gags, emesis, or grunting
Motor	Tremors, startles, twitches, coughs, sneezes, yawns, sighs, seizures	No sign of tremors, startles, twitches, coughs, sneezes, yawns, sighs, or seizures
Motor	**Fluctuating tone, uncontrolled activity**	**Consistent tone, controlled activity**
Flaccidity	Gape face, low tone in trunk, limp lower extremities and upper extremities	Muscle tone consistent in trunk and extremities and appropriate for postconceptional age
Hypertonicity	Leg extensions and sitting on air; upper extremity salutes, finger splays, and fisting; trunk arching; tongue extensions	Smooth controlled posture; smooth movements of extremities and head
Hyperflexions	Trunk, lower and/or upper extremities Frantic, diffuse activity of extremities	Motor control can be used for self-regulation—hand and foot clasp, leg and foot bracing, hand to mouth, grasping, tucking, sucking
State	**Diffused or disorganized quality of states, including range and transition between states**	**Clear states; good, calming, focused alertness**
During sleep	Twitches, sounds, whimpers, jerky movements, irregular respiratory rate, fussy, grimaces	Clear, well-defined sleep states Smooth transition between states
When awake	Abrupt state changes Eye floating, glassy eyed, staring, gaze aversion, worried or dull look, hyperalert panicked expression, weak cry, irritability	Good self-quieting and consolability Focused, clear alertness with animated expressions (e.g., frowning, cheek softening, "ooh" face, cooing, smiling) Robust crying
Attention-Interaction	**Effort to attend and interact to specific stimulus elicits stress signals of other subsystems**	**Responsive to auditory, visual, and social stimuli is clear and prolonged**
Autonomic	Irregular respiratory rate, color changes, visceral responses, coughs, yawns, sneezes, sighs, straining tremors, twitches	Actively seeks out auditory stimulus; able to shift attention smoothly from one stimulus to another
Motor state	Fluctuating tone, frantic diffuse activity Eye floating, glassy eyed, staring, worried or dull look, hyperalert panicked expression, gaze aversion, weak cry, irritability Becomes stressed if more than one type of stimulus given simultaneously Abrupt state changes	Face demonstrates bright-eyed purposeful interest varying between arousal and relaxation

Self-Regulation: Infant's efforts to achieve, maintain, or regain balance and self-organization in each subsystem as needed. Examples include motor strategies (e.g., foot clasp, leg and foot bracing, finger folding, hand clasping, hand to mouth, grasping, tucking, sucking, postural changes); state strategies (e.g., lowers state of arousal or releases energy with rhythmic, robust crying), and attention and orientation strategies, such as visual locking. The success of various strategies may vary among infants.

*Modified from the works of Heidi Als on the synactive theory of development: Als, H. (1986). A synactive model of neonatal behavioral organization: Framework for the assessment and support of the neurobehavioral development of the premature infant and his parents in the environment of the neonatal intensive care unit. *Physical and Occupational Therapy in Pediatrics. 6*, 3–53.

TABLE 21-6 Neurobehavioral Development of Preterm Infants by Gestational Age

Neurobehavioral System	Developmental Behaviors
Infants at ≤30 Weeks' Gestation	
Autonomic	May exhibit periodic breathing, apnea, and bradycardia Color changes common with stimulation Eyelids are thin; infant has minimal ability to achieve or maintain protective tightening of eyelid against bright light. Eyes flutter open, often with rapid uncoordinated eye movements or with diffuse unfocused gaze.

TABLE 21-6 Neurobehavioral Development of Preterm Infants by Gestational Age—cont'd

Neurobehavioral System	Developmental Behaviors
Motor	Reflex smiling and startle response are present.
	Muscle tone is low; limp extension of extremities and flat resting postures are predominant.
	Uncontrolled spontaneous movements such as extremity twitches and tremors are common.
	Active movements of extremities are jerky.
	Infant is unable to coordinate sucking, swallowing, and breathing.
State	Light sleep states predominate, with rapid eye movement (REM) and frequent tonguing and mouthing apparent.
	States are not yet well defined; drowsy or awake "alert" periods are brief.
Attention-interaction	Visual acuity is poor, with little accommodation.
	Apnea may result when visual stimuli are intense.
	Hearing is well developed; preference for mother's voice is possible.
	Usually easily stressed by environmental and caregiving stimuli
Self-regulation	Self-regulation efforts are immature and ineffective.
Infants at 30-33 Weeks' Gestation	
Autonomic	May exhibit periodic breathing, apnea, and bradycardia
	Reflexive ability to constrict iris emerges
	Able to keep eyelids shut, but eyelids still thin
Motor	Muscle tone improving and more flexion apparent; motor tone better in lower extremities than in upper extremities
	Motor activity becoming smoother, but startles and tremors still common.
	Improved head control is evident.
State	Active sleep predominant, but quiet sleep increasing
	Increase in alert awake time
	States more distinct as sleep-wake organization emerges
	Arousal with feeding readiness cues may be observed.
	Emerging coordination of sucking, swallowing, and breathing
Attention-interaction	Brightens to sound; preference for human voice
	May be able to visually focus briefly (with much effort) on specific stimulus
	Limited capacity for social contact
Self-regulation	Still often stressed by environmental and caregiving stimuli
	Self-regulation efforts (e.g., grasping, foot bracing, hand to mouth) increasing with variable effectiveness
Infants at 34-36 Weeks' Gestation	
Autonomic	Generally more stable heart rate, respiratory rate, and oxygen saturation
Motor	Muscle tone, activity level, and motor control continue to improve
	Able to right head forward and backward
	Decreased tremors
	Usually able to breast- or bottle-feed
State	Increase in quiet sleep with more regular respiration and decreased random activity
	Smoother transition between sleep and awake states
	Infant usually awakens to stimulation, although duration and quality of alertness may be variable
	Arousal and crying more frequent in response to discomfort, pain, or hunger
Attention-interaction	More consistent behavioral responsiveness to auditory stimuli
	Visual orientation (focus, brief tracking) present, but infant may become overstimulated or fatigued with the effort
	Increased capacity for social attentiveness and responsiveness
	May tolerate just one type of sensory or social stimulation at a time
Self-regulation	Improving efforts and success at self-consoling and self-regulation
Infants at 37-40 Weeks' Gestation	
Motor	Extremity flexor tone present; movements increasingly smooth and controlled
	Wide variety of movements are observed
	Feeds by breast or bottle
State	Well-defined range of states, with smooth transitions
	Quiet sleep increases, with equal periods of active sleep
	Sleep-wake cycles shorter with less mature sleep-wake organization than infant born at term
	Crying more closely approximates that of term infant
Attention-interaction	Increasingly consistent behavioral responsiveness to auditory stimuli; prefers human voice
	Active "looking" behaviors increase during quiet alert periods.
	Infant displays preferences for visual stimuli (usually human face) and tracks objects; best visual focus is at 8-10 inches
	More reciprocal social interaction
Self-regulation	Self-regulation efforts more organized and successful

Data from Hadley, M. A, West, D., Turner, A., & Santangelo, S. (1999). *Developmental and behavioral characteristics of preterm infants.* Petaluma, CA: NICU; and Yecco, G. J. (1993). Neurobehavioral development and developmental support of premature infants. *Journal of Perinatal and Neonatal Nursing, 7,* 56–65.

TABLE 21-7 Stages and Characteristics of Behavioral Organization in Preterm Infant

Als	Gorski, Davidson, & Brazelton
Physiologic homeostasis—stabilizing and integrating temperature control, cardiorespiratory function, digestion, and elimination. Characteristics—becomes pale, dusky, cyanotic; heart and respiratory rates change; all symptoms of disorganization of autonomic nervous system.	In-turning—physiologic stage of mere survival *Characteristics*—autonomic nervous system responses to stimuli (rapid color changes caused by swings in heart and respiratory rates); no or limited direct response; inability to arouse self spontaneously; jerky movements; asleep (and protecting the central nervous system from sensory overload) 97% of the time. Preterm infants (<32 wk) are easily physiologically overwhelmed by stimuli.
Motor development may infringe on physiologic homeostasis, resulting in defensive strategies (vomiting, color change, apnea, and bradycardia). State development becomes less diffuse and encompasses full range: sleep, awake, crying. States and state changes may affect physiologic and motor stability.	Coming out—first active response to environment may be seen as early as 34 to 35 wk (provided some physiologic stability has been achieved). *Characteristics*—remains pink with stimuli; has directed response for short periods; arouses spontaneously and maintains arousal after stimuli ceases; if interaction begins in alert state, maintains quiet alert for 5-10 min, tracks animate and inanimate stimuli; spends 10%-15% of time in alert state with predictable interaction patterns.
Alert state well differentiated from other states State changes may interfere with physiologic and motor stability.	Reciprocity—active interaction and reciprocity with environment from 36-40 wk *Characteristics*—directs response; arouses and consoles self; maintains alertness and interacts with both animate and inanimate objects; copes with external stress.

Adapted from Als, H. (1986). A synactive model of neonatal behavior organization: Framework for the assessment of neurobehavioral development in the premature infant and for support of infants and parents in the neonatal intensive care environment. *Physical and Occupational Therapy in Pediatrics, 6,* 3–55; and Gorski, P. A., Davidson, M. F., & Brazelton, T. B. (1979). Stages of behavioral organization in the high-risk neonate: Theoretical clinical considerations. *Seminars in Perinatology, 3,* 61–72.

When preterm infants were assessed and provided with developmentally supportive individualized care, Als[4] saw significantly improved outcomes, including fewer days on the ventilator, earlier feeding success, shorter hospital stay, marked reduction in the number of complications, and improved neurodevelopmental outcomes during the first 18 months of life, findings that were sustained to 8 years of age.[89]

Table 21-7 summarizes and compares the stages and characteristics of preterm behavioral organization of Gorski's in-turning, coming-out, and reciprocity model[47] with Als' synactive theory of development.

States of Arousal

State refers to the infant's degree of consciousness or arousal, with quality and consistency of state control in preterm infants generally improving as age and maturation increase. State significantly affects other areas, such as muscle tone, feeding performance, and reaction to stimuli. Caregivers need to be sensitive to an infant's state (see Table 21-4).

State is most frequently classified into six categories: state 1 (deep sleep); state 2 (light sleep); state 3 (transitional state of dozing or drowsiness); state 4 (quiet and alert); state 5 (active alert); and state 6 (crying). The smoothness or abrupt fluctuation as the infant transitions between states, both spontaneously and during handling, provides information on neural organization and control.[10] The infant who cannot be aroused, is excessively irritable, or has wide swings between sleep and cry states, with no interim alert periods, may be demonstrating immaturity or pathology. A gradual awakening with smooth transition from sleep to alertness and eventually back to sleep is one sign of maturation and neurologic integrity.

A smooth transition between states requires appropriate regulation and response to a variety of sensory inputs. The ability to modulate state is affected by intrinsic factors (e.g., pain, stress, immaturity, illness, intrauterine drug exposure) and extrinsic factors (e.g., light, noise, caregiving activities). Individual temperament may also be a variable in the infant's state of arousal; some infants are more active and demanding, whereas others are more relaxed. Sleep is essential for body and brain growth and development; supporting and protecting undisturbed sleep should be a caregiving priority.

Neuromotor Development and Interventions

Reflex Development

Neonatal reflex development has been well documented in medical and therapeutic literature. Although some occupational therapists include reflex testing in their standard NICU assessment, complete reflex testing is extremely stressful for young or acutely ill NICU infants and is unnecessary as an early routine evaluation. Self-regulatory reflexes such as suck and grasp can indicate primitive reflex integrity in young or ill infants. Selective reflex testing may be appropriate with older stable infants prior to discharge[16] or if the infant has known or suspected neuropathology or neuromuscular pathology (e.g., spina bifida, periventricular leukomalacia, congenital neuropathy). Many reflexes (e.g., grasping, sucking, head righting) can be observed within the context of normal handling, which provides functional information with less stress than generalized formal reflex testing.

Muscle Tone

Hypotonia is normal for extremely preterm infants. Muscle tone gradually increases with age, and in caudocephalic (feet to head) and distal-proximal (extremities to trunk) directions. Active muscle tone, observed during spontaneous movement or elicited by righting reactions when the infant is handled, develops before passive flexor tone is seen at rest.[26] An extremely preterm infant at term equivalency will typically demonstrate greater extension and less physiologic flexion than a newborn full-term infant. Twitches, tremors, and startles are common in preterm infants, but movements typically become smoother and tremors less prevalent as term equivalency nears.

In addition to PMA, state of arousal and medical status are significant variables when assessing muscle tone. A preterm infant may be active and feisty when awake, but hypotonic if assessed while drowsy or asleep. Muscle tone in an acutely ill infant cannot be accurately evaluated; the underlying muscle tone usually changes as the infant recovers. Many medications have neuromotor side effects. For example, phenobarbital for seizures may initially make the infant lethargic; caffeine for apnea may make the infant jittery; and midazolam for sedation may cause tremors.

The influence of evolving muscle tone on resting posture and quantity or quality of movement has implications for positioning and caregiving needs. Monitor atypical findings or asymmetric responses over time; unusual movement patterns that are not stereotypic and obligatory may resolve with maturation and physical recovery. If possible, distinguish a potential cause; for example, could an infant's asymmetry, tight retracted shoulders, or increased extensor tone be iatrogenic from poor positioning rather than neurologic in origin? Either cause will require intervention, but positional deformities have a better long-term prognosis, and positioning can be improved with future babies to avoid preventable problems.

Posture and Movement Patterns

A fetus has dynamic circumferential boundaries at all times. Flexion and symmetry are reinforced in developing neuronal pathways in utero; active fetal extension is always followed by a return to flexion because of flexible uterine constraints. An infant who has moved and developed within these constraints has a motor advantage at term birth from neuromuscular and neurologic predispositions to function in flexed postures with a midline orientation.[60,64]

An infant born very early does not have this same advantage. Extremely preterm infants have incomplete development of muscle tone, joint structures, and bone density. Muscle tone is usually hypotonic, with active extension stronger than a corresponding return to flexion. Spontaneous resting posture is often flat, extended, and asymmetric, with the head to one side (usually the right); the extremities tend to be abducted and externally rotated, resting flat on the bed surface[64] (Figure 21-12). This "frogged" posture is reinforced by the effects of gravity, hypotonia, primitive reflexes, immature neuromotor control, illness, energy depletion, and weight or torque of medical equipment. Over time, neuronal connections are reinforced that favor this flattened, externally rotated, and asymmetric resting posture as the normal baseline for these infants; active extension and arching become unopposed dominant motor patterns (Figure 21-13).

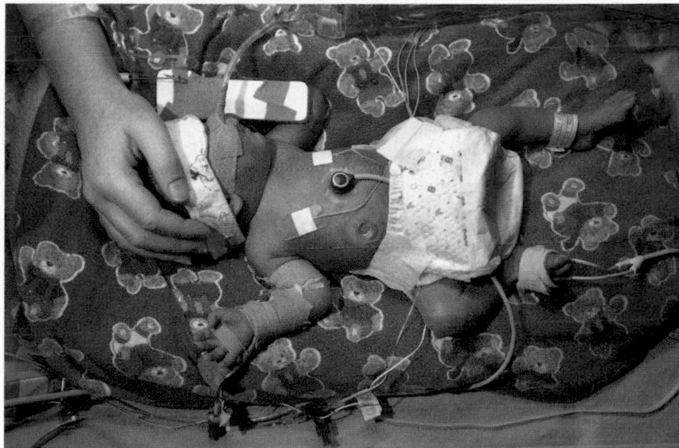

FIGURE 21-12 Hypotonic posture of premature infant. Without therapeutic positioning, the W configuration of the arms, frogged posture of the legs, and asymmetric head position may lead to positional deformities.

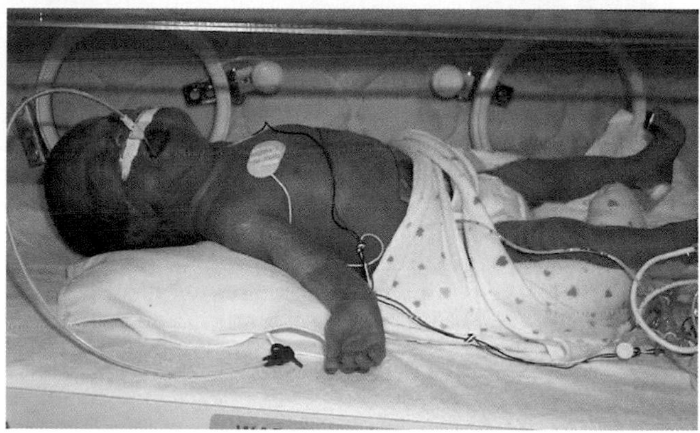

FIGURE 21-13 Active extension and arching become unopposed dominant motor patterns when therapeutic positioning is not consistent during NICU hospitalization. (Courtesy Infant Special Care Unit, University of Texas Medical Branch, Galveston, TX. Photograph by Jan Hunter).

Therapeutic Positioning in the NICU

It is well documented that lack of appropriate NICU positioning can create short-term and long-term positional deformities and functional problems for NICU infants, even in the absence of overt brain pathology (Figure 21-14). NICU positioning attempts to simulate the flexed, contained, and midline posture within flexible boundaries of the infant in utero; external supports provide a temporary substitute for an immature infant's diminished internal neuromotor control.

NICU positioning is an excellent example of how evolving knowledge and advances in technology have driven changes in developmental clinical practice. In the 1970s, few or no attempts were made to provide boundaries or positional support for infants in the NICU. In the 1980s, increased awareness of infant developmental vulnerability and environmental stressors resulted in the use of blanket rolls for boundaries, with variable effectiveness (Figure 21-15*A*). Commercially available positioning aids became available in the 1990s and increasingly replaced manually made nests of blanket rolls and sheepskin; commercial positioning aids provided greater ease and consistency of positioning among NICU staff, but still with variable

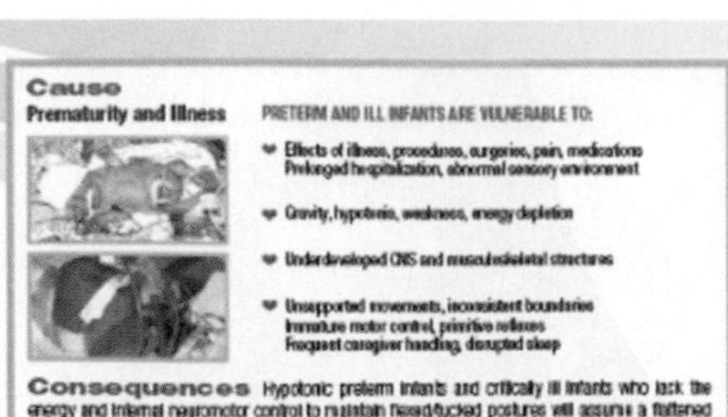

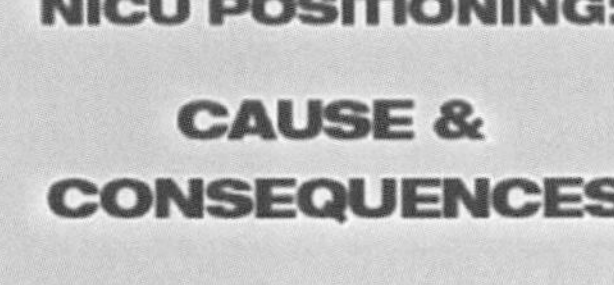

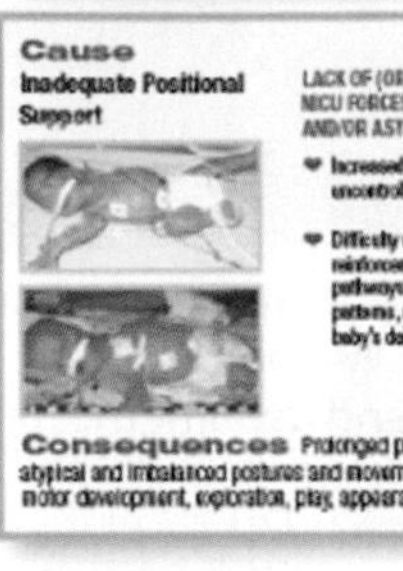

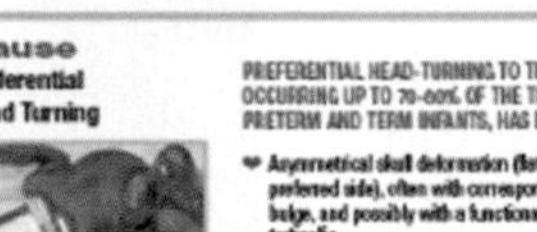

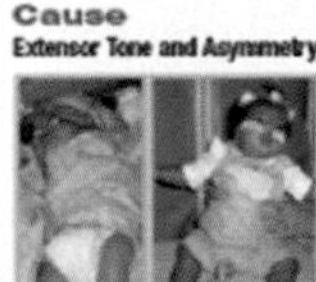

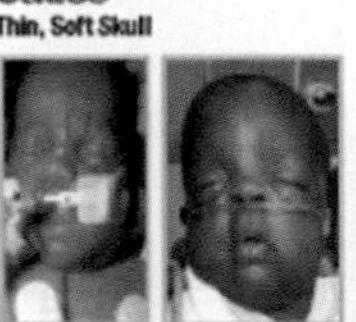

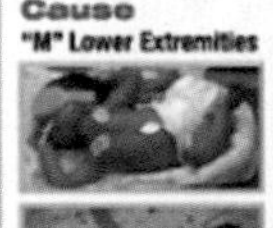

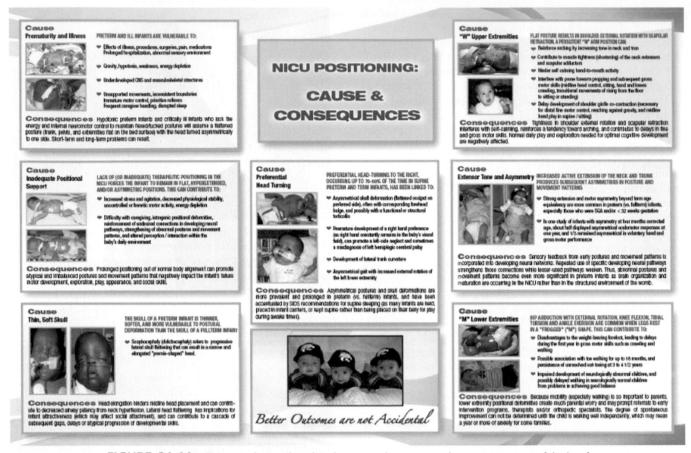

FIGURE 21-14 Illustrated are the developmental causes and consequences of lack of therapeutic positioning, with subsequent positional deformities in the NICU population. Hospital-acquired positional deformities are largely avoidable with good positioning. (Courtesy Sundance Enterprises, White Plains, NY; http://www.sundancesolutions.com.)

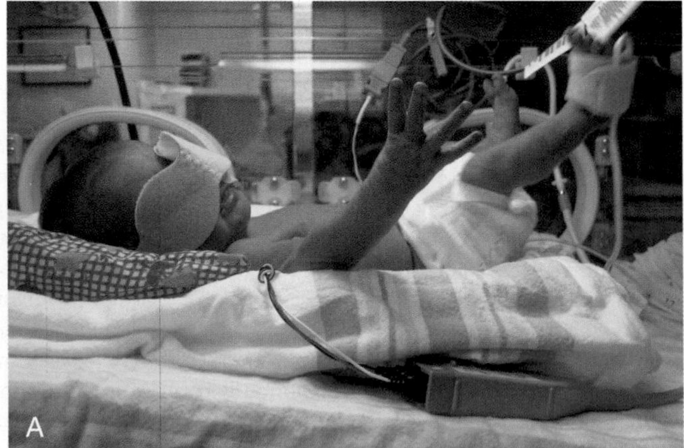

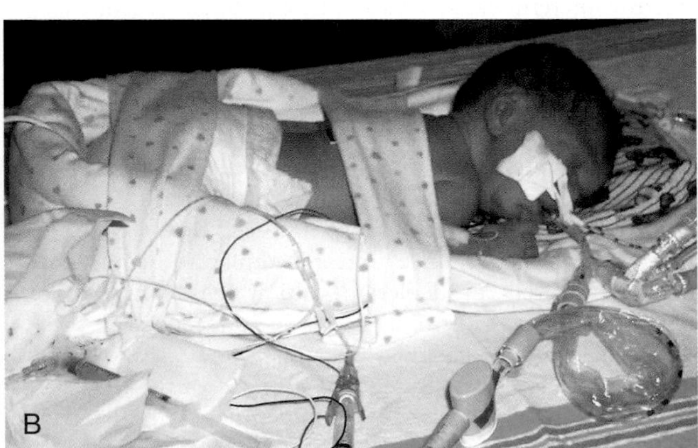

FIGURE 21-15 **A,** Blanket rolls are often too shallow and too wide to provide secure boundaries and postural support. **B,** Commercial positioning devices such as the Snuggle Up (Children's Medical Ventures, Philips Healthcare, Andover, MA) make positioning easier. This small preterm infant is supported in a side-lying position, with midline orientation and flexion of extremities. (**A** and **B** courtesy Infant Special Care Unit, University of Texas Medical Branch, Galveston, TX. Photographs by John Glow and Jan Hunter.)

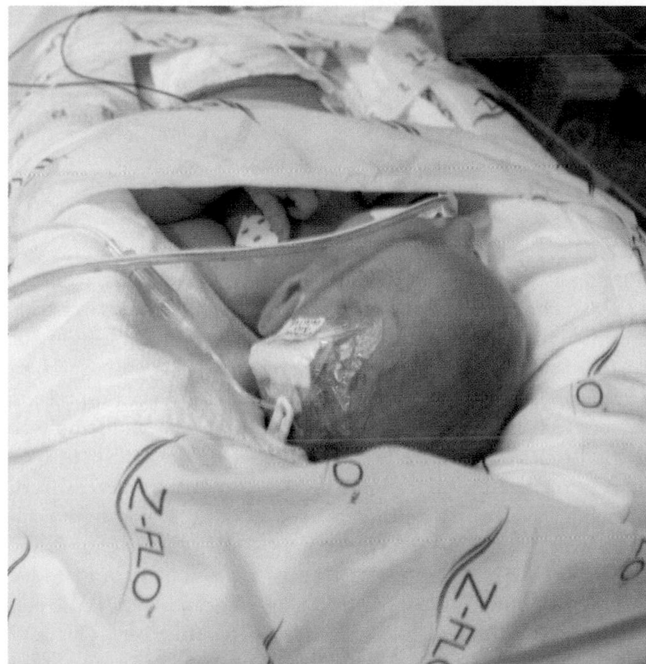

FIGURE 21-16 Postsurgical infant nested in a three-dimensional fluidized positioner that conforms to the infant, assumes the temperature of the incubator, and accommodates medical equipment. (Courtesy Sundance Enterprises, White Plains, NY; www.sundancesolutions.com.)

success in providing consistent boundaries without eliminating free movement (see Figure 21-15*B*).

NICU positioning has traditionally been a neuromotor developmental intervention to minimize positional deformities and improve muscle tone, postural alignment, movement patterns, and ultimately developmental milestones. The scope of NICU positioning focus expanded from developmental to therapeutic when fluidized positioners became available in 2007. These three-dimensional, whole-body positioners can infinitely and repeatedly conform to any body size, medical condition, and medical equipment (Figure 21-16). Empiric benefits reported by clinicians include the following: more consistent containment without limiting infant movement; increased comfort with decreased restlessness and agitation; energy conservation with frequently reduced energy requirement; more frequent and longer duration of sleep; reduced forces of friction, pressure, and shear on fragile skin because of fluidized properties; and reduced heat loss as the infant is immersed in a three-dimensional positioner that assumes the temperature of the incubator.[64]

A recent randomized clinical trial in the NICU at a major children's hospital examined sleep in infants on fluidized positioners (termed *conformational positioners* in this RCT) compared with being swaddled on a standard mattress.[137] This study demonstrated improved sleep efficiency (percentage of time asleep) as measured by sleep EEG and improved self-regulation behaviors as measured by NIDCAP evaluation (Als' synactive theory). Because sleep is elusive in the NICU,[76] any intervention that improves sleep has major implications for increased brain synaptogenesis and plasticity[50,81] (Figure 21-17).

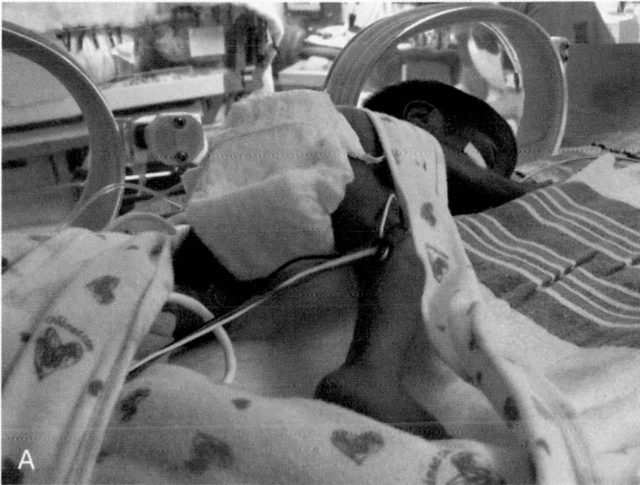

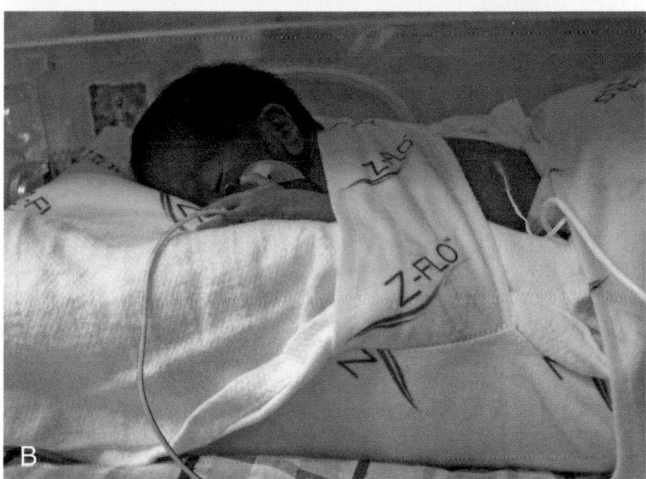

FIGURE 21-17 Continuously restless 1000-g infant, unable to settle in cloth bunting. She relaxed and fell asleep quickly after being positioned on a fluidized, full-body positioner, with a smaller pad used as a prone roll. (Courtesy Sundance Enterprises, White Plains, NY; www.sundancesolutions.com.)

Range of Motion

Passive range of motion (PROM) may be appropriate for infants who demonstrate structural or neuromuscular limitation of movement and can tolerate a rehabilitation approach. PROM incorporated into therapeutic handling is preferable to conventional ranging techniques for most infants. Hypertonicity may relax more with sustained stretch and therapeutic positioning than with repetitive PROM. PROM occasionally may be appropriate for an infant who is sedated or chemically paralyzed (and thus nonmoving) for prolonged periods. However, experience suggests that prevention of positional deformities with therapeutic positioning may be sufficient intervention for infants whose movement is temporarily restricted. Therapists should never consider PROM to be a routine NICU intervention because it is unnecessary and often stressful to the general preterm population.

Splinting

With the exception of fractures, for which immobilization is desired for healing and comfort, splinting is rarely needed with

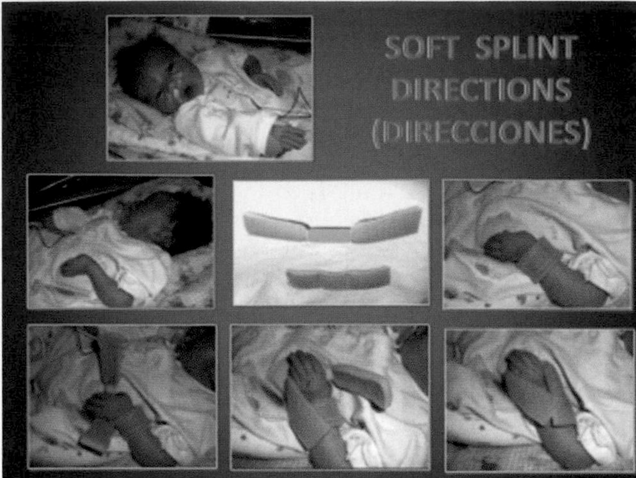

FIGURE 21-18 Newborn infant with congenital muscular dystrophy, right humeral fracture, and obvious hand deformities. Bilateral soft splints (fabricated from foam pencil grips, small Velfoam straps, and Velcro) had no pressure points. Movement was not restricted; corrected alignment actually increased the infant's active movements. (Courtesy Infant Special Care Unit, University of Texas Medical Branch, Galveston, TX. Photographs and slide by Jan Hunter.)

NICU infants. Although contractures may occur with specific diagnoses, rigid contractures are actually uncommon, and infants are notably pliable over time. Significant and rapid improvement is often seen with gentle stretch during therapeutic positioning, the effects of gravity, and spontaneous movement of the infant. Conversely, spontaneous movement is inhibited when the infant is wearing a rigid splint.

Protecting skin integrity and encouraging active movement are priorities when designing a neonatal splint. Thermoplastic material may create pressure points; adding sufficient padding may alter fit. It can also be difficult to maintain correct joint alignment on a rigid splint when extremity movement of $\frac{1}{4}$ inch can significantly change hand placement.

Less is better, and creative combinations of foams are often sufficient. Figure 21-18 illustrates bilateral hand splints made from foam pencil grips, foam straps, and a little Velcro. Alignment is corrected by tension on either strap; spontaneous movement is facilitated rather than repressed; risk for pressure is minimal; and both splints fit either hand—eliminating the potential right hand–left hand misapplication. The serial photographs were posted at bedside and given to the Spanish-speaking parents for follow-up with the local early childhood intervention program. When appropriate, splints like these rarely cause problems, although monitoring, adaptation, and education are always required.

Feeding

A Word about Breastfeeding

Although this chapter focuses on bottle feeding, breast milk is the optimal nutrition for NICU infants; any breast milk that the infant receives is valuable.[14,103] Term newborns are born with the instinctive skill and motivation to breast-feed and are able to find the breast and self-attach without assistance when skin to skin.[104]

Mothers of preterm or ill infants who are educated about the benefits of breast milk often choose to pump milk for their infants; many, however, are unable to maintain sufficient lactation for successful or exclusive breastfeeding at discharge. Early initiation and maintenance of frequent breast pumping with a hospital-grade double electric breast pump, skin-to-skin holding as soon and as often as possible, non-nutritive sucking at breast (breast pumped first, although the breast is never truly empty and some milk may be available), and establishing the basics of breastfeeding before offering a bottle are all useful for establishing and maintaining a milk supply.[40,103] Late preterm infants (34-36$\frac{6}{7}$ weeks gestation) are especially vulnerable to being discharged before breastfeeding is well established, with increased risk of significant medical complications. Breastfeeding educator (breastfeeding specialist) courses are often available through state health departments or Women, Infants, and Children (WIC) clinics; these courses are highly recommended to build knowledge, confidence, and competence. Websites such as those by the Academy of Breastfeeding (http://www.bfmed.org) can also provide useful information. Some neonatal developmental specialists may eventually choose to continue breastfeeding specialization by pursuing credentials to become an international board-certified lactation consultant (IBCLC; http://www.ilca.org).

Oral Feeding

Parents often ask when their baby can go home. For most NICU babies, the last obstacle to hospital discharge is accomplishing oral feeding. Historically, sufficient time was allowed for the preterm infant to gain endurance and for suck-swallow-breathe coordination to mature. Currently, however, oral feedings are often initiated at earlier ages or pushed more aggressively for earlier discharge.[126] Although early oral feeding may be successful for certain infants and families, others struggle when discharged and may be readmitted for dehydration or failure to gain weight.[31,117] Because preterm infants do not orally feed like term infants, the following sections establish a foundation of infant feeding basics, terminology, and mechanics that are applied in subsequent sections to oral feeding practices in the NICU.

Non-Nutritive Sucking

Non-nutritive sucking (NNS), or dry sucking without fluid, such as on a fist or pacifier, is present but disorganized in infants younger than 30 weeks; sucking rhythm generally improves by 30 to 32 weeks' postconception. Because NNS sucking does not interrupt breathing, it is usually (but not always) established before an infant has the neurologic maturation to coordinate sucking with swallowing and breathing.

NNS has been described as a self-soothing activity. Benefits of NNS have been summarized as increased oxygenation, faster transition to nipple feeding, and better bottle-feeding performance. Infants who engage in NNS during tube feeding experience less time in fussy and awake states, quicker settling after feedings, fewer defensive behaviors during tube feeding, and a significantly decreased hospital stay. No short-term negative effects have been identified.[106] In addition, NNS on a pacifier dipped in a 24% sucrose solution is advocated for the relief of procedural pain.[96]

Nutritive Sucking Patterns

Nutritive sucking is stimulated by the presence of fluid that must be swallowed; suck and swallow must be coordinated with breathing. Infants with organized sucking patterns (mature or immature) who can coordinate sucks and swallows with breathing are generally safe feeders when behavioral cues are respected. Transitional or disorganized feeding patterns are common in preterm or ill NICU infants learning to feed orally; these infants have difficulty coordinating sucks and swallows with breathing and benefit from caregiver interventions, such as slow-flow nipples and pacing to force breaks for breathing. Dysfunctional feeders demonstrate abnormal movements of the jaw and tongue; oral feeding is often possible but with atypical oral mechanics.[101] Identification of the infant's sucking pattern can guide the developmental specialist's expectations and interventions, prevent the inadvertent facilitation of increased disorganization, promote improved oral feeding mechanics, and hopefully minimize the risk of future oral aversion.

Mature sucking is an organized feeding pattern typical of healthy term infants. Sucking bursts are initially continuous for 10 to 30 sucks, with a smooth 1 : 1 : 1 or 2 : 1 : 1 suck-swallow-breathe rhythm in which respiration appears continuous and uninterrupted. Brief respiratory pauses between sucking bursts may be noted. Sucking bursts are usually longest at the beginning of a feeding (continuous sucking), followed by intermittent sucking, with more opportunities for breathing as the feeding continues. Aside from normal infant feeding techniques (e.g., adequate postural support, calm environment, burping), no therapeutic interventions are necessary. Some term newborns eat well from the start; others seem to need a few days to recover from birth, gain endurance, and develop hunger.

Instead of having the 1 : 1 : 1 or 2 : 1 : 1 suck-swallow-breathe coordination seen in term babies, infants with an immature sucking pattern often cluster three to five sucks together while holding their breath, swallow the accumulated bolus, and then cluster several rapid recovery breaths. Observed in healthy preterm infants as young as 32½ weeks, this pattern is slower and not as efficient as mature sucking, but may appear organized, because sucks and swallows alternate with breathing in a coordinated manner. Breath-holding during sucking is believed to be related to the infant's instinct to protect the airway from penetration by the liquid bolus. These infants should be allowed to set their own pace and avoid stimulating sucking when they are in the breathing pause of the cycle. If the rest pause becomes prolonged, a slight gentle outward tug on the nipple may encourage the infant to relatch and continue sucking; conversely, twirling the nipple in the infant's mouth can make the nipple difficult to grasp and can eject unwanted milk into the infants mouth, causing distress and/or aspiration. Forced oral feeding (caregiver working harder than the baby or passively milking formula into the mouth of a nonparticipatory infant) increases the risk of disorganization and aspiration. Endurance may be limited, with the remainder of a feed given by gavage tube if the infant becomes fatigued.

A transitional (disorganized) pattern, observed in some preterm infants and older medically fragile infants (up to 45 weeks' PMA), is characterized by difficulty coordinating suck and swallow with breathing.[100] An infant tries to use the continuous sucking burst of a mature pattern, but does not yet have a smooth rhythm of suck-swallow with breathing. Sucking bursts are generally six to ten sucks, but frequent and significant variation in the length of sucking bursts may occur during the same feeding. Intermittent or increasing disorganization, air hunger with apnea after longer sucking bursts, and insufficient endurance to complete the feeding are common. Disorganized transitional sucking is a frequently observed feeding pattern in NICU infants. Suck-swallow-breathe coordination can be facilitated by providing secure postural support, reducing stimuli, and using a slow-flow nipple and pacing to allow breathing pauses (Figure 21-19). An infant with chronic lung disease may benefit from temporarily increased supplemental oxygen during feeding. A cue-based feeding approach (see later) allows an infant to drive the frequency and duration of oral feedings without being force-fed.

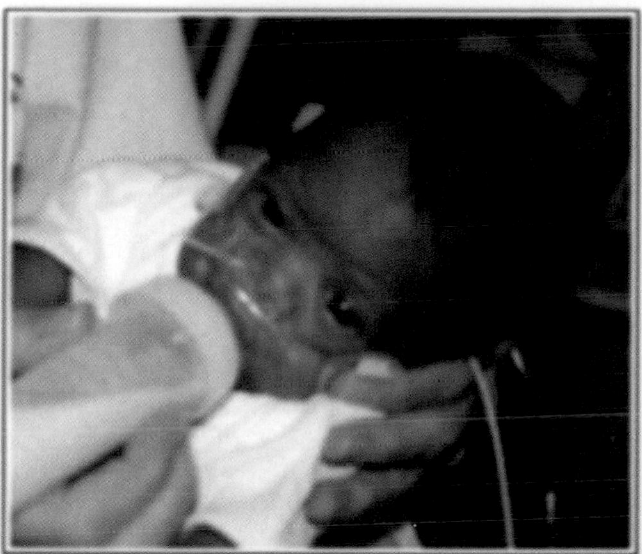

FIGURE 21-19 This infant has a transitional sucking pattern in which suck-swallow is not yet well coordinated with breathing. External pacing is provided when the caregiver tips the bottle (without removing nipple from mouth) to force a breathing break. (Courtesy Infant Special Care Unit, University of Texas Medical Branch, Galveston, TX. Photographs by Jan Hunter).

Oral motor interventions vary with each infant, but may include options such as prefeeding oral stimulation for a warm-up and use of different nipples, jaw support, inward and downward pressure on the tongue to inhibit excessive protrusion, and thickened formula for easier oral bolus control

Liquid is removed (stripped) from the nipple by a combination of suction (negative pressure) and compression (positive pressure).[62] Suction refers to negative intraoral pressure generated as the infant (1) enlarges the oral cavity by lowering the jaw and (2) prevents air entry by sealing the lips around the nipple and elevating the soft palate to close off the nasopharynx. Compression occurs when the nipple is squeezed against the premaxilla (gums) and palate by the tongue and lower jaw; compression is exerted by repetitive peristaltic motions of the tongue that strip fluid from the nipple. Compromise of either

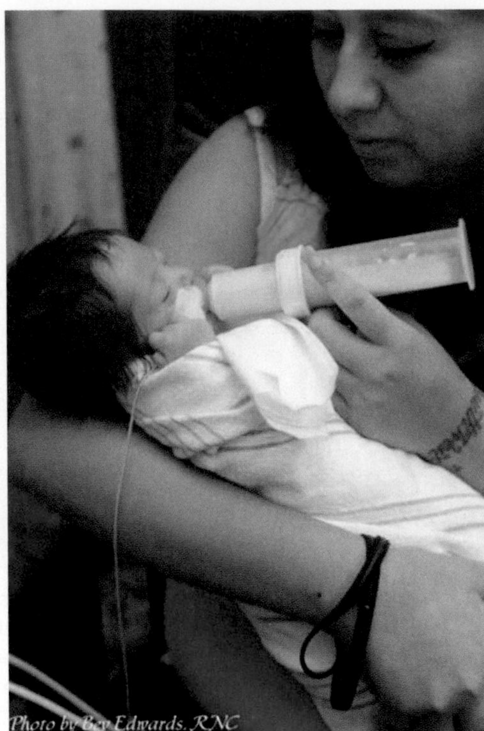

FIGURE 21-20 This infant with Down syndrome has decreased feeding endurance, with an intact swallow but weak stripping of milk from the nipple. His mother is using a Haberman feeder for added nipple length and variable flow to help compensate and improve feeding function. (Courtesy NICU, Memorial Hermann Hospital Southwest, Houston, TX. Photograph by Beverly Edwards.)

of these sucking pressure components, as in a very hypotonic infant or one with a cleft lip and palate, reduces the efficiency of stripping. An infant with poor suction or stripping may demonstrate rhythmic sucking, with relatively little milk removed from the bottle. Special nipples and bottles may be useful (Figure 21-20). Note that nipple collapse and/or vacuum pressure in the bottle may also prevent milk removal.

Oral feeding compromises oxygenation and ventilation during nutritive sucking because the airway briefly closes during every reflexive swallow.[75] This compromise is more significant during continuous sucking than during intermittent sucking and worse with an indwelling nasogastric tube than without the tube.[125] Preterm and ill infants frequently demonstrate physiologic and neurologic immaturity, respiratory compromise, disorganized sucking, and inadequate endurance.[11] Disorganized sucking and breathing often persist in the infant with chronic lung disease because the need to breathe supersedes the infant's efforts to suck.

Improvement in feeding-induced apnea, often associated with multiple swallows without breathing, appears to correlate more with advancing age (maturation) than with practice.[58] Traditionally, this has been interpreted to mean that additional time to mature is more beneficial than more frequent opportunities to "practice" oral feeding for young preterm infants.

In addition to the suck-swallow reflex, a term neonate has anatomic and physiologic safety features that offer some natural protection against aspiration. These include proportionately large soft tissue structures (tongue, epiglottis, and vocal folds), relatively small openings, shorter passageways of smaller diameter, and a higher resting position of the larynx under the base of the tongue, providing an umbrella or watershed protective effect. A preterm infant with less mature development and function of these structures may not have the same degree of protection from aspiration during feeding; trace aspiration may occur frequently, and frank aspiration often is silent—no clinical signs of choking, coughing, or color change.[38] Initiation of bottle feeding at 30 to 33 weeks' PMA has increased in some NICUs,[63,74] but the possibility of silent aspiration during bottle feeding at 30 to 32 weeks' PMA has not been studied with definitive modified barium swallow studies, and therefore the ultimate safety of these early feedings is not known.

Developmentally Supportive Feeding Interventions

Developmentally supportive feeding focuses on the infant. Neurologic maturation, medical issues, ongoing physiologic status, current stage of feeding readiness and skills, and psychosocial and interactive skills have redefined feeding success in the NICU. Quantity becomes secondary to the safety and quality of the feed.[118,123] The infant is supported during the feeding to avoid physiologic and neurobehavioral stress and instability, facilitate healthy adaptive feeding behaviors, and encourage nurturing interaction. The family develops confidence in their ability to read and respond to the infant's cues and nourish and nurture their baby as he or she learns to eat.

Because of an immature digestive system, preterm infants often struggle to achieve adequate nutrient absorption and gut tolerance of feedings.[9] These medical issues, coupled with pressure to increase intake for adequate weight gain, often cause feedings (oral or tube) to be unpleasant and stressful for the infant. Significant feeding and nutritional problems may persist long after NICU discharge.[59,117]

Late preterm infants (35-37 weeks' gestation) are expected to feed orally as competently as term infants, but they often struggle. The brain in late preterm infants remains underdeveloped. Physiologic and neuromotor immaturity, lack of endurance, poor state regulation, and medical complications can interfere with oral feeding.[86] Infants with anomalies or persistent illness who are unable to achieve oral feeding within a reasonable time may be sent home with feeding gastrostomy tubes (G-tubes). With an increased risk of disorganization and silent aspiration in the NICU population, each infant's feeding readiness and safety should guide caregiver efforts.

Oral feeding is complex, and an infant must develop many underlying skills to establish and maintain oral nutrition successfully.[11,123] Ross and Browne have identified stage progression for an infant learning to feed orally[116] (Box 21-5). These stages involve developing and maintaining stability in the physiologic, motor, and state subsystems during the work of feeding, and eventually interacting with the caregiver during feeding. (**NOTE:** Very early feedings should be nurturing, but not overtly and reciprocally social.)

The Supporting Oral Feeding in Fragile Infants (SOFFI) method is an evidence-based, clinical manual for providing quality bottle feedings for preterm, ill, and fragile infants.[102] The SOFFI method provides evidence-based text, algorithms, and reference guides for the NICU developmental specialist and bedside nurse. It is not a tool to be used during feeding itself, but rather a learning and reference tool that provides

BOX 21-5 BROSS Feeding Stages

Stage I

Stability while in bed during handling: The infant maintains stability in physiologic, motoric, and state systems while in the bed and interacting with a caregiver during routine caregiving.

1. Heart rate (HR) = 120-180 beats/min; respiratory rate (RR) = 40-60 beats/min; oxygen saturation (Sao_2) ≥ 90%
2. Able to maintain flexion of body and extremities and return to flexion after movement
3. Able to maintain body tone without flaccidity or limpness
4. Skin tone with underlying pink to slight redness overall, possible slight duskiness around eyes and mouth
5. Ability to come into an alert state emerging, with duration of <5 min
6. Mouthing on fingers and/or pacifier with support

Stage II

Stability of systems while being held; infant maintains stability in physiologic, motoric, and state systems while in the arms of a caregiver

1. Maintains stable HR, RR, and Sao_2 level
2. Able to maintain body tone without flaccidity or limpness
3. Able to remain softly rounded and maintain flexion of arms, legs, and back with support.
4. Maintains alert state for up to 10 min
5. More successful at bringing hands to face and mouth and sucking on fingers and pacifier

Stage III

Stability in arms while sucking on a pacifier—infant has a coordinated non-nutritive suck (NNS) pattern of two sucks/second

1. Maintains a stable HR, RR, and Sao_2 level
2. Maintains flexion and tone.
3. Beginning to have rhythmic sucking of pacifier or fingers, five to ten sucks/burst
4. Able to be alert and suck on fingers, pacifier for at least half of gavage feeding time

Stage IV

Obligatory—infant sucks on a nipple without stopping to breathe to the point of apnea and loss of subsystem stability unless caregiver intervenes

1. Vigorous sucking on the bottle nipple without apparent recognition of the need to integrate breathing
2. Often drops breathing rate and has a prolonged apnea spell
3. May result in a bradycardic event
4. Drop in oxygenation level if sucking and breathing are not paced by caregiver
5. Nipple expression is fairly strong, with large jaw excursions
6. Little modulation of suction and expression
7. 15-25 sucks/burst not uncommon
8. Sucking strength decreases as burst progresses
9. Will often lose motor tone if not paced by caregiver
10. Will often fall into light sleep quickly, before completing much volume

Stage V

Alternating—infant begins to alternate breathing periods with sucking bursts of 10-15 sucks/burst, followed by a breathing period

1. Alternation of sucking and breathing periods
2. Shortening of sucking bursts, down to five to ten sucks initially, then down to three to five sucks when more mature
3. May drop oxygen levels initially, until breathing every three to five sucks
4. Some variability in pattern of number of sucks per burst.
5. Appears to have less strength of suction and expression as infant tries to integrate sucking and breathing
6. Beginning to be alert prior to feeding and maintain alertness for most of the feeding
7. May use a drop in state to drowsy or light sleep as a self-regulatory compensatory skill

Stage VI

Intermittent—infant begins to integrate breathing with sucking burst, rather than alternating between breathing and sucking-swallowing; shows coordination of breathing during a sucking burst, initially has inconsistent pattern of one breath per two or three sucks, can maintain stability of subsystems

1. First coordination of sucking-swallowing-breathing
2. Brief catch breaths occur usually at least once every two or three sucks
3. Longer sucking bursts of 10-20 sucks beginning to appear
4. Oxygenation is (or oxygen levels are) stable during feeding
5. Suction becoming stronger, with collapse of nipple more common while the infant tries to integrate suction with expression
6. More efficient sucking, with greater volume
7. Length of each nutritive suck increases
8. Infant usually in alert state for entire feeding, but concentrates on feeding

Stage VII

Coordinated—infant can coordinate sucking, swallowing, and breathing, resulting in longer sucking bursts of 10-30 sucks.

1. Mature coordination of sucking-swallowing-breathing
2. Brief catch breaths occur usually at least once every one or two sucks
3. Longer sucking bursts beginning to appear, 10-30 sucks
4. Oxygenation stable during feeding
5. Suction integrated with expression, resulting in more efficient sucking
6. Greater volume consumed
7. Length of each nutritive suck burst increases
8. Infant usually maintains alert state for entire feeding, but concentrates on feeding

Stage VIII

Integrated—infant has a mature coordinated suck pattern while interacting with caregiver during the feeding.

1. Longer sucking bursts of 20-30 sucks/burst
2. Breathing occurs during sucking bursts, with 1 : 1 : 1 suck-swallow-breathe, very little variability
3. Catch breaths during sucking bursts
4. Rapid breathing between sucking bursts
5. Able to modulate suction and expression, which creates more efficient suck
6. Infant alert and demanding feedings
7. Able to integrate social interaction with caregiver during the feeding
8. Able to maintain alertness for the entire feeding; available for interaction after the feeding as well

clinicians and professional caregivers with guidance as they progress through assessment, decisions, and consequent actions. The goal of using such an all-encompassing method is to focus on the quality of the feeding rather than the volume, so that attainment of oral feeding success is done through nurturing experiences and at the infant's own pace. In turn, these methods increase the likelihood of building a foundation that will nurture continued success and reduce the risk for feeding problems in infancy and throughout early childhood.

Because premature infants rarely go home from the NICU with an integrated mastery of oral feeding (stage VIII), parents and caregivers need to be comfortable and confident in recognizing, interpreting, and responding to the infant's behaviors to support him or her appropriately through the final steps of feeding mastery at home.[124] The developmental specialist and bedside nurse educate the family to read subtle infant behaviors and teach them how to alter feeding to support the acquisition of healthy feeding behaviors.

Feeding Readiness and Cue-Based, Infant-Driven Feeding

A cue-based or infant-driven approach to oral feeding is the state-of-the-art approach. This individualized approach to feeding readiness considers factors such as the infant's medical status, neurobehavioral organization (vigor, sleep-wake cycle, ability to achieve some stable alert periods, autonomic, motor, and state stability), and feeding readiness cues (e.g., awakening or fussing prior to feedings, spontaneous rooting and sucking behaviors, gagging with gavage tube insertion).[123] Initiation of oral feeding, whether at breast or bottle, is based on when the infant shows readiness, and readiness is assessed at or surrounding each feeding time. If the infant awakens (either on his or her own or with caregiving) and shows readiness cues, he or she is given a chance to feed orally. Once the oral feeding begins, continual caregiver assessment of the infant's physiologic stability and participation in feeding determines how long the oral feeding lasts. Any volume that is not taken orally is simply given through the nasogastric tube.

For example, an infant who does not arouse with caregiving or initiate sucking on the nipple will receive a supplemental feeding by nasogastric tube; an infant who does well initially before becoming disorganized, tachypneic, or too drowsy may feed orally for a few minutes, with the remaining volume given by nasogastric tube.[102] Staff members can offer oral feedings more often but avoid prolonged sessions of trying to force-feed preset volumes. Ideally, cumulative exhaustion is avoided, with improved weight gain and smoother transition to oral feeds. Because infant-driven feedings depend on active infant participation rather than on caregiver manipulations, organization and safety are increased.

Because the infant participates during cue-based feedings, parents often experience greater success feeding their baby. Teaching parents how to reduce extraneous external stimuli, read and respect their infant's individual cues, provide secure postural support, and facilitate rest pauses or breathing breaks as needed (external pacing) boosts their confidence and increases the success of oral feeding after discharge.

Descriptive scales can be included on nursing flow sheets (now usually in the form of an electronic medical record) to document feeding readiness and performance at each feeding more consistently and objectively.[97,141] These scales allow NICU staff to document behaviors and interventions quickly so that all caregivers involved in supporting the infant's oral feeding development can have a full picture of what is occurring (Figure 21-21).

Partnering with Families in the NICU

The admission of an infant to the NICU frequently puts the infant's family in crisis, with an intense onslaught of confusing emotions. The delivery was often unexpected, and the family is now separated. The appearance of the infant can be frightening and the NICU environment overwhelming. Unknown staff and unfamiliar terminology can hinder effective communication. Some mothers have continued physical complications or illness from the pregnancy or delivery, but think that they must ignore their own healing to focus on their infants. Financial considerations, transportation or travel issues, and conflicting needs of siblings can be worrisome. Parental shock, denial, depression, and grief over loss of the ideal birth and perfect infant are compounded by concerns for the recovery of a critically ill infant.

State-of-the-art NICUs have now moved from family-centered care to family-driven care to partnering with families, in which mutual collaboration exists between caregivers and families.[27,90] The NICU environment can become comforting and inviting when attentive and compassionate caregivers welcome parents to the infant's bedside. Compassionate caregivers teach parents to understand their baby's behavioral cues and provide developmentally appropriate positioning and handling. They actively listen as parents process their shock, anger, and grief over the loss of a normal pregnancy and/or normal healthy term infant and help them heal the wounds of interrupted bonding with their infants. The concept of partnering with families in the NICU acknowledges that over time, the family has the greatest influence over an infant's health and well-being.[9] Creating an effective partnership between professionals and families has shown benefits such as decreased length of stay, increased satisfaction for staff and parents, and enhanced neurodevelopmental outcomes for infants.[36]

Facilitating attachment is a priority for all health care providers in the NICU. Early life attachment keeps the baby in the proximity of the mother to ensure infant survival, guides brain development and overall mental health, promotes emotional availability, and contributes to positive infant developmental outcomes such as cognition.[131]

A nontraditional work schedule that includes some evenings, weekends, and holidays greatly increases the developmental specialist's availability and benefit to families. Some family-friendly NICU routines and practices automatically facilitate parenting. Placing twins in adjacent bed spaces rather than in separate areas of the nursery helps create a family space. Staff efforts to make the infant as comfortable and as normal-looking as possible (e.g., positional nesting, dressing in baby clothes, adding a hair bow, providing a cute name tag) help parents look beyond the diagnosis and technology. Diligence in using an infant's name and correct gender demonstrates to the family that staff members acknowledge their baby as a real person, not just a sick patient. Caregiving can often be more flexible to accommodate parents' schedules. The inclusion of

CUE BASED FEEDING SCALES AND DOCUMENTATION TIPS

Feeding								
Readiness								
Quality								
Caregiver								
Time								
Quantity								
Nipple (circle breast or write nipple color)	Breast Nipple Color ______	Breast Nipple Color ______	Breast Nipple Color ______	Breast Nipple Color ______	Breast Nipple Color ______	Breast Nipple Color ______	Breast Nipple Color ______	Breast Nipple Color ______
Initial								

Readiness*:

Score			Description
Breastfeed	Bottle	1	Drowsy, alert or fussy prior to care. Rooting and/or hands to mouth / takes pacifier. Good tone.
		2	Drowsy or alert once handled. Some rooting or takes pacifier. Adequate tone.
	No bottle	3	Briefly alert with care. No hunger behaviors. No change in tone.
		4	Sleeping throughout care. No hunger cues. No change in tone.
Gavage Only		5	Needs increased O2 with care. A/B with care. Tachypnea over baseline with care.

Caregiver Techniques*:

Score	Description
A	Side-lying Position
B	External Pacing
C	Adding or Increasing O2 during feed
D	Imposed Breaks
E	Stimulation for / Recovery from A's / B's
F	Frequent Burping
G	Nipple Change
H	Other (Specify)

Quality Bottle*:

Score	Description
1	Nipples with a strong coordinated suck throughout feed.
2	Nipples with a strong coordinated suck initially, but fatigues with progression
3	Nipples with consistent suck, but difficulty coordinating swallow; some loss of liquid or difficulty pacing. Benefits from external pacing.
4	Nipples with a weak/inconsistent suck. Little to no rhythm. May require some rest breaks.
5	Disorganized: Unable to coordinate suck / swallow / breathe pattern despite packing. May result in frequent or significant A/B's or large amounts of liquid loss and/or tachypnea significantly above baseline with feeding.
6	Dysfunctional: Abnormal or deviant oral motor patterns evidenced by inability to extract fluid from nipple.

Quality Breastfeeding:

Score	Description
1	Latched well with a strong coordinated suck for >15 min.
2	Latched well with a strong coordinated suck initially, but fatigues with progression. Active suck for 8 - 15 min.
3	Difficulty maintaining a strong, consistent latch. May be able to intermittently nurse but only active for <15 min.
4	Latch is weak / inconsistent with a frequent need to "re-latch". Limited effort that is inconsistent in pattern. May be considered NNBF.
5	Unable to latch to breast and achieve suck / swallow / breathe pattern. May have difficulty arousing to state conducive to breastfeeding. Could result in frequent or significant A/B's and/or tachypnea significantly above baseline with feeding.

*adapted from Ludwig & Waitzman 2007

Date ______________ Signature: ______________ ______________

______________ ______________

Legend: **A/B** – Apnea/Bradycardia, **NNBF** – Non Nutritional Breastfeeding, **BF** – Breastfeed, **HFNC** – High Flow Nasal Cannula
CPAP = Continuous Positive Airway Pressure, **NPO** – Nothing By Mouth, **NG** = Nasogastric, **GA** = Gestational Age

BAYLOR UNIVERSITY MEDICAL CENTER
DALLAS, TEXAS

52606 (08/10)

CUE BASED FEEDING SCALES AND DOCUMENTATION TIPS

FIGURE 21-21 Cue-based infant feeding scales and documentation tips on nursing flow sheet, Baylor University Medical Center. (From Newland, L., L'Huillier, M., & Petrey, B. (2013). Implementation of cue based feeding in a level III NICU. *Neonatal Network, 32,* 132–137.)

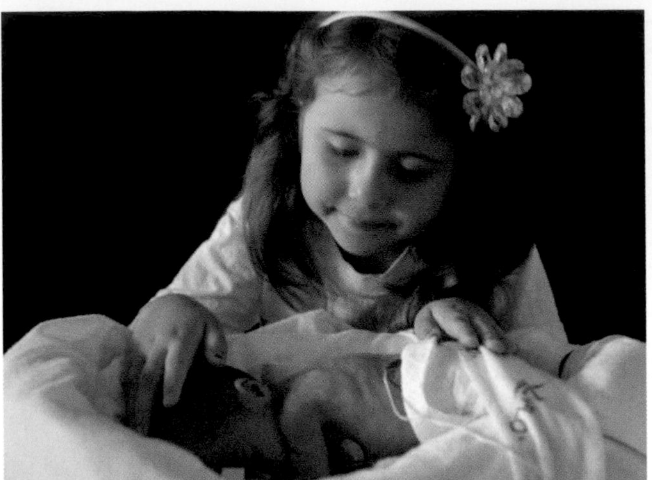

FIGURE 21-22 Family-centered care encourages and supports siblings to be an active part of their premature sibling's NICU stay. This can help relieve parental and sibling stress, as well as facilitate early attachment within the NICU setting. (Courtesy of the NICU, Memorial Hermann Hospital Southwest, Houston, TX. Photograph by Beverly Edwards.)

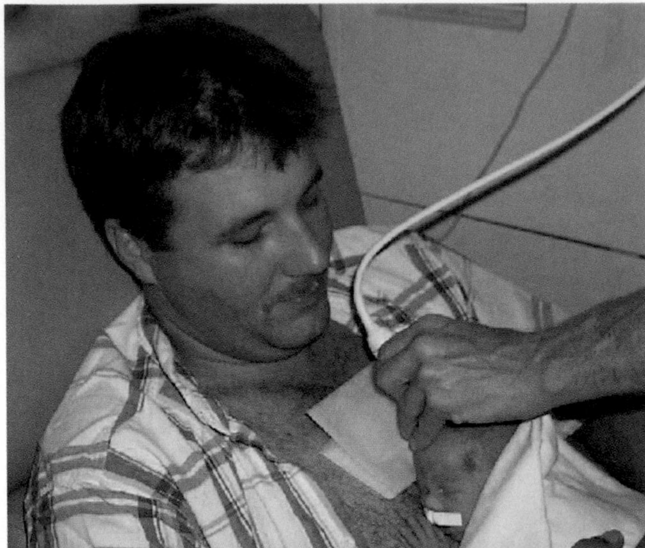

FIGURE 21-23 Infant having a head ultrasound to rule out intraventricular hemorrhage while resting comfortably on his father's chest during skin-to-skin holding. Infants tolerate many procedures better during kangaroo care. (Courtesy of the Infant Special Care Unit, University of Texas Medical Branch, Galveston, TX. Photographs by Jan Hunter).

siblings, extended family members, and other support persons should be encouraged (Figure 21-22).

Parents are encouraged to ask questions about what they understand and want to know; staff responses need to be honest, consistent, and understandable. Parents become frustrated when information appears contradictory, but anxiety from incomplete information or a perceived lack of truth is often alleviated with a sincere collaborative partnership. The former approach of "therapist as expert, child as client, parents as students" has been replaced by reciprocal dialogue; the developmental specialist talks with rather than to parents, and facilitates the family's active role with their infant and on the NICU team. Recognizing parental skills, celebrating successes, and facilitating parent's expertise are invaluable.

Awareness that gentle nurturing touch from mothers to their infants can influence pain sensitivity, affect, and growth in neonates has prompted encouragement of kangaroo care, skin-to-skin contact, and infant massage. This reciprocal tactile stimulation between mother and infant may contribute to increased maternal responsiveness and infant attachment.[32] When the quality and/or quantity of parental care toward infants is limited, such as with preterm infants in the NICU setting, these adverse experiences can lead to changes in brain architecture and function.[55]

Skin-to-Skin Care: Kangaroo Mother Care

Because the optimal caregiving environment for the infant is the mother's body, it is thought that separation from the mother plus noxious environmental and tactile stimuli in the NICU overwhelm the developing preterm infant's self-regulatory abilities.[99] Kangaroo care (KC), also called skin-to-skin care (SSC), refers to the practice of parents holding their diaper-clad premature infant on a parent's bare chest in an upright prone position; it is a fundamental component of neuroprotective and patient-family oriented care for hospitalized preterm infants[84,85] (Figure 21-23). Kangaroo care originated in Bogota, Colombia, in response to overcrowded nurseries and insufficient medical equipment but is now a global initiative.

Kangaroo care practices vary among individual NICUs according to age, weight, and acuity of the infant; skin-to-skin holding has historically been more widely accepted for stable infants not on ventilators. A Cochrane review of 16 RCTs, including 2518 infants, demonstrated a reduction in the risk of mortality, nosocomial infection and sepsis, hypothermia, and length of hospital stay. KC was also found to increase some measures of infant growth, breastfeeding, and mother-infant attachment.[39] A recent study has confirmed that SSC seems safe and effective for vulnerable preterm infants in the NICU, and SSC can be beneficial for ventilated, VLBW preterm infants.[33] These findings demonstrate a paradigm shift. Believing that "this infant is too unstable for SSC care" can be replaced by "this baby is too unstable not to implement SSC." Earlier initiation, frequency, and duration of SSC may help contribute to improved neurodevelopment of these infants.[84]

Both infant and parents benefit from skin-to-skin holding.[39,84] Physiologic benefits to the infant from skin-to-skin holding include more stable heart and breathing rates, reduced apnea, stable body temperature, improved weight gain and growth, decreased or less severe infections, and improved tolerance of procedures during skin-to-skin holding (see Figure 21-23). Infant behavioral benefits include decreased agitation, less random motor activity, reduction in stress from environmental disturbances and medical interventions, improved state control, with less crying and better self-regulation, and more mature sleep organization. An easier transition to breastfeeding, earlier hospital discharge, and a positive effect on neurodevelopmental outcomes have also been reported.

Skin-to-skin holding facilitates maternal milk production and longer duration of breastfeeding. Parents develop an increased awareness of their infant's cues of well-being or distress and increased attachment and feelings of closeness to their infant. They demonstrate more positive touch of their infant, less focus on technical care, more confidence in their own caregiving ability, and decreased maternal stress.

Establishing Your Niche in the NICU Team

A neonatal developmental specialist must master specialized knowledge and skills to work effectively and competently as part of the high-tech, neonatal care team. In addition, a few distinctions may be helpful in understanding and directing this journey.

Although developmental specialists in the NICU are currently much more common than in years past, the uniqueness of this role is neither universally understood nor applied. Staff and leadership in some NICUs may continue with a traditional therapy rehabilitation role of a consult to treat pathology but not yet appreciate the neuroprotective role of developmental support beginning at birth or the value of total team inclusion in decisions affecting infant and family support and system changes. Effort invested in educating and eliciting NICU management support for your neuroprotective developmental role will be time well spent.

Therapy supervisors may not realize that not just any therapist can rotate through the NICU according to staffing and census patterns. NICU training is extensive and productivity can be affected by indirect but very important aspects of interventions, such as collaboration or advocating for NICU developmental care. Leadership roles in developmental care include helping develop or refine policies and procedures, orienting NICU staff and physicians, developing comprehensive programs to ensure inclusion of developmentally appropriate practices and equipment, enabling consistent staff support and encouragement, and keeping current with the evidence base for neuroprotective developmentally supportive care.

Aspiring developmental specialists with previous clinical experience who are new to the NICU often have difficulty with the concept of beginning over until they realize that the NICU culture is truly unique, with its own hierarchy, set of rules, timetable, and rhythm. Furthermore, NICU infants are different from all other patient populations; direct application of interventions common for the pediatric population and adults are often not appropriate in the NICU.

For novice developmental specialists, who tend to be concrete and want a formula for success, the task of discernment can be daunting. It is advisable to evaluate the credentials of presenters and writers thoughtfully and use caution before implementation; don't be the first to jump on the bandwagon or the last to jump off. It is also necessary to learn to read neonatal literature, remaining aware that information needs to be critically analyzed rather than blindly accepted.[109]

Many new developmental specialists are tempted to rush into the many specialized training and certification courses now readily available. However, time spent in the NICU, with a focus on basics (e.g., respiratory management, nutrition and nonoral feeding, equipment, developmental care, family-centered care) before pursuit of specialty certifications, especially if there is also inexperience with critically judging literature or presentations, will greatly increase the benefits of advanced training. Time in the NICU gives the new NICU developmental specialist a chance to observe the progression of multiple infants over time, learning the wide range of normal and what is truly atypical.

Building a Successful NICU Practice

Progressing from a perceived guest to an integrated and valued team member in the NICU will take time and may not always be smooth. Staff members who do not understand the NICU developmental specialist's role or are threatened by encroachment on their turf may initially exhibit opposition and competitiveness. This is especially true with someone new and inexperienced in the NICU; for example, a new developmental specialist's academic education on infant feeding is often not convincing to the seasoned nurse who "has fed a thousand babies."

Every new person in the NICU must individually earn staff's respect, acceptance and trust, all necessary components of any successful relationship. This does not come inherent with a degree or title, but instead comes from proving to be a skilled, knowledgeable, and compassionate colleague over time, willingly learning from staff and respecting their expertise. NICU staff instinctively and vigorously try to protect their vulnerable patients; even those whose caregiving or approach to parents could be considered nondevelopmental are probably convinced that they are doing what is best for their babies. See Box 21-6 on the Evolve website.

Connection with staff on a social level is a positive start; next comes engagement of staff on a professional and educational level. Unit culture, unit leadership expectations and support, and individual mind sets of staff all affect whether education and new learning and changes in practice are desired or dreaded. Either way, education and change are mandatory for providing ongoing optimal care. The successful developmental specialist learns staff's needs, quirks, and preferences and adapts necessary education approaches over time in ways that are accepted and inspiring.

NICU staff work in a high-pressure environment in which room for error is small or nonexistent. They are (rightfully) protective of their babies and may likely rebuff or ignore a motivated energetic newcomer who jumps right in with unsolicited bedside teaching or organized in-services before making connections or earning staff trust and respect. When a new developmental specialist is proactive by being patient and skilled before pushing for changes, he or she is more likely to earn acceptance and respect. When staff attend interdisciplinary trainings together, they bond and learn to appreciate each discipline's skill set. Professional practice acts set boundaries on performing some specific tasks, but knowing why something is important and how it is done fosters mutual understanding and appreciation. It prevents the perception that you think you already know it all and offers opportunities for positive reinforcement to staff when standards or expectations are exceeded.

The outline in Box 21-7 on the Evolve website provides some practical suggestions and words of wisdom for success in facilitating professional and educational engagement with NICU staff (Figure 21-24).

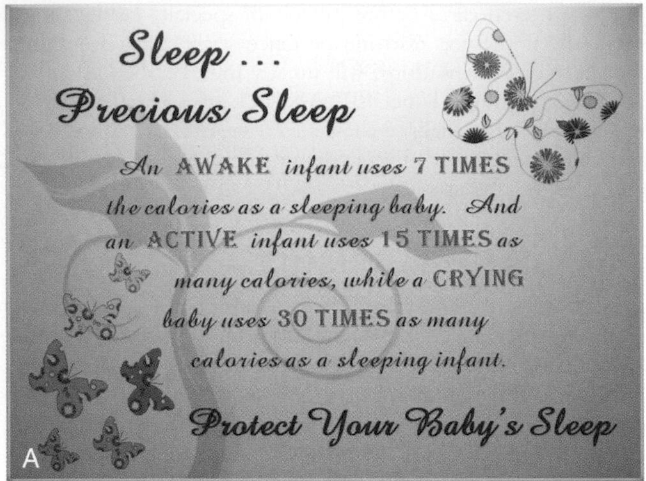

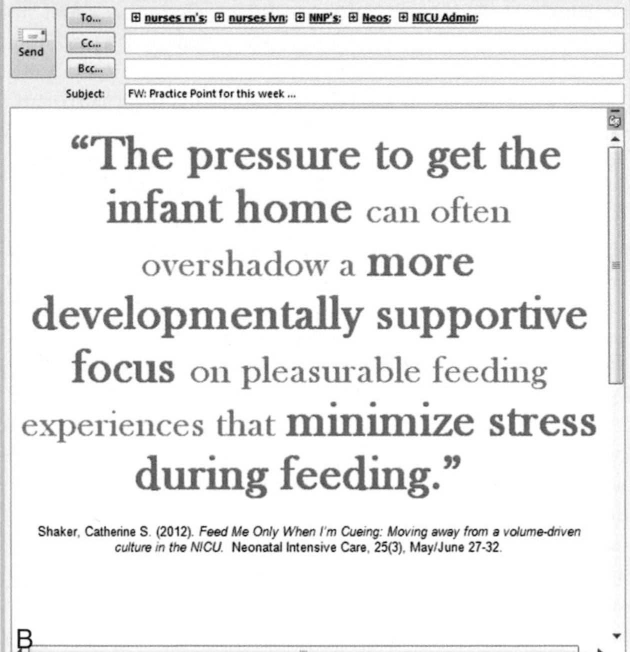

FIGURE 21-24 **A and B,** Using a poster and group e-mail to foster a climate of learning.

Reflective Practice

Finally, a staff culture of reflective practice can drive competency, motivation, and engagement in continuous learning. With reflective practice, occupational therapists consistently step back after doing something or observing an outcome, and ask what could be changed the next time for better results. Perhaps more open communication, more timely respect for the infant, or family cues could have changed the outcome. The process of reflection may allow illumination of ungrounded habits ("We've always done it this way"), bring unconscious knowledge to the forefront ("Oh! That's why this technique works"), and open dialogue that leads to change. For example, after a procedure or feeding, the developmental specialist can ask staff questions such as "How do you think that went for the baby?" or "What do you think he or she had trouble handling?" The hope is that reflection will open communication and awareness of how staff can collectively better support the infants. The term *reflective practice* was coined by Schon,[122] demonstrating the significance of the role of practice for the development of professional knowledge. Two types of reflection were identified, reflection in action and reflection on action. Reflection in action occurs while the developmental specialist is practicing, and influences the decisions made and the care given. Experienced developmental specialists are able to reflect in action by showing their ability to explore and examine responses to a situation while actually being involved in it and can adapt their actions accordingly. Reflection on action is a retrospective contemplation of practice taken to uncover the knowledge used during a particular event by becoming self-aware.[34] The key to reflection is understanding that it is not complete without action, and the goal of reflection is to challenge and ultimately change practice.[8]

Summary

Developmentally supportive care has sometimes been perceived as consisting of optional practices in a primarily technologically driven environment. However, ignorance or dismissal of the evidence that supports neuroprotective care for a preterm infant is no longer acceptable. Consistent acceptance, practice, and accountability must be established to provide the high-quality care that every infant and family deserves. Use of established guidelines, policies, and procedures to guide neonatal practice is essential. Health care professionals must be cognizant of the growing body of research regarding the impact of the NICU environment on neurodevelopmental outcomes. Recognition of neurobehavioral stability and the links to developmental care and long-term outcomes are increasing. Follow-up studies of formerly sick and premature infants are important because they are used to examine developmental outcomes, the need for developmental care from birth, and the potential costs associated with physiologic complications and sequelae that might be reduced or avoided with proper developmental care.[69]

The NICU is a complex hospital unit in which specialized care is provided to infants who are born prematurely or with significant medical problems. Neonatal developmental specialists who work in the NICU must be armed with specialized knowledge about neonatal medical conditions, intensive care equipment, necessary precautions related to handling the neonates, preterm infant development, and interventions that are neuroprotective and promote behavioral organization and interaction. This chapter described the NICU environment and emphasized how preterm neonatal neurobehavioral systems are affected by their sensory systems, especially in regard to sound and lighting conditions. The following points summarize this chapter:

- Historically, the focus of occupational therapists in the NICU was rehabilitation and developmental stimulation for older chronic infants with specific pathology or functional deficits. Currently, developmental specialists have a neuroprotective focus, beginning at birth, with any infant requiring neonatal intensive care. Examples include specialized knowledge of medical issues (e.g., conditions, procedures, equipment), neurodevelopmental organization, and the abilities and vulnerabilities of a range of infants who require the NICU.

- Developmental specialists in the NICU have advanced and specialized skills in working with families, navigating the NICU ecology, and selectively implementing hands-off (e.g., environmental modifications, change agents) and hands-on interventions (e.g., therapeutic positioning, feeding).
- Sleep protection is a top priority in the NICU. The primary activity in brain development during the last trimester is synaptogenesis, neurons connecting with other neurons at a massive rate of 1 to 2 billion connections/second. Early synaptogenesis forms the primitive neural pathways essential for developing complex brain activity and lifelong brain plasticity; during the last trimester, synaptogenesis only occurs during sleep.
- All evaluations or interventions should benefit the NICU infant. Trying an unproven technique for the practice, scheduling a baby when it is convenient for you instead of when the infant shows readiness, or seeing infants to meet productivity requirements are never acceptable practices—especially if sleep is disturbed.
- NICU positioning traditionally focused on neuromotor development of posture, muscle tone, movement patterns, positional deformities, and subsequent developmental sequelae. With recent advancements in technology, therapeutic positioning in the NICU supports and enhances the infant's energy conservation, thermoregulation, skin protection, sleep, and brain development.
- Cue-based infant-driven feeding focuses on infant readiness, participation, and physiologic and behavioral stability; the infant "drives" the volume, duration, and success of each and every feed. Cue based, infant-driven feeding is considered the state-of-the-art approach to feeding.
- See Box 21-2 for a list of common abbreviations used in the NICU.

REFERENCES

1. Aarnoudse-Moens, C. S. H., Weisglas-Kuperus, N., van Goudoever, J. B., et al. (2009). Meta-analysis of neurobehavioral outcomes in very preterm and/or very low birth weight children. *Pediatrics*, *124*, 717–728.
2. Allen, M. C., Christofalo, E. A., & Kim, C. (2011). Outcomes of preterm infants: morbidity replaces mortality. *Clinics in Perinatology*, *38*, 441–454.
3. Als, H. (1986). A synactive model of neonatal behavioral organization: Framework for the assessment and support of the neurobehavioral development of the premature infant and his parents in the environment of the neonatal intensive care unit. *Physical and Occupational Therapy in Pediatrics*, *6*, 3–53.
4. Als, H., Duffy, F. H., McAnulty, G. B., et al. (2004). Early experience alters brain function and structure. *Pediatrics*, *113*, 846–857.
5. Altimier, L. (2004). Healing environments for patients and providers. *Newborn and Infant Nursing Reviews*, *4*, 89–92.
6. Altimier, L. (2011). Mother and child integrative developmental care model: A simple approach to a complex population. *Newborn & Infant Nursing Reviews*, *11*, 105–108.
7. Altimier, L. (2012). Thermoregulation: What's new? What's not? *Newborn and Infant Nursing Reviews*, *12*, 51–63.
8. Altimier, L., & Lasater, K. (in press). *Utilizing reflective practice to obtain competency in neonatal nursing.* 2013. Newborn and Infant Nursing Reviews, *Vol 1*, 34–38.
9. Altimier, L., & Phillips, R. (2013). The neonatal integrative developmental care model: Seven neuroprotective core measures for family centered care. *Newborn and Infant Nursing Reviews*, *13*, 9–22.
10. Altimier, L., & White, R. (2014). The Neonatal intensive care unit (NICU) environment. In C. Kenner & J. W. Wright Lott (Eds.), *Comprehensive neonatal nursing care* (5th ed., pp. 722–738). New York: Springer.
11. Amaizu, I., Shulman, R. J., Schanler, R. J., et al. (2008). Maturation of oral feeding skills in preterm infants. *Acta Pediatrica*, *97*, 61–67.
12. American Academy of Pediatrics, Committee on the Fetus and Newborn. (2004). Policy statement: Age terminology during the perinatal period. *Pediatrics*, *114*, 1362–1364.
13. American Academy of Pediatrics, Committee on the Fetus and Newborn. (2012). Levels of neonatal intensive care. *Pediatrics*, *130*, 587–597.
14. American Academy of Pediatrics, Section on Breastfeeding. (2012). Breastfeeding and the use of human milk. *Pediatrics*, *129*, e827–e842.
15. American Speech-Language-Hearing Association (2004). Roles of speech-language pathologists in the neonatal intensive care unit: Technical report. Retrieved from: <www.asha.org/policy>.
16. Amiel-Tison, C. (2002). Update of the Amiel-Tison neurologic assessment for the term neonate or at 40 weeks corrected age. *Pediatric Neurology*, *27*, 196–212.
17. Axelin, A., Kiriavainen, J., Salantera, S., et al. (2010). Effects of pain management on sleep in preterm infants. *European Journal of Pain*, *14*, 752–758.
18. Aylward, G. P. (2005). Neurodevelopmental outcomes of infants born prematurely. *Journal of Developmental and Behavioral Pediatrics*, *26*, 427–440.
19. Ayres, A. (1987). *Sensory Integration and the Child* (8th ed.). Los Angeles: Western Psychological Services.
20. Barre, N., Morgan, A., Doyle, L. W., et al. (2011). Language abilities in children who were very preterm and/or very low birth weight: A meta-analysis. *Journal of Pediatrics*, *158*, 766–774.
21. Bassan, H., Feldman, H., Limperopoulos, C., et al. (2006). Periventricular hemorrhagic infarction: Risk factors and neonatal outcome. *Pediatric Neurology*, *35*, 85–92.
22. Beaino, G., Khoshnood, B., Kaminski, M., et al.; EPIPAGE Study Group. (2010). Predictors of cerebral palsy in very preterm infants: The EPIPAGE prospective population-based cohort study. *Developmental Medicine and Child Neurology*, *52*, e119–e125.
23. Bertelle, V., Sevestre, A., Laou-Hap, K., et al. (2007). Sleep in the neonatal intensive care unit. *Journal of Perinatal and Neonatal Nursing*, *21*, 140–150.
24. Bhutta, A. T., & Anand, K. J. (2002). Vulnerability of the developing brain: Neuronal mechanisms. *Clinics in Perinatology*, *29*, 357–372.
25. Blackburn, S. T. (2007). *Maternal, fetal, and neonatal physiology. A clinical perspective* (3rd ed.). Neurologic, Muscular, and Sensory Systems. St. Louis: Saunders.
26. Blackburn, S. T. (2012). Neuromuscular and sensory systems. In S. T. Blackburn (Ed.), *Maternal, fetal, and neonatal physiology: A clinical*

perspective (4th ed., pp. 546–598). St. Louis: Saunders.

27. Boykova, M., & Kenner, C. (2010). Partnerships in care: Mothers and fathers. In C. Kenner & J. McGrath (Eds.), *Developmental care of newborns and infants: A guide for health professionals* (2nd ed., pp. 145–160). Glenview, IL: National Association of Neonatal Nurses.
28. Brazelton, T., Parker, W., & Zuckerman, B. (1976). Importance of behavioral assessment of the neonate. *Current Problems in Pediatrics, 7*, 1–32.
29. Browne, J. V. (2007). Guest editorial. Evidence based developmental care for optimal babies' brain development. *Neonatal, Paediatric & Child Health Nursing, 10*(3), 2–3.
30. Browne, J. V. (2011). Developmental care for high-risk newborns: Emerging science, clinical application, and continuity from newborn intensive care unit to community. *Clinics in Perinatology, 38*, 719–729.
31. Browne, J., & Ross, E. (2011). Eating as a neurodevelopmental process for high risk newborns. *Clinics in Perinatology, 38*, 731–743.
32. Bystrova, K., Ivanova, V., Edhborg, M., et al. (2009). Early contact versus separation: Effects on mother-infant interaction one year later. *Birth (Berkeley, Calif.), 36*, 97–109.
33. Carbasse, A., Kracher, S., Hausser, M., et al. (2013). Safety and effectiveness of skin-to-skin contact in the NICU to support neurodevelopment in vulnerable preterm infants. *Journal of Perinatal and Neonatal Nursing, 27*, 255–262.
34. Carroll, M., Curtis, L., Higgins, A., et al. (2002). Is there a place for reflective practice in the nursing curriculum? *Clinical Effectiveness in Nursing, 6*, 36–41.
35. Champagne, F. A. (2012). Epigenetic influence of social experiences across the lifespan. *Developmental Psychobiology, 52*, 299–311.
36. Cleveland, L. (2008). Parenting in the neonatal intensive care unit. *Journal of Obstetrics, Gynecologic, & Neonatal Nursing, 37*, 666–691.
37. Comaru, T., & Miura, E. (2009). Postural support improves distress and pain during diaper change in preterm infants. *Journal of Perinatology, 29*, 504–507.
38. Comrie, J. D., & Helm, J. M. (1997). Common feeding problems in the intensive care nursery: Maturation, organization, evaluation and management strategies. *Seminars in Speech and Language, 18*, 239–261.
39. Conde-Agudelo, A., Belizán, J. M., & Diaz-Rossello, J. (2011). Kangaroo mother care to reduce morbidity and mortality in low birthweight infants. *Cochrane Database of Systematic Reviews*, (3), CD00277.
40. Cosimano, A., & Sandhurst, H. (2011). Strategies for successful breastfeeding in the NICU. *Neonatal Network, 30*, 340–343.
41. Coughlin, M., Gibbins, S., & Hoath, S. (2009). Core measures for developmentally supportive care in neonatal intensive care units: Theory, precedence and practice. *Journal of Advanced Nursing, 65*, 2239–2248.
42. Dreyfus, H., & Dreyfus, S. (1996). *Mind over machine: The power of human intuition and expertise in the era of the computer*. New York: Free Press.
43. Eliot, L. (1999). *What's going on in there? How the brain and mind develop in the first five years of life*. New York: Bantam Books.
44. Fielder, A. R., & Moseley, M. J. (2000). Environmental light and the preterm infant. *Seminars in Perinatology, 24*, 291–298.
45. Gardner, S. L., & Goldson, E. (2011). The neonate and the environment: Impact on development. In S. L. Merenstein & G. B. Gardner (Eds.), *Handbook of neonatal intensive care* (7th ed., pp. 270–331). St. Louis: Mosby.
46. Gibbins, S., Hoath, S. B., Coughlin, M., et al. (2008). Foundations in newborn care. the universe of developmental care: A new conceptual model for application in the neonatal intensive care unit. *Advances in Neonatal Care, 8*, 141–147.
47. Gorski, P. A., Davidson, M. F., & Brazelton, T. B. (1979). Stages of behavioral organization in the high-risk neonate: Theoretical clinical considerations. *Seminars in Perinatology, 3*, 61–72.
48. Graven, S. N. (2006). Sleep and brain development. *Clinics in Perinatology, 33*, 693–706.
49. Graven, S. N. (2011). Early visual development: Implications for the neonatal intensive care unit and care. *Clinics in Perinatology, 38*, 693–706.
50. Graven, S. N., & Browne, J. V. (2008a). Sleep and brain development: The critical role of sleep in fetal and early neonatal brain development. *Newborn & Infant Nursing Reviews, 8*, 173–179.
51. Graven, S., & Browne, J. V. (2008b). Sensory development in the fetus, neonate, and infant: Introductions and overview. *Newborn and Infant Nursing Reviews, 8*, 169–172.
52. Graven, S. N., & Philbin, J. V. (2008). Auditory development in the fetus and infant. *Newborn and Infant Nursing Reviews, 8*, 187–193.
53. Gressens, P., Rogido, M., Paindaveine, B., et al. (2002). The impact of neonatal intensive care practices on the developing brain. *Journal of Pediatrics, 14*, 646–653.
54. Grunau, R. E., Tu, M., & Whitfield, M. (2010). Cortisol, behavior, and heart rate reactivity to immunization pain at 4 months corrected age in infants born very preterm. *Clinical Journal of Pain, 26*, 698–704.
55. Gudsnuk, K. M., & Champagne, F. A. (2011). Epigenetic effects of early developmental experiences. *Clinics in Perinatology, 38*, 703–717.
56. Guyer, C., Huber, R., Fontijn, J., et al. (2012). Cycled light exposure reduces fussing and crying in very preterm infants. *Pediatrics, 130*, e145–e151.
57. Hack, M., Youngstrom, E. A., Cartar, L., et al. (2004). Behavioral outcomes and evidence of psychopathology among very low birth weight infants at age 20 years. *Pediatrics, 114*, 932–940.
58. Hawdon, J. M., Beauregard, N., Slattery, J., et al. (2000). Identification of neonates at risk of developing feeding problems in infancy. *Developmental and Medical Child Neurology, 42*, 235–239.
59. Heijst, J. J. V., Touwen, B. C. L., & Vos, J. E. (1999). Implications of a neural network model of sensorimotor development for the field of developmental neurology. *Early Human Development, 55*, 77–95.
60. Houska-Lund, C., & Durand, D. J. (2011). Skin and skin care. In S. L. Merenstein & G. B. Gardner (Eds.), *Handbook of neonatal intensive care* (7th ed., pp. 482–501). St. Louis: Mosby.
61. Hunt, A. (2008). *Pragmatic thinking and learning: Refactor your wetware*. Dallas, TX: Pragmatic Bookshelf.
62. Hunter, J. (2010). Therapeutic positioning: Neuromotor, physiologic, and sleep implications. In C. Kenner & J. McGrath (Eds.), *Developmental care of newborns and infants: A guide for health professionals* (2nd ed., pp. 285–312). Glenview, IL: National Association of Neonatal Nurses.
63. Hunter, J., & L'Huillier, M. (2007). Bottle feeding in the NICU. In L. Altimier (Ed.), *Mosby's neonatal nursing online course manual*. St. Louis: Elsevier.
64. Inder, T. E., Warfield, S. K., Wang, H., et al. (2005). Abnormal cerebral structure is present at term in premature infants. *Pediatrics, 115*, 286–294.
65. Jakobson, L. S., & Taylor, N. M. (2009). Differential vulnerability of cerebral visual functions in children born very prematurely. *Acta Pediatrica, 98*, 239–241.

66. Jerger, J., & Musiek, F. (2000). Report of the consensus conference on the diagnosis of auditory processing disorders in school-aged children. *Journal of the American Academy of Audiology, 11*, 467–474.
67. Johnson, S., Hollis, C., Kochlar, P., et al. (2010). Psychiatric disorders in extremely preterm children: Longitudinal finding at age 11 years in the EPICure study. *Journal of the American Academy of Child and Adolescent Psychiatry, 49*, 453–463.
68. Kassity-Krich, N. A., & Jones, J. E. (2014). Complementary and integrative therapies. In C. Kenner & J. W. Lott (Eds.), *Comprehensive neonatal nursing care* (pp. 773–782). New York: Springhill.
69. Kenner, C., & McGrath, J. (2010). *Developmental care of newborns and infants: A guide for health professionals* (2nd ed.). Glenview, IL: National Association of Neonatal Nurses.
70. Kenner, C., & Pressler, J. L. (2013). Trends in neonatal care delivery. In C. Kenner & J. W. Lott (Eds.), *Comprehensive neonatal nursing care* (5th ed.). New York: Springer.
71. Kranowitz, C. A. (1998). *The out-of-sync child*. New York: Berkley.
72. Krueger, C., Schue, S., & Parker, L. (2007). Neonatal intensive care unit sound levels before and after structural reconstruction. *MCN: The American Journal of Maternal Child Nursing, 32*, 358–362.
73. Laptook, A. R., O'Shea, M., Shankaran, S., et al.; NICHD Neonatal Network. (2005). Adverse neurodevelopmental outcomes among extremely low birth weight infants with a normal head ultrasound: Prevalence and antecedents. *Pediatrics, 115*, 673–680.
74. Lau, C., Smith, E. O., & Schanler, R. J. (2003). Coordination of suck-swallow and respiration in preterm infants. *Acta Paediatrica, 92*, 721–727.
75. Laudert, S., Liu, W. F., Blackington, S., et al; NIC/Q 2005 Physical Environment Exploratory Group. (2007). Implementing potentially better practices to support the neurodevelopment of infants in the NICU. *Journal of Perinatology, 27*, S75–S93.
76. Liaw, J. J., Yang, L., Chang, L. H., et al. (2009). Improving neonatal caregiving through a developmentally supportive care training program. *Applied Nursing Research, 22*, 86–93.
77. Liaw, J. J., Yang, L., Hua, Y. M., et al. (2013). Preterm infants' biobehavioral responses to caregiving and positioning over 24 hours in a neonatal unit in Taiwan. *Research in Nursing and Health, 35*, 634–646.
78. Lickliter, R. (2011). The integrated development of sensory organization. *Clinics in Perinatology, 38*, 91–603.
79. Limperopoulos, C. (2009). Autism spectrum disorders in survivors of extreme prematurity. *Clinics in Perinatology, 36*, 791–805.
80. Liu, W. F., Laudert, S., Perkins, B., et al. (2007). The development of potentially better practices to support the neurodevelopment of infants in the NICU. *Journal of Perinatology, 27*, S48–S74.
81. Loring, C., Gregory, K., Gargan, B., et al. (2012). Tub bathing improves thermoregulation of the late preterm infant. *Journal of Obstetric, Gynecologic, and Neonatal Nursing, 41*, 171–179.
82. Lubbe, W., & Kenner, C. (2008). Neonatal brain development. *Newborn and Infant Nursing Reviews, 8*, 166–167.
83. Ludington-Hoe, S. (2010). Kangaroo care is developmental care. In C. Kenner & J. McGrath (Eds.), *Developmental care of newborns and infants: A guide for health professionals* (2nd ed., pp. 349–388). Glenview, IL: National Association of Neonatal Nurses.
84. Ludington-Hoe, S. (2013). Kangaroo care as a neonatal therapy. *Newborn and Infant Nursing Reviews, 13*, 73–75.
85. Ludwig, S. M. (2007). Oral feeding and the late preterm infant. *Newborn and Infant Nursing Reviews, 7*, 72–75.
86. Hanlon, M. B., Tripp, J. H., Ellis, R. E., et al. (1997). Deglutition apnea as indicator of maturation of suckle feeding in bottle-fed infants. *Developmental Medicine and Child Neurology, 39*, 534–542.
87. Maddalena, P. (2013). Long-term outcomes of preterm birth: The role of epigenetics. *Newborn and Infant Nursing Reviews, 13*, 137–139.
88. Maquet, P., Smith, C., & Stickgold, R. (2003). *Sleep and brain plasticity*. New York: Oxford University Press.
89. McAnulty, G., et al. (2009). Individualized developmental care for a large sample of very preterm infants: Health, neurobehaviour and neurophysiology. *Acta Paediatrica, 98*, 1920–1926.
90. McGrath, J. M. (2014). Family: The essential partner in care. In C. Kenner & J. W. Lott (Eds.), *Comprehensive neonatal nursing care* (pp. 739–765). New York: Springer.
91. McGrath, J. M., Cone, S., & Samra, H. A. (2011). Neuroprotection in the preterm infant: Further understanding of the short- and long-term implications for brain development. *Newborn and Infant Nursing Reviews, 11*, 109–112.
92. Moon, C. (2011). The role of early auditory development in attachment and communication. *Clinics in Perinatology, 38*, 657–669.
93. Morag, I., & Ohlsson, A. (2013). Cycled light in the intensive care unit for preterm and low birth weight infants. *Cochrane Database of Systematic Reviews*, (8), CD006982.
94. Mueller, B. R., & Bale, T. L. (2008). Sex-specific programming of offspring emotionality after stress in early pregnancy. *Journal of Neuroscience, 28*, 9055–9065.
95. National Perinatal Association (2010). Position paper: NICU developmental care. Retrieved from: <http://nationalperinatal.org/Resources/NICU%20Development%20Care%20%2012-12-13.pdf>.
96. Naughton, K. A. (2013). The combined use of sucrose and nonnutritive sucking for procedural pain in both term and preterm neonates: An integrative review of the literature. *Advances in Neonatal Care, 13*, 9–19.
97. Newland, L., L'Huillier, M., & Petrey, B. (2013). Implementation of cue-based feeding in a Level III NICU. *Neonatal Network, 32*, 132–137.
98. Nightingale, F. (1860). *Notes on nursing: What it is and what it is not*. New York: Appleton.
99. Nyqvist, K. H., Expert Group of the International Network on Kangaroo Mother Care, Anderson, G. C., Bergman, N., et al. (2010). State of the art and recommendations. Kangaroo mother care: Application in a high-tech environment. *Acta Paediatrica, 99*, 812–819.
100. Palmer, M. M. (1993). Identification and management of the transitional suck pattern in premature infants. *Journal of Perinatal and Neonatal Nursing, 7*, 66–75.
101. Palmer, M. M., Crawley, K., & Blanco, I. A. (1993). Neonatal oral-motor assessment scale: A reliability study. *Journal of Perinatology, 13*, 28–35.
102. Philbin, M. K., & Ross, E. (2011). The SOFFI reference guide: Text, algorithms, and appendices: A manualized method for quality bottle-feedings. *The Journal of Perinatal & Neonatal Nursing, 25*, 360–380.
103. Phillips, R. (2012). The ultimate marathon: Supporting optimal milk supply for pump-dependent mothers in the NICU. Retrieved from: <https://www.theonlinelearningcenter.com/course-catalog/Product/module/8226/106>.

104. Phillips, R. (2013). Changing the culture of postpartum skin-to-skin contact to increase breastfeeding rates. Retrieved from: <https://www.theonlinelearningcenter.com/course-catalog/Product/module/8021/106>.
105. Pierrat, V., Goubet, N., Peifer, K., et al. (2007). How can we evaluate developmental care practices prior to their implementation in a neonatal intensive care unit? *Early Human Development*, *83*, 415–418.
106. Pinelli, J., & Symington, A. J. (2005). Non-nutritive sucking for promoting physiologic stability and nutrition in preterm infants. *Cochrane Database of Systematic Reviews*, Issue 4. Art. No.: CD001071. Assessed as up-to-date April 6, 2010.
107. Pitcher, J., Schneider, L. A., Drysdale, J. L., et al. (2011). Motor system development of the preterm and low birthweight infant. *Clinics in Perinatology*, *38*, 605–625.
108. Quraishy, K., Bowles, S. M., & Moore, J. (2013). A protocol for swaddled bathing in the neonatal intensive care unit. *Newborn & Infant Nursing Reviews*, *13*, 48–50.
109. Raines, D. A. (2013). Reading research articles. *Neonatal Network*, *32*, 52–54.
110. Rees, S., Harding, R., & Walker, D. (2011). The biological basis of injury and neuroprotection in the fetal and neonatal brain. *The International Journal of Developmental Neuroscience*, *29*, 551–563.
111. Reynolds, J. D., Hardy, R. J., Kennedy, K. A., et al. (1998). Lack of efficacy of light preventing retinopathy of prematurity. Light Reduction in Retinopathy of Prematurity (LIGHT-ROP) Cooperative Group. *New England Journal of Medicine*, *338*, 1572–1576.
112. Rhawn, J. (1999). Fetal brain and cognitive development. *Developmental Reviews*, *20*, 81–98.
113. Rivkees, S. A., Mayes, L., Jacobs, H., et al. (2004). Rest-activity patterns of premature infants are regulated by cycled lighting. *Pediatrics*, *113*, 833–839.
114. Rizzo, P., Rea, M., & White, R. (2010). Lighting for today's neonatal intensive care unit. *Newborn and Infant Nursing Reviews*, *10*, 107–113.
115. Robison, L. D. (2003). An organizational guide for an effective developmental program in the NICU. *Journal of Obstetric, Gynecologic, and Neonatal Nursing: JOGNN/NAACOG*, *32*, 379–386.
116. Ross, E., & Browne, J. (2002). Baby-Regulated Organization of Systems and Sucking (BROSS). Paper presented at the Physical and Developmental Environment of the High-Risk Infant, Clearwater, FL, January 28, 2002.
117. Ross, E., & Browne, J. (2013). Feeding outcomes in preterm infants after discharge from the neonatal intensive care unit (NICU): A systematic review. *Newborn and Infant Nursing Reviews*, *13*, 87–93.
118. Ross, E., & Philbin, M. K. (2011). Supporting oral feeding in fragile infants: An evidence-based method for quality bottle-feedings of preterm, ill, and fragile infants. *Journal of Perinatal and Neonatal Nursing*, *25*, 349–537.
119. Samara, M., Marlow, N., Wolke, D.; EPICure Study Group. (2008). Pervasive behavior problems at 6 years of age in a total-population sample of children born at ≤25 weeks of gestation. *Pediatrics*, *122*, 562–573.
120. Scher, M., Johnson, M., & Holditch-Davis, D. (2005). Cyclicity of neonatal sleep behaviors at 25 to 30 weeks' postconceptual age. *Pediatric Research*, *57*, 879–882.
121. Schlotz, W., & Phillips, D. I. W. (2009). Fetal origins of mental health: Evidence and mechanisms. *Brain, Behavior, and Immunity*, *23*, 905–916.
122. Schon, D. A. (1983). *The reflective practitioner*. London: Temple Smith.
123. Shaker, C. S. (2012). Feed me only when I'm cueing: Moving away from a volume-driven culture in the NICU. *Neonatal Intensive Care: The Journal of Perinatology-Neonatology*, *25*, 27–32.
124. Shaker, C. S. (2013). Cue-based co-regulated feeding in the neonatal intensive care unit: Supporting parents in learning to feed their preterm infant. *Newborn and Infant Nursing Reviews*, *13*, 51–55.
125. Shiao, S. Y. P. K., Brooker, J., & DiFiore, T. (1996). Desaturation events during oral feedings with and without a nasogastric tube in very low birth weight infants. *Heart and Lung*, *25*, 236–245.
126. Simpson, C., Schanler, R. J., & Lau, C. (2002). Early introduction of oral feeding in preterm infants. *Pediatrics*, *110*, 517–522.
127. Spruill, C. (2010). Caregiving and the caregiver. In C. Kenner & J. McGrath (Eds.), *Developmental care of newborns and infants: A guide for health professionals* (2nd ed., pp. 75–92). Glenview, IL: National Association of Neonatal Nurses.
128. Stevens, D. C., Helseth, C. C., & Kurtz, J. C. (2010). Achieving success in supporting parents and families in the neonatal intensive care unit. In C. Kenner & J. McGrath (Eds.), *Developmental care of newborns and infants: A guide for health professionals* (2nd ed., pp. 161–190). Glenview, IL: National Association of Neonatal Nurses.
129. Stokowski, L. A. (2012). Noteworthy professional news: Four levels of neonatal care. *Advances in Neonatal Care*, *12*, 326–328.
130. Stoll, B. J., Hansen, N. I., Bell, E. F., et al.; Eunice Kennedy Shriver National Institute of Child Health and Human Development Neonatal Research Network. (2010). Neonatal outcomes of extremely preterm infants from the NICHD Neonatal Research Network. *Pediatrics*, *126*, 443–456.
131. Sullivan, R., Perry, R., Sloan, A., et al. (2011). Infant bonding and attachment to the caregiver: Insights from basic and clinical science. *Clinics in Perinatology*, *38*, 643–655.
132. Sweeney, J. K., Heriza, C. B., & Blanchard, Y. (2009). Neonatal physical therapy. Part I: Clinical competencies and neonatal intensive care unit clinical training models. *Pediatric Physical Therapy*, *21*, 296–307.
133. Sweeney, J. K., Heriza, C. B., Blanchard, Y., et al. (2010). Neonatal physical therapy. Part II: Practice frameworks and evidence-based practice guidelines. *Pediatric Physical Therapy*, *22*, 2–16.
134. Taylor, H. G. (2010). Academic performance and learning disabilities. In C. Nosarti, R. M. Murray, & M. Hack (Eds.), *Neurodevelopmental outcomes of preterm birth: From childhood to adult life* (pp. 195–218). Cambridge, U.K.: Cambridge University Press.
135. Taylor, H. G., Filipek, P. A., Juranek, J., et al. (2011). Brain volumes in adolescents with very low birth weight: Effects on brain structure and associations with neuropsychological outcomes. *Developmental Neuropsychology*, *36*, 96–117.
136. Vergara, E., Anzalone, M., Bigsby, R., et al; 2005 Neonatal Intensive Care Unit Task Force. (2006). Specialized knowledge and skills for occupational therapy practice in the neonatal intensive care unit. *American Journal of Occupational Therapy*, *60*, 659–668.
137. Visscher, M. O., Lacina, L., Casper, T., et al. (in press). *Conformational positioning improves sleep in premature infants with feeding difficulties.* Journal of Pediatrics.
138. Volpe, J. J. (2008). *Neurology of the newborn* (5th ed.). Philadelphia: Elsevier.
139. Volpe, J. J. (2009). Brain injury in premature infants: A complex amalgam of destructive and developmental disturbances. *Lancet Neurology*, *8*, 110–124.

140. Wachman, E. M., & Lahav, A. (2011). The effects of noise on preterm infants in the NICU. *Archives of Disease in Childhood. Fetal and Neonatal Edition, 96*, F305–F309.
141. Waitzman, K. A., & Ludwig, S. M. (2007). Changing feeding documentation to reflect infant-driven feeding practice. *Newborn & Infant Nursing Reviews, 7*, 155–160.
142. Walden, M. (2014). Pain in the newborn and infant. In C. Kenner & J. W. Lott (Eds.), *Comprehensive neonatal nursing care* (pp. 571–586). New York: Springer.
143. White, R. (2013). The physical environment of the newborn ICU: New recommended standards and related articles. *Journal of Perinatology, 33*, S2–S16.
144. White-Traut, R., Dols, J., & McGrath, J. M. (2010). Touch and massage for high-risk infants. In C. Kenner & J. McGrath (Eds.), *Developmental care of newborns and infants: A guide for health professionals* (2nd ed., pp. 389–409). Glenview, IL: National Association of Neonatal Nurses.

CHAPTER

22 Early Intervention

Christine Teeters Myers • Jane Case-Smith • Jana Cason

KEY TERMS

Coaching models
Consultative models
Early intervention
Family-centered intervention
Individualized Family Service Plan (IFSP)
Natural environments
Part C of the Individuals with Disabilities Education Act (IDEA)
Primary service provider
Service coordinator
Telehealth

GUIDING QUESTIONS

1. What is early intervention?
2. How do federal legislation and regulations provide the framework for occupational therapy services in early intervention?
3. What is best practice in early intervention?
4. How do occupational therapists partner with families and other professionals to provide developmentally appropriate and family-centered services?
5. Which occupational therapy practices and service delivery models support early intervention in the natural environment?
6. Which strategies do occupational therapists use to promote children's performance and participation?

Definition of Early Intervention Programs

The term *early intervention* connotes different meanings to different professionals. In this chapter, *early* refers to the critical period of a child's development between birth and 3 years of age. *Intervention* refers to programs and services designed to enhance the child's development as a member of a family and support families in caring for their child. Early intervention describes services for children ages birth through 2 years who have an established risk, have a developmental delay, or are considered to be environmentally or biologically at risk. Early intervention programs serve several purposes, including enhancing the development of infants and toddlers with disabilities, minimizing their potential for developmental delay, and recognizing the significant brain development that occurs during a child's first 3 years of life.[50] Another goal of early intervention as defined in Part C of the Individuals with Disabilities Education Act (IDEA) is to enhance the capacity of families to meet the special needs of their infants and toddlers.

Legislation Related to Early Intervention

The 1980s brought widespread acceptance and support for family-centered care for children with special needs.[97] Family-centered care is based on the principle that an infant is dependent on his or her parents and other family members for daily care and meeting his or her physical and emotional needs. At the same time, the birth of an infant with special health care needs affects the entire family emotionally, socially, and economically. In 1986, amendments to the Education of the Handicapped Act (EHA) established incentives for states to develop systems of coordinated family-centered care for infants with disabilities. These incentives were strengthened in 1990, when the EHA was further amended and retitled the Individuals with Disabilities Education Act.[49] Through Part C of IDEA, states must develop and make available comprehensive services for all infants and toddlers who have developmental delays. Revisions to IDEA were made again in 1997 and 2004; the newest version is P.L. 108-446, the Individuals with Disabilities Education Improvement Act of 2004.

States that participate in Part C of IDEA are required to maintain and implement comprehensive, coordinated, multidisciplinary, interagency systems of early intervention services for infants and toddlers with disabilities and their families. Part C defines the policies and regulations that participating states must follow in establishing early intervention services and systems. The most recent regulations for Part C were released in 2011.[82] Table 22-1 summarizes the differences between Part C, which defines early intervention services for children from birth through 2 years of age, and Part B, which defines school programs for eligible students between 3 and 21 years of age (see Chapter 23). Part C is an entitlement program (acknowledges one's rights to services), and Part B defines mandated services and programs that are obligatory by law.

Importance and Outcomes of Early Intervention

The importance of early intervention is widely recognized. In particular, research on the developing brain suggests that influencing early development can significantly change a child's learning potential.[15,95,96] Neural plasticity is at its greatest in the first 3 years of life, and, although not absent in later years, neural plasticity diminishes over time. Positive early experiences shape and strengthen the brain, and social-emotional and physical health influence cognitive and communication development. Early intervention not only has the potential to affect a child's development and health, but these services may also

TABLE 22-1 Comparison of Educational Programs by Age Group

	Age (yr)		
Parameter	**0-2**	**3-5**	**6-21**
Legislation	IDEA, Part C	IDEA, Part B	IDEA, Part B
Program	Early intervention	Special education	Special education
Type	Entitlement	Mandate	Mandate
Eligibility	Noncategorical	Categorical	Categorical
Services provided	16 primary services, including occupational therapy, physical therapy, speech-language pathology, and special instruction	Related services only as support to special education	Related services only as support to special education
	Interdisciplinary and transdisciplinary assessment	Interdisciplinary and discipline-specific assessment	Discipline-specific assessment as related to education
	Individualized Family Service Plan (IFSP)	Individualized education program	Individualized education program
	Family-centered	Family-focused in theory, child-focused in practice	Child-focused, with emphasis on curricular standards
	Service coordination	Service coordination recommended but not mandated	Service coordination recommended but not mandated
	Natural settings	Home-, center-, or school-based	School-based

IDEA, Individuals with Disabilities Education Act.

reduce caregiver stress, thus increasing the capability of families to care for their child and support their child's needs.[3,43] Early intervention services also reduce the need for special education when children transition to school.[3]

In 2010, more than 340,000 children received Part C services.[19] To ensure that quality early intervention services are being provided to families and children, the Office of Special Education Programs began collecting states' early intervention data on child and family outcomes.[27,28,28a] States must report on the percentage of infants and toddlers with Individualized Family Service Plans (IFSPs) who demonstrate improvement in the following:

1. Positive social-emotional skills (including social relationships)
2. Acquisition and use of knowledge and skills (including early language and communication [and early literacy])
3. Use of appropriate behaviors to meet their needs

States must also document the percentage of families participating in Part C who report that early intervention services made improvements in the following:

1. Family's knowledge of their rights
2. Family's ability to communicate their child's needs effectively
3. Family's ability to help their child develop and learn

Nationwide data from 2011 indicated that between 71% and 76% of children from birth through 2 years showed greater than expected growth in the three child outcomes, and between 85% and 90% of families reported that early intervention services had helped them meet the family indicators above as they exited early intervention.[27,28] This chapter provides an overview of early intervention services and describes how occupational therapy services support and promote early intervention outcomes for children and families.

Occupational Therapy Services in Early Intervention Systems

Part C of IDEA considers occupational therapy to be a "primary service" for eligible infants and toddlers who qualify for early intervention services. As a primary service, occupational therapy can be provided as the only service that a child receives or in addition to other early intervention services. By its legal definition, occupational therapy includes services to address the functional needs of the child related to adaptive development (self-care); adaptive behavior and play, including social interaction; and sensory, motor, and postural development. Services include adapting the environment and selecting, designing, and fabricating assistive and orthotic devices to facilitate development and promote the acquisition of functional skills. Occupational therapy outcomes for children and families participating in IDEA Part C services include improved developmental performance, increased participation, and enhanced quality of life.[10] Activities of daily living (ADLs), rest and sleep, play, and social participation are the primary areas of occupation addressed in IDEA Part C services.

Traditionally, occupational therapists provided early intervention services with a medical orientation. That is, occupational therapy was provided in a clinic or center, and sessions usually were conducted one on one with the occupational therapist and child or in a small group with peers who were also receiving early intervention services. With the changes to IDEA 1997 requiring services to be provided in the natural environment, approximately 94% of early intervention services occur in the home or other community-based settings.[104] As a result, occupational therapists have developed models and strategies appropriate for services in homes and other community environments. Therapeutic interventions are embedded into family routines (i.e., performance patterns). Occupational therapists provide early intervention services in natural environments as part of a team, coach and consult with team members to support occupational therapy interventions, and use a family-centered approach that respects cultural differences. The following sections define the concepts that guide early intervention services and exemplify how occupational therapists apply early intervention practices.

Best Practices in Early Intervention

Partnering with Families

The early intervention system recognizes that families can be and often are knowledgeable consumers and effective change agents for their children. It also acknowledges that families need resources to support and raise a child with disabilities.[70,103] The early intervention team helps each family identify its unique resources, priorities, and concerns and identifies goals that enable them to support the child as a member of the family unit.[56]

The term *family-centeredness* encompasses several meanings—families are treated with respect; importance is placed on family strengths, not deficits; families have control and make choices regarding the care that their child receives; and families and providers work together to ensure provision of optimal early intervention services.[4,24] Within a family-centered model, occupational therapists develop goals collaboratively with the child's primary caregivers. Using a family systems perspective, the occupational therapist recognizes the influence and inter-relationships of the family within various systems, such as the extended family, neighborhood, and early intervention programs. By thinking broadly about families and their subsystems, the occupational therapist can help parents communicate their concerns and identify their priorities for the child.

Families are participants in and consumers of early intervention services.[102] The nature and extent of family involvement may vary according to family needs, values, lifestyles, and variables within the structure of the early intervention program itself. The degree of family involvement may fluctuate and change in response to external or internal factors that affect family functioning and coping. Some examples are degree of acceptance of the child's disability, job status of one or both parents, a new infant in the family, and changes in the family's support networks, such as grandparents, friends, and church groups.

To provide appropriate intervention within the family-centered model, the occupational therapist must be aware of and respect differences in beliefs and values based on culture. Multiple factors can affect family involvement, and families of children with disabilities may be under considerable stress and may be doing their best at any particular time.[42] For example, a parent who is homeless or jobless may not be concerned about occupational therapy for the child. Another parent may believe that certain skills or goals are more important than those identified by the occupational therapist. As explained in Chapter 5, family priorities need to be honored and services must follow the family's expressed priorities.

The families receiving early intervention services are highly diverse (Research Note 22-1), and acceptance of the individual

RESEARCH NOTE 22-1

Hebbeler, K., Spiker D., Bailey, D., Scarborough, A., Mallik, S., Simeonsson, R., et al. (2007). Early intervention for infants and toddlers with disabilities and their families: Participants, services, and outcomes. Final Report of the National Early Intervention Longitudinal Study (NEILS). *Menlo Park, CA: SRI International.*

Abstract

Beginning in 1996, the Office of Special Education Programs of the U.S. Department of Education sponsored research regarding early intervention (Part C). This longitudinal descriptive study was based on an ecologic model in which young children receiving early intervention (EI) services are considered to be influenced by a variety of factors, such as environment, genetics, and cultural attitudes. In particular, the interactions between child and family highly influence child outcomes. The study's purpose was to determine the characteristics of children and families who received services, types of services received, costs of services, outcomes experienced by children and families, and relationship among outcomes, services, and child-family characteristics. A nationally representative sample of 3338 children was included in the study, which drew data from a variety of sources over time—family interviews (telephone and mail), service records (i.e., IFSPs), service provider surveys, and kindergarten teacher surveys.

Implications for Practice

- The types of children and families that received EI services are highly diverse, and more than half of families are coping with multiple risk factors beyond disability or developmental delay in their children, including poverty, low level of maternal education, single-parent household, and having another child with special needs. The authors of NEILS pointed out that this diversity supports the requirement for individualized services in EI, which take into account how best to support families and are flexible regarding the needs of families and children at different points in time.
- Many of the children who receive EI services do not receive special education services in preschool or kindergarten, suggesting that for some children, disability and delay identified before 36 months may be transitory in nature. Occupational therapists need to be aware that many young children with mild impairments may need services for only a short time. In this case, EI can be considered a prevention program addressing specific developmental challenges in infancy and toddlerhood and preventing or reducing the need for additional services in the future.
- Areas of concern identified by parents and kindergarten teachers of children who received EI services included communication problems and social-emotional problems. Occupational therapists may benefit from training to address simple communication and behavioral issues within the context of different service delivery models and an understanding of when these issues need to be addressed by a professional with specialized knowledge.

- At the time of data collection (late 1990s), families were receiving typically two to four different services, with a median of 1.5 hours of scheduled service time per week. This limited amount of service time spread among several professionals supports the need for occupational therapists to incorporate families into intervention by addressing how intervention strategies will fit into family routines and daily activities in the natural environment.
- Most of the families who participate in EI identify positive outcomes associated with the program, such as knowing how to care for their child, helping their child learn and develop, learning how to work well with professionals, and feeling comfortable in asking for help and support from relatives and friends. However, ratings from low-income and minority families were lower in these areas, suggesting that EI providers, including occupational therapists, should be thoughtful of the specific needs of diverse families.

differences among families is a high priority. The occupational therapist who provides intervention in the home has an intimate view of such things as customs, eating habits, and child-rearing practices that may vary among cultures. The family's beliefs and views of disability and its cause, their view of the health care system, and their sources of medical information affect their attitude toward early intervention.[110] Based on individual cultural backgrounds, the family may view the occupational therapist as a helper or someone who interferes, and occupational therapists should reflect on how a family's cultural values and beliefs influence their participation in early intervention programs (Box 22-1). Although providers acknowledge the value of considering one's culture, research suggests that early intervention providers do not consistently develop IFSP goals that consider cultural diversity (e.g., family income, location of residence).[89] Given the importance of the IFSP in directing program implementation, this finding indicates that early intervention service providers need to make certain that they include all family-identified priorities in addition to those that relate to the child's development.

Many of the areas in which occupational therapists provide interventions and suggestions involve caregiving and are closely tied to values and beliefs about parenting and cultural views of children. Practices regarding feeding, toileting, and bathing may vary among cultures. The occupational therapist considers the family's values and cultural beliefs about these practices before making recommendations for change.[39] As part of cultural values, occupational therapists consider family rituals and meaningful aspects of family life, such as celebrations, and family traditions that support the building of family relationships and occupations (e.g., saying goodnight, buying new school shoes).[23]

Essential to family-centeredness is building ongoing relationships with families.[24] Relationships are fostered when practitioners exhibit effective listening, compassion, and empathy. Occupational therapists communicate with sensitivity their own concerns about the child's occupations and are open to the family's perceptions. Families who have children with special needs highly value services in which professionals provide clear, understandable, complete information; demonstrate respect for the child and family; provide emotional support; and provide expert, skillful intervention.[90]

BOX 22-1 Questions to Foster Cultural Competence

1. What do I know about the family's culture and beliefs about health?
   This represents the basic knowledge of cultural health practices and beliefs. Conclusions or judgments should not be formed about why these practices are present.
2. Does the family agree with these beliefs?
   Although a client may affiliate with a specific cultural group, the occupational therapist must investigate whether the cultural beliefs of health and the client's beliefs of health are similar.
3. How will these beliefs influence the intervention and outcomes of services provided?
   The occupational therapist must acknowledge and respond to the influences of cultural beliefs and practices in the intervention plan. To design a plan that conflicts with cultural beliefs would not only be counterproductive to client-centered services, but would be disrespectful of the family's belief system. If a family, in deference to the authority of the occupational therapist, follows an intervention that conflicts with cultural practices, the family may risk not receiving support and affiliation with their cultural group.
4. How can the intervention plan support culturally endorsed occupations, roles, and responsibilities to promote the family's engagement in occupation?
   The occupational therapist must consider the important occupations from a cultural perspective. Evening meals may include specific behaviors that possess strong cultural symbols for one family, but another family may view an evening meal as merely eating, with no prescribed rituals.

Adapted from Schultz-Krohn, W., & Pendleton, H. M. (2006). Application of the occupational therapy framework to physical dysfunction. In W. Schultz-Krohn & H. M. Pendleton (Eds.), *Pedretti's occupational therapy: Practice skills for physical dysfunction.* St. Louis: Mosby.

Partnering with Professionals

The success of an early intervention program depends largely on how a cooperative team of professionals develops and implements coordinated and integrated intervention plans. Teamwork is critical because the inter-related needs of a developing child and caregiving family are complex and call for the skills and resources of a team of professionals. Occupational therapists working with infants and toddlers have specialized knowledge of childhood occupations and generalized knowledge regarding young children with special needs. The emphasis of intervention is the child within the family unit, rather than the child alone, and intervention is carried out through collaboration among all professionals involved.

Although an occupational therapist may participate in various service delivery models, a transdisciplinary model in which one service provider is primary and other team members serve as consultants is considered optimal in early intervention.[59,75] In transdisciplinary early intervention, one professional, sometimes called the primary interventionist, supports and provides the functions that traditionally were performed by another professional.[59] Occupational therapists become teachers of their peers and benefit from learning about strategies and approaches used in other professions.[78] Through frequent collaboration (i.e., in-person meetings, co-treatment, and informal communication), team members build relationships characterized by mutual trust and respect, thus decreasing potential feelings of ownership over particular therapeutic approaches. Limited contact among team members may result in difficulties in supporting the roles of other team members. Coaching, described later in the chapter, is a form of early intervention consultation that allows team member to reinforce intervention strategies designed by other team members.

Coaching may be supported using telehealth, an emerging service delivery model in occupational therapy, which has become increasingly used in early intervention services.[1,11-13,44,57] Telehealth is the use of telecommunication and information technology to provide increased access to services in which provider shortages exist and facilitates consultation, collaboration, and coaching among early intervention providers and families[12] (Figure 22-1).

Opportunities for participating in collaborative activities and teaming may be challenging when providing intervention individually in homes and other community settings. Importantly, team members need to schedule meeting times to plan and communicate and develop systems for communication using e-mail, an electronic file-sharing service (e.g., Dropbox or cloud computing technology), and regularly scheduled meetings.[7]

Evaluation and Intervention Planning

Early intervention evaluation consists of a series of steps and is an ongoing, collaborative process of collecting, analyzing, and gathering information about the infant and family to identify specific needs and develop IFSP goals. The evaluation, combined with a treatment program and ongoing reassessment, is a problem-solving process that continues throughout the period during which the infant or toddler is eligible for Part C services.[73]

Two major goals in the evaluation of infants and toddlers are (1) determination of eligibility for early intervention programs and (2) development of goals and potential outcomes to guide the early intervention services.

Eligibility Determination

Certain infants and toddlers are diagnosed at birth or shortly after birth, such as children with cerebral palsy, Down syndrome, or spina bifida, and become automatically eligible for early intervention services. Infants and toddlers without a specific diagnosis who are suspected of having developmental delay are entitled to an evaluation that must be timely (completed within 45 days) and comprehensive and must include input by a multidisciplinary team. The occupational therapist is often a member of the evaluation team. Family-centered practices during the evaluation process include the following: (1) the family is treated with respect; (2) the evaluation should be individualized, flexible, and responsive to the family's culture and preferences; (3) the child and family's strengths should be emphasized rather than focusing on deficit areas; and (4) the family's expertise should be valued, and they should be included as a partner in all decision making.[31] As much as possible, the team is responsive to the family's needs and desires when determining the time and location of the evaluation and who should be present. The family's involvement is central to the evaluation process, and the family's strengths and concerns are documented.

At the time of the initial evaluation, the team introduces families to the early intervention system and to concepts such as family-centeredness and natural environments.[106] Semi-structured interviews such as the routines-based interview (RBI)[75,76] can be used to gather information about the natural environment and family priorities for intervention (see the Evolve website for an example of the RBI). The RBI includes six steps: (1) beginning statements (introduces the interview process and asks about the family's main concerns), (2) discussion about the daily routine of the child and family, (3) information about the daily routines and child's participation in these routines, (4) family's satisfaction with daily routines, (5) family's concerns and priorities, and (6) outcome writing (see later, "Writing Goals and Objectives"). The team can ask parents about their community activities, family supports, and perceived barriers to community participation.[106]

With an understanding of family priorities and context, the team administers a standardized assessment of infant cognitive, communication, motor, social-emotional, and adaptive (self-care) development. Play is often the context for or a

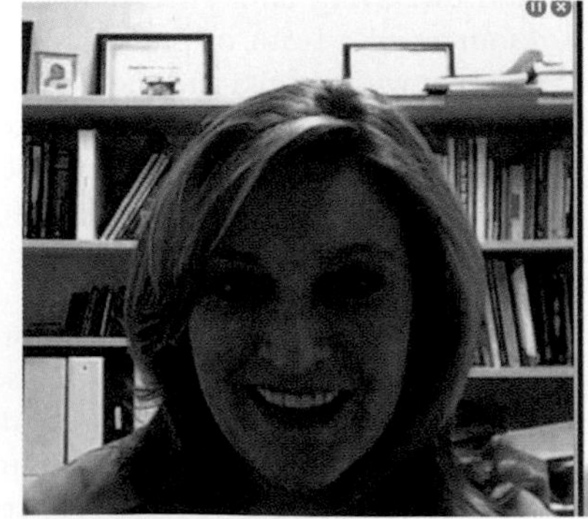
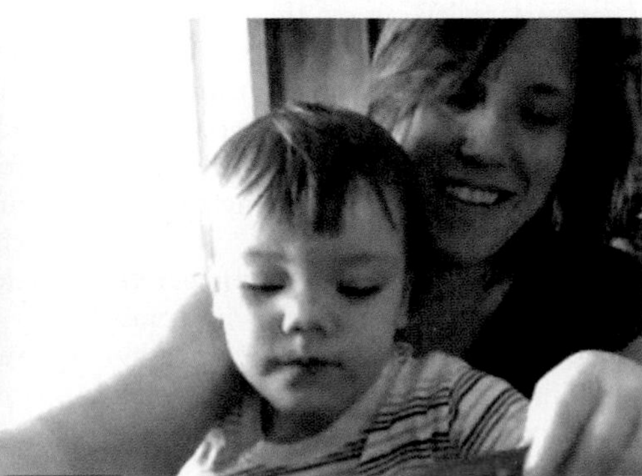

FIGURE 22-1 An occupational therapist uses telehealth technologies to coach a parent on therapeutic techniques to implement in the child's natural environment.

component of the assessment, allowing team members to determine how well the child integrates related skill areas and how he or she playfully interacts with social and physical environments. Therapists may use informal assessment through observing the child playing with caregivers, siblings, or peers.[63] The Transdisciplinary Play-Based Assessment, second edition (TPBA-2), is an example of a commonly used play-based assessment in which the child's play is facilitated and observed by the team and family.[65]

Administered frequently by early intervention teams, criterion-referenced assessments, including curriculum-based assessments, provide information about a child's ability to perform a certain set of skills that represent a developmental age range. Criterion-referenced tests can be favored over norm-referenced tests that compare a child's abilities with those of their same-age peers because children receiving early intervention services may not follow the typical ("normal") developmental sequence and may not respond to a standardized protocol. The Hawaii Early Learning Profile (HELP)[84] and the Assessment, Evaluation, and Programming System for Infants and Children, second edition (AEPS),[5] are well-used, developmental, curriculum-based assessments. The assessments chosen by teams may vary from state to state and may be specified by policies of the state agency responsible for the implementation of IDEA Part C services. Because a standardized test provides a sampling of a child's abilities and behaviors observed at a particular time and situation, from a particular perspective and with a particular instrument, Part C regulations include the term ***informed clinical opinion*** as an essential aspect of the evaluation process.[82] Practitioners' informed clinical opinions make use of qualitative and quantitative information to assist in forming determinations regarding difficult-to-measure aspects of current developmental status and the potential need for early intervention.[67] For example, an occupational therapist makes judgments about muscle tone abnormality or determines that a premature infant has oral sensitivity when fed.

Informed clinical opinion is the final opinion of the multidisciplinary team in establishing eligibility for early intervention. The team becomes informed through multiple sources, such as a review of medical records and developmental history, family interviews, child and family observations, and information from other professionals (e.g., social workers, medical providers), in addition to the findings from standardized assessments.[67] The following recommendations demonstrate the importance of integrating family-centered practices, standardized assessment, and other information sources during the evaluation of infants and young children[77]:

- The occupational therapist should base the assessment on an integrated developmental model. Parents and professionals must observe the child's range of functions in different contexts to identify how the child can best be helped, rather than simply reporting a test score.
- Assessment involves multiple sources and multiple components of information. Parents and professionals contribute to forming the total picture of the child.
- An understanding of typical child development is essential to the interpretation of developmental differences among infants and young children.
- The assessment should emphasize the child's functional capacities, such as attending, engaging, reciprocating, interacting intentionally, organizing patterns of behavior, understanding his or her environment symbolically, and having problem-solving abilities.
- The assessment process should identify the child's current abilities, strengths, and areas of need to attain desired developmental outcomes.
- The occupational therapist should not challenge young children during the assessment by separating them from their parents or caregivers. The parents' presence supports the child and begins the parent-professional collaborative process.
- An examiner who is unfamiliar to the child should not make an assessment. The occupational therapist should give the child a warm-up period. Assessment by a stranger when the parent is restricted to the role of a passive observer represents an additional challenge.
- Assessments that are limited to easily measurable areas, such as certain motor or cognitive skills, should not be considered complete.
- The occupational therapist should not consider formal or standardized tests as the determining factor in the assessment of the infant or young child. Most formal tests were developed and standardized on typically developing children and not on those with special needs.

Furthermore, many young children have difficulty attending to or complying with the basic expectations of formal tests. Formal test procedures are not the best context in which to observe functional capacities of young children. Assessments that are intended for intervention planning should use structured tests only as part of an integrated approach (Figures 22-2 and 22-3).

Once the team has defined a child's eligibility for early intervention services, further assessment is important for the occupational therapist and family to determine which intervention strategies and services are of greatest value to the child and family. At this point, evaluation becomes a comprehensive decision-making process to identify social-emotional, cognitive, adaptive, motor, and communication problems; develop goals; and define an early intervention program plan.

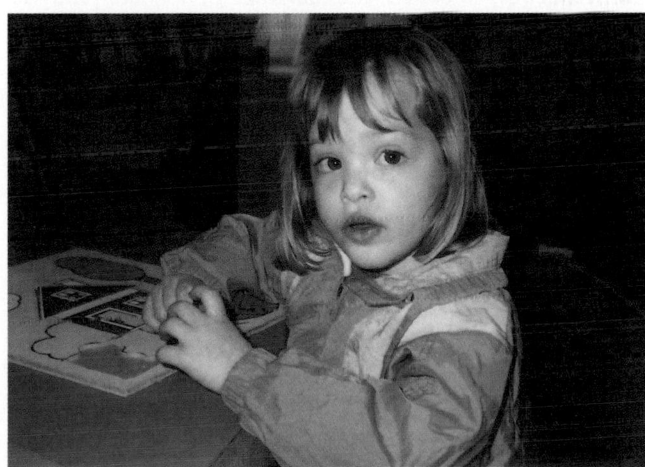

FIGURE 22-2 The occupational therapist can assess perceptual motor and motor planning skills through observation of puzzle completion.

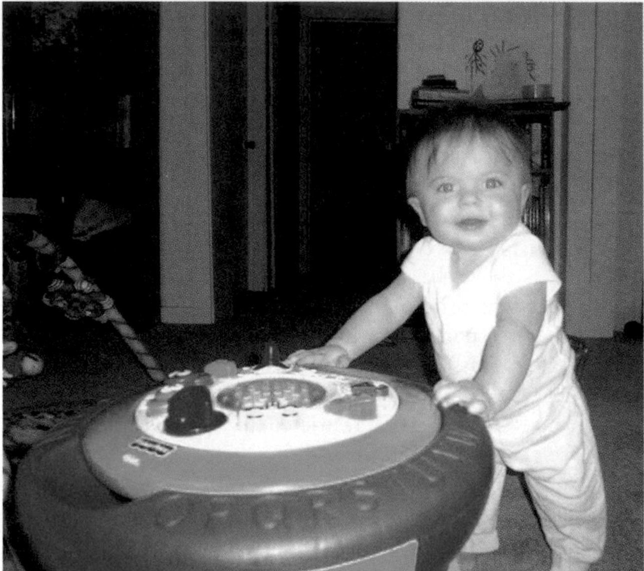

FIGURE 22-3 Important assessment data are gathered through structured observations of the child's play in his or her daily environment.

Development of the Individualized Family Service Plan

The IFSP is a map of the family's services and informs everyone who will be working with the child and family about which services will be provided, where they will be provided, and who will provide them. IDEA Part C specifies that services must be provided in the infant's or toddler's natural environments—that is, those that are natural or typical for a same-aged infant or toddler without a disability and that may include the home or community settings (34 CFR §303.26). Development of the IFSP follows completion of the initial evaluation and assessment. The IFSP defines the environments in which the child is to receive services and provides a statement of justification if services are not provided in natural environments (34 CFR §303.126). The IFSP also specifies who the provider will be; the frequency, intensity, and duration of services; and the funding sources. In some states, telehealth is used to enable service providers to participate virtually in the IFSP development process, thus supporting collaboration that may not otherwise be feasible because of travel distance or provider shortages.[13]

Occupational therapy intervention, as with other early intervention services, is based on identified concerns and expected outcomes in the IFSP. Box 22-2 lists the required components as stated in IDEA. The development of the IFSP occurs during a meeting facilitated by the service coordinator and attended by the family and at least one member of the evaluation team. It is a process in which professionals and families share information to assist the family in making decisions about the types of services that they believe will benefit them and the child. The service coordinator's role is to assist the family in accessing information and resources and coordinate implementation of the IFSP. Other service providers or anyone else the family would like to invite may also be in attendance.

BOX 22-2 Required Components of the Individualized Family Service Plan

The IFSP shall be in writing and shall contain the following (IDEA § 636):

1. A statement of the infant's or child's present level of motor, cognitive, communication, social-emotional, and adaptive development, based on objective criteria
2. A statement of the family's resources, priorities, and concerns related to enhancing the development of the infant or child
3. A statement of the major outcomes expected to be achieved for the infant or child and family and the criteria, procedures, and timelines used to determine the degree to which progress toward achieving the outcomes is being made and whether modifications or revisions of the outcomes or service are necessary
4. A statement of specific early intervention services necessary to meet the unique needs of the infant or child and family, including the frequency, intensity, and method of delivering services
5. A statement of the natural environments in which early intervention services shall appropriately be provided, including a justification of the extent, if any, to which the services will not be provided in a natural environment
6. The projected dates for initiation of service and anticipated duration of the services
7. The identification of the service coordinator from the profession most immediately relevant to the infant's or family's needs who will be responsible for implementation of the plan and coordination with other agencies and persons
8. The steps to be taken to support the transition of the child with a disability to preschool or other appropriate services

IFSP forms vary from state to state and among early intervention programs. Despite the differences in forms, each must include specific information, as specified by the IDEA regulations. The IFSP is a dynamic plan. To ensure that it meets the changing needs of the child and family, it is reviewed every 6 months or more often, if deemed necessary. During this meeting, outcomes are examined and families may opt to make changes, including the types of services the child receives.

Writing Goals and Objectives

The occupational therapist on the early intervention team focuses on outcomes from a family-centered perspective and identifies the child's occupational performance as it relates to daily family routines. Box 22-3 identifies questions to discuss with families. An outcome is a statement of changes desired by the family that can focus on any area of the child's development or family life as it relates to the child.[60] It reflects family priorities, hopes, and concerns in a broad statement that the whole team addresses. Before an outcome is developed, the early intervention team collects information about the natural environments in which families and children spend their time (e.g., using the RBI), at the home or in the community (e.g., child-care center, playground, library). The team should also assist the family in identifying the activities that they typically do or

BOX 22-3 Discussing Routines and Activities with Families When Providing Intervention in the Natural Environment

- Ask open-ended questions such as "What activities do you and your child do throughout the day or a typical week?" and "Describe how your child participates in those activities."
- Ask strengths- and interest-based questions such as "What activities go very well?" "What do you like to do together?" and "What do you wish you could do together?"
- Ask questions about activities the family might find challenging such as "What's a tough time of the day or activity for you?" and "How does your child behave and interact with others in these challenging activities?"
- Use prompts and observations to encourage the family to describe their child's engagement and participation, independence, and social interaction in various routines and activities.

Workgroup on Principles and Practices in Natural Environments, OSEP TA Community of Practice: Part C Settings. (2008, February). *Agreed upon practices for providing early intervention services in natural environments.* Retrieved from http://www.ectacenter.org/~pdfs/topics/families/AgreedUponPractices_FinalDraft2_01_08.pdf.

would like to do in those environments, such as a family who eats breakfast at the kitchen table and would like the child to participate in eating as a morning routine.[76,91] Once routines, activities, and suggested strategies have been identified, outcome statements may be written. Criteria for high-quality IFSP outcomes include the following[68]:

- The outcome statement is necessary and functional for the child's and family's life.
- The statement reflects real-life contextualized settings (e.g., not test items).
- The wording of the statement is jargon-free, clear, and simple.
- The outcome is discipline-free (e.g., not specific to occupational therapy, physical therapy, speech-language pathology, or other discipline).
- The statement avoids the use of passive words (e.g., tolerate, receive, improve, maintain).
- The wording emphasizes the positive.

"Lily will go fishing with her family and hold her own fishing pole" and "Marcus will play in the backyard getting around on his own using his walker" are examples of outcome statements that meet these criteria.[68] Other outcome statements are parent-focused and may include learning strategies to support the child or facilitate the role of a parent of a child with special needs. For example, a family-focused outcome may be a measurable outcome that relates to finding childcare for a child with special needs or understanding community resources to access appropriate services prior to exiting the early intervention program. See Box 22-3 for examples of outcome statements.

After an outcome is developed, the next step is to describe what is happening now and what will happen when the outcome is achieved. Strategies are listed to address the outcome with individuals and resources that are needed. All relevant team members should be included. For example, if the outcome is "to feed himself finger food at a family meal," the current problems might be "unable to hold food in hand and bring to mouth, cannot sit at a table, cries during meals unless parent is feeding him." The team will recognize progress when the child can sit at the table independently and pick up and eat small pieces of food. To achieve this outcome, a number of strategies are proposed. The strategies usually link to the practice areas of specific disciplines. For example, the physical therapist takes primary responsibility for developing strategies that increase the infant's stability for sitting, the speech-language pathologist for communication, and the occupational therapist for the child to increase holding the food and bringing it to his or her mouth.

Outcomes focused on participation in community activities may be particularly meaningful for families and young children.[8] Involvement in activities that occur in a setting outside the home, such as a local restaurant, place of worship, or library, may be a caregiver's main concern. Strategies could include assistive technology or equipment that helps the family manage transport (e.g., an adapted stroller), comfort (e.g., a carrying device), or behavior (e.g., recommended busy box or computer tablet activities). A worksheet that may be used to help families and other team members determine how to incorporate ideas and strategies into routines in community settings is shown in Table 22-2.

Transition Planning

As a child turns 2 years old, the early intervention team begins to develop a plan for the child's transition from the early intervention program to preschool (Part C to Part B services). The transition process for young children with disabilities and their families is often characterized by stress because of the many factors involved, such as a change of environment (e.g., receiving early intervention services at home and then moving to a preschool classroom), a change of providers (e.g., the child and family may have a close relationship with early intervention providers but will receive services from school personnel after the transition), and a difference in philosophy between early intervention programs and schools (i.e., family-centered in early intervention versus child-centered in schools).[86,92] Parents' stress may be decreased when transitions are well planned and support to families and children is provided throughout the process.[40]

Occupational therapists have an important role in transition planning because their background in understanding how different contexts may influence participation is a distinctive part of occupational therapy intervention.[79,80,85] Outcomes and strategies written on the IFSP may be used to guide the family during the transition process. For example, the family can place their child in a small play group (Case Study 22-1) to help him or her adjust to the social expectations of preschool. Potential activities in which occupational therapists may support families and children during transition include preparing caregivers for changes in roles and routines that will occur after the move to preschool, teaching caregivers how to work with their children to develop specific skills needed in preschool, and visiting the preschool classroom before the transition to assess needs for environmental modifications.[79] The occupational therapist can also support a smooth transition by making sure that the child's

TABLE 22-2 Worksheet: Plan of Strategies to Promote Tunisha's Participation in Library Story Hour

Ways to Position Tunisha	
When the Other Children ...	**Tunisha Can ...**
Sit on the floor	Sit in her floor sitter chair. Sit with you, between your legs. Be propped up in a beanbag chair. Lie on her stomach.
Sit at a table	Sit in a chair pushed up to the table and with a strap at her hips. Sit in her stroller pushed up to the table.
Stand	Sit in her stroller. Stand in front of you, with you holding her at her hips (takes two hands). Stand in front of a table with you behind her so that your leg is between her legs (to keep them apart).
Helping Tunisha Manipulate Objects or Materials	
When the Activity Requires Objects ...	**Tunisha Can ...**
Storybook stick props, rhythm band instruments, other objects	Hold objects that are large when placed in her hand (e.g., instead of using a stick on the storybook props, staple Tunisha's prop to a paper towel cardboard tube). Hold objects that can be placed on her hand or arm so that she doesn't have to grasp (e.g., bells fastened to her wrist, puppets). Hold objects using her Velcro glove.
Markers, crayons, paint brushes	Hold the object with her Velcro glove. Use fat crayons (with knobs at the top). Finger paint instead. Draw with an adult or another child helping her hold the object and move her arms.

Adapted from Campbell, P. (2004). Participation-based services: Promoting children's participation in natural settings. *Young Exceptional Children, 8*(1), 20–29.

adaptive equipment is sent to the new setting and providing team members in the new setting with a video recording of the child and caregivers doing self-care routines.[108]

Payment for Occupational Therapy Services

In general, states determine how occupational therapists are paid for their services. In some states, occupational therapists are employed by the state agency that oversees the early intervention program; in others, the occupational therapist is self-employed or employed through a private agency. In a typical scenario, the occupational therapist bills for the time spent in direct, face-to-face contact with the child, family, or other caregiver. It is important to note that "face-to-face" may be interpreted as in-person or as real-time interactions occurring through videoconferencing technology (e.g., telehealth). Billing for time spent in team meetings, on the phone with team members or family, and other indirect activities may or may not be reimbursed.

Because state funding for early intervention programs is the payment of last resort (IDEA § 635 [a][10][A]), occupational therapists are typically reimbursed through other federal programs (e.g., Medicaid) or private insurance, with families paying part of the cost of early intervention services.[34] Often the payment amount of the family share portion is determined on a sliding scale based on a family's income. Although occupational therapists working in early intervention must travel throughout the community to provide services in natural environments, travel is rarely reimbursed.[37] Early intervention services provided by telehealth technologies may be reimbursed by Medicaid, private insurance, or IDEA Part C funds.[13] Medicaid and private insurance reimbursement for services provided by telehealth vary by state. When billing for services provided by telehealth, providers may be required to use a distinct billing code that identifies the type of technology used (e.g., synchronous technology).[1,14] Occupational therapists work with administrators and service coordinators to make these issues transparent, problem-solve barriers, and optimize resources in systems that are inevitably constrained by funding.

Working in Natural Environments

To enable the child to remain an integral part of the family, and for the family to be integral parts of the neighborhood and community, services should be community-based and in locations convenient to the family.[50,103] The family should choose the natural environments that best fit their priorities and lifestyle and include typically developing children of the same age.[81] Some examples are a play group, mother's morning-out program, childcare center, playground, or park (Figure 22-4). In addition, the outcomes on the IFSP should support the provision of services in the natural environment, with outcomes linked directly to family routines and contexts.[54,55]

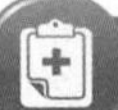

CASE STUDY 22-1 Jeremy

Background

Jeremy's pediatric neurologist referred him for a transdisciplinary assessment at 18 months of age because of motor delays caused by his mitochondrial encephalopathy. An early intervention team, which consisted of an occupational therapist, physical therapist, speech-language pathologist, and early childhood intervention specialist, assessed him in an arena assessment. Both parents participated in the assessment. Although Jeremy had received occupational therapy and physical therapy since he was 6 months old, his parents stated their desire for his inclusion with children who were typically developing and asked that therapies be integrated into his early childhood classroom.

Assessment

The team chose to administer the Battelle Developmental Inventory, second edition (BDI-2),* and the Hawaii Early Learning Profile (HELP).[84] The latter was administered through observation, direct administration of test items, and interview with the parents. The team modified portions to accommodate for Jeremy's physical limitations. Most important, the occupational therapists engaged him in play activities and used their interpretation of his interactions and movements to estimate his functional abilities.

Overall, Jeremy had very low muscle tone and poor physical endurance. He needed support for sitting and could bear only some of his weight when supported in standing. He was unable to roll or crawl. Head control was poor, with head stacking in a supported sitting position and lack of head righting in the prone position. He used his left hand very well to play with toys when he was positioned appropriately but did not use his right hand and protested when the occupational therapist attempted to evaluate his passive range of motion. Jeremy was alert and interested but was reluctant to leave his mother's lap. He said five words—mom, dad, baba for bottle, do for dog, and mo for more.

Intervention

Jeremy started in an inclusive playgroup two mornings a week. He received occupational therapy, physical therapy, and speech-language pathology on a consultative basis, with direct special instruction while in the play group. The team members agreed that Jeremy's goals included improved social interaction with peers, self-help skills, manipulation, and mobility. The team obtained adapted seating and eating utensils for him and modified group activities to enable him to participate actively and as independently as possible.

Individual Family Service Plan Review

After 6 months, the service coordinator, intervention team, and family members met to review the goals on Jeremy's IFSP and to update and modify it as needed. The family and team were pleased with Jeremy's progress and thought that he was benefiting from his intervention program. Jeremy was gaining confidence in a small group, developing good social and communication skills, and no longer tiring as easily. Jeremy's service coordinator arranged for him to participate in a special grant program at a local childcare center. He was enrolled in a class for 2-year-old children that met a few hours a week and had the support of an assistant who had been trained to facilitate the inclusion of children with special needs in the typical childcare setting. Although this facilitator had several other children to work with and was not in Jeremy's class all the time, she was available whenever he needed help or when the teacher had a question or concern. After a few months, Jeremy started attending this program twice a week; meanwhile, he continued to receive therapy services on a consultative basis at home and at the center.

Annual Reassessment

One year after entrance into the early intervention program, the intervention team reassessed Jeremy in preparation for the development of a new IFSP. They did not perform this assessment in a formal testing session but over a period of weeks as Jeremy participated in various activities with the group. In addition to the BDI-2, Jeremy's team also updated the HELP.

Results of the reassessment indicated a happy, verbal, 2-year-old child. Although he had gained in physical abilities, Jeremy needed a stroller-type wheelchair with special inserts for appropriate seating. The removable seat also acted as a floor sitter so that Jeremy could be close to the same level as his peers when they played on the floor. He demonstrated improvement in his play skills and increased spontaneous interactions with his peers—for example, he took turns and shared toys with little prompting.

Jeremy continued to participate in the class at the childcare center and no longer needed the facilitator's support. The occupational therapist and physical therapist continued to provide on-site consultation. Through a problem-solving approach, with close cooperation among the family, childcare personnel, and therapists, Jeremy thrived in the class. Strategies that supported his participation included providing wheelchair access to the playground (they had been carrying him), teaching principles of lifting and carrying, and making the stroller available to transport him from room to room so that the teacher had her hands free to keep up with other active 2-year-old children.

Summary

Jeremy is an example of a child who was able to benefit from a combination of programming that included an inclusive playgroup and typical childcare setting. His program required close cooperation among the family, early intervention personnel, and community resources. His parents look forward to his graduation to the class for 3-year-old children and increasing his typical class time to 3 days a week. They have visited the neighborhood school and plan for him to attend a regular kindergarten class when he is 5 years of age, where he will be supported by therapies. Jeremy has age-appropriate cognitive skills, and with the right kind of support and technology, he can fully participate in school and in the community.

*Newborg, J. (2005). *Battelle developmental inventory* (2nd ed.). Chicago: Riverside.

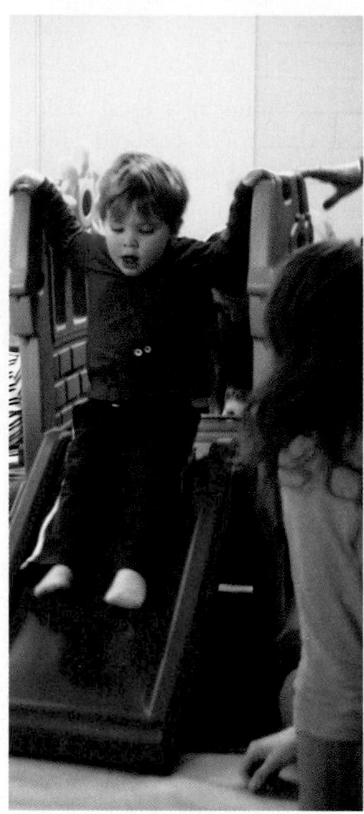

FIGURE 22-4 The occupational therapist encourages a child to participate in sensorimotor activities on the playground.

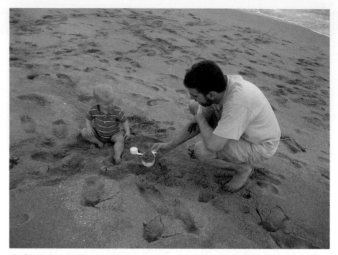

FIGURE 22-5 Family involvement supports the child in the natural environment.

Intervention in natural environments includes using toys and materials that can be found in the home and will remain available to the family or other caregivers on a consistent basis. Occupational therapists who rely on clinical equipment, whether they bring it to home visits or use it in their centers, may be selecting equipment and toys most comfortable to them but not friendly or helpful to the family.[38,78] Specialized equipment, such as suspended swings, therapy balls, or a child-sized table and chair, may be optimal for a clinic-based program to remediate sensory or motor deficits, but may not be available to families at home, caregivers at a childcare facility, or another environment in the absence of the occupational therapist. If early intervention is provided in a clinical setting, it is equally important for the occupational therapist to offer opportunities for the family and other caregivers to learn and practice therapeutic strategies and interventions to promote generalization in the natural environment.

The philosophy of inclusion extends beyond physical inclusion to mean social and emotional inclusion of the child and family.[16,103] The Division of Early Childhood of the Council for Exceptional Children (DEC) and the National Association for the Education of Young Children (NAEYC) support the philosophy of inclusion in natural environments with the following statement: "Early childhood inclusion embodies the values, policies, and practices that support the right of every infant and young child and his or her family, regardless of ability, to participate in a broad range of activities and contexts as full members of families, communities, and society. The desired results of inclusive experiences for children with and without disabilities and their families include a sense of belonging and membership, positive social relationships and friendships, and development and learning to reach their full potential"[22] (Figure 22-5).

Occupational Therapy Early Intervention Practices

Occupational therapists promote a child's development, independence, and mastery in physical, cognitive, and psychosocial functions. They guide and support families and caregivers, implement intervention strategies, and recommend technology to enhance the child's functional abilities and developmental performance. Occupational therapists also provide opportunities for children with disabilities to participate in natural learning environments with typically developing peers.

Occupational Therapy in Natural Environments

Occupational therapists provide services in a broad range of natural environments, including the homes of grandparents or relatives and other community settings when desired by families and of potential benefit to children. By providing early intervention services in natural environments, they take advantage of the actual contexts in which the occupations and co-occupations of children and families occur.[109] Examples include participation in a mothers' morning out, mother-infant play groups, petting a puppy in the park, and playing on a gym set. Occupational therapists provide services at neighborhood pools, consulting with swimming instructors, and collaborate with librarians to create storytime sessions for young children with autism. Practitioners often make recommendations for increasing the child's participation in dressing and bathing. Opportunities for learning in natural environments appear to be most effective for addressing the developmental needs of young children when the opportunities are interesting and

FIGURE 22-6 The occupational therapist uses materials in the childcare center to achieve the child's fine motor goals.

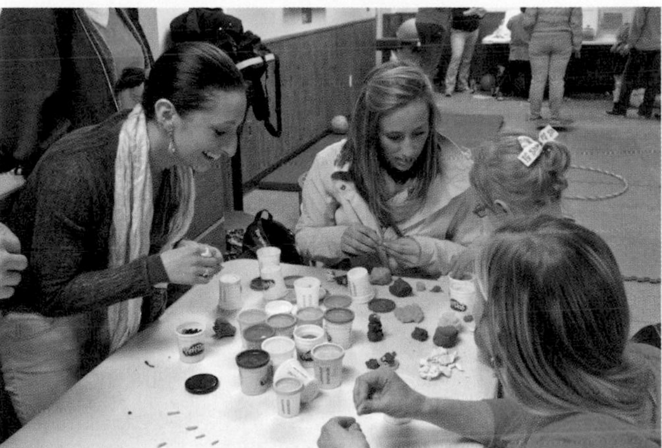

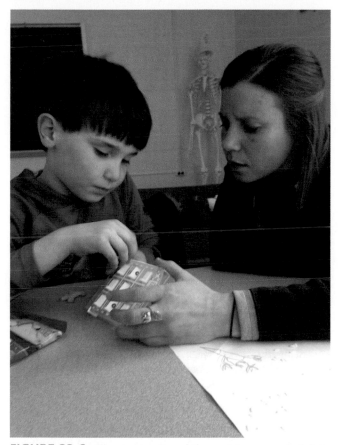

FIGURE 22-7 Inclusive settings support peer interactions and learning.

engaging and provide children with contexts for exploring, practicing, and mastering competence.[26]

Natural intervention strategies use incidental learning opportunities during the child's typical activities and interactions with peers and adults (Figure 22-6), follow the child's lead, and use natural consequences. Intervention strategies that occur in real-life settings promote the child's acquisition of functional motor, social, and communication skills (Figure 22-7).[25,74] When skills are learned in the natural setting, it is more likely that they will generalize to other activities and environments (Figures 22-8 and 22-9).[48] Two key advantages of providing occupational therapy in natural environments are that children tend to be more comfortable in familiar settings such as their homes and that teaching caregivers to implement natural learning opportunities within the daily routines of the child and family is feasible and practical[107] (Figure 22-10). Interventions in natural environments require the occupational therapist's ingenuity to develop strategies that are acceptable and supported by the caregiver(s).[8,38]

Observation of the family and child at home allows the occupational therapist to be realistic in suggesting goals that are based on the resources available, problem-solve issues unique to the home environment, and individualize the program to meet the family's interests and needs. Intervention sessions can include not only the parents but also grandparents,

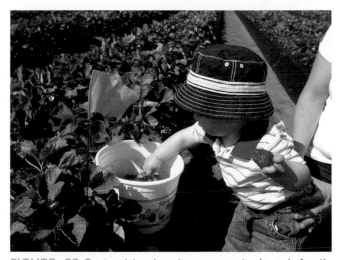

FIGURE 22-8 Participation in community-based family activities promotes developmental skills.

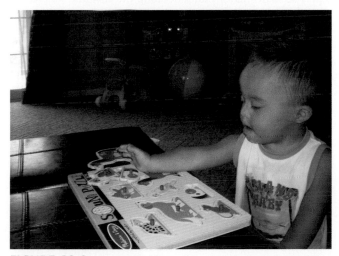

FIGURE 22-9 By using his or her own toys at home, the infant can practice with family members to improve targeted skills.

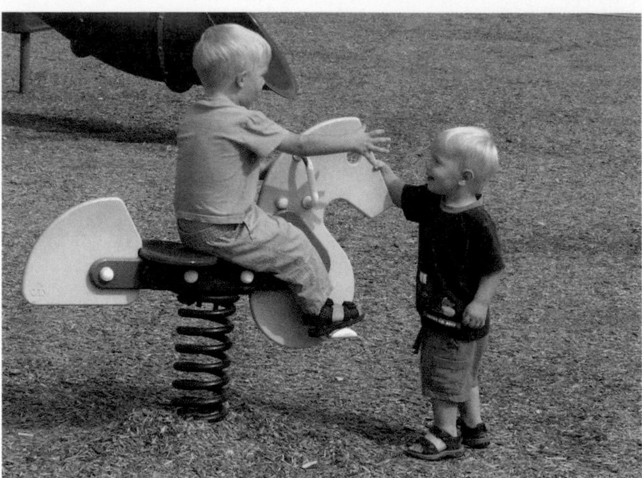

FIGURE 22-10 Play with peers in natural environments helps the child generalize newly learned skills.

childcare providers, and siblings, each of whom can promote the infant's development and participation.

Providing therapy in natural environments presents several challenges from the perspective of therapy providers, families, and governing bodies (particularly state and local agencies),[78] and research findings suggest that occupational therapists do not always consistently implement family-centered practices in the natural environment.[18,32] To provide services effectively in natural environments, occupational therapists must be creative and flexible, taking advantage of teachable moments in children's play activities. For example, the occupational therapist may have plans to use the childcare center's playground for sensory motor activities and use the activity table inside to practice fine motor skills, only to find that it is a rainy day and the children cannot go outdoors. When arriving at the classroom, she or he sees that the children are engaged in a rainy day activity of playing dress-up and immediately uses the dress-up activity as the context for the intervention, developing a play scenario that includes donning the costume selected by the targeted child.

Family-Centered Intervention

In family-centered intervention, the occupational therapist is guided by family priorities and respects the level of involvement in intervention that various family members choose to have. One important way for occupational therapists to increase the effect of services is to make the program relevant to the family's lifestyle and time commitments.[101] Therefore, occupational therapists select and recommend activities to improve behaviors and skills that the children can generalize to their daily routines at home, school, and community. Family demands and supports are always considerations when discussing home programs with parents. One mother stated the following: "There are times when even an acceptable amount of therapy becomes too much—when your child needs time just to be a child, or when you need time to be with the rest of the family. It is okay to say 'no' at those times, for a while. Your instinct will tell you when."[97] Occupational therapists support families by listening to them and giving positive feedback regarding parenting skills.[29] Because daily routines in a family with a child who has a disability can take an excessive amount of time and energy, suggestions that make routines easier or that can easily be incorporated into the daily routine are the most successful. For example, occupational therapists make suggestions for positioning and handling to enhance the efficiency of feeding and for adapting a bath seat to make bathing less taxing. The parent can incorporate therapy strategies to encourage bilateral coordination or range of motion at bath time, or an older sibling can encourage the infant to reach for toys while the mother cooks dinner. Coaching parents is one method that combines listening with teaching and encourages parents' active participation.

Coaching Families

Coaching is a family-centered approach that takes advantage of adult learning styles. Natural environments offer opportunities for occupational therapists to coach caregivers to gain self-confidence and assume responsibility in their child's daily care. Occupational therapists also coach other professionals to implement intervention strategies that they have developed. Coaching is characterized by the coach (the early interventionist), who "has specialized knowledge and skills to share about growth and development, specific intervention strategies, and enhancing the performance of young children with disabilities," and the learner (the caregiver), who "has intimate knowledge of a child's abilities, challenges, and typical performance in a given situation, ... daily routines and settings, lifestyle, family culture, ... desirable goals for [the learner] and the child" (p. 38).[93] The coach supports the learner and the child to achieve outcomes through a process described by Rush and colleagues[93]:

- Initiation: The coach or learner identifies a need, and a joint plan is developed that includes the purpose of the coaching and specific learner outcomes.
- Observation: The coach may use four possible types of observation: (1) the learner demonstrates an existing challenge or practices a new skill while the coach observes; (2) the coach models a technique, strategy, or skill while the learner observes; (3) the learner consciously thinks about how to support the child's learning while performing the activity; and (4) the coach and learner observe aspects of the environment to determine how they may influence the situation.
- Action: This includes activities that take place at times other than when the coach and learner are in contact, such as the learner's practicing the new skill or strategy or engaging in a situation that may be discussed with the coach.
- Reflection: The coach uses questioning and reflective listening and provides reflective feedback and joint problem solving to help the learner understand how to analyze practices and behaviors. The coach then reviews the discussion or observes the learner to assess the learner's understanding. The learner's strengths, competence, and mastery are acknowledged.
- Evaluation: The coach evaluates the effectiveness of the coaching process with the learner and with himself or herself. Evaluation with the learner may not take place every time the coach and learner have discussions; however, the coach should self-evaluate to determine if changes need to be made, if the coach is assisting the learner to achieve identified outcomes, or if the coaching needs to continue.

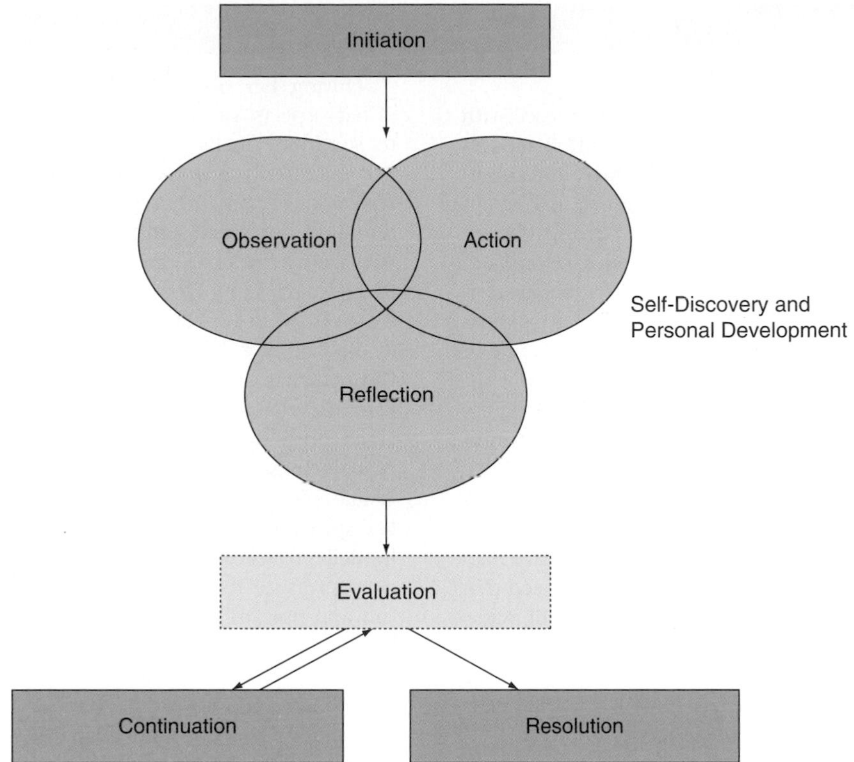

FIGURE 22-11 The coaching process. (Adapted from Rush, D. D., Shelden, M. L., & Hanft, B. E. [2003]. Coaching families and colleagues: A process for collaboration in natural settings. *Infants and Young Children, 16*(1), 33–47.)

- Continuation: The results of the coaching session are summarized and a plan is developed for what should occur before and during the following session.
- Resolution: Both the coach and learner agree that identified outcomes have been achieved. The learner has increased competence and confidence to support the child's learning opportunities in the natural environment (Figure 22-11).

Coaching may be especially helpful in a service delivery model in which one early intervention team member is the primary provider for the child and family (Case Study 22-2). In this model, the other team members provide coaching on a consultative basis for the family and also provide coaching to the primary service provider. As in any team process, coaching requires that team members use good communication skills and trust and respect one another. Opportunities for communication and collaboration are crucial to the success of coaching, thus necessitating support from early intervention programs and agencies for additional meeting times and co-visits. It is important for team members to understand that coaching is not a linear process, but rather a process in which feedback is used to refine solutions, as needed.

The occupational therapist may work with caregivers to plan and carry out therapeutic interventions for the child by integrating developmentally appropriate activities that are challenging for the child into daily routines and family-identified activity settings. For example, the occupational therapist coaches parents in methods for developing the infant's grasping competence as it relates to play with a favorite toy or finger feeding. After identifying an area of delayed performance, such as eating and participating in mealtime, the occupational therapist collaborates with caregivers to identify natural learning opportunities in which the child participates in mealtime. To promote generalization of the self-feeding performance, the occupational therapist and caregivers can use snack time activities in an environment that enables the child to focus, allows sufficient time, and uses appropriate (easy to eat) foods. The selected eating activity involves the "just-right" challenge to the child across domains (including sensory, motor, cognitive and social domains).

Most developmental skills and play occupations are learned in the context of social interaction, including give and take with another child or adult, eye contact, praise, and delight at successful attempts. Integrating therapeutic strategies into the daily routine (Figure 22-12) requires a behavior change on behalf of the caregiver. Caregivers will benefit from continued coaching with modeling and reinforcement of behaviors in addition to practicing the therapeutic strategy with the occupational therapist and receiving feedback.[66]

Use of Telehealth to Facilitate the Coaching Model

A telehealth service delivery model allows occupational therapists to use coaching within a family-centered framework. For example, an occupational therapist may use telehealth to coach a caregiver on strategies to assist a child in gaining independence in self-feeding using a spoon. Using an electronic tablet with videoconferencing software, the occupational

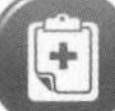

CASE STUDY 22-2 Alana

Background

Alana is a 2-year, 3-month-old child who was diagnosed with developmental delay. She receives early intervention services because of delays in motor, self-care and adaptive, and social-emotional domains. Findings from her initial assessment suggest that Alana's delays may be related to problems with sensory processing and appears to seek excessive amounts of sensory stimulation. Karen, the occupational therapist, is Alana's primary service provider. Alana's mother, Carmen, has requested that services be provided in the family's home at this time, so Karen has been making home visits once weekly. During the IFSP, the family identified that Alana has difficulty falling asleep. They would like the early intervention team to address this issue.

Intervention

At the first home visit, Carmen mentioned that Alana had been difficult to get to bed at night. Karen hypothesized that Alana's struggle to calm down in the evening and fall asleep may relate to her sensory processing difficulties. Karen initiated a coaching relationship with Carmen by asking her if she would like to work together to explore ways to help Alana sleep better. Carmen enthusiastically agreed.

Karen asked Carmen to explain what she and her husband, Ramon, had already tried with Alana during bedtime. Carmen explained that they typically gave Alana a bath, let her watch a video, and then moved into her room for some quiet time before going to bed. However, Alana, who recently switched from a crib to a toddler bed, refused to stay in bed. Instead she would pull her toys out, jump on her mattress, and run around her room, becoming increasingly active as the night wore on. Eventually, several hours later, Alana would crash on her bed and fall asleep. Carmen thought that the sleep problems were causing tension between her and Ramon because they were getting less sleep and becoming easily frustrated with each other.

Karen told Carmen that she suspected that there was a relationship between Alana's sensory processing and her difficulty falling asleep. She provided Carmen with two suggestions of strategies to incorporate increased sensory input to put into action before the next visit: (1) give Alana more opportunities for play that incorporated movement, such as climbing and crawling, before initiating the bedtime routine; and (2) use a textured bath mitt during the bath. Karen decided that it would be beneficial to observe Alana's bedtime routine, so she scheduled her next visit in the evening. When she arrived, she asked Carmen what happened when the sensory-based suggestions were implemented. Carmen reflected on the last several days and replied that it was difficult to give Alana more play time because of the late hour that the family arrived home after picking her up from day care. Carmen did think that the textured bath mitt helped calm Alana during her bath, but Alana continued to take a long time to fall asleep.

During her observation of the bedtime routine, Karen noted aspects of the routine that could be strengthened to support Alana's sensory needs and behaviors that were not necessarily sensory-based, but more likely a result of typical development in the toddler stage, such as Alana's refusal to go to bed. On arrival, Karen followed Carmen and Alana into the bedroom and Carmen turned on the video. Alana was running around the room in circles while the video, a cartoon with very little action, played. Karen asked Carmen if she had a video with characters that danced and sang. Carmen changed the video and soon Alana was dancing along with the characters. Karen explained that the dancing provided both movement and muscle work and helped meet Alana's sensory needs. After the video, she observed that Alana enjoyed her bath and sought out sensory experiences like splashing and rubbing soap on her arms and legs. Karen modeled to Carmen how to use the loofah sponge to provide deep pressure to Alana's arms, legs, and back while in the tub and how to use the towel to do the same while drying her off.

After the bath they went to Alana's room. Carmen shut the blinds and pulled the dark shades so that the room was dimly lit. Although Alana was calm when entering her room, she became increasingly active as the room got darker and the house grew quieter. Karen asked Carmen if she had an extra nightlight and Carmen placed one in the corner of Alana's room. Karen turned on Alana's small radio to the classical station at a soft volume. Karen explained that Alana might need extra visual and auditory input to help stay calm. After looking at books in bed, Carmen told Alana it was time to go to sleep. Alana began to protest, but Karen quickly suggested that they play the "Cloud Game" before going to sleep. She took Alana's pillow and placed it on Alana's back with Alana lying on her stomach. Karen pressed the pillow down firmly and told Alana "the clouds are carrying you off to sleep." Karen traded places with Carmen and encouraged Carmen to continue providing the deep pressure to Alana until Alana indicated she was ready to go to sleep.

After they left the room, Carmen called Ramon into the kitchen so that they could speak with Karen. They were both excited that Alana was asleep and how much easier it had been when using the strategies Karen suggested. Carmen and Ramon planned to implement the techniques and evaluate their effectiveness at the next visit.

Follow-Up

Karen arrived at Alana's home the next week and was greeted by Ramon. He told Karen that Alana continued to show improvement in going to sleep and was even asking to go into her bed so she could play the "Cloud Game." Karen, Carmen, and Ramon decided that further intervention regarding Alana's sleep was not needed and ended the coaching relationship for that particular need.

therapist can observe the caregiver positioning the child at mealtime and assisting the child in using a spoon, provide instruction to the caregiver on therapeutic techniques (e.g., active assistance, backward chaining, or postural supports), and observe the caregiver implementing the therapeutic techniques. The occupational therapist can provide feedback, discuss the caregiver's concerns, and problem-solve strategies for skill progression (Figure 22-13). Research suggests that the use of telehealth within early intervention services promotes family participation, supports child and family outcomes, and results in high levels of family satisfaction.[11,44,57] See Table 22-1e on the Evolve website for relevant research on telehealth and young children.

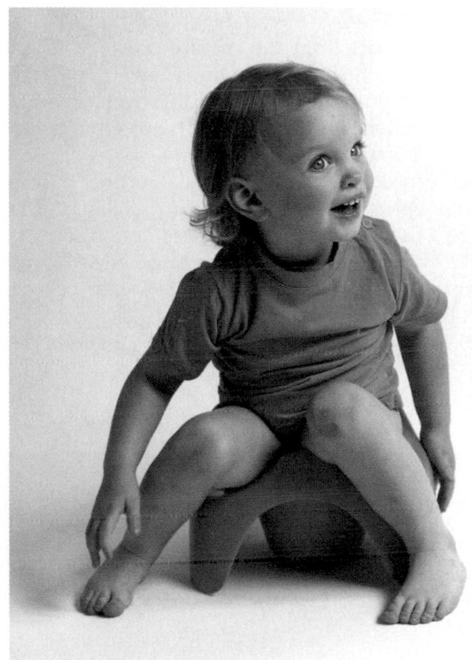

FIGURE 22-12 The occupational therapist adapts communication to promote the child's independence in using the toilet.

Telehealth also supports collaboration among specialists, remote providers, and families for the purpose of interdisciplinary evaluation, care coordination, and team-to-team consultation.[41] Evaluations by an interdisciplinary team of specialists (e.g., physicians and rehabilitation professionals) administered through telehealth technologies in collaboration with families and local providers have been perceived as effective as in-person evaluations, and a high level of satisfaction among participants (families and providers) was reported. Additionally, significant cost savings because of the decreased need for travel to specialty clinics, enhanced care coordination, family empowerment through participation in the evaluation and discussion of recommendations with providers, and mutual enhancement of professionals' skills occurred as a result of a telehealth service delivery model. Factors to consider when deciding who would benefit from telehealth services include the complexity of the child's condition; child's context and natural environments; family's preferences and access to technology (Box 22-4); nature and complexity of the interventions to be provided; requirements of the practice setting (i.e., early intervention program); and knowledge, skill, and competence of the occupational therapist[1] (see Figure 22-14).

Occupational Therapy Interventions

Primary outcomes of occupational therapy intervention for infants and toddlers are play, including object and social play; social participation, including parent-child, peer-to-peer, and group interactions; and self-care, for example, eating and sleeping. Intervention principles and strategies for each area are described in this section. See Table 22-3 for examples of evidence-based interventions for infants and toddlers.

Play is an essential element of occupational therapy with a young child and has been defined as both an intervention means (strategy to promote developmental progress) and goal (occupational outcome).[83] Therefore, occupational therapy interventions improve play outcomes and use play as a therapeutic context to promote developmental skills.

Play as an Intervention Outcome

Play is a most important child occupation. It is open-ended, self-initiated, self-directed, and unlimited in its variety. Play can

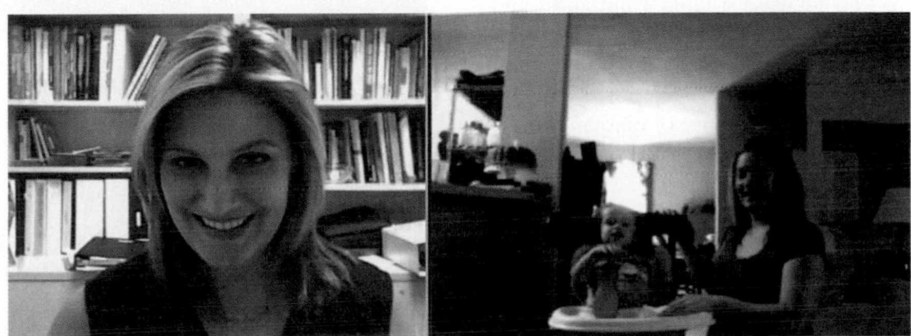

FIGURE 22-13 An occupational therapist uses telehealth technologies to coach a child's caregivers' on a backward-chaining technique to promote the child's independence with self-feeding.

BOX 22-4 Telehealth Models in Early Intervention

The remote therapist collaborates with the following:

- The child and family in the child's natural environment
- The child and family and another provider on the child's IFSP team in the child's natural environment
- The child and family (and perhaps other providers on the child's IFSP team) at a telehealth conferencing site in the child's local community
- An interpreter who is in the home with the family or who is also remote and connected with the family via videoconferencing technology
- The IFSP team to participate in an IFSP team meeting remotely

Technology Options

- Use existing technology in the natural environment (e.g., computer, electronic tablet, smartphone).
- Loan equipment to the family to support a telehealth service delivery model.
- Technology is brought into the child's natural environment by the provider to support consultation and collaboration with a remote provider.
- Leverage existing technology infrastructure available within the child's community (e.g., state telehealth network site, public health department facility, community-based site with videoconferencing equipment).
  - A telehealth network site in the community is not considered a natural environment; however, recommendations provided through telehealth by specialists and discipline-specific providers not available within the local community can be implemented by families and providers in a child's natural environment.
  - When a non-natural environment provides access to a discipline-specific provider not available in the child's local community, and all other early intervention services are provided in the child's natural environment, services will meet OSEP requirements that the *majority* of services occur in the child's natural environments.

Benefits

- Improves access to services otherwise unavailable because of provider shortages
- Facilitates family-centered service provision with the child's family and other IFSP team members receiving consultation, coaching, and support from the remote provider via telehealth technologies in the child's natural environment
- Enhances knowledge and skills of local providers through consulting and collaborating with a remote provider with discipline-specific knowledge and expertise
- If session is recorded and archived via secure platform, recording may be used as a resource for families and IFSP team members to view and practice intervention strategies and promote integration of strategies into daily routines
- Supports more efficient use of interpreters with potential cost savings because of decreased travel

be exploratory, symbolic, creative, or competitive in nature (see Chapter 17). Table 22-4 presents the developmental progression of pretend play skills as these emerge in young children.[64,83,99]

Learning how to play can be a goal of intervention, particularly for children with significant disabilities that affect multiple performance areas. Children with medically related disabilities may not develop play skills because of limited opportunity due to long hospitalizations, being connected to medical technology, or having impaired physical function. Toddlers at risk for autism may demonstrate rigid or stereotypic play that is missing important social and pretend elements. Children with motor disorders may have limited object manipulation or mobility to engage fully in sensorimotor play. Other children may experience deficits in play because of cognitive limitations or difficulties in social interactions. To increase a child's initiation and participation in play, the occupational therapist models playfulness in interactions with the child. Whether it is a game of hide and seek, knocking down a pretend wall, or digging for a treasure in sand, the activity should elicit a sense of enjoyment and fun. Chapter 17 describes interventions that promote play occupations.

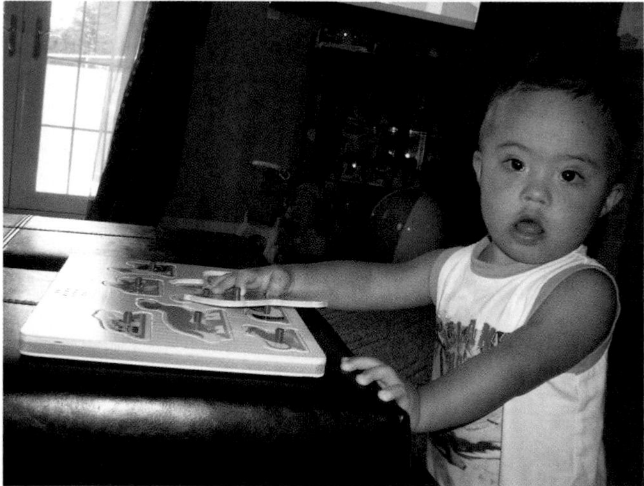

FIGURE 22-14 Using the toddler's own toys, the occupational therapist creates a social opportunity to promote joint attention while practicing perceptual motor skills.

Play as a Means to Learning Specific Skills

The child's participation in play activities allows him or her to practice mastered developmental skills and learn new skills. Skills that are the foundation for engagement in other occupations, such as the ability to manipulate objects, problem-solve, and attend to tasks, can be developed and practiced during play. Occupational therapists and caregivers create play scenarios that encourage specific skills development. Intervention activities use objects and materials typically found in the natural environment (Figure 22-14), rather than items brought into the home by the occupational therapist (e.g., therapy balls).[78] Occupational therapists can show caregivers how to

TABLE 22-3 Examples of Evidence-Based Occupational Therapy Interventions for Infants and Toddlers

Goal Area	Developmental Problem	Evidence-Based Interventions	Occupational Therapist Coaching and Family Participation
Social play	2-year-old with Down syndrome	Supported play with children with higher level development skills can increase performance.[99a] Computer or tablet activities encourage social interaction with peers.[6]	Occupational therapist helps parents create a play group for their daughter that includes other neighborhood children. Occupational therapist helps parents select computer play activities that encourage turn-taking and social interaction.
Sensorimotor play	6-month-old with cerebral palsy	Switch-operated toys increase the infant's engagement in a play activity.[6,62]	Families can obtain switch-operated toys from local adapted toy libraries. Occupational therapy clinics may lend switch-operated toys to families.
Caregiver-infant interaction	12-month-old with sensory processing problems, at risk for autism spectrum disorder	Sensitive responding to infant's cue increases the infant's responsiveness. Imitating the infant's actions can increase the infant's initiation of social gestures and responsiveness.[61]	The occupational therapist coaches parents in how to read the infant's nonverbal cues, imitate the infant's actions, and respond positively to the infant's communication attempts.
Peer interaction	28-month-old with cerebral palsy	Social toys, such as puppets and dress-up clothes, can promote social interactions among young children. Child-directed play promotes more positive social interaction than adult-directed play.[58]	Families can encourage the child's social interaction with peers using socially oriented toys such as dolls, puppets, dress-up, and toys that require sharing.
Eating	8-month-old infant born preterm with low oral muscle tone and jaw instability	Feed in an infant seat at 85 degrees upright, with small blanket rolls on the sides to support the head in midline. Using a flat latex-covered spoon with hand supporting the lower jaw can improve the infant's tongue, lip, and jaw movements for efficient suck-swallow of puréed foods.[30,33]	Mother feeds the child using the adapted infant seat. The occupational therapist coaches the mother in jaw support techniques. The occupational therapist provides the family with small flat spoons for improved suck-swallow.
Sleeping	2-year-old with self-regulatory difficulty	Limit nighttime sounds and lights; establish a nighttime routine that reinforces quiet behavior and does not reinforce active behavior. Weighted blankets may be helpful when use is carefully monitored.[53,88]	Families can establish a nighttime routine that helps the child quiet, establishes an environment that allows low arousal, and provides the child with a preferred sensory environment associated with low arousal (e.g., deep pressure, white noise, very dark).

create games and toys out of everyday objects such as plastic containers and wooden spoons, develop specific arm movements, facilitate sequential pretend play cooking or make music, and/or enhance joint attention. For example, a toddler with hemiplegic cerebral palsy plays with stuffed animals and uses his or her affected arm to stabilize the trunk when reaching into a bin to remove the toys. This activity supports a motor-based occupational therapy goal for the child to incorporate the affected arm in play and may be repeated for practice with gradual adaptation (e.g., the toddler gives the animals a hug before putting them back in the bin); it is a learning opportunity that uses play as initiated by the child with his or her own toys.

When a child has motor delays, the occupational therapist works with caregivers to determine how various age-appropriate toys, games, sensorimotor experiences, and other strategies may be incorporated into the child's daily routine to remediate motor skill deficits. For example, a family who enjoys hiking may encourage their toddler to pick up fallen leaves on the trail and put them into a small bag, an activity that encourages refined grasp and release skills. A caregiver in an infant's child-care center can play peek-a-boo with the infant to encourage reaching and grasp.

Engaging the Child in Play

To engage the infant or toddler fully in play as an outcome or intervention context for skill development, the therapists provides activities that do the following: (1) arouse and engage the child, (2) encourage and prompt practice of emerging developmental skills, (3) reinforce learning of higher level skills, and (4) promote transfer of play skills to multiple activities.

Arousal and Engagement

Occupational therapists use a variety of methods to stimulate the child's interest and motivation to engage in a play activity.

TABLE 22-4 Developmental Levels of Play Skills (0-2 years)

Play Category	Approximate Age (months)	Definition	Examples
Sensorimotor	2-4	Child explores objects, practices motor skills, enjoys sensory motor exploration	Child bounces when held, bangs rattles, mouths toys
Relational	6-10	Child relates one object to another	Child holds two objects, stacks blocks, places one object in or on another
Functional-conventional—discriminative; realistic object play	10-12	Child relates object in a social, conventional manner; uses objects for functional (real) purposes	Child places toy phone on ear, stirs with spoon in cup
Symbolic			
Pretend self; single play actions	12-18	Child relates objects to self in pretend; one-step play actions	Child pretends to drink from a cup, brush own hair
Child as agent—passive; substitute object play; multiple play actions	18-24	Child extends familiar actions to dolls, figures; can use an object as a substitute for the actual object; carries out a sequence of two or more play actions	Child feeds doll, pretends to brush teddy bear's hair, puts doll in cart to ride; pretends that a block is an airplane or a car
Child as agent—active; imaginary objects	24-30	Child includes dolls or figure action in short scenario; pretends an action without the actual object.	Child pretends that teddy bear holds a cup, doll talks on the phone; drinks from an imaginary cup
Child uses imaginary objects in complex play actions	30-36	Play is complex, with multiple steps in planned story	Child plans and carries out snack time with dolls; plays house in role as mother

Adapted from Lifter, K. (2000). Linking assessment to intervention for children with developmental disabilities or at-risk for developmental delay: The developmental play assessment (DPA) instrument. In K. Gitlin-Weiner, A Sandgrund, & C. E. Schaefer (Eds.), *Play diagnosis and assessment* (2nd ed., pp. 228–251). New York: Wiley; Takata, N. (1974). Play as a prescription. In M. Reilly (Ed.), *Play as exploratory learning* (pp. 209–246). Beverly Hills, CA: Sage.

The key to optimal arousal is a comfortable environment, with sensory elements that promote the child's self-regulation. For certain infants, self-regulation may require modifications to the environment to lower arousal, such as lowering the lighting, turning off the television,[2] or using other preferred sources of sensory input, such as rocking rhythmically to music.[72] Providing the infant's preferred types and levels of sensory input supports self-regulation and optimal arousal. An infant who has optimal arousal is alert and attentive and can engage in an activity.

Another method for engaging the child and sustaining interest is to use the child's preferred objects or activities. The caregiver can help identify toys, materials, and objects of high interest. The play activity also needs to be developmentally appropriate—that is, at the child's developmental play level. Features of a play activity that can motivate or interest a child include toys that have interactive components.[51] Toys that are known to be preferred (e.g., trains are often preferred by children with autism) and activities that are known to be personally meaningful and intrinsically motivating to that child should be included.[9,98] The meaningfulness of the play activities can be confirmed by the parents and observed in the child's level of engagement. Preferred play contexts can create and facilitate meaningful social interactions between the child with a disability and the occupational therapist or caregiver. When the child is engaged in a meaningful play activity, the occupational therapist can introduce variations to play or developmentally higher level play activities that elicit and challenge the child's emerging skills.[71]

Allow Practice of Emerging Developmental Skills

Because they are fun, play activities are easily repeated and easily varied. Engaged children may stay focused on play for long periods, allowing the type of practice that can result in skill mastery. Occupational therapists design activities to target, practice, and extend specific skills, such as building a train track on the carpet, filling a sand bucket, or making dozens of snakes out of Play-Doh. Unstructured play activities can easily be adapted or graded to promote a child's higher level response (e.g., the child can line up or stack blocks but also can create designs and build houses and bridges). A play activity that fits well into the caregiver's routine is more likely to be repeated; in this way, play skills become incorporated into the daily life of the child and family.

Reinforce Higher Level Skills

As the child plays, the occupational therapist provides appropriate (and almost universally positive) reinforcement. Because play is often internally reinforcing, the need for praise and verbal encouragement (external reinforcement) can be minimal. Often the occupational therapist's interest in and observation of the child's play are reinforcing; positive affect and enjoyment also reinforce the child's actions. Peer interaction during play can provide modeling and naturally reinforce the child's effort.[58] The occupational therapist carefully plans activities that are intrinsically reinforcing, such as climbing up and jumping into

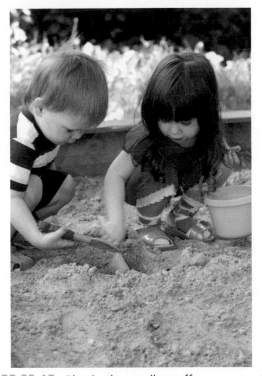

FIGURE 22-15 Play in the sandbox offers an opportunity for children to practice sensorimotor function and social play skills.

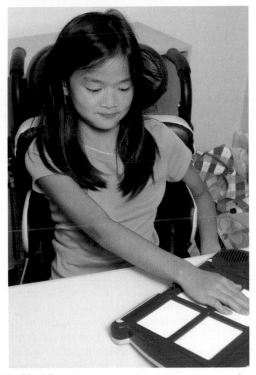

FIGURE 22-16 Adapted seating promotes good postural alignment for fine motor play at a table.

pillows, walking on a curb or the edge of a sandbox, or sharing a game with friends (Figure 22-15). In addition, the occupational therapist clinically reasons the timing of reinforcement (sometimes delayed feedback results in the sustained child performance), whether to use specific or general feedback (usually the child benefits from more specific feedback), and when to fade feedback (as the child becomes more independent, the occupational therapist or caregiver gives less feedback). Often play activities, particularly social play with peers, are intrinsically rewarding and can reinforce new skill development simply because play is fun.

Facilitate Generalization of Play Skills

The occupational therapist's goal when encouraging new skill development is that the child can generalize performance to a range of play activities and environments. Because play is usually embedded in the daily routines of young children, occupational therapists coach caregivers on how to use a variety of toys or play activities to support the child in generalizing newly learned skills. The occupational therapist works with families to determine the natural environments in which play takes place or environments in which caregivers and children spend time, such as in the backyard, the child's bedroom, or a community playground. Childcare providers may also receive support to learn strategies and approaches that will enhance the child's play and support generalization of emerging skills.

Adapting Play: Role of Assistive Technology

When a child has significant disabilities or developmental delay, the occupational therapist and family may provide adapted seating or adapted stander, adapted toys, or modify the environment to enable the child's play.[62] For children with low postural stability and limited extremity movement (e.g., a child with spinal muscular atrophy), a supportive seating device is needed to promote the child's use of the eyes and hands together in play activities. Adapted chairs (e.g., Rifton toddler chairs [Rifton Equipment, Rifton, NY]) can include head, trunk, arm, and foot supports so that the child has a stable trunk, head positioned at midline, and increased control of extremity movements (Figure 22-16). Prone standers also promote the child's alignment and postural stability to use hands and eyes for play activities. Standing with support may be the child's preferred position for interaction in play activities with peers. For toddlers with minimal arm and hand movement, the occupational therapist may suggest use of battery-operated toys with adapted switches or games on electronic tablets that use simple touch. A wide range of games that require simple motions to operate are available for tablets or computers. Tablets and battery-operated toys can be accessed with the child in a supported sitting or side-lying position. Computer play can promote social interaction between children with disabilities and their peers.[46]

Toys and materials can be adapted so that they are more accessible and easier for the child to handle. Occupational therapists or caregivers may place hook and loop fasteners on doll clothes to replace small buttons, use enlarged handles or special grips so that the child can hold a toy, or recommend use of a tray as a stabilizer for toys. Switch-activated toys can be operated by a button or squeeze switches that require a simple hand motion.[21] Families and occupational therapists collaborate when selecting assistive technology for the child because devices can be expensive and need to be appropriate for the home environment, and technology requires training for optimal use.

Social Interaction and Participation

Positive social interactions are foundational to learning and developing relationships, suggesting the importance of nourishing social emotional growth in the first years of life.[35,96] Children may have delays in social-emotional competence when they spend their first weeks of life in a neonatal intensive care unit or have significant medical and developmental problems that affect cognition, communication, and/or self-regulation. Infants and toddlers with sensory processing difficulties can be challenging for caregivers, particularly infants and toddlers who appear to have hypersensitivity to touch or sound—primary sensations of human interaction. Toddlers with autism spectrum disorder by definition have delays in social interaction skills, which include communication delays, rigid or repetitive behaviors, and difficulty understanding and responding to nonverbal communication. Social competence can also be delayed when a child has cognitive delays. The environment can also constrain social-emotional development; for example, caregivers with mental health disorders, limited social supports, and limited parenting skills can negatively affect a young child's social-emotional growth, particularly in the case of child neglect or abuse. Occupational therapists provide interventions that support the child's social-emotional development in the context of the family.

Parent-Child Interaction

Social skills are among the first skills that an infant develops; the infant demonstrates eye gaze and cuddling with caregivers in the first weeks of life and, by 6 to 8 weeks, social imitation of smiling. The purposes of infants' first social interactions are to communicate discomfort and hunger as well as pleasure. An infant who has sensory processing disorder or is at risk for autism spectrum disorder may show delays in these first social skills. For example, he or she may cry when picked up or cuddled, sleep only for short periods, feed poorly, and smile infrequently. These behaviors are difficult for caregivers to manage, can be stressful, and may have a negative effect on caregiver-child interactions.[105]

Occupational therapists facilitate caregiver-infant interaction by observing the interaction, listening to caregiver concerns, and coaching caregivers on reading cues, responding with sensitivity, and supporting the infant's communication efforts. For an infant with cerebral palsy and low muscle tone, the occupational therapist may model handling and holding that increase the infant's comfort and ability to interact (e.g., holding the infant more upright during a feeding interaction). Occupational therapists can teach caregivers massage or touch-based interventions that can calm the infant and reduce tactile hypersensitivities to promote optimal arousal.[9] Touch-based interventions with neonates are effective in promoting bonding and social-emotional development.[100]

Caregivers may desire interventions that promote their interactional skills and enhance their relationship with their child, particularly when children have delayed communication skills or demonstrate behaviors consistent with autism. Often occupational therapists coach parents using relationship-based interventions.[20,36,69] In these interventions, occupational therapists teach and encourage caregivers to become more sensitive to the child's cues and more responsive to the child's communication efforts. Nonverbal interaction and imitation of the child's actions are emphasized. Modeling and coaching are key strategies that can promote increased caregiver sensitivity and responsivity to the infant. Relationship-based interventions have shown promising positive effects on mother's responsiveness and child's self-regulation, social competence, and adaptive behavior.[9,61,69]

As infants become toddlers, most parent-child interactions occur in joint activities, requiring the young child to attend to the activity and caregiver. The caregiver reciprocally interacts with the toddler in the context of purposeful play.[61] Joint attention and sustained interaction can be limited or missing in young children with developmental delays or disabilities. Occupational therapists promote joint attention by designing a context that supports joint engagement, selecting an activity of high interest, modeling for the caregiver and child, and supporting the child's engagement with positive affect and reinforcement. For children who are hypersensitive to sound or touch, a quiet environment and less stimulating activity are carefully selected. The occupational therapist selects specific cues, prompts, and reinforcement to encourage but not overwhelm the child in the social interaction.

Peer Interaction Interventions

When toddlers approach 3 years of age, they become more interested in their peers. Occupational therapists promote peer-to-peer social interactions and social play opportunities in childcare centers, preschools, and other natural environments. These interventions use specific strategies to promote social competence in the context of naturalistic play.[9] For example, the occupational therapist selects engaging and preferred activities in natural social elements (e.g., a turn-taking game or art activity with shared materials) and with peer models who have higher level social skills. Computer and tablet activities have been shown to increase the engagement of young children and have been used with dyads or small groups of children.[6,45] Interactive or social toys, such as puppets, dress-up, dolls, trucks, and housekeeping toys, can promote social interaction in children with cognitive delays, particularly when they are paired with children who have higher level cognitive skills.[58] In these play groups, the occupational therapist models and reinforces social interaction skills and promotes interactions by designing activities that require sharing, imitation, or social interaction. Often young children need supports, such as prompting or cueing, to enter a social activity, stay in or sustain attention to the activity, or leave the activity using socially appropriate behaviors. The occupational therapist is fully engaged in the child's social interactions to provide timely cueing and reinforcement. The occupational therapist coaches caregivers in the strategies that most effectively support the child's social participation.

Adaptive Behaviors: Eating and Sleeping

Feeding and sleeping are essential daily activities that are often the focus of occupational therapy intervention. These adaptive behaviors are primary occupations of infants and toddlers and are strongly linked to health, development, and growth. Feeding and sleeping are also primary concerns of the caregivers, and infants who struggle in these areas can create high stress and great concern for caregivers. When infants struggle to eat or sleep, occupational therapists and families often prioritize interventions to improve these functional areas.

Feeding and Eating Problems

Feeding problems are common in infants with developmental disabilities and may be linked to oral sensorimotor problems, oral structural abnormalities, aspiration, self-feeding delays, failure to thrive, and selective eating.[17,47] For example, children with cerebral palsy may have difficulty with sucking, jaw stability, or coordination of swallow and breathing. Infants born prematurely may have oral sensitivity or low muscle tone, with related problems in suck-swallow-breathe coordination. Other infants may have dysregulation or irritability that affects eating and caregiver-infant interaction during feeding. Children who have multiple medical problems or cerebral palsy can have significant feeding problems in the first years of life. Infants with medical problems may not have sufficient oral motor skills for feeding by mouth, and receive nutrition first through a nasal-gastric tube and then through a gastrostomy tube. These infants miss the oral motor and oral sensory experiences needed to develop feeding competence.

Interventions to Improve Feeding Mechanics

To improve the mechanics of eating, occupational therapists develop and recommend strategies to improve the oral motor skills of sucking, chewing, and swallowing, the components of feeding competence. Infants with cerebral palsy can exhibit oral motor weakness and, as a result, struggle to eat. They benefit from additional trunk and head support during eating to optimize a coordinated suck-swallow-breathe pattern. Firm support to the head and trunk through adapted seating or therapeutic positioning can promote optimal jaw and tongue movements during eating. Infant seating that includes firm and complete trunk and head support also positions the infant for safe swallowing and facilitates higher level feeding skills. Occupational therapists may recommend adapted equipment for positioning during eating or may teach caregivers holding techniques to provide additional support of the infant's posture. Selecting specific nipples can promote improved sucking coordination, and flat spoons can enable the infant to take in food with minimal tongue and lip movement. When a child has difficulty with jaw or lip closure, or when tongue movement is insufficient for safe swallowing, occupational therapists also teach caregivers oral handling techniques that support the jaw. Chapter 14 describes occupational therapy feeding interventions in depth. In their systematic review of occupational therapy interventions for eating, Howe and Wang[47] reported that positioning,[33] oral support,[30] and pacing[52] have positive effects on infants' feeding performance.

Infants with delayed feeding skills who exhibit immature oral motor patterns or oral sensitivity may benefit from sensory strategies. Sensory strategies include full body containment (swaddling to calm the infant), gentle and firm touch pressure to the mouth or inside the mouth, and non-nutritive sucking. For infants with oral sensitivities to textures and tastes, the occupational therapist systematically introduces different textures and tastes, from most to least preferred. These sensory experiences can be paired with positive reinforcement when the child actively participates or attempts to eat. Non nutritive oral strategies can help the toddler develop the oral motor strength needed to transition to oral eating.

When toddlers begin to eat solid foods, they may continue to need external trunk and head support in addition to leg and foot support. The occupational therapist may recommend adapting a child's highchair to provide additional trunk support or may recommend purchasing adapted equipment. When recommending an adapted feeding chair, the occupational therapist considers the family's resources and priorities; he or she also identifies seating equipment that can grow with the child or be used for multiple purposes. As the child develops self-feeding skills, the occupational therapist may recommend adaptive equipment or supports to increase the child's success and can be easily implemented at home. The occupational therapist works with the family to determine which strategies are most acceptable and successful in promoting the child's self-feeding competence.

Caregiver-Infant Interaction During Feeding

Given the importance of caregiver-infant interaction during eating, occupational therapists also coach parents in methods and strategies to improve communication and interaction during feeding. Feeding a child who struggles to eat can be challenging and stressful for the caregiver.[17,94] Caregivers are anxious about the child's health and growth in addition to their own ability to feed their child. By observing a caregiver-infant interaction during feeding, the occupational therapist can make recommendations on how to hold the infant, pace the feeding, read the infant's cues, respond to nonverbal cues, and maintain the infant's engagement. Using coaching techniques, the occupational therapist observes the feeding interaction and, with the caregiver, reflects on the feeding interaction to identify goals and strategies that might improve the infant's eating success. The occupational therapist also provides emotional support to caregivers when infants need high levels of support during eating, given the frequency of feeding interactions and the consequences of poor eating on growth and health. Studies on interventions to enhance mother-infant feeding interaction have shown that the infant's feeding competency and mother-infant interaction improve.[48,87]

Sleeping and Rest

Many infants and toddlers with sensory processing problems, self-regulation difficulty, or autism spectrum disorders have sleep problems. Infants with sensory processing disorders or who are at risk for autism spectrum disorders often have disrupted sleeping patterns characterized by difficulty falling asleep or waking during the night. Between 40% and 80% of children with autism spectrum disorder have sleep problems[53] that can affect the entire family's sleep. When caregivers and children suffer chronic fatigue, family functioning and quality of life are negatively affected. Occupational therapists problem solve with families to identify how changes in routines or the sleeping environment can help children regulate their sleeping patterns.

Interventions to promote sleep generally include behavioral and sensory strategies. The occupational therapist and family develop strategies to improve sleeping patterns by discussing the nighttime routine and problem-solving antecedents and consequences of the child's behavior at bedtime and during the night. They develop a plan to reinforce the child's independence in falling asleep and to reward quiet nighttime behaviors that prevent disruption of the entire family's sleep.

Hypersensitivity and sensory modulation disorders appear to be contributing factors to sleep problems.[88] Children with autism spectrum disorder who demonstrate sensory modulation disorder appear to be more prone to sleep difficulties than those who do not have sensory modulation disorder.[88] In particular, children with high arousal who have difficulty filtering sensory stimuli appear to have difficulty lowering arousal to fall asleep. When infants or toddlers exhibit sensory modulation problems and sleeping difficulty, the occupational therapist and caregiver can identify sensory strategies to calm the child or to limit sensory stimulation at bedtime. A number of sensory strategies (e.g., rocking, music, total darkness, fan, white noise) can be tried to identify a good fit to the family's routine and nighttime patterns (Case Study 22-3). Generally, a combination of sensory and behavioral strategies is needed, as well as consistency in applying the strategies. Occupational therapists encourage good sleeping habits and help the family identify and sustain routines and patterns that allow healthy rest and sleep. Because good sleeping patterns affect not only the child's development and growth, but also the family's mental health and quality of life, sleeping routines should remain a priority for the occupational therapist and family.

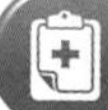

CASE STUDY 22-3 Amelia

Background

Amelia is a 24-month-old child referred to an early intervention program by her pediatrician because of concerns with gross and fine motor development, feeding, and suspected sensory processing problems. Amelia cries often in a distressful manner. Problem areas for Amelia, as reported by her mother, include uncooperative behaviors, "extreme meltdowns," whining and fussing, feeding problems associated with aversion to food textures, fearfulness, and poor balance. Although she sat independently at 6 months of age, she did not reach for and grasp an object until 8 months of age. She rolled from back to stomach at 9 months of age and began crawling at 11 months.

Assessment

An arena assessment model, with the child and primary caregiver interacting with one professional throughout the evaluation session and the other professionals observing and occasionally directly testing the child on specific skills and interviewing the caregiver, was used to determine Amelia's eligibility for services, and present levels of development and to facilitate intervention planning. The evaluation team consisted of a physical therapist and developmental interventionist. Participation by an occupational therapist was indicated; however, Amelia lives in a rural community with no access to an early intervention occupational therapist. The nearest hospital or outpatient rehabilitation clinic with an occupational therapist onsite was a 50-minute drive from the family's home.

Telehealth

The early intervention program in Amelia's area recently began using telehealth as a service delivery model to improve access to services for children living in rural and underserved areas. Amelia's mother gave consent for the use of videoconferencing to augment Amelia's early intervention services delivered in person. The physical therapist brought an electronic tablet with secure videoconferencing software to the family's home to enable the occupational therapist to participate virtually in the arena assessment.

During the assessment, Amelia was pleasant. She preferred not to be touched or held. The physical therapist took the lead in the arena assessment with the educational specialist (sometimes referred to as a developmental interventionist) assuming an observatory role. Amelia interacted with the examiner with caution after a brief period of ignoring her. Her mother remained in the room and participated in the assessment. The occupational therapist interviewed Amelia's mother via videoconferencing to obtain a sensorimotor history. Her mother reported that Amelia had difficulty with being touched and pulled away when touched. Sometimes she stiffened and arched her back when held. Amelia's mother reported that she was irritable when held and resisted having her hair or face washed. Amelia was bothered by noises, such as those from the vacuum cleaner and hair dryer. Although her aversion to sound had improved, she remained apprehensive of toys with noises. Amelia became anxious in situations with auditory and visual stimulation, such as a shopping mall. Amelia enjoyed swinging and other activities with movement.

During the arena assessment, which consisted of a criterion-referenced, five-area assessment by the early intervention team, the occupational therapist observed Amelia via videoconferencing technology. The occupational therapist noted that when handled, Amelia exhibited a mildly defensive reaction to touch. The occupational therapist asked the lead examiner (the physical therapist) to place a mitt on Amelia's foot and a piece of tape on Amelia's hand. Amelia became upset when removing the mitt from her foot and cried when a piece of tape was placed on the back of her hand. She seemed unable to plan the movements needed to remove the mitt or tape. Although she seemed to be visually oriented, visual tracking was delayed and inconsistent. Amelia enjoyed vestibular input as she was held and moved up and down or in circular motions by her mother under the direction of the lead examiner. She also enjoyed upside-down positions. Through videoconferencing, her mother completed the Infant/Toddler Sensory Profile with the occupational therapist, and Amelia's sensory responses placed her in the sensory sensitivity category.

Summary and Interpretation

The arena assessment confirmed the pediatrician's concerns associated with Amelia's gross and fine motor development, feeding, and sensory processing and established eligibility for early intervention services. Based on the occupational therapist's observations and Amelia's scores on the Infant/Toddler Sensory Profile and the motor and adaptive subtests of the criterion-referenced assessment, the occupational therapist concluded that Amelia experienced significant difficulties in receiving and modulating sensory information. This was evident particularly in her irritability and intolerance to touch and auditory stimulation. Inadequate adaptive motor

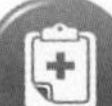

CASE STUDY 22-3 Amelia—cont'd

function and feeding difficulties stemming from aversion to textures seemed to be related to her hypersensitivity. Amelia's tactile sensitivity probably contributed to her fine motor delays. Amelia's short-term goals were: Using sensory strategies to help her prepare for activities, Amelia would demonstrate the following: (1) consuming an increased number of foods and variety of textures; (2) improved tolerance of touch, as demonstrated by improved affect when she is held or touched; and (3) improved play skills so that she could stay in a social play interaction for 10 minutes.

Intervention

The team recommended weekly occupational therapy for Amelia, which became part of her IFSP. A modified computer capable of videoconferencing and an Internet access card not accessible for other uses was loaned to the family to facilitate remote occupational therapy services, which would otherwise be unavailable to Amelia and her family because of provider shortages in her area. The occupational therapist provided sensory-based strategies and recommendations to be implemented by Amelia's parents during daily routines. Co-visits through technology occurred with the physical therapist or educational specialist who was with the family in the home. The occupational therapist, within a transdisciplinary practice model, collaborated with Amelia's parents and providers to support implementation of strategies and recommendations in Amelia's natural environments.

The occupational therapist recommended play-based activities that incorporated vestibular, proprioceptive, and tactile input (as tolerated). Intervention included coaching Amelia's parents and other providers to incorporate sensory strategies, such as crawling activities and sand and water play, and activities that encouraged the use of both hands at the midline to facilitate cooperative, bilateral hand use. The occupational therapist provided Amelia's mother with reading material and a video to help her understand how sensory processing affects behavior.

Amelia responded well to the intervention approach and began to show indications of more efficient sensory processing and the ability to modulate sensory input. Within a few weeks, Amelia began to mold to her mother when she held her and was less irritable and more relaxed in situations with auditory stimulation. After 3 months of therapy, Amelia's mother reported increased cuddling and noticeable improvement in eating. She attempted a greater variety of foods and displayed fewer aversions; feeding time was shorter; and it was no longer necessary to use the television as a diversion to get her to eat. Amelia began to interact more with her older sister and began to explore her environment. Play skills and hand use also appeared to increase.

Implications

The use of a telehealth service delivery model allowed Amelia's family to access occupational therapy services otherwise not available because of provider shortages in her area. Videoconferencing facilitated consultation, collaboration, and coaching among Amelia's early intervention providers and family and promoted improved outcomes by ensuring that the unique perspective and contributions of occupational therapy were available to Amelia's IFSP team.

Summary

- Early intervention programs serve children from birth through 2 years who have an established risk, have a developmental delay, or are at risk for developmental delay.
- A primary goal of early intervention programs is to enhance the capability of families to help their infants and toddlers develop and learn.
- Under Part C of IDEA, occupational therapy is a primary service to meet the functional needs of the child related to adaptive development; adaptive behavior and play, including social interaction; and sensory, motor, and postural development.
- Occupational therapists provide early intervention services in natural environments, are members of interprofessional teams, coach and consult with team members, and use family-centered approaches that respect cultural differences.
- Family-centered intervention means that family strengths are emphasized; families have control and make choices regarding interventions; and families and providers work together to ensure provision of optimal early intervention services.
- In early intervention, occupational therapy services are guided by the Individualized Family Service Plan, which defines the child's present level of performance; the family's resources, priorities, and concerns; a statement of major outcomes expected; the services necessary; and the natural environment in which services will be provided.
- The child's transition from early intervention to early childhood programs is carefully planned by the team; child and family supports are needed to facilitate a smooth transition.
- Natural intervention strategies use incidental learning opportunities, follow the child's lead, and use natural consequences to promote the child's acquisition of functional motor, social, and communication skills.
- Coaching, including occupational therapists coaching caregivers through telehealth, is a family-centered method of teaching that includes the occupational therapist's observation of the caregiver and the caregiver's observation of the coach, practice, reflection, and evaluation.
- Play, including adapted play, is a primary context and outcome for occupational therapy intervention.
- Occupational therapists promote social participation of young children by fostering positive parent-child interactions, using relationship-based interventions, and facilitating peer interactions in the context of social play.
- Occupational therapists provide interventions to enhance self-care and adaptive behaviors, including specific interventions to improve feeding, eating, and sleeping.

REFERENCES

1. American Occupational Therapy Association. (2013). Telehealth [position paper]. *American Journal of Occupational Therapy, 67*(Suppl.), S69–S90.
2. Anzalone, M., & Williamson, G. (2000). Sensory processing and motor performance in autism spectrum disorders. In A. M. Wetherby & B. M. Prizant (Eds.), *Autism spectrum disorder: A transactional developmental approach* (9th ed., pp. 143–166). Baltimore: Brookes.
3. Bailey, D. B., Hebbeler, K., Spiker, D., et al. (2005). Thirty-six-month outcomes for families of children who have disabilities and participated in early intervention. *Pediatrics, 116*, 1346–1352.
4. Bailey, D. B., Raspa, M., & Fox, L. C. (2012). What is the future of family outcomes and family-centered services? *Topics in Early Childhood Special Education, 31*, 216–223.
5. Bricker, D. (2002). *Assessment, Evaluation, and Programming System (AEPS) for infants and children* (2nd ed.). Baltimore: Brookes.
6. Campbell, P. H., Milbourne, S., Dugan, L. M., et al. (2006). A review of evidence on practices for teaching young children to use assistive technology devices. *Topics in Early Childhood Special Education, 26*, 3–13.
7. Campbell, P. H., & Halbert, J. (2002). Between research and practice: Provider perspectives on early intervention. *Topics in Early Childhood Special Education, 22*, 213–226.
8. Campbell, P. H. (2004). Participation-based services: Promoting children's participation in natural settings. *Young Exceptional Children, 8*(1), 20–29.
9. Case-Smith, J. (2013). Systematic review of interventions to promote social-emotional development in young children with or at risk for disabilities. *American Journal of Occupational Therapy, 67*, 395–404.
10. Case-Smith, J., Frolek Clark, G. J., & Schlabach, T. L. (2013). Systematic review of interventions used in occupational therapy to promote motor performance for children ages birth-5 years. *American Journal of Occupational Therapy, 67*, 413–424.
11. Cason, J. (2009). A pilot telerehabilitation program: Delivering early intervention services to rural families. *International Journal of Telerehabilitation, 1*, 29–38.
12. Cason, J. (2011). Telerehabilitation: An adjunct service delivery model for early intervention services. *International Journal of Telerehabilitation, 3*(1), 19–28.
13. Cason, J., Behl, D., & Ringwalt, S. (2012). Overview of states' use of telehealth for the delivery of early intervention (IDEA part C) services. *International Journal of Telerehabilitation, 4*(2), 39–46.
14. Cason, J., & Brannon, J. A. (2011). Telehealth regulatory and legal considerations: Frequently asked questions. *International Journal of Telerehabilitation, 3*(2), 15–18.
15. Center on the Developing Child at Harvard University (2010). *The foundations of lifelong health are built in early childhood.* Retrieved from: <http://www.developingchild.harvard.edu>.
16. Chai, A. Y., Zhang, C., & Bisberg, M. (2006). Rethinking natural environment practice: Implications from examining various implications and approaches. *Early Childhood Education Journal, 34*, 203–208.
17. Chatoor, I. (2002). Feeding disorders in infants and toddlers: Diagnosis and treatment. *Child and Adolescent Psychiatric Clinics of North America, 11*, 163–183.
18. Colyvas, J. L., Sawyer, L. B., & Campbell, P. H. (2010). Identifying strategies early intervention occupational therapists use to teach caregivers. *American Journal of Occupational Therapy, 64*, 776–785.
19. Danaher, J., Goode, S., & Lazara, A. (Eds.), (2011). *Part C updates* (12th ed.). Chapel Hill, NC: The University of North Carolina, FPG Child Development Institute, National Early Childhood Technical Assistance Center.
20. Daunhauer, L. A., Coster, W. J., Tickle-Degnen, L., et al. (2007). Effects of caregiver-child interactions on play occupations among young children institutionalized in Eastern Europe. *American Journal of Occupational Therapy, 61*, 429–440.
21. Deitz, J., & Swinth, Y. (2008). Accessing play through assistive technology. In L. D. Parham & L. Fazio (Eds.), *Play in occupational therapy for children* (2nd ed., pp. 395–412). St. Louis: Mosby/Elsevier.
22. DEC/NAEYC (2009). *Early childhood inclusion: A joint position statement of the Division for Early Childhood (DEC) and the National Association for the Education of Young Children (NAEYC).* Chapel Hill: The University of North Carolina, FPG Child Development Institute. Retrieved from: <http://community.fpg.unc.edu/resources/articles/Early_Childhood_Inclusion>.
23. DeGrace, B. W. (2003). Occupation-based and family-centered care: A challenge for current practice. *American Journal of Occupational Therapy, 57*, 347–350.
24. Dunst, C. J. (2002). Family-centered practices: Birth through high school. *Journal of Special Education, 36*, 139–147.
25. Dunst, C. J., Trivette, C. M., Humphries, T., et al. (2001a). Contrasting approaches to natural learning environment interventions. *Infants and Young Children, 14*(2), 48–63.
26. Dunst, C. J., Bruder, M. B., Trivette, C. M., et al. (2001b). Characteristics and consequences of everyday natural learning opportunities. *Topics in Early Childhood Special Education, 21*, 68–92.
27. Early Childhood Outcomes Center (2011a). Summary of 2011 child outcomes data. Retrieved from: <http://www.fpg.unc.edu/~eco/assets/pdfs/outcomesforchildrenfinal.pdf>.
28. Early Childhood Outcomes Center (2011b). Family data: Indicator C4 highlights. Retrieved from: <http://ecoutcomes.fpg.unc.edu/resources/family-data-indicator-c4-highlights>.

28a. Early Childhood Outcomes Center (2014). Outcomes measurement: Federal requirements. Retrieved from: <http://projects.fpg.unc.edu/~eco/pages/fed_req.cfm>.

29. Edwards, M. A., Millard, P., Praskac, L. A., et al. (2003). Occupational therapy and early intervention: A family-centered approach. *Occupational Therapy International, 10*, 239–252.
30. Einarsson-Backes, L. M., Deitz, J., Price, R., et al. (1994). The effect of oral support on sucking efficiency in preterm infants. *American Journal of Occupation Therapy, 48*, 490–498.
31. Farrell, A. F. (2009). Validating family-centeredness in early intervention evaluation reports. *Infants & Young Children, 22*, 238–252.
32. Fingerhut, P. E., Piro, J., Sutton, A., et al. (2013). Family-centered principles implemented in home-based, clinic-based, and school-based pediatric settings. *American Journal of Occupational Therapy, 67*, 228–235.
33. Gisel, E. G., Tessier, M. J., Lapierre, G., et al. (2003). Feeding management of children with severe cerebral palsy and eating impairment: An exploratory

study. *Physical & Occupational Therapy in Pediatrics, 23,* 19–44.

34. Grant, R. (2005). State strategies to contain costs in the early intervention program: Policy and evidence. *Topics in Early Childhood Special Education, 25,* 243–250.
35. Greenspan, S. I., Wieder, S., & Simons, R. (1998). *The child with special needs: Encouraging intellectual and emotional growth.* Cambridge, MA: Perseus Books.
36. Gutstein, S. E., Burgess, A. F., & Montfort, K. (2007). Evaluation of the relationship development intervention program. *Autism: The International Journal of Research and Practice, 11,* 397–411.
37. Hanft, B. E., & Anzalone, M. (2001). Issues in professional development: Preparing and supporting occupational therapists in early childhood. *Infants and Young Children, 13*(4), 67–78.
38. Hanft, B. E., & Pilkington, K. O. (2000). Therapy in natural environments: The means or end goal for early intervention? *Infants and Young Children, 12*(4), 1–13.
39. Hanson, M. J. (1998). Ethnic, cultural, and language diversity in intervention settings. In E. Lynch & M. Hanson (Eds.), *Developing cross-cultural competence* (2nd ed., pp. 3–22). Baltimore: Brookes.
40. Hanson, M. J., Beckman, P. J., Horn, E., et al. (2000). Entering preschool: Family and professional experiences in this transition process. *Journal of Early Intervention, 23,* 279–293.
41. Harper, D. (2006). Telemedicine for children with disabilities. *Children's Health Care, 35*(1), 11–27.
42. Hastings, R. P. (2002). Parental stress and behavior problems of children with developmental disability. *Journal of Intellectual and Developmental Disability, 27,* 149–160.
43. Hebbeler, K., Spiker, D., Bailey, D., et al. (2007). Early intervention for infants and toddlers with disabilities and their families: Participants, services, and outcomes. Final report of the National Early Intervention Longitudinal Study (NEILS). Retrieved from: <http://www.sri.com/neils/pdfs/NEILS_Report_02_07_Final2.pdf>.
44. Heimerl, S., & Rasch, N. (2009). Delivering developmental occupational therapy consultation services through telehealth. *Developmental Disabilities Special Interest Section Quarterly, 32*(3), 1–4.
45. Hourcade, J. P., Bullock-Rest, N. E., & Hansen, T. E. (2010). Multitouch tablet applications and activities to enhance the social skills of children with autism spectrum disorders. *Personal and Ubiquitous Computing, 16,* 157–168.
46. Howard, J., Greyrose, E., Kehr, K., et al. (1996). Teacher-facilitated microcomputer activities: Enhancing social play and affect in young children with disabilities. *Journal of Special Education Technology, 13,* 36–47.
47. Howe, T.-H., & Wang, T.-N. (2013). Systematic review of interventions used in or relevant to occupational therapy for children with feeding difficulties ages birth-5 years. *American Journal of Occupational Therapy, 67,* 405–412.
48. Humphry, R. (2002). Young children's occupations: Explicating the dynamics of developmental processes. *American Journal of Occupational Therapy, 56,* 171–179.
49. Individuals with Disabilities Education Act of 1990 Amendments (P.L. 102–119), 20 U.S.C. et seq., 1400–1485.
50. IDEA 2004 Individuals with Disabilities Education Improvement Act of 2004 (P.L. 108–446), 120 U.S.C. § 1400 et. seq. Sec. 632(4) (G),(H).
51. Ingersoll, B., Schreibman, L., & Tran, Q. H. (2003). Effect of sensory feedback on immediate object imitation in children with autism. *Journal of Autism and Developmental Disorders, 33,* 673–683.
52. Jadcherla, S. R., Stoner, E., Gupta, A., et al. (2009). Evaluation and management of neonatal dysphagia: Impact of pharyngoesophageal motility studies and multidisciplinary feeding strategy. *Journal of Pediatric Gastroenterology and Nutrition, 48,* 186–192.
53. Johnson, K. P., & Malow, B. A. (2008). Sleep in children with autism spectrum disorders. *Current Neurology and Neuroscience Reports, 8,* 155–161.
54. Jung, L. A. (2007). Writing individualized family service plan strategies that fit into the ROUTINE. *Young Exceptional Children, 10*(3), 2–9.
55. Jung, L. A., & Grisham-Brown, J. (2006). Moving from assessment information to IFSPs: Guidelines for a family-centered process. *Young Exceptional Children, 9*(2), 2–11.
56. Kaiser, A. P., & Hancock, T. B. (2003). Teaching parents new skills to support their young children's development. *Infants and Young Children, 16,* 9–21.
57. Kelso, G., Fiechtl, B., Olsen, S., et al. (2009). The feasibility of virtual home visits to provide early intervention: A pilot study. *Infants and Young Children, 22,* 332–340.
58. Kim, A., Vaughn, S., Elbaum, G., et al. (2003). Effects of toys or group composition for children with disabilities: A synthesis. *Journal of Early Intervention, 25,* 189–205.
59. King, K., Strachan, D., Tucker, M., et al. (2009). The application of a transdisciplinary model for early intervention services. *Infants and Young Children, 22,* 211–223.
60. Kramer, S., McGonigel, M., & Kaufman, R. (1991). Developing the IFSP: Outcomes, strategies, activities, and services. In M. McGonigel, R. Kaufmann, & B. Johnson (Eds.), *Guidelines and recommended practices for the individualized family service plan* (2nd ed., pp. 41–49). Bethesda, MD: Association for the Care of Children's Health.
61. Landry, W. H., Smith, K. E., Swank, P., et al. (2008). A responsive parenting intervention. The optimal timing across early childhood for impacting maternal behaviors and child outcomes. *Developmental Psychology, 44,* 1335–1353.
62. Lane, S., & Mistrett, S. (1996). Play and assistive technology issues for infants and young children with disabilities: A preliminary examination. *Focus on Autism and Other Developmental Disabilities, 11,* 96–104.
63. Lifter, K. (2000). Linking assessment to intervention for children with developmental disabilities or at-risk for developmental delay: The developmental play assessment (DPA) instrument. In K. Gitlin-Weiner, A. Sandgrund, & C. E. Schaefer (Eds.), *Play diagnosis and assessment* (2nd ed., pp. 228–251). New York: Wiley.
64. Lifter, K., Ellis, J., Cannon, B., et al. (2005). Developmental specificity in targeting and teaching play activities to children with pervasive developmental disorder. *Journal of Early Intervention, 27,* 247–267.
65. Linder, T. W. (2008). *Transdisciplinary play-based assessment: A functional approach to working with young children* (2nd ed.). Baltimore: Brookes.
66. Lorig, K. R., & Holman, H. R. (2003). Self-management education: History, definition, outcomes, and mechanisms. *Annals of Behavioral Medicine, 26*(1), 1–7.
67. Lucas, A., & Shaw, E. (2012). *Informed clinical opinion (NECTAC Notes no. 28).* Chapel Hill, NC: The University of North Carolina, FPG Child Development Institute, National Early Childhood Technical Assistance Center.
68. Lucas, A., Gillaspy, K., Peters, M. L., et al. (2012). Enhancing recognition of high-quality, functional IFSP outcomes and IEP goals: A training activity for infant and toddler service providers and ECSE teachers. Retrieved from: <http://www.ectacenter.org/~pdfs/pubs/rating-ifsp-iep-training.pdf>.

69. Mahoney, G., & Perales, F. (2005). Relationship-focused early intervention with children with pervasive developmental disorders and other disabilities: A comparative study. *Journal of Developmental and Behavioral Pediatrics, 26*, 77–85.
70. Mahoney, G., & Filer, J. (1996). How responsive is early intervention to the priorities and needs of families? *Topics in Early Childhood Special Education, 16*, 437–457.
71. Mailloux, Z., & Burke, J. (2008). Play and sensory integrative approach. In L. D. Parham & L. Fazio (Eds.), *Play in occupational therapy for children* (2nd ed., pp. 263–278). St. Louis: Mosby/Elsevier.
72. Mailloux, Z., & Roley, S. S. (2010). Sensory integration. In H. Miller Kuhaneck & R. Watling (Eds.), *Autism: A comprehensive occupational therapy approach* (3rd ed., pp. 469–508). Bethesda: AOTA Press.
73. McCormick, L. (2006). Assessment and planning: The IFSP and the IEP. In M. J. Noonan & L. McCormick (Eds.), *Young children with disabilities in natural environments* (pp. 47–75). Baltimore: Brookes.
74. McWilliam, R. A. (1996). How to provide integrated therapy. In R. A. McWilliam (Ed.), *Rethinking pull-out services in early intervention* (pp. 49–69). Baltimore: Brookes.
75. McWilliam, R. A. (2010). *Routines-based early intervention.* Baltimore: Brookes.
76. McWilliam, R. A., Casey, A. M., & Sims, J. (2009). The routines-based interview: A method for gathering information and assessing needs. *Infants and Young Children, 22*, 224–233.
77. Miller, L. J. (1994). Journey to a desirable future: A value-based model of infant and toddler assessment. *Zero to Three, 14*(6), 23–26.
78. Moore, L., Koger, D., Blumberg, S., et al. (2012). Making best practice our practice: Reflections on our journey into natural environments. *Infants and Young Children, 25*(1), 95–105.
79. Myers, C. T. (2006). Exploring occupational therapy and transitions for young children with special needs. *Physical & Occupational Therapy in Pediatrics, 26*(3), 73–88.
80. Myers, C. T. (2008). Descriptive study of occupational therapists' participation in early childhood transitions. *American Journal of Occupational Therapy, 62*, 212–220.
81. NC Department of Health & Human Services (2002). Growing up naturally: Early intervention in natural environments. Retrieved from: <http://www.beearly.nc.gov/data/files/pdf/GrowingUpNaturally.pdf>.
82. Office of Special Education Programs, U.S. Department of Education, Individuals with Disabilities Act Part C Regulations, 34 CFR Part 303. Retrieved from: <http://idea.ed.gov/part-c/regulations/1>.
83. Parham, L. D. (2008). Play and occupational therapy. In L. D. Parham & L. Fazio (Eds.), *Play in occupational therapy for children* (2nd ed., pp. 3–40). St. Louis: Mosby/Elsevier.
84. Parks, S. (2006). *Inside HELP: Administration manual for the Hawaii Early Learning Profile.* Palo Alto, CA: VORT.
85. Podvey, M. C., & Hinojosa, J. (2009). Transition from early intervention to preschool special education services: Family-centered practice that promotes positive outcomes. *Journal of Occupational Therapy, Schools, and Early Intervention, 2*(2), 73–83.
86. Podvey, M., Hinojosa, J., & Koenig, K. (2010). The transition experience to pre-school for six families with children with disabilities. *Occupational Therapy International, 17*, 177–187.
87. Pridham, K., Clark, R., Schroeder, M., et al. (2005). Effect of guided participation on feeding competencies of mothers and their premature infants. *Research in Nursing & Health, 28*, 262–267.
88. Reynolds, S., Lane, S. J., & Thacker, L. (2012). Sensory processing, physiological stress, and sleep behaviors in children with and without autism spectrum disorders. *Occupational Therapy Journal of Research, 32*, 246–257.
89. Ridgely, R., & Hallam, R. (2006). Examining the IFSPs of rural, low-income families: Are they reflective of family concerns? *Journal of Research in Childhood Education, 21*, 149–162.
90. Rosenbaum, P., King, S., Law, M., et al. (1998). Family-centered service: A conceptual framework and research review. *Physical & Occupational Therapy in Pediatrics, 18*, 1–20.
91. Rosenkoetter, S. E., & Squires, S. (2000). Writing outcomes that make a difference for children and families. *Young Exceptional Children, 4*, 2–8.
92. Rous, B., Hallam, R., Harbin, G., et al. (2007). The transition process for young children with disabilities: A conceptual framework. *Infants and Young Children, 20*, 135–148.
93. Rush, D. D., Shelden, M. L., & Hanft, B. E. (2003). Coaching families and colleagues: A process for collaboration in natural settings. *Infants and Young Children, 16*, 33–47.
94. Satter, E. (1990). The feeding relationship: Problems and interventions. *Journal of Pediatrics, 117*, S181–S189.
95. Shonkoff, J. P., & Meisels, S. J. (1990). Early childhood intervention: The evolution of a concept. In S. J. Meisels & J. P. Shonkoff (Eds.), *Handbook of early childhood intervention* (pp. 3–31). Cambridge, MA: Cambridge University Press.
96. Shonkoff, J. P., & Philips, D. A. (Eds.), (2000). *From neurons to neighborhoods: The science of early childhood development.* Washington, DC: National Academy Press.
97. Simons, R. (1985). *After the tears.* New York: Harcourt Brace Jovanovich.
98. Spitzer, S. (2008). Play in children with autism: Structure and experience. In L. D. Parham & L. Fazio (Eds.), *Play in occupational therapy for children* (2nd ed., pp. 351–374). St. Louis: Mosby/Elsevier.
99. Takata, N. (1974). Play as a prescription. In M. Reilly (Ed.), *Play as exploratory learning* (pp. 209–246). Beverly Hills, CA: Sage.
99a. Tanta, K. J., Deitz, J. C., White, O., et al. (2005). The effects of peer-play level on initiations and responses of preschool children with delayed play skills. *American Journal of Occupational Therapy, 59*, 437–445.
100. Tessier, R., Cristo, M. B., Velez, S., et al. (2003). Kangaroo mother care: A method for protecting high-risk low-birth weight and premature infants against developmental delay. *Infant Behavior and Development, 26*, 384–397.
101. Tetreault, S., Parrot, A., & Trahan, J. (2003). Home activity programs in families with children presenting with global developmental delays: Evaluation and parental perceptions. *International Journal of Rehabilitation Research, 26*, 165–173.
102. Turnbull, A. P., Turbiville, V., & Turnbull, H. R. (2000). Evolution of family-professional partnerships: Collective empowerment as the model for the early twenty-first century. In J. P. Shonkoff & S. J. Meisels (Eds.), *Handbook of early childhood intervention* (2nd ed., pp. 630–650). New York: Cambridge University Press.
103. Turnbull, A. P., Turnbull, H. R., & Blue-Banning, M. (1994). Enhancing inclusion of infants and toddlers with disabilities and their families: A theoretical and programmatic analysis. *Infants and Young Children, 7*(2), 1–14.
104. U.S. Department of Education, Office of Special Education Programs, Data Analysis System (DANS), OMB #1820-0557 (2011). Program settings where early intervention services are provided to infants and toddlers with

disabilities and their families in accordance with Part C. Retrieved from: <http://www2.ed.gov/about/offices/list/osers/osep/index.html>.

105. Weatherston, D. J., Ribaudo, J., & Glovak, S. (2002). Becoming whole: Combining infant mental health and occupational therapy on behalf of a toddler with sensory integration difficulties and his family. *Infants and Young Children, 15*(1), 19–28.

106. Woods, J. J., & Lindeman, D. P. (2008). Gathering and giving information with families. *Infants and Young Children, 21*, 272–284.

107. Woods, J. J., Wilcox, M. J., Friedman, M., et al. (2011). Collaborative consultation in natural environments: Strategies to enhance family-centered supports and services. *Language, Speech, and Hearing Services in Schools, 42*, 379–392.

108. Wooster, D. A. (2001). Early intervention programs. In M. Scaffa (Ed.), *Occupational therapy in community-based practice settings* (pp. 271–290). Philadelphia: F. A. Davis.

109. Workgroup on Principles and Practices in Natural Environments, OSEP TA Community of Practice—Part C Settings (2008). Seven key principles: Looks like/doesn't look like. Retrieved from: <http://www.nectac.org/~pdfs/topics/families/Principles_LooksLike_DoesntLookLike3_11_08.pdf>.

110. Zhang, C., & Bennett, T. (2003). Facilitating the meaningful participation of culturally and linguistically diverse families in the IFSP and IEP process. *Focus on Autism and Other Developmental Disabilities, 18*(1), 51–59.

CHAPTER

23 School-Based Occupational Therapy

Susan Bazyk • Susan Cahill

KEY TERMS

Individuals with Disabilities Education Act
Section 504 of the Rehabilitation Act
Elementary and Secondary Education Act
No Child Left Behind
Least restrictive environment
Integrated service delivery
Related services
Individualized Education Program
Health-related quality of life
School transitions
Multitiered services
Early intervening services
Co-teaching
Coaching
Response to intervention
School mental health

GUIDING QUESTIONS

1. What major legislation guides and regulates education for students with and without disabilities?
2. How do the Individuals with Disabilities Education Act (IDEA), Section 504 of the Rehabilitation Act, and Elementary and Secondary Education Act (ESEA) affect the role of occupational therapists in schools?
3. What major amendments to IDEA have been implemented over the past 3 decades?
4. What are the major provisions of Part B of IDEA—free appropriate public education (FAPE) in the least restrictive environment?
5. How do occupational therapists provide services under Part B of IDEA, including referral, evaluation, individual education program (IEP), and interventions?
6. How are occupational therapy services that support students with and without disabilities integrated into the classroom and across school environments?
7. What are examples of indirect and direct occupational therapy services?
8. How do occupational therapists under the IDEA 2004, ESEA, and No Child Left Behind Act (NCLB) provide early intervention services (EIS) and response to intervention (RtI)?
9. How do occupational therapists promote school mental health within a multitiered, public health model?

> The task of a sound education, Plato argued twenty-five centuries ago, is to teach young people to find pleasure in the right things. If children enjoyed math, they would learn math. If they enjoyed helping friends, they would grow into helpful adults. If they enjoyed Shakespeare, they would not be content watching television programs. If they enjoyed life, they would take greater pains to protect it (p. 39).[36]

Education systems worldwide have the responsibility of preparing children for adulthood, and, therefore, most professionals agree that schools must provide the intellectual and practical tools needed for successful participation in classrooms, families, future workplaces, and communities.[38] Occupational therapists help people of all ages engage in and enjoy meaningful and purposeful life activities; in schools, this means helping children participate in the academic, social, extracurricular, independent living, and vocational activities needed for student success and transition.[2,107] Given occupational therapy's focus on a broad range of occupational performance areas (e.g., education, social participation, play, leisure, work, activities of daily living [ADLs]), it is not surprising that occupational therapists enjoy a long tradition of providing services in schools and early intervention settings, making these the primary work environments for occupational therapists.[57]

Practice in schools is influenced by an educational versus medical model requiring a set of knowledge and skills unique to occupational therapy and school settings. School-based occupational therapists must combine a sound understanding of occupational therapy's domain of practice with a current understanding of the school context, which is guided by federal laws and regulations. In a U.S. survey, school-based occupational therapists identified the greatest need for knowledge and skills in the areas of federal and state regulations, role of occupational therapy, evaluation and intervention approaches, writing IEP goals, collaboration, and evaluation for assistive technology.[21] This chapter provides information to prepare occupational therapists for school-based practice.

Federal Legislation and State-Led Initiatives Influencing School-Based Practice

Federal policy, which is shaped by trends in health and education practice, directly influences services for children. In the 1930s, federal legislation establishing the rights of children

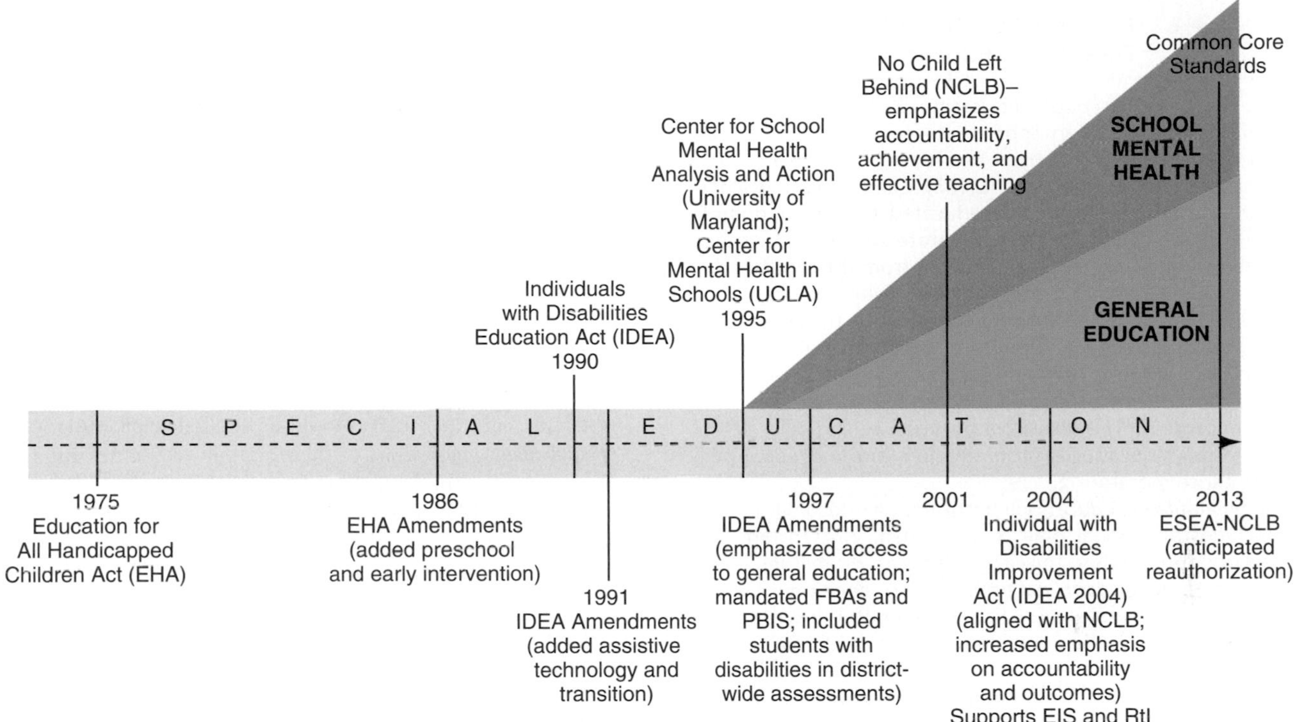

FIGURE 23-1 Timeline of important legislation and developments influencing occupational therapy's role in schools.

related to education and general well-being were established. However, it was not until 1975, with the introduction of the Education for All Handicapped Children Act (EHA; P.L. 94-142), that policy specifically addressed the needs of children with disabilities. This legislation was championed by parent advocacy groups who were seeking normalization, or opportunities for their children to participate fully in everyday routine activities.[104] The introduction of this legislation occurred at a time when it was estimated that more than 1 million children with disabilities were excluded from school, and many were institutionalized. Although occupational therapists' early work with children occurred primarily in medical rather than educational settings, a rapid shift to practicing in schools took place with the EHA legislation. Figure 23-1 depicts a timeline of important legislation, policy changes, and practice developments influencing school-based practice. The following section provides a more detailed discussion of contemporary legislation, such as IDEA, ESEA, and Section 504 of the Americans with Disabilities Act (ADA), as well as the major shifts in occupational therapy practice that have been influenced by this legislation.

Individuals with Disabilities Education Act

The EHA has been reauthorized several times, with the current iteration of the legislation known as the Individuals with Disabilities Education Act (2004; P.L. 108-446). In keeping with the intent of the original legislation, IDEA requires that states and public educational agencies provide a free appropriate public education (FAPE) to children with disabilities in the least restrictive environment (LRE). This legislation also guarantees parents and children with special needs certain rights based on a set of procedural safeguards that dictate the policies and procedures that educational teams need to follow to be in compliance with the law. Part B of IDEA specifies that an individualized education program (IEP) must be designed to include special education and related services to all students from 3 to 21 years of age if it is determined by the educational team that the student requires such services to benefit from his or her public education (§ 300.17).

According to Part B of IDEA, occupational therapy is considered a related service. Related services are described as "such developmental, corrective, and other supportive services as are required to assist a child with a disability to benefit from special education..." (IDEA 2004, Final Regulations, § 300.34, 2006). School districts are legally mandated to provide the services that a child requires to benefit from their IEP, and, therefore, occupational therapists are critical members of the educational team.

IDEA is scheduled for reauthorization every 5 to 7 years. Once it is reauthorized, the U.S. Department of Education develops rules and regulations to guide implementation. Then, state departments of education and local educational agencies (school districts, special education cooperatives) further refine the rules and regulations to establish a process of implementation. It is critical for school-based occupational therapists to be familiar with special education legislation and policy to provide educationally and functionally relevant services.[57,84] Furthermore, understanding national, state, and local policies ensures that occupational therapy practitioners can expand school-based practice to meet the needs of children with and at risk for physical, cognitive, and social-emotional problems. Most children receiving occupational therapy in schools have disabilities and receive services under IDEA. IDEA maintains that

BOX 23-1 Principles of the Individuals with Disabilities Education Act*

1. *Free appropriate public education (FAPE).* Every eligible child is entitled to an appropriate education that is free to families (supported by public funds).
2. *Least restrictive environment (LRE).* Children with disabilities are most appropriately educated with their nondisabled peers. Special classes, separate schooling, or other removal of children with disabilities from the regular educational environment is to occur only when the nature or severity of the disability of a child is such that education in regular classes with the use of supplementary aids and services cannot be achieved satisfactorily [§ 612 (a)(5)(A)].
3. *Appropriate evaluation.* All children with disabilities must be appropriately assessed for purposes of eligibility determination, educational programming, and individual performance monitoring.
4. *Individualized education program.* A document that includes an annual plan is developed, written, and (as appropriate) revised for each child with disabilities.
5. *Parent and student participation in decision making.* Parents and families must have meaningful opportunities to participate in the education of their children at school and at home.
6. *Procedural safeguards.* Safeguards are in place to ensure that the rights of children with disabilities and their parents are protected, and that students with disabilities and their parents are provided with the information they need to make decisions. In addition, procedures and mechanisms must be in place to resolve disagreements between parents and school officials.

*Formerly EHA (P.L. 94-142).

children with special needs are ensured both FAPE and LRE.[86] Four additional assurances directing the education of children with disabilities were adopted with the original law in 1975; these have remained constant, with the exception of a few subsequent amendments (Box 23-1).

Free and Appropriate Public Education

A free and appropriate public education means that special education and related services must do the following: (1) meet the standards of the state education agency (SEA), (2) be provided at public expense, (3) be under public supervision and direction, (4) include an appropriate education at all levels (preschool, elementary, and secondary levels), and (5) be provided in accordance with the child's individualized education program (IEP). *Free* means that parents will not incur any costs associated with these services, beyond typical incidental fees that are charged to all students. *Appropriate,* a term that is less objectively defined, means that children must receive the educational supports and services that adequately meet their unique needs. It does not, however, guarantee that children will receive the most advanced or innovative educational methods or have access to state-of-the-art technology and materials to meet their needs. The IEP, which legally documents the child's educational needs, also documents the individualized set of supports and services determined to be appropriate by the special education team to allow the student to benefit from his or her education and participate at school. The IEP is developed based on the contributions of the special education team, including the occupational therapist, informed by a comprehensive, multidisciplinary assessment.

Least Restrictive Environment

The LRE mandate requires that students with disabilities receive their educational program, including all their academic and related services, with children who are not disabled to the maximum extent appropriate (§ 300.114). LRE does not guarantee that all students will receive services within general education for the duration of the school day. Rather, it means that the IEP team must first consider general education as potentially meeting the student's needs, before moving on to a more restrictive setting.[51] LRE should be applied to all students with special needs, regardless of their disabilities. Removing a child from general education should only take place after it is determined that the nature of the child's disability inhibits him or her from making progress, with the addition of supports and services. IDEA states that the "removal of children with disabilities occurs only when the nature or severity of the disability of a child is such that education in regular classes with the use of supplementary aids and services cannot be achieved satisfactorily" (32 C.F.R., § 612[5][A]). All decisions regarding placement must be made on an individual basis, based on the child's unique educational needs, and reviewed annually. Placement decisions should not be based on the availability of space or resources.

Depending on the child's individual educational needs, students may receive supports and services in a variety of settings. An example of LRE is a student receiving consultative services and accommodations and modification within a general education classroom at the child's school of residency—that is, his or her home school. If the child is not able to benefit from his or her IEP at this level of LRE, he or she may receive services in a special designated classroom or a designated school building. If LRE services in these settings are not adequate, the child may receive services in a therapeutic day school, at home, in a hospital, or at a residential facility. Most children with disabilities spend at least a portion of their day with peers from general education. However, some children with very significant disabilities may not be included with peers from general education. When this is the case, it is up to the child's IEP team to document the severity of the child's educational needs and to articulate clearly why other, more inclusive settings are not adequate to meet them. Removing a child entirely from general education without the option for inclusion in at least some special classes (e.g., music class, physical education, art) or nonacademic activities (e.g., lunch, recess) should be considered by the team as the last option.

Evolution of IDEA

Although the original goal of FAPE in the LRE for children with disabilities has not changed, each reauthorization of IDEA has prompted reflection and a re-evaluation of educational services, which, in turn, has brought about important shifts in the delivery of special education and related services.

In 1986, amendments allowed states to provide preschool and early intervention services for children with disabilities from birth to age 5 years. To reflect current language, the law's name was changed to the Individuals with Disabilities

Education Act in 1990. This amendment authorized additional services (assistive technology services and devices and transition planning). The reauthorization in 1997 was significant in placing greater emphasis on delivering related services to children with disabilities within the context of the student's general education curriculum.[83,89] As a result, there has been a gradual shift in service delivery from traditional pull-out approaches to the integration of occupational therapy services into the student's classroom and other relevant school environments (e.g., lunchroom, playground, restroom).[110] This shift has required occupational therapists to become knowledgeable about the curriculum adopted in specific classrooms and within the school district so that they can better specify how a student's disability affects functioning within the educational environment and develop relevant intervention strategies. The IDEA Amendments of 1997 also focused on student outcomes by requiring students with disabilities to be included in state- and district-wide assessments.

IDEA was most recently reauthorized in 2004 as the Individuals with Disabilities Education Improvement Act. The primary goals of IDEA 2004 are to increase the focus of education on results, prevent problems through early intervention, and improve students' academic achievement, functional outcomes, and postsecondary success.[57] By focusing on accountability and improving educational outcomes, Congress intentionally aligned IDEA 2004 with NCLB (formerly ESEA) of 2002. The long-term goal of special education and related services according to IDEA is to prepare students with disabilities for further education, employment, and independent living. New provisions related to early intervention services were also emphasized in IDEA's most recent authorization. IDEA was scheduled to be reauthorized again in 2013 or 2014.

Section 504 of the Rehabilitation Act and Americans with Disabilities Act

Section 504 of the Rehabilitation Act of 1973 and Title II of the ADA 1990 complement IDEA to ensure nondiscrimination against children with disabilities in public schools.[122] Section 504 requires schools receiving federal funds to provide access to public education to qualified students with disabilities. The ADA ensures that the educational program is accessible to individuals with disabilities and may include providing specific accommodations. The definition of "disability" under Section 504 and ADA includes any student with "a physical or mental impairment that substantially limits one or more major life activities, who has record of such an impairment, or is regarded as having such an impairment" (34 C.F.R. 104.3(j)(2)(i)). Some examples of impairments that may substantially limit major life activities are mental illness, specific learning disabilities, arthritis, cancer, diabetes, and hearing impairment. Major life activities include caring for oneself, education and learning, performing manual tasks, seeing, hearing, speaking, working, walking, and breathing. Because this definition is broader than IDEA's definition of disability, students who are not IDEA-eligible may be 504-eligible for accommodations to access to the learning environment. "Under Section 504, occupational therapy can be provided alone or in combination with other education services and may be provided directly to students or as program supports to teachers working with the student" (p. 1).[3] Student eligibility for Section 504 services are documented in guidelines developed by each state and local school agency.

Sometimes students with diagnoses such as attention-deficit/hyperactivity disorder (ADHD) are not eligible for special education programs. However, these students may struggle to participate fully in classroom activities and often benefit from occupational therapy services. Occupational therapy in the schools can be provided to these students under Section 504. Because the definition of disability is broader in this civil rights act, a child may be eligible for occupational therapy even when he or she is not eligible for special education services. Although school personnel are not required to develop IEPs for students served under the Rehabilitation Act, a team should develop a written plan that states goals, services, and accommodations needed to meet those goals.[57]

Although additional federal and state funds are not provided for these laws, school districts that do not provide accommodations to students who are eligible through Section 504 and ADA can lose federal funding. Occupational therapists may assist the school team in determining the most effective and efficient solutions for meeting students' needs under Section 504 and the ADA.

Elementary and Secondary Education Act and No Child Left Behind

The ESEA of 1965 as a part of the "War on Poverty" was designed to ensure that all children have an equal opportunity to participate in and receive a good education in school.[92] This law, which is considered a key component in the education reform movement, covers all public schools in all states. In 2002, Congress amended ESEA, making major changes, and reauthorized it as NCLB (P.L. 107-110).

NCLB was mainly understood to be a general education law that emphasized increased accountability for educational outcomes on the part of school districts. Under this law, states worked to close the achievement gap by establishing high achievement standards for all students, especially those who were disadvantaged because of poverty or disability.[113] A major component of NCLB was adequate yearly progress (AYP). AYP required that school districts demonstrate that their students were meeting rigorous standards based on yearly testing and annual state and district report cards. Another major component of NCLB was the waiver system. This system allowed parents whose children were attending Title I (low-income) schools that did not make AYP for several years the option to transfer their child to a better-performing school or obtain free tutoring.[114] The final component introduced by NCLB was the requirement that public school teachers in all states meet the standards of "highly qualified." Highly qualified was defined as holding at least a bachelor's degree and having passed a state test of subject knowledge.

Since 2007, Congress has been working on the reauthorization of ESEA-NCLB.[70] However, because of political debate, the legislative process has been delayed. In order for a new bill to be passed, each branch of the legislature proposes a draft. Specific members of the House of Representatives and Senate then convene to negotiate with a combined bill. Both branches are required to vote on the proposed bill before a final bill is sent to the president for his approval.

Common Core Standards: A State-Led Initiative

NCLB caused a shift in practice by emphasizing educational accountability for all students. As a result, 45 states have voluntarily adopted the Common Core Standards (CCS) to guide the educational outcomes of all students, including those with disabilities. The development of the CCS was guided by state governors and state education commissioners. The process of developing the CCS was led by two professional organizations, the National Governors Association (NGA) and Council of Chief State School Officers (CCSSO). The CCS were drafted after a review of current state standards and research regarding what students need to know to prepare for postsecondary opportunities. In addition, the academic standards used in other high-performing countries were also influential in the development of the CCS. Input regarding the content and structure of the CCS was solicited from teachers, parents, and school administrators in the United States. As such, the CCS represent a set of clearly defined goals and expectations for children K-12 in math and English.[87] The focus of these standards is to promote college and career readiness through the development of higher order thinking skills. The CCS are to be used by teachers as a content guide and do not prescribe a specific method or form of instruction. These standards are also used to guide the education of students with disabilities and are integrated into the IEP. Students with disabilities may need support to access the rigorous content aligned with the CCS. This can be achieved through using evidence-based and individualized instructional methods, applying Universal Design for Learning (UDL) principles, supporting the use of assistive technology, and offering general accommodations.[87] In many districts, occupational therapists are encouraged to use these and other state standards as a guide for developing measurable IEP goals and educationally relevant intervention plans.

This synthesis of federal legislation and state-led initiatives provides the foundation for understanding the evolving role of occupational therapists working in schools. Changes brought about by the reauthorization of IDEA and the enactment of ESEA have been instrumental in providing opportunities for expanding occupational therapy's role in serving all children attending school.[57] In the following sections, occupational therapy's role in serving children with and without disabilities is presented, followed by a discussion of emerging roles in school mental health.

Occupational Therapy Services for Children and Youth in Schools

Occupational Therapy Domain in School-Based Practice

Education has been identified by the American Occupational Therapy Association as one of the key performance areas; it refers to the "activities needed for being a student and participating in the learning environment" (p. 620).[1] The occupation of education includes academic (e.g., math, reading, writing), nonacademic (e.g., recess, lunch, self-help skills), extracurricular (e.g., sports, band, cheerleading, clubs), and prevocational and vocational activities.[63] Consequently, in addressing a student's education, attention to a broad range of occupational performance areas, including play, leisure, social participation, ADLs, and work, is often required to help children succeed in their student role.

Occupational therapists working in schools must skillfully align their professional knowledge and skills with the definition of occupational therapy in federal and state education legislation. School districts are mandated to provide related services, including occupational therapy, when a student who receives special education requires such services to benefit from special education. "Related services" means "transportation, and such developmental, corrective, and other supportive services (including speech-language pathology and audiology services, interpreting services, psychological services, physical and occupational therapy, recreation, including therapeutic recreation, social work services, school nurse services[,] ... counseling services, including rehabilitation counseling, orientation and mobility services, and medical services, except that such medical services shall be for diagnostic and evaluation purposes only as may be required to assist a child with a disability to benefit from special education, and includes the early identification and assessment of disabling conditions in children" (§ 300.320(a)(4)). Special education and related services may be provided in a number of settings, including schools, homes, hospitals, juvenile justice centers, and alternative education settings.[2]

Occupational therapy services must be educationally, developmentally, or functionally relevant by contributing to the development or improvement of the child's academic and functional school performance. The regulations of IDEA define occupational therapy broadly as "(A) improving, developing or restoring functions impaired or lost through illness, injury or deprivation, (B) improving ability to perform tasks for independent functioning when functions are impaired or lost, and (C) preventing, through early intervention, initial or further impairment or loss of function" (§ 300.34(c)(6)). Occupational therapy services can promote self-help skills (e.g., eating, dressing), positioning (e.g., sitting appropriately in class), sensorimotor processing, fine motor performance, psychosocial function, and life skills training.[88] Services must be provided by a qualified occupational therapist or service provider under the direction or supervision of a qualified occupational therapist. Although regulations focus on what constitutes "highly qualified" teachers, requirements beyond adhering to state licensure laws have not been created for occupational therapy.[55] However, some school districts are beginning to apply teacher evaluation models,[77] such as the Danielson model, to related service providers. For example, the Danielson model provides for the examination of 22 different components of teaching. The components of teaching are broken down into four main categories: planning and preparation, classroom environment, instruction, and professional responsibilities. In practice, some of the components of the model may need to be adjusted slightly so that they are representative of therapy services. However, such models would provide a way to assess, plan for, and capture professional development.

Shifts in Occupational Therapy Service Provision

The reauthorization of IDEA in 1997 ended a long period during which special education and general education were viewed as separate programs serving separate populations.[106]

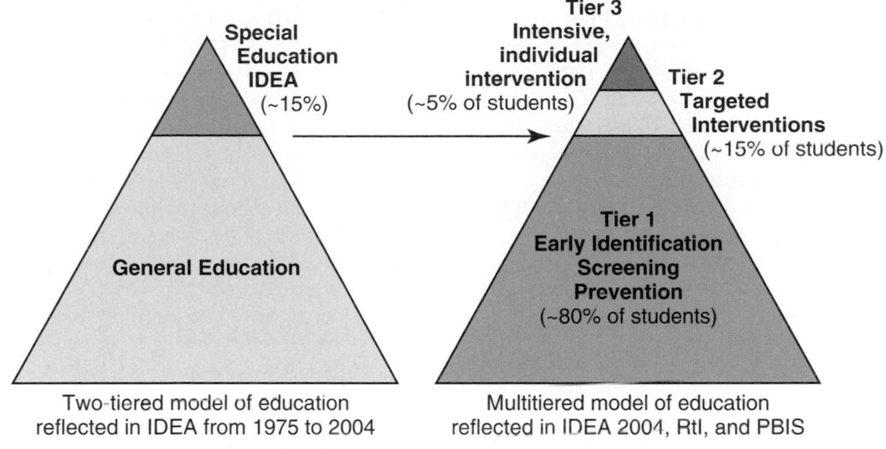

FIGURE 23-2 Tiered model of education.

IDEA 1997 placed greater emphasis on the inclusion of students with disabilities in general education by embedding special education and related services in the classroom and extracurricular activities when possible. General and special education practices have been further aligned as a result of IDEA 2004 and NCLB, providing school personnel, including occupational therapists, with increasing opportunities to expand their role in schools, particularly in the area of health promotion and prevention.[23] In addition, as a result of IDEA reauthorizations, school-based practice has advanced to include two new groups of students more fully: (1) those in general education without disabilities and (2) those with disabilities who are older than 18 years and receiving transition services.

The shift in occupational therapy services can be visualized as a movement from a two-tiered to a multitiered model of service delivery (Figure 23-2). The traditional two-tiered system represents students falling into one of two categories: children with disabilities who meet eligibility criteria as outlined in IDEA or Section 504 and receive services or students in general education who do not receive services. A concern with this system is that some children in general education with learning, behavioral, or functional difficulties do not qualify for services under IDEA. In such cases, children may experience frustration and failure before becoming eligible for special education and related services.[24] In contrast, a multitiered model of supports and services commits to the success of all students by providing early identification and intervening services.

Current practice supports occupational therapy services geared toward the development and achievement of students in general and special education by collaborating with other members of the educational team. Such practice requires that occupational therapists be knowledgeable about federal legislation and local policies, learning standards, the curricula used by their school district to achieve the standards, and the frameworks and processes used by their district to provide services to students. The following sections describe the roles and functions of occupational therapists in general and special education.

Occupational Therapy Process in General Education

To address increasing concerns among parents, teachers, and policymakers that some students have not received needed help in a timely manner, two provisions in IDEA 2004 enabled schools to provide services to students struggling with learning or behavior before being referred to special education.[86] These are early intervention services (EIS) and response to intervention (RtI).

IDEA legislation permits school districts to allocate up to 15% of their federal dollars to provide EIS to students who are in danger of school failure because of learning or behavioral concerns.[24] Comprehensive EIS are designed to help students in general education who are not eligible for special education but who need additional academic and behavioral support to succeed in school (34 CFR § 300.226). Schools are allowed to spend up to 15% of special education funds for EIS, including professional development for teachers and other staff, and to fund direct services, such as small group instruction, behavioral evaluations and supports, and information on the use of adaptive and instructional software. In cases in which the school district has a disproportionate number of minority students in special education, the school district is required to spend 15% of their funds on EIS (IDEA 2004).[56] Early intervening services include "scientifically based academic instruction and behavioral interventions, including scientifically based literacy instruction, and, where appropriate, instruction on the use of adaptive and instructional software; and providing educational and behavioral evaluations, services, and supports" (34 CFR § 300.224). Related services are specifically included in IDEA 2004 (§ 300.208) as possible EIS. In addition, under NCLB, occupational therapists may function as pupil services personnel (professionals who provide services to students) in providing EIS.

The second provision in IDEA 2004 developed to prevent school failure is the RtI process. Federal regulations (34 C.F.R. §§300.307–309) require that states adopt criteria for determining whether a child has a specific learning disability.[116] RtI is a research-based model of school-wide support services that focuses on providing high-quality instruction and intervention matched to student needs, followed by systematically evaluating their response to education and intervention.[85,100] Although originally explored as an approach assisting students with specific learning disabilities, evidence has supported its effectiveness for any student with academic or behavioral problems.[6,66]

The overall purpose of RtI is one of prevention and early intervention—to identify and address student problems early to reduce the need for more intensive services later. Typical

BOX 23-2 Response to Intervention Process

1. Identify and define problem (i.e., the discrepancy between the target student and his or her peers).
2. Analyze the problem to hypothesize causes that are related to the discrepancy.
3. Establish a student-centered performance goal.
4. Establish an intervention plan and system for monitoring progress.
5. Implement plan and monitor progress.
6. Evaluate progress using performance data.

From Illinois State Board of Education. (2008). The Illinois State Response to Intervention (RtI) Plan, January 1, 2008. Retrieved from http://www.isbe.state.il.us/pdf/rti_state_plan.pdf.

BOX 23-3 Examples of Occupational Therapy Tier 1 Supports

Recommend an evidence-based handwriting curriculum to be adopted by the school district.
Identify universal screening methods for handwriting and social-emotional skills.
Recommend changes to the physical environment to promote the access and success of all students.
Provide professional development training to teachers on how to address the sensory needs of their students in order to optimize learning and participation.

Adapted from Mallioux, Z., May-Benson, T., Summers, C., Miller, L., Brett-Green, B., Burke, J., et al. (2007). Goal attainment scaling as a measure of meaningful outcomes for children with sensory integration disorders. *American Journal of Occupational Therapy, 61,* 254-259; and McLaren, C., & Rodger, S. (2003). Goal attainment scaling: Clinical implications for paediatric occupational therapy practice. *Australian Occupational Therapy Journal, 50,* 216-224.

practices underpinning an RtI model include the following: (1) high-quality general education instruction based on scientific evidence, (2) continuous progress monitoring of student performance, (3) universal screening of academics and behavior, and (4) the use of multiple tiers of instruction that are progressively more intense, based on the student's response to intervention.[116] Many states and local districts that use RtI frameworks have adopted problem-solving teams to analyze and interpret progress-monitoring data and make decisions about when specific students would benefit from more intensive instruction.[24] Problem-solving teams typically attempt to identify the reason for the student's difficulty, develop an intervention, and plan for systematically monitoring the student's progress. This team also determines when a student changes tiers to receive more intensive services. Box 23-2 depicts a common RtI process that is used by many school-based, problem-solving teams. Most multitiered models of interventions and supports are made up of three levels: tier 1 (universal or core instruction), tier 2 (targeted intervention), and tier 3 (intensive intervention). In a three-tiered model, the first tier provides school- or classroom-wide interventions made up of high-quality instructional, behavioral, and social supports for all students.[100] Whole-class screening is used to assess whether academic and behavioral performance is appropriate for the student's age and grade. For the group of struggling students, tier 2–targeted interventions may be developed by the problem-solving team, sometimes referred to as the student support team (SST), to address specific needs. Interventions and supports at this level may include small group interventions or more intensive instruction such as tutoring. At this level, interventions reflect more intensive 1 : 1 services and supports provided within general education or special education.

Many school districts are opting to use a multitiered problem-solving framework, such as RtI, to provide EIS. RtI is designed to encourage the use of responsive instructional methods and supports to remediate a student's learning or behavioral difficulties in general education.[1,85] Many RtI frameworks consist of three instructional tiers. Tier 1 is designed to meet the needs of most students in the school or classroom, tier 2 is designed to meet the needs of small groups of students, and tier 3 is designed to meet the needs of individual students.[117]

RtI frameworks have several common characteristics.[19,24] For example, all RtI frameworks have universal screening measures embedded in the curricula to identify students who are at risk of failing. In addition, they use evidence-based interventions at all tiers of instruction and engage in continuous progress-monitoring activities to inform service delivery decisions.

Educational teams may approach special education referral differently in light of RtI.[24] Many students who are identified as being at risk for learning or behavioral needs may move through the different RtI tiers before being referred for a special education screening or evaluation. In other cases, a child might be referred to the special education team before receiving tier 2 or 3 RtI services.

RtI provides occupational therapists in school-based practice a unique opportunity to expand their role and provide services to students who are at risk and may not traditionally be part of their caseloads.[24] Depending on the state's licensure law, occupational therapists can participate at every level of RtI. Tier 2 and tier 3 services parallel the types of services that occupational therapists have traditionally provided in the schools because the focus is often on providing direct intervention or consultation to meet the needs of individual students or small groups. Tier 1 services, however, provide an opportunity for occupational therapists to effect change at the systemic level (Box 23-3).

Occupational Therapy Process in Special Education

Despite recent trends in education and federal policy, occupational therapists in school-based practice continue to spend most of their time providing services to students with special needs. In collaboration with other members of the education team, occupational therapists contribute to the referral, evaluation, intervention, and outcome processes. With these important outcomes in mind, a key question guiding the special education process should be the following: "What does the child need or want to do to be successful as a student now and to prepare for future roles?"[72] The special education process is depicted in Figure 23-3. This section describes the occupational therapy processes of referral, evaluation, and intervention.

Referral

Each school district or local education agency (LEA) has a Child Find system that locates, identifies, and evaluates all children who have disabilities and need special education.[61]

Early Intervening Services for Students Pre K through Grade 12
Screening or Child Find efforts identify students who may require interventions and supports within general education. Progress monitoring determines whether adequate progress is made or whether a referral for an evaluation to determine the need for special education is necessary.

↓

Referral
Child Find activities are conducted in order for the state to identify, locate, and evaluate all children who may need special education and related services. A referral may be made by any source including parents, school staff, or other individuals. Findings of early intervening services are reviewed as a part of the referral process.

↓

Evaluation
The child is evaluated in all areas related to the suspected disability. Results will be used to determine the child's eligibility for special education and related services.

↓

Eligibility
Based on evaluation results, a group of qualified professionals and the parents decide if the child is a "child with a disability" according to IDEA and eligible for special education and related services.

↓

IEP
Within 30 days after a child is determined eligible for special education and related services, an IEP team (including the parents and students when appropriate) must develop an IEP. The child receives sevices as soon as possible following parental consent of the IEP.

↓

Services
The school ensures that the child's IEP is being implemented as written. Teachers and service providers are responsible for carrying out his or her specific responsibilities as outlined on the IEP including accommodations, modifications, and supports.

↓

Annual Review/Re-Evaluation
The IEP is reviewed by the IEP team at least once a year, or more often if the parents or school requests a review. At least every three years the child must be reevaluated to determine if the child continues to be a "child with a disability" as defined by IDEA and what the child's educational needs are.

FIGURE 23-3 Special education process. (Adapted from Office of Special Education and Rehabilitative Services, U.S. Department of Education. [2000]. A guide to the individualized education program, pp. 5-7. Retrieved from http://www2.ed.gov/parents/needs/speced/iepguide/iepguide.pdf.)

A referral of a child suspected as having a disability may be made by any source, including parents, teachers, or other individuals. An occupational therapist evaluation may be requested at the time of initial referral if the team perceives that information provided by an occupational therapist will contribute to the evaluation process. This suggests how critical it is for school administrators and other team members to have an accurate understanding of the domain and scope of occupational therapy practice—that occupational therapists address the education, ADLs, play, leisure, work, and social participation areas of function related to the student's academic and nonacademic expectations. If team members have a narrow understanding of the scope of occupational therapy practice (e.g., occupational therapists address handwriting issues), then it is likely that the role of occupational therapy in that setting will also be narrow.[42] Efforts spent in informing principals, teachers, school

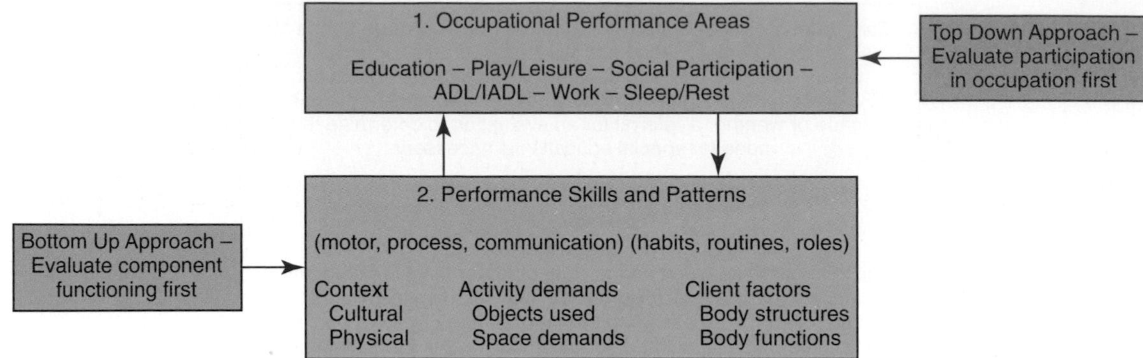

FIGURE 23-4 Top-down versus bottom-up approaches to evaluation and intervention. (Adapted from American Occupational Therapy Association. [2004]. Occupational therapy services in early intervention and school-based programs. *American Journal of Occupational Therapy, 59,* 681-685; and Coster, W. J. [1998]. Occupation-centered assessment of children. *American Journal of Occupational Therapy, 52,* 337-344.)

psychologists, and other personnel about the role of occupational therapy in special and general education ensure that students who may benefit from occupational therapy services are identified.

Evaluation

"Evaluation means procedures used in accordance with §§ 300.304-300.311 to determine whether a child has a disability and the nature and extent of the special education and related services that the child needs" (§ 300.15). After obtaining parental consent, a full and individual evaluation is completed by a multidisciplinary team to determine whether the child is eligible for special education, and, if so, it identifies educational and related service needs (§ 300.301). This multidisciplinary evaluation is needed even when the child has an obvious disability (e.g., cerebral palsy, Down syndrome) and has received therapeutic services in the past (e.g., in an early intervention program). In addition, this team determines the nature and scope of the full and individual evaluations for each child and decides whether related services evaluations, including occupational therapy, are needed.

IDEA and the Occupational Therapy Practice Framework (OTPF) define evaluation and assessment consistently.[1] Evaluation refers to the process of gathering and interpreting information about the student's strengths and educational needs. Assessment refers to the tests or measures used to obtain data about specific areas of function. IDEA specifies that school personnel evaluate referred or eligible students in all areas of suspected disability. Furthermore, a variety of assessment tools or evaluation strategies must be used to obtain relevant academic, functional, and developmental information about the student (§ 300.304(b)(1)). The evaluation must be completed within 60 days of initial parent consent, unless the state specifies otherwise.

Top-Down or Occupation-Based Approach

Although one of the main purposes of evaluation according to IDEA is to determine eligibility, which is based on qualifying as a child with a disability, the law has placed greater emphasis on assessing the child's participation needs in relevant school contexts. This thinking is in agreement with current social views regarding the evaluation of children and those adopted within the profession of occupational therapy. A top-down approach to evaluation is believed to reflect more accurately the true nature of occupational therapy and has been referred to as occupation-based evaluation.[95] A top-down approach to evaluation begins with gathering information about what the person needs and wants to do across a variety of occupational performance areas and settings (Figure 23-4).[33,39] The School Function Assessment,[34] representing a top-down strategy, is used to initiate the evaluation process. Performance skills are assessed to the extent that they are thought to limit participation in occupation. An occupational therapist's ability to implement this approach is dependent on using appropriate evaluation strategies and assessment tools, developing the knowledge and skills needed to implement these strategies, and then actually using them in practice. Refer to Box 23-1 on the Evolve website for a summary of evaluation of performance skills as related to participation in school.

Evaluation Strategies

"Occupation-based evaluation approaches help the IEP team make decisions about the student's ability to participate and perform in the school setting and identify the ways that the disability affects the student's participation in school activities and routines" (p. 35).[95] The occupational therapy evaluation focuses on strengths and weaknesses in educationally relevant occupational performance areas (e.g., education, social participation, ADLs, play, leisure, work) related to the student's suspected disability (Table 23-1). Obtaining an occupational profile initiates the evaluation process by exploring the student's educational history, interests, values, and needs. The student may be interviewed using questions such as the following:

- What do you like about school?
- What kinds of things are going well for you?
- What are some of your challenges?
- What would you like to see changed?

The occupational therapist can also observe the student during typical classroom instruction, as well as during nonacademic time (e.g., during lunchtime and recess). Such observations will assist the occupational therapist in understanding the child's interests and preferences. Observations might also help the occupational therapist gain important information about the child's social participation, as well as his or her habits and routines. The occupational therapist might also interview the teacher about classroom expectations for the student. The

TABLE 23-1 School-Related Occupational Performance Addressed During Evaluation and Intervention

Occupational Area	Examples of Participation in School-Related Occupational Performance	Examples of Occupational Therapy Intervention	School-Related Outcomes
Education	Access to and participation in classroom curriculum Organizational skills Attending to instruction Fine motor skills and hand function Written communication and handwriting	Assist with adapting assignments with high or low technology; adapt child's positioning so child can perform handwriting as effectively as possible Help manage books and notebooks, desk, homework assignments, and backpack Enable child to use self-regulatory activities to foster attending; provide strategies to enhance work completion Provide classroom materials and activities to promote fine motor skills development and in-hand manipulation skills Consult with curriculum committee in selection of a handwriting curriculum; direct services in groups or individually to assist students in letter formation; provide modifications to complete written communication including use of technology	Achieves in the learning environment, including academic (e.g., reading, math), nonacademic (e.g., recess, lunch, relationships with peers), prevocational, and vocational activities (e.g., professional and technical education)
Social participation	Successful interaction with teachers, other school personnel, and peers Ability to adapt to environmental demands	Foster appropriate interaction with peers during group interventions; attend to social interaction during lunch and recess, foster development of friends Provide strategies for coping with test anxiety; adapt procedures to reduce stressful school expectations	Develops appropriate social relationships at school with peers, teachers, and other school personnel in classroom, extracurricular activities, and preparation for work
Play and leisure	Plays with peers during recess Participates successfully in class games Develops structured extracurricular interests (e.g., sports, art, dance)	Assist in making play environments (e.g., playground) accessible; consult with school administration to ensure recess is play-based; assist students in exploring leisure interests; consult with parents to promote structured leisure participation during after-school time	Identifies and engages in age-appropriate toys, games, and play activities; participates in meaningful selection of art, music, sports, and after-school activities
Work	Prevocational	Advocate for embedding productive occupations into the school day (e.g., putting supplies away, cleaning work spaces); involve students with disabilities in work activities within the school environment (e.g., wiping down lunch tables); develop group programs to foster work skills	Develops interests, habits, and work skills needed to work or volunteer in the community after graduation from school
Activities of daily living (basic and instrumental)	Dressing (putting on and taking off coat, dressing for gym) Eating lunch and/or snack Toileting (bowel and bladder management) Basic hygiene and grooming Using communication devices Meal preparation in class Using computers Shopping Doing laundry	Provide direct intervention using a chaining approach to teach dressing or self-feeding Teach appropriate transferring strategies for wheelchair to toilet Provide group activities to promote participation in independent living skills, such as shopping, cooking, and clean up	Attends to basic self-care needs in school (e.g., eating, toileting, managing shoes and coats); uses public transportation to travel in community; develops health management routines; develops home management routines to the maximum extent possible (e.g., cleaning, shopping, meal preparation, safety and emergency responses, budgeting)

Adapted from Swinth, Y., Chandler, B., Hanft, B., Jackson, L., & Shepherd, J. (2003). *Personnel issues in school-based occupational therapy: Supply and demand, preparation, certification and licensure (COPSSE document no. IB-1)*. Gainesville, FL: University of Florida, Center on Personnel Studies in Special Education; and Kentucky Department of Education. (2006). *Resource manual for educationally related occupational therapy and physical therapy in Kentucky public schools.* Frankfort, KY: Kentucky Department of Education.

parents are also asked to identify their priorities for the child. Information obtained from the occupational profile assists the occupational therapist in developing initial impressions about the student's difficulties, which may be useful in directing the rest of the evaluation process.

In addition to observations and interviews, other useful evaluation strategies include document or chart review to obtain background information and construct an educational history. The evaluation process involves an examination of the dynamic relationship among the student's participation and performance skills, educational context, and specific educational and activity demands that may be contributing to the problems.[111] For example, to understand fully a student's difficulty with written communication during test taking, the occupational therapist may observe the student while taking a test, compare work with that of peers in the same environment, and explore curricular demands with the teacher.

Evaluation of the school environment includes the classrooms, cafeteria, playgrounds, restrooms, gymnasium, and other spaces. For children using wheelchairs or walkers, the focus of this part of the assessment may be accessibility. For children with sensory processing problems, the focus may be the degree and types of sensory stimulation in the environment. Classrooms tend to be highly visually stimulating environments, and they can be disorganizing and overwhelming to students with sensory processing problems. For children with social and emotional needs, the focus may be on aspects of the social environment and classroom routines.

To analyze educational and/or activity demands, the expected performance (as defined by the teacher and curriculum) must be understood fully. When a teacher expects neat, precisely aligned, and well-formed handwriting, a student with poor handwriting will have a significant problem in meeting that teacher's standard. As another example, some teachers show high tolerance for disruptive behavior and allow students to move freely about the room. A student with a high activity level and sensory-seeking behaviors would have greater success in a classroom in which movement was allowed, rather than one in which students were expected to remain in their seats. Often a student's goals and services are based more on the discrepancy between the student's performance and classroom teacher's expectations than on performance delays as determined by norms that reference the student's age. In addition, occupational therapists need to consider the CCS and their state's specific learning and achievement standards, which are accessible from the state's department of education website.

Assessment Measures

The occupational therapist may also decide to administer informal or formal assessment measures to obtain a full evaluation of the child's occupational performance related to curricular and extracurricular needs. However, according to IDEA, the use of assessment tools is not required if observations and interviews have provided the needed information for decision making. Because the number of standardized pediatric assessments available today has grown significantly over the past 2 decades, it is important for occupational therapists practicing in schools to make informed decisions when selecting assessments.

Pediatric assessments can be categorized as developmental, functional, and health-related quality of life (HRQL; Table 23-2).[48] Although developmental assessments may be particularly helpful when working with infants and preschoolers to identify developmental delays, they are less useful with the school-age population, for whom the emphasis shifts to functional performance and participation in context. Developmental assessments measure a child's behavior and skills rather than the ability to function as a student.[112] With a developmental approach, intervention emphasizes normalizing the underlying processes to achieve greater function.[32] Current intervention approaches, however, suggest that in addition to assessing characteristics of the individual, physical and social aspects of the environment and features of the activity also need to be considered.[33]

In contrast to developmental assessments, functional assessments measure abilities and limitations in performance of necessary daily activities.[37] Functional assessments are most aligned with an occupation-based, top-down approach. For example, the School Function Assessment (SFA)[34] and a growing number of functional, top-down assessments are now available. Although a number of occupation-based assessments have been published in the past decade, one survey found that school-based occupational therapists primarily used developmental assessments of gross and fine motor skills (e.g., Bruininks-Oseretsky Test of Motor Proficiency, Peabody Developmental Motor Scales, Beery Test of Visual Motor Integration).[23] When the findings of this survey were compared with previous research, similar trends in the use of motor and visual perception tests were found.

One of the major obstacles to using functional assessments is the dominance of the developmental model.[33] Functional assessments have only been available during the past 10 years, and time is needed for occupational therapists to become educated and skilled in using them. Most functional assessments (e.g., the SFA) are often designed so that multiple team members (parents, teachers, and therapists) knowledgeable about the student's performance can contribute to the data-gathering process, yielding a comprehensive understanding of the child. In a study of the validity and reliability of the SFA, findings have suggested that occupational therapists and teachers view students' functioning similarly.[37]

Studies have indicated that in addition to using adult informants, children can also participate actively in the evaluation process and goal setting if the procedures used are developmentally appropriate.[81] The Perceived Efficacy and Goal Setting System (PEGS)[82] is one example of such a measure. The PEGS was designed to help children with disabilities reflect on their ability to perform everyday activities and identify goals for occupational therapy intervention. Other assessment tools developed to gather information directly from the child are the School Setting Interview (SSI)[54] and the Child Occupational Self-Assessment (COSA). The information gathered from these measures on children's thoughts and feelings about their ability to fulfill childhood roles can complement results obtained from functional assessments and provide a more complete picture.[99] In addition, occupational therapists may consider using HRQL measures to obtain a clear sense of the child's life satisfaction.

Documentation of Evaluation Findings

The final step in the evaluation process involves effectively communicating the findings and recommendations in a written report. In general, an occupational therapist's evaluation report includes an overview of the student's occupational profile, assessment measures that were used, child's performance on such measures, and occupational therapist's recommendations.

TABLE 23-2 Types of Assessment Tools

Type	Description of Purpose and Implications	Assessment

Developmental	• Assess underlying performance areas to determine the following:
	  • Presence of a developmental delay
	  • Presumed cause of the functional limitations
	• Areas assessed—gross motor, fine motor, sensory, self-care, social, visual perceptual, communication, adaptive-cognitive
	• Setting—secluded testing room
	• Problem perceived to be within the child
	• Assessments tend to be norm-referenced, comparing child's performance with that of a normative sample
	• Intervention—focuses on development of isolated skills
		• Peabody Developmental Motor Scales, Second Edition (PDMS-2)
		• Bruininks-Oseretsky Test of Motor Proficiency (BOT-2)
		• Beery-Buktenica Developmental Test of Visual-Motor Integration (VMI)

Functional	• Assess function in context; focus is on personal capacities, not failure of organ function • Areas assessed—hygiene, handwriting, play, social participation, material management • Setting—natural environment; parent or teacher may provide the data • Assessments tend to be criterion-referenced, determining how a child performs in relation to a set of standards • Intervention focuses on successful participation in all school activities and settings	• WeeFIM System (Functional Independence Measure for Children) • School Function Assessment (SFA) • Children's Assessment of Participation and Enjoyment (CAPE) and Preferences for Activities of Children (PAC)—CAPE/PAC • Miller FUNction and Participation Scales (FUN Scale) • Social Skills Rating System (SSRS) • Evaluation Tool of Children's Handwriting (ETCH) • Short Child Occupational Profile (SCOPE) • Canadian Occupational Performance Measure • Evaluation of Social Interaction (ESI) • Minnesota Handwriting Assessment • The Print Tool • School Version of the Assessment of Motor and Process Skills (School AMPS) • Sensory Processing Measure (SPM)
Child-reported health-related quality of life (HRQL)	• Assess how child feels about his or her life, abilities, and overall sense of well-being • Aim is to complement functional assessments by providing more complete picture of the person • Areas assessed—person's feelings about participating in childhood roles and over-all sense of well-being	• Perceived Efficacy and Goal-Setting System (PEGS) • School Setting Interview (SSI) • Child Health Questionnaire (CHQ) • Child Occupational Self-Assessment (COSA) • Youth Quality of Life Instrument (YQOL)

Adapted from references 5, 15, 18, 22, 33, 34, 37, 40, 41, 48, 54, 60, 69, 91, and 97; and Schneider, J. W., Gurucharri, L. M., Gutierrez, A. L., & Gaebler-Spira, D. J. (2000). Health-related quality of life and functional outcome measures for children with cerebral palsy. *Developmental Medicine and Child Neurology, 43,* 601-608.

Occupational therapy documentation should reflect a top-down presentation of the student's strengths and limitations regarding participation in academic and nonacademic activities across all student environments. Performance component impairments (e.g., body structure and function) that affect participation should be reported using language understandable to all team members, including parents.

Eligibility

After the evaluation process, the team reviews all the data to determine eligibility for special education and related services. A student is eligible for special education under IDEA if he or she meets two criteria, that this is a child with a disability under one of the disability categories or is under the developmental delay category and needs special education services. The disability categories include intellectual disability, hearing impairment (including deafness), speech or language impairment, visual impairment (including blindness), serious emotional disturbance, orthopedic impairment, autism, traumatic brain injury, another health impairment, specific learning disability, deaf-blindness, or multiple disabilities (34 C.F.R. § 300.8). The term *child with a disability* for children aged 3 through 9 years may, at the discretion of the SEA and LEA and in accordance with § 300.111(b), include a child who demonstrates developmental delays as defined by the state and as measured by appropriate diagnostic instruments and procedures in one or more of the following areas—physical development, cognitive development, communication development, social or emotional development, or adaptive development—and who, by reason thereof, needs special education and related services.

If the team determines that a child is eligible for special education, the IEP process begins; the IEP team meets to develop a special education plan and determine if related services are necessary. Occupational therapy evaluation data provides the IEP team with "information related to enabling the child to be involved in and progress in the general education curriculum, or for preschool children, to participate in appropriate activities" (§ 614(b)(2)(A)(ii)). The determination of need for occupational therapy services should not be based on evaluation alone but should be driven by the student's educational program and annual goals.

A child with a disability who is not eligible for special education under IDEA may be eligible for services under Section 504 of the Rehabilitation Act of 1973. Using information from multiple sources, a multidisciplinary team determines if the child has a disability (as defined in Section 504) that substantially limits a major life activity.

Individualized Education Program

The IEP represents the formal planning process and resulting legal document that establish the services and programs that will enable the student to participate in school activities and receive an "appropriate education." Refer to Table 23-3 for a review of the IEP process. According to IDEA (34 C.F.R. §§ 300.320-300.324), the IEP is a written statement for each child with a disability that outlines the student's educational and functional needs and the supports and services required to meet those needs. It is developed, reviewed, and revised in a meeting in accordance with the guidelines of the IDEA.

The IEP team comprises at minimum the child's parents; one regular education teacher of the child; one special education teacher of the child; one special education provider, when appropriate; a representative of the public agency who has knowledge and qualifications; an individual who can interpret the instructional implications of the evaluation results (perhaps one of the other members); other individuals who have knowledge or special expertise regarding the child (e.g., related services personnel), as appropriate; and the child with a disability, when appropriate (34 C.F.R. § 300.321(a) and (b)(1)). Although related services personnel are generally considered "discretionary" team members (§ 300.321(a)(6)), if an occupational therapist is formally identified as a member of a particular IEP team or if occupational therapy is being discussed at the meeting, it is fitting and desirable that the occupational therapist attend the meeting.[57]

Collaborative Planning

The collaborative planning procedure that guides the process of developing an IEP involves many components. The

TABLE 23-3 Process Depicting the Development of the Individualized Education Program

Step	Description
Vision of Child's Needs	Interpretation of the full and individual evaluation (FIE)
1. Determine present levels of academic achievement and functional performance.	Consideration of how disability influences access to and participation in academic and functional activities
2. Describe how the student's disability affects participation in general education.	Identification of the student's strengths and needs Discussion of parent, student, and team member priorities for the child
Measurable Goals	One-year goals
Develop measurable and attainable annual goals (academic and functional)	All team members contribute to goal development Goals may be linked to state curriculum content standards Plan for measuring progress toward annual goals Related services goals must be "educationally relevant" For children with disabilities who take alternate assessments aligned to alternate achievement standards, a description of benchmarks or short-term objectives is given
Special Education and Related Services	Represents services student needs to accomplish IEP goals
Determine the special education, related services, supplemental aids and services, modifications, and supports	Team determines all needed services Services meet academic, functional, and extracurricular needs Services based on peer-reviewed research to as much as practicable Projected dates for initiating services; anticipated frequency, location, and duration of services
Statement of Accommodations	
Needed to measure academic achievement and functional performance on state and districtwide assessments	Statement of why child cannot participate in the regular assessment and why the particular alternate assessment selected is appropriate for the child
Placement in Least Restrictive Environment	Educate students with disabilities with their nondisabled peers to the maximum extent appropriate. Consider general education environment first Placement determined annually Must offer a range of service delivery options
Transition Plan	Based on age-appropriate transition assessments related to training, education, employment, and independent living skills
Beginning at 16 years of age	Identifies transition services needed to assist the child in reaching goals that may include vocational training, supported employment, independent living, work experience, community participation, or planning appropriate high school classes in preparation for college

school-based occupational therapist contributes to many of those components when participating as a member of a student's IEP team. Although the exact components may vary from state to state, depending on the special education policies and procedures adopted by the state, the following items are mandated as general requirements by IDEA (34 C.F.R. § 300.320(a))(see Table 23-3).

The first steps involve interpretation of the most recent evaluation of the child, consideration of the child's performance on any general state or districtwide assessment programs, and identification of the student's strengths and needs. These also involve discussion with the parents, educational team, and sometimes the student regarding priorities and goals. During this initial phase, it is important to "create a team 'vision' about who the student is and what a student needs to succeed in school" (p. 1).[63] This information is documented on the IEP as the present levels of academic achievement and functional performance and description of how the student's disability affects participation in general education. For a preschool student, consideration is given to whether the disability affects participation in any activity appropriate for a preschooler. Typically, all team members participate in developing this statement, which includes a summary of all evaluation results, thus giving a total picture of the student's academic and functional performance. Occupational therapists should be ready to share evaluation results, which are included in the student's present levels of performance. They should specify how the student's performance influences participation in the general education curriculum, including classroom routines and functional activities—for example, sharing the student's time delay before initiating work, percentage of time engaged in off-task behavior, or how writing speed relates to educationally relevant performance in written expression. In the case of a preschool student, the occupational therapist should document whether the performance results suggest problems that will affect the student's access to typical preschool activities. Table 23-4 provides examples of educationally relevant present levels of performance and statements of need.

The next step involves the development of measurable annual goals (academic and functional) designed to enable the student to have access to and make progress in the general education curriculum and meet the child's other educational needs that result from the child's disability (34 C.F.R. § 300.320(a)(2)(i)(B)). The goals are statements of measurable and attainable behaviors that a student is expected to demonstrate within 1 year. Many states are linking goals to the CCS or their state curriculum content standards.[55] This ensures that the goals are related directly to the learning objectives mandated by the SEA for all students. IDEA 2004 eliminated the requirement of writing short-term objectives (benchmarks) in the IEP, except for children with disabilities who take alternate assessments aligned to alternate achievement standards (§ 300.320(a)(2)(ii)). Congress opted to eliminate short-term objectives as a way to reduce paperwork and because parents are informed of short-term progress through the use of quarterly and other periodic reports. Although short-term objectives are not required for all students receiving special education, some school districts require them. At a minimum, a plan for measuring progress must be documented, specifying how the child is meeting IEP goals and when periodic progress reports will be provided (e.g., through the use of quarterly reports concurrent with the issuance of report cards; 34 C.F.R. § 300.320(a)(2)). It should be noted that the frequency of reporting progress must be at least as often as the progress reports received by the parents of nondisabled students, often on a quarterly basis. The actual progress attained toward the goals must be included. Occupational therapists are responsible for measuring progress toward annual goals and objectives when they are one of the services listed to support that student's goal. Often, several members of the IEP team share data keeping for a student's progress toward general education goals.

Goal Writing

This is a collaborative process and is completed at the IEP meeting with the input of all team members, including the parents and, in some cases, the student. Goal writing in most districts is facilitated by an online process that enables the IEP to be developed on a shared website. Student needs are prioritized and academic and functional goals are selected based on identifying skills needed to progress in the general educational environment. Team members, including occupational therapists, must relate their activities and recommendations to the

TABLE 23-4 Educationally Relevant Levels of Performance and Educational Need

Present Performance Level	Educational Need
Forms all letters correctly in isolation	Increasing speed and spacing so written words and sentences are legible
Highly sensitive to unexpected touch; will push other children when in line or moving through the hallways	Strategies and supports to tolerate being close to peers; accommodations to leave class early to avoid crowded hallways
Eyes remain fixed when reading	Accommodations and instruction to read text without skipping or rereading words
Desk and workspace cluttered; unable to locate assignments and homework	Learning to use an organizational system
Enjoys recess but tires after 5 minutes on the playground	Frequent rest breaks and strategies to understand and communicate fatigue to teaching staff
Has adequate skills for hands-on prevocational work experiences; personal hygiene not sufficient for work settings	Awareness and training for increased independence and carry-over in self-care areas

Adapted from Knippenberg, C., & Hanft, B. (2004). The key to educational relevance: Occupation throughout the school day. *School System Special Interest Section Quarterly, 11*(4), 1-4.

general education curriculum and extracurricular activities. Therefore, all team members must be knowledgeable about the classroom curriculum, behavioral expectations, and state educational standards. Target behaviors are actions and skills that students typically do or need to develop, such as participating in physical education, writing an essay, eating lunch independently, playing with friends during recess, and participating in after-school clubs.[63] Although occupational therapists may identify limitations in discrete performance skills that negatively affect school participation, such separate clinical goals should not be suggested to the IEP team. Goals need to address academic achievement and functional performance. Furthermore, the occupational therapist may think that a particular skill is a priority for a child. However, when viewing the whole child, the team may not agree. If this is the case, some negotiation among IEP team members may be needed to select priorities for the child so that appropriate goals and objectives can be developed for the student. A description of how to develop goals is provided in Box 23-4.

Once the IEP goals have been developed, the team determines the special education, related services, supplemental aids and services, modifications, and supports to be provided by the school. These pertain to the student's advancement toward the annual goals, access to the general education curriculum, and participation in nonacademic and extracurricular activities. The IEP team determines if related services are "required to assist a child with a disability to benefit from special education" (34 C.F.R. § 300.34(a)). "One of the most important clarifications that teams should understand is that students with disabilities do not attend school to receive related services; they receive services so they can attend and participate in school" (p. 6).[45] Therefore, the role of the school-based occupational therapist is not to provide a full rehabilitation program but to support the child's efforts within the academic environment and only if necessary.[43] In general, occupational therapy services under IDEA are not provided when a student has a temporary impairment (e.g., a fractured bone) or when an impairment does not interfere with the student's performance in school. For example, a bright first grader had mild left hemiparesis cerebral palsy. This student participated in all aspects of the educational program, including physical education, with few adaptations. The disability did not interfere with the student's educational program. Therefore, she was not eligible for occupational therapy in school, despite the fact that she did not have the full use of her left hand.

It is important, however, for the occupational therapist to communicate the domain and scope of occupational therapy services effectively to the entire IEP team so that an informed decision will be made regarding service provision. On the basis of evaluation findings, the occupational therapist articulates recommendations to the IEP team regarding the need for occupational therapy services to enable the child to benefit from his or her education. Therefore, it is critical that the occupational therapist understand the full scope of his or her practice and how practice is shaped within the educational context. The IEP team makes the decision about whether or not occupational therapy services are warranted based on the student's educational program and unique needs. "Occupational therapy services are appropriate when the unique skills and expertise of the occupational therapist are needed to support the priorities identified by the team" (p. 78).[49]

BOX 23-4 Steps to Developing Goals: Questions Asked by the Occupational Therapist

Collaborate with the team to identify the student's educational needs.
- What is the biggest priority?

Align educational need with Common Core Standards or other state learning standards.
- Is this priority educationally, developmentally, or functionally relevant?
- Is it an appropriate focus for occupational therapy services in the school context?

Identify the observable target behavior.
- Which behaviors need to change?
- How should the behavior be described in terms that are universally understood?

Establish a baseline for the target behaviors.
- How is the student performing right now?

Establish an outcome for the target behavior.
- Given the student's past learning trajectory, what target behavior can be accomplished in 1 year?
- Which conditions or criteria need to be in place for the student to be successful?

Determine how progress-monitoring data could be collected on target behaviors.
- How can the occupational therapist document that the student has made progress?
- What will the data collection form look like?
- How often should progress be monitored?
- Would another provider be able to collect data on this behavior?

Write the objective.
- Has the objective been written in parent-friendly language?
- Is the student the focus of the objective?
- Does the objective include one specific and observable target behavior?
- Does the objective clearly indicate positive change in the target behavior and include relevant conditions and criteria?

If the occupational therapist is to provide services to the student, it must be noted specifically in this section of the IEP along with the projected date for initiating services and anticipated frequency, location, and duration of these services. Documentation of the type of occupational therapy service delivery should ensure that a range of service approaches be available to the student—direct (to the child) and indirect (on behalf of the child) services. Based on the individualized needs of the student, direct intervention may be necessary during 1 week, whereas indirect consultation provided to the teacher on the student's behalf may be useful during the next week. In addition, flexibility in documenting time and frequency is also recommended (e.g., 2 hours/month or 1 hour/grading period), rather than specifying set weekly visits. "For example, a high school student may need 3 hours the first month to set up a prevocational program and to train the instructional team. Much smaller periods of time, such as 1 hour per month, may be needed when the OT returns in subsequent weeks to evaluate the effectiveness of the program and revise as needed" (p. 3).[94] Recommendations for duration of services, generally written as beginning and ending dates, and location of services (e.g., cafeteria, classroom, playground, hallway) must also be specified.

The occupational therapist may also participate in suggesting appropriate modifications and support based on the assessment results. As an example, the occupational therapist may suggest limiting the amount of information on the student's worksheets because of a student's poor visual figure-ground processing. If the team were to agree to the recommendation, it would be documented on the IEP. Similarly, a statement of any individual appropriate accommodations necessary to measure the academic achievement and functional performance of the child on state and districtwide assessments consistent with § 612(a)(16) of the IDEA must also be determined by the IEP team.[86] In addition, if the IEP team determines that the child must take an alternate assessment instead of the regular state or districtwide assessment of student achievement, a statement of why the child cannot participate in the regular assessment and why the alternate assessment is appropriate for the child must be documented. The occupational therapist may contribute to the team discussion about appropriate testing modification. For example, the occupational therapist may suggest testing a student with sensory sensitivities in a separate room. For a student with motor limitations and difficulty with handwriting, the occupational therapist may suggest using an electronic text format of the test that would allow the student to use a keyboard. Other typical accommodations include allowing extra time for the student to take the test and reading portions of the test to the student. Each state determines the allowable modifications.

Once the IEP team has determined what the child needs in terms of special education services, the team can determine where the services should be provided. Placement decisions are made annually based on where the IEP team has determined that the student's IEP goals can be met.[123] In accordance with LRE as defined in the IDEA, children with disabilities are required to be educated with their nondisabled peers to the maximum extent appropriate (34 C.F.R. § 300.114(A)(2)(i)). This means instruction must be available in a continuum of placement options, ranging from regular education classrooms to specialized classrooms, residential facilities, and home-based programs. Removal to separate classes is permissible only "if the nature or severity of the disability is such that education in regular classes with the use of supplementary aids and services cannot be achieved satisfactorily" (34 C.F.R. § 300.114(A(2)(ii)). On the basis of student's IEP goals, the team should consider whether supplementary aids and services provided within a general education classroom would allow the student to receive an appropriate education or whether such a placement would impede her or his learning and/or the learning of other students. If a child will not be participating fully with children without disabilities in a regular classroom in nonacademic and extracurricular activities, the team must write an explanation on the IEP as to why the child will not participate in these activities.

Full inclusion refers to a child's access to and participation in all activities of the school setting. Supports and adaptations are provided as needed to enable the child with disabilities to participate in activities with his or her peers. These services are typically provided in the child's neighborhood school. For example, Josh, a child with spina bifida and mild learning disabilities, attends his local home elementary school in a rural community. Josh is in the regular classroom for the entire day, with a classroom aide assisting him with self-care tasks, as needed. The school's special education teacher helps the classroom teacher in adapting Josh's assignments when needed.

Inclusion can consist of a variety of learning options. A student may spend a portion of the day in a resource room and a portion in regular education classes. For example, Brian, who is in the sixth grade, participates in the regular education classroom for all his classes except math and reading. For these subjects, he receives instruction from the resource room teacher because his performance in these classes is significantly lower than that of his peers, and he requires a special curriculum to progress in these areas.

Modifications and accommodations are made to support Brian's learning needs so that he can participate in learning activities. Often the regular classroom teacher groups students for science and social studies projects so that each student is given a task that he or she can manage. Because Brian has difficulty with manipulation, the teacher gives manipulation tasks to the other students in the group and often selects Brian to search the Internet or oversee final project assembly. Tests are read to Brian, and he is allowed to dictate his answers.

Finally, once the child turns 16 years old, or before that if determined appropriate by the IEP team, the IEP must include a written transition plan. It is recommended that students as young as age 14 participate in transition activities, even if they do not yet have a formal transition plan.[59] Transition is the process of beginning to plan for the student's completion of education and postgraduation life. This plan is based on age-appropriate transition assessments related to training, education, employment, and, when appropriate, independent living skills. The transition plan should include a statement of the services needed and should clearly connect the student's goals for after-school life and a planned course of studies in high school. The transition services (including courses of study) needed to assist the child in reaching those goals may include vocational training, supported employment, independent living, work experience, community participation, and planning appropriate high school classes in preparation for college. When the student reaches age 16, a statement of interagency responsibility to support his or her transition is also included in the IEP.

The literature suggests that occupational therapists are not fully participating in the development of transition plans, despite their capability to do so.[75] One reason for this may be because the beliefs of the educational staff regarding the scope of occupational therapists and their potential contributions to transition planning.[74] Although educators may be knowledgeable regarding the scope of occupational therapy,[75] occupational therapists would benefit from educating administrators and members of their local school board about the potential contributions that they could make in this regard. Occupational therapists may be involved in transition planning by completing assessments to target the student's motor and process difficulties[59] and by providing input on the student's functional capabilities related to postsecondary education, vocational planning, and community living.[6] Occupational therapists may be involved in this process by providing input on the student's functional capabilities related to vocational planning and community living.

The development of IEPs can be a daunting task because of the changing legal requirements with each reauthorization of IDEA and the changing face of each IEP team. Occupational therapists need to develop the skills to work effectively with a multitude of parents and professionals. Although IEP teams have characteristics that make them similar to other types of working teams, there are also characteristics unique to IEP teams that need to be considered by the various members. It has been suggested that IEP teams differ from other teams in the following ways[35]:

1. There is a legal framework of required relationships among partners. Federal, state, and local laws and policies spell out in some detail who must participate and what they must do. This is especially true for the school district, which has many legal responsibilities regarding the education of students with disabilities.
2. The team members share responsibility and accountability for the success of the student in meeting his or her goals.
3. The process is "results-oriented," meaning that what matters is not how happy everyone is with the process, but the success of the student's educational program.

As a result of these differences, development of the IEP involves high levels of collaboration and, at times, negotiation among and consensus building by all team members. The written IEP document is developed in a formal meeting so the contents reflect the consensus of the team. Parents and other team members, including occupational therapists, contribute equally to the process. Team members discuss the student's strengths and needs and then develop goals, outcome statements, and plans through a collaborative process. By developing the student's IEP using a team process that includes the family, the team assures the family that the IEP belongs to the student and is unique to that student's educational needs.

In addition to the required documentation for the IEP and follow-up progress reports, routine documentation of service provision is not mandated by IDEA. The occupational therapist should develop a method of documentation of services to record the student's progress toward goals, response to interventions, other changes in performance, and strategies that were promising or ineffective.[26]

Annual Review and Re-evaluation

The student's IEP must be reviewed by the IEP team at least once a year or more often if the parents or school personnel request a review. Outcomes are measured by student achievement of the IEP goals, including participation in state and districtwide assessments.[2] At the time of review, it is important to keep in mind one of the primary goals of IDEA 2004—to improve student academic achievement and functional outcomes in addition to postsecondary success. The long-term goal is for students with disabilities to leave high school prepared to work, attend higher education, and live independently.

Termination of related services may be decided at an annual review if the team determines that the related service is not necessary for the student to benefit from his or her IEP. The occupational therapist may recommend termination when the student has acquired the needed skills and uses them during school, when needed adaptations and supports are in place, or when services have failed to produce the targeted IEP outcomes despite numerous approaches and lengthy attempts.[94] When making a recommendation to terminate services, occupational therapists should be prepared to bring data to support their recommendations. The child must be re-evaluated at least every 3 years to determine if he or she continues to be a "child with a disability," as defined by IDEA, and to redefine the child's educational needs.

Data-Based Decision Making and Special Education

Data-based decision making is becoming increasingly important in school-based practice because of recent trends in education and federal policy. Occupational therapists providing services in special and general education need to be familiar with how to monitor a student's progress and objectively determine whether or not their intervention is effective in supporting a student's achievement of established outcomes. In general education, progress monitoring is used to assist problem-solving teams in determining when a student needs additional support to meet the objectives of the curriculum. Data collected through progress monitoring may be used to justify a change in the intensity, frequency, or type of service provided (e.g., moving from tier 1 services to tier 2 or 3 services).[108] In special education, progress monitoring can be used to determine whether a specific intervention strategy or accommodation is effective in supporting the student to meet his or her IEP goals. It can also be used as evidence to support the recommendation to discharge a student from occupational therapy services. This section provides an overview of progress monitoring and goal attainment scaling.

Progress Monitoring

Goal writing and progress monitoring are inextricably linked. An occupational therapist should not recommend an IEP goal or target a student behavior in RtI without having a plan to monitor the student's progress. Designing a strategy to collect data at the time of goal writing helps ensure that the target behavior is objectively defined, observable, and measurable.

The first step in monitoring progress is determining the target behavior. The target behavior should be described in specific and observable terms. The target behavior should also be sensitive to small increments of change and growth over time. Baseline data should be collected on the target behavior three to five times and during typical conditions to ensure that it is representative of the student's performance.[42]

Once baseline data are collected, a goal is established. The goal represents the desired level of change that will be achieved related to the target behavior and as a result of the intervention. For the purposes of progress monitoring, goals can be written in terms of reducing target behaviors (e.g., a reduction of talking out in class) or increasing target behaviors (e.g., an increase in time spent working on an assignment). As with other types of goals, conditions and criteria associated with performance and a time line are established.

After the goal is established, a strategy is designed to capture and document the student's response to intervention. Data are collected at regularly scheduled intervals, ranging from once a week to once a month, depending on the setting in which data are being collected, as well as the nature of the target behavior.[108] Occupational therapists may choose to use available data collection tools or develop and customize their own. Figures 23-5 and 23-6 provide examples of data collection tools. More data collection tools are available at the National Center for Response to Intervention's website (www.rti4success.org).

Upper case	A	B	C	D	E	F	G	H	I	J	K	L	M	N	O	P	Q	R	S	T	U	V	W	X	Y	Z
			X																							
Lower case	a	b	c	d	e	f	g	h	i	j	k	l	m	n	o	p	q	r	s	t	u	v	w	x	y	z
			X																							
Date of Service	March 13																									
Letters Taught	C, c, d, g, a																									
Letters Mastered	C, c																									

FIGURE 23-5 Data collection tool, example 1.

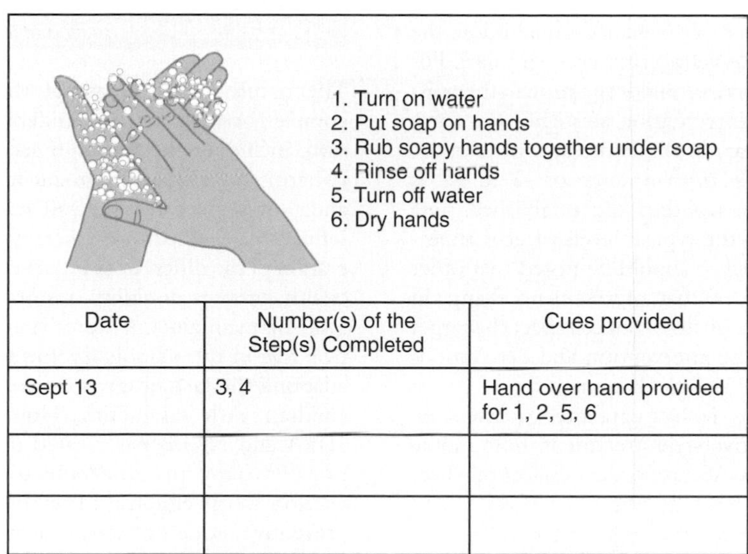
1. Turn on water
2. Put soap on hands
3. Rub soapy hands together under soap
4. Rinse off hands
5. Turn off water
6. Dry hands

Date	Number(s) of the Step(s) Completed	Cues provided
Sept 13	3, 4	Hand over hand provided for 1, 2, 5, 6

FIGURE 23-6 Data collection tool, example 2.

Progress monitoring data are analyzed after three to five measures have been collected. Progress monitoring data are typically graphed, visually analyzed, and/or compared against predefined criteria. For example, a student's goal might be to write all the uppercase letters of the alphabet independently from memory. For this student, the occupational therapist collects progress monitoring data on this goal every other week using the data collection tool in Figure 23-6. Once these data are collected, the occupational therapist charts the number of possible letters written in uppercase on the y axis and the number of weeks during the intervention period on the x axis. The occupational therapist then graphs the student's progress by plotting the number of uppercase letters that the student wrote from memory each time data were collected. If the occupational therapist is monitoring this student's progress in RtI, then he or she also plots the performance of two or three of the student's peers on the same target behavior. This comparison demonstrates whether the student's performance differs from that of other students on the same outcome (Figure 23-7). If a discrepancy is noted, and the student is not performing at the same level as his or her peers, more intensive intervention may need to be provided. On the other hand, if visual analysis of the graph and comparison to peers' performance suggests that the student has made substantial progress, the student may no longer need services. As students continue to develop and progress throughout the school year, this process of data collection may need to be repeated continually and shared with the student's educational team to ensure that he or she is responding to the instruction being provided.

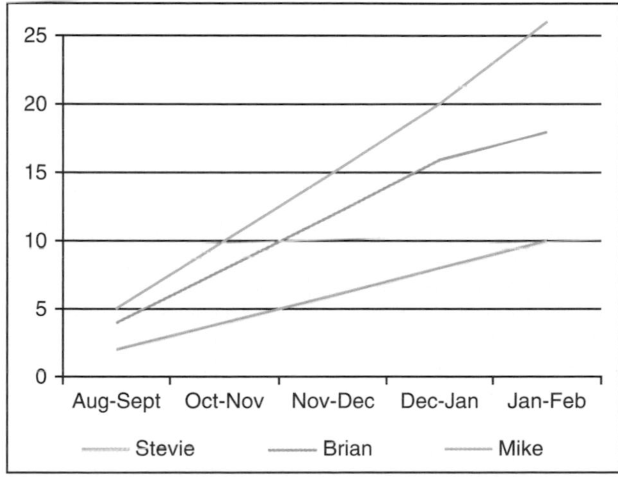

FIGURE 23-7 Progress monitoring graph used for RtI.

Goal Attainment Scaling

Goal attainment scaling (GAS) is another way to monitor progress in school-based practice. GAS is an individualized, criterion-referenced approach used to measure progress and document incremental changes on specific functional outcomes.[76,78] GAS is widely used in special education and pediatric occupational therapy.[72,78,98] The first step in using GAS is to identify the student's educational, developmental, or functional need. This can be accomplished by reviewing data from formal and informal assessment tools and collaborating with the student's IEP team. The second step is to identify the behavior that will be targeted during intervention. As with the progress monitoring method (see earlier), data need to be collected to establish a student's baseline for the target behavior. In addition, the occupational therapist defines the desired outcome of the intervention in concrete and observable terms.[98] When using GAS, occupational therapists must have an accurate sense of the student's developmental trajectory to predict the student's progression from his or her baseline performance. In addition, the scale is developed with the intervention timeline in mind. For example, in school-based practice, an occupational therapist might expect to use a set of intervention strategies for a few months, 25% of the school year, or the entire school year.

Generally, a five point scale, with a range of −2 to +2, is developed to measure progress within the established time frame.[72,78,98] Box 23-5 depicts the typical levels of goal attainment used in the scale, although it should be noted that other scales are sometimes used (e.g., 0 may represent no change in performance). These ratings are customized to reflect the target behavior that is the focus of the intervention and descriptions of the expected progression of skill development.

GAS can be used as a way to collect data after each session. Rather than writing a narrative-style treatment note, some occupational therapists use a GAS rating data collection sheet to document a student's performance during the course of the academic year (Box 23-6). When using this approach, each student goal is charted on a separate data collection sheet.

Data collected through progress monitoring and goal attainment scaling can be used to inform the decisions that occupational therapists make in school-based practice. Both methods can be applied when working with students in general or special education. In addition, both methods can provide support for an occupational therapist's recommendation to initiate, increase, decrease, or discontinue therapy services.

BOX 23-5 Typical Levels of Goal Attainment Scaling (GAS)

Rating	Description of Level
−2	Performance changed much less than expected
−1	Performance changed less than expected
0	Expected outcome or change in performance
+1	Performance changed more than expected
+2	Performance changed much more than expected

Occupational Therapy Services and Special Education

The nature of occupational therapy practice in schools is complex because of the considerable variability in service provision, including the target of services (who), place of delivery (where), types of services and how these are delivered (what and how), and scheduling of services (when). Another factor influencing occupational therapy service provision is a consideration of the different approaches to intervention—to promote health, prevent disability, restore function, adapt or modify a task, or maintain function. Traditionally, occupational therapy's role in the schools has focused on restoring function and adapting the task or environment to promote participation for children with disabilities. However, the reauthorization of IDEA and NCLB has created new opportunities for occupational therapy to contribute to health promotion and prevention in all children. The shift to include promotion and preventive models of service delivery has broadened the definition of "clients" for occupational therapists so that it includes all children and youth in general and special education.

Given the variability of services based on meeting the occupational performance needs of students in general and special education, occupational therapists must enter school practice aware of this complexity and the personal and interpersonal skills required to succeed in such an environment. For example, occupational therapists need good organizational and time management skills to develop and maintain their work schedules, given the variety of school settings and types of service needs of their particular workload. Occupational therapists must be as effective and efficient as possible in meeting the complex demands of their jobs. Providing group interventions to children with and without disabilities or embedded

BOX 23-6 Data Collection Form for Goal Attainment Scaling

	Week								
Goal	1	2	3	4	5	6	7	8	9
−2									
−1									
0									
+1									
+2									

classroom co-teaching models, for example, offer opportunities to serve integrated groups of students with services that blend promotion, prevention, and restorative intervention strategies.

Target of Services: Who Occupational Therapists Serve

General Education

Within general education, occupational therapists have opportunities to provide services to children and youth without disabilities and those at risk for developing academic and/or functional delays. With the growing movement to a three-tiered system of service provision, it is important for occupational therapists to envision, articulate, and advocate for their role in each tier. For example, occupational therapists should educate student support teams on how their services can meet the academic, health, developmental, functional, and behavioral needs of students in general education.[57] Refer to Box 23-7 for an example of how occupational therapists can promote a healthy lifestyle and prevent obesity in schools.

At tier 1 (schoolwide services), occupational therapists can assist the general education team in helping students access and participate in the curriculum by paying careful attention to areas of function within their scope of practice—education, social participation, play and leisure, ADLs, and work. For example, the occupational therapist may participate in universal screening of handwriting to identify students who are struggling, depending on whether the state allows screening.[3] This might be followed by providing a teacher in-service training presentation on multisensory strategies for teaching handwriting and joining a curriculum committee to assist in identifying an appropriate handwriting curriculum. To help foster student attendance and positive behavior, the occupational therapist might assist educators in implementing programs designed to help students regulate arousal for attending (e.g., the Alert program) in their classrooms.[121] In addition, the occupational therapist might join a school team working on a student conduct and behavior management program to become aware of issues in this area and offer strategies from an occupational therapy perspective.

BOX 23-7 Occupational Therapy Services Focusing on Health Promotion and Obesity Prevention: A School-Based, Healthy Lifestyle Initiative

Program Development

The school-based healthy lifestyle initiative consists of a multi-tiered program designed to do the following: (1) promote participation in healthy occupations, (2) support the development of volition, and (3) establish healthy performance patterns in children with and at risk for obesity. The need for the program was identified by related service providers and the school's principal after they noticed an increasing number of referrals to occupational therapy and physical therapy because of concerns related to children's overweight status. Some examples of the concerns noted by the school personnel included fatigue and inattention in class, as well as not being able to perform in physical education. They were increasingly concerned about these issues because they knew them to be symptoms of significant medical problems that children with obesity often encounter. Medical problems that are common in this population include diabetes, sleep apnea, high cholesterol levels, and high blood pressure; in addition, many children with obesity face social isolation and stigma.[103]

Prior to the introduction of the healthy lifestyle initiative, the school's principal had removed the vending machines from the school and required that parents only send healthy snacks for birthday treats. In addition, a physical therapist started a weekly open gym to allow students to participate in physical activity before the school day. Finally, local businesses were made aware of the initiative, and the school accepted donations of pedometers, other equipment, and incentives for children who participated in the program.

1. The activities included in the first tier of the program included the weekly open gym, a whole-school fitness walk, and a cook off–style competition among the different classrooms. In addition, a bulletin board space was dedicated to the initiative, and its content was changed on a weekly or biweekly basis.
2. The activities included in the second tier included training on how to develop new health-promoting habits. For example, students at this tier learned how to use and record steps with a pedometer, how to measure and record personal body mass indexes (BMIs), and how to keep food and activity logs.
3. The activities included in the third tier were designed by occupational therapy students and guided by the Model of Human Occupation. The activities at this tier centered around a collection of classroom-based groups focused on building capacity and increasing students' self-efficacy for participating in physical activities.

Program Evaluation

Although the entire school participated in this initiative, one classroom was selected to provide qualitative information for the program evaluation. Seventeen fifth-grade students participated in a picture-taking assignment that was integrated into their science class. This assignment was developed based on the Photovoice methodology.[119] Students were given disposable cameras and prompted to take pictures of things that helped them or did not help them maintain a healthy lifestyle. After the photographs were developed, students sorted their pictures and participated in two discussions that followed the typical Photovoice prompts. Students were asked to reflect on their photographs and answer the following questions:

- What do you see here?
- What is really happening?
- How does it relate to our lives?
- Why does the situation exist?
- What can we do about it?

The students who participated in this assignment were able to identify activities that promoted a healthy lifestyle and those that did not. In addition, they set goals about what they wanted to do to change specific unhealthy situations.

This program illustrates one way that occupational therapists can be involved in promoting healthy lifestyle development in children in the school context.

This program is discussed in further detail in Cahill, S., & Suarez-Balcazar, Y. (2009). Promoting children's nutrition and fitness in the urban context. *American Journal of Occupational Therapy, 63,* 113-116, and Cahill, S., & Suarez-Balcazar, Y. (2012). Using Photovoice to identify factors that influence children's health. *Internet Journal of Applied Health Sciences and Practice, 10,* 1-6.

Indirect OT services on behalf of child	Direct OT services
Planning time with school personnel	Individual or group
Educational in-service sessions	Coteaching
Participation in school-wide committee	Coaching
Consultation with teachers and other school staff	Embedded OT programs

FIGURE 23-8 Range of occupational therapy service delivery.

At tier 2 (targeted interventions for those at risk), the occupational therapist might develop a social skills group for students struggling with behavior management and social interaction with peers. Tier 3 interventions call for more individualized interventions for those not responding to tier 2 interventions. At this level, students may receive such services as a part of RtI or may be referred for special education.

With opportunities to expand occupational therapy's role in general education, occupational therapists might be questioning how they can create time to provide prevention and early intervention services. Traditionally, an occupational therapist's job expectations have been based on a caseload model of counting the number of children receiving direct intervention as part of their IEP.[4] This model often neglects to account for essential indirect services, including collaborative consultation, team meetings, and in-service trainings.[107] In contrast, the concept of workload encompasses all the direct and indirect services performed to benefit students, making a workload approach helpful for conceptualizing work patterns that optimize effectiveness and impact.[4] Occupational therapists must have the flexibility of organizing their work patterns to serve students in their LRE, collaborate with teachers and other school personnel, attend meetings, supervise and train occupational therapy assistants, plan interventions, and collect data. Careful documentation of workload using a time study may help state regulatory boards become knowledgeable about the range of occupational therapy services and encourage them to adopt a workload versus caseload system of documenting service provision. Kentucky, for example, has adopted a workload model, defining workload as "the amount of minutes per day, week, or month a therapist needs to work to adequately perform his/her duties" (p. 43).[106]

Special Education

In special education, occupational therapists provide services to children and youth with disabilities who are eligible for special education. Once the IEP team agrees that occupational therapy services are necessary to support the student's goal achievement, the occupational therapist can propose how to provide services. IDEA 2004 recognizes that services and supports need to be delivered in different ways for children with disabilities to benefit from education. Although the primary client is the child, intervention may also target general and special education teachers, other related service providers (e.g., music therapists), administrators (e.g., principals), and paraprofessionals involved in supporting the child's IEP.[26,50]

Range of Service Delivery Options: What Occupational Therapists Provide

Intervention with a variety of clients occurs as a direct result of using a range of service delivery options. Traditionally, services in schools were provided directly to the child in an isolated therapy setting, similar to clinical practice. This type of service delivery involves primarily one client, the child. However, IDEA does not mandate any one service model and allows for a range of services, including those provided directly to the child (direct), on behalf of the child (indirect), and as program supports or modifications for teachers and other staff working with the child (indirect; § 614(d)(IV)). Refer to Figure 23-8. Decisions about how occupational therapy services are provided are based on the child's needs, the educational program, and expected outcomes.[26,93] Examples of the range of services provided by an occupational therapist include working individually with children, consulting with the teacher about a student, co-leading a small group in the classroom, providing an in-service education for school personnel, and working on a curriculum or other school-level committee.[109]

Direct Services

Direct services may be provided in a variety of ways, including one to one (occupational therapist works individually with the student), small groups (lunch bunch), or large groups (in the classroom, during recess), and can take place in a variety of settings within the school (e.g., separate therapy room, special education resource room, general education classroom, cafeteria, playground). Individualized direct services in isolated settings may be useful during initial evaluation of levels of performance or during the initial stages of learning a skill. The benefit of providing services in small groups is that interaction within a group provides students with opportunities to develop and practice social skills. In addition, in an effort to meet LRE, the occupational therapist can blend students with and without disabilities in a small group intervention, targeting those at risk of delays but who are not eligible for special education. For example, an occupational therapist might co-lead groups with a special education teacher, as discussed in Box 23-8 (Figure 23-9).

Indirect Services Provided on Behalf of the Child or to Provide Program Supports

These require the therapist to work directly with a range of other clients, including regular and special educators, parents, and paraprofessionals. For example, an occupational therapist might consult with the classroom teacher to help modify instructional materials and methods for a student with physical or organizational needs requiring close interaction with the teacher. Documentation of evaluation, intervention, and outcomes is an important service and should be included in an occupational therapist's weekly schedule. Educational in-service sessions to groups of school staff (e.g., teachers, administrators, paraeducators) or parents are beneficial for providing information on discipline-specific areas of performance, such as fine motor development and handwriting, sensory

BOX 23-8 "Brownie Busters": An Occupation-Based Work Group for Children with Multiple Disabilities

Program Development

The Brownie Busters program aims to do the following: (1) provide a community-based functional curriculum for students with multiple disabilities attending elementary school; (2) provide tasks that are meaningful to elementary school students while teaching them skills needed for future employment and independence in their homes and neighborhood community; and (3) encourage collaboration among school team members, including the teacher, teacher's assistant, occupational therapist, and parents.

The foundation for the development of the 6-week Brownie Busters work group was based on literature regarding the development of work skills in children with multiple disabilities, which indicated the following: (1) preparation for employment needs to begin at an early age,[58] (2) participation in meaningful activities within an educational or work context reinforces interest,[10,67] and (3) programs for students with moderate intellectual disabilities should emphasize skills that are functional and longitudinally relevant.[81] An occupational therapist working in a large Midwestern municipal school district developed and facilitated the 1½-hour weekly groups over a period of 6 weeks. The classroom teacher, teacher's assistant, and a parent volunteer served as helpers for the groups.

The overall purpose of the Brownie Busters work group was to have the students make and sell brownie-making kits to teachers, students, and staff at their school. The groups were designed to promote the development of several independent living and work skills, including the following: planning a work task, functional reading (reading labels and recipes), safety issues related to walking in the community, grocery shopping, simple cooking (learning about ingredients and measuring, pouring, and mixing ingredients), using an oven, sanitary food handling, and selling a product.

Participants

The work group consisted of eight elementary students ages 9 to 12 years with multiple disabilities, including mild to moderate intellectual impairment and language delays. The diagnoses of the students included cerebral palsy, Down syndrome, and autism.

Group Sessions

The group sessions involved weekly discussions of basic work skills, a trip to the grocery store, making the brownie mixes, putting them in jars, decorating the jars, and selling them. Each session also involved clean up.

Qualitative Research Findings

Qualitative research methods were used to explore the meaning of group participation from the children's perspective. Each of the eight group members were interviewed during weeks 2 and 6 of the program by the occupational therapist to explore the personal meaning ascribed to the group experience. Participant observations served as the second form of data and consisted of weekly observations of the group. Based on a qualitative analysis of the interviews and participant observations, three essential themes unfolded: shopping, special ingredients, and doing everything. When asked what comes to mind or what they liked the most when they think of the occupational therapy groups, all the participants talked about walking to and shopping at the neighborhood grocery store, ingredients needed for the project, and doing the tasks necessary for making the brownie jars. By being actively involved in the shopping process, students learned first-hand about how to locate the baking ingredients needed for the brownies. The students began to take on the role of shoppers by looking for items needed for baking and using a shopping list. Students also learned about each special ingredient's unique properties by handling, measuring, and tasting it. Finally, students expressed joy in doing everything and began to function like workers—doing the task, sharing, demonstrating care with the ingredients, using sanitary strategies for handling of food, and preparing the jars to sell. Findings support the importance of occupation-based practice in fostering the link between doing and becoming.

Contributors: Eileen Dixon, MS, OTR/L, and Susan Bazyk, PhD, OTR/L, FAOTA.

processing, positioning for function, and mental health and well-being. Time spent serving on school-wide committees (e.g., positive behavioral interventions and supports [PBIS], bully prevention) is also an important indirect service, allowing occupational therapists opportunities to share expertise and become contributing members of the school community. Planning time for embedding intervention is an important indirect service and one that is not always acknowledged as an essential part of an occupational therapist's workload. However, in an outcome study of one occupational therapist's full integration of services in a kindergarten curriculum, it was found that 50% of indirect services were spent in planning integrated services.[14]

In addition to determining the most effective range of services for a child, occupational therapists are also encouraged to provide services in a flexible manner, depending on the student's stage in the therapy process and particular needs. For example, the occupational therapist may choose to work directly with a student for several weeks to teach the student how to implement the Alert Program for Self-Regulation,[121] followed by consultation with the teacher or paraprofessional to ensure generalization of the strategies in the classroom.

Integrated Service Delivery: Where Services Should be Provided

Integrated services delivery involves the provision of occupational therapy in the child's natural environment (e.g., in the classroom, on the playground, in the cafeteria, on and off the school bus), emphasizing nonintrusive methods and common goals.[14] Although sometimes viewed simply as "treatment that takes place in the classroom," integrated therapy is actually complex, requiring team collaboration and a combination of teacher education, consultation with various team members, and direct service that is skillfully embedded in the natural context.[89] IDEA does not specify the type of service delivery provided, but it does indicate that all related services be provided in the LRE to foster participation in the general education curriculum. Simply stated, integrating occupational therapy services in general education settings to the maximum extent possible is the law. Also, it is important to keep in mind that "students with disabilities do not attend school to receive related services; they receive services so they can attend and participate in school."[45] Related services must be educationally relevant, which differs from therapy that occurs in an outpatient

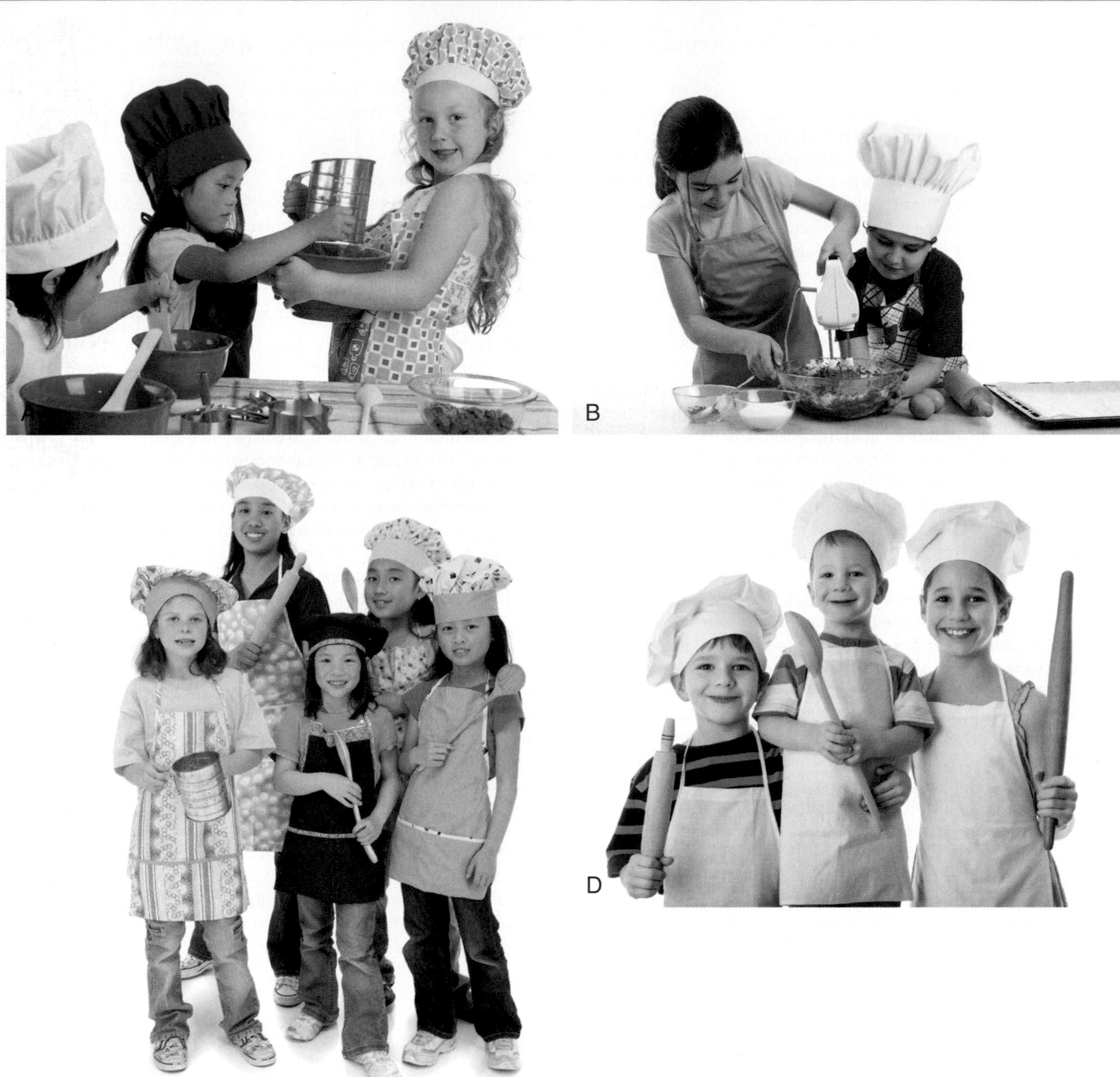

FIGURE 23-9 **A-D,** Brownie Buster group pictures.

clinic or hospital setting. It is critical for occupational therapists to articulate these differences to school staff and parents.[118] Because occupational therapy services support academic goals (e.g., handwriting, literacy) and nonacademic functional goals (e.g., organizing learning materials, using the restroom, playing during recess), the service context can include a wide range of natural settings, including classroom, playground, cafeteria, restroom, and hallways.

Another reason for providing services in an integrated setting is that theories of and research on motor control have indicated that the practice of a meaningful occupation in a natural context is most effective for achieving new skills or modifying movements.[16,73,90] Performing meaningful activities in natural settings requires children and youth to problem-solve and adapt to inherent variability, which helps reinforce learning.[90] In addition, interventions provided in natural settings during daily routines are more likely to be applied consistently, leading to functional changes.[2] Therefore, pull-out services in isolated therapy rooms filled with contrived activities and equipment are no longer considered best practice in schools. Such services may only be appropriate during initial stages of learning a task, when the student's skill level is far below the tasks presented to other students in the classroom or when the intervention activities cannot appropriately occur in a typical classroom (e.g., therapeutic use of equipment such as a swing). "Although therapists may pull students out of the classroom for brief periods to explore strategies or to introduce a new skill, time away from instruction is minimized" (p. 3).[94] McWilliam has cautioned that pull-out therapy is less effective than integrated services.[79]

Benefits

All parties benefit from integrated services. By working in natural settings, the occupational therapist learns about the curriculum, academic and behavioral expectations, teacher preferences, and unique culture of each classroom. Observing and interacting with students in the classroom and other school settings (e.g., physical education area, music, cafeteria) enables occupational therapists to analyze the relationships among the child's abilities, activity expectations, and physical and social environment fully. When the task-environment demands are greater than the student's abilities, the therapist and teacher must adapt the environment or task to foster successful participation. Integrated therapy ensures that the therapist's focus has high relevance to the performance expected in the student's classroom and other school contexts.

The therapist's presence in the classroom also benefits the instructional staff, who observe the occupational therapy model interventions that are practical and realistic.[27] With integrated services, teachers, paraeducators, administrators, and other related service providers have opportunities to learn about occupational therapists' scope of practice and skill sets. The blending of teacher education, collaborative planning, and embedded direct intervention provides a natural way for occupational therapists to contribute discipline-specific information and the strategies needed to enhance particular areas of function that are typically not within a teacher's expertise.

Students with disabilities benefit from the teacher's increased ability to implement therapy strategies when the occupational therapist is not present.[105] In a study of fine motor and emergent literacy outcomes following fully integrated occupational therapy in a kindergarten curriculum, it was found that children with and without disabilities made significant gains in fine motor and emergent literacy skills.[14] In this particular school, the principal expressed pleasure in these results, exclaiming that she was "getting the biggest bang out of her therapy buck." When providing integrated services, occupational therapists need to measure outcomes in students with and without disabilities and share these data to communicate the benefits of therapy to administrator, parents, and teachers. Figure 23-10 illustrates an occupational therapist embedding a sensorimotor activity into the classroom to foster self-regulation of attention for learning.

Challenges

Despite the well documented benefits of integrated services, successful implementation requires time and effort. Findings from several survey and qualitative studies have indicated that the greatest challenge associated with providing integrated services is time for occupational therapists, teachers, and other relevant school personnel to meet and plan embedded services.[8,20,53] Although informal collaboration with teachers in the hallways or during lunch is useful, time for regular formal meetings is essential.

Suggested Strategies for Moving Toward an Integrated Service Model

Strategies that can be used to foster the provision of integrated occupational therapy services include the following:

1. Obtain school administrative support to free teachers and OTs from their teaching and therapy schedules.

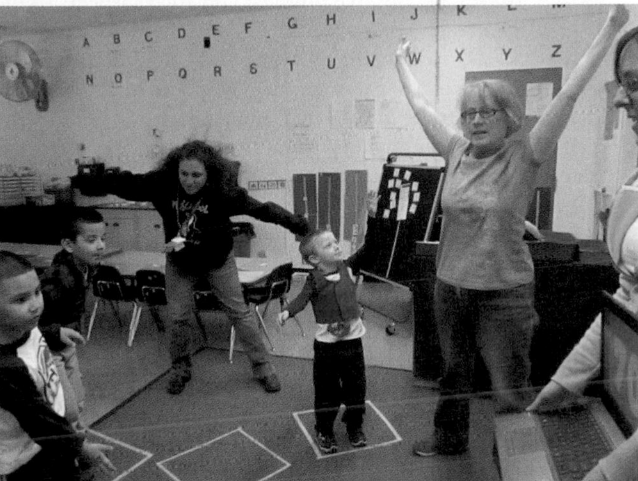

FIGURE 23-10 The occupational therapist may embed movement and/or sensory strategies to help students regulate alertness for attending.

   Bazyk and colleagues[14] found that when providing integrated services, time spent collaborating with the teacher and other personnel outweighed time spent in direct intervention by a 2 : 1 ratio. As the face of occupational therapy shifts from pull-out to embedded services, occupational therapists need to make a case for time spent in planning as a legitimate part of service because of the complexity of integrated therapy.

2. Allocate time for collaborative planning with relevant school personnel based on the specific service and setting.

   When integrating sensorimotor strategies into a preschool classroom, for example, it is important to collaborate with the teacher and paraeducator. Embedding services in the cafeteria will involve collaboration with the lunch supervisors. The need for regularly scheduled meeting times is consistently reported by therapists and teachers.[8,20,53]

3. Commit to collaboration. Develop positive relationships with teachers, paraeducators, and other relevant stakeholders (e.g., parent, mentor, physical therapist, school psychologist, speech-language pathologist, principal, cafeteria supervisor, bus driver).

   Because integration of occupational therapy services requires working closely with teachers, administrators, families, related service providers, and support staff, effective collaboration is essential. Commit to a collaborative style of interaction built on mutual trust and respect and effective communication surrounding common goals, characterized by the equal status of all parties involved in working toward a shared goal.[20] Consider developing a community of practice (CoP) to enhance collective work and impact.[120] A CoP is a group of people who are committed to a common cause, interact regularly, and share leadership and work for collective competence and impact.[120]

4. Learn about the unique classroom culture or school setting, the curriculum, and performance expectations.

   Occupational therapists need to understand school board policies, curriculum, and classroom practices of teachers to develop educationally relevant approaches to providing service. Informally observe physical and social aspects of the environment (e.g., classroom layout, teacher-student interactions). Talk with the teacher about challenges and needs specific to occupational therapy's scope of practice (e.g., issues related to social participation, attention, handwriting). When working with students in a classroom, the occupational therapist needs to have a clear understanding of classroom expectations. This includes knowledge of classroom rules, routines, and dynamics and of the general education curriculum and special education adaptations. Each classroom teacher has unique teaching and classroom management styles. Intervention techniques conducted in the classroom that may be acceptable to one teacher may not be acceptable to another teacher; they may even be considered intrusive.

5. Griswold has recommended that occupational therapists offer interventions that fit the existing classroom structure and culture.[47]

   For example, a teacher who values child-directed learning and hands-on learning centers may respond well to an occupational therapist's suggestions for activities to be included in the learning centers. Another teacher who uses a strong teacher-directed classroom may prefer to engage in team-teaching activities with the occupational therapist.

6. Provide information about occupational therapy's role and full scope of practice using informal opportunities to share information (e.g., conversations in the hallway, one-page information briefs) and formal in-service education.[53]

   Make a point to describe how occupational therapy can contribute to areas of student function beyond handwriting and sensorimotor processing, such as social participation, play, leisure, and work. Explain occupational therapists' expertise in a wide range of performance areas, including physical and motor, mental health and well-being, sensory processing, cognitive, and behavioral functioning.

7. Explore teacher preferences for integrated services.

   Be sensitive to the regular education schedule and do not disrupt the child's and the classroom schedule, if possible. Teachers may prefer to have the occupational therapist in the classroom at certain times or on certain days. These preferences should be negotiated with the teacher before intervention, and attempts should be made to schedule times for providing services to the child that coincide with targeted goal areas. For example, handwriting interventions can be integrated into the student's language arts time, and keyboarding skills can be integrated into the student's computer or language arts class. (Refer to Box 23-2 on the Evolve website, From pull-out to integrated service provision: How one school district made the transition)

Informal Strategies for Integrating Direct Services

Direct services can be embedded throughout the school day to enhance participation in a number of ways, including the following: (1) modify the physical or social environment, (2) modify the activity or task, and (3) modify the instruction.

Modifying the school environment aligns with the educational initiative called Universal Design for Learning (UDL), which focuses on fostering performance in the classroom via environmental modifications. To modify the physical environment, the occupational therapist may give the teacher materials helpful for implementing the intervention (e.g., pencil grips, slant boards, games that foster fine motor skills) or help adapt the environment so that the child can participate (e.g., establish a sensory corner, obtain supportive seating, set up a prone stander). To enable the person who is chosen to implement the strategy, the occupational therapist uses modeling and coaching as the child attempts the activities in his or her natural routine. Regular contact is necessary to update programs and supervise the manner in which the activities are implemented. Refer to Table 23-5 for examples of integrated services

TABLE 23-5 Examples of Indirect Intervention Strategies When Integrating Services

Intervention Strategies	Examples
Reframe the teacher's perspective.	Explain the functional consequences of the perceptual problems observed in children with spina bifida. Identify that a child with autism is hypersensitive to tactile and auditory stimuli. Suggest that a child's difficulty in sitting quietly is related to his or her low arousal level and need for sensory input.
Improve the student's skills.	Recommend that a student use carbon paper to monitor the amount of force applied with the pencil. Recommend that a student practice letter formation using wide-lined paper and beginning at the top of the letter. Recommend that a teacher provide standby assistance when the child practices carrying a lunch tray in the cafeteria.
Adapt the task.	Recommend that a student begin to use a computer keyboard. Introduce compensatory methods for putting on a jacket. Teach one-handed techniques during toilet training. Recommend that a student use earphones with music during written tests.
Adapt the environment.	Establish a quiet area with a tent in which students can hide and remove themselves from the stimulating environment. Suggest that excess visual stimulation be removed from the wall in front of a student.
Adapt the routine.	Recommend that a student have opportunities for exercise three times each day. Recommend that a student be given extra time to complete certain written assignments. Suggest that the student receive speech therapy after occupational therapy so that he or she can be focused and attentive during the session.

involving a combination of indirect (consultation) and direct interventions.

Formal Strategies for Integrating Direct Services

School-based occupational therapists apply a wide array of intervention methodologies based on a variety of theoretical frames of reference (e.g., sensory integration, motor learning, behavioral, biomechanical). According to IDEA 2004, and consistent with NCLB, schools are required to "ensure that such personnel have the skills and knowledge necessary to improve the academic achievement and functional performance of children with disabilities, including the use of scientifically based instructional practices, to the maximum extent possible" (§ 601(c)(5)(E)). Formal strategies for integrating occupational therapy services with emerging research evidence include co-teaching models, occupational performance coaching, and provision of specially designed programs.

Co-Teaching

Although co-teaching originally was designed as an instructional strategy for general and special educators to share teaching responsibility within an integrated classroom,[29] it has also been used by occupational therapists as a formal way to integrate services.[27,28,105] Cook and Friend have defined co-teaching as "two or more professionals delivering substantive instruction to a diverse, or blended, group of students in a single physical space" (p. 1).[29] In general, co-teaching involves collaboration to design, plan, implement, and evaluate the learning experience. In addition to working with teachers, occupational therapists may also choose to co-teach with other relevant school staff, such as the guidance counselor, health educator, or speech-language pathologist, depending on curricular need. The occupational therapist's time is scheduled for the co-teaching activities, rather than for individual sessions.

Cook and Friend have defined five variations of co-teaching: (1) one teaching and one assisting (occupational therapist takes the lead and teacher assists, or vice versa), (2) station teaching (teachers divide instructional content into two segments, teach half the content to half the class at a time, and then trade student groups and repeat the same instruction), (3) parallel teaching (teachers plan a unit of instruction and present it simultaneously to half the class, resulting in a lower student-to-teacher ratio), (4) alternative teaching (one person teaches a small group of students who need specific accommodations while the other teaches the remaining larger group), and (5) team teaching (both teachers teach at the same time, sharing the lead in the discussion).[29]

Although co-teaching may appear to require more time and effort, the benefits can outweigh the cost. The benefits of co-teaching include the following: expanded instructional options because of the combined expertise of the two teachers, improved program intensity because of a higher teacher-to-student ratio, and enhanced educational continuity for students with special needs who are not pulled out of the classroom for services.[29] Not only do the targeted students with disabilities benefit from the interventions, but students without disabilities in the class also benefit from the multidisciplinary input. For example, the classroom teacher and occupational therapist might co-plan a handwriting session. Another example might involve an occupational therapist and guidance counselor co-teaching a unit on the Zones of Regulation, a cognitive behavioral approach developed by an occupational therapist to teach children how to regulate their emotions to improve social interaction with others at school.[68]

Case-Smith and associates have examined the feasibility and effects of a 12-week, co-taught handwriting and writing program, Write Start, using a one-group, pretest–post-test design with 36 first graders.[28] The program, using a combination of station teaching and team teaching, was found to benefit students with diverse learning needs by increasing handwriting legibility and speed and writing fluency. During final interviews, the teachers and occupational therapist reported that the students received more individualized instruction and that they gained skills from working together. Specifically, the occupational therapist learned about the curriculum and behavior management approaches and the teachers learned handwriting strategies.[28]

Occupational Performance Coaching

Occupational Performance Coaching (OPC) was initially developed by Fiona Graham to provide a process for helping parents promote their child's occupational performance.[46] OPC involves three major components: emotional support, information exchange, and a structured process. Although originally developed to be applied with parents of children with disabilities, the basic elements may be used as a guide when working with teachers and other school-based personnel.

Emotional support, for example, may be provided in a way that acknowledges the interpersonal challenges associated with serving children in their specific context (e.g., classroom, cafeteria). When working with cafeteria supervisors while implementing the Creating a Comfortable Cafeteria program, it was important for the occupational therapist to acknowledge their challenges and needs. One of the biggest challenges expressed by the supervisors was dealing with the noise levels that occur when large groups of children eat together in a large room. The occupational therapist can help process reactions to and feelings about noise levels and problem-solve positive strategies for dealing with the noise levels without enforcing rules about eating in silence.

Information exchange is important to understand individual perceptions of the problem and/or occupational performance expectations. In the same cafeteria program, a discussion about noise levels resulted in supervisors talking about their personal sensory preferences for and tolerance of noise. Some cafeteria supervisors did not mind loud cafeteria environments and were happy to see children talking with each other and having fun. Others struggled with being in a loud environment.

The final component of OPC involves a clear sequence of steps including setting goals, exploring options, planning action, carrying out the plan, checking performance, and generalizing abilities. The occupational therapist's ultimate goal is guided by the dual intention to improve children's occupational performance in school contexts and assist school personnel in promoting successful participation and enjoyment. For the cafeteria program, an initial orientation session, embedded activities, and follow-up coaching were used to create a comfortable cafeteria for children with and without disabilities.

Formal Occupational Therapy–Embedded Programs

With integrated services becoming more accepted and pursued as the most preferred form of related service delivery, a growing number of occupational therapists have recently developed creative programs designed to be embedded in a variety of school contexts (e.g., classroom, cafeteria, recess) with the purpose of helping children participate in, succeed at, and enjoy learning, socializing with peers, eating a meal, and playing during recess. Table 23-6 provides a summary of some of these programs. It will be critical for occupational therapists to conduct studies that examine the feasibility and effects of embedded programs.

School Mental Health: Emerging Roles for Occupational Therapy

School Mental Health Movement

Although mental health services for children have historically been provided in hospitals and community mental health centers, the EHA of 1975 was the first federal initiative that required schools to meet the mental health needs of students with emotional disturbances, playing a key role in blurring the lines of responsibility for where such services should be provided.[11,67] Because IDEA focuses solely on students with identifiable disabilities that interfere with educational achievement, only a small percentage of children needing mental health services actually receive such care in school. Nonetheless, most children receiving mental health services obtain care in schools, making schools the "de facto mental health system for children in this country" (p. 62).[67]

"Education and mental health integration will be advanced when the goal of mental health includes effective schooling and the goal of effective schooling includes the healthy functioning of students" (p. 40).[7] Over the past 2 decades, there has been a national movement to develop and expand school mental health (SMH) services because of the high prevalence of mental health conditions among youth and an awareness that more youth can be reached in schools. This movement is also attributed to prominent federal initiatives, including the NCLB and the President's New Freedom Commission on Mental Health.[67] Schools must be active partners in the mental health of children because it is currently accepted that a major barrier to learning is the absence of essential social-emotional skills and not necessarily a lack of sufficient cognitive skills.[64] Approximately one in every five children and adolescents has a diagnosable emotional or behavioral disorder, with the most common being anxiety, depression, conduct disorders, learning disorders, and ADHD.[65] Emotional and behavioral disorders can adversely affect a child's successful participation in a range of school activities, including

TABLE 23-6 Examples of Occupational Therapy Programs Developed for Integration into Classrooms and Other School Contexts

Program	Description	Additional Information and Resources
Write Start	This is a classroom-embedded, comprehensive activity-based program for first-grade students co-taught by a trained occupational therapist and teachers focusing on handwriting and written expression. The goal is to help first-grade students become legible and fluent writers. Type of collaboration—co-teaching Length of time—12 wk, two 45-min sessions/wk Sessions include modeling of letter formation and opportunities to practice; small group activities focusing on foundation skills (visual motor integration, fine motor skills, and cognitive skills); adult modeling, monitoring, and feedback; and provision of peer supports and evaluation.	Website: http://www.write-start-handwriting.org
Zones of Regulation	This curriculum provides a systematic, cognitive behavioral approach to teach children about their emotional and sensory needs to self-regulate and control emotions and impulses, manage sensory needs, and improve the ability to problem solve conflicts. The Zones of Regulation program combines social thinking concepts and visual supports to help students identify feelings, understand how behaviors affect others, and learn tools that can be used to move to a more acceptable state. The four zones are the following: • Red zone—heightened state of alertness and intense emotions resulting in being out of control • Yellow zone—less heightened state of alertness and elevated emotions allowing for some control but that result in stress, anxiety, silliness, or nervousness • Green zone—calm state of alertness associated with being happy, content, focused, and ready to learn • Blue zone—low state of alertness that may occur when one feels sad, sick, bored, or tired Students learn strategies for regulating their emotional and sensory needs to meet the demands of the context and succeed academically and socially.	Website: http://www.zonesofregulation.com

TABLE 23-6 Examples of Occupational Therapy Programs Developed for Integration into Classrooms and Other School Contexts—cont'd

Program	Description	Additional Information and Resources
Drive-Thru Menus—relaxation and stress busters, attention, and strength	Similar to how drive thru restaurants can provide food without taking a lot of time, these drive thru menus were developed to help students engage in meaningful activities that take only a short amount of class time. Type of collaboration—consultation to educate the teacher about the program and how and when to embed it into the classroom Length of time—each activity takes about 3-5 min of class time to help students manage stress and relax or engage in active movement to attend. Program contents—each program consists of a large, laminated colorful poster with 10 activities, a DVD of the author's overview of the program, and a leader's manual that explains the purpose, how to prepare for the activity, how to do the activity, and suggested adaptations. • Relaxation menu activities use visualization and meditation to bring about a sense of peacefulness and tranquility. • Stress-buster menu activities involve active movements to relieve stress. • Strength menu activities help students who have difficulty completing fine motor tasks because of muscle weakness. • Attention menu activities help students who struggle with attention and keeping their bodies quiet enough to learn.	Websites: http://www.therapro.com/Drive-Thru-Menus-Attention-and-Strength-C307797.aspx http://www.therapro.com/Drive-Thru-Menus-Relaxation-and-Stress-Busters-C307798.aspx
Alert Program for Self-Regulation of Arousal	The Alert Program was initially developed for children with attention and learning difficulties, ages 8-12 years, but has been adapted for preschool through adult-age individuals with and without a variety of disabilities. The purpose of the program is to teach individuals (children and youth, school personnel, and parents) how to understand their unique sensory processing to help them use sensory strategies to maintain optimal states of alertness for successful functioning throughout the day. An engine analogy is used to teach children and adults how to self-regulate levels of alertness throughout the day to participate in activities they need or want to do. Three car engine levels are taught: • High—feeling hyper • Low—feeling lethargic • Just right—able to attend and focus on task at hand Five strategies for changing "engine speeds" and alertness include putting something in the mouth, move, touch, look, and listen. Children analyze how their engine speeds vary throughout the day and learn how to use sensory strategies to regulate their alertness to feel good and function well for the task at hand.	Website: http://www.alertprogram.com Products include Leaders' Guide, introductory booklet, games (Alert Bingo), and songs (Alert Program CD).

Adapted from references 8, 29, 30, 80, and 139; and from Bowen-Irish, T. (2012). *Drive-Thru Menus: Exercises for attention and strength.* Retrieved from http://www.therapro.com/Drive-Thru-Menus-Attention-and-Strength-C307797.aspx; and Bowen-Irish, T. (2012). *Drive-Thru Menus: Relaxation and stress busters.* Retrieved from http://www.therapro.com/Drive-Thru-Menus-Relaxation-and-Stress-Busters-C307798.aspx; and Bertrand, J. (2009). Interventions for children with fetal alcohol spectrum disorders (FASDs): Overview of findings for five innovative research projects. *Research in Developmental Disabilities, 30,* 986-1006.

classroom work and social participation during lunch and recess. Children with disabilities are at increased risk for developing mental and/or behavioral challenges. Almost one in three children with developmental disabilities is diagnosed with a co-occurring mental health problem.[102]

School Mental Health

SMH refers to a framework of approaches that have expanded on traditional methods addressing mental health by emphasizing promotion, prevention, positive youth development, and school-wide approaches (http://www.schoolmentalhealth.org/Resources/ESMH/DefESMH.html). This SMH framework promotes interdisciplinary collaboration among mental health providers, related service providers, teachers, and school administrators to meet the mental health needs of all students. As a result of federal support, two national technical assistance centers were developed in 1995 to promote mental health in schools—the Center for Mental Health in Schools at the

University of California at Los Angeles (UCLA) and the Center for School Mental Health Analysis and Action (CSMA) at the University of Maryland.

Mental Health Continuum

All too often, the term *mental health* is interpreted to mean services focusing on mental illness because of a long-standing emphasis on healing pathology. Evidence indicates, however, that the "absence of mental illness does not imply the presence of mental health, and the absence of [or limitations in] mental health does not imply the presence of mental illness."[62] Keyes[62] has advocated for the adoption of a two-continuum model, with mental health belonging to a continuum separate from mental illness. It is important for occupational therapists to be aware of this distinction and help school personnel, students, and families understand the emotional and behavioral indicators of mental health, as well as the symptoms associated with mental illness.[12]

Mental health is defined as a "state of successful performance of mental function, resulting in productive activities, fulfilling relationships with people, and the ability to adapt to change and cope with adversity."[115] Mental health encompasses more than demonstrating the presence of good behavior. It involves feeling good emotionally and doing well in everyday functioning.[80] The terms *mental illness* and *mental disorders* are commonly used to refer to diagnosable psychiatric conditions that significantly interfere with a person's functioning, such as bipolar disorder, schizophrenia, and dementia. The term *mental health problems* often refers to more common issues, such as anxiety and depression, which may be less severe and of shorter duration but, if left unattended, may develop into more serious conditions.[9]

Why Care About Mental Health and Happiness?

Individuals who are mentally healthy and feel happy demonstrate greater degrees of everyday functioning,[62] healthy behaviors,[96] and perceived good health.[101] Children and youth who experience positive mental health and well-being function better during academic and nonacademic times of the school day.

Use of Naturalistic Resources

Integrating mental health initiatives involves using the naturalistic resources in schools to implement and sustain effective supports for promoting positive mental health in students with and without disabilities. Although the mental health field has traditionally been viewed as the domain of mental health specialists, who provide services to individuals when mental health problems interfere with everyday functioning, it is now recognized that addressing mental health issues is far too complex to relegate to a small number of professionals and is more effectively addressed in promotional and preventive ways. Leaders in the field of SMH have been calling for a paradigm shift to better prepare all school personnel (e.g., teachers, administrators, psychologists, social workers, related service providers) to address the mental health needs of all students proactively.[64] Teachers and other front-line personnel, including occupational therapists, play a critical role in the development of children from academic and personal, social, and emotional perspectives. "An important component of integrating mental health efforts into the ongoing routines of schools is the identification and support of indigenous persons and resources within schools as agents of change" (p. 42).[7] Occupational therapists can be important change agents in integrating mental health efforts into everyday practice in schools.

Multitiered Public Health Model of School Mental Health

The failure to provide mental health services adequately for children has been viewed as a major public health concern, causing leaders in the field to propose a public health model of service delivery to address the needs of all children.[22,44] A public health model supports a system-wide shift from an individual, deficit-driven model of intervention to a school-wide, strength-based model focusing on promotion, prevention, early intervention, and integration of services for all children. Similar to RtI, addressing the mental health needs of students can be envisioned within a three-tiered framework of mental health promotion, prevention, and intensive individualized interventions[64,104] (Figure 23-11).

At the school-wide level (tier 1), services are geared toward the entire student body, including most students who do not demonstrate behavioral or mental health challenges. At this level, the emphasis is on promoting positive mental health and preventing behavioral problems. Strategies for promoting positive mental health include the following: (1) creating physical and social environments and activities that are enjoyable for all students (e.g., sensory-friendly contexts, caring adults, just right activities) and (2) embedding strategies and activities that help children and youth cope with challenges (e.g., yoga, deep breathing). Targeted intervention (tier 2) is geared toward students at risk of mental health or behavior problems (e.g., students with disabilities, those who are obese or overweight, students living in poverty). Students at this level are generally not identified as needing special education and/or mental health services and may include children with mild mental disorders, ADHD, and those living in stressful home environments. General education students demonstrating behavioral or learning difficulties because of such mental health conditions may be provided coordinated early intervention services, even if special education is not needed, according to the 2004 amendments to IDEA. For some students with mild mental health disorders, accommodations provided under Section 504 are sufficient for enhancing school functioning. When targeted interventions do not meet the needs of students, intensive interventions (tier 3) are developed to address behaviors or mental health challenges that are highly disruptive or prevent learning. All school personnel, under the leadership of professionals with a background in mental health intervention (e.g., occupational therapists, school psychologists, school nurses, guidance counselors), can embed tier 3 interventions into everyday school experiences.[12]

Role of Occupational Therapy

With occupational therapy's rich history of addressing mental health in all areas of practice, along with the call for all school personnel to address children's mental health proactively, the role of occupational therapy in SMH seems clear.[7] Occupational therapists have specialized knowledge and skills in addressing psychosocial and mental health needs of individuals

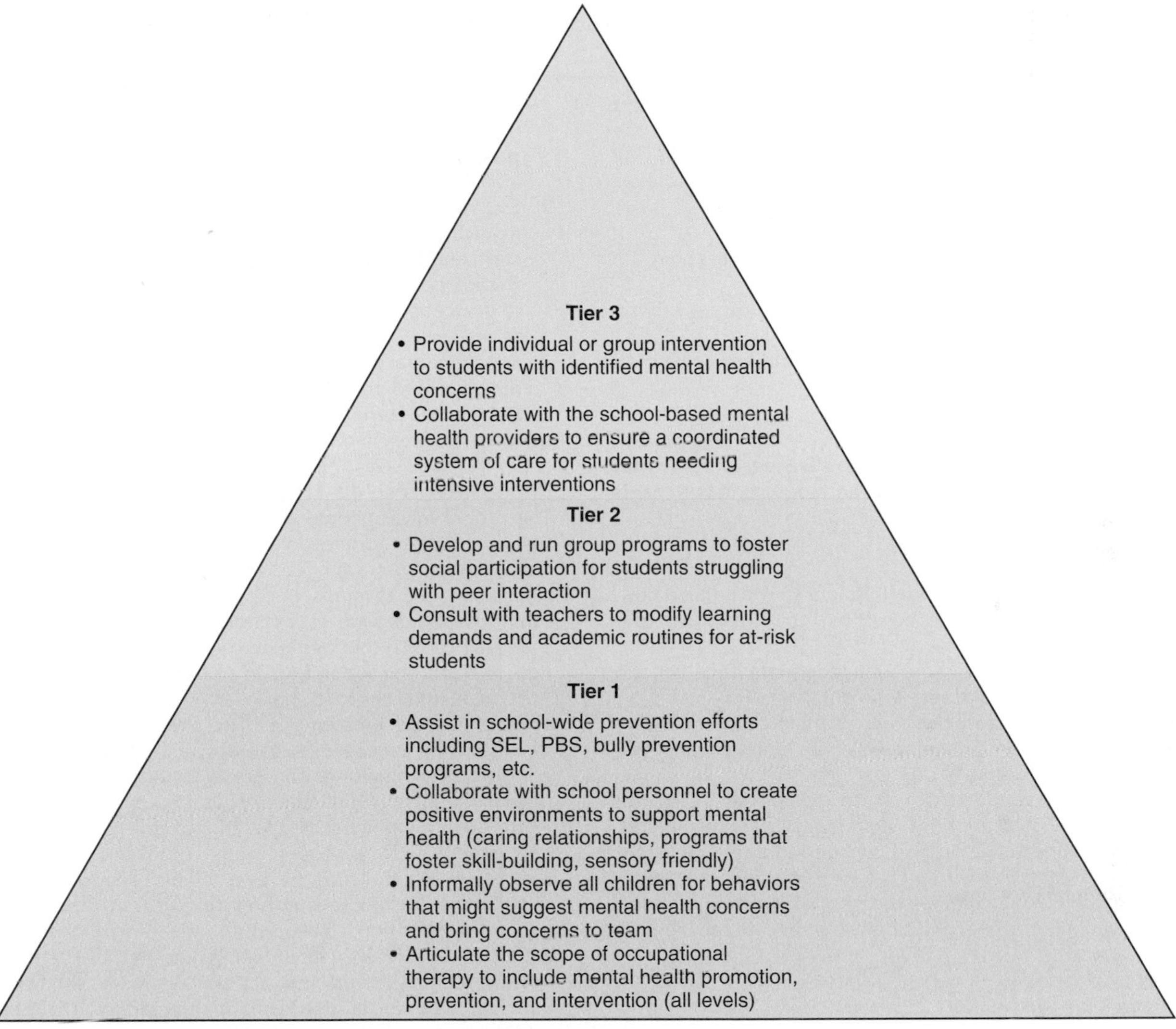

Tier 3
• Provide individual or group intervention to students with identified mental health concerns
• Collaborate with the school-based mental health providers to ensure a coordinated system of care for students needing intensive interventions
Tier 2
• Develop and run group programs to foster social participation for students struggling with peer interaction
• Consult with teachers to modify learning demands and academic routines for at-risk students
Tier 1
• Assist in school-wide prevention efforts including SEL, PBS, bully prevention programs, etc.
• Collaborate with school personnel to create positive environments to support mental health (caring relationships, programs that foster skill-building, sensory friendly)
• Informally observe all children for behaviors that might suggest mental health concerns and bring concerns to team
• Articulate the scope of occupational therapy to include mental health promotion, prevention, and intervention (all levels)

FIGURE 23-11 Public health approach to school mental health in occupational therapy.

and thus are well positioned to contribute to all three levels of promotion, prevention, and intervention. A continuum of occupational therapy's EIS, aimed at social, emotional, and mental health promotion, prevention of problem behaviors, and early detection through screening is recommended.[12]

Occupation-Based Services

Although many approaches specific to mental health promotion are important to know about and apply, all occupational therapy services share a common emphasis on the use of meaningful occupation to promote occupational performance (e.g., education, play, leisure, work, social participation, ADLs, instrumental activities of daily living, sleep, and rest) within a variety of contexts.[1] Figure 23-13 shows students engaged in an educational activity at school. The findings of a recent evidence-based literature review, for example, indicate that activity-based interventions help improve children's peer interactions, task-focused behaviors, and conformity to social norms.[13] In schools, occupation-based services can be embedded in a number of natural contexts, including the cafeteria (e.g., lunch groups), recess (e.g., game clubs), art, and physical education. Increased emphasis is placed on participation in extracurricular activities, opening the doors wider for occupational therapists to help children and youth develop and participate in structured leisure interests during after-school hours.[52,71]

What Do Lunch, Recess, and Extracurricular After-School Participation Have to Do with Mental Health Promotion?

Nonacademic aspects of the school day (lunch, recess, extracurricular after-school activities) are significant contributors to students' and schools' success. Studies have shown that increased student connection to school enhances classroom engagement, academic performance, school attendance, and completion rates and decreases dropout and problem behaviors.[17] Numerous factors are associated with students' positive attachment to school, including having good friends at school, participating in extracurricular activities, and perceiving school personnel as supportive and caring. Boxes 23-9 and 23-10 summarize major elements of occupational therapy–embedded cafeteria and recess programs aimed at helping all children and youth enjoy participation in these settings. Figure 23-12 shows students engaged in and enjoying a craft activity during recess.

BOX 23-9 Integrating Occupational Therapy into the Cafeteria: Creating a Comfortable Cafeteria Program

This 6-week program involves occupational therapy services embedded in the cafeteria 1 day/week. The purpose of the program is to create a cafeteria environment that helps all students enjoy a meal and social time with peers and adults.

Role of the Occupational Therapist

- Orient the principal, cafeteria staff, and students about the Comfortable Cafeteria Program.
- Develop and embed activities that promote mealtime enjoyment.
- Provide 6 weeks of coaching to staff to problem solve challenges and offer supports.

Vision Statement

Our school will provide pleasant and positive mealtimes so that students will enjoy eating their meal and socializing with peers and adults.

Program Principles

Based on current literature, a commitment to providing a positive mealtime experience is based on the following four principles:

1. Creating a positive environment (adequate time to eat; comfortable, clean, and safe environment)
2. Providing recess before lunch (students are more relaxed, better behaved, and eat more of their lunch when recess occurs prior to eating)
3. Respecting the importance of the social climate, which includes the integration of students of varying abilities (value the importance of the lunch period as an important time for students to relax and socialize with friends; commit to respecting and including students with varying abilities)
4. Promoting a nutritional philosophy that encourages healthy eating habits

Program Components

1. Orientation for principal and all cafeteria staff about the Comfortable Cafeteria program. This involves in-service education, needs assessment, and problem solving (1-2 hours). Orient students to the Comfortable Cafeteria program, review code of conduct, and hand out a Comfortable Cafeteria bookmark that summarizes content.
2. Six weeks of embedded occupational therapy services involving weekly themed activities, problem solving with staff, and follow-up coaching. Themes include being a good friend, positive mealtime conversations, including others and accepting differences, and trying new and nutritious foods.
3. Supplemental materials to provide social marketing for the program and reinforce weekly themes. Examples include Colorful Cafeteria posters and bookmarks and weekly newsletters for teachers and parents.

Pilot Data and Findings

This program was piloted at two elementary schools with 168 first- to third-grade students and 20 cafeteria supervisors. The program was well received by the principals, cafeteria supervisors, and students. Pre- and postsurveys of the students using visual analogue scales indicated statistically significant changes ($P \leq 0.01$) changes in perceived enjoyment and friendliness of peers and supervisors in students initially rating questions at 75 mm or lower on a 100-mm scale. These findings suggest that students with mid to lower levels of enjoyment of lunch, perceptions of supervisor or peer friendliness, and enjoyment of mealtime conversations prior to the program documented statistically significant improvements of enjoyment and friendliness at the end of the program. Survey outcomes of the cafeteria supervisors indicated positive changes in the following areas: feeling adequately trained to supervise lunch, knowing how to find resources to encourage healthy eating, having the necessary supports to be an effective cafeteria supervisor, knowing how to promote positive behavior and interact socially with children, and knowing how to resolve conflict successfully. The principal reported a decrease in the number of office referrals during lunchtime.

Contributing authors: Frances Horvath, OTR/L; Louise Demirjian, MA, OTR/L; and Susan Bazyk, PhD, OTR/L, FAOTA.

BOX 23-10 Integrating Occupational Therapy into Recess: Refreshing Recess Program

This 6-week program involves occupational therapy services embedded during recess 1 or 2 days/week. The purpose of the program is to create a recess environment that helps all students enjoy play and social time with peers and adults. Recess is important for promoting physical and mental health and academic performance. To create a positive recess environment, recess supervisors will gain the necessary knowledge and skills needed for implementation, including the following: the importance of establishing positive relationships with all students, strategies for promoting positive behavior, ideas for indoor and outdoor games, safe and enjoyable playground equipment, and supporting documents (e.g., handouts, newsletter) to reinforce best practices during recess.

Role of the Occupational Therapist

- Orient the principal, recess staff, and students about the Refreshing Recess Program.
- Develop and embed activities that promote enjoyment.
- Provide 6 weeks of coaching to staff to problem solve challenges and offer supports.

Vision Statement

Our school will provide positive play and social activities during indoor and outdoor recess so that all students have fun doing meaningful activities and enjoy time with their peers.

Program Principles

Based on current literature, a commitment to providing a positive recess experience is based on the following four principles:

1. Promote positive social interaction and friendships (encourage positive, caring relationships with children, promote the integration of students with varying abilities).
2. Promote positive behavior and the prevention of bullying (clarify expectations, model appropriate interaction and strategies for conflict management).

BOX 23-10 Integrating Occupational Therapy into Recess: Refreshing Recess Program—cont'd

3. Provide unstructured and adult-guided play opportunities (provide a balance between adult-led and child-initiated activities; children who struggle socially do better with structured group play).
4. Provide attractive and safe play materials and games.

Program Components

1. Orientation for principal and all recess staff about the Refreshing Recess program. This involves in-service education, needs assessment, and problem solving (1-2 hours). Orient students to the Refreshing Recess program, review code of conduct, and hand out a Refreshing Recess bookmark that summarizes content.
2. Six weeks of embedded OT services involving weekly themed activities, problem solving with staff and follow coaching. Weekly themes include orientation and needs assessment, fostering friendships, positive behavior supports and conflict resolution, including others and accepting differences, and bullying prevention.
3. Supplemental materials to provide social marketing for the program and reinforce weekly themes. Examples include bookmarks and weekly newsletters for teachers and parents.

Pilot Data and Findings

The program was piloted on 162 students in the third and fourth grade at one elementary school. Pre- and postsurveys of student participation demonstrated an increase in students who rated recess to be fun, who looked forward to recess, and who reported more adult-initiated games. Recess supervisor pre- and postsurvey outcomes revealed positive changes in the following areas: feeling adequately trained to supervise recess, having the necessary supports, knowing how to interact socially with children, and knowing how to resolve conflict successfully.

Contributing authors: Rebecca Mohler, MA, OTR/L; Shannon Kerns, MOT, OTR/L, & Susan Bazyk, PhD, OTR/L, FAOTA.

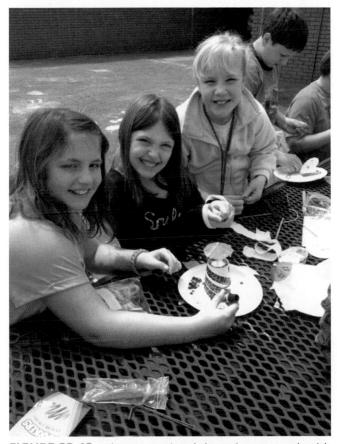

FIGURE 23-12 The occupational therapist may work with recess supervisors to help students participate in enjoyable activities.

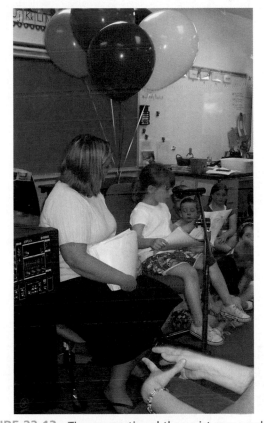

FIGURE 23-13 The occupational therapist may work with students to enhance their participation in a variety of different educational activities.

In addition to traditional occupational therapy intervention approaches, other approaches developed in the fields of public health, psychology, and education can be applied by occupational therapists, such as mental health literacy, positive youth development, social-emotional learning (SEL), and positive behavior supports (PBSs). Refer to Table 23-7 for a description of each, with supporting literature.

Within a three-tiered public health model, occupational therapists can provide a continuum of services geared toward mental health promotion, prevention, early identification, and intervention. Intervention strategies should be integrated into the student's classroom schedule, school routine, and curriculum. Sample occupational therapy activities for each tier of the public health model of SMH are depicted in Table 23-8.[24,25] These activities should be designed in accordance with research evidence as much as possible.

TABLE 23-7 Approaches Applied in School Mental Health

Approach	Description	Supporting Evidence	Implications for Occupational Therapy
Mental health literacy	*Mental health literacy,* a fairly new area of study, refers to providing all children and youth with a working knowledge of mental health as an essential part of overall health (Barry & Jenkins, 2007). It includes many components, such as learning about mental health and strategies for becoming and maintaining mental health, recognizing when a disorder is developing and where to seek help, effective self-help strategies for mild problems, and how to support others facing a mental health crisis (Jorm, 2012). Mental health first aid training courses for youth educate adults on how to provide support for adolescents showing symptoms of a mental health disorder until professional help is obtained (Kelly et al., 2011). Randomized control trials comparing mental health first aid course attendees with wait-list controls found improvements in knowledge, helping behaviors, and stigmatizing attitudes (Jorm, 2012).	Jorm, A. (2012). Mental health literacy: Empowering the community to take action for better mental health. *American Psychologist, 67,* 231-243. Kelly, C. M., Mithen, J. M., Fischer, J., A., Kitchener, B. A., Jorm, A. J., Lowe, A., & Scanlan, C. (2011). Youth mental health first aid: A description of the program and an initial evaluation. *International Journal of Mental Health Systems, 5(4),* 1-9. Pinto-Foltz, M., Logsdon, C., & Myers, J. A. (2011). Feasibility, acceptability, and initial efficacy of a knowledge-contact program to reduce mental illness stigma and improve mental health literacy in adolescents. *Social Science & Medicine, 72,* 2011-2019.	Look for opportunities to raise awareness of mental health and educate students and staff about mental health and well-being as well as mental health disorders Reinforce the attitudes and actions associated with mental health such as participating in enjoyable occupations, exercising, thinking positively, and keeping stress in check. Host Children's Mental Health Awareness Day events every May (http://www.samhsa.gov/children/) Collaborate with health educators, teachers, and school nurses to embed educational activities related to mental health literacy into the school ecology.
Positive youth development and structured leisure participation	*Positive youth development* emphasizes building and improving assets that enable youth to grow and flourish throughout life (Park, 2004). Larson (2000) emphasizes the development of initiative as a core quality of positive youth development and makes a case for participation in *structured leisure activities* (e.g., sports, arts, organized clubs) as an important context for such development. An important aspect of occupation-based practice when promoting mental health in children is attention to the development of structured leisure participation during out-of-school time. Extracurricular participation may be included as a standard item on individualized education plans. Highly structured leisure activities are associated with regular participation schedules, rule-guided interaction, direction by one or more adult leaders, an emphasis on skill development that increases in complexity and challenge, and performance that requires sustained active attention and the provision of feedback (Mahoney et al., 2005). Correlational research has demonstrated a positive relationship between participation in structured leisure and positive outcomes such as diminished delinquency, greater achievement, and increased self-efficacy and self-control (Larson, 2000).	Larson, R. W. (2000). Toward a psychology of positive youth development. *American Psychologist, 55,* 170-183. Daykin, N., Orme, J., Evans, D., Salmon, D., McEachran, M., & Brain, S. (2008). The impact of participation in performing arts on adolescent health and behavior: A systematic review of the literature. *Journal of Health Psychology, 13,* 251-264. McNeil, D. A., Wilson, B. N., Siever, J. E., Ronca, M., & Mah, J. K. (2009). Connecting children to recreational activities: Results of a cluster randomized trial. *American Journal of Health Promotion, 23,* 376-387.	Encourage students to explore and participate in out-of-school interests (arts, music, sports, clubs, etc.). Commit to helping all students engage in at least one meaningful hobby and interest. Conduct environmental scans to identify a range of extracurricular participation options for students—both school- and community-sponsored options. Provide coaching to help students with disabilities and mental health challenges successfully participate in structured leisure interests. Coaching may involve adapting entry into the activity and educating the coach or adult leader about strategies for promoting successful participation based on the individual needs of the child/youth.

Social and emotional learning (SEL) Website: www.casel.org	In 1994, *social and emotional learning* was developed as a conceptual framework to focus on the emotional needs of children and address the fragmented programs meant to address those needs.[34] SEL is defined as "the process of acquiring the skills to recognize and manage emotions, develop caring and concern for others, make responsible decisions, establish positive relationships, and handle challenging situations effectively."[15] Programs developed to enhance SEL help children recognize their emotions, think about their feelings and how one should act, and regulate their behavior based on thoughtful decision making.[26] As a national leader in the field, the Collaborative for Academic, Social, and Emotional Learning (CASEL) focuses on the development of high-quality, evidence-based SEL programs, promoting these as a necessary part of preschool through high school education. Under the leadership of CASEL, the state of Illinois, by developing social and emotional learning standards for schools, has become an example for the nation.	Carter, E. W., & Hughes, C. (2005). Increasing social interaction among adolescents with intellectual disabilities and their general education peers: Effective Interventions. *Research and Practice for Persons with Severe Disabilities, 30,* 179-193. Durlak, J. A., Weissberg, R. P., Dymnicki, A. B., Taylor, R. D., & Schellinger, K. B. (2011). The impact of enhancing students' social and emotional learning: A meta-analysis of school-based universal interventions. *Child Development, 82,* 405-432. Payton, J., Weissberg, R. P., Durlak, J. A., Dymnicki, A. B., Taylor, R. D., Schellinger, K. B., & Pachan, M. (2008). *The positive impact of social and emotional learning for kindergarten to eighth-grade students: Findings from three scientific reviews.* Chicago, IL: Collaborative for Academic, Social, and Emotional Learning.	Investigate whether the school has adopted an SEL curriculum. If so, become involved in school-wide implementation. Tune into student's feelings on a daily basis. Simply asking "How is your day going?" or "How are you feeling?" can communicate an interest in the child's emotional life. Help students develop a feeling vocabulary and use words to express feelings. Foster the ability to recognize and respond to other's emotions. Refer to Illinois' SEL academic standards in order to determine age-appropriate SEL expectations and intervention supports. Embed SEL goals and activities into all interventions.
Positive behavioral interventions and supports (PBIS) Website: www.pbis.org	Positive behavior supports (PBS) interventions and supports are designed to prevent problem behaviors by proactively altering a situation before problems escalate and by concurrently teaching appropriate alternatives. PBIS is an implementation framework designed to enhance academic and social behavior outcomes for all students by: (1) using data to inform decisions about the selection, implementation, and progress monitoring of evidence-based behavioral practices and (2) organizing resources and systems to ensure implementation fidelity. This approach recognizes that a number of relevant factors can influence a student's behavior, including those existing within the child and those reflected in the interaction between the child and the environment.[67] Schoolwide PBS systems support *all* students along a continuum of need based on the three-tiered prevention model. For students receiving services under IDEA, PBS is mandated for those whose behavior impedes the child's learning or that of others (§614(d)(3)(B)(i)).	Bradshaw, C. P., Koth, C. W., Thornton, L. A., & Leaf, P. J. (2009). Altering school climate through school-wide positive behavioral interventions and supports: Findings from a group-randomized effectiveness trial. *Prevention Science*, *10*(2), 100-115. Bradshaw, C. P., Mitchell, M. M., & Leaf, P. J. (2010). Examining the effects of schoolwide positive behavioral interventions and supports on student outcomes: Results from a randomized controlled effectiveness trial in elementary schools. *Journal of Positive Behavioral Interventions*, 161-179.	Determine whether your school has adopted PBIS as the behavioral framework. If so, explore opportunities to participate in and contribute to school-wide PBIS committees. Help create environments that focus on proactively promoting positive behavior. Collaborate with all school personnel to foster consistency in communicating behavioral expectations and reinforcing positive behaviors in classroom and nonclassroom settings.

TABLE 23-8 Some Activities Provided by Occupational Therapy Under a Public Health Model of School Mental Health

Tier	Student Populations	Suggested Intervention Strategies
Tier 3—intensive interventions for students with identified mental health challenges	Mental health challenges and disorders: • Anxiety disorders • Depression • Bipolar disorder • Schizophrenia and other thought disorders • Autism spectrum disorder • Obsessive compulsive disorder • Post-traumatic stress disorder • Severe emotional disturbance	Analyze the student's unique sensory needs and develop intervention strategies to promote sensory processing and successful function in multiple school contexts (e.g., classroom, cafeteria). Identify ways to modify or enhance school routines to reduce stress and the likelihood of behavioral outbursts. Provide individual or group intervention to students with serious emotional disturbance (SED) through special education or Section 504 to enhance participation in education, social participation, play and leisure, and ADLs. Assist teachers in modifying classroom expectations based on the student's specific behavioral or mental health needs. Collaborate with the school-based mental health providers to ensure a coordinated system of care for students needing intensive interventions. Assist in the implementation of the Functional Behavior Assessment (FBA) and development and implementation of the Behavioral Intervention Plan (BIP).
Tier 2—selective or targeted intervention for students at risk of mental health challenges	Situational stressors causing children to be at risk of mental health challenges: • Disabilities (e.g., ADHD, autism spectrum, physical disabilities) • Overweight, obesity • Poverty • Bullying	Assist in early identification of mental health problems by providing formal and/or informal screenings of psychosocial function to at-risk students (e.g., Social Skills Rating Scale). Recognize symptoms of illness at their onset and create intervention and or modifications to prevent acute illness from occurring. Evaluate social participation with peers during all school activities, including recess and lunch. Analyze the sensory, social, and cognitive demands of school tasks and recommend adaptations to support a student's participation Provide early intervening services or Section 504 accommodations for students demonstrating behavioral or learning difficulties because of mild mental health disorders or psychosocial issues. Consult with teachers to modify learning demands and academic routines to support a student's development of specific social-emotional skills. Provide parent education on how to adapt family routines or activities to support children's mental health, especially with high-risk children. Develop and run group programs to foster social participation for students struggling with peer interaction Provide psychoeducation in-services to educate teachers about the early signs of mental illness and appropriate accommodations. Provide an in-service to school personnel, including the mental health providers, about occupational therapy's unique role in the promotion of mental health and interventions for mental health dysfunction.

TABLE 23-8 Some Activities Provided by Occupational Therapy Under a Public Health Model of School Mental Health—cont'd

Tier	Student Populations	Suggested Intervention Strategies

Tier 1—school-wide, universal	All students with and without disabilities and mental health challenges	• Mental health promotion:
		  • Look for opportunities to teach students about mental health, what it is, and how to develop it (Jorm, 2012).
		  • Adapt activities and/or the environment to promote enjoyable participation throughout the day (e.g., lunch, recess, classroom). Experiencing positive emotions is thought to contribute to mental health (Fredrickson, 2004).
		• Mental health prevention: Informally observe all children for behaviors that might suggest mental health concerns or limitations in social-emotional development. Bring concerns to the educational team.
		• Positive behavioral interventions and supports (PBIS): Assist teachers and other school personnel in developing and implementing school-wide PBIS for various contexts—classroom, hallways, lunchroom, playground, and restrooms (e.g., establish clear rules, foster a positive classroom environment)
		• Provide in-service training to teachers and staff on the following topics:
		  • Sensory processing—how to adapt classroom practices based on students' varying sensory needs to enhance attending and behavior regulation (e.g., Alert Program, Zones of Regulation)
		  • Social-emotional learning (SEL)—how to embed SEL activities into classroom routines and activities (e.g., identifying feelings, thinking about how feelings influence behavior, perspective taking)
		  • Psychoeducation—educate teachers about the early signs of mental illness and proactive, strength-based prevention strategies.
		• Provide tips for promoting successful functioning throughout the school day, including transitioning to classes, organizing work spaces such as desk and locker, handling stress, and developing strategies for time management.
		  • Consult with teachers to help them recognize the student's most effective learning styles. Ensure that students are able to meet classroom demands and create modifications, if needed.
		  • Clearly articulate the scope of occupational therapy practice as including social participation, social-emotional function, and mental health (all tiers).

Adapted from Bazyk, S. (Ed.). (2011). *Mental health promotion, prevention, and intervention for children and youth: A guiding framework for occupational therapy.* Bethesda, MD: American Occupational Therapy Association; Bazyk, S., Schefkind, S., Brandenburger-Shasby, S., Olson, L., Richman, J., & Gross, M. (2008). *FAQ on school mental health for school-based occupational therapy practitioners.* Bethesda, MD: American Occupational Therapy Association; Fredrickson, 2004; and Jorm, A. (2012). Mental health literacy: Empowering the community to take action for better mental health. *American Psychologist, 67,* 231-243.

Summary

Occupational therapists must skillfully combine a sound understanding of occupational therapy's role with children with a current understanding of the evolving school context. Over the past 10 years, special and general education services have gradually aligned as a result of IDEA 2004 and ESEA, providing occupational therapists with opportunities to expand their role, particularly in the direction of promotion, prevention, and early intervention. Providing integrated services in natural contexts, collaborating effectively with school personnel and parents, shifting from caseload to workload models, developing promotional and prevention strategies, and advocating for a role in general education are among the important roles of occupational therapists. By embracing these changes and developing the knowledge and skills to work in new ways, occupational therapists can help all children participate successfully in and enjoy school.

The following summarizes the main points in this chapter:

- Legislative changes (IDEA, ESEA) and a growing emphasis on LRE have resulted in a gradual alignment of general and special education and inclusion of students with disabilities into general education settings.
- Best practice in occupational therapy involves service provision in natural school contexts including classroom, recess, cafeteria, and after-school settings.
- Integrated occupational therapy services provide opportunities to work within a multitiered model involving promotional and prevention efforts in addition to intervention for students with identified disabilities.

REFERENCES

1. American Occupational Therapy Association. (2008). Occupational therapy practice framework: Domain and process (2nd ed.). *American Journal of Occupational Therapy, 62*, 625–683.
2. American Occupational Therapy Association. (2004). Occupational therapy services in early intervention and school-based programs. *American Journal of Occupational Therapy, 59*, 681–685.
3. American Occupational Therapy Association. (2006). *FAQ on response to intervention for school-based occupational therapists and occupational therapy assistants.* Bethesda, MD: American Occupational Therapy Association.
4. American Occupational Therapy Association. (2006). *Transforming caseload to workload in school-based early intervention occupational therapy services.* Bethesda, MD: American Occupational Therapy Association.
5. Amundsen, S. (1995). *Evaluation Tool of Children's Handwriting (ETCH).* Homer, AK: OT Kids.
6. Ardoin, S. P., Witt, J. C., Connell, J. E., et al. (2005). Application of a three-tiered response to intervention model for instructional planning, decision making, and the identification of children needing services. *Journal of Psychoeducational Assessment, 23*, 362–380.
7. Atkins, M. S., Hoagwood, K. E., Kutach, K., et al. (2010). Toward the integration of education and mental health in schools. *Administration and Policy in Mental Health, 37*, 40–47.
8. Barnes, K. J., & Turner, K. D. (2001). Team collaborative practices between teachers and occupational therapists. *American Journal of Occupational Therapy, 55*, 83–89.
9. Barry, M. M., & Jenkins, R. (2007). *Implementing mental health promotion.* Edinburgh: Churchill, Livingstone, Elsevier.
10. Bazyk, S. (2005). Exploring the development of meaningful work for children and youth in Western contexts. *Work (Reading, Mass.), 24*, 11–20.
11. Bazyk, S. (2007). Addressing the mental health needs of children in schools. In L. Jackson (Ed.), *Occupational therapy services for children and youth under IDEA* (3rd ed.). Bethesda, MD: American Occupational Therapy Association.
12. Bazyk, S. (Ed.), (2011). *Mental health promotion, prevention, and intervention for children and youth: A guiding framework for occupational therapy.* Bethesda, MD: American Occupational Therapy Association.
13. Bazyk, S., & Arbesman, M. (2013). *Practice guideline: Occupational therapy's role in mental health promotion, prevention, and intervention.* Bethesda, MD: American Occupational Therapy Association.
14. Bazyk, S., Goodman, G., Michaud, P., et al. (2009). Integration of occupational therapy services in a kindergarten curriculum: A look at the outcomes. *American Journal of Occupational Therapy, 63*, 160–171.
15. Beery, K. E., Buktenica, N. A., & Beery, N. A. (2004). *Beery-Buktenica developmental test of visual-motor integration* (5th ed.). San Antonio, TX: PsychCorp.
16. Bernie, C., & Rodger, S. (2004). Cognitive strategy use in school-aged children with developmental coordination disorder. *Physical & Occupational Therapy in Pediatrics, 24*(4), 23–45.
17. Blum, R. (2005). *School connectedness: Improving the lives of students.* Baltimore: Johns Hopkins Bloomberg School of Public Health.
18. Bowyer, P., Kramer, J., Ploszaj, A., et al. (2008). *The Short Child Occupational Profile (SCOPE).* Chicago: MOHO Clearinghouse.
19. Bradly, R., Danielson, L., & Doolittle, J. (2007). Responsiveness to intervention: 1997 to 2007. *Teaching Exceptional Children, 39*, 8–12.
20. Bose, P., & Hinojosa, J. (2008). Reported experiences from occupational therapists interacting with teachers in inclusive early childhood classrooms. *American Journal of Occupational Therapy, 62*, 289–297.
21. Brandenburger-Shasby, S. (2005). School-based practice: Acquiring the knowledge and skills. *American Journal of Occupational Therapy, 59*, 88–96.
22. Bruininks, B. D., & Bruininks, R. H. (2005). *BOT-2: Bruininks-Oseretsky test of motor proficiency* (2nd ed.). San Antonio, TX: PsychCorp.
23. Burtner, P., McMain, M. P., & Crowe, T. K. (2002). Survey of occupational therapy practitioners in southwestern schools: Assessments used and preparation of students for school-based practice. *Physical and Occupational Therapy in Pediatrics, 22*(1), 25–39.
24. Cahill, S. M. (2007). A perspective on response to intervention. *Special Interest Section Quarterly: School System, 14*(3), 1–4.
25. Cahill, S., & Suarez-Balcazar, Y. (2009). Promoting children's nutrition and fitness in the urban context. *American Journal of Occupational Therapy, 63*, 113–116.
26. Carrasco, R. C., Skees-Hermes, S., Frolek-Clark, G., et al. (2007). Occupational therapy service delivery to support child and family participation in context. In L. L. Jackson (Ed.), *Occupational therapy services for children and youth under IDEA* (3rd ed.). Bethesda, MD: American Occupational Therapy Association.
27. Case-Smith, J., Holland, T., & Bishop, B. (2011). Effectiveness of an integration handwriting program for first grade students: A pilot study. *American Journal of Occupational Therapy, 65*, 670–678.
28. Case-Smith, J., Holland, T., Lane, A., et al. (2012). Effect of a co-teaching handwriting program for first graders: One group pretest-posttest design. *American Journal of Occupational Therapy, 66*, 396–405.
29. Cook, L., & Friend, M. (1995). Co-teaching: Guidelines for creating effective practices. *Focus on Exceptional Children, 28*(3), 1–16.
30. Colarusso, R. P., & Hammill, D. D. (2002). *Motor-Free Visual Perception Test* (3rd ed.). Austin, TX: Pro-Ed.
31. Collaborative for Academic, Social, and Emotional Learning (CASEL). (2006). What is Social and Emotional Learning?

<http://www.casel.org/social-and-emotional-learning>.

32. Coster, W. J. (1995). Development. In C. A. Trombly (Ed.), *Occupational therapy for physical dysfunction* (4th ed., pp. 255–264). Baltimore: Williams & Wilkins.
33. Coster, W. J. (1998). Occupation-centered assessment of children. *American Journal of Occupational Therapy, 52*, 337–344.
34. Coster, W., Deeney, T., Haltiwanger, J., et al. (1998). *School Function Assessment*. San Antonio, TX: PsychCorp.
35. Council for Exceptional Children. (1999). *IEP team guide*. Arlington, VA: Council for Exceptional Children.
36. Csikszentmihalyi, M. (1993). Activity and happiness: Towards a science of occupation. *Occupational Science: Australia, 1*, 38–42.
37. Davies, P. L., Soon, P. L., Young, M., et al. (2004). Validity and reliability of the school function assessment in elementary school students with disabilities. *Physical & Occupational Therapy in Pediatrics, 24*, 23–43.
38. Elias, M. J., Zins, J. D., Weissberg, R. P., et al. (1997). *Promoting social and emotional learning: Guidelines for educators*. Alexandria, VA: Association for Supervision and Curriculum.
39. Fisher, A. G., & Short-DeGraff, M. (1993). Improving functional assessment in occupational therapy: Recommendations and philosophy for change. *American Journal of Occupational Therapy, 47*, 199–200.
40. Fisher, A., & Griswold, L. (2010). *Evaluation of Social Interaction (ESI)*. Fort Collins, CO: Three Star Press.
41. Folio, M. R., & Fewell, R. R. (2000). *Peabody Developmental Motor Scales (PDMS-2)*. Austin, TX: Pro-Ed.
42. Frolek Clark, G., & Miller, L. (1996). Providing effective occupational therapy services: Data-based decision making in school-based practice. *American Journal of Occupational Therapy, 50*, 701–708.
43. Giangreco, M. F. (1995). Related services decision-making: A foundational component of effective education for students with disabilities. *Physical and Occupational Therapy in Pediatrics, 15*(2), 47–67.
44. Giangreco, M. F. (1996). *Vermont interdependent services team approach: A guide to coordinating education support services*. Baltimore: Paul H. Brookes.
45. Giangreco, M. F. (2001). *Guidelines for making decisions about IEP services*. Montpelier, VT: Vermont Department of Education.
46. Graham, F., Rodger, S., & Ziviani, J. (2010). Enabling occupational performance of children through coaching parents: Three case reports. *Physical & Occupational Therapy in Pediatrics, 30*(1), 4–15.
47. Griswold, L. (1993). Ethnographic analysis: A study of classroom environments. *American Journal of Occupational Therapy, 48*, 397–402.
48. Haley, S. M. (1994). Our measures reflect our practices and beliefs: A perspective on clinical measurement in pediatric physical therapy. *Pediatric Physical Therapy, 6*, 142–143.
49. Handley-More, D., & Chandler, B. E. (2007). Occupational therapy decision-making process. In L. L. Jackson (Ed.), *Occupational therapy services for children and youth under IDEA* (3rd ed.). Bethesda, MD: American Occupational Therapy Association.
50. Hanft, B. E., & Place, P. A. (1996). *The consulting therapist: A guide for OTs and PTs in Schools*. San Antonio, TX: Therapy Skill Builders.
51. Hanft, B. E., & Shepherd, J. (2008). *Collaborating for student success: A guide for school-based occupational therapy*. Bethesda, MD: American Occupational Therapy Association.
52. Hansen, D., Larson, R., & Dworkin, J. B. (2003). What adolescents learn in organized youth activities: A survey of self-reported developmental experiences. *Journal of Research on Adolescence, 13*, 25–55.
53. Hargreaves, A., Nakhooda, R., Mottay, N., et al. (2012). The collaborative relationship between teachers and occupational therapists in junior primary mainstream schools. *South African Journal of Occupational Therapy, 42*, 7–10.
54. Hoffman, O. R., Hemmingsson, H., & Kielhofner, G. (2000). *The school setting interview: A user's manual*. Chicago: University of Illinois, Department of Occupational Therapy.
55. Holbrook, M. D. (2007). A seven-step process to creating standards-based IEPs. Project forum at NASDSE. Retrieved from: <http://www.projectforum.org/docs/SevenStepProcesstoCreatingStandards-basedIEPs.pdf>.
56. Individuals With Disabilities Education Act, IDEA 2004, *Final Regulations*, § 300.34, (2006)
57. Jackson, L. L. (2007). *Occupational therapy services for children and youth under IDEA* (3rd ed.). Bethesda, MD: American Occupational Therapy Association.
58. Jackson, L. L., & Arbesman, M. (2005). *Occupational therapy practice guidelines for children with behavioral and psychosocial needs*. Bethesda, MD: American Occupational Therapy Association Press.
59. Kardos, M., & White, B. (2006). Evaluation options for secondary transition planning. *American Journal of Occupational Therapy, 60*, 333–339.
60. Keller, J., Kafkes, A., Basu, S., et al. (2005). *Child Occupational Self-Assessment (COSA)*. Chicago: MOHO Clearinghouse.
61. Kentucky Department of Education. (2006). *Resource manual for educationally related occupational therapy and physical therapy in Kentucky public schools*. Frankfort, KY: Kentucky Department of Education.
62. Keyes, C. L. (2006). Mental health in adolescence: Is America's youth flourishing? *American Journal of Orthopsychiatry, 76*, 395–402.
63. Knippenberg, C., & Hanft, B. (2004). The key to educational relevance: Occupation throughout the school day. *School System Special Interest Section Quarterly, 11*(4), 1–4.
64. Koller, J. R., & Bertel, J. M. (2006). Responding to today's mental health needs of children, families and schools: Revisiting the preservice training and preparation of school-based personnel. *Education and Treatment of Children, 29*, 197–217.
65. Koppelman, J. (2004). *Children with mental disorders: Making sense of their needs and systems that help them (NHPF issue brief no. 799)*. Washington, DC: National Health Policy Forum, George Washington University.
66. Kovaleski, J. F., Tucker, J. A., & Stevens, L. J. (1996). Bridging special and regular education: The Pennsylvania initiative. *Educational Leadership, 53*, 44–47.
67. Kutash, K., Duchnowski, A. J., & Lynn, N. (2006). *School-based mental health: An empirical guide for decision-makers*. Tampa, FL: Research and Training Center for Children's Mental Health, University of South Florida.
68. Kuypers, L. (2011). *The zones of regulation: A curriculum designed to foster self-regulation and emotional control*. San Jose, CA: Social Thinking.
69. Law, M., Baptise, S., Carswell, A., et al. (2005). *Canadian Occupational Performance Measure (COPM)*. Ottawa, ON: CAOT Publications.
70. Learning Disabilities Association (LDA). (2013). Senate moves forward on ESEA. Retrieved from: <http://www.ldaamerica.org/legislative/news-inbrief/index.asp#SenateMovesForwardESEA?utm_source=June+News-in-+Brief&utm_campaign=News-in-Brief&utm_medium=email>.
71. Mahoney, J. L., Larson, R. W., Eccles, J. S., et al. (2005). Organized activities as development contexts for children and adolescents. In J. Mahoney,

R. Larson, & J. Eccles (Eds.), *Organized activities as contexts of development: Extracurricular activities, after-school and community programs* (pp. 3–23). Mahwah, NJ: Lawrence Erlbaum.

72. Mallioux, Z., May-Benson, T., Summers, C., et al. (2007). Goal attainment scaling as a measure of meaningful outcomes for children with sensory integration disorders. *American Journal of Occupational Therapy, 61*, 254–259.
73. Mandich, A. D., Polatajko, H. J., Macnab, J. J., et al. (2001). Treatment of children with developmental coordination disorder: What is the evidence? *Physical & Occupational Therapy in Pediatrics, 20*(2/3), 51–68.
74. Mankey, T. (2011). Occupational therapists' beliefs and involvement with secondary transition planning. *Physical & Occupational Therapy in Pediatrics, 31*, 348–358.
75. Mankey, T. (2012). Educator's perceived role of occupational therapy in secondary transitions. *Journal of Occupational Therapy in Schools and Early Intervention, 5*, 105–113.
76. Marson, S., & Wei, G. (2009). A reliability analysis of goal attainment scaling (GAS) weights. *American Journal of Evaluation, 30*, 203–216.
77. McClellan, C., Atkinson, M., & Danielson, C. (2012). Teacher evaluation training and certification: Lessons learned from measures of an effective teaching project. Retrieved from: <http://www.teachscape.com/resources/teacher-effectiveness-research/2012/02/teacher-evaluator-training-and-certification.html>.
78. McLaren, C., & Rodger, S. (2003). Goal attainment scaling: Clinical implications for paediatric occupational therapy practice. *Australian Occupational Therapy Journal, 50*, 216–224.
79. McWilliam, R. A. (1995). Integration of therapy and consultative special education: A continuum in early intervention. *Infants & Young Children, 7*(4), 29–38.
80. Miles, J., Espiritu, R. C., Horen, N., et al. (2010). *A public health approach to children's mental health: A conceptual framework*. Washington, DC: Georgetown University Center for Child and Human Development, National Technical Assistance Center for Children's Mental Health.
81. Missiauna, C., & Pollock, N. (2000). Perceived efficacy and goal setting in young children. *Canadian Journal of Occupational Therapy, 67*, 101–109.
82. Missiauna, C., Pollock, N., & Law, M. (2004). *Perceived efficacy and goal setting system (PEGS)*. San Antonio, TX: PsychCorp.
83. Muhlenhaupt, M., Miller, H., Sanders, J., et al. (1998). Implications of the 1997 reauthorization of IDEA for school-based occupational therapy. *School System Special Interest Section Quarterly, 5*(3), 1–4.
84. Nanof, T. (2007). Education policy, practice, and the importance of OT in determining our role in education and early intervention. *School System Special Interest Section Quarterly, 14*(2), 1–4.
85. National Association of State Directors of Special Education (NASDSE). (2006). *Response to intervention: Policy considerations and implementation*. Alexandria, VA: NASDSE.
86. National Dissemination Center for Children with Disabilities (NICHCY). (2007). Building a legacy: A training curriculum on IDEA 2004. Retrieved from: <http://www.nichcy.org/training/contents.asp#description>.
87. National Dissemination Center for Children with Disabilities (NICHCY). NICHCY. (2008). Related services. Retrieved from: <http://www.nichcy.org/EducateChildren/IEP/Pages/RelatedServices.aspx>.
88. National Governors Association Center for Best Practices (NGA), Council of Chief State School Officers (CCSSO). (2010). *Common Core standards state initiative*. Washington DC: NGA, CCSSO.
89. Nolan, K., Mannato, L., & Wilding, G. (2004). Integrated models of pediatric physical and occupational therapy: Regional practice and related outcomes. *Pediatric Physical Therapy, 16*, 121–128.
90. O'Brien, J., & Lewin, J. E. (2008). Part 1: Translating motor control and motor learning theory into occupational therapy practice for children and youth. *OT Practice, 13*(21), CE 1–8.
91. Olsen, J., & Knapton, E. (2006). *The Print Tool* (2nd ed.). Cabin John, MD: Handwriting Without Tears.
92. Opp, A. (2007). Reauthorizing no child left behind: Opportunities for OTs. *OT Practice, 12*, 9–13.
93. Pape, L., & Ryba, K. (2004). *Practical considerations for school-based occupational therapists*. Bethesda, MD: American Occupational Therapy Association.
94. Polichino, J. E. (2001). An education-based reasoning model to support best practices for school-based OT under IDEA 97. *School System Special Interest Section Quarterly, 8*(2), 1–4.
95. Polichino, J. E., Frolek Clark, G., Swinth, Y., et al. (2007). Evaluating occupational performance in schools and early childhood settings. In L. L. Jackson (Ed.), *Occupational therapy services for children and youth under IDEA* (3rd ed.). Bethesda, MD: American Occupational Therapy Association.
96. Rasciute, S., & Downward, P. (2010). Health or happiness? What is the impact of physical activity on the individual? *Kyklos, 63*(2), 256–270.
97. Reisman, J. (1999). *Minnesota Handwriting Assessment*. San Antonio, TX: Pearson.
98. Roach, A. T., & Elliot, S. N. (2005). *Goal attainment scaling: An efficient and effective approach to monitoring student progress*. Retrieved from: <http://sspw.dpi.wi.gov/files/sspw/pdf/mhgoalscaling.pdf>.
99. Rosenbaum, P. L., & Saigal, S. (1996). Measuring health-related quality of life in pediatric populations: Conceptual issues. In B. Spilker (Ed.), *Quality of life and pharmacoeconomics in clinical trials* (2nd ed.). Philadelphia: Lippincott-Raven.
100. RTI Action Network. (2014). What is RTI? Retrieved from: <http://www.rtinetwork.org/learn/what/whatisrti>.
101. Sabatini, F. (2011). The relationship between happiness and health: Evidence from Italy. Retrieved from: <http://www.york.ac.uk/media/economics/documents/herc/wp/11_07.pdf>.
102. Schwartz, C., Garland, O., Waddell, C., et al. (2006). *Mental health and developmental disabilities in children*. Vancouver, BC: British Columbia Ministry of Children and Family Development, Children's Health Policy Centre.
103. Schwimmer, J., Burwinkle, T., & Varni, J. (2003). Health-related quality of life of severely obese children and adolescents. *Journal of the American Medical Association, 289*, 1813–1819.
104. Shapiro, J. (1994). *No pity: People with disabilities forging a new civil rights movement*. New Tork: Three Rivers Press.
105. Silverman, F. (2011). Promoting inclusion with occupational therapy: A co-teaching model. *Journal of Occupational Therapy, Schools and Early Intervention, 4*, 100–107.
106. Spencer, K. C., Turkett, A., Vaughan, R., et al. (2006). School-based practice patterns: A survey of occupational therapists in Colorado. *American Journal of Occupational Therapy, 60*, 81–90.
107. Swinth, Y. (2007). Evaluating evidence to support practice. In L. L. Jackson (Ed.), *Occupational therapy services for children and youth under IDEA* (3rd ed.). Bethesda, MD: American Occupational Therapy Association.

108. Stecker, P., Fuchs, D., & Fuchs, L. (2008). Progress monitoring as essential practice within response to intervention. *Rural Special Education Quarterly*, *27*, 10–17.
109. Swinth, Y., Chandler, B., Hanft, B., et al. (2003). *Personnel issues in school-based occupational therapy: Supply and demand, preparation, certification and licensure (COPSSE document no. IB1)*. Gainesville, FL: University of Florida, Center on Personnel Studies in Special Education.
110. Swinth, Y., & Hanft, B. (2002). School-based practice: Moving beyond 1:1 service delivery. *OT Practice*, *7*(16), 12–20.
111. Swinth, Y., Spencer, K. C., & Jackson, L. L. (2007). Occupational therapy: Effective school-based practices within a policy context (COPSSE document no. OP-3). Retrieved from: <http://copsse.education.ufl.edu/copsse/docs/OT_CP_081307/1/OT_CP_081307.pdf>.
112. Trombly, C. (1993). Anticipating the future: Assessment of occupational function. *American Journal of Occupational Therapy*, *47*, 253–257.
113. U.S. Department of Education. (2008). U.S. Secretary of Education Margaret Spellings announces proposed regulations to strengthen No Child Left Behind. Retrieved from: <http://www.ed.gov/news/pressreleases/2008/04/04222008.html>.
114. U.S. Department of Education. (2008). No Child Left Behind—2008: Summary of proposed regulations for Title I. Retrieved from: <http://www.ed.gov/policy/elsec/reg/proposal/summary.pdf>.
115. U.S. Department of Health and Human Services. (1999). *Mental health: A report of the Surgeon General—executive summary*. Rockville, MD: U.S. Department of Health and Human Services.
116. U.S. Office of Special Education Programs. (2007). Presentation: Response to intervention and early intervening programs. Retrieved from: <http://idea.ed.gov/explore/view/p/%2Croot%2Cdynamic%2CPresentation%2C28%2C>.
117. VanDerHeyden, A. M., Witt, J., & Barnett, D. (2005). The emergence and possible futures of response to intervention. *Journal of Psychoeducational Assessment*, *23*, 339–361.
118. Villeneuve, M. A., & Shulha, L. M. (2012). Learning together for effective collaboration in school-based occupational therapy practice. *Canadian Journal of Occupational Therapy*, *79*, 293–302.
119. Wang, C. (1999). Photovoice: A participatory action approach applied to women's health. *Journal of Women's Health*, *8*, 185–192.
120. Wenger, E., McDermott, R., & Snyder, W. (2002). *Cultivating communities of practice: A guide to managing knowledge*. Cambridge, MA: Harvard Business School Press.
121. Williams, M. S., & Shellenberger, S. (1996). *How does your engine run?" A leader's guide to the Alert Program for self-regulation*. Albuquerque: TherapyWorks.
122. Wright, P. W., & Wright, P. D. (2008). Key differences between Section 504, the ADA and the IDEA. Retrieved from: <http://www.wrightslaw.com/info/sec504.summ.rights.htm>.
123. Yell, M., & Katsiyannis, A. (2004). Placing students with disabilities in inclusive settings: Legal guidelines and preferred practices. *Preventing School Failure*, *49*(1), 28–35.

CHAPTER

24 Hospital and Pediatric Rehabilitation Services

Brian J. Dudgeon • Laura Crooks • Elizabeth Chappelle

KEY TERMS

Hospital-based services	Acute care
Children's hospitals	Intensive care
Evidence-based practice	Specialty units
Prioritization of care	Oncology
Documentation	Rehabilitation services
Medical teams	Outpatient services

GUIDING QUESTIONS

1. What are characteristics of children's hospitals and the functions of occupational therapists in these settings?
2. Which types of children are commonly treated in hospital-based rehabilitation units, other specialized inpatient units, and outpatient therapy services?
3. What are occupational therapy interventions in children's hospitals, and what evidence exists to support interventions for children with common diagnoses?
4. Which intervention approaches and teaching strategies are commonly used in pediatric rehabilitation?
5. How do occupational therapists establish collaborative relationships with other providers in interdisciplinary and transdisciplinary teams?
6. How do occupational therapists promote family participation in rehabilitation and address transition home as part of discharge planning?

Children receive care at a hospital for a wide variety of diagnostic and intervention reasons. Although respiratory and gastrointestinal problems are the most common reasons for hospital care,[24,27] rehabilitation services, including occupational therapy, are usually provided to children with neurologic and musculoskeletal disorders. See Box 24-1. For children who need hospitalization, issues of safety for the child and concerns about the influence of hospitalization on the child's life experiences often arise.[13] Historically, physicians and families were reluctant to hospitalize children, given the potential for psychological reactions accompanying separation from home and family. However, the need for careful, ongoing medical monitoring, specialized equipment and areas for diagnosis and treatments led to the inevitability of hospitalization for many types of conditions that can affect children. In addition to acute onset problems, chronic disease and disorders appear to be on the rise among children in the United States and other developed countries.[74] These problems may relate to children's challenges with weight management, greater inactivity, and other lifestyles that do not promote fitness.

With the unique specialized care needs of children, beginning in the late 1800s, hospitals developed to care exclusively for and manage children's health challenges. The first children's hospitals in America began in the 1850s in Philadelphia, and others soon followed. Today there are more than 150 such institutions. These community and regional efforts often led to programs that addressed not only health, but also special education needs of children. Although modern hospitals serve medical concerns almost exclusively, educational needs are still paramount in children's lives, and, not surprisingly, school-based services are often a part of children's experience with hospitalization. In addition to addressing needs for education, children's hospitals also strive to create special environments that cater to children and families.[59] Environmental features such as art, colors, and areas that are friendly, warm, and inviting allow space for play and enable families to gather and communicate. Volunteers assist with child and family services and fundraising to support costs and offset expenses for children's care. Also unique to these settings are child life specialists who attend to children's emotional and developmental needs. They may help reduce the stresses of a hospital stay by assisting families in coping with the hospital experience by providing information about play, child development, and adjustment to illness.

The demands of an evolving health care system, varied medical conditions of the children, family dynamics, and hospital's milieu all influence occupational therapy practices. This chapter describes occupational therapy services to pediatric patients in the children's hospital setting. It illustrates varied models of service delivery and explains the roles and function of hospital-based occupational therapists.

In the past, children who required hospitalization frequently had long-term stays, which included programs addressing socialization, education, and vocation.[9,21] Currently, hospital-based programs focus on acute-onset problems and provision

I wish to thank the children and families involved with Seattle Children's Hospital, Seattle, Washington, for their willingness to share their experiences. I also want to acknowledge the advice and help of colleagues from Children's Hospital of Alabama in Birmingham for the preparation of this chapter.

BOX 24-1 Habilitation Versus Rehabilitation

A primary concept in the practice of pediatric rehabilitation is the differentiation of habilitation and rehabilitation. For children, the term *habilitation* is generally used to denote attention to the child's acquisition of expected age-level skill and function. The term *rehabilitation* is used to reflect the process of an individual working to regain skills and functions that had been established but subsequently lost. For most practitioners in pediatrics, the term *rehabilitation* is used to encompass both concepts. This is true because disability, whether new or chronic, creates ongoing challenges to current function and future demands that evolve as part of growth and development. In this chapter, the term *rehabilitation* is used to express both concepts.

of specialized services for children and adolescents with disabilities that may occur infrequently but are highly complex. Hospital-based programs continue to evolve, in part because of newly identified health threats. Hospital programs now extend into the community, offering increased resources to the community and emphasizing the partnership with families in caring for a child with medical needs.

Characteristics of Children's Hospitals

Hospital-based services may include inpatient and/or outpatient care for the ill and injured, as well as prevention or wellness programs designed to reduce the need for future care needs. Hospitals in which pediatric patients are served generally fall into three categories: general hospitals, trauma centers, and children's hospitals. General hospitals strive to serve the needs of the community in which they are located. Given specific local populations, a wide variety of patients can be served in this type of hospital, which often includes those of all ages, from an infant to a geriatric population. The occupational therapist working in the general hospital setting may serve pediatric and adult patients. Hospitals that offer labor and delivery services often have neonatal intensive care services that include occupational therapy services. Some general hospitals may also have special units dedicated to serving the needs of pediatric populations; however, children with more involved or complex needs are often referred to a children's hospital.

Trauma centers are hospitals organized and certified to treat patients with more acute life-threatening injuries. Usually situated in large metropolitan areas, patients taken to trauma centers may have extensive musculoskeletal, neurologic, skin, and internal organ injuries requiring multiple specialists. As in the general hospital setting, the occupational therapist working in the trauma center may serve patients who have a variety of injuries or illnesses. Such centers often have burn units and other special trauma units or programs organized to handle the evaluations and treatments that initially focus on lifesaving and sustaining procedures and to prevent unnecessary complications (e.g., splinting, positioning, evaluating oral motor skills for feeding). As a child in such a setting becomes more stable, additional types of interventions, such as training in activities of daily living (ADLs) and age-appropriate play, can be implemented. Stress on family members from having their child in the trauma center may be compounded by having other family members also receiving care, or the hospital may be some distance from their home. Occupational therapists need to be sensitive to the stress that families experience when their children are in these centers. Once patients are stabilized, and treatment has been established, they may receive ongoing care in that particular hospital or they may be transferred to a children's hospital or general hospital closer to their own community.

Children's hospitals are specialty hospitals that offer a full range of inpatient and outpatient services for infants, children, and adolescents. The occupational therapist working with children in such a hospital may be involved with children who have a wide range of diagnoses and sometimes rarely seen conditions, and thus may have limited information available on treatment protocols or expected outcomes.

Region (Location) Served

Children's hospitals, as specialized health care institutions, tend to serve a broader geographic region than general hospitals. This may result in a child being hospitalized a significant distance from home, increasing the sense of separation from family, peers, and familiar environments. The distance between the home and hospital may affect the family's ability to visit the child and remain in contact with the those caring for the child. Frequently only one family member may be able to remain with the child. This can pose additional challenges for the family, creating not only a financial burden and psychological strains of having a child in the hospital, but the distances between family members may produce additional pressures. The size of the service area and population of the region may also mean greater cultural diversity and socioeconomic variation among those served by the hospital. Diversity in clientele requires the medical team to be sensitive to the cultural beliefs and practices of the patient and family.[72] The broader geographic region served by most children's hospitals usually requires hospital personnel to interact with a great number of practitioners and service programs across the region. This distance can pose challenges for the hospital-based occupational therapist to communicate with community-based occupational therapists regarding the child's intervention programs. Regardless of distance, hospital- and community-based occupational therapists coordinate the child's transition to home by accessing community resources and outpatient or school-based programs.

Missions of Children's Hospitals

Goals of children's hospitals often include effective advocacy for child health, conducting leading-edge pediatric research to improve on clinical outcomes, and creating and implementing a model for family-centered and community-based care. These and other program-specific missions influence the daily operations of these institutions and provide guidance about how clinical care is approached and conducted. Promotion of child health may be seen in local outreach programs in which children's hospital staff educate others in public schools and community programs regarding a wide range of children's health and safety issues. At the national level, advocacy for policies and programs to promote public health, as well as health care reforms that would enable pediatric health care coverage and the conducting of research to prevent and address pediatric health conditions, are often cited (see information provided by the National Association for Children's Hospitals and Related Institutions [NACHRI][52]).

Research on Systems and Care Outcomes

Research missions of children's hospitals and research conducted as part of clinical care can be broad or specific. They are generally motivated by particular interests and needs identified by practitioners or other advocates. Research specializations may be stand-alone efforts of the hospital faculty and staff; affiliated with local research universities; or part of regional, national, or international research programs.

Two prominent types of research conducted at children's hospitals include assessing and reducing risks of care to reduce iatrogenic causes of ill-health and developing best practices and evidence for effective outcomes with specific clinical services. NACHRI recognizes safety as a major concern and that hospitals pose risks for infection and other medical and behavioral consequences of care. For example, children's hospitals' staff recognizes that infections are sometimes transmitted by hand contact. Transmission of germs is thus carried from one patient to another, sometimes by practitioners. Effective hand washing habits have been difficult to implement, with most hospitals striving to enable and monitor such habits by reminders, providing multiple cleaning opportunities, and enforcing routines by monitoring and creating a culture of peer-to-peer feedback. Other safety measures relate to body substance isolation through conditional uses of gloves, masks, and gowns, with proper disposal of at-risk materials. Departments of risk management and infectious diseases work to identify potential risks and institute measures that prevent new and ongoing hazards, usually through repeated trainings.

Occupational therapists participate in evaluation of clinical services and client outcomes. For example, the status of ADLs and instrumental activities of daily living (IADLs), discharge placement, health-related quality of life, and well-being are some of the typical measures used to document rehabilitation outcomes.[29] Occupational therapists use research to describe medical and functional effects, validity of assessment tools related to clinical decision making, and effectiveness of specific treatment approaches or techniques. Over the past few decades, increasing emphasis has been placed on outcomes and ways to use research outcomes in evidence-based decision making.[43]

In pediatric rehabilitation, most outcomes research relates to common diagnostic groups seen in such settings. For example, Dumas and associates[20] reported functional gains demonstrated by children with a traumatic brain injury (TBI) undergoing inpatient pediatric rehabilitation. The greatest gains were made in mobility, but also in social function and self-care for all ages of children. Bedell[4] reported similar findings from a series of children treated for TBI and other acquired brain injuries, and also found that social functioning continued to be greatly impaired. Among school-age children at the time of injury, many with moderate and most with severe injury show persisting and widespread cognitive, language, academic, behavioral, and functional deficits. Although many children with such injuries are identified, referrals to therapy service may be limited[6] and recommended interventions may not be followed,[56] making associated outcomes difficult to predict.

Evidence regarding the efficacy of specific intervention strategies is lacking because it is difficult and costly to conduct research that analyzes the application of particular techniques or rehabilitation strategies. Experimental research on rehabilitation effectiveness is particularly difficult to conduct because of the heterogeneity of the participants and ethical conflicts encountered by suspending or withholding services to specific children. Randomized clinical trials can be problematic,[53] and alternate research strategies have been proposed, such as those with an emphasis on humanistic elements as part of therapeutic practice[34] and client's views about process and outcomes.[2] In a review of services and outcomes in 12 hospital-based pediatric rehabilitation programs, reporting on 814 admissions, the intensity of specific service delivery was associated with client outcomes.[11] Those receiving more occupational therapy services made the most gains in ADLs; those receiving more physical therapy services made greater mobility gains; and those receiving more speech-language services made greater communication and cognitive gains.

Family and Child-Centered Care

Family-centered care of hospitalized children is a hallmark of most children's hospitals and has led to new insights and directions for care.[22] To implement family-centered care, families are designated as a member of the health care team and encouraged to take an active part in decision making about treatments. The occupational therapist working in a hospital setting in which family-centered care has been adopted uses clear descriptions to communicate evaluation results to the family, seeks input from the family on which intervention outcomes for the child have priority, and comes to a mutually agreed-on intervention plan. As evaluations are completed and team meetings established, the family has an integral part in decision making about care.

The occupational therapist's knowledge of age-appropriate developmental tasks and understanding of the importance of purposeful activity can help the child achieve a sense of control in the foreign environment of the hospital. Occupational therapists can also help other members of the medical team understand developmental issues of concern and suggest strategies to caregivers, family members, and others to support typical development that may help the child better manage the hospitalization experience.

Accrediting and Regulatory Agencies

Pediatric rehabilitation advocates and service providers have influenced and been shaped by accreditation processes. For example, the Centers for Medicare and Medicaid Services (CMS) designate requirements for services that are organized and paid to provide "medical rehabilitation." To meet CMS guidelines for rehabilitation, rules are placed on such systems that mandate specific program emphasis, dedicated space and personnel, admission and discharge procedures, service intensity, goal setting, and monitoring of progress toward goals. Most rehabilitation programs also pursue voluntary accreditation by groups such as The Joint Commission (TJC)[39] and the Commission on Accreditation of Rehabilitation Facilities

(CARF),[12] as well as government agencies, such as the Occupational Safety and Health Administration (OSHA), that set standards regarding hospital operations. These organizations assign additional mandates that also shape program characteristics. Such guidelines may include integrated planning with community-based services and continuous quality improvement procedures. Every few years, accreditation standards and procedures based on TJC and CARF shift their emphasis and specification of essential requirements. Generally, after initial accreditation, reaccreditation reports or visits are scheduled every 3 years, and programs may be subject to periodic interim reviews and reporting about their overall performance.

Employee education regarding safety practices (e.g., risk of exposure to patient blood or other body fluids or to hazardous materials) and attention to suspected abuse are also mandated. Importantly, occupational therapists are required to report any suspicion of abuse to designated personnel within the hospital setting who, when appropriate, contact community support services, such as law enforcement personnel or Child Protective Services (CPS). Specific training in each institution regarding reporting protocols must be established and provided to the occupational therapists.

Children's hospitals are often affiliated with similar institutions, offering opportunities for consolidation of information and equipment, achievement of common goals, and program development.[70] Hospitals may be part of a medical system directed by a single administration and linking facilities that share certain resources and specialized personnel. A spectrum of care options, from acute and subacute rehabilitation, satellite outpatient clinics and programs, and home health care may be provided.

Reimbursement for Services

Inpatient services are typically funded by a combination of private insurance carriers, Medicaid or special programs within a state, and under some circumstances by Medicare. Occupational therapy has typically been recognized as a service that is reimbursed in hospitals and medical rehabilitation units, home health care, and, to a lesser extent, outpatient services. Medicare guidelines are generally universal across different states. However, each state's Medicaid rules and regulations and local insurance companies have differing provisions related to the funding of occupational therapy services and supplies or assistive devices that may be required. Local regulations must be reviewed to ensure that appropriate levels of reimbursement are available and that families are informed about service options and expected costs.

The length of stay in children's hospitals varies, from as short as a few days to weeks or perhaps months. As in other hospitals, third-party payers and other regulators strive to control costs by seeking shortened lengths of stay and transferring patients more quickly to less costly skilled nursing facilities or home care, outpatient, or school-based services. Changes within and across treatment settings can be problematic, often creating confusion in families about entitlements and expectations for services. Clearly stated goals and time frames for outcomes in each care setting are desirable.[70] Case managers who are familiar with funding rules and regulations work with families and service teams to coordinate care and prepare the family for transitions among care settings.

An issue of concern facing hospitals that provide services to children is the cost of health care. In recent years, health maintenance organizations (HMOs) and preferred provider organizations (PPOs) have proliferated, and many families are now insured in these and other managed care plans. Prospective payment systems, created within Medicare to estimate and contain costs better, can have strong impacts on reimbursement for services. This system uses preestablished rates of reimbursement for diagnostic groups using the Healthcare Common Procedure Coding System (HCPCS) for billing, which is based on the American Medical Association's Current Procedural Terminology (CPT) codes. Payers take these guidelines into consideration when authorizing care for inpatient stays. The occupational therapist should be aware of payment limitations when providing care and clearly communicate with families when establishing treatment plans and explaining the scope of services being offered.

Occupational Therapy Services in a Children's Hospital

Organization of occupational therapy and other rehabilitation services in a hospital can vary. Programs in this chapter focus on three broad types of services: acute care, rehabilitation, and outpatient clinics. Each of these services is described in more detail with case studies later in the chapter. In brief, acute care services are those wherein therapy services are ordered directly from a medical service or unit (e.g., intensive care neurology and neurosurgery, oncology or cancer care, general surgery, orthopedics, heart and pulmonary services, and, in many children's hospitals, transplantation services). Children are generally referred to acute care services for an occupational therapist's appraisal, interventions for immediate needs, and assistance in planning transition to other service settings or discharge to home. Pediatric rehabilitation services are often located in a specific location of the hospital, which may include special facilities with bedrooms and bathrooms to enable effective independence training with lifts, mobility devices, and other durable medical equipment. Spaces for individual and group intervention, socialization, and group engagements are often available as well. Outpatient services include regularly scheduled specialty clinics that address children's and family's ongoing needs and individual children's services in community-based satellite clinics.

This chapter applies a systematic approach to hospital service areas, including prioritization of care, evaluation strategies used, goal-setting guidelines, and selection of interventions. For each service area, the breadth of diagnoses and clinical approaches is described.

Functions of Occupational Therapists

A primary focus of the occupational therapist in a children's hospital is on ADLs and other instrumental tasks associated with independent living, education, and community participation. Occupational therapists use many frames of reference to develop insights about the child's function; establish intervention priorities; and guide development of goals with the child, family, and local care providers. In most forms of hospital care, the occupational therapist follows a prioritization system that focuses first on prevention of problems associated with illness, trauma or disability; then resumption of the able self; and finally restoration of lost skills and functions. Occupational therapists use learning principles[23,64,67] and clinical reasoning strategies.[50] They often use behavioral and cognitive learning principles and therapeutic use of self, blending technical competency with personal caring.

Evaluation

In almost all cases, occupational therapy services in hospital-based care are initiated through physician's orders. Often required by law or regulatory guidelines, occupational therapists respond to an initial referral or orders and then negotiate as necessary with the physician to add specific elements to assessment and intervention activities.

A review of medical records and discussions with other providers may form the initial basis for evaluation. Usually the occupational therapist uses a clinical interview and observation to initiate the assessment process, followed by physical examination and direct observation with the use of standardized tests. Once the occupational therapist formulates hypotheses about the impairment(s) and initiates intervention plans, the repeated use of clinical examination and standardized tests serves as objective measures of skill improvement. For diagnostic purposes, the occupational therapist judges a child's performance against normed scores, but for evaluative purposes, the occupational therapist usually judges a child's scores on reassessment against his or her previous performance. Selection of a specific measure should be based on its reliability, sensitivity, and appropriateness, given the child's age and diagnosis.

The therapist may organize assessment of ADLs and IADLs around checklists or other reporting tools that specify activities and methods of rating the individual's level of skill. The Functional Independence Measure (FIM; UDS-PRO) and a pediatric version, called the Wee-FIM II, were developed for children of developmental age 6 months to 7 years.[51,69] Eighteen specific ADL tasks, including communication and social cognition, are rated for dependence, based on the individual's need for adaptation and assistance from a helper. The Pediatric Evaluation of Disability Inventory—Computer Adapted Test (PEDI-CAT)[33] can be selected as a tool to report on ADLs, mobility, social function, and responsibility shift for children 7 months to 21 years of age. A wide number of tools may be used to appraise performance skills.

Determining Intervention Goals

A critical component of all intervention planning is the occupational therapist's attention to goal development and setting of outcome expectations. A collaborative process with families is essential in specifying goals, although the goals must also relate to the particular therapeutic techniques being used.[8,49]

Goals describe specific tasks that the child will perform, conditions of performance, and type and frequency of assistance needed. The occupational therapist may specify short-term goals as interim steps toward reaching long-term goals. He or she may define specific performance component targets that link to meaningful functional outcomes (e.g., achieve eye-hand coordination and manipulation skills sufficient for desktop activities and writing at school).

Functional goals include specification of skills and the expected level of independence. Levels of independence describe varying degrees of dependence on personal assistance, adaptive environments, and the use of assistive technology (AT) devices. In the case of a child with greater and long-standing disability, ADL goals may describe how he or she will manage personal care assistance to achieve a self-managed dependence. On most ADL scales, the level of independence is rated as the amount of physical and cognitive assistance needed as a proportion of the task (e.g., moderate assistance = 50%+ assistance of the amount of time required for a partial task, whole task, and task transition assistance by a care provider). However, when concerned with the integration of an individual back into his or her home, the concept of interdependence among family members may be an important consideration. Given the negative connotation associated with dependence in Western culture, a more positive term to express shared needs between family members may be termed *interreliance.* Such language is suggested to focus on the shared duties within households.

Interventions

For most children referred to occupational therapy, services are provided in a relatively brief period, requiring the occupational therapist to be highly efficient. Relatively brief intervention periods necessitate that the occupational therapist establish realistic priorities appropriate for the child's projected length of stay in the hospital. To do this, the evaluation process is streamlined, goals prioritized, and discharge plans proposed at the start of the admission and initial evaluation.

Preventing Secondary Disability and Restoring Performance

Primary prevention is a term used to denote efforts that decrease the likelihood of accidents, violence, or disease for everyone. The terms *secondary* and *tertiary prevention* refer to specific interventions, arrangement of care systems, and environmental modifications to prevent the onset of problems in at-risk populations. Children admitted to the hospital are typically at risk for developing a number of secondary disabilities. Prevention measures may include safety in positioning and movement, prevention of aspiration in swallowing, provision of orientation, and appropriate measures to reduce stresses experienced in an unfamiliar environment and prevent self-injury. Occupational therapists must be aware of risks and avoid involving the child in activities that would be harmful or perpetuate behaviors that could hamper recovery. Complications from immobilization, abnormal muscle tone, and other neuromuscular abnormalities often necessitate careful attention to maintaining range of motion, strength, and general fitness (Figure 24-1).

The occupational therapist typically addresses neuromuscular and musculoskeletal complications by using programs designed to help the client maintain or regain normal range of motion. Through the use of special handling techniques, occupational and physical therapists carry out daily programs that can involve slow stretch and joint mobilization. Occupational therapists can correct existing limitations by using a combination of these techniques and specialized positioning and splinting. The occupational therapist may also apply splints for various purposes, including maintaining positions (e.g., resting hand splint), increasing range of motion (e.g., dropout splints, dynamic splints with spring tension forces, serial casting), or promoting function (e.g., wrist cockup or tenodesis splints). See Chapter 29.

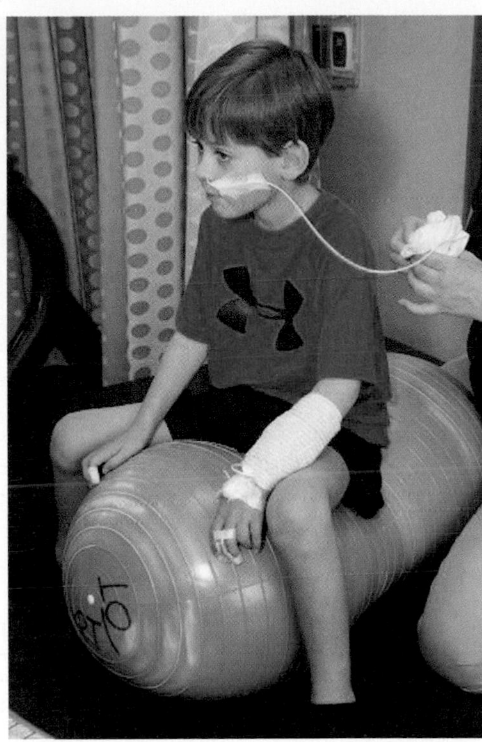

FIGURE 24-1 Dynamic sitting balance is challenged with an air-filled tube to address core trunk responses, seat and foot pressure, with visual-head orientation practice that simulate typical task demands in home or school activities.

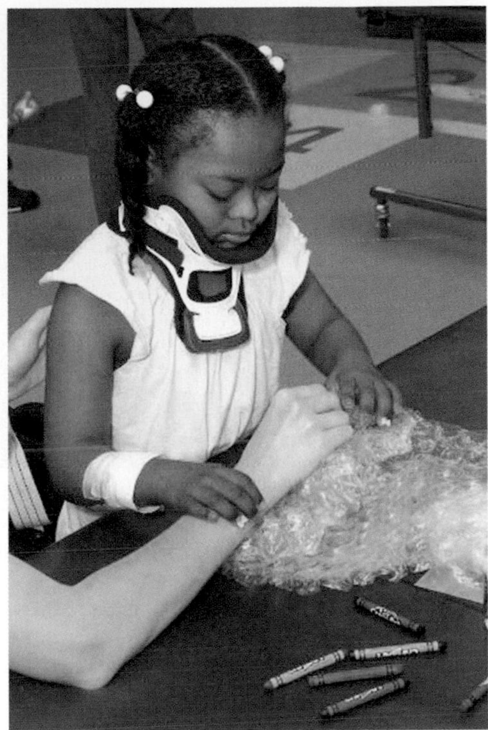

FIGURE 24-2 Visual motor skills are addressed with manipulative work using various materials and textures to promote sensory recognition, tolerances, and skilled performance.

The occupational therapist facilitates improved movement and strength by using activities and exercises that are usually incorporated into play routines. For children and adolescents with musculoskeletal and lower motor neuron or motor unit disorders, the use of progressive exercise and activity routines may be appropriate. For those with brain injury that causes upper motor neuron dysfunction, muscle tone and voluntary motor control are focused on using various sensorimotor techniques to promote postural stability, balance, visual motor skills, and fine motor performance (Figure 24-2; see Chapters 7 and 8).

Concern for wound healing and protection of insensate skin are also essential to early planning and ongoing interventions to achieve goals and education of the child and family. The entire medical team, including the occupational therapist, applies skin care, monitors the child's skin, and implements measures to prevention pressure ulcers. Pressure areas from bed positioning, static sitting, and the use of orthotics call for careful and routine skin monitoring. The child may require several days to develop a tolerance to new positioning strategies and orthotic applications. The child's skin tolerance affects decisions to change bed position, increase sitting time, and alter the wearing schedule for orthotic devices.

Individuals often experience perceptual, cognitive, and behavioral impairments after TBI, and similar concerns also arise with other diagnostic conditions. With a prevention emphasis, programs to ensure safety with physical activities and handling of objects are critical. Environmental modifications are often made to ensure the child's safety. The occupational therapist implements methods to help the child compensate for disorientation and memory loss, although restricted environments and restraints may be necessary initially. Family pictures or other familiar items from home may be used to create a stimulating and more comforting environment. When the child is more alert and aware of his or her surroundings, the occupational therapist may use an educational approach coupled with behavioral interventions. The occupational therapist should inform the child of unit rules, post these rules, and emphasize strict adherence to them. Occupational therapists may use daily orientation programs and memory books to ease the burden of confusion. It is important to teach the family about the child's perceptual and cognitive impairments and create programs to help ensure the child's orientation, safety, and comfort.

Resuming and Restoring Occupational Performance

The second level of priority for occupational therapy is a focus on resuming the use of available skills and independence in easily accomplished tasks. The occupational therapist emphasizes the able self by recommending that the child resume doing tasks on his or her own and by suggesting how others can support the child's performance of ADLs. Enabling optimal independence may be important for preventing the child or adolescent from developing dependent behaviors or learned helplessness. Efficiency demands placed on nurses often result in the child becoming a passive recipient of care. The occupational therapist should strive to provide the child with sufficient time to perform activities on his or her own. Early emphasis on providing children with opportunities to make choices about

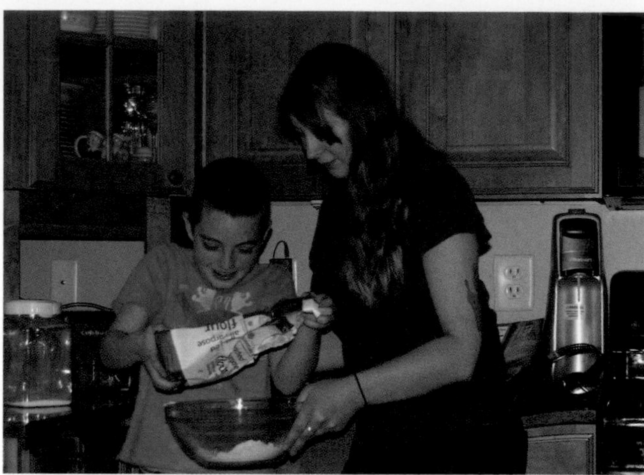

FIGURE 24-3 The occupational therapist provides the child with cues and performance feedback while he carries out an adapted IADL cooking task to address sequencing and functional bimanual performance.

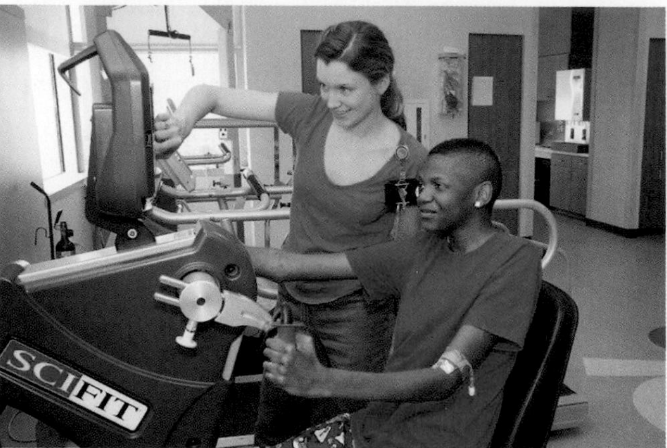

FIGURE 24-4 The therapist provides guidance in strengthening both arms using an exercise device that monitors force and repetition in a progressive manner.

the types of assistance they receive or activities they pursue may help them develop confidence in their skills and returning abilities.

Once the occupational therapist negotiates goals for ADL performance, he or she determines what the child needs to learn, how such learning will take place, and how training can best be organized within the clinical care setting. By embedding therapeutic strategies in the child or youth's natural routine, he or she may discover simple strategies to resume activity performance within a few sessions. Often the occupational therapist recommends structured routines and the use of assistive devices and other modifications to achieve performance and guide the child and other care providers in joint problem solving to determine the most effective methods of performance.

In guided learning of new performance methods, the occupational therapist uses instructional aids, such as visual supports, visual modeling, touch cues, or verbal instruction. For example, the occupational therapist may demonstrate the task to be learned and have the child imitate. The occupational therapist may also use verbal or manual guidance cues to assist learning (Figure 24-3). For some tasks, predetermined scripts or learning materials are available.[54,55]

Occupational therapy services also promote restoration of lost skills and function using biomechanical, sensorimotor, perceptual-cognitive, and rehabilitative approaches in various combinations to restore function. The occupational therapist helps the child or youth practice activities that selectively challenge an individual's skills, with the expectation that these will then transfer or generalize to occupational performance areas. Biomechanical and sensorimotor approaches include the use of therapeutic activities and exercise, splinting and positioning, facilitation of movement, and use of biomedical devices such as functional electric stimulation (Figure 24-4). Other physical agent modalities such as superficial heat or cold may also be used, whereas deep-heating techniques such as ultrasound are often avoided because children's bone epiphyseal (growth plate) areas may be damaged.[48] See Chapter 29 for additional information on physical agent modalities.

Adaptations for Activities of Daily Living Skills

Rehabilitative approaches contrast with biomechanical and sensorimotor techniques that are designed to address underlying performance skills and factors. In the rehabilitative approach, occupational therapists teach clients compensatory techniques that use existing skills to restore occupational performance. Occupational therapists teach clients to use adapted routines and AT devices and modify environments to promote optimal manipulation, mobility, cognition, and communication function. Basic principles apply to adapted performance of ADL skills, described in Table 24-1. Principles of joint protection and work simplification are commonly used; performance is geared toward functioning in a barrier-free environment with the use of familiar conveniences. Adaptations of a routine are aimed at reducing complexity, ensuring safety, and minimizing complications if errors occur.

Adaptive methods of ADL and IADL skills may include the use of different strategies and devices (see Table 24-1). A client's reliance on AT devices may be temporary or permanent. The early use of devices can increase safety or immediate function during recovery. The permanent use of devices is also common when the child exhibits residual difficulties that necessitate ongoing adaptations. When selecting devices, occupational therapists often choose to adapt existing equipment that is already familiar to them or direct the family toward the purchase of items with features that are more compatible with the child's special needs (e.g., enlarged handles on utensils, clothes with color contrast, toys with specific visual, sound, or tactile features).

Client outcomes may be optimized when occupational therapists use complementary strategies to improve the child's skills, adapt functional activities, and modify environmental contexts. For example, the occupational therapist may help the child memorize a routine so that the child can guide his or her own performance using verbal, visual, or tactile feedback. If the child cannot memorize a routine, the occupational therapist can prepare written instructions, pictorial step cues, and audiotapes with specific directions. Whole-task instruction and the use of forward- or reverse-step sequence training are commonly used methods. The occupational therapist can implement

TABLE 24-1 Rehabilitation Strategies*

Types of Limitation	Accommodations
Motor and Movement	
Limited Range of Motion	
Reach to all parts of the body and objects within the immediate environment	Extended and specially angled handles (e.g., long-handled spoon or fork, bath brush, dressing stick, or shoe horn) Use devices that extend contact and prehension, such as reachers Mount objects on the floor, wall, or table and bringing the body part to the device (e.g., boot tree for removing shoes, friction pad on floor for socks, hook on the wall to pull pants up or down, sponges mounted in the shower to wash) Replace reach requirement with use of a bidet for hygiene after toileting or manual or electric feeders operated by switches to bring food to the mouth
Limitations of hand motion reducing holding and handling of objects	Provide enlarged or differently styled handles that reduce the grasp requirement, such as a T-handled cup. Replace holding functions by the use of universal cuff or C-shaped handles. Friction surfaces may provide more secure grasp. When forearm rotation is limited, swivel spoons or angled utensils may assist bringing food to the mouth.
Gross motor movements, such as in bed mobility and elevation changes	Raise or lower surface levels to limit the extent of elevation change required. Lower the bed height to allow ease in wheelchair transfers or raise it to ease in coming up to standing from sitting. Raised chairs, toilet seats with toilet safety frames, and bath benches reduce extreme changes in elevation required in transfers.
Decreased Strength and Endurance	
Reduce the effects of gravity	Use lighter weight objects, movements in the horizontal plane, reduced friction, and, when possible, the use of body mechanics for leverage and gravity to assist movement
Efficiency of movement and reduced efforts are essential	Electrically powered devices may meet goals of work simplification. Extended handles may be necessary, but increased weight and forces required to handle and apply leverage might increase difficulty. Universal cuffs or C-cuffs limit needs for grasp and sustained holding. Use hooks and loops on clothing and adapt fasteners by using Velcro, zippers, enlarged buttons, or elastic or stretch shoelaces. Have lever handles on faucets, doors, and appliances. Use surfaces to support posture and proximal limb positions through bed positioning, seating adaptations, and the use of arm rests and table surfaces.
Limit the need to sustain static postures and prolonged holding.	Mount devices or stabilizing devices with friction from Dycem (nonslip material) or a spike board, using enlarged lightweight objects
Cardiac or pulmonary disorders limiting ADLs based on metabolic equivalents levels or by direct monitoring.	Change heights of surfaces and using devices such as sliding boards or hydraulic lifts to aid movement Schedule and pace tasks, simplifying work, using rest breaks during tasks in response to cardiopulmonary limitations
Incoordination	
Difficulty with manipulation skills	Consider range of movement required, weight and resistance of objects being handled, and positioning of the body in relation to objects used in tasks. Achieve proximal stability when executing limb movements. Stabilizing the trunk and head as one moves the arm and hand is thought to improve skilled movements. Stabilize proximal segments of the limb while manipulating the hand by resting the elbow and forearm on the table while using the wrist and fingers to manipulate objects. Friction surfaces and containers that hold objects being manipulated may also be suggested for stabilization with pads or a nonslip cup. Increased weight may dampen exaggerated movements and tremor. Select heavier objects or add weight to objects. Attach a weight to the arm or apply resistance to movement by placing devices across joints, such as using elastic sleeves or a friction feeder. Mount devices on stable surfaces and bring the body to these devices.
One-Handed Techniques	
Replacing the stabilization function of the other limb	Many tasks can easily be carried out with practice using one hand. If the hand being used was not previously the preferred or dominant hand, skilled movements may take a greater amount of time to develop. With perceptual and cognitive impairments, learning to use one hand may become particularly difficult. With hemiplegia, various dressing routines have been scripted that follow the rules of dressing the affected limb first and avoiding the use of abnormal postures.
Improving the skills of the hand being used	Assist or replace the stabilization function of the impaired or lost upper limb by mounting devices or by use of friction surfaces.
Adapting tasks that require alternating movements of two hands	Using specially designed devices or methods (e.g., a rocker knife or cutting-edged fork to help cut; buttonhook to aid in buttoning; special lacing technique to aid in shoe tying; a one-handed keyboard arrangement and training to aid in typing.

Continued

TABLE 24-1 Rehabilitation Strategies—cont'd

Types of Limitation	Accommodations
Perceptual and Cognitive Limitations (with or without movement disorders)	
Performance errors caused by faulty use of visual cues and spatial orientation	Substitute for impaired skills by using more intact sensory, perceptual, or cognitive skills (e.g., using a bell on the hemiplegic arm to draw attention if being neglected tactually or visually) Design step-by-step routines with cueing systems; repeat them in training
Sequencing errors because of memory or task attention difficulties	Use work simplification principles and modified equipment and adaptive devices as substitution strategies. Train children to rely on memorizing and reciting a verbal routine or follow audiotaped instruction, written instructions, or pictorial cues. With impaired visual perception, the child may need to learn reliance on tactile feedback cues. Use color-contrasted clothing, texture, or color-coding cues with objects. Appraise using a mirror to give the child feedback about his or her performance.
Visual Impairment	
Blindness or severe visual impairment requiring a substitute for vision by the use of other sensory skills and cognitive routines	Consistent organization of the environment and storage of items is necessary. Use tactile identifiers such as raised letters on objects and locations of more transient items described by a companion, or a standard technique, such as an analog clock location. Build sound feedback into some items to aid in orientation or search. Mobility specialists instruct use of techniques such as long canes or guide dogs for ambulation or wheelchair guidance and the use of a leader's arm for guidance in walking.

*Occupational therapists use several strategies for specific types of dysfunctions to adapt activities for children with functional limitations. In addition to these suggestions, ADL and IADL adaptations have been described (see Chapter 16) along with the uses of assistive technology (AT) (see Chapter 19).

training over several sessions that capitalize on the times when tasks are routinely performed (e.g., dressing in the morning and at night or before and after swimming). As training progresses, the occupational therapist gradually reduces the extent of external cueing from a person or instructional aids so that only a minimal amount of such support is required for safe and efficient performance. Often the team and family plan for the gradual withdrawal of aides and assistance after the child is discharged from the inpatient hospital setting. Occupational therapists teach family members or staff strategies that promote the child's participation in daily activities, including school.

To help the child generalize learning from clinic to home, he or she may visit the home. The home visits allow the child and family to survey and collaborate in planning for equipment needs, accommodations, and perhaps architectural modifications that would enable transition to home. Day or weekend home passes for the child are desirable, when possible. Feedback from the family about the time at home can be important to prioritizing goals, equipment, and family educational needs.

Documentation of Occupational Therapy Services

Documentation of patient care is an essential component of occupational therapy service provision in hospitals. Occupational therapy evaluation reports, intervention plans, patient progress notes, and discharge summaries are used to communicate occupational therapy intervention to the physician, other members of the medical team, patient and family, and reimbursement agencies. Format and frequency of documentation are determined by the policies and procedures of the hospital and occupational therapy department. Accreditation guidelines regarding documentation are provided to institutions by agencies such as TJC and CARF. Agencies that reimburse services, such as Medicaid or private insurance, also have requirements for documentation with which occupational therapists must comply.

Occupational therapy evaluation reports, intervention plans, progress notes, and discharge summaries are readily available to other health professionals in a paper-based or online medical record. Documentation of occupational therapy intervention is also made available to referring physicians or other agencies in the community, and copies become part of a permanent medical record. Regardless of the format, documentation of services must meet the criteria established by accrediting and reimbursement agencies.[40]

Scope of Occupational Therapy Services

Children are admitted to the hospital setting for many different reasons, and they can move through different care units as symptoms stabilize or effects become more apparent. Referrals to occupational therapy may be made at admission, during a stay, or near the end of a hospitalization. The occupational therapist responds to the physician's request and, when needed, may ask for greater involvement in a child's care or recommend that other services become involved as well.

Children may be admitted for acute care of their illness or injury. The occupational therapist performs an initial assessment and provides caregivers and the child with instructions, home programs, or follow-up outpatient services. The occupational therapist may also contribute to the diagnostic evaluation of a child specifically admitted for a comprehensive evaluation who is then transitioned to outpatient services. When a child requires more extensive and comprehensive therapy interventions as part of rehabilitation services, the occupational therapist evaluates the level of functioning of the child, develops an intervention plan, and involves the family in implementation of the goals and objectives.

The patient with a single injury (e.g., a hand injury) or a single episode of illness tends to have a short hospital stay, with a predictable course of treatment. Some patients admitted for an acute illness or injury may require extended rehabilitation, depending on the severity of the injury and resulting complications (see Chapter 30). TBI and spinal cord injury are two examples of injuries that require initial acute treatment and long-term rehabilitation. The length of the hospital stay for this type of patient during the acute phase of illness or injury tends to vary because the potential for complications is greater, and these patients need to be relatively stable medically before being transferred to the rehabilitative service. See Chapter 30.

Chronically ill children or adolescents may be hospitalized periodically for acute episodes of an illness or complications of an illness. Children with diabetes, cancer, or cardiac conditions are in this category. When children who are hospitalized for diagnostic testing or adjustment of medications experience a comparatively short hospital stay, the occupational therapist focuses on evaluation and intervention planning that is likely to transfer to community providers. An occupational therapy evaluation in acute care services focuses on the child's functional status within the context of the illness or injury that has resulted in hospitalization.

Organization of Hospital-Based Services

Most patient care activity in hospitals is acute care. Acute care refers to short-term medical care provided during the initial phase of an illness or injury, when the symptoms are generally the most severe. The degree of severity that categorizes an illness or injury is matched to levels of acute care designed to meet these needs. The occupational therapist providing services to children during this phase must consider the long-term implications of the illness or injury while addressing the acute needs of the patient. Families may experience increased stress during this phase and therefore may require that the information be repeated or may need more time to process the results from evaluations.

Critically ill patients who require continuous monitoring and frequent medical attention, and patients who often need special equipment to maintain or monitor vital functions, are admitted to intensive care units (ICUs) or critical care units (CCUs). Hospitals may have various levels of intensive care units, each of which is designated for a specific patient population or purpose. These can include neonatal intensive care units (NICUs), pediatric intensive care units (PICUs) for older children, and postsurgical intensive care units (SICUs). Personnel who provide care for patients in ICUs receive special training to enable them to respond quickly and effectively to meet the needs of medically unstable patients in this challenging environment (see examples in Chapter 21).

A child whose illness or injury results in hospitalization but who does not need the continuous attention, high technology, and specialized care of an ICU may be admitted to a medical or surgical acute care unit. Medical and surgical units also tend to be designated for specific types of patients. For example, children requiring neurosurgical services may be cared for on one unit, whereas children requiring orthopedic-related treatment may be served on another. Children may also be grouped according to age within the designation of these units. Placing children of similar ages together can facilitate developmentally appropriate care and allow for environments that are well designed to match children's and youth's age-based interests.

Children with infectious conditions may have a variety of diagnoses that require isolation conditions. If this is the case, these patients are often placed in special care units. Three conditions that require a child to be treated in a special care unit are (1) acute burns, (2) infectious diseases, and (3) bone marrow transplantation.

Often chronically ill patients are admitted for an exacerbation of their illnesses, for special treatments, or for complications. Diabetes, asthma, cystic fibrosis, and cancer are examples of chronic illnesses occurring in children who may require periodic hospitalizations. Patients who have progressive illness may also be seen for acute issues relating to the next stage of the disease process. For example, a youth diagnosed with Duchenne muscular dystrophy may experience a decrease in oral motor skills and subsequently be admitted for aspiration pneumonia.

Hospital-Based Therapy Teams

In hospitals, the child and family benefit from a wide range of medical care specialists and services that they can access as needed. Hospital teams are usually led by physicians who are trained as pediatricians and in other areas of practice, such as neurology, orthopedics, or developmental medicine. An important characteristic of medical teams is their dynamic nature. Because the health care disciplines represented in a specific case depend on the patient's needs, the medical team is continually changing. For example, a child with a feeding disorder who is failing to grow and gain weight may have a physician, nurse, occupational therapist, dietitian, and social worker as members of the medical team. However, a child hospitalized with multiple injuries resulting from a motor vehicle accident may have several physicians, nurses, occupational therapist, physical therapist, speech pathologist, dietitian, respiratory therapist, and social worker as members of his or her medical team. In addition, the team during one child's hospitalization may change. For example, the child admitted to the hospital for pneumonia may initially be seen by the pulmonary physician and perhaps a social worker, along with nurse(s); later the occupational therapist and speech-language pathologist may be involved when aspiration is suspected, and a physician from gastroenterology may be involved later when it is discovered that reflux is the culprit.

As a potential member of multiple medical teams within one hospital, the occupational therapist communicates and collaborates with professionals from many different health-related fields. The occupational therapist may need to redefine or explain the role of the occupational therapist continually to other team members and develop an understanding of the ways in which different team members' roles complement each other in the provision of services to children. Occupational therapists employed by hospitals face increasingly complex challenges in defining their roles in different care settings within one integrated system and participating in a variety of medical teams across the spectrum of care.

Team Interaction

Interdisciplinary care within a hospital or medical system is common and mandated by most regulatory mechanisms. The success of this collaboration often depends on a shared mission that focuses the team's energy and creativity. The team holds family conferences on admission, at key decision points during the hospitalization, and at discharge to ensure communication and clarification of care recommendations with the family and local care providers. In addition, the team conducts weekly rounds to review the progress of each child and discuss any changes in treatment plans designed for each problem.

The occupational therapist's holistic concerns related to health, function, and participation necessitate and are enriched by the collaborative relationships among team members of multiple disciplines. Partnerships between occupational therapists and occupational therapy assistants can broaden the scope and timeliness of services. The need for frequent re-evaluation and trials with new strategies necessitate dynamic and shared interventions. Team efforts are typical in medical systems. For example, occupational and physical therapists often take a joint interest in interventions to promote the child's gross and fine motor skills and make joint decisions about positioning, transfers, wheelchair seating, and functional mobility (Figure 24-5). Occupational therapists collaborate with speech-language pathologists to evaluate and plan interventions for feeding and swallowing and augmentative communication. Nurses and occupational therapists typically have collaborative roles dealing with skills such as grooming, dressing, bathing, and training in special care routines of toileting and skin care. Occupational therapists may work together with therapeutic recreation specialists and child life specialists to provide adaptive play and socialization through activity and community outings.

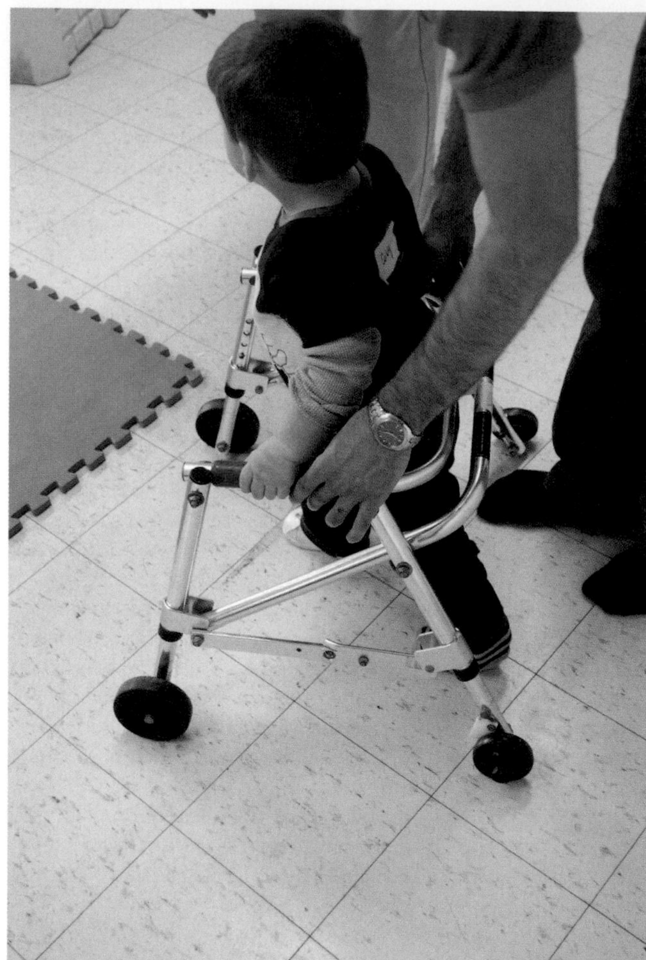

FIGURE 24-5 Functional mobility, often with walking aid devices, enables greater freedom in activity selection and accomplishment in a variety of settings.

A primary goal with children is to improve their participation and performance in educational programs. Children's hospitals typically have teachers on staff, and, in conjunction with occupational therapists and other team members, these educators and developmental specialists address skills and special needs that the child will have on returning to school. Psychologists and those who specialize in neuropsychology also provide suggestions for school placement and may work with occupational therapists to adapt learning strategies for the child as he or she returns to the classroom. Social workers often address issues of adjustment and coping with the child and family. All team members strive to be sensitive and supportive when educating family members to assume their new duties as care providers. Recommendations should seek a realistic balance within the family culture, established roles, and new responsibilities for care.

Families

The occupational therapist must recognize that families are often coping with tragic events or at least unexpected complications that seriously affect their life processes. Children and adolescents are challenged to adapt to significant functional and physical changes with bereavement,[42,46,63] and this process can be further complicated by their own cognitive or behavioral impairments.[17] An educational model may provide a helpful perspective. Recognizing that family members have a short amount of time to learn how to care for their family member who is faced with new disabilities, rehabilitation team members devote their time and attention to understanding the family's priorities and learning preferences. In nearly all cases, the typical routines of the family are severely altered by hospitalization and residual disability, resulting in worry, grief, and financial hardships that necessitate a transformation of relationships.[32] Families function in different ways, and variations in styles influence effective coping.[57] Healthy and resilient families show strong and exceptional caring, open communication, balancing of family needs, and positive problem-solving abilities.[62] Families with limited coping skills may need increased support and help in identifying resources to meet immediate needs and in coping with problems that they will face in managing the child at home. In either case, the needs of families often change during the rehabilitation process, requiring ongoing attention to maintain a collaborative partnership that can achieve the best outcomes for the child.

Acute Care Units

Intensive Care Unit Services

In the ICU, the child is often evaluated and treated at bedside because of the critical nature of the illness or injury and the need for constant monitoring of the child's physiologic status. Occupational therapy intervention in intensive care units supports medical priorities and goals for the child. It is essential that the occupational therapist be knowledgeable about the child's diagnoses and potential precautions, implications of medical procedures, use of life support or monitoring equipment, and contraindications for certain activities or positions. The occupational therapist monitors and knows immediate responses to changes in the child's vital signs, respiratory function, appearance, and symptoms.

Prolonged bed rest and immobility often occur as a result of ICU stays, during which medical technology and equipment and/or the need for restraints for the child's safety and care are in use. The average length of stay for a child in the ICU may be just a few days; however, it may be extended if the illness or injury is severe. The potential impact of extended immobility includes contractures, generalized weakness with decreased endurance, and cardiopulmonary compromise. Occupational therapists provide services to prevent these secondary problems by using graded activities and soliciting the child's participation to maintain strength and enhance functional capacities. Although the occupational therapist may have goals of increasing participation, independence, and endurance for the child, the nurse or family may believe that rest is required. Discussing the basis for the occupational therapist's intentions includes consideration of medical precautions to facilitate the team's desired outcome. Establishment of a routine, including regular therapy times within the constraints of the ICU, can also help with orientation for the patient and facilitation of regular participation. Family members or other caregivers may also be involved in carrying out interventions, such as range of motion, throughout the day. This provides them with the opportunity to become more involved in the care of their child during this portion of their hospitalization.[37,68]

Occupational therapy interventions often include positioning recommendations and use of orthotics to preserve range of motion and prevent deformity. A plan for wear or use should be established and communicated with the family and other care providers to ensure follow-through. Caregivers should also be instructed on any potential side effects, such as pressure areas with orthotics, so that interventions can be modified as needed.

Sensory deprivation and stress resulting from the ICU environment may also complicate a child's medical status and recovery. The lack of privacy, immobility, and continuous sounds and lights of the ICU provide the child with an atypical sensory experience. In addition, the ICU setting has few indicators of night and day cycles. Over a prolonged period, ICU psychoses have been reported, in which the child may have altered mental status.[3,36] Occupational therapy intervention may help counteract the effects of disorientation and sensory deprivation by fostering the establishment of a routine for the child and providing purposeful activities to facilitate cognitive, psychosocial, and motor functions.[1] Positive social interaction and the use of entertainment and play activities may be especially helpful for reducing stress and promoting engagements of young children in the ICU. Case Study 24-1 describes intervention in the ICU.

General Acute Care Unit

General acute care units tend to be designated by medical specialty. Children of various ages, with different types of conditions and treatments, may be served in the same acute care unit. Similarly, children requiring different types of surgery may be admitted to the same general surgical unit for preoperative and postoperative care. Designating units in this manner generally enables physicians and other members of the medical team to use their patient care time and equipment more efficiently.

In acute care units, children tend to be more medically stable and less dependent on life-sustaining equipment as part of their care. A lesser need for medical monitoring may enable them to benefit from greater involvement by rehabilitation specialists, including the occupational therapist, who may provide services at bedside or in the hospital's therapy clinic. Occupational therapists may be responsible for children in a variety of acute care units, requiring them to be familiar with the procedures of each unit, types of children admitted to the different units, and nurses and other hospital personnel who provide services. Case Study 24-2 describes interventions for failure to thrive.

Specialty Units

Children's hospital units are also often designated for specialty care that congregates medical and support services for diagnostic and treatment purposes. These may include a focus on orthopedics, cardiac and pulmonary services, oncology, or other hospital-specific organization of units, such as burns.

Oncology and Bone Marrow Transplantation Units

A highly specialized acute care service is the oncology unit, which may also include bone marrow transplantation services. Children served on these units may include those diagnosed with various types of cancer, immunodeficiency disorders, hemophilia, and aplastic anemia. These units and services may be housed close together and share some resources, including staff, or may be located in separate areas within the hospital setting.

The staff on the oncology unit provides care for children who are newly diagnosed with cancer and undergoing induction chemotherapy, are receiving chemotherapy courses that require close monitoring, may have complications from their treatment such as fever with neutropenia, or may have undergone high-dose radiation and surgical tumor resections. The occupational therapist working with these patients may encounter patients and families in different stages of the diagnostic and treatment continuum. Because of the chronic nature of illness for children and youth located on these units, the occupational therapist may have time to develop relationships with the child and family. Children may come in and out of the hospital throughout their treatment, and the occupational therapist may see the child for inpatient and outpatient therapy or coordinate care across services. Children may also vary greatly in their

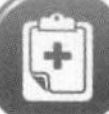

CASE STUDY 24-1 Intervention for Child in the Intensive Care Unit

Presenting Information

Michael is a 6-year-old boy admitted to the ICU with a diagnosis of necrotizing fasciitis with sepsis. He was initially seen at the general hospital in his community, approximately 2 hours' distance from the children's hospital in the area. On initial examination, Michael was found to have decreased sensation, with decreased circulation to his fingers and toes. He had a high fever (104.7°F) and was lethargic. He was airlifted to the children's hospital, and en route he began experiencing organ failure, including a cardiac arrest. His mother was able to accompany him in the airlift, but his father had to drive because of space constraints.

Background Information

Prior to his hospitalization, Michael was a typically developing young boy. He resided on a reservation with both of his parents. He attended first grade at the local elementary school, achieving average grades for his age. He also took pride in participating in the Native American dance troupe associated with his tribe and had been participating in exhibits nationally with his troupe since age 3.

Michael was playing in the park near his home with friends when he fell out of a tree and was deeply scratched by a branch. Because there was a little bleeding, he did not return home right away, but once he did return, his mother noted that the area was red and slightly warm. She cleaned the area with soap and water and placed Band-Aids on the cut. The next day, Michael had a slight fever and was complaining of generalized discomfort. By the second day, he vocalized more physical complaints, would not let anyone touch his arm, and his fever increased, even with medication and home remedies. He was taken to his family physician. By this time Michael had increased lethargy, was in and out of consciousness, and had a high fever. He was subsequently airlifted to the local pediatric hospital because of his quickly advancing disorder.

Medical and Occupational Therapy Intervention

On arrival at the children's hospital, Michael required a respirator for ventilation support, and his medical status continued to deteriorate. Evaluation revealed staphylococcal sepsis with intravascular coagulopathy, and he was admitted to the intensive care unit. During the first 48 hours, Michael continued to decline and showed evidence of organ failure. He required continuous medical interventions, including dialysis, ventilation support, and surgical intervention for increasingly necrotizing digits, including amputation of several toes and fingers.

With a focus on prevention, occupational therapy was consulted early in his care to provide positioning and maintain range of motion of affected and unaffected joints and soft tissues. The occupational therapist fabricated orthotics for both his hands and feet. He was required to wear them at all times, except during dressing changes. His parents were also instructed to carry out range of motion routines to maintain his range and participate in his care.

Although Michael's condition initially continued to deteriorate, necessitating amputation of one leg above the knee, the other at the ankle, and all but two fingers, his family held out hope that he would come through this devastating illness. The parents called in the assistance of their tribal leaders to provide guidance and use tribal medicine to enhance Western medicine techniques. Leaders were granted permission to visit Michael in the intensive care unit, with clear guidelines about acceptable procedures that could be used.

During this time, the occupational therapist continued to monitor positioning and range of motion. The occupational therapist collaborated with nursing personnel to help position Michael and his medical devices to enable his mother to rock him in a chair at bedside. As his medical condition stabilized, Michael was weaned from ventilator support and could engage in strengthening and endurance activities. Occupational therapists also began to help Michael resume personal ADLs by introducing adaptive devices to enable his independence. Michael was provided with an appropriately sized wheelchair, and gloves were adapted to ease the use of his upper limbs so that he could propel the chair around the hospital unit. As he continued to increase his strength and function, he was eventually discharged from the intensive care unit and transferred to pediatric rehabilitation services, where his functional performance challenges were further addressed by prosthetics fitting and learning adaptive methods and other compensatory strategies to restore capabilities in personal care as well as home and school functioning.

ability to participate in treatments throughout the day or during the week. Coordinating therapy with other medical interventions may enhance therapeutic benefits by providing interventions when the child's energy is highest.

A bone marrow transplantation unit has certain similarities to the oncology unit, with intensified therapies and additional toxic agents used as life-saving treatments. Bone marrow transplantations are used as part of a medical treatment protocol for a number of life-threatening childhood illnesses, including leukemia, aplastic anemia, immunodeficiency syndromes, and tumors.[73] Because of the complications of the treatment, the occupational therapist must be aware of the stages that the child is in during the transplantation process and must strictly adhere to any precautions required.[16,58,65]

Oncology Treatment

During the initial phase of treatment for cancer, children undergo a series of evaluations to determine cancer type and staging, which includes determining whether the cancer has metastasized. Patients generally receive a permanent line placement through which they receive their chemotherapy. They are often hospitalized for their induction chemotherapy, which is the initial course and may be quite intense for some children. Hospitalization is required initially to assess the effects of chemotherapy and watch for any complications. Children frequently decrease their oral intake during treatment, so nutrition and hydration need to be carefully monitored.

As treatment progresses, children are often discharged from the inpatient setting and are monitored between chemotherapy

CASE STUDY 24-2 Intervention for Child Who Fails to Thrive

Background Information

Failure to thrive (FTT) is a diagnosis given to children, frequently infants and young children, who fail to grow or gain weight. FTT may be designated as organic, arising from a diagnosable physical cause, or nonorganic, which denotes impaired growth without an apparent physical cause.[28] Children with FTT often require hospitalization and receive acute care services that address complications, including immunodeficiencies, generalized weakness, and developmental delay because of their malnutrition and behavioral difficulties.

Although organic FTT can be attributed to a specific physical disorder, nonorganic FTT is primarily (but not exclusively) associated with psychosocial factors. Disturbances in parent-child interaction and development of attachment early in life, difficult infant temperament and behavior, maternal social isolation, and financial difficulties within the family are some of the variables associated with nonorganic FTT.[51,59]

The complexity of factors implicated in FTT emphasizes the need for a coordinated team approach that offers medical, nutritional, developmental, and psychosocial intervention. As a member of the hospital-based team, the occupational therapist may contribute to the diagnosis and intervention for the child with FTT. A comprehensive occupational therapy assessment provides the medical team with information regarding the infant's developmental status, feeding behaviors, infant-caregiver interactions during play and feeding, and infant interactions with unfamiliar adults. Stewart and Meyer[66] also stressed that infant assessment emphasizes interactional issues with the caregivers, whereas the assessment of older children focuses more on behaviors in the feeding situation and attempts to differentiate between environmental factors and neuromotor difficulties that may be affecting feeding.

Occupational therapy intervention goals with a child who has FTT may include ensuring effective oral-motor and feeding skills and facilitating development. Promoting positive parent-child interaction may also be emphasized by using strategies that help the parent understand the infant or child's behavioral cues and engage them with positive and developmentally appropriate play experiences. This emphasis on positive parent-child interaction also encourages parents to develop behavioral expectations consistent with the child's level of functioning. Ongoing outpatient therapy is often necessary following discharge to support goals established on the inpatient stay and foster effective feeding behaviors.

Presenting Information

Kevin was a 3-month, 7-day-old boy brought to the emergency room by his parents because of his unresponsive behavior and concern regarding possible seizure activity. Initial diagnoses included the following: rule out abuse, severe nonorganic FTT, and other risks, including seizures. Kevin was noted to have bruising above both knees and over his right buttocks. He had diaper rash and muscular wasting around the left hip and extremities. He demonstrated poor oral feeding and was subsequently admitted to the hospital for observation and monitoring. An attending physician referred Kevin to occupational therapy on the third day of hospitalization to address oral feeding skills.

History

Kevin's parents brought him to the hospital's emergency room after a home visit by a Child Protective Services worker. On his hospital admission, his parents left and did not visit during his week-long stay at the children's hospital. His maternal great aunt visited occasionally, and she expressed interest in adopting him.

Kevin was born at term and weighed 5 pounds, 12 ounces. He went home after a 48-hour hospital stay. He was hospitalized at 2 months of age for FTT, upper respiratory tract infection, and otitis media. He was discharged to his parents with home health nursing, a Child Protective Services referral, and pediatrician follow-up. Kevin's parents had missed all follow-up appointments until they brought him to the emergency room.

Medical and Occupational Therapy Intervention

A pH probe showed severe gastroesophageal reflux. An upper gastrointestinal series was performed, which ruled out anatomic abnormality. Stool samples were analyzed and showed malabsorption, reducing substances, increased fatty acids, and *Giardia lamblia*, all of which combined to reduce his level of nutrient absorption and increase fluid loss. As a result, Kevin was severely underweight and lethargic. Treatment for the reflux included positioning on an elevated wedge and the use of thickened feeds.

Kevin was evaluated by occupational therapists using clinical observations of his oral-motor, feeding, and developmental skills. He demonstrated intact oral structures and sensation, with functional oral skills for safe oral feeding. He had small sucking pads with a weak suck and fair coordination of suck-swallow-breathe. His suck and coordination improved with support at his jaw and cheeks. Kevin's developmental skills were delayed, and he demonstrated poor state control, with high irritability.

It was the occupational therapist's impression that Kevin's weak suck, poor feeding, and irritability were from overall weakness, malnutrition, and recent intubation, rather than from a neurologic deficit. The occupational therapist developed a bedside plan of specific facilitation techniques to be used during feeding. These included jaw and cheek support, external tongue stimulation, flexion swaddling, decreasing external stimulation, upright and well-aligned feeding positioning, limiting oral feeding to 30 minutes, and turning off the continuous pump that fed Kevin through a nasal gastric tube.

After implementation of occupational therapy recommendations by nursing staff, Kevin's oral intake increased dramatically over the next 3 days, with the occupational therapist feeding him once daily to monitor progress. Once the acute feeding issues were resolved, the emphasis of occupational therapy focused on developmental activities to improve self-calming, visual tracking, and social interactions.

Kevin was referred for outpatient occupational therapy and early intervention services before discharge. Child Protective Services assumed custody of Kevin, and he was discharged to a foster home with a weight increase of 2.4 pounds (follow-up weekly weight checks were scheduled with his pediatrician). The occupational therapist provided the foster parents with a home program, including positioning, feeding, and activities to promote Kevin's play development.

sessions in outpatient visits. If the child does not have a negative reaction, or if the agents given do not have high levels of toxicity, the child may receive chemotherapy on an outpatient basis. Children receiving chemotherapy are often at high risk for infections and are susceptible to contagious diseases; therefore, they need to take precautions, particularly if they are neutropenic, which affects their ability to fight off disease. Being neutropenic is a frequent cause for admissions between chemotherapy sessions and can mean that children are readmitted multiple times throughout their treatment.

The occupational therapist working with these children should be aware of the cancer types and have general knowledge of chemotherapy drugs and their complications, radiation therapy effects, and surgical approaches that may be taken. All personnel must adhere to infection control procedures. Occupational therapists may focus on the prevention of secondary complications by implementing strengthening, range of motion, and endurance activities and resuming ADLs, feeding, or play activities with patients, depending on their needs. Children and families frequently develop a close relationship with care providers because of the physical aspects of treatment, along with the normalcy and expectation of survival that families can perceive with daily activities. Cancer survival can be a realistic outcome for many children, but residual difficulties, including post-traumatic stress disorders, may be encountered that necessitate attention years after medical treatment has been discontinued.[44]

Occasionally cure is not an option for a child and family, and the focus of treatment may change to be palliative in nature. The occupational therapist working with the dying child and his or her family must respect the cultural beliefs of the family, along with the grief process. The occupational therapist can assist with suggesting energy conservation techniques to enable the child to continue to play and interact with family members. Positioning may become particularly important as the child develops increased weakness, difficulty with breath support, or pain, and the occupational therapist can help families problem solve alternative positioning to be close to their child when comfort is of the utmost importance.[18] It is also important that the occupational therapist respect the family and child's wishes for withdrawal or discontinuation of services. Some may wish to discontinue therapy intervention, choosing to narrow the circle of support, whereas others develop a closeness with the occupational therapist throughout the treatment and want to continue contact. The occupational therapist needs to examine his or her own support systems, beliefs, and feelings around end-of-life issues to assist the child and family during this difficult time,[71] during which communication with families is essential,[35] but receipt of palliative care approaches may be limited.[41]

Transplantation Procedures, Complications, and Interventions

The procedure for bone marrow transplantation involves chemotherapy, radiation, or both before transplantation. This is followed by the intravenous infusion of the bone marrow taken from a compatible donor or from the patient before the pretransplantation regimen of chemotherapy and radiation. Children who are undergoing treatment for disease processes that do not invade the bone marrow may be eligible to undergo stem cell transplantation.[60] This involves the harvesting of stem cells throughout their initial chemotherapy treatment while in the remission stage. Although bone marrow and stem cell transplantations both involve intense chemotherapy and radiation, individuals who undergo stem cell transplantation experience lower rejection rates and fewer complications from graft-versus-host disease (GVHD). The intense chemotherapy or radiation before transplantation and underlying disease processes cause severe immunosuppression in patients, making them highly susceptible to life-threatening infections until the new bone marrow is established and the child's immunohematopoietic system is once again functioning effectively.[45,75] Continued long term effects are also a complication of transplantation. GVHD, abnormal neuroendocrine function, secondary malignancies, and avascular necrosis are some of the complications seen in pediatric patients.[59] Stretching, extremity weight bearing, and general endurance exercises improve function in children experiencing these GVHD complications.[7]

Because these children have significant compromise of their immune systems, the hospital environment is carefully designed to reduce the risk of infection significantly. Common strategies to protect bone marrow transplantation patients include room isolation, reverse isolation, and laminar airflow in a clean or sterile environment.[76] Additionally, those having access to the unit may be limited. Staff and visitors who have flu- or virus-related symptoms may not be allowed onto units serving these severely compromised patients.

Intervention by occupational therapists may include pretransplantation assessment of the child's development and functional abilities, as well as identification of limitations or problems caused by the underlying disease process. After the transplantation, the occupational therapist's goals may be as follows: (1) promote age-appropriate play, daily living, and social participation; (2) enhance coping and interaction skills; and (3) develop a plan for follow-up in the community. Case Study 24-3 describes a child from initial diagnosis and chemotherapy through the transplantation process and posttransplantation intervention.

Rehabilitation Services

Levels of rehabilitation services can be subacute, acute, and outpatient or ongoing care. Subacute rehabilitation services are typically organized within skilled nursing facilities (SNFs) or other long-term care settings. Such programs are designed for children and adolescents who are too medically fragile or dependent to be cared for at home but who are not yet able to engage in or benefit from the intensive efforts of acute rehabilitation.[31] Such settings can also address later stages of care, which may involve palliative care or extended stays. After initial hospitalization, children and adolescents with moderate to severe head injury, multitrauma, or other systemic illnesses may be admitted to an SNF with subacute rehabilitation services. In these settings, they may receive daily therapy to prevent secondary complications and work toward goals of greater independent function. This interdisciplinary care may culminate in admission to an acute rehabilitation program or planned discharge to an organized home- and community-based service system of care.

Acute rehabilitation is characterized by inpatient hospital units and services. The most common of these are dedicated

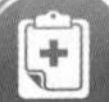

CASE STUDY 24-3 Intervention for Child with Cancer

Presenting Information

Danielle was a 21-month-old girl who was initially seen at a general hospital near her home when she experienced a decrease in standing and sitting balance. She was subsequently admitted to a pediatric tertiary care center approximately 400 miles from her rural community. Initial examination and imaging revealed a neuroblastoma in her spinal cord. Danielle was immediately placed on the pediatric oncology unit, a peripherally inserted central catheter (PICC) line was placed, and chemotherapy induction was initiated. At initial presentation, both parents flew in with Danielle, although they had separated just prior to diagnosis.

Background Information

Prior to diagnosis, Danielle was a typically developing 21-month-old girl, described by her parents as shy and reserved. She resided with her mother; her father had moved out 1 month prior to her diagnosis. Both parents were English-language learners, having immigrated from South America. They lived in a small town, with many community friends available for support. Her parents moved from a large city prior to conceiving Danielle to "obtain a simpler lifestyle." On hearing the diagnosis, the mother revealed that her grandfather had died of a glioblastoma 1 year previously.

Medical and Occupational Therapy Intervention: Oncology Phase of Treatment

Danielle was initially referred to occupational therapy immediately after diagnosis. She had initial complications coping with the increased noise and number of caregivers, along with decreased performance. She was also seen by a child life specialist for developmentally appropriate coping strategies, such as creating a calming environment and playing to facilitate release of her emotions. Danielle did not sit independently, and her overall strength was diminished.

Danielle was given chemotherapy to reduce the size of the tumor and keep it from spreading. Because of its location, tumor resection was not possible. Stem cell transplantation was discussed at initiation of treatment as the best course of possible cure for her cancer. Thus the medical plan was to reduce her tumor size, obtain remission, harvest stem cells, and prepare Danielle for transplantation. She was placed on a chemotherapy protocol recommended for her tumor type, and the family was informed of all complications, side effects, and likely outcome possibilities.

In an initial assessment, the occupational therapist evaluated Danielle's performance skills and strength. She completed family interviews to learn about the child's previous skill levels, occupations, and particular interests. A plan was made in conjunction with the parents and nurse for a daily schedule, including times when Danielle could receive therapy. She was moved to a corner room to decrease noise, and times were posted when curtains were to be drawn to allow the family private time. Pictures of caregivers, including therapists, primary nurses, and physicians, were posted for reference for Danielle and her parents.

Ongoing communication was established among all team members through online documentation and team rounds, and a care book was placed at Danielle's bedside where information and questions could be posted to facilitate communication between parents and medical personnel further. In addition, care conferences were held weekly, during which all team members, including parents, discussed and planned ongoing interventions.

Occupational therapy intervention consisted of age-appropriate play activities to facilitate strengthening and continued motor skill development. Self-feeding was encouraged and supported. The occupational therapist instructed family members and the nurses on position strategies to increase Danielle's function and enable participation. Danielle did not always participate in regular sessions because of medical treatments that resulted in nausea and neutropenic compromise, causing additional weakness and lethargy. During particularly difficult periods, intervention sessions were limited to gentle range of motion or were sometimes canceled for the day.

As medical intervention, including chemotherapy, progressed, Danielle experienced an increase in function. Her occupational therapy intervention plan was continually revised to reflect increased strength and independence. In response to chemotherapy, Danielle began to have reduced oral food intake. Strategies were implemented to help maintain oral-motor skills and optimize self-feeding.

Danielle eventually transitioned to outpatient care, where both her oncology treatment and occupational therapy continued. Because of behavior challenges, family requests, and training expertise, direct physical therapy was discontinued. Instead, a collaborative approach of consultation with the occupational therapist at regular intervals to facilitate ambulatory and lower extremity skills was established. Her parents divided care and alternated times when each parent would be present.

Once the transplantation regimen was initiated, Danielle was hospitalized for an extended stay. She underwent intensive chemotherapy and radiation to ablate her current marrow and subsequently received stem cell transplantation. During the initial stages, Danielle experienced a significant decrease in her strength and developmental skills. She had toxicity-related complications, including sloughing of her skin and mouth sores, which made participation in activities difficult. As an added complication, Danielle also experienced life-threatening pulmonary complications that required ventilation support and necessitated a 2-week stay in the intensive care unit.

Family stresses throughout this portion of her treatment were enormous, and Danielle's mother asked Danielle's maternal grandmother to come for support. Once there, interpreters were called in to translate necessary information, as the parents desired. Danielle eventually achieved slow engraftment, and transplantation-related complications diminished.

As engraftment progressed, Danielle regained her play and daily living skills, including ambulation. She was transferred to outpatient services and continued to receive occupational therapy intervention to address decreased strength and delayed motor skills. She was discharged to her community once she had completed her 90-day post-transplantation evaluation and engraftment was clear. She continued to receive ongoing occupational therapy in her community to help facilitate progress in her development.

rehabilitation units within a children's hospital. Another form of organization is the specification of beds and services for pediatric patients in a large rehabilitation hospital. Adolescents 15 years of age or older may be admitted to rehabilitation units that commonly serve adults. Children and adolescents are admitted to acute rehabilitation from other acute or transitional care medical services within the hospital, other local hospitals, or subacute rehabilitation settings. See Chapter 30. Overall, admission to pediatric rehabilitation facilities and length of inpatient stay is largely based on the child's or youth's level of function and services needed.[15]

Essential to acute rehabilitation programs is the presence of a broad range of services, including occupational therapy. The mixture and intensity of services are planned to meet systematically developed goals. Such programs are characterized as meeting three types of needs:

1. Organize and implement a planned approach for the management of recovery and rehabilitation of children post-trauma or with rapid-onset disorders.
2. Redirect care after onset of complications in children with chronic disorders.
3. Provide an environment for specialized medical or surgical procedures that involves specific care regimens and protocols.

Children and adolescents who sustain a sudden illness or injury are the most common type of admission in acute rehabilitation. Table 24-2 indicates the common problems that affect a typically developing child who experiences injury from accidents, violence, or rapid-onset disease. Acquired injuries or diseases represent a substantial health threat to children.[77] Injuries are the leading cause of death and disability among children older than 1 year of age.[25] TBIs, including closed head injury, skull fracture, and penetrating brain injuries, are an ongoing concern for children and adolescents caused by transportation-related crashes, falls, recreational injury, and violence.[47,61] Case Study 24-4 describes rehabilitation for a child with a TBI. Acute rehabilitation is also required for children who sustain spinal cord injury (SCI) and multitrauma. Environmental hazards, accidents, and abuse are also implicated in children who experience burns, near-drowning, smoke inhalation, carbon monoxide poisoning, or drug overdose.

TABLE 24-2 Rapid-Onset Conditions

Type of Onset	Examples
Accidental injury	Traumatic brain injury (e.g., closed head injury)
	Skull fracture or penetrating head injury
	Burns and smoke inhalation
	Multitrauma
	Near-drowning
	Spinal cord injury
Violence	Multitrauma
	Traumatic brain injury (e.g., gunshot wound)
	Burns, iron burns, cigarette burns, and scalding
Disease processes	Central nervous system infection (e.g., encephalitis and meningitis)
	Transverse myelitis
	Guillain-Barré syndrome
	Cancer
	Organ transplantation

Aside from known hazards, children also develop infections that involve the central nervous system (CNS); they may sustain a cerebrovascular accident or develop other neurologic disorders, such as transverse myelitis or Guillain-Barré syndrome. Cancer and its treatment may cause children and adolescents to develop problems that necessitate acute rehabilitation. All these disorders are characterized by typical development until an acute health crisis causes a severe loss of function, a likelihood of prolonged recovery with residual disability, and potential chronic health complications associated with disability. For these children and their families, the purpose of rehabilitation is to optimize recovery, prevent complications, and organize and implement an approach to initial and long-term management that optimizes function in family and community life.

Children with congenital or chronic disorders may also require acute rehabilitation. Many with genetic disorders or other congenital abnormalities or who experience chronic disease often have delayed or atypical patterns of functional skill development. These children are also at risk for complications that can create a gradual or critical loss of function. Episodes of respiratory complications, bony fractures and dislocations, skin breakdown, or other systemic complications may be associated with functional deterioration. Children with cerebral palsy, spina bifida, or other types of congenital deficits are included in this at-risk group. Similarly, those with congenital limb deficiency or arthrogryposis multiplex congenital syndrome may have reconstructive surgery necessitating acute rehabilitation. Children with osteogenesis imperfecta can have episodes of curtailed functional gains after injury, and children with juvenile rheumatoid arthritis and systemic disorders can experience periods of rapid functional decline. For these children, the goals of rehabilitation are to prevent further losses and facilitate the reacquisition of skills consistent with the pattern of functional progression that was previously shown.

A third major group of children who receive acute rehabilitation services includes those who are hospitalized for treatment with special medical, surgical, or technologic procedures. For children with cerebral palsy, the use of medical interventions such as selective dorsal rhizotomy, continuous intrathecal baclofen, or other neurosurgical techniques to reduce spasticity may involve admission to acute rehabilitation.[26] Children with severe pulmonary complications or those who become ventilator-dependent may be admitted for acute rehabilitation; their families learn how to perform care procedures and use medical technology[10]; long-term outcomes can be positive.[30] More and more children are also receiving organ transplants, which may necessitate teaching special care procedures and redeveloping fitness following a prolonged disease process. These interventions often necessitate occupational therapists, following specific evaluation and treatment protocols designed to optimize functional outcomes.

Transition from Rehabilitation to the Community

To facilitate continuity of care when the child is discharged from a pediatric rehabilitation hospitalization, the team and family develop a comprehensive plan of transition.[74] For

CASE STUDY 24-4 Intervention for Child with Traumatic Brain Injury

Presenting Information

Devon was a 6-year-old boy with a severe traumatic brain injury caused by an accidental gunshot wound to the head. Immediately following this incident, he was evacuated to the level 1 regional trauma center, where he underwent a decompressive left craniectomy for evacuation of intraparenchymal and subdural hematomas. Once stabilized and able to tolerate multiple daily therapies, Devon was transferred 13 days later to the regional children's hospital for rehabilitative services. At that time, he was delayed in following simple verbal commands, not moving the right side of his body, unable to sit unsupported and walk, and he did not speak.

Background Information

Previously healthy, Devon lived with his parents and 8-year-old brother. His brother Daniel had just finished third grade and Devon was to enter first grade in the fall. Prior to the accident, both boys were at a friend's house, where apparently they found a gun. The gun was somehow fired, and Devon was shot in the head. No one except for the children witnessed the event. The family was understandably grieving and his mom or dad had been at his side at all times during his hospitalization. His mother described Devon as a warm, loving child who knew everyone's name in the neighborhood. He loves playing with cars, riding bikes, and competing on computer-based video games.

Medical and Occupational Therapy Intervention

In addition to being cared for by the medical team and rehabilitation nurses, Devon received services from occupational therapy, physical therapy, speech therapy, recreational therapy, hospital-based school and rehabilitation psychology. Devon's family was supported by a social worker and the rehabilitation unit care coordinator.

The occupational therapist completed an initial evaluation with Devon and discussed a plan of care with Devon's family. Because Devon was not showing any movement of his right arm, the occupational therapist started a daily range of motion program to maintain full range of motion and fabricated a wrist-hand orthotic to be worn when Devon was resting in bed and at night. Once Devon tolerated this program well, the occupational therapists trained his mother and father to complete the range of motion program. As Devon began vocalizing, however, he was difficult to understand; his parents were concerned that he was unable to communicate basic needs. The occupational therapist worked with the speech therapist so that Devon would be able to point to a picture symbol board with his left hand to communicate when he was afraid, felt pain, needed to use the bathroom, and was hungry.

It was also important to Devon's family that he remain safe when he was not in therapy. The occupational therapist taught Devon how to complete his daily activities safely, with assistance and modifications as necessary, such as first dressing with sitting supports on his bed and then progressing to dressing while seated at the edge of his bed. Devon learned how to use his nonaffected left arm as his newly preferred hand to dress in loose-fitting, nonfastener clothing using one-handed techniques and with equipment to modify the task, such as elastic laces on his shoes and a ring on his zipper pull. Devon learned how to manage a spoon and a fork, eat with his left hand, and write his name. He practiced these new skills in therapy and with his family, as well as when attending the hospital schoolroom and with recreational therapy. The occupational therapist scheduled Devon for one-to-one therapy sessions twice each day and planned morning personal ADL training and afternoon therapeutic activities. In addition to structured ADL routines and orientation and memory programs, the occupational therapist also engaged him in selected activities to facilitate the use of his left arm and provide cognitive challenges in organizing steps, following sequences, and sustaining engagement in familiar and novel tasks. The occupational therapist taught Devon to carry out daily range of motion and whole-body stretches to maintain normal range and facilitate symmetric trunk and limb use.

Devon continued to have difficulty performing activities using his nondominant left hand, and left hand movements were awkward and unsuccessful. The occupational therapist cued and encouraged him to use both hands together, with the left hand assisting the right hand. This strategy improved his personal ADL performance so that the occupational therapist discontinued the use of adaptive devices, such as a button aid and rocker knife, after 2 weeks. Handwriting with the right or left hand was not satisfactory for schoolwork because of a language disorder, illegibility, and slow speed. The occupational therapist introduced a computer keyboard and initiated supplementary handwriting activities to facilitate movement and augment function.

On discharge, his parents expressed concern about him returning to school. They worried about how Devon would adjust to school. Specifically, they wanted him to perform in a regular classroom, eat lunch with his friends, and go to the bathroom by himself. The occupational therapist provided the school with results from standardized fine motor, visual perceptual, and visual motor assessments and made recommendations to the school so that they would understand what assistance Devon would need. The occupational therapist suggested accommodations for writing, cafeteria assistance, and bathroom facilities. Devon returned home with his family and continued his recovery, with outpatient therapies focusing on sensorimotor skills and school-based therapies focusing on enabling classroom participation and educational performance.

example, a child with a brain injury often requires special education services after discharge from the medical center, and readiness to return to school may be particularly problematic because of social-behavioral challenges.[5] Team and family activities and communication focus on the transition from rehabilitation to school and community as soon as discharge is considered. Transition activities include interagency team meetings at which school and rehabilitation team members are represented. Ideally, at least one interagency meeting occurs in the rehabilitation unit and at least one in the school. By sharing where the meeting is hosted, team members get a realistic picture of the child's environments. When the meeting is at the team's home site, most, if not all, team members who worked with the child can be involved.

In a visit to the school, the occupational therapist from the hospital shares information with the school-based therapists related to concerns, priorities, and results of intervention approaches (i.e., what worked and what did not). The child's rehabilitation team helps problem solve issues regarding the school's accessibility and possible modifications to the classroom and curriculum. Visits to the child's classroom can help identify accommodations that need to be in place. During these visits, the rehabilitation team can present information to the other students in the class about the child's disability, his or her rehabilitation, and types of changes that they may expect in their peer. When a child returns to his or her preinjury classroom, the hospital therapist can provide an in-service presentation about the injury so that the student's peers have expectations about his or her behavior and personality or, in the case of severe burns, about the student's appearance. In addition, before discharge, the child should visit his or her school and other important environments to determine what accommodations will need to be made.

The rehabilitation team often monitors the child's progress during the first few months after discharge. The child may continue with outpatient services while initiating school-based services. Consistency during the transition is maintained by the family members, who ultimately support the child through the transition to the home. In support of this, the teams involved provide the parents with comprehensive information about the special education system in their community, their rights as parents of a child who newly qualifies for special education services, and other community programs, supports, and resources that they can access.

Outpatient Services

Another major component of pediatric rehabilitation exists in specialized outpatient services and clinics that provide ongoing care. Typically, as part of children's hospitals or rehabilitation hospitals, interdisciplinary outpatient clinics are organized to provide monitoring and interventions for children who experience particular types of chronic health risks and disabilities. Occupational therapists often provide follow-up and follow-along attention to children and families after hospitalization, but many of these children are never hospitalized. Occupational therapists who work at these clinics often focus on the child's or adolescent's health status and development, emphasizing functional progress and participation in home, school, and community activities.

TABLE 24-3 Outpatient Clinics and Programs Often Served by Occupational Therapists

Client Disorder	Clinic or Services
Congenital disorders	Spina bifida
Neuromuscular disorders	Cerebral palsy
Developmental disabilities	Down syndrome Fetal alcohol syndrome
Rheumatologic disorders	Juvenile rheumatoid arthritis Systemic lupus erythematosus
Adolescent medicine disorders	Reflex neurovascular dystrophy
Craniofacial abnormality	Cleft lip and palate
Orthopedic disorders	Traumatic hand injury Congenital limb deficiency
Rehabilitation	Traumatic brain injury Spinal cord injury Constraint-induced movement therapy program
Muscular dystrophy	Duchenne muscular dystrophy Spinal muscle atrophy
Limb deficiency disorders	Congenital amelia Traumatic amputation
Cystic fibrosis	Cystic fibrosis
Assistive technology	Seating and positioning Wheelchair control Augmentative communication Computers and information technology Environmental controls

Outpatient clinic programs that often include occupational therapy services are listed in Table 24-3. Such programs may be scheduled weekly, monthly, quarterly, or even annually, as needed. Sometimes these programs are conducted away from the hospital facility at community sites such as schools. Occupational therapists who work in specialized hospital programs are provided with unique exposure to otherwise uncommon diagnoses and clinical procedures and can pass this experience on to other families and therapists as a conduit of information and new ideas. For example, school personnel may have limited experience with children who have arthrogryposis, brachial plexus and limb deficiency, or various forms of muscular dystrophy, whereas the hospital clinic therapists would have regular experiences with these disabling conditions. Specific study and preparation for consultation are suggested for entry-level therapists and can be an important skill for the occupational therapist to develop as part of pediatric rehabilitation,[19] particularly in working with more local, community-based therapists who may have limited experience with some diagnostic conditions and related treatment approaches that are used.

Outpatient services are important components of the total spectrum of hospital care and may be provided at the hospital, at a hospital satellite center, or as part of an interdisciplinary hospital-based clinic (e.g., rheumatology clinic, neurodevelopmental palsy clinic, special feeding clinic). Outpatient occupational therapy is generally provided for one of three purposes: (1) as part of a diagnostic assessment, (2) to provide needed intervention and assistive technology after hospital discharge,

CASE STUDY 24-5 Occupational Therapy in Spina Bifida Specialty Clinic

Stacie is an 8-year-old girl with midlumbar myelodysplasia. She ambulates with ankle-foot orthotics (AFOs) and uses Lofstrand crutches for longer distances at this time. Although she is functional for mobility in her home and at school, her future mobility demands may necessitate use of a wheelchair. She exhibits delayed coordination skills and less than expected quality and speed in handwriting tasks. Stacie uses a computer to complete some school work in her third-grade integrated classroom.

Stacie is assisted at home in dressing (managing clothing fasteners) but is otherwise independent with her morning and evening ADLs. With a neurogenic bowel and bladder, she is on a clean intermittent catheterization (CIC) program and daily bowel program (BP). Her mother has traditionally done her catheterization and is trying to transition to have her perform more of it on her own. At school, a nurse assists with her catheter routine twice daily. She is somewhat successful with her bowel program, typically having bowel movements in the morning or during the evenings at home. Timed programs include the use of diet and suppositories. Occasional bowel accidents are acknowledged, and she uses pull-ups to manage.

Although many of the activity and participation concerns with Stacie are addressed as part of school therapy and reflected in her individualized education program (IEP), the role of the specialty clinic follow-up has two major purposes. One of these is to monitor her motor skill development and status carefully. Children with spina bifida often have neurosurgical shunt placement early in life to reduce hydrocephalus. These shunts can become obstructed, and families, as well as service providers, are vigilant in attending to signs of shunt failure. Worsening of coordination and visual-perception skills can be one of these signs. The occupational therapist at the specialty clinic often performs normative hand function assessment to determine stability of performance over time. In this clinic, the occupational therapist measures grip and pinch strength and coordination testing using the Jebsen-Taylor Hand Function Test, which has norms for children, adolescents, and adults of both genders. Developmental visual-perceptual tests may also be used. In her most recent visit, Stacie's scores were similar to the prior year's findings, with her scoring about 1.5 SD below the mean on most tasks. Her grip and pinch strength were also around the 40th percentile for her age and gender.

Another role of the clinical specialist is to facilitate growth in children's ADL and IADL skill independence. Children with spina bifida have different timing and patterns of skill development that often need specific advice and the use of adaptive methods and devices.[14,41] For example, the clinical specialist may provide advice on techniques to manage orthotic and other devices, methods to develop wheelchair skills, and strategies to promote independence in bladder and bowel care programs. Stacie managed most of her personal care and participated in a few chores at home. The occupational therapist suggested that she and her family select clothes to be worn to school the night before and recommended purchasing clothes without fasteners or with a zippers and snaps. Clinical follow-up emphasized health monitoring, health promotion, and increasing her independence and participation as she transitioned to middle school.

or (3) to provide occupational therapy intervention for individuals with disabilities or other medical conditions not requiring hospitalization.

Outpatient services provided as part of an interdisciplinary specialty medical clinic usually have a specific focus (e.g., feeding clinic, behavioral disorders clinic). See Case Study 24-5. Occupational therapy services in specialty clinics are limited because children typically attend only once or twice a year. In some cases, the occupational therapist functions as a consultant, completing an assessment, and then making recommendations to the physician. In other cases, the occupational therapist is an integral part of the decision-making team and may be involved in child assessment, intervention or equipment recommendations, or the provision of orthotics and adaptive equipment.

In AT clinics, occupational therapists evaluate how the child could benefit from the use of aided and augmentative communication systems, computer access and use of information technologies, therapeutic seating, powered mobility, or other technologies that enable environmental access and control. These applications of special procedures and AT devices are characterized by preplanned and often short trials leading to the prescription of devices.[38] Efforts culminate in intensive family training and transitions to follow-up in the community, often as a partnership with local providers in the environments in which the devices are used.

Residential or intensive day treatment programs characterize another form of outpatient pediatric rehabilitation service. These extended care programs focus on direct assistance with community re-entry and participation. Simulated or actual environments become the training sites for skills that enable community participation and effective performance toward goals of independent living, education, and work activities.

Summary

The provision of occupational therapy services to children in hospitals is a specialized and challenging area of practice. Occupational therapists in hospitals must have a thorough understanding of the characteristics of health care systems, the factors and trends that affect hospitals, including legal and accreditation requirements, and the specialized needs of hospitalized children and their families. To achieve health and functional goals, the occupational therapist must also understand the roles of other professionals involved in the care of children. Occupational therapists who are employed in hospitals have the opportunity to gain expertise in assessment and intervention of children of various ages, with many different diagnoses, often within a dynamic, fast-paced environment. As hospitals broaden their range of services in response to a changing health care system, hospital-based occupational therapists will have opportunities to broaden their areas of expertise, apply different models of service delivery, and develop new practitioner roles.

- Hospital-based pediatric therapy services play a unique role in the overall management of children and adolescents with a new or chronic disability.
- In addressing acute and chronic problems, the occupational therapist's emphasis is on function and participation in life's events at home, at school, and in the community.
- New and established impairments and disabilities pose risks for further complications, which necessitate a prevention prioritization through subacute, acute, and outpatient or ongoing rehabilitation interventions.
- Medical services follow policies and regulations imposed by accreditation and regulatory agencies and third-party payers.

Collaboration with caregivers, school personnel, and community-based practitioners is critical to effective intervention and transition from hospital to home.

REFERENCES

1. Affleck, A. T., Lieberman, S., Polon, J., et al. (1986). Providing occupational therapy in an intensive care unit. *American Journal of Occupational Therapy*, *40*, 323–332.
2. Armstrong, K., & Kerns, K. A. (2002). The assessment of parent needs following paediatric traumatic brain injury. *Pediatric Rehabilitation*, *5*, 149–160.
3. Baker, C. (2004). Preventing ICU syndrome in children. *Pediatric Nursing*, *16*(10), 32–35.
4. Bedell, G. M. (2008). Functional outcomes of school-age children with acquired brain injuries at discharge from inpatient rehabilitation. *Brain Injury*, *22*, 313–324.
5. Bedell, G. M., Haley, S. M., Coster, W. J., et al. (2002). Participation readiness at discharge from inpatient rehabilitation in children and adolescents with acquired brain injuries. *Pediatric Rehabilitation*, *5*, 107–116.
6. Bennett, T. D., Niedzwecki, C. M., Korgenski, E. K., et al. (2013). Initiation of physical, occupational, and speech therapy in children with traumatic brain injury. *Archives Physical Medicine and Rehabilitation*, *94*, 1268–1276.
7. Beredjiklian, P. K., Drummond, D. S., Dormans, J. P., et al. (1998). Orthopaedic manifestations of chronic graft-versus-host disease. *Journal of Pediatric Orthopeadics*, *18*(5), 572–575.
8. Bower, E., McLellan, D. L., Arney, J., et al. (1996). A randomised controlled trial of different intensities of physiotherapy and different goal-setting procedures in 44 children with cerebral palsy. *Developmental Medicine and Child Neurology*, *38*, 226–237.
9. Burkett, K. W. (1989). Trends in pediatric rehabilitation. *Nursing Clinics of North America*, *24*, 239–255.
10. Buschbacher, R. (1995). Outcomes and problems in pediatric pulmonary rehabilitation. *American Journal of Physical Medicine and Rehabilitation*, *74*, 287–293.
11. Chen, C. C., Heinemann, A. W., Bode, R. K., et al. (2004). Impact of pediatric rehabilitation services on children's functional outcomes. *American Journal of Occupational Therapy*, *58*, 44–53.
12. Commission for the Accreditation of Rehabilitation Facilities (2009). CARF standards manual. Retrieved from: <http://www.carf.org/WorkArea/DownloadAsset.aspx?id=22717>.
13. Colville, G. (2008). The psychologic impact on children of admission to intensive care. *Pediatric Clinics North America*, *55*, 605–616.
14. Davis, B. E., Shurtleff, D. B., Walker, W. O., et al. (2006). Acquisition of autonomy in adolescents with myelomeningocele. *Developmental Medicine and Child Neurology*, *48*, 253–258.
15. DeNise-Annunziata, D. K., & Scharf, A. A. (1998). Functional status as an important predictor of length of stay in a pediatric rehabilitation hospital. *Journal of Rehabilitation Outcomes Measurement*, *2*, 12–21.
16. Diaz de Heredia, C., Moreno, A., Olive, T., et al. (1999). Role of the intensive care unit in children undergoing bone marrow transplantation with life-threatening complications. *Bone Marrow Transplantation*, *24*, 163–168.
17. Donders, J. (1993). Bereavement and mourning in pediatric rehabilitation settings. *Death Studies*, *17*, 517–527.
18. Drake, R., Frost, J., & Collins, J. J. (2003). The symptoms of dying children. *Journal of Pain and Symptom Management*, *26*, 594–603.
19. Dudgeon, B. J., & Greenberg, S. L. (1998). Preparing students for consultation roles and systems. *American Journal of Occupational Therapy*, *52*, 801–809.
20. Dumas, H. M., Haley, S. M., Ludlow, L. H., et al. (2002). Functional recovery in pediatric traumatic brain injury during inpatient rehabilitation. *American Journal of Physical Medicine and Rehabilitation*, *81*, 661–669.
21. Edwards, P. A. (1992). The evolution of rehabilitation facilities for children. *Rehabilitation Nursing*, *17*, 191–195.
22. Eckle, N., & MacLean, S. L. (2001). Assessment of family-centered care policies and practices for pediatric patients in nine US emergency departments. *Journal of Emergency Nursing*, *27*, 238–245.
23. Eliasson, A. (2005). Improving the use of hands in daily activities: Aspects of the treatment of children with cerebral palsy. *Physical and Occupational Therapy in Pediatrics*, *25*, 37–60.
24. Elixhauser, A. (2008). Hospital stays for children, 2006. HCUP statistical brief #56. Retrieved from: <http://www.hcup-us.ahrq.gov/reports/statbriefs56.pdf>.
25. Falesi, M., Berni, S., & Strambi, M. (2008). Causes of accidents in pediatric patients: What has changed through the ages. *Minerva Pediatrica*, *60*, 169–176.
26. Fleet, P. J. (2003). Rehabilitation of spasticity and related problems in childhood cerebral palsy. *Journal of Paediatrics and Child Health*, *39*, 6–14.
27. Flores, G., Abreau, M., Claisson, C. E., et al. (2003). Keeping children out of hospital: Parents' and physicians' perspectives on how pediatric hospitalizations for ambulatory care-sensitive conditions can be avoided. *Pediatrics*, *112*, 1021–1030.
28. Frank, D. A. (1985). Biologic risks in "nonorganic" failure to thrive: Diagnostic and therapeutic implications. In D. Drotar (Ed.), *New directions in failure to thrive* (pp. 17–26). New York: Plenum Press.
29. Fuhrer, M. J. (2000). Subjectifying quality of life as a medical rehabilitation outcome. *Disability Rehabilitation*, *22*, 481–489.
30. Gilgoff, R. L., & Gilgoff, I. S. (2003). Long-term follow-up of home mechanical ventilation in young children with spinal cord injury and neuromuscular conditions. *Journal of Pediatrics*, *142*, 476–480.
31. Grebin, B., & Kaplan, S. C. (1995). Toward a pediatric subacute care model: Clinical and administrative features.

Archives Physical Medicine Rehabilitation, 76(Suppl.), SC16–SC20.
32. Guerriere, D., & McKeever, P. (1997). Mothering children who survive brain injuries: Playing the hand you're dealt. *Journal of the Society of Pediatric Nurses, 2*, 105–115.
33. Haley, S. M., Coster, W. J., Dumas, H. M., et al. (2012). *PEDI-CAT (version 1.3.6)*. Boston: CRECare.
34. Halstead, L. S. (2001). The John Stanley Coulter lecture. The power of compassion and caring in rehabilitation healing. *Archives of Physical Medicine and Rehabilitation, 82*, 149–154.
35. Hays, R. M., Valentine, J., Haynes, G., et al. (2006). The Seattle Pediatric Palliative Care Project: Effects of family satisfaction and health-related quality of life. *Journal Palliative Medicine, 9*, 716–728.
36. Hewitt-Taylor, J. (1999). Children in intensive care: Physiological considerations. *Nursing in Critical Care, 4*, 40–45.
37. Hopia, H., Tomlinson, P. S., Paavilainen, E., et al. (2005). Child in hospital: Family experiences and expectations of how nurses can promote family health. *Journal Clinical Nursing, 14*, 212–222.
38. Johnson, K. L., Dudgeon, B., Kuehn, C., et al. (2007). Assistive technology use among adolescents and young adults with spina bifida. *American Journal Public Health, 97*, 330–336.
39. Joint Commission on the Accreditation of Health Care Organizations (JCAHO) (2009). *Comprehensive Accreditation Manual for Hospitals: The official handbook (CAMH)*. Oakbrook Terrace, IL: JCAHO.
40. Jongbloed, L., & Wendland, T. (2002). The impact of reimbursement systems on occupational therapy practice in Canada and the United States of America. *Canadian Journal of Occupational Therapy, 69*, 143–152.
41. Keele, L., Keenan, H. T., Sheetz, J., et al. (2013). Differences in characteristics of dying children who receive and do not receive palliative care. *Pediatrics, 132*, 72–78.
42. Kirwin, K. M., & Hamrin, V. (2005). Decreasing the risk of complicated bereavement and future psychiatric disorders in children. *Journal Child Adolescent Psychiatric Nursing, 18*(2), 62–78.
43. Law, M., & MacDermid, J. (Eds.), (2014). *Evidence-based rehabilitation: A guide to practice*. Thorofare, NJ: Slack.
44. Lee, Y., & Santacroce, S. J. (2007). Posttraumatic stress in long-term young adult survivors of childhood cancer: A questionnaire survey. *International Journal of Nursing Studies, 44*, 1406–1417.
45. Lenarsky, C. (1990). Technique of bone marrow transplantation. In F. L. Johnson & C. Pochedly (Eds.), *Bone marrow transplantation in children* (pp. 53–67). New York: Raven Press.
46. Mantymaa, M., Puura, K., Luoma, I., et al. (2003). Infant-mother interaction as a predictor of child's chronic health problems. *Child: Care, Health and Development, 29*, 181–191.
47. Mazzola, C. A., & Adelson, P. D. (2002). Critical care management of head trauma in children. *Critical Care Medicine, 30*(Suppl.), S393–S401.
48. Michlovitz, S. L. (1996). *Thermal agents in rehabilitation* (3rd ed.). Philadelphia: F. A. Davis.
49. Missiuma, C., Pollock, N., Law, M., et al. (2006). Examination of the Perceived Efficacy and Goal Setting System (PEGS) with children with disabilities, their parents and teachers. *American Journal of Occupational Therapy, 60*, 204–214.
50. Mitchell, A. W., & Batorski, R. E. (2009). A study of critical reasoning in online learning: Application of the occupational performance process. *Occupational Therapy International, 16*, 134–153.
51. Msall, M. E., DiGaudio, K. M., & Duffy, L. C. (1993). Use of functional assessment in children with developmental disabilities. *Physical Medicine and Rehabilitation Clinics of North America, 4*, 517–527.
52. National Association for Children's Hospitals and Related Institutions (NACHRI) (2009). Home page. Retrieved from: <http://www.childrenshospitals.net>.
53. Ottenbacher, K. J., & Hinderer, S. R. (2001). Evidence-based practice: Methods to evaluate individual patient improvement. *American Journal of Physical Medicine and Rehabilitation, 80*(10), 786–796.
54. Pendleton, H., & Schultz-Krohn, W. (Eds.), (2013). *Pedretti's Occupational therapy: Practice skills for physical dysfunction* (7th ed.). St. Louis: Mosby.
55. Radomski, M. V., & Trombly-Latham, C. A. (Eds.), (2008). *Occupational therapy for physical dysfunction* (6th ed.). Baltimore: Williams & Wilkins.
56. Rivara, F. P., Ennis, S. K., Mangione-Smith, R., et al. (2012). Variation in adherence to new quality of care indicators for the acute rehabilitation of children with traumatic brain injury. *Archives of Physical Medicine and Rehabilitation, 93*, 1371–1376.
57. Rivara, J. M., Jaffe, K. M., Polissar, N. L., et al. (1996). Predictors of family functioning and change 3 years after traumatic brain injury in children. *Archives of Physical Medicine and Rehabilitation, 77*, 754–764.
58. Rogers, M., Weinstock, D. M., Eagan, J., et al. (2000). Rotavirus outbreak on a pediatric oncology floor: Possible association with toys. *American Journal of Infection Control, 28*, 378–380.
59. Sanders, J. E. (1991). Long-term effects of bone marrow transplantation. *Pediatrician, 18*, 76–81.
60. Sanders, J. E. (1997). Bone marrow transplantation for pediatric malignancies. *Pediatric Oncology, 44*(4), 1005–1020.
61. Schneier, A. J., Shields, B. J., Hostetler, S. G., et al. (2006). Incidence of pediatric traumatic brain injury and associated hospital resource utilization in the United States. *Pediatrics, 118*, 483–492.
62. Schor, E. L.; American Academy of Pediatrics. (2003). Family pediatrics: Report of the Task Force on the Family. *Pediatrics, 111*(6), 1541–1571.
63. Schultz, K. (1999). Bereaved children. *Canadian Family Physician, 45*, 2914–2921.
64. Schwartz, R. K. (1991). Educational and training strategies: Therapy as learning. In C. Christiansen & C. Baum (Eds.), *Occupational therapy: Overcoming human performance deficits* (pp. 664–698). Thorofare, NJ: Slack.
65. Shaw, P. J. (2002). Suspected infection in children with cancer. *Journal of Antimicrobial Chemotherapy, 49*, 63–67.
66. Stewart, K. B., & Meyer, L. (2004). Parent-child interactions and everyday routine in young children with failure to thrive. *American Journal of Occupational Therapy, 58*, 342–346.
67. Sullivan, D., Kantak, S. S., & Burtner, P. A. (2008). Motor learning in children: Feedback effects on skills acquisition. *Physical Therapy, 88*, 720–732.
68. Tomlinson, P. S., Thomlinson, E., Peden-McAlping, C., et al. (2002). Clinical innovation for promoting family care in pediatric intensive care: Demonstration, role modeling and reflective practice. Journal of Advance Nursing, *38*, 161–170.
69. Uniform Data System, University of Buffalo (n.d). About the WeeFIM II system. Retrieved from: <http://www.udsmr.org/WebModules/WeeFIM/Wee_About.aspx>.
70. Vavili, F. (2000). Children in hospital: A design question. *World Hospitals and Health Services, 36*, 31–39, 45–46.
71. Vincent, J. L. (2001). Cultural differences in end-of-life care. *Critical Care Medicine, 29*, N52–N55.
72. Watkins, P. (2003). Ethnicity and clinical practice. *Clinical Medicine, 3*, 197–198.

73. Williams, T. E., & Safarimaryaki, S. (1990). Bone marrow transplantation for treatment of solid tumors. In F. L. Johnson & C. Pochedly (Eds.), *Bone marrow transplantation in children* (pp. 221–242). New York: Raven Press.
74. Wise, P. (2004). The transformation of child health in the United States. *Health Affairs*, *23*(5), 9–25.
75. Zander, A. R., & Aksamit, I. A. (1990). Immune recovery following bone marrow transplantation. In F. L. Johnson & C. Pochedly (Eds.), *Bone marrow transplantation in children* (pp. 87–110). New York: Raven Press.
76. Zaoutis, L. B., & Chiang, V. W. (Eds.), (2007). Infection control for pediatric hospitalists; Infection control a patient safety issue. In L. B. Zaoutis & V. W. Chiang (Eds.), *Comprehensive Pediatric Hospital Medicine.* Philadelphia: Mosby.
77. Zuckerbraun, N. S., Powell, E. C., Sheehan, K. M., et al. (2004). Community childhood injury surveillance: An emergency department-based mode. *Pediatric Emergency Care*, *20*, 361–366.

SUGGESTED READINGS

Mathews, M. D., & Alexander, M. A. (Eds.), (2010). *Pediatric rehabilitation* (4th ed.). New York: Demos Medical.

Perkin, R. M., Swift, J. D., Newton, E. A., & Anas, N. G. (Eds.), (2008). *Pediatric hospital medicine: Textbook of inpatient management* (2nd ed.). Philadelphia: Lippincott Williams & Wilkins.

CHAPTER

25 Transition to Adulthood

Dennis Cleary • Andrew Persch • Karen Spencer

KEY TERMS

- Transition services
- Transition team
- Individuals with Disabilities Education Act
- Section 504 of the Rehabilitation Act
- Americans with Disabilities Act
- Cradle to College and Career
- Common Core State Standards
- Employment First
- Project SEARCH
- Postsecondary outcomes
- Self-determination
- Emphasis on student's social competence
- Assistive technology
- Collaborative interdisciplinary and interagency teamwork

GUIDING QUESTIONS

1. What must occupational therapists know about the transition to adulthood?
2. What programs are available to support the transition from school to work?
3. What are the indicators of a successful transition to adulthood?
4. How can occupational therapists use evidence-based practices to support individuals in transition?

In the United States, individuals with disabilities may receive a free and appropriate public education through the age of 21 years. For young people 16 to 21 years of age, education is viewed as a way to develop the knowledge, skills, and experience necessary to make the critical transition from school into a variety of adult roles. On leaving high school, young adults with and without disabilities, with their parents, make decisions about their next options, including postsecondary education, paid employment, volunteer work, establishing a home, and participating in meaningful occupations and healthy relationships. When a person has a disability, this transition becomes more complex and often requires timely planning and access to a variety of supports and services that begin during and should extend after high school.

The requirement to provide transition services from school to adult life was established in 1990 by the Individuals with Disabilities Education Act (IDEA; P.L. 101-476). The most recently amended version of IDEA (P.L. 108-446) states that transition-related planning must begin for students with disabilities when they are 16 years old or earlier based on individual student needs (§ 614 (d)(1)(A)(i)(VII)). Students receiving transition-related planning and services may graduate or complete high school at around the age of 18 years with their peers who do not have disabilities. Others may continue to receive school-funded education and transition services through the age of 21. Because the legal requirement for special education and transition services ends on high school graduation, some individuals may choose to delay graduation so that they continue to receive these special education and transition services. High school exit decisions (before age 22) are based on individual student needs and goals as determined by the transition team.

Transition team is a term used throughout this chapter. The team is interdisciplinary, with team members from various professions, and may be interagency, with school employees and employees from nonschool community agencies. The transition team, sometimes called the individualized transition team, is responsible for the development of the student's Individualized Education Program (IEP) and subsequent transition services (§ 614 (d)). Regardless of the team's name, the goal remains the same, and all team members share responsibility for the student's achievement of positive post–high school outcomes.

The student is the most critical and central member of his or her transition team and is joined by an array of school and community professionals. When appropriate, the student's parent or guardian joins the team as an essential partner. It is the student's parents or other family members who usually accompany the student during the entire journey into adult life by providing essential support along the way. In contrast, professional members of the transition team are involved for only portions of the student's journey. When considered in this way, the need for professional members of the transition team to support family members in this process becomes evident.

Students who receive transition services must have a disability that fits one or more of the disability categories recognized by IDEA: intellectual disability; hearing impairment including deafness, speech, or language impairments; visual impairments (including blindness); serious emotional disturbance; orthopedic impairments; autism; traumatic brain injury; other health impairments; or specific learning disabilities (§602 (3)(A)(ii)). Furthermore, students with identified disabilities who receive specialized instruction (special education) are automatically eligible for related services such as occupational therapy.

Occupational Therapy Contributions to Transition

Occupational therapy is included as a transition service when the transition team determines that occupational therapy can help the student access, participate in, and benefit from his or her specialized education and transition services. Regardless of the student's disability label, the occupational therapist's involvement with a particular student is based on that student's demonstrated or anticipated problems in performance and participation in education and transition-related activities and contexts. These contexts may include the high school classroom, a variety of in-school environments, public transportation systems, general community, home, internship placements, community job sites, and more.

Occupational therapists working in schools understand the educational performance and participation demands, opportunities, and challenges experienced by children and youth with disabilities. Of importance, they use conditional reasoning[65] to understand and, to some extent, anticipate how a student's disability may affect his or her transition to post–high school activities and roles, including postsecondary or vocational education, employment, and community living. The occupational therapist's positive, future-oriented view of students combines a commitment to student-centered services, collaborative teamwork, and achievement of performance and participation outcomes, making him or her a valuable addition to a student's transition team.

For example, the occupational therapist may analyze a student's internship site and work with the student's job coach to make recommendations to facilitate a student's successful job performance. The student and job coach continually inform the occupational therapist about the student's job performance to monitor the effects of the recommended modifications and ultimately to measure intervention outcomes. Importantly, occupational therapy outcomes completely align with the intent of IDEA and the goals for student participation in work and community, as defined by the transition team. In summary, occupational therapists provide interventions that support students in establishing new skills, transferring skills to new contexts and activities, and modifying contexts and activities to increase performance and participation and prevent new performance problems.

This chapter connects transition policy and evidence-based practices in a way that allows occupational therapists to understand and articulate their role in the transition process and as members of a collaborative, interdisciplinary, and interagency transition team. A variety of student stories and examples are included throughout to illustrate further how occupational therapists work with transition-age youth. Occupational therapy, when added to the mix of transition services, can make a real difference in the lives of young people whose goals and dreams include some combination of post–high school employment, community living, further education or training, economic self-sufficiency, and social connections.[37]

Intersection of Policy and Scientific Evidence

The federal mandate for comprehensive school to adult life transition services was issued in 1990 following years of study by the Office of Special Education Programs in the U.S. Department of Education.[43,86] Although laws and regulations guaranteeing all children a free and appropriate public education have been in place since enactment of the Education for All Handicapped Children Act (1975; P.L. 94-142), outcome-focused research during the 1980s and 1990s revealed that educational results for youth with disabilities were disappointing at best. The extensive public investment in specialized education and related services was not consistently producing competent, well-adjusted, and self-sufficient adults. High rates of unemployment or underemployment, dependency, and social isolation characterized adults with disabilities who had been served by the special education system.[28,45,51,85]

Although important in the shaping of federal transition policy, early outcome-focused research provided almost no guidance to education and related service professionals in identifying which specific transition practices were most likely to produce the best results for youth. Transition policy, as stated in IDEA (P.L. 105-17), specified system-level processes and expected post–high school outcomes, but did not specify practices to promote those outcomes.

A growing body of evidence has shown that transition services can improve employment and life satisfaction outcomes for individuals with disabilities who receive special education services.[86] Practices with moderate to strong research evidence are most likely to produce positive postsecondary outcomes and provide local school districts with greater confidence that they can meet the intent and letter of IDEA's transition provisions. Education and related service professionals working in transition may leverage these research and policy resources to develop and implement services that prepare youth to reach their adult life goals. See Case Study 25-1.

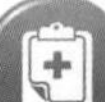

CASE STUDY 25-1 Bright Futures in Focus

Debora Davidson is an occupational therapist who works with transition-age young adults who have disabilities. She became aware that many young adults with disabilities seemed to fall through the cracks of school and VR systems and struggled to succeed after they graduated from high school. These individuals did not get jobs despite their efforts, had difficulty making friends, and had limited ability or knowledge about how to participate in their community. As an occupational therapist with over 35 years of experience in clinical, community, and educational settings, she realized that these young adults' futures were not going to improve with the current services available to them. She thought that an innovative occupational therapy approach could help improve their prognosis and help them to engage and participate in life more fully.

In June 2011, Debora left a career in academia and founded Bright Futures in Focus to help meet this untapped need to serve transition-age young adults in and around St. Louis. Debora is the creative developer and provider of clinical services for Bright Futures. She founded the practice with her husband, Ken Bolyard (LCSW, MPH) who manages the business side of the practice. Bright Futures is a small business that is fee-for-service; clients and their families pay directly for her services (Bright Futures does not accept insurance). Fee-for-service helps decrease overhead costs and allows Debora to practice occupational therapy as she thinks is appropriate for the client. She is not subject to insurance restrictions on how or what she does with clients.

Bright Futures helps transition-age young adults attain education, work, and leisure goals. Debora provides instruction and coaching to improve their skills and locates places and activities that are a fit for her clients' unique abilities and interests. She works directly with clients in their homes, workplaces, and communities.

Debora works with individuals and families to develop a vision for their future that is exciting and attainable. She helps identify local resources and suggests or develops creative options. This process is always done together with her client to ensure that his or her needs are met. Debora and the client can work together to develop solutions for immediate, short-term, and long-term challenges. Debora created the Bright Futures Service Menu, which encourages clients to prioritize areas in which they would like help (Figure 25-1). Categories in the service menu include work, education, leisure, living,

BRIGHTFUTURES
personalized transition consulting

Client Name:	Date:

Bright Futures Service Menu

Below are some examples of services that Bright Futures can provide. Please consider each item, and check the items that apply to you. Then, indicate priority by checking *high, medium,* or *low*.

WORK **I would like to....**	*Low priority*	*Medium priority*	*High priority*
Learn about skills for jobs I am interested in			
Create a resume			
Apply for jobs			
Volunteer for community agencies			
Learn about work habits and attitudes for keeping a job			
Practice the speaking skills for a job interview			
Explore different careers based on my interests, goals, and abilities			
Receive support or coaching on the job or volunteer site			
Have a consultant to work with my employer			
Start my own business			
Learn about workplace accommodations and/or job task modifications			
Other (please specify):			
EDUCATION **I would like to....**	*Low priority*	*Medium priority*	*High priority*
Organize my academic or work life			
Choose a course of study and/or institution			
Establish study habits needed for college			
Follow a schedule or routine			
Increase computer, email, or technology skills			
Use the internet to find information			
Use a planner or calendar to stay organized			
Better coordinate my educational services/ accommodations			
Find a peer mentor at my school			
Establish a transition plan for leaving or entering school			
Other (please specify):			

FIGURE 25-1 Service menu to prioritize goal setting.

Continued

CASE STUDY 25-1 Bright Futures in Focus—cont'd

LIVING SKILLS **I would like to….**	*Low priority*	*Medium priority*	*High priority*
Create a routine for daily living			
Live on my own			
Improve my self care or personal hygiene			
Use a bank account			
Take care of my home (chores, minor repairs, etc.)			
Do my own laundry			
Manage my own medicines			
Pay my own bills			
Cook my own hot meals			
Budget my money			
Use public transportation			
Learn to drive			
Plan a week of meals			
Work on childcare, pet care, of care of others			
Learn about assistive technology			
Modify my home environment to better suit my needs			
Other (please specify):			
SOCIAL/ LEISURE **I would like to….**	*Low priority*	*Medium priority*	*High priority*
Find friends to hang out with who share common interests with me			
Have fun activities that I do in my free time			
Find out about local social/leisure groups, programs, or clubs that interest me			
Plan a vacation			
Go on dates			
Develop my network of support			
Other (please specify):			
CITIZENSHIP **I would like to….**	*Low priority*	*Medium priority*	*High priority*
Register to vote			
Learn about my basic legal rights (relating to my disability, work, school, personal)			
Become more involved in my community			
Create a plan for what to do if stopped by the police			
Other (please specify):			
PERSONAL **I would like to….**	*Low priority*	*Medium priority*	*High priority*
Make healthier food choices			
Learn about energy conservation			
Make informed choices regarding sexual behavior			
Establish an exercise routine			
Set goals for myself			
Find a doctor who takes care of my health needs			
Find a lawyer to assist with long term planning or guardianship			
Find a counselor to help with my mental health needs			
Learn about how to disclose my disability in different situations (work, school, personal)			
Explore avenues for spiritual and/or religious expression			
Other (please specify):			

Bright Futures Service Menu http://b-futures.com/ Debora A. Davidson, Ph.D., OTR/L

FIGURE 25-1, cont'd

CASE STUDY 25-1 Bright Futures in Focus—cont'd

citizenship, and personal skills. The service menu allows the client to help prioritize goals to work on in occupational therapy.

The client goes through the 57 different items on the service menu and prioritizes each as high, medium, or low priority, or the client might prioritize a goal that is not listed on the service menu. The service menu is useful to ensure that the client's priorities are addressed.

After the client fills out the service menu, Debora interviews the client and family and may choose to conduct a typical occupational therapy assessment if it can provide necessary information to help the client meet his or her goals. Often the client has had negative experiences with labels and the sense of defeat that can come with standardized assessments, so Debora may choose to base goals and treatment decisions on options from the service menu and client interview rather than a standardized assessment.

After she gets to know a client, Debora locates services, programs, or community opportunities that may meet the client's specific needs and preferences, and then she and the client test these new opportunities together. Debora matches clients with paid or volunteer work opportunities in the community and provides skilled job coaching and consultation to employers. She also helps clients locate and try out social activities until they are comfortable accessing these independently. When a client is denied services or funding, she serves as a diplomatic and tenacious advocate and assists families in deciphering and completing complicated bureaucratic paperwork.

Bright Futures has a regular bowling night, free of charge, that clients are welcome to attend. This is an event that can occur in any weather, and clients are welcome to bring friends or family. It is a night of fun that offers natural opportunities to meet new people, work out transportation, practice social skills, and provide a small start to structuring a person's week. Bowling provides a topic for the young adult to talk about at family events and is an event that he or she can count on every week to meet new people, build existing friendships, and develop a hobby.

Bright Futures is different from traditional social service agencies, which offer clients a limited array of choices from which they must make a forced selection. Bright Futures starts by discovering what clients really want from life and then seeks to find ways to achieve those dreams. Debora meets with clients at times and places that are convenient to them and provides transportation to sites in the community to test out options for work, education, or social activities. She strives to use the natural resources found within the client's own community and family, promoting inclusion and a durable base of ongoing support. She facilitates clients' development of skills and habits needed for full participation and success. Clients let her know what they want to achieve, and they guide Debora's actions throughout their work together. The goal is to reach the bright future that the client desires.

Transition to Adulthood in America

Individuals with Disabilities Education Act

The Individuals with Disabilities Education Improvement Act of 2004 (P.L. 108-446), known as IDEA, is the federal law most responsible for ensuring that children and youth with disabilities have access to publicly funded, individualized education, including school to adult life transition services. Initially passed in 1975, IDEA is the law responsible for the strong presence of occupational therapists in public schools. Foundational to the IDEA are the following core beliefs expressed by the Congress and written into the law:

Disability is a natural part of the human experience and in no way diminishes the right of individuals to participate in or contribute to society. Improving educational results for children with disabilities is an essential element of our national policy of ensuring equality of opportunity, full participation, independent living, and economic self-sufficiency for individuals with disabilities (§ 601(d)(1)(A)).

Beginning with the 1997 amendments to IDEA, participation of all students within the general education context became a central focus. Specifically, students with disabilities receiving specialized instruction (special education) were expected to participate and show progress in the general curriculum alongside their same-age peers without disabilities. This means that for students with and without disabilities, the general education standards provide educational achievement and performance targets.

With specialized support, many students with disabilities can and will achieve the general education standards expected of all students. For other students with disabilities, steady progress toward general education standards is the expectation. IDEA's focus on student participation in general education has significantly raised the educational bar for the nation's children and youth with disabilities. The general education focus of IDEA challenges previously held views and practices of separate special and general education programs, staff, and curricula.[22,43,86]

Accompanying the shift toward a single general education system, special educators and related service personnel, including occupational therapists, are similarly shifting their roles and activities to support students and their teachers better within a variety of general education and transition-related contexts. Collaboration with teachers, job coaches, employers, and others characterizes the evolving role of transition-focused occupational therapists who are expected to help students achieve postsecondary education, vocational training, employment, and/or community living outcomes. Figure 25-2 depicts a student who attends a university and also works at university swim meets.

Occupational therapists working under the auspices of IDEA must understand the overarching purpose of the law and its key provisions. The full text of the IDEA law and a variety of interpretive resources are readily available at the U.S. Department of Education website (see the Evolve website) and are

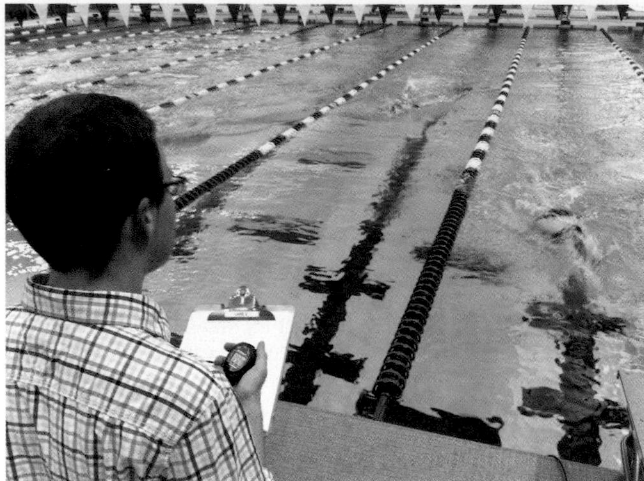

FIGURE 25-2 Intern timing college swimmers at practice.

essential reading for school-based occupational therapists. IDEA defines transition services as a coordinated set of activities for a child with a disability that:

(A) is designed to be within a results-oriented process that is focused on improving the academic and functional achievement of the child with a disability to facilitate the child's movement from school to post-school activities, including post-secondary education, vocational education, integrated employment (including supported employment), continuing and adult education, adult services, independent living, or community participation; (B) is based on the individual child's needs, taking into account the child's strengths, preferences, and interests; and (C) includes instruction, related services, community experiences, the development of employment and other post-school adult living objectives and, when appropriate, acquisition of daily living skills and functional vocational evaluation (§ 602(26)).

Section 504 of the Rehabilitation Act

Transition services may include reasonable accommodations under Section 504 of the Rehabilitation Act (as amended in 1998 by P.L. 93-516). Initially signed into law in 1973, Section 504 was among the first civil rights laws prohibiting discrimination on the basis of disability by any program or agency that receives federal funding. Section 504 defines individuals with disabilities as "persons with a physical or mental impairment which substantially limits one or more major life activities" (34 C.F.R. § 104.3 (j)(2)(i)). Subparts of the law prohibit discrimination in employment, building and program accessibility, schooling (preschool through secondary education), and postsecondary education (colleges, universities, community colleges, vocational programs).

Students who have disabilities but do not qualify for an IEP may be entitled to reasonable accommodations through Section 504. Occupational therapists are experts in identifying the need for and providing resources to create accommodations. The term *reasonable accommodation* means that an

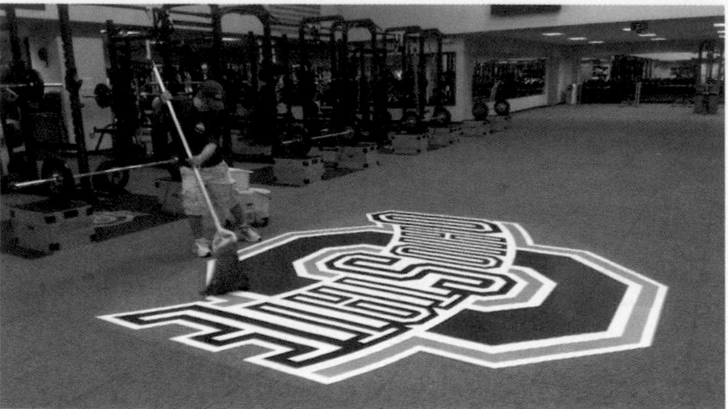

FIGURE 25-3 Intern mopping a football team's weight room.

employer (or educational institution) must take reasonable steps to accommodate an individual's disability. Examples include installing grab bars in work or learning areas, purchasing assistive technology (AT) devices to support job or school performance, ensuring that online materials are presented in an accessible format, adding an entrance ramp, or providing specific job-related training (see the Evolve website) The term *reasonable,* although somewhat vague, is used in the law to protect employers from undue hardship when accommodations are needed or requested. The law recognizes that for some employers, the resources needed to provide accommodations for an individual employee who has a disability may exceed employer resources. Most accommodations, however, are low cost, which is outweighed by the benefit of having a motivated and reliable worker who happens to have a disability.

Prevention of disability-related discrimination is at the core of the Rehabilitation Act and Section 504, but the law also created a nationwide network of state vocational rehabilitation (VR) services to enable potential workers with disabilities ultimately to enter and be successful in the workforce. Vocational rehabilitation is supported by a blend of federal and state funding and provides needed employment and independent living support for adults with disabilities. An individual who is eligible for VR services works with a VR counselor, who can serve as an important member of a school-based transition team. The VR counselor is expected to work together with school personnel to plan for the student's future job-related education and training, job placement, and independent living. VR can provide qualified individuals with needed financial support for job training, job placement services, job coaching, postsecondary education, and independent living. In all cases, VR-supported services are outcome oriented, with community employment and improved self-sufficiency as the end goal. School-based occupational therapists may work closely with VR counselors on behalf of young adults with disabilities to optimize the match between the individual and available job or postsecondary education opportunities, recommend needed accommodations, and address community and independent living needs (Figure 25-3).

Americans with Disabilities Act

The Americans with Disabilities Act (ADA) of 1990 (amended in 2008; P.L. 110-325) is a civil rights law and, like Section 504 of the Rehabilitation Act, focuses on accessibility and nondiscrimination. Unlike Section 504, ADA protections

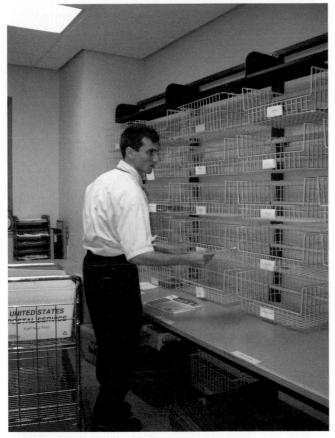

FIGURE 25-4 Intern delivering mail in clearly labeled bins.

BOX 25-1 Vision for Cradle to College and Career

- All youth have access to adequate and equitably funded quality early intervention and education that meets the diverse needs of families and children and fosters social, emotional, and developmental and educational readiness.
- Parents and students are strong stakeholders.
- Strong interagency agreements and collaboration with informal support networks are present.
- All children have the right to leave the pre-K–12 system with a diploma or credential meaningful to the individual.
- All youth are educated in a safe, supportive, and caring environment in which they feel connected and supported.
- All youth are involved in relevant and rigorous preparation activities that focus on twenty-first-century skills.
- All youth have their unique needs met and have the opportunity to be productive citizens, have choices about their outcomes, and have full access to and are involved in the community.
- All youth are engaged in meaningful, active learning school experiences that result in successful school and postschool outcomes.
- A comprehensive and coordinated system of services and supports is essential.
- All youth are working and developing to their greatest potential within an integrated, seamless lifelong system of services.
- Vocational rehabilitation is an integral, integrated, and early part of the team.

IDEA Partnership, 2013f. Retrieved August 5, 2014 from: http://ideapartnership.org.

extend beyond programs and services that receive federal funding. The ADA addresses access and discrimination in public and private schools, business establishments, and public buildings. The law also establishes clear accessibility standards for new building construction and public facilities. Occupational therapists who work with transition-age youth should become familiar with the ADA and its many provisions so they can assist employers and public facilities to eliminate barriers and provide reasonable accommodations for young adults with disabilities. Figure 25-4 shows a student sorting mail. The occupational therapist has replaced the mailboxes with larger bins and labeled with larger signs to accommodate this student in visually organizing a mail-sorting task.

Cradle to College and Career

Cradle to College and Career (CCC) is a state-led initiative that emerged in the mid-1990s in Georgia, Maryland, and Oregon to improve outcomes for at-risk students. CCC has since spread in some form to most states as part of the P-16 (preschool to college graduation) movement.[79] The CCC concept creates an educational continuum beginning at birth (cradle) that supports a student's educational needs through graduation from college or other postsecondary program and career placement. See Box 25-1.

CCC works to develop an integrated service delivery system that focuses energy and resources starting at an early age to long-term employment and life success. This focus on academic, employment, and independent living skills is important for all students, but especially for students with disabilities. As the child grows and transitions between grade levels, these services and supports must grow and adapt with the student.[32] It is never too early to focus school-based services on a student's transition to adulthood. Similarly, as students are encouraged to take responsibility for themselves and their life goals, outcomes improve.[67]

The current transition system for students may involve different agencies, such as school districts, developmental disability boards, and state rehabilitation agencies, that function in silos and do not communicate well with each other.[73] In the CCC model, schools focus energy and effort to help students succeed as they transition from one grade to the next, from one school to the next, and from high school to a postsecondary program. A student who has access to services through a VR agency or community agency must have those services linked with the student's school curriculum. The goal of CCC is to have schools work with these employment agencies and employers so that the student has the tools necessary for employment and engagement in life.[33]

Additional supports may be necessary to encourage students with disabilities or other at-risk students to continue with their education, rather than drop out of school. These supports may include services outside the traditional academic environment such as scouting, Big Brothers, Big Sisters, and volunteer experiences to provide the opportunity for students to develop many of the soft skills necessary to succeed in life that may be difficult to replicate in a typical academic setting.[20]

CCC takes a lifelong view of the student to determine what skills the student will need to be successful in life.[33] The goal is for all transitions in a student's life to be purposeful to ensure that each academic year builds on the previous year's efforts. The student and his or her transition team focus on continuity and integration as the student moves in a coordinated fashion from grade level to grade level, from school to school, and from school to career.[78]

CCC is promoted by the IDEA partnership, a group of more than 50 national associations, including the American Occupational Therapy Association (AOTA), who work together to improve outcomes for youth with disabilities.[34] The partnership seeks to build coordinated systems of service delivery that support student learning outcomes while reducing long-term costs.[35] In 2007, the estimated cost to taxpayers for someone who drops out of high school before graduating was more than $240,000 over that person's lifetime in additional health care and welfare costs and in decreased tax revenues because of lower lifetime earnings.[41] Those costs have certainly increased since 2007 in today's dollars.

Occupational therapists can play an important role in the CCC model because of the emphasis on community models and on collaboration among community agencies and schools. They are uniquely qualified to assess a student's occupational performance, design interventions within community contexts, and help students develop the skills necessary to be successful in employment and in life.

Common Core State Standards

The Common Core State Standards (CCSS) are a national curricula in English-Language Arts (ELA) and Mathematics that define the knowledge and skills that all students should master by the end of each grade level so they are ready for college and a career.[16] CCSS were developed in response to the increase in the number of high school graduates who were not prepared for the rigor of college or were not adequately prepared to enter the workforce.[14] CCSS have been approved and adopted by 45 states and are the first national curricula for the United States.[57]

The National Governor's Association developed the Common Core to raise standards so that U.S. students remain competitive with students from other countries.[1] A benefit of one national standard instead of 50 different state standards is that the expectations for high school juniors in Ohio are the same as for those for high school juniors in South Dakota, so if a student moved from South Dakota to Ohio, the standards would remain the same. States and school districts remain free to write individual curricula to meet the CCSS.[11]

The focus of the Common Core is to identify skills needed by twenty-first-century learners, with an emphasis on the application of content to real-world expectations.[74] Although it is important for students to learn their mathematics facts, the ability to apply them competently in everyday life is most essential (Box 25-2). U.S. business leaders and educational experts provided considerable input during development of the CCSS to ensure that high school students would be adequately prepared for the needs of the future workforce.

This emphasis on real-world expectations and college and career readiness is well aligned with the focus on high-quality, integrated, practical transition services for students with disabilities. Occupational therapists are well positioned to support students in this transition to college or career readiness. Public schools are a large employer of occupational therapists, but only 16% of school-based occupational therapists report that they work with adolescents and transition age-students.[37] Occupational therapists are well named and well suited to help individuals develop skills that lead to actual occupations. They offer expertise in areas essential in employment success, such as task analysis and matching the demands and abilities of the person, occupation, and environment. Figure 25-5 shows a young adult with high skills in following a written procedure, sorting, and categorizing who is working in a university laboratory.

BOX 25-2 Expected Outcomes of Common Core State Standards

Graduates will do the following:

- Demonstrate independence.
- Build strong content knowledge.
- Respond to varying demands of audience, task, purpose, and discipline.
- Comprehend as well as critique.
- Value evidence.
- Use technology and digital media strategically and capably.
- Understand other perspectives and cultures.

National Governors Association, 2013. Retrieved August 5, 2014 from: http://www.corestandards.org.

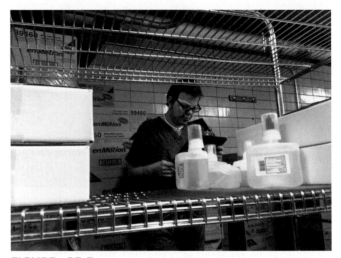

FIGURE 25-5 Intern checking inventory in university laboratory.

Employment First

Employment First is a national movement that seeks to promote community-based employment in lieu of sheltered workshops as the preferred choice for individuals with disabilities.[52] To accomplish this goal, Employment First proponents seek to change government funding structures and service delivery systems and policies so that community employment options are available and tax dollars are prioritized toward supporting community employment. Policy changes that foster community employment over sheltered work settings include government

BOX 25-3 Vocational Choices for Young Adults with Disabilities

- Internships to prepare for employment
- Supported employment
- Customized employment
- Self-employment
- Day program or sheltered workshop
- Community rehabilitation program
- Competitive employment and business models

Adapted from Wehman, P., & Brooke, V. (2013). Securing meaningful work in the community: Vocational internships, placements, and careers. In P. Wehman (Ed.), *Life beyond the classroom: Transition strategies for young people with disabilities* (pp. 310–338). Baltimore, MD: Paul H. Brookes.

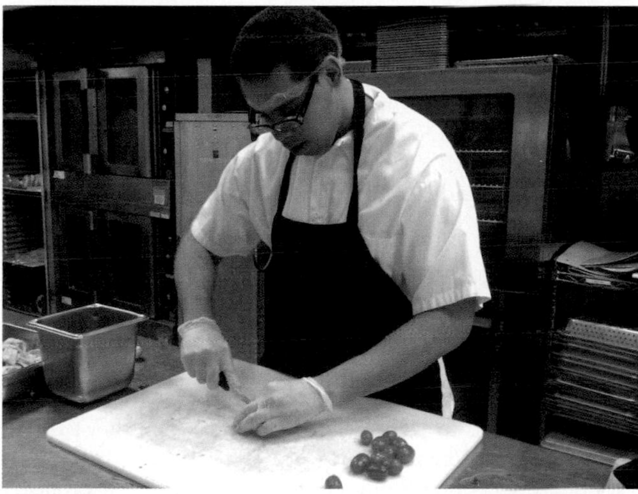

FIGURE 25-6 Intern cutting tomatoes for a salad in dorm cafeteria.

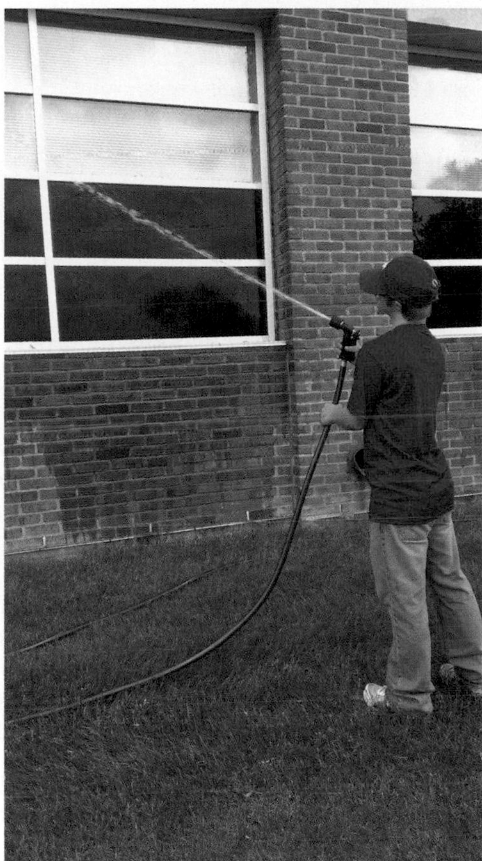

FIGURE 25-7 Intern washing windows at a college football training facility.

funding for community employment services and Medicaid buy-ins attached to the person, instead of to the sheltered workshop. The buy-in allows an individual who receives federal disability or health insurance benefits to earn an income without the risk of losing government health insurance.[66] Individuals with disabilities and their families are empowered to make employment decisions that are best for them and that encourage community employment.

Given a variety of vocational choices for young adults with disabilities (Box 25-3), Employment First prioritizes community employment. The use of internships as a primary Employment First approach has consistently resulted in positive, community-based employment outcomes. For example, Project SEARCH is a 1-year transition to community employment program that combines on-site internships, job coaching, and an employment skills curriculum.[29] Students work 20 hours/week in an unpaid internship as they develop skills on the job and in the classroom-based employment skills curriculum. Students progress through three 3-month internships during the school year, often in their last year of public education (Figure 25-6). Students build their resumés, learn to use public transportation or drive, and practice job-searching strategies with the goal of interviewing for and obtaining a paid position at the conclusion of the Project Search experience.

Cincinnati Children's hospital developed the first Project SEARCH site almost 20 years ago, and, at present, Project SEARCH has established more than 250 sites throughout the United States and in four other countries.[60] Project SEARCH is typically a partnership between a school district and the state vocational rehabilitation agency. Many Project SEARCH sites are in health care settings, with the emphasis on finding jobs that are well suited for an individual's unique talents.

Research evidence has suggested that a history of internships improves employment outcomes.[80] Internships may be chosen to suit an individual's skills or to give an individual the opportunity to learn or develop new skills. The job coach learns the job from the employer and instructs the student in how to complete the job. As the student's ability grows, the job coaching fades until the student is completing the job independently. Figure 25-7 depicts a student who has become independent in window washing for the football team's training facility. The stated goal is that 90% of Project SEARCH graduates become employed at the conclusion of the program, and each year a number of the program sites reach at least that 90% goal.[61] Figure 25-8 depicts a Project SEARCH graduate working at a university library.

Think College

Think College aspires to have individuals with intellectual disabilities attend college for the same reason that individuals without intellectual disabilities go to college: to decide on a

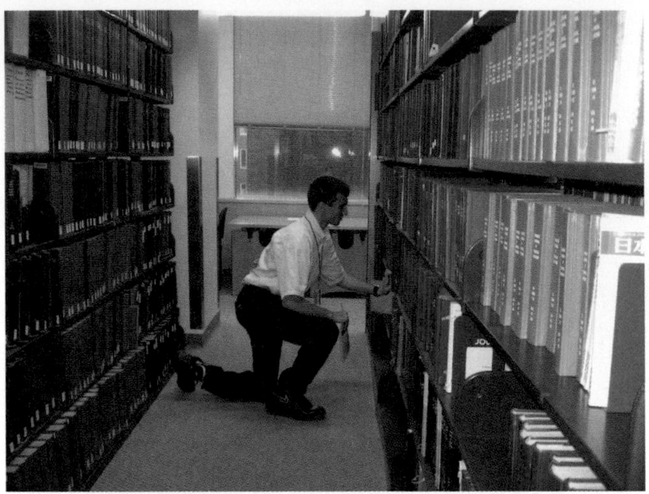

FIGURE 25-8 Intern shelving journals at a library.

career, make friends and establish connections, and improve their earning potential to "get a better job."[26] These students have been in school with their typical peers since preschool; Think College wants to know why inclusion should stop after high school. Think College promotes postsecondary opportunities for individuals with intellectual disabilities, and currently these programs are in 214 different college and university campuses in the United States.[82] Each program is different, but each offers students pathways for integration into typical campus life. Students enroll in courses, attend campus sporting and cultural events, use campus athletic and recreational facilities, and may live in campus housing. They may receive supports that are available to all students, such as those offered by the campus office of disability services or from their course instructors during typical office hours. Other students may receive additional supports, such as an academic coach or a study table specific to students in the Think College program.[54] Some programs offer additional life skills and vocational training to augment the academic program. The length of the programs varies from 1 to 4 years, and some students earn degrees or certificates. Some Think College programs are paid for by state vocational rehabilitation agencies or developmental disability funds. When public funds are not available, students and their families may choose to pay for tuition, room, and board.

Seamless Transition: Alignment of Outcomes

Two common goals of these transition programs—Cradle to College and Career, Common Core State Standards, Employment First, and Think College—are to raise expectations and improve long-term outcomes (e.g., schools, vocational rehabilitation, developmental disability) for individuals with disabilities. To achieve improved outcomes, the educational system, government developmental disability agencies and vocational rehabilitation agencies must work together, and transition planning must be in place throughout a student's schooling. The concept of a seamless transition from high school to postsecondary education and career is designed to keep the young adult on track to achieve a successful employment outcome.[12]

One example of nonseamless transition is assistive technology (AT). In most states, the school districts that purchase technology for students to use during high school require that the technology be returned when the student graduates. If that technology was beneficial to the transitioning student, doesn't it make sense for the student to own that technology? Occupational therapists can consider VR as a better funding source for AT for use in employment because the device is owned by the student. It follows that cooperation and coordination between schools and VR for the purchase of needed technology can improve employment outcomes.[73]

It is imperative that the transition from high school to postsecondary employment or academic pursuits is smooth and coordinated and that the student is well prepared for adulthood. Once a student receives his or her high school diploma, the federal mandate for educational and related services expires, and the youth moves into a system that may not have the same financial resources and expertise as that of the public schools.[49]

Transition Outcomes

In 2011, the U.S. Office of Special Education Programs reported that 6,530,552 students with disabilities were served under IDEA, Part B.[77] Of these, 2,163,479 students were aged 14 to 21 years, and 644,694 were in their last year of school. Taken together, these data reveal that roughly one third of children eligible for services under Part B of IDEA may be thought of as being of transition age—that is, being 14 to 16 years of age (depending on locality) or older and having an IEP with measurable postsecondary goals and transition services. These data also reveal that about 10% of youth with disabilities will exit the public schools any given year.

What happens to youth with disabilities when they exit the public schools? Where do they go? What do they do? What services are available? Studies have shown that postsecondary outcomes experienced by youth in transition to adulthood vary widely; some students work and/or go on to postsecondary education, but others do not go on to postsecondary education or employment.

Transition from high school to postsecondary life is often complicated by the different and sometimes competing perspectives of the various stakeholders (e.g., student, teacher, parent, community organization) involved in transition.[19] For example, special educators and related service personnel are likely to view transition to postsecondary education and/or competitive employment as the key markers of a successful transition. By contrast, vocational rehabilitation professionals (e.g., vocational counselors, job developers, job coaches) tend to emphasize the acquisition of competitive employment as the primary indicator of a successful transition to adulthood. Representatives from the state's board of developmental disabilities focus on the living arrangements, health, safety, and welfare of individuals in transition. Parents and families may prioritize health, wellness, and happiness as the most important outcomes for their child in transition. Consequently, identifying agreed-on transition outcomes may require negotiation among the students, families, and professionals involved in the transition process. Often young adults thrive in job tasks with easily learned, concrete, repetitive steps and work environments that offer opportunities to interact with peers (Figure 25-9).

Occupational therapists who understand these differences can help students and families prepare for and navigate the intricacies of the transition process. Table 25-1 summarizes the

TABLE 25-1 Interdisciplinary Transition Teams and Outcome Orientations

Organization	Personnel Involved	Outcome Orientation—Transition Target
School district	Individualized education program team Community partners	Academics Postsecondary education and/or postsecondary employment
Vocational rehabilitation (VR) agency	VR counselor Community rehabilitation provider	Employment
Board of Development Disabilities	Case manager	Health, wellness, and community living
Family	Parent Caregiver Student	Health, quality of life, independent living skills, education, employment

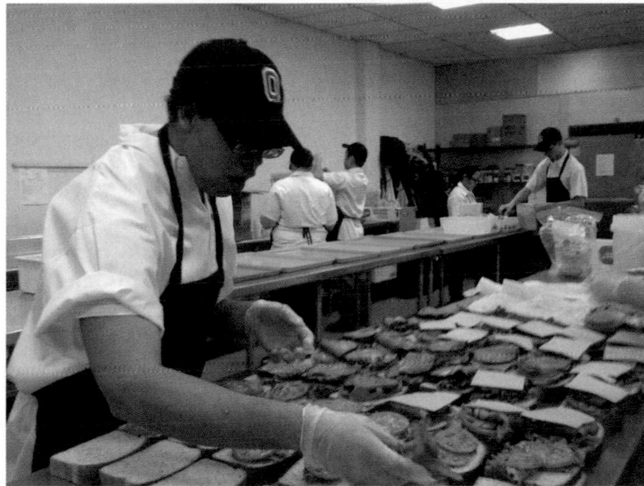

FIGURE 25-9 Intern preparing sandwiches for a university event.

different, and sometimes competing, perspectives of the stakeholders involved in the transition planning process.

Postsecondary Education Outcomes

For most adolescents and their families, matriculation to postsecondary institutions and, eventually, competitive employment remain the primary objectives of secondary education. In the context of transition outcomes, the term *postsecondary education* refers broadly to participation in three types of institutions: (1) 2-year or community colleges; (2) vocational, business, or technical schools; and (3) 4-year colleges. Understanding outcomes for youth with disabilities at these types of institutions is important for students, families, and professionals contributing to the transition planning and decision-making process.

After exiting high school, youth with disabilities pursue postsecondary education at rates lower than those without disabilities.[51] The National Longitudinal Transition Study-2 (NLTS2) followed a representative sample of more than 11,000 high school students who received special education services in high school into early adulthood to determine educational, employment, and social outcomes. The NLTS2 revealed that 60% of young adults with disabilities enroll in postsecondary education within 8 years of leaving high school.[51] By comparison, 67% of young adults without disabilities pursue postsecondary educational opportunities in the years after high school. Young adults with disabilities matriculate to postsecondary institutions at different rates, depending on their primary disability category (Table 25-2). Enrollment in postsecondary education is lowest for individuals with intellectual disabilities (28.7%), multiple disabilities (32.8%), and autism spectrum disorder (43.9%). Furthermore, the results of the NLTS2[51] indicate the following for youth with disabilities:

- They are more likely to pursue education at a 2-year institution than at a 4-year institution.
- They may take longer to matriculate to school.
- They may not consider themselves disabled by the time they enter postsecondary settings.
- They may require assistance requesting accommodations.

Postsecondary Employment Outcomes

Like postsecondary education, employment remains a key objective of youth in transition to adulthood. Employment is important for a number of reasons. Workers experience the socioeconomic benefit of earned wages and related benefits in terms of better health and quality of life. Interviews conducted as part of the NLTS2 indicated that young adults with disabilities were employed outside their homes at a rate of 60%.[51] By comparison, 66% of young adults without disabilities reported currently working. Like the picture of postsecondary education, the employment figures vary as a function of disability (see Table 25-2). Employment outside the home was lowest for individuals with deafness-blindness (30.1%), orthopedic impairment (35.0%), autism spectrum disorder (37.2%), and intellectual disabilities (38.8%). Generally, young adults with disabilities tended to work fewer hours for lower wages.[86] They also tended to retain employment for shorter periods of time, often less than 12 months.[51]

Community Participation and Inclusion

As depicted in Table 25-1, employment and education are not the only outcomes considered by an IEP team engaged in the transition planning process. For example, an adolescent may consider the acquisition of independent living skills to be his or her highest priority. According to the NLTS2[51]:

- 19% of young adults with disabilities engaged in community-based activities beyond education and employment.
- 59% of young adults with disabilities lived independently within 8 years of exiting high school.
- 59% of young adults with disabilities had checking and savings accounts.

TABLE 25-2 Outcome Data for Young Adults with Disabilities*

Disability Category	Ever Enrolled in Postsecondary Education (%)	Employed at Time of NLTS2 Interview (%)
Learning disability	66.8	67.3
Speech-language impairment	66.9	63.9
Mental retardation	28.7	38.8
Emotional disturbance	53.0	49.6
Hearing impairment	74.7	57.2
Visual impairment	71.0	43.8
Orthopedic impairment	62.0	35.0
Other health impairment	65.7	64.4
Autism	43.9	37.2
Traumatic brain injury	61.0	51.6
Multiple disabilities	32.8	39.2
Deafness-blindness	56.8	30.1

*Young adults (21-29 yr).
Adapted from Newman, L., Wagner, M., Knokey, A., Marder, C., Nagle, K., Shaver, D., et al.; National Center for Special Education Research (Eds.). (2011). *The post-high school outcomes of young adults with disabilities up to 8 years after high school: A report from the National Longitudinal Transition Study-2 (NLTS2)* (Tables 2 and 19). National Center for Special Education Research. Retreived August 5, 2014 from: http://ies.ed.gov/ncser/

- 77% of young adults with disabilities visited friends weekly outside of organized activities.
- 78% of young adults with disabilities had driving privileges.
- Many young adults with disabilities reported negative experiences, such as getting in a fight or having an encounter with law enforcement.

Participation in the meaningful activities of adulthood, such as education, employment, and community living, remains elusive for many individuals with disabilities. Recognition of these outcomes for a significant portion of young adults is the first step toward their remediation. Occupational therapists working in transition settings (e.g., schools, community) may help youth with disabilities prepare for life after high school by using evidence-based practices designed to improve these important outcomes.

Best Practices in Occupational Therapy

Federal education policy and universal commitment to civil rights and equal educational opportunity mobilized initial school to adult life transition efforts. Federal policies (e.g., IDEA) specify expected education outcomes and processes that must be followed by state and local education agencies to ensure that all children have access to a free and appropriate education. Policies, however, do not specify which research-supported practices are most likely to produce the desired outcomes.

The use of evidence-based transition practices is an expectation of the IDEA; that is, services must be based on "peer-reviewed research to the extent practicable" (§ 614 (d)(1)(A)(i)(IV)). Like special education, the occupational therapy profession is dedicated to the principles of evidence-based practice and the ongoing development of rigorous research that can lead to effective services and optimal outcomes for individuals, groups, and organizations.[42]

In recent years, scholars and practitioners have agreed that a number of evidence-based practices increase the probability of youth's success in postsecondary life. Although some are more established than others, all may be considered occupational therapy best practices when working with youth in transition. Recommended transition practices include the following:

1. Early, paid work experience
2. Student involvement in transition planning
3. Emphasis on student's social competence
4. Development of life skills
5. Use of assistive technology
6. Collaborative interdisciplinary and interagency teamwork

Early, Paid Work Experience

Work is one of the most fundamental human occupations. Identify, self-worth, health, socioeconomic status (SES), and quality of life (QoL) are strongly linked to one's ability to work independently and earn a living wage.[15,55] Beyond the functional and economic implications, work also provides a social-cognitive structure through which people interact with and experience the world.[19] Engagement in meaningful work enables the development of social networks and self-efficacy, provides a sense of belonging and security, and contributes to overall health and quality of life. People who fail to acquire and/or maintain meaningful employment experience the parallel negative effects.[68]

Work is important for individuals of all skill and ability levels. Unfortunately individuals with disabilities are employed at rates significantly lower than those of nondisabled individuals.[10] In 2011, only 17.8% of individuals with a disability were employed, compared with 63.6% for individuals without a disability.[9] The impacts of such unemployment or underemployment are significant. An estimated 21.7% of individuals with a disability (compared with 12.8% of individuals without a disability) live below the poverty line.[83] Therefore, individuals with a disability are less likely to be employed and more likely to live in poverty. It follows that individuals with disabilities who work are less likely to live in poverty and that employment is a path to socioeconomic independence for individuals with disabilities.[10,83]

Employment is also strongly related to health and quality of life. Employment status (employed, unemployed) is known to influence health in nondisabled[64,76] and disabled populations.[48,56] These studies have suggested that employed individuals tend to experience better health than unemployed individuals. This relationship may be particularly true for individuals with disabilities. Because individuals with disabilities are employed at lower rates than those without disabilities, they may experience the effects of ill health to a greater degree than nondisabled individuals. Quality of life is similarly affected by employment status. That is, employed individuals tend to experience a higher quality of life than unemployed individuals.[17,21,36,38,48,59,69]

Student engagement in paid work before his or her exit from high school is strongly associated with postsecondary employment[51] and likely leads to the benefits described in the previous paragraph. Even for students who plan to pursue postsecondary education, the ability to maintain employment is considered a critical life skill that cannot be delayed until all formal education is complete.[46]

Although secondary students secure paid work using a variety of strategies,[7] students who have disabilities may lack the skills needed to access or use conventional job search strategies effectively. For these students, supported employment provides an important, evidence-based alternative.[39,44,63] In supported employment, youth and adults receive on-the-job training and ongoing supports provided by a job coach to acquire and sustain employment in community businesses and organizations.

When an individual with a disability struggles to find or maintain employment through supported employment, the transition team may consider customized employment. As an alternative approach, customized employment "is a process for individualizing the employment relationship between a job seeker or an employee and an employer in ways that meet the needs of both."[87] In this model, an employment specialist works with the client (individual with a disability) and prospective employers in the community to match the individual strengths and needs of the job seeker with the needs of the business. Often this requires negotiating the rearranging or combining of job tasks into a job that is customized for the individual with a disability.

Enabling youth who have disabilities to secure community employment that is meaningful and individually matched to their skills and abilities is among the most important achievements of transition teams. Youth can apply for and receive VR resources to help in securing employment; these resources can support the student's job search and placement process or fund postsecondary education at a university, community college, or vocational training program as long as a career or job path is evident.[3,47] If the goal is not building skills for eventual employment, VR agencies will not fund services.

A recent review of the transition literature[46] has identified a number of work-related behaviors and experiences that relate to successful postsecondary employment outcomes. Participation in work-study programs, vocational education classes, job internships, and mentoring experiences are all known to increase the likelihood of obtaining full-time employment after high school. When students are given opportunities to practice self-management skills, such as timeliness, orderliness, and cleanliness, they are more likely to succeed in the working world. Students who learn to express their desire for work, actively pursue work, and obtain work during the high school years are likely to matriculate into postsecondary education and/or employment after transition. Occupational therapists working with transition teams can help facilitate positive outcomes by ensuring that postsecondary goals and services target these factors. See Case Study 25-2.

Student Involvement in Transition Planning

Beginning at age 16 years (age 14 in some states), IDEA requires that a student's IEP specifies measurable transition goals and needed services. Transition goals must be based on the results of age-appropriate assessments and should relate to postsecondary priorities in the areas of education, employment, and community living. Although IDEA requires that youth with disabilities be invited to IEP meetings when postsecondary goals are considered, actual participation of students with disabilities remains limited. Although almost 50% of students with disabilities provide at least some input at their most recent IEP meeting, only about 10% to 20% take leadership roles at the meeting.[84] This limited participation is of concern because a student's ability to self-direct the IEP meeting and transition planning process strongly relates to positive postsecondary outcomes.[46,86]

Over the past 2 decades, professionals, researchers, and other key stakeholders have developed a number of intervention techniques targeted at self-determination and designed to improve a student's ability to participate in the IEP meeting and transition planning process. Self-determined students do the following: (1) demonstrate self-awareness and self-advocacy, (2) make choices and decisions, (3) problem solve when issues arise, and (4) achieve self-identified goals.[88] Occupational therapists working in transition to adulthood can contribute to the development of these important skills by deploying existing, evidence-based assessment tools and curricula.

Assessment that informs the transition planning process is optimized by the inclusion of tools that enhance a student's ability to self-direct IEP meetings and make choices about postsecondary life. Box 25-4 lists recommended self-determination scales that occupational therapists can use to enhance a student's and team's awareness of strengths, weaknesses, goals, and needs. An occupational therapist who uses these tools contributes rigorous data to the transition planning process. At the same time, use of these instruments may help a student increase his or her self-awareness of personal strengths, needs, goals, and priorities.

Assessment of self-determination skills is only part of facilitating student involvement in the transition planning process. In many cases, direct instruction in required to teach individuals with disabilities to become aware of their strengths and needs and advocate for services. A number of formal, evidence-based curricula exist for just this purpose. Box 25-5 presents the information on available curricula. Occupational therapists interested in facilitating student participation in the transition planning process can incorporate these existing resources into their practice (see the Evolve website).

Emphasis on Student's Social Competence

To transition from high school to postsecondary education or employment successfully, students must understand and adapt

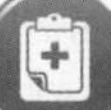

CASE STUDY 25-2 Youth with High-Functioning Autism: Planning for Postsecondary Education

Sara, a 17-year-old adolescent girl with high-functioning autism, planned to enroll in a 4-year college following graduation from high school. She did well in academic classes; however, her performance was significantly compromised whenever her routines were disturbed. Moving between classes was especially difficult for Sara. She often lost track of time during classes and was startled by the school bell that signals students to transition between classes. Because the bell was disorganizing, Sara felt unprepared to transition to her next class, and her stress disrupted her routine of writing down her assignments, organizing her materials, and inserting her ear plugs before the hallways were filled with loud students. When Sara's routine was disrupted, her performance in the next class was negatively affected. To help her prepare for transitions between classes, Sara's occupational therapist downloaded and programmed a reminders application for Sara's iPhone. The app provided vibrotactile alerts based on a schedule developed by the user. The occupational therapist developed the following alert structure to help Sara transition:

Timetable	Alert Type	Associated Behavioral Cue
Passing Time		
1 minute before class starts	iPhone vibrates 10×	Finish walking to class.
Class Time		
5 minutes before class ends	iPhone vibrates 5×	Write down assignments.
3 minutes before class ends	iPhone vibrates 3×	Organize materials for storage or place into book bag.
1 minute before class ends	iPhone vibrates 1×	Insert ear plugs.

These alerts enabled Sara to move between her classes in an orderly and timely fashion and resulted in improved academic performance.

Sara volunteered with the local animal shelter after school, which was part of her senior service requirement that she and all of her classmates had to fulfill. She used a bus app on her iPhone to track when the next bus was scheduled to arrive to minimize her wait time in the cold. She also used a checklist on her iPhone that reminded her of her assigned tasks at the animal shelter. The most challenging task for Sara was answering the animal shelter phone. The shelter administrator instructed her to answer it politely, ask basic questions of the caller, and refer the caller to the correct person. Sarah recognized that by working on this challenging task she would improve her customer interaction skills and that these would be important for most future jobs. Together, Sara, her occupational therapist, and the animal shelter manager developed a checklist of tasks for Sara to carry out. Sara videotaped the manager answering the phone and role played the most common phone scenarios. Sara found it reassuring to watch the video before her shift answering the phone. Sara had regularly scheduled video calls from the occupational therapist to ensure that she felt comfortable in her job; Sara preferred video calling so that she could show her occupational therapist the new rescue dogs that had come to the shelter that week. Sara's favorite job at the animal shelter was to train new rescued dogs to walk on a leash because she knew that dogs that could walk on a leash were more likely to be adopted. Sara loved caring for the dogs at the shelter. Although some of the tasks at the shelter were challenging, she was highly motivated and continued to gain competence in her public and phone interactions, knowing that her work in the shelter was important to finding rescued dogs a real home.

BOX 25-4 Self-Determination Scales

AIR Self-Determination Scale*

Purpose

- Profile student's level of self-determination.
- Identify strengths and needs.
- Identify goals and objectives.
- Develop strategies to improve self-determination.

ARC Self-Determination Scale†

Purpose

- Identify strengths and weaknesses of self-determination.
- Facilitate student participation in planning processes.
- Conduct self-determination research.

Online Resources

http://www.ou.edu/content/education/centers-and-partnerships/zarrow/self-determination-assessment-tools.html

*Adapted from Wolman, J. M., Campeau, P. L., DuBois, P. A., Mithaug, D. E., & Stolarski, V. S. (1994). *AIR self-determination scale and user guide.* Palo Alto, CA: American Institutes for Research.
†Adapted from Wehmeyer, M. (1995). *The ARC's self-determination scale: Procedural guidelines.* Arlington, TX: ARC National Headquarters.

BOX 25-5 Transition Curricula

Whose Future Is It Anyway?*
Purpose: Curricula designed to facilitate student participation in the transition planning process

ChoiceMaker Self-Determination Transition Curriculum†
Purpose: Formalized instruction in self-determination skills necessary for success in school and adult life

Online Resources
http://www.ou.edu/content/education/centers-and-partnerships/zarrow/self-determination-education-materials.html

*Adapted from Wehmeyer, M., Lawrence, M., Garner, N., Soukup, J., & Palmer, S. (2004). *Whose future is it anyway? A student-directed transition planning process* (2nd ed.). Lawrence, KS: Beach Center on Disability, KUCDD.
†Adapted from Martin, J. E., & Marshall, L. H. (1995). ChoiceMaker: A comprehensive self-determination transition program. *Intervention in School and Clinic, 30*(3), 147–156.

to new social environments. Social norms in employment and college settings are different from those in high school. These transitions can be difficult for many young adults and often pose serious challenges to individuals with disabilities, who may struggle with social competence.

Social competence refers to an individual's effectiveness in navigating interpersonal relationships with others at work, school, home, or public situations.[62] Social competence is largely subjective in nature and often changes, given the context in which an event occurs. A socially competent person during a rock concert would look and behave differently from a socially competent person at an opera performance. A socially competent person realizes the different expectations and decorum at each event and changes the way he or she dresses, interacts with fellow concertgoers, and responds to the music to match the event's social norms. These expectations are highly dependent on the cultural context in which the actions take place and create a feedback loop for how one is to behave in a given situation.

Once the student understands the environmental demands of a situation, he or she must have adequate social and communication skills and manage the interpersonal demands required for that situation. These social demands can be quite complicated and overwhelming for students with disabilities, who are less likely to have had social opportunities to learn, practice, and develop social competence.[53]

Occupational therapists can support a client's development of social competence by helping improve his or her social skills. This intervention focus is crucial because evidence suggests that students with disabilities who have higher levels of social skills are more likely to be employed than those who have lower levels of these skills.[80] Examples of interventions to enhance social skills follow a continuum from hands-on to advocacy, including direct instruction, peer awareness, involvement, and accommodation, and a positive climate of integration and encouragement.[4]

Occupational therapists provide direct interventions to help young adults develop social skills. Examples include training in the use of augmentative communication devices, tablet computers, and/or smartphones to improve communication output; participation in a group activities; use of social stories to prepare students for novel situations; and teaching students to self-monitor their interactions with others.[6] Peers can be effective in encouraging social participation. For example, providing peers with information about the student's disability, interests, and preferences can increase interaction between typical peers and students with disabilities.[12] The presence of trained peer mentors can increase the social participation of young adults with disabilities.[2,72] In some cases, peers are more effective than adults in helping students shape behavior, and positive peer pressure can make a difference when other interventions do not. Peer mentoring can provide natural supports in the classroom, on the job, or in the field.

This increased interaction and friendships between those with an identified disability and those without a disability can help decrease discrimination and prejudice.[23] State legislatures in most states have amended laws to change the phrase ***mental retardation*** to ***intellectual disability***, in no small part because of the efforts of a high school student.[81] This movement started in Fremd High School in Palatine, Illinois, in 2007 when Soeren Palumbo pleaded with his high school classmates in a speech not to use the term ***retardation*** ("the r word") out of respect for his sister, who had an intellectual disability. This movement, which started at one high school in Illinois, has become an international force to fight discrimination against individuals with intellectual disabilities. Each year, on the first Wednesday of March, many schools and universities encourage integration by recognizing a national day to "Spread the Word to End the Word."

The physical and social environment can also be adapted or created to increase social participation of students with disabilities. For example, school, work, or social events should always take place in accessible environments. Classrooms, lunchrooms, and extracurricular activities should be integrated so that students with disabilities have the opportunity to socialize with their typical peers, rather than be in segregated environments. Social activities outside school are the focus of Best Buddies, an affiliate program of Special Olympics, which pairs an individual with a disability with a typical peer to encourage friendship.[26] Increased social participation provides additional opportunities to practice and refine social skills important to employment and social participation.[80]

The climate of the school and work setting should be one of openness to diversity and the appreciation of differences. Teachers, therapists, paraprofessionals, job coaches, and other adults can encourage interaction between the student with a disability and his or her typical peers and co-workers. Inclusion of students with disabilities into all aspects of school, work, and social life helps raise expectations and create an environment in which differences are celebrated rather than excluded. Many organizations and employers have inclusion and diversity as part of their mission.[5] Institutions that adopt a mission of inclusion establish policies and cultural norms that welcome everyone, regardless, of gender, race, age, religion, sexual preference, veteran status, or national origin. Individuals with physical, cognitive, or psychiatric disabilities must also be seen as part of this diverse rainbow for the benefit of the individuals, the organizations, and society.

Development of Life Skills

By the time a student with disabilities enters high school, educators and therapists, with family input, must make curriculum decisions based on their vision for the student's post-transition outcome. For most professionals, this decision presents a choice between a traditional academic curriculum and a functional, life skills curriculum. A life skills curriculum is an alternative to the traditional academic curriculum designed to facilitate student development of skills necessary for success in adult life, such as the following:

- Activities of daily living (e.g., grooming, bathing)
- Community mobility and transportation (e.g., route finding, driving)
- Work skills (e.g., attention, endurance)
- Social skills (e.g., turn taking, carrying on a conversation)
- Self-determination (e.g., awareness, advocacy, problem solving)
- Functional writing and mathematics (e.g., completing a job application, writing a check)
- Independent living (e.g., budgeting, household chores)

Historically, this type of curriculum has usually been associated with students who have moderate to severe disabilities. In past years, many of these students on a functional curricular track were educated in isolation, away from peers without disabilities. Such practices conflicted with federal guidelines (IDEA 2004, NCLB 2001) that promote educating all students in natural environments and led to the stigmatization of the functional curriculum. Accordingly, the acceptability of a functional, life skills curriculum as a valid curricular choice is likely to vary across the country and among districts, cities, and states.

The functional curriculum is an important option for many young adults in transition. This is particularly true for students whose primary postsecondary target is employment and not education.[8] Occupational therapists working in transition can help teams make curricular decisions by keeping the following information in mind[8]:

- All students, whether disabled or not, must learn and master independent living skills.
- A functional, life skills curriculum is a legitimate option for students with disabilities in transition.
- The functional curriculum may be more appropriate than an academic curriculum for some students.
- Occupational therapists have expertise in life skills interventions, including assistive technologies that promote independence in instrumental activities of daily living and can contribute to the functional curriculum.

Use of Assistive Technology

Technology is evolving at an exponential rate and holds great potential to assist students with disabilities as they transition into adulthood. Adolescents and young adults are avid users and consumers of technology and are considered to be digital natives who have been raised and educated with technology.[58] Other chapters of this text describe how occupational therapists use AT to improve participation (see Chapter 19). Wheelchairs, augmentative communication devices, environmental controls, and adaptive equipment can all help improve a person's ability to navigate and participate in life. Although these supports can certainly increase independence, they also can make an individual appear disabled and different from his or her typical peers. New technologies and platforms allow students to use AT without separating them from their peers.

Concepts of universal design for learning and accessibility mandates make commercially available technology useful in supporting students in transition. Smartphones, tablets, and computers have accessible features that many consumers have found to improve efficiency and productivity. Additional applications (apps) or programs can be added to customize a device to the individual's unique needs.

Students have hundreds of different smartphone and tablet computer options from which they can choose. The operating system, size of the device, and technologic capabilities all dictate the device's functionality. Box 25-6 gives a brief overview of smartphones and tablets for occupational therapists to consider when they make technology recommendations.[18]

An advantage that tablets and smartphones have over other AT devices is that students who use this technology are using the same technology that their typical peers use, so these devices can actually become tools of inclusion. These devices can facilitate student success in academic, employment, and community engagement. For example, college students, with and without disabilities, use the following apps for their smartphones and tablet computers to support their academic success:

1. Map an app to find a college classroom.
2. Apps to audio or video record a professor's lecture can be synchronized to written notes.

BOX 25-6 Smartphone and Tablet Computer Options

Which operating system should I use?

- Android (Google) is often the least expensive device.
- iOS (Apple) has the most apps available to purchase.
- Windows (Microsoft Office) functions most like a typical computer operating system.

What hardware capability do I need?

- Amount of storage—devices with greater storage are more expensive.
- WiFi capability—will the student have access to a public WiFi network (open or closed) to be able to access the device's full capability?
- Data—will the student need the device in areas in which there is no access to a public WiFi network, and does a separate data plan need to be purchased?

What size device would be best?

- Would the use of a smartphone and a tablet cause confusion?
- Does the device need to be small enough to be kept in a pocket?
- Does the device need to be large to allow for reduced visual or fine motor capabilities?

Which built-in accessibility features will the student need?

- Does the device offer text to speech?
- Does the device offer speech to text?
- Does the device offer options for those with low vision?
- Does the device have accessible options for individuals with physical limitations?

Which apps should be purchased to make the most out of the device?

- What is the cost, and is it a one-time or ongoing cost?
- Does the app require access to the Internet to function properly?
- Does the app have an interface so it can be used on a variety of devices?

3. A built-in calendar with audio prompts can help the individual maintain the class schedule or study group meetings.
4. Reminder apps provide cognitive cues to complete assignments.
5. Spoken word to text apps help transcribe papers and assignments.
6. Text to voice apps can read assigned readings out loud.
7. Course-specific apps are available to help the student understand academic content in a different way than the professor presented it.

These devices are also useful in supporting students as they transition into competitive employment. Business is always increasing its reliance on information technology and adopting paperless workplaces. In the past, a teacher or job coach might have photographed job tasks and assembled them into a three-ring paper binder that described how to perform a particular job. These bulky binders are now being replaced by a tablet or smartphone with a series of photos or video checklist to help support a student in employment.[24] Other examples of how this technology can support employment include the following:

1. Remote job coaching. A job coach can make a video call to an employee to check on how work is progressing, and the student can show the quality of his or her work remotely.[31]
2. Telehealth. An occupational therapist can be brought in via video call (depending on state licensure requirements) to assess a task and help a student and job coach make adaptations to get the job done.[13]
3. Video modeling applications can support students as they move and learn to accomplish one task to the next on the job.[5]
4. Emotional support applications can be customized to allow students to center and calm themselves during stressful situations.[6]

Collaborative Interdisciplinary and Interagency Teamwork

Outcome-oriented, student-centered planning and services based on collaborative teamwork are at the center of high-quality transition services.[86] For transition-age students, this teamwork is accomplished by the IEP or transition team. As students with disabilities approach graduation from high school, all IEP planning and services must converge around the student's postsecondary goals and activities.[40]

When representatives from nonschool agencies join the student, family members, teachers, and related service personnel on the transition team, the interdisciplinary team becomes an interagency team. Congress, when formulating IDEA, did not intend for schools to have sole responsibility for transition processes and outcomes. Interagency linkages became part of IDEA in 1990, indicating the expectation for shared responsibility across local education agencies and adult or community programs. Establishing interagency linkages, although challenging, can be an important benefit to students with disabilities who are preparing to exit the public education system.[75]

On graduation or completion of public education programs, a student's IDEA-based entitlement to school-sponsored educational, vocational, and other services ends. In the place of one lead agency (the school system), a number of service agencies, such as the state vocational rehabilitation agency, state departments of mental health and developmental disabilities, state brain injury programs, and postsecondary education or training programs, become responsible for providing services to individuals who qualify. Those who are no longer eligible for the school's transition-focused special education or related services become responsible for identifying where to obtain the ongoing services they need and for demonstrating their eligibility to receive those services.

Interagency responsibilities and linkages should be clearly stated in IEP documents developed by the transition team. Failure to initiate and formalize these connections during high school can result in the student missing opportunities to receive important services, coping with delays in receiving services, and potentially losing skills and motivation because of these delays and missed opportunities. The importance of strong interagency linkages cannot be overstated.

For transition-age students, collaboration is viewed as an effective way for a team to come together to help them plan for and achieve desired transition outcomes in the areas of postsecondary education, community living and recreation, and employment. Collaborative teams share a sense of purpose, with shared responsibility for student outcomes.[27,71] An effective transition team is not simply a collection of individuals, each with a different set of skills. Collaboration should be evident during the planning of individualized transition services and documented in the student's IEP. Collaborative efforts and open communication are essential, given the variety of interdisciplinary team members representing the school's and community's interests.

Numerous formats exist to help the team identify potential transition outcomes.[50,70] For example, the student and team may discuss a future that includes living in an apartment or home with others who are identified or chosen by the student, use of community services (e.g., transportation, shopping, banking) and amenities (e.g., joining a health club, attending public concerts), employment (e.g., full- or part-time employment, other productive volunteer work), postsecondary education (e.g., vocational training, university enrollment), and relationships. Not surprisingly, these are goals that most people, with or without disabilities, envision for themselves or their loved ones.

While establishing a positive vision for the student's future, the team also begins to consider the student's anticipated long-term needs for resources and supports that will enable the vision to become reality. For example, a young adult with significant disabilities may require long-term job support in the form of a job coach, who provides on-the-job training and other support needed to maintain employment. Another individual with high-functioning autism may require social and academic support or accommodations to be in place and operational at the selected university before the start of the school year.

This type of planning is often termed *person-centered*[50] and involves a group of individuals who know the student well and who have come together to engage in a positive, facilitated discussion focused on the student's future. Emerging from this discussion is a comprehensive understanding of the student's unique strengths and interests, effective supports and accommodations, and potential resources and opportunities that can be incorporated into the student's transition services.

Collaborative, group-oriented planning processes have been shown to be an effective approach to student evaluation and transition planning.[30]

Summary

School-based interdisciplinary teams coordinate with community agencies to provide a range of essential services that promote positive postsecondary outcomes for individuals with disabilities. Occupational therapists understand the importance of work for fostering a person's sense of productivity, self-esteem, and self-determination and to create opportunities for social relationships and connections that support a high quality of life. Occupational therapists are well represented in the public schools, and yet only a relatively small percentage report that they work with transition-age students.[37] Occupational therapists have unique training to support individuals in transition and unique expertise on the interventions and tools needed to prepare youth and young adults to be successful in life and help them achieve that success.

The current educational and political environment has established higher expectations for postsecondary outcomes of students with disabilities. Full inclusion in postsecondary academic settings, employment, and full participation in life is the goal for all individuals with disabilities. Occupational therapists can help facilitate the successful transition of youth to adulthood. The following points summarize this chapter:

- Students with disabilities are entitled to receive transition services (e.g., special education and related services, including occupational therapy if the team determines a need) designed to help them achieve their postsecondary goals.
- In the U.S. public school system, a successful transition to adulthood is usually defined by matriculation to postsecondary education and/or employment.
- Key stakeholders, such as the student, parents, community partners, and advocates, may define additional important outcomes such as health, quality of life, friendships, and independent living skills.
- Occupational therapists are ideally positioned to provide evidence-based services to students in transition to adulthood.

REFERENCES

1. ACT. (2011). Affirming the goal: Is college and career readiness an internationally competitive standard? Retrieved from: <http://www.act.org/research/policymakers/reports/affirmingthegoal.html>.
2. Alquraini, T., & Gut, D. (2012). Critical components of successful inclusion of students with severe disabilities: Literature review. *International Journal of Special Education*, *27*(1), 42–59.
3. Bambara, L. M., Wilson, B. A., & McKenzie, M. (2007). Transition and quality of life. *Handbook of Developmental Disabilities*, 371–389.
4. Bedesem, P. L., & Dieker, L. A. (2013). Self-monitoring with a twist: Using cell phones to monitor on-task behavior. *Journal of Positive Behavior Interventions.* Published online 25 June 2013 DOI: 10.1177/1098300713492857 <http://pbi.sagepub.com/content/early/2013/06/24/1098300713492857>.
5. Bennett, K. D., Gutierrez, A., & Honsberger, T. (2013). A comparison of video prompting with and without voice-over narration on the clerical skills of adolescents with autism. *Research in Autism Spectrum Disorders*, *7*(10), 1273–1281.
6. Blood, E., Johnson, J. W., Ridenour, L., et al. (2011). Using an iPod Touch to teach social and self-management skills to an elementary student with emotional/behavioral disorders. *Education and Treatment of Children*, *34*(3), 299–321.
7. Bolles, R. N. (2011). *What color is your parachute? A practical manual for job-hunters and career-changers.* Berkeley, CA: Ten Speed Press.
8. Bouck, E. C. (2013). Secondary curriculum and transition. In P. Wehman (Ed.), *Life beyond the classroom: Transition strategies for young people with disabilities* (pp. 215–234). Baltimore: Paul H. Brookes.
9. Bureau of Labor Statistics. (2012). Persons with a disability: Labor force characteristics summary. Retrieved from: <http://www.bls.gov/news.release/disabl.nr0.htm>.
10. Butterworth, J., Smith, F. A., Hall, A. C., et al. (2012). *State data: The national report on employment services and outcomes.* Boston: Institute for Community Inclusion (UCEDD), University of Massachusetts.
11. Carmichael, S. B., Martino, G., Porter-Magee, K., et al. (2010). *The state of state standards—and the Common Core—in 2010.* Thomas B. Fordham Institute.
12. Carter, E. W., Austin, D., & Trainor, A. A. (2012). Predictors of postschool employment outcomes for young adults with severe disabilities. *Journal of Disability Policy Studies*, *23*(1), 50–63.
13. Cason, J., & Richmond, T. (2013). Telehealth opportunities in occupational therapy. In *Telerehabilitation* (pp. 139–162). New York: Springer.
14. Common Core State Standard Initiative. (2013). Standards in your state. Retrieved from: <http://www.corestandards.org/in-the-states>.
15. Corcoran, M. A. (2004). Work, occupation, and occupational therapy. *American Journal of Occupational Therapy Association*, *58*(4), 367–368.
16. Council of Chief State School Officers. (2013). *Common core state standards: Implementation tools and resources.* Council of Chief State School Officers.
17. Clayton, K. S., & Chubon, R. A. (1994). Factors associated with the quality of life of long-term spinal cord injured persons. *Archives of Physical Medicine and Rehabilitation*, *75*(6), 633–638.
18. Cleary, D. S., & Persch, A. C. (2013). IPads and iTechnology: Is it more engaging, efficient, and effective than traditional occupational therapy interventions in our schools? Retrieved from: <otwithanipad.blogspot.com>.
19. Daston, M., Riehle, J. E., Rutkowski, S., et al. (2012). *High school transition that works! Lessons learned from Project SEARCH.* Baltimore: Paul H. Brooke.
20. Duncan, A. W., & Klinger, L. G. (2010). Autism spectrum disorders: Building social skills in group, school, and community settings. *Social Work with Groups*, *33*(2–3), 175–193.
21. Eggleton, I., Robertson, S., Ryan, J., et al. (1999). The impact of employment on the quality of life of people with an intellectual disability. *Journal of Vocational Rehabilitation*, *13*, 95–107.
22. Falvey, M. A., Rosenberg, R. L., Monson, D., & Eshilian, L. (2006). Facilitating and supporting transition: Secondary school restructuring and the implementation of transition services and

programs. In P. Wehman (Ed.), *Life beyond the classroom: Transition strategies for young people with disabilities* (4th ed.). (pp. 165–182). Baltimore: Paul H. Brookes.

23. Ford, M., Acosta, A., & Sutcliffe, T. (2013). Beyond terminology: The policy impact of a grassroots movement. *Intellectual and Developmental Disabilities, 51*(2), 108–112.
24. Gentry, T., Lau, S., Molinelli, A., et al. (2012). The Apple iPod Touch as a vocational support aid for adults with autism: Three case studies. *Journal of Vocational Rehabilitation, 37*(2), 75–85.
25. Griffin, M. M., Summer, A. H., McMillan, E. D., et al. (2012). Attitudes toward including students with intellectual disabilities at college. *Journal of Policy and Practice in Intellectual Disabilities, 9*(4), 234–239.
26. Grigal, M., & Hart, D. (2010). *Think college! Postsecondary education options for students with intellectual disabilities.* Baltimore: Paul H. Brookes.
27. Hanft, B. E., & Shepherd, J. (2008). *Collaborating for student success: A guide for school-based occupational therapy.* Bethesda, MD: American Occupational Therapy Association.
28. Hasazi, S. B., Hock, M. L., & Cravedi-Cheng, L. (1992). Vermont's post-school indicators: Using satisfaction and post-school outcome data for program improvement. In F. Rusch, L. Destefano, J. Chadsey-Rusch, et al. (Eds.), *Transition from school to adult life: Models, linkages, and policy* (pp. 485–506). Pacific Grove, CA: Brooks/Cole.
29. Hendricks, D. (2010). Employment and adults with autism spectrum disorders: Challenges and strategies for success. *Journal of Vocational Rehabilitation, 32*(2), 125–134.
30. Holburn, S., & Vietze, P. M. (2002). *Person-centered planning: Research, practice, and future directions.* Baltimore: Baltimore: Paul H. Brookes.
31. Holm, M. B., & Raina, K. D. (2012). Emerging technologies for caregivers of a person with a disability. In *Multiple dimensions of caregiving and disability* (pp. 185–208). New York: Springer.
32. Idea Partnership. (2013). Needs of the field. Retrieved from: <http://www.ideapartnership.org/media/documents/CCC-Collection/ccc_needs-of-field.pdf>.
33. Idea Partnership. (2013). Grounding assumptions. Retrieved from: <http://www.ideapartnership.org/media/documents/CCC-Collection/ccc_grounding-assumptions.pdf>.
34. Idea Partnership. (2013). The partners. Retrieved from: <http://www.ideapartnership.org/the-partners.html>.
35. Idea Partnership. (2013). The partnership way. Retrieved from: <http://www.ideapartnership.org/building-connections/the-partnership-way.html>.
36. Inge, K. J. (1988). Quality of life for individuals who are labeled mentally retarded: Evaluating competitive employment versus sheltered workshop employment. *Education and Training in Mental Retardation, 23*(2), 97–104.
37. Kardos, M., & White, B. P. (2005). The role of the school-based occupational therapist in secondary education transition planning: A pilot survey study. *American Journal of Occupational Therapy, 59*, 173–180.
38. Kober, R., & Eggleton, I. R. C. (2005). The effect of different types of employment on quality of life. *Journal of Intellectual Disability Research, 49*(10), 756–760.
39. Kregel, J., & Dean, D. H. (2002). Sheltered work vs. supported employment: A direct comparison of long-term earnings outcomes for individuals with cognitive disabilities. In J. Kregel, D. H. Dean, & P. Wehman (Eds.), *Achievements and challenges in employment services for people with disabilities: The longitudinal impact of workplace supports.* Richmond, VA: Virginia Commonwealth University, Rehabilitation Research and Training Center on Workplace Supports.
40. Kohler, P. D., & Field, S. (2003). Transition-focused education: Foundation for the future. *Journal of Special Education, 37*(3), 174–183.
41. Levin, H., & Belfield, C. (2007). Educational interventions to raise high school graduation rates. In C. R. Belfield & H. M. Levin (Eds.), *The price we pay: Economic and social consequences of inadequate education* (pp. 177–199). Baltimore: Brookings Institution Press.
42. Lieberman, D., & Scheer, J. (2002). AOTA's evidence-based literature review project: An overview. *American Journal of Occupational Therapy, 56*, 344–349.
43. Lipsky, D. K., & Gartner, A. (1997). *Inclusion and school reform: Transforming America's classrooms.* Baltimore: Paul H. Brookes.
44. Mank, D., O'Neill, C., & Jansen, R. (1998). Quality in supported employment: A new demonstration of the capabilities of people with severe disabilities. *Journal of Vocational Rehabilitation, 11*, 83–95.
45. Marder, C., Cardoso, D., & Wagner, M. (2003). Employment among youth with disabilities. In M. Wagner, T. Cadwallader, & C. Marder (Eds.), Life outside the classroom for youth with disabilities. A report from the National Longitudinal Transition Study-2 (NLTS2) (pp. 5-1–5-10). Retrieved from: <http://www.nlts2.org/reports/2003_04-2/nlts2_report_2003_04-2_complete.pdf>.
46. McConnell, A. E., Martin, J. E., Juan, C. Y., et al. (2012). Identifying nonacademic behaviors associated with post-school employment and education. *Career Development and Transition for Exceptional Individuals, 36*(3), 174–187.
47. McMahan, R., & Baer, R. (2001). IDEA transition policy compliance and best practice: Perceptions of transition stakeholders. *Career Development for Exceptional Individuals, 24*(2), 169–184.
48. Miller, A., & Dishon, S. (2006). Health-related quality of life in multiple sclerosis: The impact of disability, gender and employment status. *Quality of Life Research, 15*(2), 259–271.
49. Morningstar, M. E., Bassett, D. S., Kochhar-Bryant, C., et al. (2012). Aligning transition services with secondary education reform. A position statement of the division on career development and transition. *Career Development and Transition for Exceptional Individuals, 35*(3), 132–142.
50. Mount, B. (1997). *Person-centered planning: Finding direction for change using personal futures planning* (2nd ed.). New York: Graphic Features.
51. Newman, L., Wagner, M., Knokey, A., Marder, C., et al. (Eds.), (2011). *The post-high school outcomes of young adults with disabilities up to 8 years after high school: A report from the National Longitudinal Transition Study-2 (NLTS2).* National Center for Special Education Research.
52. Niemiec, B., Lavin, D., & Owens, L. A. (2009). Establishing a national employment first agenda. *Journal of Vocational Rehabilitation, 31*(3), 139–144.
53. Orsmond, G. I., Shattuck, P. T., Cooper, B. P., et al. (2013). Social participation among young adults with an autism spectrum disorder. *Journal of Autism and Developmental Disorders, 43*(11), 2710–2719.
54. Papay, C., & Griffin, M. (2013). Developing inclusive college opportunities for students with intellectual and developmental disabilities. *Research and Practice for Persons with Severe Disabilities, 38*(2), 110–116.
55. Pedretti, L. W., Pedretti, L. W., & Early, M. B. (2001). *Occupational therapy: Practice skills for physical dysfunction.* St. Louis: Mosby.

56. Petrovski, P., & Gleeson, G. (1997). The relationship between job satisfaction and psychological health in people with an disability. *Journal of Intellectual and Developmental Disability*, *22*(3).
57. Porter, A., McMaken, J., Hwang, J., et al. (2011). Common Core Standards: The new U.S. intended curriculum. *Educational Researcher*, *40*(3), 103–116.
58. Prensky, M. (2001). Digital natives, digital immigrants. Part 1. *On the Horizon*, *9*(5), 1–6.
59. Priebe, S., Warner, R., Hubschmid, T., et al. (1998). Employment, attitudes toward work, and quality of life among people with schizophrenia in three countries. *Schizophrenia Bulletin*, *24*(3), 469–477.
60. Project SEARCH. (2013). About Project SEARCH. Retrieved from: <http://www.projectsearch.us/About.aspx>.
61. Project SEARCH. (2013). Outcome honorees. Retrieved from: <http://www.projectsearch.us/OurSUCCESSES/OutcomeHonorees.aspx>.
62. Reichow, B., & Volkmar, F. R. (2010). Social skills interventions for individuals with autism: Evaluation for evidence-based practices within a best evidence synthesis framework. *Journal of Autism and Developmental Disorders*, *40*(2), 149–166.
63. Revell, G., West, M., & Cheng, Y. (1994). Funding-supported employment: Are there better ways? In P. Wehman, J. Kregel, & M. West (Eds.), *Supported employment research: Expanding competitive employment opportunities for persons with significant disabilities* (pp. 199–211). Richmond, VA: Virginia Commonwealth University, Rehabilitation Research and Training Center on Supported Employment.
64. Ross, C. E., & Mirowsky, J. (1995). Does employment affect health? *Journal of Health and Social Behavior*, *36*, 230–243.
65. Schell, B. A., & Schell, J. W. (2008). *Clinical and professional reasoning in occupational therapy*. Philadelphia: Wolters Kluwer Health/Lippincott Williams & Wilkins.
66. Shah, M. F., Mancuso, D. C., He, L., et al. (2012). Evaluation of the Medicaid buy-in program in Washington state outcomes for workers with disabilities who purchase Medicaid coverage. *Journal of Disability Policy Studies*, *22*(4), 220–229.
67. Shogren, K. A. (2011). Culture and self-determination: A synthesis of the literature and directions for future research and practice. *Career Development for Exceptional Individuals*, *34*(2), 115–127.
68. Siegel, S. (1993). *Career ladders for challenged youths in transition from school to adult life*. Austin, TX: Pro-Ed.
69. Sinnott-Oswald, M. (1991). Supported and sheltered employment: Quality of life issues among workers with disabilities. *Education and Training in Mental Retardation*, *26*(4), 388–397.
70. Smull, M. W., & Harrison, S. (1992). *Supporting people with severe reputations in the community*. Alexandria, VA: National Association of State Mental Retardation Programs.
71. Snell, M. E., & Janney, R. E. (2005). *Collaborative teaming* (2nd ed.). Baltimore: Paul H. Brookes.
72. Stanish, H. I., & Temple, V. A. (2012). Efficacy of a peer-guided exercise programme for adolescents with intellectual disability. *Journal of Applied Research in Intellectual Disabilities*, *25*(4), 319–328.
73. Statfeld, J. L. (2001). *Transition planning*. Newark, NJ: Education Law Center.
74. Stephens, R., & Richey, M. (2013). A business view on U.S. education. *Science*, *340*, 313–314.
75. Stodden, R. A., Brown, S. E., Galloway, L. M., et al. (2004). *Essential tools: Interagency transition team development and facilitation*. Minneapolis: University of Minnesota, Institute on Community Integration, National Center on Secondary Education and Transition.
76. Stronks, K., van de Mheen, H., van den Bos, J., et al. (1997). The interrelationship between income, health and employment status. *International Journal of Epidemiology*, *26*(3), 592–600.
77. Technical Assistance and Dissemination Network. (2013). Part B, Child Count, 2011 (Microsoft Excel file). Retrieved from: <http://tadnet.public.tadnet.org/pages/712>.
78. Tennessee State Board of Education. (2009). *Annual joint report on pre-kindergarten through higher education in Tennessee*. Tennessee State Board of Education. Retrieved August 5, 2014 from: <https://www.tn.gov/thec/Legislative/Reports/reportsadd2011/JointReport2009.pdf>.
79. Test, D. W., Cease-Cook, J., Fowler, C. H., et al. (2012). College and career ready standards and secondary transition planning for students with disabilities: 101. Retrieved from: <http://nsttac.org/sites/default/files/College_and_Career_Readiness101.FINAL2.pdf>.
80. Test, D. W., Mazzotti, V. L., Mustian, A. L., et al. (2009). Evidence-based secondary transition predictors for improving postschool outcomes for students with disabilities. *Career Development for Exceptional Individuals*, *32*(3), 160–181.
81. r-word.org. (2013). R word resources. Retrieved from: <http://www.r-word.org/r-word-resources.aspx>.
82. Think College. (2013). Program database. Retrieved from: <http://www.thinkcollege.net/component/programsdatabase/?view=programsdatabase&Itemid=339>.
83. U.S. Census Bureau. (2013). *2011 American community survey 1-year estimates*. <http://www.census.gov/acs/www/>.
84. Wagner, M., Newman, L., Cameto, R., et al. (2012). A national picture of parent and youth participation in IEP and transition planning meetings. *Journal of Disability Policy Studies*, *23*(3), 140–155.
85. Ward, M. J. (1992). Introduction to secondary special education and transition issues. In F. Rusch, L. Destefano, J. Chadsey-Rusch, et al. (Eds.), *Transition from school to adult life: Models, linkages and policy* (pp. 387–389). Pacific Grove, CA: Brooks/Cole.
86. Wehman, P. (Ed.). (2013). *Life beyond the classroom: Transition strategies for young people with disabilities*. Baltimore: Paul H. Brookes.
87. Wehman, P., & Brooke, V. (2013). Securing meaningful work in the community: Vocational internships, placements, and careers. In P. Wehman (Ed.), *Life beyond the classroom: Transition strategies for young people with disabilities* (pp. 310–338). Baltimore, MD: Paul H. Brookes.
88. Wehmeyer, M. L., & Shogren, K. A. (2013). Self-determination: Getting students involved in leadership. In P. Wehman (Ed.), *Life beyond the classroom: Transition strategies for young people with disabilities* (pp. 41–68). Baltimore: Paul H. Brookes.

CHAPTER 26

Intervention for Children Who Are Blind or Who Have Visual Impairment

Kathryn M. Loukas • Patricia S. Nagaishi

KEY TERMS

- Certified low vision therapist
- Certified orientation and mobility specialist
- Certified vision rehabilitation therapist (CVRT)
- Blindness
- Visual impairment
- Visual perception
- Visual information processing
- Compensatory skills
- Assistive technology

GUIDING QUESTIONS

1. What is the definition of blindness and visual impairment in children and youth?
2. Who are the members and what are the roles of the inter-professional team who may be involved with children who are blind or visually impaired?
3. How might visual impairment affect occupational performance?
4. What are the concepts and client factors related to occupational performance of children who are blind or visually impaired?
5. Which types of assessments might be utilized in the evaluation of a child who is blind or visually impaired?
6. How might theory guide practice when working with this population?
7. What evidence supports occupational therapy intervention with infants, children, or youth with blindness/visual impairment?

"I long to accomplish a great and noble task, but it is my chief duty to accomplish humble tasks as though they were great and noble. The world is moved along, not only by the mighty shoves of its heroes, but also by the aggregate of the tiny pushes of each honest worker."

—Helen Keller[58]

Vision is the sense people use to gain understanding of the environment and the relationships among people, objects, and the surroundings. It serves as an efficient integrator of multisensory information that contributes to the development of perceptual abilities and concept formation.[20] We use vision to scan the environment (e.g., obtain information about distance, movement, spatial relations) and to discriminate features of objects and symbols (e.g., size, shape, color, orientation of letters). Because vision plays an important role in developing relationships and associations between people and objects, children with visual impairment often have delayed language. They may exhibit delayed cognitive, motor, and perceptual skills and limited self-care, play, and social participation. Occupational therapists must understand the complexity and importance of vision because of the significant impact visual impairment has on development, occupational engagement, and participation.

This chapter defines key terms related to vision and the effect of visual impairment on occupational performance; also described are assessment and evaluation measures specific to understanding children and youth with visual impairment. A description of intervention goals and strategies for children and youth with visual impairments or blindness is presented in a case study illustrating how occupational therapy interventions meet the needs of children and youth with visual impairments across different life stages (Case Study 26-1).

Terminology

In a discussion of vision, it is important to differentiate between *sight*—the ability to discriminate small objects, which is measured as visual acuity (or the resolving power of the eye to see small detail at a specified distance [i.e., 20/20 acuity is considered normal])—and *vision*—the process of taking in, processing, and integrating visual and other sensory information to form a perception.[65]

Scheiman describes an optometric model of vision comprising three interrelated components.[65] The first component consists of acuity, refraction, and eye health; the second component includes visual efficiency skills; and the third component involves visual information processing. See Table 26-1e on the Evolve website for a glossary of terms. Occupational therapy practitioners may intervene as related to each component. For example, children who exhibit deficits in acuity, refraction, and eye health may require accommodations and/or assistive devices to engage in daily activities. They may require intervention to learn to care for visual devices (e.g., glasses). Practitioners may also provide eye exercises and work closely with optometrists. The focus of occupational therapy intervention may be to enhance visual efficiency and information processing through a variety of structured visual activities.

The dynamic, complex system of visual skills, neural processing and integration, cortical interpretation, and adaptive visual-motor function develops through interactions with the world.[73]

The authors wish to thank and acknowledge the scholarly work and reference updates performed by occupational therapy graduate student Tara Kaminski.

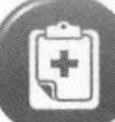

CASE STUDY 26-1 Visual Impairment Across Developmental Stages

This Case Study illustrates the evolving needs of children and youth with visual impairments and describes the role of occupational therapy. This case study applies occupational therapy concepts to intervention planning using the concepts and approaches described throughout this chapter and text to elucidate the process of occupational therapy when working with children and youth with visual impairments. The client is followed across the lifespan of childhood toward adulthood using client-centered and theoretically sound principles of intervention.

Early Childhood

Brooke was born prematurely at 32 weeks gestation, weighing 1500 grams at birth. As a result of lifesaving oxygen given to her in the neonatal intensive care unit, she had a condition called *retinopathy of prematurity.* This is a common reason for blindness or visual impairment in children in the United States.[29] Retinopathy of prematurity results from incomplete blood vessel development. As these vessels grow following premature birth, they can grow into the vitreous instead of the retinal surface. This process can pull on the retina and cause retinal detachment,[29] which was the case with Brooke. Her visual conditions included significant decrease in visual acuity at about 20/200 with corrective lenses, which corresponds to a diagnosis of legal blindness. Brooke had scarring of the retina and retinal detachment with loss of visual fields. Brooke was the oldest child of involved, concerned, and loving parents. The family lived in a small apartment outside of a small city.

Theoretical Foundation

The occupational therapy practitioner used a developmental frame of reference while integrating a dynamic systems and family-centered intervention.

Practice Setting

Early intervention (birth to 3 years of age).

Evaluation

The occupational therapist in early intervention received a referral from the pediatrician to evaluate Brooke. The evaluation began with an interprofessional arena assessment that included an occupational therapist, physical therapist, and speech and language pathologist. The team met and planned to evaluate Brooke using the Hawaii Evaluation and Learning Profile[52] and Peabody Developmental Motor Scales.[25] The occupational therapy evaluation also included an occupational profile,[4] home-based observations, and the Knox Preschool Play Scale.[39] The trio of therapists worked together as they met to interview the parent(s) and engage Brooke in playful interactions with toys and assessment objects in the therapy environment. The occupational therapist addressed areas of occupation in self-care and play with careful attention to the developmental, sensory, adaptive, and exploratory needs of the child.

Team-Based Intervention Planning

Following the evaluation, the team and family developed an individual family service plan. Using findings from the arena assessment, including those from the Hawaii Early Learning Profile and Peabody Developmental Motor Scales, observations, and interview, the team determined that Brooke had strong prelanguage and social skills. Brooke was developmentally delayed in her motor milestones and the team noticed that her parents tended to hold her versus letting her explore or move on her tummy or other positions on the floor. Cognitive development was also somewhat delayed. The team hypothesized that this was because of Brooke's inability to see objects with which to interact. The team developed goals related to play exploration, parent education, activities of daily living, rest and sleep, and sensory input. The State Center for the Blind was contacted so that services were initiated specific to the needs of children who are blind.

Description of Occupational Therapy Interventions

The occupational therapist provided family-centered intervention with Brooke, addressing concerns regarding sleep patterns by coaching them to extinguish use of sound during interruption of the night time sleep cycle.[78] The occupational therapist also addressed needs articulated by the mother regarding appropriate play in the home by bringing toys that had distinctive sensory features including tactile and auditory components. The practitioner modeled appropriate habits as she sang songs with hand motions to direct some routines such as eating and dressing; Brooke responded to this interactive, sensory motor approach. The occupational therapist used motor learning approaches (see Chapter 7) when a game challenged her emerging motor performance. Specifically, the practitioner provided short verbal directions with tactual cues as needed. The practitioner allowed Brooke to problem solve and play with a variety of toys, and the intervention occurred in the child's home (natural context). Further, the practitioner incorporated Brooke's love of stuffed animals into the games (meaning promotes motor learning).

To address development of childhood occupations,[35] the practitioner used an ecologic model, setting up an environment to promote Brooke's development of intrinsic motivation. This set up included a child-safe environment free of clutter or hazardous furniture with assorted climbing toys such as a slide, toys with tactile and auditory input, and a playhouse with play clothes, pretend food items, and other household objects. The team decided that the occupational therapy practitioner would serve as Brooke's primary therapist in early intervention services because her speech and language were strong and overall gross motor potential was evident. Working with the parents, the occupational therapist supported and encouraged healthy routines that facilitated development and adaptive functioning. The dynamic systems approach makes exceptions to strict developmental expectations. This approach includes working with the initial conditions of significant visual impairment while recognizing that Brooke may develop in some areas (such as language) much faster than others. Family-centered interventions

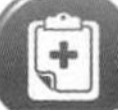

CASE STUDY 26-1 Visual Impairment Across Developmental Stages—cont'd

acknowledge the importance of family support and the home environment in services for young children (Box 26-1).

School-Age

Practice Setting

School-based practice.

Theoretical Foundation

The person-environment-occupation (PEO) model[13] uses adaptation and compensation interventions and sensory processing frame of reference[17] in an inclusive, interprofessional milieu. A remediative approach utilizing visual rehabilitation was also included in the program.

Occupational Therapy in the School Environment

As a school-aged child Brooke received occupational therapy services through the Individuals with Disabilities Education Act.[76,77] Brooke also received services through the Department of Blind Rehabilitation, including a certified vision rehabilitation therapist (CVRT) who taught Brooke to read Braille as well as other skills specific to living with blindness. Brooke learned and practiced nonvisual cane mobility with a certified orientation and mobility specialist who saw her once per month.[1] In addition, Brooke had a classroom teacher each year as well as specialist teachers in areas such as art, music, physical education, and computers.[3]

Evaluation

The occupational therapist used observations in a variety of school contexts, an occupational profile, analysis of the occupations expected in school,[4] the School Function Assessment,[16] and the Sensory Profile School Companion[18] to evaluate Brooke's school-based strengths, abilities, and adaptation needs. Formal school-based evaluations are necessary every 3 years, although goals and outcomes are documented quarterly.

Interventions for School Occupations

The occupational therapist used the PEO model to guide her thinking about the needs that Brooke had as a child with significant visual impairment/blindness. As a therapist who is consistently in the schools, the occupational therapist worked with the professionals in services for the blind to assure carryover of academic and mobility recommendations. First, the occupational therapist addressed Brooke as a *person*. Brooke was a person who sought sensory input and physical activity, particularly tactile and proprioceptive input. Brooke was also highly social, always talking and curious about the world around her. The occupational therapist influenced teachers and students to see Brooke as a person with many strengths and interests, as well as a child who is blind. Using the PEO model addressing the environment, the occupational therapist educated the school community regarding the importance of not having clutter in the halls and aisles of the classroom, as well as the importance of keeping physical obstacles in the same place. In collaboration with the CVRT, the occupational therapist implemented assistive technology such as voice-activated software to help Brooke with written work. Although Brooke was learning braille, the occupational therapist took the lead in finding auditory books and resources for Brooke. To help Brooke refrain from self-stimulation during teacher-directed learning, the occupational therapist implemented use of a sensory box in which Brooke could find stimulating items with which to fidget. The occupational therapist developed a sensory diet for the classroom and specific playground activities whereby Brooke learned to participate independently on the equipment. The occupational therapist also adapted recess games such as kick-ball with a playground ball with jingle bells inserted for Brooke to kick as well as a designated buddy runner to assist her in the game.

Brooke and the art teacher collaborated to create art that had significant tactile properties so that Brooke could feel the art. Art projects included, for example, paper mache, hanger sculpture, and others after an in-service from the occupational therapist. Brooke fully participated in the school environment according to her performance capacity in the natural context of the school.

In addition, a remediation approach of vision rehabilitation targeted maximizing Brooke's residual vision. This approach utilized vision training and specific attention to factors in her limited visual field based on experience.[74] (See Research Note 26-1.) The occupational therapist was dedicated to individualized inclusive intervention approaches and developed activities to challenge Brooke to use the vision she had. The therapist also recommended environmental adaptations throughout the school to optimize her safety and participation.

Interventions to Promote Social Participation

The occupational therapist collaborated with Brooke to develop social participation and identity building occupations. Following the therapist's recommendations and consultation, Brooke actively engaged in occupations such as horseback riding, swimming, martial arts, and wrestling. After Brooke expressed the desire to know other children who were blind or had visual impairment, the therapist encouraged the family to increase social participation by sending Brooke to a camp for children who are blind or visually impaired. Brooke was delighted because all the activities at camp were adapted for children with blindness. Brooke enjoyed meeting other children who were blind. She was curious about how they adapted to various occupations. In addition, Brooke's parents found a support network to assist them to be effective parents of a child who is blind.

Transitioning to Adult Roles

Practice Setting

School, home, and/or community.

Theoretical Foundation

The Model of Human Occupation (MOHO)[38] psychosocial and developmental frames of reference.

Challenges in Secondary Education

As Brooke entered middle and high school she encountered new areas of developmental challenge, including social relationships and preparation for adult roles and responsibility. Brooke was reading Braille fluently and achieving "on grade level" in most classes; she was involved in sports on the

Continued

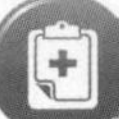

CASE STUDY 26-1 Visual Impairment Across Developmental Stages—cont'd

recreational and school team levels. Brooke began to self-advocate to meet her adaptive needs. Thus, the role of the occupational therapist changed to a consultant role and the practitioner supported Brooke's development of self and identity to prepare Brooke for independence as a young adult.[48]

Evaluation of Secondary School Students

The occupational therapist evaluated Brooke's skills and abilities with the following assessments: Occupational Circumstances Assessment Interview and Rating Scale[26]; Occupational Self-Assessment[38]; interest and role checklists[38]; Children Helping Out, Responsibilities, Expectations, and Supports (CHORES)[17]; and the Kohlman Evaluation of Living Skills[41] to assess IADL skills. At age 16 she was also given the Transition Daily Rewards and Worries Questionnaire[32] to fully address her needs in transition planning to adult life. The occupational therapist took a key role in helping Brooke transition to adult roles.[36]

Occupational Therapy Intervention

Using MOHO as the model of practice, the occupational therapy practitioner addressed the area of *volition*, as she continued a strong relationship with both Brooke and her family. During the developmental years, she influenced Brooke's athletic abilities that began with her need for and interest in physical activity. She helped Brook access the United States Association of Blind Athletes[75] to support participation in athletics using the Access Sports Model.[47,56] This model involves adapting sports targets and goals, boundaries and equipment, and/or rules. Recent legislation indicated that students with disabilities have the right to be involved in varsity and extracurricular sports, by the Disabilities Act and Interscholastic Sports,[76] which supported Brooke's motivational (volitional) involvement.

The occupational therapist consulted with the family and Brooke when examining *habituation*, to assure that she was involved in healthy routines and habits including chores and IADL activities at home and in the community to move toward independent or interdependent living. Brooke continued to work with both the CVRT and the certified orientation and mobility specialist to maximize experience, confidence, and access to the community. The occupational therapist collaborated with services for the blind to assure consistency and follow-through of recommendations and expertise. Brooke developed her own goals and took on key roles in IADLs, athletics, and school activities. The occupational therapist used the interest and role checklists to include the environment and performance capacity into her daily occupations. Brooke demonstrated some challenges in performance capacity owing to struggles with self-esteem, autonomy, and community participation, which the occupational therapist prudently addressed in intervention planning[36]. Areas of occupation addressed included education, work, leisure, instrumental activities of daily living (IADLs), and social participation. See Research Note 26-2.

BOX 26-1 Family-Centered Care

Factors Influencing Mothers' Learning

Overview: This study follows a paradigm shift away from clinic-based intervention and toward community and occupation-centered practice in early intervention. This qualitative study explored the relationship of 9 mothers and their child's occupational therapists in early intervention, specifically factors that facilitated learning. The themes that emerged included the role of parents as active partners versus passive observers and the importance of relationships and open communication in meeting the needs of mothers.

Effectiveness of Home-Based Early Intervention for Blind Infants and Preschoolers

Overview: This German study documented the positive effects of comprehensive early intervention with full-term blind children with high levels of parent involvement. The nonrandomized control trial included targeted intervention in spatial orientation, sensory awareness, and daily living skills. A specialist addressed the needs of 10 blind children with visits every 14 days for 2 years with 40 children in the control group. Children who received the specialized home-based intervention advanced in general development as compared with controls.

Harrison, C., Romer, T., Simon, M. C., & Schulze, C. (2007). Factors influencing mothers' learning from paediatric therapists: A qualitative study. *Physical & Occupational Therapy in Pediatrics, 27*(2), 77–96.

Beelmann, A., & Brambring, M. (1998). Implementation and effectiveness of a home based early intervention program for blind infants and pre-schoolers. *Research in Developmental Disabilities, 19*, 225–244.

RESEARCH NOTE 26-1

Vision Rehabilitation

Tsai, L.-T., Meng, L.-F., Wu, W.-C., Jang, Y., & Su, Y.-C. (2013). Effects of visual rehabilitation on a child with severe visual impairment. American Journal of Occupational Therapy, 67*, 437–447.*

This single case study used a research design of ABA and AB to explore the brain changes of play-based specific vision rehabilitation techniques with a 6-year-old boy with severe visual impairment. The researchers implemented and measured the effects of a chromatic luminance discrimination program and fixation training through an online game activity. The outcomes were measured using evoked potential to evaluate neural activity in the primary visual cortex. Along with neurologic changes, the authors' results indicate that this programming helped the boy detect obstacles in his environment not noticed prior to the program. The functional and neurologic changes cited in this study suggest the ability to maximize residual visual functions through experience-dependent neuroplasticity.

RESEARCH NOTE 26-2

Behaviors Associated with Future Success in Employment and Education

McConnell, A. E., Martin, J. E., Juan, C. Y., Hennessey, M. N., Terry, R. A., el-Kazimi, N. A., et al. (2012). Career development and transition for exceptional individuals. *Hammill Institute on Disabilities. Published online December 13; http://cde.sagepub.com/content/early/2012/12/13/2165143412468147.*

McConnell et al. analyzed existing research on behaviors that favorably influenced successful secondary transition of students with disabilities to adult roles. Based on a meta-analysis of 83 studies, the authors found that behaviors associated with postschool education and employment included: (a) knowledge and actions regarding their own strengths and weaknesses (insight), (b) disability awareness, (c) employment and experience, (d) goal setting and attainment, (e) persistence and proactive involvement, (h) self-advocacy, and (i) supports and utilization of resources (p. 4). Implications for occupational therapy involvement in transition planning and development of interventions related to successful transition are significant. These include educational consultation, facilitation of independence in the community, advocacy, IADL training, social participation activities, and family support.

Visual skills include fixation, tracking/pursuits, saccades, accommodation, convergence, and binocular vision. In addition, stereopsis (binocular depth perception), form perception, and field of vision depend on the coordination of accommodation and convergence.[73] Visual and sensorimotor integration involves integration of visual skills with the other sensory systems (e.g., vestibular, proprioception, auditory, tactile) that enable the child to develop functional skills (e.g., orienting responses, protective reactions, spatiotemporal orientation, eye-hand and eye-foot coordination, perceptual skills, and academic skills). At the same time, sensorimotor functions support the development of visual skills.

Visual Impairment

For the purposes of this chapter, ***visual impairment*** is defined as the loss of or deficit in visual function (i.e., vision, visual perception, interpretation of visual input) owing to pathology or processing problems in one or more components of the visual system (e.g., structures of the eye, visual pathways, and the brain) that limits the individual's ability to engage in and participate in daily occupations. The leading causes of visual impairment in young children are cortical visual impairment, retinopathy of prematurity (ROP), and optic nerve hypoplasia.[19,23,49] Other common causes include microphthalmia, anophthalmia, childhood glaucoma, retinoblastoma, and congenital cataracts, whereas less common causes include severe myopia, albinism, and nystagmus.[19]

Because the effects of visual impairment are evident in the acquisition of early milestones for occupation-based mobility, play, and hand function, children with visual impairments are often referred for developmental evaluation and intervention by pediatricians. However, children with developmental disabilities (e.g., cerebral palsy, Down syndrome) are among the most likely to receive services from occupational therapists, and 50% to 66% of children with developmental disabilities also have a significant ocular disorder or visual impairment.[49,54] Therefore occupational therapy practitioners who provide services to children with these diagnoses must recognize, understand, and address how the child's visual functioning influences occupational functioning.

In a national collaborative study that examined the developmental trajectories of a group of 186 children with visual impairment, children with visual impairment and co-occurring disabilities (e.g., intellectual disability [ID] or developmental delay) had lower developmental age scores, as measured by the Battelle Developmental Inventory, and showed a slower rate of development when compared with children with visual impairment who did not have ID, regardless of the levels of visual functioning demonstrated by the children.[34] The level of visual function was highly correlated with the presence of ID: more than half of the children with severe vision loss also had ID, whereas children with mild to moderate vision loss did not. Among the children with no ID, those with the least vision had significantly lower rates of motor and personal-social development when compared with those with the most vision. The degree of visual impairment, therefore, appears to be a factor in the development of these children, and those with better vision are more likely to have favorable developmental outcomes.[34]

The degree of visual impairment, however, is only one variable that must be considered in the individual child's developmental trajectory.[80,81] Some children with visual impairments function at least within the average range or even at the high end of developmental age norms for sighted children. Therefore the dynamic evaluation of occupational performance in relation to the demands (i.e., expectations and challenges) of the context in which the child with visual impairment functions and how these interactions change over time is presented as a more useful framework.[81] Whether the child with a visual impairment is singly impaired or has multiple disabilities, occupational therapists view the child and family in relation to their ability to participate and engage in occupations and activities that are meaningful to their everyday lives.

Children with visual impairment are often identified in the first year of life and begin to receive services from local early intervention programs, which according to best practice serve children in natural contexts such as the home or daycare. Occupational therapy practitioners are part of the interprofessional team for children who are blind or visually impaired and may work with children in the neonatal intensive care unit, early intervention sites, home care, schools, specialty schools, transition programs, vocational sites, and children's hospitals or rehabilitation centers.[15,54]

Developmental Considerations and the Impact of Visual Impairment

To evaluate the ability of children to engage in age-appropriate occupations and to design appropriate interventions, occupational therapists need to understand the development of the visual system and visual functioning. Vision is a quick, efficient integrating sense that allows immediate feedback and appreciation of both near and distant information about the environment in multiple locations.[37,72]

At 24 to 25 weeks' gestation, the major structures of the eye and the visual pathway to the level of the visual cortex are in place, but the eyelids are fused and the visual system remains immature.[30,31] Therefore infants born extremely premature are at high risk for ROP because the retina and visual cortex undergo further maturation during the last trimester of pregnancy.[30] Although improvements in neonatal and ophthalmic care have resulted in improved visual outcomes for children with ROP,[67] children with extremely low birthweight may be at higher risk for visual impairments.[68,69] By 24 to 28 weeks the eyelids are no longer fused and an immature visual response emerges, but the awake and sleep states are not well differentiated. By 30 to 34 weeks sleep and awake states become differentiated, the eyes may open, and brief visual fixation may occur. By 36 weeks the visual evoked response is similar to that of a full-term infant, and the awake state can be sustained for longer periods.[31]

At birth the infant's visual acuity is approximately 20/200 (i.e., the infant can see at 20 feet what an adult with normal vision can see at 200 feet): at 1 year, it is about 20/50, and by 2 years normal 20/20 acuity is present.[20] The maturation of the visual system in typical infants continues after birth and is a function of the transactions that occur between the infant and the environment and concurrent changes in the synaptic density of the visual cortex and other parts of the brain.[31] Vision enables an infant to explore the environment and negotiate space, to learn about the properties of objects, to interact and communicate with caregivers, and to develop the visual-perceptual skills needed for more complex activities, such as reading and writing, and for play and self-care occupations. In addition, vision is major contributor to praxis, which allows an individual to organize ideas and actions and to anticipate, monitor, and adapt to the demands of the environment.[64,68] Because many of the conditions that affect vision are congenital or have a prenatal etiology, a major system for processing and interpreting information is compromised at birth, with substantial impact on the child's subsequent development in all areas of occupation, including developing social relationships, self-care, play, activities of daily living, and academics.

Parent-Infant Attachment

Through engagement in the daily caregiving activities and routines of eating/feeding, bathing, sleep/rest, and playful interactions, the infant and the caregiver co-regulate their signals and responses, and each actively participates in these interactions. Through these interactions the infant and the caregiver develop their relationship; infant behaviors such as eye gaze and visual regard of faces, and the mother's interpretations of these behaviors, are important to this process. However, vision is not required for the basic infant behaviors that elicit caregiver responses, such as smiling and vocalizing or for infants to perceive the caregiver's responsive behaviors, such as vocalizing, cuddling, or feeding.[81] Sighted infants and infants with visual impairments engaged in similar proportions of facial expressions that were considered meaningful by their mothers, including smiling.[7]

Indeed, positive and strong attachment relationships can occur in infants with visual impairment.[80] A caregiver who is coping with learning that the infant has a visual impairment may have difficulty responding to the infant's cues, but at the same time the infant may display fewer behaviors that elicit positive responses from the caregiver, setting up a cycle of interactions that are out of sync or not mutually and emotionally satisfying. Furthermore, an infant who is visually impaired may be securely attached to a primary caregiver but have attachment behaviors that are different from those seen and expected in sighted children.[20] Vision loss itself is not necessarily a causal factor, but it may create a condition of risk for early social-emotional development and attachment.[81]

Sleep and Rest

Young children with visual impairment may experience sleep disorders that could impact the bedtime and sleep-wake routines in the household, their behavior, and performance.[20] One study examined the sleep patterns of two groups of toddlers with visual impairment ranging in age from 10 months to 39 months: one group without associated disabilities, and one group with associated disabilities.[22] The investigators found that when compared with the control group of typical sighted peers, the children with visual impairment had more difficulty falling asleep and sleeping through the night (i.e., longer time spent awake and greater number of nocturnal awakenings), and the sleep behaviors were not related to the presence of associated disabilities. Thus it is important that occupational therapists consider the daily routines of the child and family, including sleep-wake cycles, as part of the evaluation and intervention processes. See Research Note 26-3.

Exploration and Play

Vision provides children motivation to explore and seek out interactions with the physical and social worlds that contributes to the acquisition of perceptual motor skills and development across domains. Children with visual impairment, particularly those who have significantly decreased visual functioning, have a qualitatively different experience with, and level of affordances of, objects and people in their environment.[71]

Children with visual impairment often demonstrate delayed achievement of certain milestones, such as crawling and walking.[34] In a survey of 200 families, children with visual impairment demonstrated delayed gross motor development, with the most significant delays related to locomotion, such as cruising around furniture, walking independently, and negotiating stairs.[11] Among the subgroups in the sample, children with the least vision (i.e., light perception only or no light perception) had the poorest motor outcomes, followed by children with visual impairments who were born prematurely. A summary of selected studies comparing motor function, degree of visual impairment, and severity of co-occurring conditions is presented in Table 26-2e on the Evolve website.

Warren suggested that lack of vision may have an indirect rather than a direct effect on locomotion, because studies have shown significant variance among infants with visual impairment, with some achieving milestones for crawling and walking well within the normal range.[81] Specifically, vision may serve as a motivator for infants to explore interesting sights out of reach, and perhaps more important is the extent to which infants are provided with opportunities and encouragement to explore and learn.[81]

RESEARCH NOTE 26-3

Recommendations for Sleep Problems in Young Children with Blindness

Mindell and DeMarco (1997) investigated 28 blind children ages 4 to 36 months regarding sleep habits as compared with a control group of 22 sighted children.[50] The authors hypothesized that children who are blind have significantly greater sleep problems because of difficulties with circadian rhythms. According to a standardized parent questionnaire, blind children had more sleep-related problems including bedtime behavior difficulties, longer time getting to sleep, wakefulness during the night, and overall less sleep time. The authors reported that parents of blind children were more likely to use conversation, sound, or reading when the child awoke, which may have promoted the awakened behavior. A corresponding single case study by Vervloed, Hoevenaars, and Maas[78] found that parents of a 4½-year-old girl with visual impairment had significant difficulty getting the child to sleep and keeping her asleep during the night.

The parents were instructed to use graduated extinction procedures of parental attention during awakened periods during the night. This included ignoring the disrupted sleep behavior during the night. The study also incorporated an improved bedtime routine of calming activities and discontinued physical play. Parents were encouraged to use behavioral practices for 30 days, including a graduated extinction of sounds while comforting the awakened child. Results indicated that the child had improved initiation and latency of sleep 3 months following behavioral treatment.[78]

Implications for Occupational Therapy

- When children with blindness have difficulty sleeping, establishing behavior expectation may help to improve sleeping habits.
- Occupational therapists can recommend behavioral strategies combined with establishing routines to improve sleeping patterns.

Learning, Education, and Academic Performance

Children with visual impairment learn in a range of educational contexts, from general education settings to residential facilities. According to the Individuals with Disabilities Education Act[76,77] most preschoolers with visual impairment are served in early childhood special education settings. Knowledge of the typical developmental processes is critical, not only for comparison with sighted children but to provide a context for professional decision making to determine developmentally appropriate evaluation and intervention.[21] For example, children develop an understanding of the properties of the world and how things relate and work, develop logical thought and learn to problem solve, and also learn to regulate and organize executive functions such as memory, attention, and information processing. They learn by exploring and engaging in sensorimotor actions with objects, developing associations and affordances among objects, experiencing the relationship between self and others and objects in space, establishing perception and mental representations, solving complex problems, and ultimately using symbolic representation and manipulation for abstract thinking. Children with visual impairment have unique needs that must be considered when examining the development of cognition, concept development, and language. For example, the occupational therapist provides opportunities for movement, tactile exploration, and sensory experiences to stimulate cognitive associations, concept development, and language. Modifications to the environment may be needed to allow children with visual impairments to fully experience learning.

Children with visual impairment may achieve developmental milestones at a different rate and sequence than sighted children; they may achieve some developmental milestones within the same typical range.[23] Cognition and communication often develop on a later schedule, depending on factors such as age at onset, degree of visual functioning, presence of other disabilities, and the nature of the child's experiences in different contexts. Many studies found no significant differences in the cognitive/learning and communication development or school performance of children with visual impairment when compared with normative samples of typical peers.[27,42,60,61] This does not mean, however, that children with visual impairment who perform within the typical range based on standardized test scores do not have qualitative differences or needs that may affect occupational performance and require intervention.

For example, several studies reported cognitive functioning in the normal range among children with visual impairment, but some children displayed a pattern of differences in visual motor performance (see Table 26-2e on the Evolve website). In one study, although the mean scores for mental and motor development on the Bayley Scales of Infant Development II fell within the average range for a group of 54 young children with retinoblastoma (RB), visual motor performance differed relative to extent of RB (unilateral or bilateral).[61] The children with bilateral RB had significantly lower mean scores for motor development (although still within the average range), and they were more likely to be referred for intervention to address visuomotor difficulties than the children with unilateral RB.

Potential unidentified visual deficits among older children who display academic problems also need to be considered. Goldstand, Koslowe, and Parush found that among a sample of 71 seventh graders (mean age of 12.7 years; 46 proficient readers, 25 nonproficient readers) in middle school in Jerusalem, more than half the group failed an optometric vision screening measure.[33] Nonproficient readers had significantly poorer visual efficiency skills when compared with proficient readers, suggesting that basic visual skills can be important to learning to read with proficiency.

These findings suggest that visual deficits may be common among school-age children and that many of these children are in school with uncorrected visual problems. Children with visual problems often have learning problems but may not receive accommodations, remedial intervention, or related services (e.g., occupational therapy, speech-language pathology). Screening for and recognizing visual problems among children who are struggling in school can be an important role for the occupational therapist, who can make a referral to a vision care specialist for comprehensive evaluation and diagnosis. Once a child with visual problems is identified, the occupational therapist can develop appropriate compensatory and instructional strategies, accommodations, and other supports to help the child access the curriculum and improve academic performance.

Use of Information from Other Sensory Systems

It is a common assumption that children with visual impairment compensate for the loss of vision through increased use or heightened performance of the remaining senses. It is important to remember, however, that the child who is visually impaired (i.e., from birth or early infancy) is in the *process* of building experiences that affect the developing brain and therefore must learn differently than do typical children. However, infants and young children with visual impairment do make sensory associations to form perceptions through their experiences, and if the remaining sensory systems are intact and the infant is otherwise healthy, the capacity to become competent and independent can be realized.[68] Furthermore, the research suggests that visual impairment does not have a negative impact on early development of tactile and auditory perception in that infants with visual impairment demonstrate basic discrimination abilities similar to those of sighted infants.[81] As Glass noted, infants with visual impairment may have a heightened behavioral response to auditory stimuli.[62]

Although infants with visual impairment discriminate and respond to caregivers' voices or touch, their ability to connect auditory input with external objects in a specific location and to use this information to reach for objects appears to take longer to develop.[81] It is not a simple matter for an infant to know that a sound goes with a desirable object and locate it. Ross and Tobin posited that an infant may expend energy trying to interpret sounds at the expense of exploratory motor behavior.[62]

The development of occupations that use fine motor skills depends on visual monitoring. Loss or distortion of visual input makes it more difficult for children to acquire these skills, although information from the tactile system can offer some compensatory strategies.[68] Children with visual impairment can manipulate objects to detect their form and shape, and therefore their concepts of objects are developed using haptic perception. In addition, their ability to coordinate reaching with sound depends on precise tactile system perception used for exploration and concept development[45] and the use of audition to locate an object in space. Although object concept behaviors in children with visual impairment are similar to those in sighted infants through the first year and a half, performance on tasks that involve complex spatial displacements that cannot easily be tracked by audition or touch is more difficult; therefore, spatial understanding may be more of a problem than object conceptualization for children with visual impairment.[81]

The use of remaining sensory systems does not substitute for the efficiency of the visual system in integrating the child's experiences, and therefore the child with a visual impairment takes longer to develop his or her conceptual understanding of the world.[21,59] Learning is much more efficient for sighted children, who have the benefit of seeing the whole first and then discovering the different parts. As Fazzi and Klein explain, children with visual impairment must learn about things in parts based on different, discrete sensory inputs without seeing what the whole looks like first.[21] In their example, a child with a visual impairment may experience something with a furry body, a wet nose and tongue, a moving tail, and loud barking and must then integrate these pieces of sensory information to form the complete concept of "dog." Without adequate opportunities to experience all parts, the child's "picture" of the whole may be incomplete or inaccurate.

Although the child with visual impairment may gain specific information about an object's unique properties, the remaining senses do not necessarily provide him or her with sufficient information about the contexts in which the object exists.[68] For example, a child may learn about the cup he uses for drinking but may not come to understand for years that his plastic tumbler, his father's coffee mug, and the crystal wine glass used for special occasions are all variations of a class of objects used for drinking, especially if he has not had direct tactile experience with these items. If a child has limited experiences and does not have systematic introduction to objects in context, he or she will have a narrow range of schemes to work with, and these available schemes may not be fully validated by others.[59]

Sensory Modulation

Children with visual impairment and blindness often demonstrate stereotypical or repetitive behaviors, such as hand flapping, eye poking, or self-rocking.[84,85] However, occupational therapists need to be mindful that these behaviors are also seen in children with other conditions, such as autistic spectrum disorder, severe or profound intellectual disabilities, and other developmental disabilities. Therefore the presence of these behaviors (with the exception of eye poking) may not be due to blindness per se but rather to the underlying cause of the blindness, particularly in children with multiple disabilities. These stereotypic behaviors have been hypothesized to be sensory-seeking activities that may compensate for the vision loss, but another explanation may be that the behaviors emerge as a result of the severely limited repertoires of movement and behavior available to children with visual impairment.[68]

Some children with visual impairment also present with behaviors that suggest tactile hypersensitivity, postural instability, or gravitational insecurity. That is, a child may withdraw his or her hand from an object or art media, may object to being touched, may be fearful of moving through space, or may be afraid to get on playground equipment such as swings or the jungle gym. The intensity of the child's responses in these situations varies, as does the degree to which the responses interfere with the child's ability to engage in everyday occupations. Children with visual impairment who present with these behaviors may have restricted interactions with the environment and fewer typical motor and manipulative experiences that allow them to develop postural control, gross and fine motor skills, and praxis at similar levels of competence and quality as those of typical sighted children.

To understand the reasons for specific behaviors, the occupational therapist carefully evaluates the child's behaviors. For example, a child who may appear to demonstrate tactile hypersensitivity may not truly have a sensory modulation disorder or generalized hypersensitivities, but rather may need additional cues and strategies for managing new tactile experiences. The child may tolerate other tactile experiences, such as being held or wearing clothing made of different fabrics, and once the child becomes familiar with the object or material, the "defensive" reactions no longer occur. This scenario is different from that in which a child consistently demonstrates tactile hypersensitivity even to familiar tactile experiences or exhibits strong

BOX 26-2 Postural and Motor Characteristics Seen in Children with Visual Impairment

Children with visual impairment may display the following:

- Overall low muscle and postural tone, including instability in shoulder girdle and hips
- Head tilted to one side (visual or auditory accommodations)
- Head forward or hyperextended, resting on neck
- Head movements (e.g., swaying)
- Maintaining a wide base of support when standing or when walking
- Tendency to move in straight planes (e.g., decreased trunk rotation)
- High guard posture when walking

reactions to tactile stimuli beyond what could be attributed to caution or hesitance.

Children with visual impairment whose motor experiences are limited may be fearful about moving through open space (e.g., crawling across the room, walking across the playground), moving on equipment such as tricycles or swings, climbing on play structures, or going down a slide. Children with visual impairment often display characteristic postural and movement patterns (Box 26-2) that may give the appearance of or contribute to movement challenges, depending on the demonstrated level of functioning. In addition, caregivers (e.g., parents, daycare staff, teachers) who are concerned about safety may become overprotective and prevent or restrict children with visual impairment from engaging in movement and exploratory activities and experiencing the bumps and bruises that go with them, thus transmitting their fear to the child.

The integrity of the child's other sensory systems contributes to his or her ability to explore and learn from the environment, interact with family members and others, develop play skills, and master activities of daily living. Without vision, the child must use vestibular, proprioceptive, and auditory information to orient to gravity, move through space, and maintain postural alignment.[68,70] To integrate these sensory systems, the child must have opportunities to actively engage in and experience movement in a variety of situations.

Activities of Daily Living and Instrumental Activities of Daily Living

Children with visual impairment may have difficulty performing activities of daily living (ADLs), such as dressing and self-feeding. The impact of visual impairment on the development of locomotion, gross and fine motor skills, and praxis for play may also affect the child's ability to stand and lift the leg to put on a pair of pants, to direct the spoon to the plate to scoop up food, or to get into and out of the bathtub. In addition, if tactile hypersensitivity is present, the child's ability to engage in dressing, grooming, and toileting activities may be limited. If oral hypersensitivity is present, the progression to more textured foods and eating a variety of foods may be problematic. These reactions can disrupt daily routines for both the child and caregivers, as well as affect interactions with others and limit participation in learning activities at school. Negative associations with these activities can have long-lasting effects on the child's relationships with others and on occupational performance. Occupational therapy practitioners play a key role in helping children and families develop positive routines.

As children grow older and move into adolescence, participation in instrumental activities of daily living (IADLs) such as meal preparation, care of pets, and use of communication devices (i.e., Braille writers), needs to be encouraged. Supports can include adapting the task (i.e., completing the task in a different manner), changing the environment (e.g., placing materials for meal preparation in the same place), and providing adaptive equipment or technology (e.g., enlarged-print, adapted computers). A variety of commercially made technology and readily available applications for tablets and personal computers exist that may benefit the child or youth with visual impairments. (See Chapter 19 and the Evolve website for examples and resources.) The occupational therapist considers the individual's skills and abilities, environment, and the task itself when developing an intervention plan to address IADLs.

Social Participation and Communication

Patterns of interaction and communication for young children with visual impairment and their caregivers differ from those of sighted children, but can fully develop in the absence of functional vision.[81] The quality of social participation is influenced not only by the visual impairment but also the degree to which the child has acquired specific social skills. One study by Cabello and Verdugo examined the quality of social participation in different contexts (i.e., one-to-one, small group, and large group), for 64 children (4 to 18 years) with visual impairment based on teacher ratings of social skills.[10] The investigators found that visual impairment was a significant predictor for the quality of one-to-one interactions along with verbal skills, body language, and recognition and expression of emotions, whereas intellectual disability and visual impairment were significant predictors for large group interactions, with verbal skills, body language, play skills, and cooperation skills as important factors.

Specifically, young children with visual impairment may experience difficulty initiating and sustaining play and social interactions with peers. Without visual information to size up the context of the interaction and to pick up cues to respond to or imitate actions, the child with visual impairment may not have strategies to support the fluid give and take of a play scenario or social interaction.[20] The child may need explicit facilitation using physical, tactile, and verbal cues to keep up with changes that are often unpredictable, such as when play partners move to a different part of the playground or switch from sand play to ball play. In addition, the child with visual impairment may need to rely on tactile and auditory means for social referencing, and typical peers may need assistance to understand that the child's physical contact or listening is not meant to be intrusive or nonresponsive.

As children grow older, the complexity of interactions increases, and the contextual aspects of language and communication become important. Vision plays a significant role in the interpretation of facial expressions and body language and in the imitation and sustaining of the give and take of these interactions. Making eye contact, imitating facial gestures, shifting gaze, and perceiving the contextual features of visual images are often not part of the repertoire or experience of children who have vision loss at an early age.[68] The English language has many visual references that describe images, and Western culture expects individuals with visual impairment to communicate using the language of those who have sight.

Children with congenital visual impairment cannot "see" many features or qualities of objects such as a "red" button or "green" grass using the other sensory channels, nor can they see "a beautiful sunset" or "that one over there." Consequently, they can only try to imagine what it means when such descriptors or phrases are used.[68] In addition, children with visual impairment may not demonstrate the animation and nuances of facial expression because they have not experienced seeing and imitating these expressions.

These social skills difficulties may affect the child's ability to develop friendships or to fit in with the social demands and expectations of peers. When the occupational therapist, teachers, and family provide a range of opportunities and targeted strategies to support social development, these skills can fully develop and positively affect the child's participation in school, recreation, and home activities.

Occupational Therapy Evaluation

In many respects evaluation of the occupational performance of children with visual impairment encompasses the same components as in evaluation of children with other disabilities. Participation in play, self-care, school activities, and preparation for work are areas of focus for evaluation depending on the age and needs of the child. Evaluation of the performance skills (e.g., motor, process, and communication/interaction skills) that support or limit the child's ability to engage in specific activities in these areas, and the activity demands, client factors, and contexts in which the child performs these activities, is part of a comprehensive assessment. For example, a toddler with a visual impairment who has difficulty playing with toys may need evaluation of fine motor skills, tactile and proprioceptive processing, and postural control in sitting, with observations conducted in the home and day-care settings.

Standardized assessment tools for evaluating overall development in major domains (e.g., the Bayley Scales of Infant and Toddler Development, 3rd edition [Bayley III][9] or the Peabody Developmental Motor Scales, 2nd edition [PDMS-2][25]) should be used with caution because these measures were not standardized on children with visual impairment and the administration procedures do not include adaptations for this group. Therefore comparison of performance with that of sighted peers and use of the standard scores based on the normative sample are usually not appropriate. A few assessment tools (e.g., Battelle Developmental Inventory, 2nd edition)[51] are both standardized and criterion-referenced and include administration instructions for children with motor or sensory impairments.

Criterion-referenced measures, such as the Hawaii Early Learning Profile (HELP) for infants and toddlers[53] and preschoolers,[79] or play-based assessment tools, such as the Transdisciplinary Play-Based Assessment, 2nd edition,[46] may be more useful because they yield a profile of individual strengths and limitations or concerns that can be used to formulate an intervention plan. In addition, tools such as the Oregon Project Skills Inventory, 5th edition,[5] take into consideration what is known about the unique developmental trajectories of certain skills (e.g., walking independently, reaching to sound) in children with visual impairment.

An assessment tool that specifically addresses the impact of visual impairment on quality of life for students with low vision has been developed and may be of interest to occupational therapists.[14] This questionnaire was based on the Impact of Vision Impairment Profile developed for adults[43,44,82] and consists of five domains: school/specialist instruction, social interaction, community, family, and vision impairment/peer interaction. The questionnaire is helpful in identifying needs and planning intervention and its items emphasize participation in routine school and daily activities relative to social interaction, academic success, orientation and mobility skills, community acceptance, and other social opportunities.

In some instances a child who has developmental delays or difficulties may be referred for occupational therapy but has not yet been diagnosed with a visual impairment. If a child shows signs or symptoms of a vision problem and a visual impairment is suspected, the occupational therapist can assist in the diagnostic process through screening or evaluation of oculomotor skills (e.g., visual tracking, fixation, shifting gaze), focusing skills (e.g., shift from near to far), and eye teaming or binocularity (e.g., strabismus). See Table 26-1. The occupational therapist may also measure the child's visual perceptual skills (e.g., visual discrimination, visual spatial relations) and visual motor integration. Some developmental measures (e.g., Bayley III, HELP) include items that require visual attention, visual tracking, visual memory, and other vision-related areas.

Skilled observation and parent or caregiver questionnaires can be useful for gathering information about the child's temperament, self-regulation capacities, sensory processing and sensory modulation behaviors, and interaction with caregivers. In addition, interviews with the parents, teachers, or other caregivers provide information about daily routines, contexts, expectations, and resources available to support the child's participation in activities. As children get older the focus of the occupational therapy evaluation may involve collaboration with the special education or regular education teacher, education vision specialists (e.g., teacher for students with visual impairment or orientation and mobility specialist), and vision care specialists (e.g., developmental optometrist) to assess barriers in school and play settings and determine the need for adaptations for performing classroom activities, organization of desk space, or the use of assistive technology.[40,55,57] For adolescents, the occupational therapist, in collaboration with teachers, vision specialists, and the family, evaluates the individual's school, community, and work participation, in addition to leisure interests and activities. Case Study 26-1 shows the changing needs of the child and how occupational therapy services evolve over time.

Occupational Therapy Intervention

Occupational therapy for children who are blind or have significant visual impairment includes occupation-based, family-centered, developmental, visual rehabilitation, and ecologic approaches. As described in the previous sections, developmentally based oculomotor skills, visual alignment, acuity, and visual perception affect many areas of occupation.

TABLE 26-1 Signs and Symptoms of Visual Problems*

Category	Signs and Symptoms
Physical	Eyes shake or randomly wander Eyes are not able to follow moving object, face of parent Pupils of the eyes are excessively large or small Pupils of the eyes are not black; a cloudy film appears to be present Eyes are not in alignment (e.g., they are crossed or turn outward) Blurred vision or double vision Sensitivity to light
Behavioral	Needs to move closer to objects of interest; sits excessively close to the television Squinting, eyestrain, frequently rubs eyes Covers or closes one eye when looking at detail Excessive head movement Complains of discomfort or headaches when reading or doing close work Turns or tilts head when looking at detail Responds significantly better to objects on one side of the body than on the other Avoidance of or becomes tired after close work Poor attention span Complains of moving print
Performance	Appears clumsy or frequently bumps into objects when walking and running Cannot find necessary items for activities Difficulty learning left and right Has trouble learning the alphabet, recognizing words, learning basic math concepts of size, magnitude, position Difficulty with reading—reads slowly, skips lines, trouble with navigating page Difficulty with drawing, copying, writing—alignment, accuracy, reversals, organization on page, etc. Difficulty copying from board Has trouble keeping up with assignments
Social	Lack of interest in the environment Anxiety, social isolation Decreased self-confidence

*If a child shows any of the listed signs or symptoms, a referral to an eye care specialist is indicated.
Data from Takeshita, B. (n.d.). *Developing your child's vision.* Los Angeles: Center for the Partially Sighted; Scheiman, M. (2002). Optometric model of vision, parts one, two and three. In *Understanding and managing vision deficits: A guide for occupational therapists* (2nd ed., pp. 17-84). Thorofare, NJ: Slack; and Goldstand, S., Koslowe, K. D., & Parush, S. (2005). Vision, visual information processing, and academic performance among seventh-grade school children: A more significant relationship than we thought? *American Journal of Occupational Therapy, 59*, 377-389.

The outcome of occupational therapy intervention for children with visual impairment is to support participation in the daily contexts in which they function. For a 6-month-old premature infant with retinopathy of prematurity, for example, the occupational therapist may focus on establishing oral motor skills for feeding and self-soothing strategies for calming; other recommendations may include positioning strategies for feeding and caregiver-infant interactions and selecting toys that enhance the use of available vision, along with auditory and tactile channels. For a 10-year-old boy who has cerebral palsy with spastic hemiparesis and legal blindness (i.e., best corrected visual acuity of 20/200 or worse, or a visual field of 20 degrees or less in the better eye[83]), the school-based occupational therapist may focus on enhancing self-care skills, establishing organizational skills for using desk space and completing assignments, devising strategies that support the use of low vision aids, and promoting social participation in games with peers with modifications and adaptations.

Occupational therapy frames of reference that are particularly useful for intervention with children who have visual impairments may include developmental, sensory processing, motor acquisition and motor learning, visual perception, the Model of Human Occupation (MOHO), and person-environment-occupation-performance (PEOP) frameworks. Occupational therapy interventions with children and youth include emphasis on family-centered care, therapeutic use of self, therapeutic use of occupations and activities, consultation, and education. These approaches may be incorporated in different combinations and at different points during intervention in a dynamic process that changes based on the needs of the child and family, the progress and response to interventions, and the demands of the contexts involved.

The occupational therapist may be the primary practitioner for children who have visual impairments with other conditions; however, if the visual impairment is the primary or sole condition, it is more likely that an educational vision specialist (i.e., teacher of students with visual impairment, orientation and mobility specialist) is the primary interventionist, and the occupational therapist may provide consultation as needed. Generally the occupational therapist is a member of a team of professionals (e.g., general education teacher and/or special education teacher, educational vision specialist, speech-language pathologist, vision care specialist) who, along with the family, collaborate to identify the child's and family's needs and develop an intervention program to address those needs with one or more individuals providing services.

The occupational therapy practitioner often provides services to achieve the following goals.

Develop Self-Care Skills

The occupational therapist may consult with and educate those who work with the child with visual impairment to identify skill levels and explain problems affecting the child's development of self-care skills. The occupational therapist may specifically address underlying foundations and specific skills needed to perform self-care tasks, and work collaboratively with the family and the team to incorporate behavioral or learning strategies to improve self-care performance. The practitioner may suggest adaptations or modifications to the environment, recommend specialized equipment, and incorporate strategies that support independence (e.g., placing a tactile cue in specific areas of clothing to distinguish front from back or to identify color; using a divided plate or the clock orientation to serve food items).

Enhance Sensory Processing, Sensory Modulation, and Sensory Integration

Developmentally age-appropriate activities and materials that provide tactile, auditory, proprioceptive, and vestibular input can benefit the child with visual impairment and enhance or promote development of body concept, postural control, and tactile discrimination for recognizing and manipulating objects, self-regulation, and spatial relation perceptions. Sensorimotor activities can also promote bilateral hand use and praxis. Suspended equipment, scooterboards, tilt boards, obstacle courses, and other movement or balance equipment are useful, but it is also important to provide interventions using playground equipment (e.g., slides, jungle gyms, tricycles, swings) in the natural settings in which the child functions on a regular basis (Figure 26-1). Safety must be maintained in the use of equipment, and, as appropriate, the child should be allowed to control the movement and amount of input within his or her range of adaptive responses.

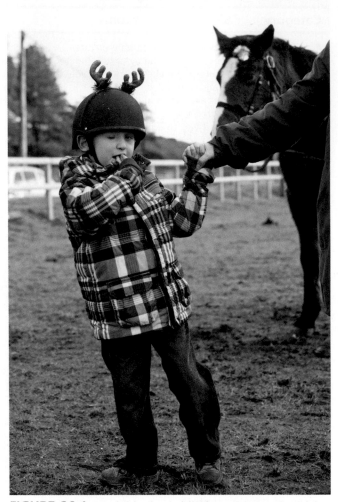

FIGURE 26-1 A child who is blind participates in equine assisted experiences.

The child with visual impairment does not see the approach of people and objects and may exhibit hypersensitivity to touch. In many instances children who have some or variable vision may have more difficulty with this than children with total blindness because children with some functional vision or low vision (i.e., best corrected visual acuity of 20/70 in the better eye[28,83]) receive unpredictable visual input from light patterns and movements. For children with total blindness, the visual input is essentially consistent. Firm touch generally is better than light touch, which can be interpreted as painful or aversive. The child with visual impairment often is more comfortable and less defensive when a verbal cue accompanies or precedes the tactile cue.

Strategies to help children modulate their reactions to tactile input include activities that encourage the child to explore and play with various materials using graded textures (e.g., sand, dried lentils, beans, and rice), activities that include vibration or proprioceptive input, and incorporation of a sensory diet at home and in the classroom. Support of the child's sensory modulation may be needed before an activity that the child finds aversive, such as art time, sand play, or eating. The child with hypersensitivity may benefit from recommendations for clothing, sleepwear, and linens. Also, if oral hypersensitivity is a factor, strategies such as introduction of graded food and liquid textures and tactile/proprioceptive activities involving the mouth (e.g., using straws with thickened liquids; blowing activities with bubbles or whistles) can be implemented. During these activities, it is important for the child with visual impairment to experience contingent responses to his or her behaviors, taking into consideration individual needs and preferences, rather than being a passive recipient of adult actions (noncontingent experiences).[12] For example, a child should not experience tactile stimulation in isolation (e.g., rubbing of different textured cloths on the arms); rather, the tactile experiences should be provided in the context of real-life activities (e.g., using a nubby towel to dry oneself after a bath) so that the child associates tactile experiences with actions and events.

Enhance Participation in Play or Productivity Through Postural Control and Movement in Space

Providing a variety of movement experiences throughout the daily routines early in life is important. Caregivers can be encouraged to use different carrying positions or carriers while

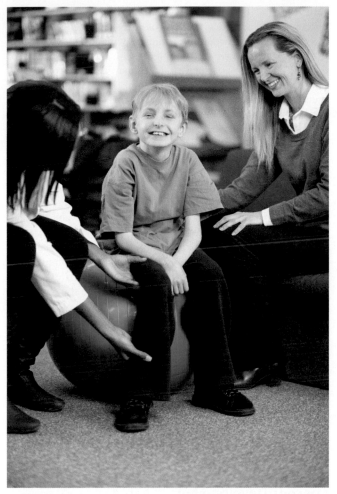
FIGURE 26-2 A child with significant visual impairment sits on a therapy ball to give him desired sensory input and to develop postural control.

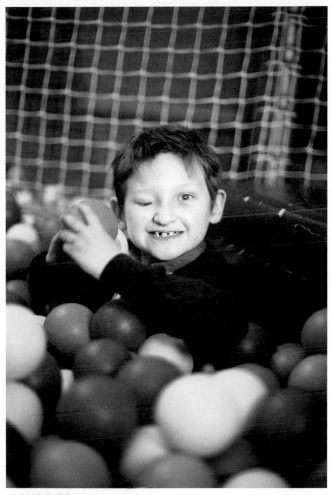
FIGURE 26-3 A child who has visual impairment enjoys time in the ball pool.

engaging in everyday activities so that infants experience movement (and vestibular and proprioceptive input) under secure conditions. Instead of passive prone positioning, in which motivation to lift the head is minimal, when visual impairment is significant, caregivers can be encouraged to engage in games that include tilting the child toward and away from them while talking to and having fun with the child, or positioning toys of interest in front of or to either side of the child and encouraging the child to reach for them.[57,71] The occupational therapist and the orientation and mobility specialist can work closely to facilitate and establish the child's ability to move through space through the use of push toys and riding toys, and by moving over surfaces of different heights, density, firmness, and/or textures (See Figures 26-2; 26-3; 26-4). In addition, motor learning principles may be applied to provide children with opportunities to practice a variety of movement strategies during different play activities, with feedback on their performance and results of their actions.

Develop Occupation-Based Mobility Through Body Awareness and Spatial Orientation

Many of the aforementioned activities can also help the child develop body awareness and directionality. Obstacle courses

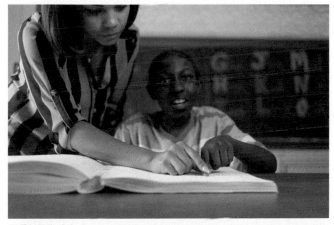
FIGURE 26-4 A child who is blind reads Braille and is assisted by professional services for the blind.

can teach the child spatial concepts such as left-right, up-down, over-under, in-out, beside, around, and behind. It is important to describe the movement or direction the child experiences to help him or her establish the association that will give meaning to the spatial concepts. Body awareness and spatial awareness are critical components that contribute to the child's development of mobility and language.[63,64,68,71]

Develop School-Based Tactile-Proprioceptive Perceptual Skills

The child with visual impairment needs to maximize tactile discrimination function to learn about the features and properties of objects; to adjust grasp according to the size, shape, and weight of an object; and to grade the amount of pressure, force, or speed needed to manipulate toys or to use tools. Tactile discrimination is also important for learning to read Braille. Finger painting, finding and identifying objects hidden in sand or beans or other media, and experiencing gradations of textures among everyday objects and materials, clothing, and surfaces are examples of activities that can increase tactile awareness and discrimination. In addition, manipulating objects and operating or using toys functionally (e.g., pushing buttons on a toy phone, playing with shape sorter toys with auditory feedback) helps children develop functional skills using tactile-proprioceptive and auditory information.

Children also need opportunities to explore and feel real-life objects to build multisensory associations and perceptions that ultimately become integrated and provide foundations for progression to more abstract representations (e.g., a real orange that is round, cold, fragrant, has an outside texture that can be peeled, can be separated into segments, tasted; a plastic orange and orange wedges used in kitchen and food play; a flat orange-shaped puzzle piece that fits into a puzzle board; a raised outline of an orange on paper for coloring). These experiences can help a child with visual impairment establish a mental image of the label "orange" and the color "orange" that is unique to each child based on characteristics that are meaningful to him or her.

Improve Manipulation and Fine Motor Skills

At first the world has to come to the child with visual impairment. A variety of toys and objects should be maintained within reach (e.g., tied to the crib, on the high chair or tabletop, on the floor). In addition, occupational therapists implement activities that promote general strength using upper extremity weight bearing.[70,71] By assessing the sensory features of the toys or objects, the occupational therapist can select objects and media appropriate for the child's ability to process the information and develop manipulation skills. For example, the occupational therapist selects objects that vary in texture, or in texture and sound, or have multisensory features (e.g., sound, texture, flashing lights) and media that are typically available in school settings (e.g., sand, paint, glue, PlayDoh). Providing opportunities for the child with visual impairment to practice in-hand manipulation with activities that involve rotation and translation of small objects can improve the dynamic use of tools. Some of the activities described previously (e.g., that address sensory integration and hypersensitivity) can also be used for sensory preparation of the hands before manipulation of objects.

Maximize Use of Functional Vision

The occupational therapist should always facilitate the child's use of whatever vision is available to him or her during intervention and everyday activities. The more a child uses visual pathways, the better vision develops.[8] Visual awareness and discrimination activities, such as color or shape recognition and matching, are important for children with functional vision. Activities such as use of a flashlight in a darkened room for tracking games or localizing targets may also improve visual skills. The occupational therapist can also promote the child's use of low vision aids recommended by the vision care specialist such as large print books or magnifiers and any other assistive technology that may be appropriate (e.g., closed-circuit television, computers with special software).

Encourage Social Participation

Children with visual impairment are at a disadvantage in social situations, particularly at school, where typical children are active and often participate in a variety of physical games. It is difficult for children with visual impairment to signal their interest in playing with peers, and reliance on others to help them with these interactions limits their ability to experience social competence.[20,37] It is important to provide the child with real-life activities, with specific instruction in social play, perhaps with one other child at first and then introducing other children as the child gains skills. Role playing, turn taking, and use of facial expressions with high affect and animation are strategies that can be used to facilitate social interactions. The child with visual impairment may need verbal or tactile cues to face people when speaking, to smile, and to maintain an upright posture with the head in midline. He or she must also learn to determine how others are reacting based on voices rather than gestures, facial expressions, or body language.

Strengthen Cognitive Skills and Concept Development

The child with visual impairment must consciously be taught to develop cognitive schemes that the sighted child picks up in a relatively casual manner. Concepts that cannot be touched or heard (e.g., clouds) need to be described and explained. To reiterate, it is beneficial to provide real-life, hands-on, multisensory experiences in a variety of meaningful contexts to help children with visual impairment establish the foundations for understanding concrete, functional, and abstract concepts.[21]

A variety of toys are available to help infants, toddlers, and preschoolers develop these skills. Toys that are of high interest and motivating can be incorporated to build intentionality, effective search strategies, and means-end understanding within everyday routines.[21] In addition, shape sorters, form boards, simple puzzles, or blocks that provide auditory feedback (e.g., music, animal sounds) when inserted into appropriate openings or when connected are useful. The occupational therapists can help children with visual impairment to develop strategies such as using one hand to locate the opening tactually and placing the shape with the other hand. For older children these goals can be accomplished through games (e.g., to promote memory, classification, sorting) using different media and many simple craft activities. The unique abilities and limitations of the child must be considered in addressing goals.

These goals require the occupational therapy practitioner to educate and consult with family members, who should be encouraged to provide the child with visual impairment opportunities for engagement in activities as they would a child without disability. Verbal and physical interaction should also be encouraged because the child may not always demonstrate behaviors that elicit interaction. Occupational therapists may consult with parents on ways to create a safe environment in which the child can play independently and make recommendations for adapting the environment to optimize independent functioning of the child.

Maximize Auditory Perceptual Abilities

The child with visual impairment must learn to identify sounds and their meanings and react to them appropriately. Sounds come from several basic sources: toys, speech, and the environment. Active, rather than passive, listening should be emphasized. Helpful activities include locating a variety of sounds in the environment, identifying sounds, and following directions from persons and recordings. In addition, the child with visual impairment must also use hearing as the primary distance sense and source for spatial information that guides his or her movement in the environment.[6] Helping children with visual impairment to use one or two sound references in their environment (e.g., the clock ticking on the wall, a bell attached to the classroom door) will be useful to enable them to know automatically where they are and where they want or need to go in a given space. Incorporate mobile objects that have sound (e.g., balls with bells inside, toy cars that make sounds), encourage children to discover interesting sounds, and vary the volume. It is just as important for children with visual impairment to register soft sounds and to filter out irrelevant auditory information, so use of toys and activities should involve grading the intensity of sensory input accordingly to avoid overwhelming or distracting the child. Also important for the child with visual impairment is the development of echolocation skills.

Supporting the Transition to Adulthood

The adolescent with visual impairment may face significant challenges in selecting an appropriate occupation,[45] although with current technology, many more opportunities are available than in the past. Although individuals with visual impairment as a group may experience unemployment or underemployment, an appropriate match between the personality and talent areas of the adolescent and the occupational choice can lead to a successful and enduring career. Lack of exposure to vocational options is a problem that the occupational therapist can address through community orientation and various activities that provide the individual with a variety of prevocational experiences.

Many IADLs, such as cooking, cleaning, and recreation, become increasingly important as the child with visual impairment reaches adolescence. The American Foundation for the Blind (http://www.afb.org) provides a comprehensive list of aids and appliances that can help the adolescent with visual impairment engage in such activities.[2] These may include a sugar meter that dispenses half a teaspoon of sugar at a time, an elbow-length oven mitt that protects against accidental burns, kits for marking canned goods, and self-threading needles. Recreational and leisure activities such as games with braille cards, low vision cards, or board games (e.g., Scrabble, Monopoly) with braille markings are available. Because many adults with severe visual impairment lead sedentary lives, it is important to instill the benefits of physical activity early in children's lives to promote healthy habits and routines. Organizations such as the United States Association for Blind Athletes (http://www.usaba.org),[75] Special Olympics (http://www.specialolympics.org), and community recreation programs offer sports and other physical activities in which children and youth with visual impairment can participate, train, and compete.

Specialized Professionals, Services, and Equipment for Children with Visual Impairment

Children with documented visual problems or who are suspected as having visual problems should have an examination by a pediatric ophthalmologist. Children with acuity, oculomotor, or eye alignment difficulties should also consider evaluation and treatment by a behavioral optometrist.[29] Occupational therapists screen for visual difficulties and provide intervention to remediate or compensate for visual impairment, in collaboration with a full medically based visual examination. Occupational therapy practitioners are uniquely trained in development and ecologic modifications for children with developmental disabilities affecting vision. However, when a child is blind or significantly visually impaired, unique and specialized technology, methodologies, resources, and supports requiring a level of specific education and training are needed. Personnel include certified low vision therapists, who evaluate and make recommendations regarding technologic supports; certified vision rehabilitation therapists (CVRT), who instruct people with blindness/visual impairment in compensatory skills and training including independent living, vocation, and education; and certified orientation and mobility specialists, who train people with significant visual impairment/blindness to access the community through nonvisual means, including the use of a white cane and leader dogs. Many of the professionals who provide services to people who are blind or visually impaired are certified in literacy braille through the National Blindness Professional Certification Board.[1] It is very important that occupational therapy practitioners recognize the need for these professionals and resources for the blind and refer children/families for these additional and essential services.

Children with severe visual impairments may rely on braille materials and talking books (e.g., those that can be listened to using devices such as compact disc and MP3 players) for their education. Braille is a system of six raised dots arranged in a cell to represent the letters of the alphabet, numbers, and words. It is produced on a special slate with a stylus or on a machine called a braillewriter. The system was developed by a young, blind French student, Louis Braille, in 1824, and was found to be more efficient than attempting to read the raised Roman alphabet. The complete Braille code consists of letters of the alphabet and contractions and words in short form.[40] Advances in technology now make it possible to use computer software and devices that incorporate Braille and/or audio formats. These devices can increase the amount and quality of written output and provide opportunities for interactive learning.

Various types of lenses are available for individuals with visual impairment, from the relatively common ones used to correct refractive errors to telescopic lenses (for viewing distant objects) and microscopic lenses (for viewing near objects) that are used as low vision aids for certain types of vision problems. Hand-held magnifiers include those that have the lens in sturdy housing (i.e., stand magnifiers) that are placed directly onto the reading material and those that can be worn around the neck. Electronic magnification systems include closed-circuit television systems, hand-held cameras that interface with a display monitor, head-mounted systems with a camera and display unit in front of each eye, small electronic systems that combine a camera and display for portable use, and miniature LCD magnifiers.[24]

Some occupational therapists are involved with low vision training (or vision therapy) to teach the child with visual impairment to use his or her available vision[8,66] in collaboration with a low vision specialist (i.e., optometrist). This may involve specific activities recommended by the low vision specialist that address problems with accommodation, vergence, visual fixation and focusing, oculomotor skills, or other vision-related problems, many of which can be incorporated into the play-based or therapeutic activities that the occupational therapist already implements. In addition, practitioners may provide a variety of adaptations and accommodations, including adjusting the intensity, position, and type of light (illumination) in the environment; minimizing glare; enhancing or maximizing contrast between objects and background or surfaces; adjusting size of objects or print; changing the spacing and positioning of objects; using color selection; and adjusting the amount of time to complete tasks.[19]

Orientation and mobility training or instruction teaches basic skills and techniques for travel in the environment such as trailing, the human (sighted) guide technique, and protective techniques.[4] In the *human guide technique*, the child who is blind takes the guide's arm and walks a half step behind and to the side of the guide to follow the guide's movements. For young children, an adapted grasp may be used, such as holding the guide's wrist (and progressing to the guide's elbow as the child gets older), or the child may hold the guide's index finger. This is preferred over the adult's holding the child's hand and pulling or leading the child. The human guide technique is safe and efficient and enables the child to interpret the guide's body movement (i.e., on uneven surfaces) and changes in direction.[6] Specific verbal and tactual cues are incorporated to negotiate stairs or narrow passages or if the child with visual impairment needs to change sides.

Trailing is a technique whereby the child with visual impairment holds his or her arm at a 45-degree angle in front and to the side of the body to follow a surface (e.g., wall) with the hand. Trailing serves several functions, including protection during movement, as a method for gathering information and locating landmarks and destinations, and for alignment.[6] The use of trailing can be enhanced when taught together with using a cane.

Echolocation is the ability to hear and interpret sound waves, which is important for orientation and travel in the environment.[6] By using clear sound signals (e.g., a clap, tongue clicking, tapping, or a hand-held clicker) the child uses echoes produced to determine the location of objects and important features (e.g., size, general shape, density) and to detect buildings, play structures, doorways, stairs, and potential obstacles (e.g., poles, trees). Echolocation serves as a means to extend the reach of the cane to gather information at much greater distances. Some children with visual impairment develop echolocation skills on their own without any instruction, whereas other children will need targeted intervention. The occupational therapist can collaborate with the orientation and mobility specialist to support recommended strategies that promote the development of echolocation skills.

Protective techniques can be taught to toddlers and preschoolers (depending on motor development, physical coordination, and attention span) and involve upper body and lower body techniques in which the arm is flexed with forearm held across the body with palm facing out at about shoulder height or at an angle in front of the face, or extended downward and diagonally across the body at the hip with palm facing the body. Another protection technique used in bending down to retrieve a dropped object is to extend the arm palm out in front of the head. The child with visual impairment can search for a lost object by touching the ground to establish a beginning point and then searching in an ever-widening concentric circle pattern. A technique for exploring a room involves searching the parameters of the room first, then mentally dividing it into grids to be searched methodically. This method can be used to introduce the child with vision impairment to a new classroom or new home set up. The use of landmarks and cues (e.g., the grass at the edge of the sidewalk) is beneficial for independent movement in the environment. These techniques help to protect against obstacles during movement, although the degree of protection is limited if it is the only technique used, and if used frequently the child may become fatigued.[6] As with trailing, these techniques are more beneficial if used in conjunction with a long cane.

The orientation and mobility specialist is typically the one who teaches human guide, trailing, and protection techniques. However, occupational therapists, as well as caregivers and others who work with children with visual impairment, should learn the basic techniques to reinforce appropriate use that supports the child's interaction with the environment. *Cane technique* is a specialized procedure that requires training from a professional, but occupational therapists can promote skills and prepare young children with visual impairment for using a mobility device, particularly when co-existing conditions also affect mobility. The occupational therapist can recommend activities and provide intervention to improve balance, coordination, postural control, praxis, and prehension. The occupational therapist (and physical therapist) can also provide input and education regarding the advantages and disadvantages of the use of commercially available infant walkers or other apparatus (e.g., infant swings, jumpers) based on the postural, motor, and sensory processing of the child. Mobile toys, such as shopping carts, push toys with long handles, ride-on toys, or large balls, can be incorporated to provide movement experiences and serve as an early navigation tool as long as they are used with safety, function, and social acceptability in mind.[6]

The orientation and mobility specialist performs evaluations to determine a child's readiness for use of a cane. Various types of mobility devices are available, including long canes (e.g., with dual handles or dual grips) and polyvinyl chloride devices (e.g., with curved tips, rollers, or wheels). Specialists disagree regarding the introduction of cane use with preschoolers, arguing for and against early use; however, a child with visual impairment who is determined to be ready and is motivated to learn to use a cane will likely benefit from early introduction to its use and move toward independent mobility.

Summary

The process of occupational therapy is unique and individualized to each client. Children with blindness or who have visual impairment present with unique client factors, life challenges, and triumphs. Many children with developmental disabilities also present with visual problems. It is important that occupational therapy practitioners recognize and refer to vision professionals who are specifically trained in services for the blind/significant visual impairment when necessary. The occupational therapy practitioner utilizes occupation-based models as well as developmental and ecologic theoretical approaches to address occupational performance for children who are blind or visually impaired. The chapter's case study followed one client through childhood and three practice settings using occupational therapy interventions grounded in theoretical perspectives. Professional reasoning and specific occupational profiles and family-centered aspects of intervention planning help the occupational therapist to provide best practice with children who are blind or have visual impairment.

Summary Points

- *Visual impairment* is defined as the loss of or deficits in visual function (i.e., vision, visual perception, interpretation of visual input) because of pathology or processing problems in one or more components of the visual system (e.g., structures of the eye, visual pathways, and the brain) that limits the individual's ability to engage in and participate in daily occupations.
- Visual impairment may interfere with a child's ability to engage in areas of occupation, which include play/leisure, eating/feeding, sleep/rest, self-care ADLs and IADLs, work/productivity, community mobility, and social participation.
- Occupational therapists collaborate with vision professionals including pediatric ophthalmologists, behavioral optometrists, certified low vision therapists, and certified orientation and mobility specialists. By understanding the important contributions of these professionals, occupational therapists make recommendations to assure children receive these essential services.
- Occupational therapy evaluation/intervention with children who are visually impaired or blind includes activities to promote development, sensory modulation, perceptual motor function, occupation-based mobility, and social participation. Full participation in life activities for people who are blind or visually impaired is the overarching goal.
- Occupational therapy practitioners using occupation-based models, including task and environment adaptation, promote the participation of infants, children, and youth with visual impairment or blindness.

REFERENCES

1. Academy for Certification of Vision Rehabilitation and Education Professionals (ACUREP). (2013). *Certified vision professionals.* Retrieved May 26 from: <http://www.acvrep.org>.
2. American Foundation for the Blind. (2008). *Statistics and sources for professionals.* From: <http://www.afb.org/section.asp?SectionIE=154DocumentID=1367#prev> Retrieved August 18, 2008.
3. American Occupational Therapy Association. (1999). *Occupational therapy services for children and youth under the Individuals with Disabilities Education Act* (2nd ed.). Bethesda, MD: AOTA.
4. American Occupational Therapy Association. (2008). The occupational therapy practice framework: Domain and process. (2nd ed.). *American Journal of Occupational Therapy, 62*(6), 625–683.
5. Angeli, S. (2003). Value of vestibular testing in young children with sensorineural hearing loss. *Archives of Otolaryngology-Head & Neck Surgery, 129*, 478–482.
6. Anthony, S. T. L., Bleier, H., Fazzi, D. L., et al. (2002). Mobility focus: Developing early skills for orientation and mobility. In R. L. Pogrund & D. L. Fazzi (Eds.), *Early focus: Working with young children who are blind or visually impaired and their families* (2nd ed., pp. 326–404). New York: AFB Press.
7. Baird, S., Mayfield, P., & Baker, P. (1997). Mothers' interpretations of the behavior of their infants with visual and other impairments during interactions. *Journal of Visual Impairment and Blindness, 91*, 467–483.
8. Baker-Nobles, L. (2005). Ocular pathology and cortical visual impairment in pediatric low vision. In M. Gentile (Ed.), *Functional visual behavior in children: An occupational therapy guide to evaluation and treatment options* (2nd ed., pp. 315–338). Bethesda, MD: AOTA.
9. Bayley, N. (2006). *Bayley scales of infant and toddler development administration manual* (3rd ed.). San Antonio, TX: Harcourt Assessment.
10. Caballo, C., & Verdugo, M. A. (2007). Social skills assessment of children and adolescents with visual impairment: Identifying relevant skills to improve quality of social relationships. *Psychological Reports, 100*, 1101–1106.
11. Celeste, M. (2002). A survey of motor development for infants and young children with visual impairment. *Journal of Visual Impairment and Blindness, 96*, 169–174.
12. Chen, D. (1999). Interactions between infants and caregivers: The context for early intervention. In D. Chen (Ed.), *Essential elements in early intervention: Visual impairment and multiple disabilities* (pp. 22–54). New York: AFB Press.
13. Christiansen, C., & Baum, C. M. (1991). *Occupational therapy: Enabling function and well-being* (2nd ed.). Thorofare, NJ: SLACK, Inc.
14. Cochrane, G., Lamoureux, E. L., & Keeffe, J. (2008). Defining the content for a new quality of life questionnaire for students with low vision (the impact of vision impairment on children: IVI_C). *Ophthalmic Epidemiology, 15*, 114–120.
15. Correa, V. I., Fazzi, D. L., & Pogrund, R. L. (2002). Team focus: Current trends, service delivery, and advocacy. In R. L. Pogrund & D. L. Fazzi (Eds.), *Early focus: Working with young children who are blind or visually impaired and their families* (2nd ed., pp. 405–441). New York: AFB Press.
16. Coster, W., Deeney, T., Haltiwanger, J., et al. (1998). *The School Function Assessment.* San Antonio, TX: The Psychological Corporation.
17. Dunn, L. (2004). Validation of the CHORES: A measure of children's participation in household tasks. *Scandinavian Journal of Occupational Therapy, 11*, 179–190.

18. Dunn, W. (1997). The impact of sensory processing on the daily lives of young children and families: A conceptual model. *Infants and Young Children, 9*(4), 23–25.
19. Erin, J. N., Fazzi, D. L., Gordon, R. L., et al. (2002). Vision focus: Understanding the medical and functional implications of vision loss. In R. L. Pogrund & D. L. Fazzi (Eds.), *Early focus: Working with young children who are blind or visually impaired and their families* (2nd ed., pp. 52–106). New York: AFB Press.
20. Fazzi, D. L. (2002). Social focus: Developing social skills and promoting positive interactions. In R. L. Pogrund & D. L. Fazzi (Eds.), *Early focus: Working with young children who are blind or visually impaired and their families* (2nd ed., pp. 188–217). New York: AFB Press.
21. Fazzi, D. L., & Klein, D. (2002). Cognitive focus: Developing cognition, concepts, and language. In R. L. Pogrund & D. L. Fazzi (Eds.), *Early focus: Working with young children who are blind or visually impaired and their families* (2nd ed., pp. 107–153). New York: AFB Press.
22. Fazzi, E., Zaccagnino, M., Gahagan, S., et al. (2008). Sleep disturbances in visual impaired toddlers. *Brain & Development, 30*, 572–578.
23. Ferrell, K. A. (1998). *Project PRISM: A longitudinal study of developmental patterns of children who are visually impaired. Executive summary (CFDA 84.0203C—Field-initiated research H025C10188)*. Washington, DC: Office of Special Education Programs, Office of Special Education and Rehabilitative Services, U.S. Department of Education.
24. Fischer, J. L., & Rosenthal, B. P. (2005). Optometric assessment and treatment of low vision in children and adults. In M. Gentile (Ed.), *Functional visual behavior in children* (2nd ed., pp. 291–314). Bethesda, MD: AOTA Press.
25. Folio, M. R., & Fewell, R. R. (2000). *Peabody Developmental Motor Scales* (2nd ed.). Austin, TX: Pro-Ed.
26. Forsyth, K., Deshpande, S., Kielhofner, G., et al. (2005). *The Occupational Circumstances Assessment Interview and Rating Scale (OCAIRS) (version 4.0)*. Chicago: Model of Human Occupation Clearinghouse, Department of Occupational therapy, College of Applied Health Sciences, University of Illinois.
27. Freeman, K., Salt, A., Prusa, A., et al. (2005). Association between congenital toxoplasmosis and parent-reported developmental outcomes, concerns, and impairment in 3 year old children. *BMC Pediatrics, 5*, 25.
28. Freeman, P. B. (2002). Low vision: Overview and review of low vision evaluation and treatment. In M. Gentile (Ed.), *Functional visual behavior in children: An occupational therapy guide to evaluation and treatment options* (2nd ed., pp. 265–289). Bethesda, MD: AOTA Press.
29. Geddie, B. E., Bina, M. J., & Miller, M. M. (2013). Vision and visual impairment. In M. L. Batshaw, N. J. Roizen, & G. R. Lotrecchiano (Eds.), *Children with disabilities* (7th ed., pp. 169–188). Baltimore, MD: Brookes Publishing.
30. Glass, P. (1995). Development of visual function in preterm infants: Implications for early intervention. *Infants & Young Children, 6*, 11–20.
31. Glass, P. (2002). Development of the visual system and implications for early intervention. *Infants & Young Children, 15*(1), 1–10.
32. Glidden, L. M., & Jobe, B. M. (2007). Measuring parental daily rewards and worries in the transition to adulthood. *American Journal on Mental Retardation, 112*, 275–278.
33. Goldstand, S., Koslowe, K. D., & Parush, S. (2005). Vision, visual-information processing, and academic performance among seventh-grade school children: A more significant relationship than we thought? *American Journal of Occupational Therapy, 59*, 377–389.
34. Hatton, D. D., Bailey, D. G., Burchinal, M. R., et al. (1997). Developmental growth curves of preschool children with vision impairments. *Child Development, 58*, 788–806.
35. Humphry, R., & Wakeford, L. (2006). An occupation-centered discussion of development and implications for practice. *American Journal of Occupational Therapy, 60*(3), 258–267.
36. Journey, B. J., & Loukas, K. M. (2009). Adolescents with disability in school-based practice: Psychosocial interventions for a successful journey into adulthood. *Journal of Occupational Therapy, Schools, & Early Intervention, 2*, 119–132.
37. Kelley, P. A., Sanspree, M. J., & Davidson, R. C. (2000). Vision impairment in children and youth. In B. Silverstone, M. A. Lang, B. P. Rosenthal, et al. (Eds.), *The Lighthouse handbook on vision impairment and vision rehabilitation* (Vol. 2, Vision rehabilitation, pp. 1137–1151). New York: Oxford University Press.
38. Kielhofner, G. (2008). *Model of Human Occupation: Theory and application* (4th ed.). Philadelphia: Lippincott Williams & Wilkins.
39. Knox, S. (2008). Development and current use of the Revised Knox Preschool Play Scale. In L. D. Parham & L. Fazio (Eds.), *Play in occupational therapy for children* (2nd ed., pp. 55–70). St Louis: Mosby.
40. Koenig, A. J., & Holbrook, M. C. (2002). Literacy focus. Developing skills and motivation for reading and writing. In R. L. Poground & D. L. Fazzi (Eds.), *Early focus: Working with young children who are blind or visually impaired and their families* (2nd ed., pp. 154–187). New York: AFB Press.
41. Kohlman Thompson, L. (1992). *The Kohlman Evaluation of Living Skills* (3rd ed.). Bethesda, MD: The American Occupational Therapy Association, Inc.
42. Kutzbach, B. R., Summers, C. G., Holleschau, A. M., et al. (2008). Neurodevelopment in children with albinism. *Ophthalmology, 115*, 1805–1808.
43. Lamoureux, E. L., Pallant, J. F., Pesudovs, K., et al. (2006). The Impact of Vision Impairment Questionnaire: An evaluation of its measurement properties using Rasch analysis. *Investigative Ophthalmology & Visual Science, 47*, 4732–4741.
44. Lamoureux, E. L., Pallant, J. F., Pesudovs, K., et al. (2007). The Impact of Vision Impairment Questionnaire: An assessment of its domain structure using confirmatory factor analysis and Rasch analysis. *Investigative Ophthalmology & Visual Science, 48*, 1001–1006.
45. Lampert, J. L. (1998). Working with students with visual impairment. In J. Case-Smith (Ed.), *Occupational therapy: Making a difference in school system practice*. Bethesda, MD: American Occupational Therapy Association.
46. Linder, T. W. (2008). *Transdisciplinary play-based assessment* (2nd ed.). Baltimore: Brookes.
47. Loukas, K. M., & Cote, T. L. (2005). Sports as occupation: A sports camp experience for children who are blind or have visual impairment. *OT Practice, March 21*, 15–19.
48. McConnell, A. E., Martin, J. E., Juan, C. Y., et al. (2012). *Career development and transition for exceptional individuals. Hammill Institute on Disabilities.* <http://cde.sagepub.com/content/early/2012/12/13/2165143412468147>.
49. Miller, M. M., & Menacker, S. J. (2007). Vision: Our window to the world. In M. L. Batshaw, L. Pellegrino, & N. Roizen (Eds.), *Children with disabilities* (6th ed., pp. 137–155). Baltimore: Brookes.
50. Mindell, J. A., & DeMarco, C. M. (1997). Sleep problems of young blind children. *Journal of Visual Impairment and Blindness, 91*(1), 33–39.

51. Newborg, J. (2005). *Battelle developmental inventory* (2nd ed.). Chicago: Riverside.
52. Parks, S. (2006). *Inside HELP: Administration and reference manual.* Palo Alto, CA: VORT Corporation.
53. Parks, S. (1999). *Inside HELP: Administration and reference manual for the Hawaii Early Learning Profile (birth-3).* Palo Alto, CA: VORT.
54. Pogrund, R. (2002). Refocus: Setting the stage for working with children who are blind or visually impaired. In R. L. Pogrund & D. L. Fazzi (Eds.), *Early focus: Working with young children who are blind or visually impaired and their families* (2nd ed., pp. 1–15). New York: AFB Press.
55. Pogrund, R. (2002). Independence focus: Promoting independence in daily living and recreational skills. In R. L. Pogrund & D. L. Fazzi (Eds.), *Early focus: Working with young children who are blind or visually impaired and their families* (2nd ed., pp. 218–249). New York: AFB Press.
56. Ponchillia, P. (2005). The access sports model: Adapting mainstream sports for individuals with visual impairments. *RE:view, 27,* 5–14.
57. Porr, S. M. (1999). The visual and auditory systems. In S. M. Porr & E. B. Rainville (Eds.), *Pediatric therapy: A systems approach* (pp. 241–266). Philadelphia: F. A. Davis.
58. Quotations. (2013). <http://www.quotationspage.com/quotes/Helen_Keller/>.
59. Recchia, S. (1997). Play and concept development in infants and young children with severe visual impairments: A constructionist view. *Journal of Visual Impairment and Blindness, 91,* 401–406.
60. Roizen, N., Kasza, K., Karrison, T., et al. (2008). Impact of visual impairment on measures of cognitive function for children with congenital toxoplasmosis: Implications for compensatory intervention strategies [Electronic version]. *Pediatrics, 118,* e379–e390.
61. Ross, G., Lipper, E. G., Abramson, D., et al. (2001). The development of young children with retinoblastoma. *Archives of Pediatric and Adolescent Medicine, 155,* 80–83.
62. Ross, S., & Tobin, M. J. (1997). Object permanence, reaching, and locomotion n infants who are blind. *Journal of Visual Impairment and Blindness, 91,* 25–32.
63. Sanspree, M. J. (2000). Pathways to habilitation: Best practices. In B. Silverstone, M. A. Lang, B. P. Rosenthal, et al. (Eds.), *The Lighthouse handbook on vision impairment and vision rehabilitation* (Vol. 2, Vision rehabilitation, pp. 1167–1182). New York: Oxford University Press.
64. Schaaf, R. C., & Smith Roley, S. (2006). Sensory integration for children with visual impairments, including blindness. In R. C. Schaaf & S. Smith Roley (Eds.), *SI: Applying clinical reasoning to practice with diverse populations* (pp. 149–169). San Antonio: TX Harcourt Assessment.
65. Scheiman, M. (2002). Optometric model of vision, parts one, two and three. In *Understanding and managing vision deficits: A guide for occupational therapists* (2nd ed., pp. 17–84). Thorofare, NJ: Slack.
66. Scheiman, M. (2002). Management of refractive, visual efficiency, and visual information processing disorders. In *Understanding and managing vision deficits: A guide for occupational therapists* (2nd ed., pp. 117–164). Thorofare, NJ: Slack.
67. Schiarti, V., Matsuba, C., Houbé, J. S., et al. (2008). Severe retinopathy of prematurity and visual outcomes in British Columbia: A 10-year analysis. *Journal of Perinatology, 28,* 1–7.
68. Smith Roley, S., & Schneck, C. (2001). Sensory integration and visual deficits, including blindness. In S. Smith Roley, E. I. Blanche, & R. C. Schaaf (Eds.), *Understanding the nature of sensory integration with diverse populations* (pp. 313–344). San Antonio, TX: Therapy Skill Builders.
69. Spencer, R. (2006). Long-term visual outcomes in extremely low-birth-weight children. (An American Ophthalmological Society thesis). *Transactions of the American Ophthalmological Society, 104,* 493–516.
70. Strickling, C. A. (1998). *Impact of vision loss on motor development: Information for occupational and physical therapists working with students with visual impairments.* Austin, TX: Texas School for the Blind and Visually Impaired.
71. Strickling, C. A., & Pogrund, R. L. (2002). Motor focus: Promoting movement experiences and motor development. In R. L. Pogrund & D. L. Fazzi (Eds.), *Early focus: Working with young children who are blind or visually impaired and their families* (2nd ed., pp. 287–325). New York: AFB Press.
72. Teplin, S. W. (1995). Visual impairment in infants and young children. *Infants & Young Children, 8*(1), 18–41.
73. Titcomb, R. E., & Okoye, R. (2005). Functional vision: A developmental, dynamic, and integrated process. In M. Gentile (Ed.), *Functional visual behavior in children: An occupational therapy guide to evaluation and treatment options* (2nd ed., pp. 1–40). Bethesda, MD: AOTA Press.
74. Tsai, L.-T., Meng, L.-F., Wu, W.-C., et al. (2013). Effects of visual rehabilitation on a child with severe visual impairment. *American Journal of Occupational Therapy, 67,* 437–447.
75. United States Association of Blind Athletes (USABA). (2014). Retrieved from: <http://www.usaba.org/>.
76. U.S. Department of Education. (2007). *27th annual report to Congress on the implementation of the Individuals with Disabilities Education Act, 2005* (Vol. 2). Washington, DC: Office of Special Education Programs, U.S. Department of Education. Retrieved August 4, 2014 from: <www.ed.gov/offices/OSERS/OSEP>.
77. U.S. Department of Education. (2014). *IDEA and IDEIA.* Retrieved from, 2014: <http://www2.ed.gov/about/offices/list/osers/osep/index.html?src=mr>.
78. Vervloed, M. P. J., Hoevenaars, E., & Maas, A. (2003). Behavioral treatment of sleep problems in a child with a visual impairment. *Journal of Visual Impairment and Blindness, 97*(1), 28–37.
79. VORT. (1995–1999). *HELP for preschoolers: Assessment & curriculum guide.* Palo Alto, CA: Author.
80. Warren, D. (1994). *Blindness in children: An individual differences approach.* New York: Cambridge University Press.
81. Warren, D. (2000). Developmental perspectives. In B. Silverstone, M. A. Lang, B. P. Rosenthal, et al. (Eds.), *The Lighthouse handbook on vision impairment and vision rehabilitation* (Vol. 1, Vision impairment, pp. 325–337). New York: Oxford University Press.
82. Weib, L. M., Hassell, J. B., & Keeffe, J. (2002). Assessment of the impact of vision impairment. *Investigative Ophthalmology & Visual Science, 43,* 927–935.
83. Yeargin-Allsopp, M., Drews-Botsch, C., & Van Naarden Braun, K. (2007). Epidemiology of developmental disabilities. In M. L. Batshaw, L. Pellegrino, & N. J. Roizen (Eds.), *Children with disabilities* (6th ed., pp. 215–243). Baltimore: Brookes.
84. Fazzi, E., Lanners, J., Danova, S., et al. (1999). Sterotyped behaviours in blind children. *Brain Development, 21*(8), 522–528.
85. McHugh, E., & Lieberman, L. (2003). The impact of developmental factors on stereotypic rocking of children with visual impairments. *Journal of Visual Impairment and Blindness, 97*(8), 453–474.

CHAPTER

27 Autism Spectrum Disorder

Heather Miller-Kuhaneck

KEY TERMS

Cognitive Orientation to Daily Occupational Performance
Family-centered care
Floortime
Positive behavioral support
Optimistic parenting
Parental stress
Coping
Self-efficacy
Social participation
Social stories
Sensory processing
Sensory integration intervention
Applied Behavioral Analysis
Reciprocal Imitation Training

GUIDING QUESTIONS

1. What is autism spectrum disorder (ASD) and how does it impact the occupational performance of individuals?
2. How does ASD in one family member affect the entire family?
3. What is an occupational therapist's role in assessment and intervention in ASD?
4. How can occupational therapists assist families to improve the occupational performance of children with ASD as well as overall family functioning?

Introduction to Autism Spectrum Disorder

Autism spectrum disorder (ASD) is a neurologic disorder seen most commonly, but not uniquely, in boys. First described 70 years ago,[110] according to the current *Diagnostic and Statistical Manual*, fifth edition (DSM-5), the symptoms of ASD cluster in two primary categories of functioning: social interaction and repetitive and restrictive behaviors.[9] Symptoms may be evident at a young age, but diagnosis is typically made during the preschool years. With a wide diversity of potential symptoms of ASD and varying levels of severity, each child presents with a unique compilation of strengths and weaknesses that will impact occupational performance for the child and family in differing ways.

History of the Diagnosis

The diagnosis of ASD has a lengthy history. Authors have speculated that case reports from the 1700s and 1800s may document individuals who had autism.[73] However, the first cases in the research literature were published in 1943 by Dr. Leo Kanner. Unfortunately for many families, Kanner considered the 11 individuals whom he labeled autistic to suffer from social withdrawal in response to poor parenting.[110] This view, broadcast in a *Time* magazine article in 1960, suggested children with autism had a "cold" mother who was able to "defrost enough to produce a child"[28,209] and even suggested "parentectomy," a treatment in which children were removed from these rejecting and unfeeling parents. This flawed accounting of the role of parenting in autism persisted for decades. See Table 27-1e on the Evolve website for resources regarding the history of the diagnosis of ASD.

In the first two editions of the DSM[4,5] ASD was not included as an accepted diagnosis, and individuals with ASD were often diagnosed with schizophrenia.[111] A diagnosis of infantile autism was defined under the umbrella term *pervasive developmental disorder* in the third edition of the DSM in 1980.[6] The label was changed to autistic disorder in 1987.[7] In the fourth edition of the DSM[8] the diagnostic criteria for autism disorders were broadened.[10] The umbrella term of pervasive developmental disorder included five individual categories: autism, Asperger's syndrome, Rett's syndrome, childhood disintegrative disorder, and pervasive developmental disorder—not otherwise specified. Researchers demonstrated that the boundaries around these categories were indistinct, and for many years researchers and professionals used the term "autism spectrum disorder" to describe the entire range of individuals who demonstrated behaviors associated with autism.

Recent Diagnostic Changes

The DSM-5[4] made significant changes to the diagnostic criteria and labeling for ASD. For example, Asperger's disorder is no longer a distinct diagnostic label. These changes have been somewhat controversial, as parents and professionals worried about the impact of these changes on individuals who could lose their diagnosis if they no longer meet the new criteria for ASD.[49] It is possible that the new diagnostic criteria may exclude up to 40% of individuals previously diagnosed under the older criteria of the DSM-IV.[143] One addition to the DSM-5 ASD diagnosis is the inclusion of criteria regarding unusual responses to sensation, an area of assessment and intervention that has historically resided primarily within the profession of occupational therapy. The opportunities for occupational therapists to emerge as leaders on the health care team in this arena are substantial.[221] Box 27-1 includes information about the current diagnostic criteria in the DSM-5. The revisions to the diagnostic criteria over time have occurred in response to

BOX 27-1 Autism Spectrum Disorder

Diagnostic Criteria

A. Persistent deficits in social communication and social interaction across multiple contexts, as manifested by the following, currently or by history (examples are illustrative, not exhaustive, see text):
   1. Deficits in social-emotional reciprocity, ranging, for example, from abnormal social approach and failure of normal back-and-forth conversation; to reduced sharing of interests, emotions, or affect; to failure to initiate or respond to social interactions.
   2. Deficits in nonverbal communicative behaviors used for social interaction, ranging, for example, from poorly integrated verbal and nonverbal communication; to abnormalities in eye contact and body language or deficits in understanding and use of gestures; to a total lack of facial expressions and nonverbal communication.
   3. Deficits in developing, maintaining, and understanding relationships, ranging, for example, from difficulties adjusting behavior to suit various social contexts; to difficulties in sharing imaginative play or in making friends; to absence of interest in peers.

Specify current severity:

Severity is based on social communication impairments and restricted, repetitive patterns of behavior.

B. Restricted, repetitive patterns of behavior, interests, or activities, as manifested by at least two of the following, currently or by history (examples are illustrative, not exhaustive, see text):
   1. Stereotyped or repetitive motor movements, use of objects, or speech (e.g., simple motor stereotypes, lining up toys or flipping objects, echolalia, idiosyncratic phrases).
   2. Insistence on sameness, inflexible adherence to routines, or ritualized patterns of verbal or nonverbal behavior (e.g., extreme distress at small changes, difficulties with transitions, rigid thinking patterns, greeting rituals, need to take same route or eat same food every day).
   3. Highly restricted, fixated interests that are abnormal in intensity or focus (e.g., strong attachment to or preoccupation with unusual objects, excessively circumscribed or perseverative interests).
   4. Hyper- or hyporeactivity to sensory input or unusual interest in sensory aspects of the environment (e.g., apparent indifference to pain/temperature, adverse response to specific sounds or textures, excessive smelling or touching of objects, visual fascination with lights or movement).

Specify current severity:

Severity is based on social communication impairments and restricted, repetitive patterns of behavior.

C. Symptoms must be present in the early developmental period (but may not become fully manifest until social demands exceed limited capacities, or may be masked by learned strategies in later life).

D. Symptoms cause clinically significant impairment in social, occupational, or other important areas of current functioning.

E. These disturbances are not better explained by intellectual disability (intellectual developmental disorder) or global developmental delay. Intellectual disability and autism spectrum disorder frequently co-occur; to make comorbid diagnoses of autism spectrum disorder and intellectual disability, social communication should be below that expected for general developmental level.

Note: Individuals with a well-established DSM-IV diagnosis of autistic disorder, Asperger's disorder, or pervasive developmental disorder not otherwise specified should be given the diagnosis of autism spectrum disorder.

From American Psychiatric Association. (2013). *Diagnostic and statistical manual of mental disorders* (5th ed.). Washington, DC: Author (pp. 50-51).

research findings and to changing needs of the medical and scientific community. Although important, these modifications have also created difficulty in determining real changes in ASD prevalence over time.

Prevalence

Research indicates a rise in the prevalence of ASD. During the 1960s and 1970s, ASD reportedly occurred in as few as one per 10,000 children.[32] Although it is likely that early prevalence studies drastically underestimated ASD rates,[190] research since the 1990s indicated a substantial increase. By 2007, the Centers for Disease Control and Prevention (CDC) reported one in 150 children with ASD, an increase from one in 166 just 2 years earlier.[42] The Centers' figures suggested an average prevalence of one in 110 children in 2009[181] and one in 88 in 2012.[16] A national survey conducted by Kogan et al. (2009) reported a prevalence of one in 91 children 3 to 17 years of age, or 1% of the population. Most recently, a prevalence rate of 1 in 50 was reported.[119]

Causal factors for the change in prevalence are unclear, and many potential mechanisms require further exploration. However, regardless of causal factors, the current reported prevalence suggests that ASD is now the second most common developmental disability in the nation. The lifetime use of services by individuals with ASD therefore reflects a large public health burden.[32,37,163] The increasing prevalence suggests considerable public health implications, including societal and familial costs associated with raising and educating a child with ASD.[74,83,153-155]

Occupational Performance in Autism Spectrum Disorder

Autism spectrum disorder may impact any and all areas of occupation but research suggests that certain types of occupational performance issues are more common than others.

Social Participation

Social issues are a hallmark of this disorder. Friendship and social inclusion requires different skills at different ages.[59] Very young children often imitate others to begin to form friendships,[220] whereas preschoolers exhibit more advanced communication skills, positive affect, conflict negotiation, and pretend play to engage in friendships with peers.[96,220] Older children and teens need shared activities, frequently sports related or online, and experiences away from adult supervision. Often children with ASD have difficulty with imitation, communication abilities, sharing similar interests with their peers, and playing with pretense and ideation. They may need supervision past an age when typically developing children require direct adult contact. For many children with ASD, therefore, forming friendships can be extremely difficult. The child's verbal and social-cognitive skills influence his or her ability to form and maintain friendships.[23,24] Although friendships of children with ASD can be both similar to and different from friendships between typically developing dyads, research suggests that children with ASD have limited friendships, may have trouble understanding what friendship means, and are lonely.[22,40,126,129] The Internet and online gaming is often one way to help children with ASD and typically developing peers develop friendships.

As children with ASD become teens and adults, social participation difficulties can continue. Many teens and young adults are underemployed or unemployed and socially isolated; furthermore, resources and programs for this age group are few.[206,207] Although many individuals desire and engage in romantic and sexual relationships, these can be difficult for some.[38,39,204] Social skill difficulties, communication problems, and sensory processing issues can hinder the development of fulfilling romantic and sexual relationships.[107,158,202] Some individuals do not understand appropriate courtship behaviors and may find themselves in trouble with the law for behaviors others consider dangerous or threatening. Limited research exists to guide professionals in determining the most successful interventions for this age group.[208] Most communities lack resources and opportunities for socialization, employment, and dating for persons with ASD. (See Figure 27-5.) One cinematic depiction of these issues, *Mozart and the Whale*, heightens awareness of the relationship, friendship, and employment issues through a story of two young adults with ASD.

Play

Children with ASD do play, although their chosen play may appear atypical.[56,198] Beginning in infancy, both extreme preoccupation with and unusual use of objects are noted.[20,169,223-225] Uncommon use of objects may include unusual visual exploration, preoccupation with object features, limited flexibility and creativity in the use of objects, and repetitive use of objects.[20,136,224] Many studies of children with ASD suggest that children engage in sensory exploration of objects beyond an age when sensorimotor play is expected[223,224] and that they engage in more exploratory and sensorimotor play than typically developing children.[55] Children with ASD also perform differently in natural free play, with brief play episodes and frequent selection of solitary sensorimotor play and functional play.[94,95]

Functional play consists of using objects as their form suggests, such as pushing a toy car, bringing a play spoon to the mouth, or pushing a train on a track. Although frequency of functional play seems similar in children with and without an ASD,[43] these groups differ in duration or the quality of the play.[223,224] Children with an ASD, when compared with language or mental age-matched controls, spend less total time in functional play,[105] and functional play is reported to be less varied and more repetitive, as would be expected considering the diagnostic criteria of the disorder.

Studies support the idea that children with ASD have specific difficulty with generating flexible and novel ideas for play and engaging in play in a way that indicates spontaneity and pleasure.[134,135] Symbolic play of children with ASD has been studied most extensively. Jarrold[104] provides a review suggesting children with an ASD are less likely to engage in pretend play and spend less total time in pretend play. However, children with an ASD are capable of pretending,[93,105,106] in particular when pretense is elicited or prompted by an adult.

Sleep

Children with ASD commonly exhibit problems with sleep. Sleep studies using parent report, sleep diaries, actigraphy (a measure of body movements during sleep), or polysomnography (a full sleep study with measurement of brain waves, heart rate, breathing, and movement) have led to findings supporting disordered sleep in ASD.[182] Children with ASD tend to have difficulty falling asleep and staying asleep and often wake early.[171,176,182,196] Studies suggest that these sleep disturbances are highly prevalent; between 40% and 73% of children with ASD are reported to have sleep difficulties.[121,176,182] Eighty percent of the parents of children with autism and 60% of the parents of children with high functioning autism reported that their own sleep was disturbed because of their child.[176] Difficulties with settling to sleep at night or with night waking are often associated with problems with bedtime routines,[171,182] and bedtime routines are difficult to develop.[128] Sleep problems in ASD have also been associated with other ASD symptoms as well as both internalizing and externalizing behavior problems,[171] suggesting the importance of sleep for both children and parents.

Activities of Daily Living

Because self-care routines are patterned behavior, children with ASD often learn and perform many self-care skills independently.[130] However, researchers have documented delayed self-care performance in children with ASD. For example, in one study, 49% of the sample of children with ASD scored 2 SD below the mean on the WeeFIM and moderately low on the Vineland Adaptive Behavior Scales.[106] Parents report their child to have difficulties with feeding and toileting in particular.[2,142] Children with ASD may have very limited diets, require special diets because of food allergies, or be placed on special diets by their parents.[137,150,161] Parents of children with ASD also reported difficulties with oral care and dental visits.[201]

Feeding, dental care, and toileting issues may relate, in part, to sensory processing difficulties. For those with sensory modulation issues, tolerating the sensory experiences that are characteristics of dressing, bathing, and toileting can create difficulty or reluctance to perform. Dressing requires toleration of fabric textures, the edges of sleeves rubbing on skin, the feel of elastic waistbands, and the rubbing of clothing tags on the back of the neck, for example. Bathing requires toleration of water temperature, the tactile experience of water moving over skin, the smell of soaps and shampoos, and the feel of towels or washcloths. In addition, washing one's hair may require leaning backward with one's eyes closed, a scary motion for someone with vestibular difficulties. Toileting requires the experience of wiping with toilet tissue, perhaps the feeling of water spray as the toilet flushes, and the noise of the flushing water.

Education

The educational needs of children with ASD are as varied as the children themselves. Given the wide range of ability, all that can be stated with certainty is that many children with ASD require accommodations to their educational program. These accommodations may be necessary for the child to fully participate in academic tasks, classroom and social activities, and the school's sensory environment. Some children with ASD (e.g., those with average or above average IQ) are fully included in general education classrooms; others receive special education services; and the most involved may be placed in separate centers specifically designed for children with ASD. Even for children with typical cognitive ability, academic achievement may not match their intellects because of social difficulties and behavioral concerns.[69] Parents may need assistance in selecting appropriate educational placements for their child, and this can be very challenging decision.[54]

Performance Patterns

Given that one of the characteristics of ASD is restricted and repetitive behaviors, it is unsurprising that children with ASD have specific needs for routine and predictability. These needs can have a significant impact on the development of family routines that work for the whole family. Families may have difficulty with various family routines, and participating in activities in and outside of the home can be particularly stressful or chaotic.[15,141,193] Families may adopt highly structured home and mealtime routines to accommodate their children's rigid behaviors, and when engaging in activities outside the home, may adopt a model of extreme flexibility.[53,130,193] Mothers report excessive planning to be one effective strategy,[123] and in general family activities often are scheduled to revolve around the needs of the child with ASD.[4,53,193] The balancing act between the need for predictable routine for the child and excessive flexibility for other family members may be particularly difficult for some families. Some families may avoid social events and activities outside the home, resulting in social isolation.[228]

Performance Skills and Client Factors

Children with ASD can have difficulties with all of the performance skills, including communication, social, emotional regulation, motor, praxis,[11,13,200,219] and sensory perceptual skills.[140,212] Difficulties with sensory processing have been documented in individuals with ASD as early as 1943, when Kanner described individuals with fear of noises from machines, who repeatedly watched bowling pins fall, who sought out movement on swings, and who mouthed objects and flicked lights[27,110] described the first sensory-based hypothesis of autism whereby they believed children were overly sensitive and therefore developed defenses to the social world. In the 1960s, Rimland developed an underarousal hypothesis suggesting that the reticular activating system was functioning improperly, impairing the child's ability to learn through pairing current and past sensory experiences.[183] Atypical brain activity with electroencephalogram recordings suggests that physiologic overarousal in autism influences many autistic behaviors.[97] In addition, chronic arousal may lead to blocking of new stimuli and related gaze aversion.[98] Ayres[14] identified common difficulties in sensory processing seen during her intervention with children with autism.

Current research suggests that a majority of individuals with ASD have various sensory processing and praxis difficulties that are present across the life span and highly variable across individuals.[25,46,75,106,195] Personal accounts suggest that individuals with ASD can articulate the impact of sensory processing difficulties on their daily lives.[77,108,118] These sensory processing deficits may be linked to social difficulties and problem behaviors in the ASDs,[17,91] motor and postural difficulties,[152] academic performance,[12] adaptive behavior,[188] daily living skills,[127] and restricted and repetitive behaviors.[44,109,222] Recent studies have also linked sensory reactivity to anxiety,[45,81] suggesting that stress responses to daily typical sensation may be atypical in the ASDs and may relate to the development of anxiety.

Research illustrates processing issues that range between behavioral hypersensitivity and hyposensitivity, as well as neurologic hyporesponsiveness and hyperresponsiveness. Poor auditory filtering and sensory seeking are both commonly reported areas of difficulty with this population.[12,127,213] The evidence appears strongest for hyporesponsivity in the ASDs.[25,189,195] It appears that habituation is intact in individuals with an ASD, whereas orienting responses may not be, at least at young ages.[71,130,195] Simple sensory recognition may be intact, whereas more complex sensory perceptual functions may not.[152]

Although sensory processing dysfunction in general is not unique to the ASDs,[21,165] specific patterns of processing may be unique. Specific sensory items have been examined to determine those that best discriminate individuals on the autism spectrum.[19,21,112,133,188,213,222] These include overreactions to sounds; overreactions to touch, tastes, and smells; atypical visual exploration of objects; poor eye contact; and lack of response to name or the inability to orient to one's name. Other important behaviors in discriminating children with ASD include excessive mouthing of objects and social touch aversions.[19]

Motor skill difficulties were somewhat ignored for many years, because often motor performance was a relative strength for individuals with ASD. However, a growing body of research has documented the motor difficulties common in this population.[29,200] Common motor concerns include poor gait, posture, balance, coordination, imitation, and praxis. Fairly consistent results suggest that imitative impairments are common in children with ASD.[200,226] Some research suggests that imitative deficits may be one of the best discriminators between individuals with and without ASD,[203] and the diagnosis of autism may be the best predictor of imitative deficits.[215] Children also demonstrate dyspraxia, that is, motor planning difficulty.[57,66,139,157]

Individuals with ASD demonstrate specific difficulties with one type of executive function called *generativity*, which is a skill in generating novel or creative thoughts and actions.[30,35,184] Poor generativity has been linked to difficulties with communication and repetitive behaviors, but occupational therapists well versed in sensory integration (SI) theory might also consider how these deficits reflect ideational praxis related to play skills and ADLs.

Family Impact

The considerable health care needs of a child with ASD, combined with the behavioral characteristics of the disorder, have a substantial impact on the entire family. Access to care varies by community, and in a survey of parents, 89% reported they were the primary case coordinator for the child with ASD.[142] More than 25% of parents report that they spend more than 10 hours per week coordinating services for their child with ASD.[120] The difficulties of coordinating care and finding appropriate care can create a significant amount of stress for the family.

Consistently parents of children with ASD report higher stress levels when compared with the parents of children with other disabilities.[153,159,194] In addition to the financial and access-to-care issues, other stressors associated with raising a child with ASD include significant and lengthy child-rearing needs and the need to have highly structured and regular routines that can restrict family lifestyle and create social isolation.[31,48,53,128,194] Responses from the 2003-2004 National Survey of Children's Health indicated that parents of children with ASD, when compared with the parents of children with attention-deficit disorder or no disability, feel a greater burden of care for their child and a lower quality of life.[132] These parents reported less community involvement, less attendance at religious services, and less child participation in organized events.

Mothers of children with ASD have reported the demands of child-rearing as overwhelming, nonstop, and often leaving them feeling powerless.[53] Maternal stress is related to child symptoms of dysregulation such as poor sleep, poor eating, and sensory sensitivity.[48] The problem behaviors in the child with ASD have been associated with higher levels of family stress; specifically, maladaptive behaviors are likely to disrupt family socialization by limiting the ability of the family to participate in social events.[48,84,88,103,210,211] Mothers of children with ASD with more common or severe restrictive repetitive behaviors or poorer adaptive behaviors report greater perceived negative impact.[31]

Mothers of children with ASD tend to carry the majority of the child-rearing burden and, therefore, often report greater levels of stress than fathers. Mothers also report a lower quality of life and poorer physical and mental health than fathers.[3,78,85,86,88] Older research that focused specifically on mothers of children with ASD found a fairly consistent stress profile in the mothers, regardless of their culture, geographic location, and age and functioning of their child with ASD.[117]

In addition to parental effects, research documents that having a sibling with a disability can impact sibling relationships.[144] Interactions between brothers and sisters provide children with their first socialization experiences, and the sibling relationship is a unique interaction that provides opportunities for social development. Sibling relationships are often the longest-lasting of all human relationships. In the ASD population, the importance of the sibling relationship increases because of the potential role of the sibling as a future caregiver. It is important to encourage and promote the development of positive, meaningful, and caring sibling and family relationships. It is also important for the coping and resiliency of the whole family that all family members are included. Sibling relationships within the family are complex and many factors interact to predict how well typically developing siblings adjust to a sibling with ASD in the family.[146]

Siblings report a variety of difficulties related to living with a sibling with ASD.[122] Some of the issues for typical siblings include loneliness, jealousy in relation to unequal parental attention, difficulty in understanding varied rules for behavior for each sibling, aggression from the sibling with ASD, and the possible need to take on a caretaking role for their sibling with ASD. However, research also shows that most siblings of children with ASD are well adjusted and may learn prosocial and positive behaviors from the experience.[144]

The Role of Occupational Therapy in Autism Spectrum Disorder

Best practice places the occupational therapist within a well-functioning and cohesive multidisciplinary team focused on assisting the family of a child with ASD as well as the child. Each team may have slightly different divisions of functions, and the role of an occupational therapist may overlap somewhat with that of a physical therapist, speech therapist, behaviorist, or teacher. Families value the contribution of occupational therapy practitioners and parents report that occupational therapy intervention is the third most commonly used intervention for individuals with ASD; intervention for SI dysfunction, also commonly provided by occupational therapists, is ranked fifth.[99]

Evaluation

The occupational therapist's evaluation of the child with ASD includes an occupational profile and assessment of occupational performance[11]; however, characteristics of ASD may require alternative assessment strategies, such as alternative communication methods. Information may need to come primarily from a parent or caregiver and through observation. Specific observational strategies to attempt to understand the importance of meaning behind unusual child behaviors may be most successful in understanding the child's occupational performance.[198]

Occupational therapists may experience difficulties using certain standardized norm-referenced assessments with this population because of child problems with communication, attention, motivation, or behavior.[1,116] Adaptations of standardized assessments frequently required to engage the child include allowing the child to become familiar with the therapist and the testing area before beginning, providing breaks between tasks, allowing parental presence, using motivators and rewards for task completion, limiting eye contact or verbal interaction, providing additional time to process verbal requests, or changing the order of item administration regarding preferred and nonpreferred tasks. Any scores obtained following modification of standardized procedures must be considered only estimates of ability, and any reports should clearly indicate which modifications were made to procedures and why.

A variety of tools have been developed specifically for children with ASD, particularly for screening or diagnosis. See Table 27-1 for an overview of potential assessment tools that may be used in evaluation of a child with ASD. Therapists should be aware that many of these tools are designed to find problems and difficulties; therefore, therapists must also be careful to take time to determine the child's strengths and abilities.

Occupational therapy evaluations must focus on function as well as determining the cause of the child's difficulties. Identifying what is currently working for the child and family can inform specific interventions for performance difficulties. For example, finding that a child has strong visual skills and ability to read written instructions may lead the therapist to suggest using clearly written instructions, perhaps with photos, to prompt the child through difficult tasks in the home or classroom. See Box 27-2 for specific classroom assessment considerations. (See Figure 27-6.)

The therapist collaborates with the family to determine which issues and difficulties are priorities for the family.

TABLE 27-1 Specific Assessment Tools Used with Children at Risk for or with Autism Spectrum Disorder

Tool Name	Authors	Publisher and Website	Type of Tool and Areas Assessed
Modified Checklist for Autism in Toddlers (MCHAT)	Robins, Fein, & Barton	Available online for free, http://www2.gsu.edu/~psydlr/Diana_L._Robins,_Ph.D._files/M-CHAT_new.pdf; http://www2.gsu.edu/~psydlr/DianaLRobins/Official_M-CHAT_Website.html	Screening for ASD in toddlers 16-30 months
Screening Tool for Autism in Toddlers and Young Children (STAT)	Stone & Ousley	Vanderbilt University, http://stat.vueinnovations.com/	Screening for ASD 24-36 months
The First Year Inventory (FYI)	Baranek, Watson, Crais, & Reznick	Information available through UNC School of Medicine, http://www.med.unc.edu/ahs/pearls/research/development-of-the-first-year-inventory	Screening for 12-month-old infants to identify those at risk of ASD
Childhood Autism Rating Scale (2nd ed.) (CARS-2)	Schopler, Van Bourgondien, Wellman, & Love	WPS http://portal.wpspublish.com/portal/page?_pageid=53,265699&_dad=portal&_schema=PORTAL	Diagnostic test for ASD
Gilliam Autism Rating Scale (3rd ed.) (GARS-3)	Gilliam	WPS http://portal.wpspublish.com/portal/page?_pageid=53,70079&_dad=portal&_schema=PORTAL	Diagnostic test for ASD
Autism Diagnostic Observation Schedule (2nd ed.) (ADOS-2)	Lord, Rutter, DiLavore, Risi, Gotham, & Bishop	WPS http://portal.wpspublish.com/portal/page?_pageid=53,288914&_dad=portal&_schema=PORTAL	Diagnostic test for ASD
Autism Diagnostic Interview—Revised (ADI-R)	Rutter, Le Couteur, & Lord	WPS http://portal.wpspublish.com/portal/page?_pageid=53,70436&_dad=portal&_schema=PORTAL	Diagnostic test for ASD and also used for research and intervention planning
Developmental, Dimensional and Diagnostic Interview (3di)	Skuse, Warrington, Bishop, Chowdhury, Lau, Mandy, & Place	Institute of Child Health, University College London http://www.ixdx.org/3di-index.html	Computer-based diagnostic test for symptoms of ASD. The authors suggest that the 3di is similar to the ADI-R but focuses on current behavior and therefore has high levels of agreement with ADOS
Diagnostic Interview for Social and Communication Disorders (DISCO)	Wing, Leekam, Libby, Gould, & Larcombe	Centre for Social and Communication Disorders http://www.autism.org.uk/our-services/diagnosing-complex-needs/the-diagnostic-interview-for-social-and-communication-disorders-disco.aspx	Diagnostic schedule for ASD and helps with assessment of individual needs
Autism Treatment Evaluation Checklist (ATEC)	Bernard Rimland & Stephen M. Edelson	Autism Research Institute http://www.autism.com/index.php/ind_atec_survey	Checklist/questionnaire completed by parents, teachers, or caretakers
Autism Screening Instrument for Educational Planning (3rd ed.) (ASIEP-3) (This includes the Autism Behavior Checklist)	Krug, Arick, & Almond	Pro-Ed http://www.proedinc.com/customer/productview.aspx?id=4217	Norm-referenced assessment to identify ASD and assist in planning educational programs
Assessment for Mothers of Children with Autism (AMCA)	Lewis, Ujcic-Snyder, Rider, & Fisher	Available through http://www.misericordia.edu/images/ot/AMCA.pdf	Interview guide for mothers of children with ASD, in relation to their stressors and coping strategies
The Motivation Assessment Scale (MAS)	Durand	Available online from http://store.monacoassociates.com/masenglishbundle.aspx For a sample one filled out with a case, see http://fba-behaviorsupport.wikispaces.com/file/view/motivation+assessment+scale.pdf	A Likert scale that examines a child's motivations for particular behaviors

McClintock, J. M., & Fraser, J. (2011). *Diagnostic instruments for autism spectrum disorder: A brief review.* New Zealand Guidelines Group. Retrieved 7-10-13 from http://www.health.govt.nz/system/files/documents/publications/asd_instruments_report.pdf; Watling, R. (2010). Behavioral and educational approaches for teaching skills to children with an autism spectrum disorder. In H. Miller-Kuhaneck & R. Watling (Eds.), *Autism: A comprehensive occupational therapy approach* (3rd ed.). Bethesda, MD: AOTA Press.

BOX 27-2 Important Considerations for Evaluating the School Environment for a Child with Autism Spectrum Disorder

- What are the expectations for this child in the classroom/school? Consider the different expectations for the teacher, parent, other professionals, and the child's peers. If there is a problem with classroom performance, whose problem is it? (Is this issue bothering the child or the teacher?)
- What does the student want to participate in at school?
  - Social activities (school dances, pep rallies, organized sporting events)
  - Recreation (recess, physical education, playground, art)
  - Communal activities (assemblies, field trips, eating in the cafeteria)
  - Creative activities (orchestra, band, chorus)
  - Civic activities (school paper, student government, school clubs)
  - Academic (labs, library)
- Is the child participating in the activities he or she desires? If not, what is getting in the way?
- Does the student have friends in the classroom or school? If not, what is hindering the development of friendships?
- How much choice is available throughout the day? How much is the student allowed choice in his or her activities and use of time?
- How predictable is the day? Does the child know the schedule and routine? How often does the routine change and how much notice is there when a change will occur?
- How does the child's performance and behavior change, based on time of day or classroom activity?
- Are there any problem behaviors in the classroom that are disruptive to the child, the classroom activities, the teacher, or peers? If so, which interventions have already been tried? What is the teacher's perception of what initiates the problem behavior?
- How are instructions given to the child in the classroom? How well are they followed?
- How is this child able to communicate or demonstrate that he or she is learning the academic content?
- Does this child use peers as a model for behavior or learning of academic content?
- How does the child respond to the classroom sensory environment?
- What are the sensory characteristics of the lunch room, playground, and gym (noise, lighting, seating, physical proximity, and number of peers), and what is required of the child socially in those settings?
- How does the teacher manage fire drills and other safety drills? What are the school lockdown procedures for a student with special needs?

The occupational therapist asks about what is working for the family and what they love and enjoy about their child. The team considers the family's perspectives, acknowledging that the family members may have very different needs and feelings about the diagnosis.[167] For certain children with ASD, safety or escapism is a concern, but this concern may not be voiced unless the therapist asks specific questions about the child's behaviors in unsafe environment (e.g., crossing the street, at the grocery store). Box 27-3 lists important questions to ask a parent about a child with ASD during an evaluation. Best practice is to presume parental competence, caring, and intelligence at all times.

BOX 27-3 Important Questions to Ask Families During an Evaluation

- What are your most pleasurable interactions with your child? Why?
- What do you love most about your child?
- What do you consider to be the strengths of your family? What works well?
- What have you already tried that works best for you?
- What routines do you have in place for your family? Are they working? With which routines are you having difficulties?
- How do you participate in family celebrations and holidays?
- Do you have any concerns for your child's safety?
- Are you satisfied with your ability to communicate and interact with your child?
- Does your child participate in decision making? How? (if age appropriate)
- If your child has siblings, what is their relationship and do you have any concerns? How do they play and interact together? How do you handle sibling conflicts?
- Do you feel satisfied with your ability to be social with others or are you feeling isolated in any way? Do you have or need respite care?
- Which interventions or accommodations have you already tried that didn't work? Why do you think that was?
- What information do you feel you need about your child?
- Are you satisfied with the services you have received so far?

From Miller-Kuhaneck, H., & Britner, P. A. (2013). A preliminary investigation of the relationship between sensory processing and social play in autism spectrum disorder. *OTJR: Occupation, Participation and Health, 33*(3):159–167.; Watling, R. (2010). Occupational therapy evaluation for individuals with an autism spectrum disorder. In H. Miller-Huhaneck & R. Watling (Eds.), Autism: A comprehensive occupational therapy approach (ed. 3, pp. 285–304). Bethesda: AOTA Press.

Family-Centered Practice

Family-centered practice stems from a set of beliefs and attitudes that value the uniqueness of every family and recognize the reality that the family is the constant in any child's life. Collaboration and family choice are key principles of family-centered care. Optimal functioning for any child occurs in a family that is supportive and involved in the child's care, and to provide the best care, the strengths and needs of all family members are considered.[113]

To communicate with families in ways that support and encourage their involvement and ability to make informed decisions about their children, the occupational therapist considers how communication reflects interpersonal power.[72,179] Expert power is the power that comes with having knowledge and skill that another does not have, and informational power comes from one person influencing another with logical information. If the caregiver changes because the occupational therapist is an expert and must know best, the occupational therapist has exerted expert power. However, if a caregiver changes because he or she has listened to the therapist and then made a decision for himself or herself, the occupational therapist has used informational power effectively. Occupational therapists working with children and families must strive to empower families to develop their own knowledge, strengths, and problem-solving abilities rather than fostering ongoing need of us and our knowledge and skill.

Coaching is a method to use informational power in a model of family-centered care. As described in Chapters 5 and 11, in coaching, the occupational therapist observes, listens, and guides the parent to learn skills helpful in managing and/or promoting skills in the child. The information is shared in such a way that allows the parent to consider it fully and make his or her own decision. Occupational therapists who listen carefully, use more indirect verbal behaviors, and allow family members to express their thoughts and feelings[36] support collaborative communication. A strategic tenet of a family-centered approach is that professionals listen actively to families and acknowledge and address families' concerns and needs. Reflection of feelings is an important skill during active listening and assists families in clarifying their concerns. By accepting families' feelings and demonstrating acceptance they may become better able to accept their own feelings. In addition, praising, encouraging, and accepting family ideas allow families to become more involved in their child's therapy and care.[36]

Another important skill in family-centered practice is to share information as one is gathering it. Particularly during initial meetings with the family, the parents may have little understanding of the role of occupational therapy. As the occupational therapist is asking questions of the family during an evaluation, it can be very helpful to also explain *why* the questions lead to understanding their child's behaviors. As the family learns more about the team's clinical reasoning, the family becomes better at providing relevant information spontaneously. In addition, occupational therapists can help families learn how to create natural learning opportunities in their day-to-day lives[62]; these successes should enable and empower, improving parental self-efficacy.[60,61] These approaches are consistent with a strengths-based approach that parents report they desire.[114]

Interventions

Occupational therapists working with children with ASD provide interventions for all areas of occupation. Because multiple chapters in this text discuss specific intervention options for pediatric occupational therapy, this section highlights intervention methods and strategies common in ASD. Interventions described in this text for social participation (see Chapter 12), self-care (see Chapters 15 and 16), educational performance (see Chapters 10, 18, and 23), play (see Chapter 17), motor skills (see Chapters 7 and 8), assistive technology (see Chapter 19), and dealing with problem behaviors (see Chapter 13) often apply to children with ASD. Clinical guidelines for the treatment of ASD have also been published (Table 27-2).

The interventions for ASD generally fall into one of two categories, adult directed and compliance based or naturalistic and more child directed and playful. Children with ASD often do not appear motivated to do the learning tasks typical of school and child growth and development. Often the activities that they are motivated to do appear strange and unusual to typically developing peers and adults. Therefore professionals need to decide whether to approach the child from a position of gaining compliance with the "work" that needs to be done or to try to achieve learning through more playful means using the child's inherent preferences.

Specific Intervention Approaches

An abundance of intervention approaches are purported to help with symptoms and behaviors of ASD. As part of our role

TABLE 27-2 Clinical Guidelines for Autism Spectrum Disorder

Type	Title	Availability
Clinical guidelines for diagnostic assessment	Autism Recognition, Referral and Diagnosis of Children and Young People on the Autism Spectrum	http://www.ncbi.nlm.nih.gov/pubmedhealth/PMH0042124/
Clinical practice guidelines, state of New York	Quick reference guide for parents and professionals Assessment and intervention for young children (age 0-3 years)	http://www.health.ny.gov/publications/4216.pdf and http://www.calaba.org/autismconsumerguidelines-docs/NYStateQuickRefGuide-Pub4216.pdf
Screening	Autism A.L.A.R.M. Guidelines	http://www.cdc.gov/ncbddd/autism/hcp-recommendations.html
Diagnosis and management	American Academy of Pediatrics	http://pediatrics.aappublications.org/content/120/5/1162.full
Occupational therapy practice	American Occupational Therapy Association	Tomchek, S. D., & Case-Smith, J. (2009). *Occupational therapy practice guidelines for children and adolescents with autism*. Bethesda (MD): American Occupational Therapy Association. See http://www.guideline.gov/content.aspx?id=15292&search=occupational+therapy
International guidelines for diagnosis	UK: Autism diagnosis in children and young people: recognition, referral and diagnosis of children and young people on the autism spectrum NZ: New Zealand Autism Spectrum Disorder Guideline	http://publications.nice.org.uk/autism-diagnosis-in-children-and-young-people-cg128 http://www.nice.org.uk/nicemedia/live/13572/56428/56428.pdf http://www.health.govt.nz/publication/new-zealand-autism-spectrum-disorder-guideline

helping families gather the information they need to make decisions, occupational therapists must be aware of these approaches and the evidence that supports or refutes them.[162] It is beyond the scope of this chapter to fully review each one, but the informed occupational therapist working with a child with ASD should feel comfortable describing these interventions and providing a family with resources to consider their purpose, effectiveness, safety, and costs (Table 27-3). A few of the approaches most commonly used by occupational therapists are highlighted in the following.

Applied Behavior Analysis

To date, many interventions used with children with an ASD are based on theories of external motivation crafted within the behavioral framework initially developed by Pavlov, Watson, and Skinner primarily through the study of animal behavior.[82,71,197,217] These early theories focused on drives as the guiding force behind human behaviors.[52] In behaviorism, the belief is that learning occurs through a change in behavior brought about by external experiences. Behavior can be

TABLE 27-3 Interventions for Children with Autism Spectrum Disorder

Intervention Name	Web Link	How Used in Occupational Therapy
Reciprocal Imitation Training (RIT)	http://www.ncbi.nlm.nih.gov/pmc/articles/PMC3686149/	Occupational therapists can use imitation to increase engagement and interaction with a child with ASD. This is particularly useful when a child is avoiding the therapist or disengaged. The occupational therapist imitates the child until the child makes some indication of connection or interaction (a look, touch, smile). For evidence of the efficacy of this type of approach, see http://psychology.msu.edu/autismlab/publications.html. The evidence for imitation models is considered to be emerging.
Relationship Development Intervention (RDI)	http://www.rdiconnect.com/pages/Home.aspx	Focuses on coping with change, being more flexible, and integrating information from multiple sources. There is currently minimal evidence of efficacy, but research is occurring. The evidence for relationship-based models is considered to be emerging.
Treatment and Education of Autistic and related Communication Handicapped Children (TEACCH)	http://www.teacch.com/	Occupational therapists can incorporate many of the visual support strategies into their sessions. See Eikeseth[67]; Mesibov & Shea, 2010 for information about the research that has been completed to examine the efficacy of this program. Efficacy is unclear at this time but one review suggests it was beneficial for improving motor skill and cognition (see http://www.effectivehealthcare.ahrq.gov/ehc/products/106/656/CER26_Autism_Report_04-14-2011.pdf). TEACCH is considered an emerging approach.
Early Start Denver Model	http://www.autismspeaks.org/what-autism/treatment/early-start-denver-model-esdm	Occupational therapists can use strategies from this model that focus on joint attention and shared interaction using a naturalistic applied behavioral approach. Well-designed studies of the Early Start model have documented effectiveness in improving IQ, language, and autism symptoms (Dawson et al., 2010). Also see http://www.effectivehealthcare.ahrq.gov/ehc/products/106/656/CER26_Autism_Report_04-14-2011.pdf. This model is considered established.
Miller Method	http://millermethod.org/	Occupational therapists can use many of the strategies to increase attention (i.e., carefully adding to the number of steps needed to achieve a desired goal or using raised surfaces to enhance attention to mobility). There is minimal evidence regarding the efficacy of the program in its entirety.
The Son-Rise Program	http://www.autismtreatmentcenter.org/	Focuses on using the child's inherent motivations to engage and interact and on helping parents be optimistic and hopeful while helping their child to learn and achieve. Very playful approach and open to including sensory-based therapy. There is currently no published evidence of efficacy for this program. See http://www.autismtreatmentcenter.org/contents/reviews_and_articles/research_project.php.

TABLE 27-3 Interventions for Children with Autism Spectrum Disorder—cont'd

Intervention Name	Web Link	How Used in Occupational Therapy
Social Communication, Emotional Regulation and Transactional Support (SCERTS)	http://scerts.com/index.php?option=com_content&view=article&id=2&Itemid=2	SCERTS is a comprehensive model to be used with a team. Occupational therapists are part of this team and are involved in the emotional regulation portion of the intervention. SCERTS can be readily combined with many other of the interventions, although it is considered to be most different from ABA. Evaluation of the SCERTS model is ongoing. See http://www.scerts.com/docs/SCERTS_EBP%20090810%20v1.pdf and http://ies.ed.gov/funding/grantsearch/details.asp?ID=978.
Pivotal Response Training (PRT)	http://www.koegelautism.com/	Occupational therapists can use specific strategies such as providing choice, using task variation, rewarding attempts, and using natural reinforcers in play-based sessions. PRT specifically teaches responsivity to multiple cues and the occupational therapist can incorporate this into activities such as visual perceptual-motor tasks (i.e., "Can you find the big, round, one? Can you find the smooth, red one?"). See http://education.ucsb.edu/autism/documents/EmpiricalSupportforPRT-ExpandedVersion.pdf for information about studies related to PRT. PRT is a well-studied approach to treatment for ASD and is considered an established approach.
Animal Assisted Therapy (AAT)	Pet Partners (formerly the Delta Society) http://www.petpartners.org/	Animals may be calming for individuals with ASD and may help increase language and social interaction. They can be used in occupational therapist sessions if the occupational therapist is trained in this approach (see Nimer & Lundahl,[164] and Sams, Fortney, & Willenbring.[191]

From Miller-Kuhaneck, H., & Gross, M. (2010). Alternative and complimentary interventions for the autism spectrum disorders. In H. Miller-Kuhaneck & R. Watling (Eds.), *Autism: A comprehensive occupational therapy approach* (3rd ed). Baltimore: AOTA; Watling, R. (2010). Behavioral and educational approaches for teaching skills to children with an autism spectrum disorder. In H. Miller-Kuhaneck & R. Watling (Eds.), *Autism: A comprehensive occupational therapy approach* (3rd ed.). Bethesda, MD: AOTA Press; also see http://www.autismspeaks.org/what-autism/treatment for summaries of many of the approaches above and http://www.nationalautismcenter.org for a national report that reviews autism interventions.

explained based on external events and behaviors and it can be modified through manipulated environmental consequences called *reinforcers* through classical or operant conditioning. Learning is defined as a change in observable behavior. Interventions based on behavioral theories are highly adult directed, focus significantly on compliance with adult demands, and often are completed in one-to-one instruction without peers. Behavioral interventionists give little consideration to the child's internal motivations for learning, the urge for mastery or competence, or the need for autonomy and choice. Although critics of these approaches[100,199] have voiced concerns, behavioral approaches have demonstrated effectiveness.[67,71,174,217] Applied behavior analysis (ABA), in particular, discrete trial training, is supported and considered to be an established approach that is commonly used by many on the health care team of a child with ASD. In ABA, the antecedents and consequences for a behavior are manipulated to influence the behavior. In very simple terms, ABA rewards desired behaviors while ignoring undesirable behaviors or providing undesirable consequences for undesired behaviors. Both positive and negative reinforcement makes the behavior more likely to occur, but positive reinforcement is the application of something pleasurable usually, whereas negative reinforcement is the removal of something unpleasant. Two types of negative reinforcement are escape and avoidance. Differential reinforcement occurs when a behavior is reinforced in some settings or situations and not in others. Reinforcement is provided in specific schedules developed by a behavioral specialist, following a functional behavior analysis or assessment. Discrete trial training (DTT) is a very specific type of ABA in which targeted skills are taught in repetitive trials using the same antecedents, behaviors, and consequences.

Positive behavioral support (PBS) is a behavioral approach developed in the 1980s based on ABA but in response to criticisms of some older ABA programs. Positive behavioral support is considered to be proactive rather than reactive in terms of problem behavior, more individualized, more respectful of an individual's right to choose activities, and better generalizable to daily life settings.[90] Positive behavioral support considers the environment in which the behavior occurs, and practitioners of PBS seek to understand the purpose of the behavior for the individual. Then once the purpose is determined, a problem-solving approach is used to find solutions for the behavior. The overall process for PBS is to establish goals, gather information about the behavior from a variety of people, analyze the patterns of the behavior, develop a plan to prevent the problem from occurring, and respond consistently if it does, and then gather data and monitor effectiveness of the plan.

Occupational therapists may use principles of ABA during intervention sessions such as assessing the functions of specific behaviors and rewarding appropriate task performance. Specific strategies used in therapy in addition to reinforcement may include prompting, shaping or chaining, and fading out (see Chapters 15 and 16). Occupational therapists may use token economy systems, sticker charts, or food rewards. They may incorporate the child's typical learned commands during intervention activities. Occupational therapists also assist is determining appropriate reinforcers with the child's team and may use this approach to gain child compliance with adult-directed activities to enhance learning of specific skills.

The Cognitive Orientation to Daily Occupational Performance Approach

The Cognitive Orientation to Daily Occupational Performance (CO-OP) approach[175] is an intervention approach designed by occupational therapists to assist children in mastering skills to achieve the performance goals they have set for themselves in collaboration with the occupational therapist. Cognitive Orientation to Daily Occupational Performance has demonstrated effectiveness for children with high-functioning ASD.[187] Cognitive theories of learning consider additional characteristics of learning that cannot be readily observed such as memory and attention. Cognitive and cognitive-behavioral approaches stress observational learning and consider the individual's internal motivations for learning as important to achieving behavioral outcomes. The CO-OP approach uses cognitive behavioral and motivation theories to guide the intervention principles. The objectives are the learning of new skills and the generalization or transfer of those skills into everyday life. Children and therapists collaborate to develop goals and then use a problem-solving, occupational therapist-guided executive function strategy termed "Goal-Plan-Do-Check." The first two steps answer the following questions for the child: What do I want to do? and How am I going to do it? Then the child tries to do the task or skill and observes how well it works. The therapist assists and collaborates throughout the process, by using child-centered assessment to assist the child in developing his or her goals and determining if the child has the motivation, knowledge, and competence to achieve the chosen goal. The therapists also discusses and refines the plan or cognitive strategies the child will use to learn the skill and achieve the goal, models strategy use, and provides feedback for performance. The therapist then works with the child to examine and consider his or her own performance and teach self-evaluation (see Chapter 10). Recent studies suggest that for children with ASD who have the language and cognitive capacity to participate in this approach, it may be effective and successful.[185-187]

Occupational Therapy-Sensory Integration (Ayres Sensory Integration) and Sensory Strategies

Ayres Sensory Integration Theory[14] suggests that all learning and development is based on a foundation of multisensory integration within the brain that often develops in children through play. Therefore occupational therapist-SI intervention uses a play-based approach. Sensory strategies developed through an understanding of occupational therapist-SI theory include modifying tasks and environment to enhance a child's comfort or toleration of an activity or experience, to improve their ability to attend and engage with others, or to alter their arousal level to provide a better platform for learning to occur. Sensory strategies can be thought of as quick fixes or over-the-counter remedies that may at times be implemented by teachers or parents with consultation from occupational therapists, whereas long-term clinic-based occupational therapist-SI intervention is believed to alter neurologic processing through brain plasticity and should be provided by a well-trained therapist who can provide the approach with fidelity to the principles. (See Chapter 9 for more information on occupational therapist-SI and sensory strategies in occupational therapist intervention with children.) (See Figure 27-1*C*.)

Occupational therapists are the experts in the intervention of sensory issues and families with children with ASD seek out occupational therapists for this expertise.[99] Treatment for sensory issues may be of primary importance in this population as they may be related to sleep problems,[115] difficulties with self-care,[106] problems with dental hygiene,[201] educational performance,[12] problem behavior,[166,214] and family occupations.[15] Knowledge of SI theory allows occupational therapists, through activity analysis, to provide suggestions and modification to a variety of tasks in the home, school, and community to allow a child to have greater comfort with, and engagement and participation in, a variety of occupations.

Floortime and the Developmental, Individual Differences, Relationship-Based Model

Developed by Stanley Greenspan, MD, a psychiatrist who worked closely with and valued occupational therapy, Floortime is a family-centered intervention approach with strategies that can easily be incorporated into naturalistic or play-based occupational therapy sessions. Three primary strategies include following the child's lead/joining in his or her world, challenging creativity and spontaneity, and expanding interaction to include sensory motor skills and emotions.

The Developmental, Individual Differences, Relationship-Based (DIR) model is a comprehensive program that considers the child's emotional developmental level, their unique strengths and needs, and their preferences. Through parent-implemented strategies, children progress through six developmental stages of self-regulation and interest in the world: intimacy, engagement and falling in love, two-way communication, complex communication, emotional ideas, and, finally, emotional and logical thinking. Occupational therapists can use the strategies of playful blocking, using child preferences in play to increase engagement and using one's own playfulness to improve interaction. Individual differences including unique sensory processing styles are considered. The parent-child relationship is encouraged and strengthened through the playful activities of Floortime. Floortime intervention therefore is a specific child-directed playful approach with the caregiver that is part of the DIR comprehensive model. The evidence for relationship-based models is considered to be emerging.[170]

Other Common Strategies

A multitude of other approaches are used with children with ASD. Many are included in Table 27-3 and are helpful to use within an occupational therapy session.[147,149,218] They exemplify the "therapeutic use of self" through playful child-therapist interactions.[149] Each session may incorporate different strategies to meet the goals for that session or activity, and it is unlikely that the therapist will use all of the strategies. The therapist's skill in careful observation and choosing which strategies work with each child within specific situations is paramount. See Box 27-4 for particular strategies and when to use them.

BOX 27-4 Specific Strategies for Occupational Therapy Sessions

Improve Engagement and Interaction, Reduce Fear or Anxiety

- Imitate the child and wait for the child to initiate interaction via eye contact, touch, or moving into closer physical proximity (reciprocal imitation training [RIT][160])
- Alter the therapist's proximity to the child[149,160]
- Reduce use of direct eye contact
- Alter the therapist's pace both motorically and verbally (ASI[149])
- Alter the therapist's voice volume or intonation (ASI[149])
- Use musical or sing-song vocalizations or word pronunciation that the child finds humorous[149]
- Use preferred objects, colors, or movements within therapy tasks. For example, hide a favorite object within Theraputty or place it on top of something to encourage climbing, under something to encourage digging, or inside something to encourage fine motor skills like opening or unbuttoning. Be sure the child sees where the object went and, if necessary, make sure that he or she will be able to get it back quickly to avoid distress and difficult behaviors. This should be a fun game. (TEACCH, PRT, RDI, DIR, SCERTS, ASI, Miller Method)
- Interact playfully (DIR, RDI, ASI, RIT, SCERTS, and others), make work into play[149]
- Create fun problems to be solved. For example, "Oh no, the pig (stuffed toy) is trapped in the mud, you have to help him get out. How can we save him?" (DIR, RDI, ASI, RIT, SCERTS, and others)
- Sing familiar songs and leave out the last word, to encourage the child to vocalize to fill in where you have omitted the word

Improve Behavior and Task Completion, Reduce Fear or Anxiety

- Use objects, visual cues, or schedules to help the child predict what will come next or what will happen. Provide a visual schedule that indicates how many times a particular action or behavior is expected. For example, place five magnetic coins on the table to be placed in the container. When the five are done, this activity is done. (TEACCH/SCERTS)
- Use the prompts that are familiar to the child (ABA)
- Know and use the child's preferred reinforcers throughout occupational therapy "work" (ABA)
- Provide clear boundaries regarding areas of the intervention space so that it is clear which type of activity occurs in each area (TEACCH)
- Provide choices or choice boards, visual schedules, or other visual materials to aid in understanding what is to be done (TEACCH)
- Provide written instructions for a child who can read (TEACCH, ABA, SCERTS)

Improve Comfort, Reduce Fear and Anxiety

- Carefully grade the introduction of novelty into a session (ASI)
- Attend to the sensory environment and the child's response (including facial expression, nonverbal responses) to the sensory environment (ASI)
- Alter lighting, noise, smells (ASI)
- Provide opportunities for deep pressure and proprioception through active play (ASI)

Improve Motor Skills/Praxis

- Create fun obstacles or challenges that encourage the movements that are therapeutically desired (e.g., require motor planning, bilateral coordination and sequencing, relate to functional goals) while engaging the child in a preferred activity of his or her choice (ASI, DIR, RDI, RIT, SCERTS, and others)
- Climb, walk, or crawl on raised surfaces to increase attention to motion. For example, climb across a wide balance beam or a horizontal ladder at 2 to 3 feet off the ground (with mats and pillows for safety and hand holding if needed). (Miller Method, ASI)
- Gradually increase motoric sequences that are completed before a desired event or object is provided. For example, place a favorite toy (or a puzzle piece) in a zip lock bag to be opened. Then wrap it in a wad of tin foil inside a zip lock bag to be opened. Then put it in a closed Tupperware, wrapped in tin foil, and inside a zip lock bag. Then in a closed Tupperware, wrapped in tin foil, inside a zip lock bag placed up a ramp, up a ladder, or through a tunnel. (Miller Method)
- Alternate preferred sensory activities with more challenging motor tasks (ASI)
- Sing about the motor activity you are doing using familiar tune. For example, using the tune of "Mary Had a Little Lamb," or "Row, Row, Row Your Boat," you can sing about Johnny's going to climb that ramp, or push, push, push that cart gently down the hall.

Improve Play and Ideational Praxis

- Use realistic props to begin to introduce role play (fireman's hats, dress-up clothing that is realistic)
- Use movie characters and stories to begin to introduce pretend play
- Promote imagination in your sessions (What would an animal look like if it were part zebra and part frog?)
- Have the child help you create a game out of unusual materials ("What could we play with this cup, this small ball, and this stuffed animal?")
- Have the child help you build an obstacle course or sensorimotor activity (ASI)
- Discuss the ways you can use certain objects based on their properties (affordances). ("Look, this is round. It can roll. These are all square shaped and they can stack. What could we do with this object?") (ASI)
- Try to add to current ideas with prompting. ("Can you think of another way to do that? How many different ways can you do that?")
- Take turns between imitating the child and having the child attempt to imitate you. Use silly motions, vocalizations, and sequences to be playful (RTI, DIR, ASI, RDI).

Specific Interventions for Areas of Occupation

Sleep

Behavioral interventions, medications, melatonin, and herbal treatments are often used for sleeping problems in children with ASD.[76] Occupational therapists combine behavioral and sensory strategies when problem solving with families who have children with poorly regulated sleeping routines. In particular, they consider the sensory environment in which sleep occurs in relation to the sensory issues of the child and the options available for providing appropriate sensation to improve sleep. Some children will need sensation to be reduced to sleep successfully, whereas others may need enhanced sensation to sleep. For most children, calming sensations are more steady and consistent and include deep pressure, neutral warmth, soft or dim sounds and lighting, and slow easy motion. Alerting sensations may include louder, brighter, more rapidly changing, or more intense sensations. Therefore to assist with sleep the auditory environment can be altered with the use of music, a white noise machine, ear plugs, or extra padding and draperies to dampen sounds. The visual environment can be altered by adding or removing wall hangings, changing patterns on drapes or bedding, providing glow-in-the-dark stars on the ceiling, using a night light, sleeping with an eye mask, or changing the colors in the room. The tactile environment can be altered by using softer bedding such as flannel or velour or heavier bedding and blankets that provide more pressure; changing sleep clothes to try different fabrics or sleeve and leg lengths; sleeping with or without socks; and providing warm baths, massage, or back rubs before bed or while falling asleep. The vestibular system can be engaged by sleeping on a waterbed or vibrating mattress or by using a rocking chair and rocking slowly before bed. For some children, chewing gum before brushing teeth and going to bed can be relaxing and help them to become calm for sleep.

Behavioral strategies can promote sleep.[156] These include, for example, unmodified or graduated extinction. In unmodified extinction parents put the child to bed at the appropriate bedtime and then ignore the child until morning (monitoring for safety). This process is meant to eliminate the reinforcer of parental attention for crying, screaming, or other bedtime behavior issues. In graduated extinction the parent ignores the behaviors at bedtime for a certain amount of time before checking on the child. The goal is for the child to develop self-soothing skills in order to fall asleep by him- or herself.

The occupational therapist can collaborate with the team and family to create consistent bedtime routines to improve sleep. Routines can include a bath, massage, and other calming activities (see Figure 27-1*A*).[151] Parents may move bedtime closer to the child's naturally established time to fall asleep and then gradually move bedtime earlier and earlier until the child is able to fall asleep at the desired bedtime. Another strategy is to remove the child from bed for a brief period of time if he or she does not fall asleep.

Extinction programs may be difficult for parents of children with ASD to follow and may need to be combined with reinforcement, for example the Excuse Me Drill.[125] First the parent teaches the child to fall asleep in the environment in which the parent wants the child to sleep (likely the child's own bedroom). Parental presence is allowed at this time, as is back rubs, rocking, singing, and so on. Next, the parent begins to reinforce appropriate bedtime behavior with their attention. In very brief bouts initially, the parent removes him- or herself with the statement, "Excuse me, I need to ___________, but I will be right back to check on you." The parent then quickly returns, praising for being good and staying quietly in bed. The duration and distance of the parent's removal is then gradually increased until the child is able to fall asleep independently in his or her room.

Activities of Daily Living and Instrumental Activities of Daily Living

Children with ASD can benefit from behavioral, cognitive, motor, and sensory strategies to improve their ability to independently perform activities of daily living (ADLs) and instrumental activities of daily living (IADLs). In addition, families often benefit from consultation to improve their use of structure and routine to assist in these endeavors.

Dressing, bathing, and toileting skills, once learned, may become established routines that children with ASD perform independently. However, for some children with motor or cognitive difficulties, learning these skills can be difficult. If cognitive issues or the development of habits and routines are the concern, visual supports and assistance for sequences may be helpful.[130] Learning from video demonstration that can be repeated many times may facilitate ADL performance. Families may need assistance with developing consistent routines to follow in the home. For children with motor delays, the occupational therapist can use motor learning strategies, the CO-OP approach, or occupational therapist-SI activities to improve praxis. For those with behavioral resistance to specific ADL tasks, implementing a behavior plan and reinforcing appropriate ADL behaviors might be most important. Behavioral approaches matched to the child's cognitive and communication skills can increase toileting independence (see Chapter 15).

For children with sensory difficulties, modification of tasks to increase comfort, reduce fear, and allow engagement in activities can help families manage their morning and evening routines with less stress. For example, a child may be more likely to learn to wipe if allowed to wear plastic gloves, or he or she may tolerate a bath or washing hair at the sink better than a shower. In addition, occupational therapist-SI may improve the related sensory issues and dyspraxia.

Feeding and eating can often be an area of difficulty for children with ASD because of their insistence on sameness and their sensory sensitivities. Occupational therapist interventions apply both behavioral and sensory strategies to address limited diet. Interventions can include changes to the feeding environment (see Figure 27-1*B*), changes to positioning the child at the table, creating a consistent feeding routine that works for the family, altering food choices based on sensory characteristics, modifying foods based on their sensory properties (texture, taste, smell) or oral motor requirements, reinforcing positive feeding behaviors, and using visual supports to promote ease of transition to the mealtime environment.[91] When using a behavioral approach, the occupational therapist might work toward increasing tolerance through repeated but gradual exposure or through food chaining (working toward acceptance of a nonpreferred or target food by starting with a preferred food and then presenting foods with one similar property to the prior accepted food in the chain). When using an SI

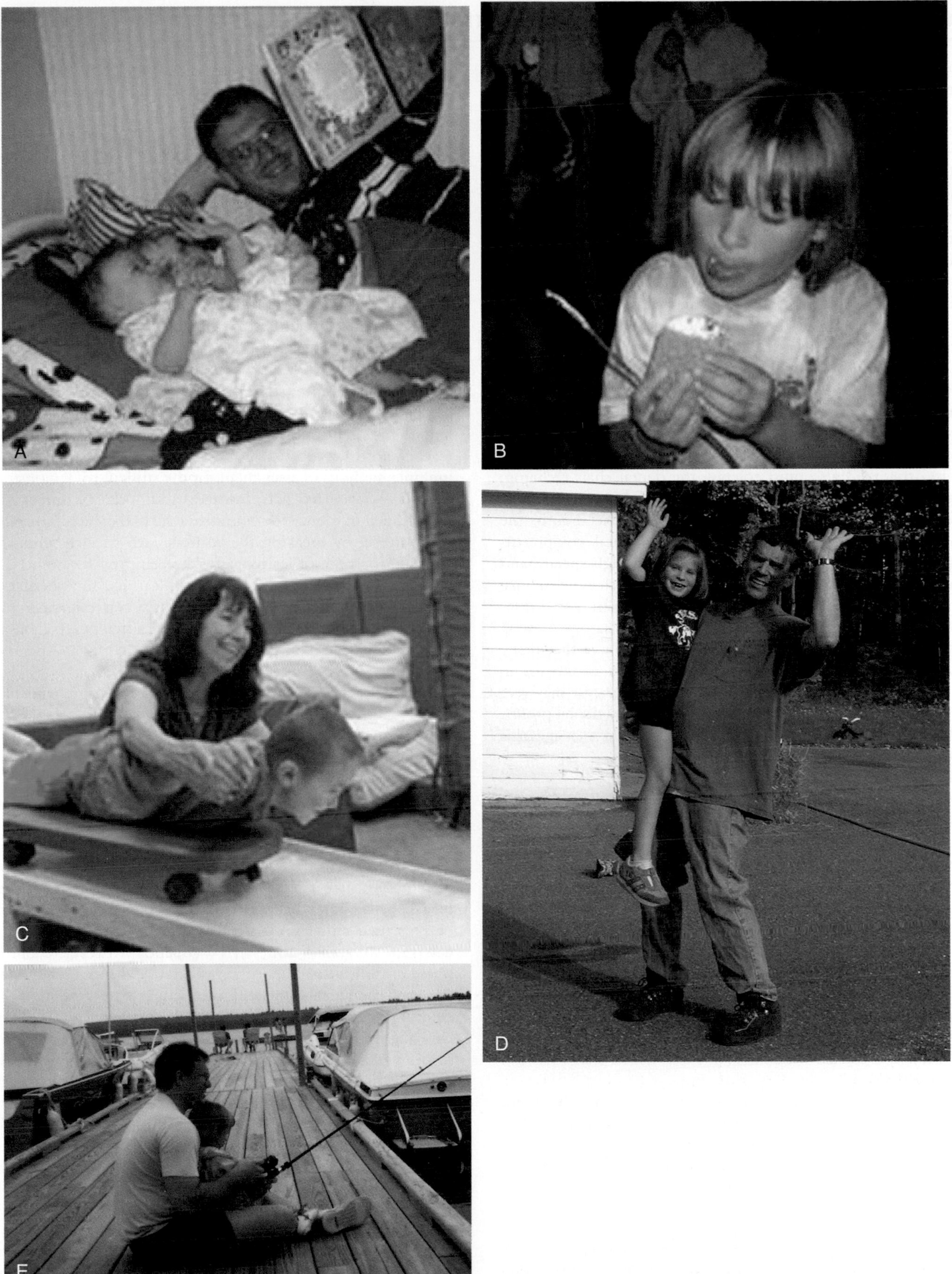

FIGURE 27-1 **A,** An important role for occupational therapists is to help families develop bedtime routines to promote sleep. **B,** Children with ASD can be picky eaters, but interventions using sensory and behavioral strategies can improve their ability to eat a wider variety of foods. **C,** Outpatient occupational therapy using ASI is highly valued by families to help children with ASD improve sensory processing and praxis. **D,** In naturalistic studies of play, children with ASD were more likely to approach adults who were smiling more and were inviting and playful. **E,** The occupational therapist can assist the family in creating meaningful shared family occupations.

approach, the occupational therapist reduces sensory sensitivities generally using deep pressure and proprioceptive activities and may first try to incorporate chewier foods or those that provide greater proprioceptive input to the oral area.

Using sensory processing and behavioral strategies, occupational therapists also provide strategies to assist families in managing oral care and visits to the dentist.[124,173] Dental visits are challenging sensory experiences in multiple sensory modalities, and many dentists are not well versed in managing children with special needs. Once the child's sensory preferences and difficulties are determined, the occupational therapist can give parents suggestions to try before and during oral care and dental visits to make the experience more comfortable for the child. In particular, children with sensory defensiveness may need supports to manage the touch to the face and tastes inside the mouth that are associated with dental hygiene and care, for example, the texture and grittiness of the tooth or polishing paste, and the toothbrush, dental tools, x-ray materials, or gloved fingers in the mouth. At the dentist's office, the child also must tolerate the dental chair reclining; bright lights shining directly into the face; the smell of the glove materials or the taste of the glove in the mouth; the paste taste or smell; the sounds of the dental equipment, especially the polishing brush, suction, and high speed hand pieces; as well as the unexpected office noises such as intercoms, door alarms, and beeps. Additionally, the hygienist's or dentist's face is often covered with a mask. Wearing a mask highlights the eyes and covers the mouth, an area that many with autism look at when speaking with others, as they often avoid direct eye contact. The occupational therapist may recommend to the parent or perhaps directly to the dental professional any of the following to help the child manage this experience:

- Use verbal preparation.
- Give a set time limit that the input will occur (i.e., "We are going to do this until the count of 20").
- Provide a timetable or a visual indication of when the procedure will be done. Ask dental staff to refrain from highly scented cleaners and air fresheners in the office area.
    - Place the chair in the fully reclined position before the patient gets into the chair, to avoid the backward motion.
    - Allow the patient to listen to music over headphones.
- Use as little touch to the face as possible. Use firm deep touch rather than light touch.
- Ask which sensory experiences (e.g., lighting) are most difficult and discuss with the family and dental staff what can be altered.
- Have the child wear the heavy x-ray vest during the entire appointment to provide extra weight and deep pressure
- Have the caregiver do oral deep pressure or vibration in the form of electric toothbrush, mini-massager, or rubbing with a toothette before the appointment.

Education

Autism spectrum disorder often adversely impacts a child's performance in academics; however, students with ASD respond well to educational settings that provide supports and accommodations tailored to meet their individual needs. Students with ASD may benefit when classroom tasks and environments are modified to improve their engagement and reduce problem behaviors. The modifications may occur in the form of academic alterations, visual supports, technological supports, behavioral supports, social supports, sensory-based modifications and strategies, or motivational supports. Teachers report that they use a multitude of strategies in the classroom for children with ASD.[89] Although the primary person responsible for the educational content is the teacher, an occupational therapist using activity analysis can provide valuable information about modifications to assist the teacher and support the student.

Academic Alterations

In a classroom that allows for differentiated curricula, teachers can determine through assessment the student's learning style or learning preference and then teach to that strength. Assessments such as the VARK (see the Evolve website) can help with this determination for students who can complete it. Concepts can be taught either through visual means, auditory means, or kinesthetic or movement methods. Tiered instruction allows teachers to teach a concept in a variety of ways and allows for multiple methods of assessment for the student to demonstrate that the concept has been learned. Additionally, content may be modified to reduce the cognitive load and enhance learning, for example, by breaking the content into smaller "chunks." The social aspect of learning can be removed for some. For example, for a young child, instead of learning the alphabet in the classroom with peers, he or she may better learn from a video of the teacher teaching about the letters, perhaps using preferred characters or puppets.

Visual Supports

Visual supports can include pictures, visual or picture schedules, choice boards, pictorial communication methods, signs, maps, timers, clocks, watches, and items as simple as checklists or written instructions for those who can read. Visual supports can also include boundaries around areas and signs or labels to explain which activity is supposed to happen in that area of the classroom. Visual supports may be real objects; for example, an occupational therapist could provide an orange and a banana when asking the child to make a choice, or can be symbolic, such as a toy banana or a line drawing or a picture of a banana. For schedules or choice boards, the items can be presented either horizontally or vertically, are often laminated for durability, and may be attached with Velcro onto a board or card. Visual supports are used to enhance communication and understanding and often help ease transitions by allowing some predictability for a child who has difficulty in knowing or understanding typical routines. They may be used to show when to start and finish an activity or to explain the sequence of multiple activities. Visual supports can help explain requirements of tasks to enhance a child's ability to complete activities. They can be used also to help identify emotions or mood, provide reminders, and teach new skill sequences. Autism Speaks has created a toolkit for parents and providers for visual supports and other accommodations for help in daily life.

Technologic Supports

Technologic supports can include devices such as communication systems, iPhones, or iPads with apps to help with academic tasks or social interactions. Technology such as computer games may assist with promoting peer interaction in the classroom. Calculators can assist those with difficulty with math skills. Those who have difficulty with handwriting may benefit from technology for keyboarding. Others may be able to use and benefit from voice recognition software, whereas still others without speech may be able to use technology for communication through speech-generating devices. (See the Evolve website for a list of preferred apps.)

Social Supports

Social supports can include but are not limited to social skills groups, peer mentoring programs, integrated play groups, scales and thermometers for emotional regulation, and assistance or guidance at recess and other less structured social times at school.[91] The occupational therapist can help facilitate games or activities at recess that will include the child with ASD and then use recess time or a social skills group at another time to teach appropriate and specific needed social skills. Peer modeling can be used for observation of appropriate behaviors and can then be reinforced using appropriate behavior plans. Occupational therapists can also be involved in school-wide programs for acceptance of difference and/or disability awareness (see Figure 27-4).

Social Stories

Developed by Carol Gray,[79,80] social stories are a teaching technique for children with ASD. They are individually written descriptions about what to expect during typical life events, individualized for each child to target specific areas of need for that child. The stories are written to create understanding and to share information, not to change behavior. They have been found effective in multiple studies to date.[33,47,168,178,205]

A social story should describe rather than direct and is written to support the child in learning about an event or a specific situation. The story has an introduction, body, and conclusion and must answer "wh" questions (i.e., who, what, where, when) about the event or behavior. The story should answer questions about what others know as well. It can be written from either first or third perspective, but with younger children, it should be written using "I." The story includes descriptive sentences, important affirmative sentences, and perspective sentences as appropriate. The story should have limited directive sentences.

Descriptive sentences state the facts. For example, one may write, "My name is ________. There are boys and girls in my class. The teacher's desk is in the front of the room. The boys and girls sit in chairs." If describing a timed event, there needs to be a way "out" if the time changes. For example, instead of writing, "I have gym class every Tuesday," one should state, "On most Tuesdays I have gym class." (Some Tuesdays there might be an assembly.) Instead of specifying, "I go home on the bus at 3:15," a social story would read, "I usually go home on the bus at 3:15." (Some days the bus might have a flat tire and be late.) Perspective sentences reflect what other people know, think, or feel. They might read, "My mother knows when it is time to go to school," "My teacher knows when it is time to go to lunch," or "The teacher will like it if I listen to her when she talks." Directive sentences remind the child of what he or she should be doing or what should be happening. They must be stated in such a way that the child will not "fail" the story if he or she is unable to do what it says. For example, one should read, "I will try to sit in my chair," rather than, "I will sit in my chair." Affirmative sentences indicate a shared value or opinion in culture. They are used only if the adult is sure they are true for the child. An example might be, "It is polite to raise my hand before speaking." Cooperative sentences describe what others will do to try to help the child. For example, a story may read, "Mom and Dad will try to remain calm while I learn to use the toilet." In a social story, the practitioner describes the situation twice as much as telling a child what to do. They must be literally correct, using "usually" and "sometimes," and mentioning changes in routines. The stories can have pictures and titles. Titles are often best expressed as questions that the story will help answer. For example, a title may be "What do children do when they ride the bus?" or "What will we do at Bob's house?" Stories can be very short (five sentences) or longer for older children. Sample social stories are available online (see the Evolve website) and there are also books for sale that provide stories for common problem events such as riding the bus.

Behavioral Supports

Therapists help to develop and support implementation of positive behavior programs in the classroom and specific behavior plans with appropriate reinforcers for the child. One of the best approaches to promote good behavior is a positive behavior plan for the classroom. Classrooms should have clear rules that promote the positive learning environment the teacher and class desire, and the behaviors desired are encouraged by positive consequences for completion such as earning free play time. Consequences for rule violations start mild and become more and more severe as the offense is repeated. Often for a child with ASD more intensive intervention is required. Typically there will be a functional behavioral analysis completed to determine the cause or the reason for the behavior. Next a behavior plan will be put in place that addresses the cause of the behavior. Occupational therapists may or may not be involved in the creation of the plan, but will likely assist in following it with the child.

Sensory Supports

Occupational therapists often provide sensory diets and sensory strategies for children with ASD in the schools. Although perhaps more difficult to implement than highly structured and standard programs, sensory diets should be individualized for the child and strategies should be implemented throughout the day based on the child's behaviors and needs, as opposed to designated by the clock. Therapists also need to be clear which frame of reference they are using when they provide sensory strategies. Sensory interventions respect the child's preferences and are not methods of desensitization to force tolerance of uncomfortable sensory experiences. The sensory strategy should not be used as a reward for good behavior if the therapist is using an SI frame of reference. However, therapists also need to be aware of the potential for sensory strategies to become an unintended reward for poor behavior, if every time the child acts out in class, he or she gets pulled out to do a preferred sensory activity.

The classroom environment is frequently brightly lit, with additional visual stimulation provided by items hanging on the walls and individuals moving about the room. Learning activities frequently provide additional touch inputs, movement experiences, and even smells. Classrooms that are noisy with poor acoustics have been associated with reduced attention, concentration, and academic performance. Individuals with ASD may react with a range of behaviors to uncomfortable stimuli, from avoidance to violent physical aggression.[145] Therapists can make recommendations to improve the match between student sensory preferences and classroom sensory

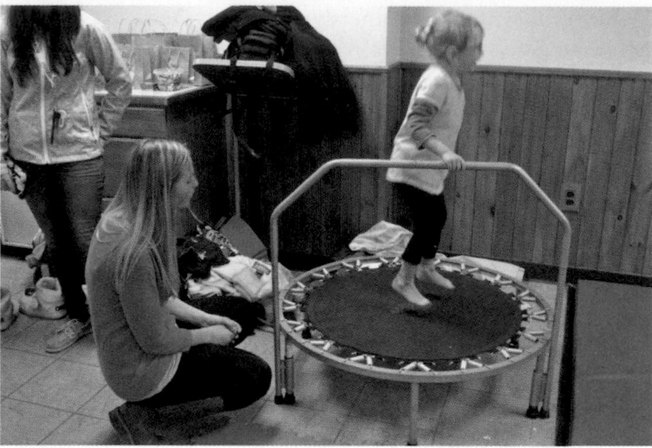

FIGURE 27-2 Sensory strategies in the home or classroom may promote better regulation of behavior and attention.

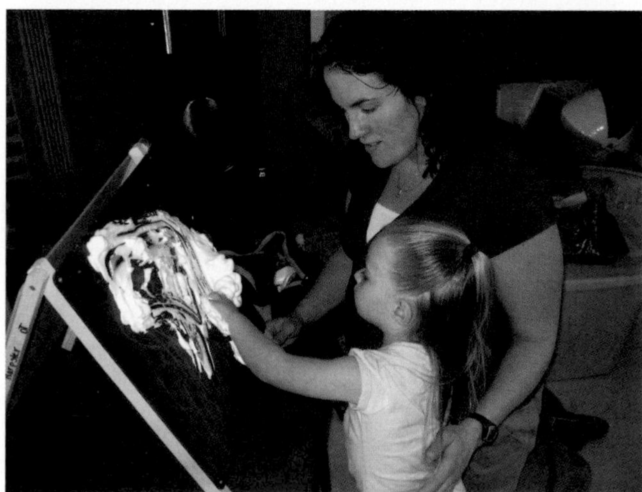

FIGURE 27-3 Sensory strategies such as those that can be used in a school or home can help a child to regulate his or her behavior and learn to explore and tolerate new experiences.

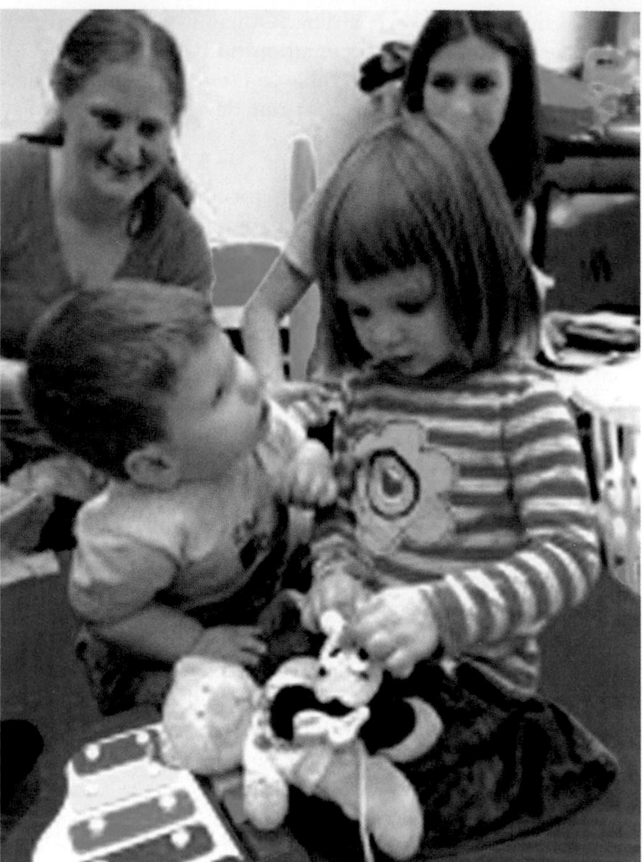

FIGURE 27-4 Peer supports can be helpful in engaging the child with ASD in play and educational activities.

environments, knowing that certain aspects of the sensory environment cannot be modified, for example, acoustics in older buildings. In those cases, other features may be modified, for example, a child could wear ear plugs or headphones in noisy environments that cannot be altered. The therapist must use knowledge about the child's sensory preferences and needs gained through evaluation and collaborate with the teacher to adapt the environment and tasks to allow the child his or her best possible performance (see Figures 27-2 and 27-3).

Motivational Supports

Motivational supports are used to increase the child's participation in educational activities the child finds undesirable. A playful and creative therapist may often gain more compliance with tasks such as writing, cutting, or using a ruler when the child's preferences are included in the task. For example, a child who loves John Deere tractors can complete matching tasks to match letters he or she needs to learn by finding them in the tractor catalog. A child who loves green frogs can be given green markers to use to write with and can write stories about frogs. A child who is passionate about trains can learn to cut squares or circles by creating trains made of colored paper as the final outcome. An additional motivational support often used by occupational therapists is providing choices between activities whenever possible.

Play

Areas of play and imitation are understudied, even though they are considered areas of core deficit in the ASDs.[227] However, a variety of intervention methods, for example, Floortime (DIR) or occupational therapist-SI, are purported to improve play in individuals with ASD. Video modeling appears to have efficacy for increasing play and interactions, play initiations, reciprocal pretend play, and independence in toy play.[92,138,172,180] Peer-mediated interventions and specifically a model called Integrated Play Groups has demonstrated effectiveness in a variety of small studies, primarily using single-subject designs.[229,230] Multiple single-subject design studies have indicated efficacy using Reciprocal Imitation Training (RIT), as applied by parents and practitioners, for developing play skills.[100-102]

A variety of studies have examined individual aspects of interventions important to the development of play skills. Use of choice, the use of preferred sensory toys or perseverative interests, the frequent variation of task demands, and the incorporation of ritualistic behaviors into interventions promote play behaviors.[18,41,58,192,216] In naturalistic studies of play, children with ASD were more likely to approach adults who were

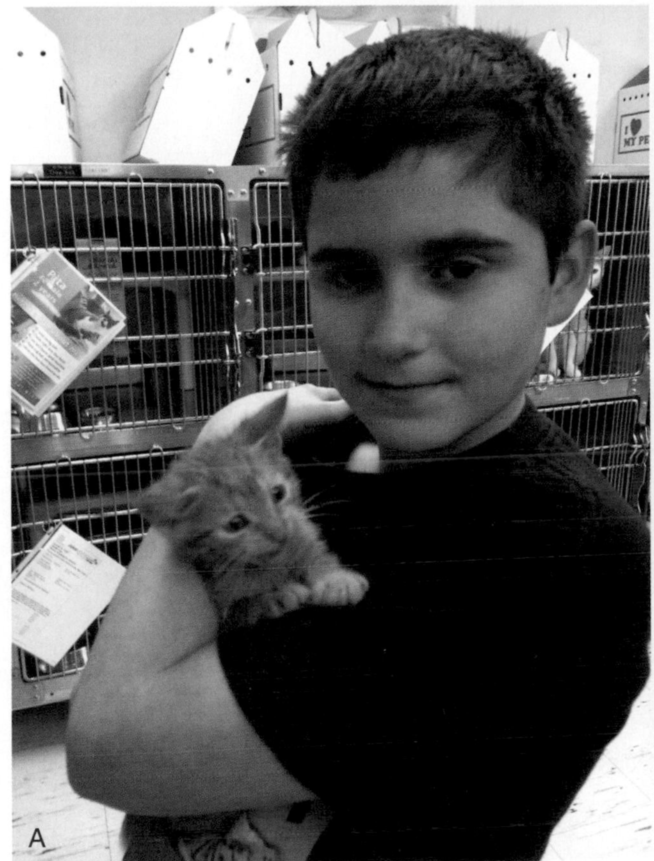

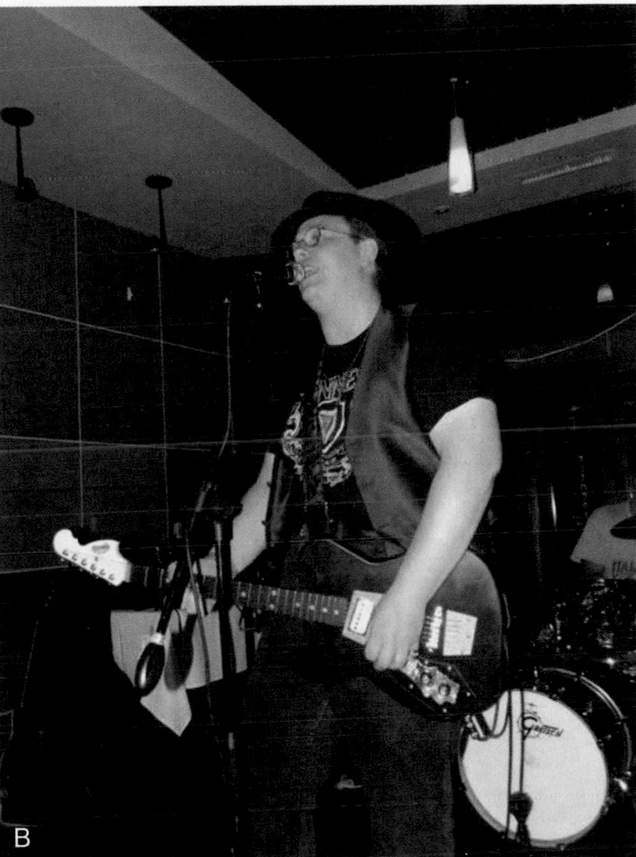

FIGURE 27-5 It is important to help families find meaningful occupations in the community for children and teens with ASD. **A,** This young boy volunteers with his mother at a local animal shelter each week. **B,** This young adult sings and plays lead guitar at local clubs and bars at his own shows and on open mike nights.

smiling more and were inviting and playful. Adult sound effects appeared particularly enticing.[160] There are also benefits when an adult imitates the child with ASD. Children with ASD respond to being imitated with greater responsiveness, more eye contact, and improved play.[50,51,68,70,160] Even brief imitative sessions can produce beneficial results.[87] These studies as a group demonstrate the importance of choice, preferred interests, affect, and the sensory properties of toys and activities to promote improved behavior and motivation, reduce the need for adult guidance or redirection, and increase interaction in children with ASD (see Figure 27-1*D*).

From the limited research, it appears that play deficits can be remediated by a variety of means. Occupational therapists can implement strategies in their sessions from many of the approaches into their playful work with children with ASD. Children with ASD may respond best, however, to playful adults and in particular to adults who imitate them at least some of the time.

Additional Intervention Concerns

Safety

Occupational therapists can assist the family in managing escapism and other safety issues through problem solving, activity analysis, and often through the use of technology. Depending on the situation, families with the financial means can install a variety of window and door alarms to alert them to the possibility of the child leaving the home. Yard fencing may be an option for some as well. GPS tracking is another option. For families with limited financial means, simple low tech solutions, such as more difficult locking mechanisms or the use of Velcro and bells to alert family members to windows or doors or cabinets being opened, can be helpful. Bed tents can provide relatively low cost relief for families of children who wander during the night. Special harnesses and mechanisms can prevent children from removing themselves from their seatbelts or child seats. Household cleaners or medicines may need to be put into different containers and kept in locked cabinets. Similar methods may be needed for knives and other sharp kitchen utensils. On some stoves the knobs may be removable. Autism Speaks has developed a list of safety products for families of individuals with ASD (see the Evolve website for a link to safety products).

Coping and Self-Efficacy

As stated, parents of children with ASD are often stressed; therefore, an important role for the occupational therapist working with a family and child with ASD may be helping the family cope. The most commonly used model of coping, the transactional model,[131] guided research for more than 20 years.

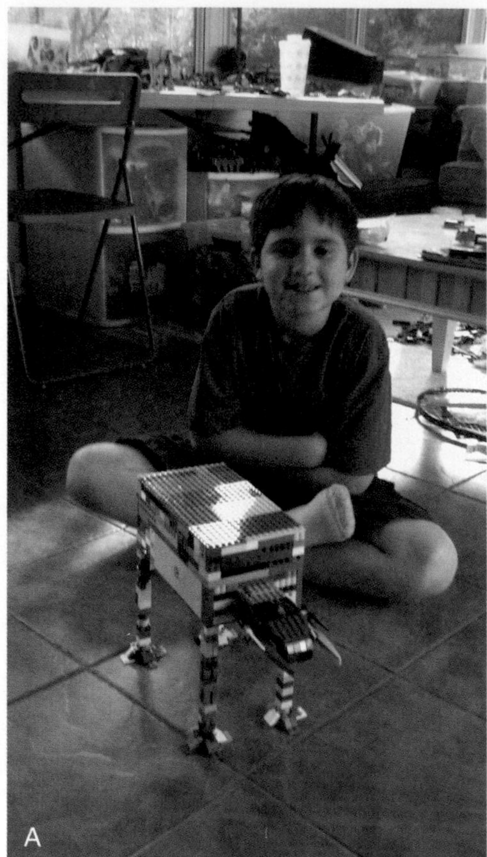

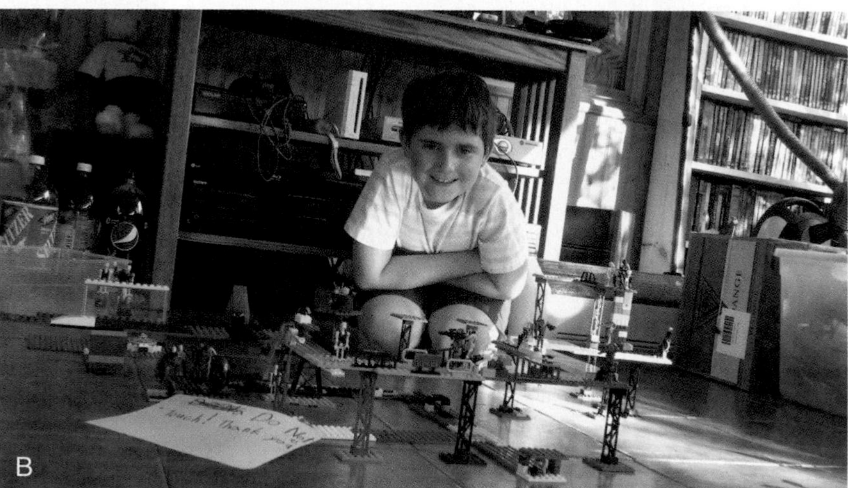

FIGURE 27-6 **A, B,** A child with ASD with special strengths in visual construction and creativity in design. An important role for occupational therapists is finding out about a child's strengths and preferences during evaluation, so that these can be used in intervention.

This model applied to parenting proposes that coping is a dynamic process, whereby following a parent appraisal that an event is stressful, the parent's coping is influenced by his or her personality, the resources available, the situation in relation to additional stressors, and the availability of coping responses. In this model, coping responses are not inherently good or bad or useful. The effectiveness of a coping response depends on the match between the actual stress and the response that is chosen to address it. Personality factors do play into coping effectiveness and psychological well-being. However, research suggests that certain coping responses may be linked to mood states.[177] For example, coping responses that were more active, such as problem-focused coping, finding and using social support, engaging in positive reframing, and compromise, were associated with a more positive daily mood, whereas coping responses such as escape, blame, withdrawal, and helplessness were associated with a more negative daily mood. Other researchers found similar results, suggesting that positive reframing is an important coping strategy for improving mental health, whereas coping strategies that could be called avoidance are associated with depression and anger.[26]

Mothers report that their coping strategies include gaining information, planning and organizing effectively, making time for their own personal needs (i.e., "me time"), and reframing the experience in a positive light, noting the joys and benefits of having a child with ASD.[123,128] Many of their reported strategies were active ones according to the preceding model, those that will help their mood and well-being. Therefore occupational therapists can assist in family coping by helping families gain or gather the information they need about ASD and intervention approaches.[123] Therapists who remain current with the latest information, research, policy changes, and clinical guidelines can also assist parents in making effective decisions about their child's care. Therapists can assist parents in creating organizational or planning methods that work for their family. Occupational therapists can assist the family in finding appropriate respite care or in developing parent-to-parent networks to share the work and allow for individual time. They can become knowledgeable about local resources for family fun and outings that are ASD friendly such as special movie nights where the theater volume is turned low and the lights are left on slightly, and malls that have initiated special times for children with ASD to visit with Santa during the holidays.

Occupational therapists can also improve parental self-efficacy by using informational power to help parents learn how to parent their child. By sharing knowledge of activity analysis, natural learning opportunities, and sensory processing, occupational therapists can empower parents to feel confident and capable of handling situations as they arise in the community, their home, or anywhere. Parents can be taught to use skills of activity analysis to attempt to understand a problem behavior for their child in the community, considering the requirements of the activity they are being asked to engage in and the environment in which they are doing so. Parents can learn to consider the sensory environment, the novelty, and the cognitive challenges provided by the activity to help prepare their child. In addition, by teaching some aspects of activity analysis, parents can learn to more readily use the natural learning opportunities provided in their day-to-day activities, to promote desired skills for their child without taking time to specifically "work" on a skill in isolation. For example, parents can be taught to look for natural opportunities during their day in which the task at hand requires a specific cognitive or motor skill or a specific social emotional behavior such as waiting, sharing, or taking turns.

Research suggests that "optimistic parenting" of a child with ASD may be quite important in managing early behavioral difficulties and keeping them from growing into larger problems.[63-65] Cognitive behavioral interventions to support parental optimism and provide positive behavioral supports (knowledge and ways to manage behaviors) appear to be successful in helping those families who need the help the most.[65] Parents need to feel able to manage their child's behavior and need to feel confident about their ability to be in the community and handle the judgments and poor behavior of others who lack understanding of ASD.

Summary

Autism spectrum disorder is a complex condition with a unique profile for each individual, and its symptoms impact multiple aspects of occupational functioning. Occupational therapists will likely address play or leisure, self-care, sleep, education, all areas of performance skills, and performance patterns, although emphasis shifts according to the practice setting and the age of the child. For some children with substantial behavioral difficulties, significant supports and intense interventions are required, whereas for other children who are high functioning, the primary focus may be enhancing social skills across a broad range of social situations. Whether or not ASD is severe, the entire family is affected. Practicing family-centered care, occupational therapists use their knowledge, expertise, and informational power to enhance families' ability to manage the difficulties and challenges that an ASD diagnosis can bring, while focusing on the family's strengths to help the family cope and engage in meaningful family occupations (see Figure 27-1*E*).

Summary Points

- Autism spectrum disorder may impact all aspects of occupational performance, but in particular social participation is often most greatly affected. Sensory issues are a common concern as well.
- A child with ASD may alter the dynamics and relationships of the entire family, and parents are often stressed and need assistance to enhance their competence, self-efficacy, and coping skills.
- Occupational therapists assess the strengths of a child with ASD and the areas of concern for the family and child and provide family-centered care to promote occupational functioning of the whole family.
- Interventions for ASD commonly include behavioral supports, sensory supports, cognitive and social supports, and the use of a variety of specific strategies and approaches that motivate the child with ASD, reduce fear and anxiety, and improve behavior, skill, and engagement.

REFERENCES

1. Akshoomoff, N. (2006). Use of the Mullen Scales of Early Learning for the assessment of young children with autism spectrum disorders. *Child Neuropsychology, 12*, 269–277.
2. Ahearn, W. H., Castine, T., Nault, K., et al. (2001). An assessment of food acceptance in children with autism or pervasive developmental disorder—not otherwise specified. *Journal of Autism and Developmental Disorders, 31*(5), 505–511.
3. Allik, H., Larsson, J., & Smedje, H. (2006). Health related quality of life in parents of school-age children with Asperger syndrome or high functioning autism. *Health and Quality of Life Outcomes, 4*, 1–8.
4. American Psychiatric Association. (1952). *Diagnostic and statistical manual for mental disorders.* Washington, DC: Author.
5. American Psychiatric Association. (1968). *Diagnostic and statistical manual for mental disorders* (2nd ed.). Washington, DC: Author.
6. American Psychiatric Association. (1980). *Diagnostic and statistical manual for mental disorders* (3rd ed.). Washington, DC: Author.
7. American Psychiatric Association. (1987). *Diagnostic and statistical manual for mental disorders* (3rd ed., rev.). Washington, DC: Author.
8. American Psychiatric Association. (1994). *Diagnostic and statistical manual for mental disorders* (4th ed.). Washington, DC: Author.
9. American Psychiatric Association. (2013). *Diagnostic and statistical manual of mental disorders* (5th ed.). Washington, DC: Author.
10. American Psychiatric Association. (2011). *History.* Retrieved from: <http://www.psych.org/MainMenu/Research/DSMIV/History_1.aspx>.
11. American Occupational Therapy Association. (2008). Occupational therapy practice framework: Domain and process (2nd ed.). *American Journal of Occupational Therapy, 62*, 625–683.
12. Ashburner, J., Ziviani, J., & Rodger, S. (2008). Sensory processing and classroom emotional, behavioral, and educational outcomes in children with autism spectrum disorder. *The American Journal of Occupational Therapy, 62*, 564–573.
13. Audet, L. (2010). The nature of pervasive developmental disorders: A holistic view. In H. Miller-Kuhaneck (Ed.), *Autism: A comprehensive occupational therapy approach* (3rd ed.). Bethesda, MD: The American Occupational Therapy Association.
14. Ayres, A. J. (1979). *Sensory integration and the child.* Los Angeles: Western Psychological Services.
15. Bagby, M. S., Dickie, V. A., & Baranek, G. T. (2011). How sensory experiences of children with and without autism affect family occupations. *American Journal of Occupational Therapy, 66*(1), 78–86.
16. Baio, J. (2012). Prevalence of autism spectrum disorders—autism and developmental disabilities monitoring

network, 14 sites, United States, 2008. *Morbidity and Mortality Weekly Report (MMWR), 61*, 1–19.
17. Baker, A. E. Z., Lane, A., Angley, M. T., et al. (2008). The relationship between sensory processing patterns and behavioural responsiveness in autistic disorder: A pilot study. *Journal of Autism and Developmental Disorders, 38*, 867–875.
18. Baker, M. J. (2000). Incorporating the thematic ritualistic behaviors of children with autism into games: Increasing social play interactions with siblings. *Journal of Positive Behavior Interventions, 2*, 66–84.
19. Baranek, G. T. (1999). Autism during infancy: A retrospective video analysis of sensory-motor and social behaviors at 9–12 months of age. *Autism: The International Journal of Research and Practice, 29*, 213–224.
20. Baranek, G. T., Danko, C. D., Skinner, M. L., et al. (2005). Video analysis of sensory-motor features in infants with fragile X syndrome at 9–12 months of age. *Journal of Autism and Developmental Disorders, 35*, 645–656.
21. Baranek, G. T., David, F. J., Poe, M. D., et al. (2006). Sensory Experiences Questionnaire: Discriminating sensory features in young children with autism, developmental delays, and typical development. *Journal of Child Psychology and Psychiatry, and Allied Disciplines, 47*, 591–601.
22. Bauminger, N., & Shulman, C. (2003). The development and maintenance of friendship in high-functioning children with autism: Maternal perceptions. *Autism: The International Journal of Research and Practice, 7*(1), 81–97.
23. Bauminger, N., Solomon, M., Aviezer, A., et al. (2008). Children with autism and their friends: A multidimensional study of friendship in high-functioning autism spectrum disorder. *Journal of Abnormal Child Psychology, 36*(2), 135–150.
24. Bauminger, N., Solomon, M., & Rogers, S. J. (2010). Predicting friendship quality in autism spectrum disorders and typical development. *Journal of Autism and Developmental Disorders, 40*(6), 751–761.
25. Ben-Sasson, A., Hen, L., Fluss, R., et al. (2009). A meta-analysis of sensory modulation symptoms in individuals with autism spectrum disorders. *Journal of Autism and Developmental Disorders, 39*, 1–11.
26. Benson, P. R. (2010). Coping, distress, and well-being in mothers of children with autism. *Research in Autism Spectrum Disorders, 4*(2), 217–228.
27. Bergman, P., & Escalona, S. K. (1949). Unusual sensitivities in very young children. *Psychoanalytic Study of the Child, 4*, 333–352.
28. Bettelheim, B. (1967). *The empty fortress: Infantile autism and the birth of the self.* New York: Free Press.
29. Bhat, A. N., Landa, R. J., & Galloway, J. C. C. (2011). Current perspectives on motor functioning in infants, children, and adults with autism spectrum disorders. *Physical Therapy, 91*, 1116–1129.
30. Bishop, D. V. M., & Norbury, C. F. (2005). Executive functions in children with communication impairments, in relation to autistic symptomatology. 1: Generativity. *Autism: The International Journal of Research and Practice, 9*(1), 7–27.
31. Bishop, S. L., Richler, J., Cain, A. C., et al. (2007). Predictors of perceived negative impact in mothers of children with autism spectrum disorder. *American Journal on Mental Retardation, 112*, 450–461.
32. Blaxill, M. F. (2004). What's going on? The question of time trends in autism. *Public Health Reports, 119*, 536–551.
33. Bledsoe, R., Myles, B. S., & Simpson, R. L. (2003). Use of a social story intervention to improve mealtime skills of an adolescent with Asperger syndrome. *Autism: The International Journal of Research and Practice, 7*(3), 289–295.
34. Blumberg, S., et al. (2013). Prevalence of autism spectrum disorders—Autism and developmental disabilities monitoring network, 14 sites, United States, 2008. *Morbidity and Mortality Weekly Report. Surveillance Summaries* (Washington, DC: 2002), *61*(3), 1–19. Retrieved from: <http://www.ncbi.nlm.nih.gov/pubmed/22456193>.
35. Boucher, J. (2007). Memory and generativity in very high functioning autism: a firsthand account, and an interpretation. *Autism: The International Journal of Research and Practice, 11*(3), 255–264.
36. Brady, S. J., Peters, D. L., Gamel-McCormick, M., et al. (2004). Types and patterns of professional-family talk in home-based early intervention. *Journal of Early Intervention, 26*, 146–159.
37. Bresnahan, M., Li, G., & Susser, E. (2009). Hidden in plain sight. *International Journal of Epidemiology, 38*, 1172–1174.
38. Byers, E. S., Nichols, S., Voyer, S. D., et al. (2012). Sexual well-being of a community sample of high-functioning adults on the autism spectrum who have been in a romantic relationship. *Autism: The International Journal of Research and Practice* [Epub ahead of print].
39. Byers, E. S., Nichols, S., & Voyer, S. D. (2013). Challenging stereotypes: Sexual functioning of single adults with high functioning autism spectrum disorder. *Journal of Autism and Developmental Disorders* [Epub ahead of print].
40. Carrington, S., Templeton, E., & Papinczak, T. (2003). Adolescents with Asperger syndrome and perceptions of friendship. *Autism: The International Journal of Research and Practice, 18*(4), 211–218.
41. Carter, C. M. (2001). Using choice with game play to increase language skills and interactive behaviors in children with autism. *Journal of Positive Behavior Interventions, 3*, 131–151.
42. Centers for Disease Control and Prevention. (2007). Prevalence of autism spectrum disorders—Autism and developmental disabilities monitoring network, 14 sites, United States, 2002. *MMWR, 56*, 12–28. Retrieved from: <http://www.cdc.gov/mmwr/preview/mmwrhtml/ss5601a2.htm>.
43. Charman, T. (1997). The relationship between joint attention and pretend play in autism. *Development and Psychopathology, 9*, 1–16.
44. Chen, Y., Rodgers, J., & McConachie, H. (2009). Restricted and repetitive behaviors, sensory processing and cognitive style in children with autism spectrum disorders. *Journal of Autism and Developmental Disorders, 39*, 635–642.
45. Corbett, B., Schupp, C., & Levine, S. (2009). Comparing cortisol, stress, and sensory sensitivity in children with autism. *Autism Research, 2*(1), 39–49.
46. Crane, L., Goddard, L., & Pring, L. (2009). Sensory processing in adults with autism spectrum disorders. *Autism: The International Journal of Research and Practice, 13*(3), 215–228.
47. Crozier, S., & Tincani, M. (2007). Effects of social stories on prosocial behavior of preschool children with autism spectrum disorders. *Journal of Autism and Developmental Disorders, 37*(9), 1803–1814.
48. Davis, N. O., & Carter, A. S. (2008). Parenting stress in mothers and fathers of toddlers with autism spectrum disorders: Associations with child characteristics. *Journal of Autism and Developmental Disorders, 38*, 1278–1291.
49. Dawson, G. (2012). *The changing definition of autism: critical issues ahead.* Retrieved from: <http://blog.autismspeaks.org/2012/01/20/the-changing-definition-of-autism-criticalissues-ahead/>.
50. Dawson, G., & Adams, A. (1984). Imitation and social responsiveness in autistic children. *Journal of Abnormal Child Psychology, 12*, 209–226.

51. Dawson, G., & Galpert, L. (1990). Mother's use of imitative play for facilitating social responsiveness and toy play in young autistic children. *Development and Psychopathology, 2*, 151–162.
52. Deci, E. L., & Moller, A. C. (2005). The concept of competence: A starting place for understanding intrinsic motivation and self-determined extrinsic motivation. In A. J. Elliot & C. J. Dweck (Eds.), *Handbook of competence and motivation* (pp. 579–597). New York: Guilford Press.
53. DeGrace, B. W. (2004). The everyday occupation of families with children with autism. *The American Journal of Occupational Therapy, 58*, 543 550.
54. Delmolino, L., & Harris, S. L. (2012). Matching children on the autism spectrum to classrooms: A guide for parents and professionals. *Journal of Autism and Developmental Disorders, 42*(6), 1197–1204.
55. Dominguez, A., Ziviani, J., & Rodger, S. (2006). Play behaviors and play object preferences of young children with autistic disorder in a clinical play environment. *Autism: The International Journal of Research and Practice, 10*, 53–69.
56. Donnelly, J., & Bovee, J. (2003). Reflections on play: Recollections from a mother and her son with Asperger syndrome. *Autism: The International Journal of Research and Practice, 7*, 471–476.
57. Dowell, L. R., Mahone, E. M., & Mostofsky, S. H. (2009). Associations between postural knowledge and basic motor skill with dyspraxia in autism: Implication for abnormalities in distributed connectivity and motor learning. *Neuropsychology, 23*, 563–570.
58. Dunlap, G., & Koegel, R. L. (1980). Motivating autistic children through stimulus variation. *Journal of Applied Behavior Analysis, 13*, 619–627.
59. Dunn, J. (2004). *Children's friendships: The beginnings of intimacy.* Oxford, UK: Blackwell.
60. Dunn, W., Cox, J., Foster, L., et al. (2012). Impact of a contextual intervention on child participation and parent competence among children with autism spectrum disorders: A pretest-posttest repeated-measures design. *The American Journal of Occupational Therapy: Official Publication of the American Occupational Therapy Association, 66*(5), 520 528.
61. Dunst, C. (2007). Early intervention for infants and toddlers with developmental disabilities. In S. L. Odom, R. H. Horner, M. E. Snell, et al. (Eds.), *Handbook of developmental disabilities* (pp. 161–180). New York: Guilford Press.
62. Dunst, C. J., Hamby, D., Trivette, C. M., et al. (2000). Everyday family and community life and children's naturally occurring learning opportunities. *Journal of Early Intervention, 23*, 151–164.
63. Durand, V. M. (2011). *Optimistic parenting: Hope and help for you and your challenging child.* Baltimore: Paul H. Brookes.
64. Durand, V. M. (2001). Future directions for children and adolescents with mental retardation. *Behavior Therapy, 32*, 633 650.
65. Durand, V. M., & Hieneman, M. (2008). *Helping parents with challenging children: Positive family intervention, facilitator's guide.* New York: Oxford University Press.
66. Dzuik, M. A., Gidley Larson, J. C., Apostu, A., et al. (2007). Dyspraxia in autism: Association with motor, social, and communicative deficits. *Developmental Medicine and Child Neurology, 49*, 734–739.
67. Eikeseth, S. (2009). Outcome of comprehensive psycho-educational interventions for young children with autism. *Research in Developmental Disabilities, 30*, 158–178.
68. Escalona, A., Field, T., Nadel, J., et al. (2002). Brief report: Imitation effects on children with autism. *Journal of Autism and Developmental Disorders, 32*, 141–144.
69. Estes, A., Rivera, V., Bryan, M., et al. (2011). Discrepancies between academic achievement and intellectual ability in higher-functioning school-aged children with autism spectrum disorder. *Journal of Autism and Developmental Disorders, 41*, 1044–1052.
70. Field, T., Sanders, C., & Nadel, J. (2001). Children with autism display more social behaviors after repeated imitation sessions. *Autism: The International Journal of Research and Practice, 5*, 317–323.
71. Foxx, R. M. (2008). Applied behavior analysis treatment of autism: The state of the art. *Child and Adolescent Psychiatric Clinics of North America, 17*, 821–834.
72. French, J. P. R., Jr., & Raven, B. (1960). The bases of social power. In D. Cartwright & A. Zander (Eds.), *Group dynamics* (pp. 607–623). New York: Harper & Row.
73. Frith, U. (2003). *Autism: Explaining the enigma* (2nd ed.). Malden, MA: Wiley-Blackwell.
74. Ganz, M. L. (2007). The lifetime distribution of the incremental societal costs of autism. *Archives of Pediatric & Adolescent Medicine, 161*, 343–349.
75. Gerrard, S., & Rugg, G. (2009). Sensory impairments and autism: A re-examination of causal modeling. *Journal of Autism and Developmental Disorders, 39*, 1449–1463.
76. Giannotti, F., Cortesi, F., Cerquiglini, A., et al. (2006). An open-label study of controlled-release melatonin in treatment of sleep disorders in children with autism. *Journal of Autism and Developmental Disorders, 36*, 741–752.
77. Grandin, T. (1997). A personal perspective on autism. In D. J. Cohen & F. R. Volkmar (Eds.), *Handbook of autism and pervasive developmental disorders* (2nd ed.). New York: Wiley.
78. Gray, D. E. (2003). Gender and coping: The parents of children with high functioning autism. *Social Science & Medicine, 56*, 631–642.
79. Gray, C. A. (1998). Social stories and comic strip conversations with students with Asperger syndrome and high-functioning autism. In E. Schopler (Ed.), *Asperger syndrome or high-functioning autism?* (pp. 167–194). New York: Plenum Press.
80. Gray, C., & White, A. L. (2002). *My social stories book.* New York: Jessica Kingsley Publishers.
81. Green, S. A., & Ben-Sasson, A. (2010). Anxiety disorders and sensory over-responsivity in children with autism spectrum disorders: Is there a causal relationship? *Journal of Autism and Developmental Disorders,* (c).
82. Green, V. A., Pituch, K. A., Itchon, J., et al. (2006). Internet survey of treatments used by parents of children with autism. *Research in Developmental Disabilities, 27*, 70–84.
83. Gurney, J. G., McPheeters, M. L., & Davis, M. M. (2006). Parental report of health conditions and health care use among children with and without autism: National Survey of Children's Health. *Archives of Pediatrics & Adolescent Medicine, 160*, 825–830.
84. Hastings, R. P. (2003). Child behavior problems and partner mental health as correlates of stress in mothers and fathers of children with autism. *Journal of Intellectual Developmental Research, 47*, 231–237.
85. Hastings, R. P., & Brown, T. (2002). Behavior problems of children with autism, parental self-efficacy, and mental health. *American Journal on Mental Retardation, 10*, 222–232.
86. Hastings, R. P., Kovshoff, H., Brown, T., et al. (2005). Coping strategies in mothers and fathers of preschool and school age children with autism. *Autism: The International Journal of Research and Practice, 9*, 377–391.
87. Heimann, M., Laberg, K. E., & Nordøen, B. (2006). Imitative

interaction increases social interest and elicited imitation in non-verbal children with autism. *Infant and Child Development, 15,* 297–309.

88. Herring, S., Gray, K., Taffe, J., et al. (2006). Behavior and emotional problems in toddlers with pervasive developmental disorders and developmental delay: Associations with parental mental health and family functioning. *Journal of Intellectual Disability Research, 50,* 874–882.
89. Hess, K. L., Morrier, M. J., Heflin, L. J., et al. (2008). Autism treatment survey: Services received by children with autism spectrum disorders in public school classrooms. *Journal of Autism and Developmental Disorders, 38,* 961–971.
90. Hieneman, M., Childs, K., & Sergay, J. (2006). *Parenting with positive behavior support.* Baltimore: Paul H. Brookes Publishing.
91. Hilton, C. L., Harper, J. D., Holmes, R., et al. (2010). Sensory responsiveness as a predictor of social severity in children with high functioning autism spectrum disorders. *Journal of Autism and Developmental Disorders, 40*(8), 937–945.
92. Hine, J. F., & Wolery, M. (2006). Using point of view video modeling to teach play to preschoolers with autism. *Topics in Early Childhood Special Education, 26,* 83–93.
93. Hobson, R. P., Lee, A., & Hobson, J. A. (2009). Qualities of symbolic play among children with autism: A social developmental perspective. *Journal of Autism and Developmental Disorders, 39,* 12–22.
94. Holmes, R. M., & Procaccino, J. K. (2009). Autistic children's play with objects, peers, and adults in a classroom setting. In C. D. Clark (Ed.), *Transactions at play: Play and culture studies* (Vol. 9, pp. 86–103). New York: University Press of America.
95. Holmes, E., & Willoughby, T. (2005). Play behaviour of children with autism spectrum disorders. *Journal of Intellectual and Developmental Disability, 30,* 156–164.
96. Howes, C. (1983). Patterns of friendship. *Child Development, 54*(4), 1041–1053.
97. Hutt, S., Hutt, C., Lee, D., et al. (1964). A behavioral and electroencephalographic study of autistic children. *Journal of Psychiatric Research, 3,* 181–197.
98. Hutt, C., & Ounsted, C. (1966). The biological significance of gaze aversion with particular reference to the syndrome of infantile autism. *Behavioral Science, 11,* 346–356.
99. Interactive Autism Network. (2010). *Interactive Autism Network Community: sensory-based therapies.* Retrieved from: <http://www.iancommunity.org/cs/what_do_we_know/sensory_based_therapies>.
100. Ingersoll, B. (2008). The social role of imitation in autism: Implications for the treatment of imitation deficits. *Infants and Young Children, 21,* 107–119.
101. Ingersoll, B., & Gergans, S. (2007). The effect of a parent-implemented imitation intervention on spontaneous imitation skills in young children with autism. *Research in Developmental Disabilities, 28,* 163–175.
102. Ingersoll, B., & Schreibman, L. (2006). Teaching reciprocal imitation skills to young children with autism using a naturalistic behavioral approach: Effects on language, pretend play, and joint attention. *Journal of Autism and Developmental Disorders, 36,* 487–505.
103. Ingersoll, B., & Hambrick, D. Z. (2011). The relationship between the broader autism phenotype, child severity, and stress and depression in parents of children with autism spectrum disorders. *Research in Autism Spectrum Disorders, 5,* 337–344.
104. Jarrold, C. (2003). A review of research into pretend play in autism. *Autism: The International Journal of Research and Practice, 7,* 379–390.
105. Jarrold, C., Boucher, J., & Smith, P. (1996). Executive function deficits and the pretend play of children with autism: a research note. *Journal of Child Psychology and Psychiatry, 35,* 1473–1482.
106. Jasmin, E., Couture, M., Mckinley, Æ. P., et al. (2009). Sensori-motor and daily living skills of preschool children with autism spectrum disorders. *Journal of Autism and Developmental Disorders,* 231–241.
107. Jobe, L. E., & Williams White, S. (2007). Loneliness, social relationships, and a broader autism phenotype in college students. *Personality and Individual Differences, 42*(8), 1479–1489.
108. Jones, R., Quigney, C., & Huws, J. (2003). First hand accounts of sensory perceptual experiences in autism: A qualitative analysis. *Journal of Intellectual & Developmental Disability, 28,* 112–121.
109. Joosten, A. V., Bundy, A. C., & Enfeld, S. L. (2009). Intrinsic and extrinsic motivation for stereotypic and repetitive behavior. *Journal of Autism and Developmental Disorders, 39,* 521–531.
110. Kanner, L. (1943). Autistic disturbances of affective contact. *The Nervous Child, 2,* 217–250.
111. Kanner, L. (1971). Follow-up study of eleven autistic children originally reported in 1943. *Journal of Autism and Childhood Schizophrenia, 1,* 119–145.
112. Kientz, M. A., & Dunn, W. (1997). A comparison of the performance of children with and without autism on the sensory profile. *American Journal of Occupational Therapy, 51,* 530–537.
113. King, S., Teplicky, R., King, G., et al. (2004). Family-centered service for children with cerebral palsy and their families: A review of the literature. *Seminars in Pediatric Neurology, 11,* 78–86.
114. Klein, S., Wynn, K., Ray, L., et al. (2011). Information sharing during diagnostic assessments: What is relevant for parents? *Physical and Occupational Therapy in Pediatrics, 31,* 120–132.
115. Klintwall, L., Holm, A., Eriksson, M., et al. (2010). Sensory abnormalities in autism: A brief report. *Research in Developmental Disabilities, 32*(2), 795–800.
116. Koegel, L. K., Koegel, R. L., & Smith, A. (1997). Variables related to differences in standardized test outcomes for children with autism. *Journal of Autism and Developmental Disorders, 27*(3), 233–243.
117. Koegel, R. L., Schreibman, L., Loos, L. M., et al. (1992). Consistent stress profiles in mothers of children with autism. *Journal of Autism and Developmental Disorders, 22,* 205–216.
118. Koenig, K. P., Stillman, W., & Kinnealy, M. (2006). *In their own voice: Facilitating participation with individuals with autistic spectrum disorders/differences (ASD).* April 27. American Occupational Therapy Association Annual Conference, Charlotte, NC.
119. Kogan, M. D., Blumberg, S. J., Schieve, L. A., et al. (2009). Prevalence of parent–reported diagnosis of autism spectrum disorder among children in the US, 2007. *Pediatrics, 124,* 1–9.
120. Kogan, M. D., Strickland, B. B., Blumberg, S. J., et al. (2008). A national profile of the health care experiences and family impact of autism spectrum disorder among children in the United States, 2005–2006. *Pediatrics, 122,* 1149–1158.
121. Krakowiak, P., Goodlin-Jones, B., Hertz-Picciotto, I., et al. (2008). Sleep problems in children with autism spectrum disorders, developmental delays, and typical development: A population-based study. *Journal of Sleep Research, 17*(2), 197–206.
122. Kuhaneck, H. M. (2009). *An examination of programmatic needs for siblings of children with an autism spectrum disorder in the state of Connecticut. Unpublished data.* Abstract

available: <http://www.uconnucedd.org/lend/pdfs/abstracts/c1/kuhaneck_abstract.pdf>.

123. Kuhaneck, H. M., Burroughs, T., Wright, J., et al. (2010). A qualitative study of coping in mothers of children with an autism spectrum disorder. *Physical & Occupational Therapy in Pediatrics*, *30*, 340–350.

124. Kuhaneck, H. M., & Chisholm, E. C. (2012). Improving dental visits for individuals with autism spectrum disorders through an understanding of sensory processing. *Special Care in Dentistry: Official Publication of the American Association of Hospital Dentists, the Academy of Dentistry for the Handicapped, and the American Society for Geriatric Dentistry*, *32*(6), 229–233.

125. Kuhn, B. (2011). The excuse-me drill: A behavioral protocol to promote independent sleep initiation skills and reduce bedtime problems in young children. In M. Perlis, M. Aloia, & B. Kuhn (Eds.), *Behavioral treatments for sleep disorders: A comprehensive primer of behavioral sleep medicine treatment protocols.* London: Academic Press.

126. Kuo, M. H., Orsmond, G. I., Cohn, E. S., et al. (2013). Friendship characteristics and activity patterns of adolescents with an autism spectrum disorder. *Autism: The International Journal of Research and Practice*, *17*(4), 481–500.

127. Lane, A. E., Young, R. L., Baker, A. E. Z., et al. (2010). Sensory processing subtypes in autism: Association with adaptive behavior. *Journal of Autism and Developmental Disorders*, *40*, 112–122.

128. Larson, E. (2006). Caregiving and autism: How does children's propensity for routinization influence participation in family activities? *OTJR: Occupation, Participation and Health*, *26*, 69–79.

129. Lasgaard, M., Nielsen, A., Eriksen, M. E., et al. (2010). Loneliness and social support in adolescent boys with autism spectrum disorders. *Journal of Autism and Developmental Disorders*, *40*(2), 218–226.

130. LaVesser, P., & Hilton, C. L. (2010). Self-care skills for children with an autism spectrum disorder. In H. M. Kuhaneck & R. Watling (Eds.), *Autism: A comprehensive occupational therapy approach* (3rd ed., pp. 427–468). Bethesda, MD: AOTA Press.

131. Lazarus, R. S., & Folkman, S. (1984). *Stress, appraisal, and coping*. New York: Springer.

132. Lee, L. C., Harrington, R. A., Louie, B. B., et al. (2008). Children with autism: Quality of life and parental concerns. *Journal of Autism and Developmental Disorders*, *38*, 1147–1160.

133. Leekam, S. R., Nieto, C., Libby, S. J., et al. (2007). Describing the sensory abnormalities of children and adults with autism. *Journal of Autism and Developmental Disorders*, *37*, 894–910. doi:10.1007/s10803-006-0218-7.

134. Lewis, V., & Boucher, J. (1991). Skill, content and generative strategies in autistic children's drawings. *British Journal of Developmental Psychology*, *9*, 393–416.

135. Lewis, V., & Boucher, J. (1995). Generativity in the play of young people with autism. *Journal of Autism and Developmental Disorders*, *25*, 105–121.

136. Libby, S., Powell, S., Messer, D., et al. (1998). Spontaneous play in children with autism: A reappraisal. *Autism: The International Journal of Research and Practice*, *28*, 487–497.

137. Lockner, D. W., Crowe, T. K., & Skipper, B. J. (2008). Dietary intake and parents' perception of mealtime behaviors in preschool-age children with autism spectrum disorder and in typically developing children. *Journal of the American Dietetic Association*, *108*(8), 1360–1363.

138. MacDonald, R., Sacramone, S., Mansfield, R., et al. (2009). Using video modeling to teach reciprocal pretend play to children with autism. *Journal of Applied Behavior Analysis*, *42*, 43–55.

139. MacNeil, L. K., & Mostofsky, S. (2012). Specificity of dyspraxia in children with autism. *Neuropsychology*, *26*(2), 165–171.

140. Mailloux, Z., & Smith Roley, S. (2010). Sensory integration. In H. Miller Kuhaneck & R. Watling (Eds.), *Autism: A comprehensive occupational therapy approach* (3rd ed., pp. 469–508). Bethesda, MD: AOTA Press.

141. Marquenie, K., Rodger, S., Mangohig, K., et al. (2011). Dinnertime and bedtime routines and rituals in families with a young child with an autism spectrum disorder. *Australian Occupational Therapy Journal*, *58*(3), 145–154.

142. McLennan, J. D., Huculak, S., & Sheehan, D. (2008). Brief report: Pilot investigation of service receipt by young children with autistic spectrum disorders. *Journal of Autism and Developmental Disorders*, *38*, 1192–1196.

143. McPartland, J. C., Reichow, B., & Volkmar, F. R. (2012). Sensitivity and specificity of proposed DSM-5 diagnostic criteria for autism spectrum disorder. *Journal of the American Academy of Child & Adolescent Psychiatry*, *51*(4), 368–383.

144. Meadan, H., Stoner, J. B., & Angell, M. E. (2009). Review of literature related to the social, emotional, and behavioral adjustment of siblings of individuals with autism spectrum disorder. *Journal of Developmental and Physical Disabilities*, *22*(1), 83–100.

145. Menzinger, B., & Jackson, R. (2009). The effect of light intensity and noise on the classroom behaviour of pupils with Asperger syndrome. *Support for Learning*, *24*, 170–175.

146. Meyer, K. A., Ingersoll, B., & Hambrick, D. Z. (2011). Factors influencing adjustment in siblings of children with autism spectrum disorders. *Research in Autism Spectrum Disorders*, *5*(4), 1413–1420.

147. Miller-Kuhaneck, H., & Glennon, T. J. (2001). Combining intervention approaches in occupational therapy for children with pervasive developmental disorders. *OT Practice CE Article*, (November), 1–8.

148. Miller-Kuhaneck, H., & Gross, M. (2010). Alternative and complimentary interventions for the autism spectrum disorders. In H. Miller-Kuhaneck & R. Watling (Eds.), *Autism: A comprehensive occupational therapy approach* (3rd ed.). Baltimore: AOTA.

149. Miller Kuhaneck, H., Spitzer, S., & Miller, E. (2010). *Activity analysis, creativity and playfulness in pediatric occupational therapy: Making play just right.* Boston: Jones & Bartlett.

150. Millward, C., Ferriter, M., Calver, S., et al. (2004). Gluten- and casein-free diets for autistic spectrum disorder. *Cochrane Database of Systematic Reviews (Online)*, (2), CD003498.

151. Mindell, J. A., Telofski, L. S., Wiegand, B., et al. (2009). A nightly bedtime routine: Impact on sleep in young children and maternal mood. *Sleep*, *32*(5), 599–606.

152. Minshew, N. J., & Hobson, J. A. (2008). Sensory sensitivities and performance on sensory perceptual tasks in high-functioning individuals with autism. *Journal of Autism and Developmental Disorders*, *38*(8), 1485–1498.

153. Montes, G., & Halterman, J. S. (2007). Psychological functioning and coping among mothers of children with autism: A population based study. *Pediatrics*, *119*, 1040–1046.

154. Montes, G., & Halterman, J. S. (2008a). Association of childhood autism spectrum disorders and loss of family income. *Pediatrics*, *121*, 821–826.

155. Montes, G., & Halterman, J. S. (2008b). Child care problems and

employment among families with preschool-aged children with autism in the United States. *Pediatrics, 122*, 202–208.

156. Morgenthaler, T. I., Owens, J., Alessi, C., et al. (2006). Practice parameters for behavioral treatment of bedtime problems and night wakings in infants and young children. *Sleep, 29*(10), 1277–1281.
157. Mostofsky, S. H., Dubey, P., Jerath, V. K., et al. (2006). Developmental dyspraxia is not limited to imitation in children with autism. *Journal of the International Neuropsychological Society, 12*, 314–326.
158. Müller, E., Schuler, A., & Yates, G. B. (2008). Social challenges and supports from the perspective of individuals with Asperger syndrome and other autism spectrum disabilities. *Autism: The International Journal of Research and Practice, 12*(2), 173–190.
159. Mugno, D., Ruta, L., D'Arrigo, V. G., et al. (2007). Impairment of quality of life in parents of children and adolescents with pervasive developmental disorder. *Health & Quality of Life Outcomes, 5*, 22–31.
160. Nadel, J., Martini, M., Field, T., et al. (2008). Children with autism approach more imitative and playful adults. *Early Child Development and Care, 178*, 461–465.
161. Nadon, G., Feldman, D. E., Dunn, W., et al. (2011). Mealtime problems in children with autism spectrum disorder and their typically developing siblings: A comparison study. *Autism: The International Journal of Research and Practice, 15*(1), 98–113.
162. National Autism Center. (2009). *Evidence-based practice autism in the schools.* Retrieved from <http://www.nationalautismcenter.org/pdf/NAC%20Ed%20Manual_FINAL.pdf>.
163. Newschaffer, C. J., Falb, M. D., & Gurney, J. G. (2005). National autism prevalence trends from United States special education data. *Pediatrics, 115*, 277–282.
164. Nimer, J., & Lundahl, B. (2007). Animal-assisted therapy: A meta-analysis. *Anthrozoos, 20*, 225–238.
165. O'Brien, J., Tsermentseli, S., Cummins, O., et al. (2009). Discriminating children with autism from children with learning difficulties with an adaptation of the Short Sensory Profile. *Early Child Development and Care, 179*(4), 383–394.
166. O'Donnell, S., Deitz, J., Kartin, D., et al. (2012). Autism Spectrum Disorders, *66*(5); O'Donnell, S., Deitz, J., Kartin, D., Nalty, T., & Dawson, G. (2012). Sensory processing, problem behavior, adaptive behavior, and cognition in preschool children with autism spectrum disorders. *American Journal of Occupational Therapy, 66*, 586–594.
167. Oppenheim, D., Dolev, S., Koren-Karie, N., et al. (2007). Parental resolution of the child's diagnosis and the parent-child relationship: Insights from the reaction to diagnosis interview. In D. Oppenheim & D. F. Goldsmith (Eds.), *Attachment theory in clinical work with children* (pp. 109–138). New York: Guilford Press.
168. Ozdemir, S. (2008). The effectiveness of social stories on decreasing disruptive behaviors of children with autism: Three case studies. *Journal of Autism and Developmental Disorders, 38*, 1689–1696.
169. Ozonoff, S., Macari, S., Young, G. S., et al. (2008). Atypical object exploration at 12 months of age is associated with autism in a prospective sample. *Autism: The International Journal of Research and Practice, 12*, 457–472.
170. Pajareya, K., & Nopmaneejumruslers, K. (2011). A pilot randomized controlled trial of DIR/Floortime™ parent training intervention for pre-school children with autistic spectrum disorders. *Autism: The International Journal of Research and Practice, 15*(5), 563–577.
171. Park, S., Cho, S.-C., Cho, I. H., et al. (2012). Sleep problems and their correlates and comorbid psychopathology of children with autism spectrum disorders. *Research in Autism Spectrum Disorders, 6*(3), 1068–1072.
172. Patterson, C. R., & Arco, L. (2007). Using video modeling for generalizing toy play in children with autism. *Behavior Modification, 31*, 660–681.
173. Peterson, E., Stein, L., & Cermak, S. (2013). Helping children with autism spectrum disorders participate in oral care. *Sensory Integration Special Interest Section Quarterly, 36*(3), 1–4.
174. Peters-Scheffer, N., Didden, R., Korzilius, H., et al. (2011). A meta-analytic study on the effectiveness of comprehensive ABA-based early intervention programs for children with autism spectrum disorders. *Research in Autism Spectrum Disorders, 5*(1), 60–69.
175. Polatajko, H. J., & Mandich, A. (2004). *Enabling occupation in children: The Cognitive Orientation to Daily Occupational Performance (CO-OP) approach.* Ottawa: CAOT Publications.
176. Polimeni, M. A., Richdale, A. L., & Francis, A. J. P. (2005). A survey of sleep problems in autism, Asperger's disorder and typically developing children. *Journal of Intellectual Disability Research: JIDR, 49*(Pt. 4), 260–268.
177. Pottie, C. G., & Ingram, K. M. (2008). Daily stress, coping, and well-being in parents of children with autism: A multilevel modeling approach. *Journal of Family Psychology, 22*(6), 855–864.
178. Quirmback, L. M., Lincoln, A. J., Feinberg-Gizzo, M. J., et al. (2009). Social stories: Mechanisms of effectiveness in increasing game play skills in children diagnosed with autism spectrum disorder using a pretest posttest repeated measures randomized control group design. *Journal of Autism and Developmental Disorders, 39*, 299–321.
179. Raven, B. H. (1965). Social influence and power. In I. D. Steiner & M. Fishbein (Eds.), *Current studies in social psychology* (pp. 371–381). New York: Holt, Rinehart & Winston.
180. Reagon, K. A., Higbee, T. S., & Endicott, K. (2006). Teaching pretend play skills to a student with autism using video modeling with a sibling as model and play partner. *Education and Treatment of Children, 29*, 517–528.
181. Rice, C., Nicholas, J., Baio, J., et al. (2010). Changes in autism spectrum disorder prevalence in 4 areas of the United States. *Disability and Health Journal, 3*, 186–201. doi:10.1016/j.dhjo.2009.10.008.
182. Richdale, A. L., & Schreck, K. A. (2009). Sleep problems in autism spectrum disorders: Prevalence, nature, & possible biopsychosocial aetiologies. *Sleep Medicine Reviews, 13*(6), 403–411.
183. Rimland, B. (1964). *Infantile autism: The syndrome and its implications for a neural theory of behavior.* New York: Appleton-Century-Crofts.
184. Robinson, S., Goddard, L., Dritschel, B., et al. (2009). Executive functions in children with autism spectrum disorders. *Brain and Cognition, 71*(3), 362–368.
185. Roger, S., & Bradenburg, J. (2009). Cognitive Orientation to (daily) Occupational Performance (CO-OP) with children with Asperger's syndrome who have motor-based occupational performance goals. *Australian Occupational Therapy Journal, 56*(1), 41–50.
186. Roger, S., Pham, C., & Mitchell, S. (2009). Cognitive strategy use by children with Asperger's syndrome during intervention for motor-based goals. *Australian Occupational Therapy Journal, 56*(2), 103–111.
187. Roger, S., & Vishram, A. (2010). Mastering social and organization goals: strategy use by two children with asperger syndrome during cognitive orientation to daily occupational performance. *Physical & Occupational Therapy in Pediatrics, 30*, 264–276.

188. Rogers, S. J., Hepburn, S. L., Stackhouse, T., et al. (2003). Imitation performance in toddlers with autism and those with other developmental disabilities. *Journal of Child Psychology & Psychiatry, 44*, 763–781.
189. Rogers, S. J., & Ozonoff, S. (2005). Annotation: what do we know about sensory dysfunction in autism? A critical review of the empirical evidence. *Journal of Child Psychology and Psychiatry, 46*, 1255–1268.
190. Rutter, M. (2005). Incidence of autism spectrum disorders: Changes over time and their meaning. *Acta Paediatrica, 94*, 2–15.
191. Sams, M. J., Fortney, E. V., & Willenbring, S. (2006). Occupational therapy incorporating animals for children with autism: a pilot investigation. *American Occupational Therapy Association, 60*, 268–274.
192. Sautter, R. A., LeBlanc, L. A., & Gillett, J. N. (2008). Using free operant preference assessments to select toys for free play between children with autism and siblings. *Research in Autism Spectrum Disorders, 2*, 17–27.
193. Schaaf, R. C., Toth-Cohen, S., Johnson, S. L., et al. (2011). The everyday routines of families of children with autism: Examining the impact of sensory processing difficulties on the family. *Autism: The International Journal of Research and Practice, 15*(3), 373–389.
194. Schieve, L. A., Blumberg, S. J., Rice, C., et al. (2007). The relationship between autism and parenting stress. *Pediatrics, 119*, 114–121.
195. Schoen, S. A., Miller, L. J., Brett-Green, B. A., et al. (2009). Physiological and behavioral differences in sensory processing: A comparison of children with autism spectrum disorder and sensory modulation disorder. *Frontiers in Integrative Neuroscience, 3*, 1–11.
196. Sivertsen, B., Posserud, M.-B., Gillberg, C., et al. (2012). Sleep problems in children with autism spectrum problems: a longitudinal population-based study. *Autism: The International Journal of Research and Practice, 16*(2), 139–150.
197. Skinner, B. F. (n.d). *A brief survey of operant behavior*. <http://www.bfskinner.org/BFSkinner/SurveyOperantBehavior.html>.
198. Spitzer, S. (2003). With and without words: Exploring occupation in relation to young children with autism. *Journal of Occupational Science, 10*, 67–79.
199. Spreckley, M., & Boyd, R. (2009). Efficacy of applied behavioral intervention in preschool children with autism for improving cognitive, language, and adaptive behavior: A systematic review and meta-analysis. *Journal of Pediatrics, 154*, 338–344.
200. Stackhouse, T. M. (2010). Motor differences in the autism spectrum disorders. In H. Miller Kuhaneck & R. Watling (Eds.), *Autism: A comprehensive occupational therapy approach* (3rd ed., pp. 163–202). Bethesda: AOTA Press.
201. Stein, L. I., Polido, J. C., & Cermak, S. A. (2012). Oral care and sensory concerns in autism. *The American Journal of Occupational Therapy, 66*, e73–e76.
202. Stokes, M., Newton, N., & Kaur, A. (2007). Stalking, and social and romantic functioning among adolescents and adults with autism spectrum disorder. *Journal of Autism and Developmental Disorders, 37*(10), 1969–1986.
203. Stone, W. L., Lemanek, K. L., Fishel, P. T., et al. (1990). Play and imitation skills in the diagnosis of autism in young children. *Pediatrics, 86*, 267–272.
204. Sullivan, A., & Caterino, L. C. (2008). Addressing the sexuality and sex education of individuals with autism spectrum disorders. *Education and Treatment of Children, 31*(3), 381–394.
205. Tarnai, B., & Wolfe, P. S. (2008). Social stories for sexuality education for persons with autism/pervasive developmental disorder. *Sexuality and Disability, 26*(1), 29–36.
206. Taylor, J. L. (2012). Transition to adulthood. *Journal of Autism and Developmental Disorders, 41*(5), 566–574.
207. Taylor, J. L., McPheeters, M. L., Sathe, N. A., et al. (2012a). A systematic review of vocational interventions for young adults with autism spectrum disorders. *Pediatrics, 130*(3), 531–538.
208. Taylor, J. L., Dove, D., Veenstra-VanderWeele, J., et al. (2012b). Interventions for adolescents and young adults with autism. *Comparative Effectiveness Review, AHRQ Publication No. 12-EHC063-EF*, (65), 1–374.
209. Thomas, C. (1960). Medicine: The child is father. *Time* magazine. July 25. Retrieved on April 18, 2009 from <http://www.time.com/time/magazine/article/0,9171,826528,00.html>.
210. Tobing, L. E., & Glenwick, D. S. (2006). Predictors and moderators of psychological distress in mothers of children with pervasive developmental disorders. *Network, 10*(4), 1–23.
211. Tomanik, S., Harris, G. E., & Hawkins, J. (2004). The relationship between behaviours exhibited by children with autism and maternal stress. *Journal of Intellectual & Developmental Disability, 29*, 16–26.
212. Tomchek, S. (2010). Sensory processing in individuals with an autism spectrum disorder. In H. Miller Kuhaneck & R. Watling (Eds.), *Autism: A comprehensive occupational therapy approach* (3rd ed., pp. 135–162). Bethesda, MD: AOTA Press.
213. Tomchek, S. D., & Dunn, W. (2007). Sensory processing in children with and without autism: A comparative study using the Short Sensory Profile. *American Journal of Occupational Therapy, 61*, 190–200.
214. Tseng, M.-H., Fu, C. P., Cermak, S. A., et al. (2011). Emotional and behavioral problems in preschool children with autism: relationship with sensory processing dysfunction. *Research in Autism Spectrum Disorders, 5*(4), 1441–1450.
215. Vanvuchelen, M., Roeyers, H., & Weerdt, W. (2007). Nature of motor imitation problems in school-aged males with autism: How congruent are the error types? *Developmental Medicine and Child Neurology, 49*, 6–12.
216. Vismara, L. A., & Lyons, G. L. (2007). Using perseverative interests to elicit joint attention behaviors in young children with autism: Theoretical and clinical implications for understanding motivation. *Journal of Positive Behavior Interventions, 9*, 214–228.
217. Virues-Ortega, J. (2010). Applied behavior analytic intervention for autism in early childhood: Meta-analysis, meta-regression and dose–response meta-analysis of multiple outcomes. *Child Psychology Review, 30*, 387–399.
218. Watling, R. (2010). Behavioral and educational approaches for teaching skills to children with an autism spectrum disorder. In H. Miller Kuhaneckm & R. Watling (Eds.), *Autism: A comprehensive occupational therapy approach* (3rd ed.). Bethesda, MD: AOTA Press.
219. Watling, R., & Miller Kuhaneck, H. (2010). Emotion regulation in the autism spectrum disorders. In H. Miller Kuhaneck & R. Watling (Eds.), *Autism: A comprehensive occupational therapy approach* (3rd ed.). Bethesda, MD: AOTA Press.
220. Whaley, K. L., & Rubenstein, T. S. (1994). How toddlers "do" friendship: A descriptive analysis of naturally occurring friendship in a group child care setting. *Journal of Social and Personal Relationships*, 383–400. doi:10.1177/0265407594113005.
221. Whitney, R. V., & Miller-Kuhaneck, H. (2012). Diagnostic Statistical Manual 5

changes to the autism diagnostic criteria: A critical moment for occupational therapists. *The Open Journal of Occupational Therapy, 1*(1).

222. Wiggins, L. D., Robins, D. L., Bakeman, R., et al. (2009). Brief report: Sensory abnormalities as distinguishing symptoms of autism spectrum disorders in young children. *Journal of Autism and Developmental Disorders, 39*, 1087–1091.
223. Williams, E. (2003). A comparative review of early forms of object-directed play and parent–infant play in typical infants and young children with autism. *Autism: The International Journal of Research and Practice, 7*, 361–377.
224. Williams, E., Costall, A., & Reddy, V. (1999). Children with autism experience problems with both objects and people. *Journal of Autism and Developmental Disorders, 29*, 367–378.
225. Williams, E., Kendall-Scott, L., & Costall, A. (2005). Parents' experiences of introducing everyday object use to their children with autism. *Autism: The International Journal of Research and Practice, 9*, 521–540.
226. Williams, J. H. G., Whiten, A., & Singh, T. (2004). A systematic review of action imitation in autistic spectrum disorder. *Journal of Autism and Developmental Disorders, 34*, 285–299.
227. Wolery, M., & Garfinkle, A. (2002). Measures in intervention research with young children who have autism. *Journal of Autism and Developmental Disorders, 32*, 463–478.
228. Woodgate, R. L., Ateah, C., & Secco, L. (2008). Living in a world of our own: The experience of parents who have a child with autism. *Qualitative Health Research, 18*(8), 1075–1083.
229. Yang, T., Wolfberg, P. J., Wu, S., et al. (2003). Supporting children on the autism spectrum in peer play at home and school: Piloting the integrated play groups model in Taiwan. *Autism: The International Journal of Research and Practice, 7*, 437–453.
230. Zercher, C., Hunt, P., Schuler, A., et al. (2001). Increasing joint attention, play and language through peer supported play. *Autism: The International Journal of Research and Practice, 5*, 373–398.

CHAPTER

28 Neuromotor: Cerebral Palsy

Patty C. Coker-Bolt • Teressa Garcia • Erin Naber

KEY TERMS

Motor control
Hemiplegia
Quadriplegia
Botulinum toxin therapy
Complementary and alternative medicine
Functional electrical stimulation
Gaming technology
Physical agent modalities
Rehabilitation robotics
Flexible and rigid taping
Adaptive recreation

GUIDING QUESTIONS

1. What are clinical characteristics associated with the different types of cerebral palsy (classification and distribution in body)?
2. How do the primary and secondary impairments associated with cerebral palsy contribute to functional limitations?
3. How are current theories of motor control applied to interventions for children with cerebral palsy?
4. How does impaired muscle tone influence activity and participation in children diagnosed with cerebral palsy?
5. How are rehabilitative and compensatory approaches applied in comprehensive services for children with cerebral palsy?

Introduction

The term *cerebral palsy* (CP) describes a group of developmental motor disorders arising from a nonprogressive lesion or disorder of the brain.[6] Associated damage to one of more areas of the brain may lead to paralysis, spasticity, or abnormal control of movement or posture. Although the injury to the brain is considered static, the pattern of motor impairment changes over time, often affecting development in all daily occupations of childhood.[3,4] The motor disorders associated with cerebral palsy can be accompanied by disturbances of sensation, cognition, communication, and perception and by a seizure disorder.[3,4] The lesion or damage in the brain may cause impairment in muscle activity in all or part of the body. Cerebral palsy typically affects the development of sensory, perceptual, and motor areas of the central nervous system. As a result, the child has difficulty integrating the information that the brain needs to correctly plan and direct movements in the trunk and extremities that are used in everyday interactions with the environment. The muscles are activated in uncoordinated and inefficient ways and are unable to work together to create smooth, effective motion.[4,8]

Prevalence and Etiology of Cerebral Palsy

Cerebral palsy is the most prevalent cause of persistent motor dysfunction in children, with a prevalence of one in 500 births to three in 1000 births.[4,28,39] The prevalence of cerebral palsy has remained stable since the 1950s, although prenatal and perinatal care has improved dramatically over the last 4 decades.[45] Societal costs for persons diagnosed with CP are substantial, and estimates of total lifetime expenditures are estimated as high as $11.5 billion.[11,37] Average lifetime expenditure per child could exceed $900,000 above ordinary costs of raising a child.[11,37]

The diagnosis of CP is approximately 1.5 times more common in males and is higher among non-Hispanic African American children and children from low to middle income families.[32] According to the United Cerebral Palsy (UCP) foundation, approximately 800,000 children and adults in the United States live with one or more symptoms of cerebral palsy.[48] The origin of brain injury may occur during the prenatal, perinatal, or postnatal period, but evidence suggests that 70% to 80% is prenatal in origin.[3,4,28] The nervous system damage that causes CP can occur before or during birth or before a child's second year, the time when myelination of the child's sensory and motor tracts and central nervous system (CNS) structures occurs rapidly.

It is increasingly apparent that CP can result from the interaction of multiple factors, and in many cases, a single cause cannot be identified.[4] Prenatal maternal infection, premature birth, low birth weight, and multiple pregnancies have been associated with cerebral palsy.[28] Prenatal factors may include genetic abnormalities or maternal health factors such as stress, malnutrition, exposure to damaging drugs, and pregnancy-induced hypertension. Some gestational conditions of the mother, such as diabetes, may cause perinatal risks to the developing infant; prematurity and low birth weight significantly increase an infant's chance of acquiring a cerebral palsy diagnosis.[44] Medical problems associated with premature birth may directly or indirectly damage the developing sensorimotor areas of the CNS. In particular, respiratory disorders can cause the premature newborn to experience hypoxemia, which deprives brain cells of the oxygen needed to function and survive. Typical postnatal causes of cerebral palsy include conditions

BOX 28-1 Risk Factors Associated with the Development of Cerebral Palsy

Prenatal
- Genetic disorders
- Maternal health factors (e.g., chronic stress, malnutrition)
- Teratogenic agents (e.g., drugs, chemical exposure, radiation)
- Placental disruption (inability of the placenta to provide the developing fetus oxygen and nutrients)
- Lack of growth factors affecting fetal growth in utero (e.g., hormones, insulin, proteins)
- RH blood type incompatibility between mother and infant

Perinatal
- Prenatal conditions (e.g., toxemia secondary to maternal diabetes)
- Medical problems associated with prematurity (e.g., compromised respiratory and cardiovascular systems, intraventricular hemorrhage [IVH], periventricular leukomalacia [PVL])
- Multiple births
- Low birth weight

Postnatal
- Severe and untreated jaundice shortly after birth
- Infections (e.g., meningitis, encephalitis, chorioamnionitis)
- Alcohol or drug intoxication transferred during breastfeeding
- Hypoxic ischemic encephalopathy (HIE)—prolonged loss of oxygen during the birthing process
- Trauma during birth or shortly after[3,4,28]

that result in significant damage to the developing CNS such as hypoxic ischemia encephalopathy resulting from lack of oxygen to the brain. Postnatal causes include infections or exposure to environmental toxins. Box 28-1 lists risk factors associated with cerebral palsy.

Practice Models to Guide Interventions for Children with Cerebral Palsy

Because children diagnosed with CP have difficulty with postural control and movement against gravity, therapists frequently use *motor control and motor learning concepts* to guide intervention of children with movement disorders. The ability to regulate movement is complex and emerges from the interaction of the child, the task, and the environment. A child generates movement to meet the demands of the task being performed in a specific environment. For example, a child selects specific movements to use a spoon to eat a bowl of soup while sitting at the kitchen table with family. The selected movements are influenced by the child's ability to feel, hold, and manipulate a spoon; the task (e.g., type of soup, size of bowl, type of spoon); and the environment (e.g., how the child is sitting, who is present at the table, environmental sounds). In everyday life, a child performs a variety of functional tasks requiring simple to complex movements. Theories of motor control and motor learning are discussed in more detail in Chapter 7.

Dynamic systems theory poses that movement is complex and multidimensional systems work in coordination to influence functional movement.[30] A good example of this is breathing, which involves linking biomechanical and musculoskeletal systems (muscles in trunk, chest, and back) to respiratory function. The head remains stable because of postural support from the trunk and pelvis, demonstrating a linkage between the function of breathing and the control of head, trunk, and pelvis. This theory suggests that impairments of any one structure (e.g., the hand or shoulder) may have significant impact on multiple systems in the body. For example, a child with CP may have shortening of elbow flexors and loss of range of motion in the ankle. This may influence the child's ability to move his or her body in an efficient manner or generate coordinated complex movement to complete a functional task (e.g., put on a shirt). In addition, dynamic systems theorists hypothesize that functional movement is influenced by psychological, environmental, social, and physical characteristics of the child in the context in which a task occurs.

Several strategic principles of dynamic systems theory include a child's ability to self-organize motor actions through repetition and practice, thus creating new patterns from refinement of motor actions. The child's physical characteristics, activity demands, and environmental factors can influence the child's functional movement. For example, a child with CP may have underlying muscle weakness or abnormal muscle tone that limits his or her ability to sustain movement against gravity.[30] Environmental supports, such as a prone stander, can allow standing. Motor behaviors move through states of stability and instability, especially when a child is learning a new motor action. Periods of instability, or transition states, are when new forms of movement are most likely to occur.[30] Chapter 7 provides an in-depth explanation of dynamic systems theory as it relates to the development of functional performance.

Reflex-hierarchic models hypothesize that motor development is based on central nervous system maturation. Motor development is "wired" in the brain, and an infant's first movements reflect lower level brain centers (i.e., the brainstem) before cortical brain functions mature allowing more controlled movement. Although this theory lacks evidence as a basis for intervention,[40,41] certain therapeutic techniques, such as the Masgutova Neurosensorimotor Reflex Integration (MNRI) method, are based on the reflex-hierarchic theory and are sometimes used for children with cerebral palsy. The MNRI method assumes that motor reflex patterns play a subordinate role in the maturation of more complex motor reflex schemes (e.g., rolling over, sitting up, crawling) and that integrating reflexes can improve functional movement. A recent systematic review of interventions for children with CP concluded that interventions focused on meaningful goal-directed activity results in better outcomes than a focus on performance components (e.g., reflex). This systematic review did not support the use of MNRI.[40,41] Consequently therapists selecting to use this approach should carefully monitor child progress and short-term outcomes to determine benefit. Most often occupational therapists use the tenets of these practice models in combination, dynamically, and tailored to meet individual needs.

Sensorimotor Function in Children with Cerebral Palsy

Posture, Postural Control, and Movement

To understand the functional movement problems that develop in children who have cerebral palsy, the occupational therapy practitioner must be familiar with the ways that people typically control their bodies and execute skilled movements. The term *posture* describes the alignment of the body's parts in relation to each other and the environment. The ability to develop a large repertoire of postures and change them easily during an activity depends on the integration of automatic, involuntary movement actions referred to as the postural mechanism. The postural mechanism includes several strategic components:

- Muscle and postural tone
- Emergence of righting, equilibrium, and protective extension reactions
- Developmental integration of early, primitive reflex movement patterns
- Intentional, voluntary movements against the forces of gravity
- The ability to combine movement patterns in the performance of functional activities

Righting reactions and equilibrium reactions allow individuals to maintain upright posture with dynamic stability. When the head is out of alignment with the body, righting reactions realign the head with the body. An individual uses equilibrium reactions or balance reactions when the body's center of gravity is moved over the base of support. Equilibrium reactions are coordinated responses of trunk, neck, and extremities as the individual moves in and out of different postures. When righting and equilibrium reactions are not sufficient to regain an upright posture, individuals use a protective extension reaction (i.e., they automatically reach outward from their bodies to catch themselves or prevent a fall). A protective response requires the motor ability to quickly extend an extremity (i.e., arm or leg).

Atypical Movement Patterns in Cerebral Palsy

Children who have CP demonstrate difficulty achieving and maintaining stable posture while lying down, sitting, and standing because of impaired patterns of muscle activation.[3,4] Poor postural alignment and stability result from the CNS's decreased ability to control co-activation and reciprocal innervation of select muscle groups. Co-activation of muscle, or simultaneous contraction of agonist and antagonist muscle groups, provides stability around a joint and stability of body posture. Reciprocal innervation in muscle groups occurs when excitatory input directs the agonist muscle to contract while inhibitory input directs the antagonist muscle to remain inactive.[28,44] These reciprocal innervations allow for extremity and trunk movement. Children who have CP may develop abnormal movement compensations and body postures as they try to overcome these motor deficits to function within their environments. Over time, movement compensations and atypical motor patterns create barriers to ongoing motor skill development. Instead of freely moving and exploring the world, as children with a normally developing sensorimotor system do, children who have CP may rely on primitive and automatic reflex movement patterns as their primary means of mobility (Boxes 28-2 and 28-3).[4,5,28]

Muscle tone is the force with which a muscle resists being lengthened; it can also be defined as the muscle's resting stiffness. It is tested by an occupational therapist's passive stretch of the muscle from the shortened to the lengthened state as the occupational therapist feels the resistance offered by the muscle to the stretch. A child's ability to perform sequential movements is supported by muscle tension (stiffness) and elasticity during the movements. Muscles must have sufficient tone to move against gravity in a smooth, coordinated motion. Emotions and mental state, including levels of alertness, fatigue, and excitement, can also influence muscle tone. Normal muscle tone develops along a continuum, with some variability among members of the typical population. The muscle's qualities of contractility and elasticity are necessary for immediate, consistent responses to the elongation and contraction experienced during movement, such as during co-activation. Muscle tone

BOX 28-2 Sensorimotor Problems in Children with Cerebral Palsy

1. Abnormal muscle tone
   - Hypertonicity—increase in resting state of muscle
   - Spasticity—velocity-dependent increase in muscle tone (occurs with active or passive movement)
   - Hypotonicity—decrease in resting state of muscle
   - Fluctuating—muscle tone changes between hypertonic and hypotonic
2. Persistence of atypical and abnormal primitive reflexes
3. Atypical righting, equilibrium, and protective responses
4. Poor sensory processing
   - Decreased processing of vestibular, visual, and proprioceptive information
   - Limited body awareness and body scheme
5. Joint hypermobility or joint stiffness
   - Reduced limb stability and poor co-contraction across joints
   - Reduced joint movement
6. Muscle weakness and poor muscle co-activation
7. Delays in typical progressing of motor movement and motor skills affecting adaptive function

BOX 28-3 Examples of Primary and Secondary Impairments in Children Diagnosed with Cerebral Palsy

Primary Impairments	Secondary Impairments
Muscle weakness or hypotonicity	Contracture in a joint (e.g., elbow, wrist, hip, knee, ankle)
Muscle tightness or hypertonicity	Poor or unsteady gait or mobility
Spasticity	Impairment of visual processing, hearing, or speech
Involuntary movement	Difficulty with bladder and bowel control
Weakness of eye muscles	Intellectual disability, learning disabilities
Abnormal muscle tone in facial musculature	Problems with breathing because of postural difficulties and weakness in trunk muscles
Impaired sensation in affected limbs	Skin integrity—increased risk of pressure sores
Possible seizure disorder	Difficulty in feeding, eating, and swallowing

allows muscles to adapt readily to the changing sensory stimuli during functional activities. Decreased muscle tone, or hypotonia, can make a child appear relaxed and even "floppy." Increased muscle tone, or hypertonia, can make a child appear stiff or rigid. In some cases of CP, an infant may initially appear hypotonic, but the muscle tone may change to hypertonia at 6 or 7 months.[4,5]

Classification and Distribution

Cerebral palsy can be classified by the location of the lesion in the CNS and by distribution of abnormal muscle tone in the trunk and extremities. Involvement of one extremity is commonly referred to a *monoplegia*, upper and lower extremities on one side of the body as *hemiplegia*, both lower extremities as *paraplegia*, all limbs as *quadriplegia*, and all limbs and head/neck as *tetraplegia*. Cerebral palsy is also classified by the nature of the movement disorder according to four main types: (1) spastic, (2) dyskinetic, (3) ataxic, and (4) mixed (Table 28-1).[4,28]

Children with spastic CP demonstrate hypertonia and muscle spasticity. Spasticity is defined as a velocity-dependent resistance to stretch.[38] Resistance to range of motion will either increase with speed of force or will increase with quick movement. The effects of spasticity are often associated with clonus, an extensor plantar response, and persistent primitive reflexes. As a child with spastic CP attempts to move, muscle tone increases and then rapidly releases, triggering a hyperactive stretch reflex in the muscle. Spasticity is associated with poor control of voluntary movement and limited ability to regulate force of movement. Distribution of spasticity can be monoplegia (rare), diplegia, hemiplegia, quadriplegia, or tetraplegia.

In dyskinetic CP, movement patterns are classified as athetoid, choreoathetoid, and dystonic, which generally affect the entire body. A child with dyskinesia exhibits excessive and abnormal movement, and often when initiating movement in one extremity, atypical and unintentional movements in other extremities result. The child with athetosis exhibits slow, writhing, involuntary motor movements in combination with abrupt, irregular, and jerky movements. Children with pure athetosis demonstrate a fluctuation of muscle tone from low to normal with little or no spasticity and poor co-activation of muscle flexors and extensors.

Children with choreoathetosis have constant fluctuations from low to high with jerky involuntary movement that may be seen more proximal to distal. Dystonic movements are sustained twisted postures that are absent at rest and triggered by movement (action). The movements follow a similar pattern, and these repetitive postures support the diagnosis of dystonia (unlike choreoathetosis, in which movement fluctuations are random).

The third type of CP, ataxia, is characterized by poor balance and coordination. Children who have ataxia may show shifts in muscle tone, with quadriplegic distribution, but to a lesser degree than those with dyskinesia. Children with ataxic type CP are more successful in directing voluntary movements but appear clumsy and show involuntary tremor. They have considerable difficulty with balance, coordination, and maintenance of stable alignment of the head, trunk, shoulders, and pelvis. These children may have poorly developed equilibrium responses and lack proximal stability in the trunk to assist with control of hand and leg movements.

Children with CP who often show combinations of high and low muscle tone problems are classified as the mixed type. Those who have spastic CP move their extremities with abrupt hypertonic motions but may also exhibit marked hypotonicity in their trunk muscles. The distribution for mixed type CP is typically quadriplegic.

Hand Skills and Upper Extremity Function

Children with CP demonstrate problems with upper limb function resulting from abnormal muscle tone and decreased ability to maintain a stable posture when attempting functional tasks.[28,29] Efficient performance of the arm and hand depends on proximal control and dynamic stability of the trunk and shoulder girdle. Children with CP demonstrate weakness in the shoulder girdle, may have contractures in their elbow, forearm, wrist, fingers, and thumb caused by hypertonicity, or may move the arm and hand in synergistic patterns, lacking the ability to isolate single joint movements. Postural instability can affect upper extremity movement also, as children with CP may need to use their upper extremity to support upright postures against gravity. When the upper extremity is fixed and used to help stabilize and compensate for trunk weakness, the arm and hand cannot be used for functional tasks (e.g., functional mobility such as pulling self from sit to stand or playing with toys at the midline of the body while challenged to sit unsupported).

Associated Problems and Functional Implications

Children with CP manifest primary impairments that are the direct result of the lesion in the CNS. Primary impairments are those that are an immediate and a direct result of the cortical

TABLE 28-1 Classification of Cerebral Palsy

Type of Movement Disorder	Area of Body Involved	Prevalence
Spastic	Diplegic: legs > arms	32%
	Quadriplegic: all four extremities	24%
	Hemiplegic: one-sided involvement, arm > leg	29%
	Double hemiplegic: both sides; one greater than other, arms > legs	24%
Dyskinetic	Choreoathetoid	14%
	Dystonic	
	Athetosis	
Ataxic		<1%
Mixed (percentages included above)		

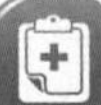

CASE STUDY 28-1 Evaluation and Classification: Ben

Ben is a 9-month-old infant referred for occupational therapy services because of developmental delay. His mother is concerned that he is "not moving like his older brother was at this age." At 9 months, he recently learned to sit independently but has difficulty rolling because of "tightness" in the left arm and leg. The occupational therapist completed a thorough evaluation including formal and informal assessment of body structure and function and developmental skills. She administered the Grasping and Visual Motor Integration subscales of the Peabody Developmental Motor Scales-2 (PDMS-2) and the Alberta Infant Motor Scales (AIMS). On each of the assessments, Ben scored below average when compared with typical age peers. He did not reach and grasp with his left arm and did not bring both hands to midline to play. He did not use both hands to hold a sippy cup and his mother reported difficulty putting on shirts and pants because of tightness in Ben's left arm and leg. During the occupational therapist's clinical observation of Ben's movement during play, she noticed that he exhibited limited control of left arm and leg movement when transitioning out of sitting, rolling, or reaching for objects. He did not use his left arm for protective reactions forward or sideways. She also noticed that his eyes were not aligned and his left eye appeared to drift laterally.

After her evaluation, the occupational therapist discussed the results of her evaluation with the referring pediatric neurologist. The neurologist ordered a magnetic resonance imaging (MRI) test to identify possible central nervous system lesion(s). The results of the MRI revealed that Ben has a lesion affecting the right primary motor cortex and internal capsule, and the neurologist confirmed a diagnosis of spastic left hemiplegic cerebral palsy.

lesion in the brain. Because the lesion occurs in immature brain structures, the progression of the child's motor development may appear to change, causing secondary impairments (see Box 28-3). Normal nervous system maturation shifts control of voluntary movement to cortical brain areas. The child who has CP exhibits some changes in movement ability that result from the expected progression of motor development skills, but these changes tend to be delayed relative to age and often show much less variety than those seen in the typically developing child. See Case Study 28-1.

Children with CP develop secondary impairments in systems or organs over time because of the effects of one or more of the primary impairments.[3,45,46] These secondary impairments may become just as debilitating as the primary impairments. Although the initial brain injury is unchanging, the results or the secondary impairments are not static and change over time with body growth and attempts to move against gravity.[4,8,28] When playing or in functional activities, children with CP move in atypical patterns that may become repetitive and fixed. The repetition of the atypical movement patterns prevents children with CP from gaining full voluntary control of their movements and can lead to diminished strength and musculoskeletal problems. The combination of impaired muscle co-activation and the use of reflexively controlled postures may lead to future contractures in the muscle, tendon, and ligamentous tissues, causing the tissues to become permanently shortened. Soft tissue changes can lead to contractures and possibly bone deformities; they can also cause spinal and joint misalignment.

In addition to the risk for joint contractures and deformities and spinal or joint misalignment, children with CP are at risk for skin breakdown and decreased bone density. Children in wheelchairs, who maintain sitting or lying for extended periods or who cannot independently shift their weight, risk skin breakdown. Children who are most vulnerable may sit with their body weight pressure on body prominences for prolonged time periods. Children in wheelchairs also experience decreased time standing or ambulating, negatively influencing the strength of the individual's bones. Children diagnosed with CP may have decreased bone mineral density and are vulnerable to pathologic fractures.[35] Occupational therapy practitioners provide opportunities for children with CP to maintain upright positions and bear weight in a variety of positions. This can be accomplished by providing children with adapted seating, such as specialized seats, prone or supine standers, and toys that promote weight bearing (e.g., scooters).

Children with CP may experience additional problems such as seizures and other medical conditions not directly related to the child's movement disorder. When postural muscles are weak, breathing can be compromised. Abnormal posture and weak muscle activity may compromise cardiac and respiratory functions and prevent these systems from working efficiently. The resulting low endurance and fatigue can influence the child's capacity for activity. The occupational therapy practitioner monitors each child's physical endurance and plans therapeutic goals to increase strength and endurance.

Cognition and Language

Because CP is caused by a focal brain lesion, language and cognition may or may not be affected, depending on which areas of the brain are affected (e.g., frontal lobe, temporal lobe). Lesions affecting the frontal lobe may affect the child's cognitive abilities, including attention, organization, problem solving, inhibition, and judgment. Lesions affecting both the primary motor and temporal lobes may affect language and speech development. Because speech requires complex movements of oral/facial structure and requires control of breathing, children and adults diagnosed with CP may have various problems with speech and language. These potential problems include decreased speech production, poor articulation, and decreased speech intelligibility. *Dysarthria* is the term used to describe a disorder of speech production secondary to decreased muscle coordination, paralysis, or weakness.

In addition to speech production disorders, children who have cerebral palsy may have changes in the quality of their voice resulting from decreased strength or control of respiratory and postural muscles. Because CP has the potential to affect areas of the brain outside of the motor system, children who have CP can have decreased expressive and receptive language skills. This means they have difficulty processing language-based information or producing responses. All of

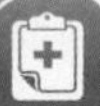

CASE STUDY 28-2 Assistive Technology to Aid Communication: Antoine

Antoine is an 8-year-old boy with a history of a seizure disorder and athetoid cerebral palsy. He uses a power wheelchair for all mobility and an augmentative communication device for communication. He attends elementary school, where he is placed in an age-appropriate classroom with accommodations and related services, including physical therapy, occupational therapy, speech-language therapy, and assistive technology. Antoine's continuous body movements make it difficult for him to complete fine motor tasks, including accessing his communication device to communicate with his teacher and friends. He gets frustrated when he knows the answer to a question but cannot communicate it to his teacher and classmates in a timely manner. He has difficulty with fine motor tasks and it takes additional time for him to complete classwork.

Antoine's therapy team discovers that a head stick helps to improve his access to his communication device and that using his head, versus his hand, is a faster and more efficient way for him to access his communication device and a word processing program on the computer. The occupational therapist worked with his art teacher to fasten a holder for tools such as a paintbrush to his head stick. Now Antoine is able to creatively express himself through a variety of media, including paint and pastels, which do not require a lot of pressure when drawing. Antoine also seems to have improved success in using the device when he grasps the armrest of his wheelchair, so his occupational therapist tries mounting a bar on his tray for him to push into to improve his trunk stability.

these potential impairments can have a significant impact on the child's participation in age-appropriate activities with peers, understanding of and response to directions, making his or her needs known, and managing his or her own care. A child's cognitive and linguistic skill level is considered when developing goals and potential outcomes (Case Study 28-2).

Sensory Functions

Children with CP may have visual or sensory impairments. Visual impairments such as blindness, uncoordinated eye movements, and eye muscle weakness affect as many as 50% of children who have CP. Children who have more severe CP are more likely to have visual impairment.[27] Regardless of the functional level of a child, vision should always be taken into consideration during fine motor tasks, play, and activities of daily living completion. Vision plays an important role in timing of grasp and release, manipulating objects, orienting materials, making eye contact, and finding needed items. Children with visual impairments may use postural adaptations, such as a head tilt or changes to the angle of gaze, to compensate for visual deficits. These deficits may be oculomotor in nature, meaning their eye muscles do not move smoothly or in sync or may move involuntarily. The term *strabismus* refers to the eyes not being aligned because of muscle imbalance. Functionally, strabismus may cause difficulty with attending to visual tasks. The child may have decreased convergence or divergence, decreased depth perception, or double vision. Other terms describing misalignment of the eyes include exotropia (one eye drifts temporally), esotropia (one eye drifts nasally), hypertropia (one eye drifts upward), and hypotropia (one eye drifts downward). *Nystagmus* refers to the eyes constantly moving in a repetitive and uncontrolled way. Functional issues associated with nystagmus include reduced acuity, difficulty fixating on a target to maintain balance, reduced target accuracy when reaching or grasping, compensatory head movements, or posturing to compensate for visual deficit.

In addition to oculomotor impairments, children may have deficits in the way the brain processes visual information. Without proper processing, a child may not understand the spatial relationships among objects, be missing part of the visual field, or not identify a partially hidden item, such as his or her coat in a closet.

Auditory reception and processing deficits have an impact on 25% of individuals with CP.[28] Hearing loss with both conductive hearing loss and sensorineural hearing impairments may occur if a child has been affected by a congenital nervous system infection.

Both vision and hearing should be tested regularly for children with CP.

Children with CP may have difficulty processing tactile and proprioceptive information (e.g., fingertip force regulation during object manipulation).[23] Children with CP may also demonstrate tactile hypersensitivities (e.g., overreacting to touch, textures, and changes in head position), causing some children to become visibly upset when handled or moved by others. When children have multiple sensory processing problems, they may have difficulty understanding and responding to the social and physical elements of their environments. Oral tactile sensitivity may be associated with abnormal oral movement patterns. Children may have aversion to certain food textures, causing disorganized oral motor control and problems coordinating chewing, sucking, and swallowing. Those with severe problems in this area may be surgically fitted with a percutaneous endoscopic gastrostomy (PEG) tube for feeding. Occupational therapy practitioners must consider a child's sensory limitations and strengths when setting intervention goals. The practitioner considers which sensory experiences are likely to improve occupational performance.

Assessment

Clinical observation of the child's occupational performance provides the occupational practitioner with data on factors influencing the child's muscle tone, reflex activity, gross and fine motor skills, sensory systems, cognition, perception, and psychosocial development. Clinical assessment data create a "picture" of the child's functioning and indicate his or her strengths and weaknesses. Observation of a child completing simple tasks such as putting on a shirt, transitioning from a

TABLE 28-2 Selected Upper Limb Assessments for Body Structure, Function, and Activity for Children with Cerebral Palsy

Assessment	Age	Domain and Activities
Melbourne Assessment of Unilateral Upper Limb Function (MUUL)[16,42]	5-15 years	Assessment of impairment and activity limitations in the upper extremity. Examiner administers 16 items that involve reach, grasp, release, and manipulation. Each item is scored according to specific criteria to rate quality of range of motion, accuracy, fluency, and dexterity, yielding a maximum possible raw score of 122.
Quality of Upper Extremity Skills Test (QUEST)[21,47]	2-13 years	A criterion-referenced observational assessment measuring 34 items in four domains (dissociated movement, grasp, weight bearing, and protective extension). Scores from each domain are summed and converted to a percentage score.
Jebson Taylor Test of Hand Function (JTTHF)[19]	6-17 years	A clinical evaluation of speed and dexterity of upper limb tasks. The seven timed subtests vary in complexity and use everyday objects to assess how a child uses grasp and release in daily tasks.

TABLE 28-3 Selected Participation and Quality of Life Measures for Children with Cerebral Palsy

Outcome Measure	Age	Domains and Relevant Items
Cerebral Palsy Quality of Life (CP QOL)—Child[49]	4-12 years Parent report; Child report 9-12 years	66 items 1. Social well-being and acceptance 2. Participation and physical health 3. Functioning 4. Emotional well-being 5. Pain and impact of disability 6. Access to services 7. Family Self-report: 53 items
Cerebral Palsy Quality of Life (CP QOL)—Teen[19]	12-18 years Child report	72 items 1. Well-being and participation 2. Communication and physical health 3. School well-being 4. Social well-being 5. Access to services 6. Family health 7. Feelings about functioning

chair to the floor, opening containers, or playing with age-appropriate toys helps the occupational therapist identify atypical postures and movements that may be limiting functional abilities. Early identification and intervention of atypical postures may minimize the use of compensatory and dysfunctional movements, which could lead to secondary impairments and decreased functional abilities for children with CP. During therapy sessions, the occupational therapist facilitates mature and typical movement patterns to promote progress in typical developmental milestones.

Thorough assessment data are essential when working as part of a service delivery team. Selection of assessment measures may be based on several factors, including the child's age, setting (e.g., home health, school system, community), and the caregiver's and child's specific concerns about functional limitations. Table 28-2 provides information on specific classification systems and assessments commonly used for children diagnosed with CP. Two assessments are designed specifically to measure quality of life and overall participation in children with CP (Table 28-3). Functional classification systems include the Gross Motor Function Classification System (GMFCS) and the Manual Ability Classification System for Children with Cerebral Palsy (MACS) (Tables 28-4 and 28-5).

The occupational therapy practitioner uses assessment information, including parent concerns and priorities, to formulate goals that match the child's needs, developmental performance, and potential outcomes. Examples include increasing a child's ability to participate in a classroom writing activity and teaching family members adaptive techniques so that they can bathe or feed a child with greater ease. Goals for the adolescent might address accessing public transportation or learning ways to perform homemaking skills. See Box 28-4 for sample goals.

Occupational Therapy Interventions

The occupational therapy practitioner plans and implements interventions to promote function and independence in children with CP. Practitioners may work one-on-one with the

TABLE 28-4 Gross Motor Function Classification System

Level	Description of Functional Abilities
Level I	Walks without limitations. Performs gross motor skills like running and jumping but speed, balance, and coordination may be impaired.
Level II	Walks with limitations. This includes on uneven surface, inclines, stairs, long distances, or in crowds or confined spaces.
Level III	Walks using a hand-held mobility device. Walks on even surfaces, indoors and outdoors with an assistive device. Children may use manual wheelchair for long distances.
Level IV	Self-mobility with limitations. Child may use powered mobility or require assistance from a caregiver. May walk short distances with a mobility device but relies primarily on wheeled mobility.
Level V	Transported in a manual wheelchair. Child has no means of independent mobility and relies on caregiver for all transportation needs.

From Palisano, R., Rosenbaum, P., Walter, S., Russell, D., Wood, E., & Galuppi, B. (1997). Development and reliability of a system to classify gross motor function in children with cerebral palsy. *Developmental Medicine & Child Neurology, 39*, 214–223.

TABLE 28-5 Manual Ability Classification System

Level	Description of Functional Abilities
Level I	Handles objects easily and successfully. At most times, handles objects with both hands. The child may have limitations in the ease of performing manual tasks requiring speed and accuracy. However, any limitations in manual abilities do not restrict independence in daily activities.
Level II	Handles most objects but with somewhat reduced quality and/or speed of achievement. The child may avoid certain activities or the activity will be achieved with some difficulty. The child develops ways of performing some manual activities that do not usually restrict independence in daily activities.
Level III	Handles objects with difficulty; needs help to prepare and/or modify activities. The child's performance is slow and achieved with limited success regarding quality and quantity. The child cannot perform certain activities and his or her degree of independence is related to the supportiveness of the environmental context. Activities are performed independently if they have been set up or adapted.
Level IV	Handles a limited selection of easily managed objects in adapted situations. The child performs parts of activities with effort and with limited success. Requires continuous support and assistance and/or adapted equipment, for even partial achievement of the activity.
Level V	Does not handle objects and has severely limited ability to perform even simple actions. Requires total assistance.

From Eliasson, A. C., Krumlinde Sundholm, L., Rösblad, B., Beckung, E., Arner, M., Öhrvall, A. M., et al. (2006). The Manual Ability Classification System (MACS) for children with cerebral palsy: Scale development and evidence of validity and reliability. *Developmental Medicine and Child Neurology, 48*, 549–554.

BOX 28-4 Sample Occupational Therapy Goals

Self-care	Child will don pullover shirt with minimal assistance, 100% trials. Child will use adaptive spoon to eat soft solid foods with modified independence.
Play	Child will show improved postural control to engage in 15-minute play activity while sitting unsupported at table with minimal physical support from occupational therapist.
Recreation	Child will successfully participate on an adaptive community sports team with same-aged peers, per parent's report.
Fine motor	Child will write first name from memory with no errors, 80% of trials. Child will isolate right index finger to successfully access games on iPad, 4 out of 5 trials.

child, lead groups of children with similar goals, or take a consultative role in assisting caregivers with problem-solving adaptive tools and strategies to encourage the child's independence. They can work with children in a variety of settings, including school, home, and the community. A recent comprehensive review of interventions used with children with CP[40] found the following interventions to be supported by current evidence, including adaptive equipment training, casting and orthotics, constraint-induced movement therapy, functional and goal-directed therapy, and bimanual training. These interventions, as well as an overview of additional interventions that occupational therapists may select to address the functional goals for children with CP, are provided in this section. The use of specific practice models is highlighted.

Adaptive Equipment Training

A variety of adaptive devices and equipment can assist a child with CP to complete activities of daily living (ADLs), instrumental activities of daily living (IADLs), play, and educational tasks. These devices serve to modify or control some of the

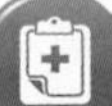

CASE STUDY 28-3 Feeding and Adaptive Equipment: Brian

Brian is an 11-year-old boy who was born at 35 weeks' gestation by emergency cesarean section. He was had global developmental delays with hypotonia and was diagnosed with quadriplegic cerebral palsy and neurodevelopmental disability.

He quickly becomes fatigued during self-feeding, and requires assistance with spoon feeding to obtain adequate nutrition. His mother reports that she often feeds him at home so he is able to eat much more quickly. She reports that he is easily distracted when eating.

During an occupational therapy assessment, Brian grasped a toddler spoon with large handle as well as a bent-handled spoon with large handle. He switched hand dominance, but performed best when using his left hand. He required moderate to maximum assistance to scoop thick foods from a scoop bowl and minimal assist to transport foods to his mouth without spilling.

Brian required repeated tactile and verbal cues to close his lips around the spoon and use his top lip to clear the spoon. He prefers to "dump" food into his mouth. He exhibited tongue thrust movements to move food laterally and posteriorly for swallowing. No coughing or choking was observed.

Brian used a straw to drink thin liquids from a juice box, but he had difficulty creating a tight seal with his lips and lost small amounts of liquid when drinking. The occupational therapist suggested an adapted straw with a larger opening to make it easier for him to drink.

Brian made gains in his ability to clear the spoon with his top lip when he was given assistance to stabilize his lower jaw and verbal cues to use his top lip to clear the spoon. He made improvements in his ability to move food from the bowl to his mouth without spilling. See Chapter 14 for additional information on feeding interventions.

degrees of freedom required for children to engage in daily activities. The occupational therapist selects a device that matches the child's motor needs while simultaneously considering his or her sensory functioning (including vision, auditory, and sensation), the environment in which it will be used, and the child's position when using it (standing, sitting, or in his or her wheelchair or bed). Other considerations are the child or family's ability to transport the adaptive equipment, the set up needed to use it, and the ease of cleaning the device.

The occupational therapist may work with interdisciplinary team members when determining the child's needs. For example when selecting a communication device for a child with quadriplegic CP and cortical visual impairment, an occupational therapist may work with a low vision therapist and speech-language pathologist to select the most appropriate device and determine the most efficient way to access the device and the optimal position to mount the device for ease of visual scanning. The occupational therapist may recommend adaptive utensils during mealtime to compensate for limited grasping patterns or nonskid material to control the child's plate on the tabletop. Dressing tasks can also be modified to optimize the child's safety, efficiency, and independence.

A large zipper pull on jeans or pants may be recommended for a child with diplegic CP and limited fine motor coordination (Case Study 28-3). The occupational therapist practitioner should become familiar with a diverse group of assistive devices so that equipment recommendations consider all occupational performance concerns and the family's financial resources. It is also common for occupational therapists to fabricate assistive devices from common household materials or splinting materials (Case Study 28-4; Figure 28-1).

Casting, Orthotics, and Splinting

Splinting or casting can be used to improve hand function, prevent joint contracture, improve hygiene, or relieve pain in a specific joint. Splinting may also be used to reduce unsafe behaviors in a child with self-injurious behaviors. Splints and orthotics can support the arm in a functional position to improve performance in activities of daily living (see Chapter 29). Serial static splints and casts are designed to lengthen tissues and correct deformity through application of gentle forces sustained for extended periods of time with the goal of reducing tightness or spasticity in a selected muscle group. Splints are remolded and casts replaced at intervals that allowed for the muscle tissue to respond to the lengthened position. The biomechanical effects of splinting and casting relate to changes in the length of muscle and connective tissues, which can reverse the effects that occur when a muscle is maintained in a shortened position. Splinting to lengthen tight and contracted muscles in children with CP is best if applied continuously for periods greater than 6 hours.[50] Casting has additional biomechanical and neurophysiologic effects, although the exact neurophysiologic effects of casting on spasticity are not well defined at this time. It is theorized that inhibition of muscle contractions allowing lengthening of muscle tissue results from decreased cutaneous sensory input from muscle receptors during the period of immobilization. The effects of neutral warmth and circumferential contact also are believed to contribute to modification of spasticity (Figure 28-2).[32]

Splints can also be used to meet the goals of the child or parent. For example, a splint may be fabricated to isolate a child's index finger to access a touch screen device or communication system. Splints have been used to compensate for hand deformities preventing the ability to grasp eating or writing utensils. Splints may also be used to aid in the ability to drive a power wheelchair such as a wrist support that allows a child to access the joystick control. Temporary splints are also fabricated by therapists to prevent movement from the hand to the mouth when children exhibit self-injurious behaviors or attempt to pull out feeding tubes, intravenous lines, or tracheostomy tubing. A systematic review of splint use in children with CP reported that splinting when combined with an active therapy program[32] can have positive effects on function. The use of splinting alone without use of other complementary interventions does not have evidence of efficacy. When an occupational therapist determines that a child would benefit from wearing an orthosis or cast, he or she needs to educate parents as to the purpose and goals for the orthosis, provide instructions for donning, doffing, and cleaning, and

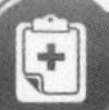

CASE STUDY 28-4 Adaptive Equipment to Improve Self-Care Skills: Nathan

Nathan is a 14-year-old boy with spastic quadriplegic cerebral palsy and normal cognition. He uses a power wheelchair. His posture is poor and he has impaired righting equilibrium and protective responses. He requires a chest strap and lateral supports on his wheelchair to assist with postural alignment and upright seating in his chair. His dynamic unsupported sitting balance is poor and his static sitting balance on the edge of his bed is fair but requires close supervision. Fine motor skills are significantly impaired with limited grip strength; his left hand is more affected than his right. Nathan has not received occupational therapy services since he was 10 years old when he and his family decided to take a break from services and explore adaptive recreational activities and aquatic therapy. Recently (at 14) he requested to return to services to become more independent in self-care. His family also recently purchased a computer tablet for him and he is interested in finding applications that will help him control his environment. At his initial evaluation the occupational therapist conducted the Canadian Occupational Performance Measure (COPM)[33] with Nathan. He identified his most important occupational performance problems as doffing his shoes, completing simple meal preparation, turning on his bedroom lights, and completing written work for school assignments. During the evaluation the occupational therapist determined that his power wheelchair was the safest place for him to complete ADLs since it offered him the best postural support.

Occupational Therapy Goals

1. While sitting with trunk supported and using adapted equipment, Nathan will successfully doff shoes within 1 minute.
2. Nathan will follow four-step instructions to prepare a simple meal with intermittent verbal cueing by the therapist.
3. Using a tablet programmed for environmental control placed on his power wheelchair, Nathan will successfully turn lights on in rooms at home, 100% of trials.
4. Nathan will dictate all appropriate school reports using adaptive word processing program with supervision and set up only.

Over the course of his 12-week admission, the occupational therapist tried and evaluated various adaptive equipment training. To increase independence in lower extremity dressing, Nathan attempted to use a reacher and long-handled shoe horn with good success. By the end of the 12 weeks, Nathan successfully unstrapped his foot supports, untied his shoes, and, using a long-handled shoe horn, doffed them. He continued to require assistance with doffing his ankle foot orthoses (AFOs) but was making progress toward independence with the strategies and adaptive equipment provided by his therapist.

To address simple meal preparation activities, the occupational therapist suggested use of an adapted cutting board that secured food and use of a rocker knife. Positioning his chair to the side of the counter to retrieve materials with his stronger arm was also beneficial. With a consult from an assistive technology specialist Nathan and the occupational therapist explored tablet applications for environmental control and found one that controlled the lights, his television, and his DVD player. The occupational therapist fabricated a mount with a Loc-Line modular hose system that allowed him to easily reposition his computer tablet or push it out of the way when not in use. The assistive technology specialist also recommended text-to-speech software and agreed that the most effective position for him to dictate school reports was in his chair, where he had the best breath support. Nathan worked with the occupational therapist to learn how to use the software and his speech-language pathologist was consulted for strategies to improve his articulation. At the end of the 12 weeks the occupational therapist reassessed his progress through structured observation and re-administered the COPM. Nathan reported improved performance and satisfaction with his performance on all the performance goals identified at admission, with the greatest change noted on meal preparation tasks. Because of his progress the occupational therapist reduced visits to one-time monthly consultative sessions for the next 6 months.

determine an optimal wearing schedule that fits the family's routines.

Constraint-Induced Movement Therapy

Constraint-induced movement therapy (CIMT) is an evidence-based intervention for children with hemiplegia that targets the functional use of the child's affected upper extremity through engagement in intensive practice, shaping and grading of targeted movements, and restricting use of the unaffected, stronger upper extremity. Children with hemiplegia often show "developmental disregard"[20]; that is, they learn to ignore the involved arm because it is inefficient. Therefore use of the involved arm is negatively reinforced despite the function that may be available. The goal of CIMT is to reverse this effect. Constraint-induced movement therapy developed out of basic experimental psychology research by Edward Taub and his colleagues on sensory contributions to motor learning in primates.[43] Constraint-induced movement therapy was initially used in the rehabilitation of patients post stroke and then developed as an intervention for children. Multiple case reports, cohort studies, and randomized control trials have reported the effectiveness of this intervention technique.[1,7,10-13,31]

Current implementation of CIMT varies, but all programs have three essential features: (1) some method of constraint of use of the unimpaired upper extremity; (2) intensive, repetitive practice of motor activities, for up to 6 hours per day, for 2 to 4 weeks; and (3) shaping of more complex, functional motor acts by identifying the component movements of a targeted task and rewarding actions that are successive approximations to the task. The literature reports a variety of constraining devices and wearing schedules, including mitts, casts, splints,

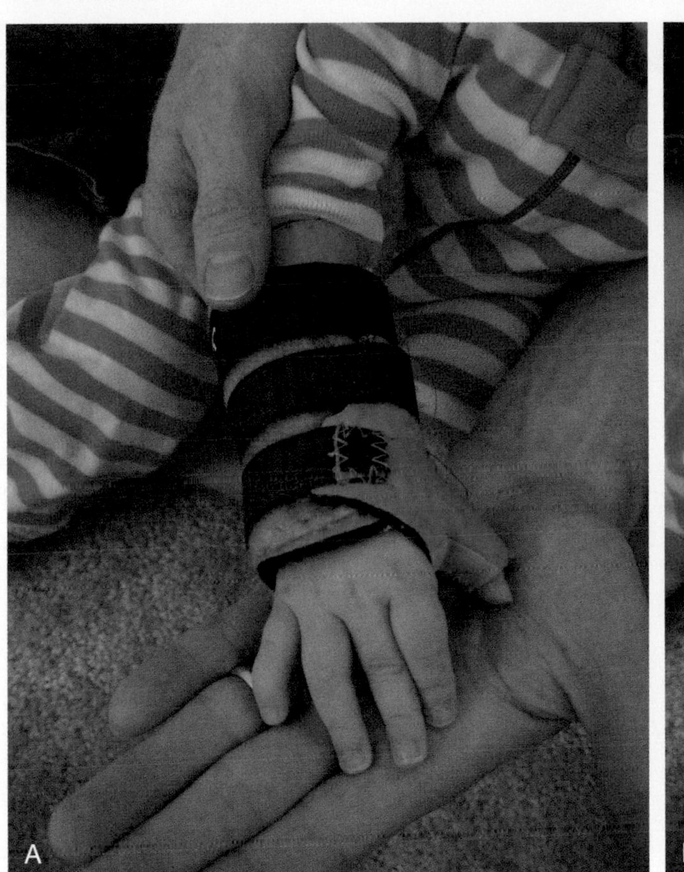

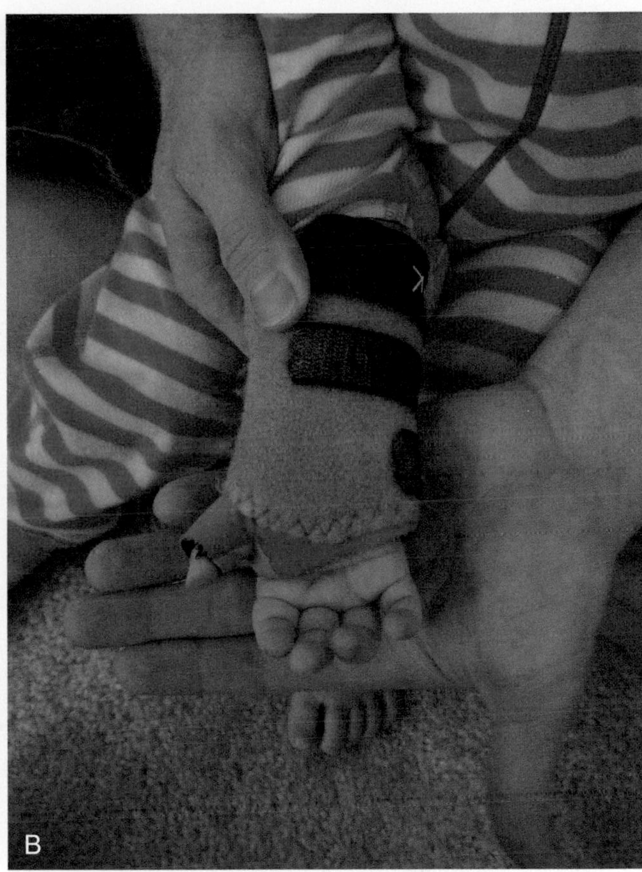

FIGURE 28-1 Example of a pre-fabricated wrist and thumb support with thermoplastic insert for a child with hemiplegia. (Photos courtesy of Kennedy Krieger Institute.)

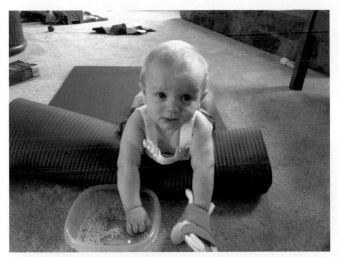

FIGURE 28-2 An example of sensory exploration during modified CIMT.

and slings. Use of constraining devices may be intermittent and they may be removed at certain times of the day or after massed practice trials are completed, or they may be applied continuously, allowing for practice and generalization of skills throughout the child's day for a set period of time.[7,31]

Constraint-induced movement therapy can be defined as either a signature CIMT or modified CIMT (m-CIMT). A signature CIMT approach has five essential components, including (1) constraint of the unaffected upper limb, (2) a high dosage of repetitive task practice (3 to 6 hours of therapy per day over several consecutive days), (3) the use of shaping techniques, (4) therapy provided in a natural setting, and (5) a transition or post-CIMT program to maintain gains acquired during CIMT program.[43] A typical signature approach provides massed practice and shaping of more mature motor movement for at least 2 consecutive weeks (14 to 21 days, dosage equal to 42 to 128 hours) by a professional with an understanding of rehabilitation techniques to improve motor function (Case Study 28-5).

Modified constraint-induced movement therapy (m-CIMT) is defined as constraint of the stronger or less affected upper limb combined with less than 3 hours per day of therapy. Most of the five essential elements of the signature approach are provided, but with modifications, including variation in where the therapy is provided (e.g., clinic or camp versus individual treatment at home) or a variation in the dosage of therapy (e.g., less concentrated, may be more distributed over several days or weeks).[43] Massed practice may be provided by a professional with training in CIMT, but not necessarily an occupational or physical therapist[14,15] (e.g., parent, daycare worker, camp counselor). Unlike occupational therapists in adult settings, pediatric therapists using CIMT embed repetitive task practice in daily functional and play activities (Figures 28-3 and 28-4).[14,15] Research questions remain about appropriate dosage, optimal age for treatment initiation, and optimal repeat intervention intervals.[43]

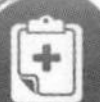

CASE STUDY 28-5 Constraint-Induced Movement Therapy: Logan

Logan is a 3½-year-old boy with hemiplegic cerebral palsy. Until he was 3 years old he received home-based services through an early intervention program. When he turned 3, he began outpatient occupational therapy services once a week. Logan's goals included increased arm strength such that he maintains a quadruped position for a minute, full arm extension to push his arm through his shirt sleeve, and pulling up his pants with both hands. Another goal is to grasp toys with his right hand and carry toys with both hands.

Occupational Therapy Goals

1. Logan will show improved upper extremity strength to play in a quadruped position for up to 10 minutes with no physical cue required from the therapist.
2. Logan will be able to push both arms through sleeves of long sleeve shirt with minimal assistance from therapist or caregiver, 100% of trials.
3. Logan will pull pants up from knees to waist after toileting with minimal assistance from therapist or caregiver, 80% of trials.

Logan participated in a constraint-induced movement therapy program at an outpatient clinic. Logan attended a program for 3 hours a day and wore a continuous cast on his unaffected, stronger arm. Activities that are motivating such as carrying a bucket loaded with balls and picking up cars and putting them on a race track are done at a high level of repetition. Imaginary play activities, such as pushing his affected arm through dress-up clothes, help him generalize these new skills to play and ADL tasks.

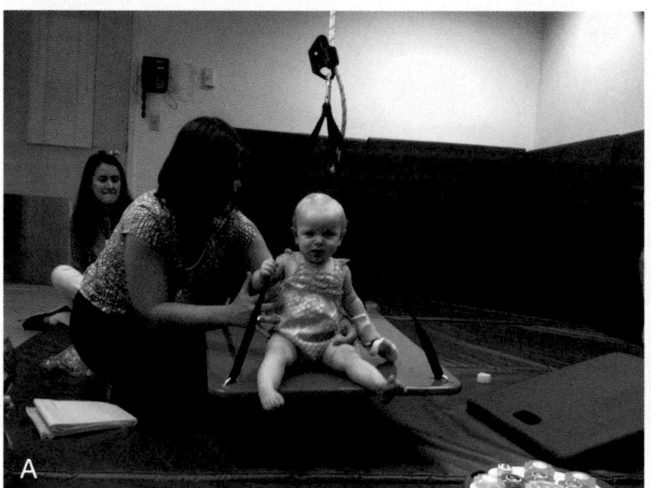

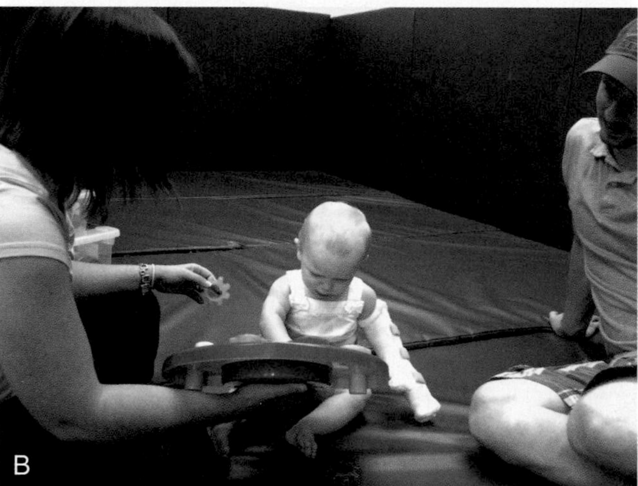

FIGURE 28-3 Example of motor based activities during modified CIMT.

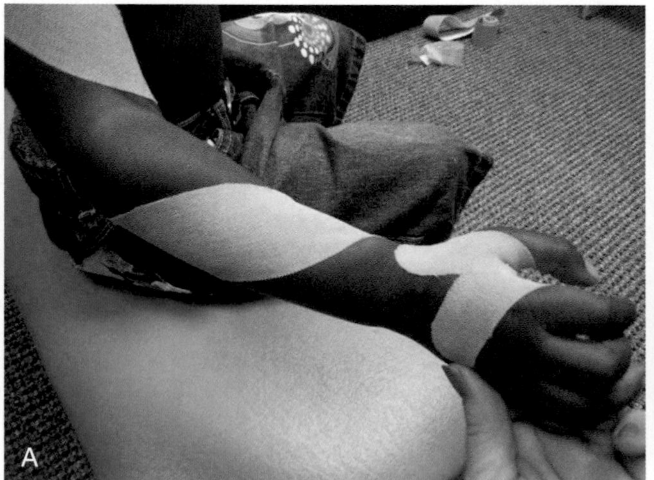

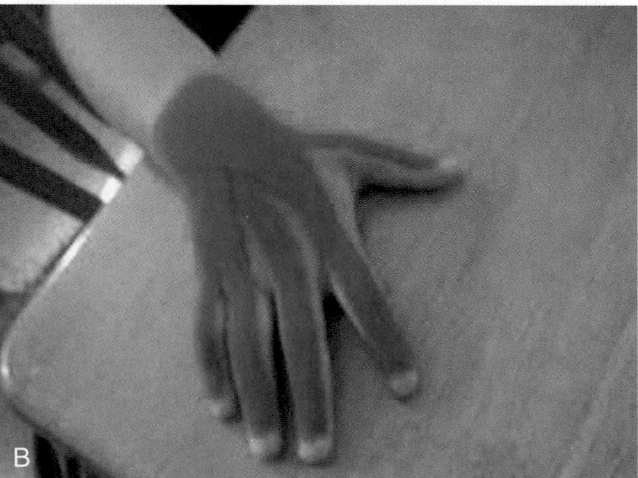

FIGURE 28-4 Two examples of kinesiology tape to improve thumb abduction needed for grasp and release. (Photos courtesy of Patty Coker-Bolt.)

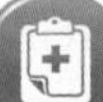

CASE STUDY 28-6 Functional Electrical Stimulation: Ava

Ava is a 17-year-old girl with hemiplegic cerebral palsy affecting her left side. Ava is learning to drive and has worked with a driver rehabilitation specialist to adapt her mini-van. As training progressed, Ava reported that she had difficulty opening the car door with her left hand when holding her backpack or her textbooks in her right hand. The occupational therapist developed a strengthening program for Ava's left hand grip and an electrical stimulation program for her left wrist extensors. Ava's electrical stimulation device was pre-programmed with the help of the therapist. During the intervention session, Ava took a photo with her camera phone of electrode placement on her left forearm. During occupational therapy, Ava demonstrated placing the pads in a correct location and collaborates with the occupational therapist to develop a list of activities to complete during electrical stimulation, which was 4 days per week for 20 minutes at home. Activities include playing games on a touch screen tablet positioned on a vertical surface, waxing her car, yoga positions in prone, and writing on a vertical surface.

Physical Agent Modalities

Various modalities target increasing muscle length and strength and reducing spasticity in children with CP to improve a child's functioning in play, ADLs, IADLs, and academics. These intervention modalities include electrical stimulation and hot/cold therapy. Heat maybe used in conjunction with a stretching program to improve muscle length and reduce pain. Electrical stimulation can be used to strengthen antagonist muscles, re-educate muscles, target pain reduction, improve coordination, increase range of motion, and reduce spasticity (Case Study 28-6).[6,51] Electrical stimulation is most effective when used with a functional activity, such as combing hair when stimulating the biceps or releasing toys into a container while stimulating wrist extensors. Use of neuromuscular electrical stimulation when applied with intensity can improve upper limb range of motion and strength, especially when paired with dynamic splinting.[51] Occupational therapy practitioners should defer to their state regulatory boards regarding guidelines for application and training requirements for using physical agent modalities (PAMs). Some states may require a physician prescription before administration. Risk for burns is an important consideration, and contraindications such as cancer apply. Practitioners should complete advanced training in physical agent modality application before using PAMs.

Therapeutic Taping and Strapping

Two types of therapeutic tape are used in rehabilitation. Therapists use ***rigid tape*** to limit movement around a joint or to protect a joint during functional movement, while flexible, elastic ***kinesiology tape*** is used to facilitate improved movement patterns.[52]

Kinesiology tape is applied directly to a child's skin and works by increasing stimulation to cutaneous mechanoreceptors that facilitate muscle contraction or inhibition (Figure 28-5). The elastic properties of the tape can also be used to reposition joints to a more appropriate alignment. Four major functions of kinesiology tape are to (1) support a weakened muscle, (2) improve circulation, (3) reduce pain, and (4) improve joint alignment.[52] Published evidence to support or refute the use of taping interventions is minimal at best and is often reported in small case studies or cohort studies without controls.[17,52] A recent case study reported significant improvements on sit-to-stand performance of a child with CP after application of elastic tape to lower extremity muscles.[17] Another

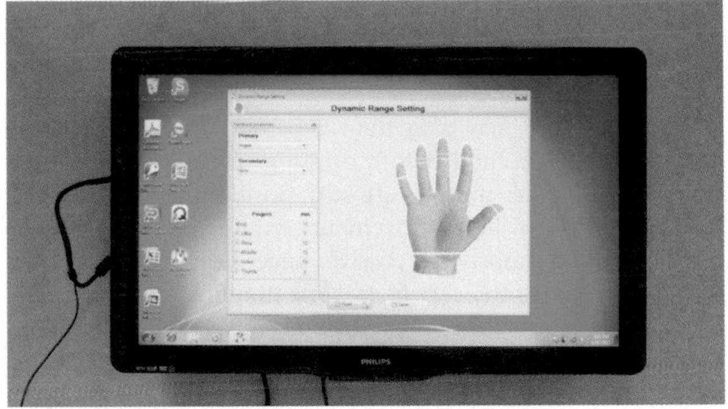

FIGURE 28-5 A screen shot of robotic device software.

report by Footer[26] examining rigid taping techniques found no improvements in postural control in a sample of 18 children with quadriplegic CP. Because of potential skin sensitivities in children, it is always important before taping a full joint, to apply a small "test" strip to the child's skin to check for negative reactions to the properties of the tape. Advanced training in kinesiology and rigid taping applications is available through continuing education courses.

Positioning, Handling, and Neurodevelopmental Treatment

Occupational therapy practitioners often employ neurodevelopmental treatment (NDT) techniques of therapeutic positioning and handling to assist children with CP to optimize their independence with functional tasks. Occupational therapists determine the safest and most efficient positioning and handling techniques to facilitate completion of ADLs and IADLs. They recommend and select wheelchairs, standers, activity chairs, commode or bath chairs, and side-lyers to aid in completing play and ADL tasks. The occupational therapist makes recommendations for positioning, seating, and mobility in collaboration with interdisciplinary team members from rehabilitation engineering, speech-language pathology, and physical therapy depending on the complexity of the child and his or her needs. For example, an occupational therapist may suggest a reclined bath chair with a seat belt to support a child with quadriplegic CP and poor head control during bathing. A school therapist may suggest a slant board and foot support to improve posture during writing tasks for a child with hemiplegic CP.

In addition to positioning in preparation for tasks, therapeutic handling can affect a child's tone throughout the body to assist with efficient muscle activation for movement. As a preparatory technique, handling techniques such as imposed rotational movement patterns, slow rocking, and bouncing facilitate or inhibit the child's muscle tone and enhance arousal level. Often children with CP have poor body awareness and a limited ability to anticipate postural changes required for movement or anticipatory control.[30] Facilitated weight bearing and weight shifting can build strength, improve co-contraction, and improve postural symmetry and alignment in children with CP. For example, an occupational therapist working with a child who tends to move in an extensor pattern may facilitate sustained flexion of the trunk and slow trunk rotation in sitting and knee flexion in quadruped in preparation for sitting in a chair for mealtime.

A practitioner may also train a parent to complete these activities with the child before dressing. If the child has high tone and his or her muscles are stiff, positioning and handling techniques may facilitate movements required for dressing and self-care tasks. Improved passive knee flexion reduces the burden of care on the caregiver while donning a child's pants. Evidence to support this intervention is mixed as recent studies have not been able to isolate the effect of treatment to this intervention.[9] Neurodevelopmental treatment research shows conflicting findings and results are difficult to interpret because researchers used a variety of outcome measures; few studies were randomized; and samples included participants with a wide range of functional abilities.[9,40]

Community Recreation

Children and teens with disabilities are at risk for limited participation in recreational and leisure activities,[8] and youths with physical disabilities experience two to three times the activity limitations that are experienced by children with other chronic conditions.[39] In addition, children with disabilities are more restricted in their participation compared with their peers. Their leisure activities tend to be limited; they attend fewer social engagements and spend less time in quiet recreation than their typically developing peers.[46] Children with disabilities tend to be involved with more informal versus formal recreation activities and participate less in physical and skill-based activities.[33,34] Occupational therapy practitioners can assist children with CP in accessing adaptive recreation options. Children's recreation and leisure participation can be divided into formal activities (e.g., structured activities with rules and often a leader) and informal activities (e.g., child-initiated, unstructured activities).[34] Occupational therapists can assist in identifying preferred formal and informal leisure and recreational activities for children with CP and also can assist in the modification of specific activities to meet the needs of the child both at home and in the community. For example, an occupational therapist may suggest the use of a tee stand for a child with hemiplegia to participate on a softball team with his or her peers or may provide a universal cuff to allow a child to participate in playing a video game at home. Occupational therapists may also guide families to appropriate community organizations that provide recreational activities for children with disabilities.

Complementary and Alternative Medicine

The National Center for Complementary and Alternative Medicine defines *complementary and alternative medicine* (CAM) as "a group of diverse medical and health care systems, practices, and products that are not generally considered part of conventional medicine."[38] Conventional medicine is practiced by holders of M.D. (medical doctor) or D.O. (Doctor of Osteopathic Medicine) degrees and by their allied health professionals such as physical therapists, psychologists, and registered nurses. Over the past several years, the use of CAM approaches, including yoga, has become more popular. According to the 2007 National Health Interview Survey, which gathered information on CAM use among more than 9000 children aged 17 and under, nearly 12% of the children had used some form of CAM during the past 12 months. The top five most commonly used forms of CAM therapy included natural products, chiropractic and osteopathy, yoga, and homeopathic treatments. Majnemer and colleagues[36] reported that 25% of the 166 adolescents with CP surveyed in their study currently use or had used some form of CAM. The most popular of these was massage. Some occupational therapy practitioners with training in these methods or advance certifications may use CAM to help children with CP engage in leisure activities to improve overall quality of life. Ultimately occupational therapists are responsible for the safety of their patients and use their clinical judgment and the best available evidence to determine use of these intervention techniques to complement service delivery.[2] Complementary and alternative medicine approaches commonly used by occupational therapists include guided imagery, myofascial release, yoga, and meditation.[2]

Robotics and Commercially Available Gaming Systems

Robotics is an emerging technology to enhance motor and cognitive performance in children diagnosed with CP. These devices typically employ robotic arms, joysticks, or other controllers to measure the patient's performance on the targeted movement. Early studies demonstrate that children using robotic devices in therapy sessions are motivated and make positive gains.[24,25] *Rehabilitation robotics* is the use of robotic devices to restore or improve function for a person with a disability. Robotics can be part of a prosthetic, used as an assistive device for some functional task, or used therapeutically to achieve a high level of repetition of movement patterns. Therapeutic robotics may be used to achieve massed practice during a therapy program. Because most devices have settings that progress and challenge movement patterns and strength, the occupational therapist can select the level of challenge most appropriate for the child.

Robotic devices range from large stationary devices with both gross and fine motor components to glove-based systems with small sensors (see Figures 28-6 and 28-7 for examples of different devices). Most robotic devices are connected to a computer so that the child can receive feedback from the game graphics on a screen or monitor (see Figure 28-6). Figure 28-7

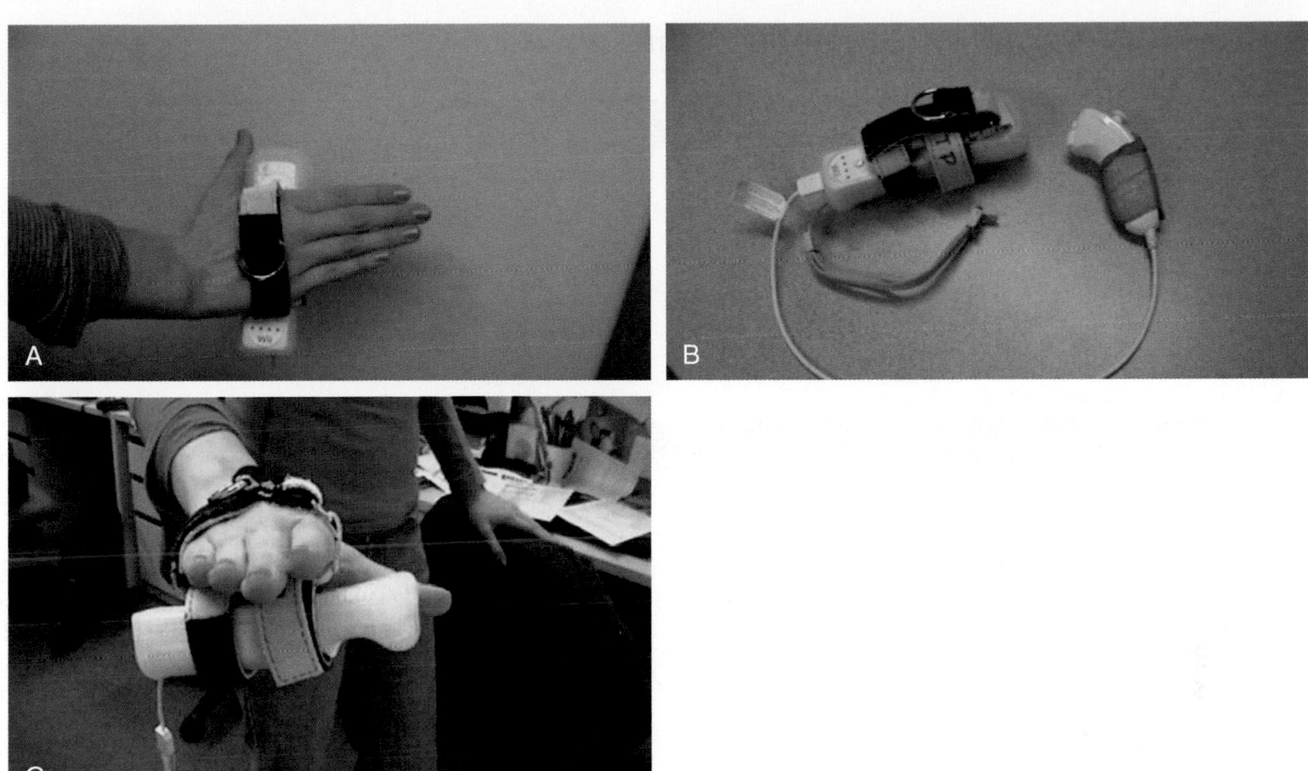

FIGURE 28-6 **A-C,** Examples of adaptive cuff and Coban grip adaptation on commercially available gaming technology. (Photo courtesy of Kennedy Krieger Institute.)

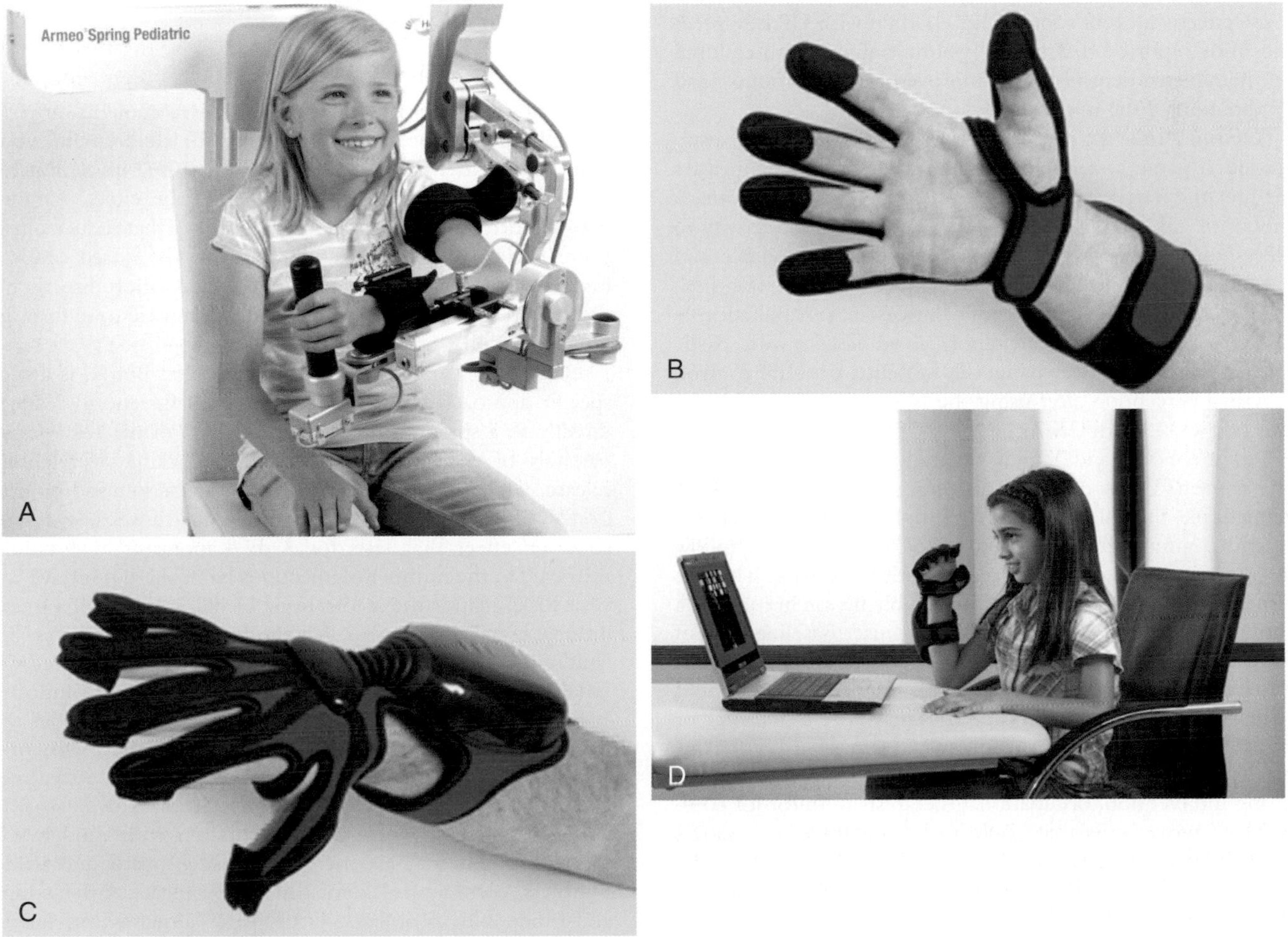

FIGURE 28-7 **A,** Armeo® Spring Exoskeleton with integrated spring mechanism. (Photo A courtesy of Hocoma, Ag, Volketswil, Switzerland.) **B-D,** Handtutor™ by Meditouch. (Photo courtesy of Meditouch, Netanya, Israel.)

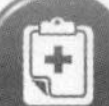

CASE STUDY 28-7 Gaming Technology: Aiden

Aiden is a 7-year-old boy with diplegic cerebral palsy. He walks with Lofstrand crutches and is working on simple snack making and lower body dressing sitting on the side of his bed. His family has a Wii gaming system at home. Although he has some trouble keeping up with his brother during outdoor play, they are evenly matched when playing these games at home. His occupational therapist develops adaptations to the Wii and makes it part of his home exercise program. With these adaptations, the Wii offers Aiden a recreational activity that also promotes arm and hand coordination and strength (see Figure 28-7).

CASE STUDY 28-8 Medical Interventions and Orthotics: Chloe

Chloe is a 10-year-old girl with spastic quadriplegic cerebral palsy and cognitive delay. Chloe has limited finger extension and significant wrist flexion contracture. Her mother reported that she recently had difficulty thoroughly washing Chloe's hands, especially her left palm. A stretching home program was trialed for 6 weeks with no changes in Chloe's functional ability to open her hand. After discussing intervention options with the physiatrist and occupational therapist, Chloe's mother agreed to botulinum neurotoxin injections to Chloe's thenar eminence and wrist flexors in conjunction with serial splinting for 2 hours during the day and all night splint wear for the next 12 weeks. Two weeks after the injection her mother noticed a significant change in the muscle tone of her left hand. Her hand was more relaxed, making it easier for her mother to open her hand for hygiene tasks and to don her splints. In addition to splinting, the therapist recommended activities to encourage hand opening, such as movement to songs that required hand opening, releasing a ball into a container, and tossing a ball to her service dog.

shows adaptations that allow children with limited hand function to use a robot arm or access gaming technology. Research on the effectiveness of robotics for children with CP is limited. One study reported that use of robotic training with children with hemiplegia demonstrated improved range of motion and coordination of the upper limb.[22]

Gaming technology refers to the use of commercially available video game systems in the clinical environment in ways that are integrated with planned therapy. In recent years, a number of gaming devices that require gross motor activity to successfully operate have become commercially available and are quickly being incorporated into clinical rehabilitation programs. Research on use of these devices in rehabilitation is limited to case reports. In one report, an adolescent with spastic diplegia showed positive changes in mobility, postural control, and visual perception after using the Nintendo Wii for 11 sessions (see Case Study 28-7).

Use of robotics and gaming technology should be selected with caution. When choosing a device or gaming system, an occupational therapist considers multiple factors. The child's age and cognitive ability suggest his or her capacity to follow directions and play games associated with the device. The size of the child's arm and hand may prohibit his or her use of a robotic device that was created for adult use. Baseline level of motor function helps determine the level of additional support or adaptations a device may require for the participant to hold the device. Visual perceptual capacities may pose a challenge or add additional frustration to game play. Games with high contrast or solid backgrounds may be easier for the child to see. During intervention, occupational therapists monitor for compensatory movements that could cause repetitive use injuries and provide breaks at regular intervals. The occupational therapist is responsible for monitoring muscle fatigue and providing the appropriate challenge based on the child's performance. Robotics, virtual reality, and commercially available gaming systems may complement an occupational therapy plan of care because they motivate the child and provide additional opportunities for massed practice.

Medical Based Interventions

Physicians may prescribe pharmaceutics, recommend surgeries, or apply specific medical interventions for children and youth with CP. Medical interventions are often used in conjunction with occupational therapy to maximize the effect. Children with spasticity may benefit from medications that reduce muscle tone. Baclofen is a medication that may be dosed orally or injected into a pump that delivers the medication directly into the cerebrospinal fluid. Baclofen reduces muscle tone throughout the person's body.

Botulinum neurotoxin, commonly called Botox, is a more specific approach to reducing tone, with injections delivered directly to a spastic muscle. The injection of the toxin causes paralysis of the targeted muscle by blocking acetylcholine release, which is necessary for muscle activation and contraction.[18,40] Botulinum injections typically take a week to demonstrate an effect that lasts for 3 to 4 months.[18,40] A child is restricted in the number of injections he or she can receive each year. Risks include the medication "bleeding" into other muscle groups, especially in areas like the hand and thumb in which children's muscle bellies are small. Injections can be paired with serial casting or splinting to maximize gains in range of motion. Evidence for the use of these injections is limited, and, as with many interventions, this technique is often paired with other techniques, making it difficult to conclude that the treatment effect is only from the injections (Case Study 28-8).

Over time and with growth, children with moderate to severe spasticity may experience increasing muscle and tendon tightness, contractures, joint dislocation (particularly at hips), and other joint problems. Orthopedic surgeries can help to ameliorate these issues when more conservative treatment such as splinting is not effective. Surgeries include tendon transfers, muscle releases, and osteotomies. In tendon transfer surgery, the insertion of a muscle is moved to change the action the muscle produces. For example, a child with weak or paralyzed hand musculature may have a wrist muscle moved to the finger flexors to assist with grasp. Other types of soft tissue surgery include muscle releases or lengthening. These procedures lengthen or release tight muscle tissue to allow increased movement of a joint. Often done in conjunction with soft tissue surgery, osteotomies are procedures in which the bone is lengthened or shortened to improve its alignment. All of these surgeries involve a period of immobilization initially, followed by early movement and occupational therapy to strengthen and promote the function made possible by the structural changes (Case Study 28-9).

CASE STUDY 28-9 Lower Extremity Tendon Transfer Surgery: Owen

Owen is a 7½-year-old boy with hemiplegic cerebral palsy and age-appropriate cognition. Owen was born at 27 weeks' gestation and had a grade 4 intraventricular hemorrhage. A magnetic resonance image revealed periventricular leukomalacia. Owen has right-sided weakness and spasticity. Recently Owen demonstrated increased tightening of his right lower extremity muscles and a leg length discrepancy with his right leg shorter than his left. Owen's balance was negatively affected by this shortening, and, subsequently, he was experiencing more trips and falls. At school Owen's occupational therapist and physical therapist noticed increased difficulty managing stairs, keeping up with his peers when walking to and from assemblies, and safely transferring in the bathroom. Owen's occupational therapist discussed adaptations with his teacher, recommending that he move his seat closer to the door and white board to decrease the length of the classroom he had to traverse and letting him leave early to walk to assemblies with a partner peer to minimize his risk of falls. After receiving training from the school occupational therapist, a classroom aide began supervising him for safety in the bathroom and provided contact guard assist as needed during toilet transfers.

His outpatient occupational therapy goals focused on bimanual coordination for fastener completion. His outpatient occupational therapist recommended that Owen position himself in long sitting on the floor against a wall while he played preferred video games at night or while doing his occupational therapy home exercise program to encourage lengthening of his hamstrings. During intervention sessions, she engaged Owen in dynamic yoga poses (such as the downward facing dog pose) that encouraged upper extremity weight bearing with hamstring and lower extremity extension. Despite these interventions and adaptations, with each growth spurt, Owen continued to experience tightening of his hamstrings and heel cords.

Occupational Therapy Goals

1. Owen will use two hands to fasten four (½-in) buttons on shirt, 80% of trials.
2. Owen will use two hands to fasten zipper on jacket, 100% of trials.

After consultation with the physiatrist and orthopedist, his family and medical team decided he would undergo right hamstring and heel cord lengthening surgery. After 2 days in the local children's hospital where the surgery was performed, Owen was transferred to a pediatric inpatient rehabilitation hospital where he received occupational therapy 3 times per week and physical therapy 6 times per week. Owen received medical orders to bear weight as tolerated on his right lower extremity. He wore a knee immobilizer on the right side; his foot and ankle were casted for 4 weeks after the surgery. His occupational therapy goals included transferring to the toilet with distant supervision, standing and performing ADLs sinkside with distant supervision, and donning his pants with supervision and adaptive equipment as needed. During occupational therapy sessions, the occupational therapist developed strategies for him to dress and bathe himself while he wore the cast and knee immobilizer. He continued to work on right upper extremity weight-bearing activities and well as fine motor activities in long sitting and standing. During physical therapy sessions he worked on sitting and standing balance, gait training, and stairs. After 2 weeks at inpatient rehabilitation, he returned home, where he received home-based occupational therapy and physical therapy services one time per week. The occupational therapist worked with Owen's caregivers to help transfer him into and out of the bathtub safely and trained them in the use of a tub bench. The practitioner worked with Owen to retrieve his clothes from his dresser and closet safely and efficiently while using a walker. The occupational therapist helped Owen prepare a simple snack at his kitchen counter to work on functional balance and practice adaptive strategies such as safely moving ingredients across counter surfaces. A home teacher provided by his school district visited two times per week to review his missed school work.

After his cast was removed, Owen returned to outpatient occupational therapy one time per week and received outpatient physical therapy three times per week. In addition to his previous goals to improve his hand skills for fastener completion, his outpatient occupational therapist added the goals of donning his new ankle foot orthosis (AFO) independently and completing all ADLs and IADLs independently while standing.

Occupational Therapy Goals

1. Owen will don elastic waist pants using adaptive equipment and modified independence, 100% of trials.
2. Owen will don AFOs independently within 2 minutes, 100% of trials.

After 4 weeks of outpatient therapy, Owen demonstrated improved standing balance and performed all ADLs and transfers safely and independently. With support of the special educator, he completed most of his missed schoolwork. With permission from his parents, the outpatient occupational therapist discussed the progress he made with the school-based therapists. Owen continued with outpatient physical therapy for the next 6 weeks in after-school sessions to work on his gait pattern. He was discharged from outpatient occupational therapy with a home exercise program.

Summary

Cerebral palsy is a condition that encompasses a group of postural control and movement disorders associated with pre-, peri-, or postnatal neurologic impairment. Occupational therapists play a vital role in helping children who have CP increase their occupational performance, functional independence, and participation in home, school, and community activities. Grounded in an understanding of motor control theory and motor skill development, occupational therapists apply positioning and handling methods to improve children's function and interaction with the environment. Occupational therapy interventions include techniques to develop postural control, righting and equilibrium reactions, and improve controlled arm and hand movement in functional daily activities. Occupational therapists can recommend and instruct children and their families in the use of assistive devices and specialized equipment to enable children with CP to engage in purposeful activities that match their occupational roles and interests.

Summary Points

- Cerebral palsy is a disorder of movement and posture associated with impairments in motor and sensory systems. Occupational therapists should consider the dynamic interplay among these systems, the impact of the environment, and the demands of the task when evaluating and providing occupational therapy intervention.
- The Gross Motor Function Classification System (GMFCS) and the Manual Ability Classification Scale (MACS) are assessments designed to quantify the level of motor function in children with CP.
- A thorough assessment of a child with CP includes both clinical observation during engagement in functional tasks (e.g., dressing) and evaluation using scales that quantify limitations in movement, activity function, and overall participation.
- Current evidence suggests that functional and goal-directed training, constraint-induced movement therapy, bimanual training, fitness training, home exercise programs, and occupational therapy following botulinum toxin injections are effective occupational therapy interventions for children with CP.[40]
- Positioning, casting, and orthotic programs help to minimize muscle tone's adverse effects on joint alignment.
- An occupational therapist may work in conjunction with several medical specialists, including a physical therapist, speech-language pathologist, neurologist, orthopedist, or physiatrist, to provide complementary intervention after a surgical or medical procedure.

REFERENCES

1. Aarts, P. B., Jongerius, P. H., Geerdink, Y. A., et al. (2010). Effectiveness of modified constraint-induced movement therapy in children with unilateral spastic cerebral palsy: a randomized controlled trial. *Neurorehabilitation and Neural Repair*, *24*(6), 509–518.
2. AOTA. (2005). *Complementary and alternative medicine (CAM) position paper*, *59*(6).
3. Batshaw, M. L. (2007). *Children with disabilities* (6th ed.). Baltimore: Paul H. Brookes.
4. Bax, M., Goldstein, M., Rosenbaum, P., et al. (2005). Proposed definition and classification of cerebral palsy. *Developmental Medicine and Child Neurology*, *47*, 571–576.
5. Benini, R., & Shevell, M. (2012). Updates in the treatment of spasticity associated with cerebral palsy. *Current Treatment Options in Neurology*, *14*(6), 650–659.
6. Bracciano, A. G. (2008). *Physical agent modalities: Theory and application for the occupational therapist* (2nd ed.). Thorofare, NJ: Slack.
7. Brady, K., & Garcia, T. (2009). Constraint induced movement therapy: Pediatric applications. *Developmental Disabilities Research Review*, *15*, 102–111.
8. Brown, M., & Gordon, W. A. (1987). Impact of impairment on activity patterns in children. *Archives of Physical Medicine and Rehabilitation*, *68*, 828–832.
9. Brown, G. T., & Burns, S. A. (2001). The efficacy of neurodevelopmental treatment in paediatrics: A systematic review. *The British Journal of Occupational Therapy*, *64*(5), 235–244.
10. Case-Smith, J., DeLuca, S. C., Stevenson, R., et al. (2012). Multicenter randomized controlled trial of pediatric constraint-induced movement therapy: 6-month follow-up. *American Journal of Occupational Therapy*, *66*(1), 15–23.
11. Centers for Disease Control. (2003). Economic costs associated with mental retardation, cerebral palsy, hearing loss, and vision impairment—United States, 2003. *Morbidity and Mortality Weekly Report*, *53*(3), 57–59.
12. Charles, J., & Gordon, A. M. (2005). A critical review of constraint-induced movement therapy and forced use in children with hemiplegia. *Neural Plasticity*, *12*, 245–261.
13. Coker, P., Karakostas, T., Dodds, C., et al. (2010). Gait characteristics of children with hemiplegic cerebral palsy before and after modified constraint-induced movement therapy. *Disability and Rehabilitation*, *32*(5), 402–408.
14. Coker, P., Lebkicker, C., & Harris, L. (2009). The effects of constraint-induced movement therapy for a child less than one year of age. *Neurorehabilitation*, *24*, 199–208.
15. Cope, S. M., Forst, H. C., Bibis, D., et al. (2008). Modified constraint-induced movement therapy for a 12-month-old child with hemiplegia: A case report. *American Journal of Occupational Therapy*, *62*, 430–437.
16. Cusick, A., Vasquez, M., Knowles, L., et al. (2005). Effect of rater training on reliability of Melbourne Assessment of Unilateral Upper Limb Function scores. *Developmental Medicine & Child Neurology*, *47*(1), 39–45.
17. Da Costa, C. S. N., Rodrigues, F. S., Leal, F. M., et al. (2013). Pilot study: Investigating the effects of kinesio taping on functional activities in children with cerebral pals. *Developmental Neurorehabilitation*, *16*(2), 121–128.
18. Dahan-Oliel, N., Kasaai, B., Montpetit, K., et al. (2012). Effectiveness and safety of botulinum toxin type a in children with musculoskeletal conditions: What is the current state of evidence? *International Journal of Pediatrics, 2012*, 1–16. Article ID 898924, 16 pages <http://dx.doi.org/10.1155/2012/898924>.
19. Davis Sears, E., & Chung, K. C. (2010). Validity and responsiveness of the Jebsen-Taylor hand function test. *Journal of Hand Surgery*, *35*(1), 30–37.
20. Deluca, S. C., Echols, K., Law, C. R., et al. (2006). Intensive pediatric constraint-induced therapy for children with cerebral palsy: Randomized,

controlled, crossover trial. *Journal of Child Neurology, 21*, 931–938.

21. DeMatteo, C., Law, M., Russell, D., et al. (1992). *QUEST: Quality of Upper Extremity Skills test manual.* Hamilton, Ontario: Neurodevelopmental Research Unit, Chedoke Campus, Chedokee-McMasters Hospital.
22. Eliasson, A. C., Bonnier, B., & Krumlinde-Sundholm, L. (2003). Clinical experience of constraint induced movement therapy in adolescents with hemiplegic cerebral palsy: A day camp model. *Developmental Medicine and Child Neurology, 45*, 357–360.
23. Eliasson, A. C., & Gordon, A. M. (2000). Impaired force coordination during object release in children with hemiplegic cerebral palsy. *Dev Med Child Neurol, 42*(4), 228–234.
24. Fasoli, S. E., Fragala-Pinkham, M., Hughes, R., et al. (2008). Upper limb robotic therapy for children with hemiplegia. *American Journal of Physical Medicine and Rehabilitation, 87*, 929–936.
25. Frascarelli, F., Masia, L., DiRosa, G., et al. (2009). The impact of robotic rehabilitation in children with acquired or congenital movement disorders. *European Journal of Physical and Rehabilitation Medicine, 45*, 135–141.
26. Footer, C. (2006). The effects of therapeutic taping on gross motor function in children with cerebral palsy. *Pediatric Physical Therapy, 18*, 245–252.
27. Ghasia, F., Brunstrom, J., Gordon, M., et al. (2008). Frequency and severity of visual sensory and motor deficits in children with cerebral palsy: Gross Motor Function Classification Scale. *Investigative Ophthalmology & Visual Science, 49*(2), 572–580.
28. Green, L., & Hurvitz, E. (2007). Cerebral palsy. *Physical Medicine and Rehabilitation Clinics in North America, 18*, 859–882.
29. Henderson, A., & Pehoski, C. (2006). *Hand function in the child* (2nd ed.). St. Louis: Mosby Elsevier.
30. Howle, J. (2002). *Neuro-developmental treatment approach: Theoretical foundations and principles of clinical practice.* Laguna Beach, CA: NDTA. Shumway-Cook, A., & Woolacott, M. (2012). *Motor control: Theory and practical applications.* Baltimore: Lippincott Williams & Wilkins.
31. Huang, H. H., Fetters, L., Hale, J., et al. (2009). Bound for success: A systematic review of constraint-induced movement therapy in children with cerebral palsy supports improved arm and hand use. *Physical Therapy, 89*(11), 1126–1141.
32. Jackman, M., Novak, I., & Lannin, N. (2013). Effectiveness of hand splints in children with cerebral palsy: A systematic review with meta-analysis. *Developmental Medicine & Child Neurology*, 1–10.
33. Law, M., Baptiste, S., Carswell, A., et al. (2005). *The Canadian Occupational Performance Measure* (4th ed.). Ottawa: Canadian Association of Occupational Therapists.
34. Law, M., King, G., King, S., et al. (2006). Patterns of participation in recreational and leisure activities among children with complex physical disabilities. *Developmental Medicine & Child Neurology, 48*, 337–342.
35. Leet, A. I., Mesfin, A., Pichard, C., et al. (2006). Fractures in children with cerebral palsy. *Journal of Pediatric Orthopaedics, 26*, 624–627.
36. Majnemer, A., Shikako-Thomas, K., Shevell, M., et al. (2013). Pursuit of complementary and alternative medicine treatments in adolescents with cerebral palsy. *Journal of Child Neurology.* Published online May 10, 2013.
37. McLellan, A., Cipparone, C., Giancola, D., et al. (2012). Medical and surgical procedures experienced by young children with cerebral palsy. *Pediatric Physical Therapy, 24*(3), 268–277.
38. National Institutes of Health National Center for Complementary and Alternative Medicine (10/13/2009). *Backgrounder: CAM use and children.* Retrieved 11/1/09, from: <http://nccam.nih.gov/health/children/#patterns>.
39. Newacheck, P. W., & Halfon, N. (1998). Prevalence and impact of disabling chronic conditions in childhood. *American Journal of Public Health, 88*, 610–617.
40. Novak, I., McIntyre, S., Morgan, C., et al. (2013). A systematic review of interventions for children with cerebral palsy: State of evidence. *Developmental Medicine and Child Neurology, 55*(10), 885–910.
41. Pilecki, W., Masgutova, S., Kowalewska, J., et al. (2012). The impact of rehabilitation carried out using the Masgutova Neurosensorimotor Reflex Integration method in children with cerebral palsy on the results of brain stem auditory potential examinations. *Advances in Clinical Experimental Medicine, 21*(3), 363–371.
42. Randall, M., Johnson, I., & Reddihough, D. (1999). *The Melbourne Assessment of Unilateral Upper Limb Function: Test administration manual.* Melbourne: Royal Children's Hospital.
43. Ramey, S., Coker-Bolt, P., & DeLuca, S. (2013). *A handbook of Pediatric Constraint-Induced Movement Therapy: A guide for occupational therapy and health care clinicians, researchers, and educators.* Bethesda, MD: American Occupational Therapy Association Press.
44. Shumway-Cook, A., & Woollacott, M. (2001). *Motor control theory and practical applications* (2nd ed.). Baltimore: Lippincott Williams & Wilkins.
45. Strauss, D., Shavelle, R., Rosenbloon, L., et al. (2007). Survival in cerebral palsy in the last 20 years: Signs of improvement? *Developmental Medicine & Child Neurology, 49*, 86–92.
46. Stevenson, C. J., Pharoah, P. O., & Stevenson, R. (1997). Cerebral palsy: The transition from youth to adulthood. *Developmental Medicine and Child Neurology, 39*, 336–342.
47. Thorley, M., Lannin, N., Cusick, A., et al. (2012). Reliability of the Quality of Upper Extremity Skills Test for children with cerebral palsy aged 2-12 years. *Physical and Occupational Therapy in Pediatrics, 32*(1), 4–21.
48. United Cerebral Palsy Cerebral Palsy Prevalence. Retrieved on July 31, 2013 from: <http://www.ucp.org/uploads/media_items/cerebral-palsy-fact-sheet.original.pdf>.
49. Waters, E., Davis, E., Boyd, R., et al. (2013). *Cerebral Palsy Quality of Life Questionnaire for Children (CP QOL-Child) Manual.* Melbourne: University of Melbourne. Retrieved on July 31, 2013, from: <http://mccaugheycentre.unimelb.edu.au/_data/assets/pdf_file/0003/712371/CPQOL_child_manual.pdf>.
50. Wilton, J. (2003). Casting, splinting, and physical and occupational therapy of hand deformity and dysfunction in cerebral palsy. *Hand Clinics, 19*, 573–584.
51. Wright, P., Durham, S., Ewins, D., et al. (2012). Neuromuscular electrical stimulation for children with cerebral palsy: A review. *Archives of Disease in Childhood, 97*, 364–371.
52. Yasukawa, A., Patel, P., & Sisung, C. (2006). Pilot study: Investigating the effects of Kinesio Taping in an acute pediatric rehabilitation setting. *American Journal of Occupational Therapy, 60*, 104–110.

CHAPTER

29 Pediatric Hand Therapy

Jenny Dorich • Karen Harpster

KEY TERMS

Activity modifications
Congenital differences
Cryotherapy
Desensitization
Dynamic splints
Energy conservation technique
Joint protection strategies
Joint tightness
Kinesiology tape
Mirror therapy
Physical agent modalities
Sensory re-education
Serial cast
Static progressive splints
Tendon tightness

GUIDING QUESTIONS

1. How do occupational therapists who specialize in pediatric hand therapy apply occupational therapy frames of reference to evaluation and intervention?
2. How do the assessment and evaluations used by occupational therapists in a pediatric hand therapy setting guide intervention planning?
3. What are the common diagnoses and associated impairments treated by pediatric hand therapists?
4. What interventions do occupational therapists implement with children who have upper extremity impairment?
5. How do occupational therapists in pediatric hand therapy apply interventions to achieve desired clinical outcomes?

The American Society of Hand Therapists (ASHT) defines the scope of hand therapy as "the art and science of rehabilitation of the upper limb, which includes the hand, wrist, elbow and shoulder girdle."[22] Hand therapy is a specialty area of practice for occupational therapists working in the pediatric setting. Occupational therapists who specialize in hand therapy have the combined knowledge of upper extremity development as well as the specialty skills of a hand therapist. Therapists are integral members of multidisciplinary care teams that include hand surgeons, nurses, physician assistants, and cast technicians. In some cases social workers, psychologists, or other medical specialists may also be members of the care team. Team members work closely together to coordinate and provide care to maximize a child's upper extremity function.

Occupational therapists specializing in pediatric hand therapy provide services to three broad categories of conditions in children and youth:

1. Congenital differences of the hand or arm
2. Upper extremity impairments resulting from an underlying disorder (e.g., cerebral palsy [CP] or rheumatoid arthritis)
3. Injuries of the arm or hand

Each type of upper extremity condition requires different considerations in designing and delivering an intervention plan as described in this chapter. In the sections that follow, assessment tools and methods, common diagnoses, and general intervention considerations for these diagnoses are explained. Conceptual frameworks, principles, and interventions with examples to illustrate intervention applications are presented.

Assessment

The International Classification of Functioning, Disability and Health (ICF)[42,106] guides the therapist's assessment of upper extremity function. The ICF defines and classifies body functions and structure, activity, and participation, incorporating contextual factors including personal and environmental factors. Occupational therapists select formal and informal assessments to evaluate these three ICF categories.

Frames of reference and conceptual principles used by hand therapists to guide assessment and the development of the plan of care include developmental, motor skill acquisition, rehabilitative, and biomechanical. These frames of references and the underlying concepts and principles used by pediatric hand therapists are explained in Table 29-1.

Operating with these frames of reference in mind, occupational therapists complete a comprehensive evaluation involving an interview, chart review, and administration of formal and informal assessments. Assessment varies according to the cause, type, and acuity of the hand condition.

The occupational therapist obtains background information from child/family interview, chart review, and clinical screening. The background information includes the following:

- A complete medical history regarding the reason for referral to occupational therapy and prior history relating to the referral
- Information regarding the child's overall health status
- Developmental history
- Information regarding other medical teams currently working with the child and the plan of care of these teams
- Family concerns and priorities that have direct impact on the child's plan of care

Knowledge of the family's and child's concerns regarding the child's condition is paramount to guiding the occupational

TABLE 29-1 Frames of Reference and Conceptual Principles Used by Hand Therapists to Guide Treatment

Age-appropriate tasks	Selecting task and environmental demands appropriate to the child's developmental levels across domains promotes successful performance.
Active learning	New skills are developed through active experimentation, experience, and repetitive practice with a variety of strategies available to perform the task. The motor skills should be challenging and at the just-right challenge level. When appropriate, the child should practice the entire task to enhance learning.
Use of purposeful, functional activities	Learning is improved when the child is performing a purposeful, functional activity rather than a repetitive, nonpurposeful task. Function activities motivate children (as opposed to repetitive, nonpurposeful activities) leading to improved performance.
Feedback to promote generalization	Providing feedback helps the child understand the results of his or her movements. Feedback should transition from feedback from the occupational therapist to internal feedback and self-evaluation by the child as the child starts to master a skill.
Practice in a variety of contexts	Varying contexts of practice will enhance the development of flexible strategies and generalization of learning to multiple environments. Learning in natural environments during daily routines is preferred.
Compensatory and/or adaptive strategies considering person, environment, occupation	The occupational therapist provides compensatory and/or adaptive strategies for patients with persistent upper extremity difficulties (e.g., chronic pain, decreased range of motion) The occupational therapist considers the context(s), activity demands, and the child's performance patterns when making adaptation and/or compensatory techniques.
Motivation	The occupational therapist considers the child's values and roles and the context in which the task will be performed to motivate the child.

therapist's plan of care. The family and child inform the occupational therapist of specific concerns regarding the child's functional skills and how the child's upper extremity impairment is impacting the child's participation in life roles. Factors such as family resources and the family structure may impact the plan of care. For instance, a family may not have the availability to come to therapy appointments as frequently as recommended by the referring practitioner, or the child's family members may not be available to provide hands-on assistance with the child's home program activities.

When the occupational therapist obtains the knowledge of these variables during the evaluation, he or she is able to develop a plan of care that is feasible within the context of the child's life.

The family's ability to cope with the child's hand condition may influence the plan of care. For example, families may be experiencing depression, anxiety, or feelings of guilt for their child's hand impairment, especially in cases of brachial plexus birth palsies (BPBP) and congenital hand anomalies.[14,49] In this situation the occupational therapist may need to coordinate support for the family from other disciplines. In trauma cases, background knowledge of the circumstances surrounding the trauma can help the therapist be sensitive to psychosocial factors associated with the trauma. For example, the injury could be the result of self-injurious behavior or an accident in which a loved one may have been lost.

Information about the child's roles and occupations are gathered through parent and child interview. Specifically, the occupational therapist inquires about play, school, work, volunteer activities, hobbies, and interests as the context for intervention. For example, children who engage in competitive sports or music often place higher demands on their extremities and require occupational therapist–directed conditioning after an injury to return to their prior level of activity.[31,84,95,117]

Initial Screening and Assessment

Each category of hand conditions carries unique considerations that influence the plan of care. These considerations can affect the timing of intervention, the intensity of therapy services, the members of the care team who are actively involved in the child's care at a particular point in time, and the level of communication needed among the occupational therapist, the child/family, and the care team. With all categories of upper extremity impairment it is essential that therapists perform a thorough assessment of the child's overall health in addition to the specific impairment for which he or she is referred to therapy. Occupational therapists also screen for any past upper extremity surgery or injury, as either could influence the expected outcomes for the current episode of care. For example, a child may have a previous joint fusion at the wrist; therefore, improved wrist range of motion (ROM) would not be an expected outcome of therapy and, furthermore, would contraindicate wrist ROM exercises. Following are specific components of the initial assessment that occupational therapists should consider specific to each category of hand condition.

Congenital Differences of the Hand or Upper Extremity

Congenital differences of the hand are a common feature of some childhood syndromes, such as VACTERL and Fanconi anemia. When a child is referred to occupational therapy for evaluation and intervention for an upper extremity congenital difference, the occupational therapist should screen the child's overall health status. When a child's congenital hand difference is one of several health concerns, the status of the child's overall health can affect the timing of therapeutic and/or surgical interventions related to the child's hand impairment. A child with congenital hand differences is also more likely to have delays in fine motor, bilateral coordination, and/or functional mobility than a child who was otherwise healthy and sustained an injury to the hand. Therefore, a screening of early developmental milestones and fine motor skills is advised so that the occupational therapist may identify if a need for additional therapy services (such as physical therapy) exists.

Underlying Disorder Affecting the Upper Extremity

Just as with congenital differences in the hand, it is not uncommon for children who are suffering from a systemic disease process that affects their upper extremity, such as CP, to have delays in meeting early developmental milestones. Occupational therapists globally screen the overall gross and fine motor skills of young children with medical conditions that are affecting the upper extremity to identify if a referral for developmental therapy is needed.

Acute Injury (Finger Fracture or Wrist Pain)

For children with acute injuries, the occupational therapist screens for the nature of the injury because certain types of trauma are more likely to develop secondary infection, for example, bite wounds.[30] The occupational therapist may be the first provider to see early signs of an infection and need to consult with the referring practitioner to coordinate care in such cases. Additionally a child with a traumatic injury may have been hospitalized and received prior care for the injury. A thorough medical history will reveal any previous care received for the injury and the outcomes from that treatment.

Clinical Assessment

When administering a comprehensive assessment, occupational therapists review the child's medical chart and interview the parents to guide the strategic elements and priorities of the assessment process. The following sections describe the components of an occupational therapy assessment in pediatric hand therapy.

Pain

Many children who are referred to hand therapy have pain. The occupational therapist screens for pain in the initial evaluation and continues to reassess pain throughout the course of care. The therapist uses the child's level of pain to guide the treatment plan. Additionally, the ongoing assessment of pain helps to guide the therapist in the progression of interventions used to achieve desired goals. For example, if a child is participating in occupational therapy following a finger fracture and having significant pain while completing active ROM exercises, the occupational therapist may wait until the child is experiencing less pain before introducing passive ROM or strengthening exercises.

To assess the location, quality, frequency, and intensity of the child's pain, the occupational therapist asks the child to point to where he or she is experiencing pain. The occupational therapist asks questions to gauge if the pain is diffuse or localized. This information can help the occupational therapist determine the appropriate intervention(s), as well as pertinent clinical findings that are reported to the referring clinician. When developmentally appropriate, the occupational therapist asks the child to describe his or her pain (i.e., sharp, dull, aching, burning, shooting, or hurting). The child's responses can provide insight into the correct diagnosis. For example, tendonitis is often characterized by a sharp or shooting pain when using the upper extremity; generalized, aching joint pain is more typical in arthritis.[81,112] The occupational therapist also asks the child how often and when the pain occurs. For example, the child may experience pain while performing specific activities or during certain periods of a day. Knowing the specific pattern of presentation guides the occupational therapist's recommendations for intervention. The intensity of pain can be quantified using a variety of self-report scales listed in Table 29-2. Quantifying the child's pain is most valuable in determining the usefulness of therapeutic intervention to decrease pain. The occupational therapist uses a pain scale appropriate to the child's age and cognition.

Occupational therapists also ask questions to determine which strategies the patient and/or family have found helpful for managing the pain. Knowledge of all aspects of the child's pain guides the occupational therapist to determine the most appropriate intervention(s) to reduce and manage the child's pain.

TABLE 29-2 Pain Scales

Pain Scale	Purpose/Description/Age Range
Faces Pain Scale—Revised (FPS-R)[12,38,41,98]	Therapist uses a card that has faces to describe pain. There are six faces and each face represents a number from 0, 2, 4, 6, 8, 10. Age range: 4-16
Oucher[10]	Consists of two scales developed for children to rate pain level. (1) The scale for younger children consists of six pictures of face to indicate pain intensity. The photographic scale should be used if the child is unable to count to 100 by ones or tens, if the child is unable to identify which of the two numbers is larger, or if the child can indicate a preference for using the photographic scale. (2) The scale for older children consists of the numbers from 0 to 100. The numeric scale should be used if the child can count to 100 by ones or tens and can identify which of any two numbers is larger. There are five versions of the Oucher scale, based on ethnic background. Age range: 3-12 years[10,11]
Visual Analog Scale (VAS)	The patient rates his or her pain using a visual representation of faces. Age range: 7 years to adult[20,57]
Numerical Rating Scale	The patient rates his or her pain on a scale from 0 to 10 where 0 is no pain and 10 is the worst possible pain. Age range: 6 years to adult[3,111]

Tenderness

The occupational therapist screens for specific patterns of tenderness when a child reports pain. If the child reports pain as occurring in a specific location of the upper extremity in response to a clinician's manual examination, then the child is reported to have tenderness. A variety of special tests are used to assess specific patterns of tenderness in the upper extremity to identify possible underlying structural concerns, such as ligamentous tear or inflamed tendon sheath. An example of a widely used assessment for tenderness is the Finklestein's test for De Quervain's tendonitis.[28] The reliability of upper extremity special tests is low[64,87,95]; therefore, they should be used in conjunction with special tests. The clinician considers the child's reported symptom pattern and strength assessment to determine the most accurate clinical presentation.

Skin

The occupational therapist performs visual inspection of the skin at the evaluation, the start of treatment, and following therapeutic interventions. The skin's appearance provides information as to what therapeutic interventions may be necessary and how well a child is tolerating specific interventions.

If the child has undergone surgery or is recovering from a traumatic injury, he or she will likely have a healing wound or scar and require therapeutic intervention for wound or scar management. Children may also have skin color changes that can reflect circulatory compromise, indicating the need to change or discontinue intervention. In addition, occupational therapists monitor skin integrity regularly when providing interventions such as therapeutic taping or splinting. Children may require a different intervention or a modification in splint design if compromised skin integrity is noted. Occupational therapists should monitor children who report excessive pain or hypersensitivity for trophic changes because complex regional pain syndrome could be a concern warranting consultation with the referring physician.

Skin assessment is reported in subjective terms. When skin is noted to have compromised integrity, the following terms apply:

1. Color: red, white, blue, mottled (i.e., blotchy), or bruised
2. Quality: moist or dry
3. Temperature: cold or warm
4. Texture: calloused, macerated (i.e., moist, soft, and separated), or lacerated (i.e., cut)

The occupational therapist may also report if the skin has a rash or an abrasion.

When a child's skin has a wound or scar, the occupational therapist performs assessment at each treatment session to determine the effectiveness of interventions being used for wound and scar management. Wound assessment includes notation of wound location, size, color, stage of healing, and exudate (i.e., drainage). Therapists closely monitor wounds for signs of infection (redness and edema in the wound bed and/or purulent [i.e., containing pus] drainage that is in excess of the inflammatory stage of wound healing) and notify the referring provider when they observe signs of a possible infection. When assessing a scar, the occupational therapist describes whether it is raised or flat, the size, height, location, pliability, and color. When a scar appears to be hypertrophic (raised or extending beyond the borders for the initial wound), and a formal assessment is needed, the occupational therapist may use the Vancouver Scar Scale (VSS) to measure changes in the four main scar characteristics (pigmentation, vascularity, pliability, and height).[5]

Edema

Edema is most common in cases of joint or tissue inflammation, such as arthritis or tendonitis, and in traumatic injury or post-surgical management of the upper extremity. Occupational therapists may document edema using subjective terms, including:

- Amount: trace, minimal, moderate, severe
- Quality: brawny (i.e., swollen and hard), pitting (i.e., swelling in which an indentation persists after pressure is applied to skin and the pressure is released)
- Location: anatomic description of the area edema is covering

More formal measurement of edema is recommended if (1) the amount of edema present is significant enough to limit the child's ROM or function, and (2) the child would benefit from treatment interventions focused on controlling the edema. Location of edema dictates the measurement tool to be used. When the edema is localized to one or a few joints, circumferential measurements are most appropriate. Edema that covers the dorsum of the hand is best measured using the figure-of-eight method.[61] In the figure-of-eight method, the occupational therapist wraps a tape measure through the palm of the hand and over the dorsum of the hand in a figure-of-eight pattern as depicted in Figure 29-1. When the edema is more

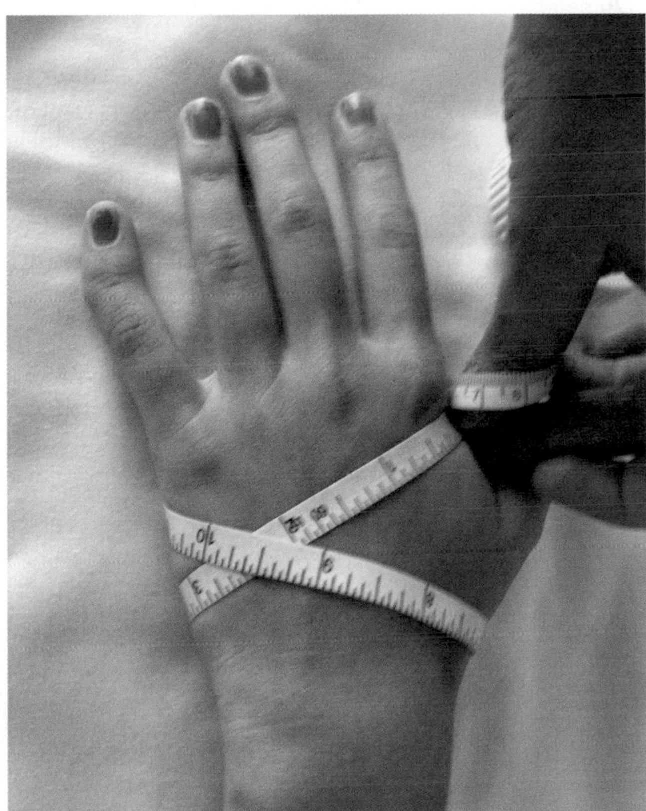

FIGURE 29-1 Figure-of-eight method for measuring edema on the dorsum of the hand.

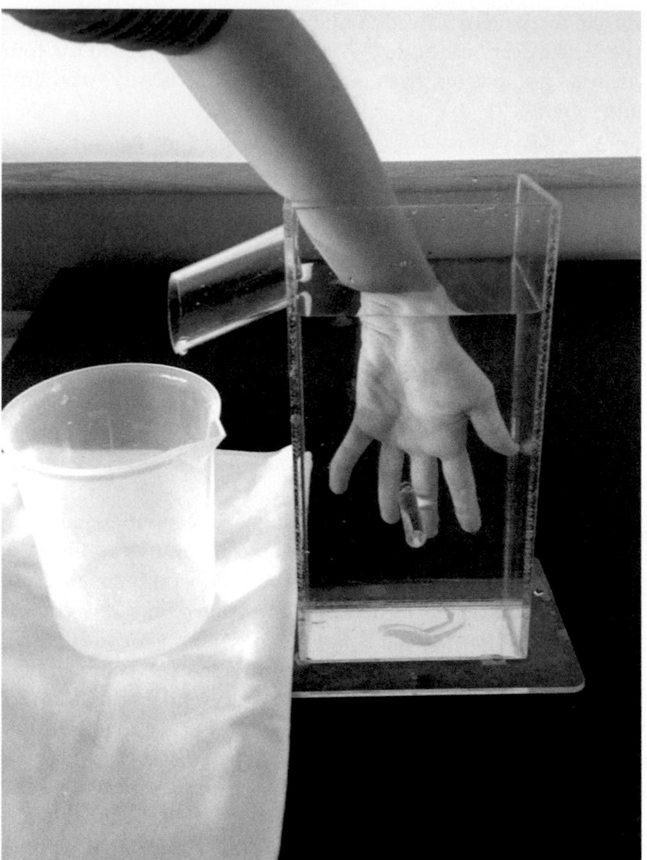

FIGURE 29-2 Assessment of hand edema with a volumeter.

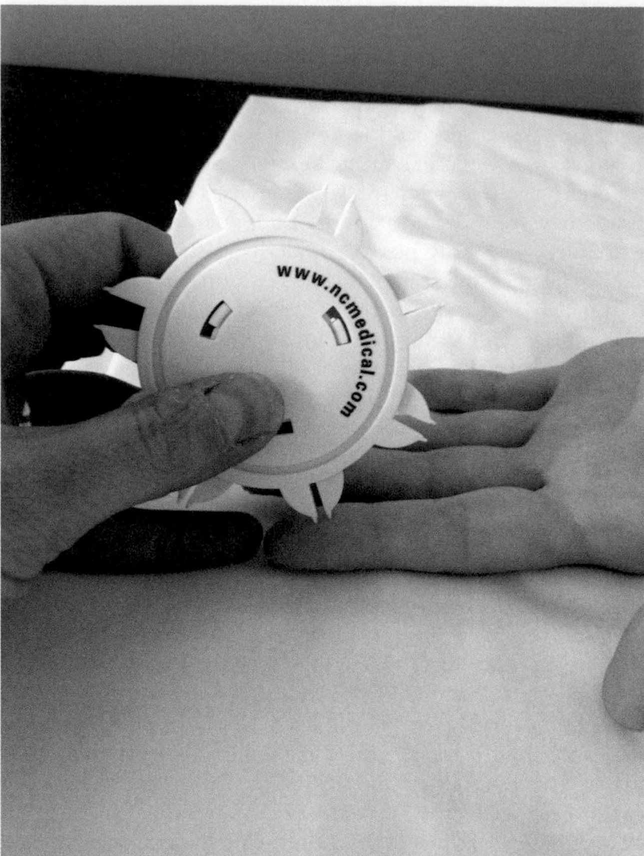

FIGURE 29-3 Two-point discrimination assessment of hand sensation with the Disk-Criminator.

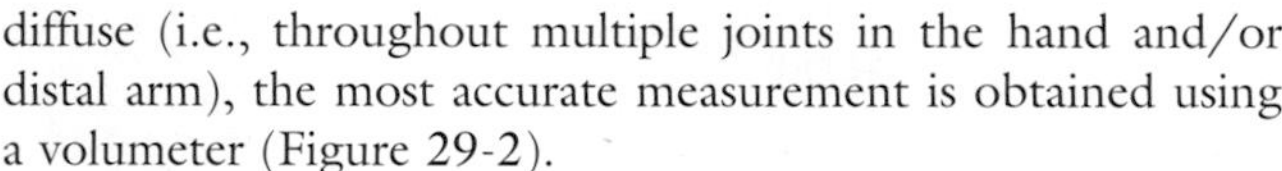

diffuse (i.e., throughout multiple joints in the hand and/or distal arm), the most accurate measurement is obtained using a volumeter (Figure 29-2).

Sensation

Occupational therapists assess sensation to detect abnormal sensory patterns that require therapeutic intervention. Assessment of sensation is important when peripheral nerve damage is reported or suspected or in cases in which extreme vascular changes have occurred. Information regarding a child's sensation is obtained through family interview, clinical observation, the wrinkle test, and other standardized assessments:

Patient and Family Interview

The occupational therapist asks the child and family about the pattern, quality, and presentation of sensory symptoms. Different patterns are indicative of specific clinical conditions. For example, if a child referred with wrist pain reports that the pattern of symptoms occurs primarily in the thumb, index, and middle finger at night and when typing or playing the piano, the occupational therapist may suspect possible median nerve compression (i.e., carpal tunnel syndrome).

Clinical Observation

The occupational therapist also observes how the child uses the arm and hand during functional tasks. The occupational therapist may note a child with normal active range of motion in the index and middle finger avoids using the index finger with fine motor tasks and instead uses the ring finger for pinch grasp. In this case, impaired sensation in the index finger may be causing this preferred pattern. For young children who are unable to explain their symptoms, the occupational therapist observes functional hand use to assess sensory function.

Wrinkle Test

The wrinkle test involves placing the child's hand in warm water for 30 minutes. When a child has peripheral nerve impairment, fingertip wrinkling is absent or diminished as compared with the unaffected hand. When sensory impairment improves, the typical wrinkling pattern returns. This is a particularly effective way to assess the presence of sensation in a child who is not able to report sensory symptoms.

Formal Assessment Tools

Two-point discrimination testing is used to assess the level of discriminative touch impairment. Therapists may use a standardized tool for assessing two point-discrimination, the two-point discriminator (Figure 29-3).[21] Occupational therapists also use Semmes Weinstein Monofilaments (SWM) to evaluate touch discrimination. Semmes Weinstein Monofilaments (Figure 29-4) are used to quantify the level of abnormal sensory discrimination and pattern of impairment. To perform two-point discrimination or sensory assessment with SWM the child must be able to reliably report the sensory information he or she is feeling. When using the Disk-Criminator, he or she reports whether one or two points are felt when touching the fingertip. With SWM, the child must point to indicate whether or not and where he or she felt the monofilaments.

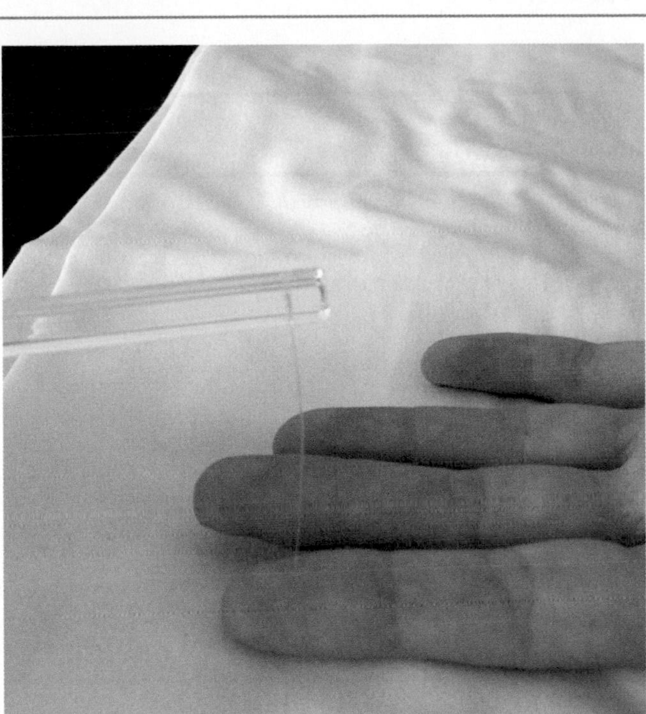

FIGURE 29-4 Assessment of hand sensation using Semmes Weinstein Monofilaments.

For both assessments, the child must also feel at ease enough in the treatment setting to close his or her eyes while the test is being administered. When performing these assessments, the child places his or her hand palm facing up and the tester alternates touching the fingertips with the testing instruments. Two-point discrimination is highly related to the sensory function required to perform certain fine motor tasks.[72] Over time, reassessment with SWM can document the progression of returning sensation.[8] For a child with sensory impairments, the interpretation scale for SWM aids in identifying the specific level of impairment and in intervention planning. Children who have sustained a nerve injury are good candidates for using this assessment tool.

Muscle Tone

Children who have an underlying neurologic disorder typically have abnormal muscle tone in their affected upper extremity. Muscle tone should be assessed through the function and feel of the upper extremity in all patients. The occupational therapist notes and describes the child's muscle tone. Generally tone is described as normal muscle, diminished (or low) muscle tone (hypotonicity), or high tone (hypertonicity). For example, a child who has spastic quadriplegic CP may have low muscle tone in core muscles and high muscle tone in his or her elbow flexors, pronators, wrist, and finger flexors. With children who have CP, the occupational therapist may use the Hypertonia Assessment Tool (HAT) to classify the type(s) of upper extremity hypertonicity.[45]

Range of Motion

Hand therapists complete a gross assessment of upper extremity AROM, including shoulder, elbow, forearm, wrist, and digits. If limitations are noted in active range of motion (AROM), the therapist completes goniometric assessment of the limited ranges.[79,89] When only one of the child's upper extremities is affected, goniometric assessment of the unaffected upper extremity can be performed to use as a guide for the child's potential ROM and to establish plan-of-care goals. If there are no precautions that preclude assessing passive range of motion (PROM) (e.g., a recent fracture) and the child tolerates passive stretch, the occupational therapist also assesses the PROM in joints in which the child has AROM limitations. The occupational therapist notes the location and intensity of any pain the child reports during ROM assessment. This is particularly useful in cases of arthritis or other conditions in which pain is a primary symptom.

Limitations in ROM can be caused by joint tightness, tendon tightness, or scar adhesions. Occupational therapists may use the following techniques to determine if underlying factors are limiting ROM. If a child presents with similar measurements for AROM and PROM in the particular movement plane for the joint, he or she may have joint tightness. For example, a child with joint tightness in the proximal interphalangeal (PIP) joint would have 40 degrees of active PIP flexion and only 40 to 45 degrees of passive PIP flexion in the same digit. When a child has tendon tightness, the available AROM and PROM at a joint vary depending on the position of joints that are more proximal to the joints being tested. Tendon tightness may occur in the intrinsic or extrinsic muscles of the hand or both. One example of tendon tightness is extrinsic flexor tightness of the finger flexors that flex the PIP and distal interphalangeal (DIP) joints of the fingers, in which case the available AROM for PIP and DIP extension decreases as the angle of wrist extension increases.

Range of motion for the child who has sustained injury or undergone surgery can be limited when scarring adheres to soft tissue structures, such as the flexor tendons, and results in tightness. When scar adhesions limit joint ROM, the child will have a significant limitation in AROM at a joint while having near normal PROM at the same joint. Gaining a complete understanding of the biomechanics underlying the limitation in the ROM guides the occupational therapist in determining the appropriate intervention plan.

When a child presents with full PROM in a joint but limited AROM, he or she has muscle weakness. For example, the child may have full passive supination but active supination only to 30 degrees. In this case the difference between PROM and AROM can reflect weakness of the muscle group (in this example, there is weakness in the supinator and/or biceps) or hypertonicity of the antagonist muscles (in this example, the pronators) that is the underlying cause of the limitation in AROM.

Standardized Assessment Tools

Occupational therapists may use standardized assessment tools, patient-reported outcome measures, and individualized performance measures throughout the intervention. Self-report and/or individualized performance measures (Table 29-3) are often used at the start of intervention to guide the plan of care. Additionally, standardized assessments (Table 29-4) may be used with patients who are surgical candidates (e.g., patients with spinal cord injury [SCI] or CP) to determine if surgery is

TABLE 29-3 Patient-Reported Outcomes

Patient-Reported Outcome Measures	Purpose/Age Range/Administration Time
Disabilities of the Arm, Shoulder, and Hand (DASH)[2,34,71]	Assesses physical function and symptoms in patients with musculoskeletal disorders of the upper extremities. It is a self-report questionnaire with 30 items. Patients rate the first 21 items related to everyday tasks from 0 (unable to perform) to 4 (no difficulty in performing); the last 9 items are related to symptoms rated from 0 (extreme) to 4 (not at all). Age range: 18 and over
Quick DASH[71]	Similar to the DASH; assesses activity of daily living; only 11 items with 2 optional four-item modules that are scored separately. Age range: 18 and over
Pediatrics Outcomes Data Collection Instrument (PODCI)[59,68,70]	Assesses upper extremity function, transfers and mobility, sports participation, pain and comfort, global function, and happiness with physical condition. Used with children with pediatric musculoskeletal conditions; each domain listed above is rated with a numerical score from 0 to 100. Age range: 19 and under
Pediatric Quality of Life Inventory (PedsQL)[67,107]	Assesses health-related quality of life in healthy children and children with acute and chronic health conditions. Age range: 2-18 years. Administration time: 5 minutes

TABLE 29-4 Standardized Assessments of Upper Extremity Function

Standardized Assessments	Purpose/Ages/Administration Time
Box and Blocks[65,84]	Assesses unilateral gross manual dexterity. The patient moves as many blocks as possible from one side of the box to the other within 60 seconds. The patient does this with both left and right hands. A higher score indicates higher dexterity. Age range: 6 years and older; administration time: 2-5 minutes
Jebsen-Taylor Hand Function Test[19,102]	Assesses a variety of hand functions used in activities of daily living. There are seven subtests, including writing, turning over index cards, picking up small items, simulated feeding, stacking checkers, picking up large objects, and picking up large, heavy objects. Tests are completed with both hands. Administration time: 30-45 minutes
9-Hole peg[86,96]	Assesses finger dexterity. The patient picks up the pegs one at a time and puts them into the holes in a square board as fast as he or she can. The patient performs the test with both hands. Age range: 18 years and up. Administration time: 5 minutes or less

a good option for achieving the child and family's goals for improved function. Standardized assessments also may be used before and after an intervention to examine the efficacy of the intervention.

Unstructured Clinical Observations

Unstructured observation of the child while engaged in age-appropriate and meaningful activities provides the occupational therapist with an understanding of how effectively the child uses the impaired upper extremity. This may be particularly helpful to occupational therapists who are working with young children who are not able to report their functional skills and limitations or children who exhibit signs of neglect with the affected upper extremity. The occupational therapist observes how the child spontaneously uses his or her affected upper extremity during play and functional tasks to determine if skills are age appropriate. For infants and toddlers, it is helpful to assess the child's use of the upper extremity during functional mobility while assessing gross motor skills (e.g., weight bearing through the upper extremity for positional changes).

Observing how the child positions and initiates use of the affected arm can provide the occupational therapist with insight into the child's true function in the affected arm. Occupational therapists observe the appearance of the child's affected arm, how the child holds the affected arm, and how the child spontaneously uses the affected arm for play or self-care activities. Observations such as the affected hand being less groomed than the unaffected (e.g., nails trimmed on the unaffected and long on the affected) or the child holding the affected arm in a protected position of shoulder adduction and internal rotation with the elbow flexed and hand held at the torso are indications that the child is protective of the affected arm and avoids using it.

For children with congenital differences of the upper extremity and other conditions affecting upper extremity function, such as CP or an SCI, it is helpful to assess the type and efficiency of the grasping patterns used. The occupational therapist documents if the child can use a pinch grasp, spherical grasp, mass grasp, or any adaptive grasping patterns, such as a scissors grasp (i.e., grasping using finger adduction) (Figure 29-5). The occupational therapist assesses the child's lateral and/or palmar pinch to determine the child's capacity for tasks requiring a pinch grasp. When children have significantly limited thumb function, they may use an adaptive scissors grasp. The occupational therapist identifies which fingers the child uses for a scissors grasp and notes the efficiency of the grasp pattern. For instance, a child born with no thumb may

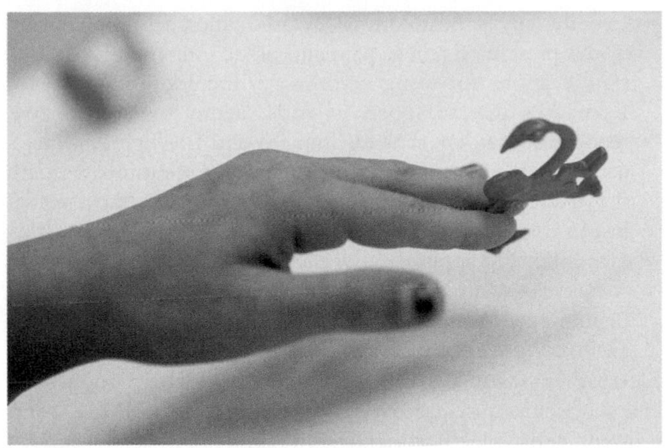

FIGURE 29-5 Example of a child using a scissors grasp of index finger and middle finger to fine motor prehension.

use a scissors grasp of the index and middle finger. This preference to use the radial side of the hand for activities requiring fine motor dexterity suggests that the child is a good candidate for a pollicization (i.e., transplantation of the digit to the location of the thumb) of the index finger. On the contrary, children who use a scissors grasp of the ring finger and small finger stand to gain less function from an index finger pollicization given their preference for ulnar grasping patterns. The occupational therapist specifically evaluates whether or not the child can demonstrate a mass digital grasp and spherical grasp. A child with limited thumb function may have limited or no spherical grasping pattern present and have difficulty with activities that require active thumb palmar abduction, such as holding a ball in the hand. The occupational therapist determines the child's overall capacity for functional grasp with the affected hand and which factors may be limiting functional performance.

For children with a history of typical upper extremity function who acquired an injury or condition affecting the arm or hand, the occupational therapist interviews the child and family to determine the child's prior level of upper extremity function. As the child engages in play or self-care tasks, the occupational therapist can observe how the child uses the affected upper extremity. Children can be highly adaptable in devising ways to work around their limitations. For example, the child may have switched to using the nondominant hand for writing, self-care, and play skills and may report minimal functional limitation yet not be returned to the baseline level of function. This provides the occupational therapist knowledge of the child's current level of function with the affected arm or hand as compared with his or her baseline performance to guide long-term goals.

Ongoing Assessment

Ongoing assessment is a component of each therapy appointment. If the child persists with ROM or strength limitations, the therapist may formally assess performance each session. Additionally, the therapist informally assesses the quality of hand function and grasping patterns at each session. Patient-reported outcome measures and goal setting assessments are completed within the first one to two sessions and periodically through the duration of the intervention to assess progress toward goals.

Intervention Principles and Strategies

The guiding frames of reference and combinations of interventions an occupational therapist uses in treating children with upper extremity impairment (see Table 29-1) varies depending on the underlying cause of the impairment, the child's cognition, the child and family's goals, and the occupational therapist's assessment of the upper extremity impairment. When pain is present (which is typical in most traumatic injuries or post-surgical cases), interventions to minimize pain are employed so that the child may be able to gain enough comfort to participate in therapy activities aimed at improving his or her upper extremity function. In addition, interventions directed at restoring or optimizing ROM are regularly used by occupational therapists with a wide variety of diagnoses. Once ROM has been maximized, interventions such as strengthening or fine motor skills training are employed to refine hand function. As the occupational therapist plans the intervention approach to take with a child, the therapist almost always incorporates the person-environment-occupation model.[58] To do so, the occupational therapist determines the occupation(s) that is important to the child and in which the child is having difficulty. The occupational therapist completes a task analysis to observe the child's performance patterns, determine his or her strengths and weaknesses, and observe the environment in which the child will be performing the task. The occupational therapist then provides the most appropriate intervention to ensure the child performs the task at the highest level of independence possible.

The following sections will discuss common interventions utilized in a pediatric hand therapy practice.

Pain Management

Pain management is often essential for children recovering from an acute upper extremity injury or with joint inflammation. Pain management is the first step toward helping a child progress toward functional goals. If the child experiences pain during the course of therapeutic interventions without relief, the occupational therapist consults with the referring practitioner or refers the family to a pain specialist.

Occupational therapists assess the child's pain to identify the most appropriate interventions to minimize or eliminate pain. Pain that occurs or increases with specific activities can be managed through activity modifications. Pain that is associated with significant inflammation in the arm or hand may improve with edema management and splinting or periods of rest to relieve pain until the inflammation subsides.

For children who are postoperative or have experienced an upper extremity trauma, pain is a typical part of the recovery process that diminishes over time. One of the most effective pain management strategies for cases of upper extremity trauma is the occupational therapist's gradual progression of therapeutic activities. For example, pain management could be as simple as the occupational therapist grading the aggressiveness of stretching and strengthening to ensure the patient is experiencing only low level discomfort. In postoperative cases or upper extremity trauma, scarring may contribute to pain with movement. Scar management strategies and static progressive splinting can improve tissue elasticity, resulting in less pain at the region of the scar.

A variety of physical agent modalities are used for pain management. Although the majority of pediatric hand therapy patients do not have pain significant enough to require the use of a modality, physical agent modalities are effective tools for pain management.

Physical Agent Modalities

Physical agent modalities (PAMs) employ a physical property, such as temperature, sound, or electricity, to achieve a specific therapeutic benefit.[99] Physical agent modalities are infrequently used in a pediatric hand therapy practice as compared with an adult population; however, when used, superficial thermal agents and electrical modalities are the most commonly applied. Ultrasound, a PAM that relies on the conversion of sound to produce a deep thermal heat, is not advised in children who are skeletally immature because it may harm growth plates in the bone.[7]

Superficial Thermal Agents

Superficial thermal agents include both heat modalities and cryotherapy (i.e., the therapeutic application of cold). See Table 29-5 for an overview of superficial thermal agents.

- Heat is typically used to achieve increased tissue extensibility or to relieve pain. Heat can also help to temporarily decrease muscle spasticity.[96] Before using a heat modality, the occupational therapist should screen for contraindications. Heat modalities should not be used in the presence of untreated infection or acute edema, immediately following vessel or nerve reconstruction, over newly placed skin grafts, or in regions of sensory impairment or malignancy.[95] Additionally, fluidotherapy and paraffin are contraindicated when a wound is present in the region to which the modality would be applied.
- Cryotherapy is most commonly used when acute inflammation is present to relieve pain and tissue inflammation. Contraindications for using cryotherapy include children with Raynaud's disease, open wounds, acute vessel or nerve reconstruction, or sensory impairment.[95] Whereas heat is usually applied at the start of a treatment session to prepare the tissue for therapeutic intervention, cryotherapy results in the tissue contracting and the patient experiencing stiffness following application of the modality. As a result, cryotherapy is usually applied after the therapy session to alleviate or minimize tissue inflammation and pain.

Electrotherapeutic Physical Agent Modalities

Electrotherapeutic PAMs used with the pediatric population include neuromuscular electrical stimulation (NMES) and transcutaneous electrical nerve stimulation (TENS).

Neuromuscular electrical stimulation has two primary treatment applications in the pediatric population: (1) to increase strength of a specific muscle or muscle group and (2) to train a muscle or muscle group to perform a specific movement. Neuromuscular electrical stimulation is most commonly used in pediatric hand therapy is to improve strength. In such cases, a gain in AROM may also be achieved at the joint controlled by the muscle group as the increased strength allows for the muscles to pull the joint through a greater arc of motion.

Common conditions that can benefit from application of NMES to improve strength and increase AROM include injury to the nerve at any level (spinal cord, brachial plexus, or peripheral nerve) and conditions in which central nervous system damage has resulted in abnormal muscle tone and movement patterns in the upper extremity (e.g., CP or traumatic brain injury). When a child has sustained an injury to the nerve, the regrowth rate is 1 inch per month. As a result, significant atrophy occurs in the muscles innervated by the nerve distal to the site of injury. When an injured nerve begins to regenerate, the occupational therapist observes trace movements in the

TABLE 29-5 Superficial Thermal Agents

Modality	Treatment Form	Description	Clinical Application
Moist heat	Heat	Delivers heat through the application of hot packs and multiple layers of toweling placed on a specific region of the upper extremity	Can be paired with a sustained stretch of a joint to achieve tissue elongation; can be replicated at home
Paraffin bath	Heat	Applies heat by child dipping his or her hand into heated paraffin wax	Can apply to the wrist and distal upper extremity; commonly used for pain management with arthritis
Fluidotherapy	Heat	A dry heat medium that is similar to a whirlpool. A fluidotherapy machine is filled with Cellux, ground corn cobs that are similar to sand in texture; the fluidotherapy unit blows these particles around the extremity placed in the unit to deliver heat.	The child may perform AROM during a fluidotherapy treatment; useful tool for desensitization
Ice packs	Cryotherapy	Delivers cold by placing ice packs on a specific region of the upper extremity	Can be replicated at home
Ice massage	Cryotherapy	A piece of ice is applied in a continuous pattern of movement (massage) directly over a specific region of the upper extremity	Particularly effective for tendonitis[62]

From Skirven, T. M., Osterman, A. L., Fedorczyk, J., & Amadio, P. C. (2011). *Rehabilitation of the hand and upper extremity.* 2-vol set: *Expert consult.* St. Louis: Mosby.

affected muscle or muscle groups. Once signs of returning motor function are observed, NMES can be used to help strengthen the atrophied muscles. When a child has a diagnosis of CP or traumatic brain injury with associated upper extremity motor impairments, NMES can be used to strengthen a weak muscle group. A common motor impairment in children with CP and upper extremity hemiparesis is muscle spasticity in the wrist and finger flexors that results in posturing (i.e., holding the affected upper extremity in wrist flexion with weaken grasp pattern). Neuromuscular electrical stimulation can be used to strengthen the weaker wrist extensor muscles, resulting in improved grasp from increased active wrist extension.

Neuromuscular electrical stimulation may also be helpful in retraining specific muscle groups. Sometimes following an injury a child will present with an imbalance in muscle groups resulting in compensatory upper extremity movement patterns. A common example is a wrist injury in which a child has significant weakness of the wrist extensors following immobilization. A common compensatory pattern for wrist extension is the use of the extensor digitorum communis to extend the wrist; that is, the child uses the muscle group that hyperextends the metacarpophalangeal (MCP) joints when he or she extends the wrist. To reduce this compensatory pattern of using a finger extensor muscle to activate wrist extension, NMES is applied on the wrist extensors with the child maintaining his or her fingers in a composite fist and extending the wrist (Figure 29-6).

Neuromuscular electrical stimulation can also be used for muscle retraining following a tendon transfer. Tendon transfers can restore or improve active muscle function in children with CP or a nerve impairment that results in permanent motor loss. For example, a child who has weak wrist extensor muscles may have a wrist flexor muscle(s) transferred to improve the power of wrist extension. Once the transfer has healed and is ready for strengthening, NMES can promote retraining of the wrist flexor to work as an extensor muscle.

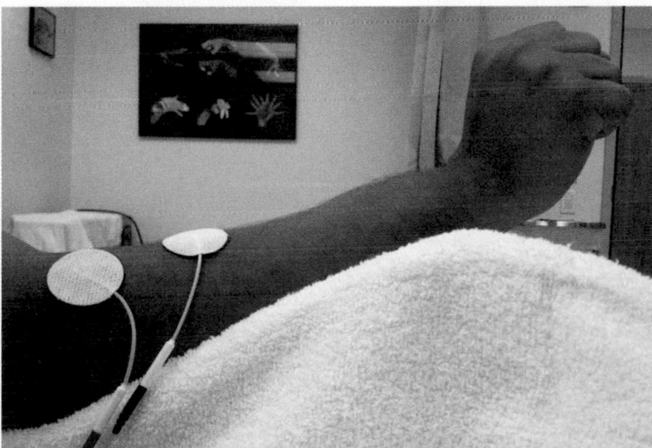

FIGURE 29-6 Neuromuscular electrical stimulation may be used to strengthen and retrain the wrist extensors (versus the extensor digitorum communes [EDC]) to extend the wrist. The child keeps the fingers in a composite fist to prevent the EDC from extending the wrist.

TENS is also used to manage pain. The majority of children in pediatric hand therapy have pain that resolves as they are healing; however, some children are unable to engage in a therapy program or use their affected upper extremity because of increased pain. When a child is having pain as a primary concern, TENS may be applied to the region of reported pain. The pain control experienced with TENS occurs primarily while the child is wearing a TENS unit.[27]

Splinting

Splinting has a wide variety of applications in pediatric hand therapy. The styles of splints most commonly used with the pediatric hand population include soft splints, static splints (splints that prevent motion in the affected joints), static progressive splints (splints that are serially modified to increase the joint angle), and dynamic splints with movable components that apply a force to a specific joint(s) for the purpose of moving that joint(s). The splints may be used for protection of the hand or arm during acute phases of healing, resting or supporting a joint for pain relief, positioning a joint for improved function, increasing ROM, or prevention of deformity in the upper extremity. When splints are used for protection (Figure 29-7), they are typically used following an injury or upper extremity surgery. A wide variety of splinting styles is used for this purpose, and the specific type and style of splint is determined by the type of injury or surgery and the specific motions that need to be prevented.

Splinting for pain relief most often occurs to treat acute pain and/or inflammation. Children with tendonitis in the upper extremity (e.g., De Quervain's tendonitis) or with a flare of arthritis symptoms in the arm or hand may benefit from splints

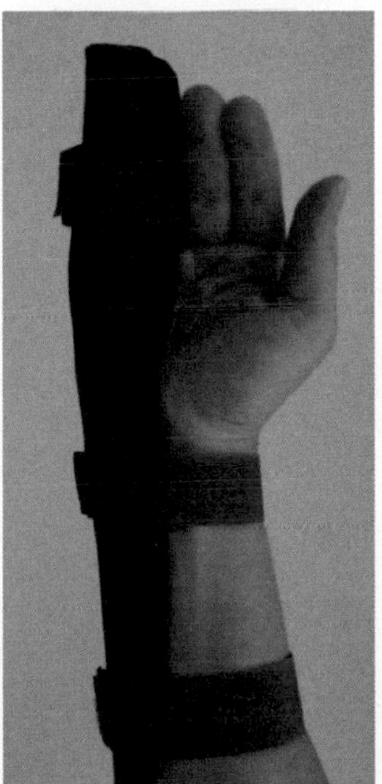

FIGURE 29-7 An ulnar gutter splint is an example of a protective splint. It is applied to protect a fracture of a digit or metacarpal in the ulnar two digits.

to rest the affected structures (e.g., joints/tendons) until their acute inflammation begins to resolve, which helps to relieve their pain.

Splints are used to improve function for children who have a condition affecting their joint stability or joint mobility. The style and type of splint appropriate for improving joint mobility is dependent on the child's specific limitations. For example, children with significant joint laxity leading to joint instability in the thumb may benefit from a splint that supports the first carpal metacarpal joint and thumb metacarpal phalangeal joints. The stability of the splint allows the child to stabilize other fingers against the thumb for improved pinch grasp and radial grasp control (Figure 29-8).[104] Additionally, children with congenital conditions, post-trauma, or systemic conditions may have limitations in joint mobility related to nerve and/or muscle impairment. Splinting in cases in which joint mobility is limited can help prevent deformity. In this case, the splint serves to position the joints in a plane in which movement is limited or missing. For example, a child with low radial nerve palsy may have no active wrist or MCP extension of the digits and no active radial abduction of the thumb until the nerve regenerates. A radial nerve palsy splint can support the wrist in extension and provide dynamic support to the digits holding them in extension while the hand is at rest and pulling them back into extension after active digit flexion. In this case the splint improves function for active grasp and release with the affected hand and prevents flexion contractures until active movement is restored.

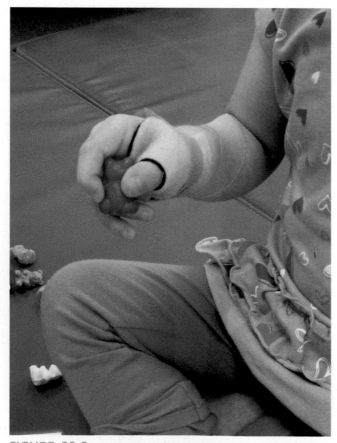

FIGURE 29-8 A McKie splint is one style of splint that provides stability to the metacarpophalangeal joint of the thumb for improved fine motor function.

Splints are used to improve ROM and correct deformity in cases of joint contracture or tendon tightness. Both static progressive splinting and dynamic splints may be appropriate to improve ROM.[60] (Both of these types of splints are discussed in following section.)

The following are styles of splints used in pediatric hand therapy:

- Occupational therapists make soft splints with neoprene or other soft material. Soft splints may be used to position the upper extremity to prevent contracture, especially in premature or young infants who are not using their upper extremities purposefully. Soft splints provide support to a joint to decrease pain or improve joint position for function. Additionally, a variety of prefabricated soft splints with or without rigid support can be ordered from vendors.
- Static splints are those that prevent motion in the affected joints. For example, a wrist and thumb spica splint immobilizes the MCP joint of the thumb, the first carpal metacarpal joint, and the wrist.
- Static progressive splinting is the application of static splint with serial adjustments to reposition the splint to change the joint angle. Static progressive splinting is used when mobility is limited by joint tightness with a soft end feel (i.e., mild to moderate resistance to passive motion in the direction of ROM limitation). An example is a static progressive elbow extension splint (Figure 29-9). Children lacking full elbow extension may be fitted with an elbow splint to increase the range of elbow extension. Children typically wear this splint when sleeping to allow for AROM and functional use of the affected arm when awake. The hand therapist routinely readjusts the splint to increase the angle of elbow extension over time. While any style of custom-fabricated splint can be serially adjusted to change the angle of positioning, prefabricated static progressive splints are also available.

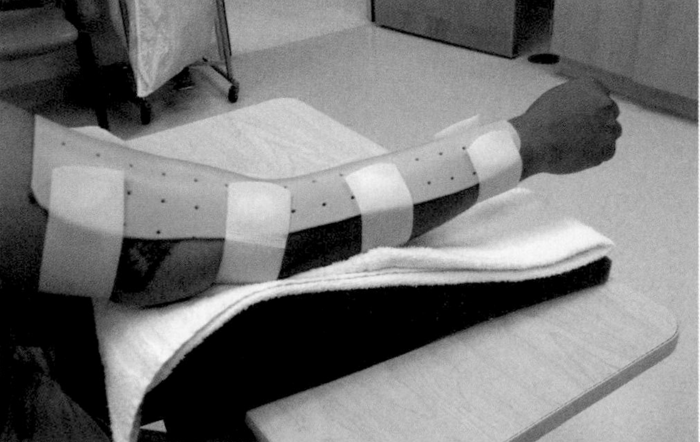

FIGURE 29-9 When a child has limited elbow extension a static elbow extension splint can be used to improve range of motion. The splint is positioned at the child's end range of extension and the child wears the splint when sleeping. The splint is readjusted for increased extension at future visits to gradually increase the stretch and the child's active elbow extension.

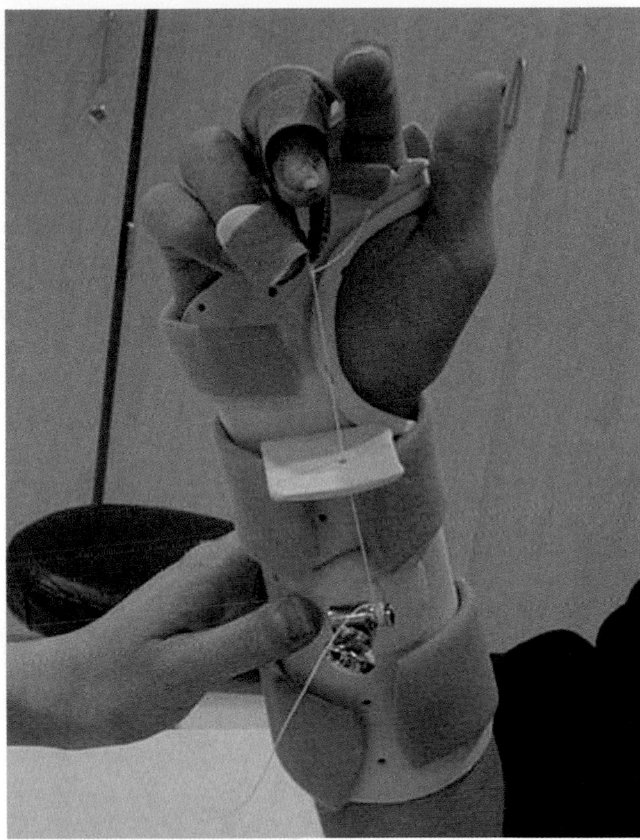

FIGURE 29-10 An example of a dynamic splint to increase proximal interphalangeal (PIP) joint flexion. The child turns the dial to gradually increase the PIP flexion stretch while wearing the splint

- Dynamic splints include components that apply a dynamic force to a joint. Dynamic splints often assist a child with a motion that is absent or very weak, for example, a splint that assists with MCP extension when a child has radial nerve palsy. Additionally, dynamic splints are also used to apply light sustained force to increase joint mobility (Figure 29-10) at a joint that is limited in active motion secondary to joint tightness. Dynamic splints can be fabricated by the occupational therapist or can be prefabricated.

Casting

Occupational therapists fabricate casts to achieve specific treatment goals. Serial casting is used to increase joint mobility and tissue extensibility for improved ROM in the child's affected upper extremity, typically when the child presents with joint tightness. Serial casting (Figure 29 11) is similar to static progressive splinting in that a series of casts are applied, with each cast increasing the angle of the affected joint(s) to obtain the desired arc of movement. The serial cast is typically applied permanently until the child returns for the next cast to be applied. A serial cast can be formed as a bivalve cast that is removable in cases in which the child may require some time out of the cast. Serial casting is an established practice to gain increased mobility following Botox or phenol injections and to decrease muscle spasticity in children who have movement limitations.[6,13,52,82]

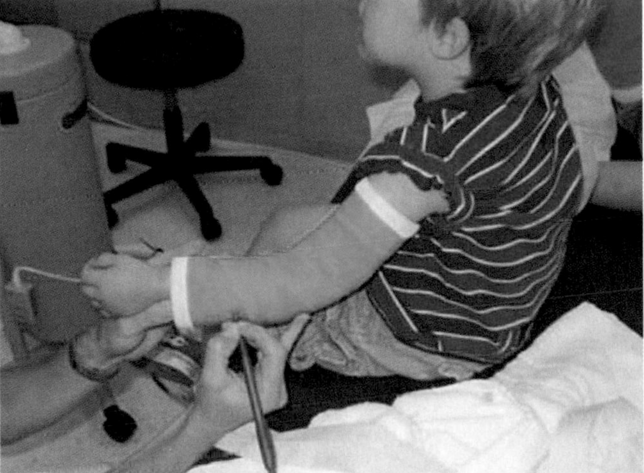

FIGURE 29-11 Serial cast for elbow extension. At each visit a new cast is applied in an increased extension stretch.

Casting is also used for children participating in constraint-induced movement therapy (CIMT). The constraint cast is applied to the less affected upper extremity to require the child to use the affected arm and hand during functional tasks. Constraint-induced movement therapy is most often implemented with children with hemiparesis resulting from conditions such as CP or a brachial plexus palsy and decreased spontaneous use of their affected arm and hand. Occupational therapists use different protocols for wearing constraint casts, including both removable and nonremovable casts.[24,39,76]

Kinesiology Tape

Kinesiology tape (KT) can be used to facilitate or inhibit specific muscles or muscle groups to decrease pain, improve ROM, enhance muscle activation, and/or relax specific muscles. It is an elastic, waterproof tape that was first used in sports therapy and has more recently been applied in the practice of pediatric hand therapy. The tape is latex-free and designed to allow skin to breathe. Kinesiotaping can enhance lymphatic drainage and improve blood flow to decrease inflammation.[50] Kinesiotaping can also improve the biomechanics of a joint; for example in the shoulder, more than one piece of KT can be used at the shoulder with tape in one region acting to inhibit specific muscles and another piece of tape placed to activate weakened muscles.[44,53,105] Studies evaluating the effectiveness of KT in treating shoulder pain in individuals with impingement syndrome showed that patients treated with KT at the shoulder had more immediate pain relief[53,105] and faster functional gains[53] compared with individuals treated without KT.

The occupational therapist may use KT to improve shoulder kinematics, particularly for children who have joint hypermobility, hemiparesis, or shoulder pain. In children with neuromuscular conditions, such as CP or SCI, KT has been found to improve postural control and upper extremity function and provide stability and joint alignment.[43,115] It is also used to improve the activation and strength of the weaker muscle

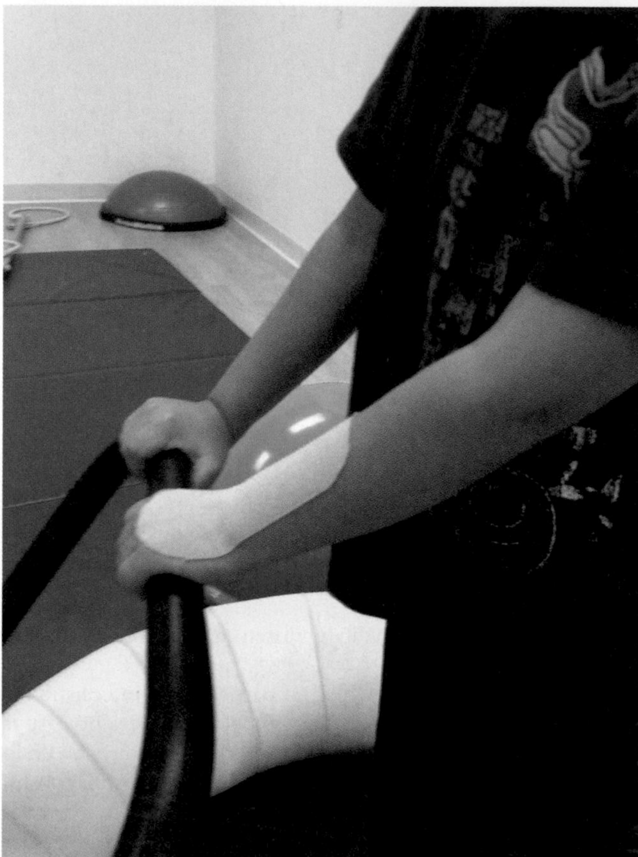

FIGURE 29-12 The child in this picture has hemiplegic cerebral palsy and weakness of the wrist extensors. The kinesiology tape is applied to facilitate the wrist extensors.

groups (Figure 29-12). The authors of this chapter have found KT to be beneficial in improving muscle activation and joint stability at the shoulder, forearm, wrist, and fingers. Children may wear KT for 3 to 5 days before a new tape application is required, and family members can be instructed in how to apply tape. The tape may be cut in specific patterns and applied in a variety of ways. The occupational therapist cuts and applies the tape in a particular pattern depending on the functional goals. Adverse effects of KT such as skin irritation[105] and muscle soreness[1] have been reported to occur infrequently (<5% of subjects). Occupational therapists may apply a small test strip of tape on the child's skin to determine if the child has adverse skin response to wearing the tape. Occupational therapists may consult *Kinesio Taping in Pediatrics: Fundamentals and Whole Body Taping*[50] for instructions on how to cut and apply tape to achieve the specific outcome desired. Therapists can obtain certification in kinesiotaping.

Child and Family Education: Activity Modification, Joint Protection, and Energy Conservation

Activity Modifications

Occupational therapists commonly use and educate the child and family about activity modifications, joint protection strategies, and energy conservation techniques for children. These strategies are often used with children who have pain that limits functional use, ROM deficit, strength impairments, or fine motor impairments in their upper extremities.

Activity modifications are adaptations made to an activity or tool in order to increase the child's ability to perform the activity or use the tool independently.[91] Using the person-environment-occupation model, the occupational therapist completes a task analysis to identify the most appropriate activity modification for the task in question. Examples of activity modifications include modified sports equipment or instruments, adapted writing utensils, assistive technology, and adaptive devices such as buttonhooks or pediatric-sized sock aids.

Joint Protection Strategies

Joint protection strategies are techniques used to decrease pain caused by the amount of strain placed on a joint during a task or the amount of work a muscle group must perform to complete the task. The occupational therapist explains the purpose and importance of joint protection strategies and interviews the child and family to determine which activities trigger joint pain. The occupational therapist reviews the child's day and pattern of symptoms to help identify the most beneficial technique(s). The occupational therapist often demonstrates the strategy and then has the child and/or family perform the strategies in the clinic setting to ensure correct application.

Energy Conservation Techniques

Children experiencing fatigue limiting their function, for example, those with systemic conditions such as juvenile idiopathic arthritis or Duchene muscular dystrophy, often benefit from energy conservation strategies. As with joint protection strategies, the occupational therapist's interview with the child and family helps to identify the child's activity demands. The occupational therapist also observes how the child performs specific activities identified as difficult or contributing to fatigue. The occupational therapist then educates the family and child on strategies used for energy conservation and helps them develop a plan for applying the strategies.

Wound Care

Pediatric hand therapists must be knowledgeable about wound care when working with children after a surgery or a traumatic upper extremity injury. Often nurses and members of the medical team manage wound care in the child's early recovery; however, sometimes children begin therapy almost immediately after surgery when pins or sutures are in place. Therefore, the occupational therapist should be knowledgeable of the pin and wound care strategies desired by the referring physician and provide family education on wound care.

In cases of significant trauma to the dermis with wound healing through tissue granulation such as abrasions in the arm or hand from shearing injuries, the time for healing often lasts several weeks and continues into the rehabilitative stages; therefore, the occupational therapist is integral in providing wound care. Similarly, when the child has a skin graft, healing requires an extended period of time. The occupational therapist monitors the health and healing of the wounds and grafts and may be involved in providing direct wound care. Skin graft precautions include avoiding sheer force over new grafts (which can be caused by edema control garments or splints) and avoiding compression that could compromise blood flow to the graft.

Scar Management

Almost all children with healing wounds in the arm or hand benefit from scar management techniques. Scarring can limit ROM, may cause pain, and can be a cosmetic concern. Once the postsurgical rehabilitation protocol allows the child to perform ROM in the joints affected by scarring, ROM exercises can be implemented to restore mobility. Scar massage is used with scars that limit AROM in a joint, lack pliability, are thick, extend the borders of the wound, or are a cosmetic concern.

Pressure on scars is an effective strategy to improve tissue extensibility and cosmesis of scars. A variety of scar pads and compressive materials are available to occupational therapists. Often, for small, minimally raised scars, compression with a soft material, such as Velfoam donned under a splint, tape, or compressive wrap, is sufficient to promote healing.[90] For scars that are more severe in terms of size or diminished pliability, a variety of specialty products are available (Figure 29-13). Occupational therapists may use gel scar pads cut to cover the region of the scar or make a custom-molded scar pad from elastomer products in combination with a splint or compressive wrap to provide adequate compression.[51] Typically, these interventions are implemented when the child is sleeping so that the upper extremity is free for functional use during the day. In cases of burns to the upper extremity or skin grafts, a period of using custom-sized compression garments is necessary for optimal scar management.[9]

Edema Control

Occupational therapists use edema control strategies when children have swelling following surgery or an upper extremity injury. Positioning and AROM are two of the most effective edema control strategies.[97] A common positioning strategy for edema is to keep the arm and hand resting above the heart. Families with young children often report that this is difficult to implement with young children because of high activity levels and resistance to prolonged periods of sitting. Occupational therapists also teach children and/or family members AROM exercises to reduce edema. Young children often respond best to performing grasp and release activities AROM exercises in an elevated position a few times throughout the day. Older children can be taught to avoid prolonged periods of full elbow extension of the affected upper extremity until edema begins to subside and, when cleared by the physician, to regularly perform AROM exercises.

When edema is moderate to severe or not responding to positioning and AROM, the occupational therapist can use compressive wraps and retrograde massage to control edema.[97] Coban wrapped distal to proximal on a digit (Figure 29-14) or compressive finger sleeves (available in sizes for larger children) can be effective in decreasing digital edema. Compressive sleeves are also available in graded sizes that can be donned over the wrist or proximal upper extremity for edema control. Retrograde therapeutic massage techniques (i.e., specific massage patterns, moving distal to proximal, to mobilize edema out of the extremity) also may be used in cases of persistent edema.[108]

Splinting is used for edema control when the swelling is associated with joint inflammation or the child is acutely ill and has limited ability to perform AROM exercises. Edema associated with systemic conditions, such as juvenile idiopathic arthritis and systemic lupus erythematosus (SLE), may improve with medication, and splinting may not be necessary. For children who experience tenosynovitis, a localized inflammation along a tendon sheath, resting the specific tendon group through splinting can reduce the inflammation.[101] Children who are medically fragile and have upper extremity edema (e.g., a child in hospital intensive care unit recovering from septic shock and vascular compromise to the hands) may benefit from splinting to alleviate edema.

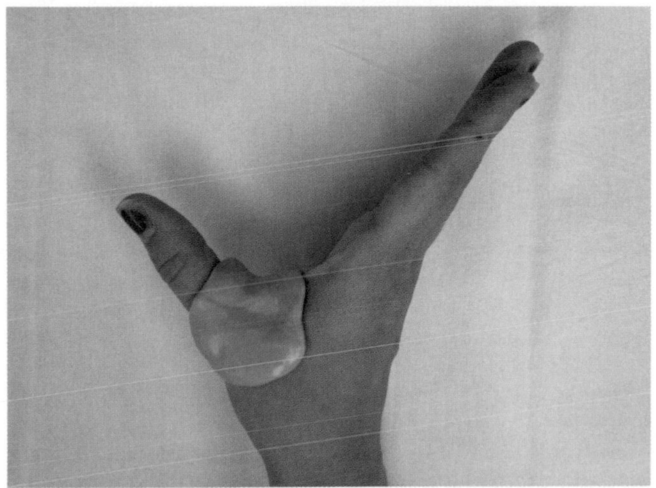

FIGURE 29-13 An example of an elastomer scar pad that a child wears when sleeping to improve scar pliability.

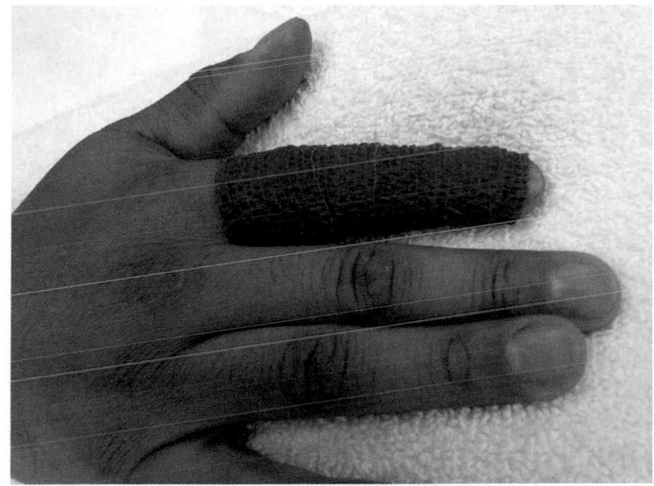

FIGURE 29-14 An example of a Coban wrap on the digit to decrease edema the finger.

Desensitization and Sensory Re-education

Desensitization and sensory re-education are two interventions occupational therapists use for children experiencing sensory impairments. Occupational therapists use desensitization strategies to reduce hypersensitivity (i.e., over-responsiveness to sensory stimulation) and facilitate the child's use of the affected arm in everyday functional activities.[94] Hypersensitivity can occur after an injury, especially if a nerve was involved. It may also occur spontaneously or after a minor injury, such as a sprain or strain to the wrist. A child may be hypersensitive to temperature, textures, and/or various grades of touch pressure. The occupational therapist desensitizes the area by using graded exposure to the types of sensory input to which the area is sensitive.[18] Using play-based activities may increase a child's tolerance for desensitization activities, especially in younger children (Figure 29-15). Behavioral reinforcement strategies can also be used to improve compliance with desensitization home program activities for children who are less motivated by play-based activities.

Sensory re-education is used when a child is experiencing sensory return after a nerve injury. The occupational therapist exposes the upper extremity to a variety of sensory activities to improve sensory discrimination. Sensory re-education is appropriate to begin when a child has a Semmes Weinstein grade of monofilament 6.65 or better.[95]

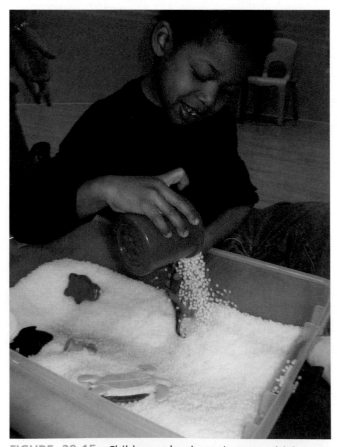

FIGURE 29-15 Children who have hypersensitivity can perform grasp release of a sensory medium or find toys hidden in a sensory medium for desensitization of the extremity.

Range of Motion Exercises

Pediatric hand therapists frequently use active, active-assistive, and PROM exercises. Occupational therapists working with children who sustained an injury or had upper extremity surgery must be familiar with the specific postsurgical protocol for progressing ROM exercises. The structures injured or repaired dictate which form of exercise is least stressful on the repair. For example, a commonly used protocol for children with flexor tendon repairs involves avoiding AROM in the early rehabilitation phase while performing passive digit flexion exercises to preserve joint mobility.[95] Therapy for upper extremity fractures begins with AROM and progresses to PROM when the referring clinician indicates fracture healing can withstand the more aggressive force.[18]

Blocking exercises (Figure 29-16) are useful when the patient demonstrates difficulty with PIP and/or DIP flexion and/or extension. This type of exercise allows for more force to be transferred to the PIP and DIP joints to achieve greater active pull at the joint. Static progressive stretches (Figure 29-17) can be used when the referring physician clears the child for PROM. To improve ROM for a child with joint or tendon tightness, static progressive exercises are often the most effective.[69]

Developmental stage and personality of the child are considered when determining activities for improving ROM. Young children rely on a family member(s) to perform active assistive range of motion (AAROM) or PROM exercises. Young children respond best to structured play activities designed to achieve active movement within the desired plane. For example, a child who needs to work on shoulder flexion and elbow extension can perform finger painting on an easel. Most school-age children can be instructed in performing a set of specific exercises and can follow through with visual and/or written instruction.

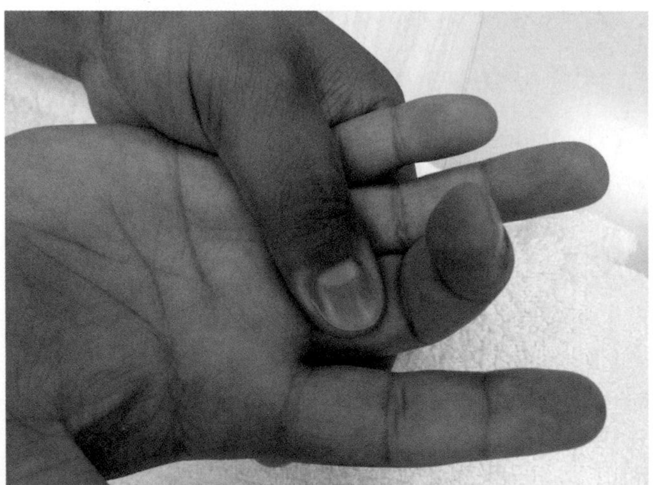

FIGURE 29-16 With a proximal interphalangeal (PIP) joint blocking exercise the therapist supports the metacarpophalangeal in neutral extension while the child flexes the PIP joint.

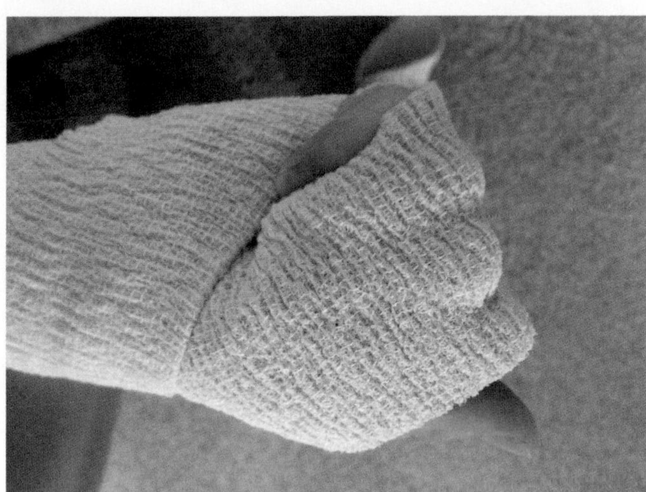

FIGURE 29-17 A flexion wrap is a static progressive exercise where the digit is wrapped into a light flexion stretch with Coban. After the child has become comfortable with the stretch, another wrap of tape is applied pulling the digit into slightly more flexion.

Strengthening

Occupational therapists grade a strengthening program from light to challenging. For the lightest form of strengthening the child might start with isometric exercises without resistance and then progress to isometric exercises with resistance for an increased challenge. Isotonic exercises may also be performed without resistance and progressed to include resistance in the form of weights or resistive bands. Occupational therapists must ensure that there are no contraindications to strengthening before progressing a child to strengthening exercises. Children with a rheumatic disease and in a stage of active joint inflammation should refrain from strengthening until the inflammation is resolved. Similarly, children recovering from surgery or an upper extremity injury must have sufficient healing to withstand resistive force to the arm and hand.

Play-based activities or exercises involving holding sustained positions may be the most effective to achieve strengthening for young children. For example, a 10-month-old recovering from brachial plexus birth palsy can strengthen his or her shoulder muscles by reaching to throw a ball into a container placed above shoulder height or by activities in quadruped.

Reducing Muscle Tone

When a child presents with hypertonia (i.e., high muscle tone) in the affected upper extremity, the occupational therapist's intervention plan should include activities to decrease the muscle tone/spasticity. Decreasing muscle spasticity helps the child gain control of movement in the upper extremity. Weight bearing through the affected arm and hand can decrease muscle spasticity.[83] Neuromuscular electrical stimulation can also be used to decrease spasticity in a specific muscle group; however, reduction in spasticity is only seen during application of the NMES.[4,37] Additionally, splinting with a night-resting hand splint following Botox injections has been shown to decrease muscle spasticity.[48]

Fine Motor Skills and Bimanual Coordination

Following reconstructive surgery of a congenital anomaly or a traumatic injury to the hand, occupational therapists focus on maximizing functional grasp patterns. When a child has fine motor impairment as a result of a recovering nerve injury or a chronic progressive condition, occupational therapists use supportive splints, activity modifications, and assistive equipment to maximize fine motor impairment. If nerve function is restored, then therapy may progress to fine motor skills training.

When children have hemiparesis resulting in limited bimanual coordination skills, occupational therapists may use CIMT and sensory-based activities to promote increased awareness and use of the affected upper extremity. Bimanual skill training activities are also effective in maximizing functional performance.[32]

Mirror Therapy

Mirror therapy (MT) is a novel therapeutic intervention first introduced by Ramachandran[89] to decrease phantom limb pain (PLP) in individuals with amputations. Since that time, MT has been reported to be effective in decreasing pain[66,73] and restoring function[74] in individuals with complex regional pain syndrome. Mirror therapy also has been found to improve motor and sensory function[114] in adults with hemiparesis after cerebral vascular accident. Gygax et al. found that children with hemiplegia achieved improved hand strength and functional ROM after 3 weeks of daily bimanual training using MT and achieved improved pinch strength after 3 weeks of daily bimanual training without the mirror.[35] Although MT is still in its infancy as an established intervention, it has promise to improve motor control and function in children with hemiparesis. Additionally, MT appears to have the potential to decrease pain and improve quality of life and function in children with phantom limb pain and complex regional pain syndrome.[114]

Interventions for Specific Conditions

This section describes the common diagnoses treated by pediatric hand therapists and presents intervention strategies for each diagnostic type.

Congenital Differences of the Upper Extremity

Although congenital differences of the hand or arm occur only in 0.2% of births,[29] they are not an uncommon diagnosis referred to a pediatric hand therapist. Upper limb development begins at 4 weeks' gestation and is complete by 8 weeks, so the majority of congenital defects of the arm and hand occur during this time of prenatal development. In addition, trauma in utero, such as vascular compromise or amniotic bands, may also result in congenital impairments of the upper extremity and typically occurs in the third trimester of prenatal development.[95]

A variety of classification scales for upper extremity congenital differences has been introduced through the years. At present, the classification developed by the International

TABLE 29-6 Embryologic Classification of Congenital Anomalies

Classification	Description	Examples
Failure of formation • Transverse • Longitudinal	Specific upper limb anatomy does not develop entirely or is entirely absent	Radial longitudinal deficiencies, ulnar longitudinal deficiencies, transverse growth arrest, phocomelia
Failure of differentiation	Characterized by a disruption in the development of the digits, metacarpals, carpals, digital or interdigital spaces	Camptodactyly, clinodactyly, syndactyly, Apert syndrome, clasped thumb, synostoses
Duplication	Specific structures in the hand are duplicated	Thumb polydactyly, supernumerary digit on ulnar side of the hand, mirror hand
Overgrowth	Enlargement in the skeletal and soft tissue structures that occurs in the digits	Macrodactyly
Undergrowth	An underdeveloped hand or absent digits	Brachydactyly
Congenital constriction band syndrome	An amniotic band wraps around the upper limb resulting in varying levels of limb abnormality distal to the level of the band	
Generalized skeletal abnormalities	Conditions in which defects of the upper extremity accompany multiple skeletal variations	Arthrogryposis, Marfan's syndrome, VATER syndrome, achondroplasia

Federation of Societies for Surgery of the Hand (IFSSH) (Table 29-6) is the most widely accepted classification scale.[16,63,102]

The occupational therapist provides conservative management and postsurgical rehabilitation in children with congenital differences of the hand and arm. Only 10% of congenital upper extremity differences require surgery; therefore, the occupational therapist's role is most often conservative.[29] Conservative interventions focus on preventing further deformity and maximizing function and include splinting, activity modifications, fine motor and upper extremity coordination skills training, therapeutic taping, and assistive equipment training. Postoperative treatment can include any of the following: splinting for positioning and protection, wound management, and scar management in the early stages of recovery. As the child heals, the occupational therapist's focus is on improving ROM, coordination, fine motor skills, and strength. In some cases, activity modifications and adaptive strategies are also used postsurgically to optimize function. See Case Study 29-1 for an example of intervention for a child with congenital differences that required surgical interventions.

Upper Extremity Impairments Caused by an Underlying Disorder

A child's upper extremity impairment can be caused by a number of underlying disorders, including neurological disorders (e.g., CP), neurodegenerative conditions (e.g., spinal muscular atrophy), rheumatic conditions (e.g., systematic lupus erythematosus), and connective tissue conditions (i.e., Ehlers Danlos syndrome). The following sections describe intervention considerations, goals, strategies, and progression for each of these conditions.

Neurologic Conditions

Children with CP or traumatic brain injury (TBI) often have associated upper extremity impairment as a result of the damage to the central nervous system. These children present with hypertonia (or, less often, hypotonia) in one or both upper extremities. A variety of therapeutic interventions may be appropriate for conservative management strategies to achieve optimal hand function or prevent deformity in these populations. The goals of therapy vary depending on the child's impairment level. For children who have the skills to manipulate objects with their affected upper extremity(ies) (Manual Ability Classification System [MACS] levels I to III), intervention strategies aim to improve functional performance. Box 29-1 shows the MACS levels. Intervention strategies can include neuromuscular retraining, serial casting, splinting, and/or CIMT, which focuses on improving sensory awareness and spontaneous use of the affected arm and hand. Intervention goals for children who do not engage in manipulating objects with their upper extremities (MACS levels IV to V) are often to prevent deformity and modify or adapt tasks.

BOX 29-1 Manual Ability Classification System Levels

Level 1	Handles objects easily and successfully. At most limitations in the ease of performing manual tasks requiring speed and accuracy
Level 2	Handles most objects, but with somewhat reduced quality and/or speed of acheivement. May avoid some tasks or use alternative ways of performance.
Level 3	Handles objects with difficulty. Needs help to prepare and/or modify activities.
Level 4	Handles a limited selection of easily managed objects in adaptive situations. Requires continuous support.
Level 5	Does not handle objects and has severely limited ability to perform even simple actions. Requires total assistance.

From http://www.macs.nu/files/MACS_identification_chart_eng.pdf.

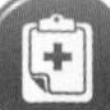

CASE STUDY 29-1 Surgical Reconstruction and Postoperative Therapy for Hypoplastic Thumb

In the following case study consider:

1. How does assessment for an infant with a congenital difference of the hand differ from the assessment of an older child?
2. How does intervention progress and what clinical parameters and family considerations and preferences guide the progression of treatment?
3. What functional differences does the child achieve following surgical reconstruction and postoperative therapy?

Connor, an 8-month-old infant, was evaluated by the orthopedic hand surgeon secondary to keeping his right thumb in his palm. The hand surgeon diagnosed him with a mild right hypoplastic thumb and referred him to occupational therapy for range of motion (ROM), splinting, and fine motor skills. The hand clinic is located 1 hour away from Connor's home. During the initial occupational therapy evaluation, the therapist interviewed the family to identify the family's concerns and priorities and assessed Connor's ROM during play-based activities. The occupational therapist noticed that Connor displayed no active palmar abduction and exhibited thumb extension to neutral when attempting to grasp with his right hand, but otherwise kept his thumb flexed in his palm. The occupational therapist:

- Fit him with a nighttime wrist and thumb spica splint with the interphalangeal joint included in full extension and thumb in palmar abduction.
- Instructed his family in passive ROM exercises for thumb extension and palmar and radial abduction.
- Provided home program activities to promote grasping toys placed in the first web space (e.g., grasping trike handle between thumb and index finger) and pinch grasp (e.g., turning book pages, picking up finger foods with a pinch grasp, and picking up small toys using thumb).

Two weeks later, the family reported that he was tolerating his night splint well and displaying no change in active ROM (AROM) during the day. The therapist fit him with a soft neoprene hand-based short opponens thumb splint for day wear to promote palmar pinch grasp by stabilizing the thumb in abduction.

Connor did not return to therapy again until he was 14 months old secondary to social factors within his family. At this time he displayed improved AROM in his right thumb but continued to hold his thumb flexed in his palm during inactivity. He had outgrown his daytime splint; therefore, he was fitted with a new neoprene hand-based short opponens splint and the family was educated in activities to promote spherical and pinch grasp for a home exercise program. Over the next 3 months, he continued to improve the AROM in his right thumb during play but only while wearing the splint. His monthly occupational therapy sessions consisted of splint modifications to accommodate for growth, activities for right thumb active pinch grasp, and AROM in extension and abduction.

At 18 months of age, Connor continued to display improved right thumb function when wearing the soft splint, but kept his right thumb resting in his palm when a splint was not applied. He needed to wear the splint to pick up finger foods with a palmar pinch grasp or attempt to hold a toy (such as small ball) with an open fist web space. Connor's family decided to return to the orthopedic hand surgeon and opted for surgical reconstruction of his right thumb. The surgeon performed a tendon transfer for right thumb opposition and a web space deepening to promote palmar abduction of the thumb and a collateral ligament reconstruction of the right thumb metacarpophalangeal (MCP) joint for increased stability of the thumb MCP joint. Connor was placed in a cast for 4 weeks after surgery and then referred to occupational therapy for postoperative therapy.

Connor was 22 months old at the time of his postoperative occupational therapy evaluation. He had a thick, raised scar in his first web space (i.e., space between his thumb and index finger) from the web space deepening and trace edema in his first web space and thenar region. He displayed a functional arc of right thumb AROM in all planes aside from not having active interphalangeal joint flexion of his right thumb. An elastomer scar pad was fashioned with the right thumb positioned in palmar abduction and the family was instructed to don it at night. The occupational therapist instructed his family in scar massage and home program activities for pinch grasp and opposition of thumb to each fingertip in his right upper extremity, including playing games to incorporate pinch grasp such as puzzles and playing with smaller toys such as small zoo animals.

Connor's family missed an appointment and returned 1 month following the occupational therapy postoperative re-evaluation. They reported that Connor continued to keep his thumb resting in neutral to slight adduction when he was not using his right hand to hold or manipulate items. The occupational therapist recommended weekly occupational therapy for right thumb AROM and fine motor skills; however, the family opted for every other week visits.

During the next 2 months, the therapist used kinesiotape to support the thumb in abduction for the first month. She used neuromuscular electrical stimulation (NMES) for training the adductor digiti minimi, the tendon transferred to perform thumb abduction. The family was educated in (1) home program activities (focusing on palmar pinch and opposition), (2) kinesiotape application, and (3) NMES. The family performed home program activities for right thumb AROM while Connor received NMES one to two times per day. He also wore tape continuously during the first month of home program activities, discontinuing it after a month per the therapist's recommendation because he was noted to have improved palmar abduction. Connor also continued with the night scar pad for his first web space that positioned the thumb in palmar abduction throughout this time.

Approximately 3 months after surgery, Connor displayed palmar abduction and opposition with his right thumb and no longer held his right thumb resting in flexion or adduction. Connor demonstrated a functional spherical grasp and palmar pinch in his right thumb. He learned to use his right hand to hold a marker for coloring and maintain grasp on the handle bar of a riding toy with an open first web space. He was discharged from therapy and all formal home exercise program activities were discontinued because his scar was flat and pliable and he displayed good right thumb function and AROM.

TABLE 29-7 Upper Extremity Surgeries for Children with Neuromuscular Impairment of the Upper Extremity

Type of Procedure	Description of Procedure	Example	Goal of Procedure
Tendon transfer	The origin of a muscle is left in place and the insertion is re-routed	Example: Green transfer (flexor carpi ulnaris [FCU] to the extensor carpi radialis or extensor carpi brevis)	To improve active motion in a specific plane. For a Green transfer the goal is to improve active wrist extension
Joint fusion	The two bones of the joint are surgically fused through surgical fixation of the bones across the joint	Wrist fusion First CMC fusion	To stabilize a joint for improved function or to improve or preserve skin integrity (ex. first CMC fusion to keep the thumb out of palm)
Tenotomy	A tendon is released from its insertion	FCU release	To release a specific tendon that is placing a very strong pull on a joint into a plane that limits function
Tendon lengthening	The length of the tendon is surgically advanced to decrease tendon tightness	Flexor tendon lengthening	To allow for improved active joint motion For example, in a flexor tendon lengthening of the long finger flexors, the patient may have improved active digit extension for increased active release of grasp

When children with CP experience muscle spasticity changes, for example, as is sometimes related to growth, they may incur secondary orthopedic impairments, including joint contractures and muscle imbalances limiting functional capacity. Surgical procedures, such as tendon transfers, joint fusions, tendon releases, and tendon lengthening (Table 29-7) are sometimes completed to improve function or correct contractures. The occupational therapist uses specific postsurgical rehabilitation protocols to guide the timing of interventions in relation to healing. In the early recovery period, the occupational therapist may fabricate splints for positioning and improving ROM, as well as educate the patient and family on scar management strategies and healing. Intervention progresses to include ROM exercises, functional skills training, and strengthening as appropriate for the surgical intervention performed.

Children with an SCI affecting C5-C8, T1 have limited arm and hand function. When an SCI is incomplete, the child may regain upper extremity function for several years as the nerves regenerate.[88] In the early phases of rehabilitation, the occupational therapist often fabricates splint(s) to prevent deformity and promote function. As the child's recovery reaches a plateau, the child may be a candidate for surgical procedures to maximize hand function. Surgical procedures, typically nerve grafts, tendon transfers, or joint fusions, are often used to restore active elbow extension, tenodesis grasp, and lateral pinch.[40,54,56]

Specific postsurgical rehabilitation protocols for SCI are used to guide the timing of interventions in relation to healing. Similar to CP and TBI patients, in the early recovery period, the occupational therapist may fabricate splints for positioning and improving ROM, as well as educate the patient and family on scar management strategies and healing. Intervention includes ROM exercises, functional skills training, and strengthening as appropriate for the surgical intervention.

Neurodegenerative Conditions

Children with degenerative neuromuscular conditions, such as Duchenne muscular dystrophy (DMD) or spinal muscular atrophy (SMA), are typically referred to therapy when their mobility and upper extremity function begin to deteriorate. Occupational therapists use splinting to preserve ROM and educate the family in stretching programs and positioning strategies to maximize function, improve comfort, and limit joint deformity. Additionally, activity modifications and assistive equipment are recommended to optimize functional independence.

Rheumatic Conditions

Pediatric rheumatic conditions encompass a wide variety of autoimmune conditions that can affect joint and soft tissue of the upper extremity. Juvenile idiopathic arthritis (JIA), SLE, and scleroderma are some of the more common diagnoses. The treatment strategies for children with pediatric rheumatic conditions are determined according to the child's stage of disease process and level of functional impairment. Intervention goals for children with active joint inflammation (i.e., joint pain and swelling) focus on limiting joint injury, preserving mobility through AROM exercises, managing pain, and enhancing function. Therapy for children with no signs of active joint inflammation and controlled disease process includes stretching for joints with limited mobility and strengthening. Because rheumatic conditions are characterized by intermittent flares in the disease process, the occupational therapist works closely with the medical care team to know the state of the child's health to guide the intervention plan. Family education on activity modification, joint protection, and energy conservation techniques remains important during all stages of the condition.

Ehlers Danlos Syndrome

Ehlers Danlos syndrome (EDS) is a genetic condition characterized by a collagen deficiency causing increased soft tissue elasticity and global joint hypermobility. Children with EDS experience joint pain and fatigue.[110] Frequently, children with EDS also have associated comorbidities, such as sleep difficulty, headaches, gastrointestinal dysmotility, and postural orthostatic tachycardia syndrome (POTS), requiring a coordinated care team to manage their multiple medical concerns. It is not uncommon for it to take years before a child is diagnosed with EDS,[93] yet the child may have endured joint pain and fatigue for several years. Therefore a hand therapist may be the first to identify or question the possibility of the diagnosis of EDS.

Whether or not the diagnosis is the primary reason for referral to a hand therapist or just suspected by the therapist, the intervention strategies for children with EDS are the same. Because of the increased joint mobility and tendency toward end range joint hyperextension, their joints are more predisposed to micro trauma, which presents as arthralgia (i.e., joint pain)[75] and sometimes localized joint swelling. Children with EDS are more likely to have pain with sustained repetitive use of their upper extremities such as while writing or playing a musical instrument. Occupational therapists use activity modifications and joint protection strategies to decrease joint strain and pain. These children may have altered proprioceptive registration[92] and benefit from proprioceptive training exercises (Figure 29-18) to learn the feel of the joint end range without going into hyperextension. Often these children use excessive force with grasp patterns on writing tools and place strain on the finger and thumb joints. Strengthening the wrist and hand muscles and adaptive writing strategies (Figure 29-19) can improve success with writing. When children continue to show joint instability, they may benefit from external supports, such as splints (Figure 29-20) or therapeutic taping, to provide joint support and limit positions that strain the joints.[75]

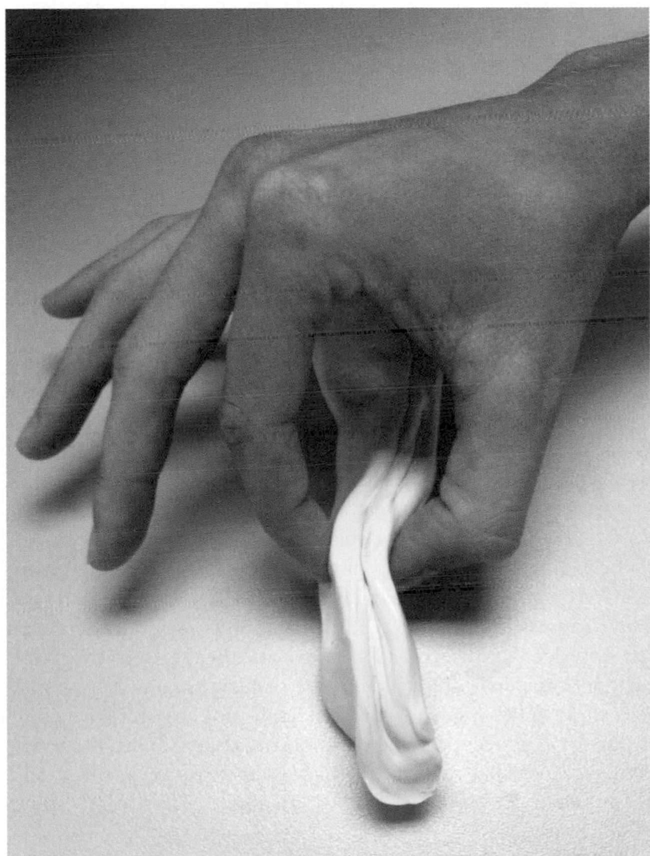

FIGURE 29-18 One example of a proprioceptive retraining exercise an occupational therapist may use is depicted. The child is learning to gauge the amount of pressure exerted when holding a writing instrument by performing tip-to-tip pinch with Theraputty and keeping the joints in flexion versus hyperextension while producing only enough force to make a small indentation in the putty.

Upper Extremity Injury

Acquired impairments of the upper extremity are the result of a trauma that results in injury to one or more of anatomic

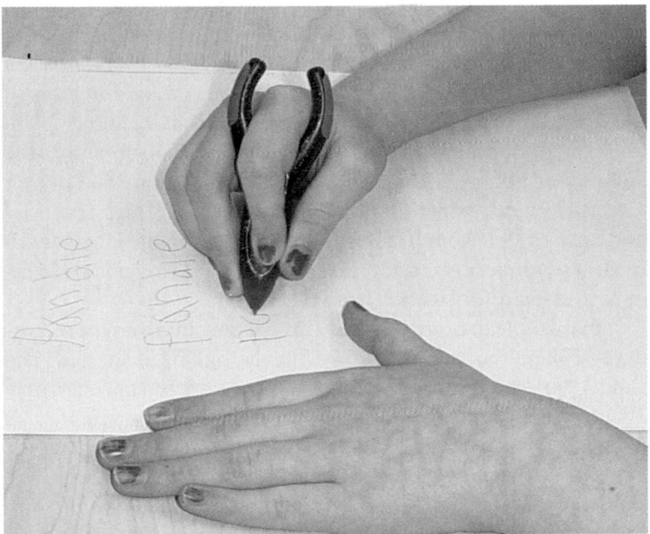

FIGURE 29-19 A Twist and Write pencil is one adaptive writing utensil that can decrease the strain on the interphalangeal joints of the hand with writing.

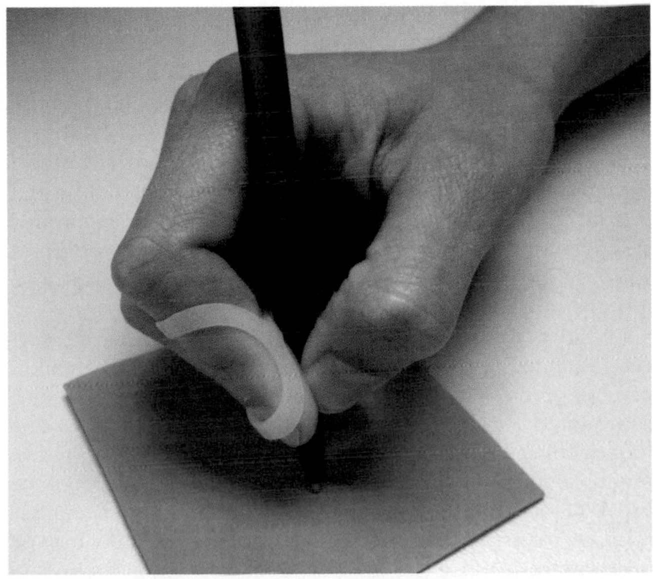

FIGURE 29-20 An Oval-8 splint placed at the distal interphalangeal (DIP) joint to prevent pain in the DIP joint that occurs with hyperextension of the index finger DIP (a common phenomenon with EDS) when writing.

substructures of the upper extremities. Brachial plexus birth palsy is type of trauma that is commonly seen in infants who are referred to therapy. Toddlers and older children can acquire injury to one or multiple structures in the upper extremities, such as the bones, nerves, or other soft tissue structures.

Brachial Plexus Birth Palsy

Brachial plexus birth palsies (BPBP) are typically the result of a shoulder traction injury (shoulder dystocia) at the time of delivery. The incidence of BPBP is 0.38 to 3 per 1000 births in the United States.[85,116] The mildest form of injury is neuropraxia, stretching of the nerve fibers. With neurapraxic injuries, the healing resolves without surgical management and typically within 2 to 3 months. When the injury involves axonal damage (axonotmesis), the nerve regenerates at the rate of 1 mm/day. When the nature of injury is axonotmesis, recovery may be incomplete and may require surgery to maximize function of the affected extremity. When the trauma has resulted in an avulsion of the cell body from the axon (neurotmesis), the nerve does not regenerate and surgery is necessary to attempt to restore nerve function. A noninvasive diagnostic test does not exist to determine the type of nerve injury in infants with BPBP, so clinicians closely monitor motor recovery to determine the need for surgical reconstruction.

Brachial plexus birth palsies can present in a variety of patterns. When the entire brachial plexus has been injured, the child's entire extremity is flaccid. This occurs in approximately 20% of patients.[23] However, the most common presentation is Erb's palsy, comprising about 38% to 73% of patients.[23] In Erb's palsy the C5/C6 nerve roots are damaged; therefore, the child has good hand function but limited shoulder function. In the classic position of the upper extremity in Erb's palsy, the arm is held with the shoulder internally rotated, elbow extended, forearm pronated, and wrist flexed.

In children with BPBP, therapy is necessary during the first few months to preserve ROM and prevent deformity. The occupational therapist also educates the family in positioning to promote the child's progression through normal developmental milestones and in sensory stimulation to the affected upper extremity to enhance sensory perception and prevent neglect of the affected upper extremity (i.e., the habit of avoiding use of the upper extremity).[77] Approximately 66% of BPBPs have complete recovery with full restoration of the upper extremity by 12 months of age, requiring therapy during this period.[77] The child's returning function should be monitored closely during the first several months because the pattern of recovery indicates whether early surgery (at around 4 to 6 months of age) is necessary.

A variety of surgeries may be performed to optimize recovery and enhance function in children with BPBP. The child's pattern of recovery helps determine which surgery is most appropriate. A nerve graft surgery, performed at around 3 to 4 months of age, is common for a child who exhibits no return in muscle function distal to specific damaged nerve roots of the brachial plexus. Surgeries such as tendon transfers, muscle releases, rotational osteotomies, and/or muscle grafts may be necessary to increase the upper extremity function for a child with incomplete recovery. These surgeries can take place over several years in the child's life and the child may benefit from occupational therapy following each surgery to promote recovery and maximize function.

Upper Extremity Fractures

Fractures can occur in any bone or multiple bones in the upper extremity. Fractures of the distal radius are the most common fracture in children.[78] Children are more likely than adults to sustain forearm shaft fractures, often fracturing both the radius and the ulna.[79] Fractures of the bone shaft take longer to heal and are more susceptible to reinjury than fractures at the epiphysis, such as distal radius fractures. As a result, fractures of the forearm are typically casted longer than a distal radius fracture. Fractures of the carpal bones are rare in children; among carpal bone fractures, the scaphoid is the most frequently fractured.[17] Metacarpal fractures are more commonly found in children over the age of 8 and are typically the result of a fight or sport injury.[113] In the fingers, fractures of the third phalanx are the most common and tend to heal well without the need for therapy.[113] Fractures elsewhere in the digits, especially if they are interarticular (i.e., in the region of the joint), are more likely to require therapy.[33] Elbow fractures, more so than fractures elsewhere in the upper extremity, may have associated nerve palsies as a result of trauma to the nerve.[46] If the elbow requires immobilization for more than 2 to 3 weeks, a child is likely to have joint stiffness and require therapy to regain mobility. Children who have an associated nerve palsy require occupational therapy interventions to address the deficits associated with the palsy. Generally, humeral shaft fractures, unless they have associated radial nerve palsy, heal well without the need for therapy.[25]

Overall, the majority of children who sustain upper extremity fractures do not require therapy. When fractures have associated trauma, such as nerve palsy, therapy may begin before the child has had his or her cast removed. Therapy goals include improving hand function and preventing deformity. If a child has hypersensitivity and/or allodynia (i.e., pain in response to a nonpainful stimulus such as a cotton ball or wind on the skin) following a fracture, early therapy is indicated to prevent complex regional pain syndrome (CRPS). Fractures that require surgery for fixation and interarticular fractures are more severe and more likely to require therapy to restore joint movement.[113] Children who avoid using their upper extremities or affected digits after sustaining fractures can benefit from therapy to restore optimal function in the affected upper extremities.

Children wear a cast or splint until the fracture has begun to heal. For children with complex fractures or nerve damage, AROM begins immediately after the cast is removed. Therapy can progress to include PROM and light strengthening as the physician indicates adequate bone healing. If the child experiences persistent stiffness, the occupational therapist may use static progressive or dynamic splinting to improve joint mobility. The occupational therapist must check with the referring care provider to ensure that healing has progressed and is sufficient to apply the force of the mobilization splint (Case Study 29-2).

Tendon and Ligament Injuries

Tendon injuries in the hand and arm can occur as the result of a laceration, a trauma that ruptures the tendon from its insertion, or a complex upper extremity trauma (e.g., crush injury). Most tendon injuries require surgical repair and a period of immobilization for healing before therapy is initiated. An exception is a mallet finger, which is an injury to the terminal extensor tendon in the digit. If treated acutely, mallet fingers

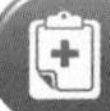

CASE STUDY 29-2 Upper Extremity Trauma: Case Study

In the following case study consider:

1. How does assessment for an upper extremity trauma advance over the course of intervention and what does it entail?
2. How does intervention progress and what clinical parameters guide the progression?
3. What role does the family have in the intervention plan, including completion of home programming?

Emily, a 4-year-old right hand–dominant girl, sustained a right supracondylar elbow fracture when she fell from monkey bars. She required closed reduction and percutaneous pinning of the fracture site and was casted 4 weeks after her surgery. Two weeks after her cast was removed she was referred to an occupational therapy because she was not using her affected arm. During her initial evaluation the occupational therapist assessed right upper extremity range of motion (ROM), sensation and grip strength and interviewed the family to identify their priorities and the child's roles and occupations. The following limitations were noted.

1. Range of motion:

Active Range of Motion	Flexion	Extension
Right elbow (affected upper extremity)	110	−15
Left elbow	135	+15

She also was lacking right thumb active palmar abduction and interphalangeal joint flexion and active flexion of the distal interphalangeal joints of the index and middle fingers. Passive range of motion (PROM) of the joints described in the preceding were within normal limits.

2. Diminished light touch sensation and report of constant tingling in her right thumb
3. Muscle atrophy in the thenar eminence and region of the first and second metacarpals
4. Grip strength of 3 pounds on her right as compared with 10 pounds on the left
5. Report of avoiding use of her right upper extremity for dressing, writing, and play

Emily was to attend kindergarten soon, and her mother was concerned that she would have difficulty writing and coloring with her right hand.

At the time of her evaluation, the occupational therapist instructed Emily and her mother in a home exercise program to be performed two times per day, including active ROM (AROM) and PROM and desensitization activities (massage and touching her right arm with different textures). Emily returned to therapy once per week for reassessment of her functional status, ROM, and sensation and progression of her home exercise program. Emily continued to avoid use of her right arm during functional tasks and had difficulty with coloring and writing in school. The occupational therapist fabricated a constraint cast for her left upper extremity. She continued to complete her home program activities for ROM and desensitization and used the constraint cast as much as possible throughout the day. At a 2-week follow-up visit, reassessment revealed that Emily had made small improvements with AROM and resolved hypersensitivity and limitations in sensory discrimination. She was using her right arm to assist with dressing, but not for writing or donning her sock. Additionally, she had decreased grip and pinch strength in her right arm as compared with the left. Therefore hand strengthening with extra soft putty for grip and pinch were added to her established home program for ROM; desensitization activities were discontinued.

She continued to return every 2 weeks for reassessment and evaluation of her home program activities. Six weeks later she displayed improved sensory return, as evidenced by prehension using opposition of her thumb to the tip of her middle finger instead of a palmar pinch grasp. Sensory assessment using Semmes Weinstein monofilaments revealed deep pressure (SW = 6.65) sensation only in her distal volar index finger and loss of protective sensation (SW = 4.56) in her thumb and proximal volar index finger. Emily and her mother reported continued functional limitations with holding a pencil/crayon and donning socks and pants with her right upper extremity. The therapist taught Emily how to hold a pencil using modifications (1-inch diameter foam pencil grip) and increased the level of resistance of putty for hand strengthening on the home program.

One month later, Emily displayed improved sensation to SW = 4.56 (loss of protective sensation) at the tip of her index finger, so she was taught to perform sensory re-education activities for stereognosis and touch localization as part of her home program.

Emily continued with monthly visits to progress her home exercise program for strengthening and sensory re-education until she was 8 months from her date of injury. At discharge she fastened buttons and zippers with her right upper extremity and she used a dynamic tripod grasp for writing/coloring with no reports of fatigue or difficulty completing her school work. Her Semmes Weinstein scores improved to normal sensation. She exhibited age-appropriate patterns and strength with her right grip and pinch.

will often heal through a period of splinting or casting.[80] The occupational therapist must follow very specific rehabilitation protocols to guide the intervention progression for tendon injuries.

Each joint in the upper extremity has ligaments that connect the bones to form the joint. These ligaments are critical for providing joint stability. Ligament injuries in children may occur in the hand, wrist, or elbow and are typically sports injuries or are the result of a fall.[55] When a ligament is injured, the joint often becomes painful, edematous, limited in ROM, and can be unstable, depending on the degree of ligament tear. If the ligament tear is a minor injury, meaning only a small portion of the ligament is torn, it is treated conservatively with a period of immobilization. More severe injuries, in which a large percentage of the ligament is torn or the ligament is completely ruptured, require surgical repair followed by

TABLE 29-8 Typical Presentation of Upper Extremity Nerve Injury and Recommended Splints

Nerve Involved	Pattern of Motor Impairment	Recommended Splints
Radial nerve	Absent or weakened: forearm supination, wrist extension, MCP extension, and thumb radial abduction	Thumb spica splint or wrist cock up splint; Benik radial nerve splint; Robinson Inrigger (adult sizes only)
Median nerve (high lesion)	Absent or weak: pronation, wrist flexion, digit flexion of the PIPs and DIPs of the IF and MF, thumb palmar abduction and opposition, thumb flexion	Thumb spica with thumb in palmar abduction
Median nerve (low lesion)	Absent or weak: thumb palmar abduction and opposition	Thumb spica with thumb in palmar abduction or short opponens splint
Ulnar nerve	Absent or weak intrinsic muscles resulting in claw positioning of RF and SF	Anticlaw splint for SF and RF (Note: If the child has MN injury, the claw deformity will also be present in the index, middle, ring, and small fingers and the anticlaw should include all four digits)

IF, Index finger; MF, middle finger; RF, ring finger; SF, small finger.

immobilization. Ligamentous injuries that are surgically repaired are more likely to require therapy to restore function than conservatively managed ligament injuries. When the child has persistent pain, joint stiffness, and/or limited function, occupational therapy is indicated.

Nerve Injuries

Primary nerve injuries are those that result from a lesion directly to the nerve, such as a laceration at the wrist severing the median nerve or a traction injury to the brachial plexus. Anatomic compression of a nerve can also result in symptoms of primary nerve injury. Carpal tunnel syndrome, which is rare in children, is compression of the median nerve as it passes under the carpal ligament. The ulnar nerve and the radial nerve also have anatomic sites of possible compression neuropathy.

Secondary nerve injuries occur as the result of an upper extremity trauma causing nerve injury. For example, the radial nerve wraps around the shaft of the humerus and may be injured by a humeral shaft fracture. Similarly, compartment syndrome is a condition in which the fascia in the arm has extreme swelling. If compartment syndrome is not surgically managed in its most acute state, the compression from the swelling can cause nerve compression or even necrosis of the nerve. When an injury to a peripheral nerve occurs in the upper extremity, a specific pattern of motor and sensory impairment occurs. Table 29-8 outlines the pattern of motor impairment and types of splints that may be used during the rehabilitation of peripheral nerve injuries in the upper extremity.

Upper extremity nerve injury can also result from a systemic process. Some systemic autoimmune conditions, such as SLE, can have associated neuropathy. Nerve damage in the arm and hand may also be the result of drug toxicity to the nerves. This can result from chemotherapy or other strong medications that children with a systemic disease process may need to take.

A child who has upper extremity nerve impairment will have loss of motor function and sensation in the innervation pattern of the nerve following the path of the nerve, distal from the site of nerve insult. Occupational therapists use ROM exercises and splinting to preserve joint mobility until AROM begins to return. Often children with nerve injuries experience pain and hypersensitivity in the affected upper extremity. In these cases occupational therapists use desensitization techniques. Occupational therapists may also use sensory retraining strategies, NMES, and strengthening in the rehabilitation of upper extremity nerve injuries.

Complex Regional Pain Syndrome

Complex regional pain syndrome (CRPS) is characterized by pain, specifically allodynia, and hyperalgesia (i.e., abnormal pain sensitivity such that an individual rates pain at a higher rate than typical for the pain stimulus). The extremity may also be edematous and have trophic changes, such as skin color changes and changes in nail growth and appearance. In progressed stages of the condition, bone density can decrease. Complex regional pain syndrome is classified as type I and type II; type I does not have an associated nerve injury and type II follows an injury to the nerve.[36]

Children with CRPS often guard against use of their affected extremities. Early therapy is recognized as a critical aspect of disease management.[47,103] Traditionally, intervention strategies included the use of weight bearing, desensitization, AROM exercises, and pain management strategies. More recently therapists have found mirror therapy[15,26] and graded motor imagery[73,74] effective with this patient population. An integrated approach of medical, psychological, and therapeutic care is most effective for recovery.[47,100,109]

Summary

Occupational therapists specializing in hand therapy use concepts and principles from developmental, motor skill acquisition, rehabilitative, and biomechanical frames of reference to guide assessment, intervention planning, and intervention. This chapter described the specific principles, strategies, and modalities for common upper extremity conditions that are used by occupational therapists specializing in pediatric hand therapy.

- Common conditions that receive occupational therapy intervention include: (1) congenital differences of the hand or arm, (2) upper extremity impairments caused by an underlying neurologic or systemic disorder, and (3) injuries of the arm or hand.

- Occupational therapists working in the pediatric hand therapy setting gather information from chart review of the medical history, child/family interview, and formal and informal assessment to guide intervention.
- In selecting an intervention the occupational therapist considers the child's developmental stage, child/family goals, the desired clinical outcomes established from the therapist's ongoing clinical assessment, and the category of hand impairment.
- Pain management is an important aspect of therapy that can have priority in the intervention sequence.
- Occupational therapists implement a wide variety of interventions for children with upper extremity conditions. These include physical agent modalities, splinting, casting, kinesiotape, mirror therapy, and activity modifications. Occupational therapists also support wound care, edema control, and scar management. An intervention session may include activities that promote sensory re-education, ROM, strengthening, manipulation, and coordination.
- Pediatric hand therapy involves a high level of coordination with surgeons, physicians, nurses, other therapists, potentially social workers, and always family members.

REFERENCES

1. Ahearn, I., Bird, S., & Gordon, M. (2011). *Kinesio tape's effect on musculature associated with upper cross syndrome*. Retrieved January 1, 2014 from: <http://www.tapingbase.nl/sites/default/files/kinesio_tapes_effect_on_musculature_associated_with_upper_cross_syndrome_syndrome.pdf>.
2. Atroshi, I., Gummesson, C., Andersson, B., et al. (2000). The disabilities of the arm, shoulder and hand (DASH) outcome questionnaire: Reliability and validity of the Swedish version evaluated in 176 patients. *Acta Orthopaedica*, *71*(6), 613–618.
3. Baeyer, C. L. (2009). Numerical rating scale for self-report of pain intensity in children and adolescents: Recent progress and further questions. *European Journal of Pain*, *13*(10), 1005–1007.
4. Bajd, T., Gregoric, M., Vodovnik, L., et al. (1985). Electrical stimulation in treating spasticity resulting from spinal cord injury. *Archives of Physical Medicine and Rehabilitation*, *66*(8), 515.
5. Baryza, M. J., & Baryza, G. A. (1995). The Vancouver Scar Scale: An administration tool and its interrater reliability. *Journal of Burn Care & Research*, *16*(5), 535–538.
6. Basciani, M., & Intiso, D. (2006). Botulinum toxin type-A and plaster cast treatment in children with upper brachial plexus palsy. *Developmental Neurorehabilitation*, *9*(2), 165–170.
7. Batavia, M. (2004). Contraindications for superficial heat and therapeutic ultrasound: Do sources agree? *Archives of Physical Medicine and Rehabilitation*, *85*(6), 1006–1012.
8. Bell-Krotoski, J., & Tomancik, E. (1987). The repeatability of testing with Semmes-Weinstein monofilaments. *The Journal of Hand Surgery*, *12*(1), 155.
9. Berman, B., Viera, M. H., Amini, S., et al. (2008). Prevention and management of hypertrophic scars and keloids after burns in children. *Journal of Craniofacial Surgery*, *19*(4), 989–1006.
10. Beyer, J. E., Denyes, M., & Villarruel, A. (1992). The creation, validation, and continuing development of the Oucher: A measure of pain intensity in children. *Journal of Pediatric Nursing*, *7*(5), 335.
11. Beyer, J. E. (1984). *The Oucher: A user's manual and technical report*. Evanston, IL: The Hospital Play Equipment Company.
12. Bieri, D., Reeve, R. A., Champion, G. D., et al. (1990). The Faces Pain Scale for the self-assessment of the severity of pain experienced by children: Development, initial validation, and preliminary investigation for ratio scale properties. *Pain*, *41*(2), 139–150.
13. Booth, M. Y., Yates, C. C., Edgar, T. S., et al. (2003). Serial casting vs. combined intervention with botulinum toxin A and serial casting in the treatment of spastic equinus in children. *Pediatric Physical Therapy*, *15*(4), 216–220.
14. Bradbury, E. (1998). Psychological issues for children and their parents. In *Congenital malformations of the hand and forearm* (pp. 49–56). London: Churchill Livingstone.
15. Cacchio, A., De Blasis, E., De Blasis, V., et al. (2009). Mirror therapy in complex regional pain syndrome type 1 of the upper limb in stroke patients. *Neurorehabilitation and Neural Repair*, *23*(8), 792–799.
16. Cheng, J., Chow, S., & Leung, P. (1987). Classification of 578 cases of congenital upper limb anomalies with the IFSSH system: A 10 years' experience. *The Journal of Hand Surgery*, *12*(6), 1055.
17. Christodoulou, A., & Colton, C. (1986). Scaphoid fractures in children. *Journal of Pediatric Orthopaedics*, *6*(1), 37–39.
18. Clark, G. L. (1997). *Hand rehabilitation: A practical guide*. London: Churchill Livingstone.
19. Davis Sears, E., & Chung, K. C. (2010). Validity and responsiveness of the Jebsen–Taylor Hand Function Test. *The Journal of Hand Surgery*, *35*(1), 30–37.
20. De Jong, A., Bremer, M., Schouten, M., et al. (2005). Reliability and validity of the pain observation scale for young children and the visual analogue scale in children with burns. *Burns: Journal of the International Society for Burn Injuries*, *31*(2), 198–204.
21. Dellon, A. (1978). The moving two-point discrimination test: Clinical evaluation of the quickly adapting fiber/receptor system. *The Journal of Hand Surgery*, *3*(5), 474.
22. Dimick, M. P., Caro, C. M., Kasch, M. C., et al. (2009). 2008 Practice analysis study of hand therapy. *Journal of Hand Therapy*, *22*(4), 361–376.
23. Dodds, S. D., & Wolfe, S. W. (2000). Perinatal brachial plexus palsy. *Current Opinion in Pediatrics*, *12*(1), 40–47.
24. Dong, V. A.-Q., Tung, I. H.-H., Siu, H. W.-Y., et al. (2013). Studies comparing the efficacy of constraint-induced movement therapy and bimanual training in children with unilateral cerebral palsy: A systematic review. *Developmental Neurorehabilitation*, *16*(2), 133–143.
25. Ekholm, R., Tidermark, J., Törnkvist, H., et al. (2006). Outcome after closed functional treatment of humeral shaft fractures. *Journal of Orthopaedic Trauma*, *20*(9), 591–596.
26. Ezendam, D., Bongers, R. M., & Jannink, M. J. (2009). Systematic review of the effectiveness of mirror therapy in upper extremity function. *Disability & Rehabilitation*, *31*(26), 2135–2149.
27. Fedorczyk, J. (1997). The role of physical agents in modulating pain. *Journal of Hand Therapy*, *10*(2), 110–121.
28. Finkelstein, H. (1930). Stenosing tenovaginitis at the radial styloid process. *Journal of Bone and Joint Surgery*, *12*, 509–540.

29. Flatt, A. E. (1994). *The care of congenital hand anomalies* (2nd ed.). St. Louis: Quality Medical Publishing.
30. Goldstein, E. J. (1992). Bite wounds and infection. *Clinical Infectious Diseases, 14*(3), 633–640.
31. Gómez, J. E. (2002). Upper extremity injuries in youth sports. *Pediatric Clinics of North America, 49*(3), 593.
32. Gordon, A. M., Hung, Y.-C., Brandao, M., et al. (2011). Bimanual training and constraint-induced movement therapy in children with hemiplegic cerebral palsy: A randomized trial. *Neurorehabilitation and Neural Repair, 25*(8), 692–702.
33. Grad, J. (1986). Children's skeletal injuries. *The Orthopedic Clinics of North America, 17*(3), 437.
34. Gummesson, C., Atroshi, I., & Ekdahl, C. (2003). The Disabilities of the Arm, Shoulder and Hand (DASH) outcome questionnaire: Longitudinal construct validity and measuring self-rated health change after surgery. *BMC Musculoskeletal Disorders, 4*(1), 11.
35. Gygax, M. J., Schneider, P., & Newman, C. J. (2011). Mirror therapy in children with hemiplegia: A pilot study. *Developmental Medicine & Child Neurology, 53*(5), 473–476.
36. Harden, R. N., & Bruehl, S. P. (2006). Diagnosis of complex regional pain syndrome: Signs, symptoms, and new empirically derived diagnostic criteria. *The Clinical Journal of Pain, 22*(5), 415–419.
37. Hesse, S., Reiter, F., Konrad, M., et al. (1998). Botulinum toxin type A and short-term electrical stimulation in the treatment of upper limb flexor spasticity after stroke: A randomized, double-blind, placebo-controlled trial. *Clinical Rehabilitation, 12*(5), 381–388.
38. Hicks, C. L., von Baeyer, C. L., Spafford, P. A., et al. (2001). The Faces Pain Scale-Revised: Toward a common metric in pediatric pain measurement. *Pain, 93*(2), 173.
39. Hoare, B., Wasiak, J., Imms, C., et al. (2007). Constraint-induced movement therapy in the treatment of the upper limb in children with hemiplegic cerebral palsy. *Cochrane Database Systems Review*, Apr 18: (2) CD004149.
40. Hoyen, H., Gonzalez, E., Williams, P., et al. (2002). Management of the paralyzed elbow in tetraplegia. *Life (Chicago, Ill.: 1978), 12*(36), 61.
41. Hunter, M., McDowell, L., Hennessy, R., et al. (2000). An evaluation of the Faces Pain Scale with young children. *Journal of Pain and Symptom Management, 20*(2), 122–129.
42. ICF, W. (2001). *International Classification of Functioning, Disability and Health* (pp. 3–25). Geneva: World Health Organization.
43. Iosa, M., Morelli, D., Nanni, M. V., et al. (2010). Functional taping: A promising technique for children with cerebral palsy. *Developmental Medicine and Child Neurology, 52*(6), 587–589.
44. Jaraczewska, E., & Long, C. (2006). Kinesio® taping in stroke: Improving functional use of the upper extremity in hemiplegia. *Topics in Stroke Rehabilitation, 13*(3), 31–42.
45. Jethwa, A., Mink, J., Macarthur, C., et al. (2010). Development of the Hypertonia Assessment Tool (HAT): A discriminative tool for hypertonia in children. *Developmental Medicine & Child Neurology, 52*(5), e83–e87.
46. Jupiter, J. B., Neff, U., Holzach, P., et al. (1985). Intercondylar fractures of the humerus: An operative approach. *The Journal of Bone and Joint Surgery. American Volume, 67*(2), 226.
47. Kachko, L., Efrat, R., Ben Ami, S., et al. (2008). Complex regional pain syndromes in children and adolescents. *Pediatrics International, 50*(4), 523–527.
48. Kanellopoulos, A., Mavrogenis, A., Mitsiokapa, E., et al. (2009). Long lasting benefits following the combination of static night upper extremity splinting with botulinum toxin A injections in cerebral palsy children. *European Journal of Physical and Rehabilitation Medicine, 45*(4), 501.
49. Karadavut, K. I., & Uneri, S. O. (2011). Burnout, depression and anxiety levels in mothers of infants with brachial plexus injury and the effects of recovery on mothers' mental health. *European Journal of Obstetrics, Gynecology, and Reproductive Biology, 157*(1), 43–47.
50. Kase, K., Yasukawa, A., & Martin, P. (2006). *Kinesio taping in pediatrics: Fundamentals and whole body taping.* Santa Fe, NM: Kinesio Taping Association.
51. Katz, B. (1992). Silastic gel sheeting is found to be effective in scar therapy. *Cosmetic Dermatology, 5*, 32–34.
52. Kay, R. M., Rethlefsen, S. A., Fern-Buneo, A., et al. (2004). Botulinum toxin as an adjunct to serial casting treatment in children with cerebral palsy. *The Journal of Bone & Joint Surgery, 86*(11), 2377–2384.
53. Kaya, E., Zinnuroglu, M., & Tugcu, I. (2011). Kinesio taping compared to physical therapy modalities for the treatment of shoulder impingement syndrome. *Clinical Rheumatology, 30*(2), 201–207.
54. Keith, M. W., & Peljovich, A. (2012). Surgical treatments to restore function control in spinal cord injury. *Spinal Cord Injuries E-Book: Handbook of Clinical Neurology Series, 109*, 167.
55. Kerssemakers, S. P., Fotiadou, A. N., de Jonge, M. C., et al. (2009). Sport injuries in the paediatric and adolescent patient: A growing problem. *Pediatric Radiology, 39*(5), 471–484.
56. Koo, B., Peljovich, A., & Bohn, A. (2008). Single-stage tendon transfer reconstruction for active pinch and grasp in tetraplegia. *Topics in Spinal Cord Injury Rehabilitation, 13*(4), 24–36.
57. Laerhoven, H. V., Zaag-Loonen, H. V. D., & Derkx, B. (2004). A comparison of Likert scale and visual analogue scales as response options in children's questionnaires. *Acta Paediatrica, 93*(6), 830–835.
58. Law, M. (2002). Participation in the occupations of everyday life. *American Journal of Occuaptional Therapy, 56*, 640–649.
59. Lerman, J. A., Sullivan, E., Barnes, D. A., et al. (2005). The Pediatric Outcomes Data Collection Instrument (PODCI) and functional assessment of patients with unilateral upper extremity deficiencies. *Journal of Pediatric Orthopaedics, 25*(3), 405–407.
60. Lucado, A. M., Li, Z., Russell, G. B., et al. (2008). Changes in impairment and function after static progressive splinting for stiffness after distal radius fracture. *Journal of Hand Therapy, 21*(4), 319–325.
61. Maihafer, G. C., Llewellyn, M. A., Pillar, W. J., Jr., et al. (2003). A comparison of the figure-of-eight method and water volumetry in measurement of hand and wrist size. *Journal of Hand Therapy, 16*(4), 305–310.
62. Manias, P., & Stasinopoulos, D. (2006). A controlled clinical pilot trial to study the effectiveness of ice as a supplement to the exercise programme for the management of lateral elbow tendinopathy. *British Journal of Sports Medicine, 40*(1), 81–85.
63. Manske, P. R., & Oberg, K. C. (2009). Classification and developmental biology of congenital anomalies of the hand and upper extremity. *The Journal of Bone & Joint Surgery, 91*(Suppl. 4), 3–18.
64. Marx, R. G., Bombardier, C., & Wright, J. G. (1999). What do we know about the reliability and validity of physical examination tests used to examine the upper extremity? *The Journal of Hand Surgery, 24*(1), 185–193.
65. Mathiowetz, V., Volland, G., Kashman, N., et al. (1985). Adult norms for the Box and Block Test of manual dexterity. *The American Journal of Occupational Therapy, 39*(6), 386–391.

66. McCabe, C. S., Haigh, R. C., Ring, E. F., et al. (2003). A controlled pilot study of the utility of mirror visual feedback in the treatment of complex regional pain syndrome (type 1). *Rheumatology (Oxford, England)*, *42*(1), 97–101.
67. McCarthy, M. L., MacKenzie, E. J., Durbin, D. R., et al. (2005). The Pediatric Quality of Life Inventory: An evaluation of its reliability and validity for children with traumatic brain injury. *Archives of Physical Medicine and Rehabilitation*, *86*(10), 1901–1909.
68. McCarthy, M. L., Silberstein, C. E., Atkins, E. A., et al. (2002). Comparing reliability and validity of pediatric instruments for measuring health and well-being of children with spastic cerebral palsy. *Developmental Medicine & Child Neurology*, *44*(7), 468–476.
69. McClure, P. W., Blackburn, L. G., & Dusold, C. (1994). The use of splints in the treatment of joint stiffness: Biologic rationale and an algorithm for making clinical decisions. *Physical Therapy*, *74*(12), 1101–1107.
70. McMulkin, M. L., Baird, G. O., Gordon, A. B., et al. (2007). The pediatric outcomes data collection instrument detects improvements for children with ambulatory cerebral palsy after orthopaedic intervention. *Journal of Pediatric Orthopaedics*, *27*(1), 1–6.
71. Mintken, P. E., Glynn, P., & Cleland, J. A. (2009). Psychometric properties of the shortened Disabilities of the Arm, Shoulder, and Hand Questionnaire (QuickDASH) and Numeric Pain Rating Scale in patients with shoulder pain. *Journal of Shoulder and Elbow Surgery*, *18*(6), 920–926.
72. Moberg, E. (1958). Objective methods for determining the functional value of sensibility in the hand. *Journal of Bone & Joint Surgery, British Volume*, *40*(3), 454–476.
73. Moseley, G. (2004). Graded motor imagery is effective for long-standing complex regional pain syndrome: A randomised controlled trial. *Pain*, *108*(1), 192–198.
74. Moseley, G. (2006). Graded motor imagery for pathologic pain: A randomized controlled trial. *Neurology*, *67*(12), 2129–2134.
75. Murray, K. J. (2006). Hypermobility disorders in children and adolescents. *Best Practice & Research Clinical Rheumatology*, *20*(2), 329–351.
76. Nascimento, L., Glória, A., & Habib, E. (2009). Effects of constraint-induced movement therapy as a rehabilitation strategy for the affected upper limb of children with hemiparesis: Systematic review of the literature. *Revista Brasileira de Fisioterapia*, *13*(2), 97–102.
77. Noetzel, M. J., Park, T. S., Robinson, S., & Kaufman, B. (2001). Prospective study of recovery following neonatal brachial plexus injury. *Journal of Child Neurology*, *16*(7), 488–492.
78. Noonan, K. J., & Price, C. T. (1998). Forearm and distal radius fractures in children. *Journal of the American Academy of Orthopaedic Surgeons*, *6*(3), 146–156.
79. Norkin, W. (2009). *Measurement of joint motion: A guide to goniometry* (4th ed.). Philadelphia: F. A. Davis.
80. Okafor, B., Mbubaegbu, C., Munshi, I., et al. (1997). Mallet deformity of the finger five-year follow-up of conservative treatment. *Journal of Bone & Joint Surgery, British Volume*, *79*(4), 544–547.
81. Omoigui, S. (2007). The biochemical origin of pain: The origin of all pain is inflammation and the inflammatory response. Part 2 of 3. Inflammatory profile of pain syndromes. *Medical Hypotheses*, *69*(6), 1169–1178.
82. Park, E. S., Rha, D.-W., Yoo, J. K., et al. (2010). Short-term effects of combined serial casting and botulinum toxin injection for spastic equinus in ambulatory children with cerebral palsy. *Yonsei Medical Journal*, *51*(4), 579–584.
83. Pin, T. W.-M. (2007). Effectiveness of static weight-bearing exercises in children with cerebral palsy. *Pediatric Physical Therapy*, *19*(1), 62–73.
84. Platz, T., Pinkowski, C., van Wijck, F., et al. (2005). Reliability and validity of arm function assessment with standardized guidelines for the Fugl-Meyer Test, Action Research Arm Test and Box and Block Test: A multicentre study. *Clinical Rehabilitation*, *19*(4), 404–411.
85. Pondaag, W., Malessy, M. J., Van Dijk, J. G., et al. (2004). Natural history of obstetric brachial plexus palsy: A systematic review. *Developmental Medicine & Child Neurology*, *46*(2), 138–144.
86. Poole, J. L., Burtner, P. A., Torres, T. A., et al. (2005). Measuring dexterity in children using the Nine-hole Peg Test. *Journal of Hand Therapy*, *18*(3), 348–351.
87. Prosser, R., Harvey, L., LaStayo, P., et al. (2011). Provocative wrist tests and MRI are of limited diagnostic value for suspected wrist ligament injuries: A cross-sectional study. *Journal of Physiotherapy*, *57*(4), 247–253.
88. Raineteau, O., & Schwab, M. E. (2001). Plasticity of motor systems after incomplete spinal cord injury. *Nature Reviews. Neuroscience*, *2*(4), 263–273.
89. Reese, N. B., & Bandy, W. D. (2009). *Joint range of motion and muscle length testing* (2nd ed.). St. Louis: Saunders.
90. Reiffel, R. S. (1995). Prevention of hypertrophic scars by long-term paper tape application. *Plastic and Reconstructive Surgery*, *96*(7), 1715–1718.
91. Roley, S., DeLany, J., Barrows, C., et al. (2008). Occupational therapy practice framework: Domain and practice. *The American Journal of Occupational Therapy: Official Publication of the American Occupational Therapy Association*, *62*(6), 625.
92. Rombaut, L., De Paepe, A., Malfait, F., et al. (2010). Joint position sense and vibratory perception sense in patients with Ehlers–Danlos syndrome type III (hypermobility type). *Clinical Rheumatology*, *29*(3), 289–295.
93. Ross, J., & Grahame, R. (2011). Joint hypermobility syndrome. *British Medical Journal*, 342.
94. Sherry, D. D., Wallace, C. A., Kelley, C., et al. (1999). Short-and long-term outcomes of children with complex regional pain syndrome type I treated with exercise therapy. *The Clinical Journal of Pain*, *15*(3), 218–223.
95. Skirven, T. M., Osterman, A. L., Fedorczyk, J., et al. (2011). *Rehabilitation of the hand and upper extremity*, 2-vol. set: *Expert consult.* St Louis: Mosby.
96. Smith, Y. A., & Hong, E. (2000). Normative and validation studies of the Nine-hole Peg Test with children. *Perceptual and Motor Skills*, *90*(3), 823–843.
97. Sorenson, M. K. (1989). The edematous hand. *Physical Therapy*, *69*(12), 1059–1064.
98. Spagrud, L. J., Piira, T., & Von Baeyer, C. L. (2003). Children's self-report of pain intensity: The Faces Pain Scale–Revised. *The American Journal of Nursing*, *103*(12), 62–64.
99. Spraggs-Young, K. et al. (2012). A position paper on the use of physical agents/modalities in hand therapy. *American Society of Hand Therapists.*
100. Stanton-Hicks, M. (2003). Complex regional pain syndrome. *Anesthesiology Clinics of North America*, *21*(4), 733.
101. Stern, P. (1990). Tendinitis, overuse syndromes, and tendon injuries. *Hand Clinics*, *6*(3), 467.
102. Swanson, A. (1976). A classification for congenital limb malformations. *The Journal of Hand Surgery*, *1*(1), 8.
103. Teasdall, R. D., Smith, B. P., & Koman, L. A. (2004). Complex regional pain syndrome (reflex sympathetic dystrophy). *Clininical Sports Medicine*, *23*(1), 145–155.
104. Ten Berge, S. R., Boonstra, A. M., Dijkstra, P. U., et al. (2012). A systematic evaluation of the effect of

thumb opponens splints on hand function in children with unilateral spastic cerebral palsy. *Clinical Rehabilitation, 26*(4), 362–371.

105. Thelen, M. D., Dauber, J. A., & Stoneman, P. D. (2008). The clinical efficacy of kinesio tape for shoulder pain: A randomized, double-blinded, clinical trial. *Journal of Orthopaedic and Sports Physical Therapy, 38*(7), 389.
106. Üstün, T. B., Chatterji, S., Bickenbach, J., et al. (2003). The International Classification of Functioning, Disability and Health: A new tool for understanding disability and health. *Disability & Rehabilitation, 25*(11–12), 565–571.
107. Varni, J. W., Burwinkle, T. M., Berrin, S. J., et al. (2006). The PedsQL in pediatric cerebral palsy: Reliability, validity, and sensitivity of the Generic Core Scales and Cerebral Palsy Module. *Developmental Medicine & Child Neurology, 48*(6), 442–449.
108. Vasudevan, S., & Melvin, J. (1979). Upper extremity edema control: Rationale of the techniques. *The American Journal of Occupational Therapy: Official Publication of the American Occupational Therapy Association, 33*(8), 520.
109. Veizi, I. E., Chelimsky, T. C., & Janata, J. W. (2012). Chronic regional pain syndrome: What specialized rehabilitation services do patients require? *Current Pain and Headache Reports, 16*(2), 139–146.
110. Voermans, N. C., Knoop, H., van de Kamp, N., et al. (2010). *Fatigue is a frequent and clinically relevant problem in Ehlers-Danlos syndrome.* Paper presented at the Seminars in Arthritis and Rheumatism.
111. von Baeyer, C. L., Spagrud, L. J., McCormick, J. C., et al. (2009). Three new datasets supporting use of the Numerical Rating Scale (NRS-11) for children's self-reports of pain intensity. *Pain, 143*(3), 223–227.
112. Werner, R. A., Franzblau, A., Gell, N., et al. (2005). A longitudinal study of industrial and clerical workers: Predictors of upper extremity tendonitis. *Journal of Occupational Rehabilitation, 15*(1), 37–46.
113. Worlock, P., & Stower, M. (1986). The incidence and pattern of hand fractures in children. *The Journal of Hand Surgery: British & European Volume, 11*(2), 198–200.
114. Wu, C.-Y., Huang, P.-C., Chen, Y.-T., et al. (2013). Effects of mirror therapy on motor and sensory recovery in chronic stroke: A randomized controlled trial. *Archives of Physical Medicine and Rehabilitation, 94*(6), 1023–1030.
115. Yasukawa, A., Patel, P., & Sisung, C. (2006). Pilot study: Investigating the effects of Kinesio Taping® in an acute pediatric rehabilitation setting. *The American Journal of Occupational Therapy, 60*(1), 104–110.
116. Zafeiriou, D. I., & Psychogiou, K. (2008). Obstetrical brachial plexus palsy. *Pediatric Neurology, 38*(4), 235–242.
117. Zetaruk, M. N. (2000). The young gymnast. *Clinics in Sports Medicine, 19*(4), 757–780.

CHAPTER

30 Trauma-Induced Conditions

Amber Lowe • Patti Sharp • Carrie Thelen • Beth Warnken

KEY TERMS

Spinal cord injury
Traumatic brain injury
Rancho Levels of Cognitive Functioning
Burn injuries
ASIA International Standards for Neurological Classification of SCI
Multidisciplinary team
Acute care
Intensive care
Rehabilitation
Community reintegration

GUIDING QUESTIONS

1. What are some examples of trauma-induced conditions in children and youth? What is the incidence and pattern of these conditions?
2. What is the impact of trauma-induced conditions on occupational performance of children and youth?
3. What are the roles of the occupational therapist across the continuum of care for specific conditions?
4. What are some examples of occupational therapy interventions at each stage of care?
5. How do therapists use therapeutic relationships, grief management, and caregiver education to assist children and youth who have experienced trauma?
6. Who are the members of a multidisciplinary team and what are the roles of specific members?

Introduction

The role of the pediatric occupational therapist to facilitate participation in age-appropriate occupations holds true when working with children with complex medical conditions from traumatic events, including any incident that causes significant injury. When a child experiences trauma, the family must adjust to and cope with differences in their loved one. Changes may range from minor deficits to significant changes in personality, appearance, and/or abilities. Regardless of the nature of the trauma or its resulting medical conditions, the therapist must be prepared for heightened emotions and rapidly changing needs of the child and caregiver post-trauma. Post-trauma, a child may receive rehabilitation services across a continuum of care, including the intensive care unit (ICU), acute care, inpatient and outpatient rehabilitation, and community reintegration services. The role of the therapist may change frequently according to the child's medical and psychosocial status. The occupational therapist's approach is determined by the child's injuries, his or her developmental stage, and the family's educational needs and priorities. This chapter describes occupational therapy services for the common trauma-induced conditions of spinal cord injury, traumatic brain injury, and burn injury.

This chapter presents background on each condition and foundational information relevant across diagnoses and the continuum of care, including therapeutic relationships, caregiver grieving, caregiver education, and multidisciplinary teamwork. Intervention, including preparatory methods, purposeful activity, occupation-based intervention, and education, are explained and illustrated. The chapter explains the stages of care with condition-specific information at each stage.

Spinal Cord Injury

The incidence of pediatric spinal cord injury (SCI) in the United States is an average of 1.99 times per 100,000, indicating approximately 1455 new injuries every year.[124] From the age of 3 years,[125] boys are more than two times as likely to experience SCI as girls.[124] The most common cause of pediatric SCI is motor vehicle accident;[124] other traumatic causes of SCI include violence, falls, and sports injuries. Non-traumatic causes of spinal cord lesion include spinal tumor, spinal procedure, or disease process such as transverse myelitis. Usually an injury is at a cervical, thoracic, or lumbar level and may be multilevel, either continuous or noncontinuous.

More than other age groups, younger children are likely to have SCI at the upper cervical level (C1-3) because of their disproportionately larger head size and ligamentous laxity.[125] Compared with other age groups, they are also more likely to experience SCI without radiographic abnormality because of greater ligamentous laxity; that is, sudden displacement of the spinal column can cause SCI without damaging vertebrae or ligaments.[53,125] After SCI, children may experience changes in muscle tone, decreased sensation, weakness, and/or paralysis below the level of injury, which is identified by the corresponding vertebra. Common medical complications include pain, latex allergy, muscle spasticity, pressure ulcers, spine deformity, hip deformity, low bone density, poor temperature regulation, autonomic dysreflexia, and decreased cardiovascular, respiratory, bowel, and bladder function.[53,125] Autonomic dysreflexia is a dangerous physiological response to noxious stimuli below the level of the SCI that causes symptoms including increased blood pressure. Until adolescence, children with SCI experience deep vein thrombosis[125] and heterotopic ossification[53] less commonly than adults with SCI.

The level of a child's injury informs a therapist as to which muscle groups and dermatomes may be affected. Children with lower-level injuries affecting their leg function have paraplegia, whereas children with higher-level injuries affecting their arms and legs have quadriplegia or tetraplegia. The *Reference Manual for the International Standards for Neurological Classification of Spinal Cord Injury* from the American Spinal Injury Association (ASIA) provides ASIA Impairment Scale (AIS) classification of injuries based on motor exam of 10 muscle groups and sensory exam of 28 sensory points.[83] For example, if no sensory or motor function is preserved in the sacral segments (S4-S5), the injury will be classified as AIS A, or complete, which is associated with the most severe injuries (Figure 30-1). This classification can help an occupational therapist to determine the extent to which muscle groups and sensation below the level of injury are affected and predicts neurologic outcome, with a better prognosis for less severe injuries.[128] Of note, the exam may be less reliable with some children because of their ability to follow directions or precision of responses.[53] Depending on the injury classification and other variables, such as medical stability and cognitive function, children with SCI have varied levels of physical function. Their function determines the extent to which they require adapted methods to participate in meaningful occupations. A child with a complete, high-level cervical injury (e.g., C2) may require a ventilator for respiratory support and have more dependent mobility needs than those with lower level injuries; he or she may use head or pneumatic switches to drive a power wheelchair and access assistive technology, including environmental controls. Environmental controls use switches or a computer interface to allow the child to operate devices or appliances, such as turning on a light or changing the channel on a television. Children with lower-level cervical injuries (e.g., C5) may be able to use hand controls instead. Children with thoracic injuries often have sufficient upper extremity strength and trunk control to self-propel manual wheelchairs and use standard methods to control their environments. Children with incomplete injuries may be able to resume functional ambulation independently or by using assistive devices.

Traumatic Brain Injury

Brain injuries are classified as traumatic when the injury is caused by an external force. Other causes of acquired brain injury include but are not limited to stroke, anoxia, arteriovenous malformation rupture, brain tumor resection, seizure activity, seizure foci resection, infections such as meningitis or encephalitis, and metabolic disorders. Because of the numerous mechanisms in which a brain injury may occur and the varying ways in which different types of brain injuries may present and recover, this chapter's focus is on traumatic brain injuries.

Typical causes of traumatic brain injury (TBI) include falls, motor vehicle accidents, sports-related injuries, nonaccidental trauma, and gunshot wounds. According to the Centers for Disease Control and Prevention (CDC), approximately 1.7 million people sustain a traumatic brain injury each year.[43] Statistics have shown that young children aged 0 to 4 years, teenagers aged 15 to 19 years, and seniors over the age of 65 are the most likely age groups to incur a traumatic brain injury. Furthermore, between the years 2002 and 2006 the CDC reported that almost half a million children aged 0 to 14 years were admitted to the emergency department because of traumatic brain injuries.[43]

Traumatic brain injuries are classified as mild, moderate, or severe and can result in deficits ranging from minor to debilitating. The Glasgow Coma Scale[120] provides an objective measurement of consciousness on a scale from 3 to 15 using observations of eye opening, verbal output, and motor responses and is used to help classify the severity of brain injuries. A mild brain injury is defined as a loss of consciousness for less than 30 minutes, a Glasgow Coma Scale score between 13 and 15, and post-traumatic amnesia that lasts for less than 24 hours.[33,79] A moderate brain injury is defined by a loss of consciousness from 30 minutes to 24 hours, a Glasgow Coma Scale score between 9 and 12, and possible observable findings on an electroencephalogram (EEG), computed tomography (CT), or magnetic resonance imaging (MRI) scans. A severe brain injury is defined as a loss of consciousness lasting more than 24 hours, a Glasgow Coma Scale score between 3 and 8, and possible significant findings on EEG, CT, or MRI scans.[33,79]

Beyond severity of injury, the functional deficits that result from brain injury are also dependent on location of injury and whether the injury was localized or diffuse. Typically children who have sustained a severe global brain injury, such as a diffuse axonal shear injury or anoxia, tend to have less optimal functional outcomes than children who have a smaller, more localized area of injury.[30,63,114] Pre-morbid factors such as family socioeconomic disadvantage, behavioral issues, and poor academic performance can also influence long-term functional outcomes of children who have sustained a TBI.[84,114] Brain injury can cause deficits in cognition: attention, language, processing speed, memory, sequencing, and pragmatics; physical functions: strength, muscle tone, sensation, and gross and fine motor skills; and behavior: emotions, behavioral regulation, social adjustment, and psychological functioning.[5]

It is helpful to use the Rancho Levels of Cognitive Functioning[54,99] when determining the occupational therapy goals and interventions for a child who has incurred a traumatic brain injury. This assessment tool describes the progression of recovery following a traumatic brain injury. The eight levels define behaviors typically observed at each stage of recovery (Table 30-1).

Using the Rancho Levels as a guide, the occupational therapist critically appraises the child's cognitive level and uses activity analysis to select and implement interventions to advance the child to the next functional level of recovery. Each child and each brain injury is unique; therefore, the rate of progression through the eight stages of recovery varies greatly. Furthermore, a child may plateau for a period of time before progressing, or, in some cases, he or she may plateau and never progress to a higher level of functioning.

Burn Injury

Approximately 450,000 individuals require medical attention for burn injuries each year.[3,93] More than half of that number is comprised of children under the age of 18, with approximately 30,000 requiring hospitalization for burn injuries.[31] The

ASIA — AMERICAN SPINAL INJURY ASSOCIATION

INTERNATIONAL STANDARDS FOR NEUROLOGICAL CLASSIFICATION OF SPINAL CORD INJURY (ISNCSCI)

ISCOS — INTERNATIONAL SPINAL CORD SOCIETY

Patient Name________________ Date/Time of Exam ________________

Examiner Name________________ Signature ________________

RIGHT

MOTOR KEY MUSCLES	SENSORY KEY SENSORY POINTS
	Light Touch (LTR) / Pin Prick (PPR)
	C2
	C3
	C4
UER (Upper Extremity Right) Elbow flexors C5	C5
Wrist extensors C6	C6
Elbow extensors C7	C7
Finger flexors C8	C8
Finger abductors (little finger) T1	T1
	T2
	T3
	T4
	T5
	T6
	T7
	T8
	T9
	T10
	T11
	T12
	L1
LER (Lower Extremity Right) Hip flexors L2	L2
Knee extensors L3	L3
Ankle dorsiflexors L4	L4
Long toe extensors L5	L5
Ankle plantar flexors S1	S1
	S2
	S3
	S4-5

Comments (Non-key Muscle? Reason for NT? Pain?):

(VAC) Voluntary anal contraction (Yes/No)

RIGHT TOTALS

(MAXIMUM) (50) (56) (56)

LEFT

SENSORY KEY SENSORY POINTS	MOTOR KEY MUSCLES
Light Touch (LTL) / Pin Prick (PPL)	
C2	
C3	
C4	
C5	C5 Elbow flexors — UEL (Upper Extremity Left)
C6	C6 Wrist extensors
C7	C7 Elbow extensors
C8	C8 Finger flexors
T1	T1 Finger abductors (little finger)
T2	
T3	
T4	
T5	
T6	
T7	
T8	
T9	
T10	
T11	
T12	
L1	
L2	L2 Hip flexors — LEL (Lower Extremity Left)
L3	L3 Knee extensors
L4	L4 Ankle dorsiflexors
L5	L5 Long toe extensors
S1	S1 Ankle plantar flexors
S2	
S3	
S4-5	

MOTOR (SCORING ON REVERSE SIDE)
0 = total paralysis
1 = palpable or visible contraction
2 = active movement, gravity eliminated
3 = active movement, against gravity
4 = active movement, against some resistance
5 = active movement, against full resistance
5* = normal corrected for pain/disuse
NT = not testable

SENSORY (SCORING ON REVERSE SIDE)
0 = absent 2 = normal
1 = altered NT = not testable

(DAP) Deep anal pressure (Yes/No)

LEFT TOTALS

(56) (56) (50) (MAXIMUM)

MOTOR SUBSCORES

UER ☐ + UEL ☐ = UEMS TOTAL ☐ LER ☐ + LEL ☐ = LEMS TOTAL ☐

MAX (25) (25) (50) MAX (25) (25) (50)

SENSORY SUBSCORES

LTR ☐ + LTL ☐ = LT TOTAL ☐ PPR ☐ + PPL ☐ = PP TOTAL ☐

MAX (56) (56) (112) MAX (56) (56) (112)

NEUROLOGICAL LEVELS Steps 1-5 for classification as on reverse — 1. SENSORY R L; 2. MOTOR R L

3. NEUROLOGICAL LEVEL OF INJURY (NLI)

4. COMPLETE OR INCOMPLETE? Incomplete = Any sensory or motor function in S4-5

5. ASIA IMPAIRMENT SCALE (AIS)

(In complete injuries only) ZONE OF PARTIAL PRESERVATION Most caudal level with any innervation — SENSORY R L; MOTOR R L

This form may be copied freely but should not be altered without permission from the American Spinal Injury Association. REV 02/13

Muscle Function Grading

0 = total paralysis
1 = palpable or visible contraction
2 = active movement, full range of motion (ROM) with gravity eliminated
3 = active movement, full ROM against gravity
4 = active movement, full ROM against gravity and moderate resistance in a muscle specific position
5 = (normal) active movement, full ROM against gravity and full resistance in a functional muscle position expected from an otherwise unimpaired person
5* = (normal) active movement, full ROM against gravity and sufficient resistance to be considered normal if identified inhibiting factors (i.e. pain, disuse) were not present
NT = not testable (i.e. due to immobilization, severe pain such that the patient cannot be graded, amputation of limb, or contracture of > 50% of the normal range of motion)

Sensory Grading

0 = Absent
1 = Altered, either decreased/impaired sensation or hypersensitivity
2 = Normal
NT = Not testable

Non Key Muscle Functions (optional)

May be used to assign a motor level to differentiate AIS B vs. C

Movement	Root level
Shoulder: Flexion, extension, abduction, adduction, internal and external rotation **Elbow:** Supination	C5
Elbow: Pronation **Wrist:** Flexion	C6
Finger: Flexion at proximal joint, extension. **Thumb:** Flexion, extension and abduction in plane of thumb	C7
Finger: Flexion at MCP joint **Thumb:** Opposition, adduction and abduction perpendicular to palm	C8
Finger: Abduction of the index finger	T1
Hip: Adduction	L2
Hip: External rotation	L3
Hip: Extension, abduction, internal rotation **Knee:** Flexion **Ankle:** Inversion and eversion **Toe:** MP and IP extension	L4
Hallux and Toe: DIP and PIP flexion and abduction	L5
Hallux: Adduction	S1

ASIA Impairment Scale (AIS)

A = Complete. No sensory or motor function is preserved in the sacral segments S4-5.

B = Sensory Incomplete. Sensory but not motor function is preserved below the neurological level and includes the sacral segments S4-5 (light touch or pin prick at S4-5 or deep anal pressure) AND no motor function is preserved more than three levels below the motor level on either side of the body.

C = Motor Incomplete. Motor function is preserved below the neurological level**, and more than half of key muscle functions below the neurological level of injury (NLI) have a muscle grade less than 3 (Grades 0-2).

D = Motor Incomplete. Motor function is preserved below the neurological level**, and at least half (half or more) of key muscle functions below the NLI have a muscle grade ≥ 3.

E = Normal. If sensation and motor function as tested with the ISNCSCI are graded as normal in all segments, and the patient had prior deficits, then the AIS grade is E. Someone without an initial SCI does not receive an AIS grade.

** For an individual to receive a grade of C or D, i.e. motor incomplete status, they must have either (1) voluntary anal sphincter contraction or (2) sacral sensory sparing with sparing of motor function more than three levels below the motor level for that side of the body. The International Standards at this time allows even non-key muscle function more than 3 levels below the motor level to be used in determining motor incomplete status (AIS B versus C).

NOTE: When assessing the extent of motor sparing below the level for distinguishing between AIS B and C, the ***motor level*** on each side is used; whereas to differentiate between AIS C and D (based on proportion of key muscle functions with strength grade 3 or greater) the ***neurological levelof injury*** is used.

ASIA — AMERICAN SPINAL INJURY ASSOCIATION

INTERNATIONAL STANDARDS FOR NEUROLOGICAL CLASSIFICATION OF SPINAL CORD INJURY

ISCOS — INTERNATIONAL SPINAL CORD SOCIETY

Steps in Classification

The following order is recommended for determining the classification of individuals with SCI.

1. Determine sensory levels for right and left sides.
The sensory level is the most caudal, intact dermatome for both pin prick and light touch sensation.

2. Determine motor levels for right and left sides.
Defined by the lowest key muscle function that has a grade of at least 3 (on supine testing), providing the key muscle functions represented by segments above that level are judged to be intact (graded as a 5).
Note: in regions where there is no myotome to test, the motor level is presumed to be the same as the sensory level, if testable motor function above that level is also normal.

3. Determine the neurological level of injury (NLI)
This refers to the most caudal segment of the cord with intact sensation and antigravity (3 or more) muscle function strength, provided that there is normal (intact) sensory and motor function rostrally respectively.
The NLI is the most cephalad of the sensory and motor levels determined in steps 1 and 2.

4. Determine whether the injury is Complete or Incomplete.
(i.e. absence or presence of sacral sparing)
*If voluntary anal contraction = **No** AND all S4-5 sensory scores = **0** AND deep anal pressure = **No**, then injury is **Complete**.*
*Otherwise, injury is **Incomplete**.*

5. Determine ASIA Impairment Scale (AIS) Grade:

Is injury Complete? **If YES, AIS=A** and can record ZPP (lowest dermatome or myotome on each side with some preservation)

NO ↓

Is injury Motor Complete? If YES, AIS=B

NO ↓ (No=voluntary anal contraction OR motor function more than three levels below the motor level on a given side, if the patient has sensory incomplete classification)

Are at least half (half or more) of the key muscles below the neurological level of injury graded 3 or better?

NO ↓ **AIS=C** **YES** ↓ **AIS=D**

If sensation and motor function is normal in all segments, AIS=E
Note: AIS E is used in follow-up testing when an individual with a documented SCI has recovered normal function. If at initial testing no deficits are found, the individual is neurologically intact; the ASIA Impairment Scale does not apply.

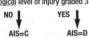

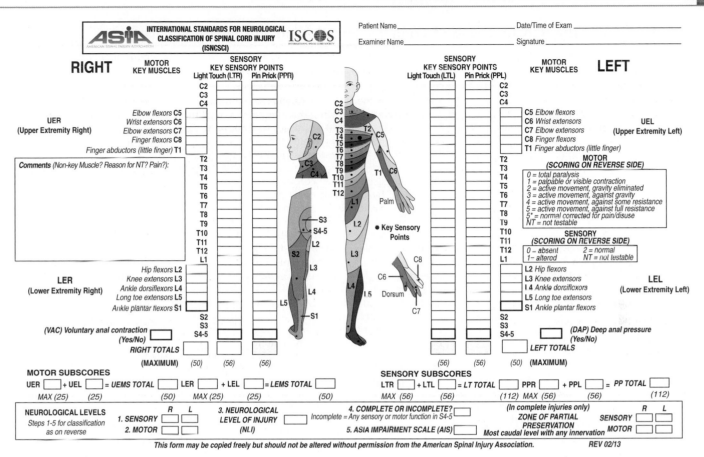

FIGURE 30-1 Exam sheet. (From American Spinal Injury Association. [2013]. *International standards for neurological classification of spinal cord injury.* Revised 2013; Atlanta, GA. Reprinted 2013.)

TABLE 30-1 The Rancho Levels of Cognitive Functioning and Typical Behaviors

Rancho Level of Cognitive Functioning	Description of Typical Behaviors
Level I : No Response	• Demonstrates no response to external stimuli
Level II: Generalized Response	• Demonstrates generalized body responses to external stimulation
Level III: Localized Response	• Demonstrates localized responses to external stimuli • May follow some basic commands
Level IV: Confused, Agitated	• Demonstrates confusion and agitation • Begins to participate in more basic activities of daily living with maximal assistance
Level V: Confused, Inappropriate, Non-agitated	• Demonstrates continued confusion • Needs step-by-step instructions for completion of self-care skills • Tends to perseverate on certain ideas or actions
Level VI: Confused, Appropriate	• Demonstrates confusion due to memory deficits • Follows daily routines with supervision or minimal verbal cues • Exhibits improved attention to functional tasks • Easily distracted by environmental stimuli • Emerging insight into physical deficits • Impulsive with actions and speech
Level VII: Automatic, Appropriate	• Emerging independence with routine tasks, functional activities • Poor insight into true physical and cognitive capabilities • Demonstrates inflexibility with thought processes and actions
Level VIII: Purposeful, Appropriate	• Realizes the physical and cognitive impact injury • Compensates for deficits to independently complete daily tasks • Demonstrates more appropriate problem-solving skills • Illustrates improved learning abilities

Adapted from Hagen et al. 1979; Rancho Los Amigos National Rehabilitation Center 2011.
Greenberg, J., Ruutiainen, A., & Kim, H. (2009). Rehabilitation of pediatric spinal cord injury: from acute medical care to rehabilitation and beyond. *Journal of Pediatric Rehabilitation Medicine: An Interdisciplinary Approach, 2*, 13–27; Rancho Los Amigos National Rehabilitation Center. (2011). The Rancho Levels of Cognitive Functioning. Retrieved April 13, 2013 from http://www.rancho.org/Research_RanchoLevels.aspx.

majority of pediatric burns (60%) are caused by kitchen or bathroom scalds, whereas 25% are caused by flame, 10% by contact with hot objects or tools, and the remaining 5% by electrical or chemical interactions.[9] Skin has two layers: the epidermis, which is thin and contains no blood vessels, and the dermis, which contains blood vessels, nerves, hair follicles, sweat glands, and fat and is responsible for cell production. The severity of complications resulting from burns is directly related to the depth of injury (Table 30-2). Burns are considered to be first degree or superficial when damage is caused only to the epidermis, second degree or partial thickness when damage enters the dermis, and third degree or deep partial or full thickness when the majority or entire dermis is damaged.

Tissue injury causing damage to deeper layers of the skin requires longer healing time and often requires surgical intervention, therefore increasing risk of infection. Burns that destroy the dermal layer of the skin most often require skin grafting, which presents risk of abnormal scar development. Sheet grafting occurs when an area of healthy skin is shaved off and placed over a same-sized wound. The healthy area is called the donor. Donor sites are similar to superficial partial thickness injuries. They generally heal within 10 to 14 days and are very painful. Donor sites may also scar. Meshed grafting is used to cover large wounds. This is when the donor skin is run through a machine for perforation so that it can cover a wound larger than the donor area. It is necessary for covering wounds when donor skin is minimal, for example, with large, full-body burns. Meshed grafting can be expanded two to nine times the original size, and the spaces in the mesh heal within 7 to 14 days. The "waffled" appearance is permanent; therefore meshed grafting is generally only used when absolutely necessary and rarely on faces or hands. For those injured on a large portion of their body with minimal donor skin, temporary wound coverage can be provided through allograft, or donor skin from a cadaver or animal, which acts as a biologic dressing and remains in place for 2 to 3 weeks. When the allograft is rejected by the body, autografting must be completed, which uses the child's own skin from an uninjured donor site on his or her body. As stated, all of these grafting procedures have a high risk of developing problematic scars.

Abnormal scar development is the cause of functional and aesthetic problems that arise from burns. With recent advances in burn care, survival rates have increased for all age groups, resulting in an increased need for effective rehabilitation. Collagen fibers that make up the skin are typically arranged in a linear fashion. When the dermal layer is damaged severely, the collagen fibers that make up the skin are overproduced and realign in a disorganized manner during the healing process, causing abnormal scarring. These hypertrophic scars are red, raised, thick, and tight in appearance. The incidence of hypertrophic scar development following burns is 67% to 90%, with increased prevalence in children and those with darker pigmented skin tones.[2,13,32,42,51,59] Unmanaged hypertrophic scars have both physical and psychosocial repercussions, including joint contracture leading to decreased function, chronic wounds and pain, social stigma associated with visible disfigurement, and overall decreased quality of life.[12,15,18,37,58,62,68,81,105] The optimal outcome for treatment of burn scars is restoration of

TABLE 30-2 Burn Depth and Intervention Implications

Degree and Thickness	Depth	Characteristics	Examples	Therapeutic Considerations
First: superficial	Epidermis	Pain, redness, itching	Sunburn	• Heals within a few days • Generally no intervention required • Monitor need for scar massage
Second: superficial partial thickness	Dermis—superficial papillary region	Pain, blistering, swelling; brief contact with burn agent	Brief contact with scalding water or curling iron, friction—road rash	• Will require heal time of 1-2 weeks • Will need scar massage and AROM • Monitor need for PROM, pressure therapy, and/or splinting
Deep second: deep partial thickness	Dermis—deeper reticular region	Relatively painless, white, leathery; significant contact with burn agent	Fire, significant contact with scalding water, friction—contact with moving treadmill	• Will likely need grafting or will require heal time of 3+ weeks • Will need PROM, scar massage, pressure, splinting, and re-teaching of skills with respect to pain and temporary limitations in joint ROM
Third: full thickness	Full dermis and/or hypodermis (muscle, bone)	Insensate, charred black or gray; prolonged contact with burn agent	Electrocution, explosions, contact with flammable chemicals, house fire entrapment	• Will need grafting, amputation, and/or complex surgical intervention • May need PROM, scar massage, and pressure depending on nature of surgery • Will likely need postoperative splinting • Will require re-teaching of skills, compensatory strategies, and/or prosthetics

tissue aesthetics and function as close to normal skin as possible. The therapist's role, as described in the following sections, is crucial during the period of active scar formation, i.e., first year following injury.

Therapeutic Relationships

Therapeutic relationships are instrumental to support the psychosocial well-being of children and their families in post-trauma care. Families may feel helpless following trauma, unfamiliar with their child's medical complications and the medical system. The therapist should assess the caregiver's readiness to learn and provide an appropriate level of information, facilitating the caregiver's increased confidence in making medical decisions and participating in his or her child's care.[24] Occupational therapists should assess and consider caregiver readiness, because encouraging caregiver participation or presenting too much information before the caregivers are ready may overwhelm them and decrease their confidence. To empower caregivers to fully participate on the medical team, occupational therapists educate caregivers using family-friendly language and methods of instruction.[14] Hands-on education may offer caregivers a sense of involvement, responsibility, confidence, and role fulfillment.

In addition to engaging with caregivers, the occupational therapist uses developmentally and cognitively appropriate strategies[5] to build rapport with the child. Children are often frightened and anxious in hospital settings; expressions of friendliness such as laughter and smiling may go a long way in building trust. If a therapy intervention is uncomfortable or difficult, the occupational therapist may promote continued rapport development by validating the child's feelings and providing him or her with age-appropriate methods for coping with the stressful situation. Another strategy is to incorporate the child's premorbid interests into therapy activities. The occupational therapist may further build trust by educating the child on the medical condition, precautions, or procedures using developmentally appropriate language. The occupational therapist who describes what he or she will be doing to a child with a low level of consciousness acknowledges the child's experience and demonstrates respect. Once the child and caregivers feel comfortable in the medical setting and trust the care team members, they become more engaged in the rehabilitation process.[5]

It is important to be mindful of the often contrasting perspectives of the health care professionals and the family. The health care team is likely meeting the child after he or she has been injured; therefore, their view of recovery progression is based on the child postinjury. In contrast, the child's and caregivers' perspectives are based on the child before his or her injury, a child to whom they want to return. Although the care team, child, and caregivers all hope to achieve recovery as close to preinjury status as possible, it is important to recognize that the child and family members have a different perspective on progress.

Grief Management

Traumatically injured children and their families experience a variety of emotions and social issues. Psychologist Ken Moses suggests impairment "shatters the dreams" a caregiver has for his or her child's future.[87] The subsequent grieving process includes states of anxiety, denial, guilt, anger, and depression. "They must go on with their lives, cope with their child as he or she is now, let go of lost dreams, and generate new dreams."[87] Moses suggests that dreams are shattered repeatedly at each stage of typical development. He conceptualizes the grieving process as dynamic, noting that caregivers may transition through grieving states in any order, rather than in a sequence, and sometimes repeat states. Every caregiver's grieving process is unique. An occupational therapist may support caregivers, acknowledge the grieving process, and gently promote progress toward desired outcomes. Two ways to promote progress are providing sensitive education and collaborating with caregivers on the occupational therapy plan of care.

Caregiver Education

The health care team must consider the family's grieving process to determine appropriate timing for delivery of delicate education topics.[115] The traumatically injured child and caregivers may be in a fragile emotional state; it is important for the occupational therapist to meet the family "where they are" in the grieving process. The occupational therapist may be cautiously hopeful with caregivers and the child, finding a careful balance between squandering hope and promising the potentially impossible.[132] The occupational therapist may also acknowledge children's and families' frustration with lack of knowledge about prognosis because there is likely not a clear-cut expected treatment outcome. It is important for the occupational therapist to continuously monitor the family's readiness to progress education.

One approach to education involves a self-management structure. The intent of self-management is to ultimately empower the child and/or caregiver to manage care responsibilities. Using this approach, the occupational therapist initially discerns the caregiver's priorities and confidence in his or her ability to manage the child's condition.[24] The occupational therapist then continually assesses the caregiver's ability to carry out health care recommendations[14] and supports the caregiver's ability to problem solve barriers.

Multidisciplinary Team

A coordinated, multidisciplinary team is comprised of health care professionals from different disciplines who are in regular collaboration with one another and the family to ensure the provision of consistent, goal-directed care.[1] This approach is essential to positive outcomes in the rehabilitation of children with trauma-induced medical conditions.[1,19,23,26,47,70,93,115,126] Professionals from each discipline develop their own treatment plans for the child, and close coordination is necessary to ensure the plans correspond with one another. Over the course of the child's recovery and according to the child's needs, certain disciplines may hold more responsibility than others for determining the course of the treatment plan. A therapist must approach team members proactively with concerns about a child's care plan. For instance, in some stages the therapist may interact with the child more frequently than the physician. In this case, the occupational therapist may inform the physician regarding barriers to progress, such as pain levels requiring pharmacologic management. Furthermore, to meet the complex needs of the child post-trauma, occupational, physical, speech, and recreational therapists need open dialog and routine collaboration, which may include transdisciplinary practices (i.e., appropriate reinforcement of each other's disciplinary goals). For example, the occupational therapist may focus on self-care while reinforcing mobility and communication, the respective primary goals of the physical therapist and speech-language pathologist. A unified approach to the child's general care plan promotes the safety of the child, models consistency of care provision among caregivers and care providers, prevents the delivery of conflicting information, and facilitates the child's ability to carry over restored skills to various contexts.[46,47,132]

The individual therapists on the care team may change as the child progresses from one stage of care to another, further emphasizing the importance of care coordination.[129] Thorough and timely team communication supports a smooth transition of care from one practitioner to another. Consistency throughout the continuum of care provides the child and caregiver with a sense of security during potentially stressful transitions.[23,115,129]

Post-Trauma Occupational Therapy Interventions

Provision of care for children post-trauma is complex and dynamic, with each child and caregiver presenting a multitude of therapy needs. To ensure holistic care and support progress, the occupational therapist uses different but intimately intertwined intervention types, including preparatory methods, purposeful activity, occupation-based intervention, and education. The occupational therapist uses preparatory methods to remediate client factors, including the injured body structures and impaired body functions. As occupational therapy intervention, preparatory methods must lead to purposeful activities or occupation-based interventions.[4] The therapist uses purposeful activities and occupation-based interventions to rehabilitate the child's participation in meaningful occupation. Both caregivers and children require educational intervention including supports and problem solving. Specific interventions post-trauma may change throughout the continuum of care (Table 30-3).

Post-Trauma Continuum of Care

Children post-trauma receive occupational therapy intervention across a continuum of care with different needs at each stage. These stages may include the intensive care unit (ICU), acute care, inpatient rehabilitation, outpatient rehabilitation, and community re-integration. Continuous assessment in each stage may include body structures (e.g., skin); mental functions, sensory functions, and pain; neuromusculoskeletal and movement-related functions (e.g., passive range of motion, strength, muscle tone, endurance, coordination); and skin functions. Although the specific interventions used may vary based on the specific trauma and resulting deficits, fundamentals for each recovery stage apply to all children's intervention

TABLE 30-3 Interventions Through the Pediatric Post-Trauma Continuum of Care

Stage of Care	Preparatory Methods	Purposeful Activities and Occupation-Based Interventions	Education	Safety Notes
Intensive care unit	• Positioning • ROM • Splinting • Soft tissue mobility • Wound care • Sensory stimulation • Medical consultation regarding medication for pain and arousal	• Promoting sleep/rest with low stimulation environment	• Education on diagnosis • Education on role of occupational therapist • Hands-on education on caring for child	• Precautions • Monitoring vitals
Acute care	• Positioning • ROM • Splinting • Soft tissue mobility • Wound care • Sensory stimulation • Scar massage • Pressure therapy • Medical consultation regarding medication for pain, arousal, and spasticity	• Trunk control work • Strengthening • Endurance • Neuromuscular re-education for coordination • Adaptive equipment training	• Education on DVT and orthostatic hypotension prevention • Education on exercises to be completed outside therapy • Education on therapeutic equipment/strategies	• Precautions • Monitoring vitals • Prevention of orthostatic hypotension
Inpatient rehabilitation	• Positioning • ROM • Splinting • Soft tissue mobility • Sensory stimulation • Scar massage • Pressure therapy • Medical consultation regarding medication for pain, arousal, and spasticity	• Postural work • Strengthening • Endurance • Neuromuscular re-education for coordination • Electrical stimulation • Adaptive equipment training • Self-care training • IADL training • Standardized assessment • Home evaluation • Community re-entry outing • Coping strategies • Social skills training • Cognitive re-training • Visual perceptual skill training • Consultation with social worker/psychologist regarding readiness for return home	• Hands-on education for care of all functional needs • Hands-on education for use of therapeutic equipment/strategies • Hands-on education on home programming • Education on importance of home programming • Education on results of standardized assessments	• Precautions • Prevention of orthostatic hypotension
Outpatient rehabilitation/community re-entry	• Positioning • ROM • Splinting • Soft tissue mobility • Sensory stimulation • Scar massage • Pressure therapy • Medical consultation regarding medication for pain, arousal, and spasticity	• Postural work • Strengthening • Endurance • Neuromuscular re-education for coordination • Electrical stimulation • Adaptive equipment training • Self-care training • IADL training • Standardized assessment • Coping strategies • Social skills training • Cognitive re-training • Cognitive strategies • Visual perceptual skill training • Consultation with school • Community integration • Referral to community resources for supports and recreational opportunities • Referral to other disciplines • Referral to certified driver rehabilitation specialist	• Hands-on education for use of therapeutic equipment/strategies • Hands-on education on home programming • Education on importance of home programming • Education on results of standardized assessments • Education on problem-solving barriers to participation and home program implementation	• Precautions

post-trauma. The following sections describe the role of the therapist at each stage of care. Further interventions specific to diagnosis at each stage of care are described to illustrate the unique needs associated with different trauma conditions.

Intensive Care Unit

In the ICU, the child's care is focused on medical recovery. The child typically presents as sedated by either a naturally occurring or pharmacologically induced coma, limiting the active engagement of the child with other people or the environment. Occupational therapy services are initiated in the ICU to prevent secondary complications from the body's state of immobility and impaired ability to maintain homeostasis.[5] The child's primary occupations at this stage, rest and sleep, are critical to healing.

Goals for ICU intervention include contracture and pressure ulcer prevention, pain management, and safety. The child's vital signs should be monitored throughout interventions to ensure stability of cardiovascular and respiratory functions. Preparatory methods to maximize range of motion include stretches, soft tissue mobilization, splinting, and positioning. Beyond contracture prevention, the occupational therapist may develop a positioning plan to prevent pressure ulcers, because unconscious children and those who have limited movement and/or sensation are at risk for skin breakdown. The occupational therapist may also use positioning plans and range of motion programs to help control pain in collaboration with physician-directed pharmacologic pain management. Pain management can also include developmentally appropriate comfort measures such as soothing music. Collaboration with nursing staff is essential for development and consistent implementation of range of motion, splinting, and positioning plans.

Ensuring the child's safety is the highest priority in treatment delivery. Therapists address safety by adhering to medically necessary movement restrictions and protective medical equipment, such as a helmet following removal of a portion of the skull. For children who become agitated the occupational therapist collaborates with the medical team to help determine the need for physician-ordered physical restraints to prevent self-injury. Examples include elbow immobilizers to prevent pulling at tubes and bed barriers such as one with zippered sides to protect the child from falls. An occupational therapist must be vigilant regarding wounds, incisions, and the placement of medical lines when transferring a child to prevent harm. It is important to be aware of seizure status and presentation as well. The occupational therapist may also help prevent critical secondary conditions, such as pressure ulcers. Maintaining awareness of all safety factors may seem overwhelming to an occupational therapist unfamiliar with this complex population. It is important to recognize one's limitations; the therapist and child benefit from use of other medical team members at key times to ensure provision of safe and appropriate care. The entire care team is committed to working closely to ensure the child's safety throughout his or her recovery.

In the ICU, the occupational therapist facilitates the caregiver's return to his or her role as the child's provider. During the assessment process, the occupational therapist seeks information from the caregiver about the child including the child's interests, premorbid levels of development and function, and family dynamics. Although the caregiver may not be an expert regarding the child's medical needs, he or she is the expert on his or her child. The occupational therapist educates the caregiver on the therapist's role to facilitate skill progression toward the child's prior level of function throughout the continuum of care. The occupational therapist also suggests ways the caregiver may collaborate with the medical care team to participate in the child's care in the hospital environment.

Children with Spinal Cord Injury in the Intensive Care Unit

Preparatory methods:

- It is estimated that 26% to 96% of clients post-SCI experience pain.[36] Neuropathic pain, which is caused by the nervous system rather than external stimuli, along with pain from injuries may limit a child's participation, making collaboration with physicians on pain management especially important.

Purposeful activities and occupation-based interventions:

- If the child is conscious, the occupational therapist can prevent the child's anxiety about mobility limitations by providing adapted call lights.

Education:

- Caregivers may benefit from general education on their child's SCI.
- Education also includes autonomic dysreflexia. Of note, children with SCI usually have lower blood pressure than those without, so elevations 20 to 40 mmHg above baseline may be a sign of autonomic dysreflexia.[53] Symptoms of autonomic dysreflexia may be managed conservatively (e.g., using removal of precipitating stimulus or positioning) and/or pharmacologically.[77]

Children with Traumatic Brain Injury in the Intensive Care Unit

Preparatory methods:

- Autonomic storming occurs in some children with brain injury and presents as cyclic symptoms that occur after a severe insult to the brain. Physical manifestations may include posturing of the limbs and trunk and increase in heart rate, respiratory rate, blood pressure, and sweating. Although the physician manages pharmacologic interventions to address autonomic storming, the occupational therapist may communicate to the medical team whether interventions are supporting improved tolerance of therapy interventions.[82]
- A low stimulation environment may promote brain healing.[5] After brain injury, loud noises, bright lights, and tactile input may overstimulate the child and lead to increased agitation and blood pressure. Increased blood pressure is dangerous to healing brain tissues because the child is already experiencing increased intracranial pressure resulting from swelling.[63,82]

Purposeful activities and occupation-based interventions:

- Depending on the child's level of consciousness, the occupational therapist may introduce appropriate sensory stimulation in a controlled manner in an effort to evoke a localized, volitional response to the environment.[5,19] Monitoring the autonomic nervous system's response to sensory stimulation can provide information on the client's potential return to consciousness.[127]

Education:

- Caregivers may benefit from general education on brain injury including how arousal, acceptance of stimulation, and body movements are impacting their child. The Rancho Levels[54,99] may facilitate understanding of the phases of recovery post brain injury and projected outcome.

Children with Burn Injury in the Intensive Care Unit

Preparatory methods:

- As the body heals from severe tissue injury, the child often seeks a position of comfort (fetal position), which unfortunately contributes to the development of contractures. Therefore the therapist must ensure that burned areas are positioned in extension to promote future function.[80] If bed positioning cannot be maintained, splinting should be used to maintain tissue length.[34]
- Splinting is also used to protect injured or exposed body structures.
- If the child has a tracheotomy, positioning the neck in adequate extension is essential to prevent contracture and has been shown to reduce the need for early reconstruction.[107]
- Passive range of motion should be completed to terminal stretch for all involved joints once per day with caution in respect to exposed body structures.[42]

Purposeful activities and occupation-based interventions:

- Despite likely low level of consciousness, it is important to acknowledge the child and his or her interests during early range of motion and dressing changes.

Education:

- Caregivers may benefit from general education on burns, including description of burn depths and locations, and how those factors may influence functional and aesthetic outcome.

Acute Care

In this stage of the continuum of care, the child who sustained a traumatically induced condition is more medically stable and hopefully starting to demonstrate an ability to interact with his or her environment. The occupational therapist continues to use preparatory methods to address injured body structures and impaired body functions, including promotion of homeostasis and prevention of secondary complications of immobility. Maintaining skin integrity is a high priority when the child experiences prolonged bed rest. The occupational therapist continually monitors if and how pain is inhibiting the child's ability to participate in functional tasks and collaborates with care team members as needed to update the pain management plan, including pharmacologic interventions and coping mechanisms. Although the body systems are functioning in a more stable manner than in the ICU, the occupational therapist continues to closely monitor vital signs during interventions.

If the child indicates wants and needs, it is important for the occupational therapist to actively engage the child in the therapy session. If the child remains relatively sedate, the occupational therapist observes the child's body language and vital signs to monitor the child's response to interventions. The occupational therapist facilitates the child's ability to resume available motor functions, including trunk control. For example, the occupational therapist assists the child to transition to different positions, including upright in bed and edge of bed sitting, and transfer to a wheelchair as appropriate. When facilitating postural control, the occupational therapist must carefully monitor for signs of pain or orthostatic hypotension, position-related low blood pressure. The child may need to slowly re-build upright tolerance.

The occupational therapist continues to build rapport with the caregiver in acute care and each subsequent stage in the continuum of care. At each stage it is also important for the occupational therapist to remain cautiously hopeful when discussing the child's prognosis and outcomes with caregivers. Information on the child's care and rehabilitation often needs to be reiterated several times throughout stages depending on caregiver readiness. New education at this stage includes the prevention of orthostatic hypotension, which is important before teaching caregivers to facilitate position changes. Caregivers may also be educated on the importance of appropriate movement to aid the prevention of deep vein thrombosis, or blood clotting, for children who are immobile for extended periods.

Children with Spinal Cord Injury in Acute Care

Preparatory methods:

- Muscle hypertonia may become more evident at this stage of recovery, in which case interventions to maximize range of motion are initiated (Figure 30-2).
- Collaboration with physicians on pharmacological management of spasticity[119] in addition to pain may support improved participation in therapy and response to interventions.

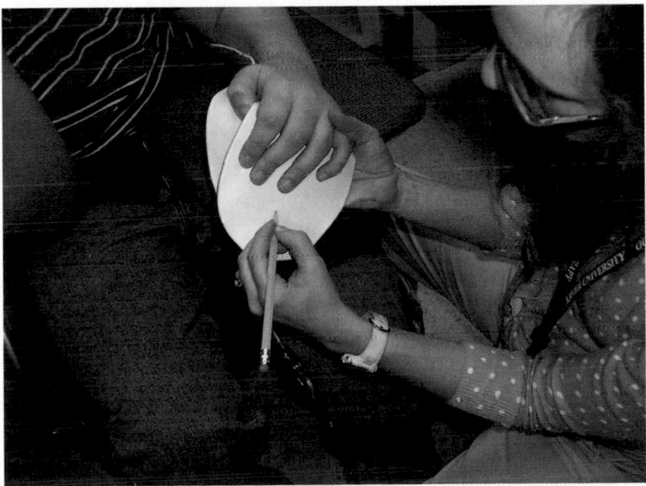

FIGURE 30-2 Occupational therapists may fabricate splints as a means to maximize range of motion and prevent deformity.

- Orthostatic hypotension may be managed conservatively (e.g., using functional electrical stimulation) and/or pharmacologically following SCI.[76]
- Vital sign instability may be caused by autonomic dysreflexia.

Purposeful activities and occupation-based interventions:

- Resumption of motor functions must remain within restrictions of spinal orthopedic equipment such as a neck or back brace. Unfortunately, this equipment may limit independent function.[21]
- Neuromuscular re-education, including hand-over-hand and sensorimotor therapeutic interventions, supports restoration of motor functions. For example, when children are beginning to re-initiate purposeful movements, they often have difficulty with precision and control. The occupational therapist can use his or her own hands, by placing them over the child's hands, as an assist to the child's action. The occupational therapist's assist to the child's movement provides the child with kinesthetic input for the movement pattern. Additionally, the occupational therapist may use vibration or muscle and tendon tapping techniques to elicit active movement in the context of a functional task and to provide the child with the sensorimotor input of how a particular action of the body should feel.
- Adaptive equipment and assistive technology should be introduced to maximize the child's function amidst new motor deficits. This may include provision of alternative call light and bed controls, abdominal binder, compression stockings, and loaner durable medical equipment, for example, wheelchair, air mattress, and commode chair. A wheelchair evaluation will determine which model and features are best for each child; optimal fit is important to maximize the child's safety and function.

Education:

- Therapists may model how to support children's ability to direct their care as appropriate. When children may have long-term movement limitations it is important to empower them to instruct those who assist them. For example, children can increase their sense of control over their bodies by communicating how they prefer to be transferred or how to position a piece of equipment most effectively for them.

Children with Traumatic Brain Injury in Acute Care

Preparatory methods:

- Muscle hypertonia may become more evident at this stage of recovery, in which case interventions to maximize range of motion are initiated.[132]
- Collaboration with physicians on pharmacologic management of muscle tone, agitation, and/or arousal in addition to pain may support improved participation in therapy and response to interventions.[132]
- Ongoing assessment of the child's mental functions is essential to monitor his or her ability to perceive or interact with the environment.[5] Examples include the ability to localize touch, blink to threat, visually track, startle to sound, localize to sound, or react to smells or tastes.
- Sensory stimulation may be used to increase or decrease alertness as appropriate to facilitate participation in functional tasks.[5]
- Physical restlessness typically increases in this stage owing to decreased pharmacologic sedation.[5] The need for safety measures, such as padding to prevent skin shearing, is continuously assessed.

Purposeful activities and occupation-based interventions:

- Once the child is able to perceive environmental stimuli, facilitation of the child's ability to interact with the environment progresses from basic functioning to more complex.[5] For example, if a child is demonstrating the ability to visually track and is initiating basic upper extremity movement, facilitating reach for a preferred object in a gravity-lessened, side-lying position may be an appropriate next step for intervention. From this position, the task can be graded in complexity in a variety of ways, including requiring the child to reach against gravity and increasing the distance of the object from the child to incorporate practice of trunk control.
- Neuromuscular re-education, including active assist of arm and hand movement and sensorimotor therapeutic interventions, supports restoration of motor functions.

Education:

- Caregivers may benefit from education on how environmental stimuli and the child's level of alertness may affect the child's ability to participate in functional tasks. The occupational therapist may then model how the caregiver can facilitate purposeful interactions.
- Caregivers may benefit from education on how the repetition of motor tasks reinforces motor learning and subsequent function.

Children with Burn Injury in Acute Care

Preparatory methods:

- Multiple changes occur at the cellular level which alter the pathology from normal wound healing to development of hypertrophic scarring. During excessive scar formation, a dysfunction of the underlying regulatory mechanisms may lead to persistent inflammation, excessive collagen synthesis, or deficient tissue degradation and remodeling.[51] This stage of active abnormal scar development peaks around 6 months postinjury and can persist an additional 12 to 18 months. Therapeutic interventions to promote optimal scar outcomes must be maintained throughout this entire period.
- Scar massage should be initiated as soon as the wound is closed to mechanically counteract the contractile forces of the healing skin. Scar massage should be completed with enough pressure to blanch the skin, and should be completed 3 to 5 minutes per area, two to three times per day.[44,103,104] Alcohol-free lotion or cream assists in skin conditioning but does not itself contribute to scar maturation or healing.
- Passive range of motion should be initiated immediately on open wounds or 5 to 10 days following graft placement and be completed in conjunction with scar massage twice per day.[42,80] It is essential to monitor for loss of range of motion as contractures are likely to begin to

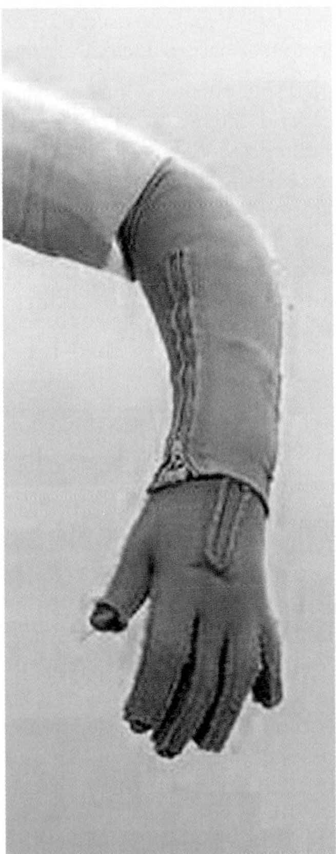

FIGURE 30-3 Pressure therapy for scar management can be accomplished through custom pressure garments or simple elastic wraps.

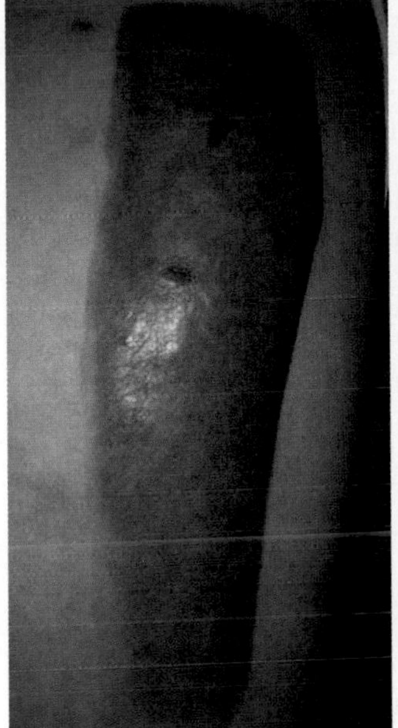
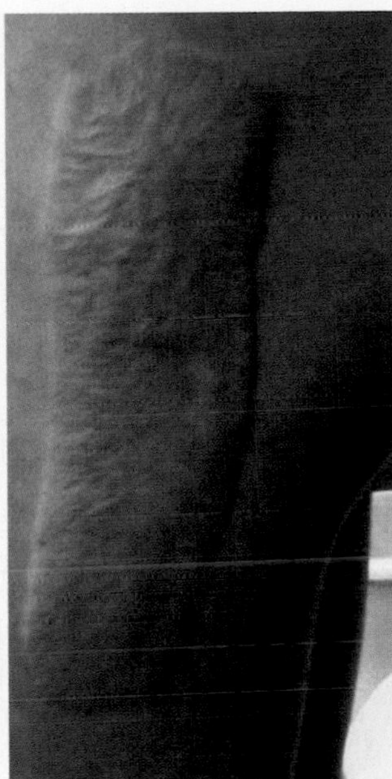

FIGURE 30-4 Scar maturation is defined by restoration of tissue aesthetics and function as close to normal skin as possible. This donor site scar was treated with massage and pressure therapy for approximately 12 months, and has regained its normal vascularity, pigmentation, and pliability. Scar height continues to persist in this client, however, and will likely remain. Every individual presents with different skin make-up and can have different responses to the standard of care.

develop at this stage owing to the heightened contractile forces of the hypertrophic scar.[121]

- When full passive range cannot be achieved within a therapy session, tissues should be placed on prolonged stretch through splinting.[8,9,11,31,42,51,80,91,94,95,102,113] Pressure therapy using compressive wraps or garments promotes optimal outcomes as soon as the healing skin can tolerate the pressure and/or shear force generated by the intervention (Figure 30-3).[11,31,42,51,73,80,91,95,102,113] Pressure therapy is initiated 5 to 10 days following wound closure or graft placement.
- Pressure wraps or garments should be fit to achieve pressure near capillary pressure (20 to 30 mmHg) to promote optimal scar outcome[9,11,17,31,41,50,80,113,123,130] and should be applied for 23 hours per day for approximately 12 months, or until scar maturation is achieved (Figure 30-4).[9,11,31,55,80,94]

Purposeful activities and occupation-based interventions:

- As the child's alertness and awareness increases, the need for pain management increases. The occupational therapist should assess the client's interests and incorporate age- and interest-appropriate distractions during painful range of motion and wound care procedures.[71,110]
- Although the child remains on bed rest for the most part, it's important to provide a glimpse of future functionality. Passive stretches may be followed by simple activities that reinforce range of motion and strength, such as tossing a ball while in bed.

Education:

- Caregivers should observe therapy sessions, which are often difficult and painful, in order to prepare themselves emotionally to complete the exercises with their child upon discharge.
- Providing samples of therapy devices (e.g., pressure garments, splints, adaptive equipment) as well as photographs of scar progression may facilitate future adherence.[64]

See Case Study 30-1.

Inpatient Rehabilitation

During inpatient rehabilitation, the child is medically stable and is physically able to tolerate a structured therapy program, which may consist of twice-daily sessions of occupational therapy, physical therapy, and speech-language pathology. If available, school services, therapeutic recreation, massage therapy, and behavioral medicine services may be included in the child's care. In this stage, the occupational therapist continues to address underlying client factors that inhibit overall function as needed.

However, the focus of therapy in this stage is to facilitate the child's independence with participation in self-care and play or leisure to prepare for the child's transition home. Self-care

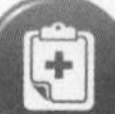

CASE STUDY 30-1 Keegan

History

Keegan is a 3-year-old boy admitted to the ICU following a car accident. He was restrained by a lap belt without a booster seat in the back seat when his mother lost control of her car, which sustained front-end impact and caught on fire. He was transported to the emergency room by ambulance where his immediate injuries were treated and later transitioned to the ICU. Before injury, Keegan was a typically developing boy who lived with his parents and older brother. He attended half-day preschool after which his grandmother cared for him. Keegan was outgoing and loved to explore the outdoors and wrestle with his brother.

Assessment

Keegan sustained a T-12 ASIA B spinal cord injury and 30% total body surface area, full-thickness burns to the neck, right shoulder, and upper extremity proximal to the elbow; he had a nasogastric feeding tube, back brace, and indwelling Foley catheter, was intubated, and was in a pharmacologically induced coma. Therapy was initiated to prevent secondary complications. Burn wound assessment revealed that full-thickness burns crossed joints including the neck and anterior axilla. Passive range of motion was measured to be normal at these joints at this point in care.

Interventions

Intensive Care Unit

The occupational therapist coordinated a positioning schedule with nursing staff to ensure Keegan was turned in bed at least every 2 hours to prevent skin breakdown and prevent deformity caused by wound contracture; he was also issued multi-podus boots to avoid direct pressure to his heels while positioning the ankles for future weight bearing. The occupational therapist educated Keegan's parents on his positioning schedule, posted in his hospital room, and on how they could help nursing staff keep track of his schedule. Following instruction, she asked that each parent demonstrate how to safely assist transitioning Keegan's position. The therapist completed passive range of motion (PROM) daily to the neck and shoulder, increasing stretch as tolerated, and provided splinting without any loss in range of motion (ROM). The surgeons performed split-thickness autografting of the burned areas following wound demarcation, and 5 days after surgery, the therapists initiated twice-daily PROM. Keegan began to demonstrate decreased shoulder and neck ROM, so the therapist initiated splinting of the shoulder into abduction and neck extension over a rolled towel when in bed. At that time, Keegan demonstrated improved medical stability; his physician ordered weaning from the coma-inducing medications and transitioned Keegan to acute care.

Acute Care

As Keegan's level of consciousness increased, he demonstrated significant difficulty tolerating therapy owing to both pain from his burn injury and neuropathic pain in his lower extremities. The occupational therapist provided his physician with input regarding potential pharmacologic pain management in hopes of balancing Keegan's tolerance for therapy with a level of alertness that allowed him to begin participating during sessions. Keegan's mother brought music from his favorite television show and the therapist began to play it during each session. When Keegan was able to follow simple commands, the occupational therapist let him know that it would hurt and assessed his active shoulder and cervical range by asking him to reach for and turn to look at different toys from home. The occupational therapist asked Keegan's brother to hold his tablet computer in a position so Keegan could only see it if he was upright; she slowly helped Keegan transition to sitting at the edge of the bed and assessed his postural control while he was watching a video clip. He cried and told the therapist not to let go, and she responded by reassuring and engaging Keegan. The occupational therapist instructed his parents on safe transfers so he could sit in a chair with supportive pillows for periods of time during the day as part of his updated positioning plan. During sessions, the therapist encouraged Keegan to perform active range as much as possible throughout stretches and let him know when she needed to passively range his joints further. She provided distraction during stretching and worked with nursing to complete ROM shortly after receiving scheduled pain medication. He then transitioned to inpatient rehabilitation.

skills addressed include bathing, dressing, feeding, functional mobility, and toileting (Figure 30-5). The occupational therapist may encourage the caregiver to bring in personal pictures or toys to motivate or comfort the child. When appropriate, siblings and other close family members may take part in therapy sessions to make the artificial hospital setting more comparable to the child's natural environment.

Therapists use a combination of restorative and adaptive treatment approaches to accommodate children's fluctuations in skill progression during the recovery process.[5,19] The restorative approach facilitates the child's performance skill progression toward his or her prior level of function. The child may reach a plateau in performance skill improvement owing to limitations in child readiness or body structure and function. For example, a child may have difficulty increasing independence with dressing because of persistent hemiplegic spasticity despite optimal pharmacologic management. At this time the occupational therapist may use an adaptive, or compensatory, approach, modifying activity demands to support increased child success. Modifying activity demands, including the use of adaptive equipment and strategies, gives children a sense of accomplishment during an otherwise potentially frustrating time (see e.g., Chapter 17, Table 17-2, and Chapter 25, Box 25-1). An occupational therapist may likely use a restorative approach with some goal-directed activities while simultaneously using an adaptive approach with other activities with the same child. The balance between approaches also depends on a variety of factors, including the child's and caregiver's priorities,

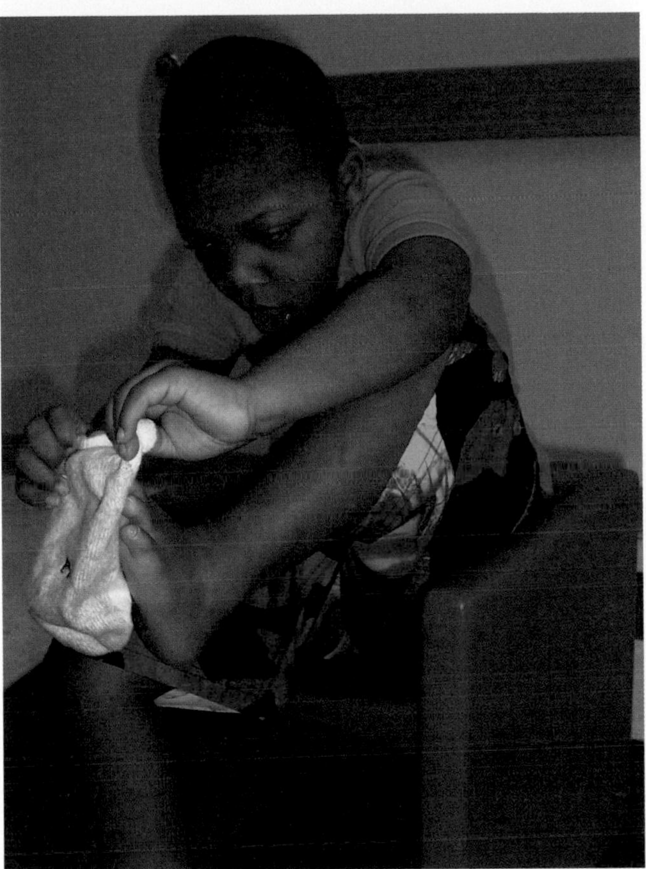

FIGURE 30-5 Self-care training is an integral focus of the inpatient rehabilitation stage of care in preparation for discharge home.

medical status, contexts for occupational performance, and current level of skill performance.

As the date of discharge becomes imminent, the inpatient rehabilitation team begins to prepare the child and caregiver for re-integration into the home, school, and community settings.[5] When necessary, an occupational or physical therapist may complete a home evaluation to provide recommendations on how to structure the home to promote safety and independence. The occupational therapist may begin to focus on school re-entry readiness and higher-level instrumental activities of daily living such as meal preparation and home management tasks given the child's functional and developmental levels. He or she may further prepare the family for return to home, school, and the community using outcome measures, hands-on caregiver education, a community re-entry outing, and collaboration with other team members on psychosocial needs.

The use of outcome measures allows for the measurement of progress during inpatient rehabilitation and helps support recommendations for school. The WeeFIM is one assessment tool used to evaluate the functional skill level of the child in various areas related to self-care, mobility, cognition, and social interaction.[88,101] The occupational therapist and multidisciplinary care team may use assessment results to determine appropriate accommodations for school and support a successful return to the classroom. To further ease the child's transition back into the natural environment, the rehabilitation team may prepare a video and/or in-service to share with the school about the child's injury and progress.

Because of the varying rate and extent of recovery associated with trauma recovery, the occupational therapist may use hands-on education to prepare the child and caregiver for a "safe" discharge to home rather than an "ideal" discharge in which the child would have returned to his or her prior level of functioning. In preparation for the return home, the caregiver must demonstrate understanding of how to manage the child's medical and functional needs, which may include medication administration, wound care, splinting and positioning schedules, and providing assistance with self-care using adaptive equipment and/or adapted strategies. Some caregivers may not be receptive to modifications or equipment that make the child appear different or "disabled." Establishing therapeutic relationships may facilitate a caregiver's ability to follow through with recommendations required for safety and participation or help determine family-centered alternatives when appropriate. For example, if a caregiver does not put a protective helmet on the child when the child is out of bed, the occupational therapist may ask open-ended questions to find out what is preventing use of the helmet, followed by delivery of necessary education and/or support of the caregiver's ability to problem solve the obstacle.

Just before the child's return to home and school, a member of the medical team (typically an occupational therapist or a recreational therapist) may complete a community re-entry outing with the child and his or her caregivers. This experience provides the therapist with insight into the child's strengths and deficits in the community; the outing also gives caregivers insight into how to navigate the community, both physically and emotionally, when their child has functional limitations. The therapist may discuss how to talk about the trauma and the functional ramifications of the injury with community members; it may empower the family to know that they are in control of how much information they give and to whom. The therapist may even role play difficult interactions the child and caregivers may encounter, especially in regard to changes in the child's appearance, behaviors, means of communication, or use of adaptive equipment.

Collaboration with a social worker and/or psychologist may be appropriate to address the child's and caregivers' emotional readiness for return to home, school, and the community.[115] During the inpatient rehabilitation stay, the lingering effects and potential permanence of the traumatic injury become more real to the caregiver. The occupational therapist may suggest coping strategies to address a caregiver's anxiety about transitioning home with a child who remains different from how he or she was before the traumatic incident. In particular, a therapist empathetically supports a caregiver whose child has not made significant improvements in function. The occupational therapist may problem solve with the caregiver how to balance the new demands of having a child with a disability and the typical demands of home, work, and family life. Furthermore, an occupational therapist must be nonjudgmental if a caregiver determines that he or she cannot care for a severely injured child with significant medical needs and chooses to pursue a long-term care placement for the child.

Often the child and caregiver have established a close working relationship with the inpatient health care providers. The occupational therapist may help ease the transition to the

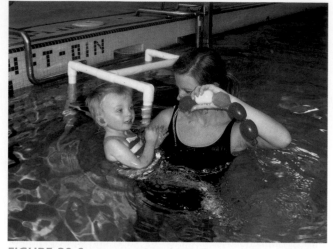

FIGURE 30-6 Aquatic therapy makes use of buoyant and resistive properties of the warm water environment to promote ROM, strengthening, and function beyond what is achievable on land for children with many conditions following trauma. This child, who presents with right hemiplegia following a TBI, is able to attain increased AROM and is more motivated than in the typical therapy environment.

outpatient stage of recovery by educating the child and the caregiver on what to expect in the school and outpatient clinic settings. He or she may also reassure the caregiver of the continuity of family-centered occupational therapy intervention throughout the stages of care.[92]

Children with Spinal Cord Injury in Inpatient Rehabilitation

Preparatory methods:

- Pain and tone management continue to be addressed by previous interventions and medical consultation as needed. In addition to previous interventions, aquatic therapy[69] (Figure 30-6), vibration input to muscles,[90] strengthening exercises, and electrical stimulation[40] may support spasticity management.
- Updated positioning schedules include a pressure relief routine because children are upright for longer periods at this stage. Pressure relief should be completed with a lateral or, preferably, anterior weight shift or pushing up on arms for 2 minutes every 15 minutes.[61] For children who cannot complete pressure relief independently, caregivers should change their position at least once an hour.[61]
- Children with active wrist extension and no active finger movement may be appropriate for promotion of a functional grasping pattern called tenodesis. The therapist uses splinting to encourage therapeutic shortening of flexor intrinsic muscles to facilitate digit flexion during wrist extension with a hand position similar to a lateral pinch grasp.[56]

Purposeful activities and occupation-based interventions:

- For small children, participation in developmentally appropriate floor play should be supported regardless of physical deficits.[65]
- Neuromuscular re-education continues to support restoration of motor functions. For example, task training, or practicing a task repeatedly, has been shown to improve function of clients with SCI[112] and may be supported by brain plasticity.[74] Of note, family-centered goal setting and specificity of task training results in improved performance of the practiced task but does not necessarily translate to other tasks.[112]
- Electrical stimulation may be used to restore coordination and strength when integrated into a functional task at a motor or sensory threshold level.[67] Electrical stimulation must be ordered by a physician and used with caution; the risk of electrical burn is significant owing to probable decreased skin sensation as well as potential intolerance, especially with the pediatric population.
- Training on optimal movement patterns promotes muscle balance and may prevent secondary injury and chronic pain. A clinical practice guideline for preserving upper extremity function published by Paralyzed Veterans of America Consortium for Spinal Cord Medicine[97] explains use of ergonomics, exercise, equipment selection and training, and environmental adaptations for prevention and management of injury and pain.
- Collaboration with nursing staff may help to facilitate the child's participation in bowel and bladder management. A bowel management program generally begins with a conservative approach (e.g., transanal irrigation or electrical stimulation of abdominal muscles), then pharmacologic, followed by a surgical approach as appropriate, with the highest level of evidence supporting pharmacologic management.[75]
- Children may be educated to perform skin inspections for pressure ulcer prevention when age appropriate.

Education:

- Information on sexual function, which may be affected by SCI, may be provided to children and adolescents in a developmentally appropriate manner.[53] For example, a teenage girl may be curious about her ability to conceive a child or want to inquire about necessary changes to her contraceptive methods without her caregivers being present.[53]
- Education on the importance of pressure relief and adherence to the bowel and bladder program is emphasized, because poor follow-through with these routines can result in re-hospitalization.

Children with Traumatic Brain Injury in Inpatient Rehabilitation

Preparatory methods:

- Arousal level and agitation can influence the child's ability to attend to and complete functional tasks.[46] Arousal, pain, and tone management continue to be addressed by previous interventions and medical consultation as needed.[46,106,132]

Purposeful activities and occupation-based interventions:

- Neuromuscular re-education continues to support restoration of motor functions. The occupational therapist promotes fine motor and visuomotor skills through activities that challenge current level of function.

- Electrical stimulation may be used to restore coordination and strength when integrated into a functional task at a motor or sensory threshold; precautions must be taken as described for children with SCI.
- Cognitive performance is a significant focus for children after TBI. Often the earlier children experience a brain injury, the poorer their cognitive prognosis, owing to a smaller foundation of typical development on which to rely during the recovery process.[5,52,132] Therefore it may be more difficult for the child to use prior experiences to restore skills postinjury.
- Cognitive re-training facilitates restoration of mental functions, including attention to task, memory, command following, sequencing, and organization. The child is given opportunities to practice adapted cognitive strategies for problem solving and safety awareness. The occupational therapist monitors, prompts, and reinforces safety awareness in a variety of contexts.[132]
- It is common for children and adolescents who have experienced a TBI to demonstrate behavioral difficulties. It may be beneficial for the occupational therapist to identify antecedents to problematic behaviors and develop strategies to promote cognitive function, executive functioning, and appropriate behavior.[63,132]
- Assessment of visual perceptual skills may be indicated at this time, as well as further cognitive and neuropsychological testing by other disciplines. Results of the assessments may support successful transition to school and subsequent improved quality of life for the child post injury.[63]

Education:

- Education on the results of standardized assessments prepares the caregiver for his or her child's return to school. If the child is able to maintain average academic performance compared with same-aged peers following a TBI, caregivers and children perceive the child to have a higher quality of life.[63]
- A child who has sustained a severe, global TBI or anoxic brain injury may not demonstrate functional progress before discharge to home. Autonomic storming, posturing, and severe agitation may remain. Significant support from the entire medical team is required to enable the caregiver to meet the medical and self-care needs of the child at home.[84]

Children with Burn Injury in Inpatient Rehabilitation

Preparatory methods:

- Aggressive range of motion and pressure therapy may continue as needed. Stretches should be completed to terminal range and held for 1 to 2 minutes because the amount of force needed for stretch is significantly more than in most diagnoses[45] (Figure 30-7). Stretches need to be completed until full active range of motion is easily achieved daily, which typically does not occur until 12 to 18 months postinjury.
- Splinting remains appropriate when full passive range of motion is not easily achieved within a therapy session. Evidence supports splinting to provide successive increase in tissue elongation, which ultimately promotes increased function.[34]

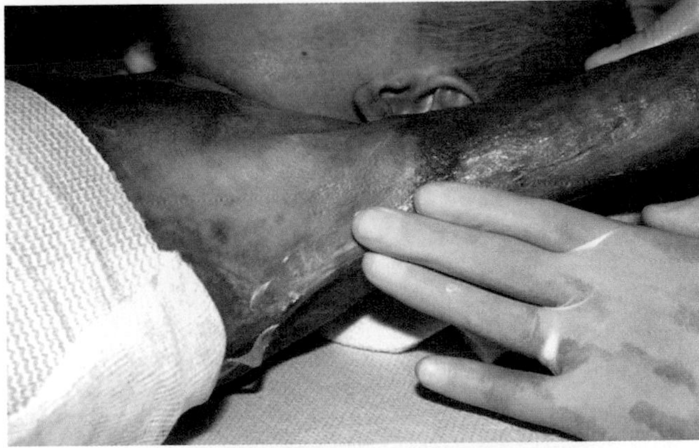

FIGURE 30-7 Healing burns and skin grafts contract with tensile force that is much stronger than normal skin during the weeks and months following injury and surgical repair. This is often seen in the inpatient rehabilitation phase. It is crucial for the therapist to complete stretches to maximal ROM twice a day, and this often takes significantly more time and force than stretches completed for other conditions.

Purposeful activities and occupation-based interventions:

- As the child regains strength and range, range of motion exercises should be followed with age- and interest-appropriate functional skills (Figure 30-8).

Education:

- Demonstration and hands-on opportunities are essential to caregivers' successful completion of the post-burn home exercise program. The occupational therapist provides home program instruction, explains its importance, facilitates practice of the home program, and gives caregivers feedback on their performance. The home program should include twice-daily range of motion and massage to all affected joints. Depending on the size of the burn, these sessions may take several hours and are often quite uncomfortable for the child. Caregivers must gain comfort and mastery with this program before discharge, as missing even a single home program session may result in a loss of range of motion.
- The occupational therapist further explains information on the child's condition. The therapist also recommends psychosocial resources and community supports as needed. Family support is essential for successful recovery from a childhood skin injury.[78]
- This period is often overwhelming and difficult for the caregivers; staff modeling of therapeutic and empathetic ways to manage the child's likely intolerance of painful interventions is crucial.

Outpatient Rehabilitation and Community Reintegration

Post-trauma, the outpatient stage of care involves addressing the child's and caregivers' needs once they have returned to their natural environments of home and community.[5] The occupational therapist examines a variety of factors during the outpatient rehabilitation evaluation. Chart review, assessment

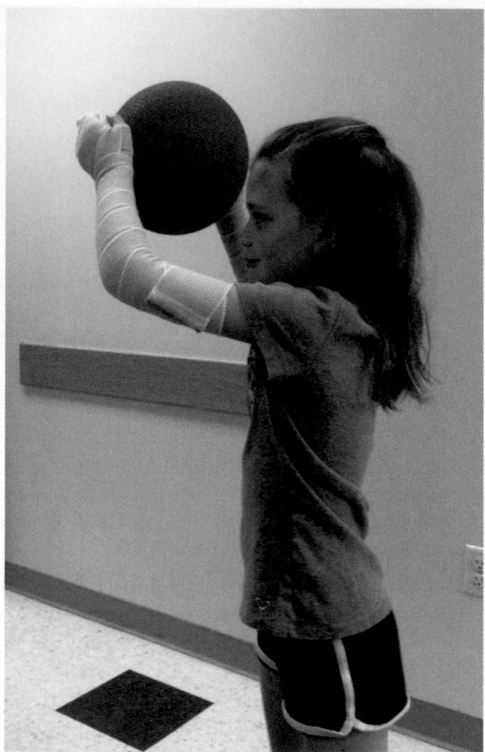

FIGURE 30-8 As strength and range of motion are regained during recovery from a burn injury, stretches should be followed with age- and interest-appropriate functional activities. This is also helpful in modeling to parents the fact that the child can participate in normal activities while wearing necessary pressure wrappings or garments.

of injured body structures and impaired body functions, and family interview are used to obtain the history and current performance, including precautions; impairments; level of participation in activities of daily living, instrumental activities of daily living, school or work, play, or leisure, and social opportunities; barriers, including context or activity demands (e.g., equipment needs); caregiver education needs; and consultation needs. The occupational therapist administers outcome measures to establish a baseline for the outpatient rehabilitation program. He or she re-administers assessments regularly to ensure efficacy of interventions, document progress, and guide occupational therapy treatment plan updates. The therapist shares results with the family and other health care team members to promote consistent, coordinated care.[63]

When appropriate, the outpatient therapist continues to use preparatory methods to address impairments that inhibit performance skills; however, the focus of therapy in this stage is on purposeful activities and occupation-based interventions.[5] The occupational therapist facilitates optimal, age-appropriate participation in self-care, school, work, and leisure. He or she collaborates with the family during occupational therapy plan of care development to create client-centered goals that address the child's short- and long-term function.

The family's priorities at initiation of outpatient rehabilitation often include safety and functional issues that have arisen since discharge home. For example, a significant number of adaptive devices issued by an inpatient therapist to clients with SCI[49] and other diagnoses are not used by the 1-year anniversary of discharge from the hospital. Families benefit from ongoing outpatient occupational therapy consultation to determine updated equipment recommendations. To address context-dependent functional issues in the outpatient setting, the occupational therapist relies on the child and caregiver to accurately report the child's participation in his or her natural environments[132] and, when appropriate, arranges the therapy space to simulate the natural environment. The occupational therapist continues to use both restorative and adaptive approaches to treatment as appropriate to maximize the child's participation while working toward return to his or her premorbid level of function.

Another common family priority post-hospital discharge is the child's school re-entry.[5] A child's re-integration into the school environment may be delayed because of medical issues and/or be gradual (i.e., initially returning to school with a partial-day schedule). In-home instruction may also be instituted. Communicating with the school may help the staff understand the child's changing needs post-discharge. Collaboration to develop school accommodations facilitates the child's optimal performance in school despite ongoing deficits post-trauma. Ongoing communication with school throughout outpatient rehabilitation promotes a consistent approach to the child's care and an ability to determine any differences in the child's function depending on context.

Once a family's daily routine, including home and school, is manageable post-discharge, the occupational therapist may facilitate community involvement. The therapist educates the child and caregiver regarding resources and opportunities for community engagement,[48,129] including adapted recreational programs and peer-based groups. The occupational therapist may deliver intervention during family outings in natural, community environments.[14] These opportunities can be a powerful way to observe how the family functions, e.g., how a family navigates in various settings and how the caregiver uses coping strategies in public places. If community outings are not feasible because of logistical or funding barriers, the occupational therapist may set up mock public environments or use a more public area of the therapy facility to accomplish community re-integration goals.

A self-management approach, including motivational interviewing (an open-ended, empathetic method of talking with caregivers) may help the practitioner identify sources of family's stress when returning home.[24] Stressors may include caring for their child without the supports of the hospital environment, equipment management, altered family dynamics, school re-entry issues, community participation barriers, schedule demands, coming to terms with their child's functional limitations, and uncertainty about the future.[48] Once identified, the occupational therapist may direct caregivers to appropriate community resources, including respite care and support groups (e.g., online, hospital-based, local, or national groups). Referral to other health care professionals, including a care coordinator, social worker, or psychologist, may also be appropriate.

Occupational therapists also use self-management to assess family readiness for change. Some education topics provided during the inpatient stage are re-stated to demonstrate continuity of care[48] and ensure caregiver understanding. New education at this stage includes home programming to support the child's progress.[14] A self-management approach may be used to support caregivers' ability to identify and problem solve barriers preventing implementation of home programs, because the occupational therapist no longer has the benefit of a controlled environment to ensure follow-through with necessary therapeutic recommendations.

As the outpatient rehabilitation episode of care continues, the caregiver's ability to manage the child's needs at home progresses. The child and his or her family members often become more cohesive and re-integrated into the community as they continue with the post-injury stage of life. The need for skilled intervention decreases as a child approaches a premorbid level of function or functional recovery slows, at which time decreasing therapy frequency or discharge from therapy may be appropriate. The Cincinnati Children's Hospital Guidelines for determining frequency of therapy[7] describe clinical reasoning to determine how frequently a child should receive therapy and when he or she should be discharged. Often survivors of pediatric trauma return to occupational therapy for future episodes of care when different functional concerns arise or new demands are placed on them throughout the life span.[23,100]

Children with Spinal Cord Injury in Outpatient Rehabilitation and Community Reintegration

Preparatory methods:

- Pain and tone management continue to be addressed by previous interventions and medical consultation as needed.

Purposeful activities and occupation-based interventions:

- Neuromuscular re-education continues to support restoration of motor functions.
- For some clients electrical stimulation may be used as adaptive equipment long-term to compensate for grasp deficits in the form of a surgically implanted or transcutaneous upper extremity neuroprosthesis.[67]
- Depending on level of injury and whether spasticity is adequately controlled, some arm and hand function may be restored surgically with tendon transfer or nerve transfer followed by neuromuscular re-education.[16,27,39]
- Common instrumental activities of daily living for children with SCI include communication device use, community mobility, meal preparation and clean up, safety procedures, health management, and shopping, as developmentally appropriate.
- A child's participation in health management may be limited by accessibility of community recreation programs. Children with SCI may benefit from development of age-appropriate and client-centered exercise programs, including upper-body ergometry via arm cycling, functional electrical stimulation, resistance strengthening, or functional strengthening. For adults with SCI, exercise has been shown to improve physical capacity, extremity strength,[57,60,98,122] respiratory strength and endurance,[109] cardiovascular function,[98] subjective well-being,[85] and upper extremity motor control and function.[72] Exercise may also prevent bone loss.[6,10] Functional electrical stimulation combined with ergometry may be an appropriate option for children.[66]
- The outpatient occupational therapist may collaborate with school therapists or teachers on classroom adaptations for children with SCI, the most common of which include writing aids; program accommodations; and physical assistance for functional mobility, health maintenance, self-care, and manipulating learning materials.[38]
- After restrictions are lifted by the physician, a teenager may resume driving with necessary car modifications as determined by a certified driving specialist.[53]
- Participation during occupational therapy is a significant predictor of functional outcomes for clients with SCI[96] therefore it is vital to maximize a child's engagement by adopting family-centered goals and integrating the child's interest into therapy interventions.
- Occupational therapy interventions increase quality of life for clients with SCI post-discharge[25] by addressing their foremost priorities, which include motor function (i.e., upper extremity function for clients with quadriplegia and functional mobility for clients with paraplegia), bowel and bladder function, and sexual function as appropriate for age.[111]

Education:

- Education must address problem-solving barriers to participation in the natural environment,[86] as well as health care topics, including safety with decreased sensation and impaired body temperature regulation.
- Referral to other health care professionals, including neuropsychologists when appropriate, may improve quality of life, because approximately 30% of individuals with SCI may be at risk for depression.[28]
- Educating on accessible community resources is also important because handicap is significantly associated with lower quality of life in clients with SCI.[35]
- Accessing social supports in the community is associated with improved physical and mental health, including improved life satisfaction and decreased pain.[89]

Children with Traumatic Brain Injury in Outpatient Rehabilitation and Community Reintegration

Preparatory methods:

- A child with a severe global injury may continue to experience significant spasticity and/or autonomic storming. Medical consultation or interventions to manage muscle tone,[132] arousal levels, and pain may continue.
- As previously discussed, if a child has become more neurologically regulated and begins to progress in recovery stages (i.e., Rancho Levels of Cognitive Functioning),[54,99] the occupational therapist may modify the therapy treatment plan to maximize purposeful engagement.

Purposeful activities and occupation-based interventions:

- Neuromuscular re-education continues to support restoration of motor functions (Figure 30-9).[5,132] For example, constraint-induced movement therapy is an intervention technique well supported in the literature to promote function of a hemiplegic upper extremity and has been used with children who have experienced a TBI (Figure 30-10).[22,108]

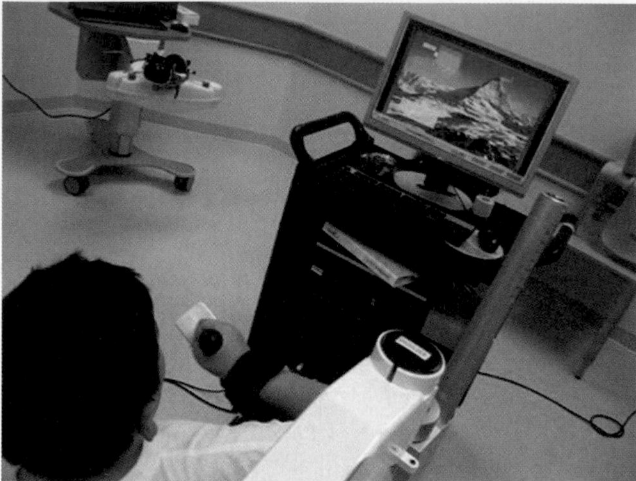

FIGURE 30-9 A supportive upper extremity mobility device can promote neuromuscular re-education through virtual reality.

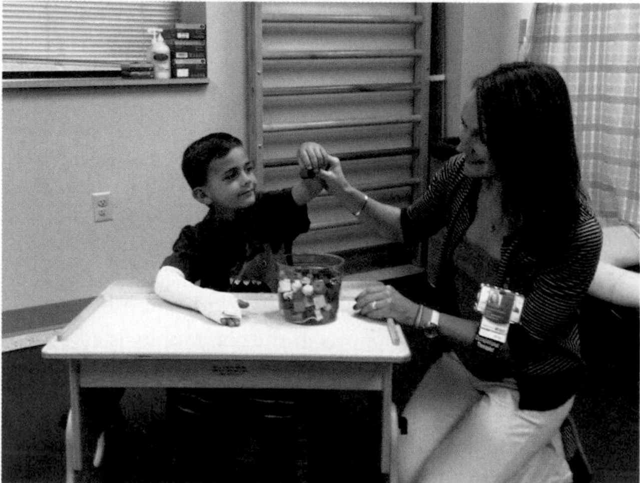

FIGURE 30-10 Constraint-induced movement therapy involves limiting use of the more functional upper extremity to promote increased strength and function of the impaired side. It is widely supported and can be used following TBI or any condition that results in hemiplegia.

- Cognitive re-training continues to support restoration of process functions.[5,19,47,132] Deficits may further emerge after school re-entry.
- Compensatory cognitive strategies may include visual schedules or reminders,[47] cueing techniques, schedule management, organization tools, and environmental modifications.[19]

Education:

- Ongoing behavioral issues are common in this population. For example, teenagers who have sustained a severe TBI demonstrate significant difficulties in behavior and mental health. These problems have significant family impact.[114] The family's ability to manage is dependent on the severity of the injury, family cohesiveness, and the resources available.[5,131,132]
- Education may include information and instruction for using adapted strategies and equipment. Caregivers are educated in methods to support the child's functional capabilities.[5,19,132]
- The caregivers may begin to seek respite opportunities because of the vast, ongoing demands on the caregiver.[93]

See Case Study 30-2.

Children with Burn Injury in Outpatient Rehabilitation and Community Reintegration

Preparatory methods:

- Range of motion exercises, scar massage, pressure therapy, and splinting must be continued to maintain or regain lost range of motion as scars mature, which typically occurs 12 to 18 months postinjury. Although these are monitored by the occupational therapist, they are the responsibility of the caregiver to perform daily.
- Supervised aerobic and progressive resistance training programs have been shown to be useful in rehabilitation following burn injuries and to significantly reduce the need for surgical reconstruction owing to joint contracture.[20,29,116-118]

Purposeful activities and occupation-based interventions:

- Therapeutic activities that follow range of motion exercises focus on resuming engagement in chosen activities and age-appropriate occupations. The occupational therapist may help facilitate the child's redefinition of self as a "burn survivor" (versus burn victim) through personal exploration.

Education:

- It is essential for the occupational therapist to continue to stress the importance of maintaining the home program during the active scarring phase, despite difficulty with child cooperation and tolerance. As always, therapeutic relationships may provide needed support and reassurance during this time.

Conclusion

Occupational therapists can be inspired by children's ability to offer a refreshing perspective on their current life situation, regardless of how daunting the circumstances may seem. A child who has been traumatically injured and his or her family must face and overcome an unexpected landmark that occurs in an instant and lasts a lifetime. They grapple with the consequences, move forward, and begin to heal their wounds, external and internal, real and metaphoric. Nothing is as motivating and inspiring as watching a child overcome horrendous obstacles in an innocent and positive way. It is difficult to match the value one can experience when a parent learns to take on the role of mom or dad again after weeks of feeling vulnerable and intimidated by his or her child's fragile medical status. The occupational therapist often has a strong impact on facilitating function during the recovery process, both the function of the child and the function of the caregivers. Few experiences are as professionally, or personally, rewarding.

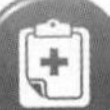

CASE STUDY 30-2 Sam

History

Sam is an 8-year-old boy who was riding his bicycle in a wind storm and was hit in the head by a large tree branch. He sustained a brain injury, including a large left frontal lobe laceration with an extensive shear injury, multiple subdural hematomas, and many regions of diffuse damage. His skull was fractured in multiple locations, along with fractures of the C7 spinous process and T1-T3 compression fractures. On admission, he underwent emergency bilateral craniectomy surgeries to relieve the intracranial pressure and address the significant subdural hemorrhaging. He spent 1 month in the ICU and was transferred to the inpatient pediatric rehabilitation unit. During his hospital stay, he experienced significant muscle spasticity managed by medication, serial casting, and splinting. His body's ability to regulate itself was inadequate, causing autonomic storming episodes with a consistent decorticate posturing pattern (tonal pattern involving intense spasticity with shoulders adducted and internally rotated, elbows flexed, forearms pronated, wrists flexed, and digits in composite flexion). He wore a back brace at all times to address his spinal stability needs and a helmet was placed on his head when out of bed. During his inpatient stages of care, his occupational therapist focused on facilitating consistent, localized responses to stimulation; decreasing his agitation via environmental adjustments and positioning methods; spasticity management via positioning and splinting during times of decreased agitation; facilitating upright and out-of-bed positioning in his wheelchair and in therapy gyms within limited tolerance; caregiver education regarding necessary adaptive equipment (fully supportive shower chair, tilt-in-space wheelchair with full support); transfers; and handling methods used to facilitate purposeful responses. In addition, hypertrophic scar development was noted on his left cheek owing to deep skin wounds sustained during the accident. These scars were managed in a manner similar to burn care, using scar massage and monitoring for the need for pressure therapy. After 3 months of hospitalization, Sam was discharged home. His recovery had stabilized and had not progressed significantly; he was fully dependent for all self-care and communication needs. Sam continued to have consistent, yet decreasing, periods of autonomic storming, hypertonicity, and agitation and was beginning to visually track for brief periods. He was assigned a home nurse who was trained in managing his care during the day while his parents worked. It was decided that he would participate in intensive occupational, physical, and speech pathology treatments on an outpatient basis.

Assessment

Sam's parents and home health nurse attended the outpatient occupational therapy evaluation. His parents reported feeling overwhelmed with Sam's care and wanting to know how the recovery process for their son would proceed. Sam was agitated and storming during the initial evaluation, making it difficult to fully assess his passive upper extremity range of motion. He postured in a modified decorticate pattern with his trunk in right rotation and pelvis in left rotation, particularly when placed in a supine position on the mat table. His parents reported that the periods of time when this posturing occurred were becoming less frequent. The occupational therapist noted that his tonal pattern decreased when he was placed in a right side-lying position, allowing his shoulders to depress and protract. The occupational therapist placed Sam in various supported positions on the mat to observe his tolerance to transitional movements, spasticity patterns, and head and trunk muscle facilitation. He did not demonstrate the ability to visually track during the evaluation; however, his parents reported that he would, at times, demonstrate purposeful visual attention in the home environment (i.e., with the television). During times of increased alertness, Sam's parents reported that he appropriately smiled to auditory input. The occupational therapist explored the family's current adaptive equipment, discussed the parents' and nurse's comfort with using the equipment, observed Sam in his wheelchair and discussed the home set up. Additionally, she asked the family questions about Sam's premorbid recreational interests, which included baseball, playing with his friends, karate, telling jokes, and spending time with his older brother.

Intervention

As outpatient therapies were initiated and his doctors refined his medications, Sam's autonomic storming episodes decreased. As this happened, bilateral upper extremity hypertonicity decreased and he presented in a hemiplegic manner. Sam's began to demonstrate purposeful use of his left upper extremity, and his right presented as flaccid proximally with simultaneous distal tightness of his long finger flexors and wrist flexors. He continued to hold his left elbow at approximately 90 degrees of flexion with internal rotation and adduction of the shoulder.

The first stage of his outpatient occupational therapy intervention facilitated his emerging purposeful left upper extremity movement. Sam was placed in a right side-lying position on the mat table to eliminate gravity to promote left upper extremity reach. For example, Sam demonstrated early motivation when exposed to a water toy. A basic button switch was connected to the water toy that poured water into a spout with activation. Initially the therapist used a hand-over-hand strategy to elicit reach in this position. From there, Sam began to visually attend to this toy and engaged in purposeful reach for the switch. The occupational therapist talked with Sam and his parents in a conversational way, making an effort to discuss with Sam professional baseball scores and tell him silly jokes. During these interactions, Sam demonstrated appropriate smiling and laughing and visually attended to the occupational therapist when she spoke.

Early outpatient sessions also included supported sitting on the edge of the mat table with a mirror in front of Sam for visual feedback to address basic head control, visual attention, and tracking. After a few weeks, he demonstrated independent head control, and trunk control became a more

Continued

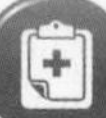

CASE STUDY 30-2 Sam—cont'd

significant focus of intervention. Functional activity was incorporated throughout each stage, engaging Sam's interests while maximizing his ability to move his left upper extremity against gravity. He reached for a baseball while seated, placed a small plastic basketball into a hoop, and participated in self-care. His parents were involved in one session per week on a common day off of work, learning how to work with Sam at home. The occupational therapist developed a splinting protocol for use with his right upper extremity at night, and functional electrical stimulation program. After a few months, Sam began to demonstrate basic reach and grasp with his more affected right side.

The occupational therapist participated in ongoing, consistent communication with other care team members regarding Sam's progress. As Sam's agitation diminished, his performance increased with left-sided functional use and fine motor skills, improved cognition, visual processing, motor planning, and emerging right-sided mobility. His self-care participation became a greater focus in occupational therapy as his independence increased. He began to assist with stand pivot transfers and used a gait trainer with physical therapy. He began attending school 2 days per week. Sam's large, tilt-in-space manual wheelchair was becoming a barrier to his function owing to components no longer needed. In therapy he trialed power wheelchairs with an equipment vendor on multiple occasions and, after educating the family and understanding his capabilities, he was deemed appropriate to use a power wheelchair. He received a new wheelchair and additional training on its use; within a few short weeks, he was able to navigate his school, home, and community environments with supervision. Sam's mindset greatly improved with his new-found independence.

Sam's outpatient rehabilitation then incorporated aquatic therapy and weekly exercises for upper extremity and trunk strength. His ataxia and right upper extremity mobility continued to improve, allowing him to focus on bimanual skills. The occupational therapist balanced the use of compensation and restoration techniques as his progress continued. Continued outpatient sessions focused on any barriers to functioning fully in the home, school, and community environments.

Summary

- Occupational therapists use restorative approaches to facilitate the child's performance skill progression toward his or her prior level of function. Alternatively, they use compensatory approaches when immediate increase in function is needed to give the child a sense of accomplishment, when a plateau in performance improvement is experienced, or when an alternative approach to increase function is needed. These approaches may be used in tandem; that is, certain child and family goals may require a restorative approach and others a compensatory approach. It is often this balance that promotes the most function and success.
- Regardless of diagnosis, the occupational therapist addresses injured body structures and impaired body functions by applying preparatory methods to promote homeostasis and prevent secondary injury. Interventions to maximize range of motion include stretches, soft tissue mobilization, splinting, and positioning and are used with children with SCI, TBI, or burn injury. Positioning is also used for pressure ulcer and pain prevention across diagnoses. For children with TBI, environmental sensory stimulation is modulated to prevent agitation. Wound care and scar massage are preparatory methods specific to children with burn injury.
- A child ideally progresses through the recovery continuum with a different therapy focus at each stage, though interventions from previous stages continue to be utilized as appropriate, e.g., splinting may be used from the ICU to outpatient rehabilitation. In the ICU, the focus is on preventing secondary complications such as pain, contracture, and pressure ulcers from the body's state of immobility and impaired ability to maintain homeostasis. The focus in acute care is on the child's ability to resume available motor functions, often beginning with basic tolerance for upright positioning and head and trunk control. The occupational therapist continues to closely monitor vital signs and tolerance of intervention. During inpatient rehabilitation the focus of therapy is to facilitate the child's independence in self-care and play or leisure activities. Caregivers require hands-on education to prepare for the child's transition back to his or her home, school, and community settings. Outpatient therapy may focus on IADL, school participation, and community re-integration.
- Coordinated care among professionals promotes the child's safety, increases the team's consistency of care provision, prevents the delivery of conflicting information, and facilitates the child's ability to carry over restored skills to various contexts. Consistency not only promotes the child's rehabilitation, but also provides the child and caregiver with a sense of security during potentially stressful transitions.
- Moses[87] suggests that a child's trauma and subsequent disability "shatter the dreams" a caregiver has for the child and begin a grieving process. A family's grieving process must be taken into account when providing education post-trauma, because a child or caregivers may be better able to take in and/or benefit from certain information in a different grieving state.
- An occupational therapist uses different methods to establish rapport with severely impaired children depending on their level of consciousness. To increase the child's comfort with and trust in the therapist, the therapist may provide the child with adaptive equipment to improve function, educate the child in directing his or her care, use developmentally appropriate comfort measures to address pain, ensure safe and consistent care provision, help create a low stimulation environment, incorporate the child's interests into all interventions, closely monitor the child's responses to interventions, and/or explain what he or she is doing with the child in a developmentally appropriate manner. For intervention directed at the caregivers, the occupational

therapist may provide an appropriate level of information, give hands-on instruction to support the ability to resume caring for the child, use family-friendly language, acknowledge their grieving process, remember their unique perspective on their child's progress, and remain cautiously hopeful.

- Rehabilitation with children differs from that with adults because of the additional consideration of each child's developmental stage. Working with children post-trauma involves focusing treatment on both the child and caregiver's priorities and needs. Compared with developmental pediatric treatment, the occupational therapist must be mindful that caregivers post-trauma are not only adjusting to sudden differences in their child, but also to differences in the breadth and depth of the caregivers' responsibilities.

REFERENCES

1. Altman, I., Swick, S., Parrot, D., et al. (2010). Effectiveness of community-based rehabilitation after traumatic brain injury for 489 program completers compared with those precipitously discharged. *Archives of Physical Medicine and Rehabilitation, 91*, 1697–1704.
2. Alster, T. S., & Tanzi, E. L. (2003). Hypertrophic scars and keloids: Etiology and management. *American Journal of Clinical Dermatology, 4*, 235–243.
3. American Burn Association (2014). *Burn Incidence and Treatment in the United States: 2013 Fact Sheet.* Retrieved July 14, 2014 from: <http://www.ameriburn.org/resources_factsheet.php>.
4. American Occupational Therapy Association. (2008). Occupational therapy practice framework: Domain and process. *American Journal of Occupational Therapy, 62*, 625–683.
5. Anderson, V., & Catroppa, C. (2006). Advances in postacute rehabilitation after childhood-acquired brain injury: A focus on cognitive, behavioral, and social domains. *American Journal of Physical Medicine and Rehabilitation, 85*, 767–778.
6. Ashe, M., Craven, C., Eng, J., et al. (2007). Prevention and treatment of bone loss after a spinal cord injury: A systematic review. *Topics in Spinal Cord Injury Rehabilitation, 13*, 123–145.
7. Bailes, A. F., Reder, R., & Burch, C. (2008). Development of guidelines for determining frequency of therapy services in a pediatric medical setting. *Pediatric Physical Therapy, 20*, 194–198.
8. Berman, B., & Flores, F. (1998). The treatment of hypertrophic scars and keloids. *European Journal of Dermatology, 8*, 591–595.
9. Berman, B., Viera, M. H., Amini, S., et al. (2008). Prevention and management of hypertrophic scars and keloids after burns in children. *Journal of Craniofacial Surgery, 19*, 989–1006.
10. Biering-Sørensen, F., Hansen, B., & Lee, B. (2009). Non-pharmacological treatment and prevention of bone loss after spinal cord injury: A systematic review. *Spinal Cord, 47*, 508–518.
11. Bloemen, M. C., van der Veer, W. M., Ulrich, M. M., et al. (2009). Prevention and curative management of hypertrophic scar formation. *Burns: Journal of the International Society for Burn Injuries, 35*, 463–475.
12. Bock, O., Schmid-Ott, G., Malewski, P., et al. (2006). Quality of life of patients with keloid and hypertrophic scarring. *Archives of Dermatology Research, 297*, 433–438.
13. Bombaro, K. M., Engrav, L. H., Carrougher, G. J., et al. (2003). What is the prevalence of hypertrophic scarring following burns? *Burns: Journal of the International Society for Burn Injuries, 29*, 299–302.
14. Braga, L. W., DaPaz Junior, A. C., & Ylvisaker, M. (2005). Direct clinician-delivered versus indirect family-supported rehabilitation of children with traumatic brain injury: A randomized controlled trial. *Brain Injury, 19*, 819–831.
15. Brown, B. C., McKenna, S. P., Siddhi, K., et al. (2008). The hidden cost of skin scars: Quality of life after skin scarring. *Journal of Plastic, Reconstructive, & Aesthetic Surgery, 61*, 1049–1058.
16. Bryden, A., Peljovich, A., Hoyen, H., et al. (2012). Surgical restoration of arm and hand function in people with tetraplegia. *Topics in Spinal Cord Injury Rehabilitation, 18*, 43–49.
17. Candy, L. H., Cecilia, L. T., & Ping, Z. Y. (2010). Effect of different pressure magnitudes on hypertrophic scar in a Chinese population. *Burns: Journal of the International Society for Burn Injuries, 36*, 1234–1241.
18. Carr, T., Harris, D., & James, C. (2000). The Derriford Appearance Scale (DAS-59): A new scale to measure individual responses to living with problems of appearance. *British Journal of Health Psychology, 5*, 201–215.
19. Catroppa, C., & Anderson, V. (2009). Traumatic brain injury in childhood: Rehabilitation considerations. *Developmental Neurorehabilitation, 12*, 53–61.
20. Celis, M. M., Suman, O. E., Huang, T. T., et al. (2003). Effect of a supervised exercise and physiotherapy program on surgical interventions in children with thermal injury. *Journal of Burn Care and Rehabilitation, 24*, 57–61.
21. Chafetz, R., Mulcahey, M., Betz, R., et al. (2007). Impact of prophylactic thoracolumbosacral orthosis bracing on functional activities and activities of daily living in the pediatric spinal cord injury population. *The Journal of Spinal Cord Medicine, 30*, S178–S183.
22. Charles, J., & Gordon, A. M. (2005). A critical review of constraint-induced movement therapy and forced use in children with hemiplegia. *Neural Plasticity, 12*, 245–261.
23. Chevignard, M. P., Brooks, N., & Truelle, J. (2010). Community integration following severe childhood traumatic brain injury. *Current Opinion in Neurology, 23*, 695–700.
24. Chronic Care: Self-Management Guideline Team, Cincinnati Children's Hospital Medical Center (2007). *Evidence-based care guideline for chronic care: Self-management.* Retrieved May 22, 2013, from: <www.cincinnatichildrens.org/svc/alpha/h/health-policy/cv-based/chronic-care.htm>.
25. Cohen, M., & Schemm, R. (2007). Client-centered occupational therapy for individuals with spinal cord injury. *Occupational Therapy in Healthcare, 21*, 1–15.
26. Commission of Accreditation of Rehabilitation Facilities (2012). *International Standards Manual for Pediatric Specialty Programs.* Tucson, AZ: Commission of Accreditation of Rehabilitation Facilities.
27. Cornwall, R., & Hausman, M. (2004). Implanted neuroprostheses for restoration of hand function in tetraplegic patients. *Journal of the American Academy of Orthopaedic Surgeons, 12*, 72–79.
28. Craig, A., Tran, Y., & Middleton, J. (2009). Psychological morbidity and spinal cord injury: A systematic review. *Spinal Cord, 47*, 108–114.
29. Cucuzzo, N. A., Ferrando, A., & Herndon, D. N. (2001). The effects of exercise programming vs traditional

outpatient therapy in the rehabilitation of severely burned children. *Journal of Burn Care and Rehabilitation, 22,* 214–220.

30. Cullen, N. K., & Weisz, K. (2011). Cognitive correlates with functional outcomes after anoxic brain injury: A case-controlled comparison with traumatic brain injury. *Brain Injury, 25,* 35–43.
31. Davoodi, P., Fernandez, J. M., & O., S. J. (2008). Postburn sequelae in the pediatric patient: Clinical presentations and treatment options. *Journal of Craniofacial Surgery, 19,* 1047–1052.
32. Deitch, E. A., Wheelahan, T. M., Rose, M. P., et al. (1983). Hypertrophic burn scars: Analysis of variables. *Journal of Trauma, 23,* 895–898.
33. Department of Defense and Department of Veterans Affairs. (2008). Departments of Defense (DoD) and Veterans Affairs (VA) code proposal. *Traumatic Brain Injury Task Force.* Retrieved May 19, 2013, from: <http://www.cdc.gov/nchs/data/icd9/Sep08TBI.pdf>.
34. Dewey, W. S., Richard, R. L., & Parry, I. S. (2011). Positioning, splinting, and contracture management. *Physical Medicine & Rehabilitation Clinics of North America, 22,* 229–247.
35. Dijkers, M. (1997). Quality of life after spinal cord injury: A meta-analysis of the effects of disablement components. *Spinal Cord, 35,* 829–840.
36. Dijkers, M., Bryce, T., & Zanca, J. (2009). Prevalence of chronic pain after traumatic spinal cord injury: A systematic review. *Journal of Rehabilitation Research & Development, 46,* 13–29.
37. Douglas, V., & Way, L. (2007). Scarring: A patient-centered approach. *Practice Nursing, 18,* 78–83.
38. Dudgeon, B., Massagli, T., & Ross, B. (1997). Educational participation of children with spinal cord injury. *American Journal of Occupational Therapy, 51,* 553–561.
39. Duff, S., Mulcahey, M., & Betz, R. (2008). Adaptation in sensorimotor control after restoration of grip and pinch in children with tetraplegia. *Topics in Spinal Cord Injury Rehabilitation, 13,* 54–71.
40. Elbasiouny, S., Moroz, D., Bakr, M., et al. (2009). Management of spasticity after spinal cord injury: Current techniques and future directions. *Neurorehabilitation & Neural Repair, 24,* 23–33.
41. Engrav, L. H., Heimbach, D. M., Rivara, F. P., et al. (2010). 12-Year within-wound study of the effectiveness of custom pressure garment therapy. *Burns: Journal of the International Society for Burn Injuries, 36,* 975–983.
42. Esselman, P. C., Thombs, B. D., Magyar-Russell, G., et al. (2006). Burn rehabilitation: State of the science. *American Journal Physical Medicine & Rehabilitation, 85,* 383–413.
43. Faul, M., Xu, L., Wald, M. M., et al. (2010). *Traumatic brain injury in the United States: Emergency department visits, hospitalizations and deaths 2002–2006.* Atlanta: Centers for Disease Control and Prevention, National Center for Injury Prevention and Control.
44. Field, T., Peck, M., Krugman, S., et al. (1998). Burn injuries benefit from massage therapy. *Journal of Burn Care & Rehabilitation, 19,* 241–244.
45. Flowers, K. R., & LaStayo, P. C. (2012). Effect of total end range time on improving passive range of motion. *Journal of Hand Therapy, 25,* 48–54.
46. Forsyth, R. (2009). Back to the future: Rehabilitation of children after brain injury. *Archives of Disease in Childhood, 95,* 554–559.
47. Galvin, J., & Mandalis, A. (2009). Executive skills and their functional implications: Approaches to rehabilitation after childhood TBI. *Developmental Neurorehabilitation, 12,* 352–360.
48. Gan, C., Gargaro, J., Brandys, C., et al. (2010). Family caregivers' support needs after brain injury: A synthesis of perspectives from caregivers, programs, and researchers. *Neurorehabilitation, 27,* 5–18.
49. Garber, S., & Gregorio, T. (1990). Upper extremity assistive devices: Assessment of use by spinal cord-injured patients with quadriplegia. *American Journal of Occupational Therapy, 44,* 126–131.
50. Garcia-Velasco, M., Ley, R., Mutch, D., et al. (1978). Compression treatment of hypertrophic scars in burned children. *Canadian Journal of Surgery, 21,* 450–452.
51. Gauglitz, G. G., Korting, H. C., Pavicic, T., et al. (2011). Hypertrophic scarring and keloids: Pathomechanisms and current and emerging treatment strategies. *Molecular Medicine, 17,* 113–125.
52. Gerrard-Morris, A., Gerry, T., Yeates, K. O., et al. (2010). Cognitive development after traumatic brain injury in young children. *Journal of the International Neuropsychological Society, 16,* 157–168.
53. Greenberg, J., Ruutiainen, A., & Kim, H. (2009). Rehabilitation of pediatric spinal cord injury: From acute medical care to rehabilitation and beyond. *Journal of Pediatric Rehabilitation Medicine: An Interdisciplinary Approach, 2,* 13–27.
54. Hagen, C., Malkmus, D., & Durham, P. (1979). *Rehabilitation of the head injured adult: Comprehensive physical management.* Downey, CA: Professional Staff Association of Rancho Los Amigos National Rehabilitation Center.
55. Haq, M. A., & Haq, A. (1990). Pressure therapy in treatment of hypertrophic scar, burn contracture and keloid: The Kenyan experience. *East African Medical Journal, 67,* 785–793.
56. Harvey, L. (1996). Principles of conservative management for a non-orthotic tenodesis grip in tetraplegics. *Journal of Hand Therapy, 9,* 238–242.
57. Harvey, L., Lin, C., Glinsky, J., et al. (2009). The effectiveness of physical interventions for people with spinal cord injuries: A systematic review. *Spinal Cord, 47,* 184–195.
58. Haverstock, B. D. (2001). Hypertrophic scars and keloids. *Clinics in Podiatric Medicine & Surgery, 18,* 147–159.
59. Herndon, D. N., & Pierre, E. J. (1998). Treatment of burns. In J. A. O'Neill, M. I. Rowe, J. L. Grosfeld, et al. (Eds.), *Pediatric surgery* (pp. 343–358). St. Louis: Mosby.
60. Hicks, A., Martin Ginis, K., Pelletier, C., et al. (2011). The effects of exercise training on physical capacity, strength, body composition and functional performance among adults with spinal cord injury: A systematic review. *Spinal Cord, 49,* 1103–1127.
61. Institute for Clinical Systems Improvement (2012). *Pressure ulcer prevention and treatment protocol: Health care protocol.* Bloomington, MN: Institute for Clinical Systems Improvement. Retrieved June 19, 2013, from: <http://www.guideline.gov/content.aspx?id=36059>.
62. Jensen, L., & Parshley, P. (1984). Postburn scar contractures: Histology and effects of pressure treatment. *Journal of Burn Care & Research, 5,* 119.
63. Johnson, A. R., DeMatt, E., & Salorio, C. F. (2009). Predictors of outcome following acquired brain injury in children. *Developmental Disabilities, Research Reviews, 15,* 124–132.
64. Johnson, J., Greenspan, B., Gorga, D., et al. (1994). Compliance with pressure garment use in burn rehabilitation. *Journal of Burn Care and Rehabilitation, 15,* 180–188.
65. Johnson, K., & Klaas, S. (2007). The changing nature of play: Implications for pediatric spinal cord injury. *The Journal of Spinal Cord Medicine, 30,* S71–S75.
66. Johnston, T., Smith, B., Oladeji, O., et al. (2008). Outcomes of a home

cycling program using functional electrical stimulation or passive motion for children with spinal cord injury: a case series. *The Journal of Spinal Cord Medicine*, *31*, 215–221.
67. Kalsi-Ryan, S., & Verrier, M. (2011). A synthesis of best evidence for the restoration of upper-extremity function in people with tetraplegia. *Physiotherapy Canada*, *63*, 474–489.
68. Kawecki, M., Bernad-Wisniewska, T., Sakiel, S., et al. (2008). Laser in the treatment of hypertrophic burn scars. *International Wound Journal*, *5*, 87–97.
69. Kesiktas, N., Paker, N., Erdogan, N., et al. (2004). The use of hydrotherapy for the management of spasticity. *Neurorehabilitation & Neural Repair*, *18*, 268–273.
70. Kim, H., & Colantonio, A. (2010). Effectiveness of rehabilitation in enhancing community integration after acute traumatic brain injury: A systematic review. *The American Journal of Occupational Therapy*, *64*, 709–719.
71. Kipping, B., Rodger, S., Miller, K., et al. (2012). Virtual reality for acute pain reduction in adolescents undergoing burn wound care: A prospective randomized controlled trial. *Burns: Journal of the International Society for Burn Injuries*, *38*, 650–657.
72. Kloosterman, M., Snoek, G., & Jannink, M. (2009). Systematic review of the effects of exercise therapy on the upper extremity of patients with spinal cord injury. *Spinal Cord*, *47*, 196–203.
73. Kloti, J., & Pochon, J. P. (1979). Long-term therapy of second and third degree burns in children using Jobst-compression suits. *Scandinavian Journal of Plastic and Reconstructive Surgery*, *13*(1), 163–166.
74. Kokotilo, K., Eng, J., & Curt, A. (2009). Reorganization and preservation of motor control of the brain in spinal cord injury: A systematic review. *Journal of Neurotrauma*, *26*, 2113–2126.
75. Krassioukov, A., Eng, J., Claxton, G., et al. (2010). Neurogenic bowel management after spinal cord injury: A systematic review of the evidence. *Spinal Cord*, *48*, 718–733.
76. Krassioukov, A., Eng, J., Warburton, D., et al. (2009). A systematic review of the management of orthostatic hypotension after spinal cord injury. *Archives of Physical Medicine & Rehabilitation*, *90*, 876–885.
77. Krassioukov, A., Warburton, D., Teasell, R., et al. (2009). A systematic review of the management of autonomic dysreflexia after spinal cord injury. *Archives of Physical Medicine & Rehabilitation*, *90*, 682–695.
78. Landolt, M. A., Grubenmann, S., & Meuli, M. (2002). Family impact greatest: Predictors of quality of life and psychological adjustment in pediatric burn survivors. *Journal of Trauma*, *53*, 1146–1151.
79. Lash, M. (Ed.), (2009). *The essential brain injury guide*. Vienna, VA: Brain Injury Association of America.
80. Latenser, B. A., & Kowal-Vern, A. (2002). Paediatric burn rehabilitation. *Pediatric Rehabilitation*, *5*(1), 3–10.
81. Leblebici, B., Turhan, N., Adam, M., et al. (2007). Clinical and epidemiologic evaluation of pressure ulcers in patients at a university hospital in Turkey. *Journal of Wound Ostomy & Continence Nursing*, *34*, 407–411.
82. Lemke, D. M. (2007). Sympathetic storming after severe traumatic brain injury. *Critical Care Nurse*, *27*, 30–37.
83. Marino, R. (Ed.), (2003). *Reference manual for the International Standards for Neurological Classification of Spinal Cord Injury*. Chicago: American Spinal Injury Association.
84. Martin, C., & Falcone, R. A. (2008). Pediatric traumatic brain injury: An update of research to understand and improve outcomes. *Current Opinion in Pediatrics*, *20*, 294–299.
85. Martin Ginis, K., Jetha, A., Mack, D., et al. (2010). Physical activity and subjective well-being among people with spinal cord injury: A meta-analysis. *Spinal Cord*, *48*, 65–72.
86. May, L., Day, R., & Warren, S. (2006). Evaluation of patient education in spinal cord injury rehabilitation: Knowledge, problem-solving and perceived importance. *Disability and Rehabilitation*, *28*, 405–413.
87. Moses, K. (1987). The impact of childhood disability: The parent's struggle. *WAYS Magazine*, *Spring*, 7–10.
88. Msall, M. E., DiGaudio, K. M., & Duffy, L. C. (1993). Use of functional assessment in children with developmental disabilities. *Physical Medicine and Rehabilitation Clinics of North America*, *4*, 517–527.
89. Muller, R., Peter, C., Cieza, A., et al. (2012). The role of social support and social skills in people with spinal cord injury: A systematic review of the literature. *Spinal Cord*, *50*, 94–106.
90. Murillo, N., Kumru, H., Vidal-Samso, J., et al. (2011). Decrease of spasticity with muscle vibration in patients with spinal cord injury. *Clinical Neurophysiology*, *122*, 1183–1189.
91. Mustoe, T. A., Cooter, R. D., Gold, M. H., et al. (2002). International clinical recommendations on scar management. *Plastic Reconstructive Surgery*, *110*, 560–571.
92. Nalder, E., Fleming, J., Foster, M., et al. (2012). Identifying factors associated with perceived success in the transition from hospital to home after brain injury. *Journal of Head Trauma Rehabilitation*, *27*, 143–153.
93. National Institutes of Health. (1999). Rehabilitation of persons with traumatic brain injury: NIH consensus development panel on rehabilitation of persons with traumatic brain injury. *Journal of the American Medical Association*, *292*, 974–983.
94. Niessen, F. B., Spauwen, P. H., Schalkwijk, J., et al. (1999). On the nature of hypertrophic scars and keloids: A review. *Plastic Reconstructive Surgery*, *104*, 1435–1458.
95. Ogawa, R. (2010). The most current algorithms for the treatment and prevention of hypertrophic scars and keloids. *Plastic Reconstructive Surgery*, *125*, 557–568.
96. Ozelie, R., Gassaway, J., Buchman, E., et al. (2012). Relationship of occupational therapy inpatient rehabilitation interventions and patient characteristics to outcomes following spinal cord injury: The SCIRehab project. *Journal of Spinal Cord Medicine*, *35*, 527–546.
97. Paralyzed Veterans of America Consortium for Spinal Cord Medicine. (2005). Preservation of upper limb function following spinal cord injury: A clinical practice guideline for health-care professionals. *Journal of Spinal Cord Medicine*, *28*, 434–470.
98. Phillips, A., Cote, A., & Warburton, D. (2011). A systematic review of exercise as a therapeutic intervention to improve arterial function in persons living with spinal cord injury. *Spinal Cord*, *49*, 702–714.
99. Rancho Los Amigos National Rehabilitation Center (2011). *The Rancho Levels of Cognitive Functioning*. Retrieved April 13, 2013, from: <http://www.rancho.org/Research_RanchoLevels.aspx>.
100. Reistetter, T. A., & Abreu, B. C. (2005). Appraising evidence on community integration following brain injury: A systematic review. *Occupational Therapy International*, *12*, 196–217.
101. Rice, S. A., Blackman, J. A., Braun, S., et al. (2005). Rehabilitation of children with traumatic brain injury: Descriptive analysis of a nationwide sample using the WeeFIM. *Archive Physical Medical Rehabilitation*, *86*, 834–836.
102. Robson, M. C., Barnett, R. A., Leitch, I. O., et al. (1992). Prevention and treatment of postburn scars and

contracture. *World Journal of Surgery, 16*, 87–96.
103. Roh, Y. S., Cho, H., Oh, J. O., et al. (2007). Effects of skin rehabilitation massage therapy on pruritus, skin status, and depression in burn survivors. *Taehan Kanho Hakhoe chi, 37*, 221–226.
104. Roques, C. (2002). Massage applied to scars. *Wound Repair & Regeneration, 10*, 126–128.
105. Rumsey, N., Clarke, A., & White, P. (2003). Exploring the psychosocial concerns of outpatients with disfiguring conditions. *Journal of Wound Care, 12*, 247–252.
106. Savage, R. C., Depompei, R., Tyler, J., et al. (2005). Paediatric traumatic brain injury: A review of pertinent issues. *Pediatric Rehabilitation, 8*, 92–103.
107. Sharp, P. A., Dougherty, M. E., & Kagan, R. J. (2007). The effect of positioning devices and pressure therapy on outcome after full-thickness burns of the neck. *Journal of Burn Care Research, 28*, 451–459.
108. Shaw, S. E., Morris, D. M., Uswatte, G., et al. (2005). Constraint-induced movement therapy for recovery of upper-limb function following traumatic brain injury. *Journal of Rehabilitation Research & Development, 42*, 769–778.
109. Sheel, A., Reid, W., Townson, A., et al. (2008). Effects of exercise training and inspiratory muscle training in spinal cord injury: A systematic review. *Journal of Spinal Cord Medicine, 31*, 500–508.
110. Sil, S., Dahlquist, L. M., & Burns, A. J. (2013). Videogame distraction reduces behavioral distress in a preschool-aged child undergoing repeated burn dressing changes: A single-subject design. *Journal of Pediatric Psychology, 38*, 330–341.
111. Simpson, L., Eng, J., Hseih, J., et al. (2012). The health and life priorities of individuals with spinal cord injury: A systematic review. *Journal of Neurotrauma, 29*, 1548–1555.
112. Spooren, A., Janssen-Potten, Y., Kerckhofs, E., et al. (2009). Outcome of motor training programmes on arm and hand functioning in patients with cervical spinal cord injury according to different levels of the ICF: A systematic review. *Journal of Rehabilitation Medicine, 41*, 497–505.
113. Staley, M., Richard, R., Billmire, D., et al. (1997). Head/face/neck burns: Therapist considerations for the pediatric patient. *Journal of Burn Care & Rehabilitation, 18*, 164–171.
114. Stancin, T., Drotar, D., Taylor, H. G., et al. (2002). Health-related quality of life of children and adolescents after traumatic brain injury. *Pediatrics, 109*, e34.
115. Stejskal, T. M. (2012). Removing barriers to rehabilitation: Theory-based family intervention in community settings after brain injury. *Neurorehabilitation, 31*, 75–83.
116. Suman, O. E., Micak, R. P., & Herndon, D. N. (2002). Effect of exercise training on pulmonary function in children with thermal injury. *Journal of Burn Care and Rehabilitation, 23*, 288–293.
117. Suman, O. E., Micak, R. P., & Herndon, D. N. (2004). Effects of exogenous growth hormone on resting pulmonary function in children with thermal injury. *Journal of Burn Care and Rehabilitation, 25*, 287–293.
118. Suman, O. E., Spies, R. J., Celis, M. M., et al. (2001). Effects of a 12-wk resistance exercise program on skeletal muscle strength in children with burn injuries. *Journal of Applied Physiology, 91*, 1168–1175.
119. Taricco, M., Adone, R., Pagliacci, C., et al. (2000). Pharmacological interventions for spasticity following spinal cord injury (Review). *Cochrane Database of Systematic Reviews*, (2), CD001131.
120. Teasdale, G., & Jennett, B. (1974). Assessment of coma and impaired consciousness: A practical scale. *Lancet, 2*, 81–84.
121. Tuan, T. L., & Nichter, L. S. (1998). The molecular basis of keloid and hypertrophic scar formation. *Molecular Medicine Today, 4*, 19–24.
122. Valent, L., Dallmeijer, A., Houdijk, H., et al. (2007). The effects of upper body exercise on the physical capacity of people with a spinal cord injury: A systematic review. *Clinical Rehabilitation, 21*, 315–330.
123. Van den Kerckhove, E., Stappaerts, K., Fieuws, S., et al. (2005). The assessment of erythema and thickness on burn related scars during pressure garment therapy as a preventive measure for hypertrophic scarring. *Burns: Journal of the International Society for Burn Injuries, 31*, 696–702.
124. Vitale, M., Goss, J., Matsumoto, H., et al. (2006). Epidemiology of pediatric spinal cord injury in the United States: Years 1997 and 2000. *Journal of Pediatric Orthopedics, 26*, 745–749.
125. Vogel, L., Betz, R., & Mulcahey, M. (2012). Spinal cord injuries in children and adolescents. In J. Verhaagen & J. McDonald (Eds.), *Handbook of Clinical Neurology*, 109 (pp. 131–148).
126. Warnken, B. (December 20, 2012). *Cincinnati Children's Hospital Medical Center best evidence statement: Coordination of outpatient rehabilitative care for patients with traumatic brain injury and their families.* Retrieved May 22, 2013, from: <http://www.cincinnatichildrens.org/svc/alpha/h/health-policy/best.htm>.
127. Wijnen, V. J. M., Heutink, M., van Boxtel, G. J. M., et al. (2006). Autonomic reactivity to sensory stimulation is related to consciousness level after severe traumatic brain injury. *Clinical Neurophysiology, 17*, 1794–1807.
128. Wilson, J., Cadotte, D., & Fehlings, M. (2012). Clinical predictors of neurological outcome, functional status, and survival after traumatic spinal cord injury: A systematic review. *Journal of Neurosurgery. Spine, 17*, 11–26.
129. Winstanley, J., Simpson, G., Tate, R., et al. (2006). Early indicators and contributors to psychological distress in relatives during rehabilitation following severe traumatic brain injury. *Journal of Head Trauma Rehabilitation, 21*, 453–466.
130. Yamaguchi, K., Gans, H., Yamaguchi, Y., et al. (1986). External compression with elastic bandages: Its effect on the peripheral blood circulation during skin traction. *Archives of Physical Medicine & Rehabilitation, 67*, 326–333.
131. Yeates, K. O., Swift, E., Taylor, G., et al. (2004). Short- and long-term social outcomes following pediatric traumatic brain injury. *Journal of the International Neuropsychological Society, 10*, 412–426.
132. Ylvisaker, M., Adelson, D., Braga, L. W., et al. (2005). Rehabilitation and ongoing support after pediatric TBI: Twenty years of progress. *Journal of Head Trauma Rehabilitation, 20*, 95–109.

Index

Page numbers followed by "f" indicate figures, "t" indicate tables, and "b" indicate boxes.

C

F

G

H

I

J

K

L

O

P

Q

R